BREASTFEEDING

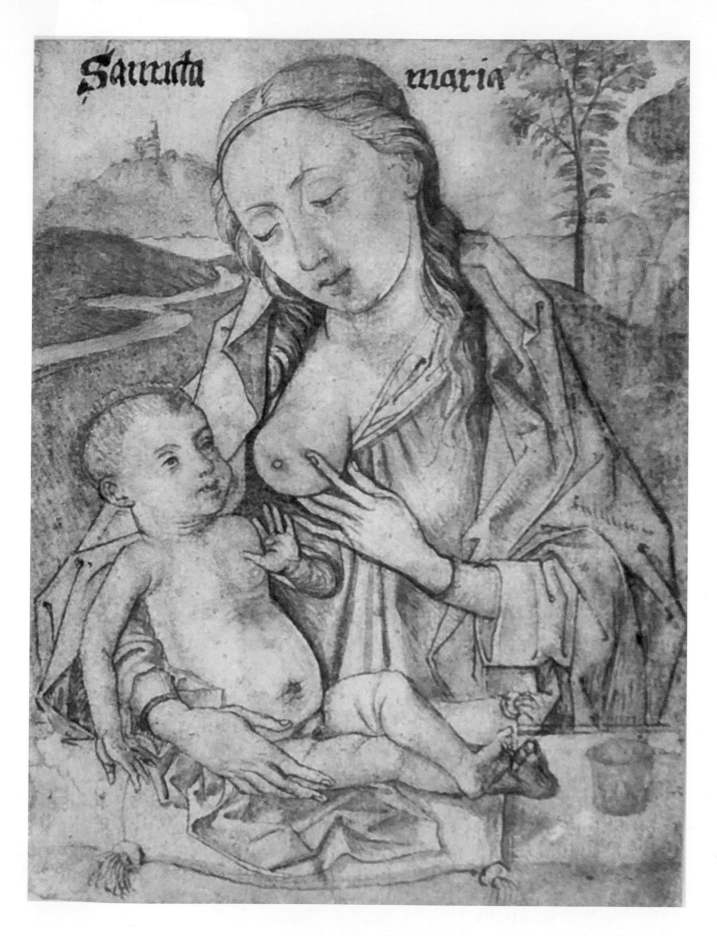

Madonna and Child, School of Bruges, Flemish, 15th century colored drawing. (*Reproduced with permission from Memorial Art Gallery of the University of Rochester.* https://mag.rochester.edu.)

NINTH EDITION

BREASTFEEDING

A GUIDE FOR THE MEDICAL PROFESSION

Edited by

RUTH A. LAWRENCE

Northumberland Trust Chair and
Distinguished Alumna Professor
Department of Pediatrics, Obstetrics and
Gynecology; University of Rochester School of
Medicine and Dentistry Rochester, New York

ROBERT M. LAWRENCE

Adjunct Clinical Professor of Pediatrics
Department of Pediatrics
University of Florida College of Medicine
Gainesville, Florida

Associate Editors

LAWRENCE NOBLE

Associate Professor, Department of Pediatrics,
Icahn School of Medicine at Mount Sinai,
New York, New York; Division of
Neonatology, Department of Pediatrics,
New York City Health + Hospitals,
Elmhurst, New York

CASEY ROSEN-CAROLE

Assistant Professor of Pediatrics and
Obstetrics and Gynecology, University of
Rochester School of Medicine and Dentistry,
Medical Director of Lactation Services and
Programs, University of Rochester Medical
Center, Rochester, New York

ALISON M. STUEBE

Professor of Maternal-Fetal Medicine,
Department of Obstetrics and Gynecology,
University of North Carolina School of
Medicine, Distinguished Professor of Infant
and Young Child Feeding, Department of
Maternal and Child Health, University of
North Carolina Gillings School of Global
Public Health, Chapel Hill, North Carolina

ELSEVIER

Elsevier
1600 John F. Kennedy Blvd.
Ste 1800
Philadelphia, PA 19103-2899

BREASTFEEDING: A GUIDE FOR THE MEDICAL PROFESSION, NINTH EDITION   ISBN: 978-0-323-68013-4

Notice

Practitioners and researchers must always rely on their own experience and knowledge in evaluating and using any information, methods, compounds or experiments described herein. Because of rapid advances in the medical sciences, in particular, independent verification of diagnoses and drug dosages should be made. To the fullest extent of the law, no responsibility is assumed by Elsevier, authors, editors, or contributors for any injury and/or damage to persons or property as a matter of products liability, negligence or otherwise, or from any use or operation of any methods, products, instructions, or ideas contained in the material herein.

Previous editions copyrighted 2016, 2011, 2005, 1999, 1994, 1989, 1985, 1980.

Library of Congress Control Number: 2020950231

Publisher: Sarah E. Barth
Director, Content Development: Rebecca Gruliow
Senior Content Development Specialist: Anne E. Snyder
Publishing Services Manager: Shereen Jameel
Project Manager: Manikandan Chandrasekaran
Cover Design and Design Direction: Ryan Cook

Printed in India

Last digit is the print number: 9 8 7 6 5 4 3 2

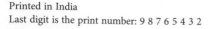

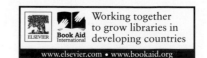

LIST OF CONTRIBUTORS

Cindy Calderon-Rodriguez, MD, FAAP
President (2019–2021) of the Puerto Rico
Chapter of the American Academy of
Pediatrics, San Juan, Puerto Rico

Melissa J. Chen, MD, MPH
Assistant Professor of Obstetrics and
Gynecology, Department of Obstetrics
and Gynecology, University of
California Davis Medical Center,
Sacramento, California

Katherine Blumoff Greenberg, MD
Associate Professor of Adolescent
Medicine and General Gynecology,
Departments of Pediatrics and
Obstetrics/Gynecology, University of
Rochester School of Medicine and
Dentistry, Rochester, New York

Ivan L. Hand, MD, FAAP
Director of Neonatology, Kings County
Hospital, Professor of Pediatrics,
SUNY Downstate School of Medicine,
Brooklyn, New York

Helen M. Johnson, MD, IBCLC
Resident Physician, Department of
Surgery, East Carolina University/
Vidant Medical Center, Greenville,
North Carolina

Robert M. Lawrence, MD, FABM
Adjunct Clinical Professor of Pediatrics,
Department of Pediatrics, University
of Florida College of Medicine,
Gainesville, Florida

Ruth A. Lawrence, MD, DD (Hon), FABM, FAAP
Northumberland Trust Chair and
Distinguished Alumna Professor,
Department of Pediatrics, Obstetrics
and Gynecology, University of
Rochester School of Medicine
and Dentistry, Rochester,
New York

Katrina B. Mitchell, MD, IBCLC, FACS
Breast Surgical Oncologist and Lactation
Consultant, Surgical Oncology, Ridley
Tree Cancer Center at Sansum Clinic,
Santa Barbara, California

Anita Noble, DNSc, CNM, CTN-A, IBCLC
Lecturer, Henrietta Szold/Hadassah-
Hebrew University, School of
Nursing, Faculty of Medicine,
Jerusalem, Israel

Lawrence Noble, MD, FAAP, FABM, IBCLC
Associate Professor, Department of
Pediatrics, Icahn School of Medicine at
Mount Sinai, New York, New York;
Division of Neonatology, Department
of Pediatrics, New York City Health +
Hospitals, Elmhurst, New York

Casey Rosen-Carole, MD, MPH, MSEd
Assistant Professor of Pediatrics and
Obstetrics and Gynecology, University
of Rochester School of Medicine and
Dentistry, Medical Director of
Lactation Services and Programs,
University of Rochester Medical
Center, Rochester, New York

Alison M. Stuebe, MD, MSc
Professor of Maternal-Fetal Medicine,
Department of Obstetrics and
Gynecology, University of North
Carolina School of Medicine,
Distinguished Professor of Infant and
Young Child Feeding, Department of
Maternal and Child Health, University
of North Carolina Gillings School of
Global Public Health, Chapel Hill,
North Carolina

FOREWORD FROM THE EIGHTH EDITION

Foreword reprinted from the 8th edition, with footnotes added for the 9th edition: The 5 years since the publication of the seventh edition of this excellent book have been a time of incredible advances in understanding several previously unknown physiologic and behavioral processes directly linked to or associated with breastfeeding and beautifully described in this new volume.

These findings change our view of the mother–infant relationship and signal an urgent need to completely review present perinatal care procedures. These new research results include the observation that when an infant suckles from the breast, there is a large outpouring of 19 different gastrointestinal hormones, including cholecystokinin, gastrin, and insulin, in both mother and infant. Several of these hormones stimulate the growth of the baby's and the mother's intestinal villi, thus increasing the surface area for the absorption of additional calories with each feeding. The stimulus for these changes is touching the nipple of the mother or the inside of the infant's mouth. The stimulus in both infant and mother results in the release of oxytocin in the periventricular area of the brain, which leads to production of these hormones via the vagus nerve. These pathways were essential for survival thousands of years ago, when periods of famine were common, before the development of modern agriculture and the storage of grain.

The discovery of the additional significance of a mother's breast and chest to the infant comes from the studies of Swedish researchers who have shown that a normal infant, placed on the mother's chest, and covered with a light blanket, will warm or maintain body temperature as well as an infant warmed with elaborate, high-tech heating devices. The same researchers found that, when infants are skin-to-skin with their mothers for the first 90 minutes after birth, they hardly cry at all compared with infants who are dried, wrapped in a towel, and placed in a bassinet. In addition, the researchers demonstrated that if a newborn is left quietly on the mother's abdomen after birth he or she will, after about 30 minutes, gradually crawl up to the mother's breast, find the nipple, self-attach, and start to suckle on his or her own.

It would appear that each of these features—the crawling ability of the infant, the absence of crying when skin-to-skin with the mother, and the warming capabilities of the mother's chest—evolved genetically more than 400,000 years ago to help preserve the infant's life.

Research findings related to the 1991 Baby Friendly Hospital Initiative (BFHI) of the World Health Organization and United Nations International Children's Emergency Fund provided insight into an additional basic process. After the introduction of the BFHI, which emphasized mother–infant contact with an opportunity for suckling in the first 30 minutes after birth and mother–infant rooming-in throughout the hospital stay, there has been a significant drop in neonatal abandonment reported in maternity hospitals in Thailand, Costa Rica, the Philippines, and St. Petersburg, Russia.

A key to understanding this behavior is the observation that, if the lips of an infant touch the mother's nipple in the first half hour of life, the mother will decide to keep the infant in her room 100 minutes longer on the second and third days of hospitalization than a mother whose infant does not touch her nipple in the first 30 minutes. It appears that these remarkable changes in maternal behavior are probably related to increased brain oxytocin levels shortly after birth. These changes, in conjunction with known sensory, physiologic, immunologic, and behavioral mechanisms, attract the mother and infant to each other and start their attachment. As pointed out back in the fifth edition, a strong, affectionate bond is most likely to develop successfully with breastfeeding, in which close contact and interaction occur repeatedly when an infant wishes and at a pace that fits the needs and wishes of the mother and the infant, resulting in gratification for both. Thus breastfeeding plays a central role in the development of a strong mother–infant attachment when begun with contact immediately after birth, which in turn has been shown to be a simple maneuver to significantly increase the success of breastfeeding. All of these exciting findings provide further evidence of why breastfeeding has been so crucial in the past and deserves strong support now.

In addition, the past few years have been associated with fundamental biochemical findings, including the importance of docosahexaenoic acid (DHA) in optimal brain development. All in all, the many new observations described in this eighth edition[*] place milk and the process of breastfeeding in a key position in the development of many critical functions in human infants and their mothers. We salute the author for her special skill in bringing together these many unique and original observations in this new and most valuable book.[†]

SUGGESTED READING

Christensson K, Cabrera T, Christensson E, et al. Separation distress call in the human neonate in the absence of maternal body contact. In: Christensson K, ed. Care of the Newborn Infant: Satisfying the Need for Comfort and Energy Conservation *[thesis]*. Stockholm: Karolinska Institute; 1994.

Christensson K, Siles C, Moreno L, et al. Temperature, metabolic adaptation and crying in healthy newborn cared for skin-to-skin or in a cot. *Acta Paediatr Scand*. 1992;81:488.

Klaus M, Klaus P. Academy of Breastfeeding Medicine Founder's Lecture 2009: maternity care re-evaluated. *Breastfeed Med*. 2010;5(3):3.

Uvnäs-Moberg K. The gastrointestinal tract in growth and reproduction. *Sci Am*. 1988;261:78.

Widström AM, Ransjo-Arvidson AB, Christensson K, et al. Gastric suction in healthy newborn infants: effects on circulation and developing feeding behavior. *Acta Paediatr Scand*. 1987;76:566.

Widström AM, Wahlberg V, Matthiesen AS, et al. Short-term effects of early suckling and touch of the nipple on maternal behavior. *Early Hum Dev*. 1990;21:153.

John H. Kennell (1922–2013)
Marshall H. Klaus (1927–2017)

---

[*] and ninth edition

[†] Ruth A. Lawrence remains the senior author and editor of this book, although her eldest son assists her and there are three new associate editors for the ninth edition. See title page and contributors.

Almost five decades ago, work began on the first edition of this text. Much has changed in the field of human lactation and in the world at large. The trickle of scientific work on the subject in 1975 has swollen into a river overflowing its banks. The Lactation Study Center at the University of Rochester has more than 50,000 documents in its database that describe peer-reviewed scientific studies and reports, and every year there are new controlled trials, systematic reviews, meta-analyses, and cost-based analyses of breastfeeding and the use of human milk. The field of lactation research has moved to the molecular and the genetic levels to analyze the chemical and component nature of breast milk and how that influences the infant's growth and development and later immunologic, allergic, metabolic, and overall health. Public health research continues to examine the short-term and long-term benefits of breast milk and breastfeeding for the infant and the mother. Clinical research seeks to apply evidenced-based data to the practice, experience, and support of breastfeeding within communities and for individual women and families. It is not simply the application of specific protocols and policies but thoughtful consideration and individualized support for the breastfeeding mother-infant dyad that leads to a mother reaching her breastfeeding goals.

The ninth edition of this text is symbolic, in that Dr. Ruth Lawrence raised nine children beginning with breastfeeding each one. This experience intimately connected her with the role and efforts required of a breastfeeding mother. It was this experience, with intellectual curiosity and recognition of the importance of breast milk and breastfeeding to the health of the maternal—infant dyad, that led to her persistence in the study of breastfeeding and the creation of nine editions. Over the years, several of her children have contributed in different ways to its publication, and now her grandchildren Madeleine Morris, Nathaniel Lawrence, and Jackson Morris have added their kind and loving assistance to the book and their "Grammy."

The intent of this volume remains to provide the basic tools of knowledge and experience that will enable a clinician to provide thoughtful counseling and guidance to the breastfeeding family that is most applicable to the particular breastfeeding dyad and the circumstances, problems, and lifestyle involved. Given the speed with which medical and scientific information about breast milk and breastfeeding is expanding, the simple presentation of current algorithms, guidelines, recommendations, and protocols will be inadequate to foster thoughtful counseling and guidance. With that challenge in mind facing the ninth edition we have invited three associate editors and several additional physicians and scientists as authors to develop this edition.

The associate editors include Dr. Casey Rosen-Carole, Medical Director of Lactation Services and Programs at the University of Rochester; Dr. Lawrence Noble, a perinatology and neonatology specialist and previously on the executive committee of the American Academy of Pediatrics' Section on Breastfeeding; and Dr. Alison Stuebe, Interim Director of the Division of Maternal-Fetal Medicine and Medical Director of Lactation Services at University of North Carolina and past president of the Academy of Breastfeeding Medicine. They are each international board-certified lactation consultants (IBCLCs) and faculty members of the Academy of Breastfeeding Medicine (FABM). See the Contents listing on page xiii for these editors' extensive contributions. The new authors also brought specific knowledge and experience related to breastfeeding and infant, maternal, and family health. Dr. Katherine Blumoff Greenberg, a specialist in adolescent medicine and LGBTQ + health, contributed to a new chapter, Chestfeeding and Lactation Care for LGBTQ+ Families (Lesbian, Gay, Bisexual, Transgender, Queer, Plus). Dr. Cindy Calderon, a pediatrician in Puerto Rico and active member of the AAP and ABM, oversaw the chapter on Infant Feeding After a Disaster. Dr. Ivan Hand, Director of Neonatology at SUNY, Downstate, King's County Hospital added his expertise to the chapter on Premature Infants and Breastfeeding. Dr. Helen Johnson and Dr. Katrina Mitchell, IBCLC and FABM, brought their experience in general surgery and expertise in breast surgery to a new separate chapter addressing Breast Conditions in the Breastfeeding Mother. Dr. Anita Noble contributed her expertise as a transcultural scientist and scholar to the chapter on the Collection and Storage of Human Milk and Human Milk Banking. Dr. Melissa Chen collaborated with Dr. Alison Stuebe for the chapter on Reproductive Function During Lactation.

Key areas on anatomy and physiology of lactation, medications in breast milk, transmission of infectious diseases through breast milk, allergy and its relationship to breastfeeding, and allergen exposure and avoidance have been updated for this edition. Important evolving topics have been expanded with the newest information, such as the cellular composition of breast milk and its importance to maternal and infant health, the microbiota of the breast and human milk and its possible roles in metabolism and infant immunity, reproductive justice and contraceptive equity, the role of patient-centered counseling as a crucial skill for clinicians communicating with women and families about infant feeding, the multifunctional role of human milk oligosaccharides in nutrition, immunity and gastrointestinal development, breastfeeding and chestfeeding in LGBTQ + families, and breastsleeping. The chapters on the breastfeeding management of infants with problems and the use of human milk for premature infants have expanded data and discussion. Four new chapters have been added to this edition: Breast Conditions in the Breastfeeding Mother; Chestfeeding and Lactation Care for LGBTQ + Families; Infant Feeding After a Disaster; and Establishing a Breastfeeding Medicine Practice or Academic Department.

With the ninth edition secure online, we have a number of individuals to thank.

We thank Jane Eggiman again for providing invaluable support as she has for past editions and Zoe Black who rescued fresh information from library archives and data bases, searching out many citations, bibliographies, and elusive details. We thank all the lactation consultants and medical doctors who have called the lactation center with their challenging clinical issues and questions. We sincerely appreciate the many physicians and scientists who continue breast milk and lactation research worldwide. We continue to be grateful to Rosemary Disney (1923–2014) for the creation of the enduring breastfeeding symbol on the cover. We are indebted to Dr. Rich Miller at the University of Rochester for his continued support of the Lactation Study Center and our work on this newest edition. We thank the team of experts at our publisher, Elsevier and especially content strategist Sarah Barth and Senior Content Development Specialist Anne Snyder for their outstanding support, patience, and perseverance in bringing the ninth edition to fruition. We are grateful to the new associate editors and the authors for their expertise, insight, professionalism, and invaluable contributions to the richness and completeness of this ninth edition. Finally, we would like to genuinely thank the readers of this ninth edition. We applaud your efforts for promotion and support of breastfeeding, lactation, and use of breast milk. We humbly offer this text as a starting point to garner existing knowledge on breastfeeding, and to stimulate novel discussion. We hope this edition will advance a continued search for new information and answers to the issues and dilemmas facing breastfeeding mothers and their infants and families.

Ruth A. Lawrence
Robert M. Lawrence

CONTENTS

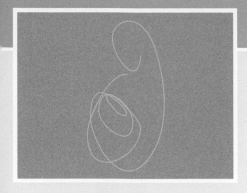

Breastfeeding in a New Era

Robert M. Lawrence and Ruth A. Lawrence

KEY POINTS

- The long history of breastfeeding has brought us to a better understanding of the crucial role of human breast milk in the nutrition and growth and development of infants and children.
- Research into lactation, breastfeeding, and human breast milk will guide how we support breastfeeding and the use of breast milk for all children. National and international legislation and policy development are necessary for the protection and promotion of breastfeeding worldwide.

- Disparities in breastfeeding exist. By addressing the inequities with a social justice framework, we can support women in reaching their individual breastfeeding goals and nations in achieving national and global targets of breastfeeding success.[13–15]

Breast milk, breastfeeding, and lactation have been described in many different ways depending on the situation and the perspective. B. D. Raphael called breastfeeding the "tender gift."[1] Various health agencies (e.g., American Academy of Pediatrics [AAP], American Public Health Association [APHA], Centers for Disease Control and Prevention [CDC], US Department of Health and Human Services [DHHS]) present the view of breastfeeding as a "public health priority."[2] George Kent says that "breastfeeding is a universal human right."[3] Deborah McCarter-Spaulding states, "Breastfeeding is, by its very definition, a family affair."[4] Paige Hall Smith postulates that "the 'right' to breastfeed is balanced with the right of women to make their own decisions about how they will feed their babies." Smith also comments that breastfeeding is a "complicated mix of food, biology, gender, caregiving and love."[5] So how did we get to this mix of conceptualizations and perspectives? Historians certainly can provide us with insight as well as discussion and debate of the contributing factors to the current state of breastfeeding and use of human milk around the world.[1,6–11] Thulier provides another perspective and a good discussion of influencing factors on breastfeeding in the United States.[12] She highlights religious, social, and medical variables on the backdrop of infant nutrition and survival, especially when lactation/breastfeeding is insufficient or fails. Breast-milk substitutes have played and continue to play a dominant role in infant-feeding practices and the "commercialization" of infant feeding. Now the use of donor human milk (DHM; through milk banks, cross-feeding, milk sharing) is taking an increasing role in infant nutrition. Governmental and nongovernmental agencies and initiatives track breastfeeding rates and strive to increase those via promotion, protection, and support of breastfeeding women and their families. The science of breast milk and lactation and the big data of public health are driving public and political action regarding procedures, policies, and legislation of infant-feeding practices.[13–15] Persistent disparities in breastfeeding success by race/ethnicity, geography, and class are pushing social justice action to improve the protection, promotion, and support of breastfeeding for all women. Seeking equity in access to care and striving for honest and fair social responsibility in health care for the least advantaged populations and individuals are key to increasing breastfeeding opportunity and success.[5,16] So, going forward, how do we navigate the numerous and perhaps competing forces in the support and promotion of breastfeeding? To do this, we need clear and meaningful communication of common goals and mutual collaboration to share lessons learned and effective interventions between the various "stakeholder" groups but especially communication with the women and families trying to make informed infant-feeding choices and working to reach their personal breastfeeding goals. Hopefully, this chapter and book will continue to serve as a guide for the medical profession in breast milk, lactation, and breastfeeding and the future of these in the health and welfare of infants and mothers.

EARLY HISTORY OF BREASTFEEDING

The world history and scientific literature, predominantly from countries other than the United States, includes many tributes to human milk. Early writings on infant care in the 1800s and early 1900s pointed out the hazards of serious infection in bottle-fed infants. Mortality charts were clear on the difference in mortality risk between breastfed and bottle-fed infants.[17] Only in recent history have the reasons for this phenomenon been identified in terms comparable with those used to define other anti-infectious properties. The identification of infants' developmental deficiencies in the immune system and specific components in human breast milk (immunoglobulins, bioactive factors [lactoferrin, lysozyme, etc.], immune cells, growth factors/hormones, cytokines, fatty acids, human milk oligosaccharides, and breast-milk microbiota) are examples of factors contributing to the immune protection of breastfed infants. It is clear that the infant receives some systemic protection transplacentally and immune system programming and local mucosal immune protection orally via the colostrum and mature milk. The environment of the intestinal tract and the microbiota of a breastfed infant continue to affect the local mucosal immunity and metabolic activation until the infant is weaned. Breastfed infants have fewer respiratory infections, occurrences of otitis media, gastrointestinal infections, and other illnesses.[18]

Colostrum

There are many culturally defined mysteries and taboos about colostrum, which go back to the dawn of civilization.[6−8,19,20] We now know of the added benefits of receiving colostrum in the first days of life because it is rich in secretory immunoglobulin A (IgA), lactoferrin, leukocytes, and epidermal growth factor. Most ancient peoples let several days pass before putting the baby to the breast, with exact times and rituals varying from group to group. Other liquids were provided in the form of herbal teas; some were pharmacologically potent, and others had no nutritional or pharmacologic worth. Culture also influenced breastfeeding.[21]

CULTURAL PRACTICES

In most cultures, mothers held their infants while seated; however, Armenian and some Asian women would lean over the supine baby, resting on a bar that ran above the cradle for support (Fig. 1.1). The infants were not lifted for the purpose of burping. Many groups carried infants on their backs and swung them into position frequently for feedings, a method that continues today with mothers caring for family and home and working outside the home. These infants are also not burped but remain semierect in the swaddling on the mother's back. The ritual of burping is actually a product of necessity in bottle-feeding because air is so easily swallowed. A review of civilized history reveals that almost every generation had to provide alternatives when the mother could not or would not nurse her infant. The ready availability of prepared formulas, paraphernalia of bottles and rubber nipples, and ease of sterilization are relatively new; the issue of alternative sources of breast milk and feeding breast-milk substitutes is not.[6,7]

Hammurabi's Code from about 1800 BC contained regulations on the practice of wet nursing, that is, nursing another woman's infant, often for hire. Throughout Europe, spouted feeding cups have been found in the graves of infants dating from about 2000 BC.

Although ancient Egyptian feeding flasks are almost unknown, specimens of Greek origin are fairly common in infant

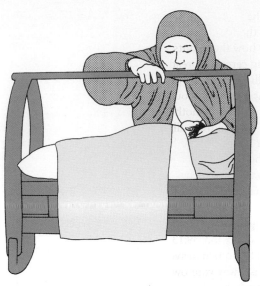

Fig. 1.1 Armenian woman suckling her child. (Redrawn from Wickes IG. A history of infant feeding. *Arch Dis Child.* 1953;28:151.)

burials. Paralleling the information about ancient feeding techniques is the problem of abandoned infants. Well-known biblical stories report such events, as do accounts from Rome during the time of the early popes. In fact, so many infants were abandoned that foundling homes were started. French foundling homes in the 1700s were staffed by wet nurses who were carefully selected, and their lives and activities were controlled to ensure adequate nourishment for the foundlings.

In Spartan times, a woman, even if she was the wife of a king, was required to nurse her eldest son; plebeians were to nurse all their children.[22] Plutarch, an ancient scribe, reported that a second son of King Themistes inherited the kingdom of Sparta only because he was nursed with his mother's milk. The eldest son had been nursed by a stranger and therefore was rejected.

No known written works describe infant feeding from ancient times to the Renaissance.[8,22] In 1472, the first pediatric incunabulum, written by Paul Bagellardus, was printed in Padua, Italy. It described the characteristics of a good wet nurse and provided counseling about hiccups, diarrhea, and vomiting. Thomas Moffat (1584) wrote of the medicinal and therapeutic use of human milk for men and women of "riper years, fallen by age or by sickness into compositions." His writings referred to the milk of the ass as being the best substitute for human milk at any age when nourishment was an issue. The milk of an ass is low in solids compared with that of most species, low in fat and protein, and high in lactose.

Wet Nurses

From AD 1500 to 1700, wealthy English women did not nurse their infants, according to Fildes,[8] who laboriously and meticulously reviewed infant-feeding history in Great Britain. Although breastfeeding was well recognized as a means of delaying another pregnancy, these women preferred to bear anywhere from 12 to 20 babies than to breastfeed them.[11]

They had a notion that breastfeeding spoiled their figures and made them old before their time. Husbands had much to say about how the infants were fed. Wet nurses were replaced by feeding cereal or bread gruel from a spoon. The death rate in foundling homes from this practice approached 100%.

The Dowager Countess of Lincoln wrote on "the duty of nursing, due by mothers to their children" in 1662.[7] She had borne 18 children, all fed by wet nurses; only one survived. When her son's wife bore a child and nursed it, the countess saw the error of her ways. She cited the biblical example of Eve, who breastfed Cain, Abel, and Seth. She deemed not breastfeeding a child to be crueler than ostriches hiding their eggs in the earth and said that a woman would have to be hardened against her young ones as though they were not hers, a reference to Job 39:13–16. The noblewoman concluded her appeal to women to avoid her mistakes: "Be not so unnatural as to thrust away your own children; be not so hardy as to venture a tender babe to a less tender breast; be not accessory to that disorder of causing a poorer woman to banish her own infant for the entertaining of a richer woman's child, as it were bidding her to unlove her own to love yours."

Toward the end of the 18th century in England, the trend of wet nursing and artificial feeding changed, partially because medical writers drew attention to health and well-being of breastfed infants and because mothers were influenced to breastfeed their young.[8]

In 18th-century France, both before and during the revolution that swept Louis XVI from the throne and brought Napoleon to power, infant feeding included maternal nursing, wet nursing, artificial feeding with the milk of animals, and feeding of pap and panada.[23] Panada is from the French *panade*, meaning bread, and means a food consisting of bread, water or other liquid, and seasoning and boiled to the consistency of pulp (Fig. 1.2). The majority of infants born to wealthy and middle-income women, especially in Paris, were placed with wet nurses. In 1718, Dionis wrote, "Today not only ladies of nobility, but yet the rich and the wives of the least of the artisans have lost the custom of nursing their infants." As early as 1705, laws controlling wet nursing required wet nurses to register, forbade them to nurse more than two infants in addition to their own, and stipulated that a crib should be available for each infant, to prevent the nurse from taking a baby to bed and chancing suffocation.[20] On the birth of the Prince of Wales (later George IV) in 1762, it was officially announced: wet nurse, Mrs. Scott; dry nurse, Mrs. Chapman; rockers, Jane Simpson and Catherine Johnson.[24]

A more extensive historical review by Apple would reveal other examples of social problems in achieving adequate care of infants.[9] Long before our modern society, some women failed to accept their biologic role as nursing mothers, and society failed to provide adequate support for nursing mothers. Breastfeeding was more common and of longer duration in stable eras and rarer in periods of "social dazzle" and lowered moral standards. Urban mothers have had greater access to alternatives (wet nurses, milk agencies, and artificial infant feedings), and rural women have had to continue to breastfeed in greater numbers.[7,9,25]

"Feeding by the Book"

In the 1920s, women were encouraged to raise their infants scientifically. "Raising by the book" was commonplace. L. Emmett Holt, MD, a renowned pediatrician, published his book *The Care and Feeding of Children*, which, although it recommended breastfeeding, interfered with "on-demand" feeding by recommending regimentation in feeding. There were 75 printings of this popular book from 1894 to the 1940s.[12] The US government published *Infant Care* in 1914 because of the high rates of infant death in the United States at that time. It was referred to as the "good book," which was the bible of child-rearing read by women from all walks of life.[26] It was republished in 1935 by the Child's Bureau of the US Department of Labor and again multiple times up through 1989, the year of the final edition.[27] The 1935 edition emphasized breastfeeding over artificial milk mixtures and recommended that when mothers could not provide breast milk to their infants of less than 6 months of age, then employing a wet nurse or obtaining breast milk from a "breast-milk agency" or from friends or relatives was preferred. For the introduction of solid foods, the 1935 text recommended cod liver oil, egg yolk, stewed fruits, and potatoes. A quote from *Parents* magazine in 1938 reflects the attitude of women's magazines in general, undermining even the staunchest breastfeeders: "You hope to nurse him, but there are an alarming number of young mothers today who are unable to breastfeed their babies and you may be one of them."[9] Apple detailed the transition from breastfeeding to raising children scientifically, by the book, and precisely as the doctor prescribes.[9]

Around the same time, the end of the 19th century and beginning of the 20th century, there were dramatic disparities in infant mortality between breastfed and artificially fed (modified animal milk) infants. This was evident in reports covering 50,000 infants, where mortality in artificially fed infants was 3 to 10 times higher than in breastfed infants in Chicago, Minnesota, other US sites, and Britain.[17,28,29] In the rest of the world, especially nonindustrialized countries, the higher mortality was associated with early weaning (<6 months of age).[30]

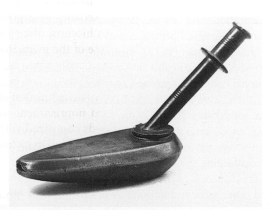

Fig. 1.2 Pewter pap spoon, circa AD 1800. Thin pap, a mixture of bread and water, was placed in a bowl. The tip of the bowl was placed in the child's mouth. Flow could be controlled by placing a finger over the open end of the hollow handle. If the contents were not taken as rapidly as desired, one could blow down the handle.

Artificial Infant Feedings

Germ theory and the process of pasteurization began to influence the preparation of artificial infant feedings. In affluent homes, home sterilizers appeared in the 1890s. Parallel to this, animal milks were being further modified (sugar-added evaporated milk, unsweetened milk in a can or condensed milk) and produced commercially. In 1855, A. V. Meig made public what was recognized as the first accurate analysis of human and cow's milk. He worked out a "formula" for a liquid infant food based on animal milk, adjusting the calories, protein, and carbohydrate content.[31] In 1865, a German chemist, Justus von Liebig, also created an infant food made of cow's milk, wheat and malt flours, and potassium bicarbonate.[32] By 1883, many other infant formulas and food products were available commercially, including 27 patented brands.[33] In the late 1800s, bottles and nipples were also improving—they were easier to clean and use, with glass bottles and rubber nipples.[6,7] Sterilization of these implements and the increasing use of refrigeration made the storage of artificial milk easier and more hygienic but did not improve the quality of their nutritional content.[32]

Decline of Breastfeeding

In 1922 Woodbury estimated that in the United States, breastfeeding was continuing at 12 months of age for 85% to 90% of children.[29] From that point, breastfeeding declined in the United States. Reports for 1965 described breastfeeding initiation rates down to 38% and breastfeeding out to 3 months of age down to 12%.[34,35] It seemed to reach a low in the 1970s; only 24% of women reportedly breastfed at least once before discharge from the hospital.[36] Presumably, this decline was due to many factors, some of which have been suggested as "raising children by the book"; the perceived science of pasteurized formulas as "safe substitutes" for breast milk; and the rise of formula companies and marketing of formula to physicians, making the formulas of economic importance to their medical practice.[12] Apple and Parfitt separately describe social and political factors contributing to the decline: the women's movement emancipating women through bottle-feeding formula, not breastfeeding; a general social approval of bottle-feeding, with the modern household of the 1950s being portrayed and characterized by a bottle-fed infant; pediatrician-recommended "regulated feeding patterns" interfering with "as-needed" or "on-demand" breastfeeding; and the overarching influence of formula companies, even including publications like *The Motherbook*, repeatedly printed by Nestle Milk Product, Inc.[37]

MODERN HISTORY OF BREASTFEEDING

So how and why did things change to bring us back to understanding the essential nature of breastfeeding for infant and maternal health and promoting, protecting, and supporting breastfeeding as it is practiced in 2020? There are as many theories as there are papers on the relatively recent history of breastfeeding.[2,4,12,38–41] (See the US and WHO data on breastfeeding rates later in this chapter.)

Variability in Breastfeeding Rates

How and why, with this increase in breastfeeding rates, did significant differences in breastfeeding rates arise in different groups? In the United States and worldwide, there arose dramatic disparity between black and white infants, urban and rural communities, and low- and middle-income countries versus high-income countries. US data from 2002 to 2014 reveal a 17-percentage-point gap in breastfeeding initiation between black and white infants.[42] Anstey et al. reported that by 2013, the exclusive breastfeeding (EBF) rate at 6 months of age was 8.5% lower, and the 12-month breastfeeding duration rate was 13.7% lower, for black infants compared with white infants.[43] There are many theories and discussions as to why this is occurring and possible solutions.[44–48] There are numerous organizations and events that have led to improving breastfeeding rates worldwide and addressing disparities in breastfeeding (Table 1.1).

Educational Influences on Breastfeeding

One of the first examples of an educational influence began in the 1940s when Edith Jackson, MD, of Yale University School of Medicine and the Grace–New Haven Hospital was awarded a federal grant to establish the first rooming-in unit in the United States. This project included the first program to prepare women for childbirth, modeled after the British obstetrician Grantly Dick-Read's *Child Birth Without Fear*.[49] This was developed with the Department of Obstetrics to reduce maternal medication during birth and keep the mother and baby alert and together. Of course, it included breastfeeding. Trainees from this program in pediatrics and obstetrics spread across the country, starting programs elsewhere.

The La Leche League (LLL) formed in 1956—for women, by mothers—to provide education, practical guidance, and support for women in their efforts to breastfeed and "mother" their children. Ward described the educational piece with the feminist component encouraging women to follow their hearts and minds with guidance from experienced mothers.[50] Mothers were empowered with new knowledge and trust from experienced mothers, and the LLL produced a book, *The Womanly Art of Breastfeeding*, and continued its expansion internationally.[51] In the 1980s, skilled lactation consultants gained increased presence, and along with the La Leche League International (LLLI), committed to a standard of competency for these health care professionals in forming the International Board of Lactation Consultant Examiners (IBLCE). In 2020 there were over 32,500 International Board–certified lactation consultants (IBCLCs) in 122 countries. The IBLCE maintains educational standards and guidelines for IBCLCs and contributes directly to the education of mothers and families about breastfeeding.

The great success of the mother-to-mother program of the LLL and other local and national women's support groups in helping women breastfeed or, as with International Childbirth Education Association (ICEA), in helping women plan and participate in childbirth is an example of the power of social relationships.[25] Raphael described the doula as a "friend from across the street" who came by at the birth of a new baby to

TABLE 1.1 Organizations, Initiatives, and Events for Breastfeeding

United States	International
1956 La Leche League (formation)	1919 International Labour Organization (ILO) Maternity Protection Convention
1966 Child Nutrition Act Special Supplemental Nutrition Program for Women, Infants, and Children (WIC)	1956 La Leche League International
1984 1st Surgeon General's Workshop on Breastfeeding	1960 International Childbirth Education Association
1985 Journal of Human Lactation first published	1979 International Code of Breast-Milk Substitutes Marketing
1985 Human Milk Bank Association of North America (HMBANA) formed	1979 International Baby Food Action Network (IBFAN)
1988 Centers for Disease Control and Prevention (CDC) breastfeeding data collection Maternity Practices in Infant Nutrition and Care (mPINC)	1981 World Health Organization (WHO) International Code of Marketing of Breastmilk Substitutes World Health Assembly endorsement
1989 WIC program—breastfeeding promotion	1985 International Lactation Consultant Association (ILCA) International Board of Lactation Consultant Examiners (IBLCE)
1990 Breastfeeding Promotion Consortium	1985 Milk Bank Network of Brazil
1993 Academy of Breastfeeding Medicine	1989 UN Convention on the Rights of the Child (CRC)
1998 United States Breastfeeding Committee	1991 World Alliance for Breastfeeding Action (WABA)
2000 Healthy People 2000—breastfeeding goals	1991 Baby-Friendly Hospital Initiative (BFHI)
2000 US Department of Health and Human Services (HHS) Blueprint for Action on Breastfeeding	1997–2003 WHO Multicentre Growth Reference Study
2002 National Advertising Council—national campaign "Babies are born to breastfeed"	2010 European Milk Bank Association (EMBA)
2005 International Breastfeeding Journal	
2006 First National Breastfeeding Coalitions Conference	
2006 Drugs and lactation database, LactMed, of the National Library of Medicine	
2006 Breastfeeding Medicine Journal	
2009 CDC National Immunization Survey—data collection on breastfeeding	
2010 HHS breastfeeding "Call to Action"	

support the mother. She would "mother the mother."[1] The doula and lactation consultants are now known as key persons for lactation education and support, especially in the first critical days and weeks after delivery.

Bryant[25] explored the social networks that exist for mothers in her study of the impact of kin, friend, and neighbor networks on infant-feeding practices in Cuban, Puerto Rican, and Anglo families in Florida. She found that these networks strongly influenced decisions about breastfeeding, bottle-feeding, the use of supplements, and the introduction of solid foods. Network members' advice and encouragement contributed to a successful lactation experience. The impact of the

health care professional is inversely proportional to the distance of the mother from her network. The health care worker must work within the cultural norms for the network. For individuals isolated from their cultural roots, the health care system may have to provide education, support, and encouragement to ensure lactation success and adherence to health care guidelines.[52]

The trend in infant feeding among mothers who participated in the Women, Infants, and Children (WIC) program in the late 1970s and early 1980s was analyzed separately by Martinez and Dodd and Martinez and Stahle from the data collected by questionnaires mailed quarterly as part of the

Ross Laboratories Mothers Survey.[53,54] The responses represented 4.8% of the total births in the United States in 1977 and 14.1% of the total births in the United States in 1980. WIC participants in 1977, including those who supplemented with formula or cow's milk, were breastfeeding in the hospital at the nadir rate of 33.6% of cases. A slight increase occurred in the frequency of breastfeeding in WIC participants; it rose to 40.4% in 1980 ($p < 0.5$). It was not until the 1990s that breastfeeding rates by WIC participants showed a sustained increase (Table 1.2). WIC data continue to be collected, and the trends have paralleled other groups. In 1992 WIC provided an enhanced food package for exclusively breastfeeding mothers.

The Food and Consumer Service (FCS) of the US Department of Agriculture (USDA) entered into a cooperative agreement with Best Start, a not-for-profit social marketing organization that promoted breastfeeding to develop a WIC breastfeeding promotion project that was national in scope and implemented at the state level. In 1997 the "Loving Support Makes Breastfeeding Work" campaign was initiated.[55] The project consisted of six components: social marketing research, a media campaign, a staff support kit, a breastfeeding resource guide, a training conference, and continuing education and technical assistance. With an annual $8 million budget for WIC, the project's goals are to increase the initiation and duration of breastfeeding among clients of WIC and expand public acceptance of and support for breastfeeding. Breastfeeding women are favored in the WIC priority system when benefits are limited; they can continue in the program for a year, but those who do not breastfeed are limited to 6 months. All pregnant participants of WIC are currently encouraged to breastfeed.

Montgomery and Splett reported the economic benefits of breastfeeding infants for mothers enrolled in WIC.[56] Comparing the costs of the WIC program and Medicaid for food and health care in Colorado, administrative and health care costs for a formula-fed infant, minus the rebate for the first 180 days of life, were $273 higher than those for the breastfed infant. These calculations did not include the pharmacy costs for illness. When these figures were translated to large WIC programs in high-cost areas (e.g., New York City, Los Angeles) and multiplied by millions of WIC participants, the savings from breastfeeding were substantial. If the goal of 90% exclusively breastfeeding women through 6 months of age in the WIC program had been reached in 2016, then total US health-related costs would have been decreased by $9.1 billion ($\sim$6.9 billion savings as a result of a reduction in early deaths, $\sim$$1.5 billion in decreased medical costs, and $\sim$$635 million in nonmedical costs).[57] Since 2000, WIC programs have energetically promoted breastfeeding, but the package for bottle-feeders has also remained popular. A new WIC package has been developed and slowly supported through the system. It increased the food allowance for lactating women. The WIC program, primarily through education, promotion, and direct support to women, has increased the numbers of WIC mothers choosing to breastfeed. The rate of breastfeeding initiation among WIC mothers has increased parallel to the national average but lagged slightly behind

TABLE 1.2 Percentage of Breastfeeding among Women, Infants, and Children (WIC) Program Participants, 1977 to 2002		
Year	In Hospital (%)	At 6 Months of Age (%)
1977	33.6	12.5
1978	34.5	9.7
1979	37.0	11.2
1980	40.4	13.1
1981	39.9	13.7
1982	45.3	16.1
1983	38.9	11.5
1984	39.1	11.9
1985	40.1	11.7
1986	38.0	10.7
1987	37.3	10.6
1988	35.3	9.2
1989	34.2	8.4
1990	33.7	8.2
1991	36.9	9.0
1992	38.8	10.1
1993	41.6	10.8
1994	44.3	11.6
1995	46.6	12.7
1996	46.6	12.9
1997	50.4	16.5
1998	56.8	18.9
1999	56.1	19.9
2000	56.8	20.1
2001	58.2	20.8
2002	58.8	22.1

Data collected from Martinez GA, Stahle DA. The recent trend in milkfeeding among WIC infants. *Am J Public Health.* 1982;72:68; Ryan AS, Rush D, Krieger FW. Recent declines in breastfeeding in the United States, 1984 through 1989. *Pediatrics.* 1991;88:719; Krieger FW. *A review of breastfeeding trends.* Presented at the Editor's Conference, New York, September 1992; Ross Laboratories Mothers Survey, unpublished data, Columbus, Ohio, 1992; Mothers Survey, Ross Products Division, Abbott Laboratories, unpublished data, 1998; Ryan AS. The resurgence of breastfeeding in the United States. *Pediatrics.* 1997;99:2 (electronic article); Mothers Survey, Ross Products Division, and Abbott Laboratories—Breastfeeding Trends 2002.

through 2015. Many local WIC programs have hired and trained peer support mothers with breastfeeding experience or another accepted source of information/education and support to help WIC clients.

Professional organizations such as the AAP, American College of Obstetrics and Gynecology (ACOG), and American Academy of Family Practice (AAFP) were slow to speak out as they wrestled with the financial contributions the formula companies made to medical education and continuing medical education (CME). In 1993 Drs. Anne Eglash and Elizabeth Williams, at an International Lactation Consultant Association meeting, initiated discussions for a multidisciplinary physician organization committed to the science of breastfeeding medicine. A core group of 12 physicians formed Physicians Advocating Breastfeeding (PHAB), which led to the formation of the Academy of Breastfeeding Medicine (ABM) in 1994. It is now a worldwide organization of medical doctors dedicated to the promotion, protection, and support of breastfeeding, uniting members of the various medical specialties with the common goals of highlighting new scientific findings and promoting the education of physicians. Other educational resources for health care professionals included the formation of several medical journals specifically for lactation and breastfeeding: the *Journal of Human Lactation* (1985), *International Breastfeeding Journal* (2005), and the *Breastfeeding Medicine Journal* (2006; see Table 1.1).

Groups Contributing to Breastfeeding Education

In 1997 the AAP made its first policy statement: "Breastfeeding and the Use of Human Milk."[58] The AAP aimed to educate all pediatricians to recommend EBF as the optimal nutrition for the growth and development of infants through approximately 6 months of age and the use of expressed human milk for premature infants and low-birth-weight infants. The AAP reviewed the few contraindications to breastfeeding and supported the gradual introduction of complementary foods at about 6 months and continued breastfeeding through at least 12 months of age. The AAP advised pediatricians on how to promote and support breastfeeding in their practice and on the transfer of medications into human milk.[59,60] Soon after that, the AAFP and ACOG issued policy statements and education for their physician members. In 2001 the AAP provided updates of previous statements about the transfer of drugs and chemicals into human milk as an educational review for pediatricians and physicians in general.[61] In 2005 the AAP published a revision of its 1997 and 2001 statements.[62] This statement reinforced the previous concepts and expanded on the specific actions to optimize breastfeeding success: breastfeeding education during pregnancy, skin-to-skin contact in the delivery room, evaluation of breastfeeding daily in the hospital, and close follow-up by the clinician in the first 2 weeks after discharge. In 2012 the AAP again expanded its recommendations on breastfeeding and the use of human milk, explicitly providing guidance on breastfeeding full-term infants, providing human milk for premature infants, the use of medication during lactation, and the increased role of the pediatrician in supporting breastfeeding women and families.[63] The US government also contributed to the education of physicians, health care professionals, and the nation on breastfeeding. In 2000 the DHHS Blueprint for Action on Breastfeeding presented a national plan for the advancement of breastfeeding through education, training, awareness, support, and research. More recently, the Office of Women's Health prepared an educational pamphlet specifically for women and families, *Your Guide to Breastfeeding*.[64] In 2020 there were dozens of other printed educational resources with regard to breastfeeding for professionals and for women and families and many more resources online. The ABM has published 32 protocols for the management of breastfeeding and one specifically outlining educational objectives and skills for physicians regarding breastfeeding. This text presents content on educating and training medical professionals in a chapter and appendix[65] (see Chapter 26, Appendix J, and https://www.bfmed.org/protocols).

Box 1.1 provides a summary of interventions for the promotion of breastfeeding presented at the Surgeon General's Workshop.[66] A federally funded national conference held in 1994 in Washington, DC, came to the same conclusions as in 1984. A conference held in Washington, DC, sponsored by the ABM and the Kellogg Foundation focused on a follow-up 25 years after the original Surgeon General's Workshop looked at disparity issues. Progress in the United States through federal activities is illustrated in Fig. 1.3.

Although these recommendations had been promoted since 1984, many hospitals and health care facilities were not adopting them. In this same time period, other groups, including the United Nations Children's Fund (formerly United Nations International Children's Emergency Fund [UNICEF]) and the World Health Organization (WHO), were working with Wellstart International and Audrey Naylor at the University of California—San Diego. They initially outlined the 10 steps for an institution to be breastfeeding-friendly and baby-friendly. A joint WHO/UNICEF statement in 1989, *Protecting, Promoting, and Supporting Breastfeeding*, describes suggested actions for breastfeeding-supportive maternity services in line with those outlined 10 steps.[67] Wellstart International, with continued support from UNICEF, developed an assessment tool for hospitals and in 1992 launched the first training of trainer/assessors for the Baby-Friendly Hospital Initiative (BFHI). Box 1.2 lists the 10 steps to becoming a designated Baby-Friendly Hospital.

In 1996 Evergreen Hospital in Kirkland, Washington, was the first Baby-Friendly Hospital designated in the United States.[68] This initiative has been reorganized and reestablished through Healthy Children, a not-for-profit organization that created Baby-Friendly USA. Worldwide, the BFHI, under the auspices of UNICEF, continues to dramatically expand the number of hospitals designated as a Baby-Friendly Hospital and offers training and assessment for professionals and hospitals. In 2009 there were over 20,000 hospitals designated "baby-friendly" in 156 countries.[69] For certification as a Baby-Friendly Hospital, the hospital must provide evidence that it has met the 10 criteria (see Box 1.2) and must demonstrate its effectiveness to a visiting team of assessors.

Role of Research in Advancing Breastfeeding

Although empiric and observational research into lactation, breast milk, and breastfeeding have occurred for centuries,

BOX 1.1 Key Elements for Promotion of Breastfeeding in the Continuum of Maternal and Infant Health Care

1. Primary care settings for women of childbearing age should have the following:
   - A supportive milieu for lactation
   - Educational opportunities (including availability of literature, personal counseling, and information about community resources) for learning about lactation and its advantages
   - Ready response to requests for further information
   - Continuity allowing for the exposure to, and development over time of, a positive attitude regarding lactation on the part of the recipient of care
2. Prenatal care settings should have the following:
   - A specific assessment at the first prenatal visit of the physical capability for, and emotional predisposition to, lactation. This assessment should include the potential role of the father of the child and other significant family members. An educational program about the advantages of, and ways of preparing for, lactation should continue throughout the pregnancy.
   - Resource personnel—such as nutritionists/dietitians, social workers, public health nurses, La Leche League members, childbirth education groups—for assistance in preparing for lactation
   - Availability and utilization of culturally suitable patient education materials
   - An established mechanism for a predelivery visit to the newborn care provider to ensure initiation and maintenance of lactation
   - A means of communicating to the in-hospital team the infant-feeding plans developed during the prenatal course
3. In-hospital settings should have the following:
   - A policy to determine a patient's infant-feeding plan on admission or during labor
   - A family-centered orientation to childbirth, including the minimum use of intrapartum medications and anesthesia
   - A medical and nursing staff informed about, and supportive of, ways to facilitate the initiation and continuation of breastfeeding (including early mother–infant contact and ready access by the mother to her baby throughout the hospital stay)
   - The availability of individualized counseling and education by a specially trained breastfeeding coordinator to facilitate lactation for those planning to breastfeed and to counsel those who have not yet decided about their method of infant feeding
   - Ongoing in-service education about lactation and ways to support it. This program should be conducted by the breastfeeding coordinator for all relevant hospital staff.
   - Proper space and equipment for breastfeeding in the postpartum and neonatal units. Attention should be given to the particular needs of women breastfeeding babies with special problems.
   - The elimination of hospital practices/policies that have the effect of inhibiting the lactation process (e.g., rules separating mother and baby)
   - The elimination of standing orders that inhibit lactation (e.g., lactation suppressants, fixed feeding schedules, maternal medications)
   - Discharge planning that includes referral to community agencies to aid in the continuing support of the lactating mother. This referral is especially important for patients discharged early.
   - A policy to limit the distribution of packages of free formula at discharge to only those mothers who are not lactating
   - The development of policies to support lactation throughout the hospital units (e.g., medicine, surgery, pediatrics, emergency room)
   - The provision of continued lactation support for those infants who must remain in the hospital after the mother's discharge
4. Postpartum ambulatory settings should have the following:
   - A capacity for telephone assistance to mothers experiencing problems with breastfeeding
   - A policy for telephone follow-up 1 to 3 days after discharge
   - A plan for an early follow-up visit (within first week after discharge)
   - The availability of lactation counseling as a means of preventing or solving lactation problems
   - Access to lay support resources for the mother
   - The presence of a supportive attitude by all staff
   - A policy to encourage bringing the infant to postpartum appointments
   - The availability of public community health nurse referral for those having problems with lactation
   - A mechanism for the smooth transition to pediatric care of the infant, including good communication between obstetric and pediatric care providers

one could consider dating the beginning of research in breast milk and breastfeeding to the mid-1800s, when A. V. Meig first provided an "accurate analysis" of human milk and cow's milk; this occurred at the same time as germ theory was being demonstrated and the process of pasteurization was introduced by Pasteur in the 1860s for use on wine and beer.[31] The

health and welfare of children came to the forefront in the 1890s with the high infant mortality rates (IMRs), and efforts to find the cause(s) and intervene began. Early public health initiatives were developed in part because the IMR in America in the early 1900s was reported as 135 deaths per 1000 live births.[70] In 1912 the Department of Labor founded

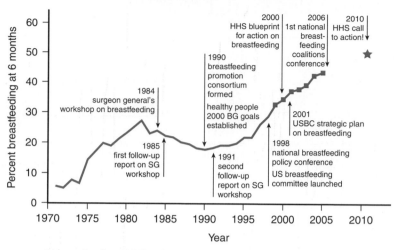

Breastfeeding progress: 1984-2009

Fig. 1.3 Federal activities in support of breastfeeding. *HHS,* US Department of Health and Human Services; *SG,* surgeon general. (Modified from Grummer-Strawn LM, Shealy KR. Progress in protecting, promoting, and supporting breastfeeding. *Breastfeed Med.* 2009;4[Suppl 1]:531.)

BOX 1.2 Toward Becoming a Baby-Friendly Hospital

10 Steps to Successful Breastfeeding

Every facility providing maternity services and care for new-born infants should do the following:

1. Have a written breastfeeding policy that is routinely communicated to all health care staff.
2. Train all health care staff members in skills necessary to implement this policy.
3. Inform all pregnant women about the benefits and management of breastfeeding.
4. Help mothers initiate breastfeeding within one hour of birth.
5. Show mothers how to breastfeed and how to maintain lactation even if they should be separated from their infants.
6. Give newborn infants no food or drink other than breast milk, unless medically indicated.
7. Practice rooming-in—allowing mothers and infants to remain together—24 hours a day.
8. Encourage breastfeeding on demand.
9. Give no artificial teats or pacifiers (also called *dummies* or *soothers*) to breastfeeding infants.
10. Foster the establishment of breastfeeding support groups and refer mothers to them on discharge from the hospital or clinic.

---

the Children's Bureau, devoted to the welfare of mothers and children.[31] In early studies of IMR by the bureau, a connection between gastrointestinal disease and mortality was found and related to feeding, poor nutrition, and poverty. Maternal education in infant feeding, nutrition, hygiene, and breastfeeding improved infant mortality.[71] Infant mortality rates and maternal mortality during childbirth were a concern worldwide, and in 1919, the International Labour Organization (ILO) held the first Maternity Protection Convention (see Table 1.1).

Empiric observations continued to influence infant care, but expert opinion dominated infant care practices (e.g., books by E. Holt, US Children's Bureau, and B. Spock).[72–74] IMRs and breastfeeding practices were tracked by the Center for Health Statistics of the US government.[34,35] Worldwide, researchers tracked the incidence and duration of breastfeeding in diverse populations and continued to analyze the composition and nutritional makeup of colostrum and milk.[75–77] In the 1970s to the 1990s, research progressed to examining the short- and long-term benefits of human breast milk and its immune-protective, nutritional, physiologic, growth-promoting, neurocognitive, and psychosocial effects on infants and children. The benefits of breastfeeding over formula-feeding were scientifically documented.[78–81]

The "definitions of breastfeeding" and the "terminology" of breastfeeding with which to examine the important variables and factors of lactation, breast milk, and breastfeeding have been continually discussed to reach a consensus and create consistency for research comparability.[82–84] (See Fig. 1.4 for a relative quantification of breast-milk consumption by the infant.) Yourkavitch and Chetwynd presented specific terminology for use in population health research, which included *breastfeeding intent* (the intended duration of breastfeeding from the mother's perspective), *breastfeeding* (feeding human milk directly from one's breast), and *breastfeeding initiation* (the time when the infant first receives a human milk feeding), among other terms.[84] Research continues to evolve in the basic science of lactation, breast milk, and the breast with new technologies (ultrasound, computerized-tomography scanning, chemical analysis and the use of cell markers) and more recently in the utilization of "omics" (genomics, transcriptomics, proteomics, metabolomics, and micro-biomics) as well as the use of epidemiology, public health, and big data.[85] This work drives our understanding of the marvel of how breast milk and lactation benefit the infant and mother. Evidence-based medicine, quality improvement, assessment of

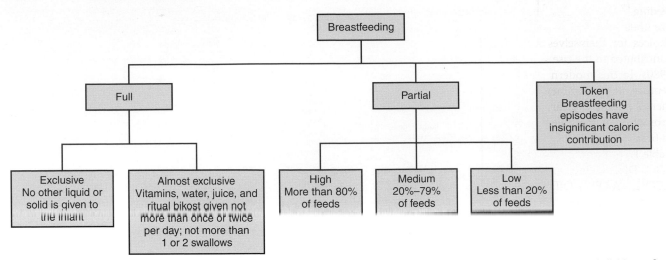

Fig. 1.4 Schema for breastfeeding definitions. (Modified from Labbok M, Krasovec K. Toward consistency in breastfeeding definitions. *Stud Fam Plan.* 1990;21:226.)

cost efficacy, tracking of population data, and measurement of intervention efficacy and the effects of policy and systems changes are informing how medicine and public health can implement changes to promote, protect, and support breastfeeding mothers and families.

Social Influences on the History of Breastfeeding

The influence of "society" on anything is not exerted in a vacuum, so previous history, science, medicine, research, public health, economics, religion, law, politics, ethics, ethnicity, gender, and culture will exert their own influences, and this is certainly true of breastfeeding. Sorting out the different competing influences is not straightforward, and there is a plethora of opinions on the relative influence of different factors.[1,8–11,20,25,37,50,86–91] Although infant feeding and breastfeeding are personal choices for mothers and families, the choice is influenced by their personal beliefs and attitudes as well as those of relatives, friends, and neighbors. The larger community exerts its influence on maternal feeding decisions through accepted practices of child care in the community; proposed roles for women in the home and community; unspoken expectations about marriage, motherhood, child care, and employment; and sometimes direct comments from neighbors, friends, and individuals in power (doctors, health care workers, teachers, etc.). Physicians and public health agencies started to have a greater influence beginning in the 1900s with the efforts to decrease infant mortality, the development of pediatrics as a specialty of infant and child health, the increase of childbirth within hospitals, and "child-rearing by the book" (e.g., Emmett Holt's *The Care and Feeding of Children* and Benjamin Spock's *The Common Sense Book of Baby and Child Care*).[12,72–74] Accepted practices of child care related to infant feeding that have changed over time and been variably perceived and accepted include Wet nursing (formal or informal) or the use of milk from "milk agencies"

and artificial infant feedings in the past and now cross-nursing, milk sharing, and the use of donor milk from milk banks and infant formula.[38] The advancing development of formula, the perceived safety of formula with the introduction of pasteurization and refrigeration, and ready availability of bottles and nipples for storage and delivery led to greater commercialization of artificial infant feeding. In the late 1800s, artificial milk and commercial infant foods, with a variety of name brands, were marketed directly to mothers as consumers.[32] Infant formulas expanded their direct effect on infant feeding in the early 1900s, with manufacturers advertising directly to physicians in Europe and the United States in the 1920s. The American Medical Association assumed "approval" for the safety and quality of formula composition with the formation of the Committee on Foods in 1929.[38] In the 1920s and 1930s, the women's movement pushed for the emancipation of women and a greater role for women in society and public compared with their diminished role at home, "tied to" breastfeeding and child care. The breast was becoming perceived as a sex symbol and example of women's oppression rather than in its normal physiologic role of lactation and nutrition.[89] By the 1940s and 1950s, infant formula use was accepted as a normal practice in infant feeding, becoming part of popular culture and adding to the decline of breastfeeding. The transition of women into a role as employed workers outside the home (especially during World War II) added to the use of formula as culturally acceptable. Breastfeeding or expressing breast milk in the workplace was not something that was accepted. By the 1950s, popular culture portrayed bottle-feeding as the norm in modern households.[37] In 1956 the LLL was formed as a group of women wanting to share breastfeeding knowledge and experience with women who wanted to breastfeed. They wanted to be a "freeing" source of knowledge and support.[50] In the 1960s, feminism evolved and championed women's freedom from a male-dominated society. This led to some women's ambivalence about a woman's role in breastfeeding and infant feeding.[89] Despite this, feminism empowered women to utilize their own knowledge and experience to make health choices for themselves and their children.[87] This partially contributed to the rise in breastfeeding in the late 1970s and 1980s. In this modern period from the 1970s into the 21st century, nongovernmental agencies and groups and governmental initiatives clearly influenced cultural support for and promotion of breastfeeding, also contributing to the increases in breastfeeding within the United States and worldwide (see Table 1.1). Some of these groups and initiatives (LLL, IBCLE, WIC, DHHS Blueprint for Action on Breastfeeding, AAP, ACOG, AAFP, Office of Women's Health National Breastfeeding Awareness Campaign, etc.) are discussed earlier in the chapter in the section on education. International organizations and initiatives that also affected cultural perspectives include the WHO International Code of Marketing of Breastmilk Substitutes; the WHO/UNICEF Innocenti Declaration on the Protection, Promotion and Support of Breastfeeding; and the Baby-Friendly Hospital Initiative.

Maternity Protection: Work and Breastfeeding

The ILO has championed maternity protection and child welfare since 1919 at its inception and at the time of the first Maternity Protection Convention. The composite of the ILO maternity protection conventions (1919, 1952, and 2000 [No. 183]) and Recommendation 2000 (No. 191) advocate for three primary provisions: (1) at least 14 weeks of maternity leave, (2) compensation at a rate of at least two thirds of previous earnings, and (3) the leave is paid for by social insurance or public funds (not the employee or employer).[92] As of 2014, 185 countries provide for some duration of maternity leave (56 countries, at least 14 weeks; 42 countries, 18 weeks or more; 60 countries, 12 to 13 weeks; 27 countries < 12 weeks); the United States and Papua Guinea do not provide nationally stipulated maternity leave. Several questions remain: Who benefits from maternity protection? How well does the national legislation provide paid maternity leave to all working mothers? How does maternity leave affect breastfeeding? How do we provide maternity protection equitably to all women? The World Alliance for Breastfeeding Action (WABA) and International Baby Food Action Network (IBFAN), among other groups, support and track country compliance with these conventions and legislation.[93,94] WABA's 2015 report on maternity protection catalogues the duration of nationally legislated maternity leave, who pays for it, other forms of leave (parental or paternity), and the regulations for breastfeeding breaks at work. The IBFAN reinforces the importance of maternity protection as a human right, maternity as a "breastfeeding right," and breastfeeding as the standard of nutrition for health and well-being stipulated in the *Universal Declaration of Human Rights*.[3,95] Approximately 830 million women lack paid coverage in law and practice, with approximately 80% of those women living in Asia and Africa. Only 74 countries provide the stipulated two thirds of earnings for at least 14 weeks; 61 countries provide 100% of previous earnings for at least 14 weeks; and in 93 countries, the maternity leave is unpaid, paid at less than

two thirds, or paid for less than 14 weeks.[95] Additionally, 107 countries provide the cash benefits through national social security plans versus some other method. The ILO estimates that only 330 million women are effectively protected and would receive cash benefits for an appropriate time if pregnant. The issue of formal versus informal workplaces is an important one. Formal workplaces with a company or business are more likely to have a stated working situation (hours, salary, benefits) with a more explicit agreement about employment. It is also more likely that such businesses will adhere to the provisions of social security, leave, and sick regulations on the national and local levels. Informal workspaces are more commonly domiciles, farms, marketplaces, or street vendors and are often in the poorest financial situations. The businesses in informal situations often do not adhere to regulatory and governmental laws. Informal employment has been reported to be as high as 95% of work/employment in southern Asia, 89% of sub-Saharan Africa, and 59% of Latin America and the Caribbean.[94] Despite the suggestion that informal work is often negotiated within traditional local cultural values (relational, trust, reciprocity, and bartering), mothers are more likely at risk of the influences of gender and power differences and susceptible to the economic effects of unpaid leave. In response to this potentially vulnerable situation, the United Nations Convention on the Elimination of All Forms of Discrimination Against Women (CEDAW) recommends that government agencies advocate for child care and other care services in the community to facilitate a return to paid work and allow improved accommodations for breastfeeding and pumping at work or in close proximity.[96] Who benefits from maternity protection? Presumably, employers benefit as a result of improved production by an already-trained workforce, less absenteeism for parents (related to their health or the infant's improved health from breastfeeding), and lowered health costs for the family. There is also the issue of recovery time and the mother's readiness to return to efficient work. Nandi et al. demonstrated in 20 low- and middle-income countries that with an additional month of maternity leave, infant mortality was lowered by 8 fewer deaths per 1000 live births.[97] In Rossin's study in the United States (which does not have national maternity leave legislation), maternity leave was associated with a small increase in birth weight, reduced occurrence of premature births, and lower infant mortality.[98]

Maternity Leave and Breastfeeding

Three different reviews of studies on maternity leave and breastfeeding report a positive association between the duration of maternity leave and breastfeeding duration.[99−101] Navarro-Rosenblatt and Garmendia noted that in the 21 studies they reviewed, the researchers did not consistently stratify by socioeconomic class, but when there was data available, black women, women in a less privileged position, and women with less education had shorter breastfeeding durations.[101] They reported that women with a maternity leave of 3 months had at least a 50% greater likelihood of having a longer duration of breastfeeding than women who had less than 3 months of maternity leave, and women with 6 months or more of maternity were 30% more likely to breastfeed for at least 6 months. Other reviews reported similar results between the duration of maternity leave and the duration of breastfeeding.[102-104] Many other studies point to "return to work" as a common and significant reason for many women to stop breastfeeding. Additional study is needed to control for potential confounding variables, job status, field of work and role, socioeconomic status, breastfeeding accommodations and protection at work, and paid work and economic considerations of the women and their families. (For more on workplace accommodations, the "business case for breastfeeding," paternity leave, and return to work while continuing breastfeeding see Chapter 18.) The ILO, in conjunction with a number of other agencies, has produced a Maternity Protection Resource Package as a reference for governments, employers, unions, and nongovernmental organizations (NGOs) regarding training, policy, and action they can initiate for maternity protection.[105]

Human Milk Banking

As acceptance of wet nursing declined in the 19th century, the advent of milk banking was begun by Theodor Escherich in Vienna in 1909, and then a second milk bank opened in Boston in 1910.[106] In the 1970s and 1980s, there was more interest in milk banks to provide human milk to premature and very low-birth-weight (VLBW) infants for the potential benefits, and five milk banks were started in England in 1975. The WHO, UNICEF, and AAP made statements in 1980 concerning the use of donated human milk in place of utilizing formula when the mother's own milk was inadequate or not available.[107] Various countries passed legislation for the establishment of milk banks, and regulations and recommendations for those were developed (United States, Canada, France, Italy, and Brazil). The Human Milk Banking Association of North America (HMBANA) was formed in 1985, the same year that Brazil created its first milk bank. There was significant growth of milk banks worldwide until the 1980s, when a number of milk banks closed due to the fear of transmission of human immunodeficiency virus (HIV) through breast milk. DHM was then considered and handled as a body fluid with potential infectious risks (hepatitis B, HIV, and human T-lymphotropic virus [HTLV] types 1 and 2). Processing of human milk underwent more formal adoption of processing guidelines, including donor screening for possible risk factors (infection, medication exposure) with an interview, serologic testing, and a physician "consent" to the donor mother's health. The HMBANA established a set of guidelines for the establishment and management of these nonprofit milk banks.[108] Human milk processing was carefully standardized, with guidelines for handling, storage, culturing for potential pathogens, pasteurization, and freezing and shipping. In the same period, the demand for human milk was increasing with the evidence that human breast milk for VLBW and premature infants had clear health benefits, particularly in protection against sepsis and NEC.[109-111] As demand increased, so did the number of milk banks, such that in 2019, the HMBANA had 29 members; Australia had 5 milk banks;

the European Milk Banking Association (EMBA) had over 241 affiliated member banks; and Brazil's network of national banks expanded to form the Global Network of Human Milk Banks, with over 230 members.

Currently, there are a number of important issues influencing the role of human milk banks in support of breastfeeding, breastfeeding women, and the optimal nutrition of all infants, including the relatively limited supply of human milk for donation; the effects of processing on DHM; the cost effectiveness of DHM banks; the allocation of pasteurized donor human milk (PDHM), predominantly occurring through local milk banks and in hospital settings; the existence of potential competition by for-profit milk banks; and the ethical and equitable distribution of DHM as a valuable resource.[112] Women lactate for a limited period of time, and of all the women who initiate breastfeeding, not all women have "excess milk" above the amount needed to feed their own child, and only a small percentage of those women donate human milk to milk banks. The practices of cross-nursing (mothers sharing the breastfeeding of infants with a relative, friend, or neighbor) and informal milk sharing, exchanging breast milk between women (even unknown to each other before sharing) are further affecting the supply available to human milk banks. This is contrasted by the increasing demand for DHM because of increasing numbers of premature and VLBW infants and the increasing recognition of situations where human milk clearly benefits sick and well infants. The increasing demand outstrips the worldwide increases in DHM production.[113] It is reported that in neonatal intensive care units worldwide, as many as 40% of infants do not have sufficient human milk for the first weeks of life.[114] There is no formal algorithm for distributing DHM, nor an organized mechanism of tracking allocation to study it and the potential for bias in an unregulated system. Parallel to the calls for the elimination of discrimination against women and the emphasis on the role of breastfeeding in reaching important Sustainable Development Goals (SDGs), there has been a "call to action for equitable access to human milk for vulnerable infants."[115] The Oxford-PATH Human Milk Working Group has proposed specific ethical considerations (vulnerability, equity and fairness, respect for autonomy, human rights) and four actions to foster equitable access to human milk. They emphasize the application of ethical principles to the ongoing development of donor milk programs; prioritization of donor milk banks within national, regional, and global maternal/infant health programs; and utilization of ongoing research to inform new strategies. Scientific inquiry continues to drive the processing of DHM to optimize its nutritional makeup, bioactive factors, and cellular composition. This includes adjustments to processing, different mechanisms of pasteurization (varying temperatures, duration of treatment, and use of pressure), fortification of DHM as needed, and the possible addition of the mother's own milk microbiota before administering DHM.[116-122] The ongoing progress in human milk banking and this call to action for equity will continue to shape breastfeeding and the use of human breast milk for the next decade.

DISPARITIES IN BREASTFEEDING

Disparities in breastfeeding have existed throughout history around the world, as have disparities in health care, and these gaps remain significant.[91,123–129] Disparity in breastfeeding may directly contribute to disparity in infant morbidity and mortality, especially through the first year of life.[129] There are numerous variables that may play a role at different times in these disparities. Nevertheless, racism, gender inequalities, and disparities related to ethnicity, nationality, politics, and poverty remain the dominant contributors to such disparities.[91,123,126] The commercialism and marketing tactics of formula companies often exacerbate preexisting disparity.[91,124,125] There are discernable inequities in the experience of adverse childhood experiences (ACEs), social determinants of health, structural racism, and lack of access to health care, which adversely affect breastfeeding and maternal and infant health, especially in communities of color or those with low socioeconomic resources.

Global Disparities in Breastfeeding

Globally, disparities in breastfeeding also exist. However, they are often hidden as a result of missing data from individual countries, the lack of an organized system of data collection, the lack of data from recent years for comparison, and the lack of data from within different areas or communities within individual countries. In the 2017 Global Breastfeeding Scorecard from the Global Breastfeeding Collective of the WHO and UNICEF, the gaps in data are dramatic, and there is significant variability in breastfeeding rates by country (Table 1.3).[130] Only 77 countries have assessed their breastfeeding programs by utilizing the indicators set out by the World Breastfeeding Trends Initiative (WBTI) in the last 5 years, and more than 100 countries have never done this. The WBTI attempts to track data on five indicators: (1) infant is put to the breast within the first hour after birth, (2) ever breastfed, (3) EBF under 6 months of age, (4) continued any breastfeeding at 12 months of age, and (5) continued breastfeeding at 24 months of age. The United States does not collect data on all these indicators but assesses (1) initiated breastfeeding, (2) any breastfeeding at 3 months and (3) 6 months, and (4) EBF at 3 months and (5) EBF at 6 months.[48] For example, the Global Breastfeeding Collective has targeted 60% EBF at under 6 months for all countries, but in 2017, the overall rate of EBF was 40%. Although 23 countries reported at least 60% EBF, rates in individual countries can be very low (e.g., the Americas). Similarly, the rate of continued breastfeeding at 12 months of age is ~74% on average, and 40% of countries report 80% breastfeeding at 12 months, whereas in the Americas, only four countries achieve such a high percentage at 12 months. The Global Breastfeeding Collective has also noted other examples of disparities worldwide: Low- and middle-income countries often have higher breastfeeding rates than high-income countries, and rural areas having higher breastfeeding rates than urban areas. In the Global Breastfeeding Scorecard of 2017, it was noted that interventions that can have a positive effect on breastfeeding rates

globally include funding directly allocated to breastfeeding education, promotion, and support; effective regulation of the marketing of breast-milk substitutes; paid maternity leave; successful implementation of Baby-Friendly Hospital initiatives; expanded community support programs; and a national focus on monitoring rates of breastfeeding and assessing national breastfeeding policies and programs.[130] Unless these interventions are applied universally with an eye to existing disparities and biases, they will not change the disparities in breastfeeding. Other authors emphasize the need for ongoing "comprehensive analysis of breastfeeding patterns" in individual countries, communities, and populations within the developing world to promote equity. They discuss the need for enhanced understanding of the local history of breastfeeding, the ongoing forces influencing breastfeeding, and the existing disparities and biases in health care to implement targeted interventions.[131]

Disparities in Breastfeeding in the United States

There have been a number of publications presenting data on breastfeeding disparity in the United States.[43,44,48] Jones et al. present data on disparities for African American women, Hispanic women, American Indian/Alaskan Native women, and Asian women through 2007.[44] African American women were 2.5 times less likely to breastfeed than white women, were 16 percentage points lower than white women in continuing breastfeeding to 6 months of age, and were more likely to give their infants formula in the first 2 days of life than any other group of women. Hispanic women generally had the highest rates of breastfeeding initiation and continuation but were also more likely to supplement with formula as early as 2 days of age and initiate sold foods before 4 months of age. There was evidence that the Hispanic group of women was heterogeneous, which may be due to their countries of origin and the degree/duration of acculturation in the United States. In this same study, American Indian and Alaskan Native women also had low rates of breastfeeding initiation and duration, second to the African American women. Asian women had higher initiation and continuation at 6 and 12 months. However, Native Hawaiian women had lower initiation rates and shorter EBF, with earlier introduction of formula.[44] Anstey et al. reported on US results from the National Immunization Survey (NIS) study for the years 2010 to 2013.[43] The gap between black and white infants for initiation of breastfeeding in this period was only slightly less (17.2-percentage-point difference) than it was in the 2003 to 2006 data. The difference in the rate of EBF at 6 months increased in this period (from 2003 to 2006 to 2010 to 2013) for black compared with white women (7.8% gap up to an 8.5% gap), as did any breastfeeding at 12 months (increased gap from 9.7 percentage points to 13.7 percentage points). Anstey et al. also noted significant differences in breastfeeding rates by state, which were worse for southern and midwestern states.[43] They noted that some barriers to breastfeeding might be overly experienced by black women (lack of breastfeeding knowledge, lack of support from peers and families, and insufficient support from

TABLE 1.3   Breastfeeding up to 24 Months by Country, 2010 to 2018 (Selected from UNICEF Infant Young Child Feeding Database, October 2019)

Country, Year of Data Collection	Early Initiation (%) (Put to Breast <1 Hour)	Ever Breastfed (%)	Exclusive Breastfeeding at 0–5 Months (%)	Continued Breastfeeding at 12–15 Months (%)	Continued Breastfeeding at 20–23 Months (%)
Sub-Saharan Africa					
Benin, 2017	54.1	96.6	41.4	91.2	42.5
Burkina Faso, 2010	55.8	99.2	47.8	84.4	80.1
Cameroon, 2014	31.2	95.6	28.0	70.3	18.5
Central African Republic, 2010	52.5	94.8	28.8	86.6	32.1
Chad, 2014	23.0	98.1	14.0	87.9	65.2
Comoros, 2012	33.7	93.0	11.4	69.7	56.7
Cote d'Ivoire, 2016	36.6	97.4	23.1	88.1	29.0
Eritrea, 2010	93.1	97.9	68.7	94.6	72.6
Ethiopia, 2016	73.3	98.8	58.5	91.8	75.5
Gabon, 2012	32.3	89.6	5.1	45.4	3.9
Ghana, 2014	55.6	98.4	52.1	94.6	50.1
Guinea, 2016	33.9	97.0	33.4	86.3	60.3
Kenya, 2014	62.2	98.7	61.4	90.4	53.1
Madagascar, 2012	65.8	99.0	41.9	89.0	83.1
Malawi, 2015	76.2	97.7	59.4	91.6	71.5
Mali, 2015	53.2	95.7	40.4	90.8	55.2
Mozambique, 2011	69.0	97.3	41.0	86.0	51.6
Namibia, 2013	71.2	95.7	46.3	64.4	21.0
Niger, 2012	52.9	98.8	23.3	92.6	50.1
Nigeria, 2016	32.8	95.0	25.2	82.9	27.8
Rwanda, 2014	80.5	98.8	86.9	95.6	87.2
South Africa, 2016	67.3	82.6	31.6	51.4	13
Senegal, 2017	33.6	98.2	42.1	94.3	40.0
Togo, 2013	60.6	98.0	57.2	94.0	61.4
Uganda, 2016	66.1	97.6	65.5	86.9	43.4
Zambia, 2013	65.8	95.5	69.9	89.8	30.4
Zimbabwe, 2015	57.6	98.1	47.1	91.1	14.2
Near East and North Africa					
Egypt, 2014	27.1	95.7	39.5	80.0	20.4
Jordan, 2017	67.0	91.7	25.4	36.2	14.9
Mauritania, 2018	67.8	94.8	40.3	91.0	39.6

(Continued)

TABLE 1.3 Breastfeeding up to 24 Months by Country, 2010 to 2018 (Selected from UNICEF Infant Young Child Feeding Database, October 2019)—cont'd

Country, Year of Data Collection	Early Initiation (%) (Put to Breast <1 Hour)	Ever Breastfed (%)	Exclusive Breastfeeding at 0–5 Months (%)	Continued Breastfeeding at 12–15 Months (%)	Continued Breastfeeding at 20–23 Months (%)
Morocco, 2017	42.6	97.1	35.0	64.9	29.7
Turkey, 2018	49.9	96.7	30.1	68.2	33.9
Yemen, 2013	52.7	96.7	9.7	71.2	45.3
Asia					
Bangladesh, 2014	50.8	96.6	55.3	96.0	87.3
Cambodia, 2014	62.6	96.2	65.2	80.0	37.1
India, 2015	41.5	95.5	54.9	86.2	71.6
Indonesia, 2017	58.2	94.9	50.7	76.5	54.6
Nepal, 2016	54.9	99.1	65.2	98.1	38.5
Pakistan, 2017	19.6	94.3	47.5	69.6	53.4
Philippines, 2017	56.9	93.2	33.0	66.0	52.3
Vietnam, 2013	26.5	96.9	24.0	65.6	21.8
Latin America and Caribbean					
Belize, 2015	68.3	92.7	33.2	51.5	35.1
Bolivia, 2016	55.0	96.8	58.3	72.2	37.9
Colombia, 2015	72.0	97.6	36.1	52.2	31.6
Dominican Republic, 2014	38.1	91.2	4.6	31.2	12.4
Ecuador, 2014	54.6	96.7	39.6	58.5	18.9
El Salvador, 2014	42.0	96.1	46.7	74.1	57.0
Guatemala, 2014	63.1	97.2	53.2	85.3	56.8
Haiti, 2016	47.4	95.2	39.9	76.9	24.9
Honduras, 2011	63.8	96.3	30.7	69.6	43.3
Nicaragua, 2011	54.4	92.3	31.7	69.9	42.0
Paraguay, 2016	49.5	96.6	29.6	48.2	21.0
Peru, 2016	49.7	98.7	66.4	80.3	48.6
Eastern Europe and Central Asia					
Armenia, 2015	40.9	96.5	44.5	36.0	21.6
Azerbaijan, 2013	19.7	94.5	12.1	42.3	16.2
Kazakhstan, 2015	83.3	97.1	37.8	59.8	21.1
Turkmenistan, 2015	73.4	98.5	58.3	64.1	19.5
Uzbekistan, 2006	NA	97.3	23.8	78.3	37.9

Data from UNICEF. UNICEF Global Database for Infant and Young Child Feeding, October 2019. http://www.data.unicef.org/resources/dataset/infant-young-child-feeding/. Accessed March 29, 2020.

health care providers) and pointed out a previous study demonstrating less access to supportive practices for breastfeeding (early initiation, rooming-in, limited use of pacifiers, and postdischarge support) in hospitals serving higher percentages of black individuals.[132] Specific hospital-related interventions to augment supportive practices for breastfeeding have been initiated in 93 hospitals in 24 southern and midwestern states under the program EMPower Breastfeeding: Enhancing Maternity Practices.[133] Johnson et al. reviewed published psychosocial interventions to enhance breastfeeding rates among African American women.[134] They also proposed analyzing and understanding the socio-historical context of breastfeeding in the United States and a framework for including interventions acting on multiple levels (individual, interpersonal, community, and policy or systems). They additionally suggested assessing the influence of ongoing discrimination, considering the social support preferred by minority women, expanding the use of media for targeted interventions, and considering socioeconomic status and its impact on the heterogeneous populations of minority women.[134] In 2019 Beauregard et al. analyzed breastfeeding data from the National Immunization Survey—Child (NIS-Child; 2016 to 2017 data) for infants born in 2015.[48] They also noted significant disparities between black infants and white infants when all infants were included in the analysis. When only infants whose mothers had initiated breastfeeding were included, the magnitude of the differences between black and white infants decreased notably for any breastfeeding at 3 months and to a lesser degree for any breastfeeding at 6 months and for EBF at 3 and 6 months (Table 1.4). Their conclusion was that the differences noted for any breastfeeding or EBF were due, to a degree, to racial and ethnic differences in the initiation of breastfeeding. Overall breastfeeding rates in the United States from NIS data are shown in Tables 1.5 and 1.6.

Breastfeeding and Social Justice

Jacqueline Wolf provides a brief history of disparities in breastfeeding and notes many of the societal battles to improve child nutrition and health that she feels led us in our first steps in social justice for breastfeeding.[91] Jones et al. specifically review racial and ethnic disparities in breastfeeding and possible influences in the United States.[44] They go beyond the statistics to review the data on common barriers to breastfeeding and a consideration of potentially effective interventions to overcome the disparities. Deborah McCarter-Spaulding examines the role of feminism in breastfeeding, acknowledging the potential for conflict among feminist theories concerning gender equality versus gender-neutral child-rearing and breastfeeding.[4] She emphasizes that disadvantaged women may be more adversely influenced in their infant-feeding choice by poverty, education, society, institutional racism, and politics. She states that health initiatives to address disparity should promote systems and policies that foster women's opportunity to make independent choices for infant feeding and breastfeeding and also foster the valuing of

healthy children and families and women's personal and public roles in society.[2] McCarter-Spaulding's emphasis on women's independence and value equally direct us to considerations of social justice.[4] Paige Hall Smith, who has written extensively on gender inequality, discusses gender inequality and its theoretical contribution to disparity in breastfeeding. She argues that the perception that breastfeeding is constraining women (when they try to breastfeed in public places, after returning to work, or if they have limited resources) is misplaced and that the constraints women experience are located in persistent systemic and societal structures of gender inequality.[135] These systemic inequalities interfere with their parenting choices and the fulfillment of their different roles in society. The failure to support women in their personal and professional roles is adversely affecting women's breastfeeding (intent, initiation, continuation [especially at time of return to work], and overall duration) such that women marginalized by education, race, income, and marital status are breastfeeding less.[136] Examination of our social responsibility to all members of society demonstrates that our failure to support all women equitably is leading to diminished breastfeeding overall. The DHHS has proposed a variety of potential solutions to promote and support breastfeeding for all women and families, including augmenting workplace flexibility (regarding parental leave and breastfeeding), increasing child-care availability and access at or close to work, improved health care systems and access for women and children who most need it, and enhanced public health and educational programs for pregnancy and breastfeeding that acknowledge the specific needs and desires of marginalized women.[128] The solutions should be offered and applied fairly to all but still be "person and family specific," similar to how "reasonable accommodations" for disabled individuals and employment are "personalized." Policies and system changes must be complemented by "changes in social norms" that value women and families in breastfeeding and child-rearing roles and provide for ongoing assessment of changes to protect against discrimination and adverse effects on women's economic and social status.[135] George Kent presents a review and summary of child feeding and human rights.[3] He elaborates on the "right to food principles for children" and considers important issues, such as food safety and security and nutrition, that contribute to the "highest attainable standard of health." As he aptly states, "human rights are universal"; therefore "Breastfeeding is the right of the mother and the child together." Joan E. Dodgson edited a special edition of the *Journal of Human Lactation* highlighting social justice and lactation. In the absence of a universal, agreed-upon definition of social justice, she emphasizes that two essential elements of social justice are fairness in providing equal access to all and the demonstration of our social responsibility to care for disadvantaged and marginalized individuals in society.[16] Paige Hall Smith, in the same issue of the *Journal of Human Lactation*, provides a conceptualized framework for applying social justice to the protection, promotion, and support of breastfeeding.[5] In this framework, synthesized from work done and in conversations with the organizing group at

TABLE 1.4 Differences in Breastfeeding Initiation and Duration at Ages 3 and 6 Months[a] Among Non-Hispanic Black and Non-Hispanic White Infants Born in 2015—Data from National Immunization Survey—Child, United States, 2016 to 2017[b]

Breastfeeding Indicator	ALL INFANTS						INFANTS WHO HAD INITIATED BREASTFEEDING					
	NON-HISPANIC WHITE		NON-HISPANIC BLACK		PERCENTAGE-POINT DIFFERENCE		NON-HISPANIC WHITE		NON-HISPANIC BLACK		PERCENTAGE-POINT DIFFERENCE	
	No.	% (95% CI)	No.	% (95% CI)	% (95% CI)		No.	% (95% CI)	No.	% (95% CI)	% (95% CI)	
Initiated breastfeeding	9907	85.9 (84.7–87.1)	1607	69.4 (65.9–73.0)	16.5 (12.7–20.2)		8729	N/A	1.159	N/A	N/A	
Any breastfeeding at age 3 mo	9907	72.7 (71.2–742)	1607	58.0 (54.2–61.71)	14.7 (10.7–18.8)		8729	84.7 (83.4–85.9)	1159	83.5 (80.3–86.71)	1.2 (−2.3–4.6)	
Exclusive breastfeeding through age 3 mo	9537	53.0 (51.4–54.7)	1573	36.0 (32.2–39.7)	17.0 (12.9–21.2)		8359	62.2 (60.5–63.9)	1125	52.3 (47.8–56.9)	9.9 (5.0–14.7)	
Any breastfeeding at age 6 mo	9907	62.0 (60.4–63.6)	1607	44.7 (40.9–48.5)	17.3 (13.1–21.4)		8729	72.2 (70.6–73.8)	1159	64.4 (60.2–68.6)	7.8 (3.3–12.3)	
Exclusive breastfeeding through age 6 mo	9537	29.5 (28.0–31.1)	1573	17.2 (14.1–20.2)	12.4 (8.9–15.8)		8359	34.7 (32.9–36.4)	1125	25.0 (20.8–29.2)	9.7 (5.1–14.2)	

CI, Confidence interval; *N/A*, not applicable.

[a]Breastfeeding initiation was determined according to the participant's response to the question, "Was [child] ever breastfed or fed breast milk?" Breastfeeding duration was determined according to the participant's response to the question "How old was [child's name] when [child 's name] completely stopped breastfeeding or being fed breast milk?" Exclusive breastfeeding was defined as only breast milk (no solids, no water, and no other liquids). To assess the duration of exclusive breastfeeding, participants were asked two questions about age: (1) "How old was [child's name] when he/she was first fed formula?" and (2) "How old was [child's name] when he/she was first fed anything other than breast milk or formula?" (This includes juke, cow's milk, sugar water, baby food, or anything else that [child] might have been given, even water.)"

[b]Based on National Immunization Survey—Child data from survey years 2016–2017, among infants born in 2015. Differences in breastfeeding rates between non-Hispanic black and non-Hispanic white infants are statistically significant (*p* < 0.05, two-sample test of proportions).

From Beauregard JL, Hamner HC, Chen J, et al. Racial disparities in breastfeeding initiation and duration among U.S. infants born in 2015. *MMWR Morb Mortal Wkly Rep.* 2019;68(34):745–748. http://doi:10.15585/mmwr.mm6834a3. PMID: 31465319.

TABLE 1.5   Breastfeeding Rates by State—Infants Born in 2004 Compared With Infants Born in 2015

OUTCOME INDICATORS

Breastfeeding Rates
(%)

State	Ever Breastfed, 2004, 2015	Breastfeeding at 6 Months, 2004, 2015	Breastfeeding at 12 Months, 2004, 2015	Exclusive Breastfeeding at 3 Months, 2004, 2015	Exclusive Breastfeeding at 6 Months, 2004, 2015
US national average	73.8, **83.2**	41.5, 57.6	20.9, **35.9**	30.5, **46.9**	11.3, 24.9
Healthy People 2020 targets, %	81.9%	60.6%	34.1%	46.2%	25.5%
Alabama	52.1, 68.1	25.4, 39.1	11.5, 24.8	19.3, 34.1	4.9, 20.6
Alaska	**84.8, 93.1**	**60.9, 69.2**	31.8, **49.7**	**47.2, 65.3**	24.3, **42.1**
Arizona	**83.5, 82.7**	46.5, 55.3	23.4, **35.5**	38.8, **51.8**	14.3, **26.3**
Arkansas	59.2, 73.8	23.2, 45.2	8.5, 24.2	15.8, 39.0	6.2, 20.4
California	**83.8, 87.2**	52.9, **66.7**	30.4, **40.2**	38.7, **53.0**	17.4, **26.3**
Colorado	**85.9, 90.9**	42.0, **63.9**	23.6, **40.0**	36.2, **57.2**	10.8, 22.4
Connecticut	79.5, **86.3**	44.6, 59.6	23.7, **39.1**	35.6, 45.5	10.1, 23.6
Delaware	63.6, 77.4	35.7, 55.6	14.6, 33.4	26.3, **47.2**	11.4, 23.6
Dist. of Columbia	68.0, **83.0**	40.0, **65.5**	21.4, **43.6**	27.8, **52.6**	9.8, **29.1**
Florida	77.9, **82.6**	37.5, 54.0	15.6, 33.5	27.8, 41.6	9.1, 21.3
Georgia	68.2, **84.0**	38.0, 55.5	16.8, **34.9**	25.6, 43.8	11.0, 22.1
Hawaii	81.0, **90.6**	50.5, **65.5**	**35.5, 47.2**	37.8, **54.2**	15.8, **32.9**
Idaho	**85.9, 90.1**	49.0, **62.1**	22.6, **39.0**	38.7, **52.6**	10.3, **28.4**
Illinois	72.5, 80.3	40.9, 53.0	17.6, 33.8	31.6, 39.6	10.0, 19.5
Indiana	64.7, 78.8	34.6, 53.5	18.0, 33.0	28.3, **47.2**	10.4, **31.7**
Iowa	74.2, 81.5	44.9, 51.4	20.0, 30.2	37.6, **51.6**	11.6, **29.5**
Kansas	74.4, **83.6**	42.2, 58.2	16.9, **36.5**	30.0, **50.4**	9.2, **26.1**
Kentucky	59.1, 73.9	26.4, 48.6	14.4, 28.2	25.3, 39.8	7.5, 21.1
Louisiana	50.7, 67.0	19.2, 39.0	8.3, 20.6	15.2, 39.4	2.8, 20.2
Maine	76.3, **85.2**	46.6, **62.1**	27.6, **41.8**	42.1, **52.5**	15.9, **34.1**
Maryland	71.0, **91.0**	40.2, **66.8**	21.2, **41.1**	32.1, **50.1**	8.6, **26.2**
Massachusetts	72.4, **87.4**	42.1, 55.6	19.0, **36.8**	32.7, **46.5**	11.9, **26.6**
Michigan	63.4, 77.7	36.4, 55.6	18.6, **34.6**	27.4, 44.1	8.3, 23.9
Minnesota	80.9, **89.2**	46.5, **65.3**	23.8, **38.9**	33.9, **56.3**	16.1, **37.2**
Mississippi	50.2, 63.2	23.3, 35.4	8.2, 18.3	19.0, 28.2	8.0, 13.0
Missouri	67.3, **82.3**	32.5, 57.8	15.8, 33.1	26.6, **52.7**	7.4, **31.3**
Montana	**87.7, 83.9**	53.8, **61.1**	28.8, **40.5**	**50.9, 56.8**	18.3, **35.7**
Nebraska	79.3, **82.2**	47.6, 57.0	21.8, **40.2**	31.7, **46.7**	9.8, 25.4
Nevada	79.7, **83.5**	45.6, 49.9	21.9, 30.6	31.9, 44.1	10.3, 20.8
New Hampshire	73.7, **87.4**	48.7, **64.7**	27.5, **45.6**	34.3, **55.9**	13.6, **30.2**
New Jersey	69.8, **82.8**	45.1, 57.6	19.4, **36.1**	27.0, 40.6	11.8, 24.4
New Mexico	80.7, **87.7**	41.2, 59.8	21.1, **35.1**	32.9, **53.0**	14.3, **27.6**

(Continued)

TABLE 1.5 Breastfeeding Rates by State—Infants Born in 2004 Compared With Infants Born in 2015—cont'd

| | OUTCOME INDICATORS | | | | |

Breastfeeding Rates (%)

State	Ever Breastfed, 2004, 2015	Breastfeeding at 6 Months, 2004, 2015	Breastfeeding at 12 Months, 2004, 2015	Exclusive Breastfeeding at 3 Months, 2004, 2015	Exclusive Breastfeeding at 6 Months, 2004, 2015
New York	73.8, **85.1**	50.0, 59.5	26.9, **38.3**	26.0, 42.8	11.4, 21.4
North Carolina	72.0, **84.9**	34.2, 58.8	18.3, 33.2	23.0, **48.1**	6.9, **27.0**
North Dakota	73.1, 81.7	45.1, 58.2	19.5, 33.4	39.4, **46.2**	15.4, **29.1**
Ohio	59.6, **81.9**	33.3, 53.1	12.9, 30.7	27.2, 44.4	9.8, 23.7
Oklahoma	67.1, 75.9	29.6, 49.0	12.7, 31.0	23.0, 44.2	10.6, 21.6
Oregon	**88.3, 89.4**	56.4, 72.5	33.5, **51.7**	41.5, **57.8**	19.9, **33.4**
Pennsylvania	66.6, **83.8**	35.2, 59.2	16.8, **39.0**	27.1, **48.9**	8.0, **25.6**
Rhode Island	69.1, 81.4	31.2, 49.6	14.0, 30.9	31.2, **47.9**	9.5, **28.9**
South Carolina	67.4, 76.4	30.0, 45.1	11.1, 28.0	26.6, 42.7	5.4, 24.4
South Dakota	71.1, **83.3**	40.5, **62.6**	23.4, **42.7**	32.2, **54.3**	12.2, **32.2**
Tennessee	71.2, 75.7	32.6, 49.8	16.6, **34.4**	26.7, 34.5	11.9, 22.7
Texas	75.4, **85.0**	37.3, 56.6	18.7, **35.2**	25.2, **48.0**	7.1, 24.1
Utah	**84.5, 89.7**	55.6, **62.5**	28.1, **40.8**	39.8, **49.7**	10.2, **27.8**
Vermont	**85.2, 89.3**	55.3, **70.9**	**34.1, 51.3**	**47.3, 62.8**	15.9, **38.0**
Virginia	79.1, 81.7	49.8, **62.5**	25.6, **39.3**	32.6, 45.6	13.4, **26.6**
Washington	**88.4, 92.4**	56.6, **72.7**	32.3, **48.2**	**49.6, 58.9**	22.5, **29.1**
West Virginia	59.3, 68.6	26.8, 40.1	14.0, 24.3	21.3, 36.3	5.2, 20.2
Wisconsin	72.1, **82.2**	39.6, 59.0	19.0, 39.3	32.5, **48.8**	13.4, **28.3**
Wyoming	80.5, **90.0**	42.9, 59.4	18.5, 38.6	36.2, **56.8**	11.4, **28.8**

Numbers in bold are those that have met the *Healthy People 2020* goals. Target %: ever breastfed—81.9%; breastfed at 6 months of age—60.6%; breastfed at 12 months of age—34.1%; exclusively breastfed through 3 months—46.2%; exclusively breastfed through 6 months of age—25. From Centers for Disease Control and Prevention. National immunization survey, 2004 births. *MMWR*. 2007;56(30):760–763; Centers for Disease Control and Prevention. Breastfeeding Report Card United States, 2018. Data from National Immunization Survey, US Department of Health and Human Services. https://www.cdc.gov/breastfeeding/data/nis_data/results.html. Accessed March 17, 2020.

the 12th Breastfeeding and Feminism International Conference in 2017, there are "7 conceptual domains" proposed: (1) the value of breastfeeding and human milk for health (and health equity); (2) the value of breastfeeding for our global environment (fit with current SDGs); (3) the right to breastfeed (beyond choice; requires protection and support); (4) supporting lactation and access to human milk for all (laws, policies, institutions, and cultural changes acting together for this aim); (5) advancing support for embodied caregiving and all caregivers (create practices and norms that value and support breastfeeding and caregiving overall); (6) removing barriers to skilled lactation support (ensuring access for marginalized individuals and groups); and (7) advancing breastfeeding as a cornerstone of health equity (requires redressing bias and oppression in social systems to achieve health equity). Powell et al. discuss breastfeeding among women with physical disabilities in the United States, identifying potential barriers to and facilitators of breastfeeding.[137] Others support the inclusion of individuals in the lesbian, gay, bisexual, transgender, and queer or questioning (LGBTQ +) community in the success of breastfeeding or chestfeeding, equity in health, and normative nurturing and caregiving.[138,139] (See Chapter 20 in this book.) The call for social justice for breastfeeding should be inclusive of any marginalized or oppressed group we can think of and even ones we have not yet recognized as such.

MEASURES OF BREASTFEEDING SUCCESS

To understand how to promote, support, and protect breastfeeding, it is important to be able to measure breastfeeding and the influence of various interventions on breastfeeding. First and foremost, we should assess the success of individual mothers and families in infant-feeding choices, including (1)

TABLE 1.6   Breastfeeding Among US Children Born 2009 to 2016, Percentage by Birth Year

| | BIRTH YEAR | | | | | | | | |
	2009	2010	2011	2012	2013	2014	2015	2016	Healthy People 2020 Targets
Ever breastfed	76.1	76.7	79.2	80.0	81.1	**82.5**	**83.2**	**83.8**	**81.9%**
	± 1.0	± 1.2	± 1.2	± 1.2	± 1.1	± 1.1	± 1.0	± 1.2	
Breastfed at 6 months	46.6	47.5	49.4	51.4	51.8	55.3	57.6	57.3	**60.6%**
	± 1.2	± 1.4	± 1.5	± 1.5	± 1.4	± 1.4	± 1.4	± 1.6	
Breastfed at 12 months	24.6	25.3	26.7	29.2	30.7	33.7	**35.9**	**36.2**	**34.1%**
	± 1.0	± 1.3	± 1.3	± 1.4	± 1.3	± 1.3	± 1.3	± 1.5	
EBF through 3 months	35.9	37.1	40.7	43.3	44.4	**46.6**	**46.9**	**47.5**	**46.2%**
	± 1.1	± 1.4	± 1.5	± 1.6	± 1.4	± 1.4	± 1.4	± 1.6	
EBF through 6 months	15.6	17.2	18.8	21.9	22.3	24.9	24.9	25.4	**25.5%**
	± 0.9	± 1.2	± 1.2	± 1.4	± 1.1	± 1.3	± 1.2	± 1.3	

EBF, Exclusive breastfeeding—only breast milk, no solids, water, or other liquid.
Data from Centers for Disease Control and Prevention National Immunization Survey (percentage ± half 95% confidence interval). Data from US territories excluded from national breastfeeding estimates to be consistent with analytical methods for *Healthy People 2020*, From Centers for Disease Control and Prevention. Breastfeeding Report Card, United States, 2018. Data from National Immunization Survey Results by Birth Year. https://www.cdc.gov/breastfeeding/data/nis_data/results.html. Accessed March 17, 2020.

making an informed decision(s) regarding infant feeding without experiencing pressure, judgment, or discrimination; (2) articulating their breastfeeding goals for intensity (exclusive, predominant, partial) and duration and their ability to adjust those goals as necessary; (3) generating a familial and community environment supportive of their breastfeeding choices; (4) successful transition of the mother/individual into her other personal and professional roles beyond pregnancy, breastfeeding, and primary child caregiver; and (5) the mother/individual viewing the infant-feeding experience positively in realizing the desired standard of health and growth and development for both the child and mother. It is essential that we understand the thoughts, feelings, and experiences of breastfeeding individuals and, in particular, what actions or interventions support them in reaching their breastfeeding goals. This requires asking mothers and parents about their experience and probing to find out the positive and negative variables affecting their breastfeeding success. It also requires surveying groups of women in different communities, groups, and areas and doing a needs assessment of barriers and effective supportive interventions within their communities.

What Women Say About Barriers and Support

A lot has been written about maternal reasons for early cessation of breastfeeding.[140–145] This has been reported for specific groups of women in the attempt to understand possible similarities and differences, including women with postpartum depressive symptoms, women of different racial and ethnic groups, women of low income, and overweight or obese women, among others.[146–149] Li et al. presented data for 1323 women—infant pairs on specific reasons mothers gave for their decision to stop breastfeeding their infants, separated

out by infant age[140] (Table 1.7). They highlighted seven main themes (lactational, psychosocial, nutritional, lifestyle, medical, milk pumping, and infant self-weaning) for the reasons and identified that lactational and nutritional factors were the most common reasons for stopping breastfeeding in the first month, with the addition of psychosocial and milk-pumping reasons in the second month. For mothers who stopped breastfeeding at 3 to 8 months postpartum, the three main reasons were as follows: breast milk alone did not satisfy the infant, the mother did not make enough milk, and the baby self-weaned or lost interest. In a subsequent analysis in 2013 of similar data, using the "same reasons" expressed by mothers, Odom et al. showed that 13 of these factors were associated with an increased odds ratio of not reaching prenatal maternal goals for the duration of breastfeeding even after adjusting for a number of potentially confounding variables.[141] These reported reasons for earlier-than-desired termination of breastfeeding included the following: my baby had trouble sucking or latching on; my nipples were sore, cracked, or bleeding; breastfeeding was too painful; my breasts were overfull or engorged; my breasts were infected or abscessed; I didn't have enough milk; breast milk alone did not satisfy my baby; I had trouble getting the milk flow to start; I thought that my baby was not gaining enough weight; a health professional said my baby was not gaining enough weight; I was sick or had to take medicine; my baby became sick and could not breastfeed; pumping milk no longer seemed worth the effort required. All of these issues are potentially amenable to education and supportive measures communicated to the mother by lactation specialists. Steube et al. performed a separate analysis of maternal survey data from the Infant Feeding Practices Study (IFPS) II, which

TABLE 1.7 Percentage of Mothers Who Indicated That Specified Reasons Were Important in Their Decision to Stop Breastfeeding, According to Infants' Age at Weaning

Reasons Cited as Important	INFANTS' AGE WHEN BREASTFEEDING WAS COMPLETELY STOPPED (MONTHS)					
	<1	1–2	3–5	6–8	≥9	Average
Lactational Factors						
My baby had trouble sucking or latching on[a]	53.7	27.1	11.0	2.6	1.5	19.2
My nipples were sore, cracked, or bleeding[a]	36.8	23.2	7.2	5.7	4.2	15.4
My breasts were overfull or engorged[a]	23.9	12.3	4.8	1.6	1.2	8.8
My breasts were infected or abscessed[a]	8.1	5.7	3.1	3.1	3.1	4.6
My breasts leaked too much[a]	14.1	8.0	3.8	1.6	1.9	5.9
Breastfeeding was too painful[a]	29.3	15.8	3.4	3.7	4.2	11.3
Psychosocial Factors						
Breastfeeding was too tiring[a]	19.8	17.2	11.0	7.8	5.3	12.2
Breastfeeding was too inconvenient[a]	20.4	22.4	18.6	12.5	4.2	15.6
I wanted to be able to leave my baby for several hours at a time[a]	11.2	24.1	18.2	15.6	7.3	15.3
I had too many household duties[a]	12.6	14.0	9.6	5.2	3.8	9.0
I wanted or needed someone else to feed my baby[a]	16.4	23.2	21.0	17.2	6.1	16.8
Someone else wanted to feed the baby[a]	13.5	15.5	12.0	5.7	3.4	10.0
I did not want to breastfeed in public[a]	14.9	18.6	15.1	4.7	4.6	11.6
Nutritional Factors						
Breast milk alone did not satisfy my baby	49.7	55.6	49.1	49.5	43.5	49.5
I thought that my baby was not gaining enough weight[a]	23.0	18.3	11.0	14.1	8.4	15.0
A health professional said my baby was not gaining enough weight[a]	19.8	15.2	8.6	9.9	5.0	11.7
I had trouble getting the milk flow to start[a]	41.4	23.2	19.6	14.6	5.7	20.9
I didn't have enough milk[a]	51.7	52.2	54.0	43.8	26.0	45.5
Lifestyle Factors						
I did not like breastfeeding[a]	16.4	10.9	6.2	3.1	1.9	7.7
I wanted to go on a weight-loss diet	6.6	7.2	10.3	10.9	6.5	8.3
I wanted to go back to my usual diet	5.5	9.5	7.2	5.2	5.0	6.5
I wanted to smoke again or more than I did while breastfeeding[a]	6.0	5.2	3.4	1.0	0.8	3.3
I wanted my body back to myself[a]	8.9	13.2	16.8	18.8	15.7	14.7
Medical Factors						
My baby became sick and could not breastfeed[a]	9.5	7.4	5.5	6.3	1.9	6.1
I was sick or had to take medicine[a]	14.4	16.3	14.8	12.5	8.0	13.2
I was not present to feed my baby for reasons other than work	3.2	6.9	5.2	5.2	2.7	4.6
I became pregnant or wanted to become pregnant again[a]	1.7	3.4	3.4	6.8	12.2	5.5
Milk-Pumping Factors						
I could not or did not want to pump or breastfeed at work[a]	11.2	22.4	21.3	13.5	4.6	14.6
Pumping milk no longer seemed worth the effort that it required[a]	16.7	21.2	23.7	17.7	11.5	18.2

(Continued)

TABLE 1.7   Percentage of Mothers Who Indicated That Specified Reasons Were Important in Their Decision to Stop Breastfeeding, According to Infants' Age at Weaning—cont'd

Reasons Cited as Important	INFANTS' AGE WHEN BREASTFEEDING WAS COMPLETELY STOPPED (MONTHS)					
	<1	1–2	3–5	6–8	≥9	Average
Infant's Self-Weaning Factors						
My baby began to bite[a]	5.2	5.7	13.4	38.5	31.7	18.9
My baby lost interest in nursing or began to wean himself or herself[a]	13.2	19.7	33.1	47.9	47.3	32.2
My baby was old enough that the difference between breast milk and formula no longer mattered[a]	5.2	11.4	16.5	26.6	28.2	17.6

[a]$p < 0.01$ for association between each reason and weaning age after adjustments for maternal age, marital status, parity, education, poverty, race, and region and Women, Infants, and Children (WIC) program participation.
From Li R, Fein SB, Chen J, et al. Why mothers stop breastfeeding: mothers' self reported reasons for stopping during the first year. *Pediatrics.* 2008;122:S69–S76.

focused on early weaning and lactation dysfunction as the major contributing factors.[142] Dysfunctional or disrupted lactation was defined as early, undesired weaning attributed to at least two of three issues: breast pain, low milk supply, and difficulty with infant latch. They estimated that disrupted lactation occurred in 12% of the 2335 women included in their analysis. Disrupted lactation was associated with mothers being overweight or obese or having depressive symptoms postpartum. This estimate of disrupted lactation fits with two previous reports of insufficient or problematic milk production in 13.1% to 13.5% of breastfeeding women who experienced early weaning.[150,151] A more recent study from Italy documented that of 552 women who completed a study of their breastfeeding experience through phone follow-up and an online survey, approximately 70% experienced breastfeeding difficulties (cracked nipples, perception of insufficient milk, pain, and fatigue).[145] Most of the difficulties occurred in the first month, and ~50% of women felt they were supported appropriately by health professionals. Specific variables (maternal perception of insufficient milk, infant's failure to grow, mastitis, and return to work) correlated with an elevated risk of non-EBF at 3 months. Taken together, these studies reinforce the frequency of mothers having some difficulty with breastfeeding and the need for "individualized" problem solving and breastfeeding support to assist mothers in reaching their breastfeeding goals. Ongoing collection of data on the issues complicating breastfeeding, globally and locally, is essential to create a baseline against which to measure the success of ongoing and future interventions of promotion, protection, and support.

Effect of BF Support Measures

Next, we should be assessing the factors that affect the breastfeeding behaviors of individuals and the community, such as available and accessible culturally appropriate breastfeeding knowledge; readily accessible assistance and support for breastfeeding questions, concerns about supply or self-efficacy, and breastfeeding difficulties; supportive cultural and social norms regarding breastfeeding within the community; direct, high-quality peer and professional lactation support and consultation; adequate, paid universal parental leave for pregnancy and lactation; "breastfeeding-friendly" inpatient and outpatient policies and systems within health care facilities; and supportive "breastfeeding-friendly" workplaces and child-care facilities. Reis-Reilly et al. present examples of solutions to address breastfeeding disparities (as might affect any of the previously mentioned factors) within the community through a collaborative public health approach of change to policy, systems, and environment.[2] Another measure, more indirect, of breastfeeding support and protection is legislation to support and protect breastfeeding in our communities and nations; to promote optimal infant, young child, and maternal nutrition; and to combat all forms of discrimination against women. All 50 states in the United States now have legislation protecting women's right to breastfeed in public, 22 states have legislation for accommodations for breastfeeding in the workplace, and another 7 states have laws about break time and a protected space for breastfeeding or expressing milk at work (Table 1.8). Internationally, this includes ongoing monitoring of activities by various agencies and national or international policy agreements, such as the United Nations CEDAW, the Convention on the Rights of the Child (CRC), and the ILO Maternity Protection Conventions (1919, No. 3; 1952, No. 103; 2000, No. 183). Each of these agreements has binding policy interventions requiring participating nations to create national laws and interventions to support and protect breastfeeding and infant nutrition.[152] Additionally, there are the "nonbinding" agreements—such as the International Code of Marketing of Breast-Milk Substitutes (World Health Assembly, 1981); Innocenti Declaration on the Protection, Promotion and Support of Breastfeeding; Breastfeeding in the 1990s: A Global Initiative (WHO/UNICEF, 1990); and the BFHI (WHO/UNICEF, 1991)—that recommend restrictions on the marketing of

TABLE 1.8 **Support Indicators in the 50 United States: Baby-Friendly Facilities, Lactation Support, State Legislation, and Coalitions[a]**

State	Percentage of Live Births Occurring at Facilities Designated as Baby-Friendly (BFHI)[b] 2018	Maternity Practices in Infant Nutrition and Care (mPINC)[c] 2015	Number of IBCLCs per 1000 Live Births, 2016[d]	Number of CLCs per 1000 Live Births, 2016[e]	Number of La Leche League Groups per 1000 Live Births, July 2016[f]	State Legislation About Breastfeeding in Public Places, July 2019[g]	State Legislation about Lactation and Employment, July 2019[g]
US, national	26.1	79	3.79	4.57	0.85	50	22 states → yes BT, space—7 states
Alabama	16.5	72	2.75	2.62	0.60	Yes	No
Alaska	3.4	82	8.08	4.35	1.15	Yes	No
Arizona	6.8	79	3.75	2.19	0.82	Yes	No
Arkansas	21.7	67	2.19	2.37	0.44	Yes	No
California	44.8	85	4.59	2.12	0.62	Yes	Yes
Colorado	48.9	85	4.69	9.57	1.34	Yes	Yes
Connecticut	46.3	83	5.62	10.01	1.79	Yes	Yes
Delaware	88.1	90	4.93	1.07	0.36	Yes	Yes
District of Columbia	49.0	82	1.98	0.94	0.42	Yes	Yes
Florida	17.5	80	2.55	5.26	0.76	Yes	No
Georgia	31.1	75	2.77	5.97	0.59	Yes	BT, space
Hawaii	12.1	80	4.57	8.21	0.60	Yes	Yes
Idaho	9.8	78	3.90	2.54	0.92	Yes	No
Illinois	22.3	81	3.34	7.68	0.78	Yes	Yes
Indiana	31.0	80	4.73	2.95	0.77	Yes	Space
Iowa	8.1	75	3.24	4.33	0.76	Yes	No
Kansas	41.1	76	4.29	1.84	1.92	Yes	No
Kentucky	24.5	73	2.88	5.86	0.29	Yes	Yes
Louisiana	41.6	76	2.29	5.17	0.62	Yes	BT, space
Maine	18.4	84	7.14	28.64	1.75	Yes	Yes
Maryland	18.2	82	5.04	1.33	0.84	Yes	No
Massachusetts	19.0	87	5.80	10.34	1.34	Yes	Yes
Michigan	30.3	78	2.97	2.71	1.00	Yes	No
Minnesota	30.6	82	4.93	9.56	0.93	Yes	Yes
Mississippi	12.5	60	1.93	2.21	0.96	Yes	No
Missouri	13.2	75	3.88	3.10	1.28	Yes	No
Montana	27.9	82	4.45	28.37	1.91	Yes	BT, space
Nebraska	12.8	71	4.39	12.79	1.28	Yes	Yes
Nevada	16.3	75	1.82	7.00	0.47	Yes	Yes
New Hampshire	49.8	90	6.76	11.84	1.53	Yes	No

(Continued)

TABLE 1.8 Support Indicators in the 50 United States: Baby-Friendly Facilities, Lactation Support, State Legislation, and Coalitions[a]—cont'd

State	Percentage of Live Births Occurring at Facilities Designated as Baby-Friendly (BFHI)[b] 2018	Maternity Practices in Infant Nutrition and Care (mPINC)[c] 2015	Number of IBCLCs per 1000 Live Births, 2016[d]	Number of CLCs per 1000 Live Births, 2016[e]	Number of La Leche League Groups per 1000 Live Births, July 2016[f]	State Legislation About Breastfeeding in Public Places, July 2019[g]	State Legislation about Lactation and Employment, July 2019[g]
New Jersey	18.9	83	3.73	3.64	1.52	Yes	Yes
New Mexico	54.3	81	4.27	1.77	0.77	Yes	BT, space
New York	21.6	82	3.74	11.40	0.81	Yes	Yes
North Carolina	37.6	78	5.16	1.19	1.21	Yes	No
North Dakota	13.8	73	2.21	13.62	0.44	Yes	No
Ohio	16.5	80	4.03	5.52	0.89	Yes	No
Oklahoma	21.7	78	3.34	3.07	0.51	Yes	BT, space
Oregon	52.6	86	8.27	0.70	1.18	Yes	Yes
Pennsylvania	25.0	78	3.42	2.92	1.08	Yes	No
Rhode Island	86.0	96	5.02	10.12	0.64	Yes	Yes
South Carolina	41.7	78	3.23	3.87	0.74	Yes	Yes
South Dakota	4.9	74	2.84	5.60	0.32	Yes	No
Tennessee	21.1	72	2.32	7.44	0.58	Yes	BT, space
Texas	20.1	77	2.50	0.98	0.43	Yes	Yes
Utah	8.6	75	2.30	1.18	0.65	Yes	Yes
Vermont	10.4	88	13.72	22.87	3.22	Yes	Yes
Virginia	12.7	80	4.71	1.22	1.32	Yes	BT, space
Washington	18.4	83	5.78	1.21	1.32	Yes	Yes
West Virginia	8.1	73	3.08	5.35	0.45	Yes	Yes
Wisconsin	16.0	82	4.40	8.68	1.04	Yes	No
Wyoming	2.4	77	2.71	22.94	1.42	Yes	No

BT, Break time; *CLC*, certified lactation counselor; *FTEs*, full-time equivalents; *IBCLC*, International Board of Certified Lactation Consultants; *mPINC*, Maternity Practices in Infant Nutrition and Care; *space*, space for breastfeeding or expressing breast milk (not a bathroom); *yes* = "reasonable accommodations for pregnancy-related conditions."

[a]All 50 states now have state coalitions for breastfeeding and websites for the coalitions.

[b]Percentage of live births occurring at hospitals or birth centers designated as Baby-Friendly Hospitals. From Baby-Friendly USA. Baby-Friendly Hospitals and Birth Centers Designated as of June 2016. http://www.babyfriendlyusa.org.

[c]From Centers for Disease Control and Prevention. National Survey: Maternity Practices in Infant Nutrition and Care (mPINC) 2015 Report. mPINC reports total scores for the state averaging all participating hospitals' scores for maintaining supportive hospital policies, appropriate infant feeding practices and adequate discharge protocols in support of breastfeeding. National Center for Chronic Disease Prevention and Health Promotion, Division of Nutrition, Physical Activity, and Obesity. https://www.cdc.gov/breastfeeding/data/mpinc/state_reports.html. Accessed March 29, 2020.

[d]From International Board of Lactation Consultant Examiners. IBCLCs by State as of January 5, 2016. http://iblce.org/wp_content/uploads/2016/01/IBCLCs-by-State-1.5.20162.pdf. Accessed March 28, 2020.

[e]From Healthy Children Project. Centers for Disease Control and Prevention, National Center for Chronic Disease Prevention and Health Promotion, Division of Nutrition, Physical Activity, and Obesity. Breastfeeding Report Card, United States, 2016. https://www.cdc.gov/breastfeeding/data/reportcard.htm. Accessed March 28, 2020.

[f]Number of La Leche League (LLL) leaders per 1000 live births as of June 2016. From La Leche League International (LLLI) database of accredited LLL Leaders, obtained from Centers for Disease Control and Prevention, National Center for Chronic Disease Prevention and Health Promotion, Division of Nutrition, Physical Activity, and Obesity. Breastfeeding Report Card. United States, 2016. https://www.cdc.gov/breastfeeding/data/reportcard.htm. Accessed March 28, 2020.

[g]From Worklife Law, University of California Hastings College of Law. 50 State Survey of Workplace Lactation Laws. July 2019. State Legislation About Breastfeeding in Public Places. http://www.PregnantAtWork.org/state-workplace-lactation-laws-testpage/. Accessed March 28, 2020. From Centers for Disease Control and Prevention. Breastfeeding Report Card United States, 2018. Data from National Immunization Survey, US Department of Health and Human Services. https://www.cdc.gov/breastfeeding/data/nis_data/results.html. Accessed March 17, 2020.

breast-milk substitutes; elaborate on the need to remove barriers to breastfeeding in health systems, workplaces, and communities; and propose steps to protect, promote, and support breastfeeding in hospital and maternity settings. The WHO already monitors, every 2 years, the countries that have implemented legislation regarding the International Code of Marketing of Breast-Milk Substitutes and legal measures to protect breastfeeding.[153] The IBFAN monitors International Code violations around the world and publishes these online with the companies involved and the specific violations.[154] In the IBFAN's 2017 report, there were 792 code violations from 79 countries ascribed to 28 companies. The WABA monitors Maternity Protection at Work, as stipulated by the ILO Maternity Protection Convention 183, Recommendation 191, by country.[93] This includes a listing by country of the duration of legislated maternity leave, who pays for the leave, other forms of leave, and breastfeeding breaks at the worksite, all of which could be a barrier or facilitate continued breastfeeding after the mother returns to work. The ILO and WABA monitor the "enforcement" and practice of maternity/paternity laws across the world.[155]

Population Data on Breastfeeding Success

Population data collection on breastfeeding has had several notable problems: (1) inconsistent and confusing definitions (for appropriate definitions, see Fig. 1.4), (2) measurement methodology that varies by country, (3) infrequency of measuring breastfeeding rates, and (4) limited ongoing support and funding for measuring breastfeeding in individual countries.

The WHO and UNICEF Global Breastfeeding Collective are attempting to standardize these variables and conditions worldwide to optimize the comparability of breastfeeding data between countries and within countries over time.[130] The collective has developed "scorecard indicators," including breastfeeding rate measures (early initiation [put to the breast <1 hour], ever/never breastfed, exclusive and predominant breastfeeding at 0 to 3 months, complementary feedings initiated at 6 to 9 months, continued breastfeeding at 12 to 15 months, and continued breastfeeding at 20 to 23 months). The collective also has eight national policy or program indicators, including (1) national funding of breastfeeding, (2) regulation of marketing of breast-milk substitutes, (3) paid maternity leave, (4) Ten Steps to Successful Breastfeeding (percentage of births in "baby-friendly" facilities), (5) breastfeeding counseling, (6) community support programs, (7) national assessment of breastfeeding policies and programs, and (8) national monitoring of breastfeeding rates. These indicators are programmatic interventions that have been documented to influence breastfeeding rates. These data are available from the UNICEF Global Database of Infant and Young Child Feeding[156] (Table 1.9; see also Table 1.3). Fig. 1.5 shows a comparison of breastfeeding rates at 2 years of age for different WHO regions by country wealth. The UNICEF Global Database of Infant and Young Child Feeding was updated October 2019 and is interactive to facilitate searching for specific data by region, country, and year, allowing comparison and analysis of progress.[156]

The United States has had its own problems with collecting data on breastfeeding rates. Historically, it has utilized a

TABLE 1.9	World Health Organization (WHO)/UNICEF Breastfeeding Statistics by Region and Year (2018)			
Region	Early Initiation of Breastfeeding (<1 hour), 2018	Exclusive Breastfeeding (0–5 months), 2018	Infants 6–8 Months of Age Fed Complementary Foods, 2018	Continued Breastfeeding at 12–23 Months, 2018
Eastern and Southern Africa	65%	55%	77%	72%
South Asia	40%	54%	52%	78%
Latin America and Caribbean	54%	38%	84%	45%
North America	N/A	35%	N/A	13%
West and Central Africa	41%	34%	68%	64%
Eastern Europe and Central Asia	57%	33%	75%	47%
East Asia and the Pacific	38%	30%	84%	60%
Middle East and North Africa	36%	30%	78%	47%
GLOBAL	**44%**	**42%**	**69%**	**65%**

N/A, Not available.

Data from UNICEF. UNICEF Global Database for Infant and Young Child Feeding, October 2019. http://www.v2-Updates-2019-October-iycf-continuum-mdd-mmf-mad-regions/copy. Accessed March 30, 2020; UNICEF. Infant and Young Child Feeding. https://data.unicef.org/topic/nutrition/infant-and-young-child-feeding/. Accessed March 30, 2020.

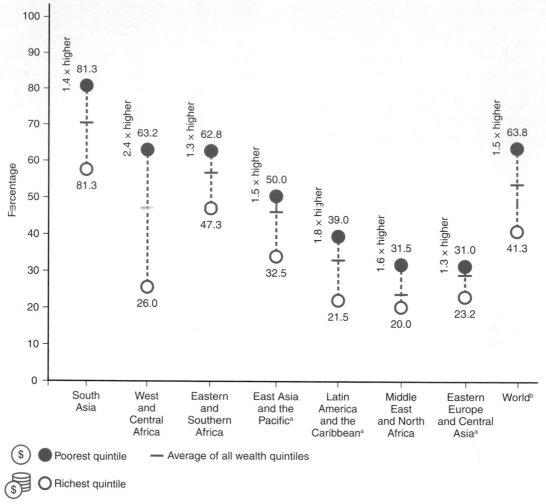

Fig. 1.5 Percentages of children still breastfeeding at 2 years of age in low- and middle-income countries, by income and region, 2017. [a]East Asia and Pacific Region does not include China. Latin America and Caribbean Region does not include Brazil. Eastern European and Central Asia Region does not include the Russian Federation, nor are these three countries included in the world[b] analysis. (Modified from UNICEF Global Database: Infant and Young Child Feeding, 2018. http://www.data.unicef.org/resources/dataset/infant-young-child-feeding/. Accessed March 29, 2020; UNICEF Nutrition Section, Programme Division, Data and Analytics Section, Division of Data, Research and Policy, and Division of Communication. Breastfeeding: A Mother's Gift, for Every Child. 2018. https://www.unicef.org/publications/index_102824.html. Accessed April 22, 2020.)

variety of programs for breastfeeding data collection, including the Ross Laboratories Mothers Surveys (1977 to 2002); the National Natality Surveys (NNS) in 1969 and 1980; the Early Childhood Longitudinal Survey, Birth Cohort (ECLS-B); the Infant Feeding Practices Survey II (IFPSII); the National Health and Nutrition Examination Survey (NHANES) of 2007; the NIS of 2006; the National Survey of Children's Health (NSCH) of 2007; the National Survey of Early Childhood Health (NSECH); the National Survey of Family Growth (NSFG); the Pediatric Nutrition Surveillance System (PedNSS); the Pregnancy Nutrition Surveillance System (PNSS); the Pregnancy Risk Assessment Monitoring System (PRAMS); the Maternity Practices in Infant Nutrition & Care (mPINC), and the WIC Participant and Program Characteristics (WPPC) of 2006. A number of these reportedly are continuing, but the most consistent and nationally representative are NHANES, NIS, mPINC, and PRAMS. PRAMS has produced data by state since 1983. Currently, PRAMS (2016 and 2017 data) provides

information on just two indicators, "ever breastfed" and "any breastfeeding at 8 weeks postpartum," for over 80% of all births in the United States.[157] mPINC collects data from hospitals by state, including hospital breastfeeding policy (and what is included and practiced in the policy), breastfeeding initiation timing, limited or no supplemental feedings, breastfeeding assistance in hospital, rooming-in practices, appropriate discharge planning and discharge packets without formula samples, and staff training. mPINC reports total scores for the state averaging all participating hospitals' scores for maintaining supportive hospital policies, appropriate infant feeding practices and adequate discharge protocols in support of breastfeeding. Results from mPINC are available by state for the proportion of hospitals achieving individual indicators and include tracking by state from year to year (2007 through 2015).[158] The CDC's Division of Nutrition, Physical Activity and Obesity has been collecting and analyzing data on breastfeeding for the last decade and publishing a "Breastfeeding

Percentage of U.S. children who were breastfed, by birth year[1,2]

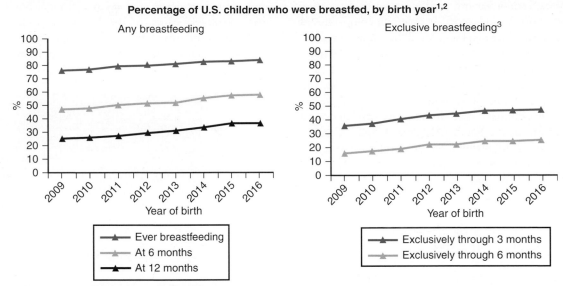

Fig. 1.6 Breastfeeding rates among US children born 2009 to 2016, National Immunization Survey. Data from US territories excluded from national breastfeeding estimates to be consistent with analytical methods for *Healthy People 2020*. EBF, Exclusive breastfeeding—only breast milk, no solids, water, or other liquid. (Modified from Centers for Disease Control and Prevention. Breastfeeding Among U.S. Children Born 2009–2016, CDC National Immunization Survey. http://www.cdc.gov/breastfeeding/data/nis_data/results.html. Accessed April 22, 2020.)

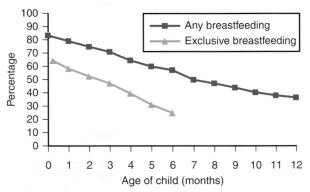

Fig. 1.7 Any and exclusive breastfeeding rates by age in children born in the United States in 2016. Data from US territories excluded from national breastfeeding estimates to be consistent with analytical methods for *Healthy People 2020*. EBF, Exclusive breastfeeding—only breast milk, no solids, water, or other liquid. (Modified from Centers for Disease Control and Prevention. Breastfeeding Among U.S. Children Born 2009–2016, CDC National Immunization Survey. http://www.cdc.gov/breastfeeding/data/nis_data/results.html. Accessed March 31, 2020.)

Report Card."[159] The breastfeeding rate indicators include ever breastfed, breastfeeding at 6 months, breastfeeding at 12 months, EBF at 3 months, and EBF at 6 months, derived from the most recent NIS data. See Table 1.6 for data on the national breastfeeding rate from 2009 through 2016. See Fig. 1.6 for a graphic representation of US national breastfeeding rates for 2009 through 2016. Fig. 1.7 graphically demonstrates breastfeeding and EBF rates by the age of the children for infants born in the United States in 2016. Table 1.5 demonstrates the increase in breastfeeding rates for all 50 states from 2004 to 2015 based on data from NIS. These indicators are different from what the UNICEF Global Breastfeeding Collective

measures. The CDC also uses different breastfeeding support indicators, including mPINC score (measuring breastfeeding-related maternity care practices at intrapartum care facilities by state); percentage of live births occurring at hospitals or birth centers designated as "Baby-Friendly" (Baby-Friendly USA data); percentage of breastfed infants receiving formula before 2 days of age (CDC NIS data); number of LLL leaders per 1000 live births (LLLI database); number of certified lactation counselors (CLCs) per 1000 live births (Healthy Children Project database of CLCs); number of IBCLCs per 1000 live births (IBLCE data); and child-care regulation that supports onsite breastfeeding (National Resource Center for Health and Safety in Child Care and Early Education). The numbers of CLCs, IBCLCs, and LLL leaders per 1000 live births provides an estimate of the available professionals trained in breastfeeding education and support available to support breastfeeding statewide (see Table 1.8). Limitations in availability and access can still be hidden within a state due to the absence of breastfeeding data in different counties, cities, or regions. The data for Baby-Friendly facility births and mPINC scores present estimates of the reach of policies and practices favoring breastfeeding care and support from birth within institutions. The CDC compares breastfeeding rates by state and territory and with *Healthy People* objectives. The Breastfeeding Report Card for the United States of 2018 utilized data from the CDC NIS for 2016 to 2017, including data on live births for the year 2016. Compared with the *Healthy People 2020* objectives, the current breastfeeding rates for the United States are exceeding the target rates for the following indicators: percentage of infants ever breastfed (83.2% vs. target 81.9%), proportion of infants breastfed at 12 months of age (35.9% vs. target 34.1%), and the proportion of infants exclusively breastfed through 3 months of age (46.9% vs. target 46.2%).[159] See Table 1.5 for US breastfeeding rates by state, a comparison of data from 2004 and 2015.

The CDC Breastfeeding Report Card is useful in comparing breastfeeding rates (five indicators) between different states as well as comparing an individual state's and the nation's progress in increasing breastfeeding rates over time. Notably, all 50 states demonstrated some improvement in their breastfeeding rates (ever breastfed, breastfeeding at 6 months and 12 months, and EBF at 3 months and 6 months) from 2004 to 2015. There are clearly states with additional room for improvement, and most of those states are in the South (Alabama, Florida, Georgia, Kentucky, Louisiana, Mississippi, South Carolina, Tennessee, and West Virginia), with a few states in the Midwest (Arkansas, Illinois, Michigan, Oklahoma).

MORTALITY STUDIES IN BREASTFED AND ARTIFICIALLY FED INFANTS

Historically, the mortality rate for breastfed infants has been lower than for artificially fed infants. Data from previous decades and other nations do show a significant difference.[17] Knodel presented a table that included rates from cities in Germany, France, England, Holland, and the United States spanning the years from 1895 to 1947[160] (Table 1.10). The mortality rate among breastfed infants is clearly lower than

that among artificially fed infants. Knodel pointed out that early neonatal deaths, in the first week or so of life, were excluded from this data. In 1922 Woodbury reported the trends in infant feeding (Fig. 1.8) and mortality rates of

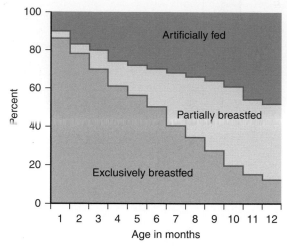

Fig. 1.8 Percentage of infants who were breastfed, partially breastfed, and artificially fed by age in months. (Modified from Woodbury RM. The relation between breast and artificial feeding and infant mortality. *Am J Hyg.* 1922;2:668.)

TABLE 1.10 Mortality Rates and Survivorship to Age 1 Year in Breastfed and Artificially Fed Infants,[a] Reports From 1895 to 1947						
		MORTALITY RATE (PER 1000)		**SURVIVORS TO AGE 1 YR (PER 1000)**		
Study Area	**Date**	**Breastfed**	**Artificially Fed**	**Breastfed**	**Artificially Fed**	**Difference**
Berlin, Germany	1895–1896	57	376	943	624	319
Bremen, Germany	1905	68	379	932	621	311
Hanover, Germany	1912	96	296	904	704	200
Boston, Mass.	1911	30	212	970	788	182
Eight US cities[b]	1911–1916	76	255	924	745	179
Paris, France	1900	140	310	860	690	170
Cologne, Germany	1908–1909	73	241	927	759	168
Amsterdam, Holland	1904	144	304	856	696	160
Liverpool, England	1905	84	134	916	866	144
Eight US cities[c]	1911–1916	76	215	924	785	139
Derby, England	1900–1903	70	198	930	802	128
Chicago, Illinois	1924–1929	2	84	998	916	82
Liverpool, England	1936–1942	10	57	990	943	47
Great Britain	1946–1947	9	18	991	982	9

[a]Most of these rates do not include deaths in the first few days or weeks of life; the mortality rate is therefore underestimated, and the survival rate is overestimated. Only the rates for the eight US cities in 1911–1916 represent the mortality rate from birth; deaths that occurred before any feeding are proportionately allocated to the two feeding categories. The rates for Berlin, Bremen, Hanover, Cologne, and the eight US cities were derived by applying life-table techniques to mortality rates given by single months of age.
[b]Comparison of breastfed infants with infants artificially fed from birth.
[c]Comparison of breastfed infants with all infants artificially fed in the period of observation.
From Knodel J. Breastfeeding and population growth. *Science.* 1977;198:1111. Copyright © 1977 by the American Association for the Advancement of Science.

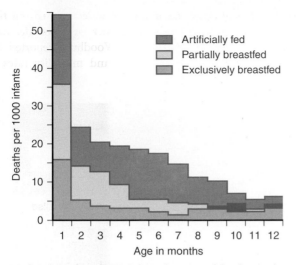

Fig. 1.9 Death rate per 1000 infants by type of feeding and age in months. (Modified from Woodbury RM. The relation between breast and artificial feeding and infant mortality. *Am J Hyg*. 1922;2:668.)

infants by type of feeding (Fig. 1.9).[29] The mortality rate was lower at all ages for breastfed infants. In the early 20th century, posters that urged mothers to breastfeed that were part of the national campaign to lower infant mortality rates were displayed everywhere by the health department, without fear of inducing guilt in mothers. Worldwide, these differences were widely publicized (Fig. 1.10). Although infant mortality gradually improved, the differences in infant mortality based on infant feeding persisted. Data from the work of Scrimshaw et al. show a mortality rate of 950 of 1000 live births in artificially fed infants and 120 of 1000 in breastfed infants.[161] The data were collected in Punjab villages from 1955 through 1959. The deaths were predominantly caused by diarrheal disease. The Pan American Health

Organization has reported similar correlations among malnutrition, infection, and mortality. In the work by Puffer and Serrano in 1973 in São Paulo, death rates among breastfed infants and proportions of mortality from diarrheal disease and malnutrition were also lower than among bottle-fed infants.[162]

Assessing the mortality rate of breastfed infants compared with bottle-fed infants is difficult today because many breastfed infants also receive supplements of formula and solid foods. The risk of death in the first year of life and in children less than 5 years old diminished in developed countries at the end of the 20th and beginning of the 21st centuries following the ongoing development of antibiotics and new immunizations and many other advances in obstetrical and pediatric care.[163] The CDC continues efforts to reduce infant mortality by specifically focusing on perinatal care, maternal and infant health, sudden infant death syndrome (SIDS) and sudden unexpected infant death (SUID), birth defects and developmental abnormalities, and injury prevention and control.[164] Improvements in under-age-5 child mortality rates worldwide have continued at a faster rate of reduction, 3.8% per year, from 2000 to 2018 compared with 1990 to 2000[165] (Fig. 1.11). The improvement in child survival in low- and middle-income countries compared with higher-income countries overall has been slower.[166,167] Sankar et al. documented, in a systematic review and meta-analysis, the association between "optimal breastfeeding practices" and lower infant and child mortality.[168] In studies around the world from 1993 to 2006, this was evident in diminished relative risk of death in infants exclusively or predominantly breastfed compared with infants receiving partial or no breast milk (Table 1.11). In some of the studies, this protection extended through 11 months of age and even out to 23 months of age. The protection also seemed to exhibit a dose response in that

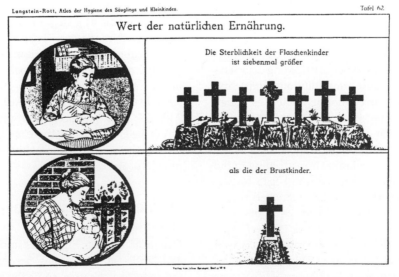

Fig. 1.10 "Value of Natural Feeding" poster used in 1918 to educate parents. The text explains that the mortality rate of bottle-fed infants (Flaschenkinder) is seven times higher than that of breastfed infants (Brustkinder). (From Langstein R. *Atlas der Hygiene des Sauglings und Kleinkindes*. Berlin: Springer-Verlag; 1918.)

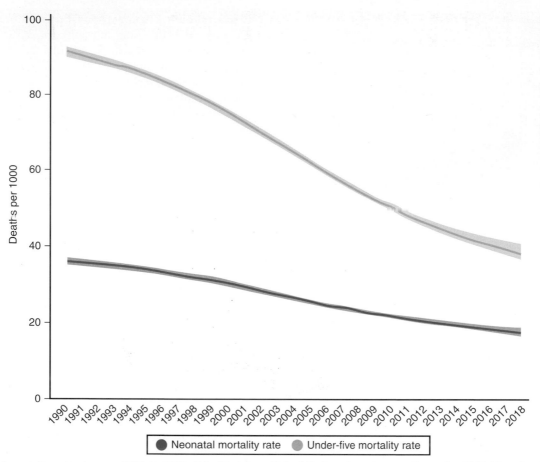

Fig. 1.11 Global mortality rates by age, 1990 to 2018. (Modified from United Nations Inter-Agency Group for Child Mortality Estimation [UN IGME]. Global Mortality Rates by Age, 1990–2018. https://data.unicef.org/topic/child-survival/under-five-mortality/. Accessed April 20, 2020.)

the increased intensity of breastfeeding (exclusive and pre-dominant) was better than partial or no breastfeeding. Even though there are multiple contributing factors for the decrease in morbidity and mortality related to infant and child diarrhea (improvements in water, sanitation, and hand-washing; increased use of oral rehydration solution, zinc, and antibiotics; and increasing use of rotavirus vaccine), there is evidence that EBF and early initiation of breastfeeding have added to the decrease.[169,170] Other investigators have demon-strated, in a recent meta-analysis, that breastfeeding decreases pneumonia-specific and all-cause morbidity and mortality, with evidence that EBF in the first 6 months of life is essential, but extending breastfeeding out to 18 months of age is also beneficial.[171] Early breastfeeding initiation has also been asso-ciated with improved infant survival. A meta-analysis by Smith et al. demonstrated that beginning breastfeeding in the first hour of life is advantageous; infants who began breast-feeding 2 to 23 hours after birth had a 33% increased risk of neonatal mortality, and if they started over 24 hours after birth, they had a 2.19-fold (95% confidence interval [CI], 1.73 to 2.77) greater risk of dying.[172] There was an increased risk of mortality (1.85; 95% CI, 1.29 to 2.67) in the compari-son of initiation of breastfeeding at < 24 hours of life versus greater than 24 hours even if all the infants in both groups were exclusively breastfed. The increased risk of neonatal

mortality was evident for delayed initiation of breastfeeding even in low-birth-weight infants (Table 1.12). Others have demonstrated an effect of early initiation of breastfeeding on breastfeeding exclusivity as well as morbidity and mortality.[173] The United Nations, UNICEF, and WHO have called nations to action regarding preventing death resulting from diarrhea and pneumonia as a steppingstone to diminishing the rate of under-age-5 mortality worldwide.[174,175] Early initiation of breastfeeding and exclusive/predominant breastfeeding are essential to achieving those goals. Even in the United States, infant mortality declined from 2005 (6.86 infant deaths per 1000 live births) to 2014 (5.82 per 1000 live births).[176] Although there have been improvements in breastfeeding rates across the United States, there is significant room for improve-ment in the early initiation of breastfeeding and EBF through 6 months of age.

Morbidity in Breastfed and Artificially Fed Infants

Demonstrating the differences in morbidity between breastfed and bottle-fed infants has become even more complex in industrialized countries since the resurgence of breastfeeding. Among the confounding variables are the inherent differences between mothers who choose to breastfeed and those who

TABLE 1.11   Review of Modern Studies: Relative Risk of Death for Breastfed Versus Nonbreastfed Infants

Author (Date)	Country	Study Design[a] and Sample Size[b]	Breastfeeding Group Classification[c]	Age[d]	All-Cause Mortality RR (95% CI)
Arifeen (2001)	Bangladesh	C	Part vs. Ex	3 d–5 mo	2.4 (1.52–3.8)
		N = 1677	No vs. Ex	3 d–5 mo	21.6 (12.3–37.9)
			No vs. Ex/Pred	3–28 d	5.66 (1.86–17.2)
			No vs. Part	3–28 d	1.46 (0.4–5.29)
Bahl (2005)	Ghana, India, Peru	Sec	Part vs. Ex	6–26 wk	1.88 (1.02–3.49)
		N = 9424	Part vs. Pred	6–26 wk	1.69 (1.1–2.61)
			No vs. Pred	6–26 wk	8.08 (4.45–4.7)
Srivastava (1994)	India	C	No vs. Ex/Pred	0–6 mo	1.62 (1.07–2.47)
		N = 500			
De Francisco (1993)	Gambia	CC	No vs. Any	12–23 mo	0.9 (0.3–2.6)
		N = 431			
Edmond (2006)	Ghana	Sec	Part vs. Ex	3–28 d	5.0 (2.86–9.09)
		N = 10,947	Part vs. Ex/Pred	3–28 d	4.55 (2.63–7.69)
Garenne (2006)	Senegal	C	No vs. Any	12–23 mo	2.0 (1.4–3.1)
		N = 3534			
Hanson (1994)	Pakistan	C	No vs. Any	6–11 mo[e]	1.59 (1.14–2.2)[e]
		N = 2166	No vs. Any	12–23 mo	2.0 (0.4–11.5)
Molbak (1994)	Guinea Bissau	C	No vs. Any	12–35 mo	3.45 (1.41–8.33)
		N = 849			
Victora (1987)	Brazil	CC	No vs. Any	6–11 mo[e]	1.59 (1.14–2.2)[e]
		N = 1071			
Yoon (1996)	Philippines	C	No vs. Any	6–11 mo[e]	1.59 (1.14–2.2)[e]
		N = 9682	No vs. Any	12–23 mo	1.4 (0.6–2.9)
Ghana VAST Study Team (1994)	Ghana	C	No vs. Any	12–24 mo	7.9 (1.2–53.2)
		N = 1099			

CI, Confidence interval; RR, relative risk.
[a]Study designs: C, cohort; CC, case control; Sec, secondary data from randomized controlled trial (RCT).
[b]Sample size: N = number of infants.
[c]Breastfeeding classification: Ex, exclusive breastfeeding (no other liquids except breast milk for first 6 months of life); Pred, predominantly breast milk (complementary foods or other liquids); Part, partial breastfeeding (not further quantified); No, no breastfeeding; Any, any breastfeeding (amount and duration not quantified).
[d]Age: da, days; wk, weeks; mo, months.
[e]Data for 6–11 months are the pooled effects of three studies (Hanson, Victora, and Yoon).
Derived from Sankar MJ, Sinha B, Chowdhury R, et al. Optimal breastfeeding practices and infant and child mortality: a systematic review and meta-analysis. *Acta Paediatr.* 2015;104:3–13. http://doi:10.1111/apa.13147.

choose to bottle-feed (age, educational level, economic status, marriage status, etc.). Although many investigators have recognized the necessity of controlling these variables, none has succeeded totally because an unavoidable factor of self-selection makes random assignment of infants impossible. There is a one-way flow of infants from the breastfed group to the bottle-fed group because a baby may change from breast to bottle but rarely from bottle to breast. Documenting breastfeeding

practices based on agreed-upon definitions is difficult when the possibility exists that some bottle-feedings are included or that solid foods have been introduced.

Differences between breastfed and bottle-fed infants in the incidence of morbidity associated with diarrhea, respiratory infections, otitis media, and pneumonia are well documented. The relationship between breastfeeding versus bottle-feeding and respiratory illness in the first year of life among nearly 2000

TABLE 1.12	Association Between Delayed Breastfeeding and Neonatal Mortality				
Infant Group (Includes Infants Who Survived 2–4 Days After Birth)	N = Number of Infants Included in Studies (Number of Studies)	Estimated Risk for Early Breastfeeding Infants[a] (Deaths per 1000 infants) Surviving 2–4 Days After Birth	Associated Risk for Delayed Breastfeeding[b] (Deaths per 1000 Infants) Surviving 2–4 Days After Birth	Relative Risk (95% CI) of Delayed Breastfeeding[b]	GRADE Quality of Evidence Estimate[c]
All infants who initiated breastfeeding	N = 136,047 (5)	Initiated at <1 hour 5.2/1000	Initiated 2–23 hours 6.9/1000	2–23 hours 1.33 (1.13–1.56)	High[d]
All infants who initiated breastfeeding	N = 136,047	Initiated at <1 hour 5.2/1000	Initiated >24 hours 11.4/1000	>24 hours 2.19 (1.73–2.77)	High[d]
All infants who initiated breastfeeding	N = 142,729 (6)	Initiated at <24 hours 7.7/1000	≥24 hours 13.1/1000	≥24 hours 1.70 (1.44–2.01)	Moderate[e]
Exclusively breastfed infants who ever breastfed	N = 65,214 (4)	Initiated at <24 hours 6.9/1000	≥24 hours 12.4/1000	≥24 hours 1.85 (1.29–2.67)	Moderate[e]
Low-birth-weight infants who initiated breastfeeding	N = 21,258	<24 hours (no estimate)	≥24 hours (no estimate)	≥24 hours 1.73 (1.38–2.18)	Moderate[e]

CI, Confidence interval.

[a]Estimated risk = median risk in the early breastfeeding group from the included studies.

[b]Associated risk = assumed risk in the early breastfeeding group and the relative effect of the intervention.

[c]GRADE Working Group grades of evidence. From Guyatt GH, Oxman AD, Vist GE, et al. GRADE: an emerging consensus on rating quality of evidence and strength of recommendations. *BMJ*. 2008;336(7650):924–926.

[d]The five studies each have a moderate risk of bias, but the strength of evidence was upgraded to "high" because of the consistency of the studies and evidence of a dose response.

[e]The studies all have a moderate risk of bias, and there was no other "modifying" evidence.

From Smith ER, Hurt L, Chowdhury R, et al. Delayed breastfeeding initiation and infant survival: a systematic review and meta-analysis. *PLoS One*. 2017;12(7):e0180722. http://doi:10.1371/journal.pone.0180722.

cohort children was reported by Watkins et al. in England.[177] There was a significant advantage to breastfeeding. Mothers who smoked were less likely to breastfeed, but even when smoking was considered, the breastfeeding advantage remained. A number of well-controlled studies of industrialized countries have shown an increased relative risk of respiratory infection with bottle-feeding compared with breastfeeding and a longer duration and greater intensity of breastfeeding (exclusive and predominant equals full breastfeeding).[178–180] A meta-analysis by Bachrach et al. in 2003 revealed that "among generally healthy infants in developed nations, more than a tripling in severe respiratory tract illnesses resulting in hospitalizations was noted for infants who were not breastfed compared with those who were exclusively breastfed for 4 months."[181] A review of 13 papers from Asia demonstrated a decreased risk of respiratory disease for exclusively breastfed infants versus formula-fed or not breastfed.[182] Similarly, there are also studies showing the benefits of breastfeeding over formula or not breastfeeding for less diarrheal illness during infancy.[176,177,179] There are now several important published reviews and meta-analyses documenting diminished morbidity and the long-term benefits of breastfeeding.[18,183–185]

SUDDEN INFANT DEATH SYNDROME

SIDS is defined as the sudden death of an infant that is unexplained after careful investigation with case review and/or autopsy and death-scene investigation. SUID (or sudden unexpected death in infancy [SUDI]) is a comprehensive and inclusive term for unexpected deaths in infancy (explained or unexplained) and includes accidental suffocation or strangulation in bed (ASSB) and other ill-defined and unspecified causes of infant death.[186] SIDS is another example of mortality that has been discussed relative to breastfeeding because of the apparent protection from breastfeeding and the intricate relationship between breastfeeding and bedsharing. The ABM published a revised protocol in 2020 on bedsharing and breastfeeding that presents a balanced discussion on the history, context, and anthropology of infant sleeping and bedsharing with and without breastfeeding and the epidemiology of bedsharing and SIDS.[186] The ABM offers current identified hazardous risk factors during bedsharing, recommendations on safe bedsharing advice, strategies to minimize the risk of bedsharing, and recommendations for breastfeeding mother–infant dyads concerning bedsharing in a home setting. These are important issues because SIDS and SUID remain

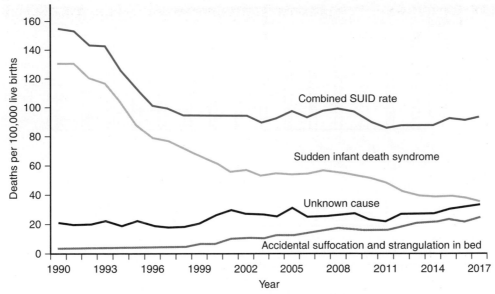

Fig. 1.12 US trends in the rates of sudden infant death syndrome (SIDS) and sudden unexpected infant death (SUID), 1990 to 2017. (Modified from Centers for Disease Control and Prevention and National Center for Health Statistics. Mortality Files. National Vital Statistics System. U.S. Trends in the rates of SIDS and SUID [1990–2017]. https://www.cdc.gov/sids/data.htm#cause. Accessed April 19, 2020.)

notable causes of infant death despite some decrease in the rates since the 1990s (Figs. 1.12 and 1.13) and an identified social responsibility to change modifiable risk factors for SIDS to protect all infants equitably.[187] This is in line with the understanding that bedsharing is a "cultural norm" in many cultures and countries across the world; bedsharing facilitates breastfeeding initiation, exclusivity, and duration; and the rates of SIDS around the world are heterogeneous and inequitable (Fig. 1.14). Maternal-infant sleep patterns and

contact while sleeping are shaped by personal, psychological, social, and practical beliefs and behaviors. Various terms for mother–infant contact during sleep are used, such as the following: *bedsharing*, indicating the infant sharing an adult bed with an adult for sleep; *co-sleeping*, which includes sleeping on a "shared surface" or sleeping in close proximity; *separate sleep*, which means room sharing without bedsharing; *solitary sleep*, which is when an infant sleeps in a separate room from parents; and "breast sleeping," which is the ongoing

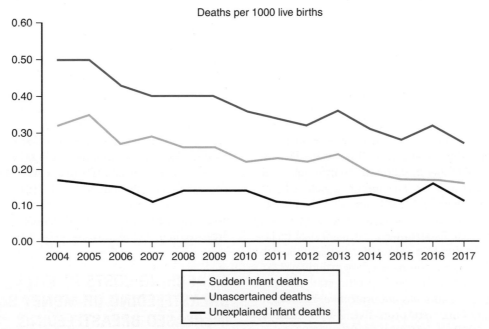

Fig. 1.13 Unexplained infant mortality rate, England and Wales, 2004 to 2017. (From Office of National Statistics. Unexplained Deaths in Infancy, England and Wales: 2017. https://www.ons.gov.uk/peoplepopulationandcommunity/birthsdeathsandmarriages/deaths/bulletins/unexplaineddeathsininfancyenglandandwales/2017. Accessed April 21, 2020.)

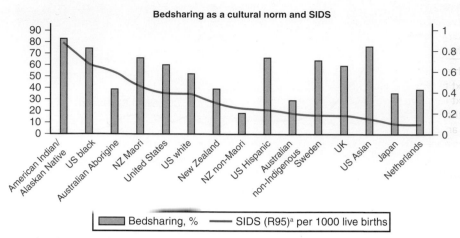

Fig. 1.14 Bedsharing as a cultural norm and sudden infant death syndrome (SIDS). (Modified from Blair PS, Ball HL, McKenna JJ, et al. Bedsharing and breastfeeding: The Academy of Breastfeeding Medicine Protocol 6, revision 2019. *Breastfeed Med.* 2020;15[1]:1–12.). [a]R95 is the problem code for SIDS which is different from R99 - Ill-defined and unspecified causes of mortality and W75 - Accidental suffocation and strangulation in bed.

intermittent contact between a breastfeeding mother and infant in which breastfeeding and sleeping are closely linked.[186,188] McKenna and Bernstraw[40] and McKenna and Mosko[71] describe the physiologic benefits to infants sleeping in proximity to their caregivers.[189,190] They have documented the physiologic changes infants experience as they move from a solitary sleep environment to co-sleeping. They monitored a group of mother–infant pairs in the sleep laboratory, using each pair as their own control (i.e., co-sleeping and sleeping separately). Infants moved from one stage of sleep to the other more frequently when co-sleeping than when sleeping alone, even when briefly waking and increasing their heart and respiratory rates. The authors commented that modern technology, including baby monitors, breathing teddy bears, and other gadgets, has replaced traditional co-sleeping.[190]

Given all the discussion and controversy about SIDS, co-sleeping, and breastfeeding, it is important to note the positive influence that breastfeeding has on the risk of SIDS. Hauck et al. performed a meta-analysis in 2011 presenting calculated summary odds ratios (SORs) of the risk of SIDS and breastfeeding from 18 case-control studies.[191] For infants receiving any breast milk, regardless of the duration, compared with artificially fed infants, the multivariable SOR was 0.55 (95% CI, 0.44 to 0.69). For infants with any breastfeeding of 2 months or longer, the univariable SOR was 0.38 (95% CI, 0.27 to 0.54). For EBF of any duration, the univariable SOR was 0.27 (95% CI, 0.24 to 0.31). The authors concluded that breastfeeding is protective against SIDS and that the protective effect is greater when the breastfeeding is exclusive. Thompson et al., in a 2017 individual participant data meta-analysis, examined the duration of breastfeeding and the risk of SIDS in eight large case-control studies including 2267 SIDS cases and 6837 control infants.[192] In this study, breastfeeding for less than 2 months was not protective. The longer durations of breastfeeding were protective: 2 to 4 months, adjusted odds ratio (aOR) = 0.60, 95% CI, 0.44 to 0.82; 4 to 6 months, aOR = 0.40, 95% CI, 0.26 to 0.63; >6 months, aOR = 0.36, 95% CI, 0.22 to 0.61. Similarly, EBF for longer

durations was also protective against SIDS: 2 to 4 months, aOR = 0.61, 95% CI, 0.42 to 0.87, and 4 to 6 months, aOR = 0.46, 95% CI, 0.29 to 0.74. The authors summarized their results as follows: A breastfeeding duration of at least 2 months was related to half the risk of SIDS, but the breastfeeding provided protection even if it was not exclusive. Other literature has identified factors and circumstances that increase the risk of SIDS during bedsharing, which have been summarized.[186,193] Even though bedsharing has not been shown to be causal of SIDS, individual countries (United States, Canada, and Germany) now advise against bedsharing. The United Kingdom and Australia have taken a different approach, emphasizing the fact that bedsharing is widespread and is culturally valued in many countries and advising medical practitioners to openly discuss risky situations for bedsharing and risk-minimization strategies to empower women and families to decide for themselves regarding infant sleeping arrangements. The ABM advises counseling all families about safe sleep, screening families for risks of infant death with bedsharing, using a nonjudgmental and open approach to conversations with families, and using planned behavior counseling. The ABM also offers public policy recommendations and future avenues of research into asphyxia, SIDS, further identifying all the risks of SIDS with bedsharing, and effective measures of communicating risk regarding bedsharing to further decrease SIDS in a socially responsible manner. For additional information on the risk factors and circumstances of bedsharing and risk-minimization strategies for bedsharing, refer to the ABM protocol on bedsharing and breastfeeding[186] (Box 1.3).

MEASURING COSTS OF NOT BREASTFEEDING OR MONEY SAVED FROM INCREASED BREASTFEEDING

As we are increasingly able to accurately "measure" the rates of breastfeeding and health outcomes, we will be better able to

---

BOX 1.3 Bedsharing Risks and Safety

Factors and Circumstances Increasing the Risk of Infant Death During Bedsharing	Factors to Improve Safe Bedsharing
• Sharing a sofa with a sleeping adult • Infant sleeping next to and adult impaired by alcohol or drugs • Infant sleeping next to an adult who smokes • Infant sleeping in the prone position • Not breastfeeding an infant • Infant sharing a chair with a sleeping adult • Infant sleeping on soft bedding • Preterm infant or low-birth-weight infant	Don't sleep with an infant on a sofa, armchair, pillow, or otherwise unsuitable surface. Place sleeping infants away from individuals impaired by alcohol or drugs. Place the infant supine for sleeping (even naps). Place infants to sleep away from secondhand smoke or a caregiver who routinely smokes (thirdhand smoke). Place the infant's bed away from walls or furniture to protect wedging of the infant's head. The infant's sleeping surface should be firm, without thick or soft covers or pillows. Don't leave the infant alone on an adult's bed. Use the "C-position"[a] for the infant with an adult as the optimal safe sleeping position.

[a]The C position is also called the "cuddle curl"; see photos at Baby Sleep Information Source, https://www.basisonline.org.uk/co-sleeping-image-archive/.
Adapted from Blair PS, Ball HL, McKenna JJ, et al. Bedsharing and breastfeeding: The Academy of Breastfeeding Medicine Protocol #6, revision 2019. *Breastfeed Med.* 2020;15(1):1–12.

---

measure the benefits of breastfeeding or the potential risks of not breastfeeding. To date, the studies on the association between lactation and maternal or infant health outcomes have been observational, and there are no published randomized controlled trials (RCTs) of the effects of breastfeeding on health outcomes.[18,183–185,194] In meta-analyses, there are a number of health outcomes that are consistently associated with breastfeeding in observational studies, albeit adjustment for potential confounders is difficult, and a causal relationship between breastfeeding and these health outcomes is not possible with the currently available literature. There are at least two online calculators for health savings related to breastfeeding: (1) the United States Breastfeeding Committee's Breastfeeding Savings Calculator, developed by Cambridge Health Alliance in a project funded by the W. K. Kellogg Foundation, and (2) Calculator for the Cost of Not Breastfeeding, created by the Alive & Thrive Organization.[195,196] Models or statistical calculators make assumptions based on apparent causality; estimates of relative risk; and estimates of the financial costs of direct health care, loss of life, health care costs for specific illnesses, and social costs of morbidity and mortality. There have been a number of cost analyses done for health outcomes for infants (acute lymphoblastic leukemia, acute otitis media, gastrointestinal infection, lower respiratory tract infection, SIDS, NEC, obesity) and mothers (breast cancer, ovarian cancer, type II diabetes mellitus, hypertension, cardiac disease, and myocardial infarction) and for specific groups (low- to middle-income countries, low-birth-weight infants and premature infants, racial and ethnic minority groups, WIC recipients).[45,197–202] Bartick et al. published a cost analysis of maternal disease with suboptimal breastfeeding comparing outcomes if 90% of mothers were able to breastfeed for 1 year versus the breastfeeding rate of 23% at 1 year, as it was in 2013.[195] This study did not show a significant difference in deaths in mothers before age 70 years, but it did show a $17.4 billion cost to society for maternal premature deaths (95% CI, $.38 to 24.68 billion). Bartick and Rheinhold also did a pediatric cost analysis for suboptimal breastfeeding in the United States.[203] They reported that if 90% of families in the United States could breastfeed exclusively for 6 months (the recommendation in 2010), it could prevent 911 excess child deaths and save $13 billion in health care costs. Colaizy et al. examined the effect of optimal breast milk (≥98% human milk vs. only premature formula [PF] or mixed diet [MD]) provision on the occurrence of NEC-related deaths and medical costs for extremely low-birth-weight (ELBW) infants.[197] Their simulation showed an estimated incidence of NEC of 1.3% for infants receiving only human milk compared with 11.1% for PF and 8.2% for MD, which would lead to 928 excess NEC cases and 121 excess deaths annually when comparing rates of human milk use for VLBW infants current in 2016 versus if 90% of VLBW infants received ≥ 98% HM. The costs related to NEC in this model would be $27.1 million in direct medical costs, $563,655 in indirect nonmedical costs, and $1.5 billion attributed to premature death. Hampson et al. performed a similar economic analysis on VLBW infants receiving a diet of exclusively human milk versus the current VLBW feeding patterns in the United States in 2016.[202] They postulated a $16,309 savings per infant for the use of a diet of exclusively human milk in VLBW infants, causing a decrease in adverse clinical events and deaths. Including broader societal costs in terms of loss of life and other health care outcomes would increase savings to $117,239 per infant. There is also evidence of how breastfeeding disparities can affect minority groups. Bartick et al. demonstrated how suboptimal breastfeeding in minorities leads to a greater "burden of disease."[45] Their analysis showed that a non-Hispanic black population (compared with a non-Hispanic white population) will have 1.7 times the number of excess cases of acute otitis media, 3.3 times the number of excess cases of NEC, and 2.2 times the number of excess deaths as a result of the current disparate rates of breastfeeding in non-Hispanic blacks. A Hispanic population compared with a non-Hispanic white population, given current published breastfeeding rates (2015) in the United States, would have 1.4 times the number of excess episodes of gastrointestinal infection and 1.5 times the number of excess child deaths. On an international level, Walters et al. utilized the Cost of Not Breastfeeding Tool available online (www.aliveandthrive.org/cost-of-not-breastfeeding/) and the current global recommendations for breastfeeding from the WHO and UNICEF.[200] The tool predicted 595,379 childhood deaths (6 to 59 months of age) resulting from diarrhea or pneumonia each year, which could be prevented with recommended breastfeeding. For women, it predicted the potential to prevent 98,243 deaths resulting from breast cancer, ovarian cancer, and type II diabetes annually related to improved breastfeeding. Estimated cost savings included $1.1 billion for treatment costs annually, $53.7 billion for premature infant and maternal deaths, and another $285.4 billion annually in cognitive losses from not breastfeeding at the recommended levels. As dramatic as these numbers are, their real utility is to inform international and national organizations of the public health implications of truly protecting, promoting, and supporting EBF and continued breastfeeding for the recommended durations. The effort and the money spent to support women to breastfeed is likely to produce some significant health benefits and provide economic savings above the initial implementation and maintenance costs of various interventions. There remains a need to balance equity with efficiency and cost effectiveness in terms of investment in and initiation of additional interventions and support for all breastfeeding families, regardless of ethnicity, race, geography, income, and so forth.

THE MAMMARY GLAND AND SCIENCE

Newer additions to research have permitted rapid advances in the understanding of the mammary gland, especially the actions of hormones and enzymes.[11] The "knock-out mouse" is a concept of using mice in which deoxyribonucleic acid (DNA) has been altered to "knock out" a specific gene that controls a specific hormone, such as one important to lactation. Observations of growth and development in these animals provide new insights into the physiology of the mammary gland. In evolutionary biology, lactogenesis is one of the most important functions for the survival of the species. Advances in molecular biology have provided biologists with a better understanding of the mechanisms that produce milk and its specific nutrient constituents. Mammary epithelial cells secrete milk. In an innovative experimental model, mammary epithelial cells are cultured in a petri dish and form a mammosphere, a micromodel of the mammary gland.[204] The advantage of bioengineering the mammary gland, initially focused on the dairy species, is to advance our knowledge and understanding of human lactation in the laboratory so that more women may nurse their infants successfully. The development, and now broader application, of "omics" to the study of human breast milk is revealing a tremendous amount about human milk bioactive factors, fatty acids, oligosaccharides, breast-milk cells, the active role they play in diverse metabolic and immune processes, and the genetic and epigenetic control of lactation.[85,205] New adaptations of radiography are revealing important aspects of the anatomy and physiology of the human breast.[206,207] The study of human breast-milk cells continues to expand, providing evidence of their origins, makeup, and functions in the mother and infant.[208] The ongoing exploration and analysis of the microbiota of the breast and human milk and its functional relationship with the immune system and gastrointestinal health is revealing new questions and avenues for research.[209,210]

SUPPORT FOR THE BREASTFEEDING WOMEN OF THE WORLD

On May 12, 1995, His Holiness John Paul II granted a Solemn Papal Audience in the Apostolic Palace of the Vatican to the participants of the Working Group on Breastfeeding: Science and Society.[211] In response to the group report, the Holy Father pronounced the following discourse (in part):

> The advantages of breastfeeding for the infant and the mother include two major benefits to the child: proper nourishment and protection against disease. This natural way of feeding can create a bond of love and security between mother and child and enable the child to assert its presence as a person through interaction with the mother. Responsible international agencies are calling on governments to ensure that women are enabled to breastfeed their children for four to six months from birth and to continue this practice, supplemented by other appropriate foods, up to the second year of life and beyond.[211]

The United Nations has put forth the new SDGs as a 15-year plan out to 2030.[212] Although at first glance these broad goals might not seem to relate to breastfeeding and human milk, just as the United Nations stands for connectedness, these goals are interconnected, and the success of all of them or even just one goal is dependent on success in each and every area. Specifically, Goals 2, End Hunger; 3, Good Health and Well-Being; 5, Gender Equality; and 10, Reduced Inequalities are directly related to breastfeeding in this new era. Breastfeeding is the essential beginning to end hunger, as the first food for all infants. Optimal nutrition by breastfeeding in the first 1000 days can diminish malnourishment, set the stage for every infant to reach their growth potential, and limit wasting and obesity. Providing adequate nutrition to the mother and family is nourishing the mother to nourish the infant. Breast milk, with its cells and bioactive factors for nutrition, growth, and immune protection, prepares and protects the gastrointestinal tract for optimal functioning and, ultimately, optimal nutrition. Enhanced nutrition leads to good health and well-being, but human breast milk directly diminishes under-age-5 mortality and has demonstrated long-term health benefits for both mother and infant. The breastfeeding targets for 2030 put forth by the UN/UNICEF Global Breastfeeding Collective are (1) a rate of 70% early initiation of breastfeeding (<1 hour of birth), (2) an EBF rate of 60% up to 6 months of age, (3) continued breastfeeding out to 12 months (80% of all children), and (4) continued breastfeeding out to 24 months (for 60% of all children). Neither ending hunger nor good health and well-being are possible without also addressing poverty, quality education, clean water and sanitation, and so forth. SDG 5, Gender Equality, and SDG 10, Reduced Inequalities, are crucial to achieving any of the other 15 goals. Gender equality (and women's empowerment) is also a Millennium Development Goal and encompasses nutrition and health, education, work and poverty, and discrimination and violence across the world. Reducing inequalities is more than improving the economy— it will also require social change (legislation, policy, representation) and eradication of discrimination and violence. Social justice is a cornerstone of equality, ensuring equity and equal access to all the positive opportunities that are necessary to achieve these goals. Just as social justice in breastfeeding is essential to women achieving their own personal breastfeeding goals, it is ultimately essential in reaching the proposed national and global breastfeeding goals.

SUMMARY

All of the topics discussed in this chapter—the long history of breastfeeding in infant nutrition and health, the progressive changes in breastfeeding and the use of DHM, our increasing scientific understanding of lactation and the essential compo-

sition and health benefits of human milk, the improvement in breastfeeding rates in the last several decades along with the general recognition of human milk as the first food for infants, and a greater realization of the role of breastfeeding in human development—bring us into a new era for breastfeeding. It is not that there are no longer barriers or obstacles to breastfeeding. It is that we recognize the barriers and difficulties, we are examining our practices for any persisting or new barriers to breastfeeding, and we are devising solutions to them. It is not that there is disagreement about human milk as the norm for human infants and for optimal nutrition; the challenge is how to effectively support every woman to reach her personal breastfeeding goals. How can we reduce inequalities and inequities in available breastfeeding services and support, which ultimately should improve breastfeeding rates overall? What more can we learn of the science of lactation and human milk that will inform how we can promote breastfeeding to augment the positive health outcomes for mothers and infants? How do we create legislation and policy that protect and facilitate breastfeeding in public, in our communities, and in the workplace? How do we optimize the practice of patient-centered and culturally sensitive communication to support women and families in their infant-feeding decisions and breastfeeding? These are only some of the questions to be answered. If we can answer these questions using a framework of social justice, and if the answers are based on evidence-based practice and research, we will create a new era of successful, life-affirming breastfeeding and the use of human milk as the first food for all infants.

The Reference list is available at www.expertconsult.com.

Anatomy of the Breast

Ruth A. Lawrence

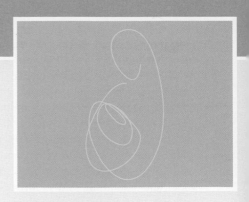

GROSS ANATOMY

The mammary gland, as the breast is medically termed, received its name from *mamma*, the Latin word for breast. The human mammary gland is the only organ that is not fully developed at birth. It experiences dramatic changes in size, shape, and function from birth through pregnancy, lactation, and ultimately involution. Mediated by large changes in gene expression,[1] there are drastic changes in composition, architecture, and function during the life cycle of the human mammary gland.[2] The gland only reaches full maturity when pregnancy occurs. This is the most significant stage of the breast because of the very high metabolic demand that uses 25% of the maternal energy intake. Pregnancy and lactation create permanent breast changes that provide a protective, yet not well understood, effect against breast malignancy. The gland undergoes three major phases of growth and development before pregnancy and lactation: in utero, during the first 2 years of life, and at puberty.

EMBRYONIC DEVELOPMENT

Early Embryonic Development

The milk streak appears in the fourth week, when the embryo is 2.5 mm long. It becomes the milk line, or ridge, during the fifth week (2.5 to 5.5 mm). Mammary glands begin to develop in the 6-week-old embryo, continuing their proliferation until milk ducts are developed by the time of birth[3] (Tables 2.1 and 2.2).

Embryologically, the mammary glands develop as ingrowths of the ectoderm into the underlying mesodermal tissue. In the human embryo, a thickened, raised area of the ectoderm can be recognized in the region of the future gland at the end of the fourth week of pregnancy.[4] The thickened ectoderm becomes depressed into the underlying mesoderm, the surface of the mammary area soon becomes flat, and it finally sinks below the level of the surrounding epidermis. The mesoderm in contact with the ingrowth of the ectoderm is compressed, and its elements become arranged in concentric layers, which at a later stage give rise to the gland's stroma. The ingrowing mass of ectodermal cells soon becomes pouch or pear shaped and then grows out into the surrounding mesoderm as a number of solid processes that represent the gland's future ducts. These processes, by dividing and branching, give rise to the future lobes and lobules and, much later, to the alveoli.

By 16 weeks' gestation, the branching stage has produced 15 to 25 epithelial strips or solid cords in the subcutaneous tissue that represent future secretory alveoli. The smooth musculature of the nipple and areola are developed. By apoptosis of the central epithelial cells, branching and canalization continue.[5]

Mid to Late Embryonic Development

By 32 weeks' gestation the primary milk ducts appear and the mammary vascular system is completely developed. From 16 to 32 weeks, the secondary mammary anlage (primordium) develops. The secondary mammary anlage then develops, with differentiation of the elements of hair follicles, sebaceous glands, and sweat glands, along with the Montgomery glands, around the alveoli. Mesenchymal cells differentiate into the smooth muscle of the nipple and areola between 12 and 16 weeks' gestation.[5] Thus far, development is independent of hormone stimulation. By 28 weeks' gestation, placental sex hormones enter the fetal circulation and induce canalization in the fetus.[5]

The lumina develop in the outgrowths, forming the lactiferous ducts and their branches. The lactiferous ducts open into a shallow epithelial depression known as the *mammary pit*. The pit becomes elevated as a result of the mesenchymal

TABLE 2.1	Embryonic Timetable of Breast Development in the Human	
Age of Embryo (wk)	**Crown-Rump Length of Embryo (mean)**	**Developmental Stage**
4	2.5 mm	Mammary streak
5	2.5–5.5 mm	Milk line, or milk ridge
6	5.5–11 mm	Parenchymal cells proliferate
7–8	11–25 mm	Mammary disk progresses to globular stage
9	25–30 mm	Cone stage: inward growth of parenchyma
10–12	30–68 mm	Epithelial buds sprout from invading parenchyma
12–13	68 mm–5 cm	Indentation buds become lobular with notching at epithelial-stromal border
15	10 cm	Buds branch into 15–25 epithelial strips
20–24	20 cm	Solid cords canalize by desquamation and lysis
24–32	30 cm	Further canalization
32–40	35–50 cm	Lobular-alveolar development

Data from Russo J, Russo IH. Development of the human mammary gland. In: Neville MC, Daniel CW, eds. *The Mammary Gland*. New York, NY: Plenum; 1987.

TABLE 2.2	Stages of Mammary Development		
Developmental Stage	**Hormonal Regulation**	**Local Factors**	**Description**
Embryogenesis	???	Fat pad necessary for ductal extension	Epithelial bud develops in 18- to 19-week fetus, extending a short distance into mammary fat pad with blind ducts that become canalized; some milk secretion may be present at birth
Pubertal development before onset of menses	Estrogen, GH	IGF-1, HGF, TGF-β, EGF	Ductal extension into the mammary fat pad; branching morphogenesis
After onset of menses	Estrogen, progesterone, PRL?		Lobular development with formation of terminal duct lobular unit
Development in pregnancy	Progesterone, PRL, placental lactogen	HER, ???	Alveolus formation; partial cellular differentiation
Transition: lactogenesis	Progesterone withdrawal, PRL, glucocorticoid	Unknown	Onset of milk secretion: stage I, midpregnancy; stage II, parturition
Lactation	PRL, oxytocin	FIL, stretch	Ongoing milk secretion, milk ejection
Involution	Withdrawal of prolactin	Milk stasis (FIL??)	Alveolar epithelium undergoes apoptosis and remodeling and gland reverts to prepregnant state

? and ??, Possibly; *???*, unknown; *EGF*, epidermal growth factor; *FIL*, feedback inhibitor of lactation; *GH*, growth hormone; *HER*, herregulin; *HGF*, human growth factor; *IGF-1*, insulin-like growth factor-1; *PRL*, prolactin; *TGF-β*, transforming growth factor-β.
From Neville MC. Breastfeeding, I: the evidence for breastfeeding: anatomy and physiology of lactation. *Pediatr Clin North Am.* 2001;48:13.

proliferation forming the nipple and areola. An inverted nipple is a result of the failure of the pit to elevate.[6] A lumen is formed in each part of the branching system of epithelial cell processes after 32 weeks' gestation. This canalization produces the primary milk ducts at this time along with further development of the mammary gland vascular system.

Near term, about 15 to 25 mammary ducts form the fetal mammary gland (Fig. 2.1). Duct and sebaceous glands coalesce near the epidermis. Parenchymal differentiation occurs with the development of lobular-alveolar structures that contain colostrum. This change occurs at 32 to 40 weeks and is called the *end-vesicle stage*.

FETAL AND PREPUBERTAL DEVELOPMENT

Fetal Development

Morphologic developments in the fetal breast tissue occur in response to hormonal stimuli, similar to those in the maternal breast.[7] From 32 to 40 weeks' gestation the mammary gland undergoes a four-fold increase in mass along with development of the nipple-areolar structure. Pigmentation of this structure also occurs at this time.

The Golgi system and abundant reticula with dilated cisternae filled with fine granular material are present in the cellular structure. Abundant mitochondria and lipid droplets are observed. Proliferation and conditioning of the epithelial cells are evident, and, in the last trimester, microvilli along the ductal lumen are accompanied by large cytoplasmic protrusions (see Table 2.2).

An extensive anatomic and histologic study of the human infant breast revealed an epithelial differentiation that followed a chronologic pattern, starting with secretory changes and apparently going through a period of apocrine metaplasia before the postsecretory changes and involution.[4] The embryonic fat probably plays a role in growth and morphogenesis of the ductal system. The male and female mammary glands develop in a similar fashion until puberty.[4]

The terminal end buds, lateral buds, and lobules of three to five alveolar buds predominate in prepubertal tissue. Lobules of alveolar buds and lobules of up to 60 ductules predominate in pubertal females. In prepuberty, these epithelium-lined ducts will bud out to form alveoli when stimulated by hormones of menarche (see Fig. 2.1).

Fully formed, the breast is made up of skin, glandular tissue, supporting connective tissue, and protective fatty tissue.

Witch's Milk

The lactiferous sinuses appear before birth as swellings of the developing ducts. Immediately after birth, the newborn's breast may even be swollen and secreting a small amount of milk, often termed *witch's milk*. This phenomenon, common among both male and female infants, is caused by the stimulation of the infant's mammary glands as a result of maternal pituitary prolactin hormones that pass across the placenta into the fetal circulation.[4]

This secretory activity subsides within 3 to 4 weeks, and then the mammary glands are inactive until shortly before the onset of puberty, when hormones begin to stimulate growth again.

Prepubertal Development

During childhood (prepuberty), the gland merely keeps pace with physical growth[2] (Figs. 2.2 and 2.3).

The molecular biology of mammary gland development depends on a combination of systemic mammotropic hormones plus local cell-to-cell interactions.[2] A variety of growth factors mediate the local cell interactions. These factors include epidermal growth factor (EGF), transforming growth factor-β (TGF-β), fibroblast growth factor (FGF), and the *Wnt* gene families. In the developing breast these factors are thought to act in concert with systemic hormones.[2]

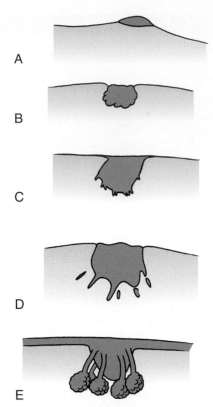

Fig. 2.1 Evolution of nipple. (A) Thickening of epidermis with formation of primary bud. (B) Growth of bud into mesenchyma. (C) Formation of solid secondary buds. (D) Formation of mammary pit and vacuolation of buds to form epithelial-lined ducts. (E) Lactiferous ducts proliferate. Areola is formed. Nipple is inverted initially. (Modified from Weatherly-White RCA. *Plastic Surgery of the Female Breast.* Hagerstown, MD: Harper & Row; 1980.)

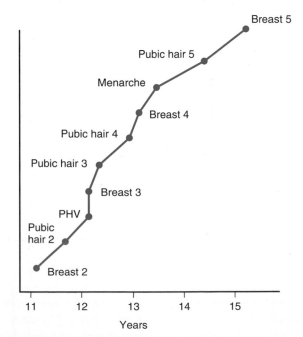

Fig. 2.2 Pubertal development in females. The sequence and mean ages of pubertal events in females, adapted from the data of Marshall and Tanner. *PHV,* Peak height velocity. (From Root AW. Endocrinology of puberty. *J Pediatr.* 1973;83:1.)

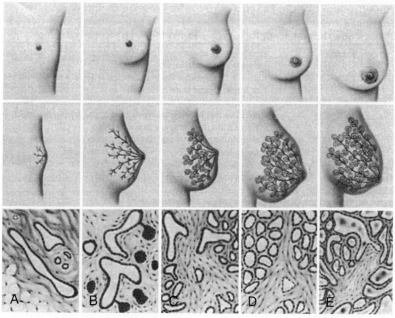

Fig. 2.3 Female breast from infancy to lactation with corresponding cross section and duct structure. (A–C) Gradual development of well-differentiated ductular and peripheral lobular-alveolar system. (D) Ductular sprouting and intensified peripheral lobular-alveolar development in pregnancy. Glandular luminal cells begin actively synthesizing milk fat and proteins near term; only small amounts are released into lumen. (E) With postpartum withdrawal of luteal and placental sex steroids and placental lactogen, prolactin is able to induce full secretory activity of alveolar cells and release of milk into alveoli and smaller ducts. (From Tanner JM. *Wachstun und Reifung des Menschen*. Stuttgart, Germany: Thieme-Verlag; 1962.)

Thelarche, or development of breast buds in females, commonly occurs between the ages of 8 and 13 years of age. Race, genetics, exercise, and body mass each can influence the age of thelarche. Concerns have been raised about earlier age of onset of thelarche. In a longitudinal cohort of 6 to 8 years of age, girls were followed from 2004 to 2011 in three geographic areas in the United States. Using Tanner staging, the age at onset of breast maturation was documented. Stage 2 onset varied by race/ethnicity, body mass index (BMI) at baseline, and site. Mean onset was 8.8, 9.3, 9.7, and 9.7 years for blacks, Hispanics, whites and non-Hispanics, and Asians, respectively. The greater the BMI, the younger the age of maturation. This study confirmed earlier onset of thelarche in girls in the last decade reported by other researchers.[8]

PUBERTAL DEVELOPMENT

Puberty stimulates rapid breast growth activated by ovulation and establishment of menses. The development of the human breast involves two distinct processes: organogenesis and milk production.[9]

Organogenesis

Organogenesis involves ductal and lobular growth and begins before and continues through puberty, resulting in growth of the breast parenchyma with its surrounding fat pad. When a girl is between 10 and 12 years of age, just before puberty, the ductal tree extends and generates its branching pattern, lengthening the existing ducts, dichotomously branching the growing ductal tips, and monopodially branching, with the growth of the lateral buds at the sides of the ducts[2] (Tables 2.2 and 2.3). During this period of rapid growth, the ducts can develop bulbous terminal end buds. The formation of alveolar buds begins within a year or two of the onset of menses.[10]

Changes During Menstruation

During the menstrual cycle, the breast changes, beginning with the follicular phase of days 3 to 14. The stroma becomes less dense. Lumina expansion takes place in the ducts. Occasionally mitosis occurs, but no secretion has been seen. In days 15 to 28, or the luteal phase, the density of the stroma progresses, and the ducts have a lumen and some secretion. From days 26 to 28 epithelial cells are reduced as apoptosis occurs, and blood flow is greatest in midcycle.[11] The sprouting of new alveolar buds continues for several years, producing alveolar lobes.[12] Mammary stem cell (MaSC) populations from the basal ductal layer are driven by the ovarian hormonal circuit, and changes in epithelial and stromal development result.[13] The mammary mini-remodeling with each cycle does not fully regress at the end of the cycle.

ANATOMIC LOCATION

The breast is located in the superficial fascia between the second rib and sixth intercostal cartilage and on the deep pectoral fascia that is superficial to the pectoralis major muscle.[2] It tends to overlap this muscle inferiorly to become superficial to the external oblique and serratus anterior muscles. The loose connective tissue between the breast and deep fascia forms the "submammary space," which allows some movement.[14] It

TABLE 2.3		**Phases of Breast Development**
Phase	**Age (yr)**	**Developmental Characteristics**
I	Puberty	Preadolescent elevation of nipple with no palpable glandular tissue or areolar pigmentation
II	11.1 ± 1.1	Presence of glandular tissue in subareolar region; nipple and breast project as single mound from chest wall
III	12.2 ± 1.09	Increase in amount of readily palpable glandular tissue, with enlargement of breast and increased diameter and pigmentation of areola; contour of breast and nipple remains in single plane
IV	13.1 ± 1.15	Enlargement of areola and increased areolar pigmentation; nipple and areola form secondary mound above breast level
V	15.3 ± 1.7	Final adolescent development of smooth contour with no projection of areola and nipple

From Macias H, Hinck L. Mammary gland development. *WIREs Dev Biol.* 2012;1:533. http://DOI:10.1002/wdev.35. Modified from Tanner JM: *Wachstun und Reifung des Menschen.* Stuttgart, Thieme-Verlag; 1962.

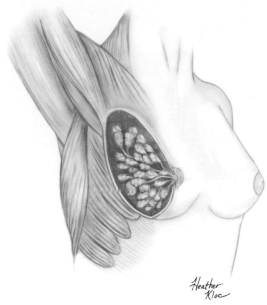

Fig. 2.5 Ramification of lactiferous ducts and mammary tissue. Ducts extend onto the upper medial aspect of the arm, to midline, and into the epigastrium. Composite drawing from mammographic studies. (Modified from Hicken NF. Mastectomy: pathologic study demonstrating why most mastectomies result in incomplete removal of the mammary gland. *Arch Surg.* 1940;40:6.)

measures 10 to 12 cm in diameter. It is located horizontally from the parasternal to midaxillary line. The central thickness of the breast is 5 to 7 cm (Fig. 2.4).

Breast Size

At puberty, the breasts of a girl enlarge to their adult size, with the left frequently slightly larger than the right.[15] In a nonpregnant woman the mature breast weighs approximately 200 g. During pregnancy, breast size and weight increase; thus when a pregnant woman is near term, the breast weighs 400 to 600 g. During lactation the breast weighs 600 to 800 g (see Fig. 2.3).

Breast development has traditionally been assessed by physical examination with Tanner staging from infancy through pregnancy (see Fig. 2.3). There is an alternative using optical spectroscopy as a noninvasive procedure if necessary.[16]

Breast Shape

The shape of breasts varies from woman to woman, just as do body build and facial characteristics. Genetic, racial, and dietary variations may be associated with discoidal, hemispheric, pear-shaped, or conical forms.[14] Typically, the breast is dome-shaped or conic in adolescence, becoming more hemispheric and finally pendulous in a parous woman.

Tail of Spence

Mammary glandular tissue projects somewhat into the axillary region. This is known as the *tail of Spence* (Fig. 2.5). Mammary tissue in the axilla, which is connected to the central duct system, becomes more obvious during pregnancy and produces milk during lactation, when it may cause various symptoms (see Chapter 16).[17] The tail of Spence is

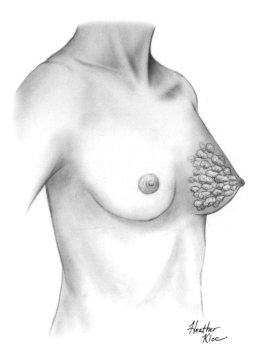

Fig. 2.4 Mammary gland in longitudinal cross section showing mature, nonlactating duct system.

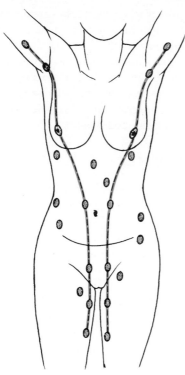

Fig. 2.6 Sites of supernumerary nipples along milk line. Ectopic nipples, areolae, or breast tissue can develop from groin to axilla and upper inner arm. They can lactate or undergo malignant change. (Modified from Weatherly-White RCA. *Plastic Surgery of the Female Breast.* Hagerstown, MD: Harper & Row; 1980.)

distinguished from a supernumerary gland because it connects to the normal duct system. Occasionally, in normal women, small masses of breast tissue may grow through the deep fascia to the muscle below. This may explain some pain distribution when the breast is engorged.

Primary Breast Structures

The three major structures of the breast are skin, subcutaneous tissue, and corpus mammae. The corpus mammae is the breast mass that remains after freeing the breast from the deep attachments and removing the skin, subcutaneous connective tissue, and adipose tissue.

The breasts of an adult woman are paired and develop from a line of glandular tissue found in the fetus and known as the *milk line.* This milk streak, or galactic band, develops from the axilla to the groin during the fifth to seventh week of embryonic life.[2] In the thoracic region, the band develops into a ridge and the rest of the band usually regresses (Fig. 2.6).

ABNORMALITIES

In some women, additional residual tissue of the galactic band remains as mammary tissue, which can develop anywhere along this line (see Fig. 2.6).

Hypermastia

Hypermastia is the presence of accessory mammary glands, which are phylogenic remnants of the embryonic mammary

ridge resulting from incomplete regression or dispersion of the primitive galactic band (see Fig. 2.6). Because of this origin, accessory nipples and glandular tissue may be found along these lines, which extend from the clavicular to the inguinal regions. Occasionally, supernumerary glands are found in the urogenital region, on the buttocks, or on the back.[18] The glands are derived from the ectoderm, and the connective tissue stroma is mesodermal in origin.

The accessory tissue may involve the corpus mammae, the areola, and the nipple.[18] Hypermastia occurs in 2% to 6% of women. The response of hypermastia to pregnancy and lactation depends on the tissue present and its location.

Box 2.1 defines other selected breast abnormalities.

Symmastia

Symmastia is a webbing across the midline between the breasts, which are usually symmetric.[4] A more common variation is the presternal confluence representing blending of breast tissue associated with large breasts. These abnormalities are ectodermal in origin and have many variations, from an empty skin web to the presence of significant glandular tissue. Little is known about their function, but several procedures exist for their surgical amelioration.[4]

Amastia and Amazia

Congenital absence of the breast is called *amastia,* which is rare. When a nipple is present but no breast tissue, the condition is called *amazia.* Another term for this condition when it occurs in addition to a normal breast is *hyperthelia.*

Polythelia

Some have suggested a relationship between polythelia (supernumerary nipple) and renal defect. Polythelia also has been associated with renal agenesis, renal cell carcinoma, obstructive disease, and supernumerary kidneys.[18] Others have described associations with congenital cardiac anomalies, pyloric stenosis, ear abnormalities, and arthrogryposis multiplex congenita.[18]

Poland Syndrome

Poland syndrome, first described in 1841 (Box 2.2), includes absence of the pectoral muscle, chest wall deformity, and breast anomalies.[5] It is now known also to include symbrachydactyly, with hypoplasia of the middle phalanges and central skin webbing. Breast hypoplasia is underdevelopment of the breast. Although 90% of cases of breast hypoplasia are

> **BOX 2.2 Types of Breast Hypoplasia, Hyperplasia, and Acquired Abnormalities**
>
> - Unilateral hypoplasia, contralateral breast normal
> - Bilateral hypoplasia with asymmetry
> - Unilateral hyperplasia, contralateral breast normal
> - Bilateral hyperplasia with asymmetry
> - Unilateral hypoplasia, contralateral breast hyperplasia
> - Unilateral hypoplasia of breast, thorax, and pectoral muscles (Poland syndrome)
> - Acquired abnormalities caused by trauma, burns, radiation treatment for hemangioma or intrathoracic disease, chest tube insertion in infancy, and preadolescent biopsy

associated with hypoplasia of the pectoral muscles, 92% of women with pectoral muscle abnormalities have normal breasts. Box 2.2 lists types of breast hypoplasia, hyperplasia (overdevelopment), and acquired breast abnormalities.

Hyperadenia

Hyperadenia is the presence of mammary tissue without nipples. The swelling and secretion of this tissue may produce pain during lactation. Occasionally, aberrant breast tissue can cause discomfort or embarrassment in adolescence and during menses, especially when located in the axilla.[18] Mammographic features of normal accessory axillary breast tissue were reviewed by Adler et al.[17] in 13 women who were diagnosed on routine mammography. Seven of these women had a mass or fullness on physical examination; one was seen postpartum because of pain; nine were asymptomatic. They ranged in age from 31 to 67 years. On radiographic study, the accessory tissue resembled the rest of the normal glandular tissue but was separate from it. It occurred on the right in 11 of the 13 women. The accessory tissue was recognized as a normal developmental variant, distinguishable from the frequent axillary tail of Spence, which represents a direct extension from the outer margin of the main mass of glandular tissue.

Evaluation and Treatment of Accessory Tissue

On mammography, accessory tissue is best visualized on oblique and exaggerated craniocaudal views and by ultrasound. In rare cases, it may be appropriate to remove the tissue surgically, a treatment well known to experienced plastic surgeons. If treatment is not initiated before pregnancy and lactation in these women, pain and swelling will be intensified and may progress to mastitis or the necessity to terminate lactation.

Further Abnormalities

Apart from physiologic variations, other conditions of abnormal anatomy include hypomastia (abnormally small breasts), hypertrophy, and inequality.

Acquired Abnormalities

The most common cause of acquired breast abnormality is iatrogenic and is most commonly caused by chest wall trauma in premature infants when chest tubes are inserted. Biopsy in prepubertal girls may remove vital tissues. Cutaneous burns to the chest wall may result in scaring and breast deformity. Sonography is often a useful method for imaging the breast and axillary tissue in an attempt to make a diagnosis without a biopsy.[19,20] With involvement of a lactation specialist, obstetrician, and surgeon, breastfeeding is possible in many situations with adequate assistance and support.

CORPUS MAMMAE

The mammary gland is an orderly conglomeration of a variable number of independent glands. It undergoes a series of changes that can be divided into developmental and differentiation phases. Surgical dissection of many postoperative specimens has contributed more precise information about the anatomic structure of the breast. The ramifications of the lactiferous ducts and stroma were carefully studied by Weatherly-White,[21] who reported that in 95% of women the ducts ascend into the axilla, occasionally following the brachial plexus and axillary vessels into the apex of the axilla. Ducts are found in the epigastric region in 15% of women. In rare cases, ducts cross the midline (see Fig. 2.6).

Morphology

The morphology of the corpus mammae includes two major divisions: the parenchyma and the stroma.[3] The parenchyma includes the ductular-lobular-alveolar structures. It is composed of the alveolar gland with treelike ductular branching alveoli, which are approximately 0.12 mm in diameter. The ducts are approximately 2 mm in diameter. The lobi, which are arranged like spokes converging on the central nipple, are 15 to 25 in number. Each lobus is divided again into 20 to 40 lobuli, and each lobulus is again subdivided into 10 to 100 alveoli, or tubulosaccular secretory units.

The stroma includes the connective tissue, fat tissue, blood vessels, nerves, and lymphatics.[2]

The mass of tissue in the breast consists of the tubuloalveolar glands embedded in fat (the adipose tissue), giving the gland its smooth, rounded contour. The mammary fat pad is essential for the proliferation and differentiation of the mammary epithelium, providing the necessary space, support, and local control for duct elongation and, ultimately, lobuloalveolar proliferation.

Each gland forms a lobe of the breast, and the lobes are separated by connective tissue septa. These septa attach to the skin. Each tubuloalveolar gland opens into a lactiferous duct, which leads into a more elastic duct. A slight constriction occurs before the duct opens onto the surface of the nipple (Fig. 2.7). Extension of ducts within the fat pad is orderly. The fat pad is critical to the development of the arborization.[22] Fat is distributed throughout the gland, buffering the alveolae and ducts. An inhibitory zone into which other ducts cannot penetrate exists around each duct, and development does not normally proceed beyond the duct end-bud stage before puberty.[2]

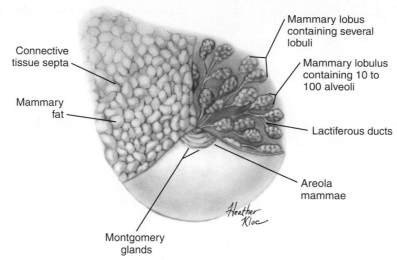

Fig. 2.7 Morphology of mature breast with dissection to reveal mammary fat and duct system.

NIPPLE AND AREOLA

The skin of the breast includes the nipple, areola, and general skin. The skin is the thin, flexible, elastic cover of the breast and is adherent to the fat-laden subcutaneous tissue. It contains hair, sebaceous glands, and apocrine sweat glands.

The Nipple

The nipple, or papilla mammae, is a conic elevation located in the center of the areola at about the fourth intercostal space, slightly below the midpoint of the breast. The nipple contains 23 to 27 milk ducts on average, with a range of 11 to 48. Each of the tubuloalveolar glands that make up the breast opens onto the nipple by a separate opening. The precise anatomy of the nipple has drawn little attention since the work of Sir Ashley Cooper in 1839.[23]

Cancer scientists are exploring the anatomy of the breast in detail to determine how cancers grow and how they spread, not to determine how the breast functions. Studies of autopsies and breasts removed for cancer in young, vital women are used.[24]

Data from mastectomy breasts have shown that collecting duct numbers in the nipple averaging 25 to 27 are greater in number than the number of nipple duct openings (6 to 8) identifiable on the nipple surface. A three-dimensional (3-D) model of the nipple from a mastectomy specimen showed three distinct populations of ducts. The largest lobe was 23% of breast volume. Half the breast was drained by three ducts and 75% by the six largest ducts. Eight small ducts drained about 1.6% of the breast volume. Seven ducts the authors called type A maintained a wide lumen up to the skin surface, 20 ducts (type B) tapered to a minute lumen in the vicinity of the skin on the apex of the nipple, and a minor duct population (type C) arose around the base of the nipple. These distinctions are not distinguishable on microscopic examination except for type C ducts.[25]

Using similar 3-D technology, Rusby et al.[24] sought clinical relevance for diagnostic techniques by accessing by cannulation of the ducts. They describe a central duct bundle narrowing to form a "waist" as the ducts enter the breast parenchyma. In a single sample 29 ducts arose from 15 orifices. At skin level, ducts are narrow, becoming larger and deeper within the nipple. Many ducts share a few common openings, confirming the apparent discrepancy between number of ducts and number of orifices. Duct diameter does not predict the penetrance of the duct deeper into the breast.

Rusby et al.[24] demonstrated that a shared opening of many ducts on the surface of the nipple and the narrow caliber of the ducts closest to the nipple lip changes the clinical interpretation of ductography, ductal lavage, and ductoscopy.

In early anatomic studies of the breast, which were done on autopsy specimens, the duct system was identified by pushing dye into the duct under pressure.[26] The duct, being elastic, can be stretched to suggest ductal sinuses, leading to the impression that the ducts have sinuses that collect milk in the areola; however, this has been shown to be incorrect.[15]

The nipple also contains smooth muscle fibers and is richly innervated with sensory nerve endings and Meissner corpuscles in the dermal papillae; it is well supplied with sebaceous and apocrine sweat glands but no hair.

Areola

The nipple is surrounded by the areola, or areola mammae, a circular pigmented area. It is usually faintly darker before pregnancy, becoming reddish brown during pregnancy, and always maintaining some darker pigmentation thereafter. The average areola measures 15 to 16 mm in diameter, although the range is great, enlarging during pregnancy and lactation.[27] The pigmentation results from many melanocytes distributed throughout the skin and glands. The understructure of the epidermis of the areola is not as elaborate as that of the nipple but is intermediate to that of the surrounding skin. The nipple and areola are extremely elastic.

Little or no true lobuloalveolar development occurs before the first pregnancy. A framework is laid down, within which the specialized secretory cells will proliferate (Fig. 2.8).[2] The

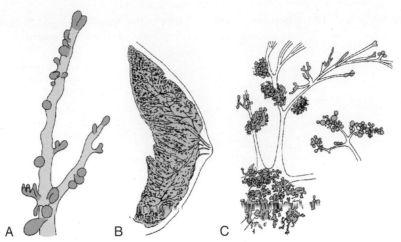

Fig. 2.8 (A) Duct end from a 15-year-old nulligravida adolescent on second day of menstruation showing typical form of puberty: a coarsely diversified system of thick, mostly well-filled ducts with round, often ball-shaped or half-ball-shaped ends. Note use of connective tissue as guiding tracts, circumvention of fat tissue, and paucity of secretory alveoli. (B) Sagittal section through milk gland of a nulligravida 19-year-old woman between menses (died of skull fracture). Note massive body of connective tissue without preserved lobes of fatty tissue and richness of connective tissue with respective richness of parenchyma. Note also the distribution of larger ducts in superficial parallel connective tissue septum of former subcutaneous fat tissue and smaller ducts in vertical septa. Thin section; drawing with Busch magnifying glasses. (C) Gland of a nulligravida 19-year-old woman (part of a 4-mm-thick section). Bushy short sprout and duct build long sprout, with the latter in acute angled bifurcation, often lying very close to each other. This demonstrates development of ductal and secretory elements during the menstrual cycle; however, connective tissue and fat are predominant. (From Dabelow A. Die Milchdrüse. In: *Handbuch der Mikroskopischen Anatomie des Menschen*. Vol 3. Part 3. Berlin, Germany: Springer-Verlag: 1957.)

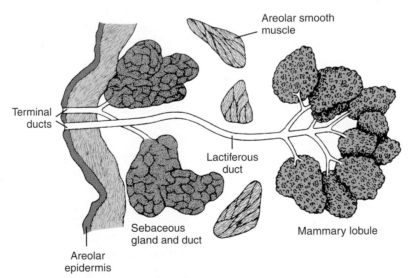

Fig. 2.9 Tubercle of Montgomery and underlying structures. Lactiferous duct may join sebaceous gland ducts and terminate at common opening in areolar epidermis as shown. (Modified from Smith DM, Peters TG, Donegan WL. Montgomery's areolar tubercle: a light microscopic study. *Arch Pathol Lab Med.* 1982;106:62.)

framework forms a vital part of the gland's overall developmental course, and maldevelopment or trauma during fetal or juvenile life can seriously reduce the size and secretory potential of the mature gland.

Montgomery Tubercles

Montgomery tubercles, containing the ductular openings of sebaceous and lactiferous glands, are present in the areola,[2] as are sweat glands and smaller, free sebaceous glands. The Montgomery glands become enlarged and look like small pimples during pregnancy and lactation (Fig. 2.9). They secrete a substance that lubricates and protects the nipples and areolae during pregnancy and lactation. A small amount of milk is also secreted from these tubercles. After lactation, these glands recede again to their former unobtrusive state.

Light microscopy has shown that Morgagni was correct in 1719 when he first described the 12 to 20 areolar glands and noted them to be sebaceous and to include lactiferous structures as well. Building on the original work, in 1837 Montgomery prepared a more detailed treatise on the tubercle itself and named it after himself. Lactiferous ducts from the deeper breast parenchyma ascended into the sebaceous glands of the tubercle (see Fig. 2.9).[2] The sebaceous gland itself was no different from those of the skin or those associated with the terminal lactiferous ducts of the nipple. The mammary duct was lined with two layers of cuboidal to columnar cells. They arose from the underlying mammary lobules through the subcutaneous tissues and into the region of the sebaceous gland. The terminal portion of the mammary duct in some cases joined the duct to the sebaceous gland and in other cases opened separately but close to it. The ducts appear to be a miniature of the major mammary system. Sebaceous and mammary ductal components underlie the areolar tubercle.[19]

Function in Breastfeeding

The areola and nipple are darker than the rest of the breast, ranging from light pink in fair-skinned women to dark brown in others. The areola's darker color may be a visual signal to newborns so that they will close their mouth on the areola, not on the nipple alone, to obtain milk.

Nipple erection is induced by tactile, sensory, and autonomic sympathetic stimuli. The corium (dermis) of the areola lacks fat but contains smooth muscle and collagenous and elastic connective tissue fibers in radial and circular arrangements. The dermis of the nipple and the areola contains many multibranched, free nerve fiber endings. Local venostasis and hyperemia occur to enhance the process of erection of the nipple because the nipple and areola are rich in arteriovenous anastomoses. The glabrous skin of the nipple is wrinkled, containing large papillae of the corium.

Each nipple contains 15 to 25 lactiferous ducts surrounded by fibromuscular tissue[3] (Figs. 2.10 through 2.13). This number often has been challenged but was finally confirmed by Taneri et al.[28] and also Rusby et al.[24] to be a mean of 23. These ducts end as small orifices near the tip of the nipple. Within the

nipple, the lactiferous ducts may merge. The ductular orifices, therefore, are sometimes fewer in number than the respective breast lobi. The ampullae function as temporary milk containers during a feeding but contain only epithelial debris in the nonlactating state.

The use of ultrasound imagery of the contralateral breast while the infant is nursing on the other breast or the other breast is being pumped has shown that the profound elasticity

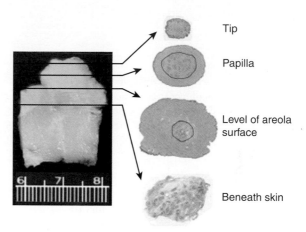

Fig. 2.11 Photograph of a sagittal section through a nipple with coronal block sections from a different nipple. The sagittal section illustrates the approximate location of tissue sections. Block sections from a coronally sectioned nipple show differences in morphology with depth. The duct bundle is *outlined in black*. The beginnings of the waist can be seen at the level of the areola. (From Rushby J, Brachtel EF, Michaelson JS, et al. Breast duct anatomy in the human nipple: three-dimensional patterns and clinical implications. *Breast Cancer Res Treat.* 2006;106:171.)

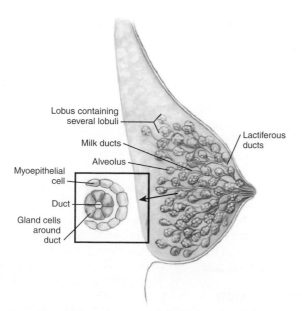

Fig. 2.10 Simplified schematic drawing of duct system with cross section of myoepithelial cells around duct opening. Myoepithelial cells contract to eject milk.

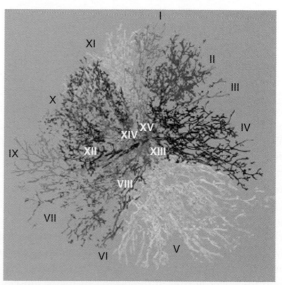

Fig. 2.12 All ducts and their branches in an autopsy breast, viewed en face. Each Roman numeral refers to a different independent duct system. (From Going JJ, Moffat DF. Escaping from flatland: clinical and biological aspects of human mammary duct anatomy in three dimensions. *J Pathol.* 2004;203:538.)

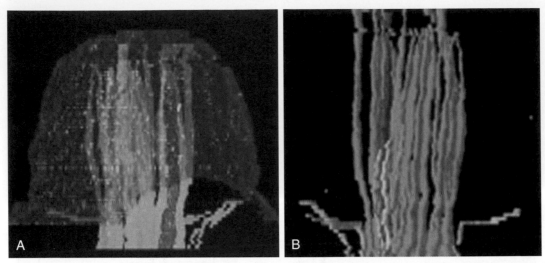

Fig. 2.13 Digital model of nipple duct anatomy. (A) Relationship of nipple duct bundle *(inner fibers)* to skin of the papilla *(outer film).* (B) Lateral view of duct bundle. Seven ducts of varying caliber extend up to the surface of the nipple (population A); 20 other ducts (population B) diminish in caliber and terminate 0.8 to 1.0 mm beneath the surface, close to skin appendages. Seven accessory ducts (population C) are shown as short fibers at base. (From Going JJ, Moffat DF. Escaping from flatland: clinical and biological aspects of human mammary duct anatomy in three dimensions. *J Pathol.* 2004;203:538.)

of the ductal system allows for an acute increase in milk duct diameter during let-down and milk production.

Contrary to the sketches of the breast in many professional and lay journals, the ducts do not form sinuses just before the nipple.[15] The concept of lactiferous sinuses was described when postmortem specimens were injected with solidifying liquid under pressure causing a ballooning of the duct. The lining of the infundibular and ampullar parts of the lactiferous ducts consists of an 8- to 10-cell layered squamous epithelium.

The bulk of the nipple is composed of smooth musculature, which represents a closing mechanism for the milk ducts of the nipple. The milk ducts in the nipple are embedded in stretchable and mobile connective tissue. The inner longitudinal muscular arrangements and the outer, more circular and radial arrangements do not obstruct the milk ducts. Tangential fibers also branch off from the more circular muscular fibers of the nipple bases to the outer circular muscular range.

The functions of the muscular fibroelastic system of the areola and nipple include decreasing the surface area of the areola, producing nipple erection, and emptying the swollen ducts during nursing. When the nipple erects because of tactile, thermal, or sexual stimulation, the system causes the nipple to become smaller, firmer, everted, and more prominent.[2]

The mammary tissues are enveloped by the superficial pectoral fascia, and the breast is fixed by fibrous bands to the overlying skin and the underlying pectoral fascia, which are known as the *ligaments of Cooper.* The glandular part of the breast is surrounded by a fat layer that seldom extends beyond the lower border of the pectoralis major muscle. The breast is attached to the muscles between the ribs, the clavicle, and the bones of the upper arm near the shoulder. The breast itself contains no supporting muscles and relies on ligaments to sustain its shape. The measurement of the glandular tissue

compared with the amount of intermingling fat tissue has been estimated by Ramsey et al.[29] using ultrasound in 21 lactating white women. The ratio was variable, ranging from 50% to 100% of the breast, proving again that size of the breast does not predict milk production. Ethnicity has little impact on breast size and production but the density of the breast is measurably less in Asian women than white or black women, according to work by Chen et al.[30] (Figs. 2.14 and 2.15).

BLOOD SUPPLY

Arterial Supply

The blood supply to the breast is from branches of the intercostal arteries and the perforating branches of the internal thoracic artery; the third, fourth, and fifth are usually most prominent. The major blood supply to the breast is provided by the internal mammary artery and the lateral thoracic artery. A small supply is obtained from the intercostal arteries and the arterial branches of the axillary and subclavian arteries, but this contribution is minimal; 60% of the total breast tissue, especially the medial and central part, receives blood from the internal mammary artery.

All the mammary branches of this artery lead transversely to the nipple and anastomoses with branches coming from the lateral thoracic artery.[11] Anastomoses with intercostal arteries are less common, but the blood supply to the nipple is extensive and close to the surface, contributing to the richer color.

Many areas of the breast are supplied by two or three arterial sources (Fig. 2.16).

Venous Supply

The venous supply parallels the arterial supply and bears similar names. The veins drain the breast and enter the fascia, muscle layers, and intercostal spaces at the same point. The

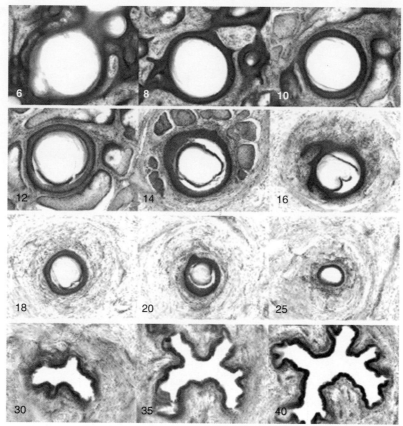

Fig. 2.14 A typical "population A" nipple duct: selected sections between 6 and 40. The duct has a wide, funnel-shaped opening onto the surface of the nipple. The lumen tapers moderately before opening out into the characteristically convoluted profile of the collecting ducts in the nipple. The lumen is plugged by keratin in section 20. (From Going JJ, Moffat DF. Escaping from flatland: clinical and biological aspects of human mammary duct anatomy in three dimensions. *J Pathol.* 2004;203:544.)

veins end in the internal thoracic and the axillary veins. Some veins may reach the external jugular vein. The veins create an anastomotic circle around the base of the papilla, called the *circulus venosis*.[7] Individual variation is common.

LYMPHATIC DRAINAGE

The lymphatic drainage of the breast has been the subject of considerable study because of the frequency of breast cancer, but it has significance for lactating breasts as well. The lymphatic drainage can be extensive. The main drainage is to axillary nodes and to the parasternal nodes along the internal thoracic artery inside the thoracic cavity. The lymphatics of the breast originate in the lymph capillaries of the mammary connective tissue, which surrounds the mammary structures, and drain through the deep substance of the breast. The subepithelial or papillary plexus of the lymphatics of the breast is confluent with the subepithelial lymphatics over the surface of the body. These valveless lymphatics communicate with subdermal lymphatic vessels and merge with the subareolar plexus.[2]

Lymphatic Components

The lymph drainage of the breast consists of the superficial or cutaneous section, the areola, and the glandular or deep-

tissue section. More than 75% of the lymph from the breast goes to the axillary nodes.[31] Other points of drainage are to pectoral nodes between the pectoralis major and minor muscles and to the subclavicular nodes in the neck deep to the clavicle. Flow from the deep subcutaneous and intramammary lymphatic vessels travels centrifugally toward the axilla and the internal mammary lymph nodes.

Some transmammary lymph drainage occurs to the opposite breast and to subdiaphragmatic lymphatics that lead ultimately to the liver and intraabdominal nodes (Fig. 2.17). There has been minimal study of lymphatic drainage of the lactating breast in spite of its importance in engorgement and mastitis.[31]

INNERVATION

The nerves of the breast are from branches of the third, fourth, fifth, and sixth intercostal nerves and consist of sensory fibers innervating the smooth muscles in the nipple and blood vessels.

The majority of the mammary nerves follow the arteries and arterioles and supply these structures. A few fibers from the perivascular networks course along the walls of the ducts. They may correspond to sensory fibers for sensing milk pressure. No innervation of mammary myoepithelial cells has been identified. It can, therefore, be concluded that secretory

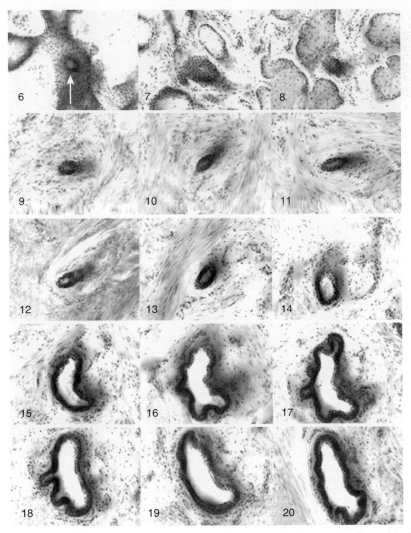

Fig. 2.15 A typical "population B" nipple duct: consecutive serial sections from 6 to 20. The duct takes origin from the deep aspect of the nipple epidermis in close proximity to skin appendages *(arrow, section 6, top left)*. It retains a minute lumen over about eight sections (800 μm) before the lumen begins to widen in sections 14 to 20. Such a duct will be difficult to cannulate. (From Going JJ, Moffat DF. Escaping from flatland: clinical and biological aspects of human mammary duct anatomy in three dimensions. *J Pathol.* 2004;203:544.)

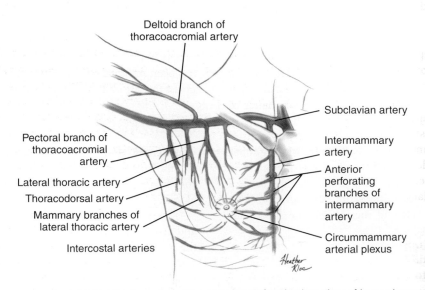

Fig. 2.16 Blood supply to mammary gland. Major blood supply is from anterior perforating branches of internal mammary artery.

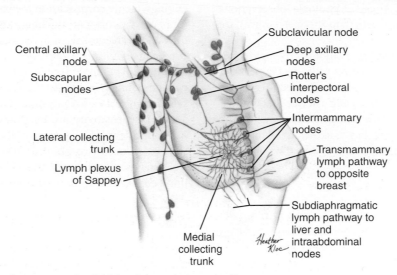

Fig. 2.17 Lymphatic drainage of mammary gland. Major drainage is toward axilla.

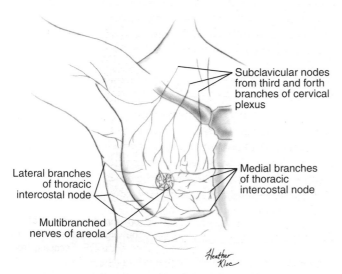

Fig. 2.18 Innervation of mammary gland. Supraclavicular nerves and lateral and medial branches of intercostal nerves provide sensory innervation. Sympathetic and motor nerves are provided by supracervical and intercostal nerves.

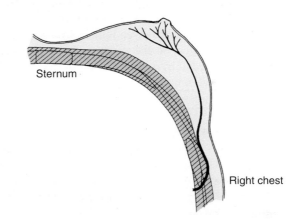

Fig. 2.19 Cross section of nerve supply of breast and nipple. Cutaneous nerves run close to deep fascia before turning outward toward skin.

activities of the acinar epithelium depend on hormonal stimulation, such as that of oxytocin and other hormones, and are not stimulated by the nervous system directly.

The supraclavicular nerves supply the sensory fibers for innervation of the upper cutaneous parts of the breast. Branches of the intercostal nerves provide the major sensory innervation of the mammary gland. The sympathetic sensory and motor fibers are derived from the supraclavicular and intercostal nerves, respectively. Sympathetic fibers run only along the mammary gland—supplying arteries to innervate the glandular body.

Innervation of the Nipple and Areola

The sensory innervation of the nipple and areola is extensive and consists of both autonomic and sensory nerves. The nipple and areola are reportedly always innervated by the anterior and lateral cutaneous branches of the third to fifth intercostal nerves,[32] which lie along the ducts to the nipple.

A detailed anatomic and clinical study of the nipple-areola complex showed that it is innervated from the lateral cutaneous branch of the fourth intercostal nerve, which penetrates the posterior aspect of the breast at the intersection of the fourth intercostal space and the pectoralis major muscle (4 o'clock on the left breast and 8 o'clock on the right breast).[2] The nerve divides into five fasciculi, one central to the nipple, two upper, and two lower branches (always at 5 and 7 o'clock, left and right side, respectively) (Figs. 2.18 and 2.19).

Innervation of the Corpus Mammae

The innervation of the corpus mammae is minimal by comparison and predominantly autonomic. No parasympathetic or cholinergic fibers supply any part of the breast. No ganglia are found in mammary tissue. Norepinephrine-containing nerve fibers are abundant among the smooth muscle cells of the nipple and at the interface between the media and adventitia of the breast arteries. Physiologic observations demonstrate that the efferent nerves to these structures are sympathetic adrenergic.

There is relatively restricted innervation to the epidermal parts of the nipple and areola, leading to lack of superficial sensory acuity. Courtiss and Goldwyn[33] measured breast sensation in a large number of women using a device that emitted a variable current producing a burning sensation when the threshold was exceeded. The areola was shown to be the most sensitive and the nipple the least sensitive, with the skin of the breast intermediate.

Hormonal Reflex

Stimulation of the sensory nerve fibers or sensory receptors does induce the release of adenohypophyseal prolactin and neurohypophyseal oxytocin by an afferent sensory reflex pathway whereby stimuli reach the hypothalamus. Sympathetic mammary stimulation causes the contraction of the small myoepithelial cells of the areola and the nipple. The locally released norepinephrine induces stimulation of the myoepithelial adrenergic receptors, causing muscular relaxation. In the absence of parasympathetic activity, a minor physiologic catecholamine inhibitory effect on the mammary myoepithelium may exist. This is overcome by oxytocin release during suckling, inducing myoepithelial contraction.

Changes in Sensitivity

The nipple and areola are sparsely innervated with neural elements at the base of the nipple and almost none in the areola.[34] A study of lactating women showed marked increase in areola and nipple sensitivity within 24 hours of birth.[34] After 1 to 6 months of breastfeeding, women were noted to have minimal two-point discrimination of the skin of the breast.[35] Thus the skin in these areas responds only to major stimuli, such as sucking.

The relatively large number of dermal nerve endings provides a high mammary responsiveness toward stimuli for elicitation of the sucking reflex. The neuroreflex induces adequate release of both prolactin and oxytocin. It appears that, in addition to the hormonal actions, breast nerves can also influence the mammary blood supply and milk secretion. Abnormalities of sensory or autonomic nerve distributions in the areola and nipple, therefore, could impair adequate lactation, especially in the functioning of the let-down reflex and the secretion of prolactin and oxytocin.

Summary

In summary, the somatic sensory cutaneous nerve supply of the breast includes the supraclavicular nerves and the thoracic intercostal nerves. The autonomic motor nerve supply of the breast is derived from the sympathetic fibers of the intercostal nerves, which supply the smooth musculature of the areola and the nipple. The autonomic supply is also derived from sympathetic fibers of the accompanying arteries, which innervate the smooth musculature of the inner glandular blood vessel walls to produce constriction. The nerve supply to the area of the areola and the nipple includes free sensory nerve endings, tactile corpuscles to the papillae of the corium of the nipple and areola, and the fibers around the larger lactiferous duct and in the dermis of the areola and peripheral breast. All cutaneous nerves run radially to the glandular body toward the nipple. The nerve supply to the inner gland is sparse and contains only sympathetic nerves accompanying blood vessels (see Fig. 2.19). Twenty-four hours postpartum, the nipple and areola sensitivity are markedly heightened but decrease in the next few days. The skin of the breast, areola, and nipple showed reduced two-point discrimination when lactation is well established. Clinical evidence supports the observation of limited nerve distribution in the breast.[36]

MICROSCOPIC ANATOMY

After many decades of neglect since the phylogenic studies of the mammary gland in the 1800s and early 1900s, the mammary gland has become one of the most studied organs because of its usefulness as a tool in developmental biology, biochemistry, endocrinology, biology, histology, oncology, toxicology, virology, and molecular biology.[37] It is clear that the microstructure of nonlactating mature breasts varies with age, the phase of the menstrual cycle, pregnancy, and lactation.

No cell can exist independent of its surrounding cells. All cells have relations with neighboring cells and with cells at distant sites. The interactions of the epithelial parenchyma and mesenchymal stroma are most important in primary and secondary induction during organogenesis.[38]

The ducts are lined with columnar epithelium of two cells thick in larger ducts and single layers in the smaller ones. Myoepithelial cells are numerous, creating a distinct layer around ducts and potential alveola.[38]

Cellular Structure of the Mammary Gland

The mammary gland consists of a branching system of excretory ducts embedded in connective tissue.[2] The gland is composed of two layers of epithelial cells: luminal epithelium and basal layer epithelium, along with a few basal (stem) cells.[39] The whole structure is surrounded by a basement membrane. In the ducts, elongated myoepithelial cells make up a continuous sheath. The luminal cell interaction with the extracellular matrix is mediated by the myoepithelium.

The integrity of the normal mammary gland is maintained by several adhesion systems.[2]

The mammary gland is composed of epithelial parenchyma and two types of mesenchymal stroma: dense mammary mesenchyma and fatty stroma. The dense mammary mesenchyma is present in the embryonic stage, in end buds of puberty, and in cancers. It determines mammary epithelium and fixes the ability of the epithelium to interact with the fatty stroma.

The fatty stroma is essential for typical mammary gland morphogenesis.[3] The two types of mammary stroma synthesize different extracellular matrix proteins. Dense mesenchyma makes fibronectin and tenascin. Fatty stroma makes laminin, proteoglycans, and fibronectin.

TABLE 2.4 Morphologic Criteria for Phase Assignment in Menstrual Cycle

Phase	Stroma	Lumen	Cell Types	Orientation of Epithelial Cells	Mitoses	Active Secretion
				EPITHELIUM		
Phase I (days 3–7)	Dense, cellular	Tight	Single predominant pale eosinophilic cell	No stratification apparent	Present, average 4/10 HPF	None
Phase II (days 8–14)	Dense, cellular-collagenous	Defined	1. Luminal columnar basophilic cell 2. Intermediate pale cell 3. Basal clear cell with hyperchromatic nucleus (myoepithelial)	Radial around lumen	Rare	None
Phase III (days 15–20)	Loose, broken	Open with some secretion	1. Luminal basophilic cell 2. Intermediate pale cell 3. Prominent vacuolization of basal clear cell (myoepithelial)	Radial around lumen	Absent	None
Phase IV (days 21–27)	Loose, edematous	Open with secretion	1. Luminal basophilic cell 2. Intermediate pale cell 3. Prominent vacuolization of basal clear cell (myoepithelial)	Radial around lumen	Absent	Active apocrine secretion from luminal cell
Phase V (days 28–29)	Dense, cellular	Distended with secretion	1. Luminal basophilic cell with scant cytoplasm 2. Extensive vacuolization of basal cells	Radial around lumen	Absent	Rare

HPF, High-powered field.
Modified from Vogel PM, Georgiade NG, Fetter BF, et al. The correlation of histologic changes in the human breast with the menstrual cycle. *Am J Pathol.* 1981;104:23.

Cellular Development of the Mammary Gland

In their structure and mode of development, the mammary glands somewhat resemble the sweat glands.[40] During embryonic life, their differentiation is similar in the two sexes. Male humans experience little additional development postnatally. Female humans, in contrast, experience extensive structural change paralleling age and the functional state of the reproductive system.

Vogel et al.[41] studied histologic changes in the normal human mammary gland in association with the menstrual cycle. They describe five phases: proliferative (days 3 to 7), follicular phase of differentiation (days 8 to 14), luteal phase of differentiation (days 15 to 20), secretory (days 21 to 27), and menstrual (days 28 to 29). Table 2.4 outlines the morphologic criteria for these phases. These findings illustrate the correlation of morphologic response to hormonal stimulus of the mammary gland during normal cycling.

The greatest development in girls is reached by the twentieth year. Gradual changes are correlated with the menstrual cycle, and major changes accompany pregnancy and lactation[2] (see Fig. 2.8).

Russo and Russo[42] describe the development of the mammary gland as "an asynchronous process of progressive invasion of the mammary stroma by a parenchyma composed of ductal elements in which the advancing ends are the club-shaped terminal end buds (TEBs) that progressively differentiate into alveolar buds (ABs) or regress to terminal ducts (TDs)" (Fig. 2.20).

MATURE MAMMARY GLAND

The mammary gland is a compound tubuloalveolar gland containing 15 to 25 irregular lobes radiating from the nipple.

Division of the Gland

Each lobe has a lactiferous duct (2 to 4 mm in diameter) lined by stratified squamous epithelium. The duct opens on the nipple and has an irregular angular outline. Beneath the areola, each duct finally emerges at the end of the nipple as a 0.4- to 0.7-mm opening. Each lobe is subdivided into lobules of various orders; the smallest are elongated tubules, the alveolar ducts, covered by small saccular evaginations, the alveoli. The interlobular connective tissue is dense; however, it is more cellular, has fewer collagenous fibers, and contains almost no fat. Greater distensibility is permitted by the looser connective tissue.

The epidermis of the nipple and areola is invaded by unusually long dermal papillae in which capillaries richly vascularize the surface and affect the richer hue. Bundles of

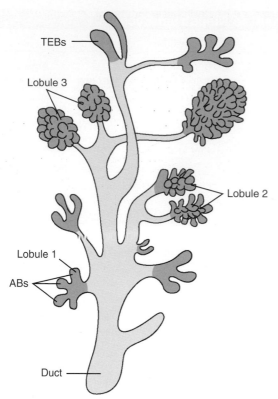

Fig. 2.20 Schematic representation depicting various topographic compartments of human mammary gland: terminal end buds *(TEBs)*; alveolar buds *(ABs)*; lobules types 1, 2, and 3; and ducts. (Modified from Russo J, Russo IH. Development of human mammary gland. In: Neville MC, Daniel CW, eds. *The Mammary Gland.* New York, NY: Plenum; 1987.)

smooth muscle, placed longitudinally along the lactiferous ducts and circumferentially within the nipple and at its base, permit the erection of the nipple. In the areola are the areolar Montgomery glands, which are intermediate in their microscopic structure between sweat glands and true mammary glands. The periphery of the areola also has sweat glands and sebaceous glands (see Fig. 2.9).

Cellular Composition

The ducts and ductules of mature women consist chiefly of two cell types: the inner lining of epithelial cells and the outer lining of myoepithelial cells. A basement membrane separates these structures from the stroma. Histochemical and immunocytochemical reagents can distinguish these elements, their positions, and their infrastructures.

Rudland[3] has reported on the histochemical organization and cellular composition of ductal buds in the developing human breast. This work suggests that cytochemical intermediates occur between epithelial and myoepithelial cells. The undifferentiated peripheral cap cells may be transitional forms of the cortical epithelial cells that will line the lumina and of the myoepithelial cells of the subtending duct.

Myoepithelial Cells

The secretory portions of the gland, the alveolar ducts and the alveoli, have cuboidal or low-columnar secretory cells, resting on basal laminae and myoepithelial cells. These myoepithelial cells enclose the alveoli in a loosely meshed network with their many starlike branchings. The myoepithelial cells are stimulated by oxytocin and sex steroids. The presence of myoepithelial cells has been used as evidence that the mammary gland is related to the sweat gland.

Epithelial Cells

In the at-rest phase, epithelial structures consist of the ducts and their branches. The presence of a few alveoli budding from the ends of ducts is still under investigation. This variance may be caused by the effect of the menstrual cycle. The swelling and engorgement accompanying the menstrual cycle are associated with hyperemia and some edema of the connective tissue. Most significant is that the gland does not have a single duct but many. Each lobe is a separate compound alveolar gland in which primary ducts join into increasingly larger ducts. These ducts drain into a lactiferous duct. Each lactiferous duct drains separately at the tip of the nipple.

Hormonal Regulation

TGF-β1, 2, and 3 are potent inhibitors of cell proliferation but play an important role in mammary gland development. They exhibit overlapping patterns of expression within the epithelium of the developing gland. TGF-β3 is detected in the myoepithelial progenitor cells of the growing end buds and the myoepithelial cells in the mature duct.[43]

MAMMARY GLAND IN PREGNANCY

Although mini-remodeling of the breast occurs at each menstrual cycle, it is not until pregnancy that complete remodeling occurs. It is transformed into a mature functional organ. The MaSC population is activated by the ovarian hormonal circuit. The levels of estrogen, progesterone, and prolactin are increased. Other hormones and growth factors regulate the mammary expansion.

Developmental Stages in Pregnancy

The first 3 to 4 weeks of pregnancy has marked ductular sprouting with some branching and lobular formation, stimulated by estrogenic release. By 5 to 8 weeks, the breast changes are physically notable with dilation of the superficial veins, heaviness, and increased pigmentation of the nipple and areola. Changes in levels of circulating hormones result in profound changes in the ductular-lobular-alveolar growth during pregnancy (Fig. 2.21).

During the first trimester, growth and branching from the terminal portion of the duct system into the adipose tissue is rapid.[44] As the epithelial structures proliferate, the adipose tissue seems to diminish. During this time, increasing infiltration of the interstitial tissue occurs with lymphocytes, plasma cells, and eosinophils. The rate of hyperplasia levels off.

In the last trimester, any enlargement is the result of parenchymal cell growth and distention of the alveoli with early colostrum, which is rich in protein and relatively low in lipid. Fat droplets gradually accumulate in the secretory

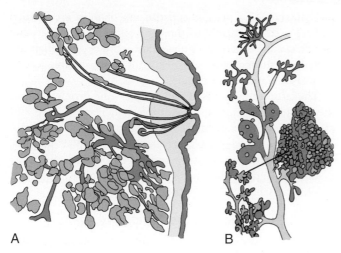

A   **B**

Fig. 2.21 (A) Milk gland of 21-year-old primigravida woman in second month of pregnancy. Development of small lobes has protruded almost to mammilla. Very regular development is shown over whole range of this thick section. Natural dimensions: 2.6 × 2.1 cm. (B) Milk gland of same 21-year-old primigravida woman. Note very different forms of sprouting. Partly atypical sprouts above diagonal line are composed from same section; bifurcations below line are in natural position. Alveoli are beginning to resemble mature gland. (From Dabelow A. Die Milchdrüse. In: *Handbuch der Mikroskopischen Anatomie des Menschen*. Vol 3. Part 3. Berlin, Germany: Springer-Verlag; 1957.)

alveolar cells. The interlobular connective tissue is noticeably decreased, and alveolar proliferation is extensive.

In experimental studies, these effects can be duplicated when estrogen and progesterone stimulate a release of prolactin-inhibiting factor. Prolactin is released in humans during pregnancy, thus stimulating epithelial growth and secretion. Prolactin levels increase over time during pregnancy.

Clinical Implications

Pregnancy-induced changes are important clinical observations usually completed by 22 weeks. The size varies markedly. Although important, breast size during pregnancy is not an accurate indicator of lactation potential. The lactation potential of women who deliver prematurely may be diminished and result in delayed secretory initiation.

Histologic Progression and Variance

The histologic appearance of the gland varies. The functional state appears to vary from dilated, thin-walled lumen to narrow-lumened, thick-walled glandular tissue. Epithelial cells vary, being flat to low columnar in shape with indistinct boundaries. Some cells protrude into the lumen of the alveoli; others are short and smooth. The lumen of the alveolus is crowded with fine granular material and lipid droplets similar to those protruding from the cells. The mammary alveoli but not the milk ducts lose the superficial layer of cells in the second trimester. The monolayer differentiates into a cell layer that accumulates eosinophilic cells, plasma cells, and leukocytes around the alveoli. Lymphocytes, round cells, and desquamated phagocytic alveolar cells are also found in the lumen.

The resting breast consists of ductal epithelial tissue with a fibrous stroma. The duct wall is lined with layers of epithelial cells. The inner layer encapsulates the ductal lumen, which is composed of cuboidal epithelial cells, some of which can actually further differentiate into milk secretory cells (lactocytes) during lactation. The outer layer, or basal layer, is made up of contractile myoepithelial cells that encircle the luminal layer and behave like smooth muscle cells (see Fig. 2.21). The basal layer lies on the basement membrane and is thought to contain MaSCs.

Role of Stem Cells

More recent studies have identified stem cells in the breast that are related to the breast's ability to expand and regress repeatedly throughout adult life. The presence of self-renewing bipotent MaSCs and unipotent progenitors have been identified in the resting epithelium. Most of the observations have been made in mice whose mammary stroma differ.[45,46]

Human mammary stroma is highly dense fibrous connective tissue that embeds in the adipose tissue. The intralobular stroma consists of mesenchymal cells. These cells are very responsive to the hormonal microenvironmental cues. They initiate and promote the various stages of mammary development as they interact with the mammary epithelium. The cellular hierarchy of the lactating breast is found in the milk itself. It includes early-stage stem cells and more differentiated myoepithelial and milk-secreting cells.[47,48]

Resulting Secretory System

By the end of pregnancy, lobular, highly branched epithelial tissue separated by some fibrous stroma is the predominant structure. Secretory differentiation has occurred in some luminal cells of the alveoli. Fat globules are visible within the cells, and alveoli are formed at the end of the duct termini, which contain the lactocytes. The lactocyte is a cuboidal polarized cell. Polarization promotes the movement of milk toward the lumen. The milk moves through the duct containing the biochemical factors secreted by lactocytes and some cells from the epithelium.

LACTATING MAMMARY GLAND

The lactating mammary gland is characterized by a large number of alveoli (Fig. 2.22). The alveoli of the lactating gland are made up of cuboidal epithelial and myoepithelial cells.[2] Only a small amount of connective tissue separates the neighboring alveoli. Under special preparations, lipid can be seen as small droplets within the cells. These droplets become larger and are discharged into the lumen.

Complex Mammary Gland Function

The functioning of the mammary gland depends on the interplay of multiple and complex nervous system and endocrine factors.[49] Some factors are involved in the development of the mammary glands to a functional state (mammogenesis),

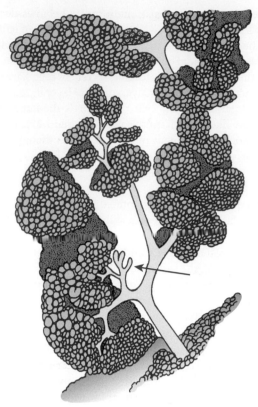

Fig. 2.22 Part of a mammary gland with significant milk obstruction in a 26-year-old woman who died from food poisoning after ingesting spoiled fish 3 weeks postpartum and who had not breastfed for 48 hours before death. In upper half, formed duct and lobes are located on alternating sides. This form results from different development of two parts of a dichotomized bifurcation: one takes over production of small lobes, and the other continues the stem. Thick section; very primitive, undeveloped sprouts *(arrow)*. (From Dabelow A: Die Milchdrüse. In: *Handbuch der Mikroskopischen Anatomie des Menschen.* Vol 3. Part 3. Berlin, Germany: Springer-Verlag; 1957.)

others in the establishment of milk secretion (lactogenesis), and others in the maintenance of lactation (galactopoiesis).[49]

Secretory Differentiation

The division and differentiation of mammary epithelial cells and presecretory alveolar cells into secretory milk-releasing alveolar cells take place in the third trimester. Stimulation of ribonucleic acid (RNA) synthesis promotes galactopoiesis and apocrine milk secretion into the alveoli. The deoxyribonucleic acid (DNA) and RNA content of the cellular nuclei increases during pregnancy and is highest at lactation (see Fig. 2.3).

Two Secretory Mechanisms

The former concepts of mammary gland secretion indicated that the mode of release was apocrine secretion. Apocrine secretion is the process by which the cell undergoes partial disintegration. A fat-filled portion projects into the lumen, the fat globule constricts at the base, and the cell replaces itself. Electron microscopy has shown that the cell has two distinct secretory products, formed and released by different mechanisms. The protein constituents of milk are formed and released identically to those of other protein-secreting glands, classified as merocrine glands. Secretory materials are passed out through the cell apex without appreciable loss of cytoplasm in merocrine glands.

The fatty components of milk arise as lipid droplets free in the cytoplasmic matrix. The droplets increase in size and move into the apex of the cell. They project into the lumen, covered by a thin layer of cytoplasm. The droplets are ultimately cast off, enveloped by a detached portion of the cell membrane and a thin rim of subjacent cytoplasm[50,51] (see Fig. 2.3 and Chapter 3 for further discussion).

Effect of Lactation on the Mammary Gland

The ultrastructure of the human mammary gland during lactogenesis was studied by Tobon and Salazar,[49] who reviewed surgical specimens from seven lactating women 1 day to 5{1/2} months postpartum. They noted widespread hypertrophy and hyperplasia of the acini accompanied by dilatation and engorgement of the lumen by milk. The vascular channels were engorged. The lactogenic epithelial cells had rich cytoplasm, prominent layers of reticulum, and enlarged oval mitochondria. The Golgi apparatus was hypertrophied. The myoepithelium was stretched and thinned to contain the filled acini.

The ratio of glandular tissue to fat tissue changes during lactation from a 1:1 ratio in the nonlactating breast to 2:1 during lactation.

Adipose Cells

Less well studied is the adipose cell, which has been recognized as important by Geddes.[34] Adipocytes have been observed to be transformed into lactocytes during pregnancy by Morroni et al.[52] using the mouse model. They then returned to adipocytes during the involuntary phase. Breast milk contains a cellular hierarchy from early-stage stem cells with embryonic-like features and multilineage differentiation potential to MaSCs from the resting breasts, cells with progenitor characteristics, to the mature myoepithelial and milk secreting cells[47,48] (see Fig. 2.3 and Chapter 3 for further discussion).

Alveolar Heterogeneity

Not all alveoli are at the same development stage; there are some nonfunctioning ducts at any given time during lactation. The signaling cascade that influences alveoli is development and differentiation patterns between different lobules. The role of vascularization may be significant in the functional heterogeneity of the lactating breast.

POSTLACTATION REGRESSION OF MAMMARY GLAND

Weaning Mechanism

If milk is not removed from the breast, the glands become greatly distended and milk production gradually ceases.[37] Part of the decrease results from the lack of stimulation of sucking, which initiates the neurohormonal reflex for maintenance of prolactin secretion.

Perhaps a stronger effect is the engorgement of the breast with compression of blood vessels, causing diminished flow. The diminished blood flow results in decreased oxytocin to the myoepithelium. The alveoli are greatly distended and the epithelium flattened. The secretion remaining in the alveolar spaces and ducts is absorbed. The alveoli gradually collapse, with an increase in perialveolar connective tissue, and shed cells accumulate in the lumen.[37]

The glandular elements gradually return to the at-rest state. Adipose tissue and macrophages increase. The gland does not return completely to the prepregnancy state in that the alveoli formed do not totally involute. Some appear as scattered, solid cords of epithelial cells.

Although the process of regression has been studied carefully in animals, little study has been done in humans. Slow weaning, which usually takes 3 months, probably has a very different timetable from abrupt weaning, in which marked involution has been intense and rapid over days or weeks. At the conclusion of weaning or involution the breast returns to a resting or nonlactating state. The structure and morphology is not the same as it was in the nulliparous stage. Some lobular structures remain in the parous gland.

Microscopic Weaning Process

Microscopically, increased autophagic and heterophagic processes occur in the first few days after weaning. Lysosomal enzymes increase, whereas nonlysosomal enzymes decrease. The gland undergoes alveolar epithelium apoptosis and remodeling, reverting back to the prepregnant state with the loss of prolactin.

The cell types that actually phagocytose the apoptotic epithelial cells are still unsettled (nonhuman research on the subject varies). Apoptotic cells may be phagocytosed by neighboring nonhematopoietic cells. The mechanisms through which involution is initiated and the gene networks involved remain under investigation.[37]

Some partially differentiated epithelial cells escape the involution and act as "memory precursor cells" in the next pregnancy.

SUMMARY

The mammary gland is the only organ that is not fully developed anatomically at birth. It undergoes dramatic ultrastructural, histologic, and anatomic changes from birth to pregnancy, lactation, and involution. The three major structures of the breast are skin, including the nipple, areola, and general skin; subcutaneous tissue; and the corpus mammae. The anatomy of the mammary gland is dynamic and experiences changes throughout the life cycle, and throughout the menstrual cycle. There is a tremendous amount more to be learned from the renewed interest in the anatomy of the breast relative to its primary role, lactation.

The Reference list is available at www.expertconsult.com.

3

Physiology of Lactation

Ruth A. Lawrence

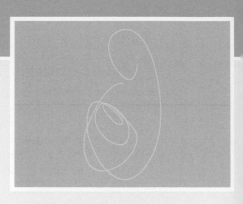

KEY POINTS

- Lactation represents the completion of the reproductive cycle and occurs as one of the major stages of mammary gland development: (1) embryogenesis; (2) mammogenesis; (3) lactogenesis, or secretory differentiation (stage 1 lactogenesis) and secretory activation (stage II lactogenesis); (4) lactation (or stage III lactogenesis), or full milk secretion; and (5) involution.
- Hormones play a central role in mammary gland development (estrogen and progesterone in particular) and in lactation (prolactin, insulin, hydrocortisone, human placental lactogen, human growth hormone, and oxytocin).
- Milk ejection is both a neural and endocrinologic process, whereby suckling stimulates sensory nerve endings in the areola and nipple, which activates the afferent neural reflex pathway via the spinal cord to the mesencephalon and then to the hypothalamus, secreting and releasing prolactin and oxytocin.
- Lactation changes the mother's metabolism greatly, redistributing the blood supply and increasing the demand for nutrients, which requires an increased metabolic rate to accommodate their production.
- Milk synthesis and secretion in the mammary alveolus include four major transcellular pathways and one paracellular pathway: (1) exocytosis of milk protein and lactose in Golgi-derived secretory vesicles, (2) milk-fat secretion via the milk-fat globule, (3) secretion of ions and water across the apical membrane, (4) pinocytosis—exocytosis of immunoglobulins, and (5) paracellular pathway for plasma components and leukocytes.

Lactation is the physiologic completion of the reproductive cycle.[1-3] Human infants at birth are the most immature and dependent of all mammals, except for marsupials. The marsupial joey is promptly attached to the teat of a mammary gland in an external pouch. The gland changes as the offspring develops, and the joey remains there until able to survive outside the pouch. In humans, throughout pregnancy, the breast develops and prepares to take over the role of fully nourishing the infant when the placenta is expelled.

There are two stages in the initiation of lactation: secretory differentiation and secretory activation. Pang and Hartmann[3] aptly describe them: "Secretory differentiation represents the stage of pregnancy when the mammary epithelial cells differentiate into lactocytes with the capacity to synthesize unique milk constituents such as lactose." They further explain that this requires the presence of a "lactogenic hormone complex." This complex of reproductive hormones includes estrogen, progesterone, prolactin, and some other metabolic hormones. Secretory activation, they note, is the initiation of copious milk secretion associated with major changes in the concentrations of many milk constituents. With the withdrawal of progesterone, secretory activation is triggered. This requires prolactin as well as insulin and cortisol. This terminology, introduced by Pang and Hartmann,[3] is being used more, but both this and the original terminology noted throughout the rest of this chapter are widely used within the related literature.

The breast is prepared for full lactation from 16 weeks' gestation without any active intervention from the mother. It is kept inactive by a balance of inhibiting hormones that suppress target-cell response. In the first few hours and days postpartum, the breast responds to changes in the hormonal milieu and to the stimulus of the newborn infant's suckling to produce and release milk.[4] The existence of mammary stem cells (MaSCs) has been speculated because the mammary gland has been regenerated by transplanting epithelial fragments in mice. Transplanted cells contributed to both luminal and myoepithelial lineages. From these, functional lobuloalveolar units during pregnancy were generated. The cells had self-renewing properties. The serial transplantations of Shackleton et al.[5] have established that single cells are multipotent and self-renewing and can generate a functional mammary gland. These cells create the potential for unlimited further understanding of the mammary gland.

Assessing the physiologic activity of the breast, accounting for both biochemical and calorimetric energy efficiencies, the human lactation process converts energy at an 80% to 85% efficiency rate.[6] Butte et al. measured and compared the energy expenditure during pregnancy and lactation. For exclusive breastfeeding, the energy cost of lactation was 2.62 MJ day^{-1} based on a mean milk production of 749 g day^{-1} and an estimated energetic efficiency of 0.80. The woman's daily energy expenditure during lactation is significantly greater than during pregnancy.

BOX 3.1 Hormone Abbreviations

Adrenocorticotropic hormone	ACTH
Epidermal growth factor	EGF
Feedback inhibitor of lactation	FIL
Follicle-stimulating hormone	FSH
Growth hormone (human growth hormone)	GH (hGH)
Heregulin	HER
Human growth factor	hGF, HGF
Human placental lactogen	hPL
Insulin-like growth factor-1	IGF-1
Prolactin	PRL
Prolactin-inhibiting factor	PIF
Thyroid-stimulating hormone	TSH
Thyrotropin-releasing hormone	TRH
Transforming growth factor beta	TGF-β

This chapter provides a review of the physiologic adaptation of the mammary gland to its role in infant survival. Several major reviews that include substantial bibliographies for readers who need the detailed reports of the original investigators are referenced. Newer scientific techniques in the study of human lactation provide more precise, more detailed, and more integrated data on which the clinician can base a physiologic approach to lactation management.

Box 3.1 lists the abbreviations for the hormones that are involved in lactation and are discussed in this chapter.[7–13]

STAGES OF MAMMARY GLAND DEVELOPMENT

The mammary gland is a unique organ in human physiology, given that it is the only organ not fully developed at birth. Rather, breast development occurs through a series of steps, beginning in the embryonic phase and ending in menopause.

APOPTOSIS IN THE MAMMARY GLAND

Epithelial apoptosis has a key role in the development and function of the mammary gland. It begins with the formation of the ducts in the embryonic phase and occurs again at puberty and within the cyclical stages of menses. Regulated apoptosis occurs at several stages of mammary development. In the embryo, epithelial buds emerge from ectoderm into mammary mesenchyme, which is the origin of the ductal tree. When the ducts later hollow out in puberty, extensive apoptosis occurs within the terminal bud.[14]

Deregulated apoptosis contributes to the malignant progression in the genesis of breast cancer. Research in apoptosis continues because it may lead to new cancer treatments, but the knowledge itself related to breast development and function will be valuable.

When suckling ceases during weaning, the alveolar component of the gland involutes by both apoptosis and tissue remodeling, which rebuilds the gland to the prepregnancy state.

Much is being learned about mammary development and function through the intense study of the breast as an experimental system. The use of novel "knockout" mouse models has been employed to study nursing failure. The apoptosis control mechanism from the perspective of the signaling pathways has also been studied. Further work at the level of the cell is under way, including extensive genetic analysis.[14]

HORMONAL CONTROL OF LACTATION

In contrast to most organs, which are fully developed at birth, the mammary gland undergoes most of its morphogenesis postnatally, in adolescence, and in adulthood.[15] Lactation is an integral part of the reproductive cycle of all mammals, including humans. The hormonal control of lactation can be described in relation to the five major stages in the development of the mammary gland: (1) embryogenesis; (2) mammogenesis, or mammary growth; (3) lactogenesis, or initiation of milk secretion; (4) lactation (stage III lactogenesis), or full milk secretion; and (5) involution (Table 3.1).[15]

Current terminology divides lactogenesis into two stages.[3] Stage I, or *secretory differentiation*, takes place during pregnancy when the gland is sufficiently developed to actually produce milk. It begins about midpregnancy (approximately 16 weeks). It can be identified by measuring the levels of plasma lactose and α-lactalbumin.[16] Should the mother deliver at this point, milk would be produced. Some mothers can express colostrum during this time. As the pregnancy proceeds, milk production is inhibited by high levels of circulating progesterone in most mammals and estrogen as well in humans.

Stage II of lactogenesis is the onset of copious milk production at delivery. In all mammals, it is associated with the drop in progesterone levels (Fig. 3.1). This drop occurs to herald delivery in some species so that milk is copious when the young are born. In humans, these levels drop during the first 4 days postpartum, which is reflected by the milk "coming in" during this time. The drop in progesterone is accompanied by the transformation of the mammary epithelium to produce increased volumes of milk, referred to by Pang and Hartmann[3] as *secretion activation*. This change includes a change in the permeability of the paracellular pathway and changes in secretion of protective factors (i.e., lactoferrin, immunoglobulins), as well as increases in all milk components that parallel increased glucose production.

During the next 10 days, the composition of the milk slowly changes to mature milk. The composition then changes slowly over the months of full exclusive breastfeeding.

EMBRYOGENESIS

Embryogenesis begins with the mammary band, which develops around the 35th embryonic day and progresses to a bud at the 49th day (see Chapter 2). The ducts continue to elongate

TABLE 3.1 Stages of Mammary Development[a]

Developmental Stage	Hormonal Regulation	Local Factors	Description
Embryogenesis	?	Fat pad necessary for ductal extension	Epithelial bud develops in 18- to 19-week-old fetus, extending short distance into mammary fat pad with blind ducts that become canalized; some milk secretion may be present at birth
Mammogenesis • Puberty • Before onset of menses • After onset of menses • Pregnancy	• Estrogen, GH • Estrogen, progesterone • ?, PRL • Progesterone, PRL, hPL	• IGF-1, hGF, TGF-β, ?, others • HER, ?, others	• Ductal extension into mammary pad; branching morphogenesis • Lobular development with formation of terminal duct lobular unit (TDLU) • Anatomic development • Alveolus formation; partial cellular differentiation
Lactogenesis	Progesterone withdrawal, PRL, glucocorticoid	Not known	Onset of milk secretion Stage I: midpregnancy Stage II: parturition
Lactation	PRL, oxytocin	FIL	Ongoing milk secretion
Involution	PRL withdrawal	Milk stasis, ?, FIL	Alveolar epithelium undergoes apoptosis and remodeling; gland reverts to prepregnant state

[a]See Box 3.1 for abbreviations.
FIL, Feedback inhibitor of lactation; *GH,* growth hormone; *HER,* heregulin; *hGF,* human growth factor; *hPL,* human placental lactogen; *IGF-1,* insulin-like growth factor-1; *PRL,* prolactin; *TGF-β,* transforming growth factor-β.
Modified from Neville MC. Breastfeeding, part I: the evidence for breastfeeding. Anatomy and physiology of lactation. *Pediatr Clin North Am.* 20014;8:13, Table 2–3; Macias H, Hinck L. Mammary gland development. *WIREs Dev Biol.* 2012;1:533. http://doi.org/10.1002/wdev.35.

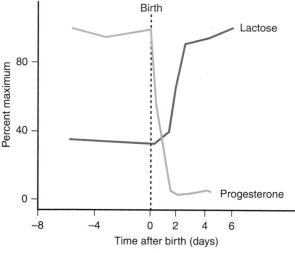

Fig. 3.1 Progesterone withdrawal initiates lactogenesis II in women. The increase in lactose concentrations associated with the increased synthesis of milk components coincides with a rapid decrease in the progesterone concentration when the placenta is removed at parturition. (From Czan KC, Henderson JJ, Kent JC, et al. Hormonal control of the lactation cycle. In: Hale TW, Hartmann PE, eds. *Textbook of Human Lactation.* Amarillo, TX: Hale Publishing LP; 2007.)

to form a mammary sprout, which invades the fat pad, branches, and canalizes, forming the rudimentary mammary ductal system present at birth. After birth, the growth of this set of small branching ducts parallels the child's linear growth but remains limited, probably controlled by growth hormone (GH) before the onset of ovarian activity.

Under the influence of sex steroids, especially the estrogens, the mammary glandular epithelium proliferates, becoming multilayered. Buds and papillae then form. The growth of the mammary gland is a gradual process that starts during puberty. The process depends on pituitary hormones. Lobuloalveolar development and ductal proliferation also depend on an intact pituitary gland.

Six Factors of Mammary Organization

Box 3.2[15–20] presents six well-documented factors that help explain the organization of mammary growth. Much of this work has resulted since the availability of "knockout" studies in mice and associated techniques.

The coordination of epithelial and stromal activity in the mammary gland is complex. Hepatocyte growth and scatter factor has been associated with the process during puberty.[20] Another growth factor, heregulin, a member of the epidermal growth factor (EGF) family, has been identified in the stroma of mammary ducts during pregnancy.

Neville[15] has diagrammed the regulation of mammary development (Fig. 3.2). She notes that the concentrations of estrogen, progesterone, and lactogenic hormone in the form of prolactin or placental lactogen (PL) greatly increase, enhance alveolar development, and result in the differentiation of alveolar cells. Although many investigators have contributed pieces to the puzzle of mammogenesis, Neville succeeded in creating the current visualization.[15]

BOX 3.2 Important Factors in the Organization of Mammary Growth

1. **Mammary ducts must grow into an adipose tissue** pad if morphogenesis is to continue. Only adipose stroma supports ductal elongation. The mammary epithelium is closely associated with the adipocyte-containing stroma in all phases of development. In midgestation during human fetal development, a fat pad is laid down as a separate condensation of mesenchyma. Rudimentary ducts expand into the fat pad but do not progress.[15] At puberty, the ducts elongate to fill the entire fat pad, terminating growth as they reach the margins of the fat pad.

2. **Estrogen is essential to mammary growth.**[3] Ductal growth does not occur in the absence of ovaries but can be stimulated when estrogen is provided. In the ovariectomized (oophorectomized) mouse, an estrogen pellet placed in the mammary tissue stimulates growth in that gland but not in the opposite gland. When the estrogen receptor is "knocked out" in the mouse, no mammary development occurs. The increase in estrogen at puberty results in mammary development. Although estrogen is essential, it is not adequate alone.[3]

3. The exact location of the estrogen receptors in human breasts is unclear. Estrogen receptors are not in the proliferating cells and have not been located in the stroma. **Cells with estrogen receptors secrete a paracrine factor** that is responsible for the proliferation of ductal cells. This paracrine factor may hold the key to understanding both normal and abnormal breast development.

4. In addition to estrogen, the **pituitary gland is necessary for breast development**. Kleinberg[17] has identified growth hormone (GH) as important to pubertal development and the development of the terminal end buds in the breast. Prolactin could not replace GH in these experiments, but insulin-like growth factor-1 (IGF-1) could. It is produced in the stromal compartment of the mammary gland under stimulation by GH, and together with estradiol from the ovaries, IGF-1 brings about ductal development at puberty.

5. **Transforming growth factor beta (TGF-β)** maintains the spacing of the mammary ducts as they branch and elongate.[15] These ducts exhibit unique behavior during growth, turning away to avoid other ducts and end buds. This avoidance behavior accounts for the orderly development of the duct system in the breast and the absence of ductal entanglements. This pattern provides ample space between ducts for later development of alveoli. TGF-β has been identified as the negative regulator and is found in many tissues, including breast tissue produced by an epithelial element. The pattern formation in ductal development depends on the localized expression of TGF-β.[18]

6. **Progesterone** secretion brings about the side branching of the mammary ducts.[19] The presence of progesterone receptors in the epithelial cells has been confirmed by studies in knockout mice in which mammary glands develop to the ductal stage but not to alveolar morphogenesis. Ormandy et al.[20] established that prolactin is necessary for full alveolar development through prolactin receptor studies in knockout mice in which mammary glands do not develop beyond the ductal stage. This was further confirmed in murine mammary cultures in which full development of the alveoli depends on prolactin. Further, when prolactin is withdrawn, apoptosis of the alveolar cells occurs.[19]

Modified from Neville MC. The physiological basis of milk secretion. Part I. Basic physiology. *Ann N Y Acad Sci.* 1990;586:1; Pang WW, Hartmann PE. Initiation of human lactation: secretory differentiation and secretory activation. *J Mammary Gland Biol Neoplasia.* 2007;12:211-221; Kleinberg DL. Early mammary development: growth hormone and IGF-1. *Mammary Gland Biol Neoplasia.* 1997;2:49; Daniel CW, Robinson S, Silberstein GB. The role of TGF-α in patterning and growth of the mammary ductal tree. *J Mammary Gland Biol Neoplasia.* 1996;1:331; Napso T, Hannah EJ, Yong J, et al. The role of placental hormones in mediating maternal adaptations to support pregnancy and lactation. *Front Physiol.* 2018;9:1; Ormandy CJ, Binart B, Kelly PA. Mammary gland development in prolactin receptor knockout mice. *J Mammary Gland Biol Neoplasia.* 1997;2:355; Fowler PA, Casey CE, Cameron GG, et al. Cyclic changes in composition and volume of the breast during the menstrual cycle, measured by magnetic resonance imaging. *Br J Obstet Gynaecol.* 1990;97:595.

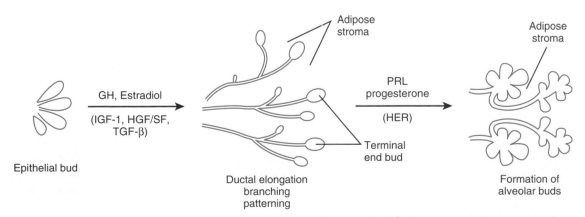

Fig. 3.2 Scheme for regulation of mammary development in the mouse. (From Neville MC. Mammary gland biology and lactation: a short course. Presented at the annual meeting of the International Society for Research on Human Milk and Lactation, Plymouth, MA; 1997.)

MAMMOGENESIS: MAMMARY GROWTH

Prepubertal Growth

Mammogenesis occurs in two phases as the gland responds to the hormones of puberty and later of pregnancy.[3] During the prepubertal phase, the primary and secondary ducts that develop in the fetus in utero continue to grow in both boys and girls in proportion to growth in general. Shortly before puberty, a more rapid expansion of the duct system begins in girls. The growth of the duct system seems to depend predominantly on estrogen and does not occur in the absence of ovaries. The complete growth of the alveoli requires stimulation by progesterone as well.

Studies of hypophysectomized animals have shown the failure of full mammary growth even with adequate estrogen and progesterone. The secretion of prolactin and somatotropin by the pituitary gland results in mammary growth. Adrenocorticotropic hormone (ACTH) and thyroid-stimulating hormone (TSH) acting on the adrenal and thyroid glands also play a minor role in the growth of the mammary gland.

Growth and development during organogenesis involve the interaction of cells with extracellular matrices and neighboring cells.[21] Necropsy breast specimens from six male and eight female infants ranging in age from 1 day to 9 months were studied to determine the process of organogenesis in humans.[22] Integrins were expressed in a pattern that correlates with morphologic and functional differentiation of the normal mammary gland. Integrins are transmembrane glycoproteins that form receptors for extracellular matrix proteins, such as fibronectin, laminin, and collagen. Integrins are widely expressed in normal tissue and are considered critical to the control of cell growth and differentiation. This suggests integrin's involvement in the functional characterization of the adhesion molecules in the breast.

Pubertal Growth

When the hypophyseal–ovarian–uterine cycle is established, a new phase of mammary growth, which includes extensive branching of the system of ducts and proliferation and canalization of the lobuloalveolar units at the distal tips of the branches, begins.[21] The organization of the stromal connective tissue forms the interlobular septa. The ducts, ductules (terminal intralobular ducts), and alveolar structures are formed by double layers of cells. One layer, the epithelial cells, circumscribes the lumen. The second layer, the myoepithelial cells, surrounds the inner epithelial cells and is bordered by a basement lamina.

Menstrual Cycle Growth

The cyclic changes of the adult mammary gland can be associated with the menstrual cycle and the hormonal changes that control that cycle. Estrogens stimulate parenchymal proliferation, with the formation of epithelial sprouts. This hyperplasia continues into the secretory phase of the cycle. Anatomically, when the corpus luteum provides increased amounts of estrogens and progesterone, there is lobular edema, thickening of the epithelial basal membrane, and secretory material in the alveolar lumen.[21] Lymphoid and plasma cells infiltrate the stroma. Clinically, mammary blood flow increases in this luteal phase. This increased flow is experienced by women as fullness, heaviness, and turgescence. The breast may become nodular because of interlobular edema and ductular-acinar growth.

After the onset of menstruation and the reduction of sex steroid levels, milk-secretory prolactin action is limited. Postmenstrual changes occur rapidly, with degeneration of glandular cells and proliferation tissue, loss of edema, and a decrease in breast size. The ovulatory cycle actually enhances mammary growth in the early years of menstruation (until

about age 30 to 35 years) because the postmenstrual regression of the glandular-alveolar growth after each cycle is not complete.[21] These changes of ductal and lobular proliferation, which occur during the follicular phase before ovulation, continue in the luteal phase and regress after the menstrual phase, exemplifying the sensitivity of this target organ to variations in the balance of hormones.

Fowler et al.[23] measured cyclic changes in the composition and volume of the breast during the menstrual cycle using nuclear magnetic resonance T1-weighted imaging. The T1 relaxation time (spin-lattice T1 relaxation) is a measure of the rate of energy loss from tissues after T1 excitation. This energy loss depends on the biophysical environment of the excited protons. A short T1, therefore, indicates the presence of lipids and organic structures that bind water tightly. A longer T1 occurs with greater hydration and with the greatest amount of cellular water. This study revealed that the lowest total breast volume and parenchymal volume of T1 and water content occurred between days 6 and 15 of the cycle. Between days 16 and 28, T1 rose sharply, and it peaked on the 25th day. The rise in parenchymal volume in the second half of the cycle resulted from not only increased tissue water but also from growth and increased tissue fluid, according to Fowler et al.[23]

Growth During Pregnancy

Hormonal influences on the breast cause profound changes during pregnancy (Figs. 3.3 and 3.4). Early in pregnancy, a marked increase in ductular sprouting, branching, and lobular formation is evoked by luteal and placental hormones.[21] PL, prolactin, and chorionic gonadotropin have been identified as contributors to the accelerated growth (see Fig. 3.4). The dichorionic ductular sprouting has been attributed to estrogen, and lobular formation to progesterone.

Prolactin is essential for complete lobular-alveolar development of the gland. Growth of the mammary lobular-alveolar system requires the "lactogenic hormone complex" of estrogen, progesterone, prolactin, and certain metabolic hormones.[24] Prolactin, as with other protein hormones, exerts its effect through receptors for the initiation of milk secretion located on the alveolar cell surfaces. The induction of milk synthesis requires insulin-induced cell division and the presence of cortisol.

From the third month of gestation, secretory material that resembles colostrum appears in the acini. Prolactin from the anterior pituitary gland stimulates the glandular production of colostrum. By the second trimester, PL begins to stimulate the secretion of colostrum. A mother who delivers after 16 weeks' gestation will secrete colostrum, even though she has had a nonviable infant. This demonstrates the effectiveness of hormonal stimulation on lactation.

An estrogen-mediated increase in prolactin secretion in pregnancy may produce as much as a 10- to 20-fold increase in plasma prolactin. This effect may be partially controlled by lactogen from the placenta, which inhibits the production of prolactin.[3] Hormonal regulation of the growth and proliferation of the mammary gland cells has been carefully studied in many species.

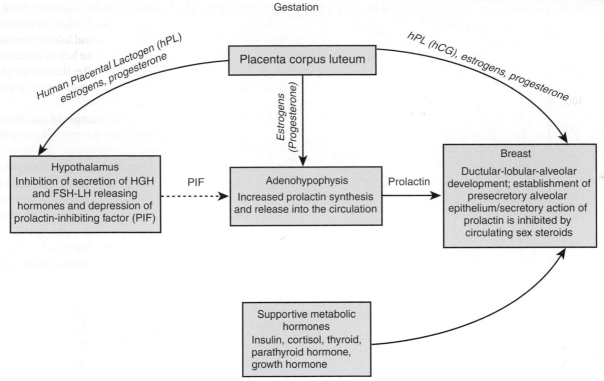

Fig. 3.3 Hormonal preparation of breast during pregnancy for lactation. (Modified from Vorherr H. *The Breast: Morphology, Physiology and Lactation.* New York: Academic Press; 1974.)

Studies of mice in which receptors for each of the hormones have been ablated demonstrate that progesterone and prolactin (or possibly placenta lactogen) are key to alveolar development in pregnancy. The major inhibitor of milk production during pregnancy has been shown to be progesterone, whereas estrogen also contributes to secretion inhibition.[21]

Hormonal Preparation of Breast for Lactation

A complex sequence of events, governed by hormonal action, prepares the breast for lactation (see Fig. 3.3). During pregnancy, 17β-estradiol stimulates the ductal system of epithelial cells to elongate. In contrast to puberty, however, when estrogens appear to directly and indirectly stimulate breast development, estrogens have no indispensable role in mammary development during pregnancy except as a prolactin potentiator: according to Neville,[12] when estrogen levels are low in pregnancy, the breast still develops. Estrogen levels are normally high in pregnancy, but not for mammogenesis. Induced lactation in the cow is dependably reproduced with 7 days of estrogen and progesterone treatment. Progesterone, in turn, induces the specific epithelial cells of the tubular invaginations to produce distinct ducts, which branch from the main tubules.[3,21]

The end result of the combined actions of estrogen and progesterone is a richly branched arborization of the gland. Highly differentiated secretory alveolar cells develop at the ends of these ducts under the influence of prolactin (Fig. 3.5).

Serum growth factor, which is present in normal human serum, and insulin can stimulate the stem cells of the gland to proliferate. These dividing cells are further directed to the

formation of alveoli by corticosteroid hormones. At least two types of cells are identified in the epithelial layer of the gland: stem cells and secretory alveolar cells. At this point in the pregnancy, prolactin influences the production of the constituents of milk.

Transforming growth factor-β (TGF-β) influences pattern formation in the developing mammary gland and may negatively regulate ductal growth as well.[18] The pattern of mammary ductal development varies widely among species and is a function of both genotype and hormonal status. Normal human breast cells secrete TGF-β and are themselves inhibited by it, suggesting an autoregulatory feedback circuit that may be modulated by estradiol. Growth and patterning of the ductal tree are regulated in part by TGF-β operating through an autocrine feedback mechanism and by paracrine circuits associated with epithelial-stromal interactions.[24]

Interplay of Prolactin and Progesterone

The high circulating levels of prolactin in pregnancy are not associated with milk production partly because of the progesterone antagonism of the stimulatory action of prolactin on casein messenger ribonucleic acid (mRNA) synthesis. During late pregnancy, the lactogenic receptors, which have similar affinities for both prolactin and human placental lactogen (hPL), are predominantly occupied by hPL. High doses of estradiol impair the incorporation of prolactin into milk secretory cells.

Prolactin is prevented from exerting its effect on milk excretion by the elevated levels of progesterone. After the drop in progesterone and estrogen at delivery, copious milk

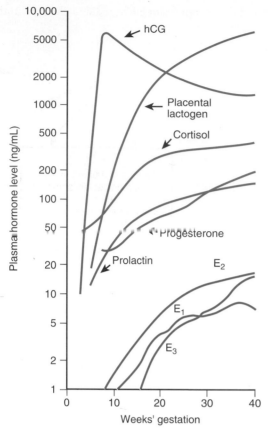

Fig. 3.4 Plasma hormone levels during pregnancy. *E1,* Estrone; *E2,* estradiol; *E3,* estriol; *hCG,* human chorionic gonadotropin. (From Neville MC, Morton J, Umemura S. The evidence for breastfeeding. *Pediatr Clin North Am.* 2001;48:42.)

secretion begins. The key hormone requirements for lactation to begin are prolactin, insulin, and hydrocortisone. A high level of plasma prolactin is essential to lactogenesis in humans as well. There is a question as to whether it is a surge in prolactin that is necessary for lactogenesis at parturition. Prolactin levels are now described as biphasic in humans for the initiation of lactogenesis at birth.[25] Prolactin stabilizes and promotes transcription of casein mRNA and stimulates the synthesis of a lactalbumin that is the regulatory protein of the lactose—synthetase enzyme system.[26] Prolactin further increases the lipoprotein lipase activity in the mammary gland. Prolactin exists in three heterogenic forms of varying biologic activity. The monomer is in the greatest quantity and is the most active form.

LACTOGENESIS—INITIATION OF MILK SECRETION

Stages of Lactogenesis

Stage I

Stage I lactogenesis starts approximately 12 weeks before parturition and is heralded by significant increases in lactose, total proteins, and immunoglobulin; decreases in sodium and chloride; and the gathering of substrate for milk production. The composition of prepartum secretion is fairly constant until delivery, as monitored by the milk protein α-lactalbumin.

Lactogenesis is initiated in the postpartum period by a fall in plasma progesterone, but prolactin levels remain high (Fig. 3.6). The initiation of the process does not depend on

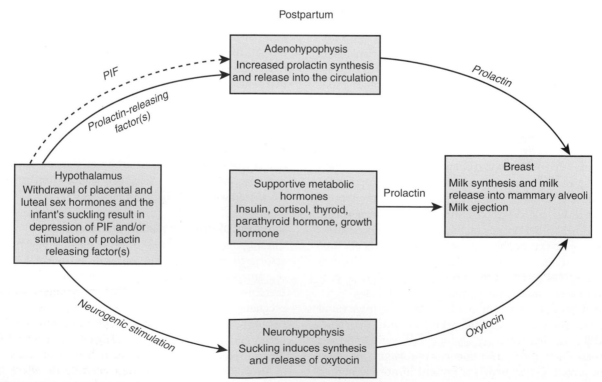

Fig. 3.5 Hormonal preparation of breast for lactation postpartum. *PIF,* Prolactin-inhibiting factor. (Modified from Vorherr H. *The Breast: Morphology, Physiology and Lactation.* New York: Academic Press; 1974.)

suckling by the infant until the third or fourth day, when the secretion declines if milk is not removed from the breast.[27]

Stage II

Stage II lactogenesis includes an increase in blood flow and oxygen and glucose uptake as well as a sharp increase in the citrate concentration, considered a reliable marker for lactogenesis stage II. Stage II at 2 to 3 days postpartum begins clinically when the secretion of milk is copious and biochemically when plasma α-lactalbumin levels peak (paralleling the period when "the milk comes in"). The major changes in milk composition continue for 10 days, when "mature milk" is established. The establishment of the mature milk supply, once called *galactopoiesis*, is now referred to as *stage III* of lactogenesis.

The profound changes in milk composition have been established for the period of transition to mature milk in relation to an increase in milk volume. Detailed studies of successfully lactating women were performed by Neville et al.,[28]

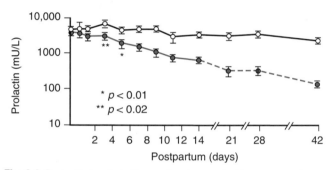

Fig. 3.6 Prolactin levels in the postpartum period in women who are lactating *(open circles)* and nonlactating *(dots)*. Levels in lactating women vary with the intensity of suckling. (From Neville MC, Morton J, Umemora S. The evidence for breastfeeding. *Pediatr Clin North Am.* 2001;48:44.)

who report that a significant fall in sodium, chloride, and protein and a rise in lactose precede the major increase in milk volume during early lactogenesis. At 46 to 96 hours postpartum, copious milk production is accompanied by an increase in citrate, glucose, free phosphate, and calcium concentrations and a decrease in pH.

The breast, one of the most complex endocrine target organs, has been prepared during pregnancy and responds to the release of prolactin by producing the constituents of milk (see Fig. 3.5). The lactogenic effects of prolactin are modulated by the complex interplay of pituitary, ovarian, thyroid, adrenal, and pancreatic hormones (Fig. 3.7).

The Science of Suckling

The ability to lactate is characteristic of all mammals, from the most primitive to the most advanced, and the instinct to feed through suckling occurs spontaneously in infants postpartum. Normal, alert newborns have been observed to "crawl" to the nipple and latch on unassisted when placed on the maternal abdomen following a normal delivery and the clamping and severing of the umbilical cord.[29] The divergence of suckling patterns, however, makes it urgent that human patterns be studied specifically. Some aquatic mammals, such as whales, nurse under water; others, such as the seal and sea lion, nurse on land. Various erect or recumbent postures are assumed by different terrestrial mammals.[30] Nursing may be continuous, as in the joey attached to a marsupial teat, or at widely different intervals characteristic of the species and parallel to the nutrient concentrations of the milk. The intervals may be a half hour for dolphins, an hour for pigs, a day for rabbits, 2 days for tree shrews, or a week for northern fur seals.

New anatomy research, gathered for the first time in 160 years since the brilliant work with dissections by Sir Ashley Cooper, has been generated in the laboratory of Peter

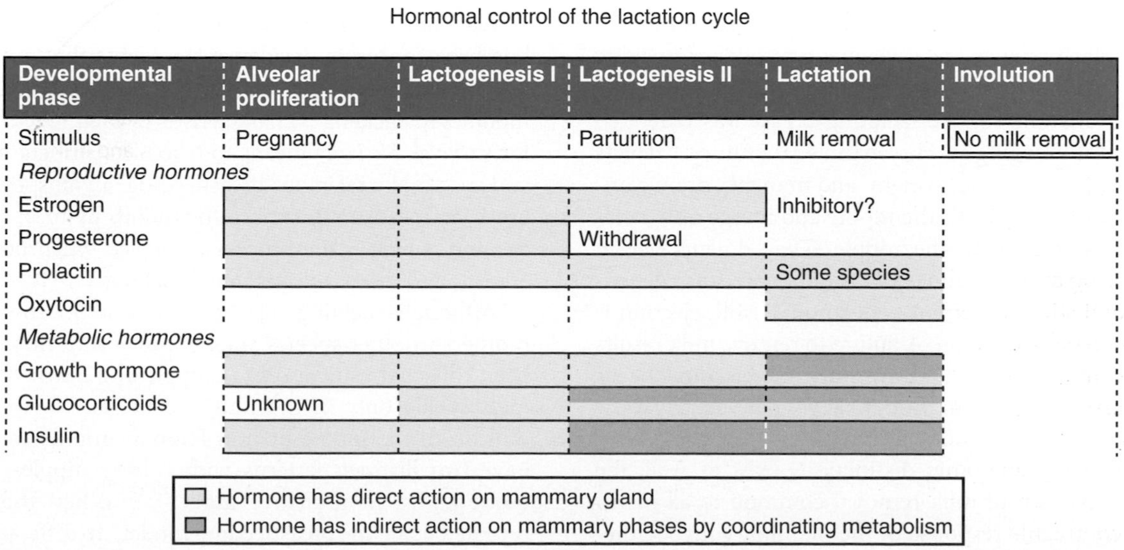

Hormonal control of the lactation cycle

Developmental phase	Alveolar proliferation	Lactogenesis I	Lactogenesis II	Lactation	Involution
Stimulus	Pregnancy		Parturition	Milk removal	No milk removal
Reproductive hormones					
Estrogen				Inhibitory?	
Progesterone			Withdrawal		
Prolactin				Some species	
Oxytocin					
Metabolic hormones					
Growth hormone					
Glucocorticoids	Unknown				
Insulin					

☐ Hormone has direct action on mammary gland
▦ Hormone has indirect action on mammary phases by coordinating metabolism

Fig. 3.7 Hormonal action necessary for phases of the lactation cycle. (From Czank C, Henderson JJ, Kent JC, et al. Hormonal control of lactation cycle. In: Hale TW, Hartmann PE, eds. *Textbook of Human Lactation.* Amarillo, TX: Hale Publishing LP; 2007:91.)

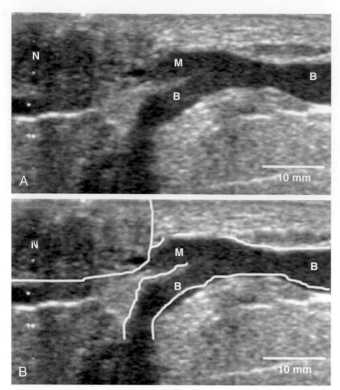

Fig. 3.8 (A and B) Ultrasound image of a main milk duct (Toshiba, Aplio). The nipple is the round hypoechoic *(dark)* structure in the left of the image *(N)*. The main duct *(M)* branches into two ducts *(B)* approximately 5 mm from the nipple. Note the small diameter of the ducts (approximately 3 mm). (From Geddes DT. Inside the lactating breast: the latest anatomy research. *J Midwifery Womens Health.* 2007;52[6], Fig. 3.)

Hartmann in Australia and his eclectic team of scientists. They have had access to the latest digital technology and have shown that the milk ducts of the breast are small (Fig. 3.8), compressible, superficial, and closely intertwined.[31] There are no "dilated sinuses" that store large amounts of milk. The amount of adipose tissue in the breast is very variable and not a measure of the amount of glandular tissue; there is twice as much glandular tissue as fat.[32] Magnetic resonance imaging has identified some central ducts in the breasts of lactating women. The anatomy of the lactating breast was redefined with ultrasound imaging in Hartmann's laboratory.[33] Ducts were found to number four to eight, and branches drain glandular tissue directly beneath the nipple and merge into a collecting duct very close to the nipple. They do increase in diameter during milk ejection. Milk production is not dependent on neural stimulation but is hormonal. Milk ejection is critical to successful lactation. A failure to remove milk results in decreased milk production. Multiple milk ejections occur during breastfeeding, even though a woman usually only senses the first milk ejection.

Although many anatomic distinctions exist as well, the principal mechanism of milk removal common to all mammals is the contractile response of the mammary myoepithelium under the hormonal influence of oxytocin released from the neurohypophysis.[34]

The key function in all species is effective control of milk delivery to the young in the right amount and at the appropriate intervals, which requires a production system, exit channels, a prehensile appendage, an expulsion mechanism, and a retention mechanism. The primary, secondary, and tertiary ducts form an uninterrupted channel for the passage of milk from the milk-producing alveoli to the prehensile appendage. A process of erection of the areolar region facilitates prehension by the young during suckling. The principal object of the suction produced by the facial musculature of the young is to draw the nipple into the mouth and retain it there. Positive pressure is used to expel milk from the gland by the contractile changes in the mammary gland provided by the myoepithelial cells. The sympathetic nervous stimuli can oppose milk ejection by increasing vasoconstrictor tone, thereby reducing the access of circulating oxytocin to the mammary myoepithelium. Sympathetic activity also can occur during conditions of apprehension or muscular exertion. The milk-ejection reflex can be blocked by emotional disturbance or reflex excitation of the neurohypophysis. The central nervous system control of milk ejection indeed suggests that restraining mechanisms exist to ensure that milk ejection can only occur under circumstances wholly conducive to the effective removal of milk by the suckling young.

In all species that have been studied, a rise in intramammary pressure and flow of milk occurs as a reflex event in suckling. The excitation of the neurohypophysis results in the release of oxytocin, which is conveyed via the bloodstream to mammary capillaries, where it evokes contraction of the myoepithelium. The successive ejection-pressure peaks, demonstrated in lactating women, can be duplicated more accurately by a series of separate oxytocin injections than by the same total dose as a single injection or by a continuous infusion of the hormone. This strongly suggests that oxytocin is released from the neurohypophysis in spurts. The study of suckling patterns in all species shows a high degree of ritualization, which in turn suggests a close neural connection between cognitive or behavioral and hormonal responses.

Attention has focused on the mechanisms that control suckling behavior, on its incidence, on events that precipitate and terminate it, on the effects of stress, and on how development modifies it. Suckling is characteristic of each species and is vital for survival. *Suckling* means to take nourishment at the breast and specifically refers to "breastfeeding" in all species. *Sucking*, however, means to draw into the mouth by means of a partial vacuum, which is the process employed when bottle-feeding. *Sucking* also means to consume by licking.

Although suckling has been studied in the young and mothers in other species, a large portion of human data has been collected using a rubber nipple and bottle. Other mammals suckle only in the nutritive mode, whether receiving milk from the nipple or not. Human infants were noted to have two distinct patterns with rubber nipples: a nutritive mode and a nonnutritive mode.[33,35] When this work was repeated using the breastfeeding model, no difference between nutritive and nonnutritive suckling rates was seen but, rather, a continuous variation of the suckling rate in response to the milk-flow rate.[36] Suckling rates in other species correlate with milk composition and species-specific feeding schedules (one suck per second in great apes and four to five sucks per second in sheep and goats).

In further experiments, an inverse linear relationship was found between milk flow and the suckling rate. Thus, the higher the milk flow, the lower the suckling rate. In human infants younger than 12 weeks of age, suckling will terminate with sleep and be reinstated on awakening, a pattern that is well described in other species. In infants older than 12 weeks, suckling is not always terminated by sleep. At 12 to 24 weeks, infants will play with the nipple, explore the mother, and not always elicit nipple attachment. Continuous measurement of milk intake during a given feeding from one breast showed a progressive reduction in intake volume per suck and an increase in the proportion of time spent pausing between bursts of sucking.

Using the miniature Doppler[37] ultrasound flow transducer, Woolridge and Baum[38] studied 32 normal mother—baby pairs from 5 to 9 days postpartum. Intakes during trials averaged 34.2 g ($\pm$ 3.7 g) on the first breast and 26.2 g ($\pm$ 3.5 g) on the second breast. At the start of feeds, the average suck volume was approximately 0.14 mL/suck, which decreased to approximately 0.10 mL/suck or less. The mean latency for the release of milk was 2.2 minutes after the infant began to suckle. The researchers also noted that on the first breast, the flow increased and stabilized after 2 minutes, with concomitant slowing and stabilizing of the sucking pattern during the remainder of the feed. On the second breast, the suck volume fell off dramatically toward the end of the feed (50% reduction from peak to end of feed; Fig. 3.9).

These observations support the theory that infants become satiated at the breast, and milk remains unconsumed in the breast. During the first month of life, infants consume a given amount of fluid with decreasing investment of time.[37] The amount of fluid per suck increases over time. The control of intake appears to come under intrinsic control of the infant during the first month of life.[39]

A cineradiographic study of breastfeeding was done by Ardran et al.[40] in 1957 and compared with a similar study of bottle-feeding.[41] The nipples and areolae of 41 breastfeeding mothers were coated with a paste of barium sulfate in lanolin, and cineradiographic films were taken with the infant at the breast. These were then reviewed meticulously. Box 3.3 lists the authors' conclusions in their original description. These observations are of historical interest, but newer techniques in imagery have more accurately described the understanding of human suckling.

The development of real-time ultrasound improved the definition of images. Several studies have been published using this noninvasive technique to observe the action of the infant's tongue and buccal mucosa and the maternal nipple areola. Using a video recorder in the 1980s that allowed frame-by-frame analysis and recorded simultaneous respiration, the pattern of suck, swallow, and breathing was documented during a period of active suckling at the breast. A suck was defined by Weber et al.[42] as the beginning of one indentation of the nipple by the tongue to the beginning of the next. Weber et al. had examined six breastfed and six bottle-fed infants between 1 and 6 days of life. Not all sucks were associated with a swallow. Box 3.4 summarizes the process.

Observations of suckling using improved techniques from 2 to 26 weeks showed that suckling starts with a series of fast

---

BOX 3.3 Radiographic Interpretation of Suckling at Breasts

1. The nipple is sucked to the back of the baby's mouth, and a teat is formed from the nipple and the adjacent areola and underlying tissues.
2. When the jaw is raised, this teat is compressed between the upper gum and the tip of the tongue resting on the lower gum. The tongue is applied to the lower surface of the teat from the front backward, pressing it against the hard palate; the teat is reduced to approximately half its former width. As the tongue moves toward the posterior edge of the hard palate, the teat shortens and becomes thicker.
3. When the jaw is lowered, the teat is again sucked to the back of the mouth and restored to its previous size.
4. Each cycle of jaw and tongue movement takes place in approximately 1.5 seconds. The pharyngeal cavity becomes airless, and the larynx closes every time the upward movement of the tongue against the teat and hard palate is completed.

BOX 3.4 Ultrasound Interpretation of Suckling at Breasts

1. The lateral margins of the tongue cup around the nipple, creating a central trough.
2. The suck is initiated by the tip of the tongue against the nipple, followed by pressure from the lower gum.
3. There is peristaltic action of the tongue toward the back of the mouth.
4. The tongue elevation continues to move the bolus of milk into the pharynx.

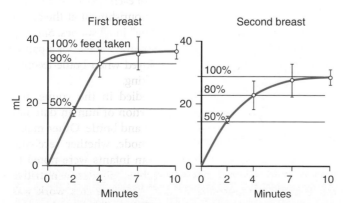

Fig. 3.9 Mother—infant pattern of milk flow. (From Lucas A, Lucas PJ, Baum JD. Pattern of milk flow in breast-fed infants. *Lancet.* 1979;2:57.)

sucking movements and then stabilizes. In a 2-week-old breastfeeding infant, sucking and breathing pattern proportions alternated smoothly at about two sucks to one breath, with swallowing occurring with every suck. Bottle-feeding patterns were variable and sometimes asynchronous with sucking and breathing.

The process of suckling has been described as a pulsating process similar to peristalsis along the rest of the gastrointestinal (GI) tract. This undulating motion, as described by cineradiography, did not involve stroking or friction, as was clearly pointed out by Woolridge.[37] The nipple should not move in and out of the infant's mouth if the breast is positioned correctly. The tip of the tongue does not move along the nipple. The positive pressure of the tongue against the teat (areola and nipple), coupled with ejection of the milk from increased intraductal pressure, evacuates the milk, not suction. The negative pressure created in the mouth holds the nipple and breast in place and reduces the "work" to refill the ducts. Visual observations and videotapes made in our laboratory to study suckling show the undulating motion of the external buccal surfaces even in newborns. Ultrasound confirms the molding of the buccal mucosa and tongue around the teat, leaving no space.

In breastfeeding, the tongue action is a "rolling," or peristaltic, action from the tip of the tongue to the base, not side to side. In bottle-feeding, the tongue action is more piston-like or squeezing. When the infant rests between sucks, the human nipple is indented by the tongue, and the latex teat is expanded in bottle-feeding (Figs. 3.10 and 3.11).

The change in nipple dimensions during suckling is detailed by Smith et al.,[43] who also used ultrasound and examined 16 term infants ages 60 to 120 days and their mothers. They demonstrated that human nipples are highly elastic and elongate during active feeding, including approximately 2 cm of areola, to form a teat approximately twice its resting length. They also showed that infants' cheeks (buccal membranes), with their thick layer of fatty tissue, known as *sucking fat pads*, act to make a passive seal to create a vacuum (as opposed to the concept that the cheeks are sucked in by the negative pressure). Milk ejection was noted to occur after maximal compression of the nipple.

Coordination of Suck and Swallow

The ability to swallow is developed in utero during the second trimester and has been well demonstrated by fetal ultrasound. Fetal swallowing of amniotic fluid is an important part of the

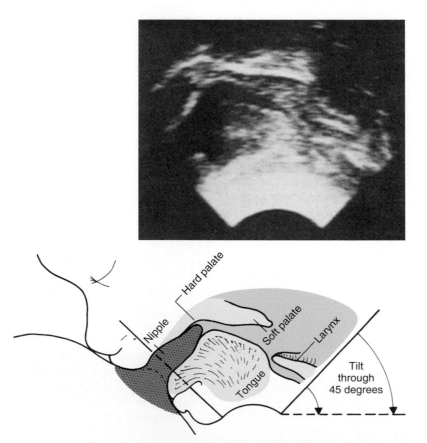

Fig. 3.10 Ultrasound of infant at breast. Still picture of ultrasound scan frame from video recording. The scanner head is at the bottom, with a sector view of 90 degrees. Below is an artist's impression of the image showing key features. The image is seen best when tilted through 45 degrees so that the infant's head is vertical. The picture corresponds to the point in the sucking cycle when the maximum point of compression of the nipple by the tongue has almost reached the tip of the nipple. Once the nipple has become fully expanded, a fresh cycle of compression will be initiated at the base of the nipple and will then move back. (From Weber F, Woolridge MW, Baum JD. An ultrasonographic study of the organization of sucking and swallowing by newborn infants. *Dev Med Child Neurol.* 1986;28:19.)

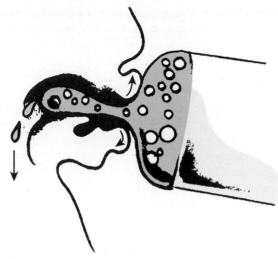

Fig. 3.11 Infant sucking on rubber nipple, which fills the mouth and thus prevents tongue action and provides flow without tongue movement. Flow occurs even if the lips are not tight around the rubber hub.

complex regulation of amniotic fluid. The suck is actually part of the oral phase of the swallow. Little was done to examine the role of swallowing on the suckling rate until Burke[44] studied the role of swallowing in the organization of suckling behavior, although with a bottle and solutions of 5% and 10% sucrose solution. The author reported two major observations: "First, the frequency of swallowing in newborns increased significantly as a function of increasing concentration and amount of sucrose solution given per criterion suck. Second, there was a significant difference in the duration of the sucking interresponse times that immediately followed the onset of swallowing and the duration of interresponse times was not associated with swallowing." These observations explain those of previous investigators regarding nutritive and nonnutritive sucking.

The coordination of sucking and swallowing was observed by ultrasound by Weber et al.[42] as a movement of the larynx. By 4 days of age, both breastfed and bottle-fed infants were swallowing with every suck. Later in the feeding, the ratio of sucks to swallows changed to 2:1 or more until sucking stopped. Swallowing occurred in the end-expiratory pause between expiration and inspiration (see Fig. 3.10). The change in the suck/swallow ratio seemed to be a function of the availability of milk.

Factors That Influence Suckling

As one manages infants with difficulty feeding, a number of rituals are often initiated to enhance infant behavior. Only a few of these have been evaluated for their effect.[45] The effect of the infant's position, that is, supine or supported upright to a 90-degree angle, was found to have no influence on the sucking pattern or pressure. The effect of temperature, however, was found to be significant. Sucking pressure decreased as environmental temperature increased from 80°F to 90°F (26.6°C to 32.2°C), which may have applications in encouraging an infant to nurse. This effect was shown to increase from the third to the fifth day of life. Higher sucking pressures have been recorded in the morning than in the afternoon.

When the size of latex nipples was studied, the large nipple elicited fewer sucks and a slower sucking rate than smaller nipples, although the volume of milk delivered was the same, in this study, with all nipple sizes. Although human nipple size cannot be altered, this knowledge may help in assessing the response of a newborn in specific situations. Increasing nipple size and decreasing sucking rate may be significant in considering using an adult finger for finger feeding.

The volume of each swallow was calculated during breastfeeding in 1905 by Süsswein,[46] who counted swallows and made test weighings. His observations were later confirmed with elaborate electronic equipment.[37] The average swallow of a newborn is 0.6 mL, which is also the exact amount drawn from a bottle equipped with an electromagnetic flowmeter transducer and a valve that responds to negative pressure at each suck in modern studies, even though the sucking mechanism between breast and bottle is different.[47] The size of the hole in the nipple influences the volume of the suck only in the valved bottle. When breastfed infants were compared with a group fed by cup from birth and a group fed by bottle, the breastfed infants had a stronger suck than either of the other two groups, who did not differ from each other in sucking skill.[29,48]

Patterns of milk intake using electronic weighings in interrupted feeds were studied. Fifty percent of a feed from each breast was consumed in 2 minutes and 80% to 90% by 4 minutes, with minimal feeding from each breast in the last 5 minutes. Bottle-fed infants, evaluated with the same technique of test weighings, took 84% of the feeding in the first 4 minutes. Bottle-feeding patterns were linear, whereas the breastfed infant had a biphasic pattern when nursed on both breasts. The total intake of the two types of feeds was similar in volume in the same 25 minutes of total time.

Fat Content and Suckling

The high concentration of fat in breast milk toward the end of a feed was hypothesized as a satiety signal to terminate the feeding. When this was studied using high- and low-fat formulas, it was found that high-fat milk did not act to cue babies to slow or stop feeding.[49] In fact, babies appeared to feed more actively on high-fat milk, sucking in longer bursts and with less resting. When human milk of low- and high-fat content was fed from bottles, switching the baby from low-fat breast milk to high-fat breast milk, the babies did not alter either the milk-intake rate or sucking patterns.

To test the hypothesis fully, a study carefully observed infants switching from the first to the second breast and back to the first breast. Infants were 2 months old and well established at exclusive breastfeeding. No significant difference was seen in the time taken to attach to the new breast and the time taken to reattach to the previously suckled breast. Mean milk intake from the first breast was 91.7 g (range 58 to 208 g), higher than that from the second breast (mean 52.5 g, range 8 to 75 g). The mean fat contents before and after nursing on the first breast were 23 and 52 g/L, whereas on the second breast, they were 24 and 48 g/L. This shows that infants will nurse when fat content is higher, contrary to the theory that increasing fat causes satiation.[48]

Studies of 3-day-old bottle-fed infants fed sucrose and glucose solutions show that they manifest tongue movements of greater amplitude when fed stronger concentrations of carbohydrate, even though they do not respond to fat content in formula. The sensory apparatus responsible for assessing sweetness is apparently competent in the newborn.

Breathing and Sucking During Feeding

Breathing and sucking during feeding were studied in normal full-term infants from 1 to 10 days of age, measuring breathing, sucking, and flow of fluid from a feeding bottle with a flow meter. No infant aspirated water, but 8 of 18 infants inhaled saline. Even from a bottle, breast milk was associated with more regular breathing than was formula feeding. It has been demonstrated in other species that newborns will become apneic when fed milk from species other than their own. The coordination of breathing and swallowing improves with an increase in milk availability and with the maturity of the infant.[41]

Suckling Patterns as Indicators of Problems or Pathology

The behavior of an infant at birth is the first opportunity to observe the infant's adeptness at suckling. In a careful analysis of videotapes of newborns in the first 90 minutes of life, Widström and Thingström-Paulsson[50] observed a consistent pattern. Licking movements preceded and followed the rooting reflex in alert infants. The tongue was placed in the bottom of the mouth cavity during distinct rooting. The authors suggest that forcing the infant to the breast might disturb reflex action and tongue position. They further observed that a healthy infant should be given the opportunity to show hunger and optimal reflexes and attach to the mother's nipple by itself.[49]

Righard and Alade[29] observed that an infant placed on the mother's abdomen will self-attach to the breast and suckle correctly in less than 50 minutes. They further reported that when the infants were separated from their mothers for delivery room procedures, the initial suckling attempts were disturbed, and many infants were too drowsy to suckle at all.[29]

Righard and Alade[51] also investigated the prognostic value of suckling technique (faulty vs. correct) during the first week after birth in relation to the long-term success of breastfeeding. For assessment of breastfeeding technique, 82 healthy mother–infant pairs were observed before discharge. The authors defined correct sucking as the infant's mouth being wide open, the tongue under the areola, and the milk expressed in slow and deep sucks. Incorrect sucking was defined as the infant positioned as if bottle-feeding, using the nipple as a teat. The oral searching reflex was defined as the infant opening the mouth wide in response to proximity of the nipple to the lips and thrusting the tongue forward in preparation to take the breast. This reflex is a part of the normal response to a circumoral stimulus, resulting in rooting by the infant, who comes forward, opens the mouth wide, and

extends the tongue when stimulated centrally on the lower lip and even the upper lip. A stimulus on the side of the mouth or cheeks elicits turning to that side.

PROLACTIN

Stricker and Grueter[52] discovered the pituitary hormone prolactin in 1928. They observed that extracts of the pituitary gland induced lactation in rabbits.

Human prolactin is a significant hormone in pregnancy and lactation.[53] Prolactin also has a range of actions in various species that is greater than any other known hormone. Prolactin has been identified in many animal species, whether they nurse their young or not. Because of the original association with lactation, the term describes its action, "support or stimulation of lactation." Prolactin, however, has been shown to control nonlactating responses in other species and has been identified with more than 300 different physiologic processes, unrelated to lactation. The study of prolactin was hampered until 1970, when it became possible to separate prolactin from human growth hormone (hGH) and isolate and characterize prolactin from human pituitary glands.

Before 1971, hGH and prolactin in humans were considered the same hormone. Until 1971, in fact, it was thought that prolactin did not exist in humans.[3] However, hGH is present in the human pituitary gland in an amount 100 times that of prolactin.[54]

Although prolactin is secreted by the anterior pituitary gland, the brain is exposed to it. Prolactin is found in the cerebrospinal fluid and may even be produced by neurons in the portal vessels of the hypothalamus. Prolactin increases the activity of tuberoinfundibular neurons, which control dopamine.[55]

Multifunctional Nature of Prolactin

Prolactin, the lactogenic hormone, is essential for glucocorticoid stimulation of the milk-protein genes.[3]

Synthesis and secretion are not restricted to the anterior pituitary gland but include multiple sites in the brain (cerebral cortex, hippocampus, amygdala, cerebellum, brainstem, and spinal cord). It is also produced in the placenta, amnion, decidua, and uterus. Evidence suggests that lymphocytes from the immune system, thymus, and spleen release bioactive prolactin. Prolactin is found in the epithelial cells of the lactating mammary gland and the milk itself. Prolactin reaches the milk by crossing the mammary epithelial cell basement membrane, attaches to a specific prolactin-binding protein, and ultimately moves by exostosis through the apical membranes into the alveolar lumen. Prolactin mRNA in milk contains more prolactin variants than serum. Milk prolactin participates in the maturation of the neuroendocrine and immune systems.

The information generated by the use of knockout mice with prolactin knockouts or prolactin-receptor knockouts has refined the understanding of mammary morphogenesis and subsequent lactogenesis.[10] It has been confirmed that prolactin does not operate alone but depends on estrogen, progesterone, and glucocorticoids, as well as insulin, thyroid hormone, parathyroid hormone, and even oxytocin (see Fig. 3.7). Prolactin also stimulates the uptake of some amino acids, the uptake of glucose, and the synthesis of milk sugar and milk fats.[1]

Plasma prolactin varies in relation to psychosocial stress. Utilizing four different real-life stress studies in a longitudinal design, Theorell[56] found that changing situations associated with passive coping are accompanied by increased plasma prolactin levels. Changing situations associated with active coping are associated with unchanged or even lowered prolactin levels. The regulation of plasma prolactin is part of a dopaminergic system (see the list of pharmacologic suppressors in the next section).

Prolactin's Effect on Milk-Protein Synthesis

In vitro, prolactin stimulates the synthesis of the mRNA of specific milk proteins by binding to membrane receptors of the mammary epithelial cells. Prolactin has been demonstrated to penetrate the cytoplasm of these cells and even their nuclei. These specific actions in the gland require the presence of extracellular calcium ions. Some prolactin actually appears in the milk substrate itself, the functional significance of which is uncertain, although it is thought to influence fluid and ion absorption from the neonatal jejunum.

The effect of the stimulation of protein synthesis by allowing the expression of milk protein genes is not a direct effect of the hormone but, rather, the consequence of the activation of sodium/potassium adenosinetriphosphatase (Na/K ATPase) in the plasma membrane.[10] The intracellular concentration of potassium is kept high, and that of sodium low, compared with the concentrations in extracellular fluid. As a result, the Na/K ratio is high both in the milk and in the intracellular fluid. Further action of prolactin has been identified in the development of the immune system in the mammary gland and, possibly more directly, in the lymphoid tissue. In conjunction with estrogen and progesterone, prolactin attracts and retains immunoglobulin A (IgA) immunoblasts from the gut-associated lymphoid tissue for the development of the immune system for the mammary gland. A very sensitive bioassay has been developed using the in vitro biologic effect of prolactin to stimulate the growth of cell cultures for malignant niobium rat lymphomas.

Variations in Prolactin Production

The baseline levels of prolactin are essentially the same in normal male and female humans (Table 3.2). Moreover, both men and women experience a rise in prolactin levels during sleep.[57] There is also a normal diurnal variation in levels in both men and women. At puberty, the increase in estrogens causes a slight but measurable increase in prolactin. Prolactin increases during the proliferative phase of the menstrual cycle but not during the secretory phase. A number of factors, including some that are significant for the nursing mother, such as psychogenic influence and stress, increase prolactin levels. Anesthesia, surgery, exercise, nipple stimulation, and sexual intercourse also produce increased amounts in both lactating and nonlactating women. Prolactin levels increase as serum osmolality increases.

Although prolactin levels in maternal serum are well established, less is known about prolactin levels in the milk and their role in the newborn. Prolactin in milk is known to be biologically potent and is absorbed by the newborn. In the intestine, prolactin influences fluid, sodium, potassium, and calcium transport. Prolactin content is highest in the early transitional milk just after the colostrum in the first postpartum week (levels of 43.1 ± 4 ng/mL). Levels drop to 11.0 ± 1.4 ng/mL in mature milk over time until approximately 40 weeks postpartum.[10]

Prolactin-Inhibiting Factor

Prolactin-inhibiting factor (PIF) controls the secretion of prolactin from the hypothalamus. Prolactin is unusual among the pituitary hormones because it is inhibited by a hypothalamic substance.[54] Catecholamine levels in the hypothalamus control the inhibiting factor, which is poured into the circulation as a result of dopaminergic impulses. Drugs and events that decrease catecholamines also decrease the inhibiting factor,

TABLE 3.2 Prolactin Levels[a]		
	Range (ng/mL)	Average (ng/mL)
Males and prepubertal and postmenopausal females	2–8	—
Females' menstrual life	8–14	10
Term pregnancy	200–500	200
Amniotic fluid	Up to 10,000	—
Lactating women	**Response to breastfeeding**	
First 10 days	Baseline 200	Rise to 400
10–90 days	60–110	70–220
90–180 days	50	100
180 days to 1 year	30–40	45–80

[a]Collation of values from multiple studies and sources.

causing a rise in prolactin. Dopamine itself can act directly on the pituitary gland to decrease prolactin secretion. Agents that increase prolactin by decreasing catecholamines, and thus the PIF level, include the phenothiazines and reserpine.

Prolactin Release and Secretion

Thyrotropin-releasing hormone (TRH) is a strong stimulator of prolactin secretion, but its physiologic role is not clear because thyrotropin levels do not rise during normal nursing. In the postpartum period, a dose of TRH will cause a marked increase in prolactin. Even a nonnursing postpartum mother will experience engorgement and milk release when stimulated with TRH. Ergot, which is frequently prescribed for postpartum patients, inhibits prolactin secretion either by direct inhibition or by its effect on the hypothalamus.

The prolactin response to breast stimulation in lactating women is not mediated by endogenous opioids. Neither baseline nor stimulated prolactin values were affected by naloxone.[58] See Box 3.5 for a list of the factors that affect prolactin release in normal humans.

The following factors affect prolactin release in normal humans:

- In pregnancy, prolactin levels begin to rise in the first trimester and continue to rise throughout gestation. In a nonnursing mother, prolactin levels drop to normal in 2 weeks, independent of therapy to suppress lactation.

BOX 3.5 Factors Affecting Prolactin Release in Humans

- Physiologic stimuli
- Nursing in postpartum women: breast stimulation
- Sleep
- Stress
- Sexual intercourse
- Pregnancy
- Pharmacologic stimuli
- Neuroleptic drugs
- Thyrotropin-releasing hormone
- Metoclopramide (procainamide derivative)
- Estrogens
- Hypoglycemia
- Phenothiazines, butyrophenones
- Norepinephrine
- Histamine
- Acetylcholine
- Pharmacologic suppressors
- Apomorphine, bromocriptine, cabergoline
- L-Dopa
- Ergot preparations (2-Br-α-ergocryptine)
- Clomiphene citrate
- Large amounts of pyridoxine
- Monoamine oxidase inhibitors
- Pramipexole
- Prostaglandins E and F2α
- Ropinirole, rotigotine, selegiline

From Cholst IN, Wardlaw SL, Newman CB, et al. Prolactin response to breast stimulation in lactating women is not mediated by endogenous opioids. *Am J Obstet Gynecol.* 1984; 150:558.

- At delivery, with the expulsion of the placenta, levels of PL, estrogens, and progesterone abruptly decline (Figs. 3.12 and 3.13).

Postpartum

PL disappears within hours. Progesterone drops over several days, and estrogens fall to baseline levels in 5 to 6 days (see Figs. 3.6 and 3.7).[59] Prolactin in nonlactating women requires 14 days to reach baseline. Progesterone is considered the key inhibiting hormone, and a decline in plasma progesterone levels is considered the lactogenic trigger for stage II lactogenesis.[3] However, progesterone does not inhibit established lactation because breast tissue does not contain progesterone-binding sites. Estrogens enhance the effect of prolactin on

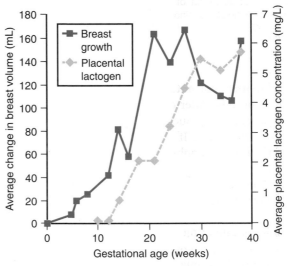

Fig. 3.12 Breast growth and placental growth are closely associated. (Modified from Cox DB, Kent JC, Casey TM, et al. Breast growth. *Exp Physiol.* 1999;84:421-434.)

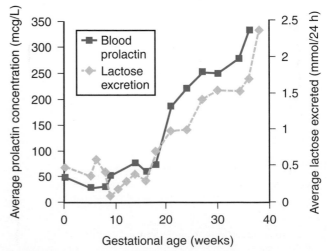

Fig. 3.13 Relationship between lactose excretion into urine and prolactin concentration in the blood during pregnancy. (Modified from Cox DB, Kent JC, Casey TM, et al. Breast growth. *Exp Physiol.* 1999;84:421-434.)

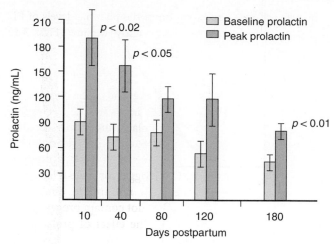

Fig. 3.14 Prolactin levels after suckling. (From Battin DA, Marrs RP, Fleiss PM, et al. Effect of suckling on serum prolactin, luteinizing hormone, follicle-stimulating hormone, and estradiol during prolonged lactation. *Obstet Gynecol.* 1985;65:785.)

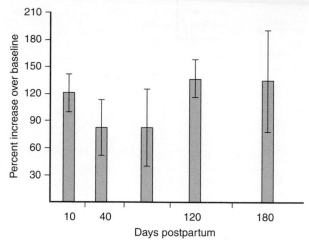

Fig. 3.15 Percentage of increase in prolactin over baseline after suckling. (From Battin DA, Marrs RP, Fleiss PM, et al. Effect of suckling on serum prolactin, luteinizing hormone, follicle-stimulating hormone, and estradiol during prolonged lactation. *Obstet Gynecol.* 1985;65:785.)

mammogenesis but antagonize prolactin by inhibiting the secretion of milk. After delivery, there are low estrogen and high prolactin levels. Suckling provides a continued stimulus for prolactin release. If prolactin, essential for lactation, is diminished by hypophysectomy or medication, lactation ceases. Baseline prolactin levels do eventually diminish to more normal levels months after parturition, although lactation may continue.[60]

Prolactin in Lactation

The surge in prolactin over baseline levels (see Fig. 3.6), however, is critical to milk production, not the baseline levels (Figs. 3.14 and 3.15). Although prolactin is necessary for milk secretion, the volume of milk secreted is not directly related to the concentration of prolactin in the plasma. Local mechanisms within the mammary gland that depend on the amount of milk removed by the infant are responsible for the day-to-day regulation of milk volume.[56] Suckling stimulates the release of adenohypophyseal prolactin and neurohypophyseal oxytocin. These hormones stimulate milk synthesis and the production of milk-ejection metabolic hormones, which are also necessary for the process of milk synthesis.[61] Thus, suckling, emptying the breast, and receiving adequate precursor nutrients are essential to effective lactation (Figs. 3.16 and 3.17).

When milk is not removed, secretion ceases in a few days, and the composition of the mammary secretion returns to a colostrum-like fluid. When the composition of the breast secretion of breastfeeding and nonbreastfeeding women was followed by Kulski and Hartmann,[62] it was the same for 3 to 4 days. Thereafter, the sodium and chloride concentrations in the nonbreastfeeding women increased rapidly.

Regulation of Milk Production

The regulation of milk production in full lactation is based primarily on infant demand.[63] Maternal nutrition, age, body

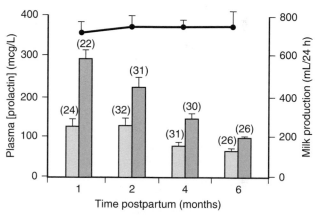

Fig. 3.16 Immunoreactive prolactin determined in plasma samples collected from 11 mothers (at 1, 2, and 4 months) and from 9 mothers (at 6 months), immediately before suckling (□, lightly shaded bar) and 45 minutes after the commencement of suckling (-, darkly shaded bar). The number of observations is shown in parentheses. Twenty-four-hour milk production (mL/24 h) of the same mothers determined by test weighing. Results are mean values (•, dark circle) + SEM. (From Cox DB, Owens RA, Hartmann PE. Blood and milk prolactin and the rate of milk synthesis in women. *Exp Physiol* 81:1007-1020, 1996.)

composition, and parity have only a secondary impact. Suckling is a powerful stimulus to prolactin synthesis and secretion, and prolactin is necessary for milk secretion.[55] The pulsatile nature of prolactin secretion makes it difficult to measure over time. Milk yield is not directly correlated to prolactin levels.

Two local mechanisms have been associated with milk-volume control. An inhibitor of milk secretion builds up as milk accumulates. The actual volume of milk secreted may be reduced if the breast is not drained adequately. Distention or stretching of the alveoli also affects the production and secretion of milk. Evidence indicates that a proteinaceous factor in

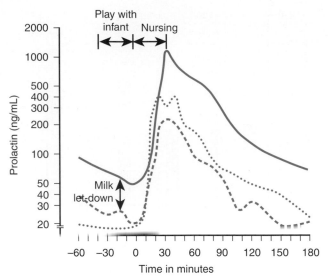

Fig. 3.17 Plasma prolactin measured by radioimmunoassay before, during, and after a period of nursing in three mothers, 22 to 26 days postpartum. Prolactin levels rose with suckling and not with infant contact. (Modified from Josimovich JB, Reynolds M, Cobo E. Lactogenic hormones, fetal nutrition, and lactation. In: Josimovich JB, Reynolds M, Cobo E, eds. *Problems of Human Reproduction.* Vol. 2. New York: John Wiley & Sons; 1974.)

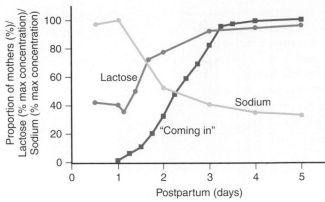

Fig. 3.18 The sense of milk "coming in." Secretory activation precedes the sense of milk "coming in." The distribution of the times when women first sensed the "coming in" of milk after normal delivery is compared with the changes in lactose and sodium concentrations of breast milk over the first postpartum days. The number of women for each time point was expressed as a cumulative percentage of the total number (*n* = 107) of women. Lactose and sodium concentrations obtained from the left and right breasts for each woman were averaged and presented as percentages of the maximum lactose and sodium concentrations over the 5 days. (From Pang WW, Hartmann PL. Initiation of human lactation: secretory differentiation and secretory activation. *J Mammary Gland Biol.* 2007;12:211-221.)

milk itself actually inhibits milk production and is associated with residual milk in the breast. This has been identified as the feedback inhibitor of lactation (FIL).

It has been assumed that prolactin levels control the rate of milk synthesis. When 24-hour milk production was measured by Cox et al.,[8] however, the results were different. The short-term rates of milk synthesis (i.e., between feeds) and the concentration of prolactin in the blood and in the milk were measured from 1 to 6 months in 11 women. The 24-hour milk production remained constant (708 ± 54.7 g per 24 hours at 1 month and 742 ± 79.4 g per 24 hours at 6 months). Marked variation in short-term milk synthesis between breasts was observed. The baseline and suckling-stimulated prolactin levels declined over time, but the peak over base remained. The concentration of prolactin in milk was related to the fullness of the breasts, being highest when the breasts were full. Cox et al.[8] found no relationship between the concentration of prolactin in the plasma and the rate of milk synthesis in either the short or long term.

Prolactin circadian rhythm persists throughout lactation. Prolactin levels are notably higher at night than during the day, despite greater nursing times during the day. The highest levels in the study by Stern and Reichlin[57] were when the least nursing occurred.

The most effective and specific stimulus to prolactin release is nursing. The stimulation is a result of nipple or breast manipulation, especially suckling, not a psychologic effect of the presence of the infant (Fig. 3.18; see also Fig. 3.17). The prolactin-release reflex during nipple stimulation is suppressed in some adult women, being evidenced only during pregnancy and lactation.[64]

During human pregnancy, when serum prolactin rises steadily to 150 to 200 ng/mL at term, there is a brief drop in levels hours before delivery and then a rise again as soon as the neonate is suckled.[63,65] The response to nipple stimulation can be abolished by applying local anesthetic.[66] On the other hand, trauma or surgery to the chest wall can initiate a prolactin rise and, in some reported cases, milk production.

Although it was initially reported that the high levels of prolactin measured in the first days and weeks of lactation dwindled to normal baseline by 6 months and showed no response to suckling stimulus, later studies clearly showed a different picture with more sensitive assays.[64] Prolactin does not drop to normal, but further stimulus causes a doubling of levels over baseline at all stages of lactation through the second year (see Table 3.2).

Prolactin Release During Milk Expression

When lactating postpartum women nurse their infants, the prolactin level increases from a high baseline level to levels several times over the mean baseline.[67] When nursing women played with but did not feed their infants, prolactin did not rise, despite the initiation of milk dripping. The substitution of a breast pump at regular intervals caused prolactin elevations similar in timing and magnitude to those induced by sucking. When normal, menstruating, nonlactating adult women were stimulated with a breast pump for 30 minutes, significant prolactin increases occurred in 7 of the 18 women. No response was obtained in normal men.

When the prolactin response was used as a measure of "success" in establishing lactation in the first week postpartum, no difference in prolactin levels was seen between women who had been considered good producers and those who were considered poor producers.[68] Mothers whose infants were in the special care unit, and who were using a breast pump to establish lactation, had minimal prolactin response to pumping but produced a mean of 86 g of milk per pumping. When prolactin levels were measured after use of the breast pump at uniform settings, all three groups were similar. This, and the work of others,[69] demonstrates that infant suckling plays a significant role in adequate milk production.

Acute prolactin and oxytocin responses were measured by Zinaman et al.,[70] who compared various mechanical pumping devices with manual expression and infant suckling. The prolactin response to mechanical expression in quantity and duration depended on the device used, with a full-size pulsatile electric pump eliciting the greatest response. This compared equally with infant suckling. There was no difference seen in oxytocin response with various devices. These data confirm that results in studies of milk production and release in humans also depend on the equipment used to stimulate the breast.[69] Eight fully lactating women were followed through the first 6 months postpartum at 10, 40, 80, 120, and 180 days, recording serum prolactin, luteinizing hormone, follicle-stimulating hormone, and estradiol (zero time only) obtained just before the initiation of suckling and during the next 120 minutes.[71] Samples were obtained at 0, +15, +30, +60, and +120 minutes. Prolactin levels were high the first 10 days (90.1 ng/mL) but slowly declined over 180 days (44.3 ng/mL). The stimulus of suckling doubled the baseline values. Mean estradiol levels were low at 10 days (7.2 pg/mL), then gradually rose to a mean of 47.3 pg/mL at 180 days postpartum in the subjects whose menses had resumed. In the amenorrhoeic subjects, the estradiol levels remained low (4.25 pg/mL), whereas baseline prolactin remained high (63.6 ng/mL). The subjects were breastfeeding on demand, averaging 11 feedings (range 8 to 16) per day at 10 days and 8 feedings (range 5 to 12) at 120 and 180 days. All infants had stopped one-night feeding, and two infants had started some solids between the third and fourth months.

When specific binding sites for prolactin were looked for in the tammar wallaby, many sites were demonstrated in the lactating mammary gland but not the inactive gland. Mammary prolactin receptors were also identified in the rabbit. Thus, the increased binding capacity would enhance tissue responsiveness, which may explain the maintenance of full lactation in the face of falling concentrations of prolactin. Prolactin also plays a critical role in increasing maternal bile secretory function postpartum.[63]

HUMAN PLACENTAL LACTOGEN AND HUMAN GROWTH HORMONE

Three main hormones are recognized in the lactogenic process: hPL, hGH, and prolactin. The progressive rise in prolactin during pregnancy parallels the rise in hPL, becoming measurable at 6 weeks' gestation and increasing to 6000 ng/mL at term (see Fig. 3.4). This parallel action contributed to the original belief that prolactin and hPL were the same.

The principal function of hPL and prolactin in humans is a lactogenic one, so no lactation ordinarily appears before delivery.[3,19] In rare cases, however, women report being able to express a few drops of colostrum before delivery.

Human Placental Lactogen

First described in 1962, hPL has been studied more than lactogens from any other species.[19] Extensive immunologic and structural homology exists between hGH and hPL, which probably explains their similar biologic activities. Concentrations of hPL increase steadily during gestation and decrease abruptly with the delivery of the placenta. A large-molecular-weight substance, hPL is derived from the chorion. Receptor sites that bind lactogen also bind protein and hGH.[19] hPL has been associated with mobilization of free fatty acids and the inhibition of peripheral glucose utilization and lactogenic action.

Human Growth Hormone

hGH is secreted from the anterior pituitary eosinophilic cells. These cells have been identified by staining techniques that distinguish them from those that produce prolactin. Toward the end of pregnancy, the cells that produce prolactin are noticeably more numerous, whereas those that produce hGH are "crowded out." The role of hGH in the maintenance of lactation is poorly defined and may be synergistic with prolactin and glucocorticoids.

Prolactin, hGH, PL, and chorionic somatotropin form a family of polypeptide hormones from the same ancestral gene, even though prolactin and hGH are produced by the pituitary and PL and chorionic somatotropin by the placenta.[72] The suckling stimulus in postpartum lactation causes a rapid increase in serum hGH and prolactin. hGH and prolactin evolve from the same precursor, and although the hormones are distinct, the acute interruption of hGH secretion does not interfere with milk secretion.

The possible role of TSH as a physiologic prolactin-releasing factor has been disproved by Gehlbach et al.,[73] who state that TSH is not responsible for the brisk release of prolactin with suckling. Normal lactation is possible in women with ateliotic dwarfism in the absence of detectable quantities of hGH. For any hormone to exert its biologic effects, however, specific receptors for the hormone must be present in the target tissue. Changes in serum concentration have no effect if receptors are not present in the mammary gland to bind the hormone.

OXYTOCIN

Oxytocin was the first hormone studied in relation to breastfeeding and to the let-down reflex. Studies first explored its role in the initiation and progression of labor. Because it was measurable, isolated in the laboratory, and finally manufactured synthetically, our knowledge of oxytocin was more extensive than it was for prolactin until the last two decades.

Oxytocin is not just a female hormone; it is produced by both male and female humans, and it is increased not just during reproduction in women. It is now credited with producing increased responsiveness to receptivity, closeness, openness to relationships, and nurturing. The oxytocin circulating during breastfeeding has been credited with producing calm, lack of stress, and an enhanced ability to interact with infants. The calm-and-connectedness response is part of a system of nerves and hormones that together trigger these effects.

Endocrinology of Oxytocin

Oxytocin is a polypeptide, found in all mammalian species, that activates receptors on the outer surface of the cell membrane.[74] Oxytocin is produced in the supraoptic and paraventricular nuclei of the hypothalamus. Receptors have been identified for oxytocin in the uterus and the breast as well as the brain. It acts via the bloodstream and as a signaling substance in the nervous system. Substances that act to stimulate the release of oxytocin include serotonin, dopamine, noradrenaline, and glutamate. Other substances, such as opiates, enkephalin, and β-endorphin, inhibit its release. Spinal anesthesia has been associated with the inhibition of oxytocin release after childbirth.[59] Estrogen can increase the number of receptors and stimulate the production of oxytocin. The release of oxytocin by repetitive soothing touches or when given via injection produces a calming reaction and lowers blood pressure and pulse rate. Uvnäs-Moberg[75] has studied oxytocin extensively and calls it the hormone of calm, love, and healing.

The polypeptide oxytocin is a messenger molecule with diverse physiologic actions as well as modes of delivery to its target sites. Oxytocin exerts effects as a hormone carried by the systemic circulation to distant targets in the uterus and the breast.[76] Oxytocin also serves as a hypophysiotropic factor, released from nerve terminals in the median eminence into the pituitary portal vasculature to affect anterior pituitary secretion. Its action here is as a peptidergic neurotransmitter or neuromodulator within the central nervous system, influencing a variety of neuroendocrine, behavioral, and autonomic functions. Its well-known role is related to reproduction and lactation, but it has other, less well explored physical and metabolic roles.[75]

STAGE III LACTOGENESIS (GALACTOPOIESIS): MAINTENANCE OF ESTABLISHED LACTATION

Early studies in the past 100 years established that milk was synthesized in the mammary gland from substances removed from the maternal arterial blood supply. Then it was confirmed that milk ejection was from the removal of stored milk and not from the rapid synthesis of milk. The enzymes and hormones involved have been identified. Understanding the molecular biochemistry and physiology of the gland has revealed the details of the production of milk. Numerous genes encode for components that are part of the intricate signaling pathways. Complex interactions of signaling molecules with epigenetic factors occur at the level of gene expression. Intracellular signaling is basic to understanding normal human mammary development.

The basic features of milk production are the identification of the cell-surface and intracellular receptors for extracellular signals (12 hormones and autocrine and paracrine factors, according to Martin and Czank[77]).

The maintenance of established milk secretion, originally called *galactopoiesis*, is now labeled *stage III lactogenesis*, or simply *lactation*. An intact hypothalamic–pituitary axis regulating prolactin and oxytocin levels is essential to the initiation and maintenance of lactation.[78] The process of lactation requires milk synthesis and milk release into the alveoli and the lactiferous sinuses. When the milk is not removed, the increased pressure lessens capillary blood flow and inhibits the lactation process. A lack of sucking stimulation means a lack of prolactin release from the pituitary gland. Basal prolactin levels that are enhanced by the spurts that result from sucking are necessary to maintain lactation in the first postpartum weeks. Without oxytocin, however, a pregnancy can be carried to term, but the woman will fail to lactate because let-down will not occur.

Sensory nerve endings, located mainly in the areola and nipple, are stimulated by suckling. The afferent neural reflex pathway, via the spinal cord to the mesencephalon and then to the hypothalamus, produces the secretion and release of prolactin and oxytocin. Hypothalamic suppression of earlier PIF secretion causes adenohypophyseal prolactin release. When prolactin is released into the circulation, it stimulates milk synthesis and secretion. A conditioned milk ejection can occur in lactating women without a concomitant release of prolactin, so the releases are indeed independent, which may be significant in treating apparent lactation failure (Fig. 3.19).

HORMONAL REGULATION OF PROLACTIN AND OXYTOCIN

The release of prolactin is inhibited by PIF.[11] PIF has not been described but is closely associated with dopamine. There is also evidence of either serotonin release of prolactin or catecholamine–serotonin control of prolactin release. TSH has also been shown to stimulate the release of prolactin. The amount of prolactin is proportional to the amount of nipple stimulation during the early stages of lactation after the first 4 days. Milk synthesis proceeds for the first 4 days whether or not the breast is stimulated. At this time, prolactin levels are the same for lactators and nonlactators[15] (Fig. 3.20).

Although both oxytocin and prolactin release are stimulated by nipple stimulation, some oxytocin is released by other sensory pathways, such as visual, tactile, olfactory, and auditory.[79] Thus, a woman may release milk on seeing, touching, hearing, smelling, or thinking about her infant. Prolactin, however, is released only on nipple stimulation so that milk production is not initiated by other sensory pathways.

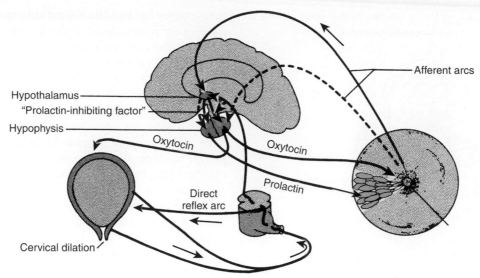

Fig. 3.19 Neuroendocrine control of milk ejection. (Modified from Vorherr H. *The Breast: Morphology, Physiology and Lactation.* New York: Academic Press; 1974.)

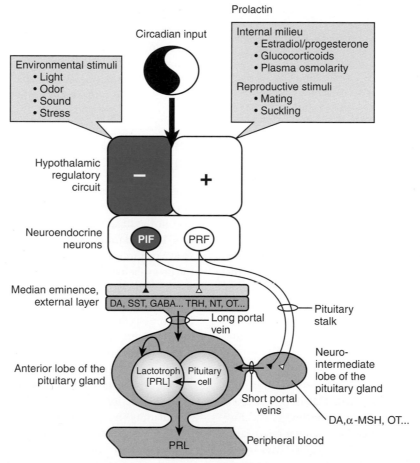

Fig. 3.20 An overview of the regulation of prolactin secretion. Prolactin secretion is paced by a light-entrained circadian rhythm, which is modified by environmental input, with the internal milieu and reproductive stimuli affecting the inhibitory or stimulatory elements of the hypothalamic regulatory circuit. The final common pathways of the central stimulatory and inhibitory control of prolactin secretion are the neuroendocrine neurons producing prolactin-inhibiting factors *(PIFs)*, such as dopamine *(DA)*, somatostatin *(SST)*, and γ-aminobutyric acid *(GABA)*, or prolactin-releasing factors *(PRFs)*, such as thyrotropin-releasing hormone *(TRH)*, oxytocin *(OT)*, and neurotensin *(NT)*. PIFs and PRFs from the neuroendocrine neurons can be released either at the median eminence into the long portal veins or at the neurointermediate lobe, which is connected to the anterior lobe of the pituitary gland by the short portal vessels. Thus, lactotrophs are regulated by bloodborne agents of central nervous system or pituitary origin (α-melanocyte –stimulating hormone) delivered to the anterior lobe by the long or short portal veins. Lactotrophs are also influenced by PRFs and PIFs released from neighboring cells (paracrine regulation) or from the lactotrophs themselves (autocrine regulation). (From Freeman ME, Kanyicska B, Lerant A, Nagy G. Prolactin: structure, function and regulation of secretion. *Physiol Rev.* 2000;80:1523-1630.)

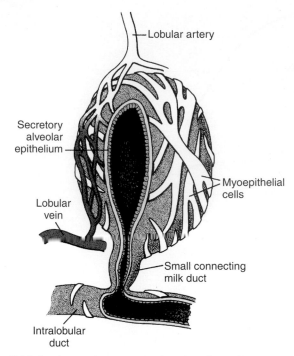

Fig. 3.21 Fundamental mammary unit at lactation, with arrangement of secretory alveoli, myoepithelial cells, and vasculature. The secretory alveolar epithelium is monolayered, and the epithelial lining of milk ducts consists of two layers. Between the bases of glandular epithelial cells and tunica propria, star-like myoepithelial mammary cells surround the alveolus in a basketlike arrangement. (Modified from Vorherr H. *The Breast: Morphology, Physiology and Lactation.* New York: Academic Press; 1974.)

Oxytocin is also released under physical stress, such as pain, exercise, cold, heat, changes in plasma osmolality, or hypovolemia, but these responses are blunted or reversed during lactation.[75,78]

When suckling occurs, oxytocin is released.[73] It enters the circulation and rapidly causes the ejection of milk from the alveoli and smaller milk ducts into the larger lactiferous ducts and sinuses. (Fig. 3.21). This is the pathway of the let-down, or ejection, reflex. Oxytocin also causes contraction of the myometrium and involution of the uterus.

Role of Suckling

After suckling is initiated, the oxytocin response is transient and intermittent rather than sustained. Plasma levels often return to basal between milk ejections, even though suckling continues. Ejection can be measured by placing a microcatheter in the mammary duct or can be noted subjectively by the mother as tingling or turgescence. The contractions last about 1 minute, with about 4 to 10 occurring in a 10-minute period. Corresponding pulses of oxytocin can be measured in the maternal bloodstream. The controls of oxytocin release are complex and are extensively described by Crowley and Armstrong.[76] That centrally released oxytocin is in control of the milk-ejection reflex was established in 1981 by Freund-Mercier and Richard.[80] They demonstrated in rats that intracerebroventricular administration of oxytocin greatly increased

the frequency and amplitude of pulsatile oxytocin release during suckling. Administration of oxytocin antagonists produced the opposite effect and suppressed responses.[79]

The human pituitary has an excessive storage capacity and contains 3000 to 9000 mU of oxytocin, but the reflex milk ejection involves the release of only 50 to 100 mU.[81,82] Except in extreme cases (Sheehan syndrome), hormone depletion is rarely an issue, but hormone release and target-organ sensitivity are. Opiate and β-endorphin released during stress are known to block stimulus-secretion coupling by dissociating electrical activity at the terminal. This inhibition is naloxone reversible.

The mammary gland, from platypus to human, has an identical fine structure consisting of alveolar tissue that has increased its surface area 10,000-fold during gestation compared with the size of the gland.[83] It continuously produces milk throughout lactation, but the most complex issue is the release of milk. Because of the substantial surface-tension forces opposing the movement of fluid in the small ducts, simple suction applied by suckling is relatively ineffective, especially in early lactation. Thus, the alveolus is enveloped in a basketlike network of myoepithelial cells that responds to oxytocin by contracting and expelling the milk into larger and larger ductules until it can be removed by the infant (see Fig. 3.21). This is a classic example of a neuroendocrine reflex, a process that is remarkably uniform in all mammals.[62]

CHANGES IN BREAST HEMODYNAMICS IN BREASTFEEDING MOTHERS

The tissue concentrations of oxyhemoglobin, deoxyhemoglobin, and total hemoglobin and the hemoglobin oxygen saturation in the breast while breastfeeding have been measured by near-infrared time-resolved spectroscopy because it is a noninvasive method of assessment during breastfeeding.[2] When both the breast being suckled and the contralateral breast were measured, both sides showed a significant decrease compared with the presuckling values. During breastfeeding, the values from both breasts fluctuated cyclically. Thus, it was documented that blood volume decreases and fluctuates during breastfeeding, as does oxygenation. The investigators speculate that this is a result of changes in pressure and resistance in blood vessels accompanying the milk-ejection reflex.[2]

Milk ejection involves both neural and endocrinologic stimulation and response. A neural afferent pathway and an endocrinologic efferent pathway are required.[65]

The ejection reflex depends on receptors located in the canalicular system of the breast. When the canaliculi are dilated or stretched, the reflex release of oxytocin is triggered. Tactile receptors for both oxytocin and reflex prolactin release are in the nipple. Neither the negative and positive pressures exerted by suckling nor the thermal changes trigger the milk-ejection reflex. Negative pressures have a minor effect, but tactile stimulation is the most important factor in milk ejection.

Studies in tactile stimulation show changes in sensitivity at puberty, during the menstrual cycle, and at parturition.[30,84]

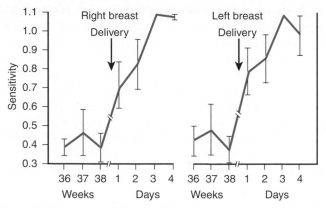

Fig. 3.22 Changes in tactile sensitivity of cutaneous breast tissue in perinatal period. Sensitivity was calculated from two-point discrimination according to the formula K − log(e). K is an arbitrary figure employed to portray a low two-point discrimination value as the peak of sensitivity. A dramatic increase in tactile sensitivity at delivery enhances the response to the suckling of the newborn. (From Robinson JE, Short RV. Changes in breast sensitivity at puberty, during the menstrual cycle, and at parturition. *Br Med J.* 1977;1:1188.)

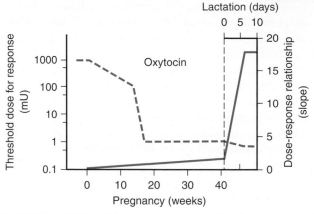

Fig. 3.23 Sensitivity of human mammary epithelium to oxytocin during pregnancy and lactation. Scale at left shows threshold dose necessary to evoke an increase in intramammary pressure; scale at right shows maximum intramammary pressure obtained. (Modified from Caldeyro-Barcia R. Milk ejection in women. In: Reynolds M, Folley SJ, eds. *Lactogenesis: The Initiation of Milk Secretion at Parturition.* Philadelphia: University of Pennsylvania Press; 1969.)

No difference exists in sensitivity between the sexes before puberty. In girls, tactile sensitivity increases after puberty and is increased at midcycle and during menstruation. (The midcycle peak is absent in women taking oral contraceptives, probably because of the suppression of ovulation.) Dramatic changes occur within 24 hours of delivery after several weeks of complete insensitivity. The nipple is the most sensitive area to both touch and pain, followed by the areola; the least sensitive area is the cutaneous breast tissue. The increased sensitivity of the breast continues several days postpartum, even when a woman does not breastfeed. Estrogen treatment suppresses the induction of prolactin release on nipple stimulation; on withdrawal of estrogen, the prolactin response returns. Increased tactile sensitivity may be the key event activating the suckling-induced release of oxytocin and prolactin at delivery (Figs. 3.22 and 3.23).

Oxytocin Challenge Tests

The clinical study of oxytocin challenge tests for use in measuring the viability of the fetus has led to the study of breast stimulus on the uterus. Numerous studies have confirmed that oxytocin levels rise significantly during nipple stimulation, with short bursts of oxytocin during accompanying uterine contractions.[30] When the effect of breast stimulation on prostaglandin secretion was tested at 38 to 40 weeks' gestation, uterine contractions occurred and prostaglandin metabolite levels increased in all cases. Shalev et al.[85] suggest that the principal action of oxytocin is to stimulate prostaglandin synthesis in uterine tissues, which then becomes the primary cause of the uterine contractions.

Oxytocin-Binding Sites

The oxytocin-binding sites are located within the basement membrane of the mammary alveolus and along the interlobular ducts. A gradual 10-fold increase occurs in the concentration of oxytocin-receptor sites in the mammary gland during pregnancy.[82] This contrasts sharply with the sudden 40-fold increase in oxytocin receptors in the uterus in the hours before delivery that then rapidly disappear. These changes in receptor availability may be why copious milk does not occur until shortly after delivery because oxytocin first facilitates delivery and then promotes milk ejection sequentially. When the increase in intramammary pressure obtained with varying doses of oxytocin in nonpregnant, pregnant, and lactating women was recorded by Caldeyro-Barcia, the amount of oxytocin required for a response dropped from 1000 mU in nonpregnancy to about 1 mU in late pregnancy and to 0.5 mU in lactation (see Fig. 3.23).[86] The maximum intramammary pressure that could be evoked increased from 1 mm Hg early in pregnancy to a peak of 10 mm Hg at 5 days postpartum. Various authors have suggested that not only the sensitivity of the myoepithelial cells but also the number of receptor sites increases during pregnancy and lactation.[87,88]

Conflicting information exists regarding the exact nature of the release of oxytocin from the pituitary. The dose–response curve of the mammary gland has a very limited dynamic range, so a bolus of 0.1 mU oxytocin (0.2 mg) given intravenously to a lactating rat fails to change intramammary pressure. An injection of 1 mU evokes an increase in pressure that begins after a delay of 10 seconds and peaks in 15 seconds at 8 to 10 mm Hg. A bolus has a greater effect than a slow push, suggesting that a pulsatile pattern of hormone release would be the most effective way of utilizing oxytocin to produce milk ejection.[64]

Plasma Oxytocin Levels

Plasma oxytocin levels measured by Lucas et al.[89] with continuous sampling every 20 seconds revealed that the hormone was released in surges and persisted in the circulation for less than 1 minute. The multiparas had a greater total response than primiparas, but with no difference between early (1 to 3 days postpartum) and late (5 to 7 days). When a similar study was done by Dawood et al.,[90] collecting samples only every 3 minutes, no pulsing was identified. Oxytocin was measurable within 2 minutes of suckling, peaked at 10 minutes, and had a bimodal curve dropping to a mean at 20 minutes, comparable with that before suckling, which followed the burping and changing of breasts at approximately 15 minutes. A secondary peak occurred at 25 minutes. They found the maximum response of intramammary pressures at the fifth to seventh day. McNeilly et al. measured the release of oxytocin in response to suckling in early and established lactation, drawing samples every 30 seconds.[91] A catheter for blood sampling was placed in the forearm 40 minutes before lactation. Oxytocin levels increased 3 to 10 minutes before suckling in response to the baby crying or becoming restless or the mother preparing herself to feed. There was no prolactin response until suckling began.

Most results clearly showed response before tactile stimuli and then a second surge in response to suckling. The levels were pulsatile during suckling and not related to milk volume, prolactin response, or the parity of the mother.

Significant elevations of the maternal oxytocin level occur at 15, 30, and 45 minutes after delivery when the infant is put skin to skin, compared with levels just before delivery during the expulsion of the placenta.[92] Levels return to baseline after 60 minutes if the infant does not suckle. When oxytocin levels were measured after initiating breast stimulation with a mechanical breast pump in early lactation (10 to 90 days), midlactation (90 to 190 days), and late lactation (180 days to 12 months), baseline levels were similar in all three periods. The stimulated plasma oxytocin levels were greater in early than late lactation, but there was always a response. Thus, the oxytocin secretory reflex appears to continue for at least the first year of lactation.

The release of oxytocin by neurohypophyseal responses during lactation has been evoked both by the infant's suckling and by mechanical dilatation of the mammary ducts. This release of oxytocin was demonstrated to be independent of vasopressin release. Conversely, further study[11,53] demonstrated that there could be stimulation of vasopressin release independent of oxytocin release.

When the levels of hGH, vasopressin, prolactin, calcitonin, gastrin, insulin, epinephrine, norepinephrine, and dopamine were measured in six lactating women during breastfeeding, Widström et al.[93] confirmed the rise in prolactin and demonstrated the progressive increase in insulin that may be secondary to prolactin rise and may participate in stimulating milk production. The gastrin level decreased, and there were no consistent findings for calcitonin, hGH, norepinephrine, or epinephrine and no change in dopamine and vasopressin. Vagally stimulated release of insulin and gastrin is antagonized when the tone of the sympathetic nervous system is increased, such as during stress, pain, or anxiety. Increased insulin also is known to stimulate the synthesis of casein and lactalbumin and thus, secondarily, milk production. It should be advantageous to breastfeed after a meal rather than before (practically, many mothers eat while feeding the infant).

Human myoepithelium, the effector tissue, is specifically stimulated by oxytocin, and the sensitivity and specificity increase throughout pregnancy. Suckling can induce milk secretion, which is under control of the adenohypophysis. In this case, oxytocin released by the neurohypophysis because of the suckling stimulus would cause both milk ejection and the release of the anterior pituitary hormones responsible for milk secretion.[94] This is probably the mechanism behind relactation and induced lactation in a woman who has never been pregnant. Mammary growth and lactogenesis may be induced by suckling, massage, and breast stimulation in many species.

Oxytocin Responsivity

Responses to oxytocin levels in the blood are well documented in animal models as well as in humans, including effects on maternal behavior, reduced blood pressure, and reduced stress responses. The relationship of oxytocin responsivity to blood pressure in breastfeeding mothers was compared with that in bottle-feeding mothers. The breastfeeding mothers had higher oxytocin levels but lower blood pressure while feeding, especially during stress. The authors concluded that oxytocin has antistress and blood-pressure-lowering effects.[95]

Alcohol has a dose-related effect on the central nervous system in inhibiting milk ejection. When intramammary pressure was measured in response to suckling by the infant while the mother received measured doses of alcohol, milk ejection was inhibited in a dose-dependent manner.[57] Doses to a maximum of 0.45 g per kilogram of body weight (blood alcohol less than 0.1%), however, had no effect on intramammary pressure. Mechanical breast stimulation for 10 minutes and concomitant administration of intravenous (IV) fluid containing normal saline, naloxone, ethanol, or a combination of ethanol and naloxone were initiated in normal nonlactating women on day 22 of the regular menstrual cycle.[96] Plasma oxytocin levels rose two-fold, with breast stimulation peaking at 10 minutes. Responses were unchanged by naloxone but were completely abolished by alcohol taken orally (approximately 110 mL of whiskey). Naloxone partially reversed the inhibiting effects of ethanol. The authors concluded that naloxone-sensitive endogenous opioids do not appear to be involved in the control of the oxytocin rise induced by breast stimulation and that opioid peptides are partly involved in the alcohol action.[95] Alcohol has been used in obstetrics to suppress premature labor in humans.

In a study of women who had received oxytocin for stimulus during labor or postpartum for control of bleeding and/or epidural analgesia compared with women who were untreated, plasma oxytocin and prolactin concentrations were measured during suckling on the second day postpartum. All subjects showed a pulsatile oxytocin pattern during the first 10 minutes of breastfeeding.[60] When women received both oxytocin and an epidural, the median oxytocin levels were the lowest. The more oxytocin they had received, the lower their endogenous oxytocin. A significant rise of prolactin occurred after 20 minutes in all women except those who had oxytocin, in whom the levels rose in 10 minutes. The rise in prolactin between 0 and

20 minutes correlated significantly with the median oxytocin and prolactin levels.[60] Thus, oxytocin infusion was observed to decrease endogenous oxytocin release dose dependently and facilitated the release of prolactin. Epidural analgesia, when combined with oxytocin, resulted in lowered endogenous oxytocin levels. The length of the breastfeeding session was increased by the prolactin levels; that is, the longer the mother breastfed, the higher the levels.

Epidural anesthesia has been demonstrated to inhibit the release of oxytocin during labor into the circulation and the brain of sheep and cows. As a consequence, maternal behavior and bonding to the young are inhibited.[60]

In this study, in the women who received only an epidural, oxytocin levels matched controls. But other studies have shown that epidurals decrease oxytocin levels.

Suckling brings about functional changes in the offspring. An infant who sucks on an artificial nipple quickly decreases the amount of body movement, increases mouth activity, and decreases crying. The suckling experience may affect infant behavior and mother–infant interaction. Nonnutritive sucking is observed in many species. In the human infant, nutritive sucking is shown to be a continuous stream of regular sucks with few, if any, pauses. Nonnutritive sucking has bursts of activity alternating with no sucking. Suckling can be altered by extraneous aural, visual, or olfactory stimuli. The response of the breast to different stimulation patterns of an electric breast pump was measured by Kent et al.[78] When cycles were 45 per minute, let-down occurred in 147 ± 13 seconds. In response to breastfeeding, let-down occurred after 56 ± 4 seconds. The volume reflected the negative pressure or vacuum applied but not the time for milk ejection.[78]

UNDERSTANDING THE MYTH OF "MILK COMING IN"

Much of lactation physiology in the human has been based on research done in the bovine and other mammals. This has led to some misinterpretation of human data. An important understanding is that despite the tendencies of other species, human secretory activation occurs after parturition rather than before. Only a small volume of colostrum is available during the first 24 to 48 hours after birth. Today, in newborn nurseries, fixation on technology and measurements has led to the determination of blood sugars and strict attention to the newborn's intake. Human newborns are born with significant stores of energy in body fat and mobilize adequate energy from these sources. This represents colostrum already secreted in the ducts and not the rapid synthesis and secretion of milk. Thus, the awaiting of milk "coming in" has been reported in the first 96 hours. Many women do not experience a sudden change but a gradual one. When the timing of "milk coming in" is compared with the actual physiologic measurements of the increase in lactose and the decrease in sodium, it is noted to lag behind these markers (see Fig. 3.18). It is thought[97] that the sensation of "milk coming in" is an "overshoot" seen more commonly in primiparas. The milk

supply then has to downregulate to match the infant's needs. Physiologically, it is not an observable event.

During active lactation, the storage time of milk in the alveoli and ducts is about an hour in the human, but it is much longer in some other species, such as rabbits and sea mammals (to a maximum of 4 days). It is important to point out that the ejection reflex (see Fig. 3.19) has been illustrated to imply that rapid synthesis and secretion occur with the activation of both oxytocin and prolactin simultaneously. That is not the case. Secretory differentiation is independent of birth; secretory activation is closely associated with birth (see Fig. 3.5). The progesterone drop in humans is associated with the delivery of the placenta (see Fig. 3.1); therefore, it is after delivery that secretory activation begins, approximately 30 to 40 hours after delivery.[3]

MATERNAL EFFECTS OF SUCKLING

Effects of suckling on the mother include the stimulation of afferent nerves for the removal of milk.[98] A reduction in sucking stimulus produces a reduction in prolactin and in milk synthesis.[93] The lactating glands adjust the milk supply to demand, probably as a result of both a local and an endocrinologic mechanism. Variations in milk secretion are rapidly reflected in anatomic changes in the mammary gland. Mammary tissue shows regression after the first week or so, if unstimulated. Tissue regression proceeds at a rate parallel to the demand for secretory tissue. Thus, when a suckling infant signals needs, the breast will respond[99] (Fig. 3.24).

The effects on maternal behavior have been attributed to lactation. Maternal behavior is more easily defined in many other species, in which early nursing is initiated by the mother, who stimulates the neonate to suckle by grooming. She then presents her mammary gland to the offspring so that the nipple is located with minimal effort. All species of lactating females have a lessened response to stress. In humans, however, nursing behavior has a strong voluntary nature. When lactating women were stressed with graded treadmill exercise, significant decreases in plasma levels of ACTH, cortisol, and epinephrine were observed compared with a matched

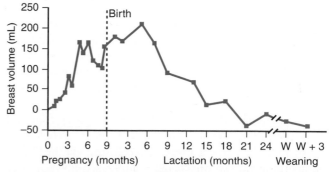

Fig. 3.24 Average change in breast volume during pregnancy, lactation, and after weaning (w) compared with preconception breast volume. (From Kent JC, Mitoulas L, Cox DB, et al. Breast volume and milk production during extended lactation. *Exp Physiol.* 1999;84:435-447.)

group of nonlactating women.[100] Plasma glucose levels did not increase in either group. Oxytocin pulse in the plasma in response to suckling was also accompanied by a decrease in plasma ACTH and cortisol in the lactating women.

Role of Oxytocin

Oxytocin administered intraventricularly to virgin rats induces maternal behavior. Local infusion of oxytocin antagonists to appropriate regions of the hypothalamus during parturition blocked the dams from pup retrieval, a measure of maternal behavior in rats. Similar observations have been made in sheep.[97] The neurophysical mechanism is under study in humans. Oxytocin promotes the development of human maternal behavior and mother—infant bonding.[101] Some effects of oxytocin in the nipple and mammary gland appear to be caused by peptides released in the nipple from axon collaterals of somatosensory afferent nerves. Oxytocin is also present in neurons projecting to many areas in the brain and exerts many central actions. In addition to maternal behavior, oxytocin causes more nonspecific behavior changes, such as sedation or antistress effects, and optimizes the transfer of energy to the mammary gland.[101]

Oxytocin also plays a direct role in the let-down process. Ultrasound observations reveal that when the mother senses let-down or when infant swallowing increases, a corresponding change in duct diameter occurs in parallel with oxytocin concentration levels. Pulses of oxytocin occur every 45 seconds or so as the ducts intermittently dilate. This is part of the overall interaction mechanism between infant suckling and milk provision, whereby the number of milk ejections influences the amount of milk consumed.[102]

Investigations of the agile wallaby, *Macropus agilis*, have revealed the let-down reflex because this species displays concurrent asynchronous lactation. The young, weighing 35 g, attach to the teat at birth. The lactating gland continues to grow for 200 days, increasing 10-fold in size. At 200 to 220 days, weighing 2500 g, the young first leaves the pouch. Twenty-six days later, a second baby is born, although the older one continues to suckle intermittently for another 160 days at the original teat. The second one attaches to an unused nipple, which begins to develop, displaying complete autonomy. Measurements of oxytocin during the initial lactation show an increase in the intraductal pressure response with a decline in sensitivity over time. This permits milk ejection in response to a small release of oxytocin to be confined to the mammary gland to which the neonate is continuously attached. The release of large quantities of oxytocin in response to the suckling of the juvenile would cause a release in both glands.

Mammals have thus evolved diverse strategies for survival. Tandem nursing in the human has not been as carefully studied, but although the milk reverts to colostrum at the birth of the new infant, no known change occurs in let-down.

Spinothalamic Tract

The spinohypothalamic tract is the most likely of the possible spinal and brainstem pathways by which the suckling stimulus reaches the forebrain. The areas of the forebrain influenced by the suckling stimulus include the hypothalamic structures that mediate oxytocin and prolactin release.[103] The inhibition of milk ejection by visual and auditory stimuli, pinealectomy, and ventrolateral midbrain lesions in lactating rats has been studied to define further the neurohormonal pathways. In these experiments, the pineal gland appeared to mediate an inhibitory visual reflex on both oxytocin release and milk ejection.[104]

A mechanism consisting of smooth muscle and elastic fibers acting as a sphincter at the end of the ducts in the nipple appears to prevent most unwanted loss of milk. Sympathetic control does not appear to be present in humans, although it is demonstrable in most other species.

As the end of pregnancy approaches, the breast is prepared to respond to the suckling offspring.[28] In humans, this is evidenced by increased sensitivity of the breast to tactile stimulation; increased responsiveness of the ductules to oxytocin, thus preparing to eject the milk; and increased responsiveness of the breast to signaling the release of prolactin to stimulate milk production. The signal for lactation occurs when the placenta is removed and the end organs in the breast can fully respond to the surge of prolactin resulting from suckling.[13]

CONCENTRATIONS OF OXYTOCIN IN MILK

Human milk samples obtained by manual expression daily from the first to the fifth postpartum day were collected immediately before and after a feeding as well as 2 hours after nursing.[105] The baseline mean oxytocin concentrations were 3.3 to 4.7 mg/mL, increasing significantly with nursing. Oxytocin in milk is fairly stable compared with that in maternal serum, which is inactivated by oxytocinase in plasma, liver, and kidney. When oxytocin was administered to rat dams, it was also found in the suckling offspring's gastric contents, where it is stable in acid. Some is absorbed into the neonatal blood, where it is unstable. The levels of oxytocin in neonatal serum are produced predominantly by the neonate itself. Whether oxytocin has a physiologic role on the gut or other hormones is unknown.

ROLE OF PROSTAGLANDINS AS MILK EJECTORS

Because prostaglandins have many physiologic effects and are known to increase mammary duct pressure, Toppozada et al.[106] investigated their role as milk ejectors. Comparison was made among three treatments: IV injections of oxytocin, prostaglandin (PG) E2 (PGE2), and 16-phenoxy-PGE2 given to one group of women on the third to sixth day postpartum; IV oxytocin, 15-methyl-PGF2α, and PGF2α tromethamine salt to a second group; and oxytocin and PGF intranasally to a third group. All combinations had some effect, with the IV route having a shorter latency period than the intranasal. PGF2α, the more potent of the prostaglandin preparations, was more potent via the nasal route than oxytocin nasally.

The response lasted 25 minutes after intranasal instillation of 400 mg. PGE2 and PGF2α, orally administered, reduce prolactin levels and appear to be successful in suppressing lactation in the immediate postpartum period when given in large doses of 2 to 4 mg or in multiple doses to a maximum of 10 times greater. Although they are produced in larger quantities by the mammary gland in vitro and in vivo, the role of prostaglandins is still not clear because these studies[105] are in conflict with previous results by Vorherr.[107] The practical application of this in-lactation failure has not been reported.

Milk-borne prostaglandins clearly survive in the environment of the infant's gastrointestinal tract and are delivered in an active form to peripheral organs. The significance of this remains under investigation.[108]

PRODUCTION OF HORMONES BY THE MAMMARY GLAND

Hormones synthesized by the mammary gland may have endocrine, autocrine, or paracrine effects within the mother. The chemical mediators known to be synthesized by the mammary gland are EGF, progesterone, prolactin, estrogens, and relaxin. Other hormones are transported to the gland.[109] These bioactive agents could have multiple roles in both the mother and the recipient infant. Insulin-like growth factors are found in high concentrations in colostrum and at lower levels in mature milk. Milk factors other than nutrients are thought to control specific developmental processes in the infant. Because infants survive and grow on formula, this latter point is difficult to prove. The actions of milk regulatory substances are much more important in at-risk infants than in full-term infants.

FEEDBACK INHIBITOR OF LACTATION (FIL)

The mammary gland is unique because, as an exocrine gland, it stores its secretion extracellularly. Storage within the gland's lumen suggests a local level of control on the rate of secretion.[15]

As stated earlier, milk is produced as long as it is removed from the mammary gland. Further, prolactin and oxytocin are responsible for the production and release of milk, allowing the infant to extract milk by suckling. The rate of milk secretion may differ between breasts if one breast is suckled more frequently or for a longer time. When lactating goats have an extra daily milking, the secretory rate is increased even if the milk is immediately replaced with an inert solution to maintain the gland's distention. The dilution of stored milk in the gland with an inert isotonic solution results in increased milk secretion, suggesting the dilution of a chemical inhibitor.

Identification of a factor that is produced and functions at the mammary level, a whey protein known as FIL, has evolved from multiple studies.[108] Wilde et al.[110] described autocrine regulation of milk secretion by a previously unknown protein in the milk. When this active whey protein, FIL, was isolated

and injected into the mammary gland of lactating goats, milk secretion was decreased temporarily.[111] FIL is able to exert reversible concentration-dependent autocrine inhibition on milk secretion in the lactating gland. It controls the secretion of all milk constituents simultaneously; that is, it affects secretion, not composition.[108]

The search for the mechanism that explains the regulation of the milk supply continues. When goats were studied, it was noted that when milk accumulated in the mammary gland, production decreased. When the milk was removed and replaced with isotonic sucrose solution to volume, the rate of milk produced increased. This finding supports the concept that it is a compound in the milk and not distention of the mammary gland that regulates synthesis. This factor, FIL, is an autocrine mechanism.

FIL cannot be the sole control of milk synthesis, or removal of milk would not stimulate milk production. Cregan and Hartmann speculate that the mechanism of local control of milk synthesis is related to the filling/emptying cycle of the alveoli[9] (see Fig. 3.21). Milk accumulation changes the morphology of the lactocytes lining the alveoli. When the luminal volume of mammospheres increased, according to Streuli and Edwards, it altered the interaction of the lactocytes with the basement membrane, inhibiting prolactin receptors and further milk synthesis.[112]

MATERNAL ADAPTATION TO LACTATION

The hormonal trigger for lactogenesis is a decrease in progesterone while prolactin levels are maintained. Postpartum prolactin levels are comparable in breastfeeding and nonbreastfeeding women for a few days (see Fig. 3.6). Thus, the basic process occurs regardless of whether breastfeeding is initiated. The mammary epithelium must be adequately prepared by the hormones of pregnancy to respond by synthesizing milk (see Figs. 3.3 and 3.7).

Each mammalian species has evolved its own lactational strategies to meet the nutritional needs of its offspring, with influences from both genetic and environmental forces. The endocrine signals promote mammary development; inhibit milk production during gestation; and then promote the development of enhanced metabolic and transport functions in adipose tissue, visceral organs, and reproductive organs.[108,113] Lactational adaptations of adipose tissue metabolism have been recognized in all species and may be most dramatic in seals, hibernating bears, and whales, which produce fat-rich milk from their fat stores while fasting. Lactation results in profound changes in adipose tissue metabolism to provide energy stores, modulate mammary development, affect appetite, and influence the function of the immune system.[3]

The substantial adaptation of the maternal intestine during lactation is the large increase in its size and complexity, which ensures adequate absorption of nutrients to meet the increased energy demand.[114] A corresponding increase occurs in liver and heart performance. In addition to extra fat demands, the calcium concentration must be sufficient to maintain maternal stores while providing for the demands of milk synthesis, which are greater than those of pregnancy.[115] The estimated calcium requirement is 12 mg/kg per day in humans. The elevation in plasma dihydroxycholecalciferol, or 1,25-(OH)2D3, during late gestation continues during early lactation. As lactation progresses beyond 3 months, plasma 1,25-(OH)2D3 levels decline. This results in decreased calcium absorption, which is offset by greater maternal bone losses and reduced urinary calcium. Glucose requirements during lactation require major adjustments in glucose production and utilization in the maternal liver, adipose tissue, bone, muscle, and other tissues. Adaptation of folic acid metabolism is equally important, although less well studied.[113]

The mechanisms by which early pregnancy and lactation decrease the incidence of breast cancer are unclear. Close examination of the more differentiated mammary cell, which is less susceptible to the loss of growth regulation, is a next step, along with examination of the role of mucin, a glycoprotein and normal differentiation antigen expressed in both milk-fat globules and mammary tumors.

DELAY IN THE ONSET OF LACTOGENESIS

Clinically, it has been observed that delayed lactogenesis occurs in women who have diabetes, are stressed during delivery, and occasionally experience retained placenta. When signs of lactogenesis are absent in the first 72 hours, a cause should be sought. In women with diabetes, extra effort should be made to ensure that the process goes well, with good hydration, adequate dietary intake, insulin control, and attention to detail. A study of the impact of cesarean delivery on lactogenesis II found that early pumping did not help and may have interfered with the volume of milk produced.[116] After stressful deliveries, it may be necessary to initiate pumping if the infant is unable to adequately stimulate the breast, but this needs further study. Again, close monitoring is essential before discharge. Retained placenta is discussed in Chapter 15. The treatment, dilatation and curettage, is definitive and dramatically therapeutic.

Anticipating problems and identifying early signals of faltering are key to ultimately improving lactogenesis.

SYNTHESIS OF HUMAN MILK

The function of the mammary gland is unique in that it produces a substance that makes tremendous demands on the maternal system without producing any physiologic advantage to the maternal organism. Because lactation is anticipated, the body prepares the breast anatomically and physiologically.[107] When lactation begins, the mother's metabolism changes greatly. The blood supply is redistributed, and the demand for nutrients increases, which requires an increased metabolic rate to accommodate their production. The mammary gland may need to produce milk at the metabolic expense of other organs. The supply of materials to the lactating breast for milk production and energy metabolism requires extensive cardiovascular

changes in the mother. There is increased mammary blood flow, increased blood flow into the gastrointestinal tract and liver, and a high cardiac output. The mammary blood flow, cardiac output, and milk secretion are suckling dependent. Suckling induces the release of anterior pituitary hormones that act directly on breast tissue.

Milk is isosmotic with plasma in all species.[11] Human milk differs from many other milks in that the concentration of major monovalent ions is lower and that of lactose is higher; in other milks, the higher the ions, the lower the lactose, and vice versa. Many disparities in the intermediary metabolism among species of animals can be linked to evolutionary adaptations involving the digestive process.[54] Nonruminants rely on glucose, derived from carbohydrate in the diet. Ruminants, because of extensive fermentation in the rumen, absorb little glucose. The microbial fermentation products, which include acetate, propionate, and butyrate, play a significant part as energy and carbon sources for tissue metabolism. Amino acids are primary substitutes for glucose in ruminants.[11]

Milk Synthesis at the Cellular Level

The biosynthesis of milk involves a cellular site where the metabolic processes occur. The epithelial cells of the gland contain stem cells and highly differentiated secretory alveolar cells at the terminal ducts. The stem cells are stimulated by hGH and insulin. Prolactin synergizes the insulin effect to stimulate the cells to secretory activity.

Prolactin binds to specific prolactin receptors on the surface of the lactocytes. There is a lactogenic signaling pathway that creates the "switching on" of the transcription of genes. These genes regulate the secretion of milk proteins, including casein and lactalbumin. The prolactin receptor is part of the cytokine-receptor family. These are activated at the onset of pregnancy and lactogenesis. The binding of prolactin to the site triggers the kinase and the chain of reactions of phosphorylation and activation of transcription[10] (Fig. 3.25).

The cells of the acini and smaller milk ducts are active in milk synthesis and milk secretion into the alveoli and smaller milk ducts. Most milk is synthesized during the process of suckling; its production is stimulated by prolactin. Cortisol plasma levels are increased during suckling as well. The secretory cells are cuboidal, changing to a cylindrical shape just before milk secretion, and cellular water uptake is increased. The cell's single nucleus is at the base in the dormant cell but migrates to the apex just before milk secretion.

The differentiated structure of the functional cell is acquired gradually during pregnancy, differing little from species to species. Very early in lactation, mammary cells show active synthesis and secretion of proteins and fat. The cells are polarized, with abundant rough endoplasmic reticulum and Golgi dictyosomes above the nucleus, which is smooth and rounded, with many mitochondria. The apical surface has microvilli, and the basal surface is extensively convoluted for the active transport of materials from the bloodstream into the cell. Fat droplets are in the cytoplasm and

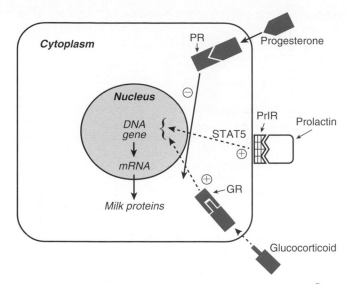

Prolactin and glucocorticoids up-regulate milk protein gene expression ⊕
Progesterone inhibits milk protein expression during pregnancy ⊖
PR = progesterone receptor, PrlR = prolactin receptor,
GR = glucocorticoid receptor

Fig. 3.25 Intracellular hormonal signaling in the lactocyte during lactation. (Adapted from Mercier JC, Gaye P. Milk protein synthesis. In: Mepham TB, ed. *Biochemistry of Lactation*. New York: Elsevier, 1983.)

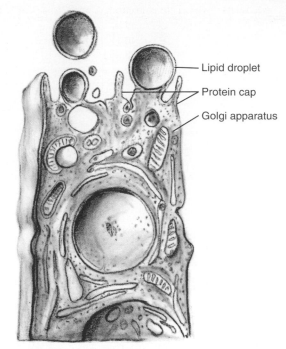

Fig. 3.26 Apocrine secretory mechanism for lipids, proteins, and lactose in milk.

bulging at the membrane. Proteins, lactose, calcium, phosphate, and citrate are packaged into secretory vesicles and pass into the lumen of the alveolus by exocytosis.

The cytoplasm is finely granular in the resting phase but striated as milk secretion begins. As secretion commences, the enlarged cell with its thickened apical membrane becomes clublike in shape. The tip pinches off, leaving the cell intact. The protein is thus free in the secreted solution, retaining a cap of membrane (Fig. 3.26).

Methods of Milk-Synthesis Measurement

Computerized breast measurement (CBM) was developed by Hartmann et al.[117] because of the inaccuracy of the established methods for measuring milk synthesis. The three other techniques utilized are (1) weighing either the infant or the mother before and after every feeding for 24 hours, (2) isotope dilution used to estimate production over a 4- or 7-day period, and (3) breast expression in which a mother removes milk from breasts (this technique does not reflect the effect of the infant on milk production by suckling). CBM is designed to measure short-term rates of milk synthesis. This technique allows the appetite of the infant to dictate the amount of milk removed from the breast while also allowing the measurement of the residual (Fig. 3.27).

CBM measures changes in breast volume without interfering with the infant's pattern of breastfeeding. CBM allows not only measurement of changes in breast volume and the volume of milk removed during a feeding but also four additional parameters.

The first is the short-term rate of milk synthesis (S) between breastfeedings. The calculation takes the increase in

breast volume from the end of one feeding (V_{B1}) to the beginning of the next (V_{B2}), divided by the time between these two measurements (T):

$$S = \frac{V_{B2} - V_{B1}}{T}$$

The second measures storage capacity (SC), which is defined by the authors as the maximum breast volume (V_{max}) minus the minimum breast volume (V_{min}) observed over a 24-hour period (see Fig. 3.27):

$$SC = V_{max} - V_{min}$$

The third measurement is the degree of fullness (F), which is the ratio of any particular breast volume (V_B) divided by the storage capacity of the breast (SC):

$$F = \frac{V_B}{SC}$$

The range of fullness (F) is from 1, when the breast is full, to 0, when it is at minimum volume, in a 24-hour period.

In addition, this CBM technology can be used to measure the increase in breast volume during pregnancy, thus measuring breast growth and breast involution after peak lactation.

The storage capacity was measured by Daly et al.[118] and varied from 80 to 600 mL. The rate of milk synthesis was minimal when the breast was full and maximum when the breast was emptied.

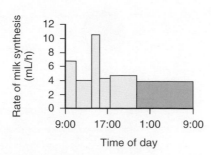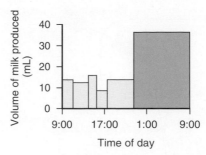

Fig. 3.27 Rate of milk synthesis and volume of milk produced in one breast by an exclusively expressing mother over a 24-hour period. The shaded columns indicate the overnight period that had the lowest rate of milk synthesis but the highest volume expressed. (From Cregan MD, Hartmann PE. Computerized breast measurement from conception to weaning: clinical implications. *J Hum Lact.* 1999;15:89.)

FUNCTION OF CELLULAR COMPONENTS OF THE LACTATING BREAST

The schema of the mammary secretory cell is represented in Figs. 3.28 and 3.29.

Nucleus

The nucleus is essential to the duplication of genetic material and the transcription of the genetic code.[119] The nucleus is also considered a regulatory organelle in cell metabolism, transmitting the design of the cell's enzymatic profile. The DNA and RNA content of the cellular nuclei increases during pregnancy and is highest during lactation.

Cytosol

The cytosol, which consists of the cytoplasm minus the mitochondrial and microsomal fractions, is also called the *particle-free supernatant.* The cytosol contains enzymes that involve key intermediates and cofactors essential to the process of milk synthesis.

Mitochondrial Proliferation

The alveolar cell population of the mammary gland must have a greatly expanded oxidative capacity during lactation. It is supplied by an increase in the size and function of the cell's mitochondrial population. Mitochondria are increased in the epithelial cell at the onset of the lactation process. Mitochondrial proliferation has been observed in all cells with a high metabolic rate and high oxygen utilization.

During the presecretory differentiation phase in late pregnancy and early lactation, each mitochondrion undergoes a type of differentiation in which the inner membrane and matrix expand greatly. As with other cells, the mitochondria are key to the respiratory activity of the cell. Mitochondria control some cellular metabolism through differential permeability to certain anions. The citrate in the mitochondria is a major source of carbon for fatty-acid biosynthesis. Mitochondria also supply the carbon for the synthesis of nonessential amino acids.

Microsomal Fraction

The microsomal fraction of the cell, which includes the Golgi apparatus, the endoplasmic reticulum, and the cell membranes, is involved in lipid synthesis. The role of the microsomal fraction is also to assemble the constituent parts (e.g., amino acids, glucose, fatty acids) into the final products of protein, carbohydrate, and fat for secretion.

INTERMEDIARY METABOLISM OF MAMMARY GLAND

The pathways identified for milk synthesis and secretion in the mammary alveolus, as described by Neville[12] include four major transcellular pathways and one paracellular pathway (Fig. 3.30):
1. Exocytosis of milk protein and lactose in Golgi-derived secretory vesicles
2. Milk fat secretion via the milk-fat globule
3. Secretion of ions and water across the apical membrane
4. Pinocytosis—exocytosis of immunoglobulins
5. Paracellular pathway for plasma components and leukocytes

CARBOHYDRATES

The major carbohydrate for most species is lactose, a disaccharide found only in milk. In addition to lactose, more than 50 oligosaccharides of different structures have been identified in human milk. One of the most important is glucose.

Glucose metabolism has a key function in milk production.[25] Glucose serves as the main source of energy for other reactions as well as a critical source of carbon. Glucose is critical to the volume of milk produced and is used in the production of lactose. The synthesis of lactose combines glucose and galactose, the latter originating from glucose-6-phosphate.[120]

Lactose synthesis is carried out by the following equations:

$$\mathrm{UDP - galactose} + N\text{-acetylglucosamine} \rightarrow \tag{3-1}$$
$$N\text{-acetyllactosamine} + \mathrm{UDP}$$

$$\mathrm{UDP - galactose + glucose \rightarrow lactose + UDP} \tag{3-2}$$

UDP is uridine diphosphogalactose. The catalyst in the first equation is a galactosyl transferase, *N*-acetyllactosamine

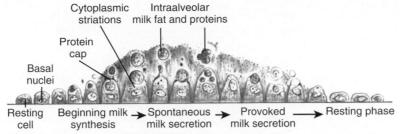

Fig. 3.28 Diagram of cycle of secretory cells from resting stage to secretion and return to resting stage. (Modified from Vorherr H. *The Breast: Morphology, Physiology and Lactation*. New York: Academic Press; 1974.)

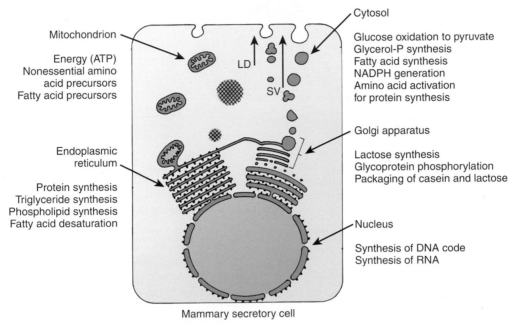

Fig. 3.29. Schema of cytologic and biochemical interrelationships of secretory cell of mammary gland. *LD,* Lipid droplet; *SV,* secretory vesicle.

synthetase. The reaction is activated by metal ions that bind to the galactosyl transferase.

Most of the intracellular glucose is derived from blood sugar. A specific whey protein, α-lactalbumin, catalyzes the lactose synthesis. It is a rate-limiting enzyme, which is inhibited by progesterone during pregnancy. In the absence of α-lactalbumin, little lactose is present. With the drop in progesterone and estrogen levels after the removal of the placenta at delivery, prolactin increases. The synthesis of α-lactalbumin becomes greater, and large amounts of lactose are produced from glucose. Progesterone regulates the onset of lactose synthesis, causing the initiation of production just as the infant needs nutrition.

Because lactose is synthesized only from glucose, maternal glucose utilization is increased by 30% in full lactation.[12]

Various aspects of lactose synthesis continue to be vigorously investigated.[3] The molecular mechanism of lactose synthesis is activated by metal ions, manganese (Mn), and calcium (Ca). Lactose synthesis takes place within the Golgi apparatus (see Fig. 3.30). The onset of copious milk secretion depends on the rapid increase of lactose synthesis. Lactose synthetase performs the rate-limiting step in lactose synthesis, which is one of the few anabolic reactions involving glucose itself rather than a phosphorylated derivative.[121] Although

progesterone, thyroxine, and lactogenic hormones are important in controlling synthesis, it is not known how they act in this system. The areas available for investigation about lactose synthesis remain vast.

FAT

Fat synthesis takes place in the endoplasmic reticulum. The alveolar cells are able to synthesize short-chain fatty acids, which are derived predominantly from acetate. Long-chain fatty acids, derived chiefly from blood plasma, are used in milk fat. Triglycerides are utilized from the plasma, as well as synthesized from intracellular glucose oxidized via the pentose pathway. The synthesis of fat from carbohydrate plays a predominant role in fat production in human milk.[122]

Two enzymes, lipoprotein lipase and palmitoyl-coenzyme A (CoA) L-glycerol-3-phosphate palmitoyl transferase, increase greatly after delivery. The lipase acts at the walls of the capillaries to catalyze the lipolysis and uptake of glycerol into the epithelial cells. The transferase catalyzes the process of synthesizing glycerides to triglycerides. It is believed that the marked increase of the lipase and transferase is stimulated by prolactin. Hormonal control of the glycerol precursors and the enzymatic release of fatty

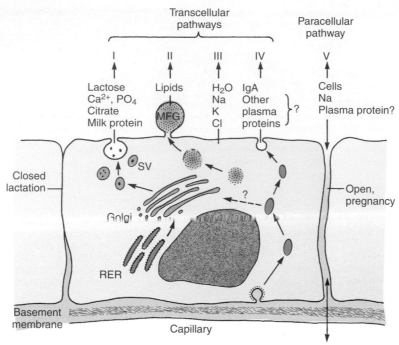

Fig. 3.30 Pathways for milk synthesis and secretion into mammary alveolus. **I,** Exocytosis of milk protein and lactose in Golgi-derived secretory vesicles. **II,** Milk-fat secretion via milk-fat globule. **III,** Secretion of ions and water across apical membrane. **IV,** Pinocytosis–exocytosis of immunoglobulins. **V,** Paracellular pathway for plasma components and leukocytes. *MFG,* Milk-fat globule; *RER;* rough endoplasmic reticulum; *SV,* secretory vesicle. (Modified from Neville MC. The physiological basis of milk secretion. Part I. Basic physiology. *Ann NY Acad Sci.* 1990;586:1.)

acids, leading to the formation of triglycerides, have been associated not only with prolactin but also with insulin, which stimulates the uptake of glucose into the mammary cells.

Esterification of fatty acids also takes place in the endoplasmic reticulum. The triglycerides subsequently accumulate into fat droplets in several cisternae. The small droplets sit on the base of the cell and coalesce to large droplets that move toward the apex of the cell. The fat droplets are engulfed in the apical membrane and project into the alveolar lumen. The discharge of fat droplets involves the bulging of the cell apex to envelop the fat globules, protein, and a small amount of cytoplasm; with the pinching off, the globule becomes detached into the lumen. The membrane of the fat globule contains all the normal plasma enzymes. The fat droplets contain predominantly polar lipid and phosphatidyl choline.

Fatty-acid synthesis involves a source of substrates and associated enzymes for their conversion to acetyl-CoA and reduced nicotinamide-adenine dinucleotide phosphate in the cytoplasm of the cell and the conversion of acetyl-CoA to malonyl-CoA. The newly synthesized fatty acid is then released from the fatty acid–synthetase complex.

Milk-Fat-Globule Membrane

The milk-fat-globule membrane in human milk serves several roles. A layer of amphophilic (bipolar) substances at the globule–skim milk interface is required for the maintenance of the emulsion stability of the fat globules.[122] This physiochemical fact applies to all emulsions and to the fat globules in the milk of all species. The globules and the milk-fat-globule membrane are compartments within the emulsion component of

milk. Once in place, the components of the milk-fat-globule membrane, which is the oil–water interfacial compartment, are more or less firmly held in place by a variety of chemical and electrical forces. The stabilizing membrane acts as a reactive barrier on the interface between the globule and milk serum.[122] It is rate controlling for the binding of enzymes and trace elements, the controlled release of the products of lipolysis, the transfer of polar materials into milk serum, the maintenance of emulsion stability by the prevention of globule fission, and the availability of fatty acids and cholesterol for micellar absorption in the small intestine. All these interactions are dynamic. The envelopment mechanism involves rapid turnover of the plasma membrane lipids and proteins during milk production.

Study of the RNA sequencing of the human fat layer transcription resulted in distinct gene-expression profiles in all stages of lactation: colostral, transitional, and mature milk production. The contribution of maternal physiology to problems with lactation is just being explored. It is known that human milk-fat globules, by enveloping cell contents as they are secreted into milk, are great sources of mammary cell RNA. Strong modulation of key genes is involved in lactose synthesis and insulin signaling. Protein tyrosine phosphatase is thought to serve as a biomarker linking insulin resistance to insufficient milk supply.

PROTEIN

Most proteins in milk are formed from free amino acids in the secretory cells of the mammary gland. The definitive data confirming the origin of milk proteins have been accumulated since 1980. The vast majority of proteins present in normal milk are specific to mammary secretions and are not identified in any quantity elsewhere in nature.[53]

Genetic Control of Protein Synthesis

The formation of milk protein and mammary enzymes is induced by prolactin and further stimulated by insulin and cortisol. De novo synthesis of protein uses both essential and non-essential plasma amino acids. Nuclear RNA, induced by prolactin, stimulates the synthesis of mRNA and transfer RNA (tRNA). The mRNA conveys the genetic information to the protein-synthesizing centers of the cells. The tRNA interprets the message to assemble the amino acids in the appropriate sequence of polypeptide chains of the specific milk proteins. The newly synthesized proteins are secreted into the milk during lactation. Casein, α-lactalbumin, and β-lactoglobulin from plasma amino acids are synthesized on the ribosomes of the endoplasmic reticulum, where they are condensed and appear as visible secretory granules moving toward the cellular apex.

The synthesis of proteins in the mammary gland follows the general pathway of all proteins under genetic control. The induction of synthesis is under hormonal control. This process involves synthesis from amino acids through the detailed system controlled by RNA and under the genetic control of DNA. Glucocorticoid is required for the expression of the casein gene in the presence of prolactin. Cortisol is the limiting factor for casein gene expression.[112] Shennan[123] has reviewed the mechanisms of mammary gland ion transport.

Golgi Complex and Protein Synthesis

After some processing, the proteins pass to the Golgi complex, where they are further glycosylated and phosphorylated and then placed in secretory vesicles for export.[12] α-lactalbumin, a protein necessary for lactose synthesis by the enzyme galactosyltransferase, is among the proteins synthesized in the mammary gland. Lactose is synthesized within the trans-Golgi complex and secreted together with the major milk proteins. The casein micelle is formed with calcium within the Golgi compartment, which presents a high concentration of calcium, phosphate, and protein via the milk. Most of the casein is bound in this manner. This pathway I (see Fig. 3.30) begins in the rough endoplasmic reticulum, where the proteins are inserted through the membrane into the lumen by exocytosis.[12]

The Golgi membrane is impermeable to lactose; thus, the sugar is osmotically active. Water is drawn into the Golgi apparatus.[112] Casein micelle formation begins in the terminal Golgi vesicles, adding calcium in the secretory vesicle. These secretory vesicles move to the plasma membrane and, through exocytosis, extrude their contents into the alveolar lumen.[124]

Human casein micelles are smaller in size (30 to 75 nm in diameter) than bovine casein (600 nm). Human milk contains only β-casein. Only 6% of the calcium in human milk is bound to casein, compared with 65% in bovine milk. The gene for human β-casein has been cloned and sequenced.[112]

Some merocrine secretion also occurs, in which proteins and other cellular constituents are secreted, leaving the cell

TABLE 3.3 Alveolar Epithelial Membrane Permeability	
Cell ↔ Alveolar Lumen	Cell → Alveolar Lumen
Glucose	Lactose
Water	Sucrose
Sodium	Citrate
Potassium	Proteins
Chloride	Fat
Iodine	Calcium
Sulfate	Phosphate

membrane intact. Protein caps, or signets, protruding into alveolar lumen, have been described on the outside of the apical membrane. Protein and lactose secreted into the lumen cannot be reabsorbed (Table 3.3).

IONS AND WATER

Sodium, potassium, chloride, magnesium, calcium, phosphate, sulfate, and citrate pass through the membrane of the alveolar cell in both directions.[27] Water also passes in both directions, predominantly from the alveolar cells but also from the interstitial fluid. Plasma water passage depends on the amount of intracellular glucose available for lactose. The aqueous phase of milk is isosmotic to plasma.[125] The major osmole of the aqueous phase of milk is lactose. The concentrations of sodium and chloride are less than those in plasma.

Human milk differs from that of many other species in that the monovalent ions are in low concentration, and lactose is in high concentration.[124] The osmolarity is the same, that is, isosmotic with plasma; thus, the higher the lactose, the lower the ions. It is presumed that the intracellular concentration of potassium is held high, and that of sodium low, by a pump on the basal membrane. The sodium and potassium ions are distributed according to the electrical potential gradient.[27] Milk is electrically positive compared with intracellular fluid. The sodium/potassium ratio is 1:3 in both milk and intracellular fluid. Vorherr[27,107] thinks that lactose secretion is responsible for the potential difference across the apical membrane, thus keeping sodium and potassium ion concentrations low.

The variation among species in the concentration of lactose and ions is caused by the rate of lactose synthesis, the permeability of the membrane, and the number of fixed negative charges on the membrane. The potential difference is higher in the human mammary gland than in any other species evaluated to date.

Infrastructure Changes for Milk Synthesis

The relationship between infrastructure and function in the mammary gland changes from pregnancy to lactation. The junction between alveolar cells has attracted much interest. Cell junctions do not merely hold cells together but enable epithelia to function as permeable barriers, allowing communication between cells and coordination of activities. The three functions of cell junctions are adhesion, occlusion, and communication, which are carried out by desmosomes, tight junctions, and gap junctions, respectively. Changes in tight junctions may provide the basis for a reduction in permeability between cells. For instance, at the initiation of lactation, a tight junction changing from "leaky" to very tight blocks the paracellular movement of lactose and ions. This requires transport across cells of these materials and the maintenance of control of high intracellular potassium and low intracellular sodium concentrations.[126]

Importance of Citrate in Lactogenesis

Citrate is thought to be the harbinger of lactogenesis. Citrate plays a central role in the metabolism of all cells, but its significance and mode of secretion remain unknown.[127] In the final stages of lactogenesis in ruminants, the previously quiescent epithelial cells suddenly start to secrete large quantities of protein, fat, and carbohydrates. The exact lactogenic trigger is unknown, although significant hormonal changes occur. In women, the onset of copious milk secretion does not begin until 3 to 4 days postpartum. Significantly, citrate levels are low at delivery and rise quickly, reaching a peak on day 4.[126] In cows and goats, copious production occurs at delivery, and the citrate levels begin to rise, increasing to 10 to 100 times the baseline values.

Citrate is the main buffer system of milk.[27] It is formed within the secretory cell, but how it is secreted into the milk is not clear. Citrate and lactose may be secreted by a similar route. After dilution of milk in the gland with isosmotic lactose, the equilibrium is restored across the apical membrane in experimental models by the entrance of sodium, potassium, and chloride into the milk. No citrate, calcium, or protein enters in excess of the normal secretion rate. Inorganic phosphate is the other major buffer system, but how it is secreted is also unknown.

Calcium, much of which is bound to casein, enters the Golgi apparatus, where it is essentially trapped with casein in the micelle, and then enters the alveolar milk by unidirectional flow.

The mammary gland is unusual among exocrine glands because the rate of secretion slows, and some secretions can be stored in its ducts.[122] Direct neural control of secretion is lacking. The parenchyma of the gland also consists of ductal tissue in addition to secretory tissue. The ductal cells, however, are impermeable to the major milk ions during lactation, so in contrast to the ductal cells of other exocrine glands (e.g., sweat, salivary), they cannot modify the secretion.

A comparison of the levels of various constituents of the milk with corresponding plasma levels can demonstrate the probable mechanism responsible for that difference in constituent levels, that is, by passive diffusion or positive or negative pump (see Table 4.18).

MILK ENZYMES

Some milk enzymes enter the alveolar milk from the mammary blood capillaries via the intercellular fluid. Others come from the breakdown of the mammary secretory cells. The milk enzymes, xanthine oxidase, aldolase, and alkaline phosphatase, are contained in the fat globule, membrane, and milk serum. The most significant enzyme, lipase, splits triglycerides.

Human milk contains both proteolytic enzymes and protease inhibitors.[128] Amylase facilitates the digestion of polysaccharides by the infant. Sulfhydryl oxidase catalyzes the oxidation of sulfhydryl groups. Glutathione peroxidase facilitates the delivery of selenium to the infant. Lysozyme and peroxidase are bactericidal.

CELLULAR COMPONENTS

Human milk has been called a *live fluid* by many and *white blood* in many ancient rites. Breast milk contains up to 4000 cells/mL, which have been identified with leukocytes and enter the milk via the paracellular pathway, pathway V.[119] The cell number is particularly high in colostrum. The cells in greatest number are the macrophages, which secrete lysozyme and lactoferrin. Lymphocytes, neutrophils, and epithelial cells are also present. Lymphocytes produce IgA and interferon.

Macrophages constitute a major cellular component in milk compared with levels in blood and can survive under conditions simulating the infant's gastrointestinal tract.[129] Because they release secretory IgA in association with phagocytosis, it is thought they play a role in host defense. Macrophage colony-stimulating factors in human milk and mammary gland epithelial cells are thought to be responsible for the expansion of the macrophages in milk.

INVOLUTION: WEANING AND APOPTOSIS

During weaning, significant increases in milk protein, chloride, and sodium concentrations and a decrease in lactose occur when milk volumes fall below 400 mL per day. Glucose and magnesium levels are unchanged.[15] This suggests that volume is regulated differently during weaning than during lactogenesis. No sentinel substance is a reliable predictor of volume in all stages, but normal ranges of milk components during full lactation are as follows: sodium, 3 to 18 mmol/L; chloride, 8 to 24 mmol/L; protein, 8 to 23 g/L; and lactose, 140 to 230 mmol/L. Values outside these ranges suggest mastitis or weaning. During gradual weaning, between 6 and 15 months postpartum, glucose, citrate, phosphate, and calcium levels decrease, whereas lipid, potassium, and magnesium increase.[2]

Postlactational involution of the mammary gland is characterized by two distinct physiologic processes.[61] First, secretory epithelial cells undergo apoptosis and programmed cell death. Second, the mammary gland's basement membrane undergoes proteolytic degradation. Apoptosis is almost absent during lactation but develops within 2 days of involution. In the initial phase of involution, apoptosis of fully differentiated mammary epithelial cells occurs without visible degradation of the extracellular matrix. The second phase consists of extracellular remodeling and altered mesenchymal-epithelial interactions, followed by apoptosis of cells no longer differentiating.[130]

During postlactational mammary gland involution, most mammary epithelium dies and is reabsorbed.

In experimental models, apoptosis has been studied at weaning by using animals, removing the pups from the breast and studying the biochemical and genetic markers. Regulation of apoptosis during mammary gland involution is multifunctional. Forced weaning is used as a tool to accelerate and synchronize the involution process, thus allowing biochemical analysis. Apoptosis phenotypes resulting from specific gene deletions have been identified when these animal mothers are unable to nurse their pups.

When suckling ceases after lactation, the alveolar component of the gland involutes through a process that involves both apoptosis and tissue remodeling, which reconstructs the gland to the prepregnancy state. In situations of forced weaning, two phases occur. An initial apoptotic phase begins within 12 hours and persists for approximately 72 hours. The second phase involves further apoptosis, matrix degradation, and gland remodeling. The first phase of involution before apoptosis is reversible, and lactation can be reinstated within 2 days. During this time, milk accumulates within the alveolar lumen, and the levels of lactogenic hormones drop. The initiation of apoptosis and the degradation of nuclear DNA into fragments is the best-understood phase of the process. The second phase begins, in which the gland remodeling takes place. The old connective tissue and the basement membrane are removed, and then the ductal component is re-formed. Apoptosis continues through this phase. High levels of tissue inhibitors of metalloproteinases are expressed, preventing excess matrix metalloproteinase activity.[14]

Significant advances have been made in the knowledge of signaling pathways that regulate epithelial cell apoptosis in the first phase. The precise nature of the triggers for apoptosis and the ultimate perpetrators of cell death are unknown. The available information suggests a complex network of signal transduction pathways that control apoptosis in the involuting mammary gland.[131]

SUMMARY

In humans, lactogenesis occurs slowly over the first few days postpartum as progesterone levels drop. Women experience "milk coming in" as a feeling of fullness between 40 and 72 hours postpartum, usually corresponding to the degree of parity, with multiparas sensing this more quickly than primiparas. The physiologic explanation of the increase in milk volume, however, suggests that the sensation of "milk coming in" is not "normal" but a sign of overshooting the mark. Some women do not sense this special fullness but are excellent milk producers. The volume of milk increases over time for the first 2 weeks, starting at less than 100 mL per day and increasing to approximately 600 mL per day at 96 hours (Fig. 3.31). This parallels the rise in citrate production, reflecting the metabolic activity of the mammary gland. Lactose, sodium chloride, and protein rise promptly, stabilizing at 24 hours and reflecting the closure of the pericellular pathway, which results in a decrease in direct flux into the milk.

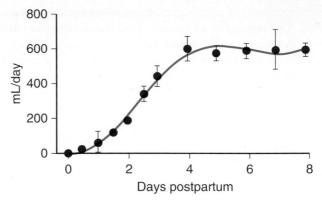

Fig. 3.31 Milk volumes during the first week postpartum. Mean values from 12 multiparous white women who test-weighed their infants before and after every feeding for the first 7 days postpartum. (Redrawn from Neville MC. Determinants of milk volume and composition. In: Jensen RG, ed. *Handbook of Milk Composition*. San Diego: Academic Press; 1995.)

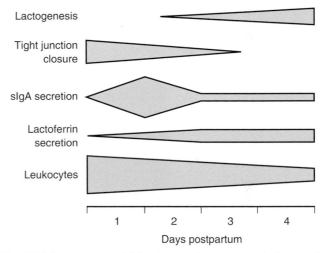

Fig. 3.32 Summary model for temporal sequence of changes in mammary gland function during lactogenesis in women. (From Neville MC. Determinants of milk volume and composition. In: Jensen RG, ed. *Handbook of Milk Composition*. San Diego: Academic Press; 1995.)

This suggests a two-step process of junctional closure followed by the onset of secretory activity.

The changes in the permeability of the tight junctions; rate of synthesis of lactose, lipids, and nutrient proteins; transport of glucose into the alveolar cells; transcytosis of secretory IgA; movement of immune cells into the alveolar lumen; and secretion of lactoferrin represent the distinct metabolic and cellular modifications. Neville[25] states, "The temporal sequence of these changes as they occur during lactogenesis suggests that they are either independently regulated or form part of an orderly cascade of temporally separate events." Fig. 3.32 graphically illustrates these changes.

The use of new molecular techniques and the use of mutant animals with transgenic technology have advanced the understanding of human milk and the physiology of lactation. The regulation of mammary gland development has been demonstrated to depend not only on various hormones but also their receptors, the signaling proteins such as protein kinases and transcription factors, as well as DNA-binding proteins. The field is advancing rapidly. Signaling pathways are being identified, and the target genes of many regulatory pathways are being sought.

The Reference list is available at www.expertconsult.com.

4

Biochemistry of Human Milk

Ruth A. Lawrence

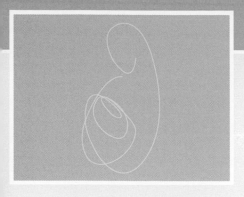

KEY POINTS

- Human milk is a highly complex composition of nutrients for infant growth, consisting primarily of fat, carbohydrates, and proteins, as well as minerals, vitamins, and other nutrients.
- The delicate balance of nutrients and the dynamic lactation process make human milk the only food substance during life that is adequate as the sole source of nutrition.

- The biochemistry of human milk changes throughout the stages of breastfeeding and as a function of infant needs and demands.
- Research continues to reveal the components of human milk and its functions and benefits for infant nutrition and lifelong health.

Human milk was considered a heavenly elixir, a living fluid. It was not until the end of the 18th century that chemical methods became available to decipher the content of milk. The biochemistry of human milk encompasses a mammoth supply of scientific data and information, most of which have been generated since 1970. Each report or study adds a tiny piece to the complex puzzle of the nutrients that make up human milk. The answers to some questions still elude us. A question as simple as the volume of milk consumed at a feeding remains a scientific challenge. The methodology must be accurate, reproducible, noninvasive, and suitable for home use night or day and must not interrupt breastfeeding. The precision analysis available for measuring the concentration of the most minuscule of elements, however, is remarkably accurate and reproducible in the laboratory. Milk has been demystified by laboratory chemistry.[1]

Advances in analytic methods bring greater sensitivity, resolving power, and speed to the analysis of milk composition. Previously unknown and unrecognized compounds have been detected. We now know milk provides both nutrients and nonnutritive signals to the neonate. With few exceptions, all milks contain the nutrients for physical growth and development. When the offspring develops rapidly, the milk is nutrient dense; when it develops slowly, the milk is more dilute. All milks contain fat, carbohydrates, and proteins, as well as minerals, vitamins, and other nutrients. The organization of milk composition includes lipids in emulsified globules coated with a membrane, colloidal dispersions of proteins as micelles, and the remainder as a true solution.[2] At no other time in life is a single food adequate as the sole source of nutrition.

The discussion in this chapter focuses predominantly on information perceived as immediately useful to the clinician. Considerable detail and species variability are overlooked to

help focus attention on details directly influencing management. Extensive and exhaustive reviews are referenced to provide the reader with easy access to greater detail and validation of the general conclusions reported here.

Human milk is not a uniform body fluid but a secretion of the mammary gland of changing composition (Fig. 4.1). The first drops at the beginning of a feeding differ from the last drops. Colostrum differs from transitional and mature milks. Milk changes with the time of day and as time goes by. As concentrations of protein, fat, carbohydrates, minerals, and cells differ, physical properties such as osmolarity and pH change. The impact of changing composition on the physiology of the infant gut is beginning to be appreciated. Many constituents have dual roles, not only nutrition but also infection protection, immunity, or a host of other effects.

The more than 200 constituents of milk include a tremendous array of molecules, descriptions of which continue to be refined as qualitative and quantitative laboratory techniques are perfected. Resolution of lipid chemicals has advanced dramatically in recent years, but new carbohydrates and proteins have been identified as well. Some of the compounds identified may well be intermediary products in the process that occurs within the mammary cells and may be only incidental in the final product.[3] Milk includes true solutions, colloids, membranes, membrane-bound globules, and living cells.

Human and bovine milks are known in the greatest detail; however, much information exists about the milk of rats and mice, as well as five other species: the water buffalo, goat, sheep, horse, and pig. Several are listed in Table 4.1. Miscellaneous data are available on the milk of 150 more species, but almost no data are available for another 4000 species. Jenness and Sloan have compiled a summary of 140 species from which a sampling has been extracted (Table 4.2). The constituents of

Formula vs. human milk

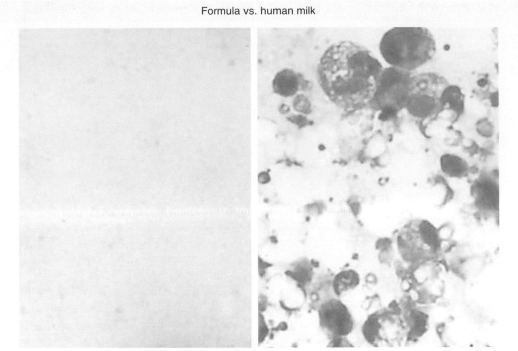

Fig. 4.1 A comparison of formula *(left)* and human milk *(right)*. Human milk is a dynamic colloidal solution of perfect nutrients and growth factors for the infant. Formula is a totally homogenized solution of nutrient chemicals. (Courtesy Nancy Wight, MD, San Diego, California.)

TABLE 4.1   Composition of Milks Obtained From Different Mammals and Growth Rate of Their Offspring

Species	Days Required to Double Birth Weight	CONTENT OF MILK (%)			
		Fat	Protein	Lactose	Ash
Human	180	3.8	0.9	7.0	0.2
Horse	60	1.9	2.5	6.2	0.5
Cow	47	3.7	3.4	4.8	0.7
Reindeer	30	16.9	11.5	2.8	—
Goat	19	4.5	2.9	4.1	0.8
Sheep	10	7.4	5.5	4.8	1.0
Rat	6	15.0	12.0	3.0	2.0

From Hambraeus L. Proprietary milk versus human breast milk in infant feeding: a critical appraisal from the nutritional point of view. *Pediatr Clin North Am.* 1977;24:17.

milk can be divided into the following groups, according to their specificity:
1. Constituents specific to both organ and species (e.g., most proteins and lipids)
2. Constituents specific to organ but not to species (e.g., lactose)
3. Constituents specific to species but not to organ (e.g., albumin, some immunoglobulins)

As Wu et al.[4] note, over 60% of studies investigating the nutrient composition of human milk occurred before 1990, and further research is clearly needed. Nevertheless, this chapter demonstrates that human milk, with its elegant complexity and dynamic mechanisms of action, remains the best option for infant nutrition.

NORMAL VARIATIONS IN HUMAN MILK

In defining the constituents of human milk, it is important to recognize that the composition varies with the stage of lactation, the time of day, the sampling time during a given feeding, maternal nutrition, and individual variation. Many early interpretations of the content of human milk were based on spot samples or even pooled samples from multiple donors at different times and stages of lactation. Samples obtained by pumping may vary from those obtained by the suckling infant because some variation exists in content among the various methods of pumping. Banked donor milk differs from freshly expressed, mature milk in nutrient content and energy value.[5]

TABLE 4.2   Constituents of Milk (g/100 g) of Specific Mammals

Mammalian Species (in Taxonomic Position)	Total Solids	Fat	Casein	Whey Protein	Total Protein	Lactose	Ash
Human	12.4	3.8	0.4	0.6	—	7.0	0.2
Baboon	14.4	5.0	—	—	1.6	7.3	0.3
Orangutan	11.5	3.5	1.1	0.4	—	6.0	0.2
Black bear	44.5	24.5	8.8	5.7	—	0.4	1.8
California sea lion	52.7	36.5	—	—	13.8	0.0	0.6
Black rhinoceros	8.1	0.0	1.1	0.3	—	6.1	0.3
Spotted dolphin	31.0	18.0	—	—	9.4	0.6	—
Domestic dog	23.5	12.9	5.8	2.1	—	3.1	1.2
Norway rat	21.0	10.3	6.4	2.0	—	2.6	1.3
Whitetail jackrabbit	40.8	13.9	19.7	4.0	—	1.7	1.5

Modified from Jenness R, Sloan RE. Composition of milk. In: Larson BL, Smith VR, eds. *Lactation, Vol. 3, Nutrition and Biochemistry of Milk/Maintenance.* New York: Academic Press; 1974.

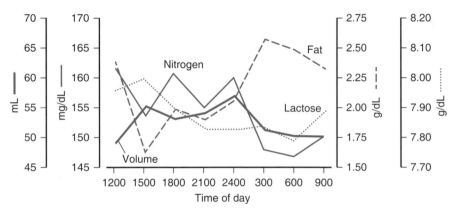

Fig. 4.2 Mean concentrations of nitrogen, lactose, and fat in human milk by time of day. (Modified from Brown KH, Black RE, Robertson AD, et al. Clinical and field studies of human lactation: methodological considerations. *Am J Clin Nutr.* 1982;35:745.)

Daytime consumption of milk in a given infant varies between 46% and 58% of the total 24-hour consumption, so that reliance on less than a 24-hour sampling may be misleading. Data from samples taken every 3 hours showed a variation in milk concentration of nitrogen, lactose, and fat, and in the volume of milk, by time of day (Fig. 4.2). Furthermore, statistically significant diurnal changes occurred in the concentration of lactose and in the volume within individual subjects, but the times of those changes were not consistent for each individual. Some individuals varied as much as two-fold in volume production from day to day. A significant difference in the concentrations of both fat and lactose and the volume of milk produced by each breast was also found. At the extreme, the less productive breast yielded only 65% of the volume of the other breast.

The variation in fat content has received some attention. Fat content changes during a given feeding, increasing as the feeding progresses, as shown in Fig. 4.3. Early studies, when

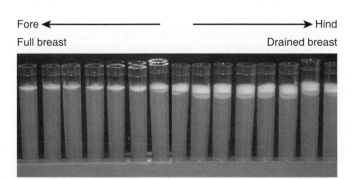

Fig. 4.3 Serial samples of breast milk collected during breast expression with an electric pump (15 minutes, samples at 1-minute intervals). The fat content increases over the course of breast expression, from *left* to *right*, from "full breast" to "drained breast" and foremilk to hindmilk. (From Jones E, King C. *Feeding and Nutrition in the Preterm Infant.* London: Churchill Livingstone; 2006.)

feeding times were controlled, reported an increase in fat content from early morning to midday. Multiple studies in different countries and different decades, summarized by Jackson et al., reveal that some of the variation is related to other factors (Fig. 4.4). Demand feeding (mothers in 1988 in Thailand) has a different circadian variation than scheduled feeding (mothers in 1932 in the United States; see Fig. 4.4). In the later part of the first year of lactation, fat content diminishes. Work done by Atkinson et al.[6] that was confirmed by other investigators showed that the nitrogen content of the milk of mothers who deliver prematurely is higher than that of those whose pregnancies reach full term. For a given volume of milk, the premature infant would receive 20% more nitrogen than the full-term infant if each were fed his or her own mother's milk. Other constituents of milk produced by mothers who deliver prematurely have also been studied. Some milk banks now provide donor milk from mothers who have delivered prematurely.

Variation by Measurement Method

An additional consideration in reviewing the information available on the levels of various constituents of milk is the technique used to derive the data. In 1975 Hambraeus reported less protein in human milk than originally calculated (see Table 4.1). The present techniques of immunoassay measure the absolute amounts; earlier figures were derived from calculations based on measurements of the nitrogen content. Of the nitrogen in human milk, 25% is nonprotein nitrogen (NPN). Cow milk has only 5% NPN.

Variation Related to Mother's Diet

A major concern about variation in the content of human milk is related to the mother's diet. Maternal diet is of particular concern when the mother is malnourished or eats an unusually restrictive diet. Malnourished mothers have approximately the same proportions of protein, fat, and carbohydrate as well-nourished mothers, but they produce less milk. Levels of water-soluble vitamins, such as ascorbic acid, thiamin, and vitamin B_{12}, are quickly affected by deficient diets. "From a nutritional perspective, infancy is a critical and vulnerable period. At no other stage in life is a single food adequate as a sole source of nutrition," writes Picciano.[7] This results from the immaturity of the tissues and organs involved in the metabolism of nutrients, which limits the ability to respond to nutrition excesses and deficiencies. The system is species-specific and depends on the presence of the self-contained enzymes and ligands to facilitate digestion at the proper stage while preserving function (e.g., secretory immunoglobulin A [sIgA]). The system continues to facilitate absorption and utilization.

In addition to variation of milk composition by genetics, diet, and lifestyle, Gómez-Gallego et al. found that mere geographic location affected the metabolic profile of breast milk and its microbiome. As a result, it is important to consider the interplay of microbes and human milk metabolites.[8]

Mother's milk is recommended for all infants under ordinary circumstances, even if the mother's diet is not perfect,

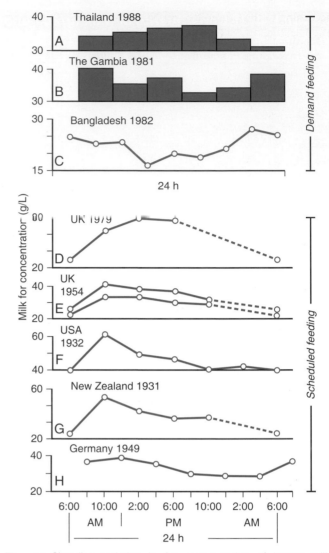

Fig. 4.4 Circadian variation in fat concentration of breast milk from published studies. (A) Thailand: Prefeed/postfeed expressed samples, 19 mothers studied for 24 hours each, infants aged 1 to 9 months. (B) The Gambia: Demand feeding, pre-/post-expressed samples, 16 mothers studied for 24 hours each, infants aged 1 to 18 months. (C) Bangladesh (Brown et al.): Samples collected at scheduled intervals by total breast extraction (breast pump), seven mothers studied for 24 hours each, infants aged 1 to 9 months. (D) United Kingdom (Jensen): Prefeed/postfeed expressed samples, one mother studied for 72 hours. (E) United Kingdom (Hytten): Samples collected by total breast extraction (breast pump). *Lower curve,* 29 mothers studied for 24 hours each, infants aged 3 to 8 days. *Upper curve,* 20 mothers studied for 24 hours each, infants aged 21 days to 4 months. (F) United States (Nims et al.): Samples collected by total breast extraction (manual), three mothers studied, but values given only for one mother, for 24 hours on six occasions and 72 hours on one occasion, infant aged 6 to 60 weeks. (G) New Zealand (Deem): Samples collected by total breast extraction (manual), 28 mothers studied for 24 hours each, infants aged 1 to 8 months. (H) Germany (Gunther and Stainier): Collection of samples by total breast extraction (manual), two mothers studied for 24 hours each, six mothers studied for 52 hours each, infants aged 8 to 11 days. (Modified from Jackson DA, Imong SM, Silprasert A, et al. Circadian variation in fat concentration of breast milk in a rural northern Thai population. *Br J Nutr.* 1988;59:349; see article for complete bibliography.)

according to the Committee on Nutrition During Pregnancy and Lactation of the Institute of Medicine.[9]

STAGES OF LACTATION

Two distinct phases of breast changes occur during pregnancy, which have been identified as mammogenesis and lactogenesis I. Mammogenesis is the developmental differentiation that begins in early pregnancy. It includes the proliferation of the ductal tree, which results in the sprouting of multiple alveoli.

Mammogenesis results in the enlargement of the breast during pregnancy as a result of the proliferation of the ductoalveolar structure. Careful study of this development has been documented utilizing computerized breast measurement, first reported by Cox et al.[10] in 1999. Computerized breast measurement is an accurate, noninvasive technology that is being used to determine changes in the size of human breasts (see Chapter 7). A longitudinal study using computerized breast measurement from before conception through pregnancy and lactation showed that growth began at week 10 of pregnancy. It was found that seven of eight women studied had an increase in breast size of about 170 mL, with considerable individual variation in the rate of change. Most women continued this growth immediately postpartum; at 1 month postpartum, they had an average 211 mL of growth. The authors correlated this growth through pregnancy with an increase in placental lactogen.[10]

Stage I lactogenesis is the onset of milk secretion and begins with the early changes in the mammary gland during pregnancy and continues until full lactation has occurred after delivery. Stage I begins when small quantities of milk components, such as casein and lactose, are secreted (prepartum milk). This amount is held in check by high levels of circulating progesterone. The first milk obtained by the newborn at birth is called *colostrum*. Lactogenesis stage II begins when the secretion of milk becomes copious. The milk produced in the first 10 days, when dramatic changes in composition and volume are occurring, is called *transitional milk*. Lactogenesis stage III begins with the establishment of mature milk production, more consistent in composition and volume, approximately days 10 to 14. (Fig. 4.5). Neville et al.[11] state that the terms *colostrum* and *transitional milk* do not describe the mammary secretion product during the first 4 days or from days 4 to 10 postpartum. It has always been recognized that the content changes rapidly in the first 4 days and then more slowly in the next 6 days or so, as a continuum. They suggest the abandonment of these terms. *Colostrum* and *transitional milk* remain convenient clinical terms.

Prepartum Milk

Prepartum milk is produced in early lactogenesis stage I before birth and is especially conspicuous in other species, such as the goat.[12] It provides evidence that the junctions between alveolar cells are "leaky" during pregnancy, allowing fluid and solutes to flow between the milk space and the interstitial fluid of the mammary gland.[13] Fig. 4.6 illustrates the

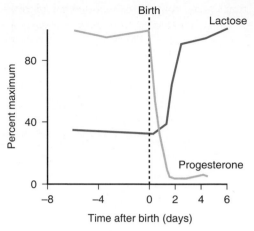

Fig. 4.5 Progesterone withdrawal initiates lactogenesis II in women. The increase in lactose concentrations associated with increased synthesis of milk components coincides with a rapid decrease in progesterone concentration when the placenta is removed at parturition. (Modified from Kulski JK, Harman PE, Martin JD, et al. Effects of bromocriptine mesylate on the composition of the mammary secretion in non-breastfeeding women. *Obstet Gynecol.* 1978;52:38; Czank C, Henderson JJ, Kent JC, et al. Hormonal control of lactation cycle. In: Hale TW, Hartmann PE, eds. *Textbook of Lactation.* Amarillo, TX: Hale Publishing; 2007.)

flow of macronutrients and some electrolytes in the breast leading to the composition of this milk in humans. The lactose concentration is directly correlated with that of potassium, but sodium and chloride are inversely related to lactose concentration. The dramatic changes in the composition of milk from prepartum to mature milk are detailed in (Tables 4.3 through 4.7). The concentration of fat in prepartum secretion is only 1 g/dL and has a different composition of lipids compared with later milk. Prepartum milk is 93% triglycerides and contains higher amounts of cell-membrane components, such as phospholipids, cholesterol, and cholesterol esters.

Colostrum

The stages in the continuum of human milk after birth in traditional nomenclature are *colostrum, transitional milk*, and *mature milk*, and their relative contents are significant for newborns and their physiologic adaption to extrauterine life.

Properties of Colostrum

The mammary secretion during the first few days consists of a yellowish, thick fluid: colostrum. The residual mixture of materials present in the mammary glands and ducts at delivery and immediately after is progressively mixed with newly secreted milk, forming colostrum. Human colostrum is known to differ from mature milk in composition, both in the nature of its components and in the relative proportions of these components. The first changes are in sodium and chloride concentrations and an increase in lactose, probably as a result of the closure of the tight junctions. The specific gravity of colostrum is 1.040 to 1.060. The mean energy value is 67 kcal/dL compared with 75 kcal/dL for mature milk. The volume varies between 2 and 20 mL per feeding in the first 3 days. The total volume per day also depends on the number

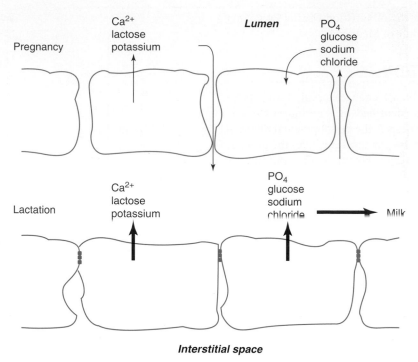

Fig. 4.6 Model for directions of major fluxes of several macronutrients during pregnancy and lactation in women. (From Neville MC. Determinants of milk volume and composition. In: Jensen RG, ed. *Handbook of Milk Composition.* San Diego: Academic Press; 1995.)

of feedings and is reported to average 100 mL in the first 24 hours (which is different from the first day, depending on the time of delivery; see Table 4.4). Tables 4.5 and 4.6 list the yield and composition of colostrum (1 to 5 days) and mature milk (14 days and beyond). The increased production of citrate is paralleled by the increase in volume (Figs. 4.7 and 4.8). The result is a decrease in sodium and chloride as a result of water dilution and an increase in lactose production over the same time.[13,14]

The antepartum milk glucose level is 0.35 ± 0.16 mmol/L (see Table 4.3). Glucose levels vary among individuals. Glucose decreases during a feed as the aqueous phase decreases and

lipid increases. In early colostrum, glucose passes into the milk via the paracellular pathway and parallels lactose. When lactation is fully established, glucose levels are unrelated to lactose levels.[9] In mature milk, the glucose level is 1.5 ± 0.4 mmol/L.

Supply as a Function of Infant Demand

Dewey et al.[15] clearly demonstrate that in a well-established milk supply, volume depends on infant demand, and the residual milk available in the breast after each feeding is comparable in both low-intake and average-intake dyads. Infant birth weight, weight at 3 months, and total time nursing were positively associated with intake. The volume also varies with

TABLE 4.3   Composition of Prepartum Human Milk[a]

Milk Component	Units	Mean ± SD (*n*)	Milk Component	Units	Mean ± SD (*n*)
Mean days prepartum		20.21 ± 12.18 (11)	Calcium	mg/dL	25.35 ± 8.48 (10)
Lipid	%	2.07 ± 0.98 (11)	Magnesium	mg/dL	5.64 ± 1.44 (10)
Lactose	mM	79.78 ± 21.68 (9)	Citrate	mM	0.40 ± 0.17 (8)
Protein	g/dL	5.44 ± 1.71 (8)	Phosphate	mg/dL	2.32 ± 0.70 (9)
Glucose	mM	0.35 ± 0.16 (8)	Ionized calcium	mM	3.25 ± 0.84 (6)
Sodium	mM	61.26 ± 25.82 (10)	pH		6.83 ± 0.18 (6)
Potassium	mM	18.30 ± 5.67 (10)	Urea	mg/dL	14.87 ± 2.40 (9)
Chloride	mM	62.21 ± 17.44 (10)	Creatinine	mg/dL	1.47 ± 0.35 (9)

SD, Standard deviation.

[a]Small samples of mammary secretion were obtained three times in prepartum period from each of 11 women. In some cases, volumes were insufficient for all analyses.

From Allen JC, Keller RP, Archer P, et al. Studies in human lactation: milk composition and daily secretion rates of macronutrients in the first year of lactation. *Am J Clin Nutr.* 1991;54:69–80.

TABLE 4.4 Average Milk Volume Outputs (mL/24 h) of Well-Nourished Mothers Who Exclusively Breastfed Their Infants

MONTH OF LACTATION

Country	No. Days Measured	Sex	<1 n	<1 mL/24 h	1–2 n	1–2 mL/24 h	2–3 n	2–3 mL/24 h	3–4 n	3–4 mL/24 h	4–5 n	4–5 mL/24 h	5–6 n	5–6 mL/24 h
US	2	M, F	—	—	3	691	5	655	3	750	—	—	—	—
US	1–2	M, F	46	681	—	—	—	—	—	—	—	—	—	—
Canada	?	M, F	—	—	—	—	—	—	33	793	31	856	28	925
Sweden	?	M, F	15	558	11	724	12	752	—	—	—	—	—	—
US	3	M, F	—	—	11	600	—	—	2	833	—	—	3	682
US	3	M, F	—	—	26	606	26	601	20	626	—	—	—	—
U.K.	4	M	—	—	27	791	23	820	18	829	5	790	1	922
		F	—	—	20	677	17	742	14	775	6	814	4	838
US	1	M, F	16	673 ± 192 SD	19	756 ± 170	16	782 ± 172	13	810 ± 142	11	805 ± 117	11	896 ± 122

MONTH OF LACTATION

Country	No. Days Measured	Sex	7	8	9	10	11	12
US	1	M, F	875 ± 142 SD	834 ± 99	774 ± 180	691 ± 233	516 ± 215	759 ± 28

SD, Standard deviation.
Modified from Ferris AM, Jensen RG. Lipids in human milk: a review. *J Pediatr Gastroenterol Nutr.* 1984;3:108.

TABLE 4.5   Yield and Composition of Human Colostrum and Milk from Days 1 to 28

Component	DAY POSTPARTUM						
	1	2	3	4	5	14	28
Yield (g/24 h)	50	190	400	625	700	1100	1250
Lactose (g/L)	20	25	31	32	33	35	35
Fat (g/L)	12	15	20	25	24	23	29
Protein (g/L)	32	17	12	11	11	8	9

Modified from Saint L, Smith M, Hartmann PE. The yield and nutrient content of colostrum and milk of women giving birth to 1 month postpartum. *Br J Nutr.* 1984;52:87.

TABLE 4.6   Composition of Human Milk from Days 1 through 36 Postpartum (Mean ± SD), British and German Donors

Day	COMPONENT (g/dL)		
	Total Protein	Lactose	Triacylglycerols
1	2.95 ± 0.86	4.07 ± 0.98	2.14 ± 0.86
3	1.99 ± 0.22	4.98 ± 0.76	3.01 ± 0.77
5	1.82 ± 0.21	5.13 ± 0.54	3.06 ± 0.45
8	1.73 ± 0.27	5.38 ± 0.97	3.73 ± 0.70
15	1.56 ± 0.42	5.42 ± 0.76	3.59 ± 0.86
22	1.51 ± 0.27	5.34 ± 0.96	3.87 ± 0.68
29	1.5 ± 0.27	4.01 ± 1.13	4.01 ± 1.13
36	1.4 ± 0.26	5.34 ± 1.31	4.01 ± 1.20

SD, Standard deviation.
Modified from Hibberd CM, Brooke DG, Carter ND, et al. Variation in the composition of breast milk during the first five weeks of lactation. *Arch Dis Child.* 1982;57:658.

the mother's parity. Women who had other pregnancies, particularly those who previously nursed infants, have colostrum more readily available at delivery, and the volume increases more rapidly.

Establishment of Bacterial Flora

Colostrum facilitates the establishment of *Lactobacillus bifidus* flora in the digestive tract. Meconium contains an essential growth factor for *L. bifidus* and is the first culture medium in the sterile intestinal lumen of the newborn infant. Oligosaccharides in colostrum serve as prebiotics for the establishment of the early infant gut microbiome. Human colostrum is rich in antibodies, which may provide protection against the bacteria and viruses that are present in the birth canal and associated with other human contact. Colostrum also contains antioxidants, which may function as traps for neutrophil-generated reactive oxygen metabolites.[16]

Comparative Composition

The yellow color of colostrum results from β-carotene. The ash content is high, and the concentrations of sodium, potassium, and chloride are greater than those of mature milk (see Tables 4.5 to 4.7). Protein, fat-soluble vitamins, and minerals are present in greater percentages than in transitional or mature milk. sIgA and lactoferrin increase in concentration. The complex sugars, oligosaccharides, also increase, adding to the infection-protection properties at this stage. It has been suggested that the mammary gland actually evolved, in part, as an inflammatory response to tissue damage and infection and that the nutritional function then followed the protective function.

The higher-protein, lower-fat, and lactose solution is rich in immunoglobulins, especially sIgA. The number of immunologically competent mononuclear cells is at its highest level. Fat, contained mainly in the core of the fat globules, increases from 2% in colostrum to 2.9% in transitional milk and to 3.6% in mature milk. Prepartum milk lipids are 93% triglycerides, increasing to 97% in colostrum, with diglycerides, monoglycerides, and free fatty acids all increasing from prepartum to

TABLE 4.7   Fat Distribution in Milk

Measurement	PREPARTUM		POSTPARTUM		
	Early	Late	Colostrum	Transitional	Mature
Fat (%)	—	2	2	2.9	3.6
Fat (g)	—	—	2.9	3.6	3.8
Lipid (g/dL)	1.15	1.28	3.16	3.49	4.14
Phospholipid (mg/dL)	37	40	35	31	27
Percentage of total lipid	3.2	3.1	1.1	0.9	0.6
Cholesterol (mg/dL)	—	—	29	20	13.5

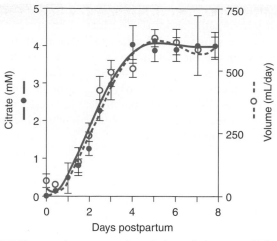

Fig. 4.7 Changes in concentration of citrate in human milk in early postpartum period compared with increase in milk volume. (From Neville MC. Determinants of milk volume and composition. In: Jensen RG, ed. *Handbook of Milk Composition*. San Diego: Academic Press; 1995.)

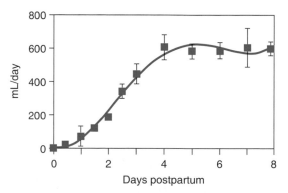

Fig. 4.8 Milk volumes during first week postpartum. Mean values from 12 multiparous white women who test-weighed their infants before and after every feeding for first 7 days postpartum. (From Neville MC, Keller R, Seacat J, et al. Studies in human lactation: milk volumes in lactating women during the onset of lactation and full lactation. *Am J Clin Nutr*. 1998;48:1375.)

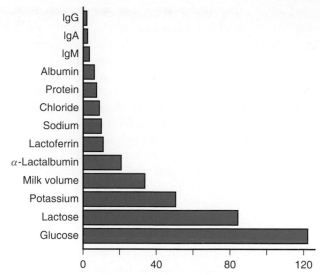

Fig. 4.9 Relative increase in yield of milk components from day 1 to day 7 postpartum. Values presented are for day 7 expressed as percentage increase over day 1. *IgA*, Immunoglobulin A; *IgG*, immunoglobulin G; *IgM*, immunoglobulin M. (Modified from Kulski JK, Hartmann PE. Changes in human milk composition during the initiation of lactation. *Aust J Exp Biol Med Sci*. 1981;59:101.)

postpartum secretions. Phospholipid levels decline during the same period. The amount of phospholipids, cholesterol, and cholesteryl esters declines from colostrum to mature milk.

Cholesterol appears to be synthesized in the mammary gland. Beyond its use in brain tissue development, the myelinization of nerves, and as the base of many enzymes, the role of cholesterol in colostrum remains elusive. Little research has been done on cholesterol in colostrum.

The progressive changes in mammary secretion in both breastfeeding and nonbreastfeeding women between 28 and 110 days before delivery and up to 5 months after delivery were followed by Kulski and Hartmann[17] to study the initiation of lactation. During late pregnancy, the secretion contained higher concentrations of proteins and lower concentrations of lactose, glucose, and urea than those contained in milk secreted when lactation was well established. The concentrations of sodium, chloride, and magnesium

were higher in colostrum than in milk, and those of potassium and calcium were lower. The osmolarity was relatively constant throughout the study. The authors described a two-phase development of lactation, with an initial phase of limited secretion in late pregnancy and a true induction of lactation in the second phase, 32 to 40 hours postpartum. Comparison with the nonlactating women revealed similar secretion during the first 3 days postpartum. This, however, was abruptly reversed during the next 6 days as mammary involution progressed. Obtaining samples in these women, however, may have served to prolong the period of production. The authors point out that although breastfeeding was not necessary for the initiation of lactation in this study, it was essential for the continuation of lactation.

The yield of milk has been calculated from absolute values to demonstrate the increase in the output of milk constituents during lactogenesis (Fig. 4.9). Dramatic increases occurred in the production of all the milk constituents. The components synthesized by the mammary epithelium (lactose, lactalbumin, and lactoferrin) increased at a rate greater than those for immunoglobulin A (IgA) or proteins derived from the serum immunoglobulin G (IgG) and immunoglobulin M (IgM). The greatest difference in yield between day 1 and day 7 postpartum was for glucose.[18]

Fat Content

A survey of the fatty acid components shows the lauric acid and myristic acid contents to be low in concentration in the first few days of milk production. When the lauric and myristic acids increased, C_{18} acids decreased. Palmitoleic acid increased at the same rate as the myristic acid. From this, it was concluded that the early fatty acids are derived from extramammary sources, but the breast quickly begins to synthesize fatty acids for the production of transitional and mature milk (see Table 4.7). The total fat content may have a predictive value. It was shown that 90% of the women whose milk contained 20 g or more of fat per feeding on the seventh day were successfully breastfeeding 3 months later. Women who had only 5 to 10 g of fat on the seventh day had an 80% dropout rate by 3 months. Colostrum's high protein and low fat are in keeping with the needs and reserves of the newborn at birth.

Nitrogen

Although the content of total nitrogen or any amino acid in breast milk in 24 hours is grossly related to the volume produced, the concentration in milligrams per deciliter (mg/dL) is not so related.[19] The relative distribution of the individual amino acids in each deciliter (100 mL) of milk differs in each mother. The colostrum may actually reflect a transitional maternal blood picture, which is associated with nitrogen metabolism of the postpartum period. The postpartum period is one of involution of body tissue and catabolism of protein in the mother (Fig. 4.10).

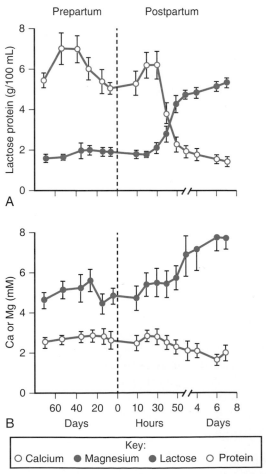

Fig. 4.10 The levels of milk constituents prepartum and postpartum change to reflect the maturation from colostrum to fully mature milk. Volume is driven by lactose production. (Modified from Dumas BR. Modifications of early milk composition during early states of lactation in nutritional adaptations of the gastrointestinal tract of the newborn. In: Kretchmer N, Minkowski A, eds. *Nutritional Adaptation of Gastrointestinal Tract of the Newborn*. Vol. 3. New York: Nestlé Vevey/Raven; 1983.)

Antioxidants

Colostrum contains at least two separate antioxidants, an ascorbate-like substance and uric acid.[16] These antioxidants may function in the colostrum as traps for neutrophil-generated, reactive oxygen metabolites. The aqueous human colostrum interferes with the oxygen metabolic and enzymatic activities of the polymorphonuclear leukocytes that are important in the reaction to acute inflammation consistent with an antiinflammatory effect.[16]

Vitamins

The mineral and vitamin reserves of the newborn infant are related to the maternal diet. A fetal supply of vitamin C, iron, and amino acids is adequate because infant blood levels exceed those of the mother. Colostrum is rich in fat-soluble vitamin A, carotenoids, and vitamin E. The average vitamin A level on the third day can be three times that of mature milk. Similarly, carotenoids in colostrum may be 10 times the level in mature milk, and vitamin E may be two to three times greater than in mature milk.

Studies that looked at multiparas versus primiparas showed that the volume of milk was significantly greater on day 5, with an earlier appearance of the casein band, in multiparas (Fig. 4.11).[20]

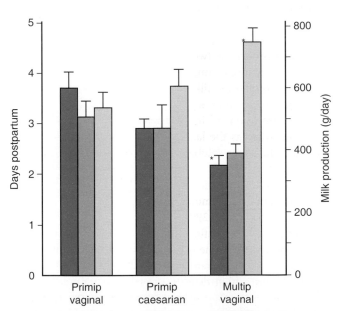

Fig. 4.11 Effect of parity on measures of lactogenesis. Data show the mean time at which fullness of the breast was observed (*dark blue bar*), the day on which the casein band first appeared (*medium blue bar*) in an electrophoretic analysis of daily milk samples, and the volume of milk produced on day 5 (*light blue bar*) by primiparous (primip) women who delivered vaginally (n = 19), primiparous women who delivered by cesarean section (n = 5), and multiparous (multip) women who delivered vaginally (n = 16). *Significant difference (p < 0.05) between multiparous and primiparous women who delivered vaginally. The distance between the error bars represents two standard errors of the mean (SEMs). (Data from Chen DC, Nommsen-Rivers L, Dewey KG, et al. Stress during labor and delivery and early lactation performance. *Am J Clin Nutr*. 1998;68:335; Neville MC, Morton J, Umemura S. Breastfeeding 2001: the evidence for breast-feeding. *Pediatr Clin North Am*. 2001;48:35.)

Sodium as a Predictor of Successful Lactogenesis

The ratio of sodium to potassium concentrations in breast milk changes over the course of lactation, decreasing as the mammary gland progresses from colostrum to transitional and mature milk production. A decrease in this ratio is an objective indicator of development toward copious milk production.[21] Early in lactogenesis, the sodium levels are high but quickly drop from 60 to 20 mmol by day 3 in women who have been fully feeding their infants. High breast-milk sodium concentrations on day 3 are suggestive of impending lactation failure.[22] Even women who remove only a small amount of milk daily for research purposes have the physiologic drop in sodium.

LACTOGENESIS STAGE II

Even though best practices recommend breastfeeding shortly after birth and frequently thereafter, Kulski et al. showed that milk removal is not needed for the programmed physiologic changes in mammary epithelium to trigger lactogenesis II.[17] Studies by Woolridge et al.[23] confirmed this when no effect of breastfeeding in the first 24 hours was observed on later milk transfer to the infants. However, the time of the first breastfeeding and the frequency of breastfeeding on day 2 are correlated with milk volume by day 5.[20]

Transitional Milk

The milk produced between the colostrum and mature milk stages is transitional milk, changing in composition from colostrum to mature milk. The transitional phase is approximately from 7 to 10 days postpartum to 2 weeks postpartum. The concentration of immunoglobulins and total protein decreases, whereas the lactose, fat, and total caloric content increase. The water-soluble vitamins increase to the levels of mature milk, and the fat-soluble vitamins decrease.

In a study of transitional milks, breast-milk samples were obtained from healthy mothers of term infants on the 1st, 3rd, 5th, 8th, 15th, 22nd, 29th, and 36th days of lactation by Hibberd et al.,[24] who defined the first day of lactation to be the 3rd day postpartum. The researchers pooled 24-hour samples for analysis, and the remainder was fed to the baby. The authors found a high degree of variability, not only among mothers but also within samples from the same mother. The maximum value in almost every case was more than twice the minimum. They were able to show, however, that the changes in composition were rapid before day 8, and then progressively less change took place until the composition was relatively stable before day 36 (see Tables 4.5 and 4.6).

Mature Milk

Human milk is a complex fluid that scientists have studied by separating the several phases by physical forces.[25] These forces include settling; short-term, low-speed centrifugation; high-speed centrifugation; and precipitation by micelle-destroying treatments, such as using the enzyme rennin (chymosin) or reducing the pH. On settling, the cream floats to the top, forming a layer of fat (about 4% by volume in human milk; Table 4.8).[26] Lipid-soluble components, such as cholesterol and phospholipid, remain with the fat. With a slow-speed spin, cellular components form a pellet. The high-speed spin brings the casein micelles into a separate phase or forms a pellet. On top of the protein pellet is a loose pellet referred to as the *fluff*, composed of membranes.[13,27] Casein precipitation (0.2% by weight) is caused by acid destruction of the micelles. The aqueous phase is whey, which also contains milk sugar, milk proteins, IgA, and the monovalent ions.

Water

In almost all mammalian milks, water is the constituent in the largest quantity, with the exception of the milk of some arctic and aquatic species, which produce milks with high-fat content (e.g., the northern fur seal produces milk with 54% fat and 65% total solids; see Table 4.2). All other constituents are dissolved, dispersed, or suspended in water. Water contributes to the temperature-regulating mechanism of the newborn because 25% of heat loss is from the evaporation of water from the lungs and skin. The lactating woman has a greatly increased obligatory water intake. If water intake is restricted during lactation, other water losses through urine and insensible loss are decreased before water for lactation is diminished. Because lactose is the regulating factor in the amount of milk produced, the secretion of water into milk is partially regulated by lactose synthesis. Investigations by Almroth show that the water requirement of infants in a hot, humid climate can be provided entirely by the water in human milk.[28]

Lipids

Intense interest in the lipids in human milk has been sparked by the reports from long-range studies of breastfed infants that show more advanced neurologic and cognitive development across the life span compared with formula-fed infants.[29] This attention has resulted from the interest in supplementing formula with various missing factors, such as cholesterol and docosahexaenoic acid (DHA).[29] Within breast milk, these compounds function in a milieu of arachidonic acid, lipases, and other enzymes, and no evidence indicates that they are effective in isolation or that more is better. The value of supplementing the mother's diet in pregnancy and lactation is an equally important question because dietary DHA levels have declined in the last half century as women have reduced eggs and animal organs in their diet (see Chapter 8).

Lipids are a chemically heterogeneous group of substances that are insoluble in water and soluble in nonpolar solvents. Lipids are separated into many classes and thousands of subclasses. The main constituents of human milk are triacylglycerols, phospholipids, and their component fatty acids, the sterols. Jensen, a renowned milk lipidologist, and his coauthors[19] remind readers, in a comprehensive review of the lipids in human milk, of the nomenclature, such as palmitic acid (16:0), oleic acid (18:1), and linoleic acid (18:2; see Box 4.1 for the recommended general nomenclature for fatty acids; Box 4.2 for a short list of saturated fatty acids in human

TABLE 4.8   Estimates of the Concentrations of Nutrients in Mature Human Milk

Nutrient	Amount in Human Milk[a] (g/L ± SD)	Nutrient	Amount in Human Milk[a] (mcg ± SD)
Lactose	72.0 ± 2.5	Calcium	280 ± 26
Protein	10.5 ± 2.0	Phosphorus	140 ± 22
Fat	39.0 ± 4.0	Magnesium	35 ± 2
		Sodium	180 ± 40
		Potassium	525 ± 35
		Chloride	420 ± 60
		Iron	380 ± 0.1[b]
		Zinc	1.2 ± 0.2
		Copper	0.19 ± 0.1[b]
		Vitamin E	2.3 ± 1.0
		Vitamin C	40 ± 10
		Thiamin	0.210 ± 0.035
		Riboflavin	0.350 ± 0.025
		Niacin	1.500 ± 0.200
		Vitamin B_6	93 ± 8[c]
		Pantothenic acid	1.800 ± 0.200
		Vitamin A, RE	670 ± 200 (2230 IU)
		Vitamin D	0.55 ± 0.10
		Vitamin K	2.1 ± 0.1
		Folate	85 ± 37[d]
		Vitamin B_{12}	0.97[e,f]
		Biotin	4 ± 1
		Iodine	110 ± 40
		Selenium	20 ± 5
		Manganese	6 ± 2
		Fluoride	16 ± 5
		Chromium	24 ± 20[b]
		Molybdenum	NR

IUs, International units; *NR*, not reported; *RE*, retinol equivalents; *SD*, standard deviation.

[a]Data from *Pediatric Nutrition Handbook*. 2nd ed. Elk Grove Village, IL: American Academy of Pediatrics; 1985: 363, unless otherwise indicated. Values are representative of amounts of nutrients present in human milk; some may differ slightly from those reported by investigators cited in the text.

[b]From Krachler M, Prohaska T, Koellensperger G, et al. Concentrations of selected trace elements in human milk and in infant formulas determined by magnetic sector field inductively coupled plasma-mass spectrometry. *Biol Trace Elem Res*. 2000;76:2.

[c]From Brown CM, Smith CM, Picciano MF. Forms of human milk folacin and variation patterns. *J Pediatr Gastroenterol Nutr*. 1986;5:278.

[d]From Sandberg DP, Begley JA, Hall CA. The content, binding, and forms of vitamin B_{12} in milk. *Am J Clin Nutr*. 1981;34:1717.

[e]SD not reported; range 0.33 to 3.20.

[f]From Styslinger L, Kirksey A. Effects of different levels of vitamin B_6 supplementation on vitamin B_6 concentrations in human milk and vitamin B_6 intakes of breastfed infants. *Am J Clin Nutr*. 1985;41:21.

From Report of Subcommittee, Institute of Medicine. *Nutrition During Lactation*. Washington, DC: National Academies Press; 1991.

milk; and Box 4.3 for a selected list of unsaturated fatty acids in human milk). The figure to the left of the colon is the number of carbons, and that to the right is the number of double bonds. Polyunsaturated fatty acids (PUFAs) have a designation for the location of the double bond; in human milk, the designation is *cis (c)*, which identifies the geometric isomer.

BOX 4.1 Nomenclature for Fatty Acids

Short-chain fatty acids (SCFAs)	5 or fewer carbons
Medium-chain fatty acids (MCFAs)	6–12 carbons
Long-chain fatty acids (LCFAs)	13–21 carbons
Very-long-chain fatty acids (VLCFAs)	22 or more carbons
Polyunsaturated fatty acids (PUFAs)	Includes LA and ALA
Long-chain polyunsaturated fatty acids (LCPUFAs)	Includes DHA and AA

AA, Arachidonic acid; *ALA*, α-linolenic acid; *DHA*, docosahexaenoic acid; *LA*, linoleic acid.

BOX 4.2 Saturated Fatty Acids

Caprylic acid	$CH_3(CH_2)_6COOH$	8:0
Capric acid	$CH_3(CH_2)_8COOH$	10:0
Lauric acid	$CH_3(CH_2)_{10}COOH$	12:0
Myristic acid	$CH_3(CH_2)_{12}COOH$	14:0
Palmitic acid	$CH_3(CH_2)_{14}COOH$	16:0
Stearic acid	$CH_3(CH_2)_{16}COOH$	18:0
Arachidic acid	$CH_3(CH_2)_{18}COOH$	20:0
Behenic acid	$CH_3(CH_2)_{20}COOH$	22:0
Lignoceric acid	$CH_3(CH_2)_{22}COOH$	24:0
Cerotic acid	$CH_3(CH_2)_{24}COOH$	26:0

BOX 4.3 Unsaturated Fatty Acids

Myristoleic acid	$CH_3(CH_2)_3\mathbf{CH}=\mathbf{CH}(CH_2)_7COOH$	14:1(9)
Palmitoleic acid	$CH_3(CH_2)_5\mathbf{CH}=\mathbf{CH}(CH_2)_7COOH$	16:1(9)
Sapienic acid	$CH_3(CH_2)_8\mathbf{CH}=\mathbf{CH}(CH_2)_4COOH$	16:1(6)
Oleic acid	$CH_3(CH_2)_7\mathbf{CH}=\mathbf{CH}(CH_2)_7COOH$	18:1(9)
Elaidic acid	$CH_3(CH_2)_7\mathbf{CH}=\mathbf{CH}(CH_2)_7COOH$	18:1 (trans-9)
Vaccenic acid	$CH_3(CH_2)_5\mathbf{CH}=\mathbf{CH}(CH_2)_9COOH$	18:1 (trans-11)
Linoleic acid (LA)	$CH_3(CH_2)_4\mathbf{CH}=\mathbf{CH}CH_2\mathbf{CH}=\mathbf{CH}(CH_2)_7COOH$	18:2(9,12)
Linoelaidic acid	$CH_3(CH_2)_4\mathbf{CH}=\mathbf{CH}CH_2\mathbf{CH}=\mathbf{CH}(CH_2)_7COOH$	18:2 (trans 9,12)
α-Linolenic acid (ALA)	$CH_3CH_2\mathbf{CH}=\mathbf{CH}CH_2\mathbf{CH}=\mathbf{CH}CH_2\mathbf{CH}=\mathbf{CH}(CH_2)_7COOH$	18:3(9,12,15)
Arachidonic acid (AA)	$CH_3(CH_2)_4\mathbf{CH}=\mathbf{CH}CH_2\mathbf{CH}=\mathbf{CH}CH_2\,\mathbf{CH}=\mathbf{CH}CH_2\mathbf{CH}=\mathbf{CH}(CH_2)_3COOH^{NIST}$	20:4(5,8,11,14)
Eicosapentaenoic acid (EPA)	$CH_3CH_2\mathbf{CH}=\mathbf{CH}CH_2\mathbf{CH}=\mathbf{CH}CH_2\mathbf{CH}=\mathbf{CH}CH_2\mathbf{CH}=\mathbf{CH}CH_2\mathbf{CH}=\mathbf{CH}(CH_2)_3COOH$	20:5(5,8,11,14,17)
Erucic acid	$CH_3(CH_2)_7\mathbf{CH}=\mathbf{CH}(CH_2)_{11}COOH$	22:1(13)
Docosahexaenoic acid (DHA)	$CH_3CH_2\mathbf{CH}=\mathbf{CH}CH_2\mathbf{CH}=\mathbf{CH}CH_2\mathbf{CH}=\mathbf{CH}\,CH_2\mathbf{CH}=\mathbf{CH}CH_2\mathbf{CH}=\mathbf{CH}CH_2\mathbf{CH}=\mathbf{CH}(CH_2)_2COOH$	22:6n-3

Lipid functions. Because milk is an exceptionally complex fluid, Jensen[30,31] and other scientists have found it helpful to classify components according to their size and concentration, with solubility in milk, or lack thereof, as additional categories (Table 4.9). The lipids fulfill a host of essential functions in growth and development,[32] provide a well-tolerated energy source, serve as carriers of messages to the infant, and provide physiologic interactions, including the following:

1. Allow maximum intestinal absorption of fatty acids
2. Contribute about 50% of calories
3. Provide essential fatty acids (EFAs) and PUFAs
4. Provide cholesterol

By percentage of concentration, the second greatest constituent in milk is the lipid fraction. Milk lipids provide the major fraction of kilocalories in human milk.[4] Lipids average 3% to 5% of human milk and occur as globules emulsified in the aqueous phase. The core or nonpolar lipids, such as triacylglycerols and cholesterol esters, are coated with bipolar materials, phospholipids, proteins, cholesterol, and enzymes. This loose layer is called the *milk-fat-globule membrane* (MFGM), which keeps the globules from coalescing and thus acts as an emulsion stabilizer.[19] Globules are 1 to 10 mm in diameter, with 1-mm globules predominating.[33]

Variations among fat constituents and concentrations. Fats are also the most variable constituents in human milk, varying in concentration over a feeding, from breast to breast, over a day's time, over time itself, and among individuals (Table 4.10).[34] This information is significant when testing milk samples for energy intake, fat-soluble constituents, and

TABLE 4.9   Compartments and Their Constituents in Mature Human Milk[a]

COMPARTMENT		MAJOR CONSTITUENTS	
Description	Content (%)	Name	Content (%)
Aqueous phase	87.0	Compounds of Ca, Mg, PO4, Na, K, Cl, CO$_2$, citrate, casein	0.2 as ash
True solution (1 nm) Whey proteins (3–9 nm)		Whey proteins: α-lactalbumin, lactoferrin, IgA, lysozyme, serum albumin	0.6
		Lactose and oligosaccharides; 7.0% and 1.0%	8.0
		Nonprotein nitrogen compounds: glucosamine, urea, amino acids, 20% of total N	35–50 mg N
		Miscellaneous: B vitamins, ascorbic acid	
Colloidal dispersion (11–55 nm, 10^{16} mL^{-1})	0.3	Caseins: beta and kappa, Ca, PO$_4$	0.2–0.3
Emulsion Fat globules (4 μm, 1.1^{10} mL^{-1})	4.0	Fat globules: triacylglycerols, sterol esters	4.0
Fat-globule-membrane interfacial layer	2.0	Milk-fat-globule membrane: proteins, phospholipids, cholesterol, enzymes, trace minerals, fat-soluble vitamins	2% of total lipid
Cells (8–40 μm, 10^4–10^5 mL^{-1})		Macrophages, neutrophils, lymphocytes, epithelial cells	

[a]All figures are approximate.
From Jensen RG. *The Lipids of Human Milk*. Boca Raton, FL: CRC; 1989.

TABLE 4.10   Factors That Influence Human Milk Fat Content and Composition

Factor	Influence
Duration of gestation	Shortened gestation increases the long-chain polyunsaturated fatty acids secreted
Stage of lactation (↑)	Phospholipid and cholesterol contents are highest in early lactation
Parity (↓)	High parity is associated with reduced endogenous fatty acid synthesis
Volume (↓)	High volume is associated with low milk fat content
Feeding (↑)	Human milk fat content progressively increases during a single nursing
Maternal diet	A diet low in fat increases endogenous synthesis of medium-chain fatty acids (C6 to C10)
Maternal energy status (↑)	A high weight gain in pregnancy is associated with increased milk fat

↑, Increase; ↓, decrease.
Modified from Picciano MF. Nutrient composition of human milk. Breastfeeding 2001, part I: the evidence for breastfeeding. *Pediatr Clin North Am*. 2001;48:53.

physiologic variation and when clinically managing lactation problems.[35] Much of the early work was based on lactation in women who "nursed by the clock" rather than tuned into infant needs. When circadian variation in fat content was studied in a rural Thai population who had practiced demand feeding for centuries, Jackson et al. found fat concentrations in feeds in the afternoon and evening (1600 to 2000 hours) were higher than those during the night (400 to 800 hours) (see Fig. 4.4). When Kent et al.[36] reexamined volume, frequency of breastfeedings, and the fat content of the milk throughout the day in 71 mother–infant dyads, they found similar trends.

They found, however, that fat content was 41.1 ± 7.8 g/L and ranged from 22.3 to 61.6 g/L. It was not related to time after birth or number of breastfeedings during the day. No effect on the average milk-fat content was related to the sex of the infant, clustered breastfeedings, or whether the infant fed at night. Fat content was higher during the day and evening compared with night and early morning. They recommended that infants be fed on demand day and night and not by schedule.

When the milk of the mothers of preterm infants was measured (6.6% ± 2.8%), the fat content was significantly higher in the evening (7.9% ± 2.9%) than in the morning ($D < 0.001$).[37]

TABLE 4.11   Lipid Class Composition of Human Milk During Lactation

Lipid Class	PERCENTAGE OF TOTAL LIPIDS AT LACTATION DAY					Immediate Extraction
	3	7	21	42	84	
Total lipid, % in milk[a]	2.04 ± 1.32	2.89 ± 0.31	3.45 ± 0.37	3.19 ± 0.43	4.87 ± 0.62	
Phospholipid	1.1	0.8	0.8	0.6	0.6	0.81
Monoacylglycerol	—	—	—	—	—	ND
Free fatty acids	—	—	—	—	—	0.08
Cholesterol (mg/dL)[b]	1.3 (34.5)	0.7 (20.2)	0.5 (17.3)	0.5 (17.3)	0.4 (19.5)	0.34
1,2-Diacylglycerol	—	—	—	—	—	0.01
1,3-Diacylglycerol	—	—	—	—	—	ND
Triacylglycerol	97.6	98.5	98.7	98.9	99.0	98.76
Cholesterol esters (mg)[c]						
Number of women	39	41	25	18	8	6

ND, Not done.

[a]Mean ± SEM.

[b]Total cholesterol content ranges from 10 to 20 mg/dL after 21 days in most milks.

[c]Not reported, but in Bitman et al. (Bitman J, Wood DL, Mehta NR, et al. Comparison of the cholesteryl ester composition of human milk from preterm and term mothers. *J Pediatr Gastroenterol Nutr.* 1986;5:780), it was 5 mg/dL at 3 days and 1 mg/dL at 21 days and thereafter.

From Jensen RG, Bitman J, Carlson SE. Milk lipids. In: Jensen RG, ed. *Handbook of Milk Composition*. San Diego: Academic Press; 1995.

It is speculated that the altered posture at night, horizontal and relatively inactive, may redistribute fat. The larger the milk consumption at a feed, the greater is the increase in fat from beginning to end of the feed. Less fat change occurs during "sleep" feeds than in the daytime. Unless 24-hour samples are collected by standardized sampling techniques, results will vary. During the course of a feeding, the fluid phase within the gland is mixed with fat droplets in increasing concentration. The fat droplets are released when the smooth muscle contracts in response to the let-down reflex.

The lipid fraction of the milk is extractable by suitable solvents and may require more than one technique to extract all the lipids.[30,31] Complete extraction in human milk is difficult because the lipids are bound to protein. Milk fats provide up to 50% of total calories.[8]

Milk-fat globul. Milk fat is dispersed in the form of droplets or globules maintained in solution by an absorbed layer or membrane. Recent research has linked milk-fat globules (MFGs) to infection prevention, neuro- and cognitive development, and immune system and microbiota maturation.[38] The protective membrane of the fat globules is made up of phospholipid complexes.

MFG composition varies significantly between mothers as well as over the course of lactation, both during single feedings and over the whole course of infant development. The variation in MFG composition is, further, a function of the nursing mother's diet, environment, genetics, and body composition as well as infant nutritional demands. More than 400 fatty acids are carried within milk fat.[38]

The rest of the phospholipids found in human milk are dispersed in the skim milk fraction. Vitamin A esters, vitamin D, vitamin K, alkyl glyceryl ethers, and glyceryl ether diesters are also in the lipid fraction but do not fall into the classes listed.

Renewed interest in defining the constituents of human milk lipid has developed as investigators look for the causes of obesity, atherosclerosis, and other degenerative diseases and their relationship to infant nutrition. A number of reports of historic value have technical problems of sampling. Because the fat content of a feeding varies with time, spot samples give spurious results. Jensen et al.[33] have reviewed the literature exhaustively and describe the fractionated lipid constituents in detail.

Most studies on the fat content of milk have been based on a geographically limited population. Milk fat changes with diet and maternal adipose stores; Yuhas et al.[39] studied milk samples from nine countries (Australia, Canada, Chile, China, Japan, Mexico, Philippines, the United Kingdom, and the United States). Saturated fatty acids were constant across countries, and monounsaturated fatty acids varied minimally. Arachidonic acid (C20: 4*n*-6) was also similar. DHA (22: 6*n*-3), however, was variable everywhere, but was dramatically different with milk from Japan having the highest values and the United States and Canada having the lowest values. Of note is the fact that the timing of collections was comparable in all countries. All samples were collected by electric pump, except in Japan where they were hand expressed.[39]

Effects of maternal diet. The average fat content of pooled 24-hour samples has been reported from multiple sources to vary in mature milk from 2.10% to 5.0% (Table 4.11). Maternal diet affects the constituents of the lipids but not the total amount of fat. A minimal increase in total lipid content of human milk was observed when an extra 1000 kcal of corn

TABLE 4.12 **Effects of Dietary Cholesterol, Phytosterol, and Polyunsaturated/Saturated (P/S) Ratio on Human Milk Sterols**

Milk Component	Maternal Ad Lib Diet (P/S 0.53; mg/100 g fat)	Low-Cholesterol/High-Phytosterol Diet (P/S 1.8; mg/100 g fat)	High-Cholesterol/Low-Phytosterol Diet (P/S 0.12; mg/100 g fat)
Cholesterol	240 ± 40	250 ± 10	250 ± 20
Phytosterol	17 ± 3	220 ± 30	70 ± 10
Dietary cholesterol	450 ± 30	130 ± 5	460 ± 90
Dietary phytosterol	23 ± 8	790 ± 17	80 ± 1
Total fat (%)	3.58 ± 0.56	2.69 ± 0.17	2.66 ± 0.16

From Lammi-Keefe CJ, Jensen RG. Lipids in human milk: a review. *J Pediatr Gastroenterol Nutr.* 1984;3:172.

oil was fed to lactating mothers. A diet rich in polyunsaturated fats will cause an increased percentage of polyunsaturated fats in the milk without altering the total fat content. When the mother is calorie deficient, depot fats are mobilized, and milk resembles depot fat. When excessive nonfat kilocalories are fed, levels of saturated fatty acids increase as lipids are synthesized from tissue stores.

When fish oil supplementation is given during pregnancy, it significantly alters the early postpartum breast-milk fatty acid composition (omega-3 PUFA). Levels of omega-3 fatty acids are increased, as are IgA and other immunomodulatory factors (CD14).[40]

A 2-week crossover study of three nursing women was done by Harzer et al.,[41] alternating high fat/low carbohydrate and the reverse. The first diet (high fat/low carbohydrate) was 50% fat, 15% protein, and 35% carbohydrate for a total of 2500 calories, which resulted in a reduction of triglycerides (4.1% to 2.6%) and an increase in lactose (5.2% to 6.4%) but no change in the protein content of the milk when compared with the low-fat/high-carbohydrate diet. Similarly, Lammi-Keefe and Jensen[42] showed changes in the percentage of fat and phytosterols in human milk with changes in maternal diet fat consumption (Table 4.12).

The US Department of Agriculture (USDA) has reported that the average American diet now includes 156 g of fat per day, up from 141 g in 1947. The significant change is from animal to vegetable fat, which is now 39% of total dietary fats, especially resulting from the switch from butter and lard. A change in fatty acid content to more long-chain fatty acids and a two-fold to three-fold increase in linoleic acid have occurred. Except for changes in the linoleic acid (18:2) content in mature milk, the fatty acid composition is remarkably uniform unless the maternal diet is unusually bizarre.

Polyunsaturated fats include C18:2 and C18:3, or linoleic and linolenic acid. The ratio of polyunsaturated to saturated fats (P/S ratio) in bovine milk is 4. The P/S ratio has shifted as a result of recent dietary changes to 1.3 from 1.35 in human milk. The P/S ratio is significant in facilitating calcium and fat absorption. Calcium absorption is depressed by a 4:5 P/S ratio and facilitated by the P/S ratio of human milk.

At least 167 fatty acids have been identified in human milk; possibly others are present in trace amounts. Bovine milk has 437 identified fatty acids. Milk from vegetarians (lacto-ovo) contained a lower proportion of fatty acids derived from animal fat and a higher proportion of PUFAs derived from dietary vegetable fat. Women who consumed 35 g or more of animal fat per day had higher C10:0, C12:0, and C18:3 (alpha-linolenic acid) but lower levels of unsaturated fats C16:0 and C18:0. Finley et al.[43] suggest that a maximum amount of C16:0 and C18:0 can be taken up from the blood and subsequently secreted into milk (Table 4.13).

The milk of strict vegetarians has extremely high levels of linoleic acid, four times that of cow's milk (see Table 4.13). Some researchers include other long-chain fatty acids (e.g., C20:2, C20:3, C24:4, C22:3) as essential nutrients because they are structural lipids in the brain and nervous tissue. The effects of maternal diet are also discussed in Chapter 8.

One important outcome of linoleic and linolenic acids is the conversion of these compounds into longer-chain polyunsaturates. These metabolites have been shown to be important for the fluidity of membrane lipids and prostaglandin synthesis. They are present in the brain and retinal cells. Long-chain polyunsaturated fatty acids (LCPUFAs) are needed for the development of the infant brain and nervous system.[43] When Gibson and Kneebore[44] studied fatty acid composition of colostrum and mature milk at 3 to 5 days and later at 6 weeks postpartum, they reported that mature milk had a higher percentage of saturated fatty acids, including medium-chain acids; lower monounsaturated fatty acids; and higher linoleic and linolenic acids and their long-chain polyunsaturated derivatives.

Infant intake of fatty acids from human milk over the first year of lactation (solids were started at 4 to 6 months) was studied by Mitoulas et al.[45] among mothers and infants in Australia. They determined the volume, fat content, and fatty acid composition of milk from each breast at each feed over 24 hours at 1, 2, 4, 6, 9, and 12 months. The volume of production was greater in the right breast (414 to 449 versus 336 to 360). Fat content varied minimally between breasts. Amounts of fat per 24 hours did not differ in the first year in the individual mothers. The overall amount of fats and arachidonic acid and DHA differed between mothers. Changes in proportions of individual fatty acids may not result in commensurate changes in 24-hour infant intakes.

TABLE 4.13 Effects of Maternal Vegetarian Diets on Saturated and Unsaturated Fatty Acids (wt%) in Human Milk Lipids (Mean ± SEM)

Lipid (%)/Fatty Acid	Vegetarian[a]	Control[a]	Vegan[b]	Vegetarian[b]	Omnivore[b]
Number	12	7	19	5	21
Saturates					
6:0	—	—	—	—	—
8:0	0.16 ± 0.03	0.22 ± 0.01	—	—	—
10:0	1.56 ± 0.13	1.57 ± 0.09	1.8 ± 0.40	1.3 ± 0.51	0.4 ± 0.23
12:0	7.07 ± 0.78	5.47 ± 0.66	6.6 ± 0.54	3.2 ± 0.49	1.7 ± 0.35
14:0	8.16 ± 1.00	6.54 ± 0.73	6.9 ± 0.58	5.2 ± 0.50	4.5 ± 0.35
16:0	15.31 ± 0.73	20.48 ± 0.64	18.1 ± 1.34	21.2 ± 1.07	25.1 ± 0.78
18:0	4.48 ± 0.37	8.14 ± 0.55	4.9 ± 0.36	7.4 ± 0.35	9.7 ± 0.68
20:0	0.54 ± 0.02	0.57 ± 0.03	—	—	—
Total	37.28	42.99			
Monounsaturates					
16:1	1.66 ± 0.14	3.35 ± 0.28	4.9 ± 0.24	2.9 ± 0.37	3.4 ± 0.35
18:1	26.89 ± 1.47	34.7 ± 0.86	32.2 ± 1.06	35.3 ± 1.94	38.7 ± 1.27
Total	28.55	38.06	37.10	38.2	42.1
Polyunsaturates					
n-6 Series					
18:2	28.82 ± 1.39	14.47 ± 1.98	23.8 ± 1.40	19.5 ± 3.62	10.9 ± 0.96
20:2	0.72 ± 0.03	0.50 ± 0.03	—	—	—
20:3	0.62 ± 0.03	0.56 ± 0.03	0.44 ± 0.03	0.42 ± 0.07	0.40 ± 0.08
20:4	0.68 ± 0.03	0.68 ± 0.03	0.32 ± 0.02	0.38 ± 0.05	0.35 ± 0.03
Total	30.84	16.21	31.4	27.5	18.4
n-3 Series					
18:3	2.76 ± 0.16	1.85 ± 0.16	1.36 ± 0.18	1.25 ± 0.22	0.49 ± 0.06
22:6	0.22 ± 0.08	0.27 ± 0.08	0.14 ± 0.06	0.30 ± 0.05	0.36 ± 0.07
Total	3.05	2.12	1.50	1.55	0.86

Dietary information

Vegetarian (col. 2): whole cereal grains, 50%–60%; soup, 5%; vegetables, 20%–25%; beans and sea vegetables, 5%–10%; macrobiotic diet for a mean of 81 months; no meat or dairy products; occasional seafood, nuts, and fruit

Vegan: No foods of animal origin

Control: typical diet in the United States

Vegetarian (col. 5): Exclude meat and fish

Omnivore: typical Western diet

SEM, Standard error of measurement.

[a]Modified from Specker BL, Wey HE, Miller D. Differences in fatty acid composition of human milk in vegetarian and nonvegetarian women: long-term effect of diet. *J Pediatr Gastroenterol Nutr*. 1987;6:764. New England donors: vegetarians, 3 to 13 months postpartum; control subjects, 1 to 5 months; capillary gas-liquid chromatography (GLC) columns.

[b]Modified from Sanders TA, Reddy S. The influence of a vegetarian diet on the fatty acid composition of human milk and the essential fatty acid status of the infant. *J Pediatr*. 1992;120:S71. British donors: 6 weeks postpartum; packed GLC columns.

From Jensen RG, Bitman J, Carlson SE. Milk lipids. In: Jensen RG, ed. *Handbook of Milk Composition*. San Diego: Academic Press; 1995.

The authors[36,45] note that their findings were similar to Jensen's work in 1995 in the United States.[19]

When this same group of investigators in Australia (Kent et al.[36] and Mitoulas et al.[45]) measured the volume of milk, frequency of feedings, and fat content at 1 to 6 months of age in a normal group of mothers using demand feeding day and night, they observed no relationship between the total number of feeds and the total volume of milk. Furthermore, fat content was 41.1 ± 7.8 g/L (range 22.3 to 61.6 g/L), and total fat was independent of the frequency of feeding. They concluded infants should be fed on demand.

Prolonged lactation has long been suspected of providing reduced nutrition. It has been established that infection protection continues, but now there is evidence that high nutrition persists as well; 34 mother–baby dyads and 27 control dyads were studied by Mandel et al.[46] The mothers who were breastfeeding beyond 1 year (12 to 39 months) were older (34.4 ± 5.1, years), lighter ($59.8 \div 8.7$ kg), and had a lower body mass index (BMI; 22.1 ± 3.0) than controls (breastfeeding 2 to 6 months; age 30.7 ± 2.9 years, weight 66.3 ± 11.8 kg, and BMI 24.5 ± 3.9). Feeding frequency per day was 5.9 ± 3.3 versus 7.36 ± 2.65 (controls). The milk of mothers who were breastfeeding beyond a year had significantly increased fat and increased energy content compared with controls.[46] More recently, researchers from Poland reported on breastmilk macronutrient content up to 48 months of lactation. Fat and protein content increased, whereas the carbohydrates decreased from 12 to 24 months and then remained stable out to 48 months. An increased amount of feeding positively increased the percentage of carbohydrates and negatively affected the amount of fat and protein.[47]

Factors affecting fatty acid composition include the stage of lactation, especially in specific fatty acids, probably because of the recruiting of body fat stores. Milk from mothers of premature infants differs from that of mothers of full-term infants in fat content, with higher levels of medium-chain fatty acids in premature milk. The significance of circadian rhythm for fatty acid composition is contradictory in the literature; therefore studies of fat content should consider this in sample collection.[48] Diet, on the other hand, has an extensive impact on the fat content of milk, with up to 85% derived from the diet in the form of chylomicrons. This has led to dietary supplementation, especially utilizing the omega-3 fatty acids.[49]

Brain development relative to lipid content of human milk. To address the issue of nutrition during brain development, it is important to consider the different periods of brain development that have been described biochemically. First, cell division occurs, with the formation of neurons and glial cells, and second, myelination. In the rat brain, 50% of polyenoic acids of the gray-matter lipids were laid down by the 15th day of life. The fatty acids characteristic of myelin lipids appeared later. Gray matter is largely composed of unmyelinated neurons, whereas white matter contains a very high proportion of myelinated conducting nerve fibers. Normal brain function depends on both. The synthesis and composition of myelin can be influenced by diet in the developing rat brain.

Myelin-specific messenger ribonucleic acid (mRNA) levels are developmentally regulated and influenced by dietary fat. The neonatal response to dietary fat is tissue specific at the mRNA level.[50]

The fatty acids characteristic of gray matter (C20:4 and C22:6) accumulate before the appearance of fatty acids characteristic of myelin (C20:1 [Paullinic acid] and C24:1 [nervonic acid]) in the developing brain. Arachidonic acid (C20:4) and DHA (C22:6) are synthesized from linoleic and linolenic acids, respectively, but the latter two must be obtained in the diet.[51]

During the first year of life, the human brain more than doubles in size, increasing from 350 to 1100 g in weight. Of this growth, 85% is cerebrum; 50% to 60% of this solid matter is lipid. Cortical total phospholipid fatty acid composition in both term and preterm infants is greatly influenced by dietary fat intake. Phospholipids make up about one-quarter of the solid matter and are integral to the vascular system on which the brain depends.[52] Brain growth is associated with an increase in the incorporation of long-chain PUFAs (e.g., arachidonic acid [AA] and DHA) into the phospholipid in the cerebral cortex.[25] The transition from colostrum to mature milk leads to an increase in sphingomyelin and a decrease in phosphatidylcholine in the milk of mothers who deliver prematurely, along with a decrease in phospholipid content. Phospholipids are essential to brain growth, especially in a premature infant. Sphingomyelin and phosphatidylcholine are a source of choline, a major constituent of membranes in the brain and nervous tissue. Extreme dietary alterations in animal experiments have demonstrated an altered PUFA composition of the developing brain.

Such studies cannot be done in humans. Farquharson et al.[52] therefore examined the necropsy specimens of cerebrocortical gray matter obtained from 20 term and 2 premature infants, all of whom died within 43 weeks of birth. All were victims of sudden death and were genetically normal. The infants had either received exclusively breast milk or exclusively formula. The latter group was divided by formula type into three groups: mixture of formulas, SMA, or CGOST (cow milk or Osterfeed). (SMA and CGOST are formulas or mixtures of formulas sold in the United Kingdom.) Breastfed infants had greater concentrations of DHA in their cerebrocortical phospholipids than formula-fed infants in all groups. A compensatory increase in *n*-6 series fatty acids (arachidonic, docosatetraenoic, and docosapentaenoic) occurred in the SMA group. No significant differences were seen between saturated and monounsaturated fatty acids. The two premature infants had the lowest levels of DHA.

Importance of infant diet. Cerebrocortical neuronal membrane glycerophospholipids are composed predominantly (95%) of phosphatidylcholine, phosphatidylethanolamine, and phosphatidylserine.[25] After birth, neuronal membranes and retinal photoreceptor cells derive most of their phospholipid DHA from diet and liver synthesis and not from fat reserves. Neither the liver nor the retinal and neuronal cells can synthesize DHA without reserves or a dietary supply. α-Linolenic acid, an EFA, is the precursor. If the enzymes are not activated or are inactivated by an excess of *n*-6 fatty acids, synthesis does not take place. Human milk provides the DHA and arachidonic acid.[53]

Dietary supplementation with fish oil in the latter part of pregnancy resulted in increased DHA status at birth when measured in the umbilical blood.[54] When postpartum women were supplemented with DHA by capsule in a blind study, breast-milk levels of DHA ranged from 0.2% to 1.7% of total fatty acids, increasing with dose. The antioxidant status of plasma AA and levels were unaffected.

Although DHA is essential to retinal development, levels peak in the retina at 36 to 38 weeks' gestation, suggesting that the most rapid rate of retinal accumulation occurs before term.[55] This further suggests that the premature infant is especially vulnerable to dietary deficiencies of DHA.

Dietary omega-3 (ω-3) fatty acids may not be essential to life, reproduction, or growth, but they are important for normal biochemical and functional development.[56] Long-chain ω-3 fatty acids, DHA in particular, form a major structural component of biologic membranes. When the ratio of omega-6 (ω-6) is high compared with ω-3, fatty acids aggravate the deficiency. Studies in monkeys have shown that DHA deficiency affects water intake and urine excretion, as well as ω-3 fatty acid levels in red blood cells.[56] Much remains to be learned about the effects of ω-3 fatty acids and DHA deficiency on developing human infants.

The EFAs, linoleic and linolenic acids, may have greater significance in the quality of the myelin laid down. Dick, observing the geographic distribution of multiple sclerosis worldwide, noted that the disease is rare in countries where breastfeeding is common.[57] He postulated that the development of myelin in infancy is critical to preventing degradation later. Dick investigated the difference between human milk and cow's milk in relation to myelin production in multiple sclerosis.

Experimental allergic encephalitis is a demyelinating condition and can be produced by shocking animals that have been sensitized to central nervous system (CNS) antigens. Newborn rats deficient in EFAs are more susceptible to this disease, which has been described as resembling multiple sclerosis pathologically.

Other influences on fat content of human milk. Infections will alter milk composition. Mastitis does not alter fat content but does lower volume and lactose and increase sodium and chloride.

Parity has been cited as a major influence on fat content, with primiparous women having more fat than multiparous women. Prentice et al. found a significant relationship between fat content and triceps skinfold thickness. The authors found seasonal changes in the Gambia, where volume and fat were lowest following the rainy season, when nutrient resources are scarce.[58]

Hyperlipoproteinemia. Milk from women with type I hyperlipoproteinemia has been investigated.[33] Because the primary deficiency is serum-stimulated lipoprotein lipase in the plasma, resulting in a reduced transfer of dietary long-chain fatty acids from blood to milk, levels of fat as fatty acids

were abnormally low (1.5%), and the amounts of 10:0 and 14:0 were higher than normal (see Chapter 15).

Cholesterol

Cholesterol is an essential component of all membranes and is required for growth, replication, and cell maintenance. Infants fed human milk have higher plasma cholesterol levels than formula-fed infants. Animal studies suggest that early postnatal ingestion of a diet high in cholesterol protects against high-cholesterol challenges later.

The cholesterol content of milk is remarkably stable at 240 mg/100 g of fat when calculated by volume of fat. The range, depending on sampling techniques, is 9 to 41 mg/dL. The amount of cholesterol changed slightly over time, decreasing 1.7-fold over the first 36 days, as reported by Harzer et al., and stabilizing at approximately day 15 postpartum at 20 mg/dL. This resulted in a change in the cholesterol/triglyceride ratio. The authors found no uniform pattern of circadian variations between mothers.[59]

Neonatal plasma cholesterol levels range between 50 and 100 mg/dL at birth, with equal distribution of low-density lipoprotein (LDL) and high-density lipoprotein (HDL). Plasma cholesterol increases rapidly over the first few days of life, with LDL predominating regardless of mode of feeding.[60] In breastfed infants, however, plasma cholesterol progressively increases compared with that in infants fed low to no cholesterol and high-PUFA formulas. This may have a lasting effect on the individual's ability to metabolize cholesterol, a point yet to be confirmed.[61] Low-birth-weight (LBW) premature infants are at risk for the stimulation of endogenous cholesterol biosynthesis, resulting in marked elevations in plasma cholesterol, as a result of intravenous nutrition.

The effect of breastfeeding on plasma cholesterol, body weight, and body length was studied longitudinally in 512 infants by Jooste et al.[62] Breastfed infants had higher plasma cholesterol than the formula-fed infants, created by a direct mechanism that persisted for as long as the infants were breastfed. Body length was similar in breastfed and formula-fed infants, but formula-fed infants weighed more.

Cholesterol as health risk. Cholesterol has been a factor of great concern because of the apparent association with risk factors for atherosclerosis and coronary heart disease. At present, commercial formulas have high P/S ratios and little or no cholesterol compared with human milk. Dietary manipulation does not change the cholesterol level in the breast milk. When the dietary cholesterol level is controlled, however, a fall in the infant's plasma cholesterol level is associated with an increase in the amount of linoleic acid present in the milk.

Kallio et al.[63] followed 193 infants from birth, measuring concentrations of cholesterol, very-low-density lipoprotein (VLDL), LDL, HDL2, and, on a limited group of 36 infants, HDL3 and apoprotein B. The largest differences in cholesterol plasma levels between exclusively breastfed and weaned infants were at 2 months (0.8 mmol/L), 4 months (0.6 mmol/L), and 6 months (0.5 mmol/L). The LDL and apoprotein B concentrations were lower in weaned infants. VLDL and HDL3 were independent of diet. The authors concluded that the low intake of cholesterol and high intake of unsaturated fatty acids greatly modify the blood lipid pattern in the first year of life.[63]

In a retrospective epidemiologic study of 5718 men in England born in the 1920s, 474 died of ischemic heart disease.[64] The infant-feeding groups were divided into those breastfed but weaned before 1 year, breastfed more than a year, and bottle-fed. The first group had the lowest death rate from ischemic heart disease and had lower total cholesterol, LDL cholesterol, and apolipoprotein B than those who were weaned after a year and especially those who were bottle-fed. In all feeding groups, serum apolipoprotein B concentrations were lower in men with higher birth weights and weights at 1 year.[65]

No long-range effect of serum cholesterol levels in infants (in the absence of genetic lipid metabolism abnormalities) has been identified, although Osborn[66] described the pathologic changes in 1500 young people (newborns to age 20). He observed the spectrum of pathologic changes from mucopolysaccharide accumulations to fully developed atherosclerotic plaques. Lesions were more frequent and severe in children who had been bottle-fed. Lesions were uncommon or mild in the breastfed children.

Animal investigations indicated that rats given high levels of cholesterol early in life were better able to cope with cholesterol in later life and maintained a lower cholesterol level.[50]

In a study of 6 breastfed and 12 formula-fed infants, ages 4 to 5 months, Wong et al.[67] measured the fractional synthesis rate. The breastfed infants had higher cholesterol intakes (18.4 ± 4.0 mg/kg per day) than formula-fed infants (only 3.4 ± 1.8 mg/kg per day). Plasma cholesterol levels were 183 ± 47 versus 112 ± 22 mg/dL; LDL cholesterol levels were 83 ± 26 versus 48 ± 16 mg/dL. An inverse relationship existed between the fractional synthesis rate of cholesterol and dietary intake of cholesterol. The authors concluded that the greater cholesterol intake of breastfed infants is associated with elevated plasma LDL cholesterol concentrations. In addition, cholesterol synthesis in human infants may be efficiently regulated by coenzyme A (CoA) reductase when infants are challenged with dietary cholesterol.

A carefully designed, well-controlled longitudinal study is needed to determine the long-range impact of cholesterol because it is a consistent constituent of human milk throughout lactation.

n-3 Fatty Acids

The n-3 fatty acids are important components of animal and plant cell membranes and are selectively distributed among the lipid classes. The role of DHA (22: n-3) in infantile nerve and brain tissue and retinal development has been discussed. It is also found in high levels in the testis and sperm. Human milk contains DHA, and studies to evaluate the effects of "fish oil" supplements to the diet suggest an elevation of the dose-dependent levels.

Eicosapentaenoic acid (EPA; 20: 5n-3) is part of another group of n-3 fatty acids, the eicosanoids, which comprise two families: the prostanoids (prostaglandins, prostacyclins, and thromboxanes) and the leukotrienes.[33] The prostanoids are mediators of inflammatory processes. Leukotrienes are key mediators of inflammation and delayed hypersensitivity. The eicosanoids are highly active lipid mediators in both physiologic and pathologic processes.[68] Eicosanoids provide cytoprotection and vasoactivity in the modulation of inflammatory and proliferative reactions. Their precursors, long-chain PUFAs, can affect the generation of eicosanoids. The role of eicosanoids in physiologic and pathophysiologic processes is beginning to be identified. It clearly goes beyond adding a little DHA to the brew. Sellmayer and Koletzko[68] reviewed this work.

In other species, restriction of n-3 fatty acids results in abnormal electroretinograms, impaired visual activity, and decreased learning ability. The influence of dietary n-3 fatty acids on visual activity development in VLBW infants was evaluated by Birch et al.,[69] using visual-evoked response and forced-choice preferential-looking procedures at 36 and 57 weeks postconception. Feeding groups were randomized to one of three diets: corn oil (only linoleic), soy oil (linoleic and linolenic), and soy/marine oil (added n-3 fatty acids). The marine oil group matched the "gold standards" of VLBW infants fed human milk. Visual activity parameters in the other infants who did not receive n-3 oils were considerably lower.

The n-3 fatty acids appear to function in the membranes of photoreceptor cells and synapses. Jensen[31] suggests a daily intake of 18: 3n-3 (0.5% of calories) with the inclusion of n-3 long-chain PUFA, which is available in human milk. Many studies affirm the value of n-3 fatty acids in the diet and as protection against heart disease, chronic inflammatory disease, and possibly cancer.[70] When synthetic DHA and AA are added to infant formula, the measurements of visual acuity do not match those of human milk. The tolerance for these formulas is still undocumented, and long-range outcomes remain unreported.

Carnitine

Carnitine is γ-trimethylamino-β-hydroxybutyrate and is essential for the catabolism of long-chain fatty acids. Only two conditions in life have been described when carnitine is indispensable: total parenteral nutrition lasting more than 3 weeks and early postnatal life. In older individuals, it is synthesized in the liver and kidney from the essential amino acids lysine and methionine. Carnitine serves as an essential carrier of acyl groups across the mitochondrial membrane to sites of oxidation and, therefore, has a central role in the mitochondrial oxidation of fatty acids in humans.[71]

Newborns undergo major metabolic changes during the transition from fetal to extrauterine life, including the rapid development of the capacity to oxidize fatty acids and ketone bodies as fuel alternatives to glucose. The fatty acids derived from high-fat milk and endogenous fat stores become the preferred fuel of the heart, brain, and tissues with high-energy demands. In addition, a dramatic increase occurs in serum fatty acids in the first hours of life. After the interruption of the fetoplacental circulation and in the absence of an exogenous supply of carnitine, neonatal plasma levels of free carnitines and acylcarnitines decrease very rapidly. Carnitine administration seems to act by increasing ketogenesis and lipolysis. When serum carnitine and ketone body concentrations were measured in breastfed and formula-fed newborn infants, lower carnitine levels were found in infants fed formulas than in those fed breast milk.

The levels of carnitine range from 70 to 95 nmol/mL in breast milk (up to 115 nmol/mL in colostrum) and from 40 to 80 nmol/mL in commercial formula (Enfamil). The bioavailability of carnitine in human milk may be a significant factor in the higher carnitine and ketone body concentrations in breastfed babies. In omnivorous mothers, carnitine levels do not vary considerably over time.[32] Levels in the milk of lacto-ovo-vegetarian mothers were always consistently lower than those of omnivores. The lower serum level of lysine in these women is a possible cause of lower carnitine.

The carnitine levels in human milk were followed for 50 days postpartum, and the mean level was found to be 62.9 nmol/mL (56.0 to 69.8 nmol/mL range) during the first 21 days and 35.2 ± 1.26 nmol/mL until days 40 to 50. Levels were not related to the volume of milk secreted.

Proteins

All varieties of milk have been evaluated for their protein contents, which vary from species to species. Proteins constitute 0.9% of the contents in human milk and range up to 20% in some rabbit species. Proteins of milk include casein, serum albumin, α-lactalbumin, β-lactoglobulins, immunoglobulins, and other glycoproteins. Eight of 20 amino acids present in milk are essential and are derived from plasma. The mammary alveolar epithelium synthesizes some nonessential amino acids. Human milk amino acids occur in proteins and peptides, as well as a small percentage in the form of free amino acids and glucosamine[72] (Table 4.14, Fig. 4.12).

TABLE 4.14   Free Amino Acid Concentrations in Human Milk

Amino Acid	Colostral Milk (μmol/dL)	Transitional Milk (μmol/dL)	Mature Milk (μmol/dL)
Glutamic acid	36–68	88–127	101–180
Glutamine	2–9	9–20	13–58
Taurine	41–45	34–50	27–67
Alanine	9–11	13–20	17–26
Threonine	5–12	7–8	6–13
Serine	12	6–11	6–14
Glycine	5–8	5–10	3–13
Aspartic acid	5–6	3–4	3–5
Leucine	3–5	2–6	2–4
Cystine	1–3	2–5	3–6
Valine	3–4	3–6	4–6
Lysine	5	1–11	2–5
Histidine	2	2–3	0.4–3
Phenylalanine	1–2	1	0.6–2
Tyrosine	2	1–2	1–2
Arginine	3–7	1–5	1–2
Isoleucine	2	1–2	1
Ornithine	1–4	1	0.5–0.9
Methionine	0.8	0.3–3	0.3–0.8
Phosphoserine	8	5	4
Phosphoethanolamine	4	8	10
α-Aminobutyrate	1	0.4–1.4	0.4–1
Tryptophan	5	1	1
Proline	—	6	2–3

From Carlson SE. Human milk nonprotein nitrogen: occurrence and possible function. *Adv Pediatr*. 1985;32:43.

Distribution of the main protein fractions in human and bovine milks

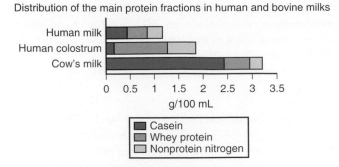

Distribution of whey protein in human and bovine milks

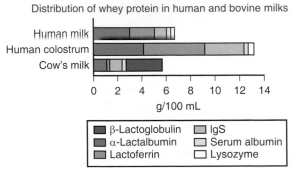

Fig. 4.12 Distribution of main protein fractions *(top)* and whey protein *(bottom)* in human and bovine milk. (Modified from Dumas BR. Modifications of early human milk composition during early states of lactation in nutritional adaptation of the gastrointestinal tract of the newborn. In: Kretchmer N, Minkowski A, eds. *Nutritional Adaptation of Gastrointestinal Tract of the Newborn.* Vol. 3. New York: Nestlé Vevey/Raven; 1983.)

Tikanoja et al.[73] reported that postprandial changes in plasma amino acids in breastfed infants were proportional to dietary intake and were highest for the branched-chain amino acids. This was also found to be true for most semi-essential and nonessential amino acids. The blood urea levels also reflect dietary intake, with values in breastfed infants being substantially lower than levels in bottle-fed infants. After a feed, the sum of plasma free amino acids rose, and the glycine/valine ratio fell. When breastfed and formula-fed infants were compared by Järvenpää et al.,[74] concentrations of citrulline, threonine, phenylalanine, and tyrosine were higher in formula-fed than in breastfed infants. Concentrations of taurine were lower in the formula-fed infants. The peak time was different for formula-fed and breastfed infants, which points out the need to standardize sampling times.

The Davis Area Research on Lactation, Infant Nutrition, and Growth (DARLING) Study was the first longitudinal study to follow a large group of mother–infant dyads to 12 months.[15] The investigators report protein intake to be positively associated with milk lipid concentrations after 16 weeks. Milk protein concentration was negatively related to milk volume at 6 and 9 months and positively related to feeding frequency at these times. Milk composition is more sensitive to maternal factors such as body composition, diet, and parity during later lactation than during the first few months.[75]

Refer to the Milk Bioactive Peptide Database (http://mbpdb.nws.oregonstate.edu) for a comprehensive database of mammalian milk proteins and peptides.[76]

Casein

Milk consists of casein, or curds, and whey proteins, or lactalbumins. The term *casein* includes a group of milk-specific proteins characterized by ester-bound phosphate, high-proline content, and low solubility at a pH of 4.0 to 5.0.[30,77] Research demonstrates that casein ingestion during infancy can have significant and long-lasting growth benefits in the first year of life and lead to better health outcomes throughout life.[78]

Caseins form complex particles or micelles, which are usually complexes of calcium caseinate and calcium phosphate. When milk clots or curdles as a result of heat, pH changes, or enzymes, the casein is transformed into an insoluble caseinate–calcium phosphate complex. Physiochemical differences exist between human and cow caseins, and indeed, even casein concentrations differ significantly between the two species: bovine milk has a much higher concentration, versus a whey:casein ratio of 60:40 in mature human milk that varies from 90:10 in early lactation changing to 50:50 in late lactation.[77] Casein has a species-specific amino acid composition.

Kunz and Lönnerdal[79] report confirming results of varying whey:casein ratio over the period of lactation and concluded that synthesis and secretion of casein and whey are affected by different mechanisms.

Utilizing a liquid chromatography with tandem mass spectrometry (LC-MS/MS) quantitative analysis, Liao et al. observed that total casein concentrations decreased over the course of a year of lactation. The individual concentrations of α-casein, β-casein, and κ-casein decreased at varying rates, with β-casein maintaining the highest concentration on average, and the whey:casein ratio in fact increased over a yearlong period, in contrast to previous research observing the opposite progression.[80] Continued quantitative analysis of human milk protein content will require a comparison of different methodologies of quantification and reanalysis.

Methionine-to-Cysteine Ratio

The cysteine content is high in human milk, whereas it is very low in cow milk. Because the methionine content is high in bovine milk, the methionine-to-cysteine ratio is two to three times greater in cow milk than in the milk of most mammals and seven times higher than in human milk. Human milk is the only mammalian milk in which the methionine-to-cysteine ratio is close to 1. Otherwise, this ratio is seen only in plant proteins.

Two significant characteristics of the amino acid composition of human milk are the ratio between the sulfur-containing amino acids methionine and cysteine and the low content of the aromatic amino acids phenylalanine and tyrosine. Newborns and especially premature infants are poorly prepared to handle phenylalanine and tyrosine because of their low levels of the specific enzymes required to metabolize them.

Taurine

Taurine is a free amino acid involved in many physiologic functions in mammals throughout life and plays a particularly critical role in the perinatal period of development.[81]

Taurine, or 2-aminoethanesulfonic acid, is a third sulfur-containing amino acid found in high concentrations in human milk (40 μmol per 100 mL) and low concentrations in cow milk (20 μmol per 100 mL).[82] It is now being added to some prepared formulas. Free taurine and glutamic acid have been measured in breast milk in high concentrations.

Taurine has been associated in the body at all ages with bile acid conjugation, and in newborns, bile acids are almost exclusively conjugated with taurine. It has been suggested that taurine may also be a neurotransmitter or neuromodulator in the brain and retina.[81] Taurine in the nutrition of human infants was reviewed by Neville et al.,[83] who report that evidence is accumulating that taurine has a more general biologic role in development, and taurine has been observed to contribute to cell-volume regulation during osmotic changes.[82]

Humans are unable to synthesize taurine to any degree as newborns and young infants and are, therefore, wholly dependent on a dietary supply. The process requires cystathionase and cysteine-sulfinic acid decarboxylase, which are enzymes that convert methionine, cysteine, or cystine to taurine. Taurine deficiency can result in slowed growth. Research has found taurine concentrations to be lower in the breast milk of vegan mothers.[81]

Differences in taurine between breast milk and formula. In studies of amino acid levels, only the concentrations of taurine in the plasma and urine of breastfed term infants were higher than those of preterm infants fed formula. The levels in term infants were higher than those of preterm infants fed pooled human milk at a fixed volume. The effects of feeding taurine-deficient formula to human infants, which occurred before the addition of taurine to infant formula, are not as severe as seen in the kitten. The presence of taurine in human milk and the predominance of taurine conjugates in the gut at birth suggest that bile acid conjugate status may be a controlling factor. When bile acid metabolism was measured in infants fed human milk, the infants consistently had higher intraluminal bile acid concentrations at all ages (1 to 5 weeks) than did formula-fed infants with and without additional taurine. Human milk also facilitated intestinal lipid absorption.[84]

Human infants conjugate bile acids predominantly with taurine at birth but quickly develop the capacity to conjugate with glycine. Those infants fed human milk continue to conjugate with taurine, whereas those fed formulas soon conjugate with glycine predominantly. In humans, the various pools of taurine in the body cannot be predicted by the measurement of plasma taurine alone.

Continued investigation of taurine. Since 1968, when scientists' attention was drawn to taurine, more than a thousand reports, including reviews, have been published. The physiologic actions of taurine have been reviewed exhaustively by Huxtable.[85] Nonmetabolic actions such as osmoregulation, calcium modulation, and interactions with phospholipid protein and zinc are reported. Taurine is also observed to be a product of metabolic action and a precursor of many other metabolic actions. Taurine does not function in isolation. Because of the growing evidence for the role of taurine during development, the requirement for taurine for the neonate remains under investigation.

Whey Proteins

When clotted milk stands, the clot contracts, leaving a clear fluid called *whey*, which contains water, electrolytes, and proteins. The ratio of whey proteins to casein is 1.5 for breast milk and 0.25 for cow's milk; that is, 40% of human milk protein is casein and 60% lactalbumin, and cow's milk is 80% casein and 20% lactalbumin.[77]

Human milk forms a flocculent suspension with zero curd tension, indicating the curds are easily digested. The total amount of protein has been recently measured to be 0.9%, which is lower than the previously reported 1.2%. The discrepancy is caused by recalculation of the data, in which the total amount of protein was determined by measuring the nitrogen content and multiplying by 6.25. Of the nitrogen content, 25% is NPN, whereas in bovine milk, 5% of the nitrogen is from NPN. Hambraeus et al.[86] have reported the composition of the NPN fraction to be urea, creatine, creatinine, uric acid, small peptides, and free amino acids.

Closer examination of the whey proteins shows α-lactalbumin and lactoferrin to be the chief fractions, with no measurable β-lactoglobulin, which is the chief constituent of cow's milk (Table 4.15). The term *lactalbumin* includes a mixture of whey proteins found in bovine milk and should not be confused with α-lactalbumin, which is a specific protein that is part of the enzyme lactose synthetase. The α-lactalbumin content parallels lactose levels in different species. Human milk is high in both lactose and α-lactalbumin. Many investigators, however, have continued to measure nitrogen compounds in human milk (see Table 4.15).

Lactoferrin

Lactoferrin is an iron-binding glycoprotein that is part of the whey fraction of proteins in human milk. Structurally, lactoferrin is a 78- to 80-kDa single peptide consisting of two globular domains, each of which binds a molecule of iron.[87] It appears in very low amounts in bovine milk. Lactoferrin ensures the infant's absorption of iron from milk and has been observed to inhibit the growth of certain iron-dependent bacteria in the gastrointestinal (GI) tract.[88] It has been suggested that lactoferrin protects against certain GI infections in breastfed infants. Giving iron to newborn infants appears to inactivate the lactoferrin by saturating it with iron and promoting the growth of *Escherichia coli* in particular. It has other functions, including cell growth regulation, deoxyribonucleic acid (DNA) binding, transcriptional activation of specific DNA sequences, activation of natural killer cells, and antitumor activity. Lactoferrin also has enzyme activity. Those identified are protease, deoxyribonuclease, ribonuclease, adenosine triphosphatase (ATPase), phosphatase, and oligosaccharide hydrolysis. The role of lactoferrin's enzymatic actions in antimicrobial function is under study.[48]

When lactoferrin is digested in the stomach by pepsin, the polypeptides produced, in particular lactoferricin, also have biologic functions, including antimicrobial, antiviral, antitumor,

TABLE 4.15 **Composition of Protein Nitrogen and Nonprotein Nitrogen in Human Milk and Cow Milk[a]**

	Human Milk		Cow Milk	
Protein nitrogen	1.43	(8.9)	5.3	(31.4)
Casein nitrogen	0.40	(2.5)	4.37	(27.3)
Whey protein nitrogen	1.03	(6.4)	0.93	(5.8)
β-Lactalbumin	0.42	(2.6)	0.17	(1.1)
Lactoferrin	0.27	(1.7)	Traces	
β-Lactoglobulin	—		0.57	(3.6)
Lysozyme	0.08	(0.5)	Traces	
Serum albumin	0.08	(0.5)	0.07	(0.4)
IgA	0.16	(1.0)	0.005	(0.03)
IgG	0.005	(0.03)	0.096	(0.06)
IgM	0.003	(0.02)	0.005	(0.03)
Nonprotein nitrogen	0.50		0.28	
Urea nitrogen	0.25		0.13	
Creatine nitrogen	0.037		0.009	
Creatinine nitrogen	0.035		0.003	
Uric acid nitrogen	0.005		0.008	
Glucosamine	0.047		?	
α-Amino nitrogen	0.13		0.048	
Ammonia nitrogen	0.002		0.006	
Nitrogen from other components	?		0.074	
Total nitrogen	1.93		5.31	

IgA, Immunoglobulin A; *IgG*, immunoglobulin G; *IgM*, immunoglobulin M.

[a]Values refer to grams of nitrogen per liter; values within parentheses refer to grams of protein per liter.
From Forsum E, Lönnerdal B. Protein evaluation of breast milk and breast milk substitutes with special reference to the nonprotein nitrogen: effect of protein intake on protein and nitrogen composition of breast milk. *Am J Clin Nutr.* 1980;33:1809.

and immunologic functions. These proteins are under continued study because of their active infection protection. Regarding the impact of storage on lactoferrin, it was noted that 5 days of refrigeration does not change levels, but 3 or more months of freezing significantly lowers the lactoferrin levels. Holder pasteurization also decreases the lactoferrin content of human milk.

Immunoglobulins

The immunoglobulins in breast milk are distinct from those of the serum. They are a key mechanism by which a mother passes immunity to the infant.[89] The main immunoglobulin in serum is IgG, which is present in the amount of 1210 mg/dL.

IgA is found in the serum at 250 mg/dL, one-fifth the level of IgG. The reverse is true of human colostrum and milk. The colostrum IgA level is 1740 mg/dL, and the milk IgA level is 100 mg/dL. Colostrum has 43 mg/dL of IgG, and milk has 4 mg/dL. The IgA and IgG in human milk are derived from serum and from synthesis in the mammary gland.

Lactation is associated with the appearance of catalytically active antibodies or abzymes (Abzs) with DNAse, RNAse, ATPase, amylolytic, protein kinase, and lipid kinase activities in breast milk. Odintsova et al.[90] have demonstrated that the immune system of clinically healthy mothers can generate IgAs with β-casein-specific serine protease-like activity.

sIgA is the principal immunoglobulin in colostrum and milk and all human secretions. sIgA contains an antigenic determinant associated with a secretory component. It is synthesized in the gland from two molecules of serum IgA linked by disulfide bonds. sIgA levels are very high in colostrum for the first few days and then decline rapidly. sIgA is stable at a low pH and resistant to proteolytic enzymes. It is present in the intestine of breastfed infants and provides a protective defense against infection by keeping viruses and bacteria from invading the mucosa. The protective qualities are further described in Chapter 5.

Nonimmunoglobulins

Human milk contains numerous nonimmunoglobulins that are being identified, with their actions isolated and quantified.[91] Mucins and sialic acid–containing glycoproteins have been isolated and demonstrated to inhibit rotavirus replication and prevent experimental gastroenteritis. The rotavirus has been observed to bind to the milk mucin complex, inhibiting its replication both in vitro and in vivo (see later discussion of oligosaccharides and glycoconjugates).

Lysozyme

Lysozyme is a specific protein and basic polypeptide with lytic properties[92] found in high concentration in egg whites and human milk but in low concentration in bovine milk. It has been identified as a nonspecific antimicrobial factor. This enzyme is bacteriolytic against *Enterobacteriaceae* and gram-positive bacteria. It has been found in concentrations up to 0.2 mg/mL. Lysozyme is stable at 100°C (212°F) and at an acid pH. Lysozyme contributes to the development and maintenance of specific intestinal flora of the breastfed infant (see later discussion of enzymes and Chapter 5, "Host-Resistance Factors and Immunologic Significance of Human Milk").

Polyamines

Polyamines are ubiquitous intracellular cationic amines recognized as participants in cell proliferation and differentiation in many tissues, especially those of intestinal tract development, absorption, and biologic activity, in both sucklings and adults of the species.[93] The synthesis of polyamines is an active process in the mammary gland throughout lactation.[94]

Putrescine, spermidine, and spermine have been identified and quantitated in human milk by Pollack et al.[93] They reported mean values per liter of 0 to 615 nmol putrescine, 73 to 3512 nmol spermidine, and 722 to 4458 nmol spermine. In contrast, levels in formula are low and dependent on the protein source. Levels of spermine and spermidine increase greatly during the first few days of lactation, plateauing at levels 12 and 8 times, respectively, the levels immediately postpartum.[6] These findings have been confirmed by Romain et al.,[95] who noted that levels in human milk remained stable throughout lactation. They demonstrated the effects of spermine or spermidine on maturation and "gut closure" and suggest a protective effect of spermine against alimentary allergies.

Nonprotein Nitrogen

NPN accounts for 18% to 30% of the total nitrogen in human milk, compared with only 3% to 5% in cow milk. The NPN fraction of human milk is traditionally identified as the acid-soluble nitrogen remaining in the supernatant after protein precipitation or as the dialyzable nitrogen after dialysis of whole milk.[94] Because large-molecular-weight glycoproteins are also soluble in the acid, the fraction should be called *acid-soluble nitrogen*.[96]

Although there are large interindividual variations, acid-soluble nitrogen ranges from 350 to 530 mg/L. The total nitrogen ranges from 1700 to 3700 mg/L, depending on length of gestation, duration of lactation, and maternal diet. Some of the nitrogen contributes to the pool available for the synthesis of nonessential amino acids in the neonate. Those compounds having more specialized roles are peptide hormone/growth factors, epidermal growth factor (EGF), amino sugars of oligosaccharides, free amino acids, amino alcohols of phospholipids, nucleic acids, nucleotides, and carnitine. Their importance is not based on the percentage of concentration because they may serve roles as catalysts. Many protein factors in human milk serve roles other than growth, such as the host resistance factors (lactoferrin, sIgA, and lysozyme).

Table 4.16 presents the significance of these compounds and their relative concentrations. The wide variety of nitrogenous compounds within the protein fraction of human milk is only beginning to be investigated and understood. This

TABLE 4.16   Levels and Significance of Nonprotein Nitrogen (NPN) Constituents of Human Milk

NPN	CONCENTRATION IN MILK		Significance
	Less Than 30 Days	More Than 30 Days	
Amino sugars			
N-Acetylglucosamine	230 mg N/L	150 mg N/L	Low oral osmotic load; controls gut colonization; constituent of gangliosides for brain development
N-Acetylneuraminic acid	63 mg N/L	3–27 mg N/L	Substrate for gut epithelium
Peptides	—	60 mg N/L	
Epidermal growth factor	88 ng/mL	—	Regulates intestinal mucosal development
Somatomedin-C/insulin-like growth factor	18 ng/mL	6–8 ng/mL	Stimulates DNA synthesis and cell division in gut
Delta sleep-inducing peptide	30 ng/mL	5 ng/mL	Diurnal pattern highest at 2 PM and 8 PM; ? influences sleep–wake patterns
Insulin	21 ng/mL	2 ng/mL	? Regulates development of gut
Free amino acids			
Taurine	41–45 μmol/dL	27–67 μmol/dL	See under "Taurine" in text
Glutamic acid/glutamine	2–9 μmol/dL	13–58 μmol/dL	Improves zinc absorption; precursor to brain glutamate
Carnitine	1.0 mg N/L	0.7 mg N/L	Brain lipid synthesis
Choline and ethanolamine	7–20 mg N/L	10–20 mg N/L	Possible growth requirement
Nucleic acid	—	19 mg N/L	Pool of DNA and RNA
Nucleotides	3 mg N/L	3 mg N/L	Growth and immune advantage
Polyamines	0.1 mg N/L	0.2 mg N/L	Increase rate of transcription, translation, and amino acid activation

DNA, Deoxyribonucleic acid; *N/L*, nitrogen per liter; *RNA*, ribonucleic acid.

information clearly widens the chemical gap between human milk and proprietary formulas. Increasing evidence suggests that the premature infant reaps even more benefit than the term infant from mother's milk, based on the investigations of NPN alone.

Although glutamic acid and taurine are the most abundant free amino acids in colostrum, taurine remains constant throughout lactation, but glutamic acid and glutamine increased from 2.5 to 20 times in the first 3 months in studies in 16 healthy lactating women.[72] The total content of free amino acids remains stable during that period, so over 50% of the total is glutamine and glutamic acid at 3 months. These components have been associated with facilitating growth and development, protecting intestinal mucosa, and potentiating immune responses.

Maternal milk production and the protein nitrogen (but not NPN) fraction of human milk are well preserved when lactating women are subjected to marginal dietary protein intakes in the short term.[96] In nitrogen-balance studies of poor Mexican women who were lactating, equilibrium was attained at 178.9 ± 25.8 mg nitrogen (1.1 g protein/kg body weight/day), which is close to current dietary standards.[97]

Interest in urea levels has been stimulated because women with various stages of renal failure were concerned about the effect of high serum levels of urea on their milk urea levels. Urea is 30% to 50% of the NPN in milk. Levels decrease from colostrum to mature milk (3.2 g/dL nitrogen in colostrum to 1.7 g/dL in milk). If the original milk urea was provided solely by passive diffusion from the maternal blood, a constant level of urea nitrogen would be anticipated at all stages of lactation instead of increasing from colostrum to mature milk.[94] There is a single clinical report of human milk analysis from a mother on chronic hemodialysis, which demonstrated elevated levels of creatinine and urea in the mother's breast milk. These levels were notably lower in post-hemodialysis samples. No data were included regarding the effect or success of breastfeeding for this mother–infant dyad.[98]

Nucleotides

Increased attention has been paid to the presence and role of nucleotides in human milk as their relative absence in bovine milk has led to experimental supplementation of some infant formulas. Nucleotides have been identified as playing key roles in biochemical processes within the cell, acting as metabolic regulators and altering enzyme activities.

A dietary requirement has not been established because they can be synthesized de novo in the adult. Human milk provides 20% of NPN as nucleotides; furthermore, human milk provides a larger percentage (30%) of nitrogen as NPN, three times more than other species. The daily intake from human milk is 1.4 to 2.1 mg of nucleotide nitrogen.[99] Cytidine, adenine, and uridine compose the majority of soluble nucleotides.

Nucleotides are compounds derived from nucleic acid by hydrolysis and consist of phosphoric acid combined with a sugar and a purine or pyrimidine derivative. The level and components of acid-soluble nucleotides of several species,

including humans, have been studied extensively. Work has shown a characteristic nucleotide composition in the milk that differs from that of the mammary gland. The large numbers of purine and pyrimidine nucleotides present in various tissues have a number of functions in the cell. They are part of nucleic acid synthesis and metabolism and are also part of milk synthesis. It is well known that adenosine triphosphate (ATP) supplies usable energy for biosynthetic reactions.

Free nucleotides in human milk have been recorded at 6.1 to 9.0 mmol/dL.[99] The levels in colostrum and mature milk are similar, although colostrum typically contains somewhat higher concentrations.[100] The conspicuous difference in the quality and quantity of nucleotides between the mammary gland and its secretion would indicate that nucleotides are secreted from the epithelial cells of the gland into the milk. Distinct species differences exist in the composition and content of nucleotides as well. Cytidine monophosphate and uracil are the nucleotides in the highest concentration in human milk, which also contains uridine diphosphate-n-acetyllactosamine and other oligosaccharides. Human milk contains only a trace of orotic acid and no guanosine diphosphate fucose. Orotic acid is the chief nucleotide of bovine milk. Nucleotide levels fall rapidly in bovine milk to minimal levels in mature bovine milk. Synthetic nucleotides produced for formula have a very different profile.

When the nitrogen fraction of human milk was further identified over time at 2, 4, 8, and 12 weeks, a variance was noted in the pattern of nucleotides (Table 4.17).[99] Levels of cytidine-5′-monophosphate and adenosine-5′-monophosphate declined from 594 to 321 mg/dL and from 244 to 143 mg/dL, respectively, whereas levels of inosine-5′-monophosphate increased from 158 to 290 mg/dL. The total nucleotide nitrogen remained constant, accounting for 0.10% to 0.15% of the total NPN. The average intake per day of a normal breastfed

TABLE 4.17 Nucleotide Content of Human Milk

Nucleotide	Mean[a] (mg/dL)
Cytidine monophosphate	461 (17.9)
Uridine monophosphate	179 (19.8)
Adenosine monophosphate	175 (12.8)
Inosine monophosphate	228 (14.5)
Guanosine monophosphate	138 (8.5)
Uridine diphosphate	174 (12.8)
Cytidine diphosphate	474 (41.5)
Adenosine diphosphate	69 (17.9)
Guanosine diphosphate	96 (8.9)

[a]Mean nucleotide content of human milk at weeks 2, 4, 8, and 12 of lactation.
Modified from Hendricks K. Nucleotide content human milk. *Semin Pediatr Gastroenterol Nutr.* 1991;2:14; Janas LM, Picciano MF. The nucleotide profile of human milk. *Pediatr Res.* 1982;16:659.

infant would be 1.4 to 2.1 mg of nucleotide nitrogen. Measurement of adenosine-5'-monophosphate and cyclic guanosine monophosphate showed variation in concentration within 15 minutes, which fluctuated throughout 24 hours.[99] Milk concentration differed widely from maternal plasma levels collected at the same time.

The biologic effects of dietary nucleotides involve the immune system, the intestinal microenvironment, and the absorption and metabolism of certain other nutrients. Given nucleotides' important roles, they are considered "semiessential" for newborns.[101] Whether inosine-5'-monophosphate contributes to the superior iron absorption is still unanswered.

Metabolic disturbances in nucleotide metabolism can result in an abnormal accumulation of specific intermediates in cells and tissues, causing a variety of diseases. An example is Lesch–Nyhan syndrome, a genetic disease characterized by mental retardation, self-mutilation, and gout, which is caused by the absence of the purine salvage enzyme. On the other hand, disturbances from a lack of nucleotides in the diet have not been identified.

Nucleotides are formed by de novo synthesis by capturing or scavenging partially degraded nucleotides or are obtained completely from the diet. Dietary nucleotides are absorbed by the action of the microvillus membrane as nucleosides. The developing neonate has a reduced capacity to synthesize or salvage nucleotides. Exogenous nucleotides are potential stimuli, modulating not only the gene control of their own metabolism but also that of a number of functions in the cardiovascular, neurologic, and immune systems.[100] Nucleotides are important as coenzymes for the processes involved in the metabolism of lipids, carbohydrates, and proteins. Nucleotides are recognized as an integral part of the immune system, acting as the host defense against bacteria, viruses, and parasites, as well as various malignancies. Nucleotides are important in the process of protein synthesis, which is enhanced in the newborn infant by a dietary supply of nucleotides. A high-protein diet (20%) does produce a significant growth increase when nucleotides are added. This result may explain the satisfactory growth pattern of breastfed infants on relatively low protein intake and the more efficient protein utilization of breastfed infants.

Study of the exact role of nucleotides continues in vivo, although some effort to supplement formula with synthetic nucleotides already occurs.

CARBOHYDRATES

The predominant carbohydrate of milk is lactose, or milk sugar. It is present in high concentration (6.8 g/dL in human milk and 4.9 g/dL in bovine milk). Lactose is a disaccharide compound of two monosaccharides, galactose and glucose. Lactose is synthesized by the mammary gland as a dynamic process.

A number of other carbohydrates are present in milk. They are classified as monosaccharides, neutral and acid oligosaccharides, and peptide-bound and protein-bound carbohydrates.

Small amounts of glucose (1.4 g/dL) and galactose (1.2 g/dL) also are present in breast milk. Other complex carbohydrates are present in free form or bound to amino acids or protein, such as n-acetylglucosamine. The concentration of oligosaccharides in human milk is about 10 times greater than that in cow's milk. These carbohydrates and glycoproteins possess bifidus factor activity. Fucose, which is not present in bovine milk, may be important to the early establishment of *L. bifidus* as gut flora. The nitrogen-containing carbohydrates are 0.7% of milk solids.

Wack et al.[102] observed that lactose concentrations increased from 66 ± 4 g/L between day 0 and 60 to 71 ± 4 g/L by day 181.

Lactose is hydrolyzed selectively by a brush-border enzyme called *lactase* located predominantly in the tip of the intestinal villi. Digestion of lactose is the rate-limiting step in its absorption. Although lactase activity develops later in fetal life than that of other disaccharidases, it is present by 24 weeks of fetal life. The lactase concentration is greatest in the proximal jejunum. Levels continue to increase throughout the last trimester, reaching concentrations at term of two to four times the levels at 2 to 11 months of age. Premature infants rapidly increase their lactase levels when given a lactose challenge. A well-fed breastfed infant ingesting 150 mL of milk/kg per day receives 10 g of lactose/kg per day, which ensures the normal unstressed infant at least 4 mg/kg per min of glucose, which is considered the optimal rate.

Lactose does appear to be specific, however, for newborn growth. It has been shown to enhance calcium absorption and has been suggested as being critical to the prevention of rickets, in view of the relatively low calcium levels in human milk. Lactose is a readily available source of galactose, which is essential to the production of the galactolipids, including cerebroside. These galactolipids are essential to CNS development.

Interesting correlations have been made between the amount of lactose in the milk of a species and the relative size of the brain (Fig. 4.13).[103] Because lactose is found only in milk and not in other animal and plant sources, its high level in human milk is even more significant. Lactose levels are relatively constant throughout the day in a given mother's milk. Even in poorly nourished mothers, the levels of lactose do not vary. Because lactose is influential in controlling volume, the total output for the day may be diminished, but the concentration of lactose in human milk will be 6.2 to 7.2 g/dL.[18] An adequate source of carbohydrate is important for optimal lactation, which suggests that excessive amounts of sugar substitutes may have an effect on volume.[104]

Oligosaccharides and Glycoconjugates

Human milk oligosaccharides (HMOs) have become an area of intense investigation and study in human milk science. They are complex sugars that provide a number of protective and early-life immune programming and prevention functions for the infant and may provide an indicator of infants' predisposition to particular diseases.[105,106] HMOs are the third-largest solid component in milk after lactose and triglycerides. They reach up to 20 g/L in early milk.[107] Of the 21

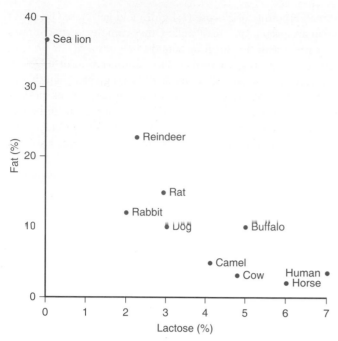

Fig. 4.13 Concentration of lactose varies with source of milk. In general, there is less lactose and more fat, which can also be used by newborn animals as an energy source. (From Kretchmer N. Lactose and lactase. *Sci Am.* 1972;227:73. Copyright © 1972 by Scientific American, Inc. All rights reserved.)

oligosaccharides studied in depth, the highest amount is present by day 4, with a gradual decrease of 20% by day 30. Nevertheless, HMO concentrations remain higher than those of milk proteins.[108]

Infants do not digest the majority of ingested HMOs; thus they reach the colon unaltered. There, they interact with intestinal microbiota and the mucosal immune system.[109] HMOs can also bind to epithelial and immune-system cells, providing proof that breast milk provides much more than just nutrition.[110] The variability in certain milk metabolites suggests possible roles in infant gut microbial development.[105]

Most of the milk oligosaccharides contain lactose at the reducing end of the structure and may also contain fucose or sialic acid at the nonreducing end. More than 200 neutral and acidic oligosaccharides have been identified.[110] One liter of milk contains 5 to 15 g of unbound oligosaccharides.[110] The high amount and structural diversity are unique to humans.[111] The structural complexity of milk oligosaccharides hampers the assignment of specific functions to single carbohydrates. Biochemically, oligosaccharides result from the sequential addition of monosaccharides to the lactose molecule in the mammary gland by glycosyltransferases.

Genetic Determinants of HMO Synthesis

The presence and quantity of different types of oligosaccharides in human milk are genetically determined,[112] and HMOs' composition mirrors the synthesizing mothers' blood group characteristics as well as nutritional and environmental variables, potentially.[108]

The *Se* gene is responsible for encoding the enzymes to synthesize α1,2-fucosylated oligosaccharides; the *Le* gene—related to Lewis blood groups—encodes the enzymes for α1,4-fucosylated oligosaccharides. An active *Se* locus means a woman can produce α1,2-fucosylated oligosaccharides and is considered a "secretor" (Se[+]), whereas a woman lacking an active *Se* locus is a "nonsecretor" (Se[−]) and does not produce milk with α1,2-fucosylated oligosaccharides. Similarly, an active *Le* locus results in the ability to produce α1,4-fucosylated oligosaccharides, making a woman "Lewis positive" (Le[+]), whereas being "Lewis negative" (Le[−]) results in a lack of α1,4-fucosylated oligosaccharides in the mother's milk.[109]

Benefits of Oligosaccharides

Neonates cannot digest oligosaccharides; however, they provide nutrition to the infants' growing gut microbiota.[105] Originally, the physiologic role of human milk and oligosaccharides had been limited to the enhancement of the growth of *L. bifidus* flora and indirectly to the protection against GI infections. It is now known that human milk oligosaccharides act as prebiotics, functioning as substrates for beneficial bacteria; soluble decoys preventing the adhesion of viruses, bacteria, and their toxins to their carbohydrate mucosal receptors; and immune modulators affecting gene expression within intestinal epithelial cells, influencing cytokine production and T-cell response and diminishing leukocyte rolling on endothelial cells and subsequent activation and infiltration.[111] An additional proinflammatory action of 3-sialyllactose has been explained as being a result of the modulation of intestinal bacterial groups and, on the other hand, to a direct stimulatory effect on CD11c + dendritic cells.[110] Sialic acid (Sia) constitutes a family of derivatives from neuraminic acid. The dominant form of Sia in humans is N-acetylneuraminic acid (Neu5Ac), which is a key precursor of neural brain glycoproteins. Evidence is accumulating that Sia-containing gangliosides contribute to brain growth and cognition.[113]

Antimicrobial effects have been demonstrated by core oligosaccharides against *Streptococcus pneumoniae*, *Helicobacter pylori*, *E. coli*, and influenza viruses. Fig. 4.14 presents HMOs' various functions.

The association between maternal maternal milk levels of two-linked fucosylated oligosaccharide and the prevention of diarrhea as a result of *Campylobacter*, caliciviruses, and all causes in breastfed infants was studied by Morrow et al.[114] Evidence was found that human milk oligosaccharides may offer clinically relevant protection against diarrhea.

Glycoproteins, glycosylated major milk proteins, include lactoferrin, immunoglobulins, and mucins. Their protective characteristics have been described as acting as receptor homologs, inhibiting the binding of enteropathogens to their host receptors. Research continues to link specific carbohydrate structures with protection against specific pathogens. These nonimmunoglobulin agents are also active against whole classes of pathogens.[2] The protective glycoconjugates and oligosaccharides are unique to human milk and to date have not been replicated synthetically. They are synthesized exclusively

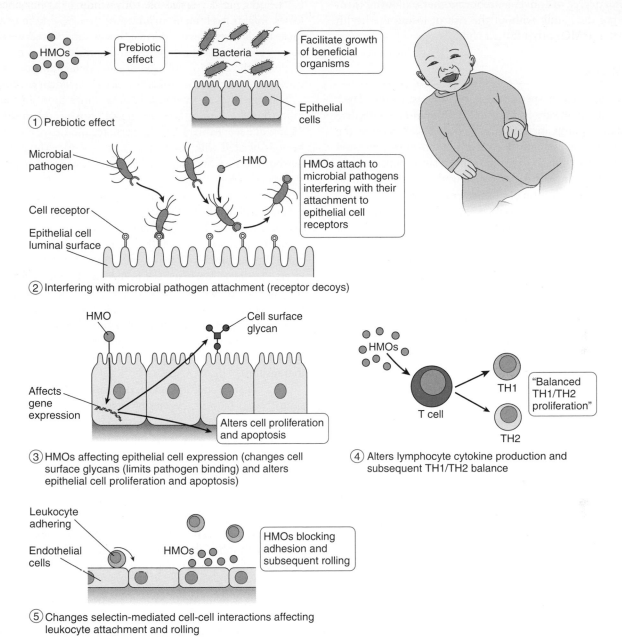

Fig. 4.14 Five potential benefits of human milk oligosaccharides *(HMOs)* on the infant's immunity. (From Bode L. Human milk oligosaccharides: Every baby needs a sugar mama. *Glycobiology* 2012;22:1147—1162, Fig. 5.)

in the mammary gland and only during lactation. Human oligosaccharides are distinct from other species with respect to quantity, quality, and diversity.[111]

HMOs, a major family of complex glycans, are relevant to clinical illness in neonates and term infants. The newly emerging technologies for the biologic testing of these molecules are opening new opportunities to identify prophylactic and therapeutic agents that inhibit a variety of pathogens.

Oligosaccharides in Formula

HMOs are both more complex and abundant than the oligosaccharides of other species' milk. As a result, infants fed with formula do not receive HMOs and their specific benefits.

Formula producers are attempting to substitute this unique human milk component by adding galactooligosaccharides and fructoololigosaccharides, which are not naturally occurring in milk. Sources of oligosaccharides for use in formulas currently include extraction from cow's milk, chemical synthesis, and production by genetically engineered microbes. To date, these are being produced in small quantities and still have to be proven as identical to or sufficiently biosimilar to achieve the benefits of HMOs in human infants.[115] The long-term health impacts of adding substitute oligosaccharides to formula have yet to be investigated.[108]

Of further note, pasteurization and even freeze-drying do not alter oligosaccharide composition.[106] As such, this provides a degree of convenience for mothers, allowing them to preserve their milk without the risk of losing the health benefits that HMOs provide their child.

MINERALS

Minerals represent a special category of constituents. Their pathways into milk vary from simple diffusion to both positive and negative pump mechanisms.[116] Table 4.18 records the measurements of the constituents in human milk compared with maternal serum. By examining this relationship, it can be estimated how the particular constituent reaches the milk, that is, by passive diffusion or positive or negative pump.

The total ash content of milk is species specific and parallels the growth rate and body structure of the offspring. Numerous metallic elements and organic and inorganic acids are present in milk as ions, unionized salts, and weakly ionized salts. Some are bound to other constituents. Sodium, potassium, calcium, and magnesium are the major cations. Phosphate, chloride, and citrate are the major anions.[117]

The monovalent ions are sodium, potassium, and chloride. The divalent ions are calcium, magnesium, citrate, phosphate, and sulfate.[118] The monovalent ions are among the most prevalent and contribute 30 mOsmol, or one-tenth of the total osmolarity of human milk.[118] The sum of the concentrations of the monovalent ions is inversely proportional to the lactose content across species. The monovalent ion concentration is regulated chiefly by the secretion mechanism in the alveolar cell, with humans having the highest lactose and lowest ion content.[27] This maintains osmolality close to that of serum.

Daily intakes of calcium, phosphorus, zinc, potassium, sodium, iron, and copper from breast milk were found to decrease significantly over the first 4 months of life, with only magnesium increasing. Despite apparently low mineral intakes, growth during this time was found to be satisfactory by Butte et al.[119] High mineral content is associated with a rapid growth rate of specific species.

Potassium and Sodium

Potassium levels are much higher than those of sodium, which are similar to the proportions in intracellular fluids (Table 4.19). Although sodium, potassium, and chloride are present as free ions, the other constituents appear as complexes and compounds. Ions can pass through the secretory cell membrane in both directions and in and out of the breast duct lumen. Intracellular sodium, chloride, and potassium are in equilibrium with the ions of the plasma and alveolar milk. An apical pumping mechanism has been calculated for chloride release, whereas sodium, potassium, and intracellular chloride pass into milk because of their electrochemical gradients. The cellular pumping mechanism maintains the ionic concentrations in the extracellular fluid and alveolar milk.

The Committee on Nutrition of the American Academy of Pediatrics[120] has stated that the daily requirement of sodium for growth is 0.5 mEq/kg per day between birth and 3 months of age, decreasing to 0.1 mEq/kg per day after 6 months of age (Table 4.20). To cover dermal losses, an additional 0.4 to 0.7 mEq/kg per day is needed, with a little for urine and stool losses. Infants fed human milk receive enough sodium to meet their needs for growth, dermal losses, and urinary losses. Studies by Keenan et al.[121] have demonstrated an apparent regulation in the levels of milk sodium and potassium concentrations by adrenocorticosteroids as well as a circadian rhythm.

Sodium levels in cow milk are 3.6 times those in human milk (human: 7 mEq/L or 15 mg/dL; bovine: 22 mEq/L or 58 mg/dL; see Table 4.19). Hypernatremic dehydration has been associated with cow's milk feedings. Experiments with newborn rats on high salt intakes have shown that hypertension can develop.

The diurnal variation in milk electrolytes was found to vary between 22% and 80%.[121] These changes varied as the lactation period progressed but were independent of the mother's diet. Sodium restriction did not influence milk levels. In a longitudinal study, sodium levels fell from 20 to 15 mEq/L in the first week. On day 8, levels were 8 mEq/L, and by the fifth week, they were stabilized at 6 mEq/L.[122] Time-dependent changes in milk composition are also reported by Allen et al. as a 25% or greater decrease in sodium, potassium, and citrate from 1 to 6 months. Calcium and glucose increase by 10% or more over this time. The authors suggest that milk composition is always in transition.[12]

At a constant sodium intake, decreasing the sodium/potassium (Na/K) ratio in the diet by increasing potassium lowers blood pressure. The dietary Na/K ratio has an important role in determining the severity, if not the development, of salt-induced hypertension. The mechanism of potassium's antihypertensive effect is unclear, but the higher potassium and lower sodium levels of breast milk appear to be physiologically beneficial.

Chloride

Little attention has been paid to the adequacy of chloride in the diet, and it has always been assumed to be sufficient until recent events focused attention on this cation.

Chloride deficiency in infants has become associated with a syndrome of failure to thrive with hypochloremia and hypokalemic metabolic alkalosis. This was first described in infants fed formula that was deficient in chloride but has also been described in a breastfed infant whose mother's milk contained less than 266 mg/L chloride (normal is greater than 400 mg/L).[102] This is a rare phenomenon caused by unexplained maternal production. This mother had previously successfully nourished five other infants.

Total Ash

Cow's milk has three times the total salt content of human milk (Table 4.21). All the minerals that appear in cow's milk also appear in human milk. The phosphorus level is six times greater in cow's milk; the calcium level is four times higher (see Table 4.21).

The renal solute load of cow milk is considerably higher than that of breast milk. This is magnified by the metabolic breakdown products of the high protein content, which are in increased amounts as well. This is shown in the high urea levels in formula-fed infants (Table 4.22). Although the mean

TABLE 4.18 Difference in Composition of Human Milk and Blood Plasma

	Specific Gravity	Osmolarity	pH	Calories (kcal/dL)	Water (g%)	Carbohydrates	Fat	PROTEIN		Iron	Na$^+$ (mg%)	K$^+$ (mg%)
								Albumin (g%)	Globulin (g%)			
Human mature milk	1031	295	7.3	65	87.5	7.0 g% (lactose)	3.7 g%	0.3	0.2	0.15 mg%	15	57
Blood plasma	1033	285	7.4	35	92	80 mg% (glucose)	200 mg%	4.5	2.5	125 µg%	320	18

	Ca^{2+} (mg%)	Mg^{2+} (mg%)	Cl$^-$ (mg%)	Phosphorus (mg%)	Sulfur (mg%)	VITAMINS					
						A^a	B$_1$ (µg%)	B$_2$ (µg%)	Niacin (µg%)	C (mg%)	D (IU/dL)
Human mature milk	35	4	43	15	14	280 IU/dL	20	50	172	5	5
Blood plasma	10	2.5	365	4	2	50 µg%	190	0.5	500	1	188

^{a}1 µg of vitamin A corresponds to the activity of 3 IU of vitamin A.
Modified from Vorheer H. *The Breasts: Morphology, Physiology, and Lactation*. New York: Academic Press; 1974.

TABLE 4.19   Minerals in Human Milk and Cow Milk (per Deciliter)

Minerals	Colostrum	Transitional	Mature	Cow's Milk
Calcium (mg)	39	46	35	130
Chlorine (mg)	85	46	40	108
Copper (µg)	40	50	40	14
Iron (µg)	70	70	100	70
Magnesium (mg)	4	4	4	12
Phosphorus (mg)	14	20	15	120
Potassium (mg)	74	64	57	145
Sodium (mg)	48	30	15	58
Sulfur (mg)	22	20	14	30
Total ash (mg)	—	—	200	700

From Food and Nutrition Board, National Research Council, National Academy of Sciences. *Recommended Dietary Allowances.* Washington, DC: US Government Printing Office; 2011.

TABLE 4.20   Recommended Dietary Intake of Electrolytes for Infants

Age	Sodium (g/d)	Potassium (g/d)	Chloride (g/d)
To 6 mo	0.12	0.4	0.18
6 mo–1 yr	0.37	0.7	0.57

From Food and Nutrition Board, National Research Council, National Academy of Sciences. *Recommended Dietary Allowances.* Washington, DC: US Government Printing Office; 2011.

TABLE 4.21   Principal Salt Constituents in Bovine and Human Milks

Constituent	Bovine (mg/dL)	Human (mg/dL)
Calcium	125	33
Magnesium	12	4
Sodium	58	15
Potassium	138	55
Chloride	103	43
Phosphorus	96	15
Citric acid	175	20–80
Sulfur (total)	30	14 ± 2.6 (4.5 mmol/L)
Carbon dioxide	20	—

From Jenness R, Sloan RE. Composition of milk. In: Larson BL, Smith VR, eds. *Lactation, Vol. 3, Nutrition and Biochemistry of Milk/Maintenance.* New York: Academic Press; 1974.

urea levels in breast milk are 37 mg/dL and only 15 mg/dL in cow milk, the blood urea levels in breastfed infants are about 22 mg/dL, whereas those of infants fed formula are 47 mg/dL and those of infants fed formula plus solids are 52 mg/dL (see Table 4.22). The plasma osmolarity of infants fed breast milk is lower and approximates the physiologic level of plasma.

Calcium-to-Phosphorus Ratio

The calcium-to-phosphorus (Ca/P) ratio is considerably lower in cow's milk (1:4) than in human milk (2:2). Many investigators have studied calcium and phosphorus values in human milk and found some variation from mother to mother and from study to study. The Ca/P ratio varied from 1.8 to 2.4, with the absolute values for calcium varying from 20 to 34 mg/dL and those for phosphorus varying from 14 to 18 mg/dL. Fetal and newborn plasma concentrations for calcium decline sharply from 10.4 mg/dL at birth to 8.5 mg/dL by day 4. Unlike calcium, phosphorus concentrations rise in the postnatal period. The drop in serum calcium levels in the bottle-fed infants was more marked than in the breastfed infants. Infant serum phosphorus concentrations rise during the postnatal period. When gestation is prolonged or the mother has preeclampsia, the concentrations are even higher at birth.

Longitudinal studies by Greer et al.,[123] measuring calcium and phosphorus in human milk and maternal and infant sera, have shown progressive increases in infant serum calcium in association with a decreasing phosphorus content of breast milk and infant serum. Maternal serum calcium also increased, although the mother's dietary intake was below recommended levels for lactating women. Calcium uptake in the maternal duodenum is enhanced during lactation.

Although the Ca/P ratio has been stressed in the past, recent investigations have not found a statistical correlation between the calcium and phosphorus contents of plasma and the corresponding breast-milk Ca/P ratio. This finding suggests that the Ca/P ratio is not critical in the low mineral loads present in breast milk. Calcium and phosphorus decrease over time during lactation.[124]

Lactating women contribute 210 mg of calcium per day in breast milk. A study of the intestinal calcium absorption of

TABLE 4.22   **Statistical Analysis by Student's *T*-Test of Blood Urea Levels in 61 Healthy Infants Age 1 to 3 Months**

Infant Group	Number	Blood Urea, Mean ± SE (mg/dL)	Individual Values >40 mg/dL	
			Number	Total Observations (%)
A: Breastfed	12	22.7 ± 1.6[a]	0	0[b]
B: Artificial milk alone	16	47.4 ± 2.0[c]	12	75[d]
C: Artificial milk + solid foods	33	51.9 ± 1.8	29	88

SE, Standard error.
[a]When compared with group B and group C: $p < 0.001$ ($t = 9.7$) and $p < 0.001$ ($t = 11.5$), respectively.
[b]When compared with group B and group C: $p < 0.001$ ($t = 6.9$) and $p < 0.001$ ($t = 15.5$), respectively.
[c]When compared with group C: $p > 0.05$ ($t = 1.6$).
[d]When compared with group C: $p > 0.05$ ($t = 1.1$).
From Davies DP, Saunders R. Blood urea: normal values in early infancy related to feeding practices. *Arch Dis Child.* 1973;48:563.

women during lactation and after weaning revealed that serum calcium and phosphorus concentrations were greater in lactating compared with nonlactating postpartum women, but levels were the same after weaning.[125] Calcitriol, however, was greater in women after weaning compared with postpartum control subjects.[126] Lactating women lost significantly more bone throughout the body and in the lumbar spine than nonlactating postpartum women in the first 6 months. After weaning, the lactating women regained significantly more bone in the lumbar spine than nonlactating women. Early resumption of menses was associated with a smaller loss and greater increase after weaning.[127] Parathyroid hormone concentrations are reported to be higher only after weaning.

Calcium supplementation does not prevent bone loss during lactation and only slightly enhances the gain in bone density after weaning.[125] Supplementation did not affect levels in the milk. Krebs et al.[128] reported that excesses of protein have a negative effect on calcium absorption in lactating women. The Ca/P ratio appears to be critical for efficient utilization. Estradiol stimulated the osteoblastic proliferation and enhanced the collagen gene expression. Calcium was shown to be well absorbed in 5- to 7-month-old breastfed infants who had begun to receive beikost (solids and semisolids).

Magnesium and Other Salts

Magnesium is present as a free ion and in complexes with casein and phosphate in caseinate micelles or citrate complexes. Cow's milk has three times as much magnesium as human milk (12 mg/dL compared with 4 mg/dL; see Table 4.21).

Generally, research has found magnesium concentrations in mature milk to be roughly 35 mg/L.[129] The bound fraction was associated with low-molecular-weight proteins, thus enhancing bioavailability.

Longitudinal magnesium concentrations were measured by Greer et al.[123] in milk and maternal sera and in the infants over a 6-month period. Progressive increases in serum magnesium level were seen in the breastfed infants in association with a decreasing phosphorus content of the milk. Butts et al. also found that magnesium concentrations in breast milk were positively associated with maternal dietary intake of magnesium.[129] Citrate is found in the milks of many species and is three to four times higher in cow's milk than in human milk (see Table 4.21). The distribution of ions and salts differs among various milks and depends on the relative concentrations of casein and citrate.

Citrate is made in the mitochondria from pyruvate and transported into the cytoplasm, where it is available for lipid synthesis and for transport into the Golgi complex.[118] Citrate levels are not often measured in human milk, although citrate may be a marker of milk-production potential (see Fig. 4.7). Levels are high the first few days and rise as calcium levels rise.

Most of the sulfur in milk is in the sulfur-containing amino acids, with only about 10% present as sulfate ion. Some organic acids are present, and they appear as anions in milk.

TRACE ELEMENTS

Table 4.23 lists the recommended daily intake of trace elements for infants.[130] Various elements are considered trace

TABLE 4.23   **Recommended Dietary Intake of Trace Elements for Infants[a]**

Age	Copper (μg/d)	Manganese (mg/d)	Fluoride (mg/d)	Chromium (μg/d)	Selenium (μg/d)	Molybdenum (μg/d)
To 6 mo	0.4–0.6	0.3–0.6	0.1–0.5	0.01–0.04	0.01–0.04	0.015–0.03
6 mo–1 yr	0.6–0.7	0.6–1.0	0.2–1.0	0.02–0.06	0.015–0.06	0.02–0.04

[a]Because the toxic levels for many trace elements may be only several times the usual intakes, the upper levels for the trace elements given in this table should not be habitually exceeded.
From Food and Nutrition Board, National Research Council, National Academy of Sciences. *Recommended Dietary Allowances.* Washington, DC: US Government Printing Office; 2011.

TABLE 4.24	Recommended Dietary Intake of Minerals for Infants[a]					
Age	Calcium (mg/d)	Phosphorus (mg/d)	Magnesium (mg/d)	Iron (mg/d)	Zinc (mg/d)	Iodine (μg/d)
To 6 mo	200	100	30	0.27	2	110
6 mo–1 yr	260	275	75	11	3	130

[a]Because little information is available on which to base allowances, these amounts are provided in the form of ranges of recommended intakes.

From Food and Nutrition Board, National Research Council, National Academy of Sciences. *Recommended Dietary Allowances.* Washington, DC: US Government Printing Office; 2011.

elements for humans, including iron, zinc, fluorine, and iodide. Copper, selenium, chromium, manganese, molybdenum, and nickel are also considered trace elements, which constitute less than 0.01% of body weight; however, their atoms are present in large numbers and play a critical role in growth and development. The technical ability to measure these elements is expanding. The effects of trace-element deficiencies in fetal and neonatal development are yet to be fully understood.

Iron

Iron is a critical element for the infant's CNS and cognitive development in the first year of life.[88] It has been determined that normal infants need 1500 mg of exogenous elemental iron in the first year of life, which can be translated into 8 to 10 mg/day (Table 4.24). Prepared infant formulas currently supply 10 to 12 mg/day. Human milk only contains between 220 and 2640 μg/L of iron, with a median of 380 μg/L,[131] which does not meet the requirements just given. Iron's bioavailability is very high, however, and breastfed infants have historically not been anemic.[88]

Feeley et al.[132] studied 102 American women by stage of lactation; 96% of the women took prenatal iron supplements. A diurnal variation was observed, and a significant decrease occurred in the iron content of their milk from 4 to 45 days postpartum. The authors estimated that fully breastfed infants would receive 0.10 mg/kg per day of iron.

Iron absorption from human milk is more efficient and has been noted to be 49% of iron available, whereas only 10% of cow's milk iron and 4% of iron in iron-fortified formulas are absorbed. The hematologic values of bottle-fed infants were abnormal, whereas those of breastfed infants were not. The breastfed infants had high ferritin levels, indicating a long-term adequacy of iron assimilation. Even when bovine lactoferrin is added to infant formula, it does not improve iron absorption because the bovine lactoferrin cannot bind to human receptors, resulting in lower iron levels.[133]

The infant who is exclusively breastfed for the first 6 months of life is not at risk for iron-deficiency anemia or the depletion of iron stores during that time.[134]

Other factors that influence iron absorption include higher amounts of vitamin C. Lactose, which promotes iron absorption, is in higher concentration in breast milk, especially compared with prepared formulas, which may not contain lactose. Calcium and phosphorus may interfere with iron absorption, as may high protein levels. Considerable doubt

still exists as to whether it is physiologically sound to increase the hemoglobin of an infant with exogenous iron, but research has found that iron supplementation can increase hemoglobin and iron storage and reduce the risk of anemia in LBW infants.[88] All mammals investigated so far have a drop in their hemoglobin levels after birth and a subsequent gradual rise to adult levels for the species.

A study of 40 normal, full-term infants followed in an Argentinian clinic found that the exclusively breastfed infants had a 27% incidence of anemia compared with a 7% rate in those who received iron-supplemented formula.[135] No storage iron was found in the breastfed infants with anemia. The average incidence of anemia in children in Argentina is 46%. The mothers had been instructed to start beef, liver, and orange juice at 6 months. Most of the iron was present in hemoglobin, the body storage of iron being a small fraction of total body iron (2.05% for breastfed infants and 2.79% for formula-fed infants).[135]

Pisacane et al.[136] studied the iron status of 30 infants breastfed until their first birthday who never received cow's milk, supplemental iron, or iron-enriched formula. Examination of their iron stores and hematocrits revealed that those exclusively breastfed for 6.5 months versus 5.5 months were less likely to have anemia.[136] None of the infants exclusively breastfed for 7 months had anemia, and all of these infants continued to have good iron status at 12 and 24 months. In a study in Peru, young exclusively breastfed infants upregulated iron absorption when iron stores were depleted.[89]

Absorption of iron from breast milk by 5- to 7-month-old infants receiving solid foods was studied using stable isotope Fe.[136] Iron was well absorbed from human milk in older infants after the introduction of solid foods to the diet.[137]

After extensive studies in Sweden and in Honduras, it was concluded that iron stores in human milk provide sufficient iron for full-term, normal birth-weight infants with good prenatal iron stores. Infants who are at risk for iron deficiency at 6 months are LBW or preterm infants or those with inadequate prenatal iron stores. At 9 months, infants with iron deficiency absorb more iron than infants with normal iron stores. No effect on weight gain was observed in infants with normal hemoglobins who received iron supplements from 4 to 9 months. Slower gain in linear growth and in head circumference, however, was seen in the infants supplemented with iron. When the hemoglobin was normal, the incidence of diarrheal disease was also greater in the supplemented group.[138,139] Further observation by Mehta et al.[88] found that exclusively breastfed LBW infants become iron-deficient at a rate of 33% by 6 months of age, and 75% can require iron supplementation as early as 10 weeks into life.

Zinc

Zinc has been identified as essential to infant and young child growth and immune system and neurobehavioral development.[140] Its chief roles described to date are as part of the enzyme structure and as an enzyme activator. Zinc has been identified as a first limiting nutrient in breast milk when anthropometric indicators of growth are correlated with zinc levels in healthy breastfed infants.[141] Zinc deficiency has been described as well, most dramatically in newborns and premature infants on hyperalimentation regimens. The chief clinical symptoms are failure to thrive and typical skin lesions. Human milk has been identified as a food with bioavailable zinc.

Zinc absorption from human milk, cow's milk, and infant formula was tested in healthy adults with labeled zinc chloride, using 65Z. The absorption was 41% from human milk, 28% from cow milk, 31% from standard infant formula, and 14% from soy formula. The dietary zinc intake of both lactating and nonlactating postpartum women was found by Moser and Reynolds[14] to be 42% of recommended allowances. No correlation was found between zinc concentrations in breast milk and maternal dietary zinc and maternal plasma and erythrocyte zinc.

Changes in hair zinc concentrations of breastfed and bottle-fed infants during the first 6 months of life were measured by MacDonald et al.[142] Only the bottle-fed boys had a significant decline in hair zinc concentration. No decline of zinc was found in any breastfed infant, which supports the concept of the superior bioavailability of zinc in breast milk.

Picciano and Guthrie[143] studied milk from 50 mothers in 350 samples. They found zinc levels to average 3.95 mg/mL and to be consistent regardless of time of day, duration of lactation, or other variables. They estimated that breastfed infants receive 0.35 mg of zinc/kg per day. They found zinc levels to decline slightly from the first to the third month postpartum (33.8 to 29.5 mmol/L). At 6 months, zinc levels are 1.1 and 0.5 mg/L at 1 year. Longitudinal changes in dietary zinc requirements for infants acquiring new lean body mass through growth were studied by Krebs and Hambidge.[144] As growth velocity declines, zinc requirements decline in the male infant from a high of 780 mg/day at 1 month to 480 mg/day in the 5th through 12th months. Meanwhile, the percentage of absorption increased over time.

Human milk was fractionated and analyzed by Fransson and Lönnerdal[145] for the distribution of zinc. Most of the zinc was found in the skim milk fraction, but significant amounts were found in the fat associated with the fat-globule membrane; less than 4% was found in the casein.

Khoshoo et al.[146] reported zinc deficiency in a full-term breastfed infant (previously reported in a breastfed premature infant). This case was diagnosed at 7 months of age by the characteristic perineal and perioral rash in an otherwise healthy, well-grown infant. The presumed cause was defective zinc uptake by the mammary gland because the milk level was only 0.13 mg/L. The infant responded promptly to oral zinc supplements.

In a 9-week-old infant with intractable diaper rash, the mother's milk was noted to have low zinc levels after the rash responded to zinc therapy.[147] She had nursed two other children without difficulty. Maternal diet does not influence zinc concentrations in the milk. Breast milk has been therapeutic in the treatment of acrodermatitis enteropathica, an inherited zinc metabolism disorder, whereas cow's milk formulas are ineffective.

Copper

Copper levels in human milk vary considerably among women and within each woman. The range is 0.09 to 0.63 mg/mL.[143] Copper levels can be higher in the morning; dietary supplements do not alter copper levels in human milk. The recommended dietary intake of copper is 0.4 to 0.6 mg/day from birth to 6 months, increasing to 0.6 to 0.7 mg/day from 6 to 12 months of age (see Table 4.23). A fully breastfed infant receives 0.05 mg of copper/kg per day based on the average volume of intake and copper content of human milk.

Most of the copper is in the skim milk fraction, with significant amounts in the fat and little in the casein.[145] Additionally, copper concentrations decrease from the colostrum (570 µg/L), to transitory milk (490 µg/L), to mature milk (150 to 230 µg/L).[131]

Copper is a component of a number of metalloenzymes. The predominant binding is observed with low-molecular-weight proteins, which enhance bioavailability.[145]

Selenium

The bioavailability of selenium depends on the sources and chemical form, and the quantitative significance is under investigation. Except for Keshan disease, a potentially fatal cardiomyopathy seen in infants in China, no convincingly associated clinical deficiency syndrome has been reported. Dietary recommendations have been based on those for adults (see Table 4.23). Dietary intakes less than the lower limits, however, should not be considered deficient, especially in breastfed infants.

Selenium concentrations in human milk are consistent in samples collected from the United States and Greece, according to work by Hadjimarkos and Shearer.[148] The mean value was 0.020 ppm, which was similar to the value from many parts of the United States, where the range was 0.007 to 0.033 ppm.

Increased selenium requirements have been observed in pregnant and lactating women. Supplementation with different compounds, such as selenium-enriched yeast and selenomethionine, significantly influenced selected indices of selenium status, including milk concentrations.[149]

Selenium is considered an essential nutrient in humans. It is an integral component of glutathione peroxidase, an enzyme known to metabolize lipid peroxides, and deficiency states have been described. Questions have been raised about the detrimental effects of high selenium intake on dentition. Smith et al.[150] assessed selenium status in infants exclusively fed human milk or infant formula for 3 months. Foremilk samples had a mean concentration of 16.3 ng/mL, hindmilk mean concentration was significantly higher, and mean formula concentration was 8.6 ng/mL. Breastfed infants have greater intakes and higher serum levels of selenium than formula-fed infants in the first 3 months.

Chromium

The concentration of chromium is highest in the organs of the newborn, and serum levels decline rapidly during the first years of life. A longitudinal study of chromium in human milk was undertaken by Kumpulainen and Vuori.[151] Mothers collected samples at 8 to 18 days, 47 to 54 days, and 128 to 159 days postpartum, representing every feed during a 24-hour period with equal portions of foremilk and hindmilk. The mean concentration was 0.39 (standard deviation [SD] = 0.15) ng/mL, and the estimated daily intake was 0.27 mg/day (SD = 0.11). The values did not change over the period of lactation. The mothers' dietary intake averaged about 30 mg/day, which is lower than the 50 to 200 mg Recommended Daily Allowance (RDA) and did not correlate with breast-milk concentrations of chromium.

When chromium metabolism was studied in 17 lactating postpartum subjects, breast-milk chromium content was independent of dietary chromium intake and serum and urinary values.[152] Chromium intake did not correlate with serum or urinary chromium.

HDL cholesterol levels can be increased with chromium supplementation. Chromium also is reported to have a favorable effect on serum lipid profiles. A deficiency of chromium in infancy may be an issue with LBW infants or those with inadequate fetal stores. Chromium is present in all tissues of the body and is present in high levels in nucleic acids.

Manganese

Inordinately high levels of manganese have been found in infant formula, but little is known about its role in infant nutrition. Manganese is a component of comparatively few metalloenzymes, including pyruvate carboxylase and mitochondrial superoxide dismutase. It does, however, activate others. Deficiencies cause impaired growth and skeletal abnormalities in all species studied. Elevated manganese levels have been associated with attention-deficit/hyperactivity disorder (ADHD), hyperactive behaviors, and low verbal and visual memory.[153] There are rare congenital metabolic disorders of manganese transport that are associated with dystonia and movement disorders.[154] In human milk, the major fraction of manganese is the 71% found in the whey, with 11% in the casein and 18% in the lipid. Most of the manganese is bound to lactoferrin in the whey fraction. Levels in human milk decreased from a mean of 6.6 μg/L in the first month of lactation to 3.5 μg/L by the third month of lactation.[155] The average intake of the breastfed infant in the first month was 2.0 μg/day.

Molybdenum

The main biochemical role of molybdenum in mammals is as a cofactor for several enzymes.[156] Deficiencies are rare as a severe autosomal-recessive inborn error of metabolism and slightly more commonly occurring in infants receiving extended total parenteral nutrition. Molybdenum levels in mature human milk were measured consistently at 1 to 2 ng/mL although there is some variability reported in mature human milk molybdenum levels.[156,157]

Nickel

Nickel is generally accepted as an essential trace element for animals, but its role in humans is undefined. Levels in human milk are stable over time at 1.2 ng/mL. The average daily intake of nickel at 1 month was 0.8 μg.[156]

Fluorine

Fluorine has been widely accepted as a significant dietary factor in decreasing dental caries, with the recommended daily intake listed in Table 4.23. The effect has been associated with the conversion of the enamel hydroxyapatite to fluorapatite with a reduction in acid solubility. The presence of fluorine during the formation of hydroxyapatite may create less soluble, more resistant crystals.

Conflicting reports of the fluorine levels in human milk have led to the belief that breastfed infants needed supplementation.[158] More accurate studies in communities where fluoride has been in the public drinking water supply show 7 mg of fluorine per liter (range 4 to 14 mg/L).[159] The American Academy of Pediatrics (AAP) no longer recommends routinely supplementing breastfed infants with fluorine[120] (see Chapter 8).

The significant development of deciduous and permanent teeth that occurs after birth depends on fetal stores of fluorine and the fluorine available in the diet. Studies comparing breastfed and bottle-fed infants show a distinct difference, with fewer dental caries and better dental health in breastfed infants. The role of fluorine and other factors, such as selenium, that predispose the breastfed infant to healthier teeth has yet to be defined completely. Nursing-bottle caries add to the total dental caries of the bottle-fed infant.

Iodine

Many individuals are iodine deficient, especially women of reproductive age. Although the cause is unknown, the lack of the use of iodized salt, the use of processed foods, and geographic location are the most likely contributors. This is of serious concern because iodine deficiency during pregnancy and lactation is associated with brain underdevelopment in the offspring. The risk is greater with the increase in environmental pollutants such as nitrate, thiocyanate, and perchlorate. Environmental chemicals such as thiocyanate, nitrate, and perchlorate compete for transport by the sodium-iodide symporter (NIS).[160] The NIS is an integral plasma membrane glycoprotein found in the thyroid gland and the breast, which mediates the iodide transport into thyroid cells, the first step in thyroid hormone synthesis. In the mammary gland, NIS

TABLE 4.25	Iodine Status Assessment: Random Urine Iodine Measurements	
Mean Urinary Iodine Concentration (g/L)	Corresponding Oral Intake (μg/dL)	Iodine Status
<20	<30	Severe deficiency
20–49	30–74	Moderate deficiency
50–99	75–149	Mild deficiency
100–199	150–299	Optimal
200–299	300–449	More than adequate
>299	>449	Possible excess

From Department of Nutrition for Health and Development. *Iodine Status Assessment: Random Urine Iodine Measurements*. Geneva: World Health Organization; 2013.

mediates the transport of iodide into milk. Thiocyanate is found in cruciferous vegetables and tobacco smoke. Nitrate is found in some drinking water and root vegetables. Perchlorate is used in industry as an oxidizer and is found naturally in arid regions such as the southwestern United States. It has been detected in many foods, drinking water, and cow's milk. The US Environmental Protection Agency (EPA) developed regulations for perchlorate in drinking water in 2011. Women in the United States are clearly exposed to perchlorate and thiocyanate, which can interfere with adequate iodine nutrition.[161] Worldwide agencies have taken similar steps.

Mothers, pregnant and lactating, should take at least 150 μg of iodine daily and use iodized table salt, according to the Council on Environmental Health of the AAP.[162] Not all supplements contain enough iodine. For example, an intake of 150 μg of potassium iodide is equivalent to only 120 μg or less of iodine. Nitrates should be avoided; they are often found in well water, which should be checked annually. Tobacco smoke and second-hand smoke contain thiocyanates, which should also be avoided.

Assessment of iodine intake is most commonly done by random urinary spot iodine assessments. The World Health Organization (WHO)[163] has adopted similar guidelines for adults and children, as shown in Table 4.25. There has been discussion that the breast-milk iodine concentration is a better indicator of adequate maternal iodine and the likelihood that the breastfed infant will receive adequate iodine via breast milk.[164,165] If there is concern about an infant's iodine nutrition, it is probably easier and more informative to measure the infant's urinary iodine level than check breast-milk levels.

pH and Osmolarity

The pH range in human milk is 6.7 to 7.4, with a mean of 7.1. The mean pH of cow's milk is 6.8. The caloric content of both human and cow's milk is 65 kcal/dL or 20 kcal/oz. The specific gravities are 1.031 and 1.032, respectively.

The osmolarity of human milk approximates that of human serum, or 286 mosmol/kg of water, whereas that for cow milk is higher at 350 mosmol. The renal solute load of human milk is considerably lower than that of cow milk. The renal solute load is roughly calculated by totaling the solutes that must be excreted by the kidney. It consists primarily of nonmetabolizable dietary components, especially electrolytes, ingested in excess of body needs, and metabolic end products, mainly from the metabolism of protein. The renal solute load can be estimated by adding the dietary intake of nitrogen and three minerals—sodium, potassium, and chloride. Each gram of protein is considered to yield 4 milliosmols (as urea), and each milliequivalent of sodium, potassium, and chloride is 1 milliosmol. The renal solute load of cow milk is 221 milliosmols, compared with 79 milliosmols for human milk. The Food and Nutrition Board of the National Academies of Sciences has reported adequate intake (AI) of total water for infants in the first year of life to be 700 to 800 mL/day.

Dearlove and Dearlove[166] investigated osmoregulation in human lactation in an effort to determine whether fluid loading was a valid clinical maneuver. It is known that an oral hypotonic fluid load results in the suppression of prolactin in adults. No changes in serum prolactin, milk yield, serum, or breast-milk osmolarity were noted, however, when normal lactating women were given a hypotonic fluid load in a controlled study. The Food and Nutrition Board of the National Academies of Sciences has reported the AI of total water for lactating women as 3.8 liters per day, which should be adequate for 97% to 99% of lactating women.[167,168] Total water includes all water contained in food, beverages, and drinking water. These reports may be accessed via http://www.nap.edu.

Carotenoids: Lutein

Carotenoids are bioactive compounds produced principally in plants and are important for the infant's visual and cognitive development.[169] They have been shown to have antioxidant and antiinflammatory effects in pregnancy and infancy. Lutein is the dominant carotenoid in the infant brain and the major carotenoid found in the retina of the eye. Its levels vary in breast milk, reflecting the mother's dietary intake. Supplementation was studied in 89 lactating women who were 4 to 6 weeks postpartum.[170] They were randomly given a placebo of 0 mg/day of lutein, 6 mg/day (low dose), or 12 mg/day (high dose). The dose was taken for 6 weeks along with their normal diet. Breast-milk levels of plasma carotenoids were measured weekly by high-performance liquid chromatography (HPLC) and at the end of the study. Infant plasma levels were measured at the end of the study, and maternal plasma levels were assessed both at the beginning and the end of the study. Dietary lutein plus zeaxanthin intake did correlate with carotenoid levels in breast milk. Maternal BMI measurements were higher in the carotenoid-supplemented groups compared with the placebo group. Other carotenoids were not affected. Supplementation with lutein in the lactating woman can increase maternal and infant plasma lutein over 3 to 6 months.

TABLE 4.26 **Vitamins and Other Constituents of Human Milk and Cow's Milk (per Deciliter)**

Milk Elements	Colostrum	Transitional	Mature	Cow's Milk
Vitamin A (μg)	151.0	88.0	75.0	41.0
Vitamin B_1 (μg)	1.9	5.9	14.0	43.0
Vitamin B_2 (μg)	30.0	37.0	40.0	145.0
Nicotinic acid (μg)	75.0	175.0	160.0	82.0
Vitamin B_6 (μg)	—	—	12.0–15.0	64.0
Pantothenic acid (μg)	183.0	288.0	246.0	340.0
Biotin (μg)	0.06	0.35	0.6	2.8
Folic acid (μg)	0.05	0.02	0.14	0.13
Vitamin B_{12} (μg)	0.05	0.04	0.1	0.6
Vitamin C (mg)	5.9	7.1	5.0	1.1
Vitamin D (μg)	—	—	0.04	0.02
Vitamin E (mg)	1.5	0.9	0.25	0.07
Vitamin K (μg)	—	—	1.5	6.0
Ash (g)	0.3	0.3	0.2	0.7
Calories (kcal)	57.0	63.0	65.0	65.0
Specific gravity	1050.0	1035.0	1031.0	1032.0
Milk (pH)	—	—	7.0	6.8

From Food and Nutrition Board, National Research Council, National Academy of Sciences. *Recommended Dietary Allowances*. 10th ed. Washington, DC: US Government Printing Office; 1989.

VITAMINS

Vitamin A

Vitamin A is critical for growth and immune system function. Hypovitaminosis A can lead to night blindness, xerophthalmia, keratomalacia, complete blindness, increased risk of diarrhea and respiratory infections, and a higher occurrence of mortality with measles infection. Mature human milk contains 75 μg/dL or 280 international units (IUs), whereas cow's milk contains only 41 μg/dL or 180 IU (Table 4.26). Thus the supply of vitamin A and its precursors, carotenoids (e.g., β-carotene), is considered adequate to meet the estimated daily requirement, which varies from 500 to 1500 IU/day if the infant consumes at least 200 mL of breast milk per day (Table 4.27).[171] Twice as much vitamin A is present in colostrum as in mature milk. During the first 6 months, the retinol equivalent (RE) content of term milk in developing countries is only 330 mg RE/L compared with 660 mg in developed countries.[172] One retinol equivalent equals 1 μg of retinol or 6 μg of carotene. The retinol content of the milk of mothers who deliver prematurely is even higher.

Vitamin A intake and serum vitamin A concentrations during pregnancy influence the composition of breast milk. Supplementing β-carotene quickly elevates β-carotene

TABLE 4.27 **Recommended Daily Dietary Allowances of Fat-Soluble Vitamins for Infants[a]**

Age	WEIGHT		HEIGHT		Protein (g)	Vitamin A (μg RE)[b]	Vitamin D (μg)[c]	Vitamin E (mg α-TE)[d]
	(kg)	(lb)	(cm)	(in)				
To 6 mo	6	13	60	24	kg × 2.2	395	7.5	3
6 mo–1 yr	9	20	71	28	kg × 1.6	375	10	4

[a]The allowances are intended to provide for individual variations among most normal persons as they live in the United States under usual environmental stresses. Diets should be based on a variety of common foods to provide other nutrients for which human requirements have been less well defined.
[b]*RE*, Retinol equivalents. 1 RE = 1 μg retinol or 6 μg carotene.
[c]As cholecalciferol, 10 μg cholecalciferol = 400 IU vitamin D.
[d]α-*TE*, α-tocopherol equivalents. 1 mg d-α-tocopherol = 1 α-TE.
From Food and Nutrition Board, National Research Council, National Academy of Sciences. *Recommended Dietary Allowances*. 10th ed. Washington, DC: US Government Printing Office; 1989.

concentrations in serum and milk, and sustained supplementation can maintain elevated retinol concentrations.[171]

Human milk is a vital source of vitamin A in developing countries and among populations with low vitamin A levels, even beyond the first year of life.[29,173,174] As a result, vitamin A supplementation has been a major project of WHO. The technologies used to test samples of milk for vitamin A before and after treatment have been studied.[175]

Vitamin D

Newborn and infant vitamin D deficiency has been linked with various clinical illnesses, including rickets, failure to thrive, type 1 diabetes, and additional immune-associated illnesses. Vitamin D has always been included in the fat-soluble vitamin group because that is the form in which it had been identified in nature. The levels in human milk were 0.05 mg/dL, previously reported in the fat fraction. Human milk was shown to have vitamin D in both the fat and the aqueous fractions. Investigators measured the water-soluble sulfate conjugate of vitamin D and evaluated the biologic activity of the water-soluble metabolites. The water-soluble fraction is considered to be inactive metabolites. When activity is calculated by an assay that measures the stimulation of intestinal calcium transport, human milk is found to contain 40 to 50 IU/L of vitamin D activity. The metabolite 25-hydroxyvitamin D_3 accounts for 75% of the activity; vitamins D_2 and D_3 account for 15%. Vitamin D sulfate, or another as-yet-unidentified water-soluble metabolite of vitamin D, has not been proven to have significant biologic activity.

A direct relationship was seen between maternal and infant levels of 25-OH-vitamin D_3 and maternal diet.[29] An additional group of infants, whose mothers' diets were unsupplemented, received 400 IU of vitamin D per day and had even higher serum concentrations of 25-OH-vitamin D_3. When mothers have been given large doses of vitamin D, the content of vitamin D and D_3 in their milk increases, as it does with exposure to sunshine. The level of 25-OH-vitamin D does not change. The majority of the activity in human milk is in the form of 25-OH-vitamin D. This may be an advantage for the breastfed infant, who utilizes this form most readily. Clearly, the levels vary and may be inadequate in human milk in some situations, especially in cold climates in the winter with little sunshine and for dark-skinned individuals.

In a review of vitamin D in adults, especially pregnant women, Hollis[176] clearly demonstrated that traditional levels of vitamin D of 400 IU/day or less are grossly inadequate today when few women get adequate sun exposure and many wear sunscreen or clothing that obstructs the exposure. Most recommendations were made before it was possible to measure circulating 25-OH-vitamin D, the true indicator of nutritional vitamin D status. The dose of 10 mg or 400 IU daily had little effect on adult 25-OH-vitamin D levels. When submariners were given 600 IU/day for several months, they failed to maintain adequate 25-OH-vitamin D levels.[177] The dose that is adequate during pregnancy is a minimum of 1000 IU daily. Doses of 10,000 IU daily in adults did not elevate circulating 25-OH-vitamin D above the normal range, and doses of 1000 IU may

not maintain normal levels. The resurgence of rickets in infants may well begin with inadequate levels in pregnancy.[178]

Cases of vitamin D–deficiency hypocalcemia and rickets in nonwhite infants have been reported in increasing numbers in exclusively breastfed infants.[179] All lactating women in this study by Chang had elevated serum parathyroid hormone levels. The epidemic of vitamin D deficiency is aggravated by the use of sunscreen, ethnic traditions of covering the body, and a lack of sunshine.[180] Serum 1,25-dihydroxyvitamin D concentrations are significantly higher in lactating compared with nonlactating women and among vegetarian compared with nonvegetarian women, as reported by Specker et al.[181] Levels of vitamin D are higher in colostrum than in mature milk.[182] Studies by Wagner et al. provided high levels of vitamin D (4000 IU/day) to mothers to increase their milk levels.[84] A study of exclusively breastfed infants was conducted, placing the infants at 1 month of age in one of four doses of vitamin D categories (200, 400, 600, 800 IU/day). At 1 month, most of the infants had levels below normal. Seventy-two percent had levels below 88.2 ± 23.0 nmol/L 25-OH-vitamin D concentrations. During the study, low levels were noted occasionally in all categories.[183]

Since 2008, the AAP has recommended that all breastfed infants receive 400 IU of vitamin D beginning at birth. Until pregnant and lactating women who are at risk for inadequate intake receive adequate supplements, it will be necessary to supplement normal breastfeeding infants.[174,184] It is certainly appropriate to provide vitamin D supplementation for both the mother and the infant to benefit each individual.[185]

The concern for the toxicity of excessive vitamin D was based on the reported relationship with cardiac disease and supravalvular aortic stenosis syndrome and William syndrome, which has been proven to be genetic. Hypervitaminosis from high levels of vitamin D has resulted from therapeutic misadventures, resulting in hypercalcemia when the circulating 25-OH-vitamin D concentrations were over 100 ng/mL (normal levels of 25-OH-vitamin D are over 15 ng/mL serum). No case of hypervitaminosis D has been reported from sun exposure, even though a half hour in the summer sun between 10 AM and 2 PM in a bathing suit (approximately 3 minimal erythemal dose exposures) will release about 50,000 IU or 1.25 mg/day of vitamin D within 24 hours in most white persons.[176]

Recent research has also begun revealing the importance of vitamin D on the mother's and infant's epigenome.[186] One of the vitamin D metabolites, 1α,25-dihydroxyvitamin D3, which binds to the vitamin D receptor, also directly affects the epigenome and transcriptome at numerous loci within the human genome. Additional study of environmental factors and measurement of epigenomic changes will likely elucidate how vitamin D can prevent rickets, osteoporosis, sarcopenia, autoimmune diseases, and possibly different types of cancer.

Vitamin E

Vitamin E has been a subject of much interest. Vitamin E includes a group of fat-soluble compounds (α-, β-, γ-, and δ-tocopherol) and their unsaturated derivatives (α-, β-, γ-, and δ-tocotrienol), of which only the isomer α-tocopherol is nutritionally valuable to humans.[187]

Vitamin E is especially critical for nervous system development and is required for muscle integrity, resistance of erythrocytes to hemolysis, and other biochemical and physiologic functions.[187] The requirement for vitamin E is related to the PUFA content of the cellular structures and of the diet (see Table 4.27). One α-tocopherol equivalent is equal to 1 mg d-α-tocopherol. One IU of vitamin E is equal to 1 mg of synthetic α-tocopherol or 0.74 mg of natural α-tocopherol acetate. Satisfactory plasma levels are 1 mg/dL, and these levels can be maintained by feedings with a vitamin E/PUFA ratio of 0.4 mg/g. The requirement for infants to age 6 months is 3 mg/day and after 6 months 4 mg/day. The requirement during lactation is 14 mg during the first 6 months and 17 mg/day after 6 months postpartum.

Levels in colostrum are 1.5 mg/dL, whereas transitional milk has 0.9 mg/dL and mature milk has 0.25 mg/dL. The difference at different stages has been found to be caused by α-tocopherol because the contents of β- and γ-tocopherol are similar. Total tocopherol in mature milk correlates with total lipid and linoleic acid contents. Significantly higher tocopherol/linoleic acid ratios are found in both colostrum and transitional milk than in mature milk.[188]

Cow's milk has 0.07 mg/dL of vitamin E (see Table 4.26). Correspondingly, serum levels in breastfed infants rise quickly at birth and maintain a normal level, whereas infants fed cow's milk have depressed levels. An IU of vitamin E is equal to 1 mg of synthetic α-tocopherol or 0.74 mg of natural α-tocopherol acetate. There are a variety of stereoisomers of α-tocopherol, of which *RRR-α*-tocopherol (*RRR-α-T*) is known to be more bioactive than *all-rac-α*-tocopherol (*all-rac-α-T*) and is the dominant form of tocopherol in human milk. There is widespread use of *all-rac-α-T* in maternal supplements. To fully understand the availability, bioactivity, and comparability of the different isomers, additional study will be necessary.[187]

An estimate of the ratio of tocopherol to linoleic acid in mature human milk is 0.79 mg α-tocopherol equivalents per gram, which is comparable to a daily requirement of 0.5 mg for term infants but may be low for premature infants, especially those receiving iron supplements. Ordinarily, this would be supplied by 4 IU of vitamin E per day. Because human milk contains 1.8 mg/L or 40 mg of vitamin E per gram of lipid, it supplies more-than-adequate levels of vitamin E.[182]

Vitamin K

Vitamin K is essential for the synthesis of blood-clotting factors, which are normal in the serum at birth. These factors decline after birth, and there is a lag in vitamin K production by intestinal flora until the growth of the necessary bacteria is well established. A developing deficiency in vitamin K can lead to various bleeding complications, of particularly grave risk is intracranial hemorrhaging, which can occur between the 2nd and 12th week and up to the 6th month of life.[189] As a result, maternal supplementation is often administered; however, this is less effective than direct vitamin K prophylaxis to the infant.[189]

It is recommended that all infants receive vitamin K at birth, regardless of feeding plans, to prevent hemorrhagic disease of the newborn caused by vitamin K deficiency in the first few days to months of life.[190,191] If the mother or family refuses the intramuscular injection for the infant, vitamin K given orally is an alternative recommended by the Canadian Pediatric Society.[192] The recommended dosing for oral vitamin K is 2 mg PO at birth and repeated at 2 to 4 weeks of age and 6 to 8 weeks of age.

Human milk contains between 2.2 and 20 nmol/L,[189] which is less than the recommended daily intake of 2 μg/day recommended for infants 0 to 6 months of age and 2.5 μg/day for infants 6 to 12 months of age (Table 4.28).[130] Canfield et al.[193] reported on the mean levels of vitamin K in colostrum (7.52 nmol/L or 3.39 μg/L) and mature milk (6.36 nmol/L or 2.87 μg/L). There was no significant change in the mean level of vitamin K in human milk from birth through 6 months postpartum. Even allowing for older infants consuming increased volumes of breast milk, breast milk does not provide sufficient vitamin K without some form of supplementation through 6 months of age.

The vitamin content of common foods has been recalculated downward so that the diets of average women are probably deficient in vitamin K. Furthermore, vitamin K levels in the serum of lactating women are not good markers of deficiency. Carboxylated prothrombin (des-γ-carboxyprothrombin) is produced in the absence of vitamin K and is a marker of vitamin K deficiency. Greer et al.[194] followed breastfed infants whose mothers were receiving 2.5 to 5.0 mg/d oral phylloquinone and found normal des-γ-carboxyprothrombin levels at birth and 4 weeks but elevations by 8 weeks. The authors recommend maternal supplementation during lactation.

The measurements of the homologs of vitamin K have been equivocal. When mothers are given a single dose of

TABLE 4.28	**Recommended Daily Dietary Allowances of Vitamins for Infants**[a]		
Age	Vitamin K (μg/d)	Biotin (μg/d)	Pantothenic Acid (mg/d)
To 6 mo	2.0	5	1.7
6 mo–1 yr	2.5	6	1.8

[a]The allowances are intended to provide for individual variations among most normal persons as they live in the United States under usual environmental stresses. Diets should be based on a variety of common foods to provide other nutrients for which human requirements have been less well defined.
From Food and Nutrition Board, National Research Council, National Academy of Sciences. *Recommended Dietary Allowances*. Washington, DC: US Government Printing Office; 2011.

20 mg of phylloquinone (K1), the milk level increases from 1.1 mcg/L to 130 mcg/L at 12 hours, dropping to 35 mcg/L by 48 hours.[189] Maternal supplementation, however, does not result in the same effects on concentration as direct infant supplementation.

When infants are given 1 mg vitamin K1 at birth, as is the practice in many countries, the concentration of K1 in both breastfed and formula-fed infants in the first week of life remains elevated. When the breastfeeding mothers were given 5 mg of oral vitamin K1 daily for 12 weeks, plasma vitamin K1 concentrations in the infant reach 2 to 3 mcg/L from the 2nd to the 12th week, whereas infants whose mothers did not receive such supplementation maintain concentrations of 0.2 to 0.4 mcg/L and can display vitamin K deficiency.[194]

Vitamin K is produced by the intestinal flora but takes several days in the previously sterile neonatal gut to be effective. Vitamin K−dependent clotting factors in term breastfed infants were normal. The prothrombin time and partial thromboplastin time were similar in breastfed and bottle-fed infants. The Normotest and Thrombotest coagulation tests were significantly prolonged in the breastfed group. The authors concluded that 5% of breastfed children have possible vitamin K deficiency.[190,195]

An association of vitamin K deficiency with home birth has been noted by various investigators, and it is suggested that the infant should receive vitamin K, if it has been omitted, immediately at the first medical contact as recommended by the AAP.[190,196,197]

Various other reports continue to document the occurrence of late-onset hemorrhagic disease of the newborn in both formula-fed and breastfed infants. Vitamin K as a single intramuscular (IM) injection at birth or 3 oral doses of vitamin K through 8 weeks of age significantly decrease the risk of hemorrhagic disease.[198] The relative risk of late-onset hemorrhagic disease of the newborn has been estimated to be 81 times greater in infants who do not receive IM vitamin K compared with infants who did receive it.[198]

Controversies will remain, but the current recommendations regarding vitamin K at birth for all infants, regardless of feeding source, remain appropriate.[190]

Vitamin C

Vitamin C (ascorbic acid) is part of several enzyme and hormone systems, as well as of intracellular chemical reactions. It is essential to collagen synthesis and has significant antioxidant properties.[199]

Human milk is an outstanding source of water-soluble vitamins (Table 4.29) and reflects maternal dietary intake (Table 4.30; see Table 4.28). Human milk contains 43 mg/dL (fresh cow's milk contains up to 21 mg) of vitamin C. Levels obtained in normal lactating women 6 months postpartum were 35 mg/L in those on normal diets and 38 mg/L in those supplemented with multivitamins containing 90 mg vitamin C.[200] Increased vitamin C has been measured in the milk within 30 minutes of a bolus of vitamin C being given to the mother.[200] Breast-milk ascorbic acid is highest in colostrum and decreases over the course of lactation. There is wide variability in the vitamin C concentrations of breast milk, ascribed to differences in maternal nutritional status and dietary intake. It has been reported that diabetes and smoking in the mother can also decrease vitamin C levels in breast milk. Levels obtained in 16 lactating women of a low socioeconomic level were 53 mg/L for unsupplemented and 65 mg/L for supplemented mothers at 1 week postpartum and 61 and 72 mg/L, respectively, at 6 weeks postpartum. Several subjects in the unsupplemented low-socioeconomic group had levels too low to provide 35 mg vitamin C per day to their infants.[201]

When lactating women were given 250, 500, or 1000 mg/day vitamin C for 2 days, milk levels remained within the range of 44 to 158 mg/L and did not differ significantly between dosages, even at 10 times the RDA.[202] The total intake of the infant through the milk ranged from 49 to 86 mg/day.[202] When women received high doses of vitamin C, levels of the vitamin excreted in the urine also increased proportionately.[203]

These findings suggest a regulatory mechanism for vitamin C levels in milk.

Vitamin B Complex
Vitamin B₁

Vitamin B_1 or thiamin is essential for the use of carbohydrates in the pyruvate metabolism (cofactor in pyruvic acid decarboxylation) and for fat synthesis. Insufficient thiamin produces insufficient carbohydrate oxidation with the accumulation of intermediary metabolites, such as lactic acid. Cases of beriberi in infants have been associated with a deficiency in the mother, and deficiency is most commonly seen in pregnant or lactating women and young children.

Vitamin B_1, or thiamin, levels increase with the duration of lactation but are lower in human milk (160 mg/dL) than in cow's milk (440 mg/dL; see Tables 4.29 and 4.30). In a study by Nail et al.,[204] levels obtained by normal lactating women showed significant increases between 1 and 6 weeks postpartum, but no difference in levels between supplemented (1.7 mg daily) and unsupplemented women was seen.

Because urinary excretion of thiamin is significantly higher in supplemented than in unsupplemented women, the amount of vitamin transferred into milk appears to be limited.[7] Thiamin intake is positively associated with breast-milk thiamin concentrations in both well-nourished and poorly nourished women. Breast-milk thiamin concentrations respond rapidly to maternal supplementation.[158]

Vitamin B₂

Vitamin B_2, or riboflavin, is significant for the newborn, in whom intestinal tract bacterial synthesis is minimal (see Tables 4.29 and 4.30). Riboflavin is involved in oxidative intracellular systems and is essential for protoplasmic growth. Riboflavin functions with the coenzymes flavin mononucleotide (FMN) and flavin adenine dinucleotide (FAD) in redox reactions for energy production. It is also involved in the activity of glutathione, which acts a free-radical scavenger. A deficiency of riboflavin affects various metabolic pathways and can cause skin conditions, peripheral neuropathy, poor growth, and diminished iron absorption.

TABLE 4.29 Estimated Secretion of Nutrients in Mature Human Milk Compared With Increments in Recommended Dietary Allowances (RDAs) for Lactating Women

A. ENERGY, PROTEIN, AND FAT-SOLUBLE VITAMINS

Measure	Energy (kcal)	Protein (g)	Vitamin A (µg RE)	Vitamin D (µg)	Vitamin E (mg of α-TE)	Vitamin K (µg)
Estimated secretion in milk[a]	420–700	6.3–10.5	400–670	0.3–0.6	1.4–2.3	1.3–2.1
Increment in RDAs[b,c] for following lactation periods						
0–6 mo	500	15	500	5	4	0
6–12 mo	500	12	400	5	3	0
Comments	Estimated 80% efficiency in conversion to milk energy	Estimated 70% efficiency in conversion to milk protein	None	Increment advised in part to maintain calcium balance	Estimated 75% absorption	No increment listed because intakes usually exceed RDA

B. WATER-SOLUBLE VITAMINS

Measure	Vitamin C (mg)	Thiamin (mg)	Riboflavin (mg)	Niacin (mg of NE)	Vitamin B6 (mg)	Folate (µg)	Vitamin B12 (µg)
Estimated secretion in milk[a]	24–40	0.13–0.21	0.21–0.35	0.9–1.5	0.06–0.09	50–83	0.6–1.0
Increment in RDAs[b,c] for following lactation periods							
0–6 mo	35	0.5	0.5	5	0.5	100	0.6
6–12 mo	30	0.5	0.4	5	0.5	80	0.6
Comments	Estimated 85% absorption	Increment higher than secretion because of increased energy needs	Estimated 70% utilization for milk production	Increment higher than secretion because of increased energy needs	Milk concentration used is for unsupplemented women	Estimated 50% absorption; RDA based on 50 rather than 83 µg/L	RDA based on 0.6 rather than 1.0 µg/L

C. MINERALS

Measure	Calcium (mg)	Phosphorus (mg)	Magnesium (mg)	Iron (mg)	Zinc (mg)	Iodine (μg)	Selenium (μg)
Estimated secretion in milk[a]	168–280	84–140	21–35	0.18–0.30	0.9–1.5[d] 0.3–0.5[e]	66–110	12–20
Increment in RDAS[b,c] for following lactation periods							
0–6 mo	400	400	75	0	7	50	20
6–12 mo	400	400	60	0	4	50	20
Comments	None	Based on desired 1:1 ratio for calcium/phosphorus intake	Estimated 50% absorption	Secretion during lactation is less than menstrual loss	Estimated 20% absorption	Based on need of infant, not maternal loss in milk	Estimated 80% absorption

α-TE, α-tocopherol equivalents; *NE*, niacin equivalents; *RE*, retinol equivalents.

[a]At volumes of 600–1000 mL/day, based on milk composition shown in Table 4.13.
[b]From Food and Nutrition Board, National Research Council, National Academy of Sciences. *Recommended Dietary Allowances.* 10th ed. Washington, DC: US Government Printing Office; 1989.
[c]Women aged 25 to 50.
[d]From 0 to 6 months.
[e]From 6 to 12 months.
From Report of Nutrition During Lactation Subcommittee, Institute of Medicine. *Nutrition During Lactation.* Washington, DC: National Academies Press; 1991.

	Vitamin C (mg/d)	Thiamin (mg/d)	Riboflavin (mg/d)	Niacin (mg/d)[b]	Vitamin B$_6$ (mg/d)	Folacin[c] (μg)	Vitamin B$_{12}$ (μg/)
TABLE 4.30 **Recommended Daily Dietary Allowances of Water-Soluble Vitamins for Infants**[a]							
Age							
To 6 mo	40	0.2	0.3	2	0.1	25	0.4
6 mo–1 yr	50	0.3	0.4	4	0.3	35	0.5

[a]The allowances are intended to provide for individual variations among most normal persons as they live in the United States under usual environmental stresses. Diets should be based on a variety of common foods to provide other nutrients for which human requirements have been less well defined.

[b]One niacin equivalent (NE) is equal to 1 mg of niacin or 60 mg of dietary tryptophan.

[c]The folacin allowances refer to dietary sources as determined by *Lactobacillus casei* assay after treatment with enzymes (conjugases) to make polyglutamyl forms of the vitamin.

From Food and Nutrition Board, National Research Council, National Academy of Sciences. *Recommended Dietary Allowances*. Washington, DC. US Government Printing Office; 2011.

Levels are 36 mg/dL in human milk and 175 mg/dL in cow milk. FAD and free riboflavin are the dominant forms of riboflavin found in breast milk. Levels obtained in normal lactating women showed significantly lower levels of riboflavin in the milk of the unsupplemented women (36.7 mg/dL) at 1 week compared with the milk of the supplemented women, who received 2 mg/day in a multivitamin (80.0 mg/dL). No significant difference was seen between 1 and 6 weeks in either group.[204]

Niacin

Niacin (nicotinamide) is an essential part of the pyridine nucleotide coenzymes and is part of the intracellular respiratory mechanisms. Human milk has 147 mg/dL, and cow's milk has 94 mg/dL (see Tables 4.29 and 4.30). Levels in human milk do respond to dietary supplementation.

Vitamin B$_6$

Vitamin B$_6$ (pyridoxine) forms the enzyme group of certain decarboxylases and transaminases involved in the metabolism of nerve tissue. The supply of vitamin B$_6$ is also vital to DNA synthesis, which is needed to form the cerebrosides in the myelination of the CNS. B$_6$ deficiency is associated with poor development, neuropathies, and seizures. Human milk has 12 to 15 mg/dL of vitamin B$_6$, and cow's milk has 64 mg/dL (see Table 4.30). Infants aged 0 to 6 months require 0.1 mg/day, and those aged 6 to 12 months require 0.3 mg/day (see Table 4.29).[132]

The principal form of vitamin B$_6$ in human milk is pyridoxal, but pyridoxine is the principal form of vitamin B$_6$ fortification in infant formulas.[205] Levels of vitamin B$_6$ in human milk vary directly with maternal intake. Concentrations among mothers consuming more than 2.5 mg of the vitamin daily (the RDA for lactating women is 2.5 mg/day) are significantly higher in the first week than those of unsupplemented mothers, 0.24 mg/L and 0.13 mg/L respectively.[132] Average maternal diets in several studies were consistently below the recommended levels of vitamin B$_6$.[206]

The accumulated stores of vitamin B$_6$ during pregnancy are significant for the maintenance of adequate vitamin B$_6$ status of infants during the early months of breastfeeding. For some infants, human milk alone without supplementary foods may be insufficient to meet vitamin B$_6$ needs after 6 months of age.[133] The recommended daily intake for infants under 6 months of age is 0.30 mg.[207]

Long-term use of oral contraceptives has been shown to result in low levels of vitamin B$_6$ in maternal serum in pregnancy and at delivery and low levels in the milk of these mothers.[206] The relationship of vitamin B$_6$ supplements to the suppression of prolactin and the treatment of galactorrhea is discussed under lactation failure (see Chapter 15). The doses used to suppress lactation (600 mg/day) far exceed the levels in multivitamins (1 to 10 mg; see Table 4.30).

Pantothenic Acid

Pantothenic acid is part of CoA, a catalyst of acetylation reactions. The reaction of CoA with acetic acid to form acetyl-CoA is central to intermediary metabolism. The levels of pantothenic acid in human milk were restudied by Johnston et al. because of the range of values in the literature. They found the mean to be 670 mg/dL in foremilk and hindmilk samples. No change occurred in concentrations from 1 to 6 months postpartum. They did find a positive correlation with dietary intake.[208]

Folacin

Folacin (folic acid, folate, vitamin B$_9$, pteroyl-L-glutamate) is part of the conversion of glycine to serine. It is also involved in the methylation of nicotinamide and homocysteine to methionine. It is essential for erythropoiesis (see Table 4.29). Folic acid has also been identified as a critical element in deficiency states during pregnancy, being associated with abruptio placentae, toxemia, neural tube defects, and intrauterine growth failure as well as megaloblastic anemia.

The folate (anionic form of folic acid) content of human milk produced by well-nourished women averages 80 to 130 mg/L (see Table 4.30).[209] These values are substantially greater than those reported in the literature previously because of difficulty in the analysis. Folate in human milk is quantitatively bound to folate-binding proteins and presents in multiple labile forms. Folate values typically increase as lactation progresses, as well as later in the day, and are even maintained as maternal stores begin to be depleted.[34]

Supplementation with folic acid in deficient mothers caused a prompt increase in levels in the milk. When mothers and their infants were evaluated, folate levels were two to three times higher in the breastfed infants than in their mothers, and a correlation was seen between levels in the milk and in the infants' plasma.[210]

Vitamin B₁₂

Vitamin B₁₂ is necessary for folate metabolism and DNA synthesis.[34] Deficiency in infancy can lead to various neurologic conditions and developmental regression. Vitamin B₁₂ also functions in transmethylations, such as the synthesis of choline from methionine, serine from glycine, and methionine from homocysteine. It is involved in pyrimidine and purine metabolism and the metabolism of folic acid. Megaloblastic anemia is a common symptom of vitamin B₁₂ deficiency.

The concentrations of vitamin B₁₂ in human milk are around 0.3 ng/mL, whereas cow's milk has 4.0 mg/mL. Well-nourished mothers on balanced diets appear to have adequate amounts for their infants.[200] Microbiologic assay has demonstrated that high concentrations of vitamin B₁₂ appear in early colostrum within 48 hours of delivery (mean 2.431 ng/mL), but within a few days, the levels fall to a range similar to the levels in normal serum.[211] Samson and McClelland measured B₁₂ levels in human milk and found a range of 33 to 320 ng/dL, with a mean of 0.97 ng/mL.[211] When nutritionally deficient, low-socioeconomic lactating women were studied by Sneed et al., supplementation with a multivitamin did result in elevated vitamin B₁₂ levels.[201] Vitamin B₁₂ concentrations in colostrum, transitional, and mature milk do not differ significantly between women receiving supplements and those not being supplemented. Dror and Allen[34] report that supplementation with oral vitamin B₁₂ during pregnancy (dose 50 μg daily) and during lactation (3 to 1000 μg daily) resulted in moderate to significant increases in breast-milk vitamin B₁₂ concentrations measured at 1 to 6 months postpartum over the B₁₂ milk levels in women receiving placebo. Maternal age, parity, BMI, smoking status, and oral contraceptive use are other possible variables influencing B₁₂ levels that have not been investigated in relation to breast-milk vitamin B₁₂ concentrations.

Although cow's milk has 5 to 10 times more vitamin B₁₂ than mature human milk, cow's milk has little vitamin B₁₂—binding capacity, which is substantial in human milk. Vitamin B₁₂ occurs exclusively in animal tissue, is bound to protein, and is minimal or absent in vegetable protein.[174]

The recommended maternal supplementation during pregnancy or lactation is approximately 2.6 to 2.8 μg/day. The recommendation for the minimum daily requirement of B₁₂ for infants is 0.3 mg/day in the first year of life, when growth is rapid (see Table 4.29). Based on their data on omnivorous and vegetarian women, Specker et al.[212] conclude that the current RDA for infants provides little margin for safety (see Table 4.30).

ENZYMES

Considerable data have been collected on the enzymatic activities of many milks. Jenness[213] reports 44 enzymes detected in bovine, human, and other milks. Xanthine oxidase, lactoperoxidase, uridine diphosphogalactose, galactosyltransferase, ribonuclease, lipase, alkaline phosphatase, acid phosphatase, and lysozyme have been isolated in crystalline form.

The role and significance of enzymes in human milk were reviewed by Hamosh,[214] who confirmed that more than 20 active human milk enzymes exist (Table 4.31). They can be categorized into three general groups by their activity: mammary gland function, which reflects physiologic changes occurring in the mammary gland itself during lactation; compensatory digestive enzymes in human milk, which have digestive functions in the neonate; and milk enzymes, important in stimulating neonatal development via other mechanisms (antiinfective and antiinflammatory).[214] Some enzyme levels are significantly higher in colostrum than in mature milk. Most are found in the whey fraction of human milk. Some enzymes, like other proteins in milk, are probably produced elsewhere and transported to the breast via the bloodstream. The evidence to support the concept that some proteins are produced by local synthesis includes the demonstration of secretory tissue in the mammary gland. Amylase levels are twice as high in milk as in serum.[215] Casein proteins have been synthesized in vitro in cell-free mammary-derived mRNA-enriched systems. Peptidomics research is demonstrating both the breakdown of specific proteins to functional peptides in the infant by enzymes contained in human milk and protection against proteolysis for other proteins.[216] The enzymes of possible importance in infant digestion are those with pancreatic analogs: amylase, lipases, protease(s), and ribonuclease.

Amylase

Amylase, the chief polysaccharide-digesting enzyme, is not developed at birth even in full-term infants, who have only 0.2% to 0.5% of adult enzymatic activity. Mammary amylase is present, however, throughout lactation, with levels higher in colostrum than in mature milk. Human milk levels of amylase are 0.5 to 1.0 g/dL. Milk levels of amylase from preterm mothers are comparable to term milk levels.

Milk levels are twice those of serum in the first 90 days and remain higher than serum over 6 months. Amylase is resistant to low pH levels and pepsin degradation.[217] When exposed to a pH of 5.3, this salivary-type amylase remains active; at a pH of 3.5, one-half the original activity is present at 2 hours, and one-third of the enzyme activity remains at 6 hours. Amylase is stable at −20°C to −70°C (−4°F to −94°F) for storage and at least for 24 hours at 15°C to 38°C (59°F to 100°F). Much milk amylase activity remains in the duodenum after a meal of human milk. This is significant for the digestion of starch because pancreatic amylase is still low in infants. Mammary amylase may be an alternate pathway of digestion of glucose polymers and of starch (Table 4.32).

Milk amylase is part of the isozyme group as salivary amylase and is thought to inhibit the growth of certain microorganisms.[218]

Lipases

Milk fat is almost completely digestible. The emulsion of fat in breast milk is greater than in cow's milk, resulting in

TABLE 4.31 Component Functions in Human Milk

Function	Component	Process
Biosynthesis of milk components in mammary gland	Phosphoglucomutase	Synthesis of lactose
	Lactose synthetase	Synthesis of lactose
	Fatty acid synthetase	Synthesis of medium-chain fatty acids
	Thioesterase	Uptake of circulating triglyceride fatty acids
	Lipoprotein lipase	Uptake of circulating triglyceride fatty acids
Digestive function in infant	Amylase	Hydrolysis of polysaccharides
	Lipase (bile salt-dependent)	Hydrolysis of triglycerides
	Proteases	Proteolysis (not verified)
	Xanthine oxidase	Carrier of iron, molybdenum
	Glutathione peroxidase	Carrier of selenium
	Alkaline phosphatase	Carrier of zinc, magnesium
Preservation of milk components	Antiprotease	Protection of bioactive proteins (i.e., enzymes and immunoglobulins)
	Sulfhydryl oxidase	Maintenance of structure and function of proteins containing disulfide bonds
Antiinfective agents	Lysozyme	Bactericidal
	Peroxidase	Bactericidal
	Lipases (lipoprotein lipase, bile salt-dependent lipase)	Release of free fatty acids that have antibacterial, antiviral, and antiprotozoan actions
Antiinflammatory agents	Vitamins A, C, and E	Scavenge oxygen radicals
	Catalase	Degrades hydrogen peroxide
	Glutathione peroxidase	Prevents lipid peroxidation
	Platelet-activating factor acetylhydrolase	Degrades platelet-activating factor
	α1-Antitrypsin	Inhibits inflammatory proteases
	α1-Antichymotrypsin	Inhibits inflammatory proteases
	Prostaglandin 1	Cytoprotective
	Prostaglandin 2	Cytoprotective
	Epidermal growth factor	Promotes gut growth and function
	Transforming growth factor-α	Promotes epithelial cell growth
	Transforming growth factor-β	Suppresses lymphocyte function
	Interleukin 10	Suppresses function of macrophages and natural killer and T cells
	Transforming growth factor-α receptors I and II	Binds to and inhibits transforming growth factor-α

From Hamosh M. Enzymes in human milk: their role in nutrient digestion, gastrointestinal function and nutrient delivery to the newborn infant. In: Lebenthal E, ed. *Textbook of Gastroenterology and Nutrition in Infancy*. 2nd ed. New York: Raven; 1989; Hamosh M. Bioactive factors in human milk. Breastfeeding 2001, part I: the evidence for breastfeeding. *Pediatr Clin North Am*. 2001;48:69.

smaller globules. Milk lipases play an active role in creating the emulsion, which yields a finer curd and facilitates the digestion of triacylglycerols. The newborn easily digests and completely uses the well-emulsified small fat globules of human milk. Free fatty acids are important sources of energy for the infant.

Lipase in human milk was first described in 1901. At least two different lipases (glycerol ester hydrolases) were described

TABLE 4.32 Characteristics of Milk Enzymes Active in Infant Digestion

Characteristic	Amylase	BSSL
High parity (≥10)	Low activity	?
Malnutrition	?	Decrease in activity
Diurnal and within feed activity	Constant	Constant
Prepartum	?	Present
Presence in preterm (PT) and term (T) milk	Equal activity PT and T	Equal activity PT and T
Pattern through lactation	Colostrum greater than milk	Colostrum lower than milk
Weaning	?	Activity constant independent of milk volume
Distribution in milk	Skim milk	Skim milk
Effect of milk storage −20°C to −70°C, 15°C to 38°C	Stable years Stable (≤24 h)	Stable years Stable (≤24 h)
Stability to low pH (passage through stomach)	pH > 3.0	pH > 3.0
Optimum pH	6.5–7.5	7.4–8.5
Enzyme characteristics	Salivary amylase isozyme	Identical with pancreatic carboxyl ester hydrolase
Evidence of activity in infant's intestine	Yes	Yes
Presence in milk of other species	?	Primates, carnivores, and rodents

BSSL, Bile salt–stimulated lipase.
From Hamosh M. Enzymes in human milk. In: Jensen RG, ed. *Handbook of Milk Composition.* San Diego: Academic Press; 1995; Hamosh M. Bioactive factors in human milk. Breastfeeding 2001, part I: the evidence for breastfeeding. *Pediatr Clin North Am.* 2001;48:69.

then. The lipases in human milk make the free fatty acids available in a large proportion even before the digestive phase of the intestine. The lipolytic milk-enzyme activity is similar to the activity of pancreatic lipase, breaking down triglycerides to free fatty acids and glycerol. One enzyme is present in the fat fraction and is inhibited by bile salts.[214]

Milk from undernourished mothers may lose some of its ability to hydrolyze milk-lipid esters over the course of lactation; this ability remains constant in well-nourished mothers.[219] This would have an effect on the utilization of the esters of lipid-soluble vitamins A, D, and E.

It appears that the function of this enzyme, inhibited by bile salts, is to facilitate the uptake by the mammary gland of fatty acids from circulating triglycerides for incorporation with milk lipids because lipase in vivo depends on added serum for activity. Its presence in milk probably represents "leakage" from the mammary gland, and it is unlikely to play a major physiologic role in the lipolysis of milk triglycerides.

Additional lipases in the skim milk fraction are stimulated by bile salts. Bile salt–stimulated lipase (BSSL) has greater activity and splits all three ester bonds of the triglyceride. This lipase is also stable in the duodenum and contributes to the hydrolysis of the triacylglycerols in the presence of the bile salts. BSSL is identical to carboxyl ester hydrolase (carboxylesterase), a pancreatic enzyme. BSSL activity is lower in colostrum than in mature milk. No correlation appears to exist between the volume of milk at various stages and the volume of enzyme secreted.[220] BSSL is present in early prepartum secretions less than 2 months before delivery and in the milk expressed during weaning. For a given well-nourished woman, levels remain stable even after prolonged lactation.[219] BSSL activity is protective against infection by virtue of the production of free fatty acids and monoglycerides, products of fat digestion that have antiinfective properties (see Table 4.32).[220]

The enzyme activity of BSSL is remarkably stable during prolonged storage of up to 2 years at either −20°C or −70°C (−4°F or −94°F). It has also been noted to be stable at 15°, 25°, and 38°C (59°, 77°, and 100°F).[35]

Contrary to earlier suggestions, no association exists between jaundice and increased levels of free fatty acids produced as a result of the high activity of milk lipase.[220]

Investigators have continued to study the action of these lipases in the presence of bile salts. The BSSL remains active during passage through the stomach because it is stable with a pH greater than 3.5 and only slowly inactivated by pepsin. The optimal bile salt concentration for activity is approximately 2 mmol/L, which is within the physiologic range in the newborn. Bile salts protect the enzyme from tryptic activity.[214]

Glucose-6-Phosphate Dehydrogenase

Glucose-6-phosphate dehydrogenase is rich in the milk of mothers with normal red blood cell dehydrogenase and absent in mothers with glucose-6-phosphate dehydrogenase deficiency. Its levels depend on the increased rate of carbohydrate metabolism in the mammary gland.[221]

Lactic and Malic Acid Dehydrogenases

Lactic and malic acid dehydrogenase levels are high in colostrum, are lower in mature milk, and are increased at the end of a feeding. The levels are higher in species with small body size; thus mice and humans have more than cows. Because no correlation exists with serum levels, these enzymes are thought to be synthesized in the mammary gland.[222] A change occurs in these enzymes during lactation.

Lactose Synthetase

Lactose synthetase catalyzes the synthesis of lactose from UDP-galactose and glucose. This enzyme has two components: A-protein, a glycoprotein, and B-protein, an α-lactalbumin. The control mechanism for lactose biosynthesis by the A-protein and α-lactalbumin ensures that lactose is synthesized in the mammary gland only in response to specific hormones.[103]

Lysozyme

Lysozyme is a thermostable, nonspecific antimicrobial factor that catalyzes the hydrolysis of β-linkage between n-acetylglucosamine and n-acetylmuramic acid in the bacterial cell wall. It is bacteriolytic toward *Enterobacteriaceae* and gram-positive bacteria and is considered to play a role in the antibacterial activity of milk as well as a significant role in the development of intestinal flora. It also hydrolyzes mucopolysaccharides. Human lysozyme is antigenically and serologically different from the bovine enzyme. The content in human milk is 3000 times that in bovine milk, and the activity is 100 times that of bovine milk. Lysozyme is considered to be a spillover product from breast epithelial cells.[223]

Phosphatases

Acid phosphatase is similar in human and bovine milk, but alkaline phosphatase is much less active in human milk, by a factor of 40. Its level increases with the increase in fat concentration and increases as the feeding progresses. In 199 samples from 20 donors, no relationship to age, nationality, or other characteristics of the donor was found. Alkaline phosphatase concentrations appeared to be related to the fat concentration in human milk. Levels increased as lactation progressed.[116]

Alkaline phosphatase is a metal-carrying enzyme with four zinc molecules and two magnesium atoms. It differs from the placental alkaline phosphatase. Serum alkaline phosphatase is increased in pregnancy. The placenta produces alkaline phosphatase, which may contribute to this increase. There is no clinical picture of altered liver function; the liver does not enlarge, and the histologic appearance is normal. The spider angiomata and palmar erythema that are sometimes observed during pregnancy are attributed to the increase in estrogen.[224]

Proteases and Antiproteases

Proteases catalyze the hydrolysis of proteins. High levels of protease are found in human milk, suggesting that enzymes may provide the breastfed infant with significant digestive assistance immediately after birth.

Several enzymes have caseinolytic activity and elastase-like activity. Beta casein and V-casein and galactothermin are probably the by-products of endogenous human milk proteolytic activity.[225] Also, small peptides of only three to eight amino acids are derived from a casein group called *β-casomorphins* with specific physiologic activity. These peptides may be associated with the sleeping patterns of neonates and even have relevance to postpartum psychosis.

Antiproteases' physiologic role is not entirely clear. The main protease inhibitors in human milk are α1-antichymotrypsin and α1-antitrypsin.[214] Trace amounts of others have been identified. One function may be to protect the mammary gland from local proteolytic activity by leukocytic and lysosomal proteases during different stages of lactogenesis. They may prevent the breakdown of proteins in stored milk.[225] The protection of immunoglobulins that are transferred intact to the neonate and the protection of growth hormones are probably other roles of the antiproteases. The presence of such inhibitors may restrain the invading bacterial enzymes in the host tissue (breast) or secretion (milk). Thus the presence of these inhibitors may protect the mammary gland and the recipient infant from infection.

Xanthine Oxidase

Xanthine oxidase catalyzes the oxidation of purines, pyrimidines, and aldehydes. Although bovine milk contains high levels, it was only after much effort that investigators were able to identify it in human milk. This enzyme's activity in human milk peaks on the third day after birth and decreases with the progression of lactation. It differs from that in bovine milk in that it is not of bacterial origin, and its activity is correlated with protein concentration.

Many enzymes are being studied in humans and other species. See Table 4.31 for a summary of the most significant enzymes. For an extensive discussion, see Hamosh.[214]

HORMONES

Protein hormones, especially prolactin, and steroid hormones, such as gestagens, estrogens, corticoids, androgens, and opiate-like peptides, can be detected in human milk and in the milk of other mammals.[226] Animal studies have shown that at least some of these hormones retain physiologic activity when ingested but not when pasteurized. Although their presence was recognized in the 1930s, advances in hormone assay techniques have brought more information to light and particularly increased related to body composition and obesity.[227,228] Hormones with simple structures, such as steroids and thyroxine (T_4), can pass easily by diffusion into the milk from circulating blood. Peptide hormones such as hypothalamic-releasing hormones, because of their small size, also would be expected to appear in milk. Of the larger-molecular-weight pituitary hormones, only prolactin has been found so far. The hormones identified in human milk include gonadotropin-releasing hormone, thyroid-releasing hormone, thyroid-stimulating hormone (TSH; thyrotropin), prolactin, gonadotropins, ovarian hormones, corticosteroids, erythropoietin (EPO), adiponectin, leptin, cyclic adenosine monophosphate, and cyclic guanosine monophosphate (Tables 4.33 and 4.34).

TABLE 4.33 Nonpeptide Hormones in Human Milk

Hormone	Concentration (ng/mL)
Thyroid	
Thyroxine (T$_4$)	1–4
	0.3–2.0
	12.0
	1.16–2.4
	0.8–2.3
Triiodothyronine (T$_3$)	0.02–0.40
	0.05–0.10
Reverse T$_3$	0.008–0.15
Adrenal gland: Cortisol	0.2–32.0 (5:10)[a] 3.7
Sexual	
Progesterone	10–40
Pregnanediol	0–450
Estrogens	15–840 (15:60)[a]
Contraceptives	Biologically significant quantities

[a]Ratio of values in colostrum/values in mature milk.
Modified from Koldovsky O, Strbak V: Hormones and growth factors in human milk. In Jensen RG, editor: *Handbook of milk composition*, San Diego, 1995, Academic Press.

TABLE 4.34 Hormonally Active Peptides in Human Milk

Peptide	Concentration	Ratio (Colostrum/ Mature Milk)
Erythropoietin	Bioassay	?
Growth factors		
Epidermal growth factor	3–107 ng/mL	2:10
Insulin	0–80 µU/mL	3:10
Insulin-like growth factor 1	1.3–7 ng/mL	2:3
Nerve growth factor	Present	
Transforming growth factor-α (TGF-α)	0–8.4 ng/mL	1
Other growth factors	Present	?
Gastrointestinal regulatory peptides		
Gastrin	10–30 pg/mL	2:3
Gastric inhibitory peptide	33–59 ng/mL	1
Gastric regulatory peptide	31–55 pg/mL; 60–430 pg/mL	2:3
Neurotensin	7–15 pg/mL	2:3
Peptide histidine methionine	3–32 pg/mL	5:10
Peptide YY	15–30 pg/mL	2:3

Modified from Koldovsky O, Strbak V. Hormones and growth factors in human milk. In: Jensen RG, ed. *Handbook of Milk Composition*. San Diego: Academic Press; 1995.

The concentration of hormones changes during lactation, with prolactin decreasing over time and triiodothyronine (T$_3$) and T$_4$ increasing. Evidence indicates that the GI tract of suckling mammals possesses the ability to absorb various proteins with substantial preservation of their immunologic properties. The absorption of large-molecular-weight hormones has been demonstrated in suckling rats and mice, with measurable amounts appearing in serum and other tissues. The potential that these hormones could be active systemically in young animals and humans is theoretically possible.[229]

Thyroid Hormones

The thyroid hormones have received considerable attention because of the apparent protection of hypothyroid infants who are breastfed. TSH content was investigated by both direct I-TSH radioimmunoassay and indirect radioimmunoassay. TSH was present in human milk in low concentrations comparable to those normally found in the serum of euthyroid adults. Experimentally, thyroidectomy of the lactating rat led to the disappearance of measurable T$_4$ and an increase in the level of TSH in the milk. In contrast, the administration of T$_3$ decreased the TSH in the rat model.

Adipokines

Given that breast milk is the optimal source of nutrition for infants and directly contributes to normal growth and development and long-term health benefits, the presence of adipokines in human breast milk is an important finding. Adipokines are produced predominantly in adipose tissue and secondarily in other tissues. It has been hypothesized that the breast, with its significant amount of adipose tissue, would likely secrete adipokines into breast milk. Adipokines apparently influence obesity, metabolic function/dysfunction, food intake, and the development of diabetes.

Various authors have reviewed the levels of the adipokines in human breast milk and tried to summarize their potential effects on the infant.[230–232] Table 4.35 lists the various adipokines. These eight hormones are produced primarily in adipose tissue in addition to some other sites. Kratzsch et al.[230] noted the variation in methodology for measurement of the adipokines; variations in measurement of skim milk versus whole milk; the limited number of studies measuring adipokines in colostrum, human milk, and infants' serum; and some discrepancies between the reported values. Notably, ghrelin has several isoforms (acylated [active form], nonacylated), as well as total ghrelin, which have been measured. Apelin also has several isoforms, a couple of which, Apelin 36 and Apelin 12, have been measured in human milk. Kratzsch et al.[230] presented an up-to-date review attempting to describe the relationship between maternal serum levels, breast-milk levels, and infant adipokine serum levels for the

TABLE 4.35   List of Adipokines, Structures, Tissues/Cells, Reported Effects, Presence, and Associations

Adipokine	Structure[a]	Tissues/Cells (+ Adipose Tissue)	Reported Effects	Presence in Breast Milk or Colostrum[b]	Associations
Leptin	167 AA peptide		Food intake, energy expenditure	C— + TransM— + HM— + Preterm— +	Total body fat mass
Ghrelin	28 AA peptide, acylated = active isoform	Stomach, Intestine, breast	Stimulates food intake, energy metabolism	C— + TransM— + HM— +	Adipogenesis
Adiponectin	244 AA protein, + isoforms	Most abundant adipose-specific protein	Insulin sensitivity, metabolic control, suppress inflammation	HM— + ? C, TransM, preterm milk	Weight gain
Resistin	114 AA peptide	Macrophages, human placenta	Antagonizes action of insulin, (subclinical) inflammation in obesity	HM— + ? C, TransM, preterm milk	Development of insulin resistance, DM, and CVD
Visfatin (Nicotinamide phosphoribosyl-transferase [NAMPT])	466 AA protein	Visceral fat tissue, leukocytes	Promotes vascular smooth muscle maturation, inhibits neutrophil apoptosis	HM— + Other milks?	Serum levels, obesity
Nesfatin-1	82 AA peptide	Central and peripheral nervous system	Regulation of energy homeostasis and food intake	C— + HM— +	Can cross the blood–brain barrier
Obestatin	23 AA peptide (derived from pre-proghrelin precursor)	Stomach, heart	Regulation of appetite, metabolism and adipogenesis	C— + HM— +	
Apelin	Group of peptides derived from a 55 AA peptide	Adipocytes, other tissues+	Decrease food intake, increase thermogenesis	Isoform 36 and Isoform 12-present in C and HM	Predictor of T2DM

CVD, Cardiovascular disease; *DM*, diabetes mellitus; *t2DM*, type 2 diabetes mellitus.
[a]*AA*, Amino acids.
[b]*C*, Colostrum; *TransM*, transitional milk; *HM*, mature human milk.

eight adipokines and any associated effects on growth or adiposity but found conflicting data in the various reports.

In an effort to assess the possible effect of adiponectin and leptin on infant composition, Gridneva et al.[228] calculated the daily intake of these adipokines using 24-hour milk intake values and an averaged human milk adipokine concentration. A higher calculated daily intake of adiponectin was associated with higher fat mass (FM), higher FM index (FMI), and %FM in the infants. A higher daily intake of skim milk leptin was associated with higher FM, FMI, and %FM. A higher calculated daily intake of whole-milk leptin at 12 months of age was associated with a greater gain in FM and %FM from 2 to 12 months.[228]

Leptin in human milk appears to not be decreased after freezing or pasteurizing milk,[233] whereas adiponectin was decreased by approximately 32% after pasteurization.[234]

Although the levels of these adipokines in human milk are important, it will be more important to understand the evidence of their serum levels in infants and the effects on infant growth, fat mass, and insulin metabolism, among others. Levels in breastfed infants should be compared with those in formula-fed infants, along with their growth and anthropomorphic measurements. It will also be interesting to compare the levels of adipokines in the mother's serum, her breast milk, and her infant, along with their growth and anthropomorphic measurements, especially in preterm versus full-term infants and appropriate-for-gestational-age infants compared with small-for-gestational-age (SGA) or large-for-gestational-age (LGA) infants. The relationship between maternal serum levels, breast-milk levels, and infant serum levels remains to be fully elucidated, along with their effects on infant growth, metabolism, obesity, and an infant's future health.

Prolactin

Prolactin has been identified as a normal constituent of human milk. Levels are high in the first few days postpartum but subsequently decline rapidly. "Prolactin-like" biologic activity is measurable in human colostrum, with the highest levels on day 1. Concentrations in the milk tend to parallel concentrations in the blood plasma among different species. Three stages of neuroendocrine development are theorized: placental, milk, and autonomous, in which the milk phase is the adaptation to extrauterine life.[214]

The exact mechanism by which prolactin enters the milk is unclear. Prolactin-binding sites have been identified within the alveolar cells.[235] The functional significance of prolactin also remains unclear. In rodents, milk prolactin influences fluid and ion absorption from the jejunum. It also may influence gonadal and adrenal function, as demonstrated in other species.

Endocrine responses in the neonate differ between breastfed and formula-fed infants.[236] In a study of 34 healthy, 6-day-old full-term infants who were formula-fed, plasma concentrations of insulin, motilin, enteroglucagon, neurotensin, and pancreatic polypeptide changed significantly after a feeding. Similar levels were measured in 43 normal breastfed infants, and little or no change was noted. Further, the basal levels of gastric inhibitory polypeptide, motilin, neurotensin, and vasoactive intestinal peptide were also higher in the bottle-fed than in the breastfed infants. Whether changes in the release of pancreatic and gut hormones affect postnatal development is yet to be determined.

Erythropoietin

Erythropoietin (EPO) is synthesized in the maternal kidney and targets bone marrow, where it stimulates erythropoiesis. The bioavailability of erythropoietin enterally is thought to be insufficient; however, it may be different for newborns when present in human milk. In the rat model, it has been shown to stimulate erythropoiesis in the suckling rat. It may have a physiologic effect on human breastfed newborns.[237]

Prostaglandins

In the investigation of the factors in human milk that may modify or supplement physiologic functions in the neonate, the role of prostaglandins comes under review. Prostaglandins include any of a class of physiologically active lipid molecules derived from AA. They are included as subclasses of eicosanoids and prostanoids. The prostanoid subclass molecules are abbreviated PGE, PGF, PGA, and PGB, with numeric subscripts according to structure.

Among the many effects of these compounds are those of vasodepression, stimulation of intestinal smooth muscle, uterine stimulation, aggregation of blood platelets, and antagonism to hormones influencing lipid metabolism.

The synthesis of prostaglandins occurs when dietary linoleic acid is converted in the body by a series of steps involving chain lengthening and dehydration to AA, the principal (but not the only) precursor of prostaglandins. Although the prostaglandins are similar in structure, the biologic effects of various prostaglandins produced from a single unsaturated fatty acid can be profoundly different and, in some cases, antagonistic based on the specific receptors within a specific tissue.

Because of the possible beneficial effects of prostaglandins on the GI tract of infants, several investigators[238,239] have measured levels in human milk. The measurements were made in colostrum, transitional milk, and mature milk, with collections of both foremilk and hindmilk. PGE and PGF have been shown to be present in breast milk in more than 100 times the concentration in adult plasma (Fig. 4.15). The ratio of the principal metabolite of PGFM to PGF itself suggests a relatively long half-life. Although prostaglandins occur in cow milk, none was measurable in cow's milk–based formulas. Two inactive metabolites were found in milk in levels similar to those in the control adult plasma.

It is thought that prostaglandins play a role in GI motility, possibly assisting peristalsis physiologically. Infantile diarrhea may occasionally be caused by excessive prostaglandin secretion into the mother's milk during menstruation, when maternal plasma levels of PGF may be raised. The difference in stool patterns between infants who are breastfed versus formula-fed may be partially attributable to the presence of prostaglandins in human milk and not in formulas.

Prostaglandins E_1, E_2, and $F_2\alpha$ (PGE_1, PGE_2, $PGF_2\alpha$) were determined in milk and plasma from the mothers of term and preterm infants by Shimizu et al.[240] They found the concentration of PGE_1 in milk to be similar to that in plasma and the concentrations of PGE_2 and $PGF_2\alpha$ to be about 1.2 to 2 times higher in milk than in plasma. Foremilk and hindmilk levels, however, were similar, as were term and preterm levels. Levels appeared to be constant throughout lactation. PGE_1 is credited with a variety of physiologic effects on the GI tract,

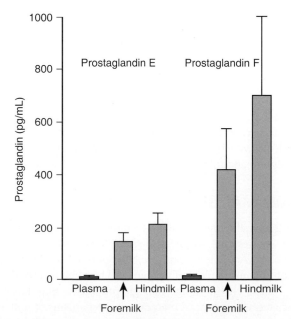

Fig. 4.15 Prostaglandins E and F (PGE, PGF; pg/mL ± standard error of the mean [SEM]) in human milk and adult plasma. (From Lucas A, Mitchell MD. Prostaglandins in human milk. *Arch Dis Child*. 1980;55:950.)

including cytoprotection and a diarrhea-producing action. Other actions are expected and yet to be identified because of prostaglandins' stability throughout lactation and lack of degradation in milk and in the lumen of the gut.

In addition, human infants may require PGE_2 for the maintenance of gastric mucosal integrity, as do adults. Therefore it is not surprising that the use of prostaglandin synthesis inhibitors, such as indomethacin for closure of a patent ductus, is associated with necrotizing enterocolitis. PGE_2 in human milk may also promote the accumulation of phospholipids in the neonatal stomach, enhancing the gastric mucosal barrier.

Relaxin

Relaxin is a hormone with a polypeptide structure similar to that of insulin. It is produced by the corpus luteum during pregnancy, as well as by the decidua and the placenta. Relaxin induces cervical softening, loosens the pelvic girdle, and decreases myometrial activity during pregnancy in many species.[241] Its role in humans remains under study.

It has been postulated that human mammary tissue is a target and a source of relaxin synthesis. Relaxin was measured by specific human relaxin radioimmunoassay in the milk and sera of women delivering at term, prematurely at 3 days, and at 6 weeks postpartum.[241] Sera and milk levels were similar in term and preterm mothers; however, at 6 weeks, relaxin concentrations in milk were higher in the preterm group. The presence in milk at 6 weeks suggests a nonluteal site of synthesis. The authors suggest that before lactation, relaxin may aid the growth and differentiation of mammary tissue, and then in the neonate, it may act directly on the GI tract.[242]

BILE SALTS

Another limiting factor in digestion in the newborn is the decreased bile salt pool and the low concentration of bile salts in the duodenum. The presence of some biologically active substances in human milk contributes to digestion in the newborn. For this reason, the role of bile salts was investigated, and cholate and chenodeoxycholate were found in all samples of milk obtained from 28 lactating women in the first postpartum week.[243] In both colostrum and milk, cholate predominated. Samples were randomly collected, and the range of concentration was wide. The ratio of maternal serum to milk levels was 1:1 for cholate and 4:1 for chenodeoxycholate. The significance of these findings is under study.

EPIDERMAL GROWTH FACTOR

EGF is a small polypeptide mitogen that has been identified in many species and isolated and characterized in human milk. Of the growth factors that have been purified to date, EGF is one of the most biologically potent and best characterized as to its physical, chemical, and biologic properties. EGF has been associated with neonatal maturation, mechanisms of milk collection, and various protective effects. It is well established that EGF stimulates the proliferation of epidermal and epithelial tissues and has significant biologic effects in the intact mammal,

particularly in the fetus and the newborn.[244] Effects verified in humans also include increased growth and maturation of the fetal pulmonary epithelium, stimulation of ornithine decarboxylase activity and DNA synthesis in the digestive tract, and acceleration of the healing of wounds of the corneal epithelium. Unrelated is the observation that EGF inhibits histamine- or pentagastrin-induced secretion of gastric acid. It has a maturational effect on duodenal mucosal cells and increased lactase activity and net calcium transport in suckling rats. EGF has been identified in plasma, saliva, urine, amniotic fluid, and milk. Human milk is known to be mitogenic for cultured cells, and it is possible that EGF is the active component related to this effect. EGF is active when administered orally, stable in acid, and resistant to trypsin digestion.

Newborn puppies fed their mother's milk were found to have hyperplasia of the enteric mucosa as compared with formula-fed littermates. Furthermore, the intestinal weight, length, and DNA and RNA content were greater in the puppies fed their mother's milk.

Previous studies specified the presence of EGF in the aqueous portion of human milk only; however, Gullett et al.[245] have established that EGF and its receptor are found in all human milk compartments: aqueous, liposomal, and membranes (MFGMs).

Studies of EGF in human milk first reported that human milk stimulates DNA synthesis in cell cultures in which growth had been arrested. The mitogenic activity of the milk was neutralized by the addition of an antibody to human EGF. These findings support the concept that EGF is a major growth-promoting agent in breast milk. Actual measurements of EGF in the milk of 11 mothers who delivered at term and 20 who delivered prematurely were also done. EGF concentrations were 68 ± 19 ng/mL (mean $\pm$ SEM) in those who delivered at term and 70 ± 5 ng/mL (mean $\pm$ SEM) in the milk of those who delivered prematurely. No significant change throughout 7 weeks and no diurnal variation were observed.[244] The total EGF content was closely correlated with the volume of milk expressed, suggesting to the authors that EGF has a passive transport from the circulation as a function of plasma concentration.

Given that EGF has significant healing effects on injured GI tract mucosa and a decreasing gestational age of neonates is associated with a higher risk of developing GI disorders, the amount of EGF in milk is significant. Concentrations of EGF in human milk from extremely preterm (23 to 27 weeks) mothers were significantly higher than values obtained from preterm and full-term mothers throughout the first month postpartum, according to studies done by Dvorak et al.[246] They also noted that transforming growth factor (TGF-α) was also elevated in this group of mothers with extremely premature infants.

Using various techniques for assay, Iacopetta et al.[247] found 30 to 40 ng/mL EGF in human milk, less than 2 ng/mL in bovine milk, and none in several bovine milk—based formulas. Little change occurred with refrigeration or freezing. The role of EGF in promoting normal growth and functional maturation of the intestinal tract continues to be under study.[248]

The Reference list is available at www.expertconsult.com.

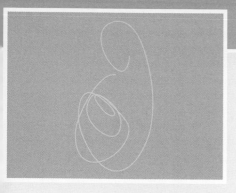

5

Host-Resistance Factors and Immunologic Significance of Human Milk

Robert M. Lawrence

KEY POINTS

- Bioactive factors in human breast milk are not only numerous but they also act in a variety of mechanisms to affect the development, growth, and ongoing health of the infant. Some of those factors also confer benefits for the mother's breast health.
- The study of the cells within breast milk has expanded to include the complete hierarchy of breast cells, hematologic cells, and the microbiota of breast milk and its effect on the infant's intestinal microbiota. Recently discovered stem cells derived from the breast are opening new areas of research into the immunologic significance of breast milk and cancer.
- The interplay between the bioactive factors, particularly human milk oligosaccharides, and the infant's intestinal

microbiota is taking on new significance for the maturation of the intestine and the "programming" of the infant's immune system.
- "Omics," including genomics, transcriptomics, proteomics, glycomics, culturomics, next-generation sequencing, and single cell analysis are some of the new research techniques facilitating the next areas of research into human milk.
- The discovery of a plethora of microRNAs (miRNAs) in various fractions of human milk is leading ongoing research into epigenetics and how these miRNAs when incorporated into the infant's cells are influencing the growth, development, metabolism, and immunity of the infant.

Some of the most dramatic and far-reaching advances in the understanding of the immunologic benefits of human milk have been made using newer techniques to demonstrate the specific contribution of the numerous "bioactive factors" contained in human milk (Table 5.1). The multifunctional capabilities of the individual factors, the interactive coordinated functioning of these factors, and the longitudinal changes in the relative concentrations of them for the duration of lactation make human milk unique. The immunologically active components of breast milk make up an important aspect of the host defenses of the mammary gland in the mother; at the same time, they complement, supplement, and stimulate the ongoing development of the infant's immune system.[1-6]

The explosion of research on all the immunologic properties and actions of breast milk in the last 10 years makes it impossible to summarize all the important aspects of what we now know about the immunologic benefits of breast milk. The recently developed technologies of genomic studies using microarrays and proteomics promise to continue this rapid expansion of knowledge on the biology of the mammary gland, human milk, and the infant's developing immune system.

The common comment about the immunologic benefits of breast milk, "It has antibodies," is a huge understatement. Antibodies in human milk play a relatively small role in the immune protection for the infant produced by breastfeeding. The intestinal microbiome, mucosal immunity, nucleotides,

probiotics and prebiotics, oligosaccharides, glycans, and cells related to the ingestion of human milk are much more important components of the infant's immune protection.[7-13] The developing immunity of infants is a dynamic process. It is made all the more complex by the contextual nature of the interactions of various components in human milk with the developing gastrointestinal (GI) tract. This directly affects both local innate immunity and systemic immunity over time.[14] This chapter emphasizes the important concepts of these immunologic benefits and refers the interested reader to the most recent literature for more extensive information on the many specific components.

OVERVIEW

The immunologic benefits of human milk can be analyzed from a variety of perspectives:

1. Reviewing the published information on the protection of infants from specific infections that compare breastfed and formula-fed infants.
2. Comparing documented deficiencies in infants' developing immune systems and the actions of bioactive factors provided in breast milk.
3. Examining the proposed function of the active components contained in human milk: antimicrobial, antiinflammatory, and immunomodulating.

TABLE 5.1   Immunologically and Pharmacologically Active Components and Hormones Observed in Human Colostrum and Milk

Soluble	Cellular	Hormones and Hormone-Like Substances
Immunologically specific	Immunologically specific	Epidermal growth factor
Immunoglobulin	T-lymphocytes	Prostaglandins
sIgA (11S), 7S IgA, IgG, IgM IgE, IgD, secretory component	B-lymphocytes	Relaxin
		Neurotensin
	Accessory Cells	Somatostatin
	Neutrophils	Bombesin
T-Cell Products	Macrophages	Gonadotropins
Histocompatibility Antigens	Epithelial cells	Ovarian steroids
		Thyroid-releasing hormone
	Additional cells	Thyroid-stimulating hormone
Nonspecific Factors	Stem cells	Thyroxine and triiodothyronine
Complement		Adrenocorticotropin
Chemotactic factors		Corticosteroids
Properdin (factor P)		Prolactin
Interferon		Erythropoietin
α-Fetoprotein		Insulin
Bifidus factor		Cytokines
Antistaphylococcal factor(s)		Interleukins
Antiadherence substances		
Epidermal growth factor		
Folate uptake enhancer		
Antiviral factor(s)		
Migration inhibition factor		
Gangliosides		
Nucleotides		
Antisecretory factor		
Spermine		
Soluble CD14		
Carrier Proteins		
Lactoferrin		
Transferrin		
Vitamin B_{12}-binding protein		
Corticoid-binding protein		
Enzymes		
Lysozyme		
Lipoprotein lipase		
Leukocyte enzymes		

Modified from Ogra PL, Fishaut M. Human breast milk. In: Remington JS, Klein JO, eds. *Infectious Diseases of the Fetus and Newborn Infant.* 4th ed. Philadelphia: Saunders; 1995.

4. Considering the nature of the different factors: soluble, cellular, and hormone-like, etc.
5. Examining the contribution of breast milk to immune protection of the mammary gland.
6. Determining the site of the postulated action of the specific factors (e.g., in the breast or in the infant) at the mucosal respiratory tract or GI tract) or systemic level.
7. Classifying the factors relative to their contribution to the constitutive defenses (innate) versus the inducible defenses (adaptive immunity) of the infant's immune system.
8. Clarifying the mechanism of action of the proposed immunologic benefit (e.g., the mucosal-associated lymphoid tissue [MALT] forms bioactive factors at the level of the mucosa, which migrate to the breast and breast milk, activating cells at those sites).
9. Considering the contribution of human milk to the development of an infant's immune system relative to potential long-term immunologic benefits, such as protection against allergy, asthma, autoimmune disease, inflammatory bowel disease (IBD), cancer, etc.
10. In the era of "omics," one can analyze the various genes that are activated, the RNA being replicated, or the proteins being produced within breast milk and analyze their potential role(s) in the immune protection of the infant.

PROTECTIVE EFFECT OF BREAST MILK

The protective effect of breast milk against infection was documented as early as 1892 in the medical literature. Data proved that milk from various species, including humans, was protective for offspring, containing antibodies against a vast number of antigens.[15]

Veterinarians have long known the urgency of offspring receiving the early milk of the mother. Death rates among human newborns not suckled at the breast in the Third World are at least five times higher than among those who receive colostrum and the mother's milk. The evidence that a lack of breastfeeding and poor environmental sanitation have a pernicious synergistic effect on infant mortality rate has been presented by Habicht et al., after studying 1262 women in Malaysia.[16]

The evidence that breastfeeding protects against infections in the digestive and respiratory tracts has been reported for several decades.[17] However, many of the older studies were criticized for flawed methodology, and because they were performed in "developing countries," where the risk for infection from poor sanitation was expected to be higher.[18,19] Various researchers have proposed specific criteria for assessing the methodology of studies reporting on the protective effects of breast milk, clearly identifying measurable outcomes and the definition of breastfeeding, with other methods to limit bias and to control for confounding variables.[20–22] More recent studies, which have incorporated many of the proposed methodologic criteria, continue to document that breastfeeding protects infants against diarrhea, respiratory infections, and

otitis media.[23–36] Individual papers report protection against urinary tract infections and neonatal sepsis.[37–39] Several papers document the decreased risk for dying in infancy associated with exclusive or predominant breastfeeding in Pakistan, Peru, Ghana, India, Nepal, and Bangladesh.[40–43] A systematic review by the Bellagio Child Survival Study Group predicted that exclusive breastfeeding for 90% of all infants through 6 months of age could prevent 13% of the childhood deaths occurring younger than 5 years of age.[44] More recent reviews on human breast milk document the evidence for protection against infectious diseases from breastfeeding for resource-rich and resource-poor countries.[45–47]

DOSE-RESPONSE RELATIONSHIP

One of the important considerations relative to measuring the immunologic benefits of breast milk is the exclusivity and duration of breastfeeding. The basic concept is identifying a dose-response relationship between the amount of breast milk received by an infant during the period of observation and the immunologic benefit gained. This is equatable to the dose-response relationship for a medication and a specific measurable effect of that medication. In the case of breast milk, the "dose" or volume of breast milk consumed by the infant will be increased by the greater exclusivity and the longer duration of breastfeeding. Drs. Labbok and Krasovec[22] carefully defined breastfeeding in terms of the patterns of breastfeeding relative to the amount of supplementation with formula or other fluids or foods (full/nearly full, medium or equal, low partial, or token) to standardize the use of equatable terms in different studies. Table 5.2 outlines these definitions of the "amount" of breastfeeding. Raisler et al. referred to a dose-response relationship when they studied the effect of "dose" of breast milk on preventing illness in more than 7000 infants.[48] "Full breastfeeding" was associated with the lowest rates of illness (diarrhea, cough, or wheeze), and even children with "most" or "equal" breastfeeding had evidence of lower odds ratios of ear infections and certain other illnesses. A number of other long-term studies demonstrated greater protection from infection with increased exclusivity of breastfeeding and durations of at least 3 months. A couple of papers demonstrated a "dose" effect relative to decreased occurrence of late-onset sepsis in very low-birth-weight (VLBW) infants associated with the infants' receiving at least 50 mL/kg per day of the mother's milk, compared with receiving other nutrition.[49,50] The current recommendations from the American Academy of Pediatrics reinforce the importance of the dose-response relationship between breastfeeding and the benefits of breastfeeding. The American Academy of Pediatrics (AAP) recommends exclusive breastfeeding for the first 6 months of life and at least partial breastfeeding after the introduction of solid foods for an additional 12 months or longer.[51–53] Another important consideration, relative to exclusive breastfeeding, is the potential effect of other foods and fluids in an infant's diet that could negatively influence immunologic benefits and infection-protective effects at the level of the GI mucosa.

TABLE 5.2 Breastfeeding Definitions

Any breastfeeding	Full breastfeeding	Exclusive human breast milk only	Infant ingests no other nutrients, supplements, or liquids
		Almost exclusive	No milk other than human milk; only minimal amounts of other substances such as water, juice, tea, or vitamins
	Partial breastfeeding	High partial	Nearly all feeds are human milk (at least 80%)
		Medium partial	A moderate amount of feeds are breast milk, in combination with other nutrient foods and nonhuman milk (20%-80% of nutritional intake is human breast milk)
		Low partial	Almost no feeds are breast milk (<20% of intake is breast milk)
	Token		Breastfeeding primarily for comfort; nonnutritive, for short periods of time, or infrequent
Never breastfed	Infant never ingested any human milk		

DEVELOPMENTAL DEFICIENCIES IN INFANTS' IMMUNE SYSTEMS

The human immune system begins forming and developing in the fetus. Newborn infants' immune systems are immature and inadequate at birth. Immune systems rapidly adapt in the postnatal period. These are related to the natural maturation of the skin and mucosal barriers and in response to the exposure of infants to inhaled and ingested antigens and microbial agents in the extrauterine environment. Infants' immune systems develop throughout at least the first 2 years of life. Overall, infants have limited abilities to respond effectively and quickly to infectious challenges, which explains their ongoing susceptibility to infections.[54-57] Box 5.1 lists most of the better understood deficiencies in infants' immune systems. An extensive discussion of these developmental immune deficiencies affecting infants is presented by Lawrence and Pane.[47] The B lymphocytes and immunoglobulin production are deficient in the amount and specificity of antibodies produced. There is limited isotype switching and slow maturation of the antibody response to specific antigens (polysaccharides).[58,59] The systemic cell-mediated immune response, including effector and memory T cells, is functionally limited in its response in infants.[60-62] Neutrophil activity in infants is also developmentally delayed, which directly contributes to infants' susceptibility to invasive bacterial infections during the first months of life.[63-66] The complement system in infants is characterized by low levels of complement components, and both the classical and alternative pathways have limitations for complement activation, although the alternative pathway is dominant in infancy.[67-70] Numerous immune components are produced in limited amounts in infancy, including complement, interferon-γ (IFN-γ), secretory immunoglobulin A (sIgA), interleukins (IL-3, IL-6, IL-10), tumor necrosis factor-α (TNF)-α, lactoferrin, and lysozyme.[71]

Relative to these various immune deficits in infants, one can find various bioactive and immunomodulating factors in breast milk that are potentially capable of complementing and enhancing the development of infants' mucosal and systemic immune systems. This concept of bioactive and immunomodulating factors in breast milk is an important area of evolving research that has been extensively reviewed in the literature.[72,73] The most intense focus of this research centers on the effects of human milk on the infant GI tract.[74-76]

BIOACTIVE FACTORS

The bioactive factors being studied are as diverse as proteins (lactoferrin, lysozyme, etc.), hormones (erythropoietin, prolactin, insulin, etc.), growth factors (epithelial growth factor, insulin-like growth factor, etc.), neuropeptides (neurotensin, somatostatin, etc.), cytokines (TNF-α, IL-6, etc.), antiinflammatory agents (enzymes, antioxidants, etc.), and nucleotides (see Table 5.1). In the past, it was adequate to point to the lists of factors (especially immunoglobulins) to "explain" the immunologic benefit of breast milk. Today, it is necessary to understand not only the "actions" of the specific factors but also how they interact with and affect the action of multiple other factors acting on the same process or system. For example, it is important to understand how sIgA interacts with or affects the actions of other bioactive factors (lactoferrin, complement, and mucins) at the level of the intestinal mucosa. The specific effects of the dynamic interactions of the numerous bioactive factors on mucosal immunity, the development of the infant's immune system, and local inflammation are only beginning to be understood.

Phagocytes (Function Matures Over the First 6 Months of Life)

Limited reserve production of phagocytes in response to infection

Poor adhesion molecule function for migration

Abnormal transendothelial migration

Inadequate chemotactic response

Qualitative deficits in hydroxyl radical production

Decreased numbers of phagocytes reaching the site of infection

Cell-Mediated Immunity

Limited numbers of mature functioning (memory) T cells (gradual acquisition of memory T cells throughout childhood)

Decreased cytokine production: interferon-α, IL-2, IL-4, IL-10

Diminished natural killer cell cytolytic activity (matures by 6 months of age)

Limited antibody-dependent cytotoxic cell activity

Poor stimulation of B cells (subsequent antibody production, isotype switching)

B Lymphocytes and Immunoglobulins

Limited amounts and repertoire of active antibody production

Poor isotype switching (primarily immunoglobulin M [IgM] and IgG1 produced in neonates)

IgG1 and IgG3 production is limited (matures at 1 to 2 years of age)

IgG2 and IgG4 production is delayed (matures at 3 to 7 years of age)

Serum IgA levels are low (less than adult levels through 6 to 8 years of age)

Deficient opsonization by immunoglobulins

Poor response to T-cell independent antigens (polysaccharides) (matures at 2 to 3 years of age)

Complement Cascade

Decreased function in both the classical and the alternative pathways

Insufficient amounts of C5a

From an evolutionary perspective, maternal antibodies are transmitted to the fetus by different pathways in different species.[77–80] An association has been recognized between the number of placental membranes and the relative importance of the placenta and colostrum as sources of antibodies. By this analysis, horses, with six placental membranes, pass little or no antibodies transplacentally and rely totally on colostrum for protection of foals. Humans and monkeys, having three placental membranes, receive more of the antibodies via the placenta and less from the colostrum. The transfer of IgG in humans is accomplished by the active transport mechanism of the immunoglobulin across the placenta. sIgAs are found in human milk and provide local protection to the mucous membranes of the GI tract. Other investigations have established that the mammary glands and their secretion of milk are important in protecting the infant not only through the colostrum but also through mature milk from birth through the early months of life.

Although the predominance of IgA in human colostrum and milk had long been described, the importance of this phenomenon was not fully appreciated until the discovery that IgA is a predominant immunoglobulin. It is present in mucosal secretions of other glands, in addition to the breast.

MUCOSAL IMMUNITY

Mucosal immunity has become the subject of extensive research.[81,82] It is clear that considerable traffic of cells occurs among mucosal, epithelial, and secretory, or lymphoid, tissue sites.[83] The data support the concept of a general system of mucosal-associated lymphoid tissue (MALT), which includes the gut, lung, mammary gland, salivary and lacrimal glands, and genital tract (Fig. 5.1). Through the immune response of MALT, a reaction to an immunogen at a mucosal site may be an effective means of producing immunity at distant sites. Antibodies against specific antigens found in milk also have been found in the saliva, which is evidence for transfer of protection to two different distant sites simultaneously. Evidence suggests that the mammary glands may act as extensions of gut-associated lymphoid tissue (GALT) and possibly the bronchiole-associated lymphoid tissue. The ability of epithelial surfaces exposed to the external environment to defend against infectious agents has been well documented for the GI, genitourinary, and respiratory tracts.[84] The sIgA and secretory IgM (sIgM) produced through the adaptive response of the mucosal-lymphoid immune system act by blocking colonization with pathogens and limiting the passage of harmful antigens across the mucosal barrier. Activated B cells and cytokines pass to the mammary gland, where they contribute to the production of sIgA in breast milk. Direct contact between the antigen and the lymphoid cells of the breast is unlikely.[85] Peyer's patches, tonsils, and other MALT structures appear to be well developed at birth.[86] Even with the Peyer's patches, tonsils, and lymphoid tissue at the mucosal level being well developed at birth, there is inadequate production of sIgA and serum IgA in infancy. A breast-feeding infant, as part of the maternal-infant dyad exposed to the same antigens by their mucosal services, can receive protective sIgA and sIgM in the mother's breast milk, produced by the mother's MALT (see Fig. 5.1).

The protective properties of human milk can be divided into cellular factors and humoral factors for facility of discussion, although they are closely related in vivo. A wide variety of soluble and cellular components and hormone-like agents have been identified in human milk and colostrum (see Table 5.1). Although the following discussion separates these elements, it is important to emphasize that the constituents of human milk are multifunctional and their functioning in vivo is interactive and probably coordinated and complementary.

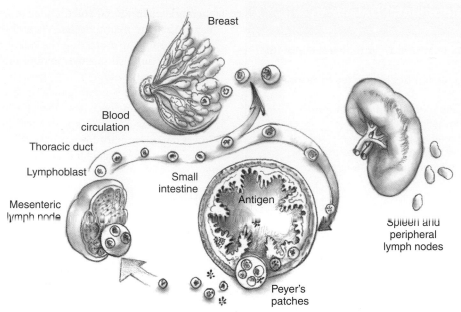

Fig. 5.1 Schema of the mechanism by which progeny of specifically sensitized lymphocytes originating from gut-associated lymphoid tissue may migrate to and infiltrate mammary gland and its secretions, supplying breast with immune cells. (Modified from Head JR, Beer AE. The immunologic role of viable leukocytic cells in mammary exosecretions. In Larson BL, ed. *Lactation.* Vol 4. *Mammary Gland/Human Lactation/Milk Synthesis.* New York: Academic Press; 1978.)

CELLULAR COMPONENTS OF HUMAN COLOSTRUM AND MILK

More than 100 years ago, cell bodies were described in the colostrum of animals. As with much older lactation research, further study of the cellular components was undertaken by the dairy industry for commercial reasons in the early 1900s. This research afforded an opportunity to make major progress in the understanding of cells in milk. Initially, it was thought that these cells represented a reaction to infection in the mammary gland and were even described as "pus cells."

It has become clear that the cells of milk are normal constituents of colostrum and milk in all species. As scientific technology evolved so has our understanding of cells in breast milk and their potential functions and roles in the mother and infant.[87–89] Histochemical staining, detection of cell surface markers, flow cytometry, and the use of genomics, proteomics, metabolomics, etc. have augmented that understanding. In the last 10 years, research in cells of human breast milk has exploded with investigation of bacterial cells, cells derived from the breast, and cells derived from blood (Fig. 5.2). The dynamic nature of the mammary gland stimulated investigation into its development from birth to adulthood, maturation through pregnancy and lactation, and subsequent postlactational involution.[90–93] The frequency, heterogeneity of the disease, and devastating consequences of breast cancer have guided study into the cellular origins of breast cancer and its evolution.[94–96] The discovery of stem cells in human breast milk has led to other paths of investigation regarding the potential uses of such stem cells, their role in the maturation and involution of the mammary gland, their function and role in the mother–infant dyad, and their relationship to breast cancer and the development of resistance to therapy in breast cancer.[97–101]

Variation in Breast Milk Cell Content

Early studies demonstrated macrophages, lymphocytes, neutrophils, and epithelial cells in breast milk totaling approximately 4000/mm.[102,103] Cell fragments and epithelial cells were examined by electron microscope in fresh samples from 30 women by Brooker.[104] He found that the membrane-bound cytoplasmic fragments in the sedimentation pellet outnumbered intact cells. The fragments were mostly from secretory cells that contained numerous cisternae of the rough endoplasmic reticulum, lipid droplets, and Golgi vesicles containing casein micelles. Secretory epithelial cells were found in all samples. Ductal epithelial cells were about 1% of the population of cells for the first week or so and then disappeared. All samples contained squamous epithelial cells, originating from lactiferous ducts and the skin of the nipple.

More recent data reinforce the concept that the cell content of human milk varies by mother, and by lactation stage (colostrum, early lactation, late lactation). The estimated range of cells is between 10,000 and 13,000,000 cells/mL (Fig. 5.3).[87,88,92,99] Hassiotou et al. reported variation in numbers of cells and cell composition with milk fat content, after removal of milk, and during occurrence of infection in the mother or infant.[88,105] With this heterogenous pattern of cells in breast milk, leukocytes remain the dominant cell type in colostrum and the milk of early lactation and epithelial cells dominate in mature milk.[88,92,99,103,105]

Leukocytes

Living leukocytes are normally present in human milk.[85] The overall concentration of these leukocytes is of the same order of magnitude as that seen in peripheral blood, although the predominant cell in milk is the macrophage rather than the neutrophil. Macrophages compose about 40% to 50% of

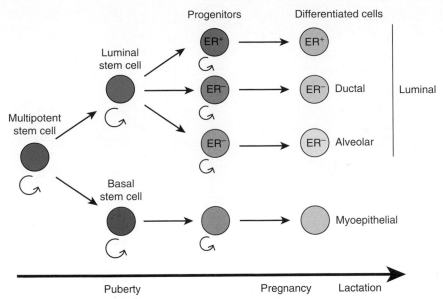

Fig. 5.2 A postulated outline of mammary epithelial cell differentiation. *ER*, estrogen receptor. From Cristea S, Polyak K. Dissecting the mammary gland one cell at a time. *Nat Commun.* 2018;9:2473–2475, Fig 1B.)

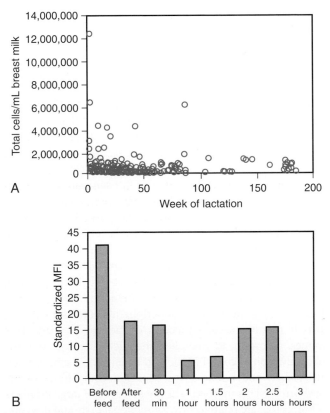

Fig. 5.3 Breast milk cell content and composition. *MFI*, mean fluorescence intensity. (From Hassiotou F, Geddes DT, Hartmann PE. Cells in human milk: state of the science. *J Human Lactation.* 2013; 29[2]:171–182.)

the leukocytes, and 2000 to 3000/mm³ are present, followed by polymorphonuclear neutrophils, also 40% to 50%.[105,106] Lymphocytes make up about 5% to 10% of the cells (200 to

300/mm³), which is a much lower concentration than in human blood.[107] The number of leukocytes found in human milk increases with mastitis and with evidence of infection in the mother or infant and then decrease to baseline at resolution.[106,108] Both large and small lymphocytes are present. By indirect immunofluorescence with anti—T-cell antibodies to identify thymus-derived lymphocytes, it has been shown that 50% of human colostral lymphocytes are T cells and up to 80% of the lymphocytes in human milk are T cells.[109] Immunofluorescence procedures to detect surface immunoglobulins characteristic of B lymphocytes identified 4% to 6% as B lymphocytes.[109,110]

The number of leukocytes and the degree of mitogenic stimulation of lymphocytes sharply decline during the first 2 or 3 months of lactation to essentially undetectable levels, according to Goldman et al.[111] (Fig. 5.4). More recent studies using new cell counting and identification techniques demonstrate that mature milk actually contains less than 2% leukocytes in a healthy mother—infant dyad.[88,105] Hassiotou et al. calculated the daily intake of leukocytes by an infant by breast milk to be hundreds to thousands based on the normal daily infant intake of milk, the reported range of total cell count in breast milk, and this 2% fraction of cells.[87,88]

Macrophages

Macrophages are large-complex phagocytes that contain lysosomes, mitochondria, pinosomes, ribosomes, and a Golgi apparatus. The monocytic phagocytes are lipid laden and were previously called the *colostral bodies of Donne*. They have the same functional and morphologic features as phagocytes from other human tissue sources. These features include ameboid movement, phagocytosis of microorganisms (fungi and bacteria), killing of bacteria, and production of complement components C3 and C4, lysosome, and

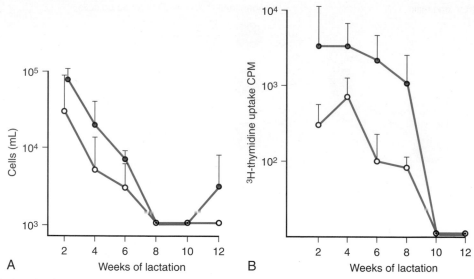

Fig. 5.4 (A) Longitudinal study of numbers of leukocytes. (B) Longitudinal study of uptake of 3H-thymidine in lymphocytes. The same subjects were examined during the second through the twelfth weeks of lactation. Data are presented as mean ± standard deviation of macrophages-neutrophils (•) and lymphocytes (o) in A and of stimulated (•) and unstimulated (o) lymphocytes in B. *CPM,* count per million lymphocytes. (From Goldman AS, Garza C, Nichols BL, et al. Immunologic factors in human milk during the first year of lactation. *J Pediatr.* 1982;100:563.)

lactoferrin. Other milk macrophage activities include the following:[112]

- Phagocytosis of latex, adherence to glass
- Secretion of lysozyme, complement components
- C3b-mediated erythrocyte adherence
- IgG-mediated erythrocyte adherence and phagocytosis
- Bacterial killing
- Inhibition of lymphocyte mitogenic response
- Release of intracellular IgA in tissue culture
- Giant cell formation
- Interaction with lymphocytes

Data suggest these macrophages also amplify T-cell reactivity by direct cellular cooperation or by antigen processing. The colostral macrophage has been suggested as a potential vehicle for the storage and transport of immunoglobulin. A significant increase in IgA and IgG synthesis by colostral lymphocytes, when incubated with supernatants of cultured macrophages, has been reported.[103]

The macrophage may also participate in the biosynthesis and excretion of lactoperoxidase and cellular growth factors that enhance growth of intestinal epithelium and maturation of intestinal brush-border enzymes.

The mobility of macrophages is inhibited by the lymphokine migration inhibitor factor, which is produced by antigen-stimulated sensitized lymphocytes. The activities of macrophages have been demonstrated in both fresh colostrum and colostral cell culture. Certain functions are altered compared with their counterpart in human peripheral blood.

Polymorphonuclear Leukocytes

The highest concentration of cells occurs in the first few days of lactation and reaches more than a million per milliliter of milk. This correlates with the period of highest basement membrane permeability in the infant's gut. Some authors propose that this decline of cells and specifically leukocytes is related to the improved intestinal barrier and diminished need for leukocytes.

Colostrum (1 to 4 days postpartum) contains 10^5 to 5×10^6 leukocytes/mL, and 40% to 60% are polymorphonuclear cells (PMNs). Mature milk (i.e., after 4 to 5 days) has fewer cells (Fig. 5.5), approximately 10^5/mL with 20% to 30% PMNs. After 6 weeks, fewer PMNs are present. The functions of the PMNs normally include microbial killing, phagocytosis, chemotactic responsiveness, stimulated hexose monophosphate shunt activity, stimulated nitroblue tetrazolium dye reduction, and stimulated oxygen consumption.[113] When milk PMNs are compared with those in the serum, their activity is often less than that of serum PMN cells. Whether milk PMNs actually perform a role in the protection of the infant has been studied by many investigators using many techniques. Briefly, animal studies have shown that (1) the mammary gland is susceptible to infection in early lactation, (2) a dramatic increase in PMNs occurs with mammary inflammation, and (3) in the presence of peripheral neutropenia during chronic mastitis, severe infection of the gland occurs. This implies, according to Buescher and Pickering, that the primary function of milk PMNs is to defend the mammary tissue, per se, and not to impart immunocompetence to the newborn.[113] This may explain the presence of large numbers of PMNs that are relatively hypofunctional early and then disappear over time. Evidence shows that neutrophils found in human milk demonstrate signs of activation, including increased expression of CD11b (an adherence glycoprotein), decreased expression of L-selectin, spontaneous production of granulocyte-macrophage colony-stimulating factor (GM-CSF), and the ability to transform into CD1+ dendritic cells (DCs).[114] Human milk macrophages have the morphology and motility of activated cells. The movement of these cells in

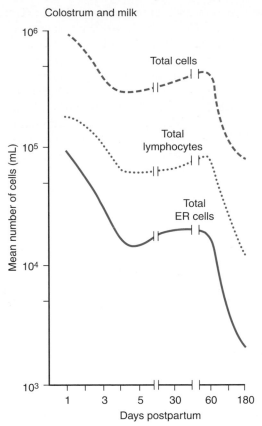

Fig. 5.5 Geometric mean concentration of total cells, lymphocytes, and erythrocyte rosette-forming cells *(ER)* in colostrum and milk of 200 lactating women. (Modified from Ogra SS, Ogra PL. Immunologic aspects of human colostrum and milk, I: distribution characteristics and concentrations of immunoglobulins at different times after the onset of lactation. *J Pediatr.* 1978;92:546.)

a three-dimensional system is greater than that of monocytes, their counterparts in peripheral blood. Such activated neutrophils may play a role in phagocytosis at the level of the mucosa of the GI tract, supplementing infants' poor ability to recruit phagocytes to that site.[115]

Lymphocytes

Both T and B lymphocytes are present in human milk and colostrum and are part of the immunologic system in human milk. T cells are 80% of the lymphocytes in breast milk. Human milk lymphocytes respond to mitogens by proliferation, with increased macrophage-lymphocyte interaction and the release of soluble mediators, including migration inhibitor factor. Cells destined to become lymphopoietic cells are derived from two separate influences, the thymus (T) and the bursa (B) or bursal equivalent tissues. The population of the B cells makes up the smaller part of the total. They synthesize IgA antibody. The term B cell is derived from its origination in a different anatomic site from the thymus; in birds, it has been identified as the bursa of Fabricius. The B cells can be identified by the presence of surface immunoglobulin markers. The B cells in human milk include cells with IgA, IgM, and IgG surface immunoglobulins. B cells transform into plasma cells and remain sessile in the tissues of the mammary gland.

T Cell System

More rapid mitotic activity occurs in the thymus gland than in any other lymphatic organ, yet 70% of the cells die within the cell substance. The thymus is the location for much of the T cell differentiation and selection and plays a major role in the development of infants' immune systems. Thymosin has been identified as a hormone produced by thymic epithelial cells to expand the peripheral lymphocyte population. After emergence from the thymus gland, T cells acquire new surface antigen markers. The T cells circulate through the lymphatic and vascular systems as long-lived lymphocytes, which are called the *recirculating pool.* They then populate restricted regions of lymph nodes, forming thymic-dependent areas.[110] It is interesting to note that exclusively breastfed infants have a significantly larger thymus than formula-fed infants at 4 and 10 months.[116] The significance of the lymphocytes in human milk in affording immunologic benefits to breastfed infants continues to be investigated. It is suggested that lymphocytes can sensitize, induce immunologic tolerance, or incite graft-versus-host reactions. According to Head and Beer, lymphocytes may be incorporated into sucklings' tissues, achieving short-term adoptive immunization of the neonate.[117] Cabinian et al. described in a mouse model breast milk T lymphocytes and cytotoxic T cells (CTLs) localizing in Peyer's patches of the mouse pup's intestine.[118]

Studies of the activities of lymphocytes have been carried out by a number of investigators who collected samples of milk from lactating women at various times postpartum, examined the number of cell types present, and then studied the activities of these cells in vitro.[85,86,119] Ogra and Ogra[120] collected samples from 200 women and measured the cell content from 1 through 180 days (see Fig. 5.5). They then compared the response of T lymphocytes in colostrum and milk with that of the T cells in the peripheral blood. T cell subpopulations also have been shown by surface epitopes to be similar to those in the peripheral blood.

The greatest number of cells appeared on the first day, with the counts ranging from 10,000 to 100,000/mm³ for total cells. By the fifth day, the count had dropped to 20% of the first day's count. In addition, the number of erythrocyte rosette-forming cells was determined by using sheep erythrocyte-rosetting technique. The erythrocyte rosette formation lymphocytes constituted a mean 100/mm³ on the first day and one-tenth of that by the fifth day.

At 180 days, total cells were 100,000/mm³, lymphocytes were 10,000/mm³, and erythrocyte rosette formation lymphocytes were 2000/mm³. The investigators compared the values with those in the peripheral blood of each mother; the levels remained essentially constant.[85] In a similar study, Bhaskaram and Reddy[120] sampled milk over time from 74 women and found comparable cell concentrations. They examined the bactericidal activity of the milk leukocytes and found it to be comparable with that of the circulating leukocytes in the blood, irrespective of the stage of lactation or state of nutrition of the mother.[120]

Ogra and Ogra also studied the lymphocyte proliferation responses of colostrum and milk to antigens.[121] Their data show response to stimulation from the viral antigens of rubella, cytomegalovirus (CMV), and mumps. Analysis of cell-mediated immunity to microbial antigens shows milk lymphocytes are limited in their potential for recognizing or responding to certain infectious agents compared with cells from the peripheral circulation. This is thought to be an intercellular action and not caused by lack of external factors. In contrast, the T cells and B cells have been shown to have unique reactivities not seen in peripheral blood.

Colostral lymphocytes are derived from mature rather than immature T-cell subsets. The distribution of T-cell subsets in colostrum includes both CD4[+] and CD8[+] cells.[122] The distribution of CD4 cells in colostrum and human milk is lower than in the serum, and fewer CD4 cells exist than CD8 cells. The percentage of CD4 cells is higher than in the serum of either postpartum donors or normal control subjects. No correlation exists with length of gestation and number of cells (normal blood usually contains twice as many CD4[+] as CD8[+] lymphocytes).[123]

Parmely et al. partially purified and propagated milk lymphocytes in vitro to study their immunologic function.[124] Milk lymphocytes responded in a unique manner to stimuli known to activate T lymphocytes from the serum. The authors found milk lymphocytes to be hyporesponsive to nonspecific mitogens and histocompatibility antigens on allogenic cells in their laboratory. They found them unresponsive to *Candida albicans*. Significant proliferation of lymphocytes occurred in response to the K1 capsular antigen of *Escherichia coli*.[125] Lymphocytes from blood failed to respond to the same antigen. This supports the concept of local mammary tissue immunity at the T-lymphocyte level.

More recent experiments in rodents have provided evidence that T lymphocytes that are reactive to transplantation alloantigens can adoptively immunize a suckling newborn. Foster nursing experiments performed in rodents have shown that newborn rats exposed to allogenic milk manifested alterations in their reactivity to skin allografts of the foster mother's strain. In animals, mothers may give their suckling newborn immunoreactive lymphocytes. The influence of maternal milk cells on the development of neonatal immunocompetence has been demonstrated in several different immunologic contexts. Congenitally, athymic nude mice nursed by their phenotypically normal mothers or normal foster mothers had increased survival. The mothers contributed their T-cell helper activity to the suckling newborn.

Colostral lymphocytes proliferate in response to various mitogens, alloantigens, and conventional antigens. Colostral cells survive in the neonatal stomach and in the gut of experimental animals, some remaining viable in the upper GI tract for a week. No evidence, however, indicates that transepithelial migration takes place when neonatal mice are foster-nursed by newly delivered animals whose colostral cells were tagged with H-thymidine.[113]

Cells in human milk have been studied using the same markers employed with cells in the peripheral blood; 80% of the lymphocytes are T cells that are equally distributed between CD4[+] and CD8[+] subpopulations, and their T-cell

receptors are principally of the α/β type. CD4[+] cells are common leukocyte cells of the helper and suppressor-inducer subsets, and CD8[+] cells are leukocytes of cytotoxic and noncytotoxic subsets. T cells in human milk are presumed activated because they display increased phenotypic markers of activation, including human leukocyte antigen (HLA)-DR and CD25 (IL-2 receptor). The majority of T cells in human milk are CD45RO[+], consistent with effector and memory T cells.[109,126] These cells are effective producers of IFN-γ, which is consistent with their phenotypic features. Here again, human milk may supplement the infant with a functioning immune cell to compensate for an identified deficiency in the infant, a paucity of memory T cells.

B Cell System

Juto studied the effect of human milk on B-cell function.[123] Cell-free, defatted, filtered colostrum, as well as mature breast milk, showed an enhancing effect on B-cell proliferation and generation of antibody secretion. This was not seen with formula. Juto[123] suggested that this could represent an important immunologic mechanism. Goldblum et al.[127] demonstrated a B-cell response in human colostrum to *E. coli* given to the mother orally, which was not accompanied by a systemic response in the mother. This suggests that the breast and breast milk reflect sites of local, humoral, or cell-mediated immunity, which were initially induced at a distant site such as the gut and transferred by reactive lymphoid cells migrating to the breast. Head and Beer provided a scheme to describe this mechanism (see Fig. 5.1).[117] The diagram depicts the progeny of specifically sensitized lymphocytes that originated in GALT, specifically Peyer's patches, as they migrate to the mammary gland. As they infiltrate the mammary gland and its secretion, they supply the breast with immune cells capable of selected immune responses. Ogra and Ogra suggest that the cells may selectively accumulate in the breast during pregnancy.[85,121] The responses of milk cells and their antibodies are not representative of an individual's total immunity.[124] Most of these immunocompetent cells, initially stimulated in GALT, recirculate to the external mucosal surface and populate the lamina propria as antibody-producing plasma cells. A substantial number of these antigen-sensitized cells selectively home-in to the stroma of the mammary glands and initiate local IgA antibody synthesis against the antigens initially encountered in the respiratory or intestinal mucosa.[121] More recent work on human milk—derived B cells demonstrates that breast milk contains activated memory B cells, different from those in the blood. These cells express mucosal adhesion molecules ($\alpha_4\beta_7^{-/+}$, $\alpha_4\beta_1^+$, CD44[+], CD62L[−]), suggesting an origin in the mammary gland, but similar to GALT-associated B cells.[128] The mucosae-associated epithelial cytokine CCL28 may contribute to migration of and retention of these cells in the mammary gland.[129] This information supports the concept of the mammary gland as an effector site of the mucosal immune system.

The accumulated epidemiologic research supports the concept that colostrum and milk provide human infants with immunologic benefits. Both T and B lymphocytes found in breast milk are reactive against organisms invading the intestinal tract. However, the proof of specific viral or bacterial protection, secondary to the action of immunologically active B cells, has not been demonstrated.

Mammary Gland Cells

The mammary gland of female mammals is a remarkable organ, only reaching full maturation after birth. It undergoes monthly changes because of the hormonal fluctuations associated with the menstrual or estrous cycle and the more remarkable changes in structure and function through pregnancy, lactation, and involution. This dramatic morphogenesis along with the gland's importance in the production of breast milk and nurturing of mammalian infants has led to renewed study of its anatomy, histology, development and functioning.[87,90–93,101] Separately the cellular origin and evolution of breast cancer is driving other avenues of research.[94–96,130,131]

The mammary gland as a functional organ consists of a number of different cell types: epithelial, adipose, immune, lymphatic, fibroblasts, vascular cells, and presumably progenitor cells/stem cells. The cells commonly identified in the greatest numbers in breast milk are epithelial cells, bacterial cells, hematogeneous immune cells, and, in fewer numbers, progenitor stem cells[87,91,92,101] (see Fig. 5.2.) Epithelial cells (ductal and alveolar, luminal-epithelial, and myoepithelial are essential to the lactating breast and can comprise over 90% of the cells in the breast milk of a healthy mother and infant.[91,105] Lactocytes are thought to predominate in mature human milk, although the exact percentage range of lactocytes varies from 10% to 28% to 11% to 99% in different studies.[87] By comparison, in cow's milk the macrophage is the predominant cell type.[87] The majority of the epithelial cells are viable in freshly acquired breast milk.[98,105] That raises the questions of why epithelial cells are present in breast milk and what function they serve. Do the cells enter breast milk as the result of apoptosis or the mechanical forces of synthesis, secretion, and ejection or expression (manual or pump) or an active process driven by gene expression to create "mobile" cells entering the breast milk with specific functions?[132] Epithelial cells are noted to form clusters in breast milk and are cultivable.[104] It is not just the luminal ductal or alveolar epithelial cells that are found in breast milk but also myoepithelial cells from the basal epithelial layers of ducts and alveoli.[91,97] How and why do basal epithelial cells enter breast milk? Notably various researchers have proposed that breast milk contains cells from the full spectrum of mammary epithelial cells differentiation. This includes multipotent stem cells, luminal and ductal stem cells, luminal and ductal progenitors, and the more differentiated epithelial cells.[87,92,93] Ongoing flow cytometry studies with cell marker identification, molecular analysis, genomics, and even single cell RNA sequencing studies are revealing new information about the mammary epithelial cell developmental stages and its cellular function and potential.[92,93]

Stem Cells

Interest in mammary stem cells (MaSCs) has blossomed since Cregan et al.[97] reported the presence of MaSCs in human breast milk. Their research was based on the demonstration of the cytokeratin 5 MaSC marker on cells isolated from human breast milk. Additional analysis showed cells from human milk with both the multipotent stem cell marker nestin and the cytokeratin 5 marker. There are several areas of interest relative to these MaSCs in humans: the potential readily availability of multipotent mesenchymal stem cells (MSCs) for autologous stem cell therapies; the identified cell markers and signaling pathways active in these cells, which could lead to more targeted breast cancer therapies; the role of stem cells in the dynamic states of the breast, especially lactation; the potential correlation between MaSCs and transplantation tolerance; and the state of microchimerism of MaSCs in the infant and the potential effects on the infant.[87,98,99,133–138]

The mammary gland is an attractive target in the search for stem cells, in that it is a dynamic, metabolically active tissue. It has the capacity to proliferate and hypertrophy through adolescent development, pregnancy, lactation, and the subsequent involution phase of the breast. Human embryonic stem cells (hESCs) have a tremendous differentiation potential, in that they can develop into every cell type in the body, different from adult stem cells, which constitute a small portion of organ cells and can mature into organ-specific cell types. Adult stem cells presumably can also produce new stem cells to maintain the population of these cells within the organ. They are said to remain quiescent within "stem cell niches" within an organ.[138] Hassiotou et al. described human breast milk stem cells (hBSCs) with evidence of pluripotency markers on these cells similar to those on hESCs.[91,98] The hBSCs were different from the hESCs in that they did not form tumors in the teratoma assay.[98] Additional analysis of hBSCs by the same group demonstrated that they are capable of differentiating into the mammary cell lineage (myoepithelial cells and lactocytes) and cells of all three germ layers (ectoderm, mesoderm, endoderm), including hepatocytes, adipocytes, chondrocytes, osteoblasts, cardiomyocytes, neurons.[88,98] Other investigators demonstrated what appear to be MSCs also in human breast milk.[99] There is a question of whether these represent true MSCs or evidence of epithelial to mesenchymal transition occurring in the breast. The full complement of stem cells or progenitor cells in human breast milk remain to be fully identified. Inman et al.[92] and Witkowska-Zimny et al.[89] reviewed the various mammary gland cells identified to date in human breast milk, including stem cells, progenitor cells, mammary epithelial cells, and even hematopoietic stem cells in small numbers (see Fig. 5.2). Subsequent research has identified signaling pathways related to stem cell propagation, including Wnt/beta-catenin, Notch, Hedgehog (Hh) transforming growth factor-β (TGF-β), phosphatase, tensin homologue, and Bmi.[138] Stem cells have many of the features of tumor cells, including self-renewal and the ability to replicate "indefinitely."[138,139] The question is what might distinguish normal progenitor cells from tumorigenic progenitor cells. Other investigators searching for such tumorigenic mammary gland stem cells identified MaSCs with the surface markers Lin⁻CD29hiCD24⁺, which were capable of generating a functional mammary gland in the mouse.[137]

The potential roles of hBSCs remain to be determined. The most likely of these roles is in the mother directly contributing to the changes from stage to stage of breast development in pregnancy to lactation. In the infant, the roles could include setting up a microchimerism state leading to local tissue homeostasis or regeneration and tolerance to various maternal antigens. The exact mechanism of acquired tolerance to noninherited maternal antigens (NIMAs) is unknown. It has been suggested that exposure of the fetus during pregnancy and exposure during breastfeeding to NIMA may be the explanation for transplantation tolerance in breastfed persons.[140–142] Breast milk contains a variety of major histocompatibility complex (MHC) antigens from the mother. Molitor et al.[141] demonstrated high levels of NIMA HLA proteins in both the cord blood and breast milk, emphasizing the potential role of human breast milk in exposing the infant to NIMAs. Dutta and Burlingham[143] propose that stem cell microchimerism in infants is related to tolerance, specifically to NIMAs.

There remains much more to be understood about the existence of human breast stem cells in human milk and their possible role in health in the infant and later in life.

SURVIVAL OF MATERNAL MILK CELLS

Large numbers of viable cells reach the infant in the daily consumption of breast milk.[87] Although it is clear that cells are provided in the colostrum and milk, the effectiveness and impact of these cells on the neonate depend on their ability to survive in the GI tract. It has been demonstrated in several species, including humans, that the pH of the stomach can be as low as 0.5, but the output of hydrochloric acid is minimal for the first few months, as is the peptic activity. Immediately after a feeding begins, the pH rises to 6.0 and returns to normal in 3 hours. The cells from milk tolerate this. Studies in rats have also shown that intact nucleated lymphoid cells are found in the stomach and intestines.[142] These cells, when removed from rat stomachs, are capable of phagocytosis. Lymphoid cells in milk have been shown to traverse the mucosal wall. In mouse models, several groups have demonstrated the transfer of cells from breast milk to the infant's tissues. Dutta and Burlingham demonstrated unspecified maternal cells by breast milk in the liver of the infant mice.[143] Hassiotou et al. reported survival of breast milk stem cells in the GI tract of infants, and passage through the bloodstream to other organs.[144] Cabinian et al. showed T lymphocytes and CTLs from breast milk localizing to Peyer's patches in the infants.[118] Additional studies are needed to confirm such results and document functionality of such transferred cells and similar transfer with mother–infant human pairs. Maternal microchimerism (the transfer and survival long term of maternal cells in the infant) is well documented to occur during pregnancy and has been proposed to lead to tolerance between the mother and infant. If this also occurs during breastfeeding, it may add to phenomena.[101]

When human milk is stored, however, the cellular components do not tolerate heating to 63°C (145.4°F), cooling to −23°C (−9.4°F), or lyophilization. Although a few cells may be identified in processed milk, they are not viable.[145]

Mammary Cells and Breast Cancer

Breast cancer is a very heterogenous disease. The World Health Organization has defined 18 different subtypes based on histologic and clinical features. There also have been 5 molecular subtypes described: luminal A, luminal B, HER2 positive [HER2+], basal-like, and normal-like. They are distinguished by the expression of estrogen receptors (ER + or −), progesterone receptors (PR + or −), HER2 expression, and gene expression signature similar to or dissimilar from "normal mammary gland tissue."[95,130] The different subtypes of breast cancer demonstrate different survival rates and response to treatment. It is this cellular and molecular heterogeneity combined with the high mortality, recurrence rates, drug resistance, and metastases, which is pushing research to characterize tumorigenesis of breast cancer. There are two main theories of breast cancer: the stem cell hierarchy model and the clonal evolution model.[137] The stem cell hierarchy model says there are "malignant" stem cells, which lead to cancer (cancer stem cells [CSCs]), resulting in a small group of tumorigenic cells and a predominance of nontumorigenic cells that differentiate from the stem cells, leading to the heterogeneity and a hierarchy of differentiated cells in the tumor. The clonal evolution model states that individual cells develop genetic and epigenetic changes over time that lead to cellular characteristics, giving them a selective advantage over other cell clones (i.e., phenotypic and functional differences facilitating tumor growth and survival). This can create a homogenous or heterogenous phenotype of cancer cells. In the CSC model, therapy could be targeted at primarily the tumorigenic cells, and in the clonal evolution model, therapy would need to target most of the cells.

The overlap between breast cancer pathogenesis and mammary gland functional biology is understanding the roles of stem cells in the breast and breast milk (hBSCs and progenitor stem cells), and the regulatory pathways, mammary gland microenvironments, hormonal effects, and noncoding RNAs that influence normal proliferation, differentiation, and apoptosis related to the normal maturation and functioning of the mammary gland.[96] Some of the regulatory/signaling pathways being studied include Wnt/Beta-catenin, Notch, Hedgehog, signal transducer, activator of transcription-5a and -5b (STAT5), and the p53 pathway. The mammary gland microenvironment as it influences normal stem cell function and differentiation involves signaling from extracellular matrix molecules, stromal-derived growth factors, proteolytic enzymes, cytokines, and steroid hormones. This same environment when altered could lead to tumorigenesis. Noncoding RNAs (transcribed from the genome, but not encoding proteins, ncRNAs) can affect gene expression by targeting mRNA and influencing cell proliferation and differentiation and stem cell maintenance within microenvironments.[96] Cataloging and comparing breast cancer phenotypes, outcomes, and cellular characteristics with the epigenomics, genomics, metabolomics, and cell lineage studies of breast cancer can lead to that enhanced understanding of breast cancer development and treatment. Ideally, this will also lead to understanding how a longer duration of breastfeeding confers protection against breast cancer.

HUMORAL FACTORS

Immunoglobulins

All classes of immunoglobulins are found in human milk. The study of immunoglobulins has been enhanced through the techniques of electrophoresis, chromatographics, and radioimmunoassay. More than 30 components have been identified; of these, 18 are associated with proteins in the maternal serum, and the others are found exclusively in milk. The concentrations are highest in the colostrum of all species, and the concentrations change as lactation proceeds.[146,147] IgA, principally sIgA, is highest in colostrum. Although postpartum levels fall throughout the next 4 weeks (Fig. 5.6), substantial levels are maintained throughout the first year, during gradual weaning between 6 and 9 months, and even during partial breastfeeding (when the infant receives solid foods) in the second year of life (Table 5.3). Specific sIgA antibodies to E. coli persist through lactation and may even increase (see Fig. 5.6).

The main immunoglobulin in human serum is IgG, and IgA content is only one-fifth the level of IgG. In milk, however, the reverse is true. IgA is the most important immunoglobulin in milk, not only in concentration but also in biologic activity. sIgA is likely synthesized in the mammary alveolar cells or by lymphocytes that have migrated from Peyer's patches in the GI tract or from lymphoid tissue in the respiratory tract via the lymphatics to the breast.[148] Cytokines cause isotype switching of local IgM$^+$ B cells to become IgA$^+$ B lymphocytes.[54,149,150] These isotype switched cells travel to the breast, where they are transformed into plasma cells producing secretory, dimeric IgA. It is through this "enteromammary" pathway that the mother provides increased amounts of sIgA to the infant against the microorganisms present in the mother's and infant's environment.[78,82] Brandtzaeg[151] has proposed a model for the transport of IgA (polymeric) and IgM (pentameric), produced by plasma cells, across the secretory epithelium. The model involves the formation of sIgA and IgM, through binding, with the secretory component attached to the epithelial membrane. This occurs in the membrane of mammary epithelial cells during lactation.[151,152]

Quantitative determinations of immunoglobulins in human milk were made from milk collected at birth to as long as 27 months postpartum by Peitersen et al.[153] and by Goldman et al.[111] The IgA content was high immediately after birth, dropping in 2 to 3 weeks, and then remaining constant. Similar observations were made on IgG levels and IgM levels. Ogra and Ogra compared serum and milk levels at various times postpartum. Samples obtained separately from the left and right breasts showed similar values.[85,121]

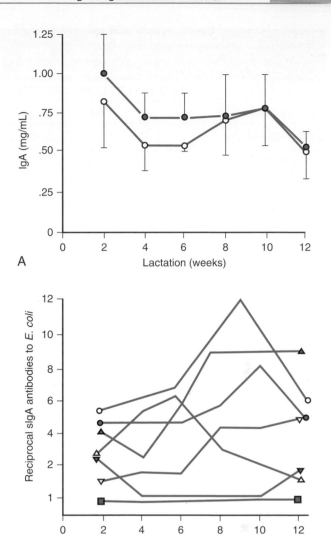

Fig. 5.6 The same subjects as in Fig. 5.5 were examined during second through twelfth weeks of lactation. (A) Longitudinal study of total immunoglobulin A *(IgA)* and secretory IgA *(sIgA)*. Total (•) and secretory IgA (o). (B) Longitudinal study of reciprocal of sIgA antibody titers to *Escherichia coli* somatic antigens in human milk. The sIgA antibody titers to *E. coli* somatic antigens from each subject are represented by a different symbol *(open circles, closed circles, diamonds,* and *squares).* (From Goldman AS, Garza C, Nichols BL, et al. Immunologic factors in human milk during the first year of lactation. *J Pediatr.* 1982;100:563.)

The levels remained constant during a given feeding and throughout a 24-hour period. In all quantitative determinations, IgA is the predominant immunoglobulin in breast milk, constituting 90% of all the immunoglobulins in colostrum and milk.

Ogra and Ogra studied the serum of postpartum lactating mothers and nonpregnant matched control subjects. They noted that the individual and mean concentrations of all immunoglobulin classes were lower in the postpartum subjects. The levels were statistically significant for IgG; they were 50 to 70 mg higher in the nonpregnant women.[85,121,154] Immunoglobulin levels, particularly IgA and IgM, are very high in colostrum and drop precipitously in the first 4 to 6 days,

TABLE 5.3 **Concentrations of Immunologic Components in Human Milk Collected During Second Year of Lactation**			
	DURATION OF LACTATION (MO)		
Component	**12**	**13–15**	**16–24**
IgA (mg/mL)			
Total	0.8 ± 0.3	1.1 ± 0.4	1.1 ± 0.3
Secretory (sIgA)	0.8 ± 0.3	1.1 ± 0.3	1.1 ± 0.2
Lactoferrin (mg/mL)	1.0 ± 0.2	1.1 ± 0.1	1.2 ± 0.1
Lysozyme (mcg/mL)	196 ± 41	244 ± 34	187 ± 33
sIgA antibodies (reciprocal titers to *E. coli* somatic antigens)	5 ± 6	9 ± 10	6 ± 3

Data are presented as the mean ± standard deviation.
From Goldman AS, Goldblum RM, Graza C. Immunologic components in human milk during the second year of lactation. *Acta Paediatr Scand.* 1983;72:461.

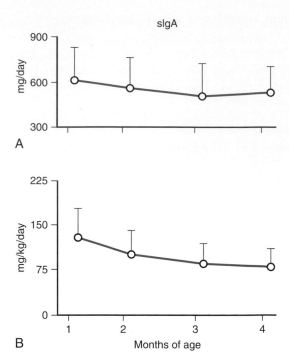

Fig. 5.7 Amounts of secretory immunoglobulin A *(sIgA)*. Total sIgA and sIgA antibodies to *Escherichia coli* somatic antigens in human milk ingested per day (A) and per kilogram per day (B). Data are presented as mean ± standard deviation. (From Butte NF, Goldblum RM, Fehl LM, et al. Daily ingestion of immunologic components in human milk during the first four months of life. *Acta Paediatr Scand.* 1984;73:296.)

but IgG does not show this decline. The volume of mammary secretion, however, increases dramatically in this same period; thus the absolute amounts of immunoglobulins remain more nearly constant than it would first appear. Local production and concentration of IgA, and probably IgM, may take place in the mammary gland at delivery.

IgE and IgD have been measured in colostrum and milk. Using radioimmunoassay techniques, colostrum was found to contain concentrations of 0.5 to 0.6 IU/mL IgE in 41% of samples and less in the remainder.[155] IgD was found in all samples in concentrations of 2 to 2000 mg/dL. Plasma levels were poorly correlated. The findings suggest possible local mammary production rather than positive transfer. The question of whether IgE or IgD antibodies in breast milk have similar specificities for antigens as the IgA antibodies in milk remains unanswered.[146] Keller et al. examined the question of local mammary IgD production, and its possible participation in a mucosal immune system, by comparing colostrum and plasma levels of total IgD with specific IgD antibodies.[119] From their work comparing colostrum-to-plasma ratios for IgG, IgD, and albumin and measuring IgD against specific antigens, the authors reported evidence for IgD participation in the response of the mucosal immune system, with increases in total IgD and IgD against specific antigens found in colostrum.

Butte et al. addressed the question of total quantities of immunologic components secreted into human milk per day and available to an infant.[156] They did so by measuring the amounts of sIgA, sIgA antibodies to *E. coli*, protein, lactoferrin, and lysozyme ingested per day and per kilogram per day in the first 4 months of life (Figs. 5.7 through 5.11). Lactoferrin, sIgA, and sIgA antibodies gradually declined in amount ingested per day and per kilogram per day. Lysozyme, in contrast, rose during the same period in total

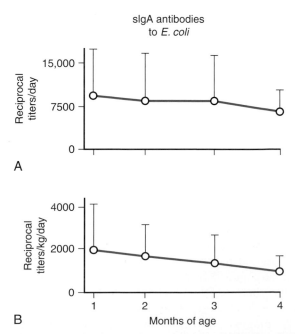

Fig. 5.8 Amounts of secretory immunoglobulin A *(sIgA)* antibodies to *Escherichia coli* somatic antigens in human milk ingested as reciprocal titers per day (A) and per kilogram per day (B). Data are presented as mean ± standard deviation. (From Butte NF, Goldblum RM, Fehl LM, et al. Daily ingestion of immunologic components in human milk during the first four months of life. *Acta Paediatr Scand.* 1984;73:296.)

amount available and amount per kilogram per day. The authors suggest that production and secretion of these immunologic factors by the mammary gland may be linked to the catabolism of the components in an infant's mucosal tissues.[156] When the concentrations of sIgA, IgG, IgM, α_1-antitrypsin, lactoferrin, lysozyme, and globulins C3 and C4 were compared in relationship to parity and age of the mother, no consistent trend was observed. When maturity of the pregnancy was considered, however, mean concentrations of all these proteins were higher, except for IgA, when the delivery was premature. Because several proteins in human milk have physiologic functions in infants, Davidson and Lönnerdal[157] examined the survival of human milk proteins through the GI tract.[157] Crossed immunoelectrophoresis showed that three human milk proteins transversed the entire intestine and were present in the feces: lactoferrin, sIgA, and α_1-antitrypsin.

Miranda et al. reported on the effect of maternal nutritional status on immunologic substances in human colostrum and milk.[158] Maternal malnutrition was characterized as lower weight-to-height ratio, creatine-to-height index, total serum proteins, and IgG and IgA. In malnourished mothers, the colostrum contained one-third the normal concentration of IgG, less than half the normal level of albumin, and lower IgA and complement C4. Lysozyme, complement C3, and IgM levels were normal. Levels improved with development of mature milk and improvement in maternal nutrition. According to one report in 2003, moderate exercise during lactation does not affect the levels of IgA, lactoferrin, or lysozyme in breast milk.[159] Immunologic components contained

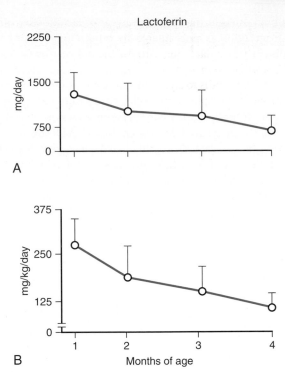

Fig. 5.10 Amount of lactoferrin in human milk ingested per day (A) and per kilogram per day (B). Data are presented as mean ± standard deviation. (From Butte NF, Goldblum RM, Fehl LM, et al. Daily ingestion of immunologic components in human milk during the first four months of life. *Acta Paediatr Scand.* 1984;73:296.)

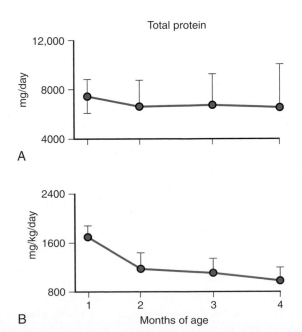

Fig. 5.9 Amount of total protein in human milk ingested per day (A) and per kilogram per day (B). Data are presented as mean ± standard deviation. (From Butte NF, Goldblum RM, Fehl LM, et al. Daily ingestion of immunologic components in human milk during the first four months of life. *Acta Paediatr Scand.* 1984;73:296.)

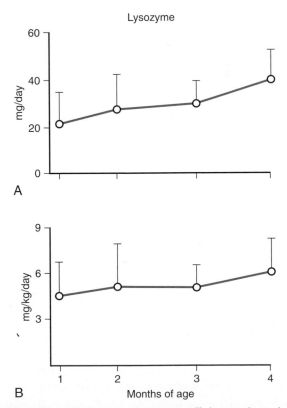

Fig. 5.11 Amount of lysozyme in human milk ingested per day (A) and per kilogram per day (B). Data are presented as mean ± SD. (From Butte NF, Goldblum RM, Fehl LM, et al. Daily ingestion of immunologic components in human milk during the first four months of life. *Acta Paediatr Scand.* 1984;73:296.)

in human milk during the second year of lactation become a significant point as more infants are nursed longer. For a longitudinal study of lactation into the second year by Goldman et al., women were included who had fully breastfed their infants for 6 months to a year and were continuing to partially breastfeed.[160] Samples were collected by fully emptying the breast by electric pump. Table 5.3 summarizes the concentrations of the measured factors in breast milk from 12 to 24 months of lactation. No leukocytes were detected. Concentrations of total IgA and sIgA, lactoferrin, and lysozyme were similar to those 7 to 12 months postpartum and during gradual weaning. sIgA antibodies to *E. coli* were produced in the second year, demonstrating significant immunologic benefit to the infant with continued breastfeeding.[160] IgA, IgM, and IgG were measured in nursing women from the beginning of lactation and simultaneously in the feces of their children by Jatsyk et al. at the Academy of Medicine in Moscow.[161] They reported IgA to be very high in the milk and rapidly increasing in the feces. IgG and IgM levels, however, were low in both milk and feces. In normal full-term bottle-fed infants, IgA appeared in the feces at 3 to 4 weeks of age, but at much lower levels than in breastfed infants. Koutras and Vigorita[162] reported that in the first 8 weeks of life increased amounts of sIgA were found in the stools of breastfed infants compared with formula-fed infants. The authors ascribed this phenomenon to the presence of sIgA in human milk and a stimulation of the local GI production of immunoglobulin.

Savilahti et al. measured serum levels of IgG, IgA, and IgM in 198 infants at 2, 4, 6, 9, and 12 months of age.[163] By 9 months, the exclusively breastfed infants had IgG and IgM levels significantly lower than those who had been weaned early (before 3.5 months) to formula. Six infants were still exclusively breastfed at 12 months, and their IgA levels had also lowered to levels found at 2 months with bottle feeders. Infection rates were similar. Two months after the children were weaned to formula, the IgG and IgM levels were comparable. Iron and zinc levels were the same in all children.

Specificity of Immunoglobulins

sIgA antibodies have been identified in human milk that recognize a large variety of microorganisms. The sIgA antibodies that recognize bacteria, viruses, parasites, and fungi are listed in Table 5.4. Some sIgA antibodies recognize various bacteria, including *E. coli*, *Shigella*, *Salmonella*, *Campylobacter pylori*, *Vibrio cholerae*, *Haemophilus influenzae*, *Streptococcus pneumoniae*, group B *Streptococcus* type III, *Staphylococcus aureus*, *Clostridium difficile*, *Clostridium botulinum*, *Klebsiella pneumoniae*, and *Listeria monocytogenes*. Some sIgA antibodies recognize *Entamoeba histolytica*, *Giardia*, *Strongyloides stercoralis*, and *C. albicans*.[54,164] The list of viruses for which sIgA antibodies exist in human milk is equally long, including enteroviruses (poliovirus, coxsackie, and echovirus), CMV, herpes simplex virus, human immunodeficiency virus (HIV), Semliki Forest virus, respiratory syncytial virus (RSV), rubella, reovirus type 3, rotavirus, measles, norovirus, and porcine coronavirus. IgG

and IgM antibodies also exist in human milk against CMV, RSV, and rubella, as well as IgE antibodies against parvovirus B19. Noguera-Obenza and Cleary reviewed the role of breast milk sIgA in providing protection for infants against various agents specifically causing bacterial enteritis.[164]

Stability of Immunoglobulins

Preservation of human milk at $-20°C$ for up to 3 months does not decrease significantly the levels of IgA, IgG, IgM, C3, C4, lactoferrin, or lysozyme.[165–168] The preservation of sIgA, IL-6, and TNF-α with freezing at $-4°C$ or $-20°C$ was recently confirmed by Hines et al.[169]

A variety of different heat treatments have been applied to milk to protect against bacterial contamination or to protect against infection with specific infectious agents (especially HIV and CMV). Heat treatments include low temperature, short time at 56°C for 15 minutes; Holder pasteurization at 62.5°C for 30 minutes; high temperature, short time at 70° to 73°C for 15 seconds; boiling at 100°C for greater than 1 minute; sterilization, variable time periods, Pretoria pasteurization at 56° to 62.5°C for approximately 15 minutes; flash heating at 56°C for approximately 6 minutes with a peak temperature at 72°C and microwave heating, with milk temperatures of 20° to 77°C for 30 seconds.[170–173] Boiling or sterilization essentially destroys 100% of immunologic activity. sIgA and lysozyme activities drop by 20% with Holder pasteurization and by 50% at 65°C. Low temperature, short time or high temperature, short time do not reduce the sIgA or lysozyme content markedly. IgG and IgM are greatly reduced by Holder pasteurization.

sIgA differs antigenically from serum IgA. IgA can be synthesized in both the nonlactating and the lactating breast. It is a compact molecule and resistant to proteolytic enzymes of the intestinal tract and the low pH of the stomach. The sIgA present in human milk is primarily manufactured by plasma cells in the mammary gland, modified in its translocation across the mammary epithelia, and only minimally produced by the cellular lymphocytes in milk. Levels in milk are 10 to 100 times higher than in serum. Levels in cow milk are very low, that is, one-tenth of the level in mature human milk (0.03 mg/dL). Later in life, the human intestinal tract's subepithelial plasma cells secrete IgA. The intestinal secretion of sIgA does not occur in the neonatal period but increases between 4 and 12 months of life.

Discussion continues as to whether any antibodies are absorbed from the intestinal tract, although it has been estimated that 10% are absorbed. Almost 75% of ingested IgA from milk survives passage through the intestinal tract and is excreted in the feces. All immunoglobulin classes have been identified in the feces.[174] A large body of evidence demonstrates the activity of the immunoglobulins, especially IgA, at the mucosal level of the GI and respiratory tracts. These antibodies provide local intestinal protection against microorganisms, which may infect the mucosa or enter the body through the gut or respiratory tract. Other roles for IgA at the level of the mucosa have been studied, including maintaining symbiotic bacterial communities, neutralizing inflammatory

TABLE 5.4 Antibodies in Human Milk

Factor	Shown, In Vitro, to Be Active Against:	Assay	Effect of Heat
Secretory IgA	Enteroviruses		
	Poliovirus types 1, 2, 3	ELISA, NA, Precipitin	Stable at 56°C for 30 min; some loss (0%–30%)
	Coxsackievirus types A$_9$, B$_3$, B$_5$	NA	Stable at 62.5°C for 30 min; destroyed by boiling
	Echovirus types 6 and 9	NA	
	Herpesvirus		
	CMV	ELISA, IFA, NA	
	Herpes simplex virus	NA	
	HIV		
	Semliki Forest virus	IFA	
	Respiratory syncytial virus	IFA	
	Rubella	IFA, HAI	
	Reovirus type 3	ELISA, NA	
	Rotavirus		
	Measles		
	Norovirus		
	Escherichia coli (EIEC, EAEC, EPEC)		
	Shigella		
	Salmonella		
	Campylobacter		
	Vibrio cholerae		
	Haemophilus influenzae type b		
	Streptococcus pneumoniae		
	Clostridium difficile		
	Clostridium botulinum (toxin B16S)		
	Clostridium perfringens enterotoxin A		
	Klebsiella pneumoniae		
	Streptococcus group B, type III		
	Listeria monocytogenes		
	Staphylococcus aureus		
	Staphylococcal toxic shock syndrome toxin-1		
	Staphylococcal enterotoxin C		
	Helicobacter pylori		
	Entamoeba histolytica		
	Strongyloides		
	Giardia		
	Candida albicans		

(Continued)

TABLE 5.4 Antibodies in Human Milk—cont'd

Factor	Shown, In Vitro, to Be Active Against:	Assay	Effect of Heat
IgM, IgG	CMV		Stable at 56°C for 30 min; IgG decreased by a third at 62.5°C for 30 min
	Respiratory syncytial virus		
	Rotavirus		
	Rubella		
IgE	Parvovirus B19	ELISA	

CMV, Cytomegalovirus; *EAEC*, enteroadherent *Escherichia coli*; *EIEC*, enteroinvasive *E. coli*; *ELISA*, enzyme-linked immunosorbent assay; *EPEC*, enteropathogenic *E. coli*; *HAI*, hemagglutination inhibition; *HIV* human immunodeficiency virus, *IFA*, immunofluorescent assay; *NA*, neutralizing assay.

microbial products, and acting to neutralize certain bacterial species without exacerbating the inflammatory response at the level of the mucosa.[175]

OTHER BIOACTIVE FACTORS

Bifidus Factor

It is well established that the predominant bacteria found in breastfed infants are bifid bacteria. Bifid bacteria are gram-positive, nonmotile, anaerobic bacilli. Many observers have shown the striking difference between the flora of the guts of breastfed and bottle-fed infants.[176] Gyorgy demonstrated the presence of a specific factor in colostrum and milk that supported the growth of *Lactobacillus bifidus*.[176] Bifidus factor has been characterized as a dialyzable, nitrogen-containing carbohydrate that contains no amino acid.

In vitro studies by Beerens et al.[177] showed the presence of a specific growth factor for *Bifidobacterium bifidum* in human milk, which they called *BB*. Other milks, including cow milk, sheep milk, pig milk, and infant formulas, did not promote the growth of this species but did show some activity supporting *Bifidobacterium infantis* and *Bifidobacterium longum*. This growth factor was found to be stable when the milk was frozen, heated, freeze-dried, and stored for 3 months. Growth-promoting factors were present for the six strains studied, which varied in their resistance to physical change. Because all of these factors were active in vitro, they did not require the presence of intestinal enzymes for activation. It has not been possible to show the presence of this growth factor in other mammalian milks; thus it may contribute to the colonization of *B. bifidum* in a breastfed infant's intestine.

Lactobacillus has been described as one of a number of probiotic bacteria that provide an immune protective benefit to their host. *Lactobacillus* reportedly stimulates antibody production and improves phagocytosis by blood leukocytes.[178,179] The use of probiotic bacteria has reportedly produced benefits in a variety of situations associated with infections. The addition of such bacteria to formula is another example of trying to make formula better by making it more like breast milk. Hatakka et al. examined the possible effect of adding probiotic bacteria to formula on the occurrence of infection in children attending daycare.[180] They reported modest reductions in the number of children with complicated respiratory infections or lower respiratory tract infections and the number of children receiving antibiotics for a respiratory infection, in the group of children receiving formula supplemented with *Lactobacillus rhamnosus* GG compared with children receiving unsupplemented formula.

Resistance Factor

It was well known in the preantibiotic era that human milk protects human infants throughout lactation against staphylococcal infection. Gyorgy identified the presence of an "anti-staphylococcal factor" in experiments with young mice that had been stressed with staphylococci.[176] This factor, with no demonstrable direct antibiotic properties, was termed *resistance factor* and described as nondialyzable, thermostable, and part of the free fatty acid (FFA) part of the phosphide fraction, probably C18:2, but distinct from linoleic acid.

Lysozyme

Human milk contains a nonspecific antimicrobial factor, lysozyme, which is a thermostable, acid-stable enzyme. This enzyme is a 130-amino-acid–containing glycoprotein that can hydrolyze the 1 to 4 linkage between N-acetylglucosamine and N-acetylmuramic acid in bacterial cell walls. It is found in large concentrations in the stools of breastfed infants and not in stools of formula-fed infants; thus it is thought to influence the flora of the intestinal tract.

Goldman et al. describe an initial fall in lysozyme levels from 85 to 90 mg/mL to 25 mg/mL at 2 to 4 weeks and then an increase during 6 months to 250 mg/mL (Fig. 5.12).[111] Lysozyme levels show an increase over time during lactation; this finding is more apparent in Indian women than in those of the Western world. Reddy et al. studied the levels of lysozyme in well-nourished and poorly nourished women in India and found no difference between them (Table 5.5).[181] As shown in this study, lysozyme levels increase during lactation. Levels in human milk are 300 times the level in cow milk. Lysozyme is bacteriostatic against Enterobacteriaceae

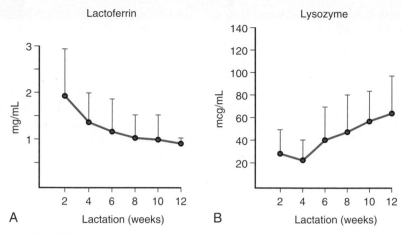

Fig. 5.12 The same subjects as in Fig. 5.5 were examined during second through twelfth weeks of lactation. Data in longitudinal studies are presented as mean ± standard deviation. (A) Concentration of lactoferrin progressively decreased through first 8 weeks (r = 0.69) (2 vs. 8 weeks; *p* < 0.02), but not thereafter. (B) In contrast, lysozyme levels steadily increased from fourth through twelfth weeks (r = 0.76) (4 vs. 12 weeks; *p* < 0.01). (From Goldman AS, Garza C, Nichols BL, et al. Immunologic factors in human milk during the first year of lactation. *J Pediatr.* 1982;100:563.)

TABLE 5.5 Antibacterial Factors in Colostrum and Mature Milk in Well-Nourished and Undernourished Indian Women

Group	Hemoglobin (g/dL)	Serum Albumin (g/dL)	IMMUNOGLOBULINS (MG/DL)			Lysozyme (mg/dL)	Lactoferrin (mg/dL)
			IgA	IgG	IgM		
Colostrum (1–5 days)							
Well-nourished women	11.5 ± 0.37	2.49 ± 0.065	335.9 ± 37.39 (17)*	5.9 ± 1.58 (17)	17.1 ± 4.29 (17)	14.2 ± 2.11 (15)	420 ± 49.0 (28)
Undernourished women	11.3 ± 0.60	2.10 ± 0.081	374.3 ± 42.13 (10)	5.3 ± 2.30 (10)	15.3 ± 2.50 (10)	16.4 ± 2.39 (21)	520 ± 69.0 (19)
Mature milk (1–6 mo)							
Well-nourished women	12.8 ± 0.43	3.39 ± 0.120	119.6 ± 7.85 (12)	2.9 ± 0.92 (12)	2.9 ± 0.92 (12)	24.8 ± 3.41 (10)	250 ± 65.0 (17)
Undernourished women	12.6 ± 0.56	3.47 ± 0.130	118.1 ± 16.2 (10)	5.8 ± 3.41 (10)	5.8 ± 3.41 (10)	23.3 ± 3.53 (23)	270 ± 92.0 (13)

*Figures in parentheses indicate number of samples analyzed.
From Reddy V, Bhaskaram C, Raghuramula N, et al. Antimicrobial factors in human milk. *Acta Paediatr Scand.* 1977;66:229.

and gram-positive bacteria.[112] It is secreted by neutrophils and some macrophages and is present in many body secretions in the adult.

In a study of immunologic components in human milk in the second year of lactation, Goldman et al. reported that concentrations of lysozyme, lactoferrin, and total IgA and sIgA were similar to those in uninterrupted lactation and in gradual weaning at 6 to 9 months.[160] sIgA antibodies to *E. coli* were also produced during the second year. The authors state that "this supports the idea that the enteromammary lymphocyte traffic pathway, which leads to the development of lymphoid cells in the mammary gland that produce IgA antibodies to enteric organisms, operates throughout lactation."[160] When cow milk formula is added to human milk, it reduces the effect of

lysozyme; however, powdered human milk fortifier (Enfamil) did not inhibit the antiinfective properties.[182]

Lactoferrin

Lactoferrin is an iron-binding protein closely related to the serum iron transport protein, transferrin, and is part of the larger transferrin protein family. Lactoferrin is found in mucosal secretions (tears, saliva, vaginal fluids, urine, nasal and bronchial secretions, bile, GI fluids) and, notably, in milk and colostrum. A bacteriostatic effect of lactoferrin is well established for a wide range of microorganisms, including gram-positive and gram-negative aerobes, anaerobes, viruses, parasites, and fungi. The original proposed mechanism of action for its bacteriostatic effect was depriving the microorganism of iron. A second antibacterial action, involving direct action with bacterial surfaces, binds negatively charged molecules (lipoteichoic acid) on the surface of gram-positive bacteria. This neutralizes the surface charge, allowing the action of other antibacterial factors (e.g., lysozyme or binding lipid A) on gram-negative bacteria, which releases the lipid, producing damage to the cell membrane. Another antibacterial action is binding bacterial adhesions blocking host cell interaction.[183] Lactoferrin can kill *C. albicans* and *C. krusei* by changing the permeability of the fungal cell surface. Lactoferrin now is considered a multifunctional, immunoregulatory protein.

The biologic role of lactoferrin has been reviewed in several publications.[104—187] They point out that lactoferrin reversibly binds two ferric ions and that its affinity for iron is 300 times greater than that of transferrin, retaining iron down to a pH of 3. Human lactoferrin is strongly basic. Lactoferrin is normally unsaturated with iron, and it is usually less than 10% saturated with iron in human milk.[187—189] Oral iron therapy for an infant can interfere with the bacteriostatic action of lactoferrin, which depends on its unsaturated state for some portion of its bacteriostatic function. Reddy et al. showed that giving iron to the mother did not interfere with the saturation of lactoferrin in the milk or, thus, its potential bacteriostatic effect.[181] Protein energy malnutrition, rather than iron supplies, influences lactoferrin synthesis in the mammary gland. Malnourished but non—iron-deficient mothers are lactoferrin deficient.

The concentration of lactoferrin is high in colostrum—600 mg/dL—then progressively declines over the next 5 months of lactation, leveling at about 180 mg/dL. Breast milk also contains small amounts of transferrin (10 to 15 mg/mL). Lactoferrin is 10% to 15% of the total protein content of human milk.[184] Lactoferrin is resistant to proteolysis, especially in its iron-saturated form. Intact lactoferrin is detectable in the stool of infants, with higher proportions of lactoferrin measurable in the stool of premature infants.[190] Both intact lactoferrin and fragments have been detected in the urine of premature infants, although absorption is less likely in full-term infants.[1] The absorption of iron from breast milk is directly enhanced by lactoferrin.[185]

Many bacteria require iron for normal growth, and one bacteriostatic effect of lactoferrin has been ascribed to its iron-binding action. In neutrophils, lactoferrin within neutrophilic granules tightly binds iron, but neutrophils with excessive iron are inefficient at destroying bacteria. Lactoferrin does not limit the growth of all microorganisms; *Helicobacter pylori* and *Neisseria, Treponema,* and *Shigella* species all have receptors for lactoferrin, directly binding iron and allowing adequate growth.

Some evidence supports various other proposed mechanisms of action for lactoferrin's antimicrobial effect. Lactoferrin has been shown to limit the formation of biofilms by specific organisms, inhibit adhesion to host cells by other organisms, and directly bind to viral particles of herpes simplex virus, HIV, and adenovirus. A proteolytic action of lactoferrin appears to inactivate virulence factors of some organisms. Separately,

lactoferrin binds directly to glycosaminoglycans (GAGs) and integrins interrupting the binding of various viruses (herpes simplex virus [HSV], HIV, adenovirus, CMV, hepatitis B virus [HBV]) to host cells. Pepsin hydrolysate products of lactoferrin (B or H) may exert a direct bactericidal effect by binding to lipopolysaccharide of gram-negative organisms and disrupting bacterial membranes.[191] Lactoferrin may cause an increased release of cytokines by cells, including anti-inflammatory cytokines such as IL-10.[192,193] Others have shown that lactoferrin suppresses the release of IL-1, IL-2, IL-6, IL-8, and TNF-α, all proinflammatory cytokines, which would be more of an immune-modulating effect. Other investigators using a recombinant human lactoferrin (talactoferrin) demonstrated evidence of lactoferrin causing increased maturation of DCs and talactoferrin causing the recruitment and activation of neutrophils and macrophages as other examples of how lactoferrin affects the innate immune protection of the growing infant.[194,195] Several other effects have been proposed for lactoferrin, including inhibition of hydroxyl radical formation, decreasing local cell damage; lipopolysaccharide binding, also leading to a diminished inflammatory response; and DNA binding, affecting transcription and possibly regulation of the production of cell products. Activation of natural killer (NK) cells, modulation of complement activity, and blocking of adhesion of enterotoxigenic *E. coli* and *Shigella flexneri* are other proposed actions of lactoferrin.[196]

A specific region of lactoferrin, near the N-terminus of the molecule, is strongly basic and is reported to mediate some of lactoferrin's antimicrobial activity. "Lactoferricins," small peptides containing this basic region and produced by proteolytic cleavage, reportedly bind to lipopolysaccharide, leading to disruption of the bacterial cell wall and cytoplasmic membrane.[191]

In another area of immune protection, lactoferrin may limit cancer development.[193] The proposed mechanisms of its anticancer effects include increasing NK cell cytotoxicity, increased production of IL-18 and inhibition of angiogenesis, augmented apoptosis of cancer cells, and initiation of cell cycle arrest in growing tumor cells.[193]

The multiple roles and proposed mechanisms of action of lactoferrin in breastfed infants continue to be more specifically elucidated.[197,198]

Interferon

Colostral cells in culture have been shown to be stimulated to secrete an IFN-like substance with strong antiviral activity up to 150 National Institutes of Health units/mL.[112] This property has not yet been identified in the supernatant of colostrum or milk. IFN-γ has been produced by T cells from human milk when stimulated in vitro. The T cells isolated from human milk were the CD45RO phenotype and have been identified as a source of IFN. Srivastava et al.[199] have measured low levels of IFN-γ in not only colostrum, but also transitional and mature milk.[199] They postulated that the low level of IFN-γ (0.7 to 2.0 pg/mL) might be adequate to protect against infection without hyperactivation of T cells. IFN is produced by NK cells and by T cells, phenotypically Thy0 and Thy1. It can cause increased expression of MHC molecules, increase macrophage function, inhibit IgE and IL-10 production, and produce antitumor and antiviral activity. The exact role of IFN-γ in breast milk has not been delineated.

Complement

The C3 and C4 components of complement, known for their ability to fuse bacteria bound to a specific antibody, are present in colostrum in low concentrations compared with their levels in serum. IgG and IgM activate complement. C3 proactivator has been described, and IgA and IgE have been identified as stimulating the system. Activated C3 has opsonic, anaphylactic, and chemotactic properties and is important for the lysis of bacteria bound to a specific antibody. No functional role for complement in breast milk has been identified.

Vitamin B₁₂—Binding Protein

Unsaturated vitamin B_{12}—binding protein of high molecular weight has been found in very high levels in human milk and in the meconium and stools of breastfed infants, compared with its levels in infant formulas and infants who are formula fed. The protein binding renders the vitamin B_{12} unavailable for bacterial growth of *E. coli* and *Bacteroides*.[200]

Glycans and Oligosaccharides

Glycans are complex carbohydrate structures attached to various other structures (a lactose moiety, a lipid component, peptides, proteins, or aminoglycans) that are present in large amounts in human milk.[201] They include glycoproteins, glycolipids (gangliosides), glycosaminoglycans, mucins, and oligosaccharides. Oligosaccharides are composed of a basic core structure derived from molecules of glucose, galactose, or *N*-acetylglucosamine (GlcNAc), fucose and/or a sialic acid derivative *N*-acetylneuraminic acid (Neu5Ac) linked together to create over 150 different compounds. Oligosaccharides compose the major portion of glycoconjugates in milk and are present in the milk-fat globule membrane and in skim milk.[10,202,203]

Gangliosides are glycolipids found in the plasma membrane of cells, especially in cells in the gray matter of the brain. More specifically, gangliosides are glycosphingolipids that contain sialic acid, hexoses, or hexose amines as the carbohydrate component and ceramide as the lipid component of the molecule. Human milk oligosaccharides (HMOs) are poorly absorbed and poorly digested and remain in the gut. Their probable functions are antipathogenic, immunomodulatory, antiinflammatory, and prebiotic.[204–206]

The predominant gangliosides in human milk are GM1, GM2, GM3, and GD3, as reported by Newburg.[203] A diverse abundance of these complex carbohydrates are synthesized by the many glycosyltransferases contained in the mammary gland. Mucin and lactadherin are two glycoproteins included in this group that have antimicrobial effects.[204] Some of these carbohydrate molecules are structurally similar to glycans on the surface of small intestine epithelial cells that act as

receptors for microorganisms. One proposed mechanism for the antimicrobial effect of these soluble substances is direct binding with the potential pathogenic organisms.[205] After studying the adhesion of S-fimbriated *E. coli* to buccal epithelial cells, Schroten et al. proposed that mucins contained in the human milk-fat globule membrane can block bacterial adhesion throughout the intestine.[206]

Gangliosides appear to be responsible for blocking the activity of heat-labile enterotoxin from *E. coli* and the toxin from *V. cholerae* in rat intestinal loop preparations.[207] Another toxin from *Campylobacter jejuni*, with similar binding specificity, also seems to be inhibited by GM1.[208] Globotriaosylceramide, another glycolipid in human milk, is the natural cell surface receptor for the toxin from *Shigella dysenteriae* and verotoxin released by enterohemorrhagic *E. coli*. The proposed mechanism of action of these glycolipids is that, by binding to the toxin, they form a stable complex that prevents the toxin from binding to the appropriate receptors on intestinal cells. However, Crane et al. proposed, from their studies, that the oligosaccharide binds to the toxin receptor to block the action of the heat-stable enterotoxin of *E. coli*.[209] Human milk gangliosides may be important in protecting infants against toxin-induced diarrhea, but this specific mechanism of action has not been demonstrated in vivo in controlled trials.[205] Evidence exists that human milk glycans inhibit a broad range of pathogens (Table 5.6).[201–210]

Human Milk Oligosaccharides

Human milk oligosaccharides (HMOs) are the third most plentiful substance in human milk (approximately 5 to 20 g/L) after lactose and lipids. HMOs remain intact even with the acidic pH in the stomach and are resistant to the brush border membrane enzymes and pancreatic enzymes. Chaturvedi et al. have reported on the survival of oligosaccharides from human milk in infants' intestines.[211] They demonstrated that the concentrations of oligosaccharides were higher in the infants' feces than in mothers' milk and higher in feces than urine. It has also been reported that HMOs can be absorbed into the blood and are excreted intact in the urine of breastfeeding infants.[212]

The major HMOs in human milk include 2′-fucosyllactose (2′FL), 3′sialyllactose (3′SL), 6′sialyllactose (6′SL), lacto-*N*-fucopentaose (LNFP, types I, II, III), and lacto-*N*-neotetraose (LNnT).[213] In human breast milk from lactating mothers of term infants, 42% to 55% of the HMOs are nonfucosylated neutral HMOs, approximately 35% to 50% are fucosylated and 12% to 14% are sialylated. The composition of HMOs in human milk are affected by maternal genetics (Secretor [Se] and Lewis [Le] blood group gene status) and geography.[214] The Se gene encodes for α1—2-fucosyltransferase (FUT2 enzyme) and the Le gene codes for α1—3/4-fucosyltransferase (FUT3 enzyme). Reportedly 30% of women worldwide lack a functional *FUT2* gene such that they lack certain fucosylated oligosaccharides that may have health consequences for their breastfed infant.[215] The *FUT2* and *FUT3* genes create four major HMO groups: Se + Le +, Se + Le−, Se−Le + and Se−Le−, each group secreting a different profile of the major HMOs.[6]

TABLE 5.6 Nonimmunoglobulin Antipathogen Factors in Human Milk

Antipathogen	Pathogen
Ganglioside GM$_1$	Cholera toxin
	Labile toxin of *Escherichia coli*
	Toxin of *Campylobacter jejuni*
Globotriaosylceramide	*Shigella* toxin I
	Shigella-like toxin of *E. coli*
GM3	Enteropathogenic *E. coli*
Fatty acids	Enveloped viruses
	Giardia lamblia
Chondroitin sulfate	HIV
Sulfatide	HIV
Glycoprotein (mucin)	Inhibition: rotavirus in vitro and in vivo
Glycoprotein (mucin, glycosaminoglycan)	HIV
Lactadherin	Rotavirus
Mucin	Adherence: S-fimbriated *E. coli*
MUC 1	Poxviruses, HIV
Glycoprotein (mannosylated)	*E. coli* intestinal adherence
Large macromolecule	Respiratory syncytial virus
Macromolecule-associated glycans	Norovirus, Pseudomonas aeruginosa
Oligosaccharides	Adherence: *Streptococcus pneumoniae* and *Haemophilus influenzae*, enteropathogenic *E. coli*
	Listeria monocytogenes
Fucosylated oligosaccharide	Adherence, invasion, *C. jejuni*, stable toxin of *E. coli* stable toxin in vivo, *Vibrio cholera*
Sialyllactose	Cholera toxin, *E. coli*, *Pseudomonas aeruginosa*, influenza virus
	Aspergillus fumigates, polyomavirus, *Helicobacter pylori*

GM, Granulocyte-macrophage; *HIV,* human immunodeficiency virus.
Modified from Newburg DS, Ruiz-Palacios GM, Morrow AL. Milk glycans protect infants against enteric pathogens. *Ann Rev Nutr.* 2005;25:37–58.

There are a few human studies that support the clinical benefit of HMOs in human breast milk. Doherty et al. report these in a systematic review: a protective effect cow's milk allergy by 18 months of age associated with lower levels of LNFP II concentrations, reduced diarrhea until 2 years of age with an abundance of fucosyloligosaccharides, diminished number of episodes of gastroenteritis and respiratory tract infections at 6 and 12 weeks of age with higher LNFP II levels and less HIV mother-to-child transmission with higher LNFP II levels.[216] A number of potential mechanisms of action for HMOs affecting the infants' immune function have been suggested: increase intestinal maturation, augment mucosal barrier function, alter goblet cell function, diminish intestinal crypt cell proliferation, promote the growth of "healthy bacteria" (*Bifidobacterium, Bacteroides),* directly or indirectly changing epithelial immune cell gene expression binding as receptor decoys to potential pathogens; blocking pathogen binding to cell-surface receptors; and altering the lymphocyte cytokine production, which could affect the Th1/Th2 response, interfere with binding of lymphocytes and neutrophils to endothelial cells and the formation of platelet-neutrophil complexes.[213,215,217]

The evidence for protection against diarrhea, the purported effects on the infant's intestinal microbiota, and the evidence that preterm infants fed human milk rather than formula are 6 to 10 times less likely to develop necrotizing enterocolitis (NEC) has led to various studies to prove the benefit of HMOs in preventing NEC. Lars Bode documents a "journey" of investigation that led to identifying an association between low levels of disialyllacto-*N*-tetraose (DSLNT) in human milk and the occurrence of NEC. The mechanism of this protection is uncertain, and additional study is ongoing.[218]

The profile of oligosaccharides found in infants is usually similar to that found in their mothers' milk. The formula-fed infants had lower concentrations of oligosaccharides, and the profiles of the oligosaccharides were different from those found in the breastfed infants. The oligosaccharides remained intact passing through the intestine. A small percentage are absorbed and excreted intact in the urine. The oligosaccharides were available at these sites to block intestinal and urinary pathogens. Two other groups of researchers have documented variation of the composition of glycans in human milk over the first 4 months of lactation and variations in the composition of glycans in diverse populations.[219,220] Others have analyzed the oligosaccharide composition of donor human milk (Holder pasteurized) and compared that to samples of human milk obtained directly from the mothers.[221] The total amount of HMO was lower in donor human milk. The concentrations of specific oligosaccharides (lacto-*N*-tetraose, lacto-*N*-neotetraose, lacto-*N*-fucopentaose I, and disialyllacto-*N*-tetraose) were significantly lower in donor milk. The concentrations of 3′-sialyllactose and 3-fucosyllactose were higher in human milk obtained directly from the mothers.[219] There is variability in the amounts of specific HMO in the milk of different mothers, at different times through each mother's period of lactation, and in human donor milk. The importance of the "match" of the mother–infant dyad based on HMO composition and quantity and the potential benefits to the infant still need to be elucidated.

Interleukins

ILs are considered a "subgroup" of cytokines.[222] Originally, when cytokines were first hypothesized, it was thought that

TABLE 5.7 Bioactivity and Concentrations of Cytokines in Human Milk

Agents	Bioactivity in Milk	Concentrations*
IL-1β	±	1130 ± 478
IL-6	+	151 ± 89
IL-7	?	79–100 ± 19[†]
IL-8	?	3684 ± 2910
IL-10	+	3400 ± 3800
TNF-α	+	620 ± 183
G-CSF	?	~358
M-CSF	+	17,120
IFN-γ	?	?
EGF	+	~200,000
TGF-α	+	~2200–7200
TGF-β₂	+	130 ± 108

CSF, Colony-stimulating factor; *EGF*, epidermal growth factor; *G*, granulocyte; *IL*, interleukin; *M*, macrophage; *TGF*, transforming growth factor; *TNF*, tumor necrosis factor.

*The concentrations of these agents were determined by enzyme-linked immunosorbent assay (ELISA) except for IL-1β and EGF by radioimmunoassay. Concentrations are expressed as pg/mL except for M-CSF (U/mL).

[†]From Ngom PT, Collinson AC, Pido-Lopez J, et al. Improved thymic function in exclusively breastfed infants is associated with higher interleukin 7 concentrations in their mothers' breastmilk. *Am J Clin Nutr.* 2004;80:722–728.

From Goldman AS, Chheda S, Garofalo R, Schmalstieg FC. Cytokines in human milk properties and potential effects upon the mammary gland and the neonate. *J Mammary Gland Biol Neoplasia.* 1996;1:251.

they were primarily produced by leukocytes and acted on other leukocytes, and therefore they could be called *interleukins*. Although much of their effect is on lymphocyte activation and differentiation, it is now known that ILs act on and are produced by a variety of cells.[107]

Goldman et al.[107] identified IL-1β, IL-6, IL-8, and IL-10 in breast milk (Table 5.7). Srivastava et al. reported measuring moderate amounts of IL-6, IL-8, and IL-10 in the different stages of breast milk.[199] Very low amounts of IL-1β were detected, especially in comparison with the amount of IL-1 receptor antagonist (RA), which presumably could block the activity of the small amount of IL-1. Hawkes et al. reported on the amount of cytokines in breast milk over the first 12 weeks of lactation.[223] The proposed "proinflammatory" cytokines, IL-1β, IL-6, and TNF-α, were present in only 7 of 36 mothers who donated samples at each point throughout the study. A broad range of concentrations of each of these cytokines was seen during the course of the study. The "antiinflammatory" cytokines, TGF-α1 and TGF-β2, were present in significant amounts in all samples. IL-2 has also been reported in breast milk in 81% of the mothers tested, with

milk (aqueous) levels correlating with plasma IL-2 levels. IL-2 was constitutively produced from 57% of milk cell samples, and IL-2 production was markedly increased by stimulation of the cells with Con A.[224]

IL-6 has been identified in breast milk by other investigators, especially in the first 2 days of life.[225,226] The authors suggest that IL-6 in human milk may augment the newborn's immune functions before the body can begin full production of cytokines. Specifically, this is accomplished by increasing antibody production, especially IgA; enhancing phagocytosis; activating T cells; and increasing α1-antitrypsin production by mononuclear phagocytes. IL-7 is a chemokine known to improve thymic output in animals and appears related to the proliferation and survival of T cells in all stages of development.[227] Ngom et al.[227] described improved thymic function in exclusively breastfed infants associated with higher IL-7 concentrations in the mother's breast milk. The breast milk of Gambian mothers contained variable levels of IL-7, but the geometric mean levels were higher in the first 8 weeks postpartum in mothers whose infants were born in the "harvest season" (January to June) compared with those mothers whose infants were born in the "hungry season." The authors postulate that IL-7 in breast milk enhances T-cell proliferation and survival and overall thymic development in the infant, leading to long-term benefits in protection from infection.

IL-8 is a chemokine capable of attracting and activating neutrophils and attracting CD45RA⁺ T cells. IL-8 is produced by mammary epithelial cells.[222,225] Srivastava et al.[199] also detected messenger ribonucleic acid (mRNA) for IL-8, suggesting that cells in breast milk were capable of producing IL-8. The exact function of IL-8 in breast milk remains to be elucidated. IL-10 is thought to have antiinflammatory effects, including decreasing the production of IFN-γ, IL-12, and other proinflammatory cytokines. It has been reported to enhance IgA, IgG, and IgM synthesis.[222]

IL-18 has been identified in colostrum, early milk, and mature milk, with the highest levels occurring in colostrum and in association with preterm deliveries and complications of pregnancy in the mothers.[228] The levels of IL-18 were correlated with soluble Fas ligand in colostrum. IL-18 was detected by immunohistochemical staining in actively secreting epithelial cells in a lactating breast. IL-18 has been shown to be produced by intestinal epithelial cells and activated macrophages. It leads to the production of other chemokines (GM-CSF, IL-2, TNF-α). It induces the expression of Fas ligand on lymphocytes. The authors suggested that IL-18, present in colostrum, may play a role in stimulating a systemic Th1 response and causing NK cell and macrophage activation in neonates.

The interaction and the direct effect of these ILs in breast milk must be clarified. The amount of T cells bearing markers of recent activation is increased in human milk compared with the results in peripheral blood of adults.[109] Wirt et al.[109] described a marked shift from virginal to antigen-primed (memory) T cells in human milk, which suggests certain functional capacities for these cells. The phenotypic pattern of T cells may result from T-cell–activating substances or selective homing of T cells to the breast. These activated T cell populations are transferred to the infant through breast milk, along with a variety of ILs at a time when infants are capable of only limited production of ILs. A complex interaction of ILs and cells in human milk and at the mucosal level may provide antimicrobial and antiinflammatory benefits to the infant.

Cytokines

Of the many bioactive substances that have been identified in human milk, cytokines are some of the most recently identified and investigated agents. Their existence has been long suspected in attempts to explain certain immunologic and protective effects of breast milk on infants. More than 300 cytokines, chemokines, and growth factors have been described, and more than 12 of these have been identified in human milk.[222–229] Cytokines are small proteins or glycoproteins that, through binding to receptors on immune and nonimmune cells, produce a broad range of effects (many still unidentified) through autocrine, paracrine, and endocrine actions. Cytokines are produced predominantly by immune cells and function in complex associations with other cytokines to stimulate and control the development and normal functioning of cells of the immune system. Chemokines are smaller proteins (8 to 12 kDa) that induce chemotaxis or cell migration of many cell types. Their activity is mediated through binding to a member of the G protein–coupled receptor superfamily. The growth factors include epidermal growth factor, neuronal growth factor, insulin-like growth factor, and vascular endothelial growth factor. Adipokines were discussed in Chapter 4.

The nomenclature and abbreviations used for cytokines are complicated and confusing. Newer systems of classification have been established according to which cells produce them or what their general functions are or based on the relative position of their cysteine residues or their receptor types (CCR, CXCR, and CX3CR).[222] Table 5.8 provides a simplified list with abbreviations. They are also classified into antiinflammatory (TGF-β, IL-7, IL-10) and the inflammatory cytokines present in breast milk (IL-1β, IL-5, IL-6, IL-8, IFN-γ, TNF-α).

Little evidence demonstrates specific in vivo activity of the different cytokines. Based on general information on the function and interaction of the particular cytokines, as well as consideration of as yet unexplained effects of breast milk, proposed functions of the cytokines include initiation of development of host defense; stimulation of host defenses; prevention of autoimmunity and antiinflammatory effects in the upper respiratory and GI tracts; and stimulation of the development of the digestive system, especially the mucosal immune system of the alimentary tract and the proximal respiratory tract. The maternal breast may respond to feedback stimulation or suppression by secreted cytokines, influencing the growth, differentiation, and secretory function of the breast. As shown in other situations, cytokines may enhance receptor expression on cells in the respiratory and GI tracts for

TABLE 5.8	Nomenclature and Abbreviations for Various Cytokines	
Nomenclature	**Abbreviations**
Interferon alpha, beta, gamma	IFN-α, -β, -γ
Granulocyte colony-stimulating factor	G-CSF
Macrophage colony-stimulating factor	M-CSF
Stem cell factor	SCF
Interleukins 1, 2, 4, 6, 8, 10	IL-1, -2, -4, -6, -8, -10
Interleukin 1 beta	IL-1β
Interleukin 1 receptor antagonist	IL-1RA
Soluble interleukin 2 receptor	sIL-2R
Transforming growth factor beta$_2$	TGF-β$_2$
Tumor necrosis factor alpha	TNF-α
Transforming growth factor alpha	TGF-α
Macrophage inflammatory protein	MIP
Regulated on activation, normal T cell expressed and secreted	RANTES
Epidermal growth factor	EGF
Growth-regulated oncogene	GRO
Monocyte chemoattractant protein 1	MCP-1
Leukocyte inhibitory factor	LIF

MHC molecules or immunoglobulins. Various cell types in the mucosal immune system may be activated or attracted to specific sites in the GI tract by the action of cytokines.

Beyond these proposed beneficial effects of cytokines, newer studies are identifying specific immunologic and protective roles for different cytokines in developing infants. For example, extensive work has been done on epidermal growth factor (EGF), and other growth factors (heparin-binding ECF [HB-EGF], granulocyte colony-stimulating factor [G-CSF], erythropoietin [EPO], and necrotizing enterocolitis EPO-like growth factors) have been studied relative to their role in preventing NEC and gut homeostasis.[230] A number of potential roles for EGF in gut homeostasis have been proposed and studied, including intestinal development, proliferation, and adaptive response to damage, repair, and regeneration and diminishing inflammatory responses to various stimuli. TGF-β has been studied for its role in initiating and stimulating IgA production early on in infancy.[231]

The actual measurement of cytokines in breast milk has been complicated by a number of factors, including different assays used (bioassays, enzyme-linked immunosorbent assay [ELISA], radioimmunoassay), binding to proteins, their existence in monomeric or polymeric forms, the presence of antagonists or receptors within breast milk, and their varying presence in colostrum, early milk, or mature milk.[232] Goldman et al.[107] reported on the bioactivity and concentration of cytokines in breast milk from their own work and that of others (see Table 5.7).[222] Srivastava et al.[199] obtained some conflicting results using different assays in colostrum, early milk, and mature milk. They confirmed the presence of macrophage colony-stimulating factor (M-CSF) throughout lactation; TGF-β1 and TGF-β2; IL-1RA, growth-regulated oncogene-α (GRO-α); monocyte chemoattractant protein-1 (MCP-1); regulated upon activation, normal T cell expressed, and secreted (RANTES); and IL-8, but reported insignificant amounts of GM-CSF, stem cell factor, leukemia inhibitory factor (LIF), macrophage inflammatory protein-1α (MIP-1α), IL-2, IL-4, IL-11, IL-12, IL-13, IL-15, soluble IL-2R (sIL-2R), and IFN-α (see Box 5.3 for nomenclature). Srivastava et al.[199] also used reverse transcriptase (RT) polymerase chain reaction (PCR) to measure the production of cytokine mRNA by cells in breast milk. They reported the presence of mRNA for MCP-1, IL-8, TGF-β1, TGF-β2, M-CSF, IL-6, IL-1β, which may be an active mechanism of putting these cytokines in breast milk. Hawkes et al. demonstrated that human milk cells from lactating women at 5 weeks postpartum are capable of active cytokine production in vitro (IL-1β, IL-6, TNF-α), with and without exposure to lipopolysaccharide.[223] Continued cytokine production by human milk cells is another explanation for the variable amounts of cytokines identified in breast milk and is further evidence that the cells are capable of responding to an infectious stimulus.

In their investigations of the possible antiinflammatory effects of breast milk, Buescher and Malinowska examined milk for the presence of soluble receptors and cytokine antagonists.[233] They demonstrated soluble intercellular adhesion molecule 1, soluble vascular cell adhesion molecule 1, and soluble E-selectin in colostrum and at lower levels in mature milk, as well as high levels of soluble TNF-α receptor I (sTNF-αRI), sTNF-αRII, and IL-1RA. In addition, they identified that most TNF-α did not exist "free" in breast milk but was associated with TNF receptors. The in vivo significance of these findings remains to be assessed.

Given the complex interaction and regulation of cytokine production and cytokines' relation to coordinated inflammatory and antiinflammatory responses in tissues, one should assume that the interaction of cytokines in breast milk and the effect of cytokines, cytokine receptors (soluble and expressed on various cell types), and cytokine antagonists on the infant will be equally complex. Presumably the health of the breastfed infant is created by a balance of the inflammatory and antiinflammatory factors maintaining the protection of the infant from exogenous factors.

A different methodology, antibody-based protein arrays, has been applied to identify cytokines in human milk.[234] Kverka et al.[234] analyzed colostrum and milk samples from the first 4 days postpartum, using two different arrays capable of detecting 42 and 79 cytokines. Three cytokines (EGF, IL-8/CXCL8, GRO/CXCL1−3) were detected in all of the tested samples; 19 cytokines were present in more than 50% of the samples. An additional 32 cytokines were identified in human milk for the first time. The concentration of cytokines varied in the different women and varied over time. Continued investigation with this and other assays will be essential to understanding the significance and specific effects of these substances in breast milk.

Nucleotides

Nucleotides, nucleosides, nucleic acids, and related metabolic products are essential to many biologic processes. Although they are not essential nutrients, because they can be synthesized endogenously and recovered from in vivo "salvage" sources, their presence in the diet may carry significant benefits under various conditions (i.e., "conditionally essential").[235−238] In situations of disease, stress, rapid growth, or limited dietary intake, supplementation of the diet with nucleotides may decrease energy expenditure to synthesize or salvage nucleotides, which optimizes the host response to these adverse situations.[236]

Nucleotides exist in relatively large amounts in human milk (15% to 20% of the nonprotein nitrogen), suggesting that they have some nutritional significance, although no clinical syndromes have been associated with nucleotide deficiency to date. Nucleotides are present in the natural milk of different species in varying amounts and composition. The nucleotide content and composition of bovine milk are particularly less and different from human milk. Infant formulas supplemented with nucleotides contain roughly the same amounts of nucleotides as human milk, from 20 to 70 mg/L.[239−241] Unsupplemented formulas contain lesser amounts of nucleotides.

Mammalian cells contain a large variety of nucleotides and related products, which have many metabolic functions, including the following:[235,238,242]

1. *Energy metabolism:* Adenosine triphosphate is a major form of available cellular energy.
2. *Nucleic acid precursors:* The monomeric units for RNA and DNA are present.
3. *Physiologic mediators:* Cyclic adenosine monophosphate (cAMP) and cyclic guanosine monophosphate (cGMP) serve as messengers for cellular processes, adenosine diphosphate is necessary for platelet aggregation, and adenosine has been shown to affect vasodilatation.
4. *Related products function as coenzymes in metabolic pathways:* Nicotinamide-adenine dinucleotide, flavin adenine dinucleotide, and coenzyme A.
5. *Related products function as intermediate carrying molecules in synthetic reactions:* Uridine diphosphate glucose in glycogen synthesis and guanosine diphosphate mannose, guanosine diphosphate-fucose, uridine diphosphate-galactose, and cytidine monophosphate sialic acid in glycoprotein synthesis.
6. *Allosteric effectors:* The intracellular concentrations of nucleotides influence the progression of certain steps of metabolic pathways.
7. *Cellular agonists:* Extracellular nucleotides influence intracellular signal transduction (e.g., cAMP and inositol-calcium pathway).

Nucleotide concentrations in cells and tissues are maintained by de novo synthesis and salvage from intermediary

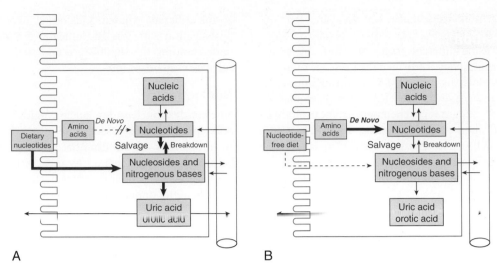

Fig. 5.13 Metabolic regulation of cellular nucleotide pools in presence and absence of nucleotide in diet. (A) Effect of dietary nucleotide activating salvage pathway. (B) De novo nucleotide synthesis is enhanced with nucleotide-free diet. (From Quan R, Barness LA. Do infants need nucleotide supplemented formula for optimal nutrition? *J Pediatr Gastroenterol Nutr.* 1990;11[4]:429.)

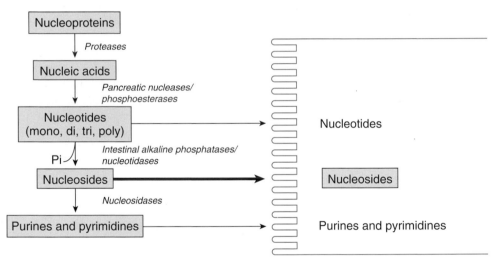

Fig. 5.14 Digestion and absorption of nucleic acids and their relational products. (From Quan R, Barness LA. Do infants need nucleotide-supplemented formula for optimal nutrition? *Pediatr Gastroenterol Nutr.* 1990;11[4]:429.)

metabolism and diet (Fig. 5.13).[243] Nucleosides are the predominant product absorbed in the small intestine. Nucleosides are probably transported by passive diffusion and a carrier-mediated process; purines and pyrimidines are transported by passive diffusion at high concentrations and by a sodium-dependent active mechanism at low concentrations (Fig. 5.14).[243] The digestion and absorption of nucleotides, nucleosides, and pyrimidines and purines also involve polymeric and monomeric nucleotides and other adducts (nucleosides in a biologically active moiety).

In early reports on the nucleotide and nucleoside content of milk, various methods of measurement were used, and the amounts were described as either the monomeric fraction of nucleotides or the total RNA. Leach et al., recognizing the complex nature of digestion and absorption of nucleotides

and related products, attempted to measure the total potentially available nucleosides (TPANs) in human milk.[241] They used solid-phase extraction, high-performance liquid chromatography analysis, and enzymatic hydrolysis of the various fractions. They analyzed breast milk samples at various stages throughout lactation (colostrum, transitional, early, and late mature milk) from 100 European women and 11 American women. They used an aqueous TPAN-fortified solution containing ribonucleosides, 5′-mononucleotides, polymeric RNA, and nucleoside-containing adducts to estimate the accuracy of their process.

The mean ranges of TPAN values were similar for European women from different countries and American women, although broad ranges were seen and the composition of individual nucleotides varied.[241] The mean TPAN

TABLE 5.9 Nucleotide and Total Potentially Available Nucleoside in Pooled Human Milk by Stage of Lactation (μmol/L)*

	Uridine	Cytidine	Guanosine	Adenosine	TPAN
Colostrum					
Site 1	27	84	22	20	153
Site 2	21	33	15	13	82
Site 3	30	82	26	26	164
Site 4	24	84	20	22	150
Mean	26	71	21	21	137
Transitional Milk					
Site 1	23	82	22	19	146
Site 2	33	76	19	17	144
Site 3	37	84	43	42	206
Site 4	36	100	36	38	210
Mean	32	86	30	29	177
Early Mature Milk					
Site 1	30	86	28	28	172
Site 2	50	79	23	21	173
Site 3	44	96	36	37	214
Site 4	67	146	91	97	402
Mean	48	102	45	46	240
Late Mature Milk					
Site 1	36	73	22	25	156
Site 2	58	106	29	27	219
Site 3	49	81	20	24	173
Site 4	45	124	40	49	259
Mean	47	96	28	31	202
Grand mean	38	88	31	32	189
SD	13	24	18	20	70
Range	21–67	33–146	19–92	13–97	84–402
American pool[†]	37	70	30	24	161

TPAN, Total potentially available nucleoside.
*Data from 100 individual samples collected at four sites and combined into 16 pooled samples (5–7 individual samples per site per stage of lactation). *Site 1,* Rouen and Mount Saint Aignau, France; *Site 2,* Mainz, Germany; *Site 3,* Bolzano, Italy; *Site 4,* Treviso, Italy.
[†]Pooled sample of milk collected from 11 American women between 2 and 4 months postpartum.
From Leach JL, Baxter JH, Molitor BE, et al. Total potentially available nucleosides of human milk by stage of lactation. *Am J Clin Nutr.* 1995;61:1224.

value was lowest in colostrum but did not show a consistent upward or downward trend in transitional, early, or late mature milk. The mean ranges of TPAN values were 82 to 164 mmol/L for colostrum, 144 to 210 mmol/L for transitional milk, 172 to 402 mmol/L for early mature milk, and 156 to 259 mmol/L for late mature milk (Table 5.9).[241] Monomeric and polymeric nucleotides were the predominant forms of TPAN in pooled samples. Cytidine, guanosine, and adenosine were found mainly in these fractions, whereas uridine was found primarily as free nucleotide and adduct (Table 5.10).[241] The methods used recovered 90% to 95% of the true TPAN values compared with the TPAN-fortified solution, although the uridine and guanosine content were underestimated. Tressler et al. measured the TPAN in pooled

TABLE 5.10 Percentage of Total Potentially Available Nucleoside in Pooled Human Milk as Adducts, Polymeric Nucleotides, Monomeric Nucleotides, and Nucleosides*

	Uridine	Cytidine	Guanosine	Adenosine	TPAN
Polymeric nucleotides	19 ± 7	57 ± 12	59 ± 21	47 ± 11	48 ± 8
Monomeric nucleotides	36 ± 12	37 ± 13	34 ± 14	35 ± 10	36 ± 10
Nucleosides	18 ± 14	5 ± 5	1 ± 2	5 ± 4	8 ± 6
Adducts[†]	27 ± 12	1 ± 1	7 ± 15	13 ± 9	9 ± 4

TPAN, Total potentially available nucleoside.

*$x \pm$ SD. Based on the mean of entire pool of human milk collected from 100 individuals at four stages of lactation at four sites.

[†]Adducts are of the form nucleoside-phosphate-phosphate-X, where X is a biologically relevant moiety (e.g., uridine diphosphate-galactose or nicotinamide-adenine dinucleotide).

From Leach JL, Baxter JH, Molitor BE, et al. Total potentially available nucleosides of human milk by stage of lactation. *Am J Clin Nutr.* 1995;61:1224.

breast milk samples from Asian women demonstrating average levels in colostrum, transitional milk, and mature milk and found it to be similar to the levels in European and American women.[244] Leach et al. concluded that their process of estimating TPANs, including sequential enzymatic hydrolyses, and measuring the entire nucleotide fraction provides a reasonable estimate of the in vivo process and the nucleotides available to the infant from human milk.[241]

Proposed effects of dietary nucleotides include effects on the immune system, iron absorption, intestinal flora, plasma lipoproteins, and growth of intestinal and hepatic cells. Effects on the immune system related to nucleotide supplementation to the diet have mainly been reported from animal studies. They include increased mortality rate from graft-versus-host disease; improved delayed-type cutaneous hypersensitivity and alloantigen-induced lymphoproliferation; reversal of malnutrition and starvation-induced immunosuppression; increased resistance to challenge with *S. aureus* and *C. albicans;* and enhanced T-cell maturation and function.[245] Spleen cells of mice fed a nucleotide-free diet produce lower levels of IL-2, express lower levels of IL-2 receptors, and have decreased NK cell activity and macrophage activity.[240,242] Presumably, these nucleotide-associated changes are related to T-helper/inducer cells and the initial phases of antigen processing and lymphocyte proliferation. In vitro and in vivo experiments documented that ingested nucleotides increased iron absorption, perhaps affecting xanthine oxidase.[243] Although in vitro studies showed that added nucleotides enhanced the growth of bifidobacteria, conflicting results have been obtained on the influence of dietary nucleotides on the fecal flora of infants receiving breast milk or nucleotide-supplemented formula.[243,246] Clinical studies in infants receiving nucleotide-supplemented formula demonstrated increased high-density lipoprotein cholesterol, lower very-low-density lipoprotein cholesterol, increased long-chain polyunsaturated fatty acids (PUFAs), and changes in red blood cell membrane phospholipid composition.[245] Supplementation studies in animals have shown enhanced GI tract growth and maturation, improved intestinal repair after diarrhea, stimulation of hepatic growth, and

augmented recovery from hepatectomy.[243] A recent review discusses the effects of dietary nucleotides on the immune system and protection against infection reported in studies in the literature.[244] Carver compared infants receiving breast milk to those receiving commercially available infant formula and formula supplemented with nucleotides at a level of 32 mg/L.[240] At 2 and 4 months, NK cell activity and IL-2 production were higher in the breastfed and nucleotide-supplemented groups compared with those receiving formula without nucleotide supplements. Infections occurred infrequently in all groups, but slightly less in the breastfed group. No differences were noted in hematologic profiles and plasma chemistry values, and no toxicity or intolerance was associated with nucleotide supplementation. The sample size was small, marked variability was seen in the IL-2 measurements, and the differences noted at 4 months were less than at 2 months. Therefore the authors concluded that dietary nucleotides may contribute to improved immunity in breastfed infants.

Brunser et al. examined the effect of a nucleotide-supplemented formula on the incidence of diarrhea in 392 infants in Chile, studied through 6 months of age.[247] Although the infants receiving the supplemented formula (20 mg/L) experienced less diarrhea, the difference in the duration of diarrhea was small. The numbers were too small to comment on the causative agents of diarrhea, although no apparent protection against any one agent was seen. The beneficial effect of nucleotides against diarrhea was proposed to be secondary to enhanced immune response to intestinal pathogens, improved intestinal integrity, or a combination of both. In a larger study of 3243 infants younger than 6 months of age, the severity of the diarrhea (duration and number of bowel movements), as well as the incidence of diarrhea, was lower in the nucleotide-supplemented group.[248] Two groups of premature infants fed either nucleotide-supplemented (20 mg/L) or unsupplemented formula were followed, and the concentration of plasma immunoglobulins throughout the first 3 months of life was measured.[236] IgG plasma concentrations were not different in the two groups during the study period. IgM plasma levels were higher in the nucleotide-supplemented group at 20 to 30 days and 3 months of life, and IgA plasma levels were significantly higher at 3 months of age in the supplemented group.

Pickering et al.[245] published a 12-month, randomized controlled study of 311 infants to examine the effect of added nucleotides at levels comparable to those of human milk on infants' immune responses to various vaccine antigens; 103 nonrandomized infants received breast milk for at least 2 months and then either human milk or a standard infant formula. Another 208 infants were randomized to receive either a standard infant formula or one supplemented with nucleotides.[245] The amount and actual nucleotide content added were based on TPANs, as measured by Leach et al., equaling 72 mg/L.[241] Overall growth and nutrition tolerance were similar in each group. The nucleotide group had significantly higher geometric mean titers of *H. influenzae* type b antibody and diphtheria antibody than the control group or the breastfed infants. No significant difference was seen between the nucleotide and control groups for the IgG response to oral poliovirus vaccine or tetanus. Infants who were breastfed for longer than 6 months had significantly higher antibody responses to oral poliovirus vaccine than children breastfed for less than 6 months or either of the two formula-fed groups. No significant differences were found between the different groups with respect to total IgG, IgA, or IgE.[245] Differences were seen in the number of children who experienced at least one episode of diarrhea: the nucleotide group (4 of 27, 15%) versus the control group (13 of 32, 41%, $p < 0.05$), and the breastfed group (6 of 27, 22%). Notably, the breastfed group was heterogeneous relative to the amount of breast milk received and the duration of feeding, whereas the nucleotide group received supplementation for the entire 12 months.[245]

Questions that remain concerning nucleotides and their proposed beneficial effects in an infant's diet include the following:

- What are the proven mechanisms of action of these proposed benefits?
- What form and concentration of nucleotides are necessary to affect these benefits?
- In what amounts do nucleotides survive pasteurization and freezing and thawing as occurs for donor banked human milk?

Debate and research to answer these and other questions concerning nucleotides will continue.

MUCOSAL IMMUNE SYSTEM

A primary function of each of the body's different mucosal surfaces is immunologic. Each distinct mucosal surface has multiple other physiologic functions, including gas exchange (in the lungs), nutrient absorption (in the gut), sensory detection (in the eyes, nose, and mouth), and reproduction (in the uterus and vagina). The thin, permeable nature of these barrier mucosal surfaces, their large surface area, and the constant exposure to microorganisms, foreign proteins, and chemicals predispose the mucosal membranes to damage and infection. During the first year(s) of life, when the infant's immune system is developing and maturing, it is doing so on a systemic and a mucosal basis, as well as involving both innate and adaptive immune mechanisms. That development must include the ability to respond to and protect against invasive pathogens, and at the same time "tolerate" the multitude of commensal organisms that reside at these surfaces. During this early development, breast milk contains numerous bioactive factors that supplement the immune protection at the mucosal level, while limiting inflammation. Additionally, these factors contribute to the immune modulation and growth stimulation of infants' mucosal and systemic immune defenses.[3,54,55,72,249,250] The mucosal immune system involves both innate mechanisms and adaptive immune mechanisms functioning in concert. The development of the mucosal immune system begins in the prenatal period and continues in the postnatal period. The functional mucosal barrier includes the action of enzymes, chemicals, acidity or pH, mucus, immunoglobulins, and indigenous flora. In as early as 8 weeks' gestational age, researchers have identified changes in the intestinal barrier with the development of enterocytes, goblet cells, and enterochromaffin cells, along with evidence of development of tight junctions between the epithelial cells.[251,252] Mucus production, which can block adherence of pathogens to epithelial cells, demonstrates both prenatal and postnatal development, beginning with evidence of expression of the MUC2 gene as early as 12 weeks' gestational age.[253] This is approximately the same time that Paneth cells appear in intestinal crypts. These cells secrete various products, including α-defensin, lysozyme, secretory phospholipase A_2, and TNF-α, which contribute to protection from pathogens, enhance stem cell protection within the epithelial layer, and influence the selection and number of commensal organisms.[254,255] sIgA and sIgM act at the epithelial surface, largely without inflammation, by limiting adherence and transmigration and facilitating phagocytosis of potential pathogens.

Mucosal-Associated Lymphoid Tissue

The well-recognized MALT is present in localized areas beneath the mucosal surfaces: tonsils and adenoids in the nasopharynx, and Peyer's patches and isolated lymphoid follicles in the intestine. Overlying the isolated lymphoid follicles of the gut are specialized epithelial cells called membrane, microfold, or multifenestrated cells (M cells). M cells come in direct contact with microorganisms and antigens because of a lack of a surface glycocalyx covering. These remarkable cells endocytose, phagocytose, and transcytose molecules and antigens, from their luminal surface to their basal surface. Antigen-presenting cells and lymphocytes process the trancytosed molecules, presenting them to submucosal aggregates of lymphocytes. The activated lymphocytes that have responded to the specifically presented antigens migrate by the lymphatics to the thoracic duct and into the blood. These lymphocytes circulate in the blood, until they return to mucosal tissues, predominantly the same ones they originated from, where they then function as effector lymphocytes in the lamina propria. This process of "directed migration" to specific sites occurs as a result of the influence of cytokines and adhesion molecules, such as chemokine CCL28 (mucosal epithelia chemokine), expressed in the colon and salivary glands, and CCL25 (thymus-expressed chemokine), which effects the site-specific migration.[83] The immune response of lymphocytes in the submucosa, and the subsequent directed migration to the same and other mucosal sites, produces a focused response to a selected repertoire of antigens at those sites. The lactating mammary gland is an essential component of MALT. A mother makes a mature effective immune response to microorganisms in her and her infant's environment through antigenic stimulation of MALT in the mother's gut and respiratory mucosa. The maternal immune response produces activated lymphocytes, cytokines, immunoglobulins, and other factors against the specific microorganism. There is a subsequent "directed migration" of these activated lymphocytes, immunoglobulins, cytokines, and bioactive factors to the breast and into the breast milk. These specific factors in the breast milk add to the protective effect of breast milk against specific microorganisms in the mother's and infant's environment. This is a well-recognized example of how breast milk can provide additional immune protection to the infant. It is also one of the reasons to continue breastfeeding when a mother or the infant has a possible infection.

The mucosal immune system undergoes significant postnatal development, in part because of the dramatic exposure of the mucosa to large numbers of microorganisms in early postnatal life. Peyer's patches are rudimentary, and few immunoglobulin-producing intestinal plasma cells are present until several weeks after birth.[86] After several weeks, germinal centers within the lymphoid follicles develop, and the number of IgM- and IgA-producing cells in the intestine increase. Immunoglobulin-producing intestinal plasma cells (primarily IgA-producing cells) in the lamina propria increase in number from 1 to 12 months of age.[256] With normal maturation of the mucosal immune system, large numbers of immunoglobulin-producing cells locate in the intestinal lamina propria. The monomeric IgA produced by these plasma cells is transported through epithelial cells to the mucosal lumen. Attachment of an epithelial glycoprotein, the membrane secretory component to two IgA molecules, leads to the formation of a dimeric molecule. The sIgA molecule is "secreted" at the mucosal surface. IgM, in the form of a pentamer, contains a polypeptide J-chain and is transported by the same mechanism.[257] A portion of the secretory component remains attached to the sIgA and IgM, which protects these molecules against proteolysis and contributes to their stability. Large amounts of sIgA and IgM are produced, in a similar fashion, by the mammary glands and delivered to the infant via breast milk. The sIgA and IgM remain stable in saliva and feces and provide specific protection by blocking adherence and entry.[258] They also facilitate inactivation, neutralization, and agglutination of a wide variety of microorganisms.

Distinct from the action of immunoglobulins, a large number of bioactive factors in breast milk act at the mucosal level to supplement the innate defenses.[259] These include lactoferrin, lysozyme, casein, oligosaccharides, glycoconjugates, and lipids. Mucin-1, lactadherin, and a glycosaminoglycan are antimicrobial components, which are part of the milk-fat globule. FFAs and monoglycerides, digested components of the milk-fat globule, can cause lysis of enveloped viruses, bacteria, fungi, and protozoa. Lauric and linoleic acids, which constitute a large percentage of the FFAs in human milk, are two such acids produced by lipolysis in the stomach.[260] Additional factors contained in breast milk with demonstrated activity at the level of the mucosa include cytokines, hormones, and growth factors. IL-10 and IFN-γ act by influencing the epithelial barrier.[261] Other factors that are considered to contribute to mucosal growth and development are TGF-α, EGF, and hormones (insulin and insulin-like growth factor). Many other factors contained in breast milk have the potential for activity at the level of the mucosa, including nutrients, vitamins, nucleotides, enzymes, and soluble molecules with receptor-like structures (soluble CD14, soluble Toll-like receptor [TLR] 2).[262–264]

TOLL-LIKE RECEPTORS

TLRs and the complex interaction between indigenous bacterial flora and the intestine are important aspects of research into the development of the mucosal immune system. Forchielli and Walker reviewed many of these immune mechanisms acting at the mucosal level.[265] TLRs are transmembrane receptors (pattern recognition receptors) capable of detecting and discriminating among various groups of potential pathogens and initiate different immune responses to them. TLRs "recognize" pathogen-associated molecular patterns, or conserved features in the pattern of molecules expressed by pathogens and commensal organisms.[266] Specific TLRs recognize a particular repertoire of patterns: TLR2 identifies bacterial lipoproteins and peptidoglycan molecules; TLR3 recognizes double-stranded DNA; and TLR4 identifies lipopolysaccharide. Ten TLRs are recognized in humans to date; some have identified legends (pathogen-associated molecular patterns from viruses, bacteria, and protozoa) to which they bind. TLRs are present on some epithelial cells but are predominantly expressed on macrophages and DCs.[267] Intestinal epithelial cells are influenced by gut flora and local immune response to express specific TLRs. The recognition of specific antigen patterns by epithelial cells, macrophages, and DCs within the gut via the different TLRs on these cells leads to the different T-lymphocyte immune responses. It has been postulated that the ongoing immune stimulation elicited by the microbial flora in the gut "programs" the host to predominately express different T-helper cell responses: T_H1-like, T_H2-like, and T_H3-like. This is referred to as *crosstalk* between the indigenous intestinal flora and the body's immune system. The T_H1-like response is described as delayed-type hypersensitivity or cellular immunity. It is characterized by the predominant release of IL-2, IL-12, and IFN-γ. The T_H2-like response is primarily involved with humoral immunity and antibody production (especially IgE) associated with ILs: IL-4, IL-5, and IL-6. The T_H3-like response is related to oral tolerance and antiinflammatory effects in association with the release of IL-10 and TGF-β. A theoretical "ideal" for this system is the ability of the host to respond to various stimuli with balanced protection against the microbial invasion, without excessive inflammation or damage to the host. An imbalanced (or poorly regulated) response of this system could result in an allergic reaction against food proteins (Th2 excess) or an autoimmune inflammatory response against self-antigens (Th1 excess).[265]

Ongoing research continues to explore these molecular mechanisms, and their potential contribution to allergy, autoimmune disease, and normal immune function development within a fetus, infant, and young child. The role of breast milk in the development of the systemic and mucosal immune systems takes on new significance when considering these concepts and mechanisms. This is especially true when examining the role of breast milk in adding to the innate and adaptive immune response at the level of the mucosa. The postulated effects of breast milk on the intestinal microbiota and the inflammatory state within the intestine also must be considered in regard to the issues of allergy, autoimmune disorders, and normal immune function development. Vorbach et al. postulated that the mammary gland evolved from a protective immune gland as part of the innate immune system.[268] They present a list of various protective molecules that are part of both mucosal secretions and human milk. They discuss how specific nutritional factors in human milk have dual functions: nutritional and protective. This highlights the dual role of the breast as a nutritional and immune organ and should stimulate further research into the breast's role in innate immunity, as a component of the mucosal immune system.

MICROBIOTA

Human Microbiota

The human microbiota includes approximately 100 trillion microbial symbionts with the human body as host symbiont or holobiont. Conceptually that means that the human body is made up of highly organized biological units with eukaryotic cells functioning as organs of the human body and the microbiota functioning within numerous microbial habitats on or in the body.[269] The human microbiota contributes in a crucial fashion to each individual human's genetic and metabolic diversity and functioning. It directly and developmentally contributes to the health and disease of the human host.[270,271] These effects are tied to different microbial habitats of the human body but especially to the microbiota of the human gut. Human milk with its own diverse microbiota and unique nutritional composition for human infants helps establish the infant's gut microbiota and directly influences the developing infant's immune system.[8,270,272]

Human Body Microbial Habitats

Many microbial habitats on and in the human body have been examined looking for core or characteristic microbiota specific to the individual site and consistent over time as the

initial step to determining how microbiome changes might affect health and disease. These habitats include the skin, ear, hair, mouth, nose, throat, GI tract (various sections), genitourinary tract, and respiratory tract, among others. These are interconnected sites that can support distinctive microbiotas and at other times exchange common organisms. Costello et al.[269] reported using 16S rRNA gene PCR-amplification and analysis to examine the microbiota of different sites of a set of seven to nine healthy adults. They demonstrated greater diversity of skin microbiota than in the gut or mouth, with high interpersonal variability and minimal temporal variability in the same individuals. They and others have documented identifiable biogeographic patterns in skin microbiota[273] and oral cavity[274,275] in gut microbiota[276] and human breast tissue.[270,277] The contributing factors to this geographic patterning remain to be clearly identified relative to the effects of age, local diet/nutrients, historical exposures, cultural factors, host genetics, immune response of host, etc. It is important to note that closely connected microbial habitats related to breast milk microbiota and the developing infant include mother's gut, skin, breast skin, breast tissue, infant's mouth, infant skin, and GI tract.

Breast Milk Is Not Sterile

Historically, mammalian milk was thought to be sterile unless the breast was infected or there was contamination during collection or storage.[278,279] In part, this was due to methodology using only "culture-dependent" techniques, the approach of looking for only pathogenic bacteria in human milk, and the fact that bacteria were often not cultured from women with clinical mastitis. There was debate about the role of bacteria in clinical mastitis (bacterial vs. nonbacterial mastitis and infectious vs. inflammatory mastitis).[280] Subsequently, culture-independent techniques for identifying bacteria were used with consistent success in identifying bacteria in human milk from both healthy women and women with apparent infection. Several summary articles present the many studies using molecular techniques to identify bacteria in breast milk.[8,272,281] The identification of lactic acid bacteria by both culture-dependent and culture-independent methods in breast milk, the skin of the breast and areola, and the infant's mouth and feces suggests that breast milk could be an important source of lactic acid bacteria for the infant. These organisms were already accepted as normal commensal organisms (*Lactobacillus, Leuconostoc, Pediococcus, Lactococcus, Bifidobacterium*, among others) in the intestines of breastfed infants. Other studies have demonstrated the consistent presence of lactic acid bacteria among others in human milk by both culture and culture-independent methods.[282–284] These data confirm that breast milk is not sterile.

Methods of Microbial Detection
Standard Culturing
The limitations of routine culturing as a method to detect the microbiota of any habitat in humans lead to the development of omics technology. This was especially true in detecting the microbiota of the human gut because many organisms within

the gut are obligate anaerobes or organisms requiring specialized nutrients or environmental conditions to grow; therefore these organisms were "uncultivable" by traditional methods. It was difficult to create the necessary conditions, as exist in the local microbial niches, for numerous very different microbial strains to grow.

Culture-Independent Microbial Detection

Culture-independent or molecular techniques were applied to the environmental detection of bacteria, including 16S rRNA gene profiling and shotgun metagenomics. 16SrRNA gene profiling relies on universal primers for amplification of various regions of the 16S rRNA gene(s) to generate data on potential operational taxonomic units (OTUs) within the specific microbial niche being studied. These data are then analyzed and classified based on known OTUs and a "profile" of the microbiota "identified" for comparison. Shotgun metagenomics is accomplished by DNA fragmentation of the microbes and sequencing of all the segments collected within a given microbial habitat. These are "similarly" analyzed by assembly-based analysis and read-based analysis for comparison to known gene sequences and functions. Metagenomics is the sequencing of the entire microbiome to identify the functional gene repertoire of the local microbiota being assessed. Metatranscriptomics is the sequencing of the entire microbial RNA pool of a given habitat. Metaproteomics is the characterization of the entire protein composition of a specific habitat microbiota at one point in time. Glycomics and glycoproteinomics is the study of the role of glycans in biologic processes and in particular the analysis of HMOs and their effects on human milk and infant gut microbiota. Metabolomics is the analysis of the metabolites produced by the microbiota within a given habitat to characterize the metabolic activities of the local microbiota. Each of these techniques gives a different view of the characteristics of the microbiota within the habitat being studied and a means for comparison, including the functional effects within the local environment (e.g., within human milk, the mother's breast or the infant's gut).[285]

Next-generation sequencing (high-efficiency, automated sequencing platforms) should be able to generate a plethora of data for higher definition analysis. This could include complete genome analysis of an entire microbiome (strain by strain). Single-cell genomics involves isolating a single microbial cell, extraction of the chromosomal DNA, and amplification of its genome. This technique can produce reference genome sequences of otherwise difficult to detect and characterize microorganisms within the microbiota. The use of targeted molecular markers that demonstrate variability for comparison at the interspecies level (e.g., internally transcribed spacer [ITS] in *Bifidobacterium*), could facilitate differentiation between similar bacterial strains in local microbial communities.[286] With all of these techniques there are strengths (process large number of samples, shorter time to results, detects uncultured bacteria, identifies abundant taxa, provides microbial signatures, facilitates clustering and functional analysis) and weaknesses (extraction and primer bias,

bioinformatics biases, viability bias and difficulty detecting minority taxa) of such methods which have to be considered.

Culturomics

Beyond these evolving molecular techniques there has been a return to advanced culturing methods (diversification and optimization of culturing conditions) in combination with matrix-assisted laser desorption ionization-time of flight (MALDI-TOF) mass spectrometry. If ready identification is not possible at this point, the addition of 16S rRNA sequencing and genome sequencing along with taxogenomics facilitates greater description of the identified bacteria. Taxogenomics is a detailed comparison between two or more genomes of the physical location of genes within the genome, analysis of the duplication of genes, functional comparison of sets or groupings of genes, and comparison of genetic distances between genes. This combination of techniques, named "culturomics," has identified many new bacterial species as part of the human microbiota, which has led to expansion of the available databases for use in identification of other microbial species.

Detecting the Human Virome

In addition to bacteria in the human microbiome, viruses are likely to be present in even greater numbers than bacteria in various human body microbial habitats given the estimated number that 10^{31} viral particles exist on earth. Methods for virus purification have been described for various human microbial habitats and the viral-like particle (VLP) sequences are identified by deep sequencing and comparison to existing open reading frame (ORF) databases.[287] These techniques facilitate the identification of new viral "pathogens," document viral evolution, characterize the integration of viral DNA into bacteria or human cells, and demonstrate the existence of complex uncultured communities of VLPs. As characterized to date the human virome is made up of readily identifiable persistent or latent human host infections (EBV, CMV, varicella-zoster virus, HSV 1, 2, HIV, hepatitis C virus, and papillomaviruses), transient infections with animal cell viruses, endogenous retroviruses, and bacteriophages infecting bacteria and archea.[288] The overwhelming majority of VLPs identified to date are phages. Similar to the bacterial composition of the microbiome, individuals harbor unique viromes that are relatively consistent over time. There is more interpersonal diversity and identifiable variables (diet, nutritional status, age, medications, immune status, and environment/geography) contributing to the diversity of the virome and to a tolerated homeostasis or dysbiosis under other circumstances. There is evidence of rapid change and variability/diversity in the human virome as a result of accumulation of base substitutions, hypervariable loci, and variation associated with diversity generating retroelements (DGRs) and clustered regularly interspaced short palindromic repeats (CRISPRs). Only a very small percentage of the identifiable VLPs in the human virome have been characterized because of limitations in methodology and database characterization of existing viruses.[288] Phages that make up much of the human virome have a tremendous potential for influencing human homeostasis (health) or dysbiosis (disease) because of their ability to infect bacteria or host cells and either kill them (lytic infection), integrate into the genome (lysogeny), or produce DNA modification by epigenetic mechanisms.

There is also ongoing study of the presence of a mycobiota/mycobiome, or all of the fungi in humans, and investigation of parasites within human milk.[289,290] Ongoing advances in the study of the human microbiota, metagenome, and virome will depend on standardization of methodologies, advances in informatics (genomic and epigenomic databases), and analysis of metagenomic data with host homeostasis and disease causality.

Microbial Niches

The human body (holobiont) is made up of numerous interconnected microbial habitats. The human milk microbiome directly connects the mother (breast microbiome) and the infant (intestinal microbiome). There is a notable overlap of microbiota from the various human microbial niches and the microbiota of the human breast and human milk.[272] The microbiota of human milk is being examined as important bioactive components in infant health with potential roles in infant gut health, and early influence on mucosal immunity and the infant's immune system. The microbiota of human breast tissue is being examined in its role in breast homeostasis and health, lactation homeostasis versus dysbiosis (mastitis), and even possible long-term effects relative to the occurrence of breast cancer.

Human Milk Microbiota

Since the identification of bacteria in the breast milk of healthy women there have been hundreds of studies on the microbiota of human milk. Heikkilä and Saris estimated from culture-detectable organisms in human milk that an infant would ingest $1 \times 10^4 - 1 \times 10^6$ bacteria per the approximately 800 mL of breast milk consumed daily.[291] Boix-Amorós et al. estimated a bacterial load, using molecular techniques to assess human milk microbiota, that equaled $10^7 - 10^8$ bacterial cells daily in 800 mL/day of breast milk ingested.[292]

The origin of bacteria in human milk has been debated whenever bacteria were identified in human milk. Juan M. Rodriguez and his collaborators have proposed several likely sources of bacteria in human milk: breast skin microbiota, infant oral microbiota, and enteromammary pathway from the maternal gut through lymph and blood to the mammary gland.[8,293]

Retrograde flow of bacteria from maternal skin and the infant's mouth into the ducts and alveoli of the mammary gland is possible based on infrared photography of milk ejection.[294] Rodríguez et al. provide ample data and discussion to support the possibility of an enteromammary pathway presenting translocated bacteria from the mother's intestine to her lactating breasts and into the human milk microbiota.[293] Jost et al. used both culture and DNA techniques to demonstrate the presence of "shared" bacteria in maternal feces, breast milk, and the infant's feces.[295]

Core Human Milk Microbiota

Data from Rodríguez et al. and Togo et al. outline the significant overlap of bacterial species in the human milk microbiota and other human microbiotas, especially the human gut microbiota.[272,293] The human milk microbiota is unique because there are approximately 300 bacterial species identified only in human breast and milk microbiota (of a total of over 800 species identified in human milk) and not in published information on other human microbial niches.[272] The complexity of the human milk microbiota is tremendous, and despite large interindividual and interpopulation variations, most research groups have tried to identify a core phyla (Proteobacteria, Firmicutes, Actinobacteria, Bacteroidetes) and genera of bacteria (Table 5.11). Hunt et al. defined a core of nine microbial genera, including *Staphylococcus, Streptococcus, Serratia, Pseudomonas, Corynebacterium, Ralstonia, Proprionibacterium, Sphingomonas,* and *Bradyrhizobiaceae*.[296] Boix-Amorós et al. described a slightly different core of seven genera: *Staphylococcus, Streptococcus, Acinetobacter, Pseudomonas, Corynebacterium, Proprionibacterium, Finegoldia,* and *Peptoniphilus*.[292] Fernández et al. summarized main species and genera identified in studies using bacterial isolation and compared those with ones identified by DNA detection.[8] Two systematic reviews provide summaries of analyses of over 200 articles in the literature on the microbiota of the human breast and human breast milk.[272,284] Togo et al., in their analysis of 142 articles on human milk microbiota, identified 17 phyla (the same 4 phyla were the most common—Proteobacteria, Firmicutes, Actinobacteria, Bacteroidetes) and listed these species as the most frequent (*Staphylococcus epidermidis, S. aureus, Streptococcus agalactiae, Cutibacterium acnes, Enterococcus faecalis, Bifidobacterium breve, E. coli, Streptococcus*

TABLE 5.11 Bacteria Commonly Found in Breast Milk

Phyla	Genera
Firmicutes	***Staphylococcus,*** * ***Streptococcus, Leuconostoc, Lactococcus,*** *Enterococcus, Clostridium, Veillonella, Gemella, Bifidobacterium, Lactobacillus*
Actinobacteria	***Corynebacterium,*** *Propionibacterium, Actinomyces*
Proteobacteria	***Pseudomonas, Serratia, Sphingomonas, Ralstonia,*** *Escherichia, Enterobacter, Acinetobacter, Bradyrhizobium*
Bacteroidetes	*Prevotella*

*Bolded bacteria are most prevalent populations detected.
Derived from Cabrera-Rubio R, Collado MC, Laitinen K, et al. The human milk microbiome changes over lactation and is shaped by maternal weight and mode of delivery. *Am J Clin Nutr.* 2012;96 (3):544–551; Fernández L, Langa S, Martín V, et al. The human milk microbiota: origin and potential roles in health and disease. *Pharmacol Res.* 2013;69(1):1–10; Hunt KM, Foster JA, Forney LJ, et al. Characterization of the diversity and temporal stability of bacterial communities in human milk. *PLoS One.* 2011;6(6):e21313.

sanguinis, Lactobacillus gasseri, Salmonela enterica).[272] Lactic acid bacteria (*Lactobacillus, Bifidobacterium,* among others), associated with milk digestion, have been found in approximately 25% of studies on the human milk microbiota, but not all. Nevertheless, four *Lactobacillus* species are common in various human anatomic niches (milk, mouth, lung, intestine, urinary tract, and vagina) (*Lactobacillus casei, L. fermentum, L. gasseri, L. rhamnosus).*[272] *Bifidobacterium (B. breve, B. longum, B. dentium)* is commonly associated with breastfeeding and with the gut microbiota of breastfed infants compared with formula-fed ones.[297] With the many differences across different studies, consideration should go into standardizing all the methodology for studying the microbiota and "omics" of human milk. Rather than a core microbiota and the importance of individual genera or species within that for the health of the mother or infant perhaps, what is crucial is a core microbiome or metagenome that maintains a homeostasis within the host (health) compared with dysbiosis (illness).[271]

Factors Contributing to the Diversity of Human Milk Microbiota

A variety of factors have been identified (beyond differences in methodology of studies) that influence the breast milk microbiota. These are summarized by Ojo-Okunola et al.,[271] including mode of delivery (cesarean section, vaginal delivery), gestational age, maternal weight (overweight, obese), antibiotic use or chemotherapy, maternal health (allergy, celiac disease, HIV), geographic location, diet and nutrition, and lactation stage (colostrum, transitional milk, mature milk). Standardization of microbiota detection and analysis and data collection regarding these many factors will be necessary to understand the importance of these variables on the human host microbiota.[271]

Human Milk Microbiota in the Setting of Mastitis

The diagnosis of mastitis is usually a clinical diagnosis.[298] There are limited situations in which culture of breast milk is necessary for diagnosis or management of mastitis. Culturing breast milk, a nonsterile fluid, in the situation of clinical mastitis has not yielded a distinct or "diagnostic" microbiome. *S. aureus, S. epidermidis, Streptococcus* (viridans group *Streptococcus* [VGS]) and gram-negative organisms are considered the dominant culture-identified pathogens in human mastitis.[299,300] Culture-independent detection methods have been applied to human milk in the setting of clinical mastitis. A couple of studies using 16S rRNA gene sequencing only on samples from women with apparent mastitis and no control group suggested that microbial diversity changed to a predominance of pathogenic organisms (*Staphylococcus, Streptococcus, Corynebacterium,* and some gram-negative organisms) and less lactic acid.[301] Mediano et al. also examined microbial diversity in milk of women with mastitis using similar 16S rRNA sequencing without an appropriate control group (such as lactating women without mastitis) and included samples from women with local breast symptoms potentially

consistent with engorgement or a blocked duct as compared with a clear clinical diagnosis of mastitis.[299,300,302] They reported a "high" diversity of bacterial species with the predominant species (*S. epidermidis, S. aureus,* viridans group *Streptococcus,* and *Corynebacterium*) similar to historical reports of culture-tested breast milk with mastitis. Two separate research groups compared healthy lactating women as controls with women with clinical mastitis using culture-independent methods.[303,304] Patel et al. used 16S rRNA gene sequencing (18 healthy controls, 16 women with subacute mastitis, and 16 women with acute mastitis), and Jiménez et al. used pyrosequencing (10 healthy women and 5 with subacute and 5 with acute lactational mastitis).[303,304] Patel et al.[304] reported that women with mastitis have lower microbial diversity with increased amounts of opportunistic pathogens and fewer obligate anaerobes (potentially commensal organisms) and by predicted functional metagenomic analysis that gene pathways of bacterial proliferation and colonization would be increased. Specific genera were augmented in the mastitis samples, including *Aeromonas, Staphylococcus, Ralstonia, Klebsiella, Serratia, Enterococcus,* and *Pseudomonas.* Jiménez et al. reported that *S. aureus* was the predominant organism identified in samples of women with acute mastitis and *S. epidermidis* dominated samples from women with subacute mastitis.[303] Fungal, protozoa, and viral DNA were detected in a majority of milk samples, but *Archaea* detection was absent from samples from women with mastitis. These and other authors refer to mastitis as dysbiosis or altered milk microbiome with a dysregulation of host-microbiota interactions leading to local inflammation and clinical disease.[8,271,272,305] The specifics of the imbalance will require further characterization at the cellular, chemical, and immunologic level by additional culturomics and culture-independent analysis, along with metagenomics, metatranscriptomics, metabolomics, etc.

Microbiota of Human Breast Tissue

The ongoing debate about commensal or pathogenic bacteria in human milk or in association with occurrences of mastitis reflects the identification of bacteria common to the alveoli and lactiferous ducts. The skin of the nipple and breast harbor a slightly different microbiota from other skin microflora and from the microbiota of human milk. The question of whether there is a distinct microbiota of breast tissue is undergoing investigation. Many of the studies included a comparison of normal breast tissue with breast tissue from surgeries performed to assess breast tumors (benign or malignant).

Core Breast Tissue Microbiota

Urbaniak et al. examined breast tissue samples from women in Canada (n = 43) and Ireland (n = 38) using culture and culture-independent techniques.[277] Tissue was from tumor tissue (benign or malignant), tissue approximately 5 cm from the tumor, and tissue from women undergoing breast reduction without a history of breast cancer. 16S rRNA and PCR amplification identified two main phyla (Proteobacteria and Firmicutes) from both groups (Canadian and Irish) and the common organisms detected from Canadian samples were *Bacillus* (11.4%), *Acinetobacter* (10%), Enterobacteriacae (unclassified), *Staphylococcus, Propionibacter,* Comamonadaceae, Gammaproteobacteria, and *Prevotella*; and in the samples from Ireland Enterobacteriaceae (unclassified) (30.8%), *Staphylococcus* (12.7%), *Listeria welshimeri* (12.1%), *Propionibacterium* (10%), and *Pseudomonas.* Bacteria were cultivable from each of the Canadian samples (Irish samples were not tested by culture), with 75 to 2000 colony-forming units (CFUs) per gram of tissue and eight strains of bacteria identified (*Bacillus* species, *Micrococcus luteus, Propionibacterium granulosum, Propionibacterium acnes, Staphylococcus* species, *Staphylococcus agalactiae* as well as *Lactobacillus* and *Bifidobacterium* in smaller numbers). There was some overlap between breast tissue and organisms commonly identified at other body sites (oral, skin, respiratory, GI tract, and vagina), but the microbiota of breast tissue was distinct, and the women were without evidence of infection. Xuan et al. tested paired samples of breast tissue (tumor tissue and adjacent "normal" tissue) from 20 US women with estrogen receptor–positive breast cancer using 16S pyrosequencing and quantitative PCR.[306] Five main phyla were identified: Proteobacteria, Firmicutes, Actinobacter, Bacteroidetes, and Verrucomicrobia, which accounted for 96.6% on average of all the sequences identified in the samples. The number of OTUs was not different in normal versus tumor tissue; however, eight OTUs were more abundant in paired normal tissue samples, and 3 OTUs were more abundant in tumor tissue samples. *Sphingomonas yanoikuyae* was the common species in 95% of normal tissue samples and *Methylobacterium radiotolerans* was the most prevalent species in the tumor tissue samples. Although *M. radiotolerans* was present in 100% of tumor samples, the absolute number of these organisms in normal and tumor tissue did not vary significantly. The authors proposed that *S. yanoiyukae* and *M. radiotolerans* might exist in similar microbial niches, whereas in tumor tissue the abundance of *S. yanoikuyae* drops off.[306] They also noted that there were 10-fold greater bacteria in tumor tissue by comparison with normal tissue while in tumor tissue the bacterial load dropped with the increasing cancer stage. In targeted gene array analysis for human antibacterial response gene activity, one-third of the antibacterial genes were downregulated in tumor tissue and none of the genes were upregulated in tumor tissue. Xuan et al. reasoned from these data that breast tissue microbiota may maintain healthy breast tissue by activation of local host inflammatory responses.[306] If a disruption occurs in the microbiota balance (dysbiosis) with decreased numbers of bacteria overall and a relative increase in *S. yanoiyukae*, less effective host inflammatory response could create a "permissive environment for breast tumorigenesis." Hieken et al. examined 33 surgical breast samples (15 from patients with invasive cancer and 13 with benign nonatypia) compared with buccal and skin swabs.[307] The microbiota of breast tissue included four main phyla (similar to the four in human milk): Firmicutes, Actinobacteria, Bacteroidetes, and Proteobacteria. The breast microbiota was distinct from that identified in skin sampling. The

makeup of the microbiota was similar for cancer versus benign tissue with evident differences occurring in the rare or less abundant lineages. Cancerous breast tissue had increased abundance of uncommon lineages: *Fusobacterium, Atopobium, Hydrogenophaga, Gluconacetobacter,* and *Lactobaccillus.* Functional Kyoto Encyclopedia of Genes and Genomes (KEGG) metabolic pathway analysis by Phylogenetic Investigation of Communities by Reconstruction of Unobserved States (PICRUSt) 16S rRNA marker gene sequences showed increased cysteine and methionine metabolism and increased glycosyltransferases and fatty acid biosynthesis in benign breast tissue while the microbiota of cancer tissue demonstrated diminished inositol phosphate metabolism.[308] Urbaniak et al.[277] analyzed surgical breast tissue from 71 Canadian women (13 benign tumors, 45 cancerous tumors, and 23 undergoing breast surgery not for tumors) using 16S rRNA amplicon sequencing.[309] Results demonstrated 61 OTUs; 28 genera; 2 predominate phyla, Proteobacteria and Firmicutes; and 4 less common phyla, Actinobacteria, Bacteroidetes, Deinococcus-Thermus, and Verrucomicrobia. The bacterial profiles were distinctly different for the healthy compared with the cancerous tissue samples. Genera in greatest abundance in the cancerous samples included *Bacillus, Staphylococcus,* Enterobacteria- ceae (unclassified), Comamonadaceae (unclassified), and Bacteroidetes. In healthy patients the most abundant genera included *Prevotella, Lactococcus, Corynebacterium, Strepto- coccus,* and *Micrococcus.* Age and menopause did not appear to be a factor in these differences. *Lactococcus* and *Streptococcus* are lactic acid bacteria that may play an anticarcinogenic role through activation of NK cells and production of antioxidant metabolites. Three isolates from the Enterobacteriaceae group and one *S. epidermidis* isolate from the breast cancer patients demonstrated the ability to cause DNA double-stranded breaks. Such double-stranded breaks are known to lead to extremely error-prone repair, which can lead to genomic instability and cancer. The authors proposed that these differences in microbiota between healthy and cancerous breast tissue could play a role in the development of breast cancer.[277]

Chan et al. characterized the microbiome of nipple aspirate fluid of breast cancer (ductal carcinoma) survivors (n = 25) compared with that of healthy control women (n = 23) along with paired breast skin samples of microbiota using 16S rRNA gene amplicon sequencing.[310] The nipple skin samples did not demonstrate a significantly different microbiota based on breast cancer history with dominant phlya, including Proteobacteria (average 36.5%), Firmicutes (average 33.4%), and Bacteroidetes (average 19.5%). The most abundant OTUs included *Alistipes* (reclassified as *Bacteroides putredinis*), Sphinogomonadaceae family, *Rhizobium,* and unclassified family of Acidobacteria. The microbiota of nipple aspirate fluid demonstrated different clustering and two distinct OTUs in different abundance. The abundant phyla included Firmicutes (averaging 42.1%), Proteobacteria (averaging 32.9%), and Bacteroidetes (averaging 14.5%). The genus *Alistipes* was identified in nipple aspirate fluid only from breast cancer survivors, whereas an unclassified genus from the *Sphingomonadaceae* family was relatively more abundant in the nipple aspirate fluid of healthy control breast tissue than in cancer survivors. Analysis of gene sequences related to KEGG metabolic pathway activity showed an abundance of activity of the "flavone and flavonol biosynthesis" pathway in nipple aspirate fluid from breast cancer tissue compared with healthy controls.

Thompson et al. used The Cancer Genome Atlas breast cancer data to analyze breast tissue microbiota and host gene expression.[311] From 668 breast tumor tissues and 72 noncancerous adjacent tissues; *Proteobacteria* were more abundant in tumor tissues and *Actinobacteria* more abundant in noncancerous tissue. Specific bacteria were identified that could play a role in tumorigenesis. Analysis of identified *Listeria fleischmannii* species demonstrated expression of gene profiles active in epithelial to mesenchymal transitions. *H. influenzae* was associated with the proliferative pathways of G2M checkpoint, E2F transcription factors, and mitotic spindle assembly consistent with tumor growth.

Banerjee et al. used whole genome and transcriptome amplification and a multipathogen microarray (PathoChip) to detect bacterial, fungal, viral, and parasitic signatures in samples of the four major types of breast cancer compared with normal controls.[312] They used 50 endocrine receptor (estrogen or progesterone) positive samples (BRER), 34 human epidermal growth factor receptor 2 (HER2) positive samples (BRHR), 24 triple-positive (estrogen, progesterone, and HER2 positive) samples (BRTP), 40 triple-negative (absence of estrogen, progesterone, and HER2 receptors) samples (BRTN), and 20 breast tissue samples from healthy control women who had breast surgeries at the University of Pennsylvania. For each of the breast cancer types, unique viral, bacterial, fungal, and parasitic signatures were identified. Unique signatures were identified more commonly in the breast cancer tissues compared with control breast tissue. Hierarchical cluster analysis demonstrated characteristic patterns associated with the triple-positive and the triple-negative breast tissue sample microbial signatures more commonly than in controls. ER-positive and HER2-positive samples manifested microbial signatures similar to the other cancer type. Seventeen viral families exhibited higher hybridization signals in the samples for the cancer types compared with controls. Three known oncogenic viruses (Polyomaviridae, Hepadnaviridae, Parapoxviridae) in unique signature patterns were detected with high signal intensity in different cancer types. Distinct bacterial signatures were identified for the different cancer types, and the hybridization signal intensity conveyed a measure of the complexity and diversity of the bacterial microbiota of breast cancer. The bacterial genera (*Brevundimonas, Mobiluncus, Actinomyces*) were identified with high hybridization signal and prevalence in all four cancer types. Unique fungal signatures, made up of 21 fungal genera in the four types of breast cancer, also showed tremendous diversity in the individual patterns detected. Yeasts (*Candida, Geotrichum, Trichosporon*), fungi (*Mucormycosis, Aspergillosis, Fonsecaea*), and dermatophytes (*Epidermophyton, Trichophyton*) infections associated with cancer were detected

among the fungal signatures. Similarly, 29 different genera of parasites were identified in the four cancer types, compared with control samples, but no single genus of parasite was found in all four cancer types. Some parasite signatures were identified in only one type of breast cancer. Specific parasites detected in the breast cancer tissue included *Trichinella, Schistosoma, Ascaris, Trichuris, Strongyloides, Leishmania,* and *Plasmodium*. The complexity of the microbial signatures (viral, bacterial, fungal, and parasitic) in different breast cancer types is tremendous, but there were some distinct microbial signatures identified in the different cancer types analyzed by Banerjee et al.[312] Additional investigation into the clinical features of different cancers, the metagenomic character of the associated microbial signature, and potential mechanisms of oncogenesis related to specific microbes will be crucial to fully understanding the role of microbiota in breast cancer.

Potential Effects of Human Breast Microbiota on the Mother's Health

The potential effects of human milk microbiota in the infant's gut have been and continue to be investigated. The effects of breast microbiota locally in the mammary gland have undergone limited evaluation. There is evidence for variation in human breast microbiota from healthy breast tissue compared with breasts affected by inflammation (mastitis, abscess) or cancer. The mechanisms of action for the mammary gland microbiota effects on local breast environment and long-term health of the breast and health of women overall require elucidation.

Sakwinska and Bosco review possible symbiotic interactions in the mammary gland between the bacteria and host cells.[305] They suggest that bacteria may interact with human milk stem cells through pattern recognition receptors (TLR4 and nucleotide-binding oligomerization domain-containing protein 2 [NOD2]) leading to cell death or cell protection. They describe possible beneficial crosstalk between bacteria and the epithelial cells of the mammary ducts and alveoli contributing to mucosal barrier immune processes of stratification (by mucins, adenosine monophosphate [AMP], and secretory IgA) and compartmentalization (via local interference with and killing of bacteria). Disturbance in the host-bacterial interactions can lead to dysbiosis with altered growth of bacterial pathogens, release of proinflammatory mediators (cytokines, chemokines, etc.), and chemoattraction of activated immune cells into the breast and human milk. Local breast dysbiosis (imbalance of microbiota and/or change in milieu) could also lead to an activation of colonizing organisms (e.g., *Staphylococcus* and *Streptococcus*) to active pathogens participating in acute or chronic local damage and inflammation. Conversely, the use of probiotic bacterial strains (*Lactobacillus fermentum* or *L. salivarius*) similar to ones in human milk microbiota to treat or prevent lactational mastitis has had some success.[313,314] In either situation the exact mechanisms of bacterial and mammary host cell interactions in eubiosis or dysbiosis need to be better characterized.

Breast Tissue Microbiota and Breast Cancer

Beyond multiple individual studies describing the microbiota of breast and breast cancer tissue (referred to earlier), several recent reviews have tried to summarize what we understand about the relationship between the microbiota of the breast and breast cancer.[312,315–317] In terms of general mechanisms by which the human microbiome might lead to cancer development, these have only been presumed and not proven. Given the diversity of microbiota in breast tissue samples, normal tissue versus different forms of breast cancer, the presence of individual bacterial strains is likely to be less important compared with the metagenomic, metatranscriptomic, and metabolomic environment generated by the combined local microbiota. Several general mechanisms are likely to play a role in the carcinogenic potential of the human microbiome: chronic inflammation, altered immune response, altered barrier integrity (between host and microbiota), genomic stability, DNA damage, epigenetic effects, and metabolic function. The local microbiota can change the balance of host cell proliferation and death, stimulate poorly regulated innate and adaptive immune responses, and affect the balance of reactive oxygen species. Certain groups of organisms (*E. coli* and *S. epidermidis*) can produce genotoxins (colibactin), which could lead to genomic instability. Changes in the local metabolism as a result of metabolomic changes in estrogen and progesterone metabolism, cysteine and methionine metabolism, glucosyltransferases, fatty acid biosynthesis, and butyrate metabolism could also lead to additional oncogenic effects. Large-scale studies correlating clinical features of breast cancer with metagenomic, metatranscriptomic, and metabolomic analysis in groups of patients with cancer compared with healthy controls will be crucial to clarifying the role that the breast tissue microbiome has in breast cancer oncogenesis.

Microbiota of Infant Gastrointestinal Tract

Of the various microbial niches encompassed by the human body, the gut microbiota contains the highest density of microbial cells. The mother's composite microbiota has a direct influence on their infant's microbiota, along with a number of environmental factors. Food is presumed to be the most important influence on the intestinal microbiota and particularly the different effect of breast milk versus cow's milk or formula. There is increasing data that the early infant gut microbiota has long-term effects on later child and adult health or disease. Dysbiosis, a disruption of the "healthy" or "established" gut microbiota, leads to interference with normal growth, development, and health in the infant. There is now a focus on how to maintain the balance of the intestinal microbiota and interventions to affect its composition and metabolic functioning through the use of probiotics and/or prebiotics. The most important caution regarding the data on the infant's intestinal microbiota relative to the potential long-term effects on the infant's health is the need to consider the methodologies, contributing variables, timing of microbiota development and potential confounders when comparing data or drawing conclusions about its effects.

Factors Affecting the Infant Gut Microbiota

There is some evidence that prenatal microbial sources, bacteria from the uterus, placenta, umbilical cord, and amniotic fluid initiate the colonization of the fetus. There are, however, concerns regarding the data because the reported bacterial counts are low and the studies lack control data and adequate rigor to guard against possible contamination of samples.[270] There is good data regarding perinatal (mode of delivery, gestational age) and postnatal (infant feeding mode, maternal diet, family lifestyle variables, geographic location, host genetics, and weaning vs. introduction of complementary foods) factors affecting the development of the infant's intestinal microbiota. Early neonatal gut colonization can occur by vagina-associated microorganisms (*Lactobacillus, Prevotella*).[318] Infants born by cesarean section (C-section) are more likely to contact microorganisms from maternal skin and the hospital environment. Proteobacteria and Firmicutes were reported to predominate in neonate's feces in the first days after C-section, with Actinobacteria being identified on days 7 to 15 after delivery. Infants delivered by C-section were more likely to be colonized with *Clostridium sensu stricto* and *C. difficile*, have a more heterogenous microbiota make-up, and be less often colonized with *Bifidobacterium* and *Bacteroides* compared with vaginally born infants.[319] There is conflicting evidence for how long such microbial differences persist after delivery: years versus the immediate neonatal period.[320] Gestational age affects gut colonization as preterm infants demonstrate delay in colonization with *Bifidobacterium* and *Bacteroides* and tend to have higher levels of Enterobacteriaceae, *Enterococcus*, and various pathogenic bacteria (*Staphylococcus, Enterococcus, Clostridium*) compared with full-term infants. Separate from specifically the gestational age, it is possible that the medical interventions (long hospitalizations with exposures to ventilators and other equipment, artificial feedings or parenteral nutrition, antibiotics and other medications, etc.) to care for premature infants are more important factors influencing the gut microbiome. There is a large amount of interindividual variability observed in premature infants. The make-up of the preterm's intestinal microbiota has been associated with an increased risk for NEC or sepsis.[321–324] Infant feeding is another major driver of early microbial gut colonization.[325] The combination of nutrients, probiotics, prebiotics (especially HMOs), and immune active components (sIgA, lactoferrin, etc.) promote intestinal microbiota, which favors bifidobacteria and lactobacilli and fewer potential pathogens. The microbiota of breastfed infants is less diverse than that of formula-fed infants. The higher level of diversity in intestinal microbiota of formula-fed infants also leads to earlier achievement of an adult-like microbiota composition.[319] The predominant microorganisms in formula-fed infants tend to include staphylococci, bacteroides, clostridia, enterococci, and enterobacteria.[326] Additionally, weaning affects the gut microbiota, in the transition from exclusive milk feeding to dependency on complementary foods. There is increasing diversity and predominance of different organisms as the gut microbiota moves from the infant to the toddler stage and later to adult-like microbiota from 1 to 4 years of age.[270] Other variables considered to affect the infant's gut microbiota include mother's diet and mother's weight gain or obesity during pregnancy and/or postpartum, although data on this are conflicting. Family lifestyle and geographic location also appear to play a role in the development of the infant's gut intestinal flora. There are a variety of studies linking ethnicity, host genetics, and diet as potential geographic-related influences on the gut microbiome.[270] Clearly, continued work is needed in assessing the contribution of these many potential factors influencing the infant's gut microbiota. The significant interindividual variability of the gut microbiota will likely relate to the relative influence of these contributing factors.

Core Infant Gastrointestinal Tract Microbiota

There is a core microbiota for breast milk described in the literature (see Table 5.11). It is more difficult to describe a core gut microbiota of the "normal" or "healthy" infant because the gut microbiota demonstrates high interindividual variability, and a dynamic evolution over time in response to numerous influences. There is also significant variability in the results reported from different studies on infant intestinal microbiota as it evolves over the infant's life—weeks, to months, to years. Proteobacteria (mainly Enterobacteriaceae) and Actinobacteria dominate neonatal intestinal microbiota during early weeks, giving way to bifidobacteria with a decline in Enterobacteriaceae. Bifidobacterium is clearly the dominant colonizer of the breastfed infant's intestine. Later transition includes a decrease in Proteobacteria and Actinobacteria and increase in Firmicutes and Bacteroides as the microbiota transitions to the greater diversity and relative stability of the adult gut microbiota.[327]

Vallès et al. described a "core infant gut microbiota" in six main functional groups: (1) Enterobacteriales, (2) Bacteroidales and Verrucomicrobiales, (3) Selenomonadales and Clostridiales genera Pseudoflavonifractor and Subdoligranulum and deltaproteobacteria Desulfovibrio, (4) all Pasteurellales, (5) most of the Clostridiales, and (6) Clostridiales genera Anaerostipes and Faecalibacterium and the Lactobacillales and all Actinobacteria.[328] It is notable the dominant genera (Bifidobacterium, Veillonella, Streptococcus, Citrobacter, Escherichia, Bacteroides, Clostridium) of the infant gut microbiota are also present in large quantities in the adult gut microbiota. Not surprisingly, there are additional genera common to both adult and infant gut microbiota in significantly different amounts. Bifidobacterium is one of the dominant organisms of the infant gut microbiota, identified by both culture-dependent and culture-independent methods. Of the 59 different taxa of the genus Bifidobacterium, there are 5 that are readily isolated from human fecal samples: B. bifidum PRL2010, Bifidobacterium catenulatum, Bifidobacterium adolescentis 22L, B. breve 12L, and Bifidobacterium longum subspecie infantis ATCC15697. B. longum subspecie infantis, specifically cultured from infant feces, demonstrates genes (fucosidase, sialidase, β-hexosaminidase, and β-galactosidase) encoding for enzymes involved in the degradation of important HMOs and mucins that facilitate its thriving in the GI

tract. Cross-feeding of different bacteria within the microbiota by competition for or cooperative sharing of nutrients leads to the establishment of a "fit," thriving community of microorganisms.[329] Turroni et al.[329] review some of these cross-feeding activities between Bifidobacterium and other members of the community. Clostridium genera are members of the infant gut microbiota, including C. perfringens and C. difficile, known pathogenic organisms associated with bacteremia and pseudomembranous colitis in high-density and intestinal commensals in the Ruminococcaceae and Lachnospiraceae families known to produce short-chain fatty acids (SCFAs).[330] Decreased numbers of Ruminococcaceae and Lachnospiraceae lead to diminished SCFAs and are associated with low butyrate in the feces and development of IBD. Bacteroides genus colonizes the gut through specific microbe-host immune interactions and metabolic activities, such as metabolization of HMOs and mucin complex plant polysaccharides, and deconjugation of bile acids.[331] The less common Veillonella genus is characterized as saccharolytic, using products of carbohydrate fermentation of other intestinal bacteria to produce propionate. Propionate is a beneficial SCFA with antiinflammatory and energy homeostasis influences in the gut.[332] The genus Lactobacillus, present in relatively lower numbers, have been detected in meconium and early on after vaginal delivery versus less often after C-section. As a lactic acid bacillus, Lactobacillus has been determined capable of HMO metabolism to secure its niche in the neonatal intestine. Akkermansia muciniphila is present in low levels in the infant's gut soon after birth. It increases in relative abundance with age and after weaning and has been correlated with intestinal integrity.[333]

Potential Effects of Microbiota on Infant Health

A number of research groups have summarized the potential effects of the intestinal microbiota in early life on infant and childhood health.[270,334-336] Notably, the infant's intestinal microbiota has dynamic effects on gut immunity and maturation, and on systemic immune development.[9] In combination with the bioactive markers and cells within breast milk, the human milk facilitates microbiota's dynamic protection of the intestine and the infant in the early high-risk neonatal period. Specific proposed mechanisms of how probiotic bacteria and prebiotic substances contribute to an infant's developing immune system include competition with pathogenic bacteria for colonization, strengthening the tight junctions to enhance the mucosal barrier, producing antimicrobial bacteriocidins, stimulating mucus production, stimulating peristalsis, influencing the secretion of sIgA, stimulating the crosstalk interaction between intestinal cells and colonizing bacteria affect the mucosal immune development, and increasing the production of certain cytokines (IL-10 and IFN-γ).[337-339] The infant's intestinal microbiota primes a balanced innate and adaptive immunity and a balanced Th1 and Th2 response. The early colonizers in breastfed infants, in particular Firmicutes, Bacteroides, Enterobacteriaceae, Veillonella, and Bifidobacterium, create an anaerobic lactic acid and SCFA-abundant environment, which leads to colonization resistance of potential pathogens. Protection from breast milk's bioactive factors adds to colonization resistance and dampens any inflammatory response at the same time. The effect of the intestinal microbiota on the host includes creating a balance of immune cell populations and regulatory T cells (Treg), stimulating development of Peyer's patches and the MALT and maturation of the intestinal barrier (intestinal epithelial cells, M cells, Paneth cells, and goblet cells). Microbial-associated molecular patterns (MAMPs) directly influence the crosstalk between host and microbiota. This includes TLR signaling effecting tolerogenic DCs and increasing the balance of Tregs. When "primed" DCs sense particular types of pattern recognition receptors (PRRs) in the intestinal microbiota, this leads to stimulated Th1 response, secretion of antiinflammatory cytokines (IL-10), and a maintenance of mucosal homeostasis.[335] Intestinal immune tolerance is generated by multiple mechanisms, in particular regulatory T cells. The specific intestinal commensal bacteria (*Lactobacillus, Bifidobacterium, Bacteroides, Clostridium*, and *Streptococcus*) with the metabolic products of these bacteria (butyric acid and propionic acid) appear to program the Treg cells in the intestine.[340] Human breast milk with all its antimicrobial and antiinflammatory factors protects the infant during this growth and maturation period occurring in the intestine and systemically. HMOs play a crucial role in establishing the intestinal microbiota (*Bifidobacterium, Lactobacillus, Bacteroides*, and *Staphylococcus*) and acting as "decoy receptors" interfering with the binding of pathogens to the intestinal epithelium. The HMOs serve as substrate for the favored microbiota that produce by fermentation lactate, acetate, butyrate, and other SCFAs. Butyrate is antiinflammatory by suppression of nuclear factor-κB (NF-κB) and by stimulating mucin synthesis. The SCFAs are also substrate for colonocytes and other commensal bacteria adding to the intestinal homeostasis.[334]

Zhuang et al.[336] review the potential effects of the infant intestinal microbiota on childhood health. They compare eubiosis or symbiosis with dysbiosis and the maintenance of health versus disease states. Dysbiosis refers to microbial imbalance or maladaptation within the intestine. The established or "healthy" microbiota is altered or displaced such that the normally dominant species become underrepresented and potentially pathogenic microorganisms become dominant. In some situations, this has been described as small intestinal bacterial overgrowth or small intestine fungal overgrowth. Whether the dysbiosis is mechanistically the result of a relative abundance of specific organisms, a change in the ratio of competing organisms, a less diverse microbiota, a less stable microbiota, a change in the metabolome of the intestine, or epigenetic changes occurring locally or systemically remains to be determined in the different disease states. Zhuang et al.[336] discuss the intestinal microbiota and various disease conditions: late-onset sepsis, necrotizing enterocolitis, eczema, asthma, food allergy, type 1 diabetes mellitus, obesity, irritable bowel syndrome (IBS), IBD, and neuropsychiatric disorders (autism and attention deficit disorder). Table 5.12 presents specific considerations of mechanisms of pathophysiology, possible organisms involved in the dysbiosis and potential contributing factors to selected diseases.

Modification of Intestinal Microbiota

Probiotics have been broadly defined as microorganisms that can coexist within a host while affording benefits for the organisms and the host. Prebiotics are substances that (through different mechanisms) increase the growth and survival of probiotic bacteria within the host. Commonly recognized probiotic bacteria are *L. rhamnosus* GG, *B. infantis, Streptococcus thermophilus, Bacillus subtilis*, and *B. bifidum*. Many more organisms are considered to be probiotics, some of which are commercially available.[341−344] Prebiotics are predominantly nondigestible oligosaccharides that ferment within the colon, changing the ambient pH and producing SCFAs. Human breast milk, with its significant composition of oligosaccharides (HMOs), functions as a prebiotic source for an infant, facilitating the growth of bifidobacteria and lactobacilli in particular.[345,346] Ongoing research is exploring the potentially mutually beneficial relationship between the microbes and the host. Researchers are paying particular attention to nutrition (the availability of nutrients, energy sources, and synthesis of vitamins as influenced by the microbes), the developing GI tract (including angiogenesis and mucosal barrier repair), the maturation of mucosal immunity, both the innate system and adaptive system, and the bioavailability and metabolism of drugs and chemicals in the GI tract.[12,337,338,347−353]

Both probiotics and prebiotics, when introduced orally, can modify the intestinal microbiota depending on local conditions; the question remains whether it is a temporary or longer lasting modification. There are hopes that probiotics can modify disease such as allergies, GI infections, obesity, IBD, and IBS.[343]

Although hopes are high for the therapeutic use of probiotics, the efficacy of different strains or combinations of strains needs to be determined, and the timing of application and the safety of preparations require more study.

Antibiotics when directed against a specific infection with a known microorganism can be efficacious and beneficial. They can also alter the intestinal microbiota, which can affect digestion and absorption of vitamins and nutrients, alter the local immune response, and create resistant organisms. Antibiotics are reported to increase the risk for developing diabetes, asthma, obesity, and antibiotic-associated infections (antibiotic-associated diarrhea, *C. difficile*).

Dietary modifications also create short- and long-term effects on the intestinal microbiota. This is most commonly evident with the introduction of complementary foods in infancy.[354] It is also demonstrated in dietary modifications to treat diseases such as diabetes, diarrhea, and Crohn's disease. Additional studies are needed to further the understanding of how various diets (i.e., combinations of foods, nutrients, and vitamins) affect the microbiota.

Fecal microbiota transplantation (FMT) is a new intervention to affect the intestinal microbiota, currently used to treat resistant/persistent *C. difficile* infection. A fecal suspension

TABLE 5.12 Intestinal Microbiota Changes and Pediatric Diseases

Pediatric Disease	Disease Mechanism	Microorganisms	Contributing Factors	References
Necrotizing enterocolitis (NEC)	Low microbial diversity, overgrowth of pathogenic bacteria, reduced levels of "protective" bacteria?	Abundance of Proteobacteria, or *Sphingomonas;* relative paucity of Firmicutes and Bacteroidetes	Prematurity, hypoxia, difficult delivery, feeding difficulty, formula feeding, antibiotics, histamine 2 blockers	Pammi et al. *Microbiome,* 2017; Neu, Pammi. *Semin Fetal Neonatal Med,* 2018
Late-onset sepsis (LOS)	Less diverse microbiota, predominance of pathogens, bacterial translocation	Lower levels of *Bacteroides* and *Bifidobacterium,* predominance of *Enterobacterium*	NEC, bacterial translocation, preterm formula	Mai et al. *PLoS One,* 2013; Miller et al. *Nutrients,* 2018; Collins et al. *Arch Dis Child Fetal Neonatal Ed,* 2018
Eczema	Mechanism? Abundant pathogenic bacteria? Inflammation/atopy	*Enterococcus, Shigella* genera; *Ruminococcus gnavus, Faecalibacterium prausnitzii*	Genetics/family history	Kau et al. *Nature,* 2011; Greer et al. *Pediatrics,* 2019
Asthma	Dysbiosis, T-cell dysfunction—hyperactivation of the Th2 arm of immunity	?	Genetics, exposure to antibiotics, pets or livestock in pregnancy, antibiotics in early life, formula feeding	Kemter, Nagler. *J Clin Invest,* 2019; Greer et al. *Pediatrics,* 2019
Food allergy	Decreased diversity of intestinal microbiota, increased *Bacteroides*	Diminished Firmicutes and Clostridia	Genetics	Plunkett, Nagler. *J Immunol,* 2017; Greer et al. *Pediatrics,* 2019
Type 1 diabetes mellitus	Less diverse and less stable microbiota, dysbiosis, β cell autoimmunity	Change in proportion of Firmicutes to Bacteroidetes	Genetics, mode of delivery, diet in early life, antibiotic usage	Hummel et al. *Diabetes Care,* 2017; Hu et al. *Pharmacol Res,* 2017
Obesity	Dietary energy usage, promotion of fat deposition, systemic inflammation activation	Increased colonization with *Staphylococcus aureus, Bacteroides fragilis* and increased body mass index	Genetics, type 2 diabetes	Scheepers et al. *Int J Obesity,* 2015; Wang et al. *Science,* 2017
Irritable bowel syndrome	Multifactorial, dysbiosis or small intestine bacterial overgrowth at diagnosis	?	Gastroenteritis, antibiotic use	Simren et al. *Gut,* 2013; Jalanka-Tuovinen et al. *Gut,* 2014
Inflammatory bowel disease (IBD), Crohn's disease (CD), ulcerative colitis (UC)	Dysbiosis, ? T cell activation, interleukins IL-23/Th17 pathway, microbial recognition and autophagy?	Loss of Bacteroidetes and Firmicutes phyla; increase Proteobacteria	Genetics, gut microbial flora, immune response?	Khor et al. *Nature,* 2011
Neuropsychiatric disorders (schizophrenia, cognitive dysfunction, depression)	Humoral and neural pathways of gut-brain communication, epigenetic changes?	?	Genetics, intestinal microbiota essential for healthy functional microglia?	Cryan and Dinan. *Neuropsychopharmacology,* 2015; Cenit et al. *World J Gastroenterol,* 2017
Autism	Epigenetics?	Altered levels of Firmicutes and Bacteroidetes	Genetics, epigenetics	Tomova et al. *Physiol Behav,* 2015
Attention deficit hyperactivity disorder	Epigenetics	?	Epigenetics, environment	Cenit et al. *Eur Child Adolesc Psychiatry,* 2017

Zhuang L, Chen H, Zhang S, et al. Intestinal microbiota in early life and its implications on childhood health. *Genomics Proteomics Bioinforma.* 2019;17:13–25. doi:10.1016/j.gpb.2018.10.002.

from a "healthy" donor is introduced into a recipient patient to modify the function and diversity of that patient's intestinal microbiota and hopefully suppress or eliminate colonization with *C. difficile*. The FMT is achieved via colonoscopy, nasogastric or nasoduodenal tube, enemas, or oral capsules.[355] Again, with FMT, the specific microbial and functional profile of the transplanted microbiota (as for probiotic preparations) needs to be carefully characterized and the short and long-term effects fully assessed.

Microbiota Summary

It is clear that the intestinal microbiota is essential to the maturation of the GI tract and the infant's developing immune system. Human breast milk is an important determining factor in the make-up of the microbiota. The microbiota, in combination with many of the bioactive factors in breast milk, is crucial to maintaining a eubiotic state in the intestinal tract and programming both immunity and metabolic functioning of the infant into the future.[7,8,13,14,353,356,357]

GENETICS AND EPIGENETICS

General Features of Epigenetics

As research pushes to identify all the benefits of human breast milk for the developing infant and corroborate the etiologic effect of factors in breast milk that lead to specific outcomes in neonates, the how and why of these effects become more important. The high level of variability in breast milk composition and the potential link between breast milk variation and neonatal outcomes suggest genetic or epigenetic effects or both. Baumgartel and Conley presented a systematic review of publications of genetic studies that used RNA and DNA found in human breast milk and the potential effects on breast milk compositional variability and neonatal outcomes.[133] They identified 13 articles that focused on gene expression and three articles on epigenetics. A number of methods for the analyses of genes were used in these studies: northern blot, RT-PCR, spectrophotometry, microarrays, and Western blots. Bisulfite conversion, PCR amplification, and pyrosequencing were used for epigenetic analysis. In addition to "cataloguing" these studies, the authors outlined the limitations of these studies. They made recommendations for the methodology of future studies on breast milk concerning gene expression and epigenetic effects. The related gene products examined in these studies included important proteins contained in breast milk (β-casein, α-lactalbumin, M-ficolin, and parathyroid hormone–related protein), transporter proteins, cytokines, and ILs. The epigenetic studies examined methylation of specific genes; for example, kallikrein-related peptidase 6 (KLK6), retinol binding protein (RBP1), and glutathione S-transferase (GSTP1), among others. This small collection of studies only emphasizes how much work there is to do to understand the genetics and epigenetics of breast milk and breastfeeding.

The complexity of the breast, its various stages of development, the stages of lactation, and the variable composition of human breast milk suggest a complex interplay between genetic, epigenetic, environmental, and lifestyle factors. These all affect milk production and influence the benefits of lactation for the mother and infant. Epigenetics may play a pivotal role in our understanding of the benefits of breastfeeding. The word *epigenetics* means "atop" or "surrounding" genetics. Various definitions of epigenetics enhance our understanding of its essential features: (1) "changes in gene function which do not alter the underlying structure of DNA but result in genes being switched on or off in a reversible way" and (2) "stable heritable phenotype resulting from changes in a chromosome without alterations in the DNA sequence."[358,359] Broadly, this implies any mitotically or meiotically heritable change that leads to different gene expression without actually changing the DNA sequence. The true implication is that each individual "adapts" to the environment through some of these epigenetic mechanisms, leading to potentially different health outcomes for the individual.

Berger et al.[358] discuss three "categories of signals" leading to the epigenetic change, which becomes a stably heritable state: epigenator, epigenetic initiator, and epigenetic maintainer. The epigenator is an external or environmental signal that affects the cell, leading to the activation of the initiator. The intracellular epigenetic initiator "selects" the location of chromosomal/chromatin change, which leads to a change in gene expression. The epigenetic maintainer preserves the new epigenetic chromatin state. The major epigenetic mechanisms for changing gene expression and maintaining it are DNA methylation, histone modification, chromatin remodeling, and long noncoding RNAs (ncRNA) and microRNA (miRNA). DNA methylation and histone modification can influence the transcription of specific genes. ncRNAs can affect either transcription (production of an RNA copy of specific genes) or interference with translation (the production of an amino acid sequence from messenger RNA [mRNA]). DNA methylation often results in the "silencing" of the affected gene. Methylation in humans happens at a cytosine next to a guanine nucleotide (CpG site). The critical periods for the occurrence of DNA methylation are early in gestation and early in infancy. "Genomic imprinting" is a specific example of DNA methylation. Imprinting is the inactivation of one of the two copies of a gene inherited from one's parents, leading to the expression of the other copy of the gene. Imprinting has been described in a percentage of children with Beckwith-Wiedemann syndrome; a change in DNA methylation leads to genomic imprinting and, subsequently, the disorder. As noted in adults and children, there are genes involved in DNA methylation regulation that are mutated in acute myeloid leukemia.[359] Histone modification changes how the DNA and proteins are "packaged" to form chromatin. Either the chromatin is formed in the "inactive form," leading to transcriptional repression, or in the "active form," leading to active transcription and gene expression.

Human Milk MicroRNAs

Verduci et al. summarized a number of possible epigenetic effects of human breast milk components on specified health outcomes.[360] They describe in vitro animal studies correlating specific breast milk components with variable gene expression and potential health outcomes. These include lactoferrin or human milk microbiota reducing NF-κB expression and leading to less NEC; prostaglandin J decreasing the expression of cholesterol biosynthesis enzymes and prevention of nonalcoholic fatty liver disease; and long-chain PUFA n-3 causing diminished expression of hepatic hydroxymethyl glutaryl coenzyme A (HMG-CoA) reductase, limiting the development of high total blood cholesterol in adult mice. They also note several human milk epigenetic effects hypothesized in humans: prostaglandin J, which leads to increased perioxisome proliferator-activated receptor-γ (PPARγ) and less obesity in adolescents; and undigestible oligosaccharides, which promote the growth of various commensal bacteria and lead to diminished inflammation through the inhibition of NF-κB activation of B cells. Each of these is an example of the types of epigenetic changes that could occur in humans as a result of exposure to specific factors in human breast milk. Verduci et al. refer to dietary factors leading to changes in gene expression as "nutritional epigenetics or nutritional hypothesis."[360]

Kosaka et al. described the existence of microRNA in breast milk and its potential as an immune regulatory agent through transfer from mother to infant.[361] After the extraction of RNA from human breast milk, they performed a miRNA microarray analysis. They identified specific miRNAs as abundant in human milk. These were related to T- and B-cell maturation and regulation, neutrophil proliferation, and activation and regulation of TLRs. They also demonstrated that extracted human milk miRNA was resistant to degradation by low pH (pH 1), freezing and thawing, and RNase digestion. As a result, it is highly likely that infants ingest a good amount of miRNA. More recently, miRNAs have been identified in abundance in cells and lipid fractions of human milk more so than the fat-free fraction of human milk.[362] mRNAs were not detectable in infant formulas, which are initially treated with centrifugation to remove cells and much of the lipid fraction. Cow's milk has numerous miRNAs, as does the milk of many other mammals.[363] There is significant overlap in the most abundant microRNAs identified in human milk compared with the milk of cows, pigs, and pandas. MicroRNAs are also identified in multiple body fluids, with human breast milk having a relative abundance compared with other body fluids.[364] Several research groups have reported on the numerous microRNAs contained in human milk and their potential role as epigenetic regulators in infant health and disease.[365–368] Most of the microRNA is carried in extracellular vesicles, milk fat globules (MFGs), and the cell fraction of human milk with small amounts in the "skim milk" fraction.[367] Extracellular vesicles have been described as made up of three groups: exosomes (30 to 100 nm in diameter), microvesicles (100 to 200 nm) formed from plasma membrane, and apoptotic bodies (> 1000 nm) formed from blebs during apoptosis. The milk exosomes come from four main cellular sources: direct exosome separation from mammary epithelial cells, indirect exosome sequestration from MFGs, exosomes released from immune-associated cells in milk, and exosomes from nonimmune cells (e.g., milk stem cells).[368] The exosomes have a lipid bilayer membrane that confers additional protection for the microRNA. There is evidence that the exosomes are taken up into cells by various endocytic paths, including clathrin-dependent endocytosis, caveolin-mediated uptake, micropinocytosis, phagocytosis, and lipid-raft mediated internalization.[369] miRNAs within exosomes can enter intestinal epithelial cells and reach the systemic circulation. Milk-derived, lactation-specific miRNAs can reach the systemic circulation of the infant recipient and affect regulatory function.[367] The transfer of miRNAs from bovine milk is also reported in adults consuming cow's milk. Research is only beginning into how lactation-specific miRNas are distributed into milk exosomes and their potential roles in epigenetic changes of different molecular, cellular, and development functions in the recipient infants. Alsaweed et al.[367] reported on the top 20 highly expressed known and novel miRNAs they identified in human milk samples, many of which are involved in milk synthesis, production of triacylglycerol in milk fat, and fatty acid synthesis. They additionally predicted from these miRNAs using computational models probable targets of the miRNAs in immune responses, development, growth, metabolic processes, reproduction, and developmental functions.[367] Melnick and Schmitz[368] outlined a model of milk-mediated epigenetic regulation based on DNA methyltransferases-targeted demethylation, leading to upregulation of gene expression for transcriptional factors (NRF2, SREBP1, FOXP3, and NR4A3) and key metabolic regulators (INS, IGF1, CAV1, GLUT1, and LCT). They postulated a second model of milk-mediated activation of the *fat mass— and obesity-associated protein* (FTO) gene expression via RNA m^{6}A demethylation, which could effect hyperphagia, feeding reward, adipogenesis, and intestinal growth.[368] They additionally discuss how specific miRNAs may target specific metabolic and growth processes for health or disease (miRNA-148a and miRNA-29 and myogenesis; miRNA-148a and miRNA-21 and osteogenesis; miRNA-148a and epidermal differentiation; miRNA-29 and diabetes; miRNA-21 and miRNA-148a and cancer; miRNA-148a and Parkinson's disease). Melnick and Schmitz proposed a potential health hazard for adipogenesis, diabetogenesis, neurodegenerative changes, and carcinogenesis in the ongoing consumption of cow's milk through life and ongoing exposure to milk miRNA—mediated epigenetic signaling and especially so in the milk from cows selected for enhanced lactation performance related to epigenetic changes in mammary gland epithelial cells of cows.[368]

It is clear that miRNAs in human breast milk can function in cell-to-cell communication from mother to infant, affecting the expression of specific genes in the infant. Complete understanding of the roles of genetics and epigenetics in the explanation of specific benefits of breast milk for the infant and maternal health remains in the future, with the success of ongoing research.

EFFECTIVENESS OF HUMAN MILK IN CONTROLLING INFECTION

The properties of human milk do appear to control or limit infections in infants. Hundreds of articles have been written about the protective effect of breastfeeding, including the recent Agency for Healthcare Research and Quality (AHRQ) publication "Breastfeeding and Maternal and Infant Health Outcomes in Developed Countries from 2007."[46,370,371] Using evidence-based analyses, the report documents the decreased risk for acute otitis media, GI infections, and lower respiratory tract diseases in breastfed infants in developed countries.

Protection Against Bacterial Infection

Breast milk IgA has antitoxin activity against enterotoxins of *E. coli* and *V. cholerae* that may be significant in preventing infantile diarrhea. Antibodies against O antigen of some of the most common serotypes of *E. coli* were found in high titers in breast milk samples collected from healthy mothers in Sweden. The infants who had consumed reasonable amounts of breast milk with high titers of *E. coli* antibodies had antibodies in their stool.[372] Protection against cholera in breastfed children by antibodies in breast milk was studied by Glass et al.[196] A prospective study in Bangladesh showed cholera antibody levels to vary in the colostrum and milk. The correlation among colonization, disease, and milk antibodies led the authors to conclude that breast milk antibodies against cholera do not protect children from colonization with *V. cholerae*, but they do protect against disease.

Salmonella infection was similarly studied by France et al. to evaluate the immunologic mechanisms in host colostrum and milk specific for salmonellae.[373] Vigorous responses of colostral and milk cells against these organisms and nonspecific opsonizing capacity of the aqueous phase of colostrum and milk were demonstrated.

Gothefors et al. showed that *E. coli* isolated from stools of breastfed infants differed from strains found in formula-fed infants in two respects.[374] First, *E. coli* strains were more sensitive to the bactericidal effect of human serum. Second, and more often, spontaneously agglutinated bacteria from other sites, such as the prepuce or periurethral area, were less sensitive in breastfed infants. These findings support the theory that breast milk favors proliferation of mutant strains, which have decreased virulence. This mutation of bacterial strains is another way breastfeeding may protect against infection.

It has been suggested that "milk immunization" is a dynamic process, because a mother's milk has been found to contain antibodies to virtually all her infant's strains of intestinal bacteria. The mother, exposed to the infant's microorganisms through either the breast or the gut, responds immunologically to those microorganisms. In this way the mother directly provides protection for her immunologically immature infant.

The orderly review of data on the presence of antibodies in human milk has produced a substantial list of affected organisms. In addition to *E. coli*, antibodies to *B. fragilis, Clostridium tetani, Haemophilus pertussis, Diplococcus pneumoniae, Corynebacterium diphtheriae, Salmonella, Shigella, Chlamydia trachomatis, V. cholerae, S. aureus,* and several strains of *Streptococcus* (see Table 5.3) have been identified. Noguera-Obenza and Cleary[164] have summarized the contribution of sIgA in breast milk to protecting infants from bacterial enteritis.

A study in Oslo by Hanson[372] of an outbreak of severe diarrhea caused by *E. coli* strain 0111 showed that six severely ill children were formula fed. Two infants who were breastfed had *E. coli* strain 0111 in their stools but showed few symptoms. Their mothers had no detectable antibodies for strain 0111 in their milk, which would suggest that other factors in human milk protect the infant from serious illness when no antibodies are in the milk. Hanson also reported the results of another study in which, after colonization with a specific strain of *E. coli*, mothers had large numbers of lymphoid cells in their milk with antibodies to that *E. coli*. The mothers' serum showed no such response. This supports the concept that antigen-triggered lymphoid cells from Peyer's patches seek out lymphoid-rich tissue, producing IgA in the mammary gland. The mother is immunized in the gut at the same time as her milk. It has also been shown that *E. coli* enteritis can be cured by feeding human milk. Others have reviewed the nonantibody antimicrobial factors in human milk (Tables 5.13, 5.14, and 5.15).[164,262]

Schlesinger and Covelli studied possible cell-mediated immunity in breastfed infants.[375] They showed that tuberculin-positive nursing mothers had reactive T cells in their colostrum and early milk. Furthermore, 8 of 13 infants nursed by tuberculin-positive mothers had tuberculin-reactive peripheral blood T cells after 4 weeks. Cord blood had no such activity. No clinical or research data suggesting a protective effect of this apparently induced tuberculin reactivity in infants are available.

Protection Against Viral Infection

Protection against viruses has been the subject of similar studies. Breast milk contains antibodies against poliovirus, coxsackievirus, echovirus, enterovirus, influenza virus, reovirus, RSV, rotavirus, and rhinovirus.[376,377] It has been confirmed that human milk inhibits the growth of these viruses in tissue culture. Nonspecific substances in human milk are active against arbovirus and murine leukemia virus, according to work by Fieldsteel.[378]

A high degree of antiviral activity against Japanese B encephalitis virus, as well as the two leukemia viruses, has been found in human milk. The factor was found in the fat fraction and was not destroyed by extended heating, which distinguishes it from antibodies. May believes the nonimmunoglobulin macromolecule antiviral activity in human milk is caused by specific fatty acids and monoglycerides (see Table 5.14).[370] It is important to recognize that factors other than immunoglobulins are contained in breast milk, which can play a role in the protection of the breastfeeding infant from viral infections.[379]

TABLE 5.13   Nonantibody, Antibacterial Protective Factors in Human Milk

Factors	Proposed Mechanisms of Action	Organisms Affected	Effect of Heat
Bifidus factor	Inhibits replication of certain bacteria in GI tract by causing proliferation of lactobacilli	Enterobacteriaceae, including shigellae, salmonellae, and some *Escherichia coli*	Stable to boiling
Complement components	Opsonic, chemotactic, and bacteriolytic activity	*E. coli*	Destroyed by heating at 56°C for 30 min
Lysozyme	With IgA, peroxide, or ascorbate, causes lysis of bacteria	*E. coli*, salmonellae	Some loss (0%–23%) at 62.5°C for 30 min; essentially destroyed by boiling for 15 min
Lactoferrin (nutrient binders)	Binds ferric iron	*E. coli, Candida albicans*	Two thirds destroyed at 62.5°C for 30 min
Lactoperoxidase	Oxidizes bacteria	*E. coli, Salmonella typhimurium*	Presumably destroyed by boiling
Nonantibody proteins: Receptor-like glycolipid or glycoprotein	Inhibit bacterial adherence	*Vibrio cholerae*	Stable to boiling for 15 min
Gangliosides (GM1-like)	Interfere with attachment of enterotoxin to GM1 cell membrane ganglioside receptors	*E. coli* and *V. cholerae* enterotoxins	Stable to boiling
Nonlactose carbohydrate factors	Prevent action of stable toxin	*E. coli* stable toxin	Stable at 85°C for 30 min
Milk cells (macrophages, polymorphonuclear leukocytes, B- and T-lymphocytes)	By phagocytosis and killing: *E. coli, S. aureus, S. enteritidis*		
	By sensitized lymphocytes: *E. coli*		Destroyed at 62.5°C for 30 min
	By phagocytosis: *C. albicans* lymphocyte stimulation by *E. coli* K antigen		

Modified from May JT. Antimicrobial properties and microbial contaminants of breast milk: an update. *Aust Paediatr J.* 1984;20:265; and Pickering LK, Kohl S. Human milk humoral immunity and infant defense mechanisms. In: Howell RR, Morriss RH, Pickering LK, eds. *Human Milk and Infant Nutrition and Health*, Springfield, IL: Charles C Thomas; 1986.

Specimens of human colostrum have been found to contain neutralizing activity against RSV. RSV has become a major threat in infancy and is the most common reason for hospitalization in infancy in some developed countries. It has a high mortality rate. Epidemics have occurred in special care nurseries. Statistically significant data collected by Downham et al. showed that, compared with uninfected control subjects who were breastfed (46 of 167), few breastfed babies (8 of 115) were among the infants hospitalized for RSV infection.[380] Fishaut et al. studied the immune response to RSV prospectively in 26 nursing mothers over several months.[381] Antiviral IgM and IgG were rarely found in colostrum or milk. RSV-specific IgA, however, was identified in 40% to 75% of specimens. Two mothers with the disease had specific IgG, IgM, and IgA antibodies in serum and nasopharyngeal secretions, but only IgA was found in their milk. This confirms that IgA antibodies to specific respiratory tract pathogens are present in the products of lactation. Because RSV appears to replicate only in the respiratory tract, the authors suggest that viral-specific antibody activity in the mammary gland may be derived from the bronchiole-associated lymphoid tissue.

Antiprotozoan Factors

In human milk, bile salt-stimulated lipase has been found to be the major factor inactivating protozoans (see Table 5.15). The mechanism by which lipase acts is not known, although it may generate fatty acids and monoglycerides, which inactivate enveloped bacteria, viruses, or protozoa. A nonimmunoglobulin, nonlipase, heat-stable factor has been identified in human milk that can inactivate *Giardia lamblia*.

TABLE 5.14 Nonantibody, Antiviral, and Antiprotozoan Factors in Human Milk

Factors	Proposed Mechanisms of Action	Organisms Affected	Effect of Heat
Lipids (unsaturated fatty acids and monoglycerides)	Inactivate lipid-enveloped virus	Herpes simplex	Stable to boiling for 30 min
		Semliki Forest virus	
		Influenza	
		Ross River virus	
Macromolecules	Inhibit attachment and penetration	Herpes simplex	Most stable at 56°C for 30 min
		Coxsackievirus B_4	Destroyed by boiling for 30 min
		CMV	
		Rotavirus	
α_2-Macroglobulin protein	Inhibits hemagglutinin activity	Influenza	Stable to boiling for 15 min
		Parainfluenza	
α_1-Antitrypsin	Trypsin-dependent inhibition	Rotavirus	Stable to boiling for 10 min
Bile salt-stimulated lipase	May generate fatty acids and monoglycerides that inactivate organisms	Giardia lamblia	
		Entamoeba histolytica	
Nonlipase macromolecule	Unknown	G. lamblia	
Milk cells	Induce interferon by virus or phytohemagglutinin; induce lymphokine by phytohemagglutinin; induce cytokine by herpes simplex virus; lymphocyte stimulation by rubella, CMV, herpesvirus, measles, mumps		Destroyed at 62.5°C for 30 min

Modified from May JT. Antimicrobial properties and microbial contaminants of breast milk: an update. *Aust Paediatr J.* 1984;20:265; and Pickering LK, Kohl S. Human milk humoral immunity and infant defense mechanisms. In: Howell RR, et al., eds. *Human Milk and Infant Nutrition and Health*, Springfield, IL: Charles C Thomas; 1986.

TABLE 5.15 Antiprotozoan Factors in Human Milk

Factor	Organisms Affected (In Vitro)	Effect of Heat
Bile salt-stimulated lipase	Giardia lamblia	Destroyed at 62.5°C for 1 min
	Entamoeba histolytica	
	Trichomonas vaginalis	
Nonimmunoglobulin, nonlipase macromolecule	G. lamblia	Stable to boiling for 20 min

Modified from May JT. Antimicrobial properties and microbial contaminants of breast milk: an update. *Aust Paediatr J.* 1984;20:265.

ANTIINFLAMMATORY PROPERTIES

Human milk protects against many intestinal and respiratory pathogens with minimal evidence of inflammation. Goldman et al. hypothesize that human milk is poor in initiators and mediators of inflammation, but rich in antiinflammatory agents.[382] Several major biochemical pathways of inflammation, including the coagulation system, the fibrinolytic system, and complement, are poorly represented in human milk. Table 5.16 outlines the antiinflammatory properties of various constituents and the paucity of certain proinflammatory mediators in breast milk.

The interaction of factors in the milk with one another or with host defenses cannot be entirely predicted by examining each factor separately. When the decreased response of human milk leukocytes to chemoattractant peptides was demonstrated by Thorpe et al., the failure of the response of human milk leukocytes was not caused by alterations in

TABLE 5.16   Antiinflammatory Features of Human Milk

Paucity of Initiators and Mediators

Foreign antigens

Immunoglobulin G (IgG) antibodies

Complement system

Fibrinolytic system

Coagulation system

Kallikrein system

Antiinflammatory Agents

Lactoferrin	Inhibits complement
Secretory IgA	Prevents bacterial adherence
	Inhibits neutrophil chemotaxis
	Limits antigen penetration
Lysozyme	Inhibits neutrophil chemotaxis, generation of toxic oxygen radicals
Catalase	Destroys hydrogen peroxide
α-Tocopherol	Scavengers of oxygen radicals
Cysteine	
Ascorbic acid	
Histaminase	Degrades histamine
Arylsulfatase	Degrades leukotrienes
α_1-Antichymotrypsin	Neutralizes enzymes that act in inflammation
α_1-Antitrypsin	Neutralizes proteases that act in inflammation
Prostaglandins (E_2, $F_2\alpha$)	Cytoprotective: Inhibit neutrophil degranulation, lymphocyte activation
Pregnancy-associated α_2-glycoprotein	Inhibits lymphocyte blastogenesis
Oligosaccharides	Inhibits microbial attachment
Epidermal growth factors	Strengthens mucosal barriers

Special Features of Leukocytes

No basophils, mast cells, eosinophils, or platelets

T lymphocytes respond poorly to allogeneic cells

Low natural killer cell activity or antibody-dependent cytotoxicity

Poor response of neutrophils and macrophages to chemoattractants

maternal peripheral blood leukocytes.[383] This suggests that inhibitors are in the milk, and that human milk leukocytes may be modified in the mammary gland to protect through noninflammatory mechanisms. Only low numbers of basophils, mast cells, eosinophils, and CTLs are present in breast milk. Many other studies have documented the decreased function of milk polymorphonuclear leukocytes and macrophages in both colostrum and mature milk.[384]

The antioxidant properties of human colostrum were demonstrated by Buescher and McIlheran using aqueous human colostrum on human PMNs.[385] The colostrum significantly interfered with PMN oxygen metabolic and enzymatic activities, which are important in the mediation of acute inflammation.

Antioxidants in breast milk can also contribute to the overall antiinflammatory effect of breast milk. Demonstrated antioxidants contained in breast milk include an ascorbate-like compound, uric acid, α-tocopherol, β-carotene, and L-histidine, all of which scavenge oxygen radicals. Blood levels of α-tocopherol and β-carotene are higher in breastfed than unsupplemented formula-fed infants. Catalase, glutathione peroxidase, and lactoferrin are functionally antioxidants. Antioxidant activity has been demonstrated in colostrum and, at lower levels, in mature human milk.

Additionally, specific cytokines that can exhibit antiinflammatory effects have been identified in human colostrum and milk: TGF-β$_1$, TGF-β$_2$, and IL-10.[386-388] A cytokine antagonist, IL-1RA, and soluble receptors for TNF-α which can exert antiinflammatory effects by binding to IL-1α, IL-1β and TNF-α and TNF-β are found in colostrum and milk.[233]

Both human colostrum and milk cause a diminished influx of PMNs to a local site of inflammation in two different in vivo models of inflammation in rats.[389-391]

The inflammatory response can be protective for the host at the same time because it can produce the symptoms of clinical illness. Breast milk contains a large variety of antimicrobial factors that exert their protective effect without causing significant inflammation (e.g., sIgA, oligosaccharides, lactoferrin, and nucleotides). Many other cells and factors in breast milk participate in a complex interaction to both protect the infant and limit the potential damaging effects of an uncontrolled inflammatory response. Further study into the dynamic interplay of the many factors in breast milk with developing infants' mucosal barriers and immune system is needed to fully understand the protective immune response and the antiinflammatory benefits of human milk.

ALLERGIC PROTECTIVE PROPERTIES (SEE CHAPTER 17 ON HUMAN MILK AS PROPHYLAXIS IN ALLERGY)

In discussing the allergic protective properties of human milk, it is difficult to identify specific protective factors that are proved to protect against allergy. It is equally difficult to discuss the proposed mechanisms of protection because the exact mechanism of "tolerance" remains theoretical, and the relative importance of contributing factors to hypersensitivity must still be adequately defined. Some of the important variables concerning tolerance and sensitization are genetic background of the host, nature and dose of the antigen, frequency of exposure, timing (age) at first and subsequent exposures, immunologic status of the host, and route of exposure.

During the neonatal period, the small intestine has increased permeability to macromolecules. Infants have more serum and secretory antibodies against dietary proteins than children or adults. Production of IgA in the intestinal tract is delayed until 6 weeks to 3 months of age. IgA in colostrum and breast milk prevents the absorption of foreign macromolecules when an infant's immune system is immature. Mucin, oligosaccharides, and other factors within breast milk may affect antigen presentation. Protein of breast milk is species specific and therefore nonallergenic for human infants unless there is a specific abnormality of the infant's immune response. No antibody response has been demonstrated to occur with human milk in infants. It has also been shown that macromolecules in breast milk are not absorbed.

Indirect evidence regarding an allergic-like response can be inferred from the demonstration of an infant's response to cow milk protein. Within 18 days of taking cow milk, the infant will begin to develop antibodies. Since the advent of prepared formulas, in which the protein has been denatured by heating and drying, the incidence of cow milk allergy in breastfed children has been considered to be approximately 0.5% to 1% and in formula-fed infants approximately 2% to 7% from different sources.[392-394] The most reliable means of diagnosing cow milk allergy is by challenging with isolated cow milk protein. Although circulating antibodies and coproantibodies have been identified, these are not reliable techniques to make the diagnosis of cow's milk protein allergy for a clinician involved in patient care.

The allergic syndromes that have been associated with cow milk allergy include gastroenteropathy; atopic dermatitis; allergic rhinitis; chronic pulmonary disease; asthma; eosinophilia; failure to thrive; and sudden infant death syndrome, or cot death, which has in some cases been attributed to anaphylaxis to cow milk.[395,396] GI symptoms have received the greatest attention and include spitting-up, colic, diarrhea, blood in the stools, frank vomiting, weight loss, malabsorption, colitis, and failure to thrive. Cow milk has been associated with GI protein and blood loss. The diagnosis is best made by elimination of cow milk from the diet and, when appropriate, challenge tests. Cutaneous testing is of little help. Cow milk allergy has been described in breastfed infants, and exclusive breastfeeding alone is not sufficient for an infant at high risk for becoming sensitized to cow milk proteins.[397]

Murray showed the association of nasal secretion eosinophilia with infants freely fed cow milk or solid foods, compared with eosinophilia in strictly breastfed infants.[398] In infants receiving cow milk, 32% had high eosinophilic secretions. Only 11% of breastfed infants had eosinophils present in nasal secretions.

Not surprisingly, many different antigenic specificities are recognized when the colostrum or milk of one species is fed to or injected into another species. Cow milk is high on the list of food allergens, particularly in children. Sensitivity to cow milk is responsible for at least 20% of all pediatric allergic conditions, according to Gerrard et al.[399] Evidence indicates that IgA antibodies play an important role in confining food antigens to the gut. Food antigens given to bottle-fed infants before they can make their own IgA, and when they are deprived of that in human milk and plasma cells, may be expected to be more readily absorbed.

Glaser first made the association between the drop in breastfeeding and the rise in allergy. He pioneered the theory of prophylactic management of allergy.[400] Allergy in infancy is associated with a familial history of atopic disease and elevated cord blood IgE levels. The introduction of "foreign" proteins to an infant's diet, and even to the mother's diet, in the breastfeeding dyad can lead to allergic symptoms in the infant. Exclusive breastfeeding does not protect high-risk children from allergic symptoms, not even if the mother also adheres closely to a restrictive diet that excludes common allergens.[401]

A large body of literature examines whether breastfeeding protects against atopic disease. In 1988 Kramer[21] defined 12 standards for methodology and the study of allergy and breastfeeding. The standards clarified the definitions of breastfeeding, measurable outcomes, and the diagnostic criteria for specific allergic syndromes, defined children at high risk for atopic disease, and addressed methods to decrease bias and control for confounding variables. Several recent large meta-analyses have been performed assessing the protective effect of breastfeeding against allergic rhinitis, atopic dermatitis, and asthma.[402–404] Exclusive breastfeeding for at least 3 months was associated with lower rates of atopic dermatitis in children with a family history of atopy. Exclusive breastfeeding in the first months of life was protective against asthma during childhood (odds ratio 0.70; 95% confidence interval, 0.60 to 0.81).

The American Academy of Pediatrics' Committee on Nutrition and Section on Allergy and Immunology reviewed data on breastfeeding and its potential protection against allergy in 2019. The published results are reviewed in Chapter 17.

PROTECTION AGAINST CHRONIC DISEASE IN CHILDHOOD

The major elements in human milk related to the infant's immune system are direct-acting antimicrobial factors, anti-inflammatory factors, and immunomodulating bioactive compounds.[405] Epidemiologic studies have produced compelling information that suggests that breastfeeding for 4 months or longer can provide some immunologic protection against some childhood-onset diseases.[406]

In 1991 Viirtanen et al. reported a prospective long-term study among children in Finland that showed a significantly lower incidence of type 1 diabetes in those at-risk children who had been breastfed for 4 months or longer.[407] Other epidemiologic studies have demonstrated a decreased incidence of type 1 insulin-dependent diabetes mellitus in breastfed children.[408,409] These clinical observations have been supported in the laboratory by studies of diet control in diabetic mice. The isolation of a bovine albumin peptide as a possible trigger of type 1 insulin-dependent diabetes mellitus makes further study imperative.[410] Based on limited data, the AHRQ report from 2007 cautiously concluded that breastfeeding for

at least 3 months reduced the risk for type 1 diabetes, compared with breastfeeding for less than 3 months. For type 2 diabetes, the same report concluded that breastfeeding in infancy produced a decreased risk, compared with not breastfeeding.

The review of the national perinatal collaborative study by Davis et al. showed a protective effect against development of childhood cancer by being breastfed for 4 months or longer for children followed for 10 years.[411] The effect was greater for acute leukemia and lymphoma. The role of infant feeding practices showed a similar effect of breastfeeding as protective in postponing or decreasing the occurrence of IBD in childhood.[412,413] Ciccu et al. reported a decreased risk for celiac disease in breastfed infants.[414] The AHRQ report concluded that an association exists between breastfeeding for at least 6 months and a decreased risk for developing acute lymphocytic leukemia and acute myelogenous leukemia. Maternal renal allografts have a better survival rate in individuals who were breastfed in infancy, compared with those who were not breastfed.[415,416] The mechanism of these apparent long-term immunologic benefits remains unclear, although theories abound. Given the potential for confounding factors and bias in large long-term studies, confirmation of these proposed benefits by additional, carefully controlled trials is required.

SUMMARY

An increasing amount of accumulated epidemiologic literature, using improved methodology and statistics, demonstrates the protective benefits of human milk for infants. A large number of bioactive factors have been identified and measured in breast milk during the period of lactation. Additional research is needed to clarify the interactions and the mechanisms of action of the many bioactive factors in human milk and then correlate these immunomodulatory actions with specific protective benefits for the infant. Our understanding of the cellular nature of the breast and breast milk is informing new studies on the role of these cells in breast cancer, breast health, protection at the level of the infant's intestinal tract and the infant's overall immune defenses. The dramatic increase in research on breast milk microbiota and the infant microbiota and separately on miRNAs and epigenetic changes as potential mechanisms for breast milk's long-term effects on infant and child health continues. Hopefully, new studies will clarify our understanding of how the specific components in human milk directly affect the health of the infant and mother.

The Reference list is available at www.expertconsult.com.

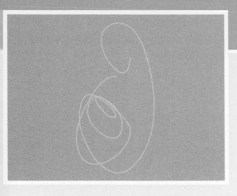

6

Population Health and Informed Feeding Decisions

Alison M. Stuebe

KEY POINTS

- Breastfeeding is a women's health issue. Disruption of breastfeeding is associated with higher rates of maternal breast and ovarian cancer, diabetes, hypertension, myocardial infarction, and stroke.
- Breastfeeding is also a children's health issue. Not being breastfed is associated with higher rates of infectious morbidity, childhood leukemia, sudden infant death syndrome, and necrotizing enterocolitis, as well as higher rates of obesity and diabetes and lower IQ.
- On a population level, suboptimal breastfeeding is associated with substantial health costs, premature loss of life, and reduced cognitive development.
- Most major medical organizations recommend 6 months of exclusive breastfeeding, with continued breastfeeding through 1 to 2 years or longer as mutually desired.

- Informing families about the health importance of breastfeeding is necessary, but not sufficient, to affect infant feeding behavior.
- Provider—patient communication can support breastfeeding by fostering relationships, validating emotions, sharing information and treatment recommendations, enabling self-management, and managing uncertainty.
- It can be helpful to apply tenets of social cognitive theory, which considers both cognitive and environmental influences on behavior, to address the multiple factors that affect infant feeding.
- Infant feeding decisions reflect multiple trade-offs that mothers negotiate to balance care for themselves and their infants. Efforts to make breastfeeding easier for mothers, as well as to promote health benefits, will enable more mothers and infants to breastfeed.

In human physiology, lactation follows pregnancy. Multiple studies have demonstrated that disruption of this physiology is associated with adverse outcomes for mothers and infants. For mothers, greater duration and intensity of lactation is associated with reduced risk for breast cancer, ovarian cancer, and cardiometabolic disease, among other health conditions.[1] For infants, breastfeeding is associated with reduced risk for infectious disease, autoimmune conditions, and sudden infant death syndrome (SIDS).

Sharing this information is an important part of anticipatory guidance in maternity care to enable families to make an informed decision regarding how to nourish and nurture the infant. This counseling is particularly important in light of aggressive and misleading marketing of infant formula.[2] Formula companies rely on disruption of breastfeeding to sell their product; every time a baby goes to breast, the formula industry loses a sale.[3] At the same time, individual mothers weigh multiple factors when deciding whether and how long to breastfeed, and patient-centered, respectful conversations that seek to understand her individual context are essential to support an informed decision.

BREASTFEEDING AND MATERNAL HEALTH

Although breastfeeding promotion typically has focused on the infant effects of ingesting human milk, lactation has substantial effects on maternal physiology, and these effects likely mediate associations between breastfeeding and women's health.

Breast Cancer

The mammary gland does not completely differentiate until pregnancy and lactation have occurred. During puberty, exposure to estrogen and progesterone stimulates development of breast tissue, with elaboration of ducts and lobules with each menstrual cycle. During pregnancy, sustained exposure to estrogen and progesterone, as well as growth hormone, human placental lactogen, and prolactin, result in secretory differentiation, with the appearance of lactocytes that are capable of producing milk.[4] After birth, withdrawal of progesterone and stimulation of the breast by the infant prompt secretory activation and the production of mature milk. With weaning, the breast involutes and returns to its prepregnant state.

Completion of this differentiation may explain the reduced risk for breast cancer among women who have lactated for longer periods. In a meta-analysis that included more than 250,000 women, ever breastfeeding was associated with a lower risk for breast cancer (pooled odds ratio [OR], 0.78, 95% confidence interval [CI] 0.74 to 0.82). This association was particularly pronounced for luminal triple-negative breast cancers,[1] which have the highest mortality risk and which disproportionately affect black women.[5]

In an analysis of the AMBER consortium, pregnancy without breastfeeding was associated with an increased risk for estrogen receptor—negative breast cancer among black women; each pregnancy without breastfeeding was associated with an increase in risk.[6] These findings underscore the urgency of dismantling structural barriers to breastfeeding for women of color.

Ovarian Cancer

Longer durations of breastfeeding are consistently associated with lower risk for ovarian cancer.[1,7,8] Several mechanisms have been proposed, including anovulation as a result of lactational amenorrhea and the effects of breastfeeding on gonadotropin homeostasis.[7] An immunologic mechanism also has been proposed, based on sensitization to MUC-1 antigen, which is present in breast epithelium and in ovarian cancer epithelium. Women who have breastfed have higher levels of anti—MUC-1 antibodies, with the highest levels found among women who have breastfed and have had mastitis, and higher levels of MUC-1 antibody are associated with lower ovarian cancer risk.[9,10]

Cardiometabolic Disease

Breastfeeding imposes a substantial metabolic load on maternal physiology; exclusive breastfeeding requires 597 to 716 kcal (2.5 to 3.0 megajoule [MJ]) per day.[11] This metabolic demand may facilitate mobilization of gestational weight gain[12] and "reset" maternal metabolic changes of pregnancy.[13]

The impact of lactation on weight trajectory is modified by maternal dietary intake, and in observational studies, associations between lactation and weight loss are inconsistent.

A meta-analysis of 16 cohort studies including 47,655 women found insufficient evidence to conclude that breastfeeding per se increased postpartum weight loss.[1]

However, greater breastfeeding duration and intensity is associated with reduced risk for type 2 diabetes and hypertension[1] and reduced risk for progression from gestational diabetes to type 2 diabetes.[14] Women with gestational diabetes who are breastfeeding at the time of their postpartum glucose tolerance test have lower glucose levels and are less likely to meet criteria for type 2 diabetes.[15,16] These associations may reflect the effects of lactation on maternal physiology or the extent to which underlying maternal insulin resistance is associated with early weaning.[17]

Longer breastfeeding is similarly associated with reduced hypertension risk[1,18] and reduced risk for myocardial infarction,[19] cardiovascular disease,[20] and stroke.[21] These findings suggest that enabling breastfeeding is an essential part of improving women's cardiovascular health.

Depression

Although it is conventional wisdom that breastfeeding prevents depression, the relationship between breastfeeding and maternal mood is complex. Systematic reviews of the literature have found that prenatal depression and anxiety are risk factors for early weaning, and breastfeeding difficulties often presage or co-present with mood disorders.[22,23]

BREASTFEEDING AND INFANT HEALTH

For mammals, species-specific milk plays a fundamental role in the transition to extrauterine life and the development of

TABLE 6.1	Relative or Absolute Contraindications to Breastfeeding	
	Infant	**Mother**
Infant should not be fed mother's milk	Classic galactosemia	HTLV I or II Untreated brucellosis Illicit substance use: PCP, cocaine, methamphetamines, etc.) Medications: Chemotherapy, radioactive compounds (see Chapter 11)
Infant should not be fed at breast, but expressed milk can be provided		Active HSV lesion on breast Varicella diagnosed 5 days before through 2 days after birth H1N1 virus and febrile
Breastfeeding recommendations vary[b]		Untreated tuberculosis[a] HIV[b]
Counsel mother to reduce or discontinue use while breastfeeding		Marijuana Nicotine (including e-cigarettes) Alcohol > 2 oz liquor, 8 oz wine, or 2 beers

HIV, Human immunodeficiency virus; *HSV,* herpes simplex virus; *HTLV,* human T-cell lymphotropic virus; *PCP,* phencyclidine.
[a]*US guidelines:* Mother and infant should be separated until mother has been treated for 2 weeks; expressed milk may be provided to the infant during this time. *World Health Organization (WHO) guidelines:* If mother is diagnosed with tuberculosis and started treatment <2 months before birth, mother should be reassured that breastfeeding is safe and infant should be treated with isoniazid (INH) for 6 months, followed by bacillus Calmette—Guérin vaccination (see Chapter 12).
[b]Per WHO guidelines, national authorities should decide whether maternal and child health programs will principally support breastfeeding and antiretroviral treatment as the way to ensure infants born to HIV-infected mothers the greatest chance of HIV-free survival. In high-income countries where replacement feeding can be prepared safely, breastfeeding is typically not recommended.

gut and immune physiology.[24] Moreover, feeding at breast, as opposed to from an artificial teat, can entrain mother—infant interaction and facilitate development of satiety cues. Thus what the infant is fed and how the infant is fed have significant implications for both acute and long-term health outcomes.

Infectious Morbidity

Lactation plays a central role in protecting the neonate, through both specific and innate immune mechanisms. The lactating mother produces immunoglobulin A (IgA) antibodies specific to her environment and life experience,[25] conferring production from infections. In addition, oligosaccharides, lactoferrin, and other innate immune molecules provide protection.[26] In low- and middle-income controls, never breastfeeding is associated with an eight-fold increase in mortality because of infection in the first 6 months of life compared with exclusive breastfeeding (OR 0.12, 95% CI 0.04 to 0.31).[27]

Breastfeeding is similarly associated with reductions in infectious morbidity in high-income countries. In a meta-analysis of studies including more than 16,000 infants, exclusive breastfeeding for the first 6 months of life was associated with reduced odds of otitis media by age 2 (OR 0.57, 95% CI 0.44 to 0.75); ever breastfeeding was associated with a more modest reduction in risk (OR 0.67, 95% CI 0.56 to 0.80).[28]

Risk for gastroenteritis is also reduced among breastfed infants: 4 months of exclusive breastfeeding, with continued breastfeeding through 6 months, is associated with an adjusted OR of 0.41 (95% CI 0.26 to 0.64).[29] Being breastfed is also associated with reduced odds of lower respiratory tract infections: 4 months of exclusive breastfeeding with continuation through 6 months was associated with an adjusted OR (aOR) of 0.50 (95% CI 0.32 to 0.79) for the first 6 months and 0.46 (95% CI 0.31 to 0.69) for 7 to 12 months of life.[29]

Childhood Leukemia

Longer durations of breastfeeding are consistently associated with a reduced risk for childhood leukemia. A meta-analysis found that 14% to 19% of all childhood leukemia cases may be prevented by breastfeeding for 6 months or more.[30]

Sudden Infant Death Syndrome

Not breastfeeding is a risk factor for SIDS. In a participant-level meta-analysis,[31] any breastfeeding for longer than 2 months was protective compared with never breastfeeding (2 to 4 months: aOR 0.60, 95% CI 0.44 to 0.82; 4 to 6 months: aOR 0.40, 95% CI 0.26 to 0.63; and longer than 6 months: aOR 0.36, 95% CI 0.22 to 0.61); the association strengthened with exclusive breastfeeding (exclusive 2 to 4 months: aOR 0.61, 95% CI 0.42 to 0.87; 4 to 6 months: aOR 0.46, 95% CI 0.29 to 0.74). Recommendations to breastfeed therefore should be incorporated into public health campaigns to reduce SIDS risk.

TABLE 6.2 Number of Annual Deaths of Women and Children Attributable to Not Breastfeeding by Region and Country Income Group

Regions	Due to Child Diarrhea (0—23 mo)	Due to child ARI/ pneumonia (0—23)	Total Child Deaths	Due to Breast Cancer in Mothers	Due to Ovarian Cancer in Mothers	Due to Type 2 Diabetes in Mothers	Total Number of Maternal Deaths
East Asia and Pacific	13,932	39,680	53,613	11,898	5,922	19,964	37,785
Europe and Central Asia	2,132	5,302	7,434	3,007	1,877	2,683	7,567
Middle East and North Africa	6,455	15,272	21,727	1,801	606	5,261	7,668
Latin America and Caribbean	3,938	10,897	14,835	4,292	2,092	11,503	17,887
North America	0	0	0	0	0	0	0
South Asia	66,530	96,350	162,880	3,444	1,677	10,791	15,913
Sub-Saharan Africa	132,828	202,064	334,892	2,626	1,471	8,028	12,125
High income	11	95	106	704	471	654	1,829
Upper middle-income	10,928	33,952	44,879	15,677	7,619	29,414	52,711
Lower middle-income	147,999	233,025	381,024	9,313	4,763	25,323	39,399
Low income	66,877	102,493	169,370	1,374	791	2,839	5,004
Total	225,815	369,565	595,379	27,069	13,644	58,230	98,943

ARI, Acute respiratory infection.
From Walters DD, Phan LTH, Mathisen R. The cost of not breastfeeding: global results from a new tool. *Health Policy Plan.* 2019;34(6):407—417. PMC6735804.

Allergic Disease

Being breastfed is associated with a reduced risk for asthma and recent wheezing illness. In a meta-analysis,[32] the strongest association was found for the first 2 years of life (ever breastfed vs. never breastfed, OR 0.65, 95% CI 0.51 to 0.82; ≥ 3 vs. <3 months exclusive 0.62, 95% CI 0.51 to 0.74). For children aged 7 years or older, ever having been breastfed was associated with a modest reduction in risk (OR 0.86, 95% CI 0.77 to 0.96). A second meta-analysis evaluated associations with asthma, eczema, allergic rhinitis, and food allergy and found serious limitations in the evidence, with the exception of exclusive breastfeeding for longer than 4 months and eczema before age 2 (OR 0.74, 95% CI 0.57 to 0.97).[33] A 2019 report by the American Academy of Pediatrics found that in the first 2 years of life, more than 3 to 4 months of exclusive breastfeeding is associated with a reduced risk for eczema and that any breastfeeding longer than 3 to 4 months is associated with a reduced risk for wheezing. Longer durations of any breastfeeding were also associated with reduced risk for asthma. Infant feeding was not related to risk for food allergy.[34]

Type 1 Diabetes

Feeding of breast milk substitutes has been proposed to increase type 1 diabetes risk through exposure to cow's milk protein antigen in early life. To test this hypothesis, the Trial to Reduce IDDM in the Genetically at Risk (TRIGR) study randomized infants with high-risk human leukocyte antigen

TABLE 6.3 Global and Regional Economic Losses From Mortality and Cognitive Losses and Total Attributable to Not Breastfeeding by Region and by Country Income Group[a]

	From Child Mortality ($US Billion)	From Maternal Mortality ($US Billion)	From Cognitive Losses ($US Billion)	Total Cost (Health, Mortality, and Cognitive) ($US Billion)	Total Cost as % of GNI
East Asia and Pacific	10.39 (2.71, 49.67)	0.66 (0.55, 0.80)	74.76 (19.46, 357.66)	86.12 (23.04, 408.45)	0.59 (0.16, 2.78)
Europe and Central Asia	1.35 (0.35, 6.38)	0.25 (0.21, 0.29)	14.76 (3.86, 70.15)	16.27 (4.37, 76.71)	0.42 (0.11, 1.97)
Middle East and North Africa	3.76 (0.98, 17.99)	0.03 (0.03, 0.04)	18.65 (4.85, 89.38)	22.57 (5.98, 107.54)	0.91 (0.24, 4.32)
Latin America and Caribbean	4.08 (1.07, 19.35)	0.28 (0.23, 0.34)	32.25 (8.41, 154.02)	36.85 (9.94, 173.95)	0.70 (0.19, 3.32)
North America	0.00 (0.00, 0.00)	0.00 (0.00, 0.00)	114.94 (29.87, 551.37)	114.97 (29.90, 551.40)	0.63 (0.16, 3.04)
South Asia	10.58 (2.75, 50.59)	0.02 (0.02, 0.02)	11.73 (3.05, 56.12)	22.49 (5.99, 106.90)	0.84 (0.22, 3.99)
Sub-Saharan Africa	23.56 (6.59, 101.00)	0.02 (0.01, 0.02)	18.31 (5.05, 80.05)	42.06 (11.82, 181.25)	2.58 (0.72, 11.11)
Low and middle income	53.57 (14.41, 244.27)	1.08 (0.90, 1.30)	162.55 (42.62, 769.48)	218.27 (59.01, 1,016.13)	0.83 (0.22, 3.86)
High income	0.15 (0.04, 0.71)	0.18 (0.15, 0.22)	122.84 (31.92, 589.28)	123.06 (32.03, 590.06)	0.25 (0.06, 1.20)
Upper middle income	14.44 (3.81, 67.79)	0.95 (0.80, 1.16)	114.07 (29.74, 544.54)	130.07 (34.95, 614.10)	0.65 (0.17, 3.07)
Lower middle income	35.19 (9.53, 158.64)	0.12 (0.10, 0.14)	44.73 (11.88, 207.87)	80.47 (21.94, 367.09)	1.36 (0.37, 6.20)
Low income	3.95 (1.07, 17.83)	0.01 (0.00, 0.01)	3.74 (1.01, 17.07)	7.73 (2.12, 34.95)	1.99 (0.54, 8.98)
Total	53.72 (14.45, 244.99)	1.26 (1.06, 1.52)	285.39 (74.55, 1,358.75)	341.33 (91.04, 1,606.19)	0.70 (0.19, 3.29)

GNI, Gross national income.

[a]Default scenario (not in parentheses) based on discount rate on benefits of 3% and long-term gross domestic product (GDP) growth rate assumption of 3%. Figures in parentheses are lower and higher bound estimates based on assumptions of 1.5% discount rate on benefits and 5% long-term GDP growth rate for the figure on the left and 5% discount rate on benefits and 1.5% long-term GDP growth rate for the figure on the right.

From Walters DD, Phan LTH, Mathisen R. The cost of not breastfeeding: global results from a new tool. *Health Policy Plan.* 2019;34(6):407-417. PMC6735804.

(HLA) types to weaning to cow's milk formula or hydrolyzed formula. They found no difference in development of beta-cell autoimmunity[35] or type 1 diabetes.[36]

Whereas hydrolyzed formula does not reduce risk for type 1 diabetes, a systematic review found limited evidence that never being fed human milk was associated with a higher risk for type 1 diabetes, and moderate evidence that shorter durations of human milk feeding were associated with a higher risk for type 1 diabetes.[37]

Long-Term Outcomes: Cardiometabolic Disease and Cognition

Among adults, having been breastfed in infancy is associated with reduced risks for type 2 diabetes (pooled OR 0.65, 95% CI 0.49 to 0.86) and obesity or overweight (pooled OR 0.74, 95% CI 0.70 to 0.78).[38] Longer breastfeeding is also associated with a modest increase in IQ (pooled difference 2.62 points, 95% CI 1.25 to 3.98) with adjustment for maternal IQ.[39]

Necrotizing Enterocolitis

For infants born preterm, a diet comprised of mother's own milk is associated with reduced risk for necrotizing enterocolitis.[40] When mother's own milk is not available, donor human milk is recommended as standard of care for preterm infants.[41] Sharing this information with mothers of preterm infants has been shown to increase uptake of breastfeeding without increasing maternal anxiety.[42,43]

CONTRAINDICATIONS TO BREASTFEEDING

There are relatively few contraindications to breastfeeding (Table 6.1). For the infant, classic galactosemia is not compatible with being fed human milk. For some other metabolic disorders, such as phenylketonuria, infants can be breastfed in combination with specialized formula. Mother's milk should not be provided to the infant in the setting of human T-cell lymphotropic virus (HTLV) type I and type II, untreated brucellosis, or use of illicit substances such as cocaine, methamphetamines, or phencyclidine (PCP). Most medications are compatible with breastfeeding, with the exception of chemotherapy and some radioactive compounds. The selection of medications for the breastfeeding mother is covered in detail in Chapter 11. For some infectious diseases, direct breastfeeding is not recommended during the acute phase, but expressed milk can be provided to the infant; these include varicella diagnosed between 5 days before and 2 days after birth, active herpes simplex virus, H1N1 influenza and, in the United States, tuberculosis. Recommendations regarding human immunodeficiency virus (HIV) vary. The World Health Organization recommends that national authorities determine whether breastfeeding and antiretroviral treatment or replacement feeding is the best strategy to ensure infants born to HIV-infected mothers the greatest chance of HIV-free survival. In high-income settings, replacement feeding is recommended, although guidelines are beginning to support mothers making a shared decision regarding breastfeeding with antiretroviral therapy for mother and infant (see Chapter 12). For women using marijuana, nicotine, or

TABLE 6.4 Key Functions of Provider–Patient Communication

Relational	Examples of Language to Discuss Breastfeeding
Fostering healing provider–patient relationships	What have you heard about breastfeeding? How did feeding go with your last baby?
Validating and responding to emotions	What is going well? What's difficult? How can I help you today?
Task-Driven	
Exchanging and managing information	What have you heard about skin to skin? About the early days of breastfeeding? About feeding on cue?
Making treatment decisions	What are your goals for feeding your baby? How have your goals changed over time? What help might make it easier for you? To what extent is breastfeeding making it more or less enjoyable to nurture your baby?
Enabling patient self-management	What have you heard about engorgement? About pain with latch? About expressing at work or school? What has been helpful to you so far?
Managing uncertainty	We know a great deal about how lactation works in dairy animals, but much less about how it works in mothers. In addition, many health care providers are parents, and all of us have been babies. Often, that means the health care team relies on personal experience to give advice. Please let me know if what I'm suggesting doesn't match what you've heard from others.

Modified from Duggan A, Street RL. Interpersonal communication in health and illness. In: Glanz K, Rimer BK, Viswanath K, eds. *Health Behavior: Theory, Research, and Practice.* 5th ed. San Francisco, CA: Jossey-Bass; 2015:243–267.

TABLE 6.5   Major Constructs for Social Cognitive Theory

Cognitive influences on behavior: Personal abilities for processing information, applying knowledge, and changing preferences

Construct	Definition	Explanation
Self-efficacy	A person's confidence in his or her ability to perform a behavior that leads to an outcome.	Self-efficacy is a core SCT construct. Confidence is enhanced through mastery experiences, social modeling, verbal persuasion, and practice under stress-free conditions.
Collective efficacy	Belief in the ability of a group of individuals to perform concerted actions to achieve an outcome.	Because people operate individually and collectively, self-efficacy can be both a personal and a social construct. Group efficacy is enhanced by shared goals, communication, teamwork, and prior success.
Outcome expectations	Outcomes arise from actions. Outcome expectations are judgments about the likely consequences of actions.	Outcome expectations, either positive or negative, are a core SCT construct. Expected consequences can be divided into physical (e.g., use of condoms protects against STDs), social (reactions from others: such as interest, approval, recognition, status), and self-evaluative (reactions to one's own behavior based on internal personal standards).
Knowledge	Knowledge is an understanding of the health risks and benefits of different health practices and the information necessary to perform a behavior.	Knowledge of risks and benefits is a precondition for change. Information is also needed to perform certain behaviors; for example, to cook a healthy meal one needs to know a recipe, where to purchase healthy ingredients, and methods of preparation.

Environmental influences on behavior: Physical and social factors in an individual's environment that affect a person's behavior

Construct	Definition	Explanation
Observational learning	A type of learning in which a person learns new information and behaviors by observing the behaviors of others and the consequences of others' behaviors.	Accomplished by observing an influential role model or peer-leader performing a behavior and achieving an outcome. Methods include observation made in the context of peer-led education, mass media, behavioral journalism, and dramatic performances.
Normative beliefs	Cultural norms and beliefs about the social acceptability and perceived prevalence of a behavior.	Interventions seek to correct normative beliefs (e.g., adolescents' common misperceptions about how many of their peers smoke cigarettes) through discussions of perceptions vs. actual data.
Social support	The perception of encouragement and support a person receives from his or her social network.	Interventions seek to provide informational, instrumental, or emotional support (through, e.g., program flyers, offers to babysit, or a sympathetic conversation) for behavior changes.
Barriers and opportunities	Attributes of the social or physical environment that make behaviors harder or easier to perform.	Interventions seek to facilitate behavior change by increasing opportunities to safely engage in and master the behavior, or by removing impediments to developing the behavior.

Supporting behavioral factors: Actions taken by individuals that can be classified as either health-enhancing (leading to improved health) or health-compromising (leading to poorer health)

Construct	Definition	Explanation
Behavioral skills	The abilities needed to successfully perform a behavior.	Many behaviors require developing a repertoire of specific skills to be successfully enacted. Examples include avoiding high-risk situations, playing a sport, or preparing a healthy meal. Knowledge and skills together make up what is called behavioral capability.
Intentions	The goals of adding new behaviors or modifying existing behaviors, both proximal and distal.	Intentions serve as self-incentives and guides to health behaviors. Attaining specific behaviors is often accomplished by writing or verbalizing goals, setting target dates and activities for skill mastery, and monitoring progress.
Reinforcement and punishment	Behavior can be increased or attenuated through provision or removal of rewards or punishments.	Rewards and punishments can be either tangible (e.g., money, goods, physical ailments, weight gain) or social (e.g., praise, approval, attention, exclusion, or ridicule).

SCT, Social Cognitive Theory; *STD,* sexually transmitted disease.
From Kelder SH, Hoelscher D, Perry C. How individuals, environments and health behaviors interact: social cognitive theory. In: Glanz K, Rimer BK, Viswanath K, eds. *Health Behavior: Theory, Research, and Practice.* 5th ed. San Francisco, CA: Jossey-Bass; 2015:159–181.

alcohol, the risks of infant exposure must be weighed against the risks of replacement feeding (see Chapter 11).

POPULATION HEALTH IMPACT

Given the multiple associations between breastfeeding and health outcomes, enabling breastfeeding has tremendous potential to affect population health. In 2016 *The Lancet* Breastfeeding Series synthesized literature on breastfeeding and health outcomes for children and international data on breastfeeding rates. Victora et al.[44] found that scaling up breastfeeding to near-universal levels globally would prevent 823,000 deaths in children younger than 5 years of age each year. For mothers, the study by *The Lancet* considered only breast cancer and estimated prevention of 22,216 deaths, or 10% of breast cancer deaths annually.

In a US model, Bartick et al.[45] considered the costs attributable to suboptimal breastfeeding for mothers and infants. Disease outcomes modeled included maternal breast and ovarian cancer, diabetes, hypertension, and heart disease, as well as child outcomes of leukemia, otitis media, inflammatory bowel disease, gastrointestinal infection, lower respiratory tract infection, obesity, SIDS, and necrotizing enterocolitis. They found that suboptimal breastfeeding rates were associated with an annual excess of 3340 maternal deaths (95% CI 1886 to 4785) and 721 pediatric deaths (95% CI 543 to 899). Excess annual medical costs totaled $604,873,116 for children and $2,417,207,838 for mothers.

A global model (Tables 6.2 and 6.3) considered costs for children (diarrhea, acute respiratory infection, child obesity, cognitive function) and mothers (breast cancer, ovarian cancer, and type 2 diabetes) and found that not breastfeeding was responsible for 595,379 child deaths and 98,943 maternal deaths each year.[46] Health costs were estimated at $1.1 billion annually, and costs related to cognitive loss were estimated at $285 billion. The financial impact varied by region, ranging from 0.42% to 2.58% of gross national income per capita. The authors concluded, "The substantial human and economic costs of not breastfeeding in countries with low breastfeeding rates can to some extent be reversed with government, donor and civil society action to increase the financing envelope available for the evidence-based high-impact breastfeeding and nutrition interventions and policies."

FROM POPULATION TO PATIENT: COUNSELING THE FEEDING DECISION

Given the wide range of health outcomes affected by breastfeeding, major medical organizations recommend exclusive breastfeeding for the first 6 months of life, with continued breastfeeding as complementary foods are introduced through 1 to 2 years or longer as mutually desired.[47–51] Globally, the vast majority of women initiate breastfeeding; however, exclusivity and duration fall short of these consensus recommendations.

Theories of Health Behavior Change

Knowledge alone is not sufficient to change behavior.[52] Theories of health behavior have identified multiple factors that affect whether an individual is willing and able to engage in a particular health behavior, ranging from individual-level considerations to national and even international policies that affect the individual's context. This theoretical framework is supported by studies of maternal feeding decisions: in a meta-synthesis, Nelson found that most women know "breastfeeding is best"; their feeding decisions stemmed from multiple other domains.[53] Themes included feeling pressured to make a particular choice by health professionals and/or family members, concerns about breastfeeding in public, discomfort associated with so much physical contact with the infant, confidence—or lack of confidence—based on prior experience, the need for ongoing support, and concerns about constraints on personal lifestyle and independence.

In clinical care, the patient-provider interaction is a critical domain for motivating and supporting health behaviors such as breastfeeding. Duggan and Street[54] identify six key functions of provider–patient communication (Table 6.4). The first two functions are relational. Patients want providers to be respectful, friendly, interested, nonjudgmental, and sensitive, and to address their needs holistically.[55] They also want providers to validate their emotions and assist them to cope with setbacks and uncertainty. Provider–patient communication also serves task-driven functions. Exchanging and managing information enables the provider and patient to reach a shared understanding of the patient's circumstances; this requires more than a simple transmission of information from the provider to the patient. From this shared

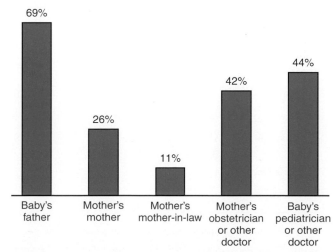

Fig. 6.1 Percent of pregnant women indicating that the opinion of selected individuals is especially important in her decision about how to feed her baby. (Data from Infant Feeding Practices Study II, Table 1.34. https://www.cdc.gov/breastfeeding/pdf/ifps/data/ifps2_tables_ch1.pdf. Accessed May 16, 2020.)

understanding, the patient and provider can make a shared treatment decision, recognizing that the patient's desire to be responsible for the final decision varies. The provider also enables the patient to self-manage the health condition and helps the patient manage uncertainty.

These concepts apply to conversations about infant feeding. A rote statement by the provider that "breast is best" (or that not breastfeeding is risky) is unlikely to have an impact on a patient's feeding decision. Effective counseling begins with establishing a relationship with the patient. Open-ended questions, such as "What have you heard about breastfeeding?" or, "How did feeding go with your last baby?" demonstrate interest and indicate respect for her lived experience. Many mothers wean earlier than desired, and validating

TABLE 6.6   Maternal Perception of Family Members' and Providers Opinion About Infant Feeding and Odds of Not Initiating Breastfeeding

	n (2041)	% Not Initiating	Adjusted Odds Ratio[a]	95% CI
Feeding Preference by Family Members				
Infant's Father				
Breastfeeding only	1,141	1.9	Reference	
Formula only	135	82.2	110.4	52.0–234.4
Breastfeeding + formula	350	10.0	3.2	1.7–5.9
No opinion or do not know	415	26.8	7.6	4.5–12.7
Maternal Grandmother				
Breastfeeding only	814	1.6	Reference	
Formula only	161	55.3	15.9	7.0–36.0
Breastfeeding + formula	317	8.2	2.0	0.9–4.5
No opinion or do not know	749	20.2	5.4	2.6–11.0
Paternal Grandmother				
Breastfeeding only	595	3.4	Reference	
Formula only	119	39.5	0.5	0.2–1.4
Breastfeeding + formula	261	8.4	1.4	0.6–3.3
No opinion or do not know	1,066	17.8	1.4	0.8–2.7
Feeding Preference by Providers				
Infant's Doctor				
Breastfeeding only	919	4.8	Reference	
Formula only	25	88.0	2.0	0.2–18.8
Breastfeeding + formula	247	17.8	2.7	1.2–6.2
No opinion or do not know	850	19.9	1.9	1.0–3.7
Mother's Doctor				
Breastfeeding only	882	5.0	Reference	
Formula only	29	75.9	5.4	0.8–38.3
Breastfeeding + formula	242	17.8	1.3	0.5–3.0
No opinion or do not know	888	19.1	1.3	0.7–2.6

[a]All sociodemographic covariates, the family, and the health care provider's opinions were entered simultaneously into the model. Covariates included maternal age; parity; marital status; education; household poverty level; participation in the Special Supplemental Nutrition Program for Women, Infants, and Children (WIC); and ethnicity.

From Odom EC, Li R, Scanlon KS, et al. Association of family and health care provider opinion on infant feeding with mother's breastfeeding decision. *J Acad Nutr Diet*. 2014;114(8):1203–1207. PMC4443256.

TABLE 6.7 Results From a Metasynthesis of Qualitative Studies of Breastfeeding Support Among Women

Categories and Themes	Examples of Quotations
EXAMPLES OF QUOTATIONS FROM REVIEWED ARTICLES	
Authentic Presence	
Being there for me	I know she's there for me whenever I want her....I don't know her (peer supporter), but I seem to feel I can rely on her all the time
Empathetic Approach	Well, I think the, just the... they were so warm... you felt total trust in the fact they knew what they were talking about, and they knew what I was going through
Taking time, touching base	It seemed important to her... she took time to talk to me, asked me questions, and she gave me suggestions
Providing affirmation	She would just say: "You're doing fine, you're doing fine" when I was thinking that I was doing something wrong
Being responsive, sharing the experience	I got help when I needed it and not just about breastfeeding Even just sitting there, having a cup of tea while I was trying to feed, was the most help I could want. So I wasn't on my own You think nobody understands. It's so nice to have somebody to talk to, because it does encourage you, because they have done it and they will come out and help you
Having a Relationship	But her coming around is also relationship-based. She's not coming round just to do her duty, she comes to build a relationship and that actually makes you feel comfortable around her, to actually talk to her and open up to her
Facilitative Style	
Realistic information	A balanced discussion of the advantages and disadvantages of different feeding options would be most useful...A presentation of both sides-breast versus bottle Focusing to a greater extent on how to overcome common difficulties, albeit in an "it does get better" framework
Accurately and sufficiently detailed information	Answer(ing) all my questions for me It would have been more helpful if I had information on possible baby behaviors and many different stories on breastfeeding patterns so I would not have been so uncertain for the first days
Encouragement for breastfeeding	I am surprised to find that I hardly know any people who breastfed their babies, so it was difficult to have a role model. I feel that more should be done at parent craft classes to encourage mothers to breastfeed
Encourage dialogue	They give you a whole bunch of papers, then they say, "Here, read this." That's your education. I think it would be best if they went over it with you. Just not like you're illiterate, but go over it with you instead of just expecting you to go home and read it
Offering practical help and being proactive	It was the first time. We just couldn't seem to get it right. I felt like all thumbs. Then a nurse came in and told me to put his stomach next to mine. She moved him around so he could get my breast. What a difference that made. Such a little thing.
Reductionist Approach	
Conflicting information and advice	Every single midwife who came in had an entirely different opinion on what to do and it was just, it was far too confusing
Standard information	They tell you in health talk. "They use medical jargon", and "Her explanations were real technical. I guess I felt a bit rushed." There are a lot of things I asked them (nurses) not to do. I know they have rules, but it means a lot to me to do it my way...to feed him when he's hungry, not when they say it's time
Didactic approach	No one asked me what I wanted Some aren't interested in what others have told you I wasn't ready for her telling me how to express. I wasn't at the stage where I wanted to know about that. I felt things were going well...she was determined to tell me

(Continued)

TABLE 6.7   Results From a Metasynthesis of Qualitative Studies of Breastfeeding Support Among Women—cont'd

EXAMPLES OF QUOTATIONS FROM REVIEWED ARTICLES

Categories and Themes	Examples of Quotations
Disconnected Encounters	
Undermining and blaming	I had great difficulty getting him to latch on or suck, and I very much felt the midwives blamed me for this. When I said to one, "it isn't easy", she replied, "Of course it's easy, all the other mothers can do it!"
Feeling Pressured	It's really drummed into people, you know, breastfeeding is best, you shouldn't bottle feed and I just when I changed her over to the bottle I just felt guilty because everyone there's so much hype about breastfeeding, and she is just as happy, if not more, on the bottle. You know, I don't think they should drum it into you as much. You know "you should breastfeed." It's your decision, it's up to every individual
	She [health-visitor] said "Well, that's 2 weeks, and she hasn't made up her birthweight. It just means we'll have to take the child to care if you're going to persist with this breastfeeding." I thought that was a terrible thing to say
Communicating temporal pressure; they do not give you the time	They are so busy, they don't have the time to sit and help you do it. They really don't. They are rushed off their feet, and are quite harassed, and I was quite willing to give up
	From day 1, I thought I would breastfeed, but when I went into the hospital, and I wasn't getting much help, I just thought, "Stuff it…I didn't even know how to start myself, and the nurse showed me once, but after that I still couldn't do it…and I started getting myself depressed and anxious, and I thought, "No, I won't be able to cope"
Insensitive and invasive touch	They're trying to grab, grab onto your breast. And trying to get it into his mouth

From Schmeid V, Beake S, Sheehan A, et al. Women's perceptions and experiences of breastfeeding support: a metasynthesis. Birth. 2011; 38(1): 49–60.

emotions about a difficult prior breastfeeding experience is important to build a trusting relationship. With respect to task-driven functions, information about the health importance of breastfeeding should be aligned with the patient's stated interests and priorities. Exclusive breastfeeding requires a substantial commitment of time and energy, and the mother is uniquely positioned to determine what is "worth it" given her life circumstances and context. Anticipatory guidance, such as engorgement, leaking, positioning and latch, and sustaining breastfeeding when separated from the infant, can facilitate self-management of common breastfeeding concerns. Finally, when challenges are encountered, clinicians can help women manage uncertainty and take a stepwise approach to working through difficulties.

In the rare case when breastfeeding is contraindicated (see Table 6.1), the mother may be disappointed that she will not be able to breastfeed or will need to wean earlier than planned. Open-ended questions, such as "What are your thoughts about not breastfeeding?" may be helpful to inform discussion. Opportunities for nurturing at the breast, such as skin-to-skin care, can be explored. Mothers may also wish to consider donor human milk.

Although good provider–patient communication is necessary, it is not sufficient to enable sustained breastfeeding. Bandura's social cognitive theory offers a helpful construct for considering the multiple factors that have an impact on the process of adopting a new health behavior[56] (Table 6.5).

This theory incorporates cognitive influences, environmental influences, and supporting behavioral factors that affect behavior change. Within the cognitive domain, knowledge of risks and benefits is a precondition for change, but alone, such knowledge is insufficient. In addition, self-efficacy is needed, as well as an expectation that the desired behavior will improve outcomes. Bandura's work also addresses the role of physical and social factors that affect behavior, including opportunities to observe the behavior, cultural norms, encouragement from within the individual's social network, and barriers and opportunities to perform the behavior. Finally, behavioral factors include learned skills, intentions, and rewards or punishments for performing the behavior.

Providers can incorporate these domains into their counseling and education. To address self-efficacy, it can be helpful to discuss breastfeeding as a learned behavior. Like learning to ride a bicycle, it takes time and patience to move from the somewhat frantic wobbling of a first time off training wheels to an efficient and enjoyable mode of transportation. Setting realistic expectations can prepare families for early challenges. Connecting families with opportunities for observational learning and social support is key; local breastfeeding mothers' groups often welcome expectant mothers and provide opportunities to see and interact with other breastfeeding women. Partners, grandparents, and other support persons should be invited to prenatal visits and breastfeeding classes so that their questions and concerns can be addressed and they can learn how to support the mother—baby dyad. To facilitate learning skills, practicing breastfeeding positioning with dolls or other props may be helpful. During the maternity stay, supporting the mother and her support person(s) to position and attach can ensure that hands-on support is available after discharge. To support intentions, mothers can be encouraged to review their progress every 5 to 7 days and evaluate which strategies are helpful and which are not. Finally, providers may consider reinforcements for sustaining breastfeeding. Pediatrician Jenny Thomas gives "Got Breastmilk" t-shirts to 1-year-olds in her practice who have breastfed for 12 months, and posts their photographs in a prominent location in the her office.[57]

Provider Opinions and Counseling

Physicians and other health care providers can encourage women to initiate and sustain breastfeeding by sharing information on its importance for maternal and child health.

Mothers value their provider's opinion; in a study that compared perceptions of mothers and of providers, 39% of mothers thought their obstetric clinician's advice on breastfeeding duration was very important, but only 8% of obstetric clinicians thought their opinion was important.[58]

In the Infant Feeding Practices Study II (IFPS II), more pregnant women rated their health care provider's opinion on infant feeding as "very important" than their mother or mother-in-law's opinion (Fig. 6.1). Indeed, when a mother in IFPS II perceived that her infant's physician favors mixed feeding or is unaware of the provider's opinion, she was less likely to initiate breastfeeding than when her infant's doctor recommends exclusive breastfeeding.[59] A similar pattern was found for the mother's provider, although the association was not significant when adjusted for family opinions and sociodemographic factors (Table 6.6).

Delivery of prenatal breastfeeding counseling varies. In an analysis of data from the 2010 Pregnancy Risk Assessment

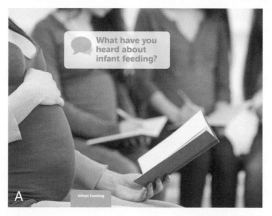

What have you heard about infant feeding?
Have you or anyone that you've known breastfed before?

MAIN MESSAGE

Each of us have a unique opinions on infant feeding formed from our own experiences and those of others we know. As part of your healthcare team, we want you to know the facts.

POINTS TO COVER

• Knowing the facts will help you **make informed choices** that are best for your family. Together, we can help you meet your own personal infant feeding goals.

• Take a look at the facts on pages 4 and 5 of the booklet - do any of these facts surprise you? Let's talk about the ones that caught your attention.

ⓘ *Refer to Pages 4-5 of the patient booklet, "Find Out the Facts!" Allow time for review and discussion. Share with her that these facts are based on the most common misbeliefs parents have - she is not alone.*

ⓘ **TEACHABLE MOMENT**

This discussion is perhaps the most important part of this counseling curriculum. **Please allow adequate time for her feelings to be revealed.** *Establish a mutual trust through* **unbiased active listening.** *What you learn will help you tailor the education you provide to her unique needs.*

• *Listen attentively and thank her for sharing what she's heard about breastfeeding.*

• *Be sure to **validate** her experience and **affirm** that you heard what she shared.*

• *Remember **there are no right or wrong opinions** - corrections may stifle expression.*

• ***Do not judge** her comments from your own experience or perception. Just listen and affirm.*

• *Remember, skin-to-skin, rooming-in, and feeding on cue are important best practices for **all babies,** regardless of how they are fed.*

B

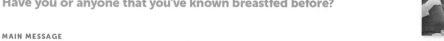

Fig. 6.2 Patient-facing and provider-facing content from Ready, Set Baby. (A) A flip-chart educational tool pairs an open-ended question for the family with (B) talking points to cover for the health educator. (From Carolina Global Breastfeeding Institute. Ready, Set, Baby: a guide to welcoming your new family member. Patient Booklet and Educator Flipchart. Version 3, 2018. Chapel Hill, NC: Carolina Global Breastfeeding Institute.)

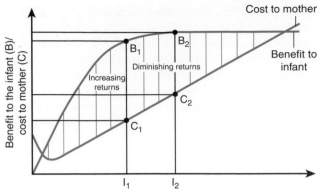

Fig. 6.3 Theoretical mother–infant trade-offs in infant feeding. (From Tully KP, Ball HL. Trade-offs underlying maternal breastfeeding decisions: a conceptual model. *Matern Child Nutr.* 2013;9[1]:90–98.)

Monitoring System, 17% of women in the United States reported that breastfeeding was not addressed during prenatal care.[60] In this sample, women who were more likely to report being counseled on breastfeeding were younger, Hispanic or non-Hispanic black, primiparous, overweight, not privately insured, not married, and received Special Supplemental Nutrition Program for Women, Infants, and Children (WIC) services during pregnancy. As the authors acknowledge, a limitation of the study was that it assessed whether breastfeeding was addressed, but did not assess the quality of the counseling provided. The groups that were more likely to report receiving counseling had lower rates of breastfeeding initiation and continuation in 2010, underscoring that a discussion during prenatal care is not sufficient to overcome structural barriers and enable women to initiate and sustain breastfeeding.

The quality of counseling also varies. In an analysis of transcripts of initial prenatal visits at an urban, hospital-based prenatal clinic, breastfeeding was addressed in just 29%

of visits, and the mean duration of the breastfeeding discussion was 39 seconds.[61] Certified nurse midwives were more likely than obstetric residents to discuss breastfeeding and to use a facilitative approach that validated patient concerns and explored solutions.

The value of such conversation-based, facilitative discussions is supported by a meta-synthesis of qualitative studies of breastfeeding support.[62] Women valued an authentic presence, characterized by a trusting relationship with the caregiver, and a facilitative style that centered education on the learner and encouraged dialogue. In contrast, women disliked reductionist interactions that presented standard information and described disconnected encounters that undermined or blamed the woman (Table 6.7).

The Carolina Global Breastfeeding Institute has developed Ready, Set, Baby, a free visually based curriculum for prenatal conversations about infant feeding.[63] The curriculum includes a patient booklet and a flip chart with patient-facing prompts for conversation and instructor-facing guidance on key concepts to share (Fig. 6.2). The tool includes specific guidance on active listening, validation, and nonjudgement, consistent with key tenets of patient-provider communication. In a pre-post study, completion of the curriculum increased knowledge about baby-friendly practices, feeding cues, and the health importance of breastfeeding and strengthened infant feeding intention. Materials are available in multiple languages for download from https://sph.unc.edu/cgbi/resources-ready-set-baby/.

Consistent with tenets of provider–patient communication and social cognitive theory, facilitative, conversation-based counseling along with hands-on support also appears to be more effective than simply providing standardized advice. In a randomized controlled trial in New York City, women were allocated to one-on-one counseling from an international board-certified lactation consultant (IBCLC), electronic prompts to the patient's provider to discuss breastfeeding during prenatal care, or both.[64] Compared with the control group, women allocated to IBCLC

BOX 6.1 Language to Consider When Counseling the Mother Who Is Struggling With Breastfeeding

- Remember that breastfeeding is a part of motherhood, not the point of motherhood.
- You are uniquely qualified to weigh the health importance of breastfeeding with the demands of sustaining breastfeeding for you and your baby. Every 5 to 7 days, pause to think about how breastfeeding is going and decide whether it is what makes sense for you and your baby.
- You can nurture your baby at the breast no matter how much milk you make.
- A supplemental nursing system (SNS) is helpful for some mothers. With an SNS, you can stimulate your breasts while supplementing your baby. Try this for a few feedings to see you it works for you. You also might try using hand expression to transfer more of your milk to your baby at an at-breast feeding, rather than pumping after nursing. If your baby is being supplemented routinely, consider providing the supplement first, and then offering the breast for dessert, so your baby can fall asleep satisfied at the breast.
- There are many ways to nurture a baby—try different approaches until you find a way that feels right for you. Above all, make sure to enjoy your baby. Make sure to balance enjoying your baby with making milk!
- Moms often ask whether they will have trouble making milk in a future pregnancy. Moms who have struggled with one baby are more likely to face challenges the next time around, but there are many factors that affect breastfeeding. It can be helpful to meet with a lactation consultant or breastfeeding medicine specialist during your next pregnancy so that you have a plan in place.

counseling and support were more likely to be breastfeeding at high intensity at 3 months; the prompts alone had no effect on feeding outcomes. Of note, in qualitative feedback, providers reported that they lacked the knowledge and counseling skills to respond to patient questions about infant feeding.[65]

Context and Trade-Offs

Even when families receive evidence-based information and support delivered with attention to key tenets of patient–provider communication, some mothers decide not to breastfeed, to mix feed, or to discontinue breastfeeding earlier than recommended by medical authorities. Shared decision making does not mean that the patient decides to follow the recommendation of the health care provider; rather, shared decision making brings together at least two experts, the patient and the provider.

While breastfeeding is often portrayed as a mutually rewarding and joyous endeavor, the costs and benefits to mother and infant differ. Tully and Ball[66] present decision-making about breastfeeding in the context of maternal–offspring conflict, noting that returns may diminish over time (Fig. 6.3). They propose that strategies to both reduce costs and increase benefits are needed to facilitate longer durations of breastfeeding.

Acknowledging these trade-offs has the potential to address issues of guilt and shame around the infant feeding decisions of individual mothers. On a population level, higher breastfeeding rates are associated with better health outcomes for mothers and for infants. However, different dyads encounter different costs to sustain breastfeeding. In some cases, social constraints such as lack of access to paid leave or caregiving demands for other family members preclude breastfeeding. Providers should be informed about legal protections and policies and share this information with patients to address structural barriers. For mother–infant dyads struggling with pain or milk supply problems, the clinician's first recourse is to work with the family to implement corrective measures. However, sometimes lactation, like any other bodily process, does not function. As Marianne Neifert has written:[67]

The bold claims made about the infallibility of lactation are not cited about any other physiologic processes. A health care professional would never tell a diabetic woman that "every pancreas can make insulin" or insist to a devastated infertility patient that "every woman can get pregnant." The fact is that lactation, like all physiologic functions, sometimes fails because of various medical causes.

Provider–patient communication is perhaps most important when counseling the mother for whom breastfeeding is coming undone (Box 6.1). It may be helpful to advise that breastfeeding is a part of motherhood, not the point of motherhood. If the effort required to sustain breastfeeding is interfering with the mother's ability to care for herself or her child, then for them, breastfeeding may not be "best." The mother is the only person who can say with certainty what is "worth it."

For the mother who is not able to meet all of the infant's nutritional needs, it may be helpful to try out options for supplementing at breast, such as with a supplemental nursing system (SNS). Some women love the SNS; others may find it cumbersome or intrusive. When maternal production does not match infant needs, it may be helpful to consider starting with supplementation, and then offering the breast "for dessert." This strategy can avoid a prolonged struggle between a hungry baby and a tearful mother that is resolved when another caregiver "rescues" the feeding with a bottle of donor milk or formula. These strategies can be offered to families as "options on the menu" to support a sustainable, nurturing relationship at breast.

More broadly, clinicians can advocate for policies and protections that remove societal barriers and lower the costs of breastfeeding for all women. As Bernice Hausman writes,[68] "Changing the bottle-feeding culture that we live in is a political enterprise that cannot be accomplished solely by advertising risks to replacement feeding or heralding the medicinal qualities of breast milk."

The Reference list is available at www.expertconsult.com.

7

Practical Management of the Nursing "Dyad"

Casey Rosen-Carole and Alison M. Stuebe

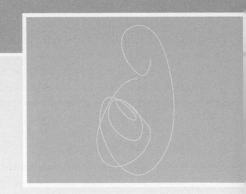

KEY POINTS

- Breastfeeding units are best conceived of as physiologically interrelated, or "dyads," although each family may include multiple interdependent dyads (e.g., those with multiples or more than one lactating parent).
- Supporting lactation and breastfeeding requires understanding a rich tapestry, including the physiology of milk production, the mechanics of milk transfer, normal infant

- behavior and growth, and the multiple social forces that enable or prevent achieving parental goals.
- Solving problems in lactation depends on addressing three components for each dyad: milk production (the mother), milk transfer, and infant oral function and growth.

Management of lactation begins with understanding the dyadic process of milk production, latching on, suckling, and milk transfer (see Chapter 3). For millennia, women have fed their young at the breast. Support for these women was, and is, culturally mediated. In some areas of the world, women support each other; in other areas, this cultural practice has been erased. Especially in areas lacking strong cultural support for breastfeeding, the medical provider plays a critical role in enabling human lactation.

Successful nursing depends on the interaction of mother and infant (the "dyad"), with appropriate support from other parents, the family, available health care resources, and the community. Because mothers and infants vary, there is not a simple set of rules that will guarantee success. In fact, lactation may not be limited to a mother and infant: gender nonconforming families may include several parents who desire to lactate, induce lactation, or feed donor milk to their children. Twins and triplets with differing health status may add complications in terms of milk production, timing, and transfer. Therefore lactation should be evaluated just like any other physiologic process—providers must understand the anatomy and physiology of lactation, assess and manage problems, and use complex decision-making procedures to enable the best outcomes.[1] Different from other processes is the analysis of the dyadic interplay of two physiologies involved in milk transfer. Unfortunately, many physicians have not received formal education about breastfeeding; thus they gain information from a variety of sources, including personal experiences, and may generalize from these sources without complete knowledge.[2-4]

This chapter addresses the basic management of breastfeeding, including common and less common issues that may arise. Because it is not written for a lay audience, other books may be used for patient education, including K. Huggins's *The Nursing Mother's Companion*, now in its 8th edition after more than

30 years of inspiring mothers to breastfeed.[5] *The Womanly Art of Breastfeeding* from La Leche League International is also available.[6] The World Health Organization (WHO) and United Nations Children's Fund (UNICEF) have a variety of country-specific resources and publications in multiple languages to support breastfeeding around the world. The references for this chapter are not an exhaustive list of all material written on the topic; rather, they are intended to assist a reader in locating research that supports the evidence-based concepts described here. This chapter is divided into two major parts. The first part describes routine management of lactation perinatally: (1) prenatal period; (2) immediate postpartum, or hospital, period; and (3) postnatal, or posthospital, period. The second part provides a structure for the diagnosis and management of breastfeeding problems.

BASIC PRACTICAL MANAGEMENT OF LACTATION

Current Practices in the United States and Internationally

Although recommendations on infant feeding are clear, infant feeding practices continue to depart substantially from these guidelines. Infant feeding and care practices in the United States were assessed by the US Department of Health and Human Services and published as a supplement to *Pediatrics* in 2008.[7] This publication documents various aspects of infant feeding, as reported by more than 2000 women nationally for 1 year postpartum in 2004, and compares results with a similar study in 1993. In this cohort, approximately half of breastfed infants had received infant formula in the birth hospitalization, and nearly half were being fed solid foods before the age of 4 months.[6] The most frequently reported reason for weaning at any age was the maternal perception that the child was not satisfied by breast milk alone.[8,9] In addition, a new trend emerged: approximately 6% of women fed their children expressed breast milk without ever putting their child to the breast, a trend that continues and is arguably increasing in the United States.[10] *The Lancet* 2016 series on breastfeeding included a more global perspective and reported that high-income countries had shorter breastfeeding duration than low- or middle-income countries, but that only 37% of infants younger than 6 months were exclusively breastfed even in these latter categories.[11] In addition, people with lower incomes tended to breastfeed longer than their wealthier counterparts in all country groupings, although in the United States, this social gradient reversed in the 1960s.

It is therefore important to note that practices surrounding infant feeding vary widely. Although we have learned much about appropriate management, there remain large gaps in the literature. Therefore medical providers should be transparent with families about what is anecdotal about advice as opposed to what is evidence based. In addition, when formulating support plans, it is critical to acknowledge the variety of cultural influences on the management of breastfeeding, including geography, religion, and other social pressures from family or employers. Given that about 1 in 3 women worldwide has experienced physical and/or sexual violence, concerns for privacy, safety, and touch (both by the infant and by the provider) should be kept in mind.[12] Women who have experienced intimate partner violence may be less likely to initiate breastfeeding and will need their providers to be carefully attuned to their medical and psychosocial needs.[13] (See also Breastfeeding Among Trauma Survivors, Chapter 15.)

The key to counseling the nursing couple lies in supporting parental decision-making, enabling a sense of confidence, and providing rapid access to support when required. Then, when a problem arises, a mechanism is already in place for a mother to receive help from her provider's office before the problem creates a serious medical complication.

PRENATAL BREASTFEEDING EDUCATION AND MANAGEMENT

Decision to Breastfeed and Informed Consent

Most decisions regarding breastfeeding initiation are made in the preconception or prenatal period; few women who intend to formula-feed change their minds at birth.[14–16] Therefore, ideally, education regarding breastfeeding should occur early in life or in the preconception period. Family planning counseling may provide obstetric providers with a brief moment to discuss breastfeeding in relation to a normal breast exam.

Support

Along with the medical provider, a breastfeeding family is likely to need and use support from other places, including family, friends, lactation consultants, employers, support groups, and online/technology-mediated support (see Chapter 16). In general, such supports should be encouraged and online resources

fact-checked. Bringing a support person along for a visit is likely to be helpful when counseling about breastfeeding or managing breastfeeding problems.[17]

Prenatal Period

It is most effective to prepare for breastfeeding well in advance of delivery, if possible, in preconception or at the first prenatal visit. The Academy of Breastfeeding Medicine (ABM) provides a helpful protocol titled "Breastfeeding Promotion in the Prenatal Setting."[3] Particularly with first children, it is appropriate to suggest to the parents that they select a pediatric care provider early. Some pediatric providers offer a prenatal visit to discuss infant feeding, care concerns, and child-rearing questions. In some places, the medical profession has been hesitant to take anything but a neutral position in discussions of breastfeeding for fear of pressuring mothers or creating guilt. Manufacturers of infant formula have capitalized on this and created advertising campaigns designed to further polarize parents toward victimization.[3] Despite this, the ethical principle of autonomy makes clear a provider's duty with respect to parents: evidence is clear that breast-milk substitutes (infant formula) carry risk; breastfeeding is an important health care decision with implications for lifelong health, and parents have the right to be advised and make informed choices. Finally, as support for breastfeeding has increased, so, too, have negative emotions experienced by mothers who are using infant formula.[18] Studies from around the world show that parents use informal information sources to learn best formula-feeding practices and that many practices are therefore unsafe.[19] The prenatal discussion should therefore include discussions of benefits and risks of infant feeding options, answers to any questions the parents may have about the lactation process and a mother's ability to make milk, and medically approved resources to support further learning.

Breast and Nipple Exam

An examination of the breasts is part of good prenatal care and an excellent opportunity to discuss breastfeeding. For detailed information on breast and nipple examination, see Chapter 25.

Resources Versus Discussion

Although a provider may give literature on breastfeeding or suggest reading sources for the patient, decision-making will be enhanced by open discussion with a knowledgeable provider. Childbirth preparation programs in the community and breastfeeding classes offered by lactation consultants or peer counselors may help prepare families for breastfeeding. However, the role of the care provider in promoting and supporting breastfeeding remains important, both by making a clear recommendation to breastfeed, where appropriate, and in ensuring best practices are followed after birth to support the family's choice.[20,21] A 2017 Cochrane review found that support improved exclusivity and duration at 6 weeks and 6 months postpartum.[17]

Although decisions to breastfeed include consideration of the health of the infant and mother, concerns about breastfeeding reported prenatally include medical as well as social concerns and are reported similarly around the world.[22–25] Authors have suggested prenatal counseling toolkits, including the "Ready, Set, BABY" counseling approach, and have found increases in breastfeeding intention.[26] The American College of Obstetrics and Gynecology has a toolkit with patient handouts and resources, and the WHO/UNICEF offers online access to handouts in different languages.[27] Table 7.1 reviews the most commonly expressed concerns in the prenatal period, along with counseling points for providers. (See Chapter 6 for making an informed decision, and see Chapter 16 for managing common concerns about the nipples and breasts.)

Hand Expression Prenatally

Prenatal hand expression has been discouraged because of the concern for the stimulation of uterine contraction, early labor, and prepartum mastitis. However, no significant harms were found in the Diabetes and Antenatal Milk Expressing (DAME) trial by Forster et al.[28] In this multicenter randomized controlled trial (RCT), 635 women with diabetes in pregnancy were randomized to hand expression twice daily starting at 36 weeks' gestation or standard care. There were no between-group differences in birth characteristics or infant admission to the neonatal intensive care unit (NICU), and there was a beneficial effect on exclusive breast-milk feeding in the first 24 hours of hospitalization after birth; however, there was no difference in exclusive breastfeeding across the birth hospitalization or in any or exclusive breastfeeding at 3 months. Given the concerns raised in studies on breast and nipple preparation, maternal experience is important to consider. In a qualitative study among 19 primiparous women recruited from a US midwifery practice, Demirci et al. found that twice-daily prenatal hand expression was considered easy to fit into their lives and increased their confidence in breastfeeding.[29]

Nipple Stimulation and Labor Management

Breast stimulation triggers the release of oxytocin from the posterior pituitary and has been used to augment or induce labor. In a Cochrane meta-analysis comparing breast stimulation with usual care, women allocated to breast stimulation were more likely to labor within 72 hours and less likely to have a postpartum hemorrhage; of note, in subgroup analyses, breast stimulation was effective for women with a favorable cervix but not for women with an unfavorable cervix.[30]

In an RCT in India ($n = 199$), primiparous women were allocated to breast massage for 15 to 20 minutes three times a day or usual care.[31] Women allocated to breast massage were less likely to birth by cesarean (8% vs. 20.4%). In a study in Turkey of women with a Bishop's score of 6 or higher ($n = 390$), nipple stimulation was performed for 4 to 5 minutes every 30 minutes; there were no C-sections in the nipple-stimulation group, and only 9.2% of primiparas and 4.6% of multiparas required synthetic oxytocin. In the control group, 8.5% of women underwent C-section, and oxytocin was required in 92.3% of primiparas and 86.2% of multiparas.[32] Tachystole and bradycardia have been described secondary to nipple stimulation in a case report; terbutaline

was administered, with recovery of the fetal heart tracing and subsequent uncomplicated vaginal birth.[33]

In a small feasibility study ($n = 16$) of 1 hour of nipple stimulation on 3 consecutive days, salivary oxytocin levels were highest on day 3; a subsequent study comparing women performing nipple stimulation with controls found that oxytocin increased from day 1 to day 3 in the nipple-stimulation group but not in the control group; however, there was no difference in onset of labor between the two groups.[34,35]

Nipple stimulation or infant suckling has also been studied for the management of the third stage of labor and reduction of postpartum hemorrhage. A Cochrane review found insufficient evidence on the effect of nipple stimulation for reducing maternal morbidity or postpartum blood loss.[36] A subsequently published randomized clinical trial compared intermittent breast stimulation to an infusion of 30 IU oxytocin per 1000 mL infusate (maximum rate of 10 mL (0.3 IU) per minute) after delivery.[37] There were no differences in the duration of the third stage, estimated blood loss, or change in hemoglobin from before delivery to 24 hours after delivery; however, maternal satisfaction was higher and pain was lower in the nipple-stimulation group. Of note, none of the women in the study held their infant skin to skin or breastfed during the third stage, which limits the generalizability of the results.

Summary of Appropriate Prenatal Management

1. During preconception or at the first prenatal visit, begin to explore patient knowledge and attitudes about breastfeeding. During the first trimester, perform a breast examination and address any concerns. Continue (or begin) the discussion about how the infant is to be fed and the benefits of breastfeeding.
2. Inquire about other influences on breastfeeding. Encourage the participation of fathers, other parents, or support people at visits. Consider referring families to a prenatal pediatric visit, childbirth classes, or breastfeeding classes. Knowledge of community resources is vital. At each prenatal visit, offer information about breastfeeding and address any concerns.
3. In the second trimester, discuss the importance of skin-to-skin contact after birth, rooming-in, and feeding on cue, and address any concerns.
4. If a patient has risk factors for delayed lactogenesis 2 or low milk supply, consider encouraging antenatal milk expression, and support the patient to make plans for early follow-up after discharge with a pediatric provider.
5. To address prenatal anticipatory guidance, hand expression, and postpartum care, consider adding a board-certified lactation consultant to your staff.

Immediate Postpartum/Hospital Management

Birth practices, doulas, and medications in labor are addressed in Chapter 15.

Immediate Postpartum Period/The First Hour

Immediately after the placenta has separated, the establishment of lactation begins. Breastfeeding is thus considered the

TABLE 7.1 Mothers' Expressed Concerns About Breastfeeding When Interviewed Prenatally, Along With Counseling Points

Prenatal Concern	Evidence	Prenatal Counseling Points
Will I make enough milk?/Will baby latch and grow?	Because of the difficulty with measurement and diagnosis of low milk supply, studies vary on the prevalence of this issue. Estimates vary, but between 8% and 30% of mothers experience low milk supply in the first 2 weeks postpartum.[201] Risk factors for low milk supply include (1) anatomic/medical concerns, such as mammary hypoplasia or no breast changes in pregnancy; (2) early disruption of milk removal through separation and supplementation with infant formula; and (3) conditions related to delayed lactogenesis 2 (after 72 hours) and milk supply (including hypertension, gestational diabetes, maternal age >30, primiparity, maternal body mass index >25, excess maternal gestational weight gain, infant birth weight >3600 g, preterm birth [and possible timing of antenatal steroids], and infrequent feeding or latch difficulties after birth.[202–205] In addition, environmental and medical exposures, such as medications, tobacco smoking, smoke exposure, and alcohol use, may affect milk supply (see Chapter 11).	• Most women make enough breast milk, and most babies will learn to latch. • There are effective interventions to support milk production, such as skin to skin, rooming-in, and frequent feeding on cue. • Identify postpartum supports for families so that they may access them when a concern arises. • If a mother is at risk for low milk supply, she should be counseled to limit her risk factors when possible (e.g., tobacco, unnecessary medications); may consider antenatal colostrum expression to improve confidence, time to lactogenesis 2, and milk supply (see section on antenatal hand expression later in the chapter)[a]; and should have close postpartum follow-up with trained lactation consultants.
Will it hurt?	Although many women are told that breastfeeding is a joyful experience and shouldn't hurt, estimates suggest that from 10% to 96% of mothers report pain while breastfeeding.[b] As lactation consultants and experienced breastfeeding women know, seemingly small changes in positioning and offering the breast can make large impacts on maternal pain. In addition, because support for breastfeeding varies and the natural history of ankyloglossia without frenotomy is poorly understood, it is unclear how many women who stop breastfeeding as a result of nipple pain have had remediable causes.	• The goal of breastfeeding is to establish an effective, pain-free latch. • Nipple pain while breastfeeding may occur, but there are interventions that may help, such as latch support, diagnosis and management of infant ankyloglossia, and treatment of infections, should they arise. • If your baby is latched and it hurts, you are not "doing it wrong"—your body is trying to tell you something. If you're walking down the street and there's a pebble in your shoe, you're not walking wrong—your foot is telling you to remove the pebble. Similarly, if your baby's latch is not comfortable, your breast is telling you to adjust your baby's position.
What is the effect on the mother's lifestyle, work, and sleep?	Breastfeeding requires a significant investment of time and effort. Reallocation of other maternal duties toward the home, other children, finances, food, and society may be an effective way of ensuring that breastfeeding mothers do not become overwhelmed. However, this varies significantly between cultures and families. In addition, paid parental leave policies vary substantially around the world; thus the financial landscape of making the decision to breastfeed differs.[206] Data support that it is possible to maintain lactation while separated from an infant (e.g., for work, to share infant feeding, etc.). Pumping or expression of milk in any location must be safe, clean, private, and available when mothers need to express milk. Some countries have labor laws supporting a mother's right to express milk at work, but	• Help families to understand the importance of breastfeeding initiation, even if they are concerned about their ability to continue because of work or other concerns. • The family may plan to share other maternal duties regarding the home, other children, finances, food, and society while breastfeeding. • Teaching a mother to maintain lactation while separated from her infant is best practice and one of the tenets of the 10 steps. • The health care provider can help to advocate for mothers who need support from their employers, notifying them of the benefits of having a breastfeeding employee (see Chapter 18) and any existing laws supporting mothers' rights to express milk at work. • Breastfeeding has not been shown to make babies temperamentally dependent.

(Continued)

TABLE 7.1   Mothers' Expressed Concerns About Breastfeeding When Interviewed Prenatally, Along With Counseling Points—cont'd

Prenatal Concern	Evidence	Prenatal Counseling Points
	these are usually incompletely enforced, and mothers may continue to struggle against unfair labor practices. In these situations, health care providers may be allies to help families reach their breastfeeding goals. In unsupportive environments, employment may be a reason for both not initiating breastfeeding and for limiting the duration of breastfeeding (see Chapter 18). Breastfeeding has not been shown to cause infants to be "needy" or overly dependent on their mothers but, rather, to create a secure attachment that leads to independence later in life.[c] Most studies examining the role of breastfeeding on sleep have found either no effect of breastfeeding on the quantity of sleep or that breastfeeding mothers have qualitatively deeper sleep in the immediate postpartum period and overall longer duration of sleep than families who feed formula.[d,207]	• Breastfeeding has not been shown to worsen maternal sleep; some small studies suggest that it may improve sleep.
What is the effect on the mother's breast shape and size?	Data indicate that breasts are affected by heredity, age, pregnancy, higher body mass index, significant weight loss (>50 lb), larger bra cup size, and smoking history. Weight gain during pregnancy and lack of regular upper body exercise were not found to be related to breast shape.[208] Pregnancy enlarges the breasts temporarily, as does early lactation, but the effect is temporary.	• Pregnancy and other causes are more likely to change the ongoing shape of maternal breasts than lactation. • Changes resulting from lactation are temporary. • Breastfeeding decreases the risk of breast cancer, which also contributes to the risk of long-term breast changes.
Safety/breast exposure	Some women may have safety concerns about breastfeeding in public, whereas others may face social stigma, embarrassment, or abuse. These experiences vary geographically and culturally. Publicity campaigns, "latch-ins," and increased reporting have changed the culture in some areas but not others. Medical providers must be attuned to community practices, prejudices, and consequences associated with breastfeeding in public in their area.	• Discuss with pregnant women openly about their concerns about breastfeeding in public, and reassure, citing legislation protecting the right to breastfeed in public, when able. • When breastfeeding in public may not be safe, considering breastfeeding covers, wearing loose/accessible clothing, or predetermining safe locations to breastfeed may help a mother to plan how to feed her baby outside of the house.

[a]Demirci J, Schmella M, Glasser M, et al. Delayed lactogenesis II and potential utility of antenatal milk expression in women developing late-onset preeclampsia: a case series. *BMC Pregnancy Childbirth.* 2018;18(1):68. http://doi:10.1186/s12884-018-1693-5; Demirci JR, Glasser M, Fichner J, et al. "It gave me so much confidence": first-time U.S. mothers' experiences with antenatal milk expression. *Matern Child Nutr.* 2019;15(4):e12824. http://doi:10.1111/mcn.12824. Epub 2019 May 23.
[b]Dennis CL, Jackson K, Watson J. Interventions for treating painful nipples among breastfeeding women. *Cochrane Database Syst Rev.* 2014;12:CD007366. http://doi:10.1002/14651858.CD007366.pub2; Puapornpong P, Paritakul P, Suksamarnwong M, et al. Nipple pain incidence, the predisposing factors, the recovery period after care management, and the exclusive breastfeeding outcome. *Breastfeed Med.* 2017;12: 169–173. http://doi:10.1089/bfm.2016.0194. Epub 2017 Apr 1.
[c]Gibbs BG, Forste R, Lybbert E. Breastfeeding, parenting, and infant attachment behaviors. *Matern Child Health J.* 2018;22(4):579–588. http://doi:10.1007/s10995-018-2427-z.
[d]Brown A, Harries V. Infant sleep and night feeding patterns during later infancy: association with breastfeeding frequency, daytime complementary food intake, and infant weight. *Breastfeed Med.* 2015;10(5):246–252. http://doi:10.1089/bfm.2014.0153.

completion of the reproductive cycle. This is a critical period because mothers who receive the proper support after birth are more likely to successfully establish an effective latch and milk supply.

Every birthing center, certified as part of the "Baby-Friendly Hospital Initiative" or not, should provide the basic management recommended by the 10 evidence-based steps to support breastfeeding (see Chapter 1).[38,39] After birth, the infant should immediately be placed on the mother's chest or abdomen, to root for and seek the breast (i.e., the "breast crawl," see later discussion). The normal infant behaviors of latching will generally begin within 30 to 60 minutes of birth. Even if the mother does not ask, the obstetrician and delivery room staff should suggest and facilitate it. Data confirm the view that delivery room or birthing center protocols that interrupt interaction and suckling between mother and infant increase the stress of patients and have a negative impact on long-term lactation success.[40,41]

In the mother, oxytocin levels at 15, 30, and 45 minutes after delivery are significantly elevated, coinciding both with breastfeeding and with the expulsion of the placenta. Oxytocin has been associated with positive maternal feelings and with maternal bonding; thus it is appropriate to optimize mother–infant interaction at this point of high oxytocin levels by facilitating suckling.[41,42] Skin-to-skin contact after birth has been associated with other important maternal factors, including moderating the effect of birth trauma; functional magnetic resonance imaging (fMRI) demonstrated stimulation of bonding centers in the brain, improved confidence, reduced postpartum bleeding, and decreased depression.[43–45]

In the infant, skin-to-skin contact after birth performs an organizing function, which has been well documented in research on kangaroo care. A Cochrane review that included 38 trials with 3472 mother–infant pairs across 21 countries concluded that early skin-to-skin contact for healthy newborns resulted in lower infant crying time, improved thermoregulation, lower heart rate, and lower rates of hypoglycemia, in addition to improved breastfeeding duration and exclusivity.[45]

For preterm, low-birth-weight, or sick infants, this effect may be even more pronounced. Skin-to-skin holding during the time of critical care (NICU) has demonstrated improved physiologic stability and neurosensory integration, lowered morbidities, and improved parental attachment. Ten- and 20-year follow-up studies have shown lasting effects on cognition, social behaviors, and motor skills.[46]

The Breast Crawl

As noted earlier, healthy newborns placed on the mother's abdomen will find their way to the breast and latch on if unimpeded. This "breast crawl" is based in mammalian neurophysiology and will be demonstrated as an innate behavior of healthy newborns if not interrupted. It is a fundamental component of establishing the confidence and learning associated with latching on and also positively affects the maternal milk supply. A video and textual description are available online at http://breastcrawl.org.

For this first breastfeeding, the infant should be placed prone on the mother, who is supine ("tummy to tummy"). The head, body, and back of the baby should be dried during skin-to-skin time, and dry blankets should replace wet ones to cover the baby (and mother, if desired). At this time, the infant is alert, opening its eyes, and adjusting to the world. The odor of the breast, maternal heat and heartbeat, and infant vernix all combine to help the infant orient to the breast. In this position, the infant's legs are able to massage

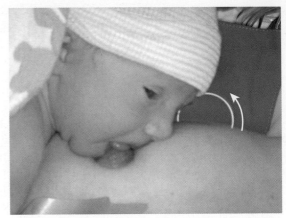

Fig. 7.1 Hand massage and licking: innate infant responses to skin-to-skin care immediately after birth. (From Leifer G, Keenan-Lindsay L. *Leifer's Introduction to Maternity and Pediatric Nursing in Canada.* St. Louis: Elsevier; 2020.)

the uterus while pushing the infant up toward the breast. After crawling, a few rest breaks, massaging the breasts, and licking the nipple (Fig. 7.1), the infant will generally gape and extend the tongue under the nipple to draw the breast into the mouth. If an infant is not able to or has not been allowed to crawl up to the breast, then the mother should be assisted to try different positions. The infant should be presented squarely to the breast and should not have to turn its head toward the breast. The mother may need assistance in holding her breast so as to present the nipple squarely into the infant's mouth, which is stimulated to open by stroking the center of the lower lip with the nipple. When the nipple touches the lower lip, the infant will open widely and extend the tongue under the nipple. The breast will be drawn into the mouth, the nipple and areola elongated into a teat, and the suckling reflex initiated.

Potential Obstacles to First Latch

A few possible obstacles exist to immediate nursing: (1) a heavily medicated mother or unanticipated cesarean with general anesthesia, (2) a sick infant (e.g., respiratory distress, low Apgar scores, prematurity), and (3) a stable premature or late preterm infant (i.e., hypotonic or at high risk of decompensation). In these cases, the following recommendations may be helpful:

- **If the mother and infant are stable,** skin-to-skin and latching should be attempted with continuous assistance, and hand expression should follow, with the colostrum being given to the infant by syringe, cup, or swab.
- **If the dyad is separated,** hand expression should proceed as soon as the mother is awake and alert, and the colostrum should be brought to the infant; this both stimulates the physiology of lactation and protects the infant with the metabolic and immune stability afforded by colostrum. (See Appendix E on the manual expression of breast milk.)
- **If the mother is unconscious and separated from her infant,** and she plans to breastfeed or her plans are unknown,

hand expression should begin as soon as is feasible, ideally within 1 hour of delivery. The mother should then be regularly expressed (pump or hand) every 3 hours until she is awake and able to express milk or transition to breastfeeding independently. Maternal medications should be reviewed for safety with breastfeeding (see Chapter 11 on medications and Chapter 15 on medical complications of mothers).

- **If the mother is unconscious, the infant is stable and not fully separated from her,** and the mother's medications do not preclude breastfeeding, the infant may feed directly from the breast, with assistance, until the mother is awake and able to breastfeed independently.

Other, more rare concerns include a tracheoesophageal fistula or choanal atresia. The concern for an infant with a tracheoesophageal fistula is important, but nonacidified breast milk has not been shown to cause injury to lung tissue.[47] If polyhydramnios or excess secretions are present at birth, a tube may be passed to the stomach to make sure the esophagus is patent. Choanal atresia is another anomaly that would be of concern, wherein infants will be unable to sustain a suck on the breast or bottle, which will prompt investigation.

Environment

In hospitals, both mother and infant will do better if there is an atmosphere of tranquility in the room, although this is significantly culturally mediated.[48] Another risk to the infant is thermal stress. If the room is cool, warmed dry blankets may be used, and a hat could cover the infant's head. Alternatively, it may be necessary to provide a radiant warmer over the infant and mother, given that both should be naked for skin-to-skin contact. Some mothers have shaking chills following the strenuous event of labor and cannot provide adequate warmth for the infant without some external source of heat or a blanket. It is well described that inadequately drying or warming an infant may lead to a cascade of events, from hypothermia to hypoglycemia, tachypnea, mild acidosis, and even sepsis evaluation and separation from the parents. Hypothermia is therefore more easily prevented than treated.

Supervision and Sudden Unexpected Postnatal Collapse

Supervision of the mother–infant dyad after birth is important to the health of the newborn, if not of the mother. *Sudden unexpected postnatal collapse* (SUPC) refers to a life-threatening incident during hospitalization following birth that may or may not result in death. Infants appear to be at the highest risk for SUPC during the first 2 hours of life, while in a prone position and unsupervised (such as during skin-to-skin care or unsupervised breastfeeding.[49] Paul et al. report on a quality improvement bundle designed to prevent SUPC while encouraging appropriate breastfeeding care, including skin-to-skin care.[50] They reported no SUPC events after implementing a standardized assessment tool and measurement of oxygen saturation levels with prescribed responses during skin-to-skin care. The center's rate of SUPC fell from 0.54/1000 to 0/13,964 after intervention. Routine oxygen monitoring is both expensive and impractical for many centers around the world, and no RCTs have proven benefit. In addition, reviews of implementation of the 10 steps show an overall decrease in sudden unexpected infant death in the first 6 days after birth.[51] Based on the current evidence, we therefore suggest that mother–infant dyads be observed continuously during skin to skin and breastfeeding in the first 2 hours after birth and that risk assessment tools be incorporated into care to identify which mothers may need longer periods of observation.

Family Bonding

If possible, the mother, other parent or support person, and infant should remain together for at least the next hour. The first hour for the infant is usually one of quiet alertness, a state that will usually recur only briefly again in the next few days.

Early Term/Postnatal Distress

Infants who are early term (37 to 38 weeks) or have had a difficult delivery (e.g., failure to progress, vacuum delivery, unanticipated cesarean, maternal infection) may demonstrate feeding difficulties.[52] In particular, perinatal hypoxia, as noted by low Apgar scores, may be associated with subtle difficulties in suck. One analysis showed that the rhythms of nonnutritive sucking in infants with a history of perinatal distress were significantly different from the rhythms of normal control subjects even when no gross neurologic signs were present.[53] See Chapters 13 and 14 for information on assisting infants with complications.

Ocular Gonorrhea Prophylaxis

Ocular gonorrhea prophylaxis remains an important intervention to reduce gonococcal ophthalmia neonatorum.[54] However, providers should consider delaying the instillation of prophylactic eyedrops or ointment until after the first 1 to 2 hours after birth. If the drops are put into the eyes, blepharospasm may prevent the infant from opening the eyes and will mar eye-to-eye contact and further adaptation of the neonate. Only if there is a known risk for gonorrhea should the treatment be immediately applied. Protocols in delivery rooms for nursing procedures and even some legislation has included the prompt administration of treatment within 1 hour of birth or before leaving the delivery area, which is not based on medical necessity but, rather, hospital management and nursing control.

Baths

The impact of the timing of an infant's first bath on breastfeeding has been researched. Initial findings showed increased breastfeeding initiation with delaying the first bath, although later studies have not replicated this finding.[55–57] This may be a result of significant study heterogeneity in baseline timing of the bath between study populations. For example, one recent study showed improved breastfeeding exclusivity with delaying the bath to 13 hours of life, but the starting bath time was between 1 and 3 hours after birth.[58] It is well known that interrupting breastfeeding in this earlier timeframe can interrupt first latch and therefore reduce breastfeeding success. Studies that did not show an improvement in breastfeeding exclusivity had baseline bath starting times later than 6 hours.

Infants have shown less hypothermia with delayed baths and immersion-style bathing rather than nearly immediate sponge-bathing. In some areas, parents prefer to participate in giving the first bath in the room, and this may function as a learning opportunity for discharge education.[59] This, coupled with the improved breastfeeding outcomes, suggests that the standard of care is moving toward later, immersion-style baths in the parent's room, if bathing is done at all. There are significant cultural variations and traditions surrounding infant bathing after birth and skin care. Because of high infant mortality rates worldwide and the need for a focus on thermoregulation, the WHO recommends drying and rubbing the newborn after birth but delaying the bath for 24 hours.[60]

Assisting With Latch

Although healthy newborns can latch themselves after birth and skin-to-skin time, some infants may need more assistance, especially in the days following. There are many positions that are used for breastfeeding, and over the course of the first week, mothers should be instructed in several so that they may find what is most comfortable for them and their infants. The elements described herein are most important for newborns and young infants and are progressively less important over time: infants and toddlers may empty the breast comfortably in many positions. All positions should follow the same basic principles to ensure effectiveness (milk transfer) and comfort (lack of maternal pain or infant fussing). Table 7.2 describes the elements of an effective latch. In teaching families, it can help to remind them that these are the same as are required for an adult drinking a glass of water: lining up straight (body positioned straight toward the water), head straight (no head turning to allow for swallowing), arms wide (to ensure closeness with the glass), and head tilted back (when the head is brought straight again, this simulates nipple to nose). Ultrasound studies have been done to observe the oral mechanics involved in milk expression while nursing, helping to confirm the rationale for these positions.[61] Fig. 7.2 shows an ultrasound image of an infant at the breast, and Fig. 7.3 depicts latching at the breast. Images of various positions for the infant and mother to facilitate latching on are shown in Fig. 7.4A to E.

Shortly after birth, **lying down** may be preferable for the mother. The mother may lie back (fully or partially) (**laid back** position) and latch with the infant lying on top of her or lie on her side, with the infant placed on its side, facing the breast. Breast support may be provided with the hands or bedding (small towel, blanket, or pillow). In any position, pillows help sustain the mother's position, especially on her back, arms, and between her knees (if side-lying). The pillow between the knees while lying down may prevent her from rolling over should she drift asleep.

When a mother is sitting up, the **cradle position,** with the mother bringing the infant to the breast while cradling the

TABLE 7.2 Elements of Effective Latch in Any Position

Positioning	Rationale	Assistance
Body: Infant abdomen touching maternal abdomen ("tummy to tummy")	Ensures infant and maternal proximity, encourages skin to skin while learning to latch, aids in aligning the infant to the breast so that the head may approach the breast properly	• Unwrap baby. • Laid-back: Place baby facedown on mother. • Cross-cradle: place baby with abdomen touching mother's horizontally.
Arms: Infant arms around breast	To manage infants' sometimes active arms, many mothers are encouraged to "tuck in" the arms between the mother and infant. Pinning down the arms in this manner creates distance between the mother and infant, which may result in a shallower latch. Also, it can require the infant to turn their head to latch, limiting milk transfer.	• Avoid tucking or "pinning" arms between mother and infant. • Respond to earlier feeding cues so that arms are less active. • If arm holding is necessary, the father/other parent or helper may assist.
Head: Aligned straight to mother's breast/not turned	Having a turned head while latching creates a side-looking rooting, shallower gape, less nipple stretch, and poor milk transfer. This may be uncomfortable for both mother and infant.	• Turning the infant's body to face the mother is often all that is required to correct a turned head. • In the "football" position/under the arm, pillows under the mother's arm and behind her back will assist the head alignment.
Head: Nipple to infant's nose (see Fig. 7.3)	This allows the infant to create a natural head tilt, which enables maternal nipple stretching and effective infant swallowing. In this position, the infant's lips should be flanged open (rolled outward) so that more of the mucus membrane of the mouth is touching the nipple rather than the lip itself.	• If the mother positions with the nipple at the infant mouth, demonstrate moving the infant slightly so that the nipple starts pointing at the infant's nose. • Infants who push back from the breast are often responding to being placed directly in front of the nipple or with the nipple below the mouth.

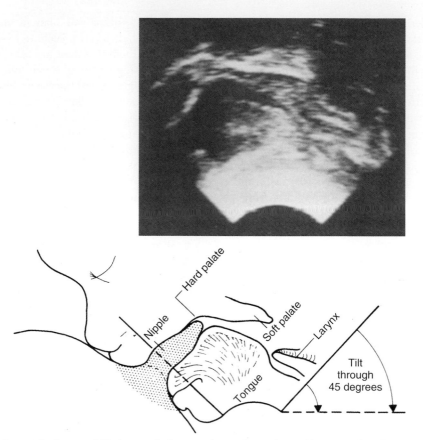

Fig. 7.2 Ultrasound of an infant at the breast. Still picture of ultrasound scan frame from video recording. The scanner head is at the bottom, with a sector view of 90 degrees. Below is an artist's impression of the image showing key features. The image is seen best when tilted through 45 degrees so that the infant's head is vertical. The picture corresponds to the point in the sucking cycle when the maximum point of compression of the nipple by the tongue has almost reached the tip of the nipple. Once the nipple has become fully expanded, a fresh cycle of compression will be initiated at the base of the nipple and will then move back. (From Weber F, Woolridge MW, Baum JD. An ultrasonographic study of the organization of sucking and swallowing by newborn infants. *Dev Med Child Neurol.* 1986;28:19.)

infant in her bent elbow, is the most common and natural position, especially once a mother is home.

The **cross-cradle** or **cross-over hold** works best with the mother sitting erect with one to two pillows in her lap so that the baby is just at the level of the breast and not above the breast. The infant is held with the opposite arm so that the infant's head and shoulders are held. The thumb is below one ear, and the fingers are below the other ear. With the head tipped back slightly and the infant brought to the breast, the nipple can stroke the infant's lower lip.

The **football hold** refers to the infant being tucked under the arm so that the mother supports the infant's head with her hand and the infant is supported by the mother's arm or pillows under the arm. The infant must be squarely facing the breast. The **side-lying** position is where both mother and infant are lying on their sides on the same horizontal surface, with the infant directly facing the breast. The breast may be supported by a towel or pillow, and the mother's hand supports the infant's upper back, neck, and head as needed.

Traditional cradle and football positions were called into question by Colson et al., who observed less effective breast-feeding and declining duration with these positions, despite maternal training.[62] They studied 40 mothers and infants in England and France by watching videotaped feeds during the first month postpartum. Primitive neonatal reflexes were described and compared, along with their impact on latching (stimulating or inhibiting latch). They found that more stimulating reflexes were expressed by infants who were fed in a semireclined posture rather than an upright or side-lying position. When mothers chose their own body positions, they selected semiinclined positions, in which the infant displayed antigravity reflexes that helped them to latch. Gravity pulled the infant's chin and tongue forward, triggering mouth opening to achieve attachment. This is also the basis for Pamela Douglas's "Gestalt Breastfeeding" method, which attempts to return mothers from a "checklist" version of latching to a more natural, infant-led approach.[63] These training methods are available online, at a cost. At the very least, these suggest that alternatives to side-lying and sitting upright are viable positions to initiate lactation.[62]

Introducing all the possible positions is overwhelming at first and should be avoided. With a little practice, mothers will find what works best. Visual demonstration of the latch is available online. "Fifteen-Minute Helper" is a physician-produced video for the physician audience created by Jane Morten, MD, from Stanford University.[64]

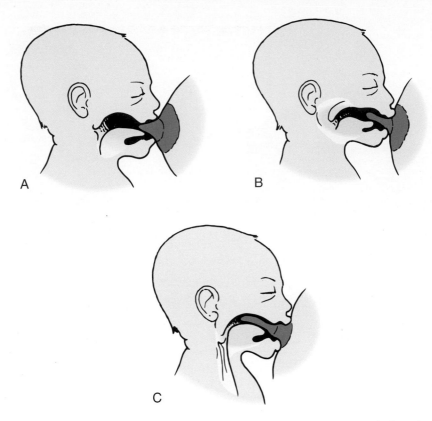

Fig. 7.3 (A) As the infant grasps the breast, the tongue moves forward to draw in the nipple. (B) The nipple and areola move toward the palate as the glottis still permits breathing. (C) The tongue moves along the nipple, pressing it against the hard palate and creating pressure. Ductules under the areola are milked, and flow begins as a result of peristaltic movement of the tongue. The glottis closes. Swallow follows.

Hand Positions

Two natural hand positions for the mother to introduce the breast are used most often. With attention to a few details, either position works (one is not right and the other wrong). The mother should be encouraged to use the hand position that is most natural and comfortable for her. The **scissor grasp** involves placement of the thumb and index finger above the areola and the other three fingers below the breast for support, thus allowing some compression of the areola. Care should be taken that the hand is not in the infant's way of getting sufficient areola into the mouth (Fig. 7.5). This grip has been used for centuries and was shown in sketches and paintings of ancient times. It may work better than the palmar grasp if the hand is large or the breast small.

The **palmar grasp** is the placement of all the fingers under the breast and only the thumb above (Fig. 7.6). This has been called the **C-hold** or **V-hold,** depending on the size of the breast and the size of the hand. This gives firm support to the breast. It permits directing the breast squarely into the infant's mouth and avoids the need to press the breast away from the infant's nose. The palmar grasp is similar to the prehensile grasp of apes when they nurse their young.

Apes, however, are unable to assume another hand posture neurologically or anatomically. If too much pressure is exerted by the human thumb, the nipple will be tipped upward (Fig. 7.7B), causing abrasion of the underside of the nipple. It is preferable that the nipple be directed horizontally as it is placed in the mouth (see Fig. 7.7A), with the infant's head tilted up (some describe this as "aiming the nipple at the baby's palate").

Days in the Hospital

All hospitals should incorporate the WHO/UNICEF 10 steps, which are the best current evidence for in-hospital breastfeeding support. Ideally, hospitals should become Baby-Friendly because it provides routine oversight and review of practices, enabling a hospital to be continuously self-reflective. If a birth takes place at home or in a birthing center, staff with a rich understanding of breastfeeding should be made available. The value of a well-trained, knowledgeable, and empathetic nursing staff should not be underestimated. The knowledge and attitude of the staff have been two of the most important variables in successful breastfeeding. This style of postpartum care better prepares parents for discharge because they will gain the confidence to know and respond to their infants' cues.

Providers should ensure safe rooming-in: that patients are encouraged to have their infants with them at all times, except as required for medical complications, necessary procedures that cannot be done in the room, or parental exhaustion risking the well-being of the infant or parents. An experienced nursing staff is critical to the management of the nursing family in the first few days postpartum. Advice should be reasonable and consistent, following evidence and best practices. Care teams should be educated in these practices yearly and should be aware of the potential to cause parental confusion

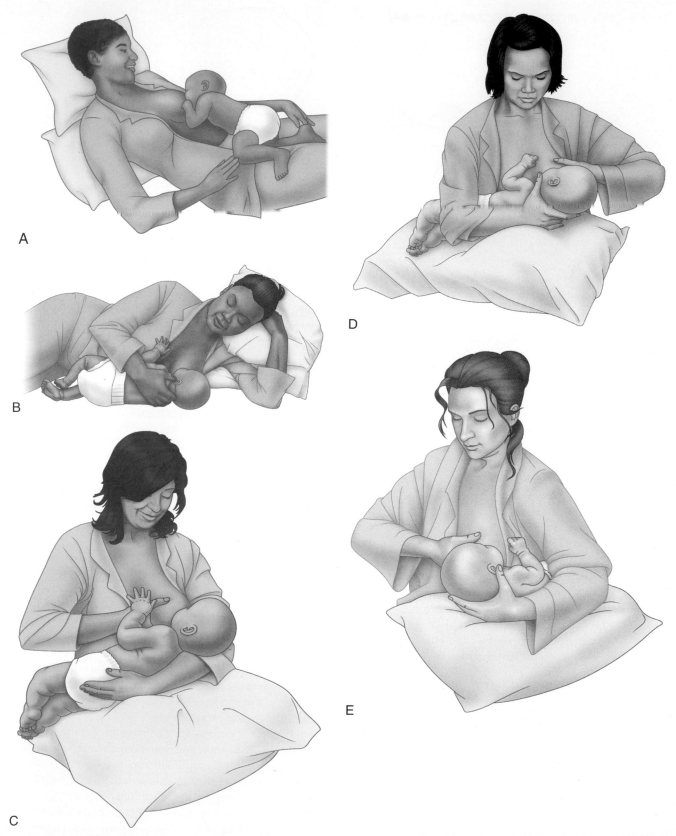

Fig. 7.4 Different positions used for breastfeeding. (A) Laid-back breastfeeding position. (B) Side-lying position. (C) Cradle position for breastfeeding. (D) Cross-cradle position. (E) Football-hold position. (Reprinted with permission from Carolina Global Breastfeeding Institute. Ready, Set, Baby. A Guide to Welcoming Your New Family Member. Patient Booklet and Educator Flipchart. Version 3, 2018, p. 12. https://sph.unc.edu/cgbi/ready-set-baby. Image credits: A, La Leche League International; B, C, D: Region of Peel Health Services of Ontario.)

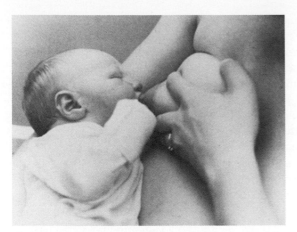

Fig. 7.5 Scissor grasp, presenting breast while supporting infant.

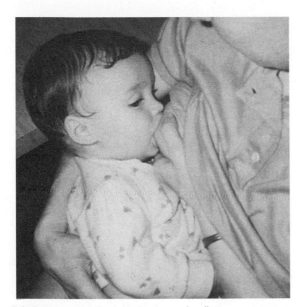

Fig. 7.6 Palmar grasp for initiating breastfeeding.

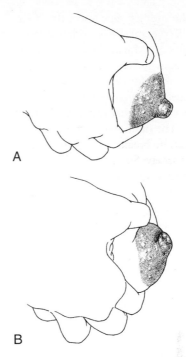

Fig. 7.7 Palmar grasp (C-hold). (A) When the palm and fingers cup the breast with support and the thumb rests lightly above the areola, the nipple projects straight ahead or slightly downward (correct). (B) When the fingers come forward and the thumb presses firmly above, the nipple tips up and causes improper positioning. Improper positioning is a common cause of nipple abrasion (lower half) and pain with suckling. (Modified from Higgins K. *The Nursing Mother's Companion*. 2nd ed. Boston: Harvard Common Press; 1990.)

BOX 7.1 Signs of Hunger in an Infant

1. Begins to stir
2. Brings hand(s) to mouth
3. Shows increasing efforts to root
4. Increasing activity, arms and legs flexed, hands in fists
5. If not picked up, progresses to frantic movements, whimpering
6. Cries (a late sign of hunger)

---

by providing different advice than other staff assisting with breastfeeding. When too many individuals are involved in postpartum care, mothers are easily overwhelmed with information, especially if each person says something different. The hospital should provide at least one staff member who is also a board-certified licensed lactation consultant for every 15 postpartum patients.

Key points in management should include the following[65]:

1. **Rooming-in:** A mother and infant should be housed together unless there is a medical contraindication. Delay the bath and perform it in the room when possible. The policy of the nursery should be to have all breastfed infants taken to their mothers when they awaken during the night, if they are not already rooming-in.
2. **Feeding on cue:** Feed whenever the infant shows signs of hunger (Box 7.1). In keeping with the Baby-Friendly Hospital Initiative (see Chapter 1), infants should be nursed on cue around the clock and receive no other food or drink unless medically indicated.

3. **Assist with latching:**
   a. Help the mother find a comfortable position. No rules should exist about sitting up or lying down on her side or on her back. Use pillows to support maternal position. If needed, help the mother find a comfortable hold for her breast.
   b. Help the mother position the infant so that she may bring her baby to the breast. Avoid pushing the infant's head toward the breast because the infant will push back, often arching away from the breast. Holding or pushing the infant's head has been associated with persistent arching by the infant (arching reflex).
   c. When waking an infant to initiate feeding, unwrap the blanket if wrapped, place the infant skin to skin, and use a gentle stimulus.

d. Help the mother reposition the infant on the second breast if the infant is still interested after releasing the first side. Moving may be difficult for the mother immediately postpartum.

e. It is common for the infant to fall asleep at the breast. Nonnutritive suckling while asleep may result in a shallow latch, which can cause nipple discomfort and trauma. The mother should be shown how to un-latch the infant by breaking suction with her finger.

f. Signs of satiety: Sounds of swallowing dwindle and stop, nonnutritive suckling occurs in brief bursts, the arms and legs relax, and the infant falls asleep and usually releases the nipple.

4. **Timing of feeds:** Stopwatch timing is not appropriate. It takes 2 to 3 minutes for the let-down reflex to produce milk in the early days, so the feeding must allow for the let-down. It is helpful for some mothers to have guidelines or estimates from which to work. Usually, infants nurse for about 10 to 15 minutes per breast in the first days, 8 to 12 times per day. Nursing continually hour after hour without a stretch of sleep should prompt evaluation for poor milk transfer or low milk supply.

5. **Caring for the mother/visiting hours/naps:** With hospital or home, liberal visiting hours may limit parental sleep and recovery from the labor of birth. Adequate rest is essential to successful lactation. In the early days of the Rooming-In Unit at the Yale–New Haven Hospital, Barnes et al. insisted that all postpartum mothers have a nap after lunch.[66] Every day, the shades were drawn, and traffic was decreased on the unit for an hour. This has been reinstituted in some hospitals and birthing centers as an afternoon "quiet time" and is part of mothering the mother. Many traditional cultures continue practices of mothering the mother after a birth: mothers are supported to rest, fed, groomed, and protected after delivery, sometimes for weeks.

6. **Rooming-in is the standard of care for all infants, regardless of feeding method.** As noted in the Baby-Friendly USA interim guidelines (Step 7, Guideline 7.1), "When a mother requests that her infant be cared for in the nursery, the health care staff should sensitively engage her in a conversation to learn more about her understanding of the importance of rooming-in and the reasons for the request. Staff should work to resolve any medical reasons, safety-related reasons, or maternal concerns. If the mother still requests or if it is determined that the infant is best cared for in the nursery, the process and informed decision should be documented."[39]

Infant in the Hospital

Feeding characteristics: Can infants be said to have a feeding "type"? In 1953 Dr. Edith Jackson, with Barnes and other colleagues from the Yale Rooming-In Unit, prepared a classic description of the management of breastfeeding that remains an insightful look at the behaviors and needs associated with establishing lactation in a hospital setting.[66] Infants were described as barracudas, excited ineffectives, procrastinators, gourmets or mouthers, and resters. This construct was found to correlate with breastfeeding duration in a study done in 2004 by Mizuno et al. with 1474 Japanese mothers.[67] Although it seems clear that infants have different feeding styles, and families should be educated to be attuned to their infant's eating patterns and cues, these types of descriptors also likely correspond to different feeding problems that we understand better today. Teaching a family that their feeding problem is a result of their child's personality may undermine both the diagnosis and management of that problem, as well as the bonding relationship. For instance, infants who have severe tongue restriction and who are causing maternal nipple damage and are said to be barracudas," who always want to nurse and have no regard for the mother's pain. Mothers dread feedings and their infants as a result. Or a child with frank failure to thrive as a result of inadequate maternal milk supply is called *lazy*, thus delaying appropriate diagnosis and management of both the mother and infant. A procrastinator or rester may have had a difficult birth, an excited ineffective may be overly hungry, and so forth. In fact, a qualitative analysis of postpartum audio recordings of interactions between health professionals and mothers while discussing breastfeeding found that many negative interpretations of infant behavior took place, and these influenced how mothers perceived their infants.[68] Also concerning were the findings in a descriptive study of 87 low-risk mothers and infants >34 weeks' gestation in New South Wales.[69] Lucas et al. found that mothers with a body mass index (BMI) over 25 who described their infants as "vigorous nursers" (i.e., barracudas) were less likely to exclusively directly breastfeed at 1 month postpartum. They hypothesized that this was a result of the perception of inadequate milk supply and continuing discomfort with latch, both of which raise the concern for ongoing medical or educational issues with breastfeeding rather than the infant's behavior.

It is therefore preferable to emphasize actionable observational findings over personality characteristics or "types." For example:

- Instead of calling a baby a "procrastinator," say: "I see your infant is falling asleep at the breast; this may happen when an infant is full or when they are tired out from trying to get milk. Let's figure out which one."
- Instead of calling a baby a "barracuda" or "piranha," say: "I see your baby is working very hard to nurse and causing you pain; let's see if we can make this better for you both."

Fixing a medical problem associated with difficult nursing situations often changes infant behaviors at the breast. Alternatively, the baby's nursing method may match well with maternal supply and anatomy, and a mother may be reassured when it goes well.

Timing of Feeds

The role of the clock. In heavily industrialized cultures, living with close attention to schedules (i.e., "living by the clock") has become necessary. Therefore families who are more familiar with schedules than they are with newborns may have trouble when advised to feed a newborn by their cues. Anthropologist Millard examined pediatric advice on breastfeeding from textbooks written from 1897 to 1987 and noted a focus on timing, coupled with a heavy distrust of maternal and infant knowing.[70] It has taken some time for the medical community to move from this undermining approach toward a more biophysical and supportive one. In breastfeeding, providers can help families break their bonds to timing and move to the central issues of successful breastfeeding, responding to the mother's body and the infant's cues.

Feeding frequency. A comparison of mammalian care patterns and composition of milk shows an inverse relationship between protein concentration and frequency of feedings. From this, it might be deduced that a human infant might need to be fed more frequently than every 4 hours (Table 7.3).

New mothers may be insecure and concerned about the lack of scheduling, especially when an ad lib program of feeding has been suggested. Other mothers may thrive on random scheduling. When rigid feeding schedules are proposed, this undermines the appropriate establishment of lactation.[71] A Cochrane review notes that feeding on cue is currently the standard of care, and there is no sufficient evidence to recommend scheduled feedings instead.[72] Three- to 4-hour feeding programs were originally based on the feedings of bottle-fed infants, whose slow emptying time of the stomach with formulas requires up to 4 hours. The emptying time for breast milk is about 1½ hours; thus frequent feedings are not unusual. Pediatric textbooks at the beginning of the 20th century described 10 to 12 feedings per day as normal.[71] In one study of 71 mother–infant pairs, feeding frequency was independent of timed fat content and, rather, varied by time of day, which breast was used, which breast had been used last, whether both breasts were offered, and whether the infant fed at night.[73]

Infants who sleep 5 to 6 hours at a stretch at night may make up for skipped feedings during the day. When milk intake and feeding patterns of 45 thriving, ad-lib feeding, exclusively breastfed infants were documented from birth for the first 4 months of life by Butte et al., two feeding patterns emerged.[74] In one, the authors describe the feedings as distributed throughout the 24-hour day. In the other, feedings were excluded from midnight to 6 AM. Total intake was the same in 24 hours. Milk volume per feeding decreased over the day. Frequency and duration declined over the 4-month period. Weight gain was similar in the two groups. This suggests that there is not a perfect pattern for all infants, and milk intake can self-regulate when exclusive breastfeeding is going well, regardless of the pattern.

Patterns of intake. The pattern of intake during a feeding is different between breastfed and bottle-fed infants. A bottle-feeding infant sucks steadily in a linear pattern, receiving 81% of the feed in 10 minutes. Howie et al. showed that a breastfed infant has a biphasic pattern, which includes the first 4 minutes on the first breast and the first 4 minutes on the second breast (this latter between 15 and 19 minutes into the feed).[75,76] The infant receives 84% of the total volume in those 8 minutes. In another study, 50% of the feed on each breast was consumed in 2 minutes and 80% to 90% by 5 minutes. Milk flow was minimal during the last 5 minutes. All these observations were made on the fifth to seventh day of life (Fig. 7.8). Donna Geddes and Peter Hartmann confirmed this using submental ultrasound and intraoral vacuum measurement during nursing and found that infants become more efficient at milk transfer over time, having a total feed duration of 14 minutes at less than 1 month and 10 minutes at 4 months of age.[77]

Providers and lactation consultants have recommended different patterns of nursing to promote milk supply and transfer; some of these recommendations may disrupt physiologic feeding. For example, "switch nursing" refers to removing the infant from the first side offered before they have emptied the breast—for example, feeding 5 minutes on the right side, then switching to the left for 5 minutes, then back to the right, then back to the left (see Fig. 7.8). When mothers fed 10 minutes on each breast (10 + 10), they produced the same amount of milk as they did when nursing for 5 minutes on a side and switching back (5+5+5+5). The suckling-induced prolactin was similar with both patterns as well. A major concern of

TABLE 7.3	Mammalian Care Patterns and Composition of Species Milk						
	Pinnipedia: Seal, Sea Lion	Tree Shrew	Rabbit	Rat	Black Rhinoceros[a]	Chimpanzee	Human
Infant care pattern	Return to ocean after birth	—	Cache	Carry, hibernate	—	Carry	?
Feeding interval	Once a week	48 h	24 h	Continuous	—	Continuous	?
Composition of Milk							
Total solids (%)	62–65	20	33–40	21	8.1	11.9	12.4
Protein (%)	8–14	11	14–23	10	0.0	3.7	3.8
Fat (%)	53	6.5	18	8	1.4	1.2	1.2
Carbohydrate (%)	0–0.90	3.2	2.0	2.6	6.1	7.0	7.0

[a]The rhinoceros has an anatomic variation in the stomach that provides four pouches that fill during a feeding and provide a constant trickle of milk to the central groove leading to the small intestine, thus creating a constant feed.

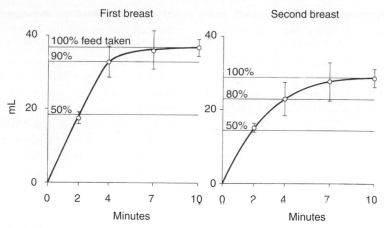

Fig. 7.8 Mother–infant pattern of milk flow. (From Lucas A, Lucas PJ, Baum JD. Pattern of milk flow in breast-fed infants. *Lancet.* 1979;2:57.)

switch nursing is not feeding long enough on either breast to obtain the full calories of hindmilk. Even if this improves volume, total calories may be decreased. The infants do not nurse for a full 20 minutes in some cases, and the nutritive feeding time is less than 15 minutes. The duration of feeding should be determined by the infant's response and not by time. Enough time must be spent on a single breast to ensure that the infant gets the fat-rich, calorie-rich hindmilk. Another suggestion offered to parents is to offer the "third side," which means after the infant has transferred what they can from the two breasts, putting them back to the first side again. This is done when the infant is still showing signs of hunger after what should be a "full feeding." Howie et al.'s study (discussed previously) may help to explain why this rarely results in significant milk transfer. In our experience, test weights after this "third side" reveal little to no milk transfer.[76] Rather, infants fall asleep, tired and unable to get a full feed.

Lactogenesis 2 and milk volume in the hospital. In the immediate postpartum period, the strongest indicator of the development of an adequate milk supply is the history of breast changes during pregnancy. The next strongest indicator for an adequate milk supply is the timing of lactogenesis 2. Risk factors for delayed lactogenesis 2 are outlined in Table 7.4, and if these are identified prenatally, then antenatal milk expression may be considered, although evidence is currently weak. After birth, early feeding, or expression if the infant is ill or separated from the mother, is paramount. Although initiation in the first 6 hours was initially posited as an appropriate target, several studies have demonstrated that expressing milk in the first hour results in higher milk volumes and decreased time to lactogenesis 2.[78–80]

Hand expression has been posited as the preferred method of colostrum expression, although a small RCT ($n = 26$) comparing hand and electric expression in mothers of very low-birth-weight infants in the first week of life found increased volumes per day in the electric expression group, including in the first week. Interestingly, cumulative volumes on days 14 and 28 did not differ. Pumping frequency was also important: on multivariate regression, each added pumping session was associated with 25 mL more in daily milk volume in the first 28 days.[81]

After lactogenesis 2, milk volume will depend on feeding frequency, along with any underlying maternal or infant risk factors (see later discussion on low milk supply). In the case of maternal–infant separation, there is evidence to suggest that after lactogenesis 2, well-fitting double electric hospital-grade pumps and pumping both breasts at the same time is the superior method for producing milk.[82,83]

Manual expression (see Appendix E). Because double electric pumps and electricity are not always available, or the lack of running water may make them unhygienic, all mothers should be instructed in hand expression of milk before discharge. In addition to ensuring milk removal in cases of separation or poor infant transfer, this technique improves confidence in milk supply and allows the mother to relieve engorgement. Discharging a mother who is able to express milk is also an essential step in the Baby-Friendly Hospital Initiative, "teaching mother to maintain lactation when separated from her infant," regardless of the type of expression.

Expression of milk is a procedure best done by the mother, and a skilled and experienced person should be available to teach this technique. The mother should support the breast with her fingers and place her thumbs distally and massage gently toward the areola, rotating gradually around the breast to include all quadrants. Then, once the peripheral lobules have been softened, areolar expression should be used to encourage complete emptying of the collecting ducts in the areola. Placing the thumb and forefinger at the margins of the areola and pressing back in toward the chest and then bringing the fingers together, rhythmically simulating the action of the infant's jaw, will start the flow and soften the tense tissue. In women with significant engorgement, it may be helpful to use an electric pump, set at low pressure and rate, which is effective because of its gentle milking action (see Chapter 22). The breast should be massaged distally before and during pumping as well. See the later discussion for more information on breast pumps.

Weight Loss

Breastfed newborns physiologically lose 7% to 8% of birth weight in the first week of life. Much of this loss takes place in the first 24 hours as a normal post-birth diuresis, and therefore percent weight loss has been noted to be higher in infants

TABLE 7.4 Delayed and Failed Lactogenesis, Risk Factors (17% to 44% of women)

PREDICTORS FOR DELAYED LACTOGENESIS 2 (>72 H POSTPARTUM)

	Strong Evidence	Some Evidence
Maternal factors	• Age >30 • Primiparity • First breastfeeding experience • Prepregnancy BMI >25 • Excess gestational weight gain • Gestational diabetes • Polycystic ovarian syndrome	• Prenatal care provider/doula • Alcohol use in pregnancy • Flat or inverted nipples • Hypertension • Hormonal contraceptive use in the first week postpartum • Maternal tobacco exposure • Breast surgery/injury • Hypothyroidism or hypopituitarism • Postpartum depression (EPDS ≥10)
Labor	• Long labor duration (stage 2) • Stressful labor and delivery • Cesarean delivery • Retained placental fragments	• Preeclampsia • Preterm birth, timing of antenatal steroids • Labor pain medication • Oxytocin use
Infant		• Infant birthweight • Infant Apgar score <8 • Excess infant weight loss
Breastfeeding	• Delayed first feed, infrequent feeding or latch difficulties after birth	• Nipple pain while breastfeeding • Early supplementation (within 48 h of birth)

RISK FACTORS FOR FAILED LACTOGENESIS

	Strong Evidence	Some Evidence
Mother	• Postpartum hemorrhage with Sheehan's syndrome • Mammary hypoplasia or insufficient glandular tissue • Ovarian theca-lutein cyst • Retained placental fragments • History of intracranial irradiation causing hypopituitarism	• Hypothyroidism • Hypopituitarism • Breast surgery

BMI, Body mass index; *EDPS,* Edinburgh Postnatal Depression Scale.
Derived from Brownell E, Howard CR, Lawrence RA, Dozier AM. Delayed onset lactogenesis II predicts the cessation of any or exclusive breastfeeding. *J Pediatr.* 2012;161(4), 608–614. http://doi:10.1016/j.jpeds.2012.03.035; Cregan MD, De Mello TR, Kershaw D, et al. Initiation of lactation in women after preterm delivery. *Acta Obstet Gynecol Scand.* 2002;81(9):870–877. http://doi:aog810913 [pii]; Demirci J, Schmella M, Glasser M, et al. Delayed lactogenesis II and potential utility of antenatal milk expression in women developing late-onset preeclampsia: a case series. *BMC Pregnancy Childbirth.* 2018;18(1):68. http://doi:10.1186/s12884-018-1693-5; Demirci JR, Glasser M, Fichner J, et al. "It gave me so much confidence": first-time U.S. mothers' experiences with antenatal milk expression. *Matern Child Nutr.* 2019;15(4):e12824. http://doi:10.1111/mcn.12824. Epub 2019 May 23; Hurst NM. Recognizing and treating delayed or failed lactogenesis II. *J Midwifery Womens Health.* 2007;52(6):588–594. http://doi:10.1016/j.jmwh.2007.05.005; Nommsen-Rivers LA, et al. Delayed onset of lactogenesis among first-time mothers is related to maternal obesity and factors associated with ineffective breastfeeding. *Am J Clin Nutr.* 2010;92(3):574–584. http://doi:10.3945/ajcn.2010.29192; Rocha BO, Machado MP, Bastos LL, et al. Risk factors for delayed onset of lactogenesis ii among primiparous mothers from a Brazilian Baby-Friendly hospital. *J Hum Lact.* 2020;36(1):146–156. http://doi:10.1177/0890334419835174. Epub 2019 Mar 22.

of mothers who have received intravenous fluids during labor or who have had a cesarean section. Because of this, weight loss closer to 10% of birthweight may be seen and be normal. The infant may be closely followed without supplementation as long as breastfeeding is going well, signs of lactogenesis 2 are apparent, the infant is behaving normally, and the infant is voiding and stooling well. Some have suggested that a "dry weight" taken 24 hours after birth (after the initial diuresis) may prove a more reliable measure of breastfeeding-related weight loss than the current standard of percent loss of birth weight. Nevertheless, excess weight loss is a relatively early indicator of breastfeeding difficulty and constitutes a risk to the infant; it should be noted and evaluated. The most

common reasons for excess infant weight loss after birth are delayed lactogenesis 2 in the mother (see Table 7.4 for risk factors) and inability to transfer milk (such as with ankyloglossia, discussed later in the chapter, and premature infants, as discussed in Chapter 14).

In response to the need for more clarity on normal infant weight loss and appropriate timing of interventions, much work has been done by Valerie Flaherman's group in the Kaiser network of California. Flaherman et al. analyzed cohort data of 161,471 term newborns, of which 108,907 were exclusively breastfed (83,433 delivered vaginally; 25,474 by C-section).[84] Differential loss by delivery mode was evident in 6 hours and persisted over time. Only 5% of vaginally delivered infants and more than 10% of C-section–delivered infants had lost more than 10% of their birth weight in 48 hours. The group created hourly nomograms from these data, which have been externally validated in a geographically distinct area. The nomograms are provided in Appendix F and have been made available online by Penn State Hershey Medical Center, along with a calculator for newborn weight (Newborn Weight Tool [NEWT]) to aid in the identification of neonates on a trajectory for greater weight loss and possible morbidities.[85]

Although supplementation itself will interfere with the establishment of breastfeeding, it may be indicated for infants with excessive weight loss.[1] A Flaherman et al. cohort study of 83,344 infants ≥ 36 weeks' gestation at birth and exclusively breastfed during the hospital stay determined that excess weight loss at discharge predicted cessation of *exclusive* breastfeeding at 1 month.[86] Furthermore, those with a worsening course of weight loss throughout the hospitalization were more likely to have worse outcomes. A worsening trajectory in this study was defined as increasing in the category of weight-loss percentile, that is, from <50th percentile weight loss to 50 to 74th, 75 to 89th, 90 to 94th, or 95 to 100th. These results point to the fact that breastfeeding problems at birth (which may immediately or eventually require formula supplementation) may be detected early based on the infant weight-loss trajectory. In other words, formula supplementation in the hospital may be a marker of underlying problems, rather than the cause of later problems.

Early limited formula (ELF) supplementation with extensively hydrolyzed formula has been explored for infants with weight loss ≥ 5% on the second postnatal day. Although a small pilot study (n = 40) found that ELF improved breastfeeding outcomes, a follow-up RCT with a larger sample size (n = 164) did not find any difference in breastfeeding outcomes at 1 month.[87,88] In an exploratory analysis of gut flora (n = 15 infants), the authors found that early limited supplementation with hydrolyzed formula did not affect the abundance of *Lactobacillus* or *Bifidobacterium*.[89] In follow-up through 1 year, dyads randomized to ELF discontinued breastfeeding earlier than those randomized to routine care (intent-to-treat hazard ratio [HR] 0.65, 95% confidence interval [CI] 0.43 to 0.97).[90]

Voiding and Stooling

In addition to monitoring weight, voiding and stooling can be used as barometers of breastfeeding adequacy, although they have been shown to have low specificity.[91,92] In the first week of life, voiding will indicate postnatal diuresis and hydration status, whereas an increase in stooling and color and consistency change to yellow and seedy may signal the onset of lactogenesis 2 and appropriate milk transfer. Some will use the saying "4 stools by day 4" as a way of teaching parents the importance of looking for this sign. After the first week of life, many infants will stool with each feeding, a sign of the gastrocolic reflex. The infant should have at least 6 voids and 3 to 6 stools per day. After the first month, the frequency of stooling decreases substantially, and it may be normal to stool "7 times

per day or once every 7 days." If an exclusively breastfed infant is well appearing, nursing well, and gaining weight, they should be evaluated when they haven't passed a stool in 5 to 7 days. If the infant is uncomfortable at any time before this, they should be evaluated by a provider.

Interventions That Interfere With Normal Infant Breastfeeding Behaviors

As outlined in the 10 steps, there are many things health care providers may do, or not do, that can interfere with normal breastfeeding. The provision of early formula supplementation without a medical indication in the hospital is associated with less successful lactation. Pre-lacteal feeds, including water, sugar water, or formula, are not indicated and may be harmful. Interrupting skin-to-skin contact and separating mother and infant disrupt the normal physiology of breastfeeding and the learning process of cue-based feeding. Introducing pacifiers and other nipples has been inconsistently associated with breastfeeding outcomes. Their use may either develop skills in the infant that are different from those needed at the breast or mask early hunger cues, which delays feeding and makes latching more difficult—it is hard for babies to learn when they are overly hungry.

GOING HOME FROM THE HOSPITAL OR BIRTHING CENTER

If delivering in a hospital or birthing facility in the United States, uncomplicated maternity patients who have birthed vaginally are discharged in 24 to 48 hours. This is certainly before lactation is well established and generally before engorgement peaks. In some cases, in which maternity floors were run so rigidly that ad lib breastfeeding was an impossible feat, it was suggested that a mother go home and get away from the negative hospital atmosphere to a place where she could relax and concentrate on feeding the infant and resting. A Baby-Friendly–certified hospital will avoid these problems but does not protect against a lack of local support services after discharge. Clearly, this depends largely on the location of childbirth. At the very least, it is clear that after discharge, mothers will need ongoing support for successful breastfeeding. Although no one solution has been proven superior for supporting breastfeeding families above others, many have shown efficacy.[17] These include in-home supports, text- and phone-based support, and office-based support. Programs that have a longitudinal component (i.e., starting in prenatal care) and include lay support, a face-to-face component, and scheduled contacts in the range of four to eight contacts may be superior to others.

Dr. Dana Raphael, an anthropologist and lifelong breastfeeding advocate, once stated: "The common denominator for success in breastfeeding is the assurance of some degree of help from some specific person for a definite period of time after childbirth."[93] In her 1973 book *The Tender Gift: Breast Feeding*, she coined the term *doula* and described the positive impact on breastfeeding of a confident, calm person to care for the mother and infant in the first weeks after birth. Although providers are rarely the doula, they can be sure that a family understands the need and can suggest family or community resources to fill this role.

Other important supports in the community include primary care providers, lactation consultants, and home visiting programs. A lactation consultant should be available in the office or the community. The office practice should be available by telephone. Ideally, a nurse or provider will make a home visit in the first week. In some countries, this occurs automatically after birth (e.g., United Kingdom). For others, it requires a referral for a high-risk situation (e.g., United States). Home visiting support has shown a positive effect on breastfeeding when studied on many continents.[17] However, at the level of meta-analysis and systematic review, the data were considered insufficient for any routine recommendation.[94]

Predicting Risk of Breastfeeding Cessation

If providers are able to anticipate the risk of breastfeeding cessation after delivery, they can arrange for more robust follow-up, thereby identifying and addressing problems early. Several methodologies have been proposed, including Flaherman et al.'s prediction based on weight trajectory (see previous discussion).[86,88]

The Breastfeeding Assessment Score (BAS) has been proposed as a measure to identify the risk for the cessation of breastfeeding within the first 2 weeks postpartum.[95] Eight variables apparently predictive of breastfeeding cessation on logistical modeling—including maternal age, previous breastfeeding experience, latching difficulty, breastfeeding interval, and number of bottles of formula—are scored 0 to 2. Two points are removed for previous breast surgery, maternal hypertension during pregnancy, and vacuum vaginal delivery. The lower the score, the greater the risk for early cessation (Tables 7.5 and 7.6). This score was evaluated by systematic review and meta-analysis for accuracy and external validity; a BAS score <8 predicted breastfeeding cessation by 14 days with 80% sensitivity and 50% specificity.[96] Given study heterogeneity, if this score is used, the authors recommend local calibration. For the timing of visits to the baby's provider, the WHO recommends that a mother and infant be assessed at 48 to 72 hours after birth, between 7 and 14 days, and again at 6 weeks.[60] For a home birth, the WHO recommends a home visit as soon as possible, within a day of birth, at day 3, and another visit before the end of the first week. It is clear that these timeframes should be shortened if a problem exists, especially for a weight check or hyperbilirubinemia. When the provider has been specially trained in lactation, the breastfeeding outcome for mothers and infants shows more prolonged breastfeeding and increased exclusivity.[97] Studies have demonstrated the value of postresidency training in breastfeeding when practitioners did not receive such training in residency (see Chapter 26).

Weight Gain

Weight gain after the first week of life should be 15 to 30 g daily (0.5 to 1 oz). Birth weight should be regained in 2 weeks,

TABLE 7.5 Breastfeeding Assessment Score[a]

Variable	SCORE		
	0	1	2
Maternal age (yr)	<21	21–24	>24
Previous breastfeeding experience	Failure	None	Success
Latching difficulty	Every feeding	Half the feeding	<3 feedings
Breastfeeding interval, every hour	>6	3–6	<3
No. of bottles of formula before enrollment	>2	1	0

[a]Two points should be subtracted for the presence of each of the variables of previous breast surgery, maternal hypertension during pregnancy, or vacuum vaginal delivery.
From Hall RT, Mercer AM, Teasly SL, et al. A breast-feeding assessment score to evaluate the risk for cessation of breastfeeding by 7 to 10 days of age. *J Pediatr*. 2002;141:659–664.

TABLE 7.6 Breastfeeding Cessation Rates (%) at 7 to 10 Days by Breastfeeding Score

Score	No. of Patients	CESSATION RATE	
		Predicted	Actual
10	173	3.2	1.7
9	288	5.1	5.6
8	244	8.1	7.4
7	183	12.7	16.4
6	101	19.2	17.8
5	49	28.1	26.5
4	18	39.0	33.3
3	13	51.2	38.5
2	5	63.2	80.0
1	1	73.8	100.0
<1	0	—	—

From Hall RT, Mercer AM, Teasly SL, et al. A breast-feeding assessment score to evaluate the risk for cessation of breastfeeding by 7 to 10 days of age. *J Pediatr*. 2002;141:659–664.

at most. The WHO growth charts for infants 0 to 2 years old are based on internationally representative samples of breastfed infants followed longitudinally and are therefore appropriate for monitoring an infant's growth past the neonatal period (see Appendix F).

First Visit to the Obstetric Provider

Recommendations vary between countries regarding the timing and frequency of maternal follow-up after birth.[98]

Whereas the National Institute of Health Care Excellence (NICE) guidelines (United Kingdom) recommend that women be seen at 24 hours, 2 to 7 days, and between 2 and 8 weeks, until 2018, the standard of care in the United States was a single visit at 6 weeks postpartum. For mothers facing breastfeeding challenges, a 6-week visit was often too little and far too late. Recognizing the challenges that women face in the weeks following birth, the American College of Obstetricians and Gynecologists issued new recommendations in 2018 for post-partum care.[99] The college reconceptualized postpartum care as an ongoing process spanning the 12 weeks after birth and suggested that all women have contact with their postpartum care provider within 3 weeks, as well as receive ongoing care and support until fully recovered from birth.

It may be helpful to begin these visits by asking, "What is going well?" Women face multiple physical and emotional challenges in the weeks following birth, and understanding what is working well can help to frame solutions for areas that are challenging. Topics to address include comfort during feeding, confidence in milk production, social support, and plans for return to work or school. Postpartum depression and anxiety are common, affecting as many as 1 in 5 women, and often co-present with breastfeeding difficulties. Routine screening with a validated instrument is recommended, alongside open-ended questions (Box 7.2).

PART 2: DIAGNOSING BREASTFEEDING PROBLEMS

Three (or More) Facets

Because breastfeeding physiology is (at least) a dyadic process, the pathology is similarly complicated. It is therefore useful to consider three facets to every breastfeeding problem: the mother, milk transfer/latch, and the infant. Problems may exist at all three levels or may begin with one area of this spectrum and proceed to affect the others. For instance, an infant with a tongue-tie may cause maternal pain and have difficulty

> **BOX 7.2 Questions to Consider During Obstetric Visits**
> - What is going well with you and your baby?
> - How is breastfeeding going?
> - What is making it easier? What is making it harder?
> - Who is your "village"? (i.e., the people who are helping you to cope)
> - How is your support system helping?
> - Have you noticed your breasts soften with feeding?
> - Have you noticed your baby swallowing during the feeding?
> - Do you have nipples that turn white during/after feeding or pumping?
> - Do you have broken skin, blisters, or other lesions on your nipples?
> - What are your plans for returning to work or school?
> - Are you able to sleep when the baby sleeps?
> - Have you been having a lot of scary thoughts or worries about your baby?

transferring milk; low milk transfer causes negative feedback and may reduce milk supply (Fig. 7.9). Alternatively, a mother with low milk supply may transfer inadequate milk to her child, who may then suffer from poor weight gain or hyperbilirubinemia. The management of these issues must also take into account all levels of the paradigm. To treat the dyad with low maternal milk supply and infant poor weight gain, one must ensure that the mother is fully promoting her milk supply, consider galactagogues, address any milk-transfer concerns of the infant, and adequately (but not overly) supplement the infant to ensure growth. In the case of twins, triplets, two lactating parents, or parents who are pumping, this evaluation will become increasingly more complicated.

Although, of course, all problems are interrelated, in the rest of the chapter, we describe the evaluation and management of maternal, milk-transfer, and infant-side problems, starting with an overview of the information needed to make an assessment.

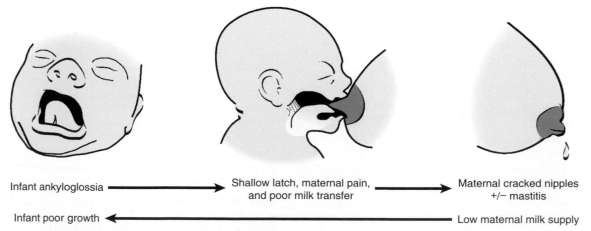

Infant ankyloglossia ⟶ Shallow latch, maternal pain, and poor milk transfer ⟶ Maternal cracked nipples +/− mastitis

Infant poor growth ⟵ Low maternal milk supply

Fig. 7.9 The three levels of breastfeeding problems and their interdependence. Infant tongue-tie can cause maternal pain and poor milk transfer, which then in turn may cause low milk supply and/or maternal mastitis, which in turn can lead to poor infant growth. (Used with permission from Ryan Healey.)

OVERVIEW

To collect the information necessary to evaluate a breastfeeding problem, it is helpful to know the following about the total breastfeeding experience:

1. Chief complaint, history of present illness: What are your goals for breastfeeding?
2. Supply and latch:
   a. How many times a day is the infant(s) feeding at the breast?
   b. How many times a day is the infant receiving another form of feeding (bottle, cup, syringe, etc.), if at all?
      i. How much is being given in the bottle? When?
      ii. Is it the mother's own milk, infant formula, or donor milk (where from)?
   c. Total daily amount of infant formula used, if any
   d. Total pumping/expressing per day and amounts
   e. How much of the mother's own milk is stored, if any?
3. Maternal pain history, past medical/surgical history, breast changes in pregnancy, birth history, medications, family history of breastfeeding or low milk supply, supports, and depression and safety/abuse screening. Asking specifically about fertility treatments is important because some patients do not necessarily consider this to fit in the previous categories.
4. Infant pain/discomfort history, past medical/surgical history, birth history, medications, family history of tongue-tie or speech delays, sleep location

MATERNAL PROBLEMS

Maternal problems with breastfeeding in the initial postpartum period are generally related to engorgement, painful nipples, and lactogenesis 2 or milk supply. Medical problems of mothers impacting lactation are covered in Chapter 15. Breast conditions are covered in detail in Chapter 16. In this chapter, we cover common problems, such as rest and early milk production, as well as more uncommon problems with milk ejection and milk supply.

Adequate Rest

If nursing is not going well, it may be both a cause and effect of maternal fatigue and frank exhaustion. Moreover, for women with health conditions, such as bipolar disorder or epilepsy, consolidated sleep is medically necessary to reduce the risk of seizure or mania (see Chapter 15). The mother may need help identifying ways she can recruit help with the infant, other children, the home, or financially so that she can rest. It may be helpful for mothers to try to nap when the infant is napping, especially during the day. Despite this rather routinely given advice, it is important to note that a lack of *consolidated* sleep, rather than short overall duration of sleep, appears to be the underlying cause of postpartum fatigue.[100] This suggests that "sleeping when the baby sleeps" during the day may not alleviate exhaustion. Families may find it helpful to "sleep in shifts," designating a 4- to 6-hour

block when another caregiver assumes responsibility for the infant while the mother sleeps; the infant can be brought to her to feed while side-lying, without requiring her to fully awaken (see Chapter 15, Practical Demands of Breastfeeding). In some cases, it may include a feed with pumped breast milk given by bottle or cup feeding while the mother sleeps undisturbed for a few hours. Notably, in observational studies, there are no differences in objective or subjective measures of maternal sleep when infants are breastfed, mixed-fed, or formula-fed.[101]

Fatigue both contributes to and may precipitate postpartum depression.[102,103] See Chapter 15 for more on postpartum depression.

Engorgement

Engorgement is common in the early postpartum period. The mainstay of management is breast emptying and promoting maternal comfort. This is covered in detail in Chapter 16.

Medications

Acetaminophen or ibuprofen may give the mother some relief and is safe for the nursing infant. Most medications are safe for breastfeeding and should be timed so that the least amount possible reaches the mother's milk and the baby. Medications are covered in detail in Chapter 11.

Drainage of the Breasts and Milk Supply

It is important to maintain drainage of the ducts during this period of engorgement to prevent back pressure in the ducts from developing and eventually depressing milk production. Intraductal pressure can eventually lead to atrophy of both the secreting and the myoepithelial cells and a diminishing milk supply. The best treatment is breastfeeding frequently around the clock because suckling by the infant is the most effective mechanism for the removal of milk. Relief is based on the establishment of flow. The infant may have trouble grasping or may not be interested in nursing frequently in the first few days, so manual expression may also be necessary. Engorgement at this stage is vascular; thus hand expressing or pumping briefly to stimulate the breast, if the infant is not nursing adequately, is appropriate. Pumping "to relieve engorgement" will yield little milk and may traumatize the hypervascular breast. ABM Clinical Protocol 20 (see Appendix I) discusses the diagnosis and management of engorgement.[104]

Nipple Pain

Although many women are told that breastfeeding shouldn't hurt, between 10% and 96% of mothers report pain of some kind while breastfeeding.[105,106] The initial grasp of the nipple and first suckles typically cause discomfort in the first few days of lactation because it is a new experience for the mother. This is not a cause for alarm but does require reassurance. The sensation is created by the stretching of the nipple and the negative pressure on the ductules, which are not yet filled with milk. Later, when lactation is well established and the let-down reflex has matured, mothers describe a turgescence, which is the increased fluid pressure being relieved by suckling. If the pain persists throughout the feeding, the situation demands immediate attention.

Nipple pain was studied in 1,649 singleton pregnant women in Thailand who presented for a 1-week postpartum visit to a breastfeeding clinic.[106] The incidence of nipple pain at 7 days postpartum was 9.6%, with poor positioning accounting for 72.3% of cases. Tongue-tie accounted for 23.2% of cases, and oversupply accounted for 4.4%. Interestingly, after management, nipple pain resolved in 1 to 2 weeks, and there were no differences in exclusive breastfeeding at 6 weeks between those women who had treated nipple pain and those without nipple pain. This highlights the need for timely and comprehensive assessment for persistent pain while breastfeeding (see Chapter 16).

Routine Nipple Care

The breast will be moist with milk right after a feeding. This should not be wiped away but allowed to dry on the skin. The mother may therefore expose her breasts to air briefly after each feeding. Nipple sizes, creams, trauma, infections, and vasospasms are covered in detail in Chapter 16.

Nipple Shields

A nipple shield is a device made of silicone that is worn over the nipple and areola while an infant is suckling. Concerns about nipple shields are based on the concern for limited milk transfer, thereby putting an infant's growth and maternal milk supply at risk, and the consequent work involved with weaning an infant off the shield. Although nipple shields may be overused, there appear to be instances in which they can be helpful, such as when the infant is not able to latch at all, struggles to maintain a latch, or is causing severe maternal nipple discomfort. A thorough breastfeeding consultation should take place before a shield is used. Shields are covered in detail in Chapter 16.

Milk Supply and Rates of Breast-Milk Production

After the immediate postpartum period and lactogenesis 2, milk supply transitions to local control and is therefore largely dependent on breast drainage. Milk production is therefore influenced by the frequency, intensity, and duration of suckling by the infant, along with any expression of milk. "Empty breast" is an expression used to teach and assess, rather than being a physiologically attainable goal. Rather, the rate of synthesis of breast milk appears constant, as confirmed by topographic imaging. Sequential breast-volume measurements have been used to study short-term rates of milk synthesis.[107] By using a rapid, computerized breast-measurement system, a close correlation was established between the amount of milk the infant consumed and the change in breast volume. The rates of production measured varied between 11 and 58 mL/h. At some point, this technique may be applied to the clinical assessment of milk production. This technology and the work of others have led to new insights into lactation physiology.[108] Mothers know that the breasts fill gradually to a certain degree

between feedings. When feedings are delayed or missed, breasts can be uncomfortable, with relief achieved when the infant nurses. It is well established that there is both autocrine and paracrine regulation of milk synthesis, along with an emerging understanding of the various factors involved in feedback inhibition resulting from milk stasis.[108] This feedback inhibition of lactation is further discussed in Chapter 3. Stress, lack of support, and acute illness have been associated with decreased volumes, especially in relation to poor let-down.

Inadequate Milk Supply: Perceived and Actual

Perceived lack of milk is the most common reason women report for early termination of lactation. As stated previously, anticipatory care on discharge from the hospital or birthing center should include how to identify appropriate milk production: signs of lactogenesis 2, infant hunger and satiety cues, and infant voiding and stooling patterns (see Chapter 3). Estimates vary but suggest that between 8% and 30% of mothers have a perceived low milk supply. Comparisons of perceived low milk supply and actual insufficient milk supply have not been found to associate.[109–112]

With increasing advocacy for exclusive breastfeeding, the risk is therefore in reassuring mothers who should not be reassured—that is, when there is an actual milk-supply or milk-transfer problem. This has been the focus of significant media attention in the United States, with widely publicized cases of failure to thrive in infants who were reassured by medical providers. To prevent missing cases in which breastfeeding is not going well, careful attention must be paid to signs of adequate milk production and transfer. Several screening instruments have been developed. See the earlier section on predicting the risk of breastfeeding cessation. Communication between the maternity center and the dyad's outpatient providers is essential, with early follow-up to evaluate milk intake and weight trajectory.

Drug-Enhanced Lactation
Oxytocin

The most direct therapy to enhance let-down is oxytocin. It is unlikely to help with milk production, as shown in a small RCT ($n = 51$) in which no benefit was found for oxytocin use versus placebo in mothers expressing milk for preterm infants.[113] The mothers who used oxytocin had an initially faster production, with later convergence of the two groups. Therefore oxytocin use should only be considered in disorders of let-down. For this use, there is no evidentiary base. Oxytocin is no longer available as a packaged nasal spray and must be obtained by a compounding prescription as Pitocin, a synthetic oxytocin. The available preparation is intended for intramuscular or intravenous (IV) use and contains only 10 units of oxytocin hormone per milliliter. The original nasal spray brand, Syntocinon, contained 40 units/mL. The currently available prescription is written for a 15-mL nasal spray or nasal dropper using standard oxytocin. The dose is reportedly one or two sprays or four to six drops in the nares, followed by feeding or pumping within 2 to 3 minutes. The dose may be repeated in the other nares if let-down falters or the infant is nursed on the other breast. In most cases, it is effective within one or two feedings. Let-down will usually continue without medication, although some concern for dependency has been raised. To avoid this, we recommend ensuring that the primary cause of inhibited let-down be addressed and that other methods of association also be used, such as meditation or guided relaxation.

Metoclopramide

The efficacy of metoclopramide in enhancing milk production has been reported in women pumping for infants unable to nurse or in women whose infants have significant failure to thrive because of inadequate milk supply.[114] The dose is 10–15 mg of metoclopramide three times per day until milk volume increases (i.e., 4 to 6 days, then taper over 4 to 6 days). When the infant is actively suckling, this stimulus is usually adequate. Mothers with underlying hormonal or genetic causes of low milk supply may find that their milk supply decreases again when the drug is discontinued. The original studies did not explore long-term use. Metoclopramide is used in adults for various forms of reflux for 4 to 12 weeks. The amount transferred to the infant through breast milk is reported as only 28 to 157 mg/L (1 to 13 mg/kg per day). Side effects do occur in mothers and tend to be dose related (i.e., greater than 40 mg/day in adults). Mothers may experience diarrhea, sedation, nausea, or a triggering of anxiety or depression. No symptoms have been observed in neonates, although some may receive doses that are pharmacologically active (0.1 to 0.5 mg/kg per day is the dose for reflux in infants). Torsades de pointes has been reported to be unrelated to dose. Tardive dyskinesia is associated with large or chronic doses of metoclopramide. It is not recommended for long-term use. Caution should be used in hypertensive women.

Domperidone

Domperidone, which is not approved for use by the US Food and Drug Administration (FDA) in the United States, is available in Canada and other countries under the names Motilidone and Motilium.[115] It has the most evidence for improving milk supply in postpartum women and can be used long term without the concerns for tardive dyskinesia raised with metoclopramide.[112,116] It has been reported anecdotally that 10 to 20 mg three to four times per day will increase prolactin levels and increase milk production. Any mother contemplating using domperidone should check with her physician because it can prolong the QT interval. Screening for any medical conditions, such as a personal or family history of cardiac arrhythmias or concurrent use of other medications that may prolong the QT interval or inhibit the metabolism of domperidone (e.g., macrolide antibiotics and triazole antifungals), is essential. Its risk–benefit relationship must be carefully weighed for each breastfeeding mother and family.

Herbals

Because of complications with available pharmacologic agents, there is a resurgence in interest in herbal preparations for breastfeeding. Many herbal preparations have been used as galactagogues for centuries, although data from controlled studies are limited. Fenugreek is one of the more commonly available and used galactagogues. It is a known component of curries and may be used as a flavoring agent. A recent network meta-analysis found it to be superior to placebo in five studies with 122 participants.[117] As a galactagogue, large amounts of fenugreek (three capsules three times per day) may be required, with the advice generally being to "take enough that mother starts to smell of 'maple syrup' or curry." Fenugreek dosing varies a lot in published reports, often 1 to 6 grams a day. It has a cross-allergy to peanuts and may cause fussiness in the infant. Further discussion can be found in Chapter 11. One small RCT done with mothers of preterm infants tested an herbal tea mixture containing 1% stinging nettle and six other herbs; it showed an 80% improvement in milk supply for the treatment group compared with 34% in the placebo group and 30% in the control group.[118] Another small, double-blinded RCT of silymarin-phosphatidylserine and *Galega* found improvement in milk supply in mothers of preterm infants over placebo.[119] These data show that as rigorous scientific techniques are applied to the study of herbal galactagogues, we are likely to find suitable alternatives to pharmacologic agents. Moreover, herbals tend to carry fewer side effects; because many of the tested herbs are used in teas or at doses similar to those consumed as foods, they may be better tolerated by patients. Unfortunately, they do not tend to be covered by insurance and may be costly in some countries. In other countries, they may already form part of the normative postpartum diet.

"Oversupply" of Milk, Hyperlactation, and Plugged Ducts

Oversupply of milk is a situation often encountered but not studied or written about in medical references. In the Infant Feeding Practices Study II, 23.9% of mothers who had stopped breastfeeding in less than a month said it was because their breasts were too full or engorged, and 14.1% said they leaked.[7] These reasons persisted to some degree to 9 months. In clinical scenarios, we have seen mothers who desired to wean because they were unable to control oversupply. Recurrent plugged ducts may occur with oversupply or simply with a change in nursing routine or inadequate drainage. These are also uncomfortable for nursing mothers. Hyperlactation and plugged ducts are covered in detail in Chapter 16.

Milk Leakage

For some mothers, leakage of breast milk feels uncomfortable. For others, not leaking may give the impression of low supply. Mothers should be reassured that leaking is individual and not necessarily predictive of supply. Breast pads may be helpful, and some women use breast shells that catch leaked milk. During engorgement, shells may worsen obstruction and edema. If used, they should be emptied every hour if the milk will be fed to the infant.

Let-Down Reflex

A mother may produce the milk, but if she does not excrete it, further production is suppressed. Much has been written on

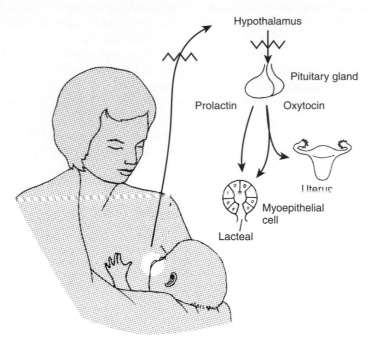

Fig. 7.10 Diagram of ejection-reflex arc. When the infant suckles the breast, mechanoreceptors in the nipple and areola are stimulated, which sends a stimulus along nerve pathways to the hypothalamus, which stimulates the posterior pituitary gland to release oxytocin. Oxytocin is carried via the bloodstream to the breast and uterus. Oxytocin stimulates myoepithelial cells in the breast to contract and eject milk from the alveolus. Prolactin is responsible for milk production in the alveolus. Prolactin is secreted by the anterior pituitary gland in response to suckling. Stress, such as pain and anxiety, can inhibit let-down reflex. The sight or cry of an infant can stimulate the release of oxytocin but not prolactin.

the let-down reflex by physiologists, endocrinologists, biochemists, pathologists, anatomists, psychologists, psychiatrists, obstetricians, and pediatricians. It is a complex function that depends on hormones, nerves, and glands, which can be inhibited most easily by psychological block or pain (Fig. 7.10).[120] See Chapter 3 for more discussion of the let-down reflex.

Practical Aspects of Milk-Ejection Reflex

Early in lactation, if engorgement is marked, the ejection reflex may be inhibited. This may be a result of maternal pain, periductal edema causing duct collapse, or possibly because of congested blood flow to the target organ, the myoepithelial cell. It is plausible that when suckling is initiated and oxytocin is released into the bloodstream, the ejection reflex message is delayed in reaching the myoepithelial cell with the message because of the vascular congestion. Regardless of the underlying mechanics, preparing the breast with warm soaks, gentle massage, and manual expression of a little milk may facilitate let-down. This may be a result of decreased edema and improved blood flow.

Distraction, stress, and pain have also been shown to interrupt let-down. Newton studied the milk-ejection reflex and clearly showed the effect of painful distraction on the let-down reflex.[121] In the clinical experiment, distractions included immersing the feet in ice water; being asked mathematic questions in rapid series, which resulted in an electric shock if a wrong answer was given; or having painful traction on the big toe (Table 7.7). Each caused decreased milk transfer, which could be restimulated with an injection of oxytocin (this was compared with a saline injection to limit confounding caused

TABLE 7.7 Milk-Ejection Reflex[a]	
Maternal Disturbance	**Mean Amount of Milk Obtained by Infant (g)**
No distractions (no injection)	168
Distraction (saline injection)	99
Distraction (oxytocin injection)	153

[a]Interrupted milk flow can be restarted with hormone injection. Modified from Newton M, Newton N. The let-down reflex in human lactation. *J Pediatr.* 1977;91:1.

by the pain of injection). In practice, pain, stress, and mental anguish can interfere with let-down.

When simple adjustments, such as making the mother more comfortable, playing soft music, or leaving the mother in a quiet room, do not work, other techniques should be tried. There are emerging studies on the use of meditation for relaxation during milk expression. Gentle stroking of the breast may help to decrease anxiety and stimulate flow. The use of tactile warmth, as opposed to cold, may improve release. Ice in the form of a painful cold stimulus to the feet was shown to interrupt let-down, but its use on the breasts and nipples is not studied.[121]

Side Effects Associated With Let-Down and Breastfeeding

The let-down reflex has been associated with several secondary effects, including headache, nausea, hot flashes, night sweats, hives, itching, and dysphoria. Headache, which occurs transiently at the time of initial let-down and then when changing breasts, appears to be related to surges in oxytocin.

Nausea has also been associated with let-down and specifically with the release of oxytocin. Women compare it with the waves of nausea of pregnancy. Treatment is taking food before initiating the let-down and breastfeeding. Dry crackers work well. The symptom is more effectively prevented than cured. Usually the symptom disappears in 3 to 4 weeks. Wearing pressure wristbands, which are effective for motion sickness, can be effective if applied before starting to nurse.

Marshall et al. used thermal probes on the mother and infant to document hot flashes. Skin conductance increased, followed by increased skin temperature.[122] Women also experienced night sweats and hot flashes during lactation, especially in the early weeks postpartum. They were most notable during night feedings. The phenomenon is also associated with oxytocin releases.

Generalized body itching and hives have also been seen with breastfeeding, generally just after let-down. Frank lactational anaphylaxis has also been described and has been theorized to occur because of the postpartum drop in progesterone, which facilitates an exaggerated histamine response. Antihistamines have been tried for prophylaxis, and some women have been advised to wean, if severe.[123–125] See Chapter 15 on anaphylaxis and breastfeeding.

Let-down may be so strong that it feels painful, particularly among women with oversupply. Therapeutic breast massage may be helpful.[126]

Dysphoric Milk-Ejection Reflex

Another unfortunate side effect from let-down is the dysphoric milk-ejection reflex (D-MER), which has been described in case reports. Ureno et al. have published a small case series and a descriptive study.[127,128] There is limited research, but this is a clinically defined phenomenon in which mothers become acutely saddened, tearful, or depressed with milk ejection. These waves of negative emotions have been reported to last until the infant begins to vigorously suck, and they may remit or decrease in intensity over the first 3 months of lactation. Some authors have suggested that it results from a severe drop in dopamine. Ameliorating factors have included distraction, chocolate ice cream, herbals (e.g., *Rhodiola rhodia*), Sudafed, bupropion, and smoking cigarettes. Clearly, smoking cigarettes should not be recommended, and all treatments should be evaluated for their effect on the individual case of maternal lactation and infant health. However, these findings may help us to better understand the etiology.

The management of D-MER should begin with normalization because it tends to be accompanied by substantial guilt for feeling negatively toward a supposedly joyful bonding experience. Patients may be advised to seek the company of others, use distractions (e.g., television, reading, enjoyable snacks, video games, meditation, visualization, and deep breathing). Ultimately, the mother is uniquely qualified to determine whether continued breastfeeding versus weaning is best for her and her child.

Phantom Let-Down

Postlactation phantom let-down is described by women who breastfed their children but are no longer lactating. It is described as the sensation of let-down, including the tingling and turgescence, when they hear a newborn baby cry, visit the nursery, or have some other encounter with infants. It is usually bilateral and transient. It does not produce milk. If it were to do so, the women should be evaluated for a prolactinoma. Women well past menopause have described being able to induce the sensation. No treatment is usually necessary, although vitamin E has been suggested for other breast pain at 800 mg/day for a week and then reduced to 400 mg/day until the pain is gone (courtesy Kathy Leeper, MD, Milkworks, Lincoln, Nebraska).

Nipple Biting

Blanching of the nipples may cause burning pain during suckling. A vigorous nurser or a baby with tongue-tie can cause blanching of the nipple from pressure. Later in lactation (i.e., after 4 months, when teething begins), infants may bite down to relieve gum pain and cause nipple blanching and burning pain. The mother should be instructed to keep her finger ready to break the suction if the pain becomes extreme or biting becomes frequent. Vasospasm, a painful nipple blanching with no apparent mechanical cause, is covered in Chapter 16.

MILK TRANSFER/OBSERVING A LATCH OR PUMP SESSION

The category of milk transfer refers to the complex trajectory of milk flow (after the production cycle) from the nipple to the infant's oral cavity and gastrointestinal tract. In other words, it refers to how milk gets from mother to baby. At the center of these difficulties is the technique of the "latch," when an infant establishes an effective connection to the mother's breast.

Latch

To solve any breastfeeding problem, it is essential to observe a mother feeding her infant. This may be left out of the evaluation only in cases in which a mother prefers to express and bottle-feed an infant; in these cases, directly observed milk expression is important to evaluate flange fit and ensure appropriate pump settings.

Often the problem is a simple one, such as poor positioning and alignment, with a mother so uncomfortable that the let-down reflex will not trigger, or perhaps an infant with a poor suck or poor latch. In these cases and others, the diagnosis can be made most easily by direct observation. Therefore understanding the mechanism of suckling in the neonate is essential to recognizing ineffective sucking. This is described in detail in Chapter 3 on physiology and is briefly reviewed here. As the breast is offered to the infant, the mouth opens wide, and the tongue is extended as the nipple is drawn into the mouth (Fig. 7.11; see Fig. 7.3). In a rhythmic motion, the tongue moves up against the hard palate as it draws the nipple and areola into the mouth, creating an elongated teat, such that the

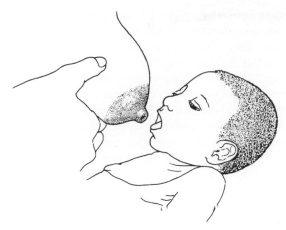

Fig. 7.11 Latch-on response. In response to stimulating the infant's lower lip with the nipple, the mouth opens wide. This response has been called the *oral searching reflex*. It is part of the circumoral rooting reflex. (From Righard L, Alade MO. Sucking technique and its effect on success of breastfeeding. *Birth*. 1992;19:185.)

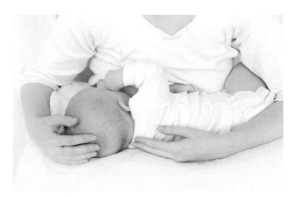

Fig. 7.12 Use of pillow to support mother and infant in cross-cradle hold.

end of the nipple is at the soft palate. The cheeks fill the mouth because of the sucking fat pads and provide further negative pressure because they do not collapse. As has been described by ultrasound studies, the tongue undulates in a peristaltic motion along the nipple while remaining in place, compressing the collecting ductules in the areola and "milking" them toward the nipple. The swallowing reflex is triggered, and the peristaltic wave continues to the posterior tongue and pharynx and down the esophagus, all the way down the gastrointestinal tract. Potential problems that can be identified by visually inspecting a latch therefore include refusal to latch, poor alignment/positioning (Fig. 7.12), discoordinate suck, suck/swallow difficulties, failure to sustain negative pressure, bottle nipple preference, maternal pain, poorly flanged lips, chomping suck, small gape, and infant falling asleep at the breast. (See Table 7.8 for a complete description of these, along with management pearls. This is not meant to be a complete list of what is observable but, rather, commonly seen issues.)

The Reliance of Milk Volume on Milk Transfer and Infant Cues

It is difficult to overfeed a breastfeeding infant. The wide range in breast-milk volume in well-nourished mothers was

shown by Dewey and Lönnerdal to be caused by a variation in infant demand rather than an inadequacy of milk production. They stimulated milk production with postfeeding pumping for 2 weeks and asked the mothers to continue feeding their infants on cue. The infants failed to take more than before mothers stimulated an oversupply. Although milk production was augmented by pumping, the infants regulated their own intake.[129]

Underfeeding is a more common concern, particularly when the family is learning infant cues or the infant has poor weight gain. When a family expresses concerns about frequent feedings and worries about the adequacy of breastfeeding, they may find that keeping a record of feeding times and duration, as well as sleep and wakeful times, is helpful. This may be done on paper (Table 7.9) or on several smartphone applications. This approach serves to refocus attention on the infant and cues and not on the clock. A follow-up plan specific to the mother–infant dyad can be created. The family may be surprised to find that an infant is developing a schedule. Often, the infant is sleeping longer than they thought. The chart may also be reassuring to the provider: timing of feeds can be related to lactogenesis 2, and therefore weight loss may be predicted to plateau in a certain timeframe. In other cases, a diary will highlight a problem not previously identified, such as overly frequent feeds (more than 12 times per day) in an infant who is not gaining well, associated with few episodes of quiet alert time. This is a classic scenario of a child who is attempting, but failing, to increase milk transfer from the breast.

Infant Weight, Milk Transfer, and Frequency of Feeds

Infant weight has been associated with the volume of milk intake. Greater suckling strength, frequency, and duration of feedings apparently play a part in weight gain, according to cross-cultural studies. A study of 71 mother–infant pairs, in which the infants were 1 to 6 months of age and exclusively breastfed on cue, test weighed the infants before and after each feeding in 24 hours and collected milk samples. The frequency of feeds varied from 11 ± 3 times in 24 hours (range 6 to 18), and the volume was 76.0 ± 12.6 g (range 0 to 240 g). The volumes of the left and right breast were different. The fat content was 41.1 ± 7.8 g/L (range 22.3 to 61.6 g/L) and was independent of frequency, as was volume per 24 hours.[73] Importantly, nighttime feedings made a substantial contribution to daily volumes. The authors concluded that given the variation between mothers, feeding on cue is more likely to be attuned to the needs of the specific dyad than using guidance based on averages.

Test Weights

Weighing the infant before and after feedings provides information to the family and provider on how much milk the infant has transferred from breastfeeding (Table 7.10). This may create or allay anxiety, depending on the situation. However, multiple studies have found that test weights in general improve breastfeeding confidence.[130–132]

TABLE 7.8   Latch Problems Described, Along With Clinical Management Pearls

Latch Problem Visualized	Description	Clinical Management Pearl
Refusal to latch	Refusal to latch may occur at any age. In early infancy, it often represents a problem with breastfeeding, whereas in later infancy, it may represent a behavioral "nursing strike," mouth or ear pain, or weaning attempt. In early breastfeeding, infants may be properly aligned but will open their mouths and turn their heads side to side, fussing and not latching. These infants may be unable to create and maintain negative pressure (e.g., tongue restricted), unable to transfer milk, prefer a bottle, or need to burp. This may also result from being overly hungry.	• To remedy refusal to latch, working with a calm infant is essential. The infant should be fed if necessary, via cup or bottle, and may be placed skin to skin and soothed by the mother. • Working with an infant with refusal to latch involves feeding at early cues and supporting a positive relationship at the breast, and it may involve many tools, such as a breast pump to facilitate let-down, a nipple shield to assist those with oral structure problems, or a supplemental nursing system to increase stamina and reward. • If refusal happens in the middle of a feed, patting the back to help express a burp may be helpful. • For bottle preference, see below.
Poor alignment/ positioning	This is a broad category and the subject of many teaching tools. Here, we will present some of the more common signs *at the level of the latch itself* of when positioning may be the culprit. First, when an infant throws the head backward while a mother is attempting to breastfeeding, this tends to be a result of either pressure on the back of the head (arching reflex stimulation) or because the infant is being forced to look down to latch. Second, in a "symmetric" latch (straight on instead of head tilted back, nipple to nose), having the infant looking to the side or with the arms tucked leads to a shallow latch because of the distance created between the infant and the breast. This may be painful and is most often ineffective. Third, a fussy infant who is refusing to latch may be doing so because its legs and lower back are poorly supported.	• Ensure proper positioning and alignment. Teaching families the analogy to an adult drinking water can be helpful to attune them to the needs of their infant. • A small mouthed latch may be the result of positioning problems. • Giving attention to supporting the infant so that the infant feels secure is essential.
Discoordinate suck	If an infant has a fluttering tongue that is discoordinated, it may not be as productive in stimulating ejection or sufficiently transferring milk. This may happen in the case of premature infants; those with hypoxia at birth, hypotonia, or tongue-tie; or illness such as sepsis, hypoglycemia, or jaundice. It is palpable during physical examination when an infant who should have an intact suck reflex does not draw in the examiner's finger and begin a repeated peristaltic motion exerting pressure. Rather, the tongue may move side to side, flutter, wobble, or push out, and the gums may "chomp" in a chewing motion. Limited suction will be felt on the finger, and the latch will be easily broken. Neonates may also have trouble organizing suck if they are overly hungry, one of the reasons behind rooming-in: if a child is over-soothed in a nursery so that parents can sleep, then brought back to the mother overly hungry, that infant is likely to have trouble organizing a suck.	• If the cause is prematurity, parents should be encouraged to keep trying. In our experience, some premature infants take up to 2 weeks after their due date to fully coordinate an efficient latch. • Infant should be evaluated for tongue restriction (see Chapter 13). • An overly hungry child who cannot coordinate to latch should be fed with a small amount (e.g., ¼ to ½ of a feed for the age) of expressed milk by cup, syringe, or bottle to calm them, and then latch may be attempted again.
Oral aversion	A child who thrusts out their tongue against the examiner's finger, clamps down their mouth against the examination, or cries when the mouth is approached may be exhibiting signs of oral aversion. This is likely to be more common in medically complex children.	• Infant should be fed by preferred methods to ensure growth. • Feeding therapy with a speech-language or occupational therapist is recommended to slowly desensitize the child and teach proper oro-motor skills.[209]

(Continued)

TABLE 7.8   Latch Problems Described, Along With Clinical Management Pearls—cont'd

Latch Problem Visualized	Description	Clinical Management Pearl
Suck/Swallow difficulties and choking, coughing	If the infant cannot coordinate suck and swallow, choking may occur, as in the case of prematurity and neurologic insult. Sometimes, if let-down is strong, the first rush of milk will cause choking. Usually the flow moderates in the next few days. As long as the mother doesn't continue to stimulate an oversupply, this problem is temporary or is limited to times when the infant has not been nursed for an unusually long interval.	• With infants who are neurologically immature paired with mothers with strong let-down, practice at a breast that has been drained first by pumping or hand expression will decrease the flow to the infant and allow practice at the breast. • In the case of strong let-down causing choking/gagging at the beginning of a feed, stopping and starting again should solve the problem. • If the mother's milk continues to flow abundantly with first let-down, she may need to express manually (and save) the first few milliliters to avoid choking the infant. This may also be accomplished with a breast shell or silicone suction hand pump. • Positioning the infant over the breast with the mother on her back may also diminish the flow via gravity in these special cases.[62]
Failure to maintain negative pressure/keep the nipple in the mouth/clicking	There are several reasons for the frequent breaking of a latch or failure to keep the nipple in the infant's mouth. One is, as above, too strong of a flow for the infant to manage without breaking suction. Another is weakness of the oral musculature, especially the cheeks. This will be made apparent by dimpling of the cheeks, suggesting that strength is not sufficient to maintain negative pressure. Dimpling of the cheeks and clicking are also found with restrictive ankyloglossia, wherein the infant's tongue is unable to sufficiently extend and expand to cup the nipple (to maintain negative pressure), and peristalsis is limited, which necessitates the recruitment of other oral musculature to create milk transfer. If an infant's jaw is slightly receding, the nipple may also not stay in place.	• Some therapists recommend cheek or chin support while feeding infants with hypotonia. This should be done gently because forceful support can create a negative feeding experience (see Fig. 1 in Appendix I, ABM Clinical Protocol 16: Breastfeeding the Hypotonic Infant). • Infant should be evaluated for tongue restriction. • The laid-back or "football" position has been found to be helpful for some mothers with this difficulty. • For a receding jaw, gentle support from the mother's index finger at the angle of the jaw, bringing it forward, may help. She may always have to support the breast with her hand (see Chapter 13).
Nipple preference (aka, "confusion")	Although it is possible that some infants are "confused" when being fed at the breast after being fed a bottle, in our experience, this manifests itself more as a "preference." Infants who do not know how to breastfeed (i.e., missed teaching opportunities because of illness) or who cannot transfer milk from the breast (e.g., those with a tongue restriction) may become anxious when presented with a breast while they are hungry, especially if feeding is well established with another modality. This can quickly lead to negative breastfeeding experiences and breast aversion. The suck from a bottle is notably different from suckling at the breast: the relatively inflexible silicone nipple may keep the tongue from its usual rhythmic action, the infant may learn to put their tongue against the holes of the nipple to slow a fast flow from the bottle, or the shallow position of the bottle teat may cause the infant to gag when presented with an elongated maternal nipple. When infants use the same tongue action needed for a bottle teat (negative pressure by dropping of the back of the tongue) while at the breast, they may even push the human nipple out of the mouth.	• Avoid introducing alternative feeding methods, if medically necessary, until breastfeeding is well established. • If a child appears anxious at the breast because of bottle nipple preference, ensure that they are not overly hungry, calm with ¼ to ½ of a feed by bottle, and then try again. • Attempt to feed at the very first hunger cue: rapid eye movement sleep, begin skin to skin, feed at the breast with a bottle if necessary to teach the infant that this is a safe and warm feeding space. • Some mothers have found a nipple shield useful when a child has a bottle nipple preference. • Infant should be evaluated for tongue restriction.

(Continued)

TABLE 7.8 Latch Problems Described, Along With Clinical Management Pearls—cont'd

Latch Problem Visualized	Description	Clinical Management Pearl
Maternal pain	Maternal pain is often, but not always, the result of poor alignment and positioning, which results in small gape and shallow latch.	• The mother should be encouraged to reposition herself, with guidance, until she is able to find a comfortable latch. • Ensure adequate support (see Fig. 7.12). • Consider infant-led laid-back breastfeeding. • If mother is unable to achieve a more comfortable latch with assistance, she should be evaluated for nipple pathology or allodynia, and infant should be evaluated for tongue restriction.
Poorly flanged lips	The infant's lips should be relaxed and rolled outward in a "flanged" position, which allows for the mucous membranes of the lips to touch the areola. If the areola is dry, the lips may be slightly drawn in. However, if a child has one or two lips persistently rolled under, it may be a sign that the lips are compensating for a restricted tongue that is unable to create a seal with the nipple. There are no good studies of low-lying maxillary frenula ("lip ties'), which are likely a rare cause of latch difficulties and are discussed fully in Chapter 13.	• The mother may use her finger to gently pull out the infant's upper and lower lips if they are rolled under. • A persistently rolling lip may be caused by a tight maxillary frenulum or may be compensating for a restricted tongue; the infant should be evaluated.
Chomping, "biting" suck	Lactation specialists will describe a child's suck as "chomping" or "biting" when an infant's jaw moves up and down in a piston, rather than rocking, manner. This is evident especially after let-down because the suck is slower but is similar to nonnutritive sucking. It is often, but not always, described as painful for mothers. It is often ineffective at transferring milk.	• The infant's tongue should be evaluated for restriction. • Maternal milk supply should be assessed and protected by expression or pumping if the infant is not able to drain the breast. • A laid-back or "football" position may be helpful. • Occupational therapists, craniosacral therapists, and chiropractors will sometimes treat children with this type of suck for "tightness" of the head and neck. There is some literature on this, although it is at the level of case reports currently. The International Chiropractic Pediatric Association has a certification process for those working with children, and evidence is available on the association's website.
Small gape	Mothers may allow their infants to draw the nipple into their mouths using a small, closed-mouth sucking motion. After adjustments, this may eventually result in a good latch, but more often, it is shallow and painful. Infants may need to be retaught how to latch by stimulating a gape response.	• To reteach how to initiate a latch, it is best to start at early hunger cues, during a time of day when the infant is usually alert. • Instruction is likely to be most successful after observing a mother's own technique. They can then be taught methods to widen the gape or latch angle. • After positioning, the mother may stroke the infant from nose to lower lip in a straight line. The infant will respond to the lower lip stimulus by opening its mouth wide (see Fig. 7.11). The mother then needs to quickly move the infant toward her breast to take advantage of the reflex.
Infant falls asleep at the breast without relaxing	When infants fall asleep at the breast quickly, or after a long time, but remain tense and wake shortly after still hungry, this should raise a concern over poor milk transfer. There are several signs that may observed to demonstrate milk transfer, although they shouldn't be relied upon fully: some infants may nurse for even	• Pre- and postfeed weights are critical to determine milk transfer in cases like these. • The mother may pump or hand express after the feeding to determine if this is a milk-supply issue or exclusively a milk-transfer problem.

(Continued)

TABLE 7.8   Latch Problems Described, Along With Clinical Management Pearls—cont'd

Latch Problem Visualized	Description	Clinical Management Pearl
	long periods of time, appear to swallow, then fall asleep tired but underfed. In these cases, it is likely they are swallowing some milk and some saliva. Infants should be observed for rocker motion of the masseter muscle during suckling, sounds of swallowing, and a ratio of sucks to swallows moving to 1:1 or 2:1 as a feeding progresses. Suck/swallow ratios above this (e.g., 3:1 or 4:1 and more) suggest milk-transfer problems.	• Infants in these cases are often gaining weight poorly, and falling asleep is a sign of impending hypoglycemia, so the infant should most often be supplemented with the pumped milk, donor milk, or formula as soon as possible. • The infant should be evaluated for tongue restriction.

TABLE 7.9   Example of Newborn Feeding Diary

Feeding Time	Method (breast, bottle, other)	Wet Diapers	Stools	Sleep
10 AM	Breastfed both sides, 20 min	1	2	10:30 AM–12 PM
12:20 PM	Bottle of breast milk 50 mL	1	0	2–4 PM

A test weight should only be performed after lactogenesis 2 because of the low volumes of colostrum. If test weighing is done, scales accurate to at least 1 g or better will give a more reliable estimate of milk transferred.[133] With the development of similar equipment, scales may be practical for home use in some situations (as in a preterm infant discharged from the hospital with nasogastric tube feeds and breastfeeding). When ordinary balance scales are used, such as when a parent holds the infant before and after a feed, the margin of error has been shown to be greatest with the smaller volumes. In volumes of milk less than 60 mL, the error can be ± 20%.

EXPRESSION OF MILK TO FEED

Women express their own milk for various reasons, such as when pumping for a sick newborn or for feeding the infant while the mother is at work, school, or other activities. It may be done temporarily because of maternal illness or the need to take a contraindicated drug.

Feeding of expressed milk has increased over time as pumps have become more widely available. In a US study, 85% of breastfeeding mothers fed at least some expressed milk.[134] Some women exclusively express milk and bottle-feed; however, this practice has been associated with earlier discontinuation of breastfeeding in multiple studies.[135–137] More frequent pumping is also associated with earlier cessation of exclusive and any breastfeeding.[138]

A longitudinal qualitative study characterized reasons for pumping as anticipated or unanticipated and as elective or nonelective (Fig. 7.13).[139] Reasons also varied over time, from early infancy, when women expressed milk to establish supply or compensate for infant difficulties feeding at the breast, to mid-infancy or later, when women expressed milk to provide for human milk when the mother and child were separated for work or school. Given the various reasons that women express and bottle-feed, the authors speculate that "long-term

feeding outcomes are not hindered by high-frequency pumping, per se, but by high-frequency pumping that results from constraints to or difficulty with feeding at the breast."[138]

The experience and health impact of feeding expressed breast milk versus feeding at the breast requires consideration of multiple dimensions (Fig. 7.14), including the extent to which the mother relies on the pump to extract milk, the proportion of infant feeds that are human milk, and the proportion of infant feeds that are from bottles versus from the breast.[140]

These questions are not captured as part of national surveillance in the United States; a more comprehensive Questionnaire on Infant Feeding has been proposed that assesses at-the-breast and expressed-milk feedings, as well as feeding of donor milk.[141]

There is emerging evidence that feeding expressed breast milk is associated with different health outcomes than direct breastfeeding. Boone et al. found that among exclusively breastfed infants, being fed expressed breast milk was associated with higher odds of one or more episodes of otitis media than being fed at the breast.[142] Expressed-milk feeding may also affect infant weight gain and satiety. In an analysis of the Infant Feeding Practices Study II, infants who were fed expressed breast milk gained more weight than infants who were fed at the breast.[143] When followed up at age 6, maternal encouragement to empty bottles at 6 months was associated with pressure to eat and reduced satiety responsiveness.[144]

Milk expression followed by heat treatment can be considered for mothers living with HIV (Box 7.3).[145] Flash heating involves expressing milk into a glass jar, placing the jar in a pan of water that is two finger-breadths above the level of the milk, and heating the water to a rolling boil. The milk is then removed from the heat and allowed to cool before feeding. This technique has been shown to inactivate HIV.[146] Flash-heat-treated milk had low rates of bacterial growth during storage at room temperature for 0 to 8 hours, and immunoglobulins remained active after heat treatment.[147,148] The practice has been shown

TABLE 7.10 **Supplementation Worksheet to Guide Decision Making Around Supplementation and Return to Exclusivity if Possible**

SUPPLEMENTATION WORKSHEET FOR PROVIDERS

Steps	Relevant Questions to Consider	Notes
1	**Is supplementation required?**	
	YES NO	WHY?
	Consider:	
	1. _____% weight loss since birth	
	2. _____% ile by Newborn Weight Loss Tool (NEWT)	
	3. *Trend* by NEWT	
2	**Why/How is breastfeeding not going well?**	Is it: 1. Mother's health/milk *production* 2. The latch/milk *transfer* 3. Infant health problem
3	**How much is the infant getting in a typical feed?**	
	Equation: Prefeed weight − postfeed weight (+ discarded liquids and solids from diaper, if applicable) = approximate amount ingested by infant	Use same-day or recent measurements. Ask: Was this a typical feed?
	Prefeed weight, kg	
	Postfeed weight, kg	Weighed with same clothes and diaper
	Weight of wet diaper − weight of regular diaper (amount of liquid and solids in diaper), kg	(Only if a diaper was changed)
	Pre- and postfeed weight difference (add back weight of liquid and solids, if applicable) _____ kg × 1000 = _____ mL	This is the approximate amount ingested by the infant for one feed.
	Equation: Ingested amount × Times fed per 24 h = 24 h intake	Parent will approximate times fed per day OR keep records.
	This baby had approximately: _____ mL ingested in 24 h	
4	**How much does the infant need to grow?**	
	Approximate amounts: 140–200 mL/kg/24 h for the first 3 months of life[a]	Calculate range, choose higher volumes for children with failure to thrive.
	Equation: _____ kg baby × _____ mL/kg/24 h = _____ Needed mL in 24 h	Compare with what baby approximately ingests in 24 h (above).
	Equation: Needed mL − Ingested mL = _____ **mL supplementation in 24 h**	To grow appropriately. This is approximate.
5	**How will supplementation be given?**	
	Types of supplementation:	**Methods of supplementation**
	1. Mom's own milk (expressed breast milk) 2. Banked breast milk 3. Partially hydrolyzed formula 4. Other formula, Why? **Consider:** Is the family "milk sharing"? If so, explain details of informal milk sharing.	**Useful for neonates:** Spoon, cup, finger, syringe **Useful for older infants:** 1. Cup 2. Supplemental feeding system (feeding tube to the nipple) 3. Bottle (slow flow, paced bottle feeding; see Fig. 7.15.)

(Continued)

TABLE 7.10   Supplementation Worksheet to Guide Decision Making Around Supplementation and Return to Exclusivity if Possible—cont'd

	SUPPLEMENTATION WORKSHEET FOR PROVIDERS	
Steps	Relevant Questions to Consider	Notes
6	**What can be done to remedy the cause of poor growth or weight loss?**	
	Origin of problem(s):	Actions to consider:
	1. Mother's health/milk *production*	
	Increase milk supply.	Pump/Express after feeds Pump/Express every 2 hours Pump/Express during long nursing breaks Treat underlying maternal health problem(s) Consider galactagogues
	2. The latch/milk *transfer*	
	Assist with latch mechanics.	Nipple-to-nose positioning Feed on demand Clip tongue-tie Lactation consult
	Soothe sore nipples.	Express breast milk every 2 hours Take a break from nursing on the affected side Air dry nipples; apply breast milk
	3. Infant health	
	Refer to a lactation specialist.	IBCLC, CLC, lactation medicine specialist, feeding therapist, counselor
	Refer to a different specialist (supply or milk transfer may not be the primary problem).	Consider ENT, GI, allergy, cardiology
7	**How can this mother–baby dyad return to exclusive or near-exclusive breastfeeding? What are the goals and follow-up plans?**	
	Early follow-up	Phone (within 48 h) In person (depending on infant weight and hydration status)
	Frequent weight checks	Who How Where

CLC, Certified lactation consultant; *ENT,* ear, nose, and throat; *GI,* gastrointestinal; *IBCLC,* International Board Certified Lactation Consultant.
[a]DiMaggio DM, Cox A, Porto AF. Updates in infant nutrition. *Pediatrics Rev.* 2017;38(10):449–462. http://doi:10.1542/pir.2016-0239.
Copyright Casey Rosen-Carole, MD.

to be feasible in a research study; however, qualitative research has identified multiple barriers to implementation.[149,150]

Breast Pumps

Teaching with hand and electrical pumps is important in areas in which they are commonly used. The use of these pumps is not intuitive, and improper flange fit can result in pain, nipple damage, and lower milk production. In most cases, the introduction to the breast pump can wait until breastfeeding is well established, and a pump may never need to be used if the mother and child will not be separated. Reasons for early introduction of a pump may include the following: mother and infant separation that is likely to be ongoing (e.g., in the case of infant illness), the mother needs help feeding (e.g., multiples, exhaustion, depression, and need for sleep), or the mother will be returning to work early and desires to start storing milk.

As stated previously, after lactogenesis 2, a well-fitting double electric hospital-grade pump is the superior method for producing milk on an ongoing basis. Because there are ever-increasing brands and types of breast pumps, we review only the basic components of pumps here (see Chapter 22, Collection and Storage of Human Milk).

1. Types: Hand, single electric, and double electric pumps are sold, which can be plugged in or battery operated. Two new pumps are battery operated and fit within a brassiere, although they are currently expensive, have difficulty with fit, and have potentially lower pressures. There are also silicone suction-cup-style milk collectors that some refer to as "pumps," although they are used to

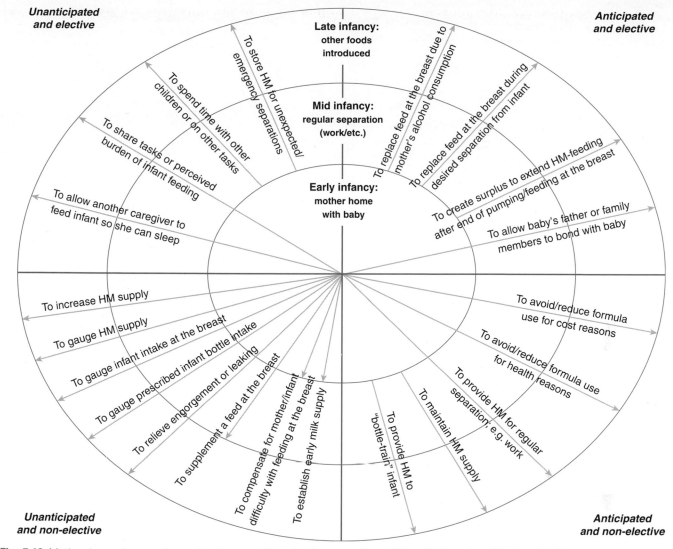

Fig. 7.13 Mothers' experiences of pumping human milk in the first year. (From Felice JP, Geraghty SR, Quaglieri CW, et al. "Breastfeeding" without baby: A longitudinal, qualitative investigation of how mothers perceive, feel about, and practice human milk expression. *Matern Child Nutr.* 2017;13[3].)

passively collect milk and use pressures at approximately 10% of those of electric pumps. Hospital-grade pumps are created to have no milk/pump interface so that they may be used by multiple users. They are also intended to mimic the suck and frequencies of a full-term infant; this is potentially why they may be superior to personal-use double electric pumps for producing milk in pump-dependent situations.[83] Variations in frequency, vacuum, and compression of the breast near the areola have been developed to improve milk extraction and comfort. Although comparative data are largely lacking, some evidence supports the use of the initiation phase and maintenance phase of the Medela pump for mothers of preterm infants, mimicking the natural differences in infant suck patterns as they mature.[82] Hand pumps can be used but exert only negative pressure on the areola and limit the ability to use massage at the same time. This being said, some women prefer hand pumps. Given the importance of let-down, it is possible that personal

control of suction pressure, or preference for the pump, is important in these cases.

2. Flanges and flange fit: Although various flange styles are being produced, there is a lack of comparative evidence. Most flanges involve a funnel shape leading to a circular rim, or step-off, which enables the nipple to stretch into the flange in response to increasing pressure. Generally, this tunnel is straight, which may cause mothers to need to lean forward so that milk does not pool near the nipple and drip out of the sides; this may result in back pain. Sometimes, the tunnel is curved (i.e., Pumpin Pals), without a rigid step-off. Anecdotally, these flanges have been reported to increase comfort and milk supply in some but decrease milk supply in others. This is perhaps a result of differing amounts of nipple stretch produced in different women if a rim or step-off is not present. Some flanges have incorporated soft silicone siding and integrated some areolar compression, and there is some emerging evidence on the comfort and efficacy of this

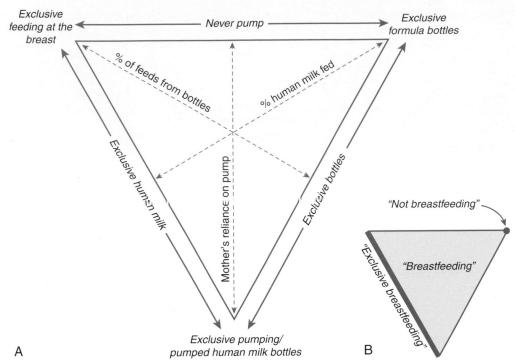

Fig. 7.14 A framework for characterizing the American mother—infant dyad with respect to the use of human milk, infant formula, bottles, and breastfeeding. (A) New framework for categorizing mother—infant use of human milk versus formula and bottles versus breastfeeding. (B) How the current terminology fits current practices of feeding human milk. (From Felice JP, Rasmussen KM. Breasts, pumps and bottles, and unanswered questions. *Breastfeed Med.* 2015;10[9]:412—415.)

BOX 7.3 Circumstances in Which to Consider Heat-Treated, Expressed Breast Milk

Mothers known to be living with HIV may consider expressing and heat-treating breast milk as an interim feeding strategy:

- in special circumstances, such as when the infant has low birth weight or is otherwise ill in the neonatal period and unable to breastfeed; or
- when the mother is unwell and temporarily unable to breastfeed or has a temporary breast health problem, such as mastitis; or
- to assist mothers in stopping breastfeeding; or
- if antiretroviral (ARV) drugs are temporarily not available.

World Health Organization and United Nations Children's Fund. *Guideline: Updates on HIV and Infant Feeding: The Duration of Breastfeeding, and Support from Health Services to Improve Feeding Practices Among Mothers Living With HIV.* Geneva: World Health Organization; 2016.

technique.[151] Mothers should be advised that interchanging pump flange kits can alter the minimum and maximum suction pressure for a given breast pump.[152]

3. Three-way component, tubing, bottle, and valve: After the flange, there is generally a three-way component. This allows negative pressure to be delivered from the tubing connected to the central component and breast milk to enter the bottle. There is also a one-way valve that allows milk to flow into bottles but not in the reverse direction. This valve is a potential source of wear and buildup of biofilms and should be monitored for the need for replacement. Sometimes there is another component of the three-way valve that involves a chamber and a soft silicone diaphragm; this enables a closed system so that milk does not reflux into the tubing. It may also change the pressure curve by altering the resistance.

4. Pressures/Vacuum: Different pumps enable different amounts of vacuum pressure, and sufficient pressure is largely responsible for volume. The comfort of the mother must be balanced with this, and evidence shows that women prefer pressures of approximately 200 mm Hg.[87] Many pumps reach or exceed 250 mm Hg, and using pressures that are too high may cause pain, inhibit let-down, cause acute or chronic nipple damage, or collapse ducts with negative pressure, thereby decreasing milk supply.

5. Cycles/Frequency: A cycle time of 105 to 120 cycles per minute to initiate let-down and 47 to 55 cycles per minute to express milk may be most efficient.[87] Some pumps do not enable a mother to choose her cycle length, and as pressure increases, the cycle frequency decreases, and the draw time lengthens. These pumps generally have a let-down function with high-frequency, low-pressure operation. The lengthened draw time may not be ideal for women with damaged or sensitive nipples. On the other hand, pumps that allow cycle and pressure settings may be overwhelming because of the variety of possible combinations.

6. Timing: In general, women should start by expressing or feeding from both sides at least 8 times in a 24-hour period. This may need to be higher in women with multiples or could be lower in women with oversupply. If pumping exclusively, this can be adjusted after the mother determines her output, a comfortable schedule, and goals. An overnight sleep period of approximately 4 to 6 hours should be instituted to allow for sleep. Mothers should generally expect to get their highest production in the early morning. Pumping both sides at the same time reduces total expression time and likely increases the total volume expressed.

7. Power pumping: This refers to a session in which the pump is put on and taken off over the course of a time period. Typically, it starts with a 10- to 20-minute pump session, and then the mother removes the pump for 10 minutes and reapplies it for 10 minutes in sequence for a full hour. It is meant to simulate a cluster-feed and is based on the principle that 80% of milk volume is taken in the first 5 minutes of a feed, after the first let-down. It attempts to stimulate many let-downs and may thereby improve milk volumes. Although power pumping is commonly recommended, it has not been studied. It is labor-intensive and can add a burden to an already stressed family. It may also cause nipple damage, especially with poor flange fit.

8. Milk storage: After proper handwashing and expressing, milk should be stored in containers made for the purpose. If these are not available, glass containers or food-grade BPA-free plastic containers are preferable. Breast milk can be stored at room temperature (27 to 32°C [80 to 90 °F]) for approximately 4 hours, or 6 to 8 hours if temperatures are cooler. In a closed container with an ice pack (15°C [59 °F]), milk is likely to be safe for 24 hours. Refrigerated milk (4°C [39 °F]) can be safely stored for 4 to 8 days and frozen for 6 to 12 months at less than −20°C (−4 °F). (See Appendix I, ABM Protocol 8,[153] which summarizes recommendations for human milk storage, milk warming, and feeding.)

9. Cleaning: The US-based Centers for Disease Control and Prevention recommends disassembling and washing pump parts in warm, soapy water or a dishwasher after each use.[154] Sanitizing by steaming or boiling may offer added protection for infants at risk for poor immunity: those less than 3 months, premature, or immunosuppressed. If properly used, the tubing should not need to be washed, and water introduced into the tubing may precipitate fungal infections. Some mothers with heavy pumping schedules store their breast pump parts assembled in the refrigerator between uses, then wash at the end of the day. Given the bactericidal activity of refrigerated milk, especially under 24 hours, this is likely to be safe. However, care should be taken to disassemble and scrub at the end of the day. There is no evidence to support best practices for breast-pump washing or sanitizing.

10. Choosing a pump: Interpretation of studies comparing different pump types is difficult, given that the research is often funded by a pump manufacturer. Based on a Cochrane review of best evidence, the success of a method for breast-milk expression depends largely on the need that it is addressing, and Dr. Paula Meier has a publication providing education and guidance for the health care professional who counsels their patients on pumps.[83,155] In addition, nutrient content may vary by pump type, and breast massage ("hands-on pumping") has shown higher fat content in pumped milk. Warming and relaxation may also help with let-down and pumped volumes.

ONE-BREAST/TWO-BREAST FEEDINGS

Parents have long been instructed in various ways regarding whether to use both breasts at each feed and how long to offer each breast. These recommendations were largely based on theories or tradition until studies were done in the 1990s. A case report of Woolridge and Fisher describes an infant with failure to thrive, colic, and green and frothy stools when fed by switching away from the first breast after 10 minutes of feeding.[156] The authors demonstrated that this mother did not produce high-fat milk until well into the feeding, and thus switching to the second side deprived the infant of fat-rich, calorie-rich milk ("hindmilk"). Confining the feeding to a single breast solved the problem. The authors also pointed out that consuming volumes of low-fat milk meant relatively high-lactose milk, which may have caused diarrhea and further calorie loss. When a later study by Woolridge et al. compared the two patterns of feeding in 12 mother–infant pairs, the authors found that the two patterns led to different milk volumes and mean feed-fat concentrations.[157] The mean fat intake in 24 hours, however, was the same. Infants appeared to regulate their fat intake quickly.

In a nonrandomized study by Evans et al., an experimental group of 150 newly delivered mothers was compared with a control group of 152 mothers over 8 days. The experimental group was instructed to breastfeed by favoring one breast per feeding, allowing the infant to "finish" and offering the second side only if the infant was still hungry. They were told to alternate the breast offered first.[158] The control group (n = 152) offered both breasts equally with each feed, switching off the first breast before the infant was fully "finished" on that side so that the total time breastfeeding was evenly divided. There was less engorgement (61% vs. 74%) and less colic (12% vs. 23%) in the one-breast-favoring group, but the groups showed no difference in infant weight gain, duration of breastfeeding, or mastitis incidence. In addition, 63% of mothers in the experimental group reported needing to feed the infant on the second side to relieve their infant's hunger. An investigation in Sweden reported no clinical differences at 1 month between mothers instructed to feed either at one or two breasts; they, too, noted that many infants whose mothers were instructed to favor one breast only required feeding on the other side as a result of hunger.[159]

The best reasoning therefore indicates that infants should feed on one breast until they "finish," rather than being switched to the second breast based on timing in the feed, such as "halfway" or "10 minutes." This may enable them to consume the higher-fat milk of the first breast, whereas offering the second breast will contribute their volume intake, if necessary. In other words, a mother should initiate a feeding and continue until the infant discontinues feeding on that side. If, after burping, the infant wants more, the mother offers the second side. To relieve engorgement and maintain supply, the next feeding time is started on the opposite breast.

In our clinical experience, there are some mother—infant dyads for whom breastfeeding on one breast is sufficient even from lactogenesis 2. As the previously noted study by Evans et al. indicates, this may be in as many as 27% of dyads.[158] For others, enforcing one-breast feedings may limit needed calories, increase hunger, and limit growth. Additionally, enforced one-breast feedings before lactogenesis 2 may decrease the stimulation needed to generate milk production. Most successful nursing mothers adapt to their own infants' cues instead of following arbitrary rules.

The identification of a factor that exerts a direct and local inhibitory action on further milk synthesis may explain why it is possible to nurse only on one breast as a cultural mode (e.g., Tanka people of southern China). In situations in which the infant rejects one breast, some inhibition of milk production may precipitate the rejection.[160] The inhibitory factor decreases the production in the unused breast while the suckled or pumped breast continues to function and sustain the infant's growth. Many mothers are able to continue nursing on one breast indefinitely.[161,162] This has been suggested in cases of nipple retraction, unilateral recurrent mastitis resistant to repeated antibiotic therapy, or with scarring (e.g., after lumpectomies for cancer). There would be a concern only in the case of mammary hypoplasia (inadequate glandular tissue).

BREAST REJECTION OR NURSING "STRIKES"

Infants have been observed to reject the breast intermittently, most often at 3 to 4 months, and then to go back after several feedings or a day or so. This may be a result of oral pain, ear pain, a change in routine, the flavor of the milk, or a behavioral "nursing strike." A bottle can be substituted, or cup feedings, if the situation becomes extreme, as described in Chapter 14. (Nursing strikes are also discussed in Chapter 9.) Total rejection of both breasts may follow the return of menstruation. A mother may notice that the infant will reject the breast for a day or so with each period. Other infants seem unaffected. Strong foods in the diet may cause rejection of milk, which usually occurs 8 to 12 hours after ingestion and disappears by 24 hours after ingestion. It may result from a change in milk flavor. On systematic review, moderate evidence indicates that alcohol, anise/caraway, carrot, eucalyptus, vanilla, garlic, and mint can be detected in breast milk by infants.[163] A dietary history, including beverages and herbs, is an important part of discovering problems.

INFANT-SIDE PROBLEMS

Ankyloglossia (Tongue-Tie)

With maternal pain or poor milk transfer that is not improved with lactation assistance (positioning, waking infant, teaching cues, etc.), ankyloglossia should be considered. *Ankyloglossia*, or *tongue-tie*, refers to a lingual frenulum that is positioned toward the tip of the tongue or is restricted in function. This condition, including the upper lip, buccal ties, and suck dysfunction, is discussed fully in Chapter 13.

Supplementary Feedings

It is agreed that the normal, full-term infant whose mother has an adequate supply does not require routine supplemental feedings. Even in hot, dry climates, water supplements are not necessary.[164–167] Supplementing when medically unnecessary has been shown to increase exposure to the risks of formula (see Chapter 18) and decrease the duration of breastfeeding. During hospitalization, giving a substitute bottle may disrupt infants' breastfeeding learning, especially if they have suck dysfunction. Other risks of supplementation include the introduction of bovine protein and the allergic response as a result of early exposure to foreign protein. Supplements interrupt the delicate balance of immune modulation and early intestinal priming and clearly change the gut flora. When lactation is going well, supplements are not needed, and when it is not going well, a bottle of infant formula without careful assessment and treatment of the underlying problem may aggravate the situation.

At any time, supplementation with formula may be a parent's choice, generally as a result of fatigue, the need to share feedings, or a concern for infant satiety. Supplementation for these latter causes can result from a misunderstanding of lactation physiology; many parents who supplement for these reasons refer to the desire to "both breastfeed and bottle-feed formula." Some may even consider infant formula as a healthy addition to their infant's diet. In addition to educating the family in the prenatal and immediate postpartum periods, it is important that they are informed that using infant formula may limit their ability to establish and maintain a milk supply. Confirming what we know about lactation physiology, Brownell et al. and Dozier et al. used population-level data to find that a period of exclusivity of 9 weeks was required to reach 3 months of breastfeeding duration, and 17 weeks was the minimum threshold of exclusivity needed to maintain any breastfeeding at 1 year.[168,169] Because this sample was not largely representative, these findings should be interpreted with caution. Mothers should be given resources to contact in the case of maternal pain leading to supplementation; these causes should be quickly treated so that mothers may resume breastfeeding.

The medical need for supplementation is a marker of impending trouble, which requires an evaluation of maternal milk supply, milk transfer, and infant growth. Such an assessment should be done by an experienced provider or lactation consultant. Common causes of medically indicated supplementation include hypoglycemia, dehydration, and jaundice in the early neonatal period and slow weight gain or failure to thrive in later periods of infancy. Indications for supplementation and management strategies are noted Appendix I, ABM Clinical Protocol 3, "Supplementary Feedings in the Healthy, Term Breastfed Neonate, Revised 2017."[170]

When breastfeeding is not going well, the negative effects of supplementation may skew families and providers against supplementation when it may be medically appropriate and may even prolong breastfeeding. Howard et al. attempted to elucidate whether supplementation itself or the method of supplementation negatively affected breastfeeding.[171] In a randomized clinical trial, they studied 700 breastfed newborns for 52 weeks, comparing pacifier and bottle use versus cup feeding. Any supplementation was associated with decreased breastfeeding duration, and there was no difference in breastfeeding outcomes for the overall population of infants fed by cup versus bottle. However, for infants born by C-section and those infants who needed more than two supplements, cup feeding had a positive effect on breastfeeding. This suggests that for those who require supplementation, using methods other than bottle-feeding may improve breastfeeding outcomes.

Ideally, supplements should be by physician order and be documented in the chart, including volume, content, timing, and medical indications. This will prevent overuse of infant formula in nonmedically indicated scenarios and reminds caregivers about appropriate counseling of families who request formula use. When breastfed infants are supplemented, amounts appropriate to their gestational age should be used, rather than arbitrary amounts (such as "1 ounce after each feed"). After lactogenesis 2, pre- and postfeed weights can be used to calculate an estimated daily intake, which can then be compared with the fluid requirements of the age group. Table 7.10 provides a helpful worksheet to calculate amounts and create a plan. If available, the mother's own expressed milk should be used for supplementation, or donor milk should be used. After this, hydrolyzed infant formula may be used for short-term supplementation, or regular formula may be used if supplementation is ongoing. In the newborn period, a cup or spoon may be more hygienic and the least impactful of supplementation devices. If supplementation needs are large or ongoing, a bottle or supplemental nursing system may be more appropriate. A slow-flow nipple should be used, and infants should be allowed opportunities to rest and burp. "Paced bottle-feeding" is a method in which the infant is fed with the bottle teat half-full of milk in a horizontal position, which allows the infant to use more dynamic suck mechanics while bottle-feeding, rather than being a passive recipient of flowing milk (Fig. 7.15). This is theoretically beneficial, although it has not been studied. Some use this term to recommend frequently removing the bottle nipple from the child's mouth every few sucks, which can result in severe crying and fussing. Forcing a hungry infant to take multiple "pauses" while crying through a feed should be avoided. Feeding should not be a stressful event for the infant, no matter the delivery mechanism.

The final step in supplementation considerations is how to return to exclusivity at the breast, if that is the mother's goal. This requires attention to maternal milk supply (i.e., through

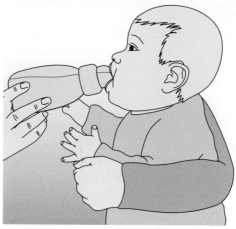

Fig. 7.15 Positioning for paced bottle-feeding. Note that the infant is propped, and the bottle is held approximately horizontally.

expressing milk or galactagogues), continuing to have the breast be a happy place where the infant enjoys being (through skin-to-skin contact), and clear criteria for when supplementation may be discontinued (i.e., based on infant growth or maternal pumping amounts).

"Nipple Confusion" and Bottle-Feeding

Nipple confusion refers to when an infant is fussy at or refuses the breast after being introduced to a bottle. It has been suggested to occur in some sensitive infants whose suckling is not well established. This term has been critiqued by those who point out that infants are unlikely to be "confused" but, rather, show an early preference for the bottle, have learned a different method of sucking, are incapable of transferring milk from the breast, or are overfed by formula supplementation and therefore not interested in breastfeeding.

Many infants will switch back and forth between bottle and breast effortlessly, which makes it difficult to predict which infant will struggle with breastfeeding as a consequence of being introduced to a bottle. However, in our clinical experience, those at high risk include infants with tongue-tie, NICU graduates who have been underexposed to breastfeeding, infants started early on nipple shields, or those with suck dysfunction (who may need supplementation because of poor milk transfer). If supplementation is required in these cases, cup feeding in the short term or the use of a supplemental nursing system for longer-term supplementation may be considered. For more discussion on the promotion of feeding at the breast in the NICU, see Chapters 13 and 14.

Exclusive Breastfeeding for 6 Months

There is some controversy among pediatricians and breastfeeding advocates regarding the appropriate time to introduce solid foods: whether it should be closer to 4 or 6 months for the maintenance of appropriate iron balance and to decrease the risk for allergies. A Cochrane review on the subject was done by Kramer and Kakuma and found that exclusive breastfeeding for 6 months had incremental benefits over 4 months in the reduction of gastrointestinal morbidity, had no increased risk of allergic disease, and prolonged lactational amenorrhea.[172] However, a reduced level of iron has been observed in low-income countries. The WHO recommends breastfeeding exclusively for 6 months. Although the American Academy of Pediatrics (AAP) recommends iron supplementation for exclusively breastfed infants at 4 months of age, the AAP Section on Breastfeeding disagrees, noting that the physiologic nadir of hemoglobin has not been shown to be harmful, nor has its treatment shown benefits. Additionally, delayed cord clamping is now the standard of care in many countries and may improve the iron status of infants during this nadir.[173,174] Infants who are born premature or are at risk of nutritional deficiency should be treated with elemental iron.

Solid Foods

Breast milk supplies the appropriate nutrients and water for the first 6 months of life. At approximately 6 months, a normal infant begins to deplete iron stores and begins to show signs of interest in foods. This is probably an appropriate time to start solid foods, especially iron-containing ones (e.g., meats, prunes, legumes, greens). This permits the entire process of weaning to cup and solid foods to be gradual. An infant does not need teeth to eat baby food and, conversely, does not have to be weaned from the breast because teeth have erupted. By 6 months, the number of feedings usually decreases. The timing and volume begin to cycle to a schedule that resembles three meals per day and some snacks.

Carrying, Holding, and Attachment

In many cultures around the world, infants are carried with the mother night and day. Conversely, in some cultures, infants are tightly swaddled and put down because carrying young infants has been considered as predisposing to spoiling. In the immediate postpartum period, being held skin to skin has positive effects on breastfeeding and the physiologic stability of infants.[45] In preterm infants, being held skin to skin reduces the length of the hospital stay and has short- and long-term health, behavioral, and parenting effects measurable 20 years later.[46] After discharge, benefits from holding can be seen. In an RCT of primiparous breastfeeding women, Hunziker and Barr showed that increased carrying reduced infant crying.[175] An interesting analysis of toddler attachment and breastfeeding in 9800 children aged 9 months to kindergarten controlled for a broad array of parenting behaviors to determine if there was a direct link between breastfeeding and attachment.[176] The authors found that children breastfed for 6 months or longer had higher attachment security as toddlers and no increase in temperamental dependency (separation-distress proneness). This means that breastfeeding itself may confer increased attachment, regardless of other parenting behaviors, and does not predispose to clinging, spoiling, or separation distress.

Sleeping

Immediate Postpartum Sleep and Support

The first concern for infant and maternal sleep in the immediate postpartum period is when and how it will take place.

Parents are exhausted, and in some cases, visitation schedules are intense. In other cases, infants and mothers are partially separated so that the mother may recover from childbirth (i.e., the postpartum "hotels" in Korea, Taiwan, or Israel). In a society in which extended families are not present to assist, nighttime care and feeding fall squarely on the shoulders of the parents (often the mother), who must learn how to function during the day as well as provide appropriate care at night. Each of these models may interrupt breastfeeding success. Therefore help over the night is a key role for partners, fathers, or other caregivers. There are some cultural traditions that support breastfeeding as well as a mother's need for sleep, commonly referred to as *lying-in*. There is historical evidence of long-standing traditions of lying-in all over the world, and some of these traditions are still observed. One example is the Chinese "sitting the month," in which mothers are isolated and have restrictions and recommendations surrounding foods, visitors, and personal hygiene. There are more, or less, restrictive types of these practices. They could be at once lauded for their focus on maternal and infant health and breastfeeding and also be criticized for the lack of freedom they afford for the mother's choices and independence.

Sleep Location

Sleep practices are highly culturally dependent and vary significantly around the world. For older infants and children, sleeping in a "family bed" or in an individual bed have both been shown to have acceptable outcomes for attachment and child health. The decision of whether to bed-share therefore should be respected by providers. Most parents will note that their infant will sleep longer if allowed to sleep with the mother. Co-sleeping has been shown to increase the number of nighttime feeds, milk supply, and breastfeeding duration. Unfortunately, bedsharing is associated with a higher risk of suffocation and sudden infant death syndrome (SIDS). This is particularly true in areas in which parents sleep together in a shared bed with a nonfirm mattress, as opposed to in a hammock, on a mat, or on the floor. The concern for suffocation and SIDS has led the AAP to recommend against bedsharing in all its forms. Sleeping with an infant is nevertheless common: in a sample from 32 birth hospitals including 3218 mothers in the United States from 2011 to 2014, 21% reported bedsharing with an infant.[177] In this sample, mothers who bed-shared were more likely to report partial breastfeeding (adjusted odds ratio [OR] 1.75, 95% CI 1.33 to 2.31) or exclusive breastfeeding (adjusted OR 2.46, 95% CI 1.76 to 3.45) than those who did not bed-share.

This seeming paradox, that bedsharing increases the risk of unexpected infant death, yet breastfeeding is enabled by bedsharing and reduces the risk of SIDS, has led to a fierce debate among and between maternal-child health advocates. For instance, whereas the AAP recommends against bedsharing in any form, this is in opposition to the UNICEF UK infant sleep recommendation and the ABM recommendation, which both focus on parental education to reduce *hazardous* co-sleeping situations.[178] Similarly, La Leche League International has educational materials for parents based on

"The Safe Sleep Seven," that is, ways to remember and reduce potential co-sleeping hazards.[6]

Breastsleeping

In response to this impasse, James McKenna and Lee Gettler, prominent anthropologists at Notre Dame University and directors of the Mother–Baby Behavioral Sleep Laboratory and the Hormones, Health and Human Behavior Laboratory, respectively, have proposed the term "breastsleeping" as reflective of co-sleeping in the context of exclusive breastfeeding and in the absence of any other risk factors (Table 7.11). They propose that this concept be used to acknowledge the evolutionarily complex "'suite' of co-evolving traits," which includes immediate and sustained maternal-infant contact, breastfeeding, and parental investment and nurturing behaviors. Focusing on breastsleeping in research and clinical environments may allow us to develop better answers to which babies are at highest and lowest risk for SIDS.[179]

The ABM has developed a protocol regarding the issue of safe sleep while promoting breastfeeding, which addresses parental counseling and risk reduction.[178] Essentially, there is insufficient data to universally recommend against bedsharing to reduce the risk of SIDS. Using current data to recommend against bedsharing in all forms has similar logic to noticing that toddlers choke on certain foods and saying that they therefore should not eat. Thus parents should be counseled to protect breastfeeding and reduce hazardous sleeping situations, as outlined in Table 7.11.

Timing of Neonatal and Infant Sleep

For an infant, whose fetal life was spent moving largely when the mother was less active (i.e., at night), sleeping through the night has been assumed to be an important developmental milestone dependent on maturation. This was investigated in a small study ($n = 26$) with first-time parents of exclusively breastfed infants who were taught to "sleep train" their newborns by feeding at 10 PM and midnight and delaying other overnight feeds while using other methods to soothe.[180] At 3 at 8 weeks, the treatment-group infants slept longer at night and fed more during the day. Milk intakes for 24 hours between the two groups were not different. The authors concluded that parents can teach their breastfed infants to lengthen nighttime sleep periods. This was a small study, and more research is needed before recommending sleep training of neonates. Additionally, in a group of 715 mothers of 6- to 12-month-olds, increased daytime feeding was associated with reduced nighttime feeding but not with reduced nighttime awakening.[181]

Because of parental exhaustion, many trials have sought to develop programming to support increased sleep for parents. Thus far, psychosocial interventions have shown minimal impact on nighttime waking or overall rest.[182] Parents should therefore be encouraged to develop management plans that they find most comfortable.

Milk Composition and Sleep

Milk composition may influence infant sleep latency. Tryptophan concentrations are higher in human milk than in formula, and tryptophan is known to increase sleep in adults. When breastfed and formula-fed infants were compared using formulas with different levels of tryptophan, infants had shorter sleep latency with high levels of tryptophan.[183] Researchers have also found lower levels of melatonin in daytime milk as compared with milk collected at night. Melatonin appears to be stable in human milk for 4 to 24 hours after freezing and defrosting and is therefore available in pumped milk as well.[184] More research is needed before making conclusions about milk composition and infant sleep.

Colic and Crying

Colic has the same etymologic origin in Latin and Middle English as the word *colon,* and used as such, it refers to the spasmodic contraction of smooth muscle in the abdomen, causing pain and discomfort. When the term *colic* is used in reference to infants, it describes a syndrome in which the infant has unexplained paroxysms of irritability, fussing, and crying for a prolonged period, often at the same time of day, in the early months of life. The infant usually draws the legs up as if in pain and has a red or flushed face. Infantile colic has been reported to occur equally among breastfed and formula-fed infants. In one Danish cohort of 62,761 infants, those born before 32 weeks' gestation and those born small for gestational age were found to have higher odds of colic.[185] Premature infants may present these symptoms closer to their adjusted age, rather than chronologic age.

The Rome IV criteria are used for diagnosis of colic in children under 5 months of age and include the following: (1) the aforementioned irritability without obvious cause; (2) crying for more than 3 hours per day, more than 3 days per week for more than 1 week; and (3) the absence of failure to thrive. Symptoms usually self-resolve by 3 months of age.[186] It is considered a "benign" condition because of the lack of impact on growth and long-term neurodevelopment, but it is nevertheless very impactful for families who must live through it. Although parenting style may contribute to infant crying, and parental expectations may over- or undervalue that crying, the symptoms of infantile colic are generally much more severe than any normal fussing.

Characteristically, an infant will cry and scream as if in pain for 3 to 4 hours at a stretch, often between 6 and 10 PM. The infant will nurse frequently and then scream and pull away from the breast as if in pain, only to cry a few minutes later. The infant may respond to gentle rocking when held against a warm shoulder. If the infant is put down, the screaming starts again. If the nursing mother holds the infant, the infant is frantic unless nursed and yet does not need to be fed. This may disturb a new mother, who wonders why she cannot console her infant: Is her milk weak? Does it disagree with her infant? Is she an inadequate mother? None of these is true, but smelling the mother's milk makes the infant behave as if it needs to nurse. Sometimes the infant can be comforted by another adult, such as the father, grandmother, or other caregiver. Picking up the infant does not spoil the child, and rocking and cuddling are appropriate. Warm pressure may help; a warm hot water bottle or warm shoulder with some pressure or

TABLE 7.11   Modifiable and Nonmodifiable Risk Factors for Sudden Infant Death Syndrome and Suffocation in Breastfed Infants and Their Relationship With Breastfeeding

Risk or Protective Factor	Direction of Effect	Impact on Breastfeeding	Risk Reduction
Modifiable			
Supine sleep position	Strong protective	None	• All infants should be placed on their backs to sleep.
Bedsharing	Controversial effect	Significant. Bedsharing may improve breastfeeding duration and exclusivity. Possibly modifiable by ensuring bed sharing is safer.	• Firm mattress • No loose bedding • Infant on mother's side only • No pets • No smokers • No cracks, not between mother and the wall • No other children or pets • Mother not taking medications that create drowsiness or using alcohol • Potentially modifiable: maternal obesity
Loose bedding, soft sleep surfaces, entrapment hazards or cord risks	Strong risk	None	• Loose bedding and soft sleep surfaces should be avoided. • Entrapment hazards and cords should be kept far from the sleep area.
Maternal smoking in breastfeeding	Strong risk	Smoking reduces breastfeeding duration, possibly through impacts on milk supply.	• Mothers who smoke and breastfeed should never sleep with their infants. • Resources to quit smoking should be offered.
Pacifier use	Controversial effect	Potentially limits duration and exclusivity.	• Pacifier at bedtime may be offered after breastfeeding is well established and if parent desires.
Immunizations	Strong protective	None	• All infants should be immunized per Centers for Disease Control and Prevention guidelines
Nonmodifiable			
Maternal smoking in pregnancy	Strong risk	Smoking in pregnancy has been shown to reduce breastfeeding duration, possibly through impacts on milk supply.	• Suggest smoking cessation in pregnancy.
Preterm birth, low birth weight, poor prenatal care, low socioeconomic status of the family, young parents, low educational level of parents	Strong risk	Many, including decreased duration and exclusivity	• Significant improvements in policies and social supports are necessary to prevent these causes.
Short periods between pregnancies, multiple pregnancy, drug intake during pregnancy	Strong risk	Many, including decreased duration and exclusivity	• Strengthened preconception care, drug-treatment resources • Significant improvements in policies and social supports are necessary to prevent these causes.
Winter months, male sex	Strong risk	None	• None
Overheating, head covering	Strong risk	None	• Avoid overheating; some evidence suggests a fan in the infant's room in summer may be protective.

(Continued)

TABLE 7.11 Modifiable and Nonmodifiable Risk Factors for Sudden Infant Death Syndrome and Suffocation in Breastfed Infants and Their Relationship With Breastfeeding—cont'd

Risk or Protective Factor	Direction of Effect	Impact on Breastfeeding	Risk Reduction
Infection	Strong risk	Is more common in infants fed formula	• Promote breastfeeding • Promote handwashing • Early identification and management of group B *Strep* • Ensure parental education about fever and infant behavior • Ensure access to care

Carlin RF, Moon RY. Risk factors, protective factors, and current recommendations to reduce sudden infant death syndrome: a review. *JAMA Pediatr.* 2017;171(2):175–180. http://doi:10.1001/jamapediatrics.2016.3345; Harper RM, Kinney HC, Fleming PJ, et al. Sleep influences on homeostatic functions: implications for sudden infant death syndrome. *Respir Physiol.* 2000;119(2–3):123–132.

massage is comforting. The use of rhythmic incessant sounds or lights (e.g., vacuum cleaner, white noise, washing machine, "shhh" noises) has variable success.

In general, the level of quality of research on colic has failed to identify a specific cause or appropriate treatments for this condition, although the role of probiotics is promising. A carefully taken history and physical examination will rule out other pathologic conditions, which may be found in about 5% of infants with symptoms of colic. Providers should consider at least the following: otitis media, anal fissure, hair tourniquet, hunger, reflux, milk protein allergy, hernia, or nonaccidental trauma. Medications have been studied. Conflicting data exist for simethicone, whereas dicyclomine hydrochloride and cimetropium bromide cause unacceptable side effects.[186] A 2017 systematic review and meta-analysis of five RCTs found that supplementation of breastfed infants with colic with the probiotic *Lactobacillus reuteri* resulted in a greater chance of 50% reduction in crying time as compared with placebo.[187] There were no adverse events. A Cochrane review confirms this possibility but calls for more research.[188]

Importantly, parents require understanding and support to get through this difficult time. Families should be informed that putting the child down in a safe space to take a break for themselves and seek support may help to prevent unintentional injury to the child or exhaustion in themselves. Normalizing their experiences of frustration, fear, failure, anger, and anxiety may help them to feel heard as they wait for the symptoms of colic to abate.

The sleep-tight method of calming crying and colicky infants was developed by Dr. Harvey Karp, who produced an illustrative video demonstrating the technique.[189] He compares the first few months of life to the "fourth trimester" and suggests that creating a "womb-like" atmosphere is very calming. His "five S" system consists of the following:

Swaddling: Tight swaddling provides the continuous touching and support the infant experienced while in the mother's womb.

Side/stomach position: Place the baby, while holding her, either on her left side to assist in digestion or on her stomach to provide reassuring support. Once the baby is happily asleep, you can safely put her in her crib on her back.

Shushing sounds: These sounds imitate the continual whooshing sound made by the blood flowing through arteries

near the womb. This white noise can be in the form of a vacuum cleaner, a hair dryer, or a fan.

Swinging: Newborns are used to the swinging motions that were present when they were in utero. Rocking, car rides, and other swinging movements can help.

Sucking: "Sucking has its effects deep within the nervous system and triggers the calming reflex and releases natural chemicals within the brain"; this "S" can be accomplished with breast, bottle, pacifier, or even a finger, according to Karp.[189]

The "five S" system was studied in an RCT to reduce post-vaccination pain in 2- and 4-month-old infants ($n = 230$) and showed reduced crying time over sucrose or standard-of-care comfort.[190] Of note, oversoothing of a newborn may delay the interpretation of feeding cues and result in fewer feedings than are necessary to establish milk supply and adequate infant growth. It is therefore important to ensure that neonates who have not yet regained birth weight are unwrapped to have skin-to-skin time and opportunities to nurse every 2 to 3 hours.

Cow's Milk Protein Allergy, Non-Immunoglobulin E (IgE)—Mediated Food Sensitivities, and Food-Protein—Induced Enterocolitis Syndrome (FPIES)

Breastfed infants who present with severe fussiness, mucus or blood in the stool, eczema, and/or reflux may be reacting to food proteins passed through maternal milk. This is covered in detail in Chapter 17.

Esophageal Reflux

Many infants will spit up milk after eating. This is called *physiologic reflux* and is rarely a cause of distress. Parents may be reassured. *Pathologic reflux,* on the other hand, causes infant distress, pain, poor appetite, and sometimes failure to thrive. Although less common than in bottle-fed infants, esophageal reflux can occur in breastfed infants; reflux is covered in detail in Chapter 13.

Other Food Avoidances in Breastfeeding, Elimination Diets

Maternal dietary restrictions and food taboos after birth have been common around the world and across cultures. In some cases, these are based on cultural beliefs of what foods will help with postpartum recovery, and in others, they are related to theoretical infant health consequences. As studies from Canada and Korea show, there may be significant social pressure to modify the maternal diet, although there is limited medical guidance for these mothers.[191,192] Evidence supportive of an association between maternal food intake and infant health has been of limited scope and methodology.[192] For example, in one study in which associations were found between certain foods (cruciferous vegetables, onions, cow's milk, and chocolate) and colic, mothers self-reported breastfeeding, colic symptoms, and diet by recall after 4 months, which is subject to significant bias.[193] In addition, the types of food to which infants are said to be sensitive varies significantly geographically, sometimes in direct contradiction. Because of these concerns, a Cochrane review and meta-analysis was completed in 2018 and found insufficient data to recommend a specific dietary restriction for the avoidance or treatment of infant colic.[194]

It is important to note that concern over maternal diet may create significant stress or even cause mothers to not initiate or to stop breastfeeding. Its theoretical benefits should therefore be carefully weighed against potential harms. If a maternal food is consistently and clearly related to a strong reaction in a child, and it is not a dietary hardship for the mother to avoid this food, then she may be encouraged to do so. In clinical and anecdotal experience, foods that seem poorly tolerated are different for different infants.

Pacifiers, Dummies

Infants are born with some self-comforting mechanisms, including resuming the fetal position and sucking a thumb, finger, or fist. A bottle-fed infant may have nonnutritive sucking with a pacifier and avoid overeating. However, pacifiers in breastfed infants risk interfering with breastfeeding. This may be a result of the different mechanism of suck it promotes or because it delays feeding past early hunger cues, resulting in an overly hungry baby who cannot settle to breastfeed. Pacifiers have become the subject of controversy for full-term, healthy infants. Restricting artificial nipples has been a central tenet of the UNICEF 10 steps to support breastfeeding, although this was revised with the latest guidelines.[38,39] This is because in the past 10 years, studies have not found an association with early weaning or have reported the reverse. Two competing systematic reviews with meta-analyses have concluded in opposition to each other: a Cochrane review found no valid data to support the restriction of pacifier use, and a review from Sao Paolo, Brazil, and Yale University found an increased risk of exclusive breastfeeding cessation with the introduction of pacifiers.[195,196] In ill or preterm newborns, some studies have suggested that pacifier use reduces pain and may help with oral skills as these infants transition to oral feeds, even when breastfeeding. Literature in dentistry has found associations between pacifier use and malocclusion, after controlling for breastfeeding.[197,198]

The Task Force on Sudden Infant Death of the AAP has recommended pacifier use at sleep times, making the suggestion that pacifiers be introduced immediately in bottle-fed babies but delayed until breastfeeding is well established in breastfed infants.[199] A Cochrane review of pacifiers and sudden infant death has not found sufficient evidence to support or refute this recommendation.[200] Breastfeeding has been recognized as a protection against SIDS (see Chapter 15), and therefore the potential risk to breastfeeding should be weighed against the potential benefit of offering a pacifier.

Based on the difficulties in interpreting the data, parents should be informed of potential risks and benefits and supported in their decisions.[39,199] If breastfeeding, they should be educated that early feeding cues may be missed and to cease pacifier use if the infant begins to be fussy at the breast. A pacifier should not be introduced by hospital staff unless the mother requests it, is counseled on their use, and concerns are addressed.

Vomiting Blood

A breastfed baby who vomits blood may be vomiting maternal blood ingested from a cracked nipple or duct, or their own blood (see Chapter 16). If there is a clear cause, the cause should be remedied and the provider notified. If it is necessary to differentiate whose blood was vomited (i.e., the infant or the mother is unwell), this can be differentiated by the Apt test to measure fetal or adult hemoglobin. Blood is suspended in a small amount of saline solution and an equal amount of 10% sodium hydroxide added; adult hemoglobin turns brown, whereas fetal hemoglobin stays pink. Breastfeeding can usually continue with maternal milk if the infant will comfortably nurse and the cause of the bleeding has been addressed.

Greenish or brown milk is occasionally described in the first few days if the mother is pumping or her infant vomits. It usually results from old blood in the ducts, a residual of rapid growth and vascularization during pregnancy. This milk is usually harmless and clears spontaneously in a day or two. It usually goes unnoticed if the infant is nursing well at the breast. If being pumped, it may be used, unless an infection is suspected. Breastfeeding does not need to be interrupted. This has been referred to as *rusty pipe syndrome*. See Chapter 16 for more details on differently colored milk.

The Reference list is available at www.expertconsult.com.

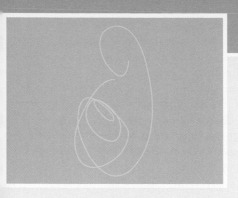

8

Maternal Nutrition and Supplements for Mother and Infant

Ruth A. Lawrence

KEY POINTS

- Exclusive breastfeeding for 4 to 6 months is capable of nourishing an infant for appropriate growth and development even when the mother's nutrition is "less than perfect."
- The quantity of breast milk produced can be affected by maternal dehydration (when severe, >10% weight loss) or severe maternal malnutrition, but the quality of breast milk as adequate nutrition for the infant is maintained.
- Maternal conditions that are associated with macro- or micronutrient deficiencies should be noted (e.g., smoking, exclusion diets [dairy], vegan diet with marked limitations, malabsorption, bariatric surgery, etc.) and supplements provided during lactation to replenish maternal stores of deficient nutrients.

- Once lactation is well established through 4 to 6 weeks, maternal exercise and controlled weight loss (0.5 to 2 kg of weight per week) will not affect the quantity or quality of breast-milk production or infant growth. Diets for weight loss should include balanced, varied foods rich in calcium, zinc, magnesium, vitamin B_6, and folate, with a minimum energy intake of approximately 1800 kcal. Calcium and multivitamin—mineral supplements may be necessary to replace stores if the diet is marginal.

NUTRITION FOR BREASTFEEDING

Lactation is the physiologic completion of the reproductive cycle. The maternal body prepares during pregnancy for lactation, not only by developing the breast to produce milk but also by storing additional nutrients and energy for milk production. The transition to fully sustaining an infant by breastfeeding should not be complex or require major nutritional adjustments for a woman. After delivery, mothers usually note an increase in appetite and thirst and a change in some dietary preferences. In some cultures, anthropologists have noted that, traditionally, the birth of a baby means that members of the community take gifts of special foods—usually high in protein, nutrients, and calories—for the mother to ensure she will make good milk for the infant. This tradition may have affected some early studies in which relatively malnourished women were noted to produce milk comparable with that produced by well-nourished women in industrialized countries.

After an exhaustive study of the world's literature and current scientific evidence, the Subcommittee on Nutrition During Lactation of the Committee on Nutritional Status During Pregnancy and Lactation of the Food and Nutrition Board of the Institute of Medicine at the National Academy of Sciences published its first report.[1] The subcommittee stated that breastfeeding is recommended for all infants in the United States under ordinary circumstances. Women living in a wide variety of circumstances in the United States and elsewhere are capable of fully nourishing their infants by breastfeeding them. Furthermore, exclusive breastfeeding is preferred for the first 4 to 6 months. The report further stated that mothers with less-than-perfect diets could make nutritionally adequate milk.

The overwhelming evidence indicates that women are able to "produce milk of sufficient quantity and quality to support growth and promote the health of infants—even when the mother's supply of nutrients is limited."[1] Nonetheless, the depletion of the mother's nutrient stores is a risk if efforts to achieve adequate food intake are not made to replace maternal stores.

Most materials written for nursing mothers regarding maternal diet during lactation set up complicated "rules" about dietary intake that fail to consider the mother's dietary stores, normal dietary preferences, and cultural patterns. Thus one barrier to breastfeeding for some women is the "diet rules" they see as being too hard to follow or too restrictive.[2] All over the world, women produce adequate and even abundant milk on apparently inadequate diets.[3] Women in cultures with modest but adequate diets produce milk without any obvious detriment to themselves and with none of the fatigue and loss of well-being that some well-fed Western mothers experience. Insufficient milk is a problem in Western cultures and rarely in developing countries.[4]

IMPACT OF MATERNAL DIET ON MILK PRODUCTION

Although much has been learned about dietary requirements for lactation by studying women from many cultures and various levels of nutrition, some of the information is conflicting, principally because of varying sampling techniques and the improvement over time in laboratory analysis. Extensive reviews of the current literature on various nutrients in human milk and the influence of maternal dietary intake have been referenced.[5-13] Those readers needing access to the original studies are referred to the bibliographies from these reviews, which include hundreds of items, a listing beyond the scope of this text.

Milk Volume

The volume of milk produced varies over the duration of lactation from the first few weeks to 6 months and beyond but is remarkably predictable except during extreme malnutrition or severe dehydration. In periods of acute water deprivation, manifested in a healthy mother by an acute bout of vomiting and diarrhea, the volume of milk will diminish only after the maternal urine output has been significantly compromised (10% dehydration or greater).

Of practical significance for counseling healthy women in the industrialized world is the work of Butte et al.[14] investigating the effect of maternal diet and body composition on lactational performance; 45 healthy lactating women were followed for 4 months from delivery with detailed measurements of milk production, dietary intake, and maternal body composition. The overall mean energy intake was 2186 ± 463 kcal/day. Milk production averaged 751, 725, 723, and 740 g/day for months 1, 2, 3, and 4, respectively. The average maternal weight reduction was from 64.6 to 59.3 kg. Energy was calculated to be sufficient for maintenance and activity, yet the mothers achieved gradual weight reduction. The authors conclude that energy intakes of approximately 15% less than those currently recommended are compatible with full lactation, full activity, and gradual weight reduction to prepregnant weight (Tables 8.1 and 8.2). Diets otherwise contained recommended daily allowances for lactation.

Malnutrition, however, is complex, and single-nutrient deficiencies are rare. Malnutrition does seem to influence the total volume of milk produced. Extreme cases, such as famines, cause milk supply to dwindle and cease, with the ultimate starvation of the infant. The classic study is the report by Smith on the effects of maternal undernutrition on the newborn infant in the Hunger Winter in Holland in 1944 to 1945.[15] It was reported that the volume of milk was slightly diminished, but the duration of lactation was not affected. The latter is a testimony to courage rather than diet. Analysis of milk produced showed no significant deviations from the normal chemical structure. Milk was produced at the expense of maternal tissue.

These data from the Dutch famine in the 1940s during World War II were reexamined by Stein et al., who pointed out that women who conceived during the famine did develop some maternal stores in anticipation of lactation that were not accounted for by the fetus, placenta, or amniotic fluid, even though the newborns were, on average, a pound lighter at birth.[16] They reported fetal weight down by 10% but maternal weight down by only 4%. This demonstrates the mother's body's strong biologic "mandate" to prepare for lactation during pregnancy.

There is a wide range of volume of milk intake among healthy breastfed infants, averaging 750 to 800 g/day and ranging from 450 to 1200 g/day.[14] Any factor that influences the frequency, intensity, or duration of suckling by an infant influences the volume.[17] In a study of wet nurses in the 1920s, Macy et al. reported human milk production capacity at 3500 mL/day when serving as a wet nurse for multiple children.[18] Compared with the 800 mL from mothers with singletons, studies of mothers producing for multiples, done by Saint et al., confirmed production of 2 to 3 L/day for twins and triplets.[19] At 3 months of age for all populations, the volume averages 770 g/day (range 500 to 1200 g/day).[20] The self-regulation of milk supply by the infant has been confirmed by

TABLE 8.1   Milk Production Over First 4 Months of Lactation

	Month 1 (*n* = 37)	Month 2 (*n* = 40)	Month 3 (*n* = 37)	Month 4 (*n* = 41)
Human milk[a] (g/day)	751 (130)[b]	725 (131)	723 (114)	740 (128)
Feedings (no./day)	8.3 (1.9)	7.2 (1.9)	6.8 (1.9)	6.7 (1.8)
Total nitrogen (mg/g)	2.17 (0.30)	1.94 (0.24)	1.84 (0.19)	1.80 (0.21)
Protein nitrogen (mg/g)	1.61 (0.24)	1.42 (0.17)	1.34 (0.15)	1.31 (0.17)
Nonprotein nitrogen (mg/g)	0.56 (0.28)	0.52 (0.20)	0.50 (0.13)	0.48 (0.14)
Fat (mg/g)	36.2 (7.5)	34.4 (6.8)	32.2 (7.8)	34.8 (10.8)
Energy (kcal/g)	0.68 (0.08)	0.64 (0.08)	0.62 (0.09)	0.64 (0.10)

[a]At the onset of the study, milk was estimated by deuterium dilution, a technique that was later determined to be inaccurate. For this reason, data are missing at 17 time points during the first 3 months.
[b]Mean (standard deviation [SD]).
From Butte NF, Garza C, Stuff JE, et al. Effect of maternal diet and body composition on lactational performance. *Am J Clin Nutr*. 1984;39:296.

TABLE 8.2 Anthropometric Changes in Mothers During Lactation

Parameter	Postpartum	Month 1	Month 2	Month 3	Month 4
Weight (kg)	64.6 (9.1)[a]	61.3 (9.5)	60.7 (10.0)	60.2 (10.4)	59.3 (10.5)
Weight/height (kg/cm)[b]	0.40 (0.04)	0.37 (0.05)	0.37 (0.05)	0.37 (0.05)	0.36 (0.06)
Weight/prepregnancy weight[c]	1.16 (0.06)	1.08 (0.05)	1.07 (0.05)	1.06 (0.05)	1.05 (0.07)
Weight change (kg/mo)		−3.83 (2.26)	−0.59 (1.20)	−0.62 (1.12)	−0.80 (1.86)
Triceps (mm)	16.3 (5.1)	16.9 (4.6)	17.0 (4.7)	17.3 (5.3)	17.2 (5.2)
Subscapular (mm)	18.2 (7.1)	16.8 (6.4)	16.4 (7.4)	15.7 (7.2)	15.1 (7.3)
Biceps (mm)	7.8 (3.9)	6.9 (3.2)	6.9 (3.3)	7.3 (4.6)	6.8 (3.4)
Suprailiac (mm)	26.1 (8.5)	25.7 (6.9)	25.2 (7.6)	23.1 (8.1)	22.2 (8.0)
Sum skinfolds (mm)	68.4 (20.2)	66.3 (18.9)	65.5 (20.6)	63.4 (22.9)	61.7 (21.8)
Midarm circumference (cm)	26.9 (3.5)	26.7 (2.6)	26.8 (3.2)	26.6 (2.9)	26.7 (3.6)

[a]Mean (standard deviation [SD]).
[b]Maternal height = 163.0 cm (6.3 cm).
[c]Prepregnancy weight gain = 14.4 kg (3.3 kg).
From Butte NF, Garza C, Stuff JE, et al. Effect of maternal diet and body composition on lactational performance. *Am J Clin Nutr*. 1984;39:296.

a study by Dewey et al. in which additional milk was pumped after each feeding for 2 weeks, thus increasing the milk supply. The infants, however, remained at baseline consumption during the pumping.[21] The residual milk supply of healthy women (i.e., that which can be extracted after a full feeding) is about 100 g/day, even when an infant consumes comparatively low volumes of milk.[17,21,22]

Topographic computer imaging of the breast has been used to study breast production and storage capacities in the laboratory of Peter Hartmann. Using "moiré patterns" projected onto the breast, it has been possible to calculate the volume of milk produced. As the breast expands with increasing milk, the moiré patterns change. By correlating the maternal weights before and after a feeding and the imagery patterns, data were converted to accurate milk volumes. This technique has remarkable potential for clinical use. Hartmann reports the normal range of milk production from 1 to 6 months postpartum to be between 440 and 1220 g/day for mothers who gave birth at full term.[23]

Prentice and Prentice described "energy-sparing adaptations" that were associated with normal lactation when energy intake is limited. These were decreases in basal metabolic rate, thermogenesis, and physical activity.[24]

When well-nourished mothers reduced their intake by 32% for 1 week, consuming no less than 1500 kcal/day, no reduction in milk volume occurred, although plasma prolactin levels increased. Mothers who consumed less than 1500 kcal/day for a week did experience decreased milk volumes compared with those of the control group and the group consuming more than 1500 kcal.

Exercise, manual labor, and losing weight do not usually alter an established milk volume. Milk production will increase with infant demand, but infant demand will only increase with growth, which depends on sufficient nourishment.[20]

Energy Supplementation and Lactation Performance

When women received supplements during the last trimester of pregnancy, no effect was noted in their milk production. This suggests that short-term supplementation may be ineffective or that the effect of supplementation may be more psychological than physiologic. Other studies that provided supplementation of a maximum of 900 kcal/day for 2 weeks resulted in an increase in milk production (662 to 787 g/day).[25] No increase in infant weight compared with the control group's infants was seen in this period of 2 weeks.

The problem of insufficient milk supply for a baby is reported in well-nourished as well as poorly nourished populations, but in cross-cultural studies, it appears to be unrelated to maternal nutrition status.[26] In countries where food supplies vary with the season, milk supplies drop 1 dL/day during periods of progressively greater food shortages. Studies continue on the lactation performance of poorly nourished women around the world, including Myanmar, Burma, and Gambia, as well as among Navajo people. The results continue to reflect an impact on quantity, not quality, of milk.[27–30]

The interrelationship of milk volume, nutrient concentration, and total nutrient intake by the infant must be considered.[21] The reason for low protein content in a given sample may be a lack of protein stores, a lack of total energy content, or a lack of vitamin B_6, a requirement of normal protein metabolism.

Of concern, however, is the report of dietary supplementation of Gambian nursing mothers in whom lactational performance was not affected by increased calories (700 kcal/day).[29] The supplement produced a slight initial improvement in maternal body weight and subcutaneous fat but not in milk output. Whether the mothers utilized the increased energy to work harder or whether the infants did not stimulate increased milk production is unresolved. Food supplementation of lactating women in areas where malnutrition is prevalent has generally had little, if any, impact on milk volume.[1] Such supplementation improves maternal health and is more likely to benefit the mother than the infant, except where milk composition had been affected by specific deficiencies.

Protein Content

Since the work of Hambraeus reestablished the norms for protein in human milk to be 0.8 to 0.9 g/dL in well-nourished mothers, figures from previous studies have been recalculated to consider that all nitrogen in human milk is not protein.[31] Twenty-five percent of the nitrogen is nonprotein nitrogen (NPN) in human milk, and only 5% of the nitrogen is NPN in bovine milk.[32] The protein content of milk from poorly nourished mothers is surprisingly high, and malnutrition has little effect on protein concentration. An increase in dietary protein increases volume but not overall protein content, given the normal variations seen in healthy, well-nourished women.

Observations made over a 20-month period of continued lactation showed that milk quality did not change, although the quantity decreased slightly, which has been attributed to the decreasing demand of a child who is receiving other nourishment. Therefore the total protein available with the decreased volume of milk and increased weight of the child decreased from 2.2 g/kg of body weight to 0.45 g/kg. The need for additional protein sources from other foods for the child after 1 year of age becomes obvious.[33]

The composition of human milk is maintained even with less-than-recommended dietary intake of macronutrients. The concentrations of major minerals, including calcium, phosphorus, magnesium, sodium, and potassium, are not affected by diet. Maternal dietary intakes of selenium and iodine, however, are positively affected: an increase in the diet increases the level in the milk.[34,35] The proportion of different fatty acids in human milk varies with the maternal dietary intake.[36]

In the Congo (formerly Zaire), 83 lactating mothers with protein malnutrition were given 500 kcal (2093 kilojoules [kJ]) and 18 g of protein as a cow-milk supplement for 2 months, after which their nutritional status improved significantly.[37] The volume of milk did not change (607 versus 604 mL). Their breastfed infants, however, did show significant improvement in their mean serum albumin levels, and their growth matched that of healthy infants of the same age.

The effect of very-low-protein (8% of energy) and very-high-protein (20% of energy) diets on the protein and nitrogen composition of breast milk in three healthy Swedish women "in full lactation" was significant.[38] High-protein diets produced higher production and greater concentrations of total nitrogen, true protein, and NPN. The increased NPN was caused by increased urea levels and free amino acids. The 24-hour outputs of lactoferrin, lactalbumin, and serum albumin were not significantly higher.

When marginally nourished women were provided a mixed-protein diet predominantly from plant sources up to 1.2 g/kg per day, equilibrium was achieved at a protein intake of 1.1 g/kg. In a study of healthy women given marginal protein intakes, Motil et al. reported that maternal milk production and the protein nitrogen, but not the NPN, fraction of human milk were relatively well preserved in the short term.[39] The practical significance, except as related to fad diets, of these results is limited because the diets were extreme and were maintained for only 4 days. The fact that milk production and protein nitrogen were maintained despite marginal protein intake is important. Taurine, an amino acid found only in animal products, is the second most abundant free amino acid in human milk. Even milk of women who have no animal foods in their diet contains some taurine, at levels (33 mg/dL) that are lower than those in women who consume animal products (54 mg/dL).[40] Taurine is singularly important as the principal protein in the human brain. Cow milk does not contain taurine.

Fat, Cholesterol, and Omega-3 Fatty Acids

Mature human milk contains approximately 50% of its energy as fat. This fat is necessary for the tremendous growth of the newborn and is essential to the structural development of the brain, retina, and other tissues. Both omega-6 (n-6 or ω-6) and omega-3 (n-3 or ω-3) fatty acids are essential components of the phospholipids of cell membranes. They are critical to the fluidity, permeability, and activity of membrane-bound enzymes and receptors. During the first 4 to 6 months of life, an infant accumulates 1300 to 1600 g of lipids.

Considerable attention has been focused on the impact of dietary fat and cholesterol on the composition of human milk. Fat is the main source of kilocalories in human milk for the infant. The fatty acid composition of the triglycerides, which make up more than 98% of the lipid component of human milk, can be affected by maternal diet. Diets with different lipid composition, caloric content, proportion of calories from fat, and fatty acid composition have been studied.

In a classic work that was carefully controlled, Insull et al.[36] fed lactating women in a metabolic ward diets that differed in caloric content, proportion of calories from fat, and fatty acid composition. Neither milk volume nor total milk fat was affected by diet. When the high-calorie, no-fat diet was fed, milk triglycerides were higher in fatty acids 12:0 and 14:0 and lower in 18:0 and 18:1, which indicated that when fatty acids were synthesized from carbohydrate, more intermediate-chain fatty acids were produced. With the low-calorie, no-fat diet, the fatty acid composition of the milk resembled the maintenance diet and the depot fat. When corn oil was the fat source, milk levels of 18:2 and 18:3 were higher, with a major increase in linoleic acid, than when lard or butter was used. Multiple studies have shown that medium-chain fatty acids, lauric and myristic acid (12:0 and 14:0), are not affected by diet, indicating synthesis by the mammary gland.[5,41,42]

Trans fatty acids are produced in hydrogenation reactions and appear in human milk as a reflection of dietary intake, so women who eat margarine rather than butter have high levels in their milk. Elaidic acid (18:1 trans) is found in margarine, for instance. Because of the high level of trans fatty acids in hydrogenated vegetable oils such as margarine, the milk of women in the United States is high in trans fatty acids, whereas the milk of women in West Germany who do not use margarine is low in trans fatty acids.[43]

The concern about fat composition in terms of the ratio of polyunsaturated fatty acid (PUFA) to saturated fatty acid (P/S ratio) and the high level of cholesterol normally found in breast milk have led to monitoring mothers on altered lipid intakes. Lactating women were placed on one of two experimental diets after a period of a study of their normal Australian diet, which included 400 to 600 mg of cholesterol per day and fat that was rich in saturated fatty acids.[44] Following this baseline study, the mothers were given either diet A, with 580 mg cholesterol and a high level of saturated fats, or diet B, with 110 mg cholesterol and a higher level of polyunsaturated fats from vegetable oils. A second study, by the same authors, was carried out with these two diets high in either saturated or unsaturated fats, but the cholesterol remained the same, 345 to 380 mg/day.[44]

The increase in PUFA in the diet rapidly increased the levels of linoleate in the milk to twice the previous level, at the expense of myristate and palmitate. Protein levels remained the same in the milk throughout the study. Infant plasma cholesterol levels decreased in response to an increase in the concentration of linoleate in the milk. The significant dietary change seemed to depend on the consumption of high PUFA and low cholesterol to alter the levels in the milk and thus in the infant's plasma (Table 8.3).[44]

Low-cholesterol diets lowered the maternal blood cholesterol but not the triglyceride levels. The cholesterol level of the milk, however, was unaffected in any diet combination.[45] Cholesterol levels remain relatively stable throughout at least 16 weeks of lactation. The presence or absence of phytosterols influences both the accuracy of analysis (i.e., overestimated level of cholesterol) and the physiologic significance of cholesterol. Phytosterols are those sterols derived from plant sources. They are distinguishable from cholesterol, which is of animal origin. During a given feeding, the concentration of cholesterol in the milk may increase more than 60%, although the total for the feeding is constant. The effect of maternal diet on cholesterol and phytosterol levels in human milk was measured by Mellies et al., who reported no change in cholesterol but a dramatic increase in phytosterols on high-cholesterol

and high-phytosterol diets.[46] The level of phytosterol in infant plasma did not change, however. These observations further confirm that cholesterol is synthesized at least in part in the mammary gland, whereas phytosterol is not.

Thus no evidence is available that concentrations of cholesterol and phospholipids can be changed by diet. Milk cholesterol is stable at 100 to 150 mg/L even in hypercholesterolemic women and increases only in severe cases of pathologic hypercholesterolemia, according to Jensen.[47] The fat-globule membrane contains both cholesterol and phospholipids, and their secretion rates are related to the total quantity and are not influenced by diet. This supports the conclusion that cholesterol is essential to the diet of the infant.

Where maternal undernutrition is commonplace, the percentage of maternal body fat may influence the concentration of fat in the milk.[24] Milk-fat concentrations in Gambian women were positively correlated with maternal skinfold thickness and decreased over the course of lactation.[29] In lactation beyond 6 months, similar correlations were noted in the United States by Nommsen et al.[48] Other investigators studying the impact of weight loss noted that the rate of post-pregnancy weight loss affected the level of elaidic acid in milk and levels of trans fatty acid.[49] This is explained by the mobilization of fatty acids from maternal adipose tissue.

The synthesis of fatty acids up to the carbon number of 16, as well as the direct desaturation of stearic acid into oleic acid, can take place in the mammary gland, whereas longer-chain fatty acids come directly from plasma triglycerides (see Chapter 4, Biochemistry).[50] The intake of both carbohydrate and fat must be considered when evaluating maternal diet because high-carbohydrate diets increase lauric acid and myristic acid, and moderate levels of carbohydrate influence linoleic acid.

When serum lipids are measured in African women accustomed to a low-fat intake, the levels are relatively low, and the women are virtually free of coronary heart disease. Among long-lactating (1 to 2 years minimum) African mothers, the amount of fat in their daily milk is of the same order as that ingested in their standard diet.[51] Despite this, they are not significantly hypolipidemic when compared with nonlactators.

Human milk samples obtained from women living in five different regions of China showed the great diversity of milk

TABLE 8.3   Lipid Concentrations of Mature Human Milk

Study	Plan	DIET Saturation of Fat[a]	Cholesterol (mg/day)	LIPID CONCENTRATION IN MILK Cholesterol (mg/dL)	Triglyceride (g/dL)	Phospholipid (mg P/dL)
I (n = 7)	A	S	580	18.1 ± 2.7[b]	3.42 ± 0.61	4.04 ± 0.71
	B	P	110	19.3 ± 3.6	3.57 ± 0.82	4.18 ± 0.91
II (n = 3)	C	S	380	23.3 ± 2.3	4.11 ± 0.42	
	D	P	345	21.3 ± 2.4	4.12 ± 0.56	

[a]S, Rich in saturated fatty acids (P/S ratio ∼0.07); P, rich in polyunsaturated fatty acids (P/S ∼1.3).
[b]Mean ± standard error of measurement (SEM).
From Potter JM, Nestel PJ. The effects of dietary fatty acids and cholesterol on the milk lipids of lactating women and the plasma cholesterol of breast-fed infants. *Am J Clin Nutr.* 1976;29:54.

fatty acids. The docosahexaenoic acid (DHA) concentrations in women from the marine region were twice as high as those from rural areas.[52] The milk concentrations of DHA varied greatly (0.44 ± 0.29 to 2.78 ± 1.20 g/100 g total fat), with pastoral regions being lowest and the marine region highest. Seafood consumption was high in the marine group. Similarly, arachidonic acid (AA), when stated as a ratio (AA/DHA, g/g), was 2.77 in pastoral areas and 0.42 in the marine region. AA has been associated with infant growth and DHA with brain and retinal growth. Similar findings are reported in Alaskan Inuit people who have a diet high in fish and fish oil. When women's diets were supplemented with fish and fish oils, the blood concentrations of DHA in the maternal plasma and red blood cells (RBCs) were increased.[53] Infants showed a 35% DHA increase in RBCs and a 45% increase in plasma, which supports the concept that maternal diet can influence the DHA levels in newborns. The fatty acid patterns of human milk correlate with the current American diet, which has a high P/S ratio; there is a shift toward higher levels of C18:2 fatty acids, linoleic acid, and C18:3 linolenic acid.[45,47,54] Depot fat reflects dietary fatty acid patterns and thus the pool for mammary gland synthesis of milk fats. The mammary gland can dehydrogenate saturated and monosaturated fatty acids.[55]

Diet composition affects milk-fat synthesis. When a woman is in energy balance, the fatty acids from the diet account for approximately 30% of the total fatty acids in her milk.

The habitual diet of healthy primiparas in Finland was associated with breast milk containing 3.8% fat.[56] Their diet was 16% protein, 39% fat, and 45% carbohydrate. Half the fatty acids of the diet and the milk were saturated, and one-third were monoenoic. PUFAs were 15% of the diet and 13% of the breast milk, with a P/S ratio of 0.3 for both. The maternal diet had no effect on the total fat content of the milk, except for the low level of oleic acid, which is apparently peculiar to Finnish breast milk.

DHA, a long-chain fatty acid (22:6, n-3), has attracted attention because deficiency has been associated with visual impairment in the offspring of rhesus monkeys. Essential n-3 fatty acids in pregnant women have been linked to visual acuity and neural development in their term infants. Some pregnant women in the United States have been found to be deficient in DHA.[57] A descriptive meta-analysis of 106 studies worldwide was culled to 65 to include only those utilizing modern analysis methods to obtain fatty acid profiles. The highest DHA concentrations were found in coastal populations and associated with the consumption of fish. DHA was 0.32% ± 0.22% and 0.47% ± 0.13% for AA, representing the mean concentrations worldwide. Omega-3 DHA is important to the fetus and to the offspring through breast-feeding, and emerging science suggests it may protect against preterm delivery, as well as postpartum depression.[58]

Fish Consumption During Lactation

Maternal fish consumption during pregnancy has been correlated with cognitive and visual abilities in offspring. Maternal

n-3 long-chain polyunsaturated fatty acid (LCPUFA) supplementation during pregnancy was evaluated in a study that compared early childhood cognitive and visual development in mothers with and without supplementation. A systematic review and meta-analysis of randomized controlled trials (RCTs) failed to prove or disprove that n-3 LCPUFA supplementation in pregnancy improves cognitive and visual development of the children.[59]

Fish oil is an excellent dietary source of DHA, and women who consistently eat fish have higher levels in their milk. In a study, Finley et al.[41] found that vegetarians have higher DHA levels in their milk than omnivore control subjects. Many formulas have been supplemented with synthetically derived DHA in an effort to mimic human milk. They do not, however, contain cholesterol, and no data support the concept that synthetically derived DHA is as effective as natural DHA in human milk.

A strong association exists between the body fat of the mother and the lipids in her milk. Lovelady et al. found that the best predictor of milk lipids was overall "fatness" rather than the distribution of that fat.[60] Dietary fat was not associated with milk fat in the women with a higher percentage of body fat (27% or more body fat) but was positively correlated with diet in lean women (less than 27% body fat).

When healthy pregnant women are supplemented with fish-oil capsules from the 30th week of gestation, the fatty acid compositions of the phospholipids isolated from umbilical plasma and umbilical vessel walls differ from those of unsupplemented mothers, with more n-3 and less n-6 fatty acids.[61] This suggests that DHA status can be altered at birth.

In one study, lactating women were given supplements of different doses of fish-oil concentrates rich in n-3 fatty acids, including DHA.[62] Receiving 5 g/day for 28 days, 10 g/day for 14 days, and 47 g/day for 8 days, each experienced significant dose-dependent increases in DHA in their milk and plasma. Baseline levels in milk were 0.1% of total fatty acids, and levels rose from 0.8% to as high as 4.8% on the 47-g/day diet. This suggests that relatively small supplements of DHA can enhance levels in the milk. Preformed dietary DHA is known to be better synthesized into nervous tissue than that synthesized from linolenic acid, and other essential fatty acids can inhibit this transformation to DHA. The consumption of fish during pregnancy and lactation is an important dietary consideration in preference to fish-oil capsules. The concern rests with possible mercury contamination. Fish, however, provides lean protein; an abundance of vitamin B, zinc, iodine, and selenium; and naturally rich sources of long-chain n-3 fatty acids and vitamin D. It has been recorded that women who do not eat fish during pregnancy put their infants at risk for suboptimal visual, cognitive, motor, and behavior skill outcomes.[57] International studies have shown the value of fish in pregnancy and lactation. In the Danish National Cohort Study, a higher fish intake by mothers and a longer duration of breastfeeding (10 months or more vs. ≤ 1 month) were associated with higher child development scores.[63] In a US study, maternal intake of >2 servings of fish per week was associated with enhanced child cognitive testing, and higher

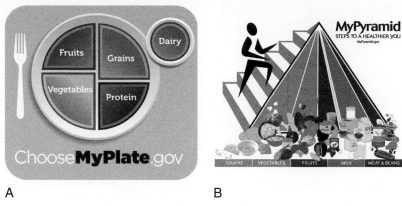

Fig. 8.1 ChooseMyPlate (A) and MyPyramid (B) are tools for ensuring adequate nutrition in both children and adults. See ChooseMyPlate.gov and Nutrition.gov for more information. (From the US Department of Agriculture.)

mean maternal mercury levels were associated with poorer testing scores.[64] The US Department of Agriculture (USDA) has put forth ChooseMyPlate and MyPyramid tools to help mothers and families select foods and diets with adequate nutrition for children and adults (Fig. 8.1). The US Food and Drug Administration (FDA) has stated that although fish oil supplements are beneficial for those who cannot eat fish, fish has the full range of nutrients. The FDA, in revised 2019 guidelines, recommends a minimum of two meals of fish per week (8 to 12 ounces) during lactation.[65]

The FDA additionally recommends that the fish should be less likely to contain mercury and provide a listing on its website of "best choices" of fish. Studies of linoleic acid supplementation from 20 weeks' gestation in normal women showed that levels increased in those with low linoleic acid levels to match those with high levels, but the neonatal linoleic acid status did not change.[66] Linoleic acid supplementation did result in significantly higher total amounts of n-6 long-chain polyenes in umbilical plasma. Linoleic acid (18:2, n-6) is essential to the maintenance of the epidermal water barrier and is the ultimate dietary precursor of eicosanoids, which include leukotrienes, prostaglandins, and thromboxanes. Linoleic acid is not synthesized by humans and must be supplied by diet.

A diet deficient in n-3 fatty acids leads to a triad of signs in the rhesus monkey: visual impairment, electroretinographic abnormalities, and polydipsia. Profound biochemical changes in the fatty acid composition of the membranes of the retina, brain, and other organs are seen experimentally. Low concentrations of n-3 fatty acids occur at birth in the placenta, RBCs, and neural tissues when the mothers are fed deficient diets. Studies in monkeys confirm that the most critical period of life for providing n-3 fatty acids is during pregnancy and during lactation in early infancy.[53] In humans, supplementation of the maternal diet with fish and fish oils has increased the levels of n-3 fatty acids, especially DHA. Humans can synthesize DHA from linolenic acid, but this is limited in both infants and adults. Supplementing with linolenic acid does not significantly increase DHA in the blood.[36] No evidence suggests that supplements in normal women with good diets are beneficial. Excesses of DHA affect AA levels and interfere

with the AA:DHA ratio. The content of conjugated linoleic isomer and trans vaccenic acid in human milk was found to be higher in women who consumed organic dairy and organic meat products. The health effects of conjugated linoleic isomer and trans vaccenic acid on human newborns continue to be investigated, but the effects in animals and in human adults show immunomodulating properties, such as with influenza and other viruses.

Lactose

In human milk, the principal carbohydrate is lactose, present at approximately 70 g/L and second only to water as a major constituent. The milk of all species is isotonic with maternal plasma, and 60% to 70% of the osmotic pressure is created by lactose. Lactose provides twice the energy value per molecule or unit of osmotic pressure. Because milk volume is driven by available lactose, its concentration is stable.[21] Changes in the carbohydrate levels in the diet have been studied. A comparison of mothers on diets with three different levels of carbohydrate shows that the amounts of protein, fat, and carbohydrate in their milk are similar. No evidence indicates that dietary manipulations affect lactose levels in human milk.

Water

No data support the assumption that increasing fluid intake will increase milk volume, and restricting fluids has not been shown to decrease milk volume.[67] Data on the topic are limited and have been reviewed, demonstrating a high level of bias.[68] Forcing fluids, however, has been shown to affect milk production negatively in a controlled crossover-design study of breastfeeding mothers. Thus women taking excessive fluids produced less milk, suggesting that drinking to thirst and heeding body cues is more physiologic than prescribing a specific amount of fluid per day.[69] This observation was first demonstrated in a 1939 study that concluded, "Forced, excessive drinking is therefore neither necessary nor beneficial as far as the nursing is concerned and may even be harmful." Hypogalactia cannot be arrested by forced drinking beyond the natural dictates of thirst. Urine output in these studies was proportional to intake.[70] A similar study of 210 postpartum mothers, half of whom drank ad lib, taking an average of

69 oz daily, while the other half were forced to take 6 pt and averaged 107 oz daily, showed that the mothers forced to drink beyond thirst produced less milk, and their babies gained weight less well.[67]

From a practical standpoint, mothers have increased thirst. When fluids are restricted, mothers will experience a decrease in urine output, not in milk. Sharply decreasing fluids to prevent engorgement in the mother who is not lactating is ineffectual and only adds another inconvenience and discomfort.

Kilocalories

The caloric content, sample by sample, of milk from well-nourished mothers does vary but averages 75 kcal/dL. Because fat is the chief source of kilocalories, the fat content has the greatest impact on total kilocalories, with lactose and protein also contributing to the total. Thus, in malnourished mothers with low fat stores, the caloric content may be reduced.

Body fat increases during pregnancy and decreases during lactation. Changes in the adipose depot primarily result from a change in fat-cell size, not number. Adipose tissue fatty acid synthesis remains low throughout pregnancy, as does lipoprotein lipase activity. Conversely, mammary lipoprotein lipase activity increases and remains high during lactation.[71]

How does this correlate with the caloric needs of the mother to produce milk? The calculations for energy requirements have been made by comparing the energy intake of nursing mothers and nonnursing mothers who were matched for other variables. Nursing mothers consumed 2460 kcal daily, and nonnursing mothers consumed 1880 kcal, a net difference of 580 kcal.

Lactation will not produce a net drain on the mother if the amount of energy available and the requirement of any given nutrient are replaced in the diet. There is only a small kilocalorie energy cost for milk production because the breasts work at remarkable efficiency.[72] During pregnancy, fat and other nutrients are stored for the fetus and in preparation for lactation. Lactation is subsidized, as is fetal growth, by maternal stores, even though the diet on any given day may be relatively deficient in a specific nutrient. This can be clarified by Fig. 8.2, which shows that diet and stores are available for milk, as well as for the maintenance of the mother.

A study of 26 healthy, normotensive, nonsmoking, euthyroid women—12 of whom were breastfeeding, 7 bottle-feeding, and 7 nonpregnant and nonlactating control subjects—was reported by Illingworth et al.[73] Energy expenditure at rest and in response to a meal and to an infusion of noradrenaline was measured. During lactation, the resting metabolic rate was unaltered, but a reduced response to infusion of noradrenaline and to a meal was observed. These responses returned to normal control values in these women postlactation. Women who bottle-fed were similar to control subjects. The woman's metabolic efficiency is greatly enhanced during lactation and results in a reduction in the nonlactational component of maternal energy expenditure (Fig. 8.3).

When comparing dietary intake during lactation at 6 weeks postpartum to the intake of a comparable group of nonpregnant women and a group of nonlactating but

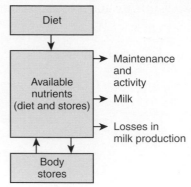

Fig. 8.2 Energy utilization during lactation, showing availability of body stores and dietary sources.

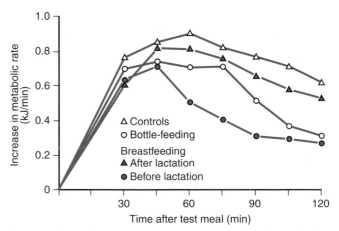

Fig. 8.3 Metabolic response to test meal while breastfeeding compared with response of women who bottle-feed and nonpregnant control subjects. (From Illingworth PJ, Jung RT, Howie PW, et al. Diminution in energy expenditure during lactation. *Br Med J.* 1986; 292:437.)

postpartum women using a 7-day food diary and questionnaire, total daily intakes and meal patterns were not different between body-weight-matched lactators and nonlactators. The lactating women, however, consumed a significantly smaller percentage of the Recommended Dietary Allowances (RDAs) per day and were much calmer both before and after meals. The lactating women did not increase their daily intake over their prepregnancy diet.[74]

The total amount of nutrients that the lactating mother secretes in her milk is directly related to the extent and duration of lactation.[1] Furthermore, lactating women who consume a well-balanced diet with adequate calories (2700 kcal/day) meet the RDAs for all nutrients, with the exception of calcium and zinc, according to assessments of the average American diet for young women. This is based on the nutrient density (nutrient intake per 1000 kcal) of the average woman's diet in the United States.[75] Nutrient densities for proteins, minerals, and vitamins have been determined from nationally representative samples of women aged 19 to 50 years of age. The nutrient values at three different levels of energy are calculated (nutrient density × kcal of energy = total intake). The levels of energy used are 2700 kcal, the recommendation for lactating women; 2200 kcal,

BOX 8.1 Dietary Reference Intakes (DRIs)

- The **Estimated Average Requirement** (EAR) is the average daily nutrient intake level that can be expected to satisfy the needs of 50% of the healthy people in that age group and gender group based on a review of the scientific literature.
- The **Recommended Dietary Allowance** (RDA) is the daily dietary intake level of a nutrient considered sufficient by the Food and Nutrition Board of the Institute of Medicine to meet the requirements of 97.5% of healthy individuals in each life-stage group and gender group. The definition implies that the intake level would cause a harmful nutrient deficiency in just 2.5%. It is calculated based on the EAR and is usually approximately 20% higher than the EAR. It is calculated as follows: RDA = EAR + 2 SD_{EAR} (2 standard deviations of the EAR).
- **Adequate intake** (AI) is used where no RDA has been established, but the amount established is somewhat less firmly believed to be adequate for everyone in the demographic group.
- **Tolerable upper intake levels** (ULs) are proposed to caution against excessive intake of nutrients (e.g., vitamin A) that can be harmful in large amounts. This is the highest level of daily nutrient consumption that is considered to be safe for, and likely to cause no side effects in, 97.5% of healthy individuals in each life-stage and sex group. The definition implies that the intake level would cause a harmful nutrient excess in just 2.5% of individuals.

From US Department of Health and Human Services and US Food and Drug Administration. Food Labeling: Revision of the Nutrition and Supplement Facts Labels. *Fed. Reg.* May 27, 2016;81. https://www.govinfo.gov/content/pkg/FR-2016-05-27/pdf/2016–11867.pdf. Accessed November 15, 2019.

as reported by lactating women as actual consumption; and 1800 kcal, the minimal level a lactating woman should consider in a restricted diet. See Box 8.1 for descriptions of Dietary Reference Intakes (DRIs).[76] The relative nutrient deficiencies are identified next.

For the lactating woman, a 2700-kcal diet may be deficient in calcium and zinc; the 2200-kcal diet is deficient in calcium, magnesium, zinc, thiamin, vitamin B_6, and vitamin E; and the 1800-kcal diet is deficient in all the previously mentioned nutrient levels plus riboflavin, folate, phosphorus, and iron unless special attention is paid to intake of these nutrients (Tables 8.4 through 8.7).

Women should be encouraged to follow dietary guidelines, especially in terms of fruits, vegetables, and whole grains; calcium-rich dairy products; and protein-rich foods. Vitamin and mineral supplements are not recommended for lactating women. If, however, dietary review suggests intake is lower than recommended, the woman should be encouraged to consume more foods rich in those nutrients. A woman with serious dietary problems leading to a low intake of one or more nutrients should be encouraged by counseling to correct her dietary deficiencies. Nutrient supplements are recommended only as a last resort.

Table 8.8 lists measures for improving the nutrient intake of women with restrictive eating patterns. Overt signs of deficiency are rare in the United States, even for the nutrients with small safety margins.

Prebiotics and Probiotics

Human milk contains substantial quantities of prebiotics. Exploration of prebiotics and probiotics has been motivated by the formula industry in its efforts to try to make infant formulas more like human milk. A probiotic is defined as an oral supplement or a food product containing a sufficient amount of viable microorganisms to alter the microflora of the host, with the potential for health benefits. A prebiotic, as defined by the American Academy of Pediatricians (AAP), is a nondigestible food ingredient that benefits the host by selectively favoring growth and activity of one or more indigenous probiotic bacteria. A synbiotic is a product that contains both probiotics and prebiotics, in theory acting synergistically. A postbiotic is a metabolic by-product generated by probiotic microorganisms that influences the host's biologic function. The microorganisms commonly recognized as human milk probiotics are *Lactobacillus*, *Bifidobacterium*, and *Streptococcus*, typically producing lactic acid. They dominate the microorganisms in the gastrointestinal tract. Human milk oligosaccharides (HMOs) are recognized as prebiotics for many probiotic organisms.[77] Commercially available prebiotics are oligosaccharides, which are added to formula, foods, and beverages. The commercialization of these products in formula has yet to be confirmed to improve infants' defense systems and has yet to be proven as safe. They are promoted as developing the immune system but possibly result in immune dysregulation in susceptible individuals. Breastfed infants are naturally provided the constituents to protect the gastrointestinal tract, encourage the growth of *Lactobacillus* and other probiotic bacteria, and suppress pathogens. Breastfed infants who have been given antibiotics will physiologically recolonize their guts when given human milk, which also contains a robust supply of *Lactobacillus*, among other probiotic organisms.

Vitamins
Water-Soluble Vitamins

Water-soluble vitamins move with ease from serum to milk; thus their dietary fluctuation is more apparent. Levels of water-soluble vitamins in milk are raised or lowered by changes in the maternal diet. The body's requirement for vitamin C increases under stress, including lactation. Furthermore, the vitamin C content of human organs at autopsy is much higher in the neonate than at any other time of life. This is true of all the major organs, including the brain.

The influence of maternal intake of vitamin C on the concentration of vitamin C in human milk and on the intake of vitamin C by the infant has been carefully measured in 25 well-nourished lactating women.[78] Supplements ranged from 0 to 1000 mg vitamin C daily (more than 10 times the RDA).

TABLE 8.4 Dietary Reference Intakes: Recommended Intakes for Individual Vitamins (Food and Nutrition Board, Institute of Medicine, National Academies)

Life-Stage Group	Vitamin A (μg/day)[a]	Vitamin C (mg/day)	Vitamin D (μg/day)[b,c]	Vitamin E (mg/day)[d]	Vitamin K (μg/day)	Thiamin (mg/day)	Riboflavin (mg/day)	Niacin (mg/day)[e]	Vitamin B_6 (mg/day)	Folate (μg/day)[f]	Vitamin B12 (μg/day)	Pantothenic Acid (mg/day)	Biotin (μg/day)	Choline (mg/day)[g]
Females														
9–13 yr	600	45	5*	11	60*	0.9	0.9	12	1.0	300	1.8	4*	20*	375*
14–18 yr	700	65	5*	15	75*	1.0	1.0	14	1.2	400	2.4	5*	25*	400*
19–30 yr	700	75	5*	15	90*	1.1	1.1	14	1.3	400	2.4	5*	30*	425*
31–50 yr	700	75	5*	15	90*	1.1	1.1	14	1.3	400	2.4	5*	30*	425*
51–70 yr	700	75	10*	15	90*	1.1	1.1	14	1.5	400	2.4	5*	30*	425*
> 70 yr	700	75	15*	15	90*	1.1	1.1	14	1.5	400	2.4	5*	30*	425*
Pregnancy														
14–18 yr	750	80	5*	15	75*	1.4	1.4	18	1.9	600	2.6	6*	30*	450*
19–30 yr	770	85	5*	15	90*	1.4	1.4	18	1.9	600	2.6	6*	30*	450*
31–50 yr	770	85	5*	15	90*	1.4	1.4	18	1.9	600	2.6	6*	30*	450*
Lactation														
14–18 yr	1200	115	5*	19	75*	1.4	1.6	17	2	500	2.8	7*	35*	550*
19–30 yr	1300	120	5*	19	90*	1.4	1.6	17	2	500	2.8	7*	35*	550*
31–50 yr	1300	120	5*	19	90*	1.4	1.6	17	2	500	2.8	7*	35*	550*

Note: This table (taken from the Dietary Reference Intake [DRI] reports; see http://www.nap.edu) presents Recommended Dietary Allowances (RDAs) in bold type and adequate intakes (AIs) in ordinary type followed by an asterisk (*). RDAs and AIs may both be used as goals for individual intake. RDAs are set to meet the needs of almost all (97% to 98%) individuals in a group. For healthy breastfed infants, the AI is the mean intake. The AI for other life stages and gender groups is believed to cover needs of all individuals in the group, but a lack of data or uncertainty in the data prevent being able to specify with confidence the percentage of individuals covered by this intake.

[a] As retinol activity equivalents (RAEs): 1 RAE = 1 μg retinol, 12 μg β-carotene, 24 μg α-carotene, or 24 μg β-cryptoxanthin. The RAE for dietary provitamir A carotenoids is two-fold greater than retinol equivalents (REs), whereas the RAE for preformed vitamin A is the same as that for RE.

[b] As cholecalciferol: 1 μg cholecalciferol = 40 IU vitamin D.

[c] In the absence of adequate exposure to sunlight.

[d] As α-Tocopherol. α-Tocopherol includes *RRR*-α-tocopherol, the only form of α-tocopherol that occurs naturally in foods, and the 2*R*-stereoisomeric forms of α-tocopherol (*RRR*-, *RSR*-, *RRS*-, and *RSS*-α-tocopherol) that occur in fortified foods and supplements. It does not include the 2*S*-stereoisomeric forms of α-tocopherol (*SRR*-, *SSR*-, *SRS*-, and *SSS*-α- tocopherol), also found in fortified foods and supplements.

[e] As niacin equivalents (NEs): 1 mg of niacin = 60 mg of tryptophan; 0 to 6 months = preformed niacin (not NE).

[f] As dietary folate equivalents (DFEs): 1 DFE = 1 μg food folate = 0.6 μg of folic acid from fortified food or as a supplement consumed with food = 0.5 μg of a supplement taken on an empty stomach.

[g] Although AIs have been set for choline, there are few data to assess whether a dietary supply of choline is needed at all stages of the life cycle, and it may be that the choline requirement can be met by endogenous synthesis at some of these stages.

TABLE 8.5 Dietary Reference Intakes: Recommended Intakes for Individual Macronutrients (Food and Nutrition Board, Institute of Medicine, National Academies)

Life Stage Group	Total Water[a] (L/day)	Carbohydrate[b] (g/day)	Total Fiber (g/day)	Fat (g/day)	Linoleic Acid (g/day)	α-Linolenic Acid (g/day)	Protein[c] (g/day)
Females							
9–13 yr	2.1	130	26	ND	10	1.0	34
14–18 yr	2.3	130	26	ND	11	1.1	46
19–30 yr	2.7	130	25	ND	12	1.1	46
31–50 yr	2.7	130	25	ND	12	1.1	46
51–70 yr	2.7	130	21	ND	11	1.1	46
> 70 yr	2.7	130	21	ND	11	1.1	46
Pregnancy							
14–18 yr	3.0	175	28	ND	13	1.4	71
19–30 yr	3.0	175	28	ND	13	1.4	71
31–50 yr	3.0	175	28	ND	13	1.4	71
Lactation							
14–18 yr	3.8	210	29	ND	13	1.3	71
19–30 yr	3.8	210	29	ND	13	1.3	71
31–50 yr	3.8	210	29	ND	13	1.3	71

ND, Not determinable.

[a]Total water includes all water contained in food, beverages, and drinking water. The values presented are adequate intakes (AIs).

[b]Carbohydrate values presented are recommended dietary allowances (RDAs).

[c]Protein is based on g protein per kg of body weight for the reference body weight. The values presented are the recommended dietary allowances (RDAs).

Sources: Institute of Medicine. Dietary Reference Intakes for Energy, Carbohydrate, Fiber, Fat, Fatty Acids, Cholesterol, Protein and Amino Acids. Washington, DC: The National Academies Press; 2005. https://doi.org/10.17226/10490.

Concentrations in milk ranged from 44 to 158 mg/L and were not correlated significantly with maternal intakes, which ranged from 156 (0 mg supplement) to 1123 mg (1000 mg supplement). Dietary vitamin C had no effect on the volume of milk produced. Maternal excretion of vitamin C in urine was correlated with maternal intake. Regardless of the level of maternal intake of vitamin C, the mean vitamin C concentration in breast milk was twice that recommended for infant formula. Vitamin C levels in human milk did not increase in response to increasing maternal intake despite 10-fold increases, whereas urinary excretion did suggest that mammary tissue becomes saturated.

It is postulated that a regulatory mechanism functioning in the breast prevents an elevation in the concentration of vitamin C beyond a certain level in milk.[78] Vitamin C levels were at the same or higher levels in exclusively breastfed infants at 6 and 9 months of age compared with levels of supplemented bottle-fed control infants.[79] Levels in the infants were dependent on maternal nutrition and vitamin C levels in milk. Low levels of vitamin C are recorded in 6% of well-nourished, healthy mothers. In malnourished women, tissue stores may take time to replenish, which explains why 35-mg/day supplementation failed to increase low plasma levels. Data from multiple studies suggest that there is a level above which further vitamin C supplementation will not affect milk vitamin C levels.[80]

The level of B vitamins, also water soluble, reflects dietary intake. The serum levels are affected acutely by maternal diet, and therefore B_{12} can enter breast milk. Infantile beriberi is not unheard of in seemingly normal infants nursed by apparently well-nourished mothers with thiamin-deficient diets. The influence of maternal diet has been pointed out dramatically in reported cases of megaloblastic anemia, methylmalonic aciduria, and homocystinuria in the breastfed infants of strict vegetarians.[81,82] Vitamin B_{12} exists in all animal protein but not in vegetable protein. A strict vegetarian would require vitamin B_{12} supplements during pregnancy and lactation.[83] Vitamin B_{12} deficiency in infants has also been seen in New Delhi, where malnourished mothers produced vitamin B_{12}–deficient milk. These infants also had megaloblastic anemia.

Infants of vegetarians who have low vitamin B_{12} serum and milk levels have methylmalonic acid in their urine inversely proportional to their vitamin B_{12} levels, even though they are asymptomatic.[84] Other authors have concluded that the current RDA for infants provides little margin of safety: 0.3 or 0.05 mg/kg body weight is close to the intake below which infant urinary methylmalonic acid measures are elevated.[81,82]

TABLE 8.6 Dietary Reference Intakes: Tolerable Upper Intake Levels[a]—Elements (Food and Nutrition Board, Institute of Medicine, National Academies)

Life-Stage Group	Arsenic[b]	Boron (mg/day)	Calcium (g/day)	Chromium	Copper (μg/day)	Fluoride (mg/day)	Iodine (μg/day)	Iron (mg/day)	Magnesium (mg/day)[c]	Manganese (mg/day)	Molybdenum (μg/day)	Nickel (mg/day)	Phosphorus (g/day)	Potassium	Selenium (μg/day)	Silicon[d]	Sulfate	Vanadium (mg/day)[e]	Zinc (mg/day)	Sodium (g/day)	Chloride (g/day)
Pregnancy																					
14–18 yr	ND[f]	17	2.5	ND	8000	10	900	45	350	9	1700	1.0	3.5	ND	400	NE	ND	ND	34	2.3	3.6
19–50 yr	ND	20	2.5	ND	10,000	10	1100	45	350	11	2000	1.0	3.5	ND	400	NE	ND	ND	40	2.3	3.6
Lactation																					
14–18 yr	ND	17	2.5	ND	8000	10	900	45	350	9	1700	1.0	4	ND	400	NE	ND	ND	34	2.3	3.6
19–50 yr	ND	20	2.5	ND	10,000	10	1100	45	350	11	2000	1.0	4	ND	400	NE	ND	ND	40	2.3	3.6

ND, Not determinable.

[a]Upper limit (UL) = the maximum level of daily nutrient intake that is likely to pose no risk of adverse effects. Unless otherwise specified, the UL represents total intake from food, water, and supplements. Because of a lack of suitable data, ULs could not be established for arsenic, chromium, silicon, potassium, and sulfate. In the absence of ULs, extra caution may be warranted in consuming levels above recommended intakes.

[b]Although the UL was not determined for arsenic, there is no justification for adding arsenic to food or supplements.

[c]The ULs for magnesium represent intake from a pharmacologic agent only and do not include intake from food and water.

[d]Although silicon has not been shown to cause adverse effects in humans, there is no justification for adding silicon to supplements.

[e]Although vanadium in food has not been shown to cause adverse effects in humans, there is no justification for adding vanadium to food, and vanadium supplements should be used with caution. The UL is based on adverse effects in laboratory animals, and these data could be used to set a UL for adults but not children and adolescents.

[f]ND as a result of a lack of data of adverse effects in this age group and concern with regard to lack of ability to handle excess amounts. Source of intake should be from food only to prevent high levels of intake.

TABLE 8.7 Dietary Reference Intakes: Estimated Average Requirements for Groups (Food and Nutrition Board, Institute of Medicine, National Academies)

Life-Stage Group	CHO (g/day)	Protein (g/day)	Vitamin A (μg/day)[a]	Vitamin C (mg/day)	Vitamin E (mg/day)[b]	Thiamin (mg/day)	Riboflavin (mg/day)	Niacin (mg/day)[c]	Vitamin B6 (mg/day)	Folate (μg/day)[d]	Vitamin B12 (μg/day)	Copper (μg/day)	Iodine (μg/day)	Iron (mg/day)	Magnesium (mg/day)	Molybdenum (μg/day)	Phosphorus (mg/day)	Selenium (μg/day)	Zinc (mg/day)
Females																			
9–13 yr	100	28	420	39	9	0.7	0.8	9	0.8	250	1.5	540	73	5.7	200	26	1055	35	7.0
14–18 yr	100	38	485	56	12	0.9	0.9	11	1.0	330	2.0	685	95	7.9	300	33	1055	45	7.3
19–30 yr	100	38	500	60	12	0.9	0.9	11	1.1	320	2.0	700	95	8.1	255	34	580	45	6.8
31–50 yr	100	38	500	60	12	0.9	0.9	11	1.1	320	2.0	700	95	8.1	265	34	580	45	6.8
51–70 yr	100	38	500	60	12	0.9	0.9	11	1.3	320	2.0	700	95	5	265	34	580	45	6.8
> 70 yr	100	38	500	60	12	0.9	0.9	11	1.3	320	2.0	700	95	5	265	34	580	45	6.8
Pregnancy																			
14–18 yr	135	50	530	66	12	1.2	1.2	14	1.6	520	2.2	785	160	23	335	40	1055		
19–30 yr	135	50	550	70	12	1.2	1.2	14	1.6	520	2.2	800	160	22	290	40	580		
31–50 yr	135	50	550	70	12	1.2	1.2	14	1.6	520	2.2	800	160	22	300	40	580		
Lactation																			
14–18 yr	160	60	885	96	16	1.2	1.3	13	1.7	450	2.4	985	209	7	300	35	1055		
19–30 yr	160	60	900	100	16	1.2	1.3	13	1.7	450	2.4	1000	209	6.5	255	36	580		
31–50 yr	160	60	900	100	16	1.2	1.3	13	1.7	450	2.4	1000	209	6.5	265	36	580		

Note: This table presents estimated average requirement (EARs), which serve two purposes: for assessing the adequacy of population intakes and as the basis for calculating Recommended Dietary Allowances (RDAs) for individuals for those nutrients. EARs have not been established for vitamin D, vitamin K, pantothenic acid, biotin, choline, calcium, chromium, fluoride, manganese, or other nutrients not yet evaluated via the Dietary Reference Intake (DRI) process.

[a] As retinol activity equivalents (RAEs): 1 RAE = 1 mg retinol, 12 mg β-carotene, 24 mg α-carotene, or 24 mg β-cryptoxanthin. The RAE for dietary provitamin A carotenoids is two-fold greater than retinol equivalents (REs), whereas the RAE for preformed vitamin A is the same as that for RE.

[b] As α-Tocopherol. α-Tocopherol includes *RRR*-α-tocopherol, the only form of α-tocopherol that occurs naturally in foods, and the 2*R*-stereoisomeric forms of α-tocopherol (*RRR*-, *RSR*-, *RRS*-, and *RSS*-α-tocopherol) that occur in fortified foods and supplements. It does not include the 2*S*-stereoisomeric forms of α-tocopherol (*SRR*-, *SSR*-, *SRS*-, and *SSS*-α-tocopherol), also found in fortified foods and supplements.

[c] As niacin equivalents (NEs): 1 mg of niacin = 60 mg of tryptophan.

[d] As dietary folate equivalents (DFEs): 1 DFE = 1 mg food folate = 0.6 g of folic acid from fortified food or as a supplement consumed with food = 0.5 mg of a supplement taken on an empty stomach.

Sources: Dietary Reference Intakes for Calcium, Phosphorous, Magnesium, Vitamin D, and Fluoride (1997); Dietary Reference Intakes for Thiamin, Riboflavin, Niacin, Vitamin B6, Folate, Vitamin B12, Pantothenic Acid, Biotin, and Choline (1998); Dietary Reference Intakes for Vitamin C, Vitamin E, Selenium, and Carotenoids (2000); Dietary Reference Intakes for Vitamin A, Vitamin K, Arsenic, Boron, Chromium, Copper, Iodine, Iron, Manganese, Molybdenum, Nickel, Silicon, Vanadium, and Zinc (2001), and Dietary Reference Intakes for Energy, Carbohydrate, Fiber, Fat, Fatty Acids, Cholesterol, Protein, and Amino Acids (2002). These reports may be accessed via http://www.nap.edu. Copyright 2002 by the National Academy of Sciences. All rights reserved.

TABLE 8.8	Suggested Measures for Improving Nutrient Intake of Women With Restrictive Eating Patterns
Type of Restrictive Eating Pattern	**Corrective Measures**
Excessive restriction of food intake (i.e., ingestion of less than 1800 kcal/day), which ordinarily leads to unsatisfactory intake of nutrients compared with amounts needed by lactating women	Encourage increased intake of nutrient-rich foods to achieve energy intake of at least 1800 kcal/day; if mother insists on curbing food intake sharply, promote substitution of foods rich in vitamins, minerals, and protein for those lower in nutritive value; in individual cases, it may be advisable to recommend a balanced multivitamin–mineral supplement and discourage the use of liquid weight-loss diets and appetite suppressants.
Complete vegetarianism—that is, avoidance of all animal foods, including meat, fish, dairy products, and eggs	Advise intake of regular source of vitamin B_{12}, such as special vitamin B_{12}—containing plant food products or a 2.5-μg vitamin B_{12} supplement daily
Avoidance of milk, cheese, or other calcium-rich dairy products	Encourage increased intake of other culturally appropriate dietary calcium sources, such as collard greens for Blacks from southeastern United States; provide information on appropriate use of low-lactose dairy products if milk is being avoided because of lactose intolerance; if correction by diet cannot be achieved, it may be advisable to recommend 1000–1300 mg of elemental calcium per day taken with meals.
Avoidance of vitamin D–fortified foods, such as fortified milk or cereal, combined with limited exposure to ultraviolet light	Recommend 10 μg of supplemental vitamin D per day.

From the Institute of Medicine. Dietary Reference Intakes for Energy, Carbohydrate, Fiber, Fat, Fatty Acids, Cholesterol, Protein, and Amino Acids. Washington, DC: The National Academies Press; 2005. https://doi.org/10.17226/10490.

Thiamine (vitamin B_1) has been studied infrequently, but maternal supplementation does not increase milk levels beyond a certain limit. Urinary excretion of thiamine is significantly higher in supplemented compared with unsupplemented women. In malnourished women, evidence indicates that supplementation does increase thiamine levels in milk. It is recommended that thiamine intake be at least 1.3 mg/day (the RDA for nonpregnant, nonlactating women of 1.1 mg/day plus an increment for milk secretion of 0.2 mg/day) when the calorie intake is less than 2200 kcal/day. (See Table 8.7 for estimated average requirements.)

Riboflavin (vitamin B_2) requirements of lactating women in a controlled study in Gambia showed the minimum to be 2.5 mg/day to maintain normal biochemical status in the mother and adequate levels of vitamin B_2 in her milk.[85] This level is higher than what is recommended in the United States and the United Kingdom.

The niacin (vitamin B_3) content of human milk has been reported to parallel dietary intake. In unsupplemented diets, low vitamin B_3 levels usually parallel low levels of other B vitamins and low protein intakes.

Pyridoxine (vitamin B_6) intake and milk levels were studied in healthy lactating women. There were marked diurnal variations of vitamin B_6 levels, with peaks occurring in those mothers taking supplements 3 to 5 hours after a dose. Those taking less than 2.5 mg/day had much lower milk levels. Vitamin B_6 concentrations in human milk change rapidly with maternal intake.[86] When supplemented, the level in the milk is a direct reflection of the amount ingested. Plasma pyridoxal-5'-phosphate levels and birth weight are strong predictors of infant growth.[87]

When lactating mothers received supplements of vitamin B_6 ranging from 0 to 20 mg pyridoxine hydrochloride, the levels of vitamin B_6 measurable in the milk paralleled the intake, with levels peaking 5 hours after ingesting the supplement. When maternal intakes of vitamin B_6 approximated 2.0 mg/day, breastfed infants were unlikely to receive the current RDA of 0.3 mg vitamin B_6 per day. The AAP Committee on Nutrition[88] recommends a minimum of 0.35 mg vitamin B_6/100 kcal milk from birth to 12 months. The RDA for vitamin B_6 for lactating women is 0.5 mg daily. Vitamin B_6 is the vitamin in milk that is most likely to be deficient because pyridoxine levels in milk are closely influenced by dietary intake.[86,87] Supplementing with an additional 2.5 mg/day results in levels twice as high as in unsupplemented women.[86] The increment in the RDA for vitamin B_6 in lactation is more than five times the estimated secretion of this vitamin in milk,[1] which varies between 0.01 and 0.02 mg/L early in lactation to 0.10 to 0.25 mg/L in mature milk. The recommendation is to advise diets rich in vitamin B_6, such as poultry, meat, fish, and some legumes, and reserve supplementation for special-risk cases.

Pantothenic acid (vitamin B_5) levels in milk are correlated with maternal intake for the preceding day, although some pantothenic acid is stored in the body. Studies of malnourished women show increased levels in milk after supplementation. The pantothenic acid content of human milk (2 to 2.5 mg/L) does not vary appreciably with dietary variations in well-nourished mothers, but the overall intake over time does influence milk levels.[89]

Biotin is reported in few studies, but the findings are consistent that levels range from 5 to 12 μg/L, with supplementation even up to 250 mg/day having little effect except when levels are significantly below this range.

Pregnant and lactating women are at risk for suboptimal folate status because of the increased dietary requirement to facilitate enhanced anabolic activity. Until megaloblastic anemia develops, no validated, quick, nonintrusive tests exist to assess functional folate status. Milk folate levels are maintained at the expense of maternal reserves, thereby protecting the nursling. O'Connor[90] provides an extensive review of the issues.

Folate supplementation in well-nourished women does not affect the level of folate in the milk, although studies involving women with low folate (less than 60% RDA) show they responded to supplementation with increased levels in their milk. Differences in assay methods have produced inconsistencies among studies. Milk levels normally range between 40 and 70 mg/L and increase slightly in the early weeks of lactation. The daily dose during lactation should be 500 μg/day.

The effect of the stage of lactation on levels of vitamins B_1, B_2, B_3, B_6, and B_{12} and ascorbic acid has been reported. The values remained fairly constant throughout, except for those of vitamin B_3, which increased slightly over time. The relationship to socioeconomic group showed an increase in vitamin B_3 and B_6 levels with increased status. Vitamin B_1 was higher in poorer mothers. Tables 8.9 and 8.10 summarize the effects of diet on vitamin levels in maternal milk.

Fat-Soluble Vitamins

Fat-soluble compounds are generally transported into milk via the fat, and levels are less easily improved by dietary change. Because vitamins A and D are stored in tissues, the impact of dietary supplementation is more difficult to measure. Milk levels do not change until a certain level is achieved in the stores. High dietary levels of β-carotene do not appear to result in excessive levels of either vitamin A or β-carotene. An increase in vitamin A in the diet of undernourished women does increase its level in milk.

Vitamin A. When malnourished mothers were given a single oral megadose of 209 mmol of vitamin A and the control subjects were given none, serum retinol (vitamin A_1) levels increased in the supplemented mothers and remained significantly higher for at least 3 months. Breast-milk levels were higher (11.3 vs. 2.9 mmol/L) and remained so for 6 months. An associated observation was the reduction in the duration

TABLE 8.9   Water-Soluble Vitamins in Human Milk

Vitamin	Recognizable Clinical Deficiency in Infant	EFFECT OF MATERNAL SUPPLEMENTS		Effect of Dietary Intake on Milk Content
		In Malnourished	In Well Nourished	
Ascorbic acid (C)	Rare	Yes	Minimal	Limited at 50 mg/L
Thiamin (B_1)	Yes	Yes	Limited	Yes, up to 200 μg/L
Riboflavin (B_2)	Yes	Yes	Yes	Yes
Niacin (B_3)	Unknown	Yes	Yes	Yes
Pantothenic acid	Unknown	Yes	No	Yes
Pyridoxine (B_6)	Yes	Yes	Yes	Yes
Biotin	Yes	Yes	No	Limited
Folate	Unknown	Yes	No	No
Cyanocobalamin (B_{12})	Rare	Yes	No	Yes

TABLE 8.10   Fat-Soluble Vitamins in Human Milk

Vitamin	Recognizable Clinical Deficiency in Infant	EFFECT OF MATERNAL SUPPLEMENTS		Effect of Dietary Intake on Milk Content
		In Malnourished	In Well Nourished	
D	Yes	Yes	Yes	Yes
K	Yes	Yes	Variable	Probable
A	Unknown	Yes	Minimal	Yes
E	Unknown	Unknown	Yes	Unknown

Prepared from Subcommittee on Nutrition During Lactation, Committee on Nutritional Status During Pregnancy and Lactation, Food and Nutrition Board, Institute of Medicine, National Academy of Sciences. *Nutrition During Lactation.* Washington, DC: The National Academies Press; 1991.

of respiratory tract infections and febrile illnesses in the infants of the supplemented mothers.[91] This observation was confirmed by Stoltzfus et al., who did a randomized, double-blind study giving women 312 mmol of vitamin A as retinyl palmitate or placebo orally.[92] Maternal levels in the supplemented group were significantly higher at 6 months than in the group given the placebo. Among the infants at 6 months, 36% of the placebo group and 15% of the vitamin A group had low retinol concentrations. Their relative dose response demonstrating low vitamin A stores was 23% in the placebo group and 10% in the treated group. This confirmed the value of high-single-dose vitamin A in lactating women, according to the authors.

Maternal postpartum vitamin A supplementation (VAS) was subjected to a systematic review of RCTs by Gogia and Sachelev in 2010.[93] No evidence of a reduction in mortality or morbidity was found; low birth weight was not measured. Imdad et al. published a systematic review and meta-analysis of VAS directly to infants and its effects on morbidity and mortality. They reported that VAS for infants is associated with a clinically important reduction in morbidity and mortality for children. Recommendations for VAS in children should be separate from VAS in mothers.[94] Policy formulation should be based on improvement of maternal benefits (morbidity and mortality), maternal safety, and cost-effectiveness.[95]

Vitamin D. Many women have surprisingly inadequate vitamin D levels.[96] Vitamin D had been considered to be at a stable level in milk that was unaffected by diet. However, studies involving maternal levels and infant levels have demonstrated low milk levels.[97] When mothers were given 0, 500, and 2500 IU ergocalciferol daily, they produced milk with 39, 218, and 3040 mg/mL vitamin D. The effect on levels of 25-hydroxyvitamin D was less dramatic.[97] The physiologic significance to the infant was disputed because the major source of antirachitic sterols was thought to be sunlight, not milk. The role of water-soluble vitamin D in human milk has not been confirmed. Infants born to mothers with inadequate vitamin D stores need a regular supply of vitamin D through diet, supplements, and exposure to ultraviolet light.[96]

Infant levels of vitamin D have been found to be low. Because of the report of clinical rickets in breastfed infants in a sunny climate, the AAP[98] and the Centers for Disease Control and Prevention (CDC) have determined that breastfed infants should be supplemented regardless of maternal vitamin D status and exposure to sunlight. This mandate has been supported by dermatologists, who have recommended no sun exposure and the use of sunscreen in infancy. The best estimate of adequate exposure to sunlight for white infants was 30 minutes per week clothed only in a diaper or 2 hours per week fully clothed and with the head and hands exposed.

Multiple studies have demonstrated that maternal 25-hydroxyvitamin D levels can be raised by supplementation.[99] For women at risk of vitamin D deficiency (dark skin, limited sun exposure, inflammatory bowel disease or limited fat absorption, obese, or gastric bypass surgery), this supplementation should begin during pregnancy to prevent low cholecalciferol levels and continue through lactation to ensure adequate levels in their milk. Supplementing mothers is preferred to supplementing the breastfed infant because the mother is also in deficit.[100]

Vitamin D deficiency in infants is not breast-milk deficiency but the deficiency of sunlight. Societal changes have diminished infant sun exposure, including the avoidance of sunlight, the use of sunscreen, the migration to northern latitudes by dark-skinned individuals, and the use of total body clothing for religious reasons by individuals migrating to northern climates. Replacing this natural source of vitamin D has been a challenge but requires actual supplementation.

While recommending vitamin D supplementation across the board, the AAP[98] and the CDC have not considered maternal supplementation partially because of possible toxicity, although doses of 4000 IU/day for up to 5 months have been shown to be safe in a wide population of adults. To achieve normal vitamin D status in breastfeeding mother–infant pairs, high-dose maternal vitamin D was utilized by Wagner and Greer.[96] A dose of 1600 IU vitamin D per day for 3 months has minimal effect on vitamin D levels in mother or infant; 3600 IU/day provided clinically relevant increases in the nutritional vitamin D_2 status of both the mother and her infant. In the absence of sunshine or in dark-skinned individuals, 4000 IU/day appears to be the minimal maternal dose to achieve clinical results. Deficit mothers may need up to 4000 IU/day. Because laboratory vitamin D is easily obtained, doses can be based on individual needs (Table 8.11).

Dark-skinned infants reared in climates where sunlight is minimal may be at significant risk for rickets when breastfed unless attention is given to the possible need for supplementation of vitamin D.[101] Although rickets was considered a disease of the past, the disease has reemerged since the 1980s partially because of the high risk for premature infants, especially micropremature infants, but also because of the increase in breastfeeding, especially by women who avoid dairy products, which are the major food source of vitamin D supplementation.[102] It is just not about rickets anymore, but any signs of vitamin D deficiency, which begins with decreased absorption of intestinal calcium and urinary loss of phosphorus but normal calcium levels in infants. The progression of deficiency shows bone demineralization and elevated alkaline phosphatase, followed by hypocalcemia and hypophosphatemia and frank rickets. Vitamin D deficiency has also been associated with significant disease states, including autoimmune diseases through vitamin D (e.g., rheumatoid arthritis, systemic lupus erythematosus,

TABLE 8.11 Serum 25-Hydroxyvitamin D Reference Range Recommendations

ng/mL	Interpretation
Serum 25-hydroxyvitamin D	
<20	Moderate risk of deficiency
20–29	Low risk of deficiency
30–60	Adequate
>60	Potentially harmful

multiple sclerosis, diabetes mellitus type 1, Crohn disease); cancers, such as breast, prostate, colon, and skin; cardiovascular disease; and insulin resistance. Insufficient vitamin D levels in pregnancy have been linked to higher levels of body fat in the child at 6 years of age.[103]

The recommendation is for all breastfed infants and any infant receiving less than 500 mL of fortified formula per day to receive 400 units of vitamin D daily beginning at birth.[98] Liquid preparations of vitamin D (400 units/mL and 400 units in one drop) only are available because a breastfed infant does not need other vitamins unless the mother is deficient.[99]

Vitamin E. Vitamin E refers to at least eight chemical forms of α-tocopherol and α-tocotrienol with antioxidant activities. α-Tocopherol is in human plasma and breast milk and functions as a nutrient in humans. Levels of α-tocopherol are highest in the colostrum (2 to 50 micromol/L) when the neonate is most dependent on its physiologic effect as an antioxidant and in the prevention of hemolytic anemia attributed to vitamin E deficiency. α-tocopherol levels decline in transitional (7 to 14 micromol/L) and mature milk (3 to 9 micromol/L), and levels are highest in hindmilk compared with foremilk.[104] Maternal intake during pregnancy does affect neonatal levels and levels in colostrum. Vitamin E deficiency in adults and children is defined as a serum α-tocopherol level of <12 micromol/L. Clinical manifestations (spinocerebellar ataxia, skeletal myopathy, and pigmented retinopathy) of vitamin E deficiency appear to be rare except in premature and very-low-birth-weight infants, which can manifest with hemolysis, retinal damage, and infection.[105] Dietary food sources include green leafy vegetables; nuts; wheat germ oil; and soybean, canola, corn, and other vegetable oils. The recommended daily allowance for lactating women is 16 mg compared with 4 to 5 mg/day for infants up to 12 months of age. Maternal supplementation with prenatal vitamins can increase milk vitamin E levels and the vitamin E status of breastfed infants.[104] There have been studies on single-dose vitamin E maternal supplementation, which does increase levels of vitamin E in colostrum and mature milk.[106,107] The potential long-term benefits and potential for toxicity for mothers or infants of such supplementation have not been studied. Low-dose daily maternal vitamin E intake can influence the levels of vitamin E in the milk. However, no evidence indicates that vitamin E deficiency occurs in individuals with normal fat absorption.[1] To compensate for maternal losses in milk and maintain stores, 4-mg α-tocopherol equivalents (16 mg vitamin E) per day are recommended for lactating women.[75]

Vitamin K. The most critical need for vitamin K in the infant is during the birth process and in the first few days of life, when the risk for bleeding, especially intracranial bleeding, is greatest.[108] Maternal dietary intake is most critical during the last trimester. Transplacental passage of vitamin K is slow, and cord blood levels are almost imperceptible. The synthesis of menaquinones by bacteria in the breastfed infant gut is minimal because lactobacilli do not synthesize them. Studies on supplementation of lactating women have shown that small doses are inadequate to raise the maternal level. Greer et al.[109] have shown that the average woman's intake is now 0.8 to 1.03 mg/kg per day. The content of human milk is 0.1 to 0.2 mg/dL, which does not supply the daily requirement of 1 mg/kg per day. Maternal supplements of 5 mg/day of vitamin K increase breast-milk concentration to 4.5 to 6.0 mg/dL, thus increasing serum concentrations in exclusively breastfed infants.

After the intramuscular (IM) injection of 1 mg of vitamin K at birth, no further recommendations for vitamin K supplements are made for healthy breastfeeding infants and their mothers. If the infant receives an oral preparation at birth, the dose of 2 mg should be repeated at 7 and 28 days of age.

Levels of proteins induced by vitamin K absence (PIVKAs; under-γ-carboxylated prothrombin produced in the absence of vitamin K) are a marker of K deficiency. The cord blood of full-term infants often has high PIVKA levels (0.1 AU/mL), correlating with low vitamin K. Levels of vitamin K in the infant are undetectable at 4 weeks after IM vitamin K administration at birth, but in some infants, they become elevated by 8 weeks. This has led to the recommendation that mothers be supplemented with 90 μg of vitamin K daily through the first 3 months of lactation.[108]

The consensus is that late vitamin K–deficiency bleeding should be prevented by prophylaxis (Box 8.2). After a study of different oral schedules in Australia, Germany, the Netherlands, and Switzerland, it was confirmed that oral doses of 1 mg vitamin K for the infant are less effective than IM dosing. It takes at least 6 hours after an IM dose of vitamin K to improve clotting.[110] If parents refuse IM vitamin K, some experts recommend 2 to 4 mg PO vitamin K after the first feeding, then 2 mg at 2 to 4 weeks and again at 6 to 8 weeks; or 2 to 4 mg PO vitamin K after the first feeding, then 2 mg within the first week and weekly while breastfeeding; or 2 mg PO vitamin K after the first feeding, then 2 mg within the first week, followed by 25 mcg daily for 13 weeks. There are no RCTs supporting these regimens.[111]

BOX 8.2 Administration of Vitamin K to Newborns

Because parenteral vitamin K prevents a life-threatening disease of the newborn and the risks of cancer are unproven and unlikely, the American Academy of Pediatrics recommends the following:
1. Vitamin K_1 should be given to all newborns as a single, intramuscular dose of 0.5 to 1 mg.
2. Further research on the efficacy, safety, and bioavailability of oral formulations of vitamin K is warranted.
3. An oral dosage form is not currently available in the United States but ought to be developed and licensed. If an appropriate oral form is developed and licensed in the United States, it should be given at birth (2.0 mg) and should be administered again at 1 to 2 weeks and at 4 weeks of age to breastfed infants. If diarrhea occurs in an exclusively breastfed infant, the dose should be repeated.

The least invasive method would be to increase the milk levels by supplementing the mother. In the 1950s, efforts to increase vitamin K and prothrombin levels at birth by giving mothers a large dose of vitamin K in labor failed to change the incidence of hemorrhagic disease in newborns. However, maternal supplementation during lactation is effective in raising vitamin K levels for the mother. Vitamin K is transferred into human milk, but at very low levels, and it requires other factors (bile salts, etc.) to enhance absorption. Although the amount of vitamin K available in infant formulas is very high, no toxicity has yet been demonstrated.

Vitamins Summary

Although dietary supplements improve the milk quality and quantity in malnourished women, a balanced diet without excessive supplementation is the most physiologic and economical way to ensure good milk. Nutrients, especially vitamins, are excreted in the urine only when taken in excess. The AAP Committee on Nutrition recommends 400 mg vitamin D for breastfeeding infants beginning at birth in the absence of adequate sun exposure.[88] Maternal supplementation is under study. Vitamin K at birth for the infant is essential. The AAP recommends a single dose of vitamin K (0.5 to 1.0 mg IM) at the time of delivery.[98]

Minerals

Calcium

Calcium has been associated with bone growth, and concern has been expressed because the total calcium in breast milk is low. The available information is inadequate to determine the true requirement for lactation.[7] Studies with radioactive calcium in nonpregnant adults have shown that losses occur into the gut and through the kidney. Absorption and retention of calcium also depend on the reserves in the body. Long-term shortage causes an economy of utilization, and the apparent requirement is lower.[112] During lactation, absorption and retention are greater.

Serum calcium and phosphorus concentrations are greater in lactating women compared with nonlactating women.[97] Lactation stimulates increases in fractional calcium absorption and serum calcitriol. This is most apparent after weaning. Alterations in absorption, metabolism, and excretion may conserve calcium during lactation.[113] Women with low calcium intakes have no direct benefit from supplementation as a protective mechanism to maintain breast milk calcium or maternal bone mineral content.[114,115] Urinary calcium was found to be higher in the supplemented group. Specific risk factors that have the greatest predictability for osteoporosis include a positive family history of osteoporosis, fair complexion, lower body mass and height, not breastfeeding their infants, smoking, and fat deposits.[116] Scanning transmission techniques showed that lactating women mobilize 2% of their skeletal calcium in 100 days of nursing. The calcium content of milk appears to be maintained despite greatly deficient intake, probably because of skeletal stores.[117] The milk calcium levels are the same in mothers of rachitic and nonrachitic infants. This is most important for women younger than age 25 because the calcium content of bones is expected to increase until age 25 to 30.[118] Peak bone mass is achieved during the childbearing years.

Estradiol concentrations are related to bone mineral density because estradiol stimulates osteoblastic proliferation and enhances collagen gene expression. The relatively low estrogen levels during lactation increase bone mobilization. Prolonged amenorrhea is associated with increased mobilization, and the greatest reduction in bone mass occurs early in lactation. Prolactin has a synergistic effect on mobilization. The ratio of dietary calcium to dietary protein has also been identified as important; that is, women with high-protein diets must also have high calcium intake. Recovery after weaning is reported to be negatively affected by parity.

The Recommended Dietary Intake (RDI) for calcium is higher for women younger than age 18, even when prepregnant, than for older women (1300 mg calcium compared with 1000 mg recommended for nonpregnant women 18 to 50 years old and 1200 mg/day for women greater than 50 years old).[118] Calcium status is only one of many possible factors in the etiology of osteoporosis. Dietary guidance during lactation should include recommendations for the replacement of stores. Women who have lactated are not more prone to osteoporosis than nonlactators or nulliparas.[119,120] Postweaning bone regeneration is accelerated for the first 4 to 6 months after lactation ceases. Postweaning bone density is then often greater than prepregnancy.

There is no additional requirement for calcium while lactating. The requirement of 1000 mg/day for women 18 to 50 years old and 1300 mg/day for women 14 to 18 years old is adequate intake (AI). The same calcium supplementation for women, based on age, should continue postweaning.

Sodium, Potassium, and Chlorine

The breast milk concentration of sodium is the most variable of all the minerals, fluctuating as much as 10-fold during normal lactation and diurnally, separate from the effects of mastitis, emotional stress, or involution. Maternal sodium or potassium intake has no immediate influence, either high or low, on postprandial milk sodium or potassium concentrations.[121] Dietary potassium may influence milk potassium more significantly. The potassium RDI in lactation is 5.1 g/day. With increasing numbers of women with cardiac and renal disease choosing to lactate, potassium amounts in the diet are more relevant, in addition to concerns about necessary medications that are known to deplete potassium levels.

The chlorine level in breast milk is not thought to be affected by maternal diet. A chlorine deficiency reported in a breastfed infant was associated with normal maternal serum and dietary intake but with deficient levels in the milk (less than 2 mEq/L).[122] Normal is greater than 8 mEq/L. This deficit in the milk was assumed to be a defect of breast function. The daily requirement for sodium is 2300 mg/day.

The concentration of electrolytes (sodium, potassium, chloride) in milk is determined by an electrical potential gradient in the secretory cell rather than by maternal nutritional status.[1]

Iron

The iron content of milk is not readily affected by the iron content of the diet or the maternal serum iron level. Increases in dietary iron that increase serum levels do not increase iron in the milk. It is important, however, for the mother to replace her iron stores postpartum.[123] It has not been established that increases in tissue iron are advantageous. Iron that is added to human milk will bind to lactoferrin and may interfere with its function. Infants exclusively breastfed for 7 months or longer were not found to be anemic at 12 or 24 months.[123] Half the infants breastfed for a shorter period were anemic at 12 months because additional dietary iron from solids was not provided.

A large study involving children from Sweden and Honduras examined whether iron supplements affect growth and morbidity.[124] Children were assigned to supplements or a placebo. If the hemoglobin was less than 110 g/L at onset, iron had a therapeutic effect. Growth measurements were significantly lower in length and head circumference in those who received iron. Those who had hemoglobin greater than 110 g/L and received iron had more diarrhea. The authors suggest that iron not be given unless it is needed. In another observational study involving more than 900 children at 8 and 12 months, infant intake of >600 mL of cow's milk or formula and intake of >6 breastfeeds per day was associated with lower intakes of solids and iron intake of less than the reference nutrient intake recommendation. The authors recommend more iron-containing solids and less milk for this age group.[125]

Iron supplementation appears to be safe, according to Friel et al.,[126] who conducted a double-blind, RCT of iron supplementation in early infancy in a total of 77 healthy term breastfed infants using 7.5 mg/day of elemental iron as ferrous sulfate or a placebo from 1 to 6 months of age. Iron supplementation produced higher hemoglobin and mean corpuscular volume at 6 months of age, as well as higher visual acuity and psychomotor development index at 13 months of age.

Dietary iron for lactating women is set at 9 mg/day, which is offset by the suppression of menses during lactation. The requirement for iron is 1.8 times higher for vegetarian mothers because of the lower bioavailability of iron from vegetarian sources.[127]

Phosphorus, Magnesium, Zinc, and Copper

Phosphorus, magnesium, zinc, and copper levels in milk are not affected by dietary administration of these elements.[128] Again, however, it is important for the mother to maintain and replenish her stores.[123]

According to the RDA, many lactating women are receiving marginal amounts of magnesium.[127] The amount recommended for lactation is two to three times the amount estimated to be in the milk, or 310 to 320 mg/day.

Zinc has an RDA during lactation of 4 to 13 times higher than the amount estimated to be in the milk, on the basis that it is poorly absorbed (20%). Studies done with stable isotopes in lactating women show that absorption was 59% to 84% of intake. Zinc absorption during pregnancy increases dramatically and decreases slightly during lactation, but it is double the

prepregnant rates, presumably in response to the demand by the breast for milk synthesis.[129] Milk levels are unaffected by supplementation and gradually decline over time from 4.7 to ± 1.74 mg/L on day 1 to 2.65 ± 1.06 mg/L on day 28 and 0.46 ± 0.36 mg/L at 6 months.[130] Supplementation does result in increased maternal absorption and increased plasma levels.

Prolactin is a zinc-binding hormone that is associated with the initiation and maintenance of lactation. Zinc is also thought to be involved with the synthesis, storage, and secretion of prolactin. Increasing zinc availability is thought to inhibit the formation and secretion of prolactin from the pituitary. The relationships among plasma zinc, prolactin, milk transfer, and milk zinc were studied by O'Brien et al.[131] No differences in milk transfer or prolactin levels were found between those who were zinc supplemented and those who were not. Low zinc levels are seen in those with a history of long-term alcohol ingestion. Their daily requirement is doubled.

Although no major health risks have been associated with low zinc intakes, zinc is known to be important to immune function.[132] The RDA for zinc is 12 to 13 mg/day during pregnancy and lactation. The recommended intake for infants 0 to 6 months of age is 2 to 4 mg/day.

Iron supplementation has no significant effect on levels of copper, selenium, and zinc in the mother's serum and breast milk.[133]

Selenium

A correlation exists between selenium in human milk and maternal dietary intake.[134] Maternal plasma levels vary with the form of selenium supplementation (selenomethionine or selenium-enriched yeast).[135] The original source of selenium is the soil, and levels vary geographically. It is transferred to plants and works up the food chain. Breastfed infants are known to have higher intake and utilization than infants fed formula or cow's milk because of bioavailability.[34] Many selenoproteins have been identified, but glutathione peroxidase is involved with producing a variety of organic hydroperoxides or reactive oxygen radicals in the liver. Although selenium toxicity is possible, deficiency from low intake is a problem.[134] Two diseases showing selenium deficiency are Keshan disease and Kashin–Beck disease, which are associated with the accumulation of lipid peroxides. Dietary studies have shown that intake can affect the mother's plasma and milk levels.[34] The RDI is 70 μg daily during lactation, compared with 55 μg for nonlactators.[136]

Chromium

Breast-milk levels of chromium are reported to be 3.54 ± 40 nmol/L (0.18 ng/mL) and to be independent of dietary intake.[137] Total absorption for lactating women was 0.79 ± 0.08 mmol/dL, which was greater than that of nonlactators. Serum levels were correlated with urinary chromium excretion, a good indicator of serum levels. The estimated RDA for breastfed infants is 10 μg/day, which is much greater than the levels measured in the study by Anderson et al.[137] The adequate daily intake for infants and children <12 months old is

0.2 to 5.5 μg/day.[138] The RDA for adults is 45 μg/day during lactation and 25 μg/day for nonlactating women of the same age.

Iodine

Iodine in milk does depend on dietary content. The breast can raise the concentration of iodine in the milk above that in the blood, and thus there is an increased danger in giving radioactive iodine to the lactating woman. With iodized salt, bread dough, conditioners, and the common use of iodine-containing cleansers, excessive iodine intake is a risk. There are varied food sources of iodine, such as seaweed, cod, yogurt, iodized salt, milk, fish sticks, enriched bread, fruit cocktail, shrimp, chocolate ice cream, macaroni, eggs, and tuna (all containing greater than 10% of the recommended daily value). The question of possible iodine deficiency, however, has been raised in breastfed infants around the globe as well as in the United States.[139] A systematic review of iodine nutrition status in lactating mothers living in countries with various types of iodine-fortification programs reported deficiency in lactating women.[140] The urinary iodine concentration (UIC; accepted as a measure of iodine deficiency when <100 μg/L) was utilized to assess iodine deficiency. The mean or median UIC was reported as deficient in lactating women in a number of countries with mandatory iodine-fortification programs (India, Denmark, Mali, New Zealand, Australia, Slovakia, Sudan, and Turkey). Separately, the median or mean UIC was deficient in countries with voluntary fortification programs (Switzerland, Australia, New Zealand, Ireland, and Germany).[139] Universal salt iodization programs are likely more feasible and cost-effective in most countries as long as the supplementation is adjusted to meet the local/regional needs and follow-up testing documents low levels of deficiency in the majority of the population, with special attention to infants and lactating mothers. A study of women in Boston found a mean breast milk concentration of 155 μg/L, with a mean urinary iodine level of 144 μg/L; 47% of the women had milk insufficient in iodine.[141] Smoking is also recognized to reduce iodine concentrations in breast milk to a mean level of 26 μg/L. The authors suggest that lactating women should take iodine supplements, such as an iodine-containing vitamin preparation with at least 150 μg per dose. The daily requirement is 290 μg; however, more than 450 μg daily is considered excessive.[139] Urinary iodine concentrations optimally are 100 to 199 μg/L, with a corresponding intake of 150 to 299 μg/day. Infants need 110 μg/day.

Milk iodine concentrations are higher now than those reported in the 1930s. Mean breast-milk iodide levels ranged from 29 to 490 mg/L, averaging 178 mg/L, above the RDA for infants. In a study of pregnant and lactating women in Bangkok, iodine levels were 170.6 and 138.0, respectively, following supplementation with 200 mg iodine daily. Cord-blood thyroid-stimulating hormone (TSH) was reduced with supplementation during pregnancy. Median breast milk iodine concentrations were higher in lactating women supplemented with iodine compared with the nonsupplemented group. This demonstrated that maternal supplementation in pregnancy and lactation could improve the cord-blood TSH

levels, the breast-milk iodine concentration, and subsequently the thyroid function of the infants in iodine-poor regions.[142]

Fluorine

Human milk contains 16 ± 5 mg fluoride per liter and reflects, to some degree, the level in the water supply. The risk for excessive fluoride has been pointed out by Walton and Messer,[143] who report dental mottling and milk fluorosis in supplemented breastfed infants. The AAP Committee on Nutrition states that fluoride supplements may be unnecessary when mothers/infants live in areas with adequately fluoridated water, as recommended by the US Department of Health and Human Services (0.7 mg/L). This amount provides enough fluoride to prevent tooth decay in children and adults while decreasing the risk of dental fluorosis.[144] If the water is not fluoridated or the mother drinks fluoride-free bottled water, she should be supplemented.

The fluoride concentrations of infant foods and drinks have been found to vary widely, ranging from 0.01 to 0.72 mg/kg, so no need exists for supplementation if the diet is well balanced when solid foods are initiated.[145]

Minerals Summary

Table 8.12 summarizes constituent levels in human milk and changes over time.

MATERNAL NUTRITION: IMMUNOLOGIC SUBSTANCES

Substances in colostrum and mature milk confer important infection protection in breastfed infants. Maternal malnutrition was associated with lower levels of immunoglobulins G and A (IgG, IgA) in a group of Colombian women studied by Miranda et al.[146] The colostrum contained only one-third the normal levels of IgG and less than half the normal albumin. Significant reductions in IgA and complement C4 were observed in colostrum, but lysozyme, C3, and immunoglobulin M (IgM) were normal. Titers against respiratory syncytial virus were unaffected by nutritional status. The protective deficiencies improved in mature milk over time and with improvement of nutritional status. The total leukocyte concentrations and their bactericidal capacity were similar in well-nourished and undernourished women.[147]

Prentice et al. measured breast-milk antimicrobial factors of rural Gambian mothers. The concentrations and daily secretions of all immunoproteins, except lysozyme, decreased during the first year and then remained steady. Compared with breast-milk levels in Western women, levels of IgG, IgM, C3, and C4 were higher in Gambian women; IgA and lactoferrin were similar; and lysozyme was lower. Dietary supplementation in Gambian women did not raise the breast-milk immunoproteins in this study.[148] Separately, there is literature on the effect of mothers being overweight or obese and the immunologic properties and composition of their breast milk. In particular, the inflammatory cytokines, adipokines (leptin, adiponectin), are present in different amounts in the breast milk of overweight/obese women, and there is an

TABLE 8.12 Representative Values for Constituents of Human Milk[a]

Constituent (per Liter)[a]	Early Milk (<28 days Postpartum)	Mature Milk (≥28 days Postpartum)
Energy (kcal)		650–700
Carbohydrate		
Lactose (g)	20–30	67
Glucose (g)	0.2–1.0	0.2–0.3
Oligosaccharides (g)	22–24	12–14
Total nitrogen (g)	3.0	1.9
Nonprotein nitrogen (g)	0.5	0.45
Protein nitrogen (g)	2.5	1.45
Total protein (g)	16	9–12.6
Total casein (g)		
β-Casein (g)	3.8	5.7
κ-Casein (g)	2.6	4.4
Whey proteins		6.7
α-Lactalbumin (g)	3.62	3.26
Lactoferrin (g)	3.53	1.94
Serum albumin (g)	0.39	0.41
Serum IgA (g)	2.0	1.0
IgM (g)	0.12	0.2
IgG (g)	0.34	0.05
Amino acids (g)[b]		
Alanine	0.65–1.71	0.26–0.42
Arginine	1.16–1.42	0.25–0.40
Aspartic acid	1.18–3.52	0.54–0.92
Cystine	0.47–1.41	0.11–0.23
Glutamic acid + glutamine	2.03–4.75	1.26–1.97
Glycine	0.36–1.42	0.10–0.27
Histidine	0.41–0.67	0.15–0.25
Isoleucine	0.43–1.27	0.33–0.57
Leucine	1.48–2.80	0.82–0.94
Lysine	0.72–2.06	0.30–0.90
Methionine	0.16–0.45	0.09–0.19
Phenylalanine	0.50–1.52	0.26–0.36
Proline	0.93–2.51	0.57–1.05
Serine	1.27–2.59	0.42–0.62
Threonine	0.65–1.94	0.32–0.42
Tryptophan	0.25–0.42	0.09–0.17
Tyrosine	0.76–0.54	0.31–0.47
Valine	0.88–1.66	0.35–0.51

(Continued)

TABLE 8.12   Representative Values for Constituents of Human Milk[a]—cont'd

Constituent (per Liter)[a]	Early Milk (<28 days Postpartum)	Mature Milk (≥28 days Postpartum)
Total lipids (%)	2	3.5
Triglyceride (% total lipids)	97–98	97–98
Cholesterol[c] (% total lipids)	0.7–1.3	0.4–0.5
Phospholipids (% total lipids)	1.1	0.6–0.8
Fatty acids (weight %)	88	88
Total % saturated fatty acids	43–44	44–45
C12:0		5
C14:0		0
C16:0		20
C18:0		8
Total % monounsaturated fatty acids		40
C18: 1ω-9	32	31
Total % polyunsaturated fatty acids (PUFAs)	13	14–15
Total ω-3	1.5	1.5
C18: 3ω-3	0.7	0.9
C20: 5ω-3	0.2	0.1
C22: 6ω-3	0.5	0.2
Total ω-6	11.6	13.06
C18: 2ω-6	8.9	11.3
C20: 4ω-6	0.7	0.5
C22: 4ω-6	0.2	0.1
Water-Soluble Vitamins		
Ascorbic acid (mg)		80–100
Thiamin (μg)	20	200
Riboflavin (μg)		400–600
Niacin (mg)	0.5	1.8–6.0
Vitamin B$_6$ (mg)		0.09–0.31
Folate (μg)		80–140
Vitamin B$_{12}$ (μg)		0.5–1.0
Pantothenic acid (mg)		2.0–2.5
Biotin (μg)		5–9
Fat-Soluble Vitamins		
Retinol (mg)	2	0.3–0.6
Carotenoids (mg)	2	0.2–0.6
Vitamin K (μg)	2–5	2–3
Vitamin D (μg)		0.33
Vitamin E (mg)	8–12	3–8

(Continued)

TABLE 8.12 Representative Values for Constituents of Human Milk[a]—cont'd

Constituent (per Liter)[a]	Early Milk (<28 days Postpartum)	Mature Milk (≥28 days Postpartum)
Major Minerals		
Calcium (mg)	250	200–250
Magnesium (mg)	30–35	30–35
Phosphorus (mg)	120–160	120–140
Sodium (mg)	300–400	120–250
Potassium (mg)	600–700	400–550
Chloride (mg)	600–800	400–450
Trace Minerals		
Iron (mg)	0.5–1.0	0.3–0.9
Zinc (mg)	8–12	1–3
Copper (mg)	0.5–0.8	0.2–0.4
Manganese (mg)	5–6	3
Selenium (mg)	40	7–33
Iodine (mg)		150
Fluoride (mg)		4–15

IgA, Immunoglobulin A; *IgG,* immunoglobulin G; *IgM,* immunoglobulin M; *ω-3,* omega-3; *ω-6,* omega-6. The values are expressed per liter of milk as a percentage on the basis of milk volume or weight of total lipids. Values as mean values or ranges of means.

[a]All nutrient values except for amino acids are modified from Picciano MF. Appendix: representative values for constituents of human milk. *Pediatr Clin North Am.* 2001;48:263.

[b]Modified from George DR, De Francesca BA. Human milk in comparison to cow milk. In Lebenthal E, ed. *Textbook of Gastroenterology and Nutrition in Infancy and Childhood.* 2nd ed. New York: Raven Press; 1989: 242–243.

[c]The cholesterol content of human milk ranges from 100 to 200 mg/L in most samples of human milk after day 21 of lactation.

influence on the levels of 29 other immunologic constituents of human milk.[149] The authors, Erliana and Fly, concluded there is insufficient evidence to recommend that overweight/obese women not breastfeed, although they do recommend limiting excessive calorie intake during pregnancy and following a healthy weight-loss program after lactation is well established at 6 to 8 weeks postpartum.[150]

The Subcommittee on Nutrition During Lactation has concluded that the effects of maternal nutritional status on the immunologic system in human milk are controversial.[1] Clearly, further investigation into the immunologic effects of maternal nutrition (malnutrition, overweight/obesity, and calorie-restriction eating plans) on the mother's milk composition is necessary before more specific recommendations can be made.

RECOMMENDATIONS FOR NUTRITIONAL SUPPORT DURING LACTATION

The previous section noted that the quantity, protein content, and calcium content of milk are relatively independent of maternal nutritional status and diet. The contents of the amino acids lysine and methionine, certain fatty acids, and water-soluble vitamin vary with maternal dietary intake. It is important to point out that stores of calcium, minerals, and fat-

soluble vitamins need to be replenished.[151] Much of the data collected on breast-milk composition have varied, depending on the method used in collection. The daily intakes thought necessary for infants were determined by feeding infants processed human milk in a bottle, which is not a physiologic standard.[150] It is known, for example, that putting the entire sample in one container removes the natural variation in fat from beginning to end of the feeding.

The Subcommittee on Nutrition During Lactation and the Food and Nutrition Board of the Institute of Medicine recommend a balanced diet comparable to one for the nonlactating postpartum mother, with a few additions.[1,75] Although the calculated caloric cost of producing 1 L of milk is 940 kcal, during pregnancy, most women store 2 to 4 kg of extra tissue in the physiologic preparation for lactation.[75] Thus it is probably necessary to add only 500 kcal to the diet during lactation, except in women with known high metabolic rates.

Preparation for lactation begins in pregnancy, if not before. The major daily dietary increases for pregnancy are an increase in intake by 300 kcal; 20 g of protein; a 20% increase in all vitamins and minerals except folic acid, which is doubled; and a 33% increase in calcium, phosphorus, and magnesium. In comparing the RDAs for lactating women with those for nonlactating adult women, the increases suggested should provide ample nutrition and replace stores (see Table 8.7).

When dietary supplements are suggested, questions arise about increased costs. It has been reported in the literature for several decades that healthier diets cost more than unhealthy diets. Darmon and Drewnowski have published a review and analysis of disparities in diet quality and health based on a comparison of food prices and diet cost.[152] They demonstrated, again, that foods of lower nutritional value cost less per calorie. Despite the availability of some lower-cost nutrient-dense foods, these were reported as "less palatable" and less culturally acceptable among different groups of consumers. The authors propose identifying both the foods and the "diet patterns" that are "nutrient rich, affordable and appealing" as essential to supporting healthy choices. This is especially true for pregnant or lactating women, who need foods that satisfy hunger, fit their budget, are accessible, are personally and culturally acceptable, and are feasible to obtain and prepare.

After the report of the Subcommittee on Nutrition During Lactation,[1] an additional report was prepared, "Nutrition During Pregnancy and Lactation: An Implementation Guide From the Institute of Medicine."[153] These publications remain practical guides for primary care providers and include a sample nutrition screening questionnaire, indications for supplementation, nutritional assessment guidelines, and how and when to refer patients to registered dietitians.

The subcommittee did not propose a food guide because it recognized that diverse ways are available to meet nutrient needs and that culturally appropriate foods are important, especially in the perinatal period. It did offer the following recommendations:[152]

- Avoid diets and medications that promise rapid weight loss.
- Eat a wide variety of breads and cereal grains, fruits, vegetables, milk products, and meats or meat alternatives each day.
- Consume three or more servings of milk products daily.
- Make a greater effort to eat vitamin A–rich vegetables or fruits often. Examples of foods high in vitamin A include carrots, spinach or other cooked greens, sweet potatoes, and cantaloupe.
- Be sure to drink when thirsty. Lactation requires more fluid than usual.
- If you drink coffee or other caffeinated beverages, such as cola, do so in moderation. Two servings daily are unlikely to harm the infant. Caffeine passes into the milk.

Nutritional guidelines exist for many countries around the world and include recommendations for pregnancy and lactation. The Food and Agricultural Organization of the United Nations and UNICEF are additional resources for finding country-specific nutritional recommendations.[154,155]

Malnutrition: Special Supplementation for the Lactating Woman

It has been suggested that supplementing the diet of malnourished mothers with a special formula would be the best way to achieve ideal nourishment for mother and child. Infants will then gain the additional advantages of human milk, such as protection against infection. Such formulas have been devised. Gonzalez-Cossio et al. demonstrated that high-energy maternal nutritional supplementation increased milk production and the duration of exclusive breastfeeding of undernourished women.[156] When nutritional supplements are recommended, ideally, they are given to the mother. Such studies have been repeated in many geographic areas, with conflicting results. The results confirm that the provision of supplemental food to the malnourished mother can improve infant birth weight and improve milk production and the duration of exclusive breastfeeding among specific subgroups of malnourished women. In contrast, supplements taken by well-nourished women do not show any benefits from supplementation.[151,155] There are no systematic reviews or meta-analyses on the topic.

With the ready availability of well-balanced nutritional supplements today in the form of stable powders, it should not be difficult to initiate a high-protein, vitamin-enriched diet supplementation that is also palatable for a mother who is at nutritional risk. The Women, Infants, and Children (WIC) program provides dietary counseling and supplementation for mothers at the poverty level to encourage these mothers to breastfeed and to give them nutritional support while doing so. Infants in WIC programs receive the greatest benefit from being breastfed. The present WIC supplements focus on improving maternal diet and were expanded and diversified in 2009.

Given the negative effects of malnutrition on breast milk's infection-protection properties and on galactopoietic hormones (corticosteroids are greatly increased, and prolactin is decreased), nourishing the mother is the most effective way of benefiting the infant rather than supplementing the infant to meet growth standards.

The impact of dietary supplementation on lactating women with restricted diets has been reported to be inconsistent with respect to lactational amenorrhea.[157] Most recently, a study in Sri Lankan women did not show an effect on menstruation or ovulation with supplementation.[25] However, the study did result in a longer duration of full breastfeeding in supplemented women, which may have had an effect in suppressing ovulation. No difference was seen between supplemented and unsupplemented women regarding lactational amenorrhea.[157]

Allergy

There is a significant history of detection of nonhuman proteins in human breast milk over several decades.[158] These proteins are part of the human milk proteome and demonstrate that milk proteins reach the milk by synthesis by mammary cells, exocytotic fusion release from breast cells, or transcytosis from the blood to the mammary gland.[159] The importance of nonhuman proteins in human milk remains to be fully determined, but their presence has raised concerns about their role in infant allergy.[160] Zhu et al. identified 109 nonhuman peptides in human milk, which could be grouped into 36 nonhuman proteins, including bovine caseins (α-S1-, α-S2-, β-, κ-caseins) and β-lactoglobulin.[158] Other investigators have identified proteins from eggs, peanuts, and wheat.[161] Notably, 90% of all food allergies are ascribed to eight groups of allergenic foods: cow's milk, eggs, fish, crustacean shellfish, tree nuts, peanuts, wheat, and soybean.[162] Specific nutritional interventions have been explored relative to the development of atopic disease in infants and children.[160,162] The most recent review and report by the Committee on Nutrition and Section on Allergy and Immunology of the AAP summarized data from the original report by these groups in 2008 and included data from newer systematic reviews, meta-analyses, and RCTs from 2008 through 2017.[162] They summarize a lot of data and make specific statements about maternal dietary restrictions during pregnancy and lactation and the role of breastfeeding in prevention of atopic disease. The available data do not support maternal dietary restrictions during pregnancy or lactation to prevent atopic disease. They highlight the role of breastfeeding in preventing atopic disease in five main points: (1) evidence supports that exclusive breastfeeding for 3 to 4 months decreases the incidence of eczema in children less than 2 years old, (2) exclusive breastfeeding beyond 3 to 4 months does not add short- or long-term effects against developing atopic disease, (3) breastfeeding beyond 3 to 4 months of age is protective against wheezing in the first 2 years of life, (4) there is new evidence that a longer duration of breastfeeding versus less breastfeeding protects against asthma even beyond 5 years of age, and (5) it is not evident that breastfeeding protects against the development of specific food allergies. The authors make recommendations, developed from evidence-based data, regarding the timing of initiation of allergenic foods.[162] There remains considerable opportunity to study the potential benefits of breastfeeding, and specifically exclusive breastfeeding, and the introduction of complementary foods and protection against atopic disease.

Vegetarian Diets

The growing interest in vegetarianism has necessitated a better understanding of the several types of diets and their potential for adequate nutrients and growth, as well as the motivation for these diets (Table 8.13).[163] There is much more information available on plant-based nutritional plans, but it is appropriate for health care professionals to become more knowledgeable to serve as a resource to patients.[164,165] There is variability in the reasons for choosing a vegetarian diet, as well as different types of vegetarian diets and variation in dietary practices among vegetarians; therefore individual assessment of the dietary intakes of vegetarians, especially during pregnancy and lactation, is appropriate.[166]

Reports of malnutrition among breastfed infants of vegetarian mothers usually focus on the very strict groups, such as vegans and those on macrobiotic diets. The dietary risks involved are predominantly with the B vitamins because these vitamins are usually associated with protein, which is also proportionally lower from vegetable sources. An additional concern is the availability of various amino acids in specific concentrations to utilize them for protein synthesis.[167] The net protein utilization of a food may be considerably lower than the total protein content; therefore, when using vegetable sources of protein, it is important to use foods with "complementary protein" in the same meal. Vegetarian cookbooks emphasize the use of complementary proteins. Throughout history, culturally traditional meals have ensured a combination of complementary proteins.

Vitamin B_{12} deficiency has been described in vegans because of the absence of animal protein. It is advisable in these cases to supplement the diets of pregnant or lactating women and of infants or growing children with up to 4 mg/day of vitamin B_{12}. It has been shown that fermented soybean foods do contain vitamin B_{12}, as do the single-cell proteins, such as yeast, because even single-cell animal species contain small amounts of vitamin B_{12}. In a study of vegetarian mothers and their infants, a large proportion of the infants had elevated methylmalonic acid levels, indicative of vitamin B_{12} deficiency.[84] A significant number of vegetarian

TABLE 8.13   Vegetarianism and Associated Risks

Type of Vegetarian	Diet Includes	Diet Avoids	Risks
Semivegetarian	Vegetables, milk products, seafood, poultry	Red meat	Minerals[a]
Ovolactovegetarian	Vegetables, milk products, eggs	Flesh foods (meat, seafood, poultry)	Minerals,[a] especially zinc
Lactovegetarian	Vegetables, milk products	Flesh foods, eggs	Minerals,[a] especially zinc, protein[b]
Ovovegetarian	Vegetables, eggs	Flesh foods, milk products	Minerals,[a] especially iron and zinc, protein,[b] riboflavin, vitamin D, vitamin B_{12}
Vegan	Only vegetables	Flesh foods, milk products, eggs	Minerals,[a] protein,[b] riboflavin, vitamin D, vitamin B_{12}
Macrobiotic	Gradual progression to a diet of only cereals		Advanced-stage nutritionally inadequate

[a]Excessive dietary phytates and dietary fiber inhibit absorption of minerals such as iron, zinc, and calcium. *Phytates* are organic chemicals present in many vegetables and unleavened bread that bind with minerals.
[b]Diets not using complementary proteins may be deficient in net protein because the net protein utilization is low.

women, both lactators and nonlactators, had elevated methylmalonic acid levels and low vitamin B_{12} levels. Vitamin B_{12} deficiency in vegetarians occurs across different types of vegetarian diets and was associated with low vitamin B_{12} levels in human milk in 15% to 20% of a sample of 74 lactating women in the United States.[168,169] Almost 85% of the women identified as B_{12} deficient in this study were taking larger doses of vitamin B_{12} supplements compared with the RDA. Pregnant and lactating women on any type of vegetarian diet should be screened for vitamin B_{12} deficiency and supplemented as needed.[170]

As noted previously, vegetarians have lower levels of DHA.[55] A comparison of the umbilical cord blood of infants born to South Asian vegetarian women showed less DHA in the plasma and cord-blood phospholipids than in infants born to omnivores. Early onset of labor; incidence of cesarean delivery; lower birth weight, head circumference, and length, after adjusting for maternal height; duration of gestation; parity; smoking; and the sex of infant were also related to DHA levels. The total n-3 fatty acid requirements may be higher for vegetarians than for nonvegetarians because vegetarians must rely on the conversion of alpha-linolenic acid (ALA) to eicosapentaenoic acid (EPA) and DHA.[171,172] A study of the milk from vegetarian mothers compared with that from nonvegetarian mothers looked at fat and fatty acid composition. Those fats and fatty acids produced de novo by the breast were not different.[173] The precursors of AA were higher in vegetarians, yet the AA level in the milk was lower and continued to decrease the longer the vegetarian diet was maintained. Linoleic acid was greater among vegetarians. The amounts of DHA were not different. Among 34 breastfed infants at 7 months in the Tufts study, 3 were below the 10th percentile for height and weight, 1 had low weight for length, and 3 had high weight for length, whereas of the 51 who were not breastfed, 6 were below the 10th percentile, 2 had low weight for length, and 4 had high weight for length.[41]

Other reports of growth curves in vegetarian children in the first few years show them to be shorter and leaner than standard, with the greatest effect among those whose mothers were on the most restricted diets.[174] Studies of children from birth to 10 years in the Netherlands reared in a macrobiotic tradition showed the greatest growth retardation, with fat and muscle wasting and slower psychomotor development between 6 and 18 months of age.[175] The breast milk of their mothers, who breastfed an average of 13.6 months, contained less vitamin B_{12}, calcium, and magnesium compared with matched omnivorous control subjects. Breastfed vegetarian infants are usually on the norms for growth, with the exception of those receiving minimal vitamin D and calcium, as reported in dark-skinned mothers in cloudy climates. The mean serum 1,25-dihydroxyvitamin D concentrations were 37% higher in lactating vegetarian women than nonvegetarian women. The serum parathyroid hormone was elevated in all lactators compared with nonlactators. It is postulated that the low calcium in the vegetarian diet stimulates the elevated 1,25-dihydroxyvitamin D level, and this in turn stimulates the increased absorption of calcium to meet the needs of milk production.[176]

Four vegetarian children between 8 and 24 months of age were reported by Hellebostad et al.[177] to have rickets from vitamin D deficiency (three with tetany and seizures) and vitamin B_{12} deficiency. All the infants were initially breastfed by mothers whose diets were low in vitamin D, high in fiber and phytate (which interferes with enterohepatic circulation of vitamin D), and low in calcium and phosphate.

Cereals are the primary source of dietary zinc in vegetarian diets. The bioavailability of zinc is affected by the presence of phytates, fiber, calcium, or other zinc-absorption inhibitors, which results in poor absorption of zinc in vegetarian diets.[127] Vitamins B_6 and B_{12}, vitamin A, and calcium, because of a high content of oxalic acid, are poorly absorbed. Selenium is dependent on the selenium content of the soil, as is zinc. Increased dietary sources or supplementation of these vitamins are required in vegetarians.

General recommendations for lactating vegetarian women are as follows:
1. Supplement with soy flour, molasses, and nuts.
2. Use complementary protein combinations.
3. Avoid excessive phytates and bran.
4. Watch protein and iron intake. Calcium should be supplemented if bone mineralization decreases because the milk levels will be adequate.
5. Supplement with 10 µg vitamin D plus adequate sunshine.
6. Know that vitamins B_{12} and B_2 (riboflavin) are low in vegetarian diets and should be supplemented.

If the mother does not supplement herself, then supplementation for the infant would be appropriate.

Supplementation of Breastfed Infants' Diets

For newborn infants, human milk is the ideal food, containing all the necessary nutrients. In establishing dietary norms for infants fed cow's milk, many nutrients identified as being needed in the diet were found to exist in greater amounts in cow's milk than in human milk. This does not consider the probability that the nutrient may be in a more bioavailable form in human milk. The specific items in question are protein, sodium, iron, vitamin D, and fluorine.

When a breastfed infant must be supplemented with formula, however, it is preferable that a formula low in iron be used to avoid providing excessive iron that will bind with lactoferrin and interfere with its infection protective activity.

The AAP Committee on Nutrition has noted that iron deficiency is rare in breastfed infants and attributes this to increased absorption and the absence of microscopic blood loss into the gastrointestinal tract, which is seen in bottle-fed infants. The Section on Breastfeeding of the AAP recommends a source of iron in solid foods (fortified infant cereal) at 6 months of age for breastfed infants.[98]

The AAP no longer recommends fluoride supplements in all breastfed infants. Many breastfed infants have done without fluorine supplementation and have had no adverse dental problems, but the decision should be based on individual determinants, including family dental history and the level of fluoride in the water supply, which is ideally between 0.7 and 1.0 ppm. If the level is less than 0.3 ppm, 0.25 mg of daily fluoride should be given. Maternal supplementation may be the better choice in this case.

The AAP now recommends 400 IU vitamin D daily for all breastfed infants starting at birth unless they are also receiving 500 mL fortified formula daily. Maternal supplementation is a preferred alternative. The Section on Breastfeeding of the AAP, however, tailors the recommendation to the dyad, using supplements of vitamin D to the infant as a last resort.

Exercise While Breastfeeding

There are usually no contraindications to exercise during lactation. The most common obstacle is having sufficient time. The availability of home exercise equipment does offer an option for home programs. Exercise baby carriages, which have large wheels for greater speed and rough terrain, are another option. Because they tip somewhat easily, infants may need a helmet and a safety strap. A safety strap that attaches to the runner's wrist prevents the vehicle from getting away. These carriages are excellent for brisk walks as well.

The impact of programmed exercise on milk volume, milk composition, and ultimately milk acceptability has been studied.[178] Women who exercise excessively, especially those who jog, may have trouble maintaining their milk supply. This difficulty has been attributed to any activity that results in persistent motion of the breasts and excessive friction of clothing against the nipples. A firm athletic brassiere made of cotton will reduce this effect. No data are available on the impact of jogging with or without support on later breast sagging.

The production of lactic acid during exercise has been studied in relation to lactation by Wallace et al., who had mothers report whether their infants refused to nurse or fussed when breastfed after exercise.[179] The study demonstrated that seven healthy lactating women who normally spent more than 30 minutes in aerobic activity (jogging, running, swimming, biking, and aerobics), as well as some who did calisthenics and racket sports, had an increase in their blood lactic acid levels after exercise. When a standardized treadmill exercise was used to maximal voluntary effort, the blood lactic acid level increased at 10 minutes compared with that of the at-rest sample, but the level at 30 minutes had returned almost to at-rest levels. Milk samples at 10 and 30 minutes continued to have elevated lactic acid, although wide variation was seen among subjects.

In a larger sample, when 26 women between 2 and 6 months postpartum who normally exercised during pregnancy and postpartum were exercised on a standardized treadmill to maximal voluntary effort, the levels of lactic acid were correlated to infant acceptance of the milk. The breasts were wiped with a dry towel before milk collection. Milk samples collected before exercise and at 10 and 30 minutes after exercise revealed an increase in lactic acid levels over baseline at both 10 and 30 minutes. In a double-blind order of samples, the infants were offered milk by dropper and were less likely to accept samples with high lactic acid.[180] The authors

noted that the levels of lactic acid were high enough for adults to detect when offered water solutions at the same concentrations (1.6 mmol). Human milk is sweet, but lactic acid is known to be bitter/sour. Infants have been noted to make a puckering facial expression to a sour taste as early as a few hours of age.[181] Studies of sucking in newborns have shown more rapid rates with sweet than sour, with some change in heart rate, respiratory rate, and sucking patterns.[182] The lactic acid level can remain elevated in the milk for as long as 90 minutes, according to Wallace and Rabin.[183]

When exercise studies were undertaken by Wallace and Rabin comparing the effects of a typical workout and a standard maximal exercise regimen, significant differences were noted. The milk lactate level before exercise was 0.61 ± 0.14 mM, and that after typical exercise was 1.06 ± 33 mM. After maximal exercise in the same women, the level was 2.88 ± 0.80 mM.[183] Seventeen percent of the subjects had lactate levels above the reported adult taste threshold of 1.6 mmol. Milk rejection probably is a function of lactate concentration in the milk and infants' sensitivity to taste. Women who exercised with full breasts developed a peak postexercise lactate concentration at 10 minutes, whereas women who exercised with empty breasts did not peak for 30 minutes.[180] Many of the studies reported may not have measured peak lactate when samples were collected only at 10 minutes.

Mothers have reported that their infants may reject their milk after exercising. Women reported to the Lactation Study Center that their infants were fussy and colicky for as long as 4 to 6 hours after the mother's strenuous exercise. Exercise generates sweat that is high in sodium and chloride, and lactic acid may change the pH. Although these studies are ongoing, the following precautions might be recommended when breastfeeding after strenuous exercise:

- Shower, or at least wash the breast of perspiration.
- Manually express 3 to 5 mL of milk from each breast and discard.
- If the infant displays a puckering facial expression, postpone feeding or replace feeding with previously pumped milk.

Levels of prolactin and adrenal activation have been studied in eumenorrheic and amenorrheic women who exercise regularly. Prolactin levels after exercise are elevated for 20 to 40 minutes.[178] The effect appears to be unrelated to anaerobiosis. The hypothalamic–pituitary–adrenal axis is known to be activated under the influence of various forms of stress, including exercise. How this activation might affect milk production or oxytocin-stimulated milk let-down after exercise has yet to be determined.

Serum prolactin and growth hormone increased severalfold during prolonged acute exercise in normal women and runners with and without menses, demonstrating that a threshold of exercise intensity must be reached for this reaction to occur.[184] There was no correlation to menstrual dysfunction.

When the lactation performances of eight physically fit, exercising women were compared with those of sedentary control subjects, no significant differences in milk volume or composition were observed despite wide variations in energy intake and expenditure.[60] Exercising women compensated by increasing energy intake; thus no net difference (in plasma hormones, milk energy or milk lipid, or protein or lactose content) was seen between the groups. It has been reported that lactating women exercising on a regular basis expended an average of 2630 kcal/day exclusive of milk energy output, compared with the 1800 to 1900 kcal/day expenditures of women who did not exercise.[1]

Dewey et al.[185] studied the impact of regular exercise on the volume and composition of breast milk and further confirmed that breastfeeding women can safely exercise. Although previous studies were done on exercising fit women, this study randomly assigned sedentary women to exercise with supervised aerobic exercise to 60% to 70% of the heart rate reserve for 45 minutes per day, 5 days a week, for 12 weeks. The control group remained breastfeeding but sedentary. Measurements of energy expended, dietary intake, body composition, and milk volume and composition were collected at 6 to 8 weeks, 12 to 14 weeks, and 18 to 20 weeks postpartum. Maximum oxygen uptake and plasma prolactin response in 2 hours after nursing were measured at the first and last assessment times. No significant differences were seen in maternal weight and fat losses, volume or composition of milk, infant weight gain, or plasma prolactin response between exercising and sedentary women. No women reported difficulty nursing after moderate exercise. The authors did note that the 300-kcal/day mean extra energy expenditure of the exercise group at midpoint in the study decreased toward the end as they cut back on other activities to compensate.[185] This suggests that high levels of energy expenditure may be difficult to sustain while lactating because of fatigue and time limitations (Figs. 8.4 and 8.5).

Lovelady et al.[60,186] further evaluated this same study group, who were randomly assigned to exercise or to remain sedentary. Exercise marginally increased levels of high-density lipoprotein cholesterol but did not affect other lipid concentrations. Further, the at-rest metabolic rate did not change over time. Weight and body fat percentage declined similarly in both groups. No difference was found between exercising and sedentary groups regarding insulin, glucose, or thermal response. The authors concluded that sedentary women can initiate moderate exercise programs during lactation but that exercise does not increase weight loss or fat loss without dietary control, that is, by avoiding compensatory increased intake. In a similar randomized study of 33 women, Potter et al.[187] and Prentice and Prentice[24] reported that moderate exercise is enough to improve cardiovascular fitness without marked changes in energy expenditure, dietary intake, and body weight, and composition does not jeopardize lactation performance.

Maternal exercise did not alter the mineral content of the milk in a randomized crossover trial measuring phosphorus, calcium, magnesium, sodium, and potassium. Samples were drawn before and during rest periods after 10, 30, and 60 minutes of maximal graded exercise. Thus, with the exception of a temporary rise in milk lactate after prolonged heavy exercise, exercise has no apparent impact on milk composition.[188]

Dieting While Breastfeeding

The Subcommittee on Nutrition During Lactation[1] stated in its report that the average rate of weight loss postpartum while maintaining adequate milk volume is 0.5 to 1.0 kg (1 to 2 lb) per month. In individuals who are significantly overweight, a weight loss of up to 1 to 2 kg (about 4 to 5 lb) per month should not affect milk volume, although weight gain and feeding pattern should be monitored in the infant. The

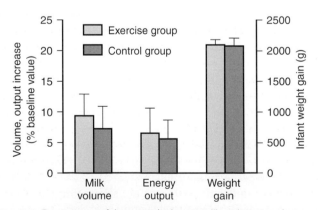

Fig. 8.4 Percentage of increase in breast-milk volume and energy output and absolute increase in infants' weight in exercise and control groups during a 12-week study. Values shown are means ± standard error (SE). To convert kilocalories to megajoules, multiply by 0.004186. None of the differences between the groups were significant. The 95% confidence intervals were as follows: for the percentage of change in milk volume, 2% to 17% for the exercise group and −1% to 16% for the control group (p = 0.66); for the percentage of change in energy output in breast milk, −2% to 15% for the exercise group and −1% to 12% for the control group (p = 0.85); and for infant weight gain, 1871 to 2279 g for the exercise group and 1733 to 2355 g for the control group (p = 0.86). (Modified from Dewey KG, Lovelady CA, Nommsen-Rivers LA, et al. A randomized study of the effects of aerobic exercise by lactating women on breast-milk volume and composition. *N Engl J Med.* 1994;330:449.)

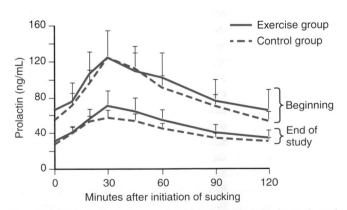

Fig. 8.5 Plasma prolactin response to nursing in control and exercise groups at beginning (top two lines on graph) and end (bottom two lines) of study. Values shown are mean ± standard error (SE). Study began 6 to 8 weeks postpartum and ended 18 to 20 weeks postpartum. The change in the area under the curve from the beginning to the end of the study was not significantly different between the two groups (p = 0.38). (Modified from Dewey KG, Lovelady CA, Nommsen-Rivers LA, et al. A randomized study of the effects of aerobic exercise by lactating women on breast-milk volume and composition. *N Engl J Med.* 1994;330:449.)

subcommittee[1] considers rapid weight loss, that is, more than 2 kg per month after the first month, ill-advised. In addition, because no data exist about curtailing maternal energy intake during the first 2 to 3 weeks postpartum, dieting immediately postpartum is not recommended and could be associated with poor milk supply. Energy intake must be balanced with the level of physical activity. The subcommittee does not recommend intakes of less than 1500 kcal/day; however, brief fasts, perhaps for religious reasons, of less than a day are unlikely to affect milk supply. Liquid diets or weight-loss medications are not recommended. In studies of food-deprived rats, a clear correlation exists between adequate milk production and adequate food intake. This finding was amplified if the diet was also restricted during pregnancy.

Weight Loss While Breastfeeding

Studies of weight loss report conflicting data on the benefit of lactation for postpartum weight loss. A prospective longitudinal study reported on 470 women where exclusive breastfeeding was not associated with changes in postpartum maternal weight of body fat percentage.[189] In a systematic review and meta-analysis from 2015, breastfeeding for 3 to 6 months had a negative influence on postpartum weight retention, but with >6 months of breastfeeding, there was little or no influence.[190] Another systematic review and critical evaluation by Neville et al. evaluated 37 prospective studies and 8 retrospective studies.[191] In 27 studies, there was little or no association between weight change and breastfeeding. In 4 of 5 studies assessed to be of "high methodologic quality," weight loss was associated with breastfeeding. Several studies have reported that the duration of breastfeeding rather than the "category of breastfeeding" (exclusive, predominant, complementary, or nonbreastfeeding) was associated with maternal weight loss.[192,193] The numerous other potential contributing factors to weight loss or gain make the study and analysis of postpartum weight difficult. Many women in developed countries experience an appetite surge during lactation and may experience no weight loss in the first months beyond the weight lost in the first weeks. They may not return to prepregnancy weight for 6 months. Women who are prone to gaining weight may be more apt to gain on an unregulated diet. Maternal nutrition status in the United States, as measured by anthropometric indices prenatally and postpartum, is unrelated to milk volume, according to the studies of Butte et al.[14] and Dewey.[157] The total energy expenditure of sedentary women, including those housebound with a new baby, averages 1800 kcal/day, exclusive of the energy put into the milk produced.[5]

In a study of 411 postpartum women, no consistent relationship was reported between mode of feeding (i.e., breast or bottle) and postpartum weight loss.[187] Despite the energy deficiency of breastfeeding women, the trend was toward greater weight loss in nonlactators. Women who gained more during pregnancy lost more postpartum weight regardless of their pregnancy weight. No dietary intake was recorded because the data were collected retrospectively.

The Stockholm Pregnancy and Weight Development Study prospectively investigated trends in eating patterns, physical activity, and sociodemographic factors in relation to postpartum body weight development, following 1423 pregnant women.[194] Weight retention 1 year postpartum was greater in women who increased their energy intake during and after pregnancy. Weight retention also increased in those who not only increased their snacking to three or more times per day but also decreased their lunch frequency. A sedentary lifestyle was correlated with a weight gain of 5 kg or more over prepartum weight. The authors summarized their findings as being related most closely to a change in lifestyle after pregnancy.[194]

The tremendous variability in women's responses to the stress of reproduction and lactation suggests that there is very low stress per unit time. Thus many different variables exist during the perinatal period to rebalance the energy equation, according to Prentice and Prentice.[24] Some women are energy sparing and some energy profligate. Although generally beneficial, the interaction between exercise and skeletal integrity is influenced by hormonal status and many exercise variables.

During lactation, many women do not need additional dietary supplements as often recommended, according to work by Hartmann et al.[195] They reported considerable variation among individual women for the energy output in milk and the energy mobilized from maternal stores for milk synthesis, and they recommend that energy should be calculated for each mother depending on her energy stores and milk demands. Even a low-fat diet could be appropriate to maximize the de novo synthesis of fatty acids for milk triacylglycerols, if one were sure there was adequate intake of long-chain PUFAs and basic nutrients. Further, they demonstrated that a perceived inability to make milk was usually a function of inappropriate suckling, scheduled feeds, and other lactation management issues, not a lack of substrate (Table 8.14).

Weight loss during lactation is greatest between 3 and 6 months. Dietary advice for women who choose to diet while lactating should include the following:[1]

- The diet must include balanced, varied foods rich in calcium, zinc, magnesium, vitamin B_6, and folate.
- The minimum energy intake should be 1800 kcal.
- Calcium and multivitamin–mineral supplements may be necessary to replace stores if the diet is marginal.

FOODS TO AVOID

The concern about foods causing gas in breastfed babies has no scientific basis. The normal intestinal flora produces gas from the action on fiber in the intestinal tract. Neither the fiber nor the gas is absorbed from the intestinal tract, and they do not enter the milk, even though they may cause the mother some discomfort. The acid content of the maternal diet also does not affect the milk because it does not change the pH of the maternal plasma. Essential oils are present in foods such as garlic and some spices that have characteristic odors and flavors. These oils may pass into the milk, and occasionally an infant objects to their presence.

TABLE 8.14   Dietary Reference Intakes: Additional Macronutrient Recommendations

Macronutrient	Recommendation
Dietary cholesterol	As low as possible while consuming a nutritionally adequate diet
Trans fatty acids	As low as possible while consuming a nutritionally adequate diet
Saturated fatty acids	As low as possible while consuming a nutritionally adequate diet
Added sugars	Limit to no more than 25% of total energy

From Food and Nutrition Board, Institute of Medicine, National Academies. Dietary Reference Intakes for Energy, Carbohydrate, Fiber, Fat, Fatty Acids, Cholesterol, Protein, and Amino Acids, Washington, DC: Food and Nutrition Board, Institute of Medicine, National Academies; 2002.

Twenty-four-hour colic studies by Mennella and Beauchamp[196,197] show that the diet of the lactating woman alters the sensory qualities of her milk. They found that garlic ingestion significantly and consistently increased the intensity of the milk odor as perceived by blinded adult panelists. The odor was not apparent at 1 hour, peaked at 2 hours, and decreased thereafter. Similar observations have been made in other species. Garlic is one of the most potent of the volatile sulfur-containing foods (onions, broccoli, etc.). Garlic consumption by the mother increased the length of time spent suckling and the rate of suckling of the next feeding.[197] This behavior is usually associated with a tendency of the breast to make more milk. The authors suggest that the mouth movements made during sucking facilitated the retronasal perception of the garlic volatile oils in the milk. This study reports only the first 4 hours postingestion and makes no reference to the period between 4 and 24 hours after ingestion, a time occasionally associated with colic in breastfed infants after ingestion of certain foods by the mothers (often called *24-hour colic*).

When these mothers and infants were tested over an 11-day period, those infants who had garlic previously showed no response to reexposure; that is, suckling pattern and volume ingested were unchanged.[198] A garlic odor of amniotic fluid has been noted when the mother consumed garlic before delivery or amniocentesis. These investigators also report that alcohol, mint, and cheese flavors are transmitted to milk.

Animal studies show that odors in utero and early in life are associated with a preference for them after birth. Breastfed infants experience a wide variety of odors and flavors during maternal lactation, which may enhance their weaning to solid foods. This suggests that infants fed standard formulas experience a constant set of flavors, thus missing significant sensory experiences. In experiments with rats, Mennella and Beauchamp[197] found that a mother's milk contains gustatory cues reflecting the flavor of the mother's diet and that these cues are enough to influence dietary preferences at weaning.

Extensive clinical experience suggests, however, that some infants do not tolerate certain foods in the mother's diet, particularly specific vegetables and fruits. Garlic and onions may cause 24-hour colic in some infants. Cabbage, turnips, broccoli, or beans may bother others, making them "colicky" for 24 hours. The same has been said of rhubarb, apricots, and prunes. If a mother questions the effect of a food, she should avoid it or document its effect carefully by watching for colic in the 24 hours after ingestion. A heavy diet of melon, peaches, and other fresh fruits has been known to cause colic and diarrhea in the infant. Red pepper, which contains capsaicin and related compounds, has been reported to cause dermatitis in breastfed infants within an hour of milk ingestion.[199] The rash can last 12 to 48 hours and differs from the contact dermatitis known to occur from capsaicin applied directly. When hot peppers are prepared with bare hands, an intensely painful reaction can occur. In countries where red pepper dishes such as kimchi are common (Korea), a perianal rash has long been seen in breastfed infants whose mothers ingested these specific spice-containing dishes.

Food Additives

Artificial sweeteners are the most common food additives. Saccharin and cyclamate are not known to be teratogenic, but the remote relationship to cancer in rats has led to the recommendation that they be used in moderation. The same pertains during lactation. Cyclamate is a cyclohexylamine, an indirectly acting sympathomimetic amine that has been banned from use.

Aspartame is a dipeptide sweetener, aspartyl-L-phenylalanine methyl ester, that metabolizes to phenylalanine and aspartic acid. Thus it poses a risk to those with phenylketonuria. Normal individuals can consume 50 mg/kg per day without adverse effects. In large doses of 75 mg/kg per day, individuals increase their excretion of formate and methanol. When given aspartame, lactating women were noted to have phenylalanine levels four times the normal in their plasma.[200] Milk levels of phenylalanine and tyrosine were only slightly elevated. Aspartame in moderation during lactation is presumed safe unless the infant has phenylketonuria.

COLOR OF MILK AND MATERNAL DIET

The color of mature human milk is bluish white (foremilk), initially changing to creamy white (hindmilk). The color of colostrum is yellow to yellow-orange. Mothers occasionally report changes in the color of their milk. Most of these changes can be traced to pigments consumed in the diet, medications, or herbal remedies. The infant's urine may also turn color.

Pink or Pink-Orange Milk

Pink-orange milk was traced to Sunkist orange soda, which contains red and yellow dyes. A case of a breastfed infant with pink to orange urine was reported by Roseman.[201] This combination of food dyes is also used in other brands of soda, fruit drinks, and gelatin desserts. Even fresh beets can change the urine of both mother and infant to a red-pink hue.

Green Milk

Several cases of green milk have been reported to the Lactation Study Center at the University of Rochester. A careful search of the diet for the offending substance was made in each case. The effects of ingestion and avoidance of the identified culprit were then tested to confirm the association with the milk's color. Several items have been clearly identified. Gatorade energy drink (green variants), kelp and other forms of seaweed (especially in tablet form), and natural vitamins from health food sources have been associated with one or more cases of green milk and usually green urine.

Black Milk

Minocycline hydrochloride therapy was associated with black milk galactorrhea in a 24-year-old woman who received the compound for pustulocystic acne for 4 years.[202] Examination of the fluid revealed that the macrophages contained hemosiderin, thus causing the black color. This drug is known to cause black pigmentation of the skin. A second case was reported in a 29-year-old woman who had weaned but could express black milk 3 weeks after beginning oral minocycline therapy. Hunt et al.[203] found iron-staining pigment particles in the macrophages and suggested it was an iron chelate of minocycline.

Summary

Recommendations for maternal supplementation during lactation are unnecessary unless the mother's diet is deficient. Continuing prenatal vitamins postpartum is usually adequate. For malnourished women, supplementation may be appropriate after a personalized assessment of maternal deficiencies and intake. For lactating mothers adhering to the more restrictive vegetarian diets, the use of complementary protein combinations; supplementation with D and B vitamins; and attention to protein, iron, and calcium intake are appropriate. Having adequate vitamin D stores during pregnancy and lactation is important. Continued studies are being conducted to determine the efficacy of large doses of vitamin D for mothers so that supplementing infants can be avoided.

Supplements for breastfeeding infants are likely unnecessary in exclusively breastfed infants unless a deficiency is identified. The AAP does recommend vitamin D 400 mg beginning at birth. Iron needs should be addressed with appropriate solid foods (iron rich or iron fortified) after 6 months of exclusive breastfeeding. Fluoride supplementation is unnecessary if the mother is adequately resourced; if not, the mother should take fluoride.

There are no contraindications to exercise during lactation. Limiting caloric intake or dieting after establishing lactation through 6 to 8 weeks postpartum is also acceptable with attention to caloric intake, macro- and micronutrient intake, and monitoring of milk production along with infant growth. Weight loss in a scenario of dieting during lactation should average 0.5 to 2 kg of weight per month based on the mother's delivery weight and body mass index.

The Reference list is available at www.expertconsult.com.

9

Weaning

Ruth A. Lawrence

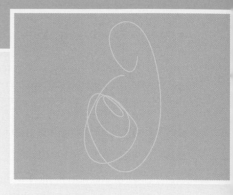

KEY POINTS

- Simply stated, weaning is the transition of the infant from dependence on mother's milk to reliance on other sources of nourishment for nutrition, health and growth, and development.
- Current recommendations are for 6 months of exclusive breastfeeding and initiation of complementary foods at 4

to 7 months of age with continued breastfeeding through 12 months and beyond.
- The "how to" for transition to complementary feeding is best outlined in the guiding principles of complementary feeding for the breastfed infant published by Pan American Health Organization (see Box 9.1).

What does *weaning* mean? Textbooks on pediatrics and mothers' manuals imply that it is the process by which one changes from one method of feeding to another. Raphael[1] states that the first introduction of solid foods is the true beginning of weaning. The term *weaning* is derived from the Anglo-Saxon *wenian*, which means "to become accustomed to something different." It does not mean the total cessation of breastfeeding but the addition of other things. If one consults the dictionary, however, one learns that to *wean* is to transfer the young of any animal from dependence on its mother's milk to another form of nourishment. A *weanling* is a child or animal who is newly weaned. The World Health Organization (WHO) in some of its publications uses "weaning" in a narrow sense as the complete stopping of breastfeeding. Complementary foods are nutrient-containing solids or liquids that are introduced during the transition period of weaning. During weaning, the infant transitions from complete dependence on breast milk for all its nutritional needs to ingesting solid and liquid forms of nutrition commonly used, acceptable, and readily available within an infant's household, family, community, and culture.

Weaning from a physiologic point of view is a complex process involving nutritional, microbiologic, immunologic, biochemical, and psychologic adjustments. This should be a safe process, maintaining optimal nutrition, growth, and development. Conceptually, early nutritional exposures are associated with both the infant's immediate health and later health through a process of "programming" the gastrointestinal tract, metabolism, and endocrinologic balance of the infant for later functioning in life. The practice of weaning within a family or community also depends on traditions, ethnical origins, and scientific beliefs consistent with perceptions of this stage of life.[2] A qualitative review of the literature on maternal infant feeding practices in the process of weaning revealed

three predominant themes: (1) infant physical and behavioral cues suggesting readiness to wean; (2) mother's knowledge, skills, and coping strategies to demonstrate "good mothering"; and (3) community pressure and inconsistent advice led to generational feeding and adoption of already established cultural feeding practices. The mothers made choices regarding feeding and weaning based on their perceptions of healthy infant feeding and successful parenting. Additional investigation of these factors will be essential to effectively supporting mothers and families in their infant feeding practices, including weaning.[3]

INFANT'S NEED

When discussing the process of weaning a human infant, one might say it is the transition of the infant from dependence on mother's milk to other sources of nourishment. If one were to determine the appropriate time for this to take place, it would be based on nutritional needs and developmental goals. Observations among other mammals suggest that achievement of a degree of maturity that allows a pup to forage for food is a trigger for initiating weaning by the mother.

The search for the appropriate weaning time for human infants has produced a number of extremes, from the regimen of J.R. Sackett in 1953 of introducing solids on the second day of life to withholding all solid foods until the infant had sufficient teeth to chew thoroughly, a method described by Bartholomäus Mettinger, a German physician, in 1473.[4] The birth of the infant food industry began with German chemist Justis von Leitbig in 1867. He marketed "the perfect infant food" to the public at the turn of the twentieth century, a mixture of wheat flour, malt flour, and cow milk. Abraham Jacobi, called the father of American pediatrics, advised no solids for a year and no vegetables before 2 years of age. Even early on the

---

BOX 9.1 Guiding Principles for Complementary Feeding of the Breastfed Child

1. *Duration of Exclusive Breastfeeding and Age of Introduction of Complementary Foods.* Practice exclusive breastfeeding from birth to 6 months of age, and introduce complementary foods at 6 months of age (180 days) while continuing to breastfeed.

2. *Maintenance of Breastfeeding.* Continue frequent, on-demand breastfeeding until 2 years of age or beyond.

3. *Responsive Feeding.* Practice responsive feeding, applying the principles of psychosocial care. Specifically: (1) Feed infants directly and assist older children when they feed themselves, being sensitive to their hunger and satiety cues; (2) feed slowly and patiently, and encourage children to eat, but do not force them; (3) if children refuse many foods, experiment with different food combinations, tastes, textures, and methods of encouragement; (4) minimize distractions during meals if the child loses interest easily; (5) remember that feeding times are periods of learning and love—talk to children during feeding, with eye to eye contact.

4. *Safe Preparation and Storage of Complementary Foods.* Practice good hygiene and proper food handling by (1) washing caregivers' and children's hands before food preparation and eating, (2) storing foods safely and serving foods immediately after preparation, (3) using clean utensils to prepare and serve food, (4) using clean cups and bowls when feeding children, and (5) avoiding the use of feeding bottles, which are difficult to keep clean.

5. *Amount of Complementary Food Needed.* Start at 6 months of age with small amounts of food and increase the quantity as the child gets older, while maintaining frequent breastfeeding. The energy needs from complementary foods for infants with "average" breast milk intake in developing countries are approximately 200 kcal per day at 6 to 8 months of age, 300 kcal per day at 9 to 11 months of age, and 550 kcal per day at 12 to 23 months of age. In industrialized countries these estimates differ somewhat (130, 310, and 580 kcal/day at 6 to 8, 9 to 11, and 12 to 23 months, respectively) because of differences in average breast milk intake.

6. *Food Consistency.* Gradually increase food consistency and variety as the infant gets older, adapting to the infant's requirements and abilities. Infants can eat pureed, mashed, and semi-solid foods beginning at 6 months. By 8 months most infants can also eat "finger foods" (snacks that can be eaten by children alone). By 12 months, most children can eat the same types of foods as consumed by the rest of the family (keeping in mind the need for nutrient-dense foods, as explained in no. 8). Avoid foods that may cause choking (i.e., items that have a shape and/or consistency that may cause them to become lodged in the trachea, such as nuts, grapes, raw carrots).

7. *Meal Frequency and Energy Density.* Increase the number of times that the child is fed complementary foods as he or she gets older. The appropriate number of feedings depends on the energy density of the local foods and the usual amounts consumed at each feeding. For the average healthy breastfed infant, meals of complementary foods should be provided two or three times per day at 6 to 8 months of age and three or four times per day at 9 to 11 and 12 to 24 months of age, with additional nutritious snacks (such as a piece of fruit or bread or chapatti with nut paste) offered one or two times per day, as desired. Snacks are defined as foods eaten between meals—usually self-fed, convenient, and easy to prepare. If energy density or amount of food per meal is low, or the child is no longer breastfed, more frequent meals may be required.

8. *Nutrient Content of Complementary Foods.* Feed a variety of foods to ensure that nutrient needs are met. Meat, poultry, fish, or eggs should be eaten daily, or as often as possible. Vegetarian diets cannot meet nutrient needs at this age unless nutrient supplements or fortified products are used (see no. 9). Vitamin A–rich fruits and vegetables should be eaten daily. Provide diets with adequate fat content. Avoid giving drinks with low nutrient value, such as tea, coffee, and sugary drinks such as soda. Limit the amount of juice offered so as to avoid displacing more nutrient-rich foods.

9. *Use of Vitamin-Mineral Supplements or Fortified Products for Infant and Mother.* Use fortified complementary foods or vitamin-mineral supplements for the infant, as needed. In some populations, breastfeeding mothers may also need vitamin mineral supplements or fortified products, both for their own health and to ensure normal concentrations of certain nutrients (particularly vitamins) in their breast milk. (Such products also may be beneficial for prepregnant and pregnant women.)

10. *Feeding During and After Illness.* Increase fluid intake during illness, including more frequent breastfeeding, and encourage the child to eat soft, varied, appetizing, favorite foods. After illness, give food more often than usual and encourage the child to eat more.

From Dewey KG; Pan American Health Organization. *Guiding Principles for Complementary Feeding of the Breastfed Child.* Washington, DC: Pan American Health Organization; 2002.)

---

recommendations concerning weaning varied by culture, ethnic group, medical intervention, and financial considerations.

Acknowledging that humans are primates, Dettwyler recognized that lactation and weaning occur according to certain regular patterns in nonhuman primates.[2] She searched for a natural age of weaning for human infants uninfluenced by culture and trends. Evaluating various "rules of thumb" for determining weaning age by biologic references, she found them inappropriate. Breastfeeding from an anthropologic point of view is both a biologic process and a culturalized

activity. In primitive cultures, the age of weaning from the breast was between 2 and 5 years, averaging 3 to 4 years.

If the definition of weaning is used to mean the cessation of all feedings at the breast, the age at weaning in nonhuman primates and other mammals is a function of genetics and instinct. Primates have a longer gestation, greater infant dependency, longer life spans, and larger brains per unit of body size than other mammals. Dettwyler[2] suggests that a possible formula for weaning is the ratio of present weight to birth weight as 4:1; that is, the offspring weans when four times the birth weight is achieved, usually between 2 and 3 years for well-fed healthy human infants.

In using weaning according to attainment of one-third the adult weight as the rule of thumb, Dettwyler notes the variations in size of human adults by ethnic and cultural groups. The average weight of an adult woman is 54 kg (119 lb); one-third is 18 kg (39½ lb), a weight achieved between 4 and 7 years for girls. The average weight of an adult man is 59 kg (130 lb); one-third is 19.3 kg (42½ lb). This would mean boys would be nursed longer. The present tendency for obesity in the developed world would accentuate these calculations.

When length of gestation is used as the determinant for weaning time, the weaning to gestation ratio can be determined. The ratio across primate species varies from 0.41 in the *Galago demidovii*, a small-bodied primate, to 6.40 in the *Pan troglodytes* (chimpanzee). The former primates nurse less than half the length of pregnancy (11/45 days); chimpanzees nurse 1460 days (228-day gestation). Gorillas nurse for 1583 days (256-day gestation). Because the human is closest to the chimpanzee and gorilla, six times the gestation period might be a more physiologic norm: 54 months, or 4½ years.[2]

When the eruption of the first permanent molar is used as the indicator for complete weaning, it estimates weaning at 5½ to 6 years in humans. Tooth eruption is genetically controlled and comparatively unaffected by diet or disease. Six years is also identified as the time of achieving an adult level of immunocompetence in humans.

The range of calculated ages for weaning derived from these formula ranges from 2.3 years to 6 or 7 years. Before the widespread availability of foods suitable for infants and of artificial formulas, infants were traditionally breastfed for 3 to 4 years (Fig. 9.1).

Other species gradually introduce other foods and teach their offspring how to obtain them on their own. Usually the mothers in most species make the determination for final termination and no longer permit the young to nurse. There seems to be a close correlation between age of weaning and age of reproductive maturity measured either as first ovulation (menarche) or average age of first breeding. Dettwyler[5] notes that these markers are also related to body size, with larger bodied species breastfeeding longer.

CULTURAL PATTERNS OF WEANING

Among humans, many cultural influences mandate weaning time and process.[6] Public and social pressures have influenced weaning for some families in industrialized society. Few traditional societies wean before 1 year of age, and some do not begin until 2 years of age (Fig. 9.2). In ancient Hebrew tradition (c. 536 BC), breastfeeding duration according to the Talmud was at least 3 years. Aristotle suggested that women should breastfeed while no menstruation was occurring, failing to recognize that one influences the other (lactation suppresses menstruation). The Romans recommended breastfeeding at least to the age of 3 years. In the Muslim world, especially Africa and the Sudan, however, weaning of children is by the Islamic teaching of the Koran, which advises breastfeeding until at least 2 years of age, with many breastfeeding to age 4 or 5. Before 1979, the average time of complete cessation worldwide was 4.2 years. Hervada and Newman[7] provide a historic review of weaning that also presents recent concerns about iron

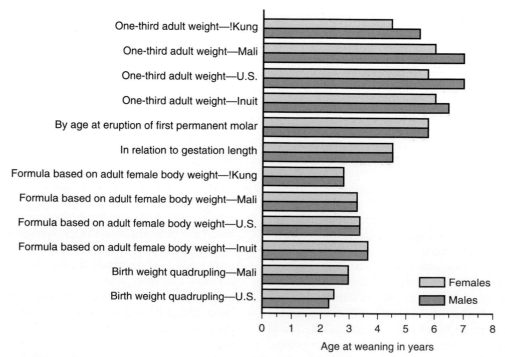

Fig. 9.1 Natural age at weaning according to technique used. (Modified from Dettwyler KA. A time to wean. In: Stuart-MacAdam P, Dettwyler KA, eds. *Breastfeeding: Biocultural Perspectives.* New York: Aldine de Gruyter; 1995.)

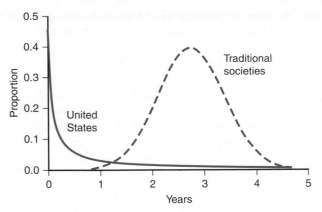

Fig. 9.2 Comparison of age at weaning in United States and 64 traditional societies. (Modified from Dettwyler KA. A time to wean. In: Stuart-MacAdam P, Dettwyler KA, eds. *Breastfeeding: Biocultural Perspectives.* New York: Aldine de Gruyter; 1995.)

TABLE 9.1	**Recommendations on Duration of Breastfeeding**	
WHO	Exclusive for 6 months	Continue 2 years and beyond
AAP	Exclusive for 6 months	Continue 1 year and as long as mother/infant wish
AAFP	Approximately 6 months exclusive	Continue 1 year/ mutually desired
ACOG	Approximately 6 months exclusive	As long as possible
Healthy People 2010	75% at birth	25% at 6 months
Healthy People 2020	Exclusive for 6 months	Continue for 1 year

AAFP, American Academy of Family Practice; *AAP,* American Academy of Pediatrics; *ACOG,* American College of Obstetrics and Gynecology; *WHO,* World Health Organization.
Modified from Dettwyler KA. A time to wean: the hominid blueprint for the natural age of weaning in modern human populations. In: Stuart-MacAdam P, Dettwyler KA, eds. *Breastfeeding: Biocultural Perspectives.* New York: Aldine de Gruyter; 1995.

deficiency and other problems more common to formula-fed infants.

Breastfeeding benefits for an older infant also have been evaluated. In the developing world, breastfeeding continues for at least 1 to 2 years after introduction of solid foods. Major benefits include not only the nutrients but also protective, digestive, and trophic agents that extend the period of infertility in the mother and reduce the incidence and severity of infectious diseases for the infant. A review of middle-class breastfed infants between the ages of 16 and 30 months in the United States revealed a decrease in the number of infections and improved overall health compared with those children no longer breastfed.[6]

Nutritionally, it is appropriate to begin iron-containing foods at 6 months, the time the stores from birth are diminishing. The requirement at this age exceeds that supplied by human milk. An additional source of protein becomes necessary toward the end of the first year of life because the grams of protein needed per kilogram of body weight can no longer be supplied by milk alone as the infant grows heavier. The content of protein in the milk begins to drop slightly after 9 months of lactation. A human infant also needs bulk, or roughage, in the diet. The exact time this need becomes apparent is not known, but it may well be by the end of the first year.

Developmentally, an infant is ready to learn to chew solids instead of suckle liquids at approximately 6 months. It has been suggested that there is a "critical period of development" during which infants can and must learn to chew.[8] Chewing is an entirely different motion of the tongue and mouth from sucking. The sucking fat pads in the cheeks begin to disappear at the end of the first year. The rooting reflex has been lost. Even though all the teeth are not in, the development of good dentition requires chewing exercise.

Various health organizations have made recommendations for the duration of breastfeeding based on evidence-based literature regarding breastfeeding, exclusive breastfeeding, and transition to complementary foods and infant nutrition, growth and development, health benefits, and risks and morbidity and

mortality (Table 9.1). Despite all the investigation, literature, and debate, the question remains whether such "broad" recommendations regarding the optimal duration of exclusive breastfeeding as a definitive time of 6 months should be applicable to the diverse populations across the world. Probably the most convincing data for such broad recommendations comes from the research for the WHO Child Growth Standards and the WHO study of nutrient adequacy of exclusive breastfeeding.[9-11] Using the data collected for growth of breastfeeding infants within 6 countries with sufficient socioeconomic status to ensure adequate nutrition through 36 months of life, growth patterns were analyzed. The growth patterns from the different countries in this study (Brazil, Ghana, India, Norway, Oman, and the United States) were so similar they were "superimposable" and individual country data could be excluded without significantly changing the composite curves (length/height, weight for age) the study generated. The implication is that the genetic potential for growth of children from diverse backgrounds is similar as long as the infants were exclusively breastfed for 4 to 6 months with continued breastfeeding through 12 months simultaneously with the introduction of complementary feeds and received nutritionally adequate intake for continued growth. Exclusive/predominantly breastfeeding occurred in 74.7% of the children for the first 4 months, 99.5% of children began complementary foods by 6 months of age and 68.3% of the children were partially breastfed until 12 months of age.

ROLE OF DEVELOPMENT IN INITIATION OF WEANING

Although the developmental milestones of infant behavior are noted to influence the introduction of weaning foods, the development of the gastrointestinal tract plays an equal role. Even the taste buds, which can be identified at the seventh week of fetal life as collections of elongated cells on the dorsal surface of the tongue, are fully innervated over the next weeks. The fetus is known to suck and swallow in utero; sucking is discussed in Chapters 3 and 7.

When taste becomes a factor in feeding is not known, although a lack of discrimination has been noted in the first weeks of life: infants have consumed formula with high salt or absence of chloride with morbid results. Because of the variation in the composition of mother's milk over a feeding, over a day, and from time to time according to maternal dietary intake, a breastfed infant has a richer range of experience in tasting than a formula-fed infant. Breastfed infants are, therefore, more accustomed to new taste experiences.[12] Similarly, chronic feeding problems in infants are rare in breastfed infants.[13–15] Conversely, formula-fed infants monotonously receive the same tastes, flavors, and consistencies for weeks, months, and years.

Both sucking and chewing are complex movements, having reflexive as well as learned components. The development of the chew-swallow reflex is necessary for the successful introduction of solids. This skill develops sequentially with neuronal development and then is a learned behavior conditioned by oral stimulation.[16] Before this point, when a spoon is introduced, the infant purses the lips and pushes the tongue against the spoon. By 4 to 6 months, the tongue is depressed in response to the spoon and the food accepted, and by 7 to 9 months, rhythmic biting movements occur regardless of the presence of teeth. Biting and masticatory strength and efficiency progress throughout infancy. If a stimulus is not applied when the neural development is taking place, the chewing reflex will not develop and the infant will always be a poor chewer. For a human infant, nursing also plays a role as a comfort and emotional support, a mechanism often referred to as *comfort nursing*. Inadequate nipple contact may lead to thumb sucking or the substitute use of a pacifier.

In summary, an infant is ready to explore new feeding experiences at approximately 6 months. Feeding is an important social as well as nutritional encounter. Eating solids and learning to drink from a cup are important behavioral and social achievements as well. This readiness does not mean the infant is taken from the breast, but that the diet is expanded and now includes solid foods, other liquids, and breast milk. Although a range of qualitative, quantitative, and temporal practices for weaning are known, the optimal approach matches the needs and requirements of a given child with the functions and capacities of his or her developing body.

INTRODUCTION OF SOLIDS

The WHO, the Canadian Pediatric Society, the Paediatric Society of New Zealand, and similar groups in England and Scotland[11,13,14,17] emphasize that weaning is not the termination of breastfeeding but the addition of other liquids and solids while continuing breastfeeding. The key recommendation on length of exclusive breastfeeding from the WHO[17] reads as follows:

> To strengthen activities and develop new approaches to protect, promote and support exclusive breastfeeding for six months as a global public health recommendation, taking into account the findings of the WHO expert consultation on optimal duration of exclusive breastfeeding, and to provide safe and appropriate complementary foods, with continued breastfeeding for up to two years of age or beyond, emphasizing channels of social dissemination of these concepts in order to lead communities to adhere to these practices.

The intake of complementary foods may add nutrients in a less bioavailable form, and it decreases the bioavailability of nutrients in human milk and the intake of other important factors in human milk. Investigators have shown that when solid foods are introduced in the diet of breastfed infants, energy intake per kilogram of body weight does not increase.[18] Solid foods displaced energy intake from human milk in 6-month-old infants even though they were breastfed on demand.[19]

When to Wean

Recommendations for the optimal time to introduce complementary foods to the breastfed infant remain controversial. The Section on Breastfeeding of the American Academy of Pediatrics (AAP) supports the introduction of solids at 6 months in concert with the WHO and United Nations International Education Fund (UNICEF).[20] This recommendation was in response to a systematic review of published reports in developed and underdeveloped countries conducted by Kramer and Kakuma[21] that included controlled clinical trials and observational studies in many languages. From 2668 reports, only 23 citations met criteria of an internal comparison group. Rigorous assessment of health outcomes included growth, iron and zinc status, infectious morbidity, atopic disease, neuromotor development, rate of maternal weight loss, and duration of lactational amenorrhea.[21]

This discussion of the weanling's dilemma (i.e., the choice between the known protective effects of exclusive breastfeeding against infectious morbidity, reducing atopy, and the theoretical insufficiency of breast milk alone as nutrition) continues. This is because there are numerous other variables that influence breastfeeding duration such as demographic factors of race, age, marital status, education, and socioeconomics and biologic variables, including issues of sufficient or insufficient milk supply, infant health problems, maternal obesity, and the physical challenges of breastfeeding, maternal smoking, parity, and method of delivery. Social variables, including paid work, family support, and professional support, play a role in duration of breastfeeding decisions, accomplishment, and psychological variables of maternal intention, paternal and family interest and support, and confidence in breastfeeding success. These variables were highlighted in a systematic review in 2009 reinforcing the need for further study regarding optimizing duration of breastfeeding for each individual woman and placing emphasis on support of the mother and family in achieving their breastfeeding goals.[22]

In summary, exclusive breastfeeding for 6 months supported appropriate gain in weight and length and adequate iron and zinc status when the mother is well nourished, reduced infection rates, provided some reduction in atopy, and had a significant advantage in achieving some developmental milestones. WHO-UNICEF, the AAP, and many other organizations have reached the same conclusion and recommend exclusive breastfeeding for 6 months (see Table 9.1).

Nutritional Needs During Weaning

Fewtrell et al.[23] recommend that nutrient intake during introduction of complementary feeds in a healthy full-term infant should be calculated as "the difference between nutrients provided by breast milk and the estimated total needs." Various organizations offer recommendations on nutrient needs during weaning and complementary feeding.[11,24–26]

Protein

In information collected by Dewey et al.[27] in 1994 on well-nourished breastfed infants, no "faltering" in growth pattern could be identified. In a review of protein and energy during weaning, Axelsson and Räihä[28] conclude that 1.65 g/kg per day from 5 to 9 months and 1.48 g/kg per day from 9 to 12 months are appropriate. The growth of exclusively breastfed infants, from 4 to 6 months of age, matched or exceeded that of randomly selected breastfed infants given 20% added protein. The exclusively breastfed group received 0.98 g/kg per day, whereas the supplemented group received 1.18 g/kg per day. Thus protein intake is not a limiting factor with respect to growth that would mandate weaning from the breast. On review of protein requirements for infants and children established by the WHO, they were higher than necessary for breastfed infants. Formula-fed infants require more protein because of comparatively poor utilization.[29]

Iron and Zinc

The challenge of meeting nutrient needs of infants and young children when complementary foods are added is great. It is a period of high nutrient density requirement, especially iron and zinc. In countries where cereal-based porridges with low nutrient density are the weaning foods, deficiencies are common. Iron and zinc need to be accounted for (Table 9.2).

The duration for which the iron endowment at birth remains adequate varies based on maternal iron status in pregnancy and other factors causing lower iron stores in the infant (infants of diabetic mothers, low-birth-weight infants). Some exclusively breastfed infants will benefit from additional iron (1 mg/kg per day) at 4 to 6 months.[30,31] Partially breastfed infants who consume over half of their daily milk intake as formula and are not on iron-fortified complementary foods should receive iron supplements until they have an adequate source from complementary foods.

When iron was added to the diet at 4 months by giving iron-rich solids to infants who did not have iron-deficiency anemia, the length growth was less than in unsupplemented control infants. Head growth was also slower in iron-supplemented infants. No improvement in weight gain was observed, and the treated infants had more occurrences of diarrhea if their hemoglobin levels were normal. More boys than girls had iron deficiency anemia at 9 months according to Dewey et al.[30]

The data on zinc are meager. The concentrations of zinc in milk decline after the first few months of lactation and are independent of maternal zinc intake.[32] Hepatic stores will sustain levels in the infant early on, but exogenous zinc in the diet will be required after 6 months of age (recommended dietary allowance [RDA] 3 mg/day between 7 to 36 months of age).[33]

Energy Requirements During Weaning

Breastfed infants self-regulate their total energy intake when other foods are introduced. No advantage to introducing complementary foods before 6 months has been seen relative to caloric need, growth, or activity. A review by Foote and Marriott[34] expresses the concern that some infants might need additional nutrients. They point out that the energy density of the food should exceed that of breast milk (4.2 kJ/g or

TABLE 9.2	Nutrient Density (mg/100 kcal) of Milk During Weaning								
	WEEK								
	0	2	4	6	8	10	12	PTM*	R†
Protein	1.5	1.2	1.3	1.0	1.3	1.2	1.9	1.8	2.7
Na	24.0	17.0	20.0	13.0	24.0	25.0	46.0	25.0	53.0
Ca	38.0	30.0	33.0	21.0	30.0	26.0	38.0	34.5	140.0
Zn	0.21	0.17	0.19	0.09	0.10	0.10	0.11	3.8	0.5

*Nutrient densities of milk from women who deliver premature infants.
†Nutrient densities calculated to achieve intrauterine growth rates assuming that the caloric requirement of low-birth-weight infants is 130 kcal/kg.
PTM, Preterm milk; R, rate. From Garza C, Johnson CA, Smith E, et al. Changes in the nutrient composition of human milk during gradual weaning. Am J Clin Nutr. 1983;37:61.

0.55 to 0.80 kcal/g). They also warn that foods with high phytate levels can interfere with mineral absorption and recommend the avoidance of juices and other drinks. Giving infants solids by 4 months is associated with less positive health outcomes such as increased body fat, higher body mass index, and a greater incidence of wheezing and respiratory illness in childhood, according to Fewtrell et al.[35] Other authors report no effect of age at weaning and infant growth.[36]

Feeding Infants and Toddlers Study

In the study of nutrient intakes and food choices of 3000 infants and toddlers participating in the Feeding Infants and Toddlers Study (FITS), there were 150 participants in the Special Supplemental Nutrition Program for Women, Infants, and Children (WIC) nutrition program.[37] It was observed that infants in the WIC program were less likely to have ever been breastfed and were more likely to be taking formula.[38] The mean usual intake of nutrients exceeded adequate intakes. Mean energy intake was excessive, with little consumption of fruits and vegetables. In the entire study of 3000 infants, 76% were fully or partially breastfed at birth, dropping to 30% at 6 months and to 16% at 1 year. Average duration of breastfeeding was 5.5 months. From 4 to 6 months, more than 65% had been given solids, not all of which were nutrient dense. Sweetened juices, French fries, hot dogs, potato chips, popcorn, pizza, and candy were reported in up to 9% of infants aged 7 to 8 months old.

Other Variables

Exposure to Taste

An infant's first flavor experiences probably occur in utero. When garlic was ingested by mothers before amniocentesis or delivery, the amniotic fluid smelled of garlic.[39] The normal fetus ingests amniotic fluid in utero and thus experiences those flavors. When breastfed, the infant continues to experience those flavors as a bridging experience to solid foods.[12]

Not surprisingly, breastfed infants consume cereal prepared with their mother's milk more eagerly and in greater volume than when it is prepared with water. In a carefully controlled experiment, infants were fed the cereals by their mothers, who wore facial masks but no perfume to avoid affecting the infant's interest in the food.[39] The infant's interest was reflected in opening of the mouth sooner, fewer negative facial expressions, and greater intake. Mennella and Beauchamp[39] suggest that from the perspective of flavors, weaning means "to accustom," which actually describes what occurs with breastfeeding: the flavors in the milk accustom the infant to new flavors in the transition to solid foods. Putting mother's milk in the bland cereal is part of the bridging. Infants whose mothers have a more varied diet during pregnancy and lactation tend to adapt to solid foods more readily, according to these investigations.[40]

Weaning to a Cup

Weaning to a cup is a natural transfer because infants learn to drink from a cup by 7 to 9 months. The use of fruit juice in the cup was originally encouraged for its vitamin C content.

Fruit juice may be replacing milk, however, in the diets of young children.[41] This is a concern because milk is an important source of protein and calcium, whereas nutrients in fruit juices are limited predominantly to carbohydrates, calories, and varying amounts of vitamin C. Juices are also replacing fruit in the diet. Excessive fruit juice consumption reportedly leads to short stature and failure to thrive in some infants, chronic diarrhea in some, and obesity in others.[42] The trend often begins when fruit juice is put in a nursing bottle. The pediatrician should be alert to the exact content of the weaning foods, ensuring adequate protein, calcium, vitamins, and fiber, and to the development of feeding skills, including feeding from a cup and from a spoon.

MOTHERS' CHOICES

In practice, human mothers are often the determinants of weaning time, as is true for other species. Some mothers want to nurse for a few weeks and wean to a bottle to go to work. Other mothers wean at 3 months to be free again.[43,44] A large number of variables are associated with the duration of breastfeeding and the "reason for weaning."[17,45−47] Mothers' self-reported reasons for stopping breastfeeding include inconvenience or fatigue, concerns about milk supply, return to work or school, perception that the infant was not satisfied by breast milk, baby lost interest or weaned herself or himself, and the baby was biting, to name the most common.[47,48] To a large degree these reasons overlap with maternal reasons for "earlier than desired" cessation of breastfeeding as reported by a number of groups.[46−51] "Disrupted lactation" or lactation dysfunction as defined by Stuebe et al.[46] includes two of three "physiologic reasons" for early cessation: pain, difficulty with latch, and low milk supply. In addition to the difficulties with lactation/breastfeeding and concerns regarding the infant's or mother's health (medication use), the effort associated with breastfeeding or milk pumping plays a prominent role. There are certainly occasions when it seems (to the mother) that it is the infant who stops breastfeeding or weans herself or himself. A newer term, "baby-led weaning," first used by Gill Rapley, refers to the concept that infants as young as 6 months can play a role in their own food intake. This fits more with infant behavior in choosing the complementary foods they want, amounts of food and timing or rhythm of eating.[52−54] The important point in weaning is to make it a gradual and manageable adjustment for both mother and infant.

Currently, health goals for the United States recommend that mothers nurse exclusively for at least 6 months,[55] continuing breastfeeding while adding weaning foods until 1 year and then for as long thereafter as mother and child wish. Specific Healthy People 2020 Objectives include increasing the proportion of infants who are exclusively breastfed at 3 and 6 months and any ongoing breastfeeding at 6 and 12 months.

Historically, maternal worries about the demands of breastfeeding had a negative effect on the duration. If mothers worried about the demands of breastfeeding, they were more likely to perceive problems with scheduling breastfeeding when they returned to work. Mothers who worried about lack of family support to breastfeed were more apt to worry about the demands of breastfeeding. Those women who saw the practical advantages of breastfeeding did not perceive returning to work as presenting a problem and nursed longer. Medical illness, sore nipples, fatigue, or breast infections were less influential in weaning depending on the woman's intent and reasons for breastfeeding. In this current era of more women working outside the home and having careers; work and "scheduling life" have a larger role in most mothers' decision to wean.[7] Refer to Chapter 18 for further discussion on establishing a proper balance between work and motherly responsibilities.

Achieving Breastfeeding Goals

Stuebe[56] suggests that obstetricians are uniquely positioned to provide anticipatory guidance, support normal lactation physiologic processes, and evaluate and treat breastfeeding complications, thus enabling more women to achieve their breastfeeding goals. Ideally, health care professionals can assist and inform mothers as the mothers develop their breastfeeding goals. Beyond knowledge about the risks and benefits of breastfeeding and exposure to breastfeeding by other women throughout their lives, the mother's own beliefs, perceptions, and preferences along with those of the baby's father, the family, and their friends and community will inform the mother's choices. Mothers should be able to choose what breastfeeding support they would like and from whom to achieve their goals. Breastfeeding self-efficacy development is part of the process of learning about breastfeeding and determining one's breastfeeding goals.[57] Additional discussion about what the mother perceives as potential barriers to her breastfeeding goals can add to the mother's self-efficacy.[58]

Why Women Wean

In 2001, using the National Survey of Family Growth to analyze breastfeeding behaviors of a national probability sample of 6733 first-time mothers in the United States from 15 to 44 years of age, Taylor et al.[59] found 3267 women who breastfed. Among these women, 46%, 68%, 78%, and 85% had weaned by 3, 6, 9, and 12 months, respectively. The reason 1091 women stopped breastfeeding was because their infant was "old enough to wean." This reason was claimed by 15%, 34%, 54% and 78% at the same 3-month intervals. White and Hispanic women had similar weaning patterns. For black women who stopped because their child was "old enough to wean," greater numbers weaned sooner (22%, 46%, 68%, and 86% stopped at 3, 6, 9, and 12 months, respectively). Physical and medical problems were the next most common reasons (26.9%), followed with "job or schedule" (17.9%), and "preferred to bottle feed" (15.3%) (Table 9.3). Differences by race revealed black women stopped because they "preferred to bottle feed." Hispanic women had a few more infants who refused the breast (3.7%) compared with black women (0.5%) and white women (2.1%). In 2006 to 2007 the Infant Feeding Practices Study II (IFPS II), a mail survey supported by the

TABLE 9.3	Reasons Women Stopped Breastfeeding Their First Child (n = 3267)*							
	Total	RACE/ETHNICITY		HISPANIC VS. WHITE			BLACK VS. WHITE	
Reason	Sample (%)	Hispanic (%)	Black (%)	White (%)	Unadjusted OR (95% CI)[†]	Adjusted OR (95% CI) [†,‡]	Unadjusted OR (95% CI) [†]	Adjusted OR (95% CI) [†,‡]
Baby old enough to wean	35.7	34.7	30.4	37.0	1.00	1.00	1.00	1.00
Job/schedule	17.9	14.9	17.5	19.0	0.70 (0.52−0.94)	1.04 (0.77−1.42)	1.01 (0.70−1.47)	1.10 (0.74−1.65)
Physical/ medical problem	26.9	25.6	23.6	27.9	0.87 (0.66−1.15)	0.61 (0.44−0.85)	0.97 (0.68−1.38)	0.75 (0.52−1.08)
Preferred to bottle feed	15.3	20.2	25.8	11.8	1.62 (1.20−2.18)	1.17 (0.85−1.62)	2.80 (1.96−3.99)	2.18 (1.55−3.05)
Baby refused	2.2	3.7	0.5	2.1	1.86 (1.00−3.46)	1.86 (1.05−3.30)	0.18 (0.04−0.86)	0.16 (0.03−0.82)

*The 90 women who were still breastfeeding at the time of the interview and the 131 women who categorized their race as "other" (211 total; 10 women were in both groups) were not included in the analyses. The 25 women (0.8%) who answered "other" as a reason for not breastfeeding (including the baby's father or someone else discouraged breastfeeding, fears about breastfeeding, and others) were not included in the analyses. The reference group is women who stopped breastfeeding because the baby was "old enough to wean" (final n = 3000).
[†]NSFG sampling weights applied.
[‡]Adjusted for maternal demographics (age, race, marital status, education, poverty level).
CI, Confidence interval; NSFG, National Survey of Family Growth; OR, odds ratio.
Taylor JS, Risica RM, Cabral HJ. Why primiparous mothers do not breastfeed in the United States: a national survey. Acta Paediatr. 2003;92:1308.

Division of Nutrition of the Centers for Disease Control and Prevention (CDC), was focused on why women stop breastfeeding. In a forced answer questionnaire the statements were slightly different but the three top explanations were that the infant was not satisfied, the child was old enough to wean, and concern about nutritional issues (Table 9.4). In the first 2 months, mothers were concerned that the milk was inadequate nutritionally or there were concerns about breastfeeding. After 2 months, however, mothers' reasons for stopping breastfeeding were concerns that infants' behaviors indicated "self-weaning"—43.5% reported breast milk alone did not satisfy the infant, 47.3% reported the infant "lost interest" in nursing or "weaned herself or himself," and 31.7% reported the infant began to bite. Later, weaning took place for reported social reasons such as work or maternal freedom. When infants were approximately 1 year old, the misconception that it was the age to wean was a factor. Clearly, each of these issues could be addressed through adequate counseling.

When data were extracted from the Pregnancy Risk Assessment Monitoring System (PRAMS) from the United

TABLE 9.4 Percentage of Mothers Who Indicated That Specified Reasons Were Important in Their Decision to Stop Breastfeeding, According to Infants' Age at Weaning

| Reasons Cited as Important | INFANTS' AGE WHEN BREASTFEEDING WAS COMPLETELY STOPPED (MO) | | | | | |
	<1	1–2	3–5	6–8	≥9	Average
Lactational Factor						
My baby had trouble sucking or latching on*	51.7	27.1	11.0	2.6	1.5	19.2
My nipples were sore, cracked, or bleeding*	36.8	23.2	7.2	5.7	4.2	15.4
My breasts were overfull or engorged*	23.9	12.3	4.8	1.6	1.2	8.8
My breasts were infected or abscessed*	8.1	5.7	3.1	3.1	3.1	4.6
My breasts leaked too much*	14.1	8.0	3.8	1.6	1.9	5.9
Breastfeeding was too painful*	29.3	15.8	3.4	3.7	4.2	11.3
Psychosocial Factor						
Breastfeeding was too tiring*	19.8	17.2	11.0	7.8	5.3	12.2
Breastfeeding was too inconvenient*	20.4	22.4	18.6	12.5	4.2	15.6
I wanted to be able to leave my baby for several hours at a time*	11.2	24.1	18.2	15.6	7.3	15.3
I had too many household duties*	12.6	14.0	9.6	5.2	18	9.0
I wanted or needed someone else to feed my baby*	16.4	23.2	21.0	17.2	6.1	16.8
Someone else wanted to feed the baby*	13.5	15.5	120	5.7	3.4	10.0
I did not want to breastfeed in public*	14.9	18.6	15.1	4.7	4.6	11.6
Nutritional Factor						
Breast milk alone did not satisfy my baby*	49.0	55.6	49.1	49.5	43.5	49.5
I thought that my baby was not gaining enough weight*	23.0	18.3	11.0	14.1	8.4	15.0
A health professional said my baby was not gaining enough weight*	19.8	15.2	8.6	9.9	5.0	11.7
I had trouble getting the milk flow to start*	41.4	23.2	19.6	14.6	5.7	20.9
I didn't have enough milk*	51.7	52.2	54.0	41.8	26.0	45.5
Lifestyle Factor						
I did not like breastfeeding*	16.4	10.9	6.2	1.1	1.9	7.7
I wanted to go on a weight-loss diet*	6.6	7.2	10.3	10.9	6.5	8.3
I wanted to go back to my usual diet*	5.5	9.5	7.2	5.2	5.0	6.5
I wanted to smoke again or more than I did while breastfeeding	6.0	5.2	3.4	1.0	0.8	3.3
I wanted my body back to myself*	8.9	13.2	16.8	18.8	15.7	14.7

(Continued)

TABLE 9.4 **Percentage of Mothers Who Indicated That Specified Reasons Were Important in Their Decision to Stop Breastfeeding, According to Infants' Age at Weaning—cont'd**

Reasons Cited as Important	INFANTS' AGE WHEN BREASTFEEDING WAS COMPLETELY STOPPED (MO)					
	<1	1–2	3–5	6–8	≥9	Average
Medical Factor						
My baby became sick and could not breastfeed*	9.5	7.4	5.5	6.3	19	6.1
I was sick or had to take medicine	14.4	16.3	14.8	12.5	8.0	11.2
I was not present to feed my baby for reasons other than work	3.2	6.9	5.2	5.2	2.7	4.6
I became pregnant or wanted to become pregnant again*	1.7	3.4	3.4	6.8	12.2	5.5
Milk-Pumping Factor						
I could not, or did not want to, pump or breastfeed at work*	11.2	22.4	21.3	13.5	4.6	14.6
Pumping milk no longer seemed worth the effort that it required*	16.7	21.2	23.1	17.7	11.5	18.2
Infant's Self-Weaning Factor						
My baby began to bite*	5.2	5.7	13.4	38.5	31.7	18.9
My baby lost interest in nursing or began to wean himself or herself*	13.2	19.7	33.1	47.9	47.3	32.2
My baby was old enough that the difference between breast milk and formula no longer mattered*	5.2	11.4	16.5	26.6	28.2	17.6

*$p < 0.01$ for association between each reason and weaning age after adjustments for maternal age; marital status; parity; education; poverty; Special Supplemental Nutrition Program for Women, Infants, and Children (WIC) participation; race; and region.
From Li J, Fein SB, Chen J, et al. Why mothers stop breastfeeding: mothers' self-reported reasons for stopping during the first year. *Pediatrics.* 2008;122:S69–S76.

States to examine breastfeeding behaviors, periods of vulnerability for breastfeeding cessation, and predelivery intentions, it was clear that younger women with limited economic resources stopped early.[60] Those who planned to breastfeed were more likely to continue than those who did not plan ahead to breastfeed. Early postpartum cessation was due to physical discomforts of breastfeeding and the uncertainty about milk supply. Professional intervention early might well change these figures.

A longitudinal observational study involving appropriate controls and mothers who delivered healthy term infants at Yale New Haven Hospital and planned to take them to the clinic showed that a mother's knowledge and problems with lactation were not associated with early stopping of breastfeeding.[61] Those who lacked confidence in their success and those who thought the baby preferred formula were most likely to stop in 2 weeks. The rates of discontinuation were 27%, 37%, 70%, and 89% by 1, 2, 8, and 16 weeks, cumulatively. In this population of minority women, 91% of whom were already enrolled in WIC. The authors recommended that the focus needs to shift from increasing knowledge and problem management to enhancing a mother's confidence and correcting misconceptions about an infant's preferences. In an analysis of data from the Western Australian Pregnancy Cohort Study of 2420 women, the probability of early weaning is increased by the occurrence of stressful life events during pregnancy such as separation, divorce, financial stresses, and residential moves. This was independent of hospital care and delivery issues.[62]

Causes of Earlier Weaning

Reasons why mothers wean sooner than they had planned were analyzed from 1177 mothers over 18 years of age who responded to monthly surveys from the Infant Feeding Practices Study II (IFPS II) conducted by the US Food and Drug Administration (FDA) and the CDC.[49] Sixty percent of these mothers stopped sooner than they had planned. The major reasons given were (1) difficulties breastfeeding, (2) concern for infant nutrition and weight gain, (3) maternal illness or need to take medicine, and (4) the time and effort associated with pumping. The authors suggested continued professional intervention as a possible solution (Table 9.5).

In a subsequent study from the IFPS II that included 1334 mothers who reported a 7-day food frequency questionnaire monthly, determination was made of the exact time mothers were introducing solids. Of those in the study, 24.3% of breastfed, 52.7% of formula-fed, and 50.2% of mixed-fed infants started introducing solids before 4 months.[29] The mean age of introduction was 11.8 weeks, and 9.1% of mothers who were formula feeding started before 4 weeks. It was claimed that a doctor suggested it for 55.5% of mothers and 46.4% of mothers were told that solids would help the baby sleep. The odds of these behaviors were higher for formula-fed

TABLE 9.5   Sociodemographic Characteristics of Mothers Who Met and Did Not Meet Their Intention for Breastfeeding Duration

Characteristic	Overall (*N* = 1177)	Did Not Meet Intentions (*n* = 708)	Met Intentions (*n* = 471)	*p*
Age (yr)				0.18
18–24	21.6	23.4	18.9	
25–29	34.0	34.4	33.3	
30–34	28.9	27.8	30.6	
≥ 35	15.6	14.5	17.2	
Marital status				0.0000
Married	79.4	76.1	84.3	
Not married	20.7	23.9	15.7	
Parity				0.001
Primiparous	32.4	64.0	73.0	
Multiparous	67.6	36.0	27.0	
Education				0.0001
High school or less	18.2	19.8	15.7	
Some college	40.7	44.3	35.2	
College graduate	41.1	35.8	49.0	
Income (% of poverty)				0.14
<185	38.2	39.0	37.2	
185–350	34.1	35.4	32.1	
≥350	27.7	25.6	30.8	
WIC participant				0.003
No	63.0	59.5	68.2	
Yes	37.0	40.5	31.9	
Race				0.10
White	84.8	86.4	82.4	
Black	4.0	3.4	4.9	
Hispanic	7.1	5.8	8.9	
Other	4.2	4.4	3.8	
Prenatal breastfeeding intention: mean ± SD no. of months	8.3 ± 4.0	8.4 ± 4.1	8.1 ± 3.7	0.16

Data are presented as % of mean ± SD. *p* value was determined by using the χ^2 test for all control variables except prenatal breastfeeding intention, which was determined by using a *t* test. *SD*, Standard deviation; *WIC*, Special Supplemental Nutrition Program for Women, Infants, and Children.

From Odom EC, Li R, Scanlon KS, et al. Reasons for earlier than desired cessation of breastfeeding. *Pediatrics.* 2013;131:e726–e732, Table 9.1.

infants (Table 9.6). Breastfeeding mothers tend to feel more satisfied with the infant feeding experience.

Undesired Weaning

"Undesired" early weaning emphasizes that women do set breastfeeding goals and then have to contend with numerous factors and barriers that could interfere with achieving those goals (Table 9.7). In a study noted previously, by Stuebe et al.,[46] 2335 women who initiated breastfeeding were assessed by questionnaire looking for "lactation dysfunction" as the primary cause of early weaning. Lactation dysfunction included the physiologic problems associated with lactation: pain, difficulty with latch, and low milk supply. The study documented 1 in 8 mothers (12/100 women, 95% confidence

TABLE 9.6 Percentage of Infants First Introduced to Solid Food by Age and Milk Feeding at Time of Introduction

	AGE						
	0–6 Weeks (1 month)	7–11 Weeks (2 months)	12–16 Weeks (3 months)	17–20 Weeks (4 months)	21–25 Weeks (5 months)	≥26 Weeks (5 months)	Mean Age at Introduction, wk (SD)
n	104	120	315	457	243	95	1334
Total	7.8	9.0	23.6	34.3	18.2	7.1	17.7 (6.3)
Milk Feeding Type at Time of Solid Food Introduction							
Breast milk	4.5	2.7	17.1	36.1	27.8	11.8	19.9 (5.8)
Formula	11.2	13.5	28.0	34.0	9.3	3.9	15.8 (6.2)*
Mixed	8.3	13.3	28.6	31.2	15.0	3.7	16.6 (5.9)*

SD, standard deviation.

*$p < 0.05$ for association between type of milk feeding and mean age at solid food introduction (compared with breast milk).

From Clayton HB, Li R, Perrine CG, et al. Prevalence and reasons for introducing infants early to solid foods: variations by milk feeding type. *Pediatrics*. 2013;131:e1108–e1114, Table 10.2.

TABLE 9.7 Main Reasons for Premature Weaning

Reason	N	%
Not enough, inadequate, or "weak" milk	307	30.9
Child refused breast	177	17.8
Illness of child	159	16.0
Mother needed to go to work	149	15.0
Correct age for bottle-feeding	139	14.0
Other reasons	64	6.3
Total	995	100.0

From Gunn TR. The incidence of breastfeeding and the reasons for weaning. *NZ Med J*. 1984;97:360.

interval [CI] 11, 13) who self-reported early, undesired weaning attributed to physiologic difficulties, "disrupted lactation." The prevalence of disrupted lactation was higher among young, unmarried, nonprofessional women without a college degree. Obesity and symptoms of maternal depression were associated with increased odds of disrupted lactation, independent of other potential confounders. The study design did not facilitate the detection of other reported barriers to achieving breastfeeding goals; for example, poor maternity care practices, uneven training for health professionals, lack of access to postpartum support and limited maternity leave. Although the authors allowed that there could be other sociodemographic factors contributing to the difficulties with lactation beyond the physiologic ones identified, this study underscores the need for ready access to well-informed, high-quality lactation support. In a maternity survey from England, 3840 women reported the timing of their

breastfeeding cessation.[63] Thirteen percent (n = 486) had stopped breastfeeding by 10 days postpartum and of the 3354 women who continued beyond 10 days 17% of those had stopped by 6 weeks. This questionnaire study focused on "breastfeeding support" and found in multivariate analysis that the need for help and advice in breastfeeding had an increased odds ratio of cessation at 10 days or 6 weeks. Additionally, they found a need for both non–health professional breastfeeding support (peers or volunteers) and lactation specialist support (breastfeeding clinics) among the women who stopped breastfeeding by 6 weeks postpartum.

A systematic review from 2009 found strong evidence for six determinants of early weaning: younger maternal age, less maternal education, low socioeconomic status, maternal smoking, lack of information on breastfeeding, and less access to professional lactation advice.[64] A more recent systematic review from 2019 identified the two most common reasons for early breastfeeding cessation as perceived inadequate milk supply and maternal breast or nipple pain.[50]

Obviously, the factors that could interfere with achieving individual and community-wide breastfeeding goals are multiple and varied. Despite the need for ongoing research, the CDC's "Guide to Strategies to Support Breastfeeding Mothers and Babies" is an excellent resource for practical and effective interventions collected from the literature.[65]

WEANING PROCESS

Gradually replacing one feeding at a time with solids or liquids in a bottle or cup, depending on an infant's age and stage of development, is usually preferable.[66,67] After the adjustment has been made to one substitute feeding, a second feeding is replaced with a substitute, usually at the opposite time of day. This process is continued until only the morning and night feedings remain. Then these two are gradually stopped. The morning and night feedings can be maintained for some months, and often an infant is nursed well beyond the second year, especially at these times. Mothers who wish to wean partially as early as 3 months may continue the morning and night nursing. This schedule is especially suited to the working mother. The decline in lactation and the regression of the mammary gland occur slowly with gradual weaning.

When an infant is fully breastfeeding and solids are initiated, a feeding of solids is given during the day and breastfeeding continues on demand. As solids are increased and a three-meals-per-day schedule is reached, breastfeeding continues on demand, although nursing opportunities may be fewer or briefer. No nursing need be intentionally omitted in this scheme, although it is important to give the scheduled solids before breastfeeding the infant.

Composition of Milk With Abrupt Weaning

Study of the composition of milk during abrupt weaning revealed that the secretory capability of the mammary gland of women changed dramatically after complete cessation of breastfeeding but the involuting gland remained partially functional for approximately 45 days.[68] After termination that occurred in 1 day, sample collections were attempted for each breast by manual expression at the same time on days 1, 2, 4, 8, 16, 21, 31, 42, and 45. The concentrations of lactose and potassium decreased, whereas those of sodium, chloride, fat, and total protein increased progressively over 42 days. The milk became notably salty, but the infants continued to drink the salty fluid. The increase in protein was related to increases in the concentrations of lactoferrin, immunoglobulin A (IgA), IgG, IgM, albumin, lactalbumin, and casein. Concentrations from each breast were similar throughout.

The involution in other species is rapid. For example, complete reabsorption occurs in 7 days in cows. The threshold dose of oxytocin required to elicit milk ejection increased progressively for at least 30 days after termination of breastfeeding. It is thought that a psychological nursing stimulus contributes to this effect in humans because they continue contact with their infants, whereas other species are separated. Experimental animals given oxytocin after weaning also show a delay in involution.

Weaning Ages and Techniques

Weaning ages and techniques in a sample of American women who practiced extended breastfeeding were reported by Sugarman and Kendall-Tackett.[69] Women were recruited from La Leche League meetings in the area and nationally, using survey forms (closed-end, self-administered, 96-item questionnaires). Based on 134 mothers and 211 children, the weaning age ranged from 1 month to 7 years 4 months. For those who weaned three children, as well as the entire sample, the tendency was to nurse the youngest child for the longest period, perhaps because it was not supplanted by a sibling.

Reasons for weaning were predominantly child-led for approximately 60% of children, but weaning was the mother's decision in up to 15.8% in the youngest child (Tables 9.8 and 9.9). Those who were still nursing responded to the question,

TABLE 9.8 Reasons for Weaning and Types of Methods

	Child A* (*n* = 25)	Child B* (*n* = 125)	Child C* (*n* = 69)
Reasons for Weaning (%)			
Lack of information	5.3	4.2	8.7
Lack of support or opposition	2.6	4.2	8.7
Next pregnancy affected taste or supply of milk	7.9	14.3	8.7
Next pregnancy affected mother's motivation	5.3	21.8	24.6
Illness or separation from child	5.3	5.9	11.6
Child-led, happened naturally	63.2	57.1	52.2
Mother's decision that child was ready	15.0	13.4	10.1
Mother's decision based on family circumstance	7.9	5.0	4.3
Other	0.0	5.9	1.4
How Weaning Was Accomplished (Mean %)			
Sudden	12.8	7.6	8.8
Gradual	56.4	60.2	45.6
Child-led	53.3	56.7	54.1
Mother deliberately weaned	2.6	11.0	13.2
Mother encouraged weaning by talking to child	23.1	31.4	20.6
Substituted thumb, pacifier	2.6	3.4	1.5
Other	1.7	1.8	1.7
Number of reasons (mean)	1.8	1.8	1.7

*A, B, and C represent three consecutive children in a family, child A being the youngest and C the oldest of the three children.
From Sugarman M, Kendall-Tackett KA. Weaning ages in a sample of American women who practice extended breast feeding. *Clin Pediatr* 1995;34:642.

"Have you thought about weaning this child?" predominantly with a "no" (see Table 9.9).

A normal, well-adjusted mother may experience some depression and sadness at the reality of the last feeding.[70] It may be difficult to deal with this experience. It is important to recognize this as a physiologic phenomenon and as an

TABLE 9.9   Reasons for Weaning or Not Weaning (Have You Thought About Weaning This Child?)

Response	Frequency (%)
No, weaning should be child-led	75.9
No, enjoy the nursing relationship	72.3
Yes, for a specific reason (pregnancy, returning to work)	4.8
Yes, child is ready/child is biting	7.8
Yes, because of pressure	3.6
Yes, child is nursing too frequently for age	3.6

From Sugarman M, Kendall-Tackett KA. Weaning ages in a sample of American women who practice extended breastfeeding. *Clin Pediatr.* 1995;34:642.

emotional one. If a mother is forced by circumstances beyond her control to wean early, she may need understanding and encouragement to cope with the disappointment. If she had pressure from friends or relatives to breastfeed, she may need to face what she considers failure and recognize that one can bottle feed and still mother very well.

Historically, weaning has varied from strict to permissive schedules depending on cultural norms.[5] Rigid feeding schedules were associated with early weaning.[71] Weaning has varied from early strict denial of breast milk to slow and gentle withdrawal of breastfeeding. In the twentieth century, the age considered proper in many societies for weaning gradually shortened from 2 or 3 or 4 years of age to as soon as 6 to 8 months of age or younger. Public opinion has overlooked an infant's needs in favor of what are considered the mother's rights. It is not necessary to have a specific plan for weaning in the early weeks of nursing unless constraints on the mother's time are an issue. Weaning should be done with an infant's needs as a guide.[6] If an infant younger than 1 year of age rejects the breast, it is unusual but not abnormal and should not be considered by the mother as a personal rejection. Some bottle-fed infants throw down the bottle at 9 months as well.

Studies of Weaning Practices

Studies of weaning practices are few. There is no evidence-based data on the "how to" wean relative to the introduction of complementary foods and the gradual decrease in intake of breast milk. There are studies on the timing of introduction of complementary foods, factors influencing that decision, and various growth and nutritional outcomes based on the age of introduction. In a study from the United States with 1482 infants 6 to 36 months of age in the National Health and Nutrition Examination Survey (2009 to 2014), 16.3% initiated complementary foods at younger than 4 months, 38.3% between 4 and less than 6 months, 32.5% between 6 and less than 7 months, and 12.9.% at 7 months of age and older.

Infants who never breastfed or stopped breastfeeding before 4 months of age were more likely to be introduced to complementary foods than in children who breastfed longer than 4 months.[72] In a study from two European countries (Poland and Austria) of 5815 children 12 to 36 months of age, complementary foods were initiated before 4 months in 3% of children, at 4 to 6 months in 65%, and after 6 months in 32.1% of infants.[73] No description of "how to" was included. Data from 5 countries (Belgium, Germany, Italy, Poland, and Spain) show that approximately 25% of children began complementary foods before 4 months of age and over 90% of infants had eaten solid food by 6 months of age. The weaning age in this study was lower for formula-fed infants compared with breastfed infants at 4 (37.2% vs. 17.2%) and at 6 months (96.2% vs. 87.1%). A systematic review concerning the age of introduction of complementary foods for healthy full-term infants showed an equal number of studies (13 and 13) supporting beginning complementary foods before 6 months and after 6 months based on growth and nutritional parameters and another seven studies that supported the initiation of complementary foods at 4 to 6 months. They also noted some studies that identified "subgroups" within the studies who "may require" complementary feeding before 6 months to avoid growth or nutritional deficiencies (caloric intake, iron deficiency, zinc deficiency). They concluded that it may not be appropriate to make broad recommendations for infant feeding practices with the variation in maternal nutritional status and nutritional quality of traditional or common complementary foods.[19]

Given the importance of this period of life for the infant (growth, development, nutrition, maturation of the gastrointestinal system, and immunologic functionality), the implications for the future ("healthy eating behaviors," microbiome, long-term health status [weight/obesity, cardiovascular, diabetes, allergy, etc.]), and the establishment of familial and ethnic social eating patterns, weaning is an important topic for families and health care professionals.[74]

Several summaries from health organizations provide some practical specifics regarding weaning and introduction of complementary foods. The National Institute of Child Health and Human Development published a summary of important considerations for maternal nutrition and optimal infant feeding practices.[75] The WHO has a number of appropriate publications including, "Infant and Young Child Feeding," a model chapter for textbooks that includes practical information and guidance on the quality, frequency, and amount of food to offer children 6 to 23 months of age who are breastfed on demand, appropriate foods for complementary feeding, "principles" for complementary feeding of the breastfed child, and a food intake reference tool for children 6 to 23 months of age.[76] The Italian Society of Gastroenterology, Hepatology and Pediatric Nutrition and the Italian Society of Allergology and Pediatric Immunology published their recommendations on complementary feeding for healthy, full-term infants.[77] They discuss important issues in weaning and complementary foods (allergy, chronic disease, micronutrients and macronutrients, and baby-led weaning) but do not address a practical "how to." Campoy et al.[78]

address the when, what, and why of complementary feeding in developed countries. Here again the practicalities of how are not directly addressed, but they do elaborate on the important physiologic and neurologic changes that should occur to establish the optimal time to begin complementary feeding for individual children. They outline and discuss the current recommendations for complementary food nutrient requirements. They discuss issues around timing, baby-led weaning, introduction of potentially allergenic foods (peanuts, gluten, cow's milk), and introduction of pureed, lumpy, and solid foods.

Separately the concern regarding commercially prepared infant foods compared with homemade complementary foods has not been adequately addressed in randomized clinical trials. However, there is evidence that homemade or commercial foods can be selected/prepared for lower sugar and salt content[79] and commercially prepared foods do affect individual taste and food preferences and decreased fruit and vegetable intake in infancy.[80]

Probably the closest outline of "how to" for complementary feeding and weaning was produced by K.G. Dewey and the Pan American Health Organization in Guiding Principles for Complementary Feeding of the Breastfed Child[26] (Box 9.1).

Associations With Longer Breastfeeding

In most studies, those who breastfeed longer tend to be older than 25 years, well-educated, middle class, self-educated about lactation, and enjoy breastfeeding.[81] Worldwide the duration of breastfeeding is longer, between 2 and 4 years in length.

The problem of recall bias when reporting breastfeeding duration was investigated by Huttly et al.,[82] who compared responses given at 11, 23, and 47 months postpartum by the mothers of 1000 children; 24% misclassified weaning time at 23 months and 30% at 4 years. Those in the better educated, higher socioeconomic group were more apt to report longer breastfeeding.

The mean monthly bias introduced was to reduce breastfeeding by 2 months. In worldwide epidemiologic studies, the interruption of breastfeeding because of pregnancy may play a significant role in the timing of weaning. In Third World countries, infant death also lowers the duration of breastfeeding inversely to the mother's education; that is, the less educated the mother, the greater the risk for infant death from infection and accident.

INFANT-INITIATED WEANING

Infant-initiated weaning in the first year of life was investigated by Clarke and Harmon,[83] who studied 50 healthy breastfed infants who were totally weaned; 46% of the group of infants initiated the weaning. This is often mistakenly referred to as *self-weaning* because there is always an infant and mother involved in the transition. The onset was usually between 5 and 9 months of age, with a median age of 6 months. Mothers described the behavior as an increased interest in exploring the environment and in other foods and a decreased interest in breastfeeding.

The duration of infant-initiated weaning is approximately 1 month and is an interactive process that requires "at a minimum maternal complicity." It can lead to relatively easy mutual weaning. It can usually be reversed or delayed, however, by a mother's efforts to continue breastfeeding.

Refusal to Breastfeed: "Nursing Strike"

Sudden onset of refusal to nurse can occur at any time and often is taken by the mother as a personal rejection, who promptly follows through by weaning completely.[48]

Often these mothers consider the refusal to mean that they do not have enough milk or that something is wrong with their milk. This behavior has been called *nursing strike* and has been noted to be temporary.[84] The various causes associated with this abrupt behavior include the following:

- Onset of menses in the mother
- Dietary indiscretion by the mother
- Change in maternal soap, perfume, or deodorant
- Stress in the mother
- Earache or nasal obstruction in the infant
- Teething
- Episode of biting with startle and pain reaction by the mother

If a reason is identified that is possibly associated and can be changed, nursing should resume. It may take extra effort to reestablish the relationship. Suggestions that may be made to the mother include the following:

- Make feeding special and quiet, with no distractions and no other people in the room.
- Increase amount of cuddling, stroking, and soothing the baby. Walk with the infant cradled in the arms or an infant sling.
- Offer the breast when the infant is sleepy.
- Do not starve the child into submission.
- If simple remedial steps do not result in a return to nursing, the physician should see the child to rule out otitis media, fever, infection, thrush, and so on.
- If biting was the associated event, keep finger ready to break suction should it occur again to avoid startling the infant.

Baby-Led Weaning

Baby-led weaning (BLW), as a phrase, was first coined by Gill Rapley in 2008.[52] It is more applicable to the introduction of solid foods or complementary feeding and refers to the belief that infants as young as 6 months of age can participate in choices related to what foods and the amounts of food the infant eats, when they eat, and the "rhythm" or pattern of eating. Dogan et al.[85] refer to baby-led complementary feeding in a randomized controlled trial ($n = 280$ 5- to 6-month-old infants) comparing "traditional spoon feeding" with BLW in which infants were given a "choice" in foods eaten versus a caregiver choosing the food and feeding by spoon. The authors found no difference in the risk for iron deficiency, reported episodes of choking, or growth in the two groups.[85]

There are several literature reviews that offer limited comparable studies or data.[53] D'Auria et al.[86] provide a nice description of studies included in their review and outline some notable unresolved issues from the literature (standardized definition of BLW and recommended safe practices, accurate quantification of energy and nutrient intake to compare with growth or biomarkers of nutritional status, and short- and long-term outcomes).[86]

EMERGENCY WEANING

Occasionally, sudden weaning is necessary because of severe illness in the mother or some prolonged separation of mother and infant. Sudden illness in the infant does not require weaning, and, in fact, weaning is contraindicated. This is difficult for both. After abrupt weaning the mammary glands remain partially functional for more than a month.

Changes in the composition of the mammary secretion of women after abrupt termination of breastfeeding have been investigated in seven women before and after termination. The concentrations of lactose and potassium decreased, whereas sodium, chloride, fat, and total protein increased progressively for 42 days.[68] The increase in protein represents an increase in the concentration of lactoferrin, IgA, IgG, IgM, albumin, α-lactalbumin, and casein. This represents a notable change in secretion with abrupt weaning compared with a couple of small studies of breast milk composition during "natural" weaning. Neville et al.[87] described changes in breast milk concentrations of protein, lactose, chloride, and sodium when during weaning the milk volume declined to below 400 mL/day. Garza et al.[81] reported on six exclusively breastfeeding women enrolled to study gradual weaning at approximately 5 to 7 months postpartum. Breast milk preweaning was compared with breast milk obtained at 2-week intervals (2 to 12 weeks) after weaning was initiated. At 12 weeks, protein (142%), sodium (220%), and iron (172%) concentrations had increased compared with baseline values.[81] Zinc fell to 58% of the baseline value, calcium concentration did not change at 12 weeks after weaning, and fat composition had increased over the 10 weeks but was back at baseline at 12 weeks.[81]

Despite these variable changes in breast milk during weaning in these studies, there were no reports of infants having difficulty during the weaning period or after.

Depending on an infant's age, mother's illness, the reason for separation, and the current feeding plan, a surrogate mother/adult may need to provide some feedings by bottle, cup, or spoon to facilitate a smooth transition. Maintenance of lactation and safely saving available breast milk is essential in this period until it is clear the situation warrants actual weaning from breastfeeding and breast milk. In some cases, an older infant (> 6 months) may take only solids and refuse other liquids for days. Again, depending on the situation, it may be appropriate to facilitate relactation when the period of separation is over.

MILK FEVER

The mother may experience "milk fever" at any time in abrupt weaning. The mother in the meantime may have considerable discomfort. The degree of engorgement may be significant if weaning occurs at a time of high milk production. This illness is characterized by fever, chills, and malaise, resembling a flu-like syndrome. It is thought to be caused by the sudden reabsorption of milk products into the system. Milk fever usually lasts 3 to 4 days and should not be confused with other more serious illnesses.

The hormonal change resulting from sudden weaning early in lactation is more distinct and likely to occur because the prolactin levels from suckling are higher immediately postpartum (see Chapter 3). Prolactin has been associated with a feeling of well-being; thus its decrease may be associated with relative depression. Patients with psychiatric disorders have been observed to cope postpartum until they wean the infant from the breast. It is important to provide an adequate social and medical support system during weaning for the mother who is prone to depression or psychiatric problems. Maternal suicide and injury to the infant by the mother have been reported in such a scenario.

GROWTH AND WEANING

Are Growth Parameters and Illness Influenced by Weaning?

Most current writings on weaning refer to the problems in underdeveloped countries when infants are weaned early to overdiluted cow milk or to artificial formulas that do not contain the antiinfective properties of human milk for human infants. "Weanling diarrhea" is a clinical syndrome (different causes: infectious, contaminated water, improper dilution of formula, etc.) associated with weaning from the breast in the past.

Diarrheas contribute to the malnutrition seen in underdeveloped countries because of the resultant lack of appetite and increased metabolic losses. In resource-poor countries, morbidity and mortality rates in infancy rise sharply at the time of weaning from human milk because of the occurrence of infections. Malnutrition is also a major threat to the weanling in the developing world. Rickets, iron deficiency, and protein energy malnutrition are the three major nutritional threats after weaning. Second to these are the risks for zinc deficiency and allergy, which affect a wider group of children. If weaning is temporally associated with diarrhea, infection, protein energy malnutrition, rickets, iron deficiency, or zinc deficiency, it is more likely to be associated with poor growth or failure to thrive. In well-nourished mothers and their infants, diarrhea does not occur from controlled gradual weaning unless the infant has a cow milk allergy, metabolic disorder, or some other illness.

The current recommendations for exclusive breastfeeding through 6 months of age with introduction of complementary foods in an infant's diet at 6 months of age by the WHO/UNICEF are based on studies that support that there is ongoing uninterrupted weight, height, and head circumference growth. A systematic review and analysis by Vail et al.[36] reported that weaning between 3 and 6 months of age had "neutral effects" on infant growth in resource-rich countries. They recommend study of other health outcomes for the infant and mother to further guide recommendations about the optimal age at weaning.

Data from over 1600 infants from five prospective randomized trials completed in the United Kingdom were used to determine the influence of weaning at younger than 12 weeks versus after 12 weeks of age on growth and health outcomes (diarrhea, vomiting, chest infections, atopy, and sleep) up to 18 months of age. The infants included term appropriate gestational age (AGA), term small for gestational age (SGA), and preterm infants. Early weaned infants were larger at 12 weeks, but the growth trajectories of the two groups (weaning ≤ 12 weeks vs. >12 weeks) were equal at 18 months. Health outcomes were not different in those weaned before and after 12 weeks.[88]

CHANGES IN MILK COMPOSITION DURING GRADUAL WEANING

Changes in the nutrient composition of human milk during gradual weaning were studied by Garza et al.[81] in six fully lactating women recruited at 5 to 7 months postpartum (see Table 9.2). The weaning consisted of decreasing the frequency and duration of breastfeeding by one-third each month for a period of 3 months. Milk was collected at 2-week intervals. Volume decreased to 67%, 40%, and 20% of baseline each month. The concentrations of protein and sodium were increased to 142% and 220% of baseline, respectively, by the twelfth week of weaning. Changes in fat composition were linear through the tenth week but at the twelfth week were similar to baseline. Iron was increased 172%, calcium was unchanged, and zinc fell to 58%. Similar observations have been made in bovine milk. Milk produced during either rapid or gradual weaning is characterized by a decreasing concentration of lactose. Fat accounts for an increasing percentage of calories (up 80%), and protein remains stable at 6% of calories.

The immunologic components in human milk were also measured, and the concentrations of certain components of the immunologic system are maintained during gradual weaning.[89] The effect of gradual weaning differs from that of abrupt weaning, in which the concentrations of all components rise dramatically. Measurements at 4, 8, and 12 weeks showed a decrease in the milk volume of 67%, 40%, and 20% as the levels of IgA and secretory IgA rose slightly. Lysozyme and lactoferrin rose slightly. The total intake of protective factors is stable temporarily (increased concentration in spite of decreased volume).

Lipase activities in human milk during weaning were studied by Freed et al.[90] Bile salt–stimulated lipase slowly decreased throughout weaning, whereas lipoprotein lipase became substantially lower or absent compared with colostrum. Lipase activity continues but decreases with the decrease in milk volume.

The caloric needs for infants have been overestimated in the past. Continued growth occurs on lower volumes of human milk than formula, with breastfed infants refusing additional milk even when a woman increases her volume by pumping.[91] The energy requirement is 115 kcal/kg per day in the first 2 months of life, after which requirements decline rapidly, reaching a low of 85 kcal/kg per day at 6 months. Between 6 and 12 months of age, requirements gradually increase with increased activity to 100 kcal/kg per day. These figures are a radical departure from those recommended in the past. Most studies of energy intakes show, at all ages, that boys have greater intake and greater rates of growth than girls and are usually weaned sooner.[92] Beyond caloric needs, illness (frequent, recurrent infections) and social deprivation can adversely affect infant and child growth. In one example study, of 819 extremely poor Ethiopian children, 325 (39.7%) were stunted, 135 (16.5%) were underweight, and 27 (3.3%) were wasted. The results demonstrated that stunting and being underweight were negatively associated with developmental skills. Even considering the effects of stunting and being underweight on the developmental outcomes, it was noted that limited play activities, limited child-to-child interactions, and mother–child relationships negatively affected growth and development.[93]

PHYSICIAN'S ROLE IN WEANING

A physician's responsibility in weaning is to advise the mother concerning the initiation of the appropriate solid foods, which probably should begin at 6 months of age and usually not before. Introduction of a cup as a developmental step should usually begin by 7 months. Eating finger foods and learning self-feeding are the next steps for the child.

None of the previously mentioned factors means termination of breastfeeding, but rather the gradual developmental progression of feeding. Breastfeeding continues "on demand." As other foods are introduced and feeding begins to cluster into three meals and some "snacks," breastfeedings will be decreased eventually to two or three per day in the second year.

The nourishment value is not a key issue of continued nursing after 1 year if other foods are adequate, although very valuable nutrition and immunoprotection continue to be provided. A physician's role is to ensure adequate nutrition and to be available for advice for as long as breastfeeding continues.

No detriment to continued or extended nursing is known, and there is some indication that nursing a few times per day or during times of stress is beneficial to the mother–infant relationship when the child is older than 1 year of age. The objections raised to extended breastfeeding are usually based on custom or personal taste. It is important for a clinician to avoid judgmental counseling based only on personal biases. Lay publications on the subject may help guide a mother who is nursing a toddler.[94]

A physician may need to help the mother work through her own feelings about nursing her infant beyond the first year. Many women have been overwhelmed by friendly advice from lay experts about infants who nurse for several years. Beyond a year, weaning is rarely child initiated until age 4. The child may not lose interest, so the final steps in termination may require maternal intervention if weaning is desired sooner. A mother is not a poor parent if she begins to feel resentful toward nursing. Planning appropriate alternatives to breastfeeding sessions that are to be eliminated is helpful in turning a child's attention toward the new event instead of toward the loss of an old and cherished one, feeding at the breast. A mother may need to be helped to see how to avoid situations that easily predispose to nursing. She needs to know that it is acceptable to set some rules and to have some limitations and control over the breastfeeding.

If the mother becomes pregnant, she should decide when she wants to wean or whether she will continue to nurse through pregnancy and then tandem-nurse the new baby (see Chapter 21). For the child, it is important to avoid abrupt weaning or weaning to make room for the new baby, who will now take the child's place. Weaning well before delivery is usually less traumatic for the child than at delivery time. At delivery, however, a new infant is fed first to ensure that the newborn receives adequate colostrum.

UNDERSTANDING THE REASONS TO WEAN

The motivation to wean an infant may be multifactorial for a mother and family. It may be suggested by the father, grandmother, or members of the mother's social circle. The physician should be aware of and understand the multiple possible reasons but should not initiate a plan to wean except for medical reasons. The physician may initiate discussion about it to ensure the mother has given weaning some thought and has her own plan, which hopefully is compatible with her breastfeeding goals.

Reasons for weaning have been analyzed by a number of investigators. Factor analysis of a longitudinal database was done by Kirkland and Fein.[95] Mother's concerns about her milk supply, wanting to leave the infant, and wanting someone else to feed the infant were the major reasons for weaning in this group who weaned between 6 to 12 months postpartum. Concern about the appropriate age for breastfeeding cessation was a prominent concern toward the later months. Parents may find nursing an older baby or a toddler distasteful. Mothers are encouraged to anticipate and plan for weaning; it can be gradual, taking advantage of developmental progress and new interests of the toddler. It is wise to avoid associating sleeping with a feeding as the time to wean approaches because it may be more difficult to make the break. The father can play a vital role in nonnutritive cuddling, beginning from birth, and can be especially helpful in easing an infant through weaning, particularly when night feedings have become the custom. Not all parents perceive weaning, night feedings, and taking an infant to the parents' bed in the same light. Reasons given why women in Dunedin, New Zealand, elected to wean their infants early included concern about their milk supply and other maternal problems. One of the most significant factors in lactation termination in that study was mismanagement of breastfeeding by health professionals.[96] A similar study in Sweden reported that 66% of the mothers weaned because they thought their milk was drying up. Additional reasons given included anxiety of all kinds, lack of motivation, stress, tiredness, and work outside the home.[97]

A primary cause of failing milk supply reported by most investigators is inadequate help or instructions about milk production from medical personnel. In a study of 700 mother–baby dyads, Howard et al.[98] showed a clear relationship to early weaning, decreased exclusive breastfeeding, and the early introduction of a pacifier. Therefore understanding the various possible reasons for weaning and the clear need for guidance and support regarding how to breastfeed with "problems" and how to manage milk supply should motivate physicians and health care professionals to be knowledgeable and competent in problem solving these issues that lead to early weaning.

Concerns Regarding Co-Sleeping or Bedsharing While Breastfeeding

Questions or concerns around sudden infant death syndrome (SIDS) and co-sleeping or bedsharing should not be a reason for weaning. The AAP Committee on Sudden Infant Death Syndrome (SIDS) has banned co-sleeping. Not all physicians view these matters equally, but they should avoid imposing personal views on patients and share the AAP SIDS statement.[99] The Academy of Breastfeeding Medicine (ABM) has a revised version of their Protocol #6 Bedsharing and Breastfeeding, 2019.[100] ABM emphasizes that current evidence does not document that bedsharing by breastfeeding infants causes SIDS without the presence of other risk factors or a hazardous situation. Physicians should be able to make a balanced presentation of the available information about the risks and benefits of bedsharing and the issues of separate sleep and its effect on breastfeeding relative to weaning and duration of breastfeeding. The mother's knowledge, beliefs, preferences, and living/family situation should be included in this nonjudgmental open discussion. The ABM offers risk minimization strategies for families in which bedsharing is a high risk, including promotion and support of breastfeeding, referral of family members for smoking cessation and alcohol or drug treatment, discussion of specific high-risk situations (sofa-sharing, chair sleeping, smoke exposure of the infant, infant sleeping next to an impaired adult), and safe sleeping alternatives, suggesting sidecars or in-bed devices and recommending room-sharing if and when bedsharing cannot be safely done in the home. Safe sleeping environment and co-sleeping practices are discussed in detail in Chapter 7 (Practical Management of the Mother-Infant Nursing Couple).

Other Common Reasons for Weaning

Regarding weaning in resource-poor countries, the decision was thought to be made on the basis of traditional beliefs, nutritional status of the child, maternal beliefs and preferences, or reasons similar to those reported in resource-rich countries.[19,63,69,72–74] When the reasons for termination of breastfeeding were studied in over 1600 children in West Africa, however, illness in the child, a new pregnancy, and illness in the mother were found to be the most common precipitating events early on compared with children weaned because they were "healthy" or "old enough."[101] Martines et al.[102] reported on reasons for early termination of breast-feeding in urban poor in Brazil, and mothers' concerns about infant growth and that their breast milk was inadequate were the two most common reasons reported by mothers. A report from China detailed that the reasons that 180 mothers stopped breastfeeding before their infants were 6 months old were insufficient milk supply, medical reasons, lactational factors (breast pain, mastitis), and return to work.[103] Physicians should be aware and open to the numerous reasons women report for early cessation of breastfeeding and be aware of the mother's and her family's culture and background to counsel mothers appropriately.

CLOSET NURSING

A physician should be fully informed about the physiologic and psychological aspects of breastfeeding. A trusted physician communicates well with patients and is kept informed by the parents. Unfortunately, many mothers are driven to "closet nursing" by insensitive, uninformed relatives and friends and even health care providers. Closet nursing is nursing privately at home in secret. The practice propagates ignorance about breastfeeding duration and influences not only other mothers but also physicians who are unaware and custody court judges who are led to think extended nursing is abnormal. Worldwide, normal, healthy children are breastfed until they are 2 to 4 years old. The benefits of human milk continue. Research documents health protection and improved development for at least 2 years. It has not been evaluated beyond that except for the positive emotional and bonding experience associated with long-term nursing.[68,88,104]

Because breastfeeding surveys are not carried out much beyond a child reaching 1 year old, data are scarce. Dettwyler[5] set up a voluntary survey of children who had been breastfed more than 3 years, amassing 1280 children in 5 years between 1995 and 2000. The average age of weaning in this special group was 4.24 years (range 3 to 9.17 years).[5] Half of the children were weaned between 3 and 4 years. Child-led weaning occurred at 4.39 years and mother-led weaning at 3.83 years. Those who voluntarily participated were middle to upper class women who worked outside the home, were highly educated, and were of European-American ethnicity. Two thirds of the mothers became pregnant while nursing and then tandem nursed the two. The average length of tandem nursing was 1.62 years.

Although not necessarily common in the United States, worldwide, breastfeeding a child more than 2 years is in no way unusual or unexpected.

WORKING MOTHERS AND WEANING

Some breastfeeding mothers choose to return to work. Whether the reason is money, career, or personal satisfaction is not relevant to management. It takes tremendous commitment to work and breastfeed, but it can be done, it has been done, and it will be done. Although an early return to work may be driven by necessity, legislated and paid maternity leave is a factor that is contributing to breastfeeding moms returning to work outside the home.[105-107] Legislated breastfeeding accommodations in the workplace is a separate issue that is facilitating the mother's adjustment to returning to work and her likelihood of continuing breastfeeding. Many resources are now available for mothers and for businesses to accommodate, facilitate, and support breastfeeding in the workplace. (See Chapter 18.)

Usually the biggest problem a mother faces is coping with people who do not understand why she bothers or why she "needs" to breastfeed or pump and save breast milk while at work. An understanding physician who provides the reassurance and support necessary to manage is a great asset. A mother may go home for a feeding in the middle of the day, pump milk to leave for the infant to have from a bottle, or give a substitute bottle. Chapter 22 offers suggestions for collecting milk.

Some infants quickly learn the mother's schedule and will sleep while she is away and feed more frequently during the evening and night to make up for it. It takes some personal adjustment to plan ahead and a babysitter who is patient and cooperative. Many infants are tended in daycare centers, which requires packing up and transporting the infant to other surroundings.

A mother needs to be alert to the infant's needs and can plan to leave feedings ready when she is away, even if she had hoped the infant would sleep through the day. If a mother works long hours or has an inflexible schedule, it may be necessary to wean the infant to morning and night feedings at the breast. This arrangement still provides the special benefits of human milk as well as the closeness that an infant needs; thus it is worth the effort. Chapter 18 discusses maternal employment.

LEGAL ISSUES

In the present turmoil of family life, with many marriages ending in separation or divorce in which parents are separating when the children are still young, several custody cases have been based on the court's or judge's perception of what is a normal duration of breastfeeding and what constitutes an excessive duration and poor maternal childcare. A number of cases in the United States have come to the attention of the Lactation Study Center in which the father has sought custody on the basis of prolonged breastfeeding, when the child nursed for comfort to approximately age 4. In most cases the judge found in favor of the mother. In one case in Rochester, New York, the judge found in favor of the father when an expert witness, a local psychologist, declared in court that "you have to be crazy to nurse that long." No amount of scientific evidence could counter this inappropriate remark (personal communication).

No evidence shows that breastfeeding a child beyond infancy is harmful. In fact, breastfeeding benefits toddlers and young children both nutritionally and psychologically. Breastfeeding is neither child abuse nor neglect, and no reported legal decisions made to date claim that it is.[108]

Present day society is not knowledgeable about, or supportive of, extended breastfeeding. Breastfeeding past infancy is as old as mankind and was common in Western cultures until 100 years ago with the advent of artificial feeding and its commercialization.

Other issues of parental rights have surfaced in cases of child custody and visitation rights when the child is younger than 2 years of age and breastfeeding. Usually the argument over separation of the mother from her breastfeeding infant is part of a larger problem. Physicians called on to give expert testimony need to review carefully all the issues because rarely is the breastfeeding question the only concern related to custody. It also would seem appropriate that judges review the entire case and qualifications of the respective parents and refrain from basing their decision on a single issue. It is also advisable for expert witnesses to be fully informed on a subject about which they will testify and to avoid extending their comments beyond their area of expertise.

Developmental psychologist Ainsworth[109] has studied the maturation of the child and summarized the literature, which shows that infants with a strong attachment to their mothers through breastfeeding are psychologically independent at 2 years of age. These children have more mastery of themselves at age 5 and less anxiety entering school than bottle-fed children.

WHY DO SOME WOMEN NOT BREASTFEED?

Given the tremendous benefits to mother and infant of breastfeeding, why do some women choose not to breastfeed? Studies in our laboratory in the 1990s among young women in the WIC program prenatally indicated that although they knew that mother's milk was best and why, they did not plan to breastfeed because there were too many rules. Prenatal classes about infant feeding given at WIC made formula feeding look easy and breastfeeding complicated. The perceived complexity included dietary restrictions, breast holding hand grips and body positions, and the limitations concerning alcohol, caffeine, and medications. They found it overwhelming and certainly not physiologic or natural.

Using the data from the National Survey of Family Growth to analyze the breastfeeding behaviors of a national probability sample of 6733 first-time mothers aged 15 to 44 years, Taylor et al.[59] measured the reasons for never breastfeeding. The most common reason mothers gave was "preferred to bottle feed" (66.3%). The next most common reason was a "physical or medical problem" (14.9%). For women giving physical or medical problem as the reason, no one problem stood out, and most were probably surmountable. Job or schedule was a distant third as a reason (9.8%). "Did not know how to breastfeed" was given by 4.7% of women even though more than 97% had received prenatal care. According to the survey, 1.8% of the babies refused the breast. The authors stated that provider encouragement increased breastfeeding initiation among women of all social and ethnic backgrounds. They found that most women have decided about breastfeeding by the third trimester; thus providers of prenatal care should have a significant role in breastfeeding promotion. "Preferred to bottle feed" was interpreted by Taylor et al.[59] as representing an intrinsic decision on the part of the mother or an amalgam of many indistinct social and cultural pressures. Atchan et al.[110] reported a range of reasons women offered in their decision not to breastfeed: convenience, dislike of the "breastfeeding act," embarrassment at feeding in public, personal health concerns, fear of pain, partner involvement/approval, early return to work, previous experience with breastfeeding, preference, and comparability/superiority of formula. Attitudes of health professionals and lack of needed support as reasons to not breastfeed point to the work that is still needed to truly support all mothers in their choice of infant feeding and breastfeeding.

SUMMARY

Weaning is a complex process involving nutritional, microbiologic, immunologic, biochemical, and psychologic adjustments in the transitioning from a reliance on human breast milk for nutrition to other nutrient-rich and calorie-rich solids and liquids while maintaining optimal nutrition, growth, and development of the infant. During this transition the needs of the infant and mother should balance out and fit with the mother's beliefs, perceptions, and preferences. There is a tremendous amount of data on the benefits of exclusive breastfeeding through 6 months, although a single recommendation for the optimal time for transitioning to complementary foods remains uncertain. Breastfeeding, through 12 months or longer, should continue while complementary foods are introduced. The reasons why women cease breastfeeding remain complex and numerous. These need to be better understood on the individual and public health level to use effective interventions of promotion and support to help women achieve their breastfeeding goals and improve breastfeeding rates. Just as each infant has individualized needs for energy and micronutrients and macronutrients, the process of weaning and transition to complementary foods must be individualized to the specific infant, mother, family community, and culture.

The guiding principles for complementary feeding of the breastfed infant from the Pan American Health Organization remains the best "how to" resource for weaning and transition to complementary foods.

The Reference list is available at www.expertconsult.com.

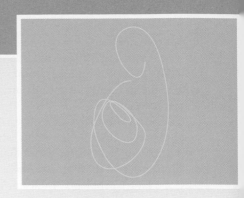

10

Normal Growth, Growth Faltering, and Obesity in Breastfed Infants

Robert M. Lawrence and Ruth A. Lawrence

KEY POINTS

- Optimal growth can be achieved only through the interaction of genetic potential and optimal nutrition at the appropriate times (intrauterine, infancy, childhood, and adolescence) to immediately effect timely active growth and "program" organogenesis and metabolism to optimize future growth and health.
- The World Health Organization (WHO) growth standards represent appropriate growth references for assessing the optimal growth of breastfeeding infants and children through 24 months of age. These standards are also appropriate for human variation in growth related to genetics, ethnicity, and culture when breastfeeding and complementary feeding are optimized.
- The continued use of Centers for Disease Control and Prevention (CDC) charts from 24 to 59 months is recommended because the charts extend out to 20 years, whereas WHO charts cover only 0 to 59 months. Switching at 24 months is explained because of the transition at 24 months from measuring recumbent length to standing height. Nevertheless, the WHO charts reflect optimal growth and the CDC charts reflect population averages.
- Recognition of growth faltering in a breastfeeding infant by comparison of an individual child's growth to the WHO growth standards for breastfeeding infants should be a call for assessment of the situation and intervention

to optimize nutrition, allowing the infant to return to appropriate growth. Direct observation of breastfeeding by the mother and child is essential to identifying breastfeeding difficulties and potential solutions.
- If the infant with growth faltering is hungry and is not getting adequate nutrition, feeding the baby is the next crucial step. The questions why, what, how much, and how should guide the feeding intervention and ideally generate a plan back to easier breastfeeding and optimal nutrition.
- Childhood obesity is a complex condition generated through the interaction of genetics and environment. There are numerous potentially contributing factors acting in the prenatal, intrauterine, and postnatal periods. Body mass index is the accepted practical estimate of adiposity, overweight, and obesity.
- At this juncture, data are not clear that breastfeeding has any more than a small effect on decreasing obesity in the breastfed infant. Nevertheless, a few appropriate recommendations to minimize obesity in infants and children include exclusive breastfeeding from birth to 6 months of age, introduction of appropriate complementary foods at 4 to 6 months of age, continued use of human milk though 12 to 36 months of age, and overall limiting cow's milk intake for any age child.

NORMAL GROWTH

The focus on growth evaluations in childhood have relied on averages: averages of the fat, the thin, the tall, the short, the sick, and the well. The important scientific question is to identify ideal growth in optimally fed children anywhere in the world. Breastfeeding is the biologic norm for optimal nutrition for the first 4 to 6 months of life, with complementary feeds added at 6 months of age within an environment supportive for unrestricted growth.

General Considerations

The growth of exclusively breastfed infants has become the focus of much interest among pediatricians, researchers, and nutritionists. Historically, the Boyd-Orr cohort study in the

1920s and 1930s showed that breastfed children were taller in childhood and adulthood.[1] Stature was associated with health and life expectancy. Adult leg length is very sensitive to environmental factors and diet in early childhood because this is the time of most rapid leg growth. Leg length has been used as the best measurement of growth progress. After infancy, chest growth is rapid before puberty and is sensitive to stress and illness.

A number of long-range follow-up studies were initiated to address the issues of growth during the critical first year of life, when brain growth is greater than it ever will be again in postnatal life. The issues of malnutrition and stunting continued to plague children worldwide. An interest in height and weight increments and ratios is only part of the concern about obesity and the long-range issues of adiposity. Does breastfeeding protect against adult obesity? Does human milk protect against hypercholesterolemia or dyslipidemia in adult life? The questions are clear, but the answers are not unless one assumes the teleologic approach: human milk is ideal for human infants, with its low protein, controlled calories, and persistent unchangeable cholesterol.

Other questions were raised regarding optimal growth: "Is it safe to overfeed an infant with formula?" "Is it safe to deprive an infant of cholesterol during a period of critical brain growth when brain growth depends on cholesterol?" and "When infants are deprived of cholesterol in early infancy, are they less able to tolerate it later?" This question is significant because infant formulas do not contain cholesterol deliberately.

Antiquated data and anthropometric standards based on that data have led to the belief that the growth curves and tables of normal height and weight do not reflect the growth of most healthy, well-fed breastfeeding infants.[2] Reliability of weight gain as a measure of growth has developed because it is a measurement easily obtained. Measurement of length, however, is considered a better standard.[3] Weight gain and linear growth are not always correlated. Furthermore, during infancy and childhood, the lower leg grows at a higher rate than the rest of the body. Knee-heel length can be expressed as a percentage of total length and increases with age: 25% at birth, 27% at 12 months, and 31% in adult life. During several decades of formula feeding, "normal" growth curves were developed based only on formula-fed infants. These curves reflected how children grew "on average" of tall and short, fat and thin, and sick and well children. The curves did not reflect optimal growth of infants and children afforded optimal nutrition in a nurturing environment to achieve their growth potential.

The First 1000 Days: Nutrition and Growth

Along with recognizing the effects of malnutrition in infancy and early childhood leading to increased mortality in children younger than 5 years and morbidities associated with stunting and malnutrition, several other issues are clear. There is a crucial window for brain growth in the first several years of life and the effects early malnutrition might have on that growth. Early-life obesity leads to obesity in adolescents and adults with all the associated morbidities. Maternal prenatal nutrition also seems to influence growth in infancy and early childhood with a real potential for affecting longer term health. The first 1000 days of life (280 days + 365 days + 355 days = 1000), roughly the time from conception through an infant's second birthday, coincides with the brain's essential early growth and development and the establishment of physical growth, immune function, and other metabolic features consistent with long-term health or disease. In fact, the first 1000 days of life are susceptible to two major threats undernutrition/malnutrition (related to poverty, food insecurity, poor sanitation, etc.) and "overnutrition" and the risk for obesity (related to food excess, unbalanced diets, and inadequate nutritional understanding/education).[4–7] The United Nations International Children Education Fund (UNICEF), the World

Health Organization (WHO), and World Bank Group track malnutrition worldwide in its various forms: stunting, wasting, and overweight.[8] Inroads have been made for "good nutrition" since 2000, with declines worldwide in malnutrition.[8] Current estimates for 2018 include 149 million children under 5 affected by stunting, 49 million children under 5 with wasting, and 40 million children under 5 years of age estimated to be overweight. These dire estimates exist despite the recommendations that exclusive breastfeeding should be provided for the first 6 months of life and continued through 12 to 24 months of age or longer, that whole cow milk be diminished or removed from an infant's diet, and the introduction of appropriate complementary solid foods should occur at 6 months of age and older. Despite these recommendations by various health groups, including the WHO and UNICEF, the question remains concerning implementation, uptake, and support of these recommendations by governments, physicians, health care workers, and families.

Comparison of Formula-Fed Versus Breastfed Growth

Formula-fed infants gain more rapidly in weight and length during the first months of life than do breastfed infants.[9] Therefore evaluating an infant's physical growth by standards set by bottle-fed infants predisposes one to the diagnosis of failure to thrive for breastfed infants.

Forman et al.[10] reported a longitudinal study of breastfed and bottle-fed infants during the first few months of life that demonstrated the 10th and 90th percentile values for weight and length of the two groups were similar at birth, and the 10th percentile values of the two groups were similar at age 112 days. The significant difference was in the values for the 90th percentile. Bottle-fed infants were above this percentile in substantially greater numbers. These differences were attributed to caloric intake rather than the difference in composition of the diet. Fomon et al.[11] showed that the bottle-fed infant not only gains more in weight and length, but also gains more weight for a unit of length. Per the authors and others, this gain reflects the overfeeding of the bottle-fed infants.

Most studies of growth in breastfed infants have been plagued with the problem of variation in the definition of "breastfed" (exclusive, almost exclusive, partial breastfeeding, token), the amount of formula supplementation, and the occurrence of partial weaning.

The effects on growth of specific protein and energy intake in 4- to 6-month-old infants who were either breastfed or formula fed with high and low protein were measured by Axelsson et al.[12] No significant differences were found in the growth rate of crown-heel length and head circumference or weight gain. The authors concluded that the differences in protein intake between breastfed and formula-fed infants without differences in growth indicate that the formulas may provide a protein intake in excess of the needs. When milk intake and growth in exclusively breastfed infants were carefully documented in the first 4 months by Butte et al.,[13] energy and protein intakes were substantially less than current nutrient allowances. Infant growth progressed satisfactorily when compared with National Center for Health Statistics (NCHS) standards, despite that energy ingested by breastfed infants dropped from 110 ± 24 kcal/kg per day at 1 month to 71 ± 17 kcal/kg per day at 4 months.[13] Similarly, protein intake decreased from 1.6 ± 0.3 g/kg per day at 1 month to 0.9 ± 0.2 g/kg per day at 4 months. Reevaluation of protein and energy requirements is essential.

Weight-for-length and weight gain were significantly correlated with total energy intake but not with activity level during the first 6 months of life in breastfed infants studied by Dewey et al.[14,15] Energy intake was considerably lower than recommended—85 to 89 kcal/kg per day—when compared with the 115 kcal/kg per day recommended dietary allowances of the National Academy of Sciences in 1980.[16] Presently energy recommendations for infants 0–3 months of age suggested by the National Academy of Medicine (formerly the Institute of Medicine) are expressed as $(89 \times \text{weight[kg]} - 100) + 175$ kcal.

Infants who consumed the most breast milk became the fattest. A 4-kg infant would require 105 kcal/kg per day.

When patterns of growth are examined in the infants of marginally nourished mothers, weight gain is comparable to a reference population but does not permit recovery of weight differential at birth, which occurs in infants who are small for gestational age (SGA).[17] The intakes of energy and protein by individual infants were reflected in their weight gain but were below internationally recommended norms.[18] Maternal milk alone, when produced in sufficient amounts, can maintain normal growth up to the sixth month of life. Exclusive breastfeeding in Chilean infants of low-middle and low socioeconomic families produced the highest weight gain and practically no illness or hospitalization.[19]

In the Copenhagen Cohort Study in 1994, exclusively breastfed term infants had a mean intake of 781 and 855 mL/24 hours at 2 and 4 months, respectively.[20] The median fat concentration of human milk was 39.2 g/L and was positively associated with maternal weight gain during pregnancy. This supports the concept that maternal fat stores laid down during pregnancy are easier to mobilize during lactation than other fat stores. This may limit milk fat when pregnancy fat stores are exhausted.

In addition to recognizing the importance of genetic, metabolic, and environmental influences in producing significant differences in growth patterns, Barness suggests that recommendations for nutrition of healthy neonates may be too high for some and too low for others.[21] However, the benchmark for nutritional requirements of the full-term infant remains milk from the infant's healthy, well-nourished mother.

Gain in physical growth is not as critical as gain in brain growth, but measurements of brain growth are only indirectly implied from growth of the head. In evaluating any infant's progress, head circumference is an important consideration, especially in the first year of life. Deceleration in the rate of increase in head circumference occurs over the first year. The head circumference increases approximately 7.5 cm (3 inches) in the first year of life and another 7.5 cm in the next 16 years of life. When growth failure includes failure of head growth, the growth failure is severe. However, many other factors independent of body growth influence head growth.

Weight Loss in the First Week of Life (Formula-Fed Versus Breastfed Infants)

A weight loss of 3% to 5% is usually accepted as the norm for formula-fed infants in the first week of life, although supporting information in pediatric textbooks is meager. A loss of 5% to 7% is average for breastfed infants, with a nadir of weight loss at 2 to 4 days of life. When the weight loss continues to progress toward 10% or more or the weight loss continues to drop after day 3 or 4 of life, the clinician should be alerted to this and the breastfeeding process and milk ingestion carefully assessed, adjustments made, and intake followed to document a reversal of the weight loss. Macdonald et al. documented this difference in weight loss between formula-fed and breastfed infants ($n = 937$, 45% breastfed, 42% formula fed, and 13% mixed feeding), noting the median weight loss for formula-fed infants was 3.5% of birth weight and 6.6% for breastfed infants.[22] Weight loss for breastfed infants at the 95th centile (11.8% loss) and the 97.5th centile (12.8% loss) exceeded 10%, although it was rare for a formula-fed infant to lose 10% of birth weight. There were distinct differences in the time to recovery of birth weight: for breastfed infants median 8.3 days, 95th centile 18.7 days, 97.5th centile 21 days; formula-fed infants median 6.5 days, 95th centile 14.5 days and 97.5th centile 16.7 days. Additional studies confirmed these weight loss differences between formula-fed and breastfed infants and pointed to specific variables associated with "excess weight loss," including cesarean birth, absence of labor before delivery, lower gestational age, higher birth weight, intrapartum fluid balance, and delayed lactogenesis.[23–25] Systematic reviews reinforced the information, although there were concerns about methodologic flaws, such as gaps in data, poorly documented feeding groups, etc.[26] For the breastfed infants, there was also evidence of supplementation with formula because of the concern for weight loss or concern for delayed lactogenesis. Along with this came concerns of interrupting exclusive breastfeeding and precipitation of stopping breast- feeding.

One group from the Northern Kaiser Permanente Hospitals studied early weight loss in both breastfed and formula-fed infants in an hour-by-hour analysis in hopes of facilitating detection of those infants at risk for an adverse outcome and in need of early intervention/assistance. Flaherman et al. published data for 108,907 exclusively breastfed newborns, with 83,433 by vaginal delivery and 25,474 delivered by cesarean.[27] They reported that almost 5% of vaginally delivered infants and over 10% of infants from cesarean deliveries lost 10% or more of their birthweight 48 hours after delivery. Over 25% of infants from cesarean deliveries had lost more than 10% of their birth weight by 72 hours of age. They developed nomograms of early weight loss by hour over the first 72 hours, separately for vaginal and cesarean deliveries. (See Appendix F.) Subsequently Drs. Paul, Flaherman, and Schaefer in collaboration with a group of US academic centers created a tool for assessing and tracking breastfed infant weight loss in the first 72 to 96 hours of life. An online calculator (Newborn Weight Tool, NEWT, https://www.newbornweight.org) is available for doing this.[28] In subsequent work the same group developed similar nomograms for formula-fed newborns.[29] They have gone on to validate the use of these nomograms and track early weight loss with breastfeeding outcomes through 1 month of age and health care usage relative to feeding mode and early weight loss.[30−32]

It is impossible to predict which infants will be adversely affected by "excessive" early weight loss or the amount of weight loss or the timing of weight loss in an individual infant. It is possible to recognize risk factors for excessive weight loss, and it is possible to diagnose delayed lactogenesis and identify infants in need of supplementation. The Academy of Breastfeeding Medicine (ABM) has reviewed the issue of supplementary feedings for the healthy term infant, indications for supplementation, nonindications, ways to prevent the need for supplementation, and how to supplement and support continued breastfeeding if possible in their protocol on supplementation.[33]

They emphasize not blindly pushing on with breastfeeding, but rather pausing to truly assess the mother's milk production, goals for breastfeeding, and evidence that the infant is or is not receiving adequate milk. Dr. B. Phillip and Dr. C. Rosen-Carole, faculty members of the ABM, offer their approach to this dilemma in an online discussion at Baby-Friendly USA (https://www.babyfriendlyusa.org/news/what-should-happen-when-baby-does-not-get-enough-milk-from-mom/).[34] Assess the infant by looking for signs that the infant is sleeping normally, easily takes to the breast, and appears satisfied with the feedings, demonstrating both early feeding cues and satiety without fussiness or hypersomnolence, good activity, and good urine output and stool frequency. There should be no signs or symptoms of dehydration, no excessive weight loss (use the nomograms or online NEWT weight tool [see Appendix F]), and no evidence of hypoglycemia, abnormal electrolytes, or hyperbilirubinemia. Assess the mother's milk production (breast fullness, let-down, milk leaking, and prefeeding and postfeeding breast changes), breast glandular sufficiency, history of breast pathologic condition or prior surgeries that might interfere with milk production/delivery. Check for temporary cessation of breastfeeding or separation of mother and baby without ongoing available breast milk for the infant, possible interference with milk production by maternal medications, or intolerable pain during feeding without relief from appropriate interventions. Always directly observe the mother and infant breastfeeding, checking positioning and latch and observing for success or difficulty. If the infant is not getting enough milk, the infant should be fed. Act to ensure the safe feeding of the infant at the same time as respecting the mother's (and family's) desires and plans for breastfeeding. If the mother is committed to breastfeeding, "bridge the gap," "feed the baby," "support the mother," and "don't undermine breastfeeding."[34] Supplementing, if necessary, then becomes part of appropriate medical care by (1) thinking about why the baby is being supplemented (indication[s] and expected outcome measures), (2) considering how much to supplement, (3) deciding what to supplement with (expressed breastmilk, donor breast milk, or formula), (4) deciding how to feed the infant (cup, syringe, bottle, or supplemental nursing system), (5) continuing or reinitiate breastfeeding (continue breast milk expression and use or storage), and (6) planning for follow-up and documentation of successful feeding and weight gain by the infant.[34]

Growth of Breastfed Infants

Dewey et al. suggested that new, separate growth charts are needed for breastfed infants.[15,35,36] The Davis Area Research on Lactation, Infant Nutrition, and Growth (DARLING) Study collected data prospectively on growth patterns, nutrient intake, morbidity, and activity levels of matched cohorts of infants who were either exclusively breastfed or bottle fed during the first 12 months of life. Measurements were followed beyond 12 months to 18, 21, 24, and 36 months as well. Growth in length and head circumference did not differ significantly between the two groups; however, weight gain was slower among breastfed infants after approximately 3 months of age. These weight gain differences continued even after solid foods were added at 6 months in both groups. Breastfed infants were leaner than their counterparts. The slower growth rates and lower energy intake of the breastfed infants were associated with normal or accelerated development and less morbidity from infectious illnesses. The authors concluded that it is normal for breastfed infants to gain at this pace, which is less rapid than that indicated by the scales developed for bottle-fed infants.[35]

When the growth patterns of a large sample of breastfed infants were pooled from the United States, Canada, and Europe, Dewey et al. reported that results were consistent across studies.[15,35,36] Breastfed infants grew more rapidly in weight during the first 2 months and less rapidly over 3 to 12 months. Head circumference was well above the WHO/Centers for Disease Control and Prevention (CDC) median throughout the first year. Length-for-age did not decline, nor did the weight-for-age and weight-for-length scores as breastfeeding increased in duration.

Garza et al. reviewed growth patterns of breastfed infants. Breastfed infants clearly consumed less energy than recommended by WHO in the second 3-month period by choice and not because the mother could not produce more milk.[37] Dewey et al. first pointed this out when they had mothers pump to increase their production and found the infants self-regulated to the original intake measured before the pumping program in spite of the fact that the mother was producing more milk.[14,38] Many researchers at that time recommended separate growth curves for exclusively breastfed infants.

International Growth Standards

It became clear that growth curves developed by the CDC were averages taken from bottle-fed infants, mostly overfed, fat and thin, tall and short, sick and well. They reflected how children grew on the average as predominantly formula-fed infants. The WHO convened an international committee of experts to develop a model for how breastfed children should grow. Data were collected from six countries of widely divergent populations from stable families who breastfed exclusively for 6 months and continued breastmilk for a minimum of a year and longer. The infants had access to health care and good housing. This multicenter growth reference study involved 8440 children 0 to 5 years of age from Brazil, Ghana, India, Norway, Oman, and the United States (Sacramento, California).[39,40] The sample had ethnic or genetic variability in addition to cultural variation in how the children were nurtured, strengthening the standard's universal applicability. One remarkable observation was that all the children grow at the same pace; curves could be superimposed, regardless of racial or ethnic background or geographic region. The observations confirmed the thought that children in a healthy environment can achieve their genetic growth potential regardless of poverty, ethnicity, or culture. The charts differ from the CDC growth charts, especially for the first 2 years of life, in which formula-fed infants show greater weight gain, which averages that the formula-fed infant is 600 to 650 g heavier at 12 months of age. Differences in length are minimal, and, therefore, breastfed infants are lower in weight-for-length measurements and other indices of fatness. Breastfed individuals are not shorter in adult life but are less likely to be obese. Assessment of sex differences and heterogeneity in motor milestone attainment among populations in the multicenter study supports the appropriateness of pooling data from all sites and both sexes for the purpose of an international standard. Six gross motor milestones were used: sitting without support, hands-and-knees crawling, standing with assistance, walking with assistance, standing alone, and walking alone. The WHO child growth standards depict normal growth under optimal environmental conditions for nutrition and growth and can be used to assess children everywhere, regardless of ethnicity, socioeconomic status, and type of feeding. They represent how children should grow globally.[41,42]

The recommendation for use of the WHO charts by the CDC states the following for infants under 24 months: use the WHO growth charts recognizing the values 2 standard deviations above and below the median, or the 2.3rd and 97.7th percentiles (labeled) as the 2nd and 98th percentile for possible recognition of children whose growth indicates an adverse health condition. The rationale for this use is recognition that breastfeeding is the recommended standard for infant feeding and, unlike the CDC charts, the WHO growth charts reflect patterns of breastfed infants for at least 4 months and still breastfeeding at 12 months, and all the data are based on a high-quality study (Multicentre Growth Reference Study [MGRS]).[43]

The continued use of CDC charts from 24 to 59 months is recommended because the charts extend out to 20 years, whereas WHO charts cover 0 to 59 months. Switching at 24 months is explained because of the transition at 24 months from measuring recumbent length to standing height. Nevertheless, the WHO charts reflect optimal growth whereas the CDC charts reflect population averages.

Impact of Weaning Foods on Growth

Weaning foods is a term used by breastfeeding practitioners, but the infant nutrition community uses the term *complementary foods*; foods that complement breast milk. As an infant approaches 6 months of age, the stores of iron are diminishing and iron in human milk is not sufficient to meet needs; likewise, the once high levels of stored zinc are diminishing and the levels of zinc in human milk are decreasing. Thus complementary foods need to contain iron and zinc, as most meats and fortified cereals do.[44] Krebs et al. found low measurements of iron and zinc levels in breastfeeding infants at 6 months; when meat was added as a weaning food, levels increased toward normal.[45] Routine assessment of iron and zinc levels increased toward normal. Routine assessment of iron and zinc levels is not practical; therefore the Committee on Nutrition recommends fortified cereal or infant-style meats as weaning food.[46]

The transition from breast milk to a reliance on the calories and nutrients of complementary foods also depends on the infant's developmental readiness to eat solid or semisolid foods. Some of the signs of developmental readiness include ability to sit without support, good head control, opening of the mouth when food is presented, and decreased extrusion reflex. Other signs of readiness are behaviors that demonstrate being unsatisfied after breast milk or formula feeding, demonstrated interest in what the caregiver is eating, and displaying cues that they are done eating by turning their head away or refusing additional food.

The timing of initiation of weaning foods before 6 months of age has shown that as energy intake increases from solid foods, energy intake from breast milk decreases. The downward trend of weight-to-age and weight-to-length ratios continues with the addition of solids, which would not be expected if growth faltering were the basis for the decline.[37] Breastfed infants apparently self-regulate when offered solids in part by leaving some solids uneaten. When breastfed infants were given solids between 4 and 7 months, their weight-for-age and weight-for-length were consistently lower than those for infants introduced to solids at 8 months or older. Length-for-age was similar between the two groups.

Does the growth rate of exclusively breastfed infants reflect a need for increased protein?[47] This question has challenged the wisdom of exclusive breastfeeding. A group of exclusively breastfed infants were matched with a second group who received prepared solid foods, including egg yolk, beginning at 4 months of age.[38] Neither weight gain nor length gain from 4 to 6 months differed between the groups. The solid-food group received 20% higher protein intake as well as higher intakes of iron, zinc, calcium, vitamin A, and riboflavin. The authors concluded that protein intake is not a limiting factor in the growth of breastfed infants.[38,47]

Similarly, Cohen et al.[48] demonstrated that breastfed infants given solids at 4 months self-regulated so that the energy intake and protein intake were the same in both the supplemented group and the unsupplemented group. When Motil et al. calculated the gross efficiency of nutrient usage for each infant in a longitudinal study of breastfed and bottle-fed infants, length and weight gains and lean body mass and body fat accretion during the first 24 weeks of life were similar.[49] The formula-fed infants had received significantly higher nitrogen and energy. The gross efficiency of dietary energy usage for lean body mass deposition was two times greater in breastfed than bottle-fed infants. No association was found between lean body mass deposition and dietary protein intake. This confirms previous studies that human milk protein does not limit growth.[49] Breastfed infants self-regulate their energy intake at lower levels than formula-fed infants. Body temperature and metabolic rates are lower in breastfed infants.[50]

Recommendations for Optimal Duration of Exclusive Breastfeeding

Recommendations for optimal duration of exclusive breastfeeding have been controversial.[50] The WHO has revised its recommendation for both developed and developing countries to promote exclusive breastfeeding for 6 months.[40] Kramer and Kakuman provide a comprehensive review of the literature, including both controlled clinical trials and observational studies in any language comparing exclusive breastfeeding to exclusive breastfeeding for less time with mixed feeding for at least 6 months.[51] The health outcomes reported included growth, iron and zinc status, infectious morbidity, atopic disease, neuromotor development, rate of postpartum maternal weight loss, and duration of lactational amenorrhea. The conclusions were that exclusive breastfeeding for 6 months resulted in lower risk for gastrointestinal infection and no growth deficits. In concert with the WHO, the section on breastfeeding of the American Academy of Pediatrics (AAP) promotes exclusive breastfeeding for 6 months. The WHO recommends the need for animal source foods and fruits and vegetables in the initial period of 6 to 9 months of age, as demonstrated in the MGRS.[39,41,42]

Prolonged Breastfeeding

Considerable controversy surrounds the question of prolonged breastfeeding. Although the value of prolonged breastfeeding has not been challenged in industrialized countries, it has in developing countries. When the fat and energy content were measured in 34 mothers of healthy term infants who had been lactating for more than a year (12 to 39 months) and compared with the milk of control mothers who had been lactating for 2 to 6 months, levels were significantly increased in fat and energy content. The elevated levels did not correlate with maternal age, diet, body mass index (BMI), or number of daily feedings.[52] Another analysis of breast-milk macronutrient content in prolonged lactation (women breastfeeding for ≥ 18 months) demonstrated that fat and protein increased and carbohydrates decreased compared with expressed milk of mothers breastfeeding for less than 12 months.[53] Some studies showed that small, undergrown infants are breastfed longer.[54,55] Careful assessments reveal that larger infants are weaned earlier. A cautious review of available studies suggests that prolonged breastfeeding does

not cause malnutrition; rather, the small and undergrown infants are kept at the breast longer. Child size appears to be related to the decision to wean so that, in general, large healthy infants are weaned completely from the breast earlier.[54] Thus smaller infants being breastfed longer is not the cause of the undergrowth. The effect of prolonged breastfeeding on growth has been an issue of concern and been evaluated, especially in developing countries.[10,35] In a review of 13 studies, Grummer-Strawn pointed out in 1993 that 8 reported a negative relationship, 2 had a positive relationship, and 3 had mixed results.[56] Grummer-Strawn identified the flaws in study design and suggested that until better information is available, women should nurse as long as possible because the benefits to infant health (infection protection) exceed the risks in these geographic areas.[56] Kramer et al. used three analytic approaches (intention-to-treat, observational [as fed], and instrumental variable [randomization as the instrument to create more than 12 months of breastfeeding]) to examine the relationship between prolonged lactation and infant growth.[57] The observational approach of analysis of the data from the same children indicated an opposite causal inference compared with the other two approaches. The authors concluded that slower previous growth may have led to prolonged breastfeeding and is an example of apparent reverse causality. Hopefully, future study will accurately define the issue of causality related to prolonged breastfeeding and infant growth.

Catch-Up Growth in Small-for-Gestational-Age Infants

SGA infants have been identified as being at risk for continued growth failure in extrauterine life, learning difficulties, and behavioral problems. Lucas et al.[58] explored the influence of early nutrition on growth in the first year of life in full-term SGA infants, comparing those receiving breast milk with those receiving formula. This was a subset of a study on early carnitine supplementation. An equal number of breastfed and formula-fed infants received carnitine. Additional demographic, social, clinical, and anthropometric data were collected. Breastfeeding was associated with a greater increase in weight at 2 weeks and 3 months of age, which persisted beyond the actual breastfeeding period. The authors reported greater catch-up growth in head measurement and a greater increase in body length in the breastfed infant. They suggest that breastfeeding promotes faster catch-up growth, and breastfed infants have the potential for improved catch-up growth in developmental parameters as well.[58]

In a study designed to examine the role of zinc supplementation in catch-up growth in SGA infants, Castillo-Duran et al. reported that infants who were exclusively breastfed had increased growth compared with those who were formula fed and supplemented with zinc.[59] A recent study of premature SGA infants demonstrated the benefits of an exclusive human milk–based diet. The 18 SGA infants demonstrated good catch-up growth at 2 years of age without evidence of insulin resistance of increased adiposity compared with the 33 premature infants who were appropriate for gestational age.[60] One systematic review by Santiago et al., reported from an analysis of seven articles of term infants, SGA, and breastfed (compared with high-calorie formula feeding) that the breastfed infants' catch-up growth was without body composition alteration or increased insulin resistance.[61] They did report variability in type of evaluations completed and age of the infants at time of assessment. Campisi et al. reported in their systematic review that there was significant variability in the definitions of SGA, catch-up growth, and measured growth outcomes such that their conclusions were regarding the need for standardization of definitions, measurement, and follow-up.[62] They did recommend the use of international standards for fetal growth and infant size to facilitate agreed-on definitions and measurements.[63] Other groups have recommended nutritional assessment in a practical approach applicable to preterm infants and SGA infants. They propose specific anthropometric measurements (weight gain velocity, body weight, body length, head circumference, mid-upper arm circumference, skinfolds, weight-to-length ratio, BMI, ponderal index) and biochemical markers (glucose, iron, ferritin, protein, BUN, serum prealbumin), serum transferrin, retinol-binding protein, serum calcium, phosphate, alkaline phosphatase, urinary calcium, and phosphate markers) to be tracked.[64] They include references to the use of these measurements, techniques and instrumentation, and reference values.[65,66]

Cognitive and Motor Development

Cognitive and motor development are intimately tied to growth in infants and children and essential to any definition of optimal growth and basic measurement of achieving human potential. Cognitive development in the first 7 years of life was related to breastfeeding practices of a birth cohort in New Zealand.[67] The researchers took into account maternal intelligence, maternal education, maternal training in child rearing, childhood experiences, family socioeconomic status, birth weight, and gestational age. The breastfed children had slightly higher test scores on the Peabody Picture Vocabulary Test, the 5-year measure on the Stanford Binet Intelligence Scale, and the 7-year measure on the Wechsler Child Intelligence Scale. Measures of language development were equally influenced. This very small improvement in scores persisted when adjustments were made for all variables. The scores were also influenced by length of breastfeeding less than and longer than 4 months.

An additional study on the same birth cohort was done to assess breastfeeding and subsequent social adjustment in 6- to 8-year-old children. Fergusson et al. studied prospectively 1024 children who were part of the Christchurch Child Development Study. They used the maternal and teacher ratings of childhood conduct disorders.[68] A statistically significant tendency for conduct disorder scores declined with increasing duration of breastfeeding; that is, breastfed children were less prone to conduct disorders than bottle-fed children. Breastfed children, however, tended to come from slightly more socially advantaged, economically privileged

homes that were more stable. The analysis failed to examine early mother–infant interaction patterns.

This cohort of 1000 individuals now has been reported as an 18-year longitudinal study by Horwood and Fergusson.[69] A small but detectable increase in child cognitive and educational achievement in the children who had been breastfed as infants was still seen. The results were confirmed in standardized tests, teacher ratings, and academic outcomes in high school and young adulthood.

De Andraca and Uauy[70] reviewed the factors in human milk and the breastfeeding process that affect optimal mental and visual development. The complex relationships point to a clear advantage to breastfeeding.

The relationship of infant-feeding practices and dependent variables to the subsequent cognitive abilities were reported from the Yale Harvard Research Project in Tunisia.[71] Within the underprivileged group, they found that breastfeeding promoted not only physical growth but also sensor motor development as assessed by Bayley motor and mental scales. No great differences were found in the ability to sit alone or to take first steps, but especially among boys in the lower socioeconomic group, significant superiority of breastfed infants at 8, 14, and 16 months of age was observed in the Bayley mental scales. In this study, all infants were from the same social and intellectual strata.

The question of whether breastfeeding influences a child's developmental outcome has appeared in modern literature since Hoefer and Hardy first reported in 1929 that breastfed infants were more active and achieved motor milestones earlier than bottle-fed infants.[72] These authors described enhanced learning ability and higher intelligence quotient (IQ) scores at 7 to 13 years of age in children exclusively breastfed for 4 to 9 months. Although socioeconomic status and mothers' education were not reported, it is an interesting historic note that it was the well-educated, higher socioeconomic mothers who could afford to bottle feed in the 1920s and 1930s and into the 1940s. In an attempt to clarify the relationship to maternal status, Taylor and Wadsworth took the negative hypothesis but were unable to eliminate the possibility that breastfeeding had a positive effect on intellectual development at 5 years of age.[73]

In a national study of 13,135 children in England, Scotland, and Wales, a positive correlation between duration of breastfeeding and performance in tests of vocabulary and visuomotor coordination was found; these behavior scores remained steady when tested against intervening social and biologic variables. This British 1946 cohort study continued. They showed that breastfeeding was significantly and positively associated with educational attainment and cognition at age 15 years and with adult social class. Breastfeeding did not affect verbal memory independently at 53 years of age in this longitudinal cohort. Breastfeeding clearly has long-term potential impact across life's course according to the authors.[74]

The advantage of human milk for at-risk infants has been investigated by Lucas et al., who raised public awareness when their results were reported in newspapers internationally in 1992.[75,76] The initial cohort of 771 infants whose birth weights were less than 1850 g were given their mothers' milk; these infants had a mean 8-point advantage on the Bayley Mental Developmental Index compared with infants who did not receive their mothers' milk.[75] Both groups received nutrition by feeding tube for the first month of life. A 4.3-point advantage remained when outcome was adjusted for demographic and perinatal factors. The same advantage was found using an IQ equivalent test, which is a fundamentally different test. The same group of infants was tested regularly, and results at age 7½ to 8 years showed a 10-point advantage in IQ testing even when controlled for maternal social class and education.

This report precipitated a torrent of responses from other investigators, who provided support for and against the conclusion that breast milk is effective in improving the outcome of high-risk infants.[77–79] A systematic review and meta-analysis of 17 studies demonstrated by a random effects model that breastfed infants achieved a higher IQ (mean difference 3.44 [95% confidence interval (CI), 2.30 to 4.58]) and controlling for maternal IQ demonstrated a smaller benefit (2.62 [95% CI, 1.25 to 3.98]).[80] Evidence from a randomized trial demonstrated that children breastfed exclusively for up to 3 months had IQs that were on average 2.1 points higher compared with the others breastfed for a shorter period (95% CI, 0.24 to 3.9). Analysis on data of children breastfed for 4 to 6 months showed higher IQ by 2.6 points (95% CI, 0.87 to 4.27) and the benefit for children breastfed even longer (> 6 months) was higher by 3.8 points (95% CI, 2.11 to 5.45).[81] This evidence showed that longer duration of exclusive breastfeeding has a dose effect on IQ and similarly, there is evidence of a dose effect of breastfeeding/use of human milk in preterm infant neurodevelopment.[82] These and other studies suggest a causal effect of breastmilk on intelligence.[81–83]

To determine the effect of breastfeeding on optimal visual development, Birch et al.[84] studied term and preterm infants fed human milk or corn oil–based formula with no added omega-3 essential fatty acids. Visual testing using visual-evoked potential and forced-choice preferential looking activity was performed at 4 months' adjusted age; infants given human milk scored better. This was confirmed at 36 months using random dot stereo acuity and letter-matching ability. Results correlated with a measure of dietary omega-3 sufficiency index from the infants' red blood cells at 4 months.

GROWTH FALTERING (FAILURE TO THRIVE)

Definition

Failure to thrive is an imprecise, archaic term. Failure to thrive is a symptom and not a diagnosis. The causes of failure to thrive in children have been associated with malfunctions of many organ systems and with nutritional, environmental, social, and psychologic factors. Failure to thrive while breastfeeding has often been inappropriately considered in the same terms as failure associated with other sources of nourishment and involving other age groups.[85] Growth or weight

faltering is another term proposed to diminish the strong negative connotations of failure.[85] Growth faltering while breastfeeding is a phenomenon associated with the first year of life and more likely younger than 6 months. Exclusive breastfeeding is appropriate for the first 6 months, and then solids should be added. Therefore the symptom is no longer exclusively associated with lactation, except in rare cases in which the infant is breastfed beyond 9 months with no solids added.

The term failure to thrive has been loosely used to describe all infants who show some degree of growth faltering.[86] (Here these two terms will be used interchangeably.) Severe malnutrition or insufficient caloric intake for energy expenditure impairs overall growth, which has an impact on weight first, length usually second, and head circumference third (relatively spared except in extreme malnutrition). It is a syndromic classification that has been used to describe infants whose gain in weight, length, or both fails to occur in a normal progressive fashion. For the breastfed infant, it may be a matter of using an inappropriate growth chart or comparing a slower gaining breastfed infant to the excessive weight-gain patterns of bottle-fed infants.

The current recommendations for diagnosis and treatment of failure to thrive emphasize the assessment of and therapy for malnutrition and its complications and the context in which they occur.[50] The AAP suggests that the needs of each child who is not thriving should be evaluated according to four parameters: medical, nutritional, developmental, and social. The entire family should be included in the assessment as part of the infant's environment for growth. The ecologic context in which such a situation occurs in countries where food is plentiful suggests the cause of deficiency is poverty and food insecurity. This approach is appropriate for children beyond infancy but not for the newborn and early months of life when the child is breastfed.

The disorder for an infant is defined as failure to thrive when the infant continues to lose weight after 10 days of life, does not regain birth weight by 3 weeks of age, or gains at a rate below the 10th percentile for weight gain beyond 1 month of age. Various growth standards are available depending on the situation and the age of the infant.[28,43,63] Weight loss (5% to 7% of birth weight for a breastfed infant) in the first 10 to 14 days of life can be normal but may be an appropriate reason to assess the breastfeeding mother—infant dyad regarding milk production and intake. (See section on early weight loss earlier in this chapter and Appendix F.) Unlike a bottle-fed infant, who can be placed in a hospital where professionals can feed him or her, a breastfed infant needs to be evaluated in the home setting and observed nursing at the breast unless urgent intervention is indicated. If the infant requires hospitalization, the breastfeeding mother is included in the assessment of feeding, including examination of the breasts for signs of milk production and response to feeding, expressing, and/or pumping.

Human growth has been considered a continuous process, characterized by changing velocity of growth at different ages. Despite there being guides for median daily weight gain at different ages, the median daily weight gain often should be measured over slightly longer periods (e.g., 3, 5, 7, or 14 days depending on the situation) and not day to day. (Table 10.1 presents median daily weight gain based on age of the child.) Lampl et al. made serial measurements of length in normal infants weekly, semiweekly, and daily during the infants' first 21 months.[87] They show clearly that growth in length occurs by discontinuous, periodic, saltatory spurts. Furthermore, these bursts were 0.5 to 2.5 cm (0.2 to 1 inch) of length or height during intervals separated by no measurable change (2 to 63 days' duration). The authors suggest that 90% to 95% of normal development during infancy is growth free.[87] Length accretion is distinctly a salutatory process of incremental bursts punctuating background stasis. Thus evaluation of length requires more than one measurement and the careful consideration of an experienced physician familiar with growth parameters. In standard textbooks, the term failure to thrive has been replaced with malnourished or suffering from protein energy malnutrition but is used for children older than a year and no longer depending solely on breast milk for their entire caloric needs.

As increasingly more women breastfeed, increasing numbers of cases of failure to thrive appear in the literature. No statistical data on incidence rates are available because no large prospective study has been done.[88] Only in extreme cases are infants hospitalized, but the number of these cases is increasing as well, partly because of a failure to recognize poor weight gain or weight faltering earlier and to further evaluate the issues and make appropriate interventions for improved caloric intake.

With the introduction of the WHO growth standards based on normal healthy breastfed infants instead of on overfed formula-fed infants, the diagnosis of failure to thrive should be less frequent. An occasional child is clearly not gaining weight nor growing because of a lack of enough breast milk. That lack of weight gain may be related to a confluence of factors, including but not limited to breastfeeding difficulties related to latch, breast pain, and low milk production; contributing factors such as maternal fatigue, overtaxing family/household responsibilities, mother's return to work or school; and the mother's or family's perception of insufficient milk supply. The question that arises is "Does early breastfeeding cessation represent actual failure to thrive by the infant, lactogenesis failure, or simply breastfeeding difficulty and lack of adequate support for the

breastfeeding mother–infant dyad?" Steube et al. reported a prevalence of 12 per 100 women in the Infant Feeding Practices Study II in the United States who reported "lactation dysfunction," which the authors defined as undesired, early weaning from breastfeeding and two of three common problems (breast pain, low milk supply, and difficulty with infant latch).[89] They also reported three significant risk factors for early weaning being women who were overweight, obese, or manifested with depressive symptoms at 2 months postpartum. Feenstra et al. reported from Denmark on data from a postal survey from 1437 mothers with full-term singleton infants.[90] Up to 40% of the women reported "early breastfeeding problems," the most prominent of which were difficulty with latch and sore or cracked nipples. Pain was often reported with breastfeeding problems with no specific diagnosis for the pain. In another study from the United States of 7942 participants enrolled in a peer counseling breastfeeding support group the most common reasons for stopping breastfeeding were mother's choice (39%) and low milk supply (21%).[91] The most common reasons for stopping in participants who stopped the earliest were "breastfeeding challenges," low milk supply, and "mother's preference."[91] Neither failure to thrive by the infant nor lactogenesis failure were discussed in any of these studies.

L. Gatti did a literature review of original research papers on human milk, milk supply, and perceived milk supply.[92] She reported that a 35% of all women who wean early report "perceived insufficient milk supply," although neither the mother nor clinicians and researchers reportedly assessed the actual milk production. Early breastfeeding behaviors of the mother–infant dyad and potential factors associated with perceived insufficient milk supply and socioeconomic or demographic factors were not carefully analyzed and reported in the selected research papers. A couple of other systematic reviews report mixed results of the influence of maternal confidence on exclusive breastfeeding duration and the various factors associated with breastfeeding cessation (maternal young age, low level of education, return to work within 12 weeks postpartum cesarean delivery, depression, and perceived inadequate milk supply.[93,94] It remains difficult to determine if failure to grow by a breastfeeding infant is a common occurrence or significant public health concern.

True failure to thrive with the resultant insufficient caloric and protein intake for an individual infant's energy and

TABLE 10.1	**Daily Weight Gain and Recommended Caloric Intake Allowances for Children Younger Than 1 Year of Age**	
Age (mo)	Median Daily Weight Gain (g)	Recommended Daily Allowance (kcal/kg per day)
0–3	26–31	108
3–6	17–18	108
6–9	12–13	98
9–12	9	98

From National Research Council, Food and Nutrition Board, National Academy of Sciences. *Recommended Dietary Allowances.* 10th ed. Washington, DC: US Government Printing Office; 1989.

growth needs can occur for reasons of medical illness in the infant. Undesired early weaning most likely represents a mixture of situations and contributing factors, only some of which are failure to thrive for the infant. Nevertheless, in any situation with poor infant growth, pain while breastfeeding, or perceived low milk supply, additional assessment and breastfeeding support and education are indicated.

Underlying metabolic disorders causing lack of metabolism of nutrients or lack of absorption are uncommon. Children with congenital anomalies of the first arch, such as cleft lip and/or cleft palate, are at risk but should be identified before hospital discharge and scheduled to receive close follow-up. Congenital illness or infection affecting major organs (lung, liver, heart, kidney, etc.) can affect both caloric and nutrient intake and need. Children with developmental delay may present after a month or so when they cannot maintain adequate suckling and the mothers' milk supply dwindles with diminishing stimulation/milk removal. It is appropriate to evaluate an infant for lead intoxication when there is insufficient growth or developmental delay. Psychosocial risk factors include unusual health and nutrition beliefs of the family, including fear of obesity or other diseases that have been associated with rigid and restricted feeding patterns.

Diagnosis

The problem of slow or inadequate weight gain has confounded even the physicians most committed to breastfeeding. It should be approached with the same orderly diagnostic process used to address any medical problem. Thus a complete history, including the details of the breastfeeds, a physical examination of the infant, an examination of the maternal breast, observation of the feeding, and appropriate laboratory work are indicated. Organizing the data collected by this process will help identify the maternal and infant causes separately.

Slow Gaining Versus Failure to Thrive

Some helpful distinctions exist between a breastfed infant who is slow to gain weight and the infant who is failing to thrive while breastfeeding versus excess weight loss in the first 2 to 4 weeks of life.[95] Assessing ongoing growth by serial weights, lengths, and head circumferences should be included in the routine "well baby" evaluation of all breastfed infants, beginning with the first visit. With serial measurements the infant's demonstrated weight gain over a specific number of days can be compared with the median daily weight gain for age (Table 10.1).[31,34] With early discharge often occurring less than 48 hours after birth, the first outpatient visit may need to be within 48 hours of discharge from the hospital, depending on an infant's gestational age, weight loss before discharge, and history of jaundice and in response to the mother's experience or needs. The pediatric office or clinic should have a failsafe system of follow-up for all newborns that includes access by telephone. The pediatric office also should be alert to the close follow-up of primiparas, especially those mothers who are older and well educated. A study of delayed lactogenesis and excess neonatal weight loss by Dewey et al.[38] revealed the high correlation not to ethnic groups, but to age and advanced education, noting increased problems with the early periods of breastfeeding. In the absence of reliable phone contact, visiting nurse involvement may be appropriate. Although many hospitals provide breastfeeding warm lines that mothers can call for information and help, the family must make the transition from the birthplace to the primary care provider promptly, especially for parents of a first baby who have no previous office contact. New parents often do not recognize when there is a problem.

The feeding pattern of an infant with slow weight gain is usually frequent feedings with evidence of a good suck (see Table 10.2). The mother's breasts are full before feeding, and she can describe a let-down during the feeding. At least six diapers per day are wet, urine is pale and dilute, and stools are

TABLE 10.2 Parameters for Evaluation of Breastfed Infants

Infant Who Is Slow to Gain Weight	Infant With Failure to Thrive
Alert healthy appearance	Apathetic or crying
Good muscle tone	Poor tone
Good skin turgor	Poor turgor
At least six wet diapers/day	Few wet diapers
Pale, dilute urine	"Strong" urine
Stools frequent, seedy (or if infrequent, large and soft)	Stools infrequent, scanty
Eight or more feedings/day, lasting 15–20 minutes	Fewer than eight feedings, often brief
Well-established let-down reflex	No signs of functioning let-down reflex
Weight gain consistent but slow	Weight erratic; may seem to lose weight at different points of assessment

Phillip B, Rosen-Carole C. What SHOULD happen when baby does not get enough milk from mom? https://www.babyfriendlyusa.org/news/what-should-happen-when-baby-does-not-get-enough-milk-from-mom/. December 3, 2019. Accessed February 20, 2020.

BOX 10.1   Conditions Associated With or Causing Disorders of Sucking and Swallowing

Absent or Diminished Suck

Maternal anesthesia or analgesia
Anoxia or hypoxia
Prematurity
Trisomy 21
Trisomy 13-15
Hypothyroidism
Neuromuscular abnormalities
Kernicterus
Werdnig-Hoffmann disease
Neonatal myasthenia gravis
Congenital muscular dystrophy
Central nervous system infections
Toxoplasmosis
Cytomegalovirus infection
Bacterial meningitis

Mechanical Factors Interfering With Sucking

Macroglossia
Cleft lip
Fusion of gums
Tumors of mouth or gums
Temporomandibular ankylosis or hypoplasia

Disorders of Swallowing Mechanism (Not Including Esophageal Abnormalities)

Choanal atresia
Cleft palate
Micrognathia
Postintubation dysphagia
Palatal paralysis
Pharyngeal tumors
Pharyngeal diverticula
Familial dysautonomia

loose and seedy. Weight gain is slow but consistent. If the infant is gaining extremely slowly but is alert, bright, responsive, and developing along the appropriate level, the infant is a "slow gainer." In contrast, the infant with true failure to thrive is usually apathetic or weakly crying with poor tone and poor turgor. Few diapers are wet (none is ever soaked) and urine is "strong." Stools are infrequent and scanty. Feedings are often by schedule but always fewer than eight per day and brief. No signs of a good let-down reflex are found. True failure to thrive is potentially serious; early recognition is essential if the integrity of both brain growth and breastfeeding is to be safely preserved.

Although slow gaining may be familial or genetic (small parents), it is always appropriate to be sure the process of breastfeeding is optimized.[46] Attention to adequate fat in the milk is important, especially because mothers have often been encouraged to "switch nurse," that is, switch back and forth between breasts in each feeding to build up an adequate milk supply. The switch-nursing process interrupts the release of fat and the production of fat-rich hindmilk. If the mother is interrupting the feeding to go to the other side, a period of

feeding exclusively on one breast during each feeding may change the gaining pattern. If necessary, the level of fat in the milk can be checked by doing a "creamatocrit," comparing milk before and after the switch from one breast to the other (see Chapter 22). By weighing the infant before and after a feeding with a digital readout scale, an accurate measurement of breast milk intake can be recorded. A slow gainer will have good intake during the individual feeding.

In a schema for classifying failure to thrive at the breast, the causes associated with infant behavior and problems are distinguished from those related to maternal problems (Fig. 10.1). The causes in the infant can be further evaluated by looking at net intake, which may be associated with poor feeding, poor net intake from additional losses, or high energy needs. The maternal causes can be divided into poor production of milk and poor release of milk. When a poor let-down reflex continues long enough, it will eventually cause a decrease in milk production. Several factors may affect the outcome, and more than one management change may be indicated in supporting breastfeeding and suggesting changes to the mother.

Evaluation of Infant

Examination of the infant should suggest any underlying physical problems, such as hypothyroidism, congenital heart disease, mechanical abnormalities of the mouth (e.g., cleft palate), or major neurologic disturbances.[96] An infant's ability to root, suck, and coordinate swallowing should be observed (Box 10.1). Today, a greater risk for missing subtle structural problems exists because infants spend much of their hospital life out of the newborn nursery away from the eyes of experienced nurses and are discharged before problems manifest.

The routine observation of a feeding by an infant's physician should be part of the discharge examination from the hospital. If this is not practical, such an examination should be incorporated into the first office or clinic visit within the first week of life. The mother should be asked to let you see how the baby feeds. The focus, however, should be to watch the positioning of the mother and the infant, placement of the mother's hands, and initiation of latch-on (see Chapter 7). A small number of infants will be identified with physical abnormalities or conditions that interfere with feeding and that need early medical attention (see Box 10.1).

Lukefahr identified 38 infants younger than 6 months of age in a suburban pediatric practice as having failure to thrive while breastfeeding.[97] Only 2 of 28 infants (7.1%) who presented in the first 4 weeks had underlying illnesses (salt-losing adrenogenital syndrome and congenital hypotonia); 5 of the 10 presenting between 1 and 6 months had underlying disease (all of whom actually presented with a problem by 4 months). This report stresses the importance of ruling out underlying disease and the urgency of having a pediatrician evaluate a child when the symptom of poor weight gain is first suspected, thus avoiding the serious complications of dehydration and metabolic disorders that may result when "home remedies" for lactation problems are used.

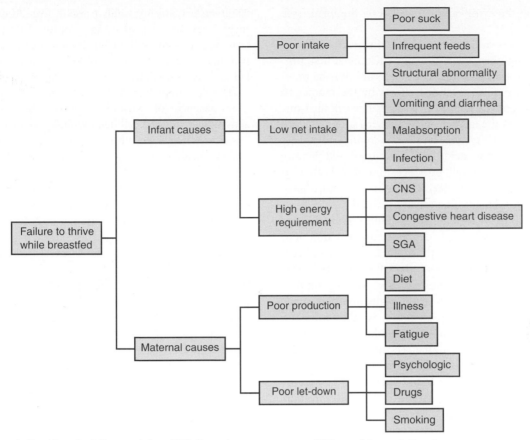

Fig. 10.1 Diagnostic flowchart for failure to thrive. *CNS*, Central nervous system; *SGA*, small for gestational age.

Oral motor problems: feeding skills disorder. Growth failure secondary to feeding skills disorder is the terminology proposed by Ramsay et al. and others to replace nonorganic failure to thrive.[98,99] The authors describe a series of children who were referred for nonorganic failure to thrive who had displayed subtle problems since birth. The criteria include early abnormal feeding-related symptoms present shortly after birth, such as impaired oral function, suggesting the infants are minimally neurologically abnormal, sometimes associated with borderline low Apgar scores. Difficulties during earlier stages of feeding development not only may interfere with the development of more mature feeding skills, but also may contribute eventually to difficulties in mother–infant interaction. The common finding among all infants with failure to thrive was underlying feeding-related symptoms that were neurophysiologic but manifested in different degrees of oral sensorimotor (and pharyngeal) impairment. The neurologic impairment may vary from obvious cerebral palsy to symptoms that are not apparent on casual observation but lead to abnormal feeding-related symptoms in early life. When the mother copes and adapts feeding to the infant, the disorder may go unnoticed until solid foods are added. Diagnosis requires oral sensorimotor assessments and a focused neurologic examination sensitive enough to measure minimal neurologic impairment in an apparently healthy child who is failing to gain. Prenatal, perinatal, and early postnatal history are also critically important to identifying risk factors and potential contributing causes of impairment.

Small-for-gestational-age infant. The SGA infant will be identified if gestational age and birth weight are scrutinized. This infant is small at birth in comparison to newborn standards for weight for specific gestational time in utero or postconceptional age. An SGA infant has a large nutritional deficit from intrauterine failure to grow. The cause of the intrauterine problem should be assessed: placental insufficiency, maternal disease, toxemia, heavy smoking, or intrauterine infection, such as toxoplasmosis, etc. SGA can be symmetric, involving weight, length, and head circumference each being the same relative amount lower than the accepted standards or just weight (asymmetric).

SGA infants may be difficult to feed initially by any method and often require tube feedings for a few days. Their caloric needs parallel the needs of an infant of appropriate weight for gestational age rather than their actual low weight. SGA infants should be placed on frequent feedings, every 2 to 3 hours by day and every 4 hours at night. They should be awakened for feedings if they sleep long periods. If they have not been nursing well, the breast may not be stimulated to produce to its full capability. The mother may need to express milk manually or mechanically pump milk to enhance her production. Her milk may then be given by a passive means such as a tube, a small cup, or the lactation supplementing device, which provides additional stimulus to the breast while providing the extra calories needed by the infant (see Chapter 19).

An infant who is sufficiently starved in utero may have a degree of inanition that prevents active suckling at first, predisposing to further starvation. The successful nursing of an SGA infant may require extended efforts by the mother to ensure adequate growth. Such efforts are well worth the trouble if one considers the impact of intrauterine growth failure on the central nervous system. It is to the infant's advantage to have the critical amino acids, such as taurine, and the mix of fatty acids that human milk provides, for optimal catch-up brain growth.[100] As noted earlier, SGA infants are more likely to close the growth gap more rapidly if breastfed.[58]

Jaundice. An infant with an elevated bilirubin level from any cause may be neurologically depressed and lethargic and, therefore, may not nurse well. If the infant appears jaundiced, laboratory evaluation to determine the cause and its appropriate treatment should be undertaken. Visible jaundice under 24 hours of age requires a full evaluation and is not related to breastfeeding. When an infant is taken from the breast at 2 or 3 days of age because of jaundice, this interferes with the establishment of lactation at a critical time, especially for a primipara. Management of the jaundiced infant depends on adequate calories, hydration, and the active passage of stools, which is the means by which the body excretes the bilirubin in meconium and stools.

"Breastfeeding jaundice," which is related to underfeeding or starvation, does not develop until the infant is 3 or more days old, so other causes must be sought if the jaundice appears earlier. In addition, care must be taken to help the mother continue to stimulate milk production with manual expression or pumping to avoid inducing iatrogenic lactation failure. (See Chapter 13 for discussion of hyperbilirubinemia.)

Metabolic screen. Most hospitals provide, often because the law mandates it, screening for rare genetic metabolic disorders, including galactosemia, phenylketonuria, maple syrup urine disease, and disorders of metabolism of other amino acids. If these simple screening tests were not performed or their validity is in doubt, they should be done again. Usually the service is available in the state or county laboratory. Thyroid screening for abnormal thyroxine (T_4) or thyroid-stimulating hormone also should be performed. Mass screening programs for neonatal thyroid disease have identified cases of deficiency that, even in retrospect, were not in evidence at birth or early on; the infant showed none of the characteristic findings of hypothyroidism, such as thick, coarse features; hoarse cry; slow pulse; macroglossia; umbilical hernia; and jaundice. In the neonate, hypothyroidism is often associated with failure to thrive if undiagnosed and untreated.

Galactosemia. Galactosemia, which is a hereditary disorder of the metabolism of galactose-1-phosphate, is manifest by renal disease and liver dysfunction after ingestion of lactose. The lack of galactose-1-phosphate uridyltransferase activity may be relative or partial. The clinical symptoms may be fulminating, with severe jaundice, hepatosplenomegaly, weight loss, vomiting, and diarrhea, or may be more subtle.

Cataracts are not invariably present. In mild cases, failure to thrive may be the presenting symptom. A urine screen for reducing substances (by Clinitest and not Dextrostix, which will identify only glucose) should be done on all infants who fail to thrive, especially if there is hepatomegaly or jaundice.

The definitive diagnosis is the identification of absence or near absence of galactose-1-phosphate uridyltransferase activity in red blood cell hemolysates. Even though a routine initial metabolic screen for galactosemia was done on the second or third day of life, a urine screen should be considered. The treatment is a lactose-free diet, which would mandate prompt weaning from breast milk to prevent further insult to the liver, kidneys, and brain. This is one of the few indications for prompt weaning from human milk. A formula free of lactose (e.g., Isomil, Nutramigen) is indicated. No medical indications exist, however, to use a lactose-free formula for a normal breastfeeding infant either to supplement or to wean from breast milk, which contains lactose. (Refer to pediatric texts on neonatal metabolic disorders for a full description of galactosemia; see also Chapter 13.)

Vomiting and diarrhea. Vomiting and diarrhea are unusual in a breastfed infant. Spitting up small amounts of milk after feedings is sometimes observed in otherwise normal infants and is of no consequence if it does not affect overall weight gain. Although pyloric stenosis is reportedly less common in breastfed infants, this phenomenon should be ruled out in any infant who vomits consistently after feeding, has diminished urine and stools, and shows no weight gain or loses weight. Usually these infants do well initially and then the vomiting becomes progressive at 4 to 8 weeks of age.

Vomiting may be a manifesting symptom for various metabolic disorders. Thus metabolic disorders should be considered in the differential diagnosis. All possible metabolic disorders, such as congenital adrenal hyperplasia, are not routinely screened. These infants may present with vomiting and weight loss in the first week or two of life or with an acute episode of sepsis. The usual causes of vomiting, as well as the causes peculiar to breast milk, should be considered. Maternal diet should be checked for unusual foods. In families at high risk for allergy, intake by the mother of known family food allergens may cause symptoms in the infant. Diarrhea may be caused by foods in the mother's diet or her use of cathartics, such as phenolphthalein.

Chronic infections. Chronic fetal infection in utero, which predisposes the infant to intrauterine growth failure, may continue to cause growth problems postnatally in the presence of adequate kilocalories. Chronic viral infections include cytomegalovirus, hepatitis, acquired immunodeficiency syndrome (AIDS), or other less common viruses (see Chapter 12).

Acute infections. An infant who is not growing well may have an infection in the gastrointestinal tract; therefore the nature of the stools is important. The urinary tract may be another site of infection not readily identified. If, however, the initial evaluation includes a urinalysis with microscopic evaluation and a white blood cell count and differential count, this can usually be ruled out (see Chapter 12).

High energy requirements. When the metabolic rate of an infant is increased, weight gain will be diminished or absent. When the infant is hyperactive with a strong startle reflex and sleeps poorly, consideration should be given to stimulants present in the milk as well as to neurologic disorders. When a mother drinks coffee, tea (including herbal teas), cola, or other carbonated beverages with added caffeine, the accumulated caffeine may be enough to make the infant irritable and hyperactive and affect feeding. The best treatment is to replace the caffeine-containing beverages (see Chapter 11). Some disorders of the central nervous system are associated with hyperactivity. Infants with severe congenital heart disease are "working" to breathe and oxygenate and often have greatly increased metabolic rates. For management of these special infants at the breast, see Chapter 13.

Observation of Nursing Process

In addition to establishing that no obvious physical or metabolic reasons exist for the failure to gain weight, an infant should be observed suckling at the breast. Does the infant get a good latch and suck vigorously? If not, what interferes? A receding chin, a weak suck, lack of coordination, the breast obstructing breathing, and mouthing of the nipple or other ineffectual sucking motions are some of the possibilities. If the problem is the suckling process, the infant may need assistance. This cause is more common with infants who have had some experience with bottles or rubber nipples or who use a pacifier. Small or slightly premature infants who were started on bottle feedings have trouble "relearning" the proper sucking motion with the tongue (see Chapter 7).

Bottle-feedings and pacifiers may have to be discontinued until the infant is more experienced at the breast. This may require a program of manually expressing milk to soften the areola, having milk at the nipple to entice the infant, and gently offering the nipple and areola well compressed between two fingers. If the infant has a receding chin or a relaxed jaw, it may help to have the mother hold the lower jaw forward by supporting the angle of the jaw with her thumb. The physician should examine the infant carefully to be sure the jaw is not dislocated, especially if a vertex delivery was done in the posterior position. The physician can easily move the jaw forward to relocate it.

Positioning the infant for the breast so the child directly faces the breast, straddling the mother's leg in a semi-upright position, may work best. This is the position twins may assume when nursing simultaneously when they are 3 to 4 months old. Although it is not recommended routinely, for an infant with a receding chin or a cleft, having the mother lean slightly forward for latch-on may help. She should then bring the infant upward as she sits back for the feeding.

It may be necessary to assist both mother and baby with presentation of the breast and latch. If the infant by 2 weeks of age cannot maintain the breast in the mouth without the mother holding it, it is an indication of improper suckling and warrants additional evaluation of the infant. In that situation, the infant may need to be repositioned with the ventral surface squarely facing the mother's chest wall—that is,

tummy to tummy—and the breast presented by the mother with her hand positioned with thumb on top and fingers below the breast. (See discussion in Chapter 7.) The mother may have to maintain support throughout the feeding. Failure to maintain the breast in the mouth has neurologic implications for long-term follow-up.

When infants have trouble maintaining the latch when the flow of milk is excessive and causes choking, the mother may try lying flat on her back holding the infant over the breast, which she supports with her hand. The flow becomes manageable and the infant's mouth relaxes and draws in the breast.

A good check of adequate let-down is to observe the opposite breast as the baby nurses to see if milk flows. It also can be tested by seeing if milk is flowing when nursing is interrupted abruptly. If let-down was good, milk will continue to flow, at least drop by drop, for a few moments from the breast that had been suckled. A mother can be trained to listen for the infant's swallowing. During proper suckling, the masseter muscle in the jaw is in full view and is contracting visibly and rhythmically. Swallowing can be seen and heard. The ratio of suck to swallow is 1:1 or 2:1. Occasionally, infants do not suck vigorously at the breast but occasionally use rapid shallow sucks called "flutter sucking" with little or no swallowing. These infants can be gradually taught to suck effectively. Correct positioning of the breast directly in the infant's mouth and holding the breast firmly in position with all the fingers under the breast and only the thumb above allows the infant to grasp properly without sucking the tongue or lower lip. Nipple shields usually make the situation worse.

The most productive part of the diagnostic workup is often observation of the baby at the breast. For this reason, this critical responsibility should not be passed on to others but should be performed personally by the physician as well as a certified lactation consultant.

The five general types of nursing patterns described in Chapter 7 should be kept in mind. If the mother understands that it is acceptable for the infant to drop off to sleep and snack later, she may not hesitate to follow this lead, thus providing a more adequate feeding.

Some infants will not settle down and nurse well if there is too much activity or noise in the room. Some need to be tightly swaddled; others fall asleep and need to be unwrapped and stimulated to provide adequate suckling time. Frequent feedings, using both breasts, may be the answer in some cases. In others, there may be too many ineffective feedings, which are wearing the mother out; a change that lengthens the time between feedings but also lengthens the time at the breast may help, especially if it is quiet and the mother's position allows her to nap while feeding. Concentrating on using one breast at a feeding, emptying the hindmilk with its higher fat content may be the most effective change in adding to the infant's caloric intake.

Psychosocial Failure to Thrive

In the study of undernutrition in bottle-fed infants and infants beyond the suckling age, terminology has received more attention than the underlying issues. Thus the emphasis has been on "organic" versus "nonorganic" failure to thrive. A disorder of maternal–infant bonding has become synonymous with maternal deprivation. *Reactive attachment disorder* has been the term applied when bonding or attachment difficulties lead to growth faltering. When an infant does not have an organic disorder that explains the growth failure, the patient is diagnosed as having psychosocial failure to thrive. Often the typical psychosocial and nutritional pattern reported in psychosocial failure to thrive includes evidence of a chaotic/overly stressful family life, emotional deprivation, and inadequate nutrition. To effectively support and assist the mother and family it is important to understand the underlying reasons for the stress(es), the emotional upset, and the issues regarding nutrition in the home. Domestic violence and postnatal depression are common underlying situations.

Prolonged Exclusive Breastfeeding

Prolonged exclusive breastfeeding may occasionally result in a unique deficit in the developmental process of eating. Exclusive breastfeeding is not nutritionally adequate in the second half of the first year, especially beyond 12 months, although nursing can safely continue for several years when combined with adequate solids that provide appropriate amounts of protein, iron, and zinc. The syndrome of the breastfed infant in the second 6 months of life with frequent breastfeeding, poor intake of complementary foods, and poor growth was labeled a manifestation of "vulnerable child syndrome" by O'Connor and Szekely.[101] These children are described to have good weight gain for 5 to 6 months, but by 8 months their weight/height score has decreased dramatically. The intake of solid foods is minimal; these infants refuse solids, aggressively spitting food out. The breastfeeding pattern is usually every 1 to 2 hours during the day and frequently at night. Further investigation revealed numerous household stressors, sometimes lack of understanding of the nutritional role of breastfeeding and complementary foods at this age, or the mother's need to maintain control of nutrition/feeding by breastfeeding.

Growth Faltering

The growth of predominantly breastfed infants who live in underprivileged populations in developing countries has been reported to falter between 4 and 6 months of age, but the reason has never been well understood. This growth faltering was reported by different research groups in Mexico City, Brazil, and four prospective cohorts studied in Ghana, Malawi, and Burkina Faso.[102–104] In developed countries, energy intake declines between 4 and 6 months but growth does not falter. To determine whether growth faltering in this age-group was due to inadequate intake of human milk, the nutrient intakes of 30 Otami Indian infants from farms in Capulhuac, Mexico, were studied from 4 to 6 months.[105] Growth velocities were not correlated with nutrient intakes. The children's growth faltered despite energy intakes comparable with those of children in more supportive and protected environments. The energy requirements of these children were significantly higher. Some infants in developed countries may live in equally challenging environments leading to an increased energy requirement. Others looked at the growth reference standards used for this apparent "growth faltering" and suggested that the standards may not reflect the growth of exclusively/predominantly breastfed infants.[106] This was one more issue that led to the development of the WHO child growth standards for breastfed infants.[107]

At this point in time, if "growth faltering" is observed in one or more breastfed children while using the WHO growth standards for infants and children, assessment for extenuating circumstances and energy expenditure and consumption should be undertaken.[108] Interventions to improve the caloric consumption and nutrient intake (protein, iron, zinc) are appropriate during this important window of opportunity for nutrition and growth in infants and children.[109]

Health Beliefs

Parental misconception and health beliefs concerning what constitutes a normal diet for infants have been reported by Pugliese et al.[110] as a cause for failure to thrive. They reported seven infants from 7 to 22 months of age with poor weight gain and linear growth who received only 60% to 94% of minimum caloric intake for their age and sex. The parents explained that they wanted to avoid obesity, atherosclerosis, or junk food habits. It also has been shown that parental health beliefs and expectations have led to short stature and delayed puberty in older children.

Fruit Juice Excess

The custom of excessive use of fruit juices in recent decades has replaced the use of water for additional fluids after 6 months of life when the infant is learning to drink from a cup or a straw. The attractive packaging has contributed to this trend. Excessive fruit juice diminishes appetite, resulting in decreased dietary intake of nutrient-dense foods and a decrease in weight gain and ultimately in linear growth. An excess of fruit juice may be a cause of failure to thrive in older infants. Decrease in total high-energy intake is combined with malabsorption of fructose and diarrhea from sorbitol, thus compounding the problem.[111] Excessive fruit juice intake in infancy is a major nutrition problem because juice has low nutrient value but high calories. The AAP has developed a guideline with restrictions on the use of fruit juices. For older children, their high caloric content may be a contributor to obesity.

Maternal Causes

Questions about a mother's health, dietary habits, sleep pattern, smoking habits, medication intake, the events that occur during nursing, and the psychosocial atmosphere in the home are an important part of the history (Fig. 10.2).

Anatomic Causes

Lactation failure from insufficient glandular development of the breast has been described by Neifert et al. and Seacat and

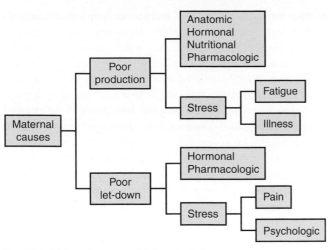

Fig. 10.2 Maternal causes of failure to thrive.

Neifert, who report three cases in which the breast tissue was asymmetric.[112,113] Transillumination confirmed a minimally active gland. One family showed a history of similar failure. All three women benefited psychologically from the diagnosis and chose to continue to breastfeed and supplement. The authors have since identified 14 more women who had anatomic deficiency but normal prolactin levels and failed to respond to a thorough team approach to lactation support.[113] Retained placenta is also a cause of early lactation failure that is quickly identified by a complete history of postpartum breast change and patterns of lochia that an obstetrician associates with retained tissue (see Chapter 15). If prolactin response to stimulus is adequate, ultrasonography can determine the presence of adequate mammary tissue and ductal arborization.[89,114] There are various case reports describing women with insufficient glandular tissue who successfully fed their infants with partial breastfeeding and supplementation because of their commitment to breastfeeding and their plan for infant feeding.[89,114]

One-Breast Versus Two-Breast Feeding

An infant whose failure to thrive was traced to inadequate fat intake associated with using both breasts without completely emptying either, with each feed resulting in low fat (and relatively high lactose by comparison) intake, caused the debate regarding using one or two breasts during each feeding to be rekindled. When this infant was fed at one breast per feeding, the low-density caloric feeding changed to high-fat feeding, resulting in decreased stooling and increased weight gain. Some women require more time to release fat into the milk and limiting the feeding to one breast increases emptying the breast and the hindmilk, leading to enhanced fat content. In some cases, this is true, and it is further verified by an infant fed at both breasts having many loose stools because of the high lactose and considerable gassy discomfort that also resolves with the change to single-breast feeds.

In early lactation, when milk supply is being established, mothers may be encouraged to nurse on both breasts at each feed to provide frequent stimulus. A clinician, however, should obtain a thorough history of feeding frequency and distribution between breasts, especially when the infant is well hydrated, has many stools, and may or may not be fussy but fails to gain weight, remaining less than birth weight for several weeks. The need for higher fat content in the feeding may be a consideration in the slow-gaining baby as well. An adjustment in feeding to enhance the fat content should be tried. Usually limiting each feeding to one breast will do that (see Chapter 7). However, some women have smaller storage capacity than others, as demonstrated with ultrasound imagery by Hartmann et al.[115] These women need to feed from both breasts at each feed but completely emptying each to ensure that the infant gets the "hind" milk with higher percent fat. Storage capacity ranges from 100 to more than 250 mL per breast.[115,116] There is evidence in the literature that milk intake by infants fed as needed relates to the appetite of the infant and not to the amount of milk present in the breasts. Daly and others demonstrated that the change in breast volume from before to after a breastfeed was closely related to the volume of milk the infant consumed as determined by test weighing of the infant (r=0.93).[117,118] They also measured the rate of milk synthesis between breastfeeds, for six women varied from 11 to 58 mL/hour. These results show that the amount of milk available in the breast is not necessarily an important determinant of the amount of milk removed by the infant at a breastfeeding. When assessing milk synthesis in a mother, measurement of milk production for each breast is indicated.[119] Daly et al.[120] also showed that short-term rates of milk synthesis varied markedly between the breasts of individual mothers. It was clear from this work that variations in the short-term rates of milk synthesis and responsiveness of milk synthesis to the degree of breast emptying provided mechanisms whereby maternal milk supply could be directly linked to infant demand.[120] When assessing the infant's nutritional intake, it is the overall milk volume per day ingested without distinction between the amount produced by each breast.

Poor Milk Production

Diets. Although it has been demonstrated that malnourished mothers can produce milk for their infants, marginal diets in Western cultures do affect some mothers' ability to nourish an infant. A case of failure to thrive in a breastfed infant associated with maternal dietary protein and energy restriction was reported.[121] The mother, at 8 months postpartum, independently reduced her dietary energy to 20 kcal/kg per day and her protein to 0.7 g/kg per day to treat cholecystitis medically and avoid surgery. At 12 months, her infant's growth curves had fallen below the 5th percentile in both weight and length, although the infant had been receiving solid foods since 24 weeks of age. The authors concluded the failure to thrive was directly related to severe maternal restriction.[121] Dietary analysis and maternal anthropometry showed that women who gained adequate weight and skin thickness during pregnancy had increased milk production and weight gain in their infants for the first 6 months of life.[18]

If a mother is restricting intake deliberately or inadvertently, she should be instructed to meet the dietary requirement for lactating women (a minimum of 1800 kcal/day for adequate nutrient intake) (see Chapter 8). She does not have to drink milk, but the necessary dietary constituents should be in the diet through cheese, eggs, ice cream, or other sources of calcium and protein. Studies of hormones triggered while eating have shown that more milk is produced if a mother eats just before or during breastfeeding. Prescribing brewer's yeast as a dietary supplement has been observed to provide improvement in milk production beyond that accounted for by mere addition of the same nutrients. Some mothers report a feeling of well-being from taking yeast that they do not obtain from taking daily vitamins. Concern has been expressed regarding the effect of increased vitamin B_6 on prolactin production, but doses that suppress lactation are 60 times the commonly prescribed therapeutic dose.

Maternal Illness. The presence of infection or other illness in a mother may affect milk production, and the cause of the illness should be identified and treated. Urinary tract infection, endometritis, or upper respiratory tract infection may need treatment with antibiotics. The antibiotic prescribed also should be appropriate for the infant because it will pass into the milk. Metabolic disorders such as thyroid disease also should be considered. Postpartum hypothyroid disease is increasingly being recognized as screening tests of T_4 and thyroid-stimulating hormone are being done when a mother complains of severe "baby blues" or fatigue. Adequate treatment with thyroid hormone will result in increased milk supply.

Fatigue. Fatigue is a very common cause of inadequate milk supply. Fatigue may be caused by lack of sleep because the infant demands considerable attention at night, but generally it is more subtle. The pressures of the rest of the family for meals or services or the self-inflicted demands of a job, career, or social commitments may be the cause. The mother must be placed on a medically mandated strict rest regimen that is respected by family and friends. In the first month, while lactation is being established, fatigue is devastating to milk production. The infant then becomes hungry more often, cries, and demands more frequent feeding; thus a vicious circle is established. In later months of lactation, a mother becomes quickly aware of the impact of protracted fatigue on the nursing experience and usually will take steps to increase her rest.

Poor release of milk. Interference with the let-down reflex may cause a well-nourished lactating mother to fail to satisfy her infant. The collecting ducts may be full, but if the let-down or ejection reflex is not triggered, the process will be at a standstill. The infant becomes frustrated and pulls away crying or screaming. Interference with the ejection reflex, such as pain, fatigue, stress, smoking, and general environmental chaos, is predominantly situational and rarely hormonal (see Chapter 7).

Smoking may interfere with the let-down reflex. Mothers should be discouraged from ever smoking in the same room with the infant because of the occurrence of second-hand smoke predisposing to the early and frequent respiratory infections in infants of smokers. Smokers are less likely to breastfeed, and if they do choose to breastfeed, they tend to wean earlier because of insufficient milk. Trouble with milk production may be related to the nicotine. This has been observed in many situations, and there is a study that demonstrated a clear relationship between smoking and the amount of milk produced.[122] The infants of these mothers grew more slowly.[123–125] An epidemiologic review showed that women who smoke are both less likely to intend to breastfeed and less likely to initiate breastfeeding. Women who smoke are likely to breastfeed for a shorter duration than nonsmokers.[123] That same review by Donath and Amir[100] discussed several publications revealing a dose-response relationship between the number of cigarettes smoked each day and breastfeeding intention, initiation, and duration that persists after adjusting for potential confounding factors. Psychosocial intent and motivation are more likely reasons for the apparent association between smoking and shorter duration of breastfeeding than a physiologic explanation.[124,125] Avoiding smoking for 2 hours before a feeding will improve the let-down reflex and minimize the amount of nicotine in the milk. Given the value of breastfeeding to the infant, especially in reducing the risk for sudden infant death syndrome, it is important that smokers try to reduce the smoke exposure but still breastfeed (see Chapter 15).

Experimentally, alcohol has been shown to interfere with oxytocin release in laboratory animals, but the dosage used correlates with moderate to heavy drinking in humans. Studies following the offspring of women who drink heavily have shown some delay in gross motor activity at 1 year using the Bayley developmental scales.[126] Other studies have suggested that alcohol changes the flavor of the milk and that infants nurse less well at a feeding immediately after the mother has had a drink.[127,128] This is contrary to observations over the years in countries where wine and beer are common beverages and are considered galactagogues (see Chapter 11).

The clinician should consider the impact of smoking or alcohol use in the context of reviewing inadequate milk production.

Medications that the mother may be taking should be evaluated. Although L-dopa and ergot preparations are known to inhibit prolactin release, other medications not clearly implicated may have the same effect (see Chapter 11).

The most common cause for the failure of the ejection reflex is psychologic inhibition. In a few cases the cause of the psychologic stress may be obvious, such as a family member who openly disapproves of breastfeeding, but in most cases the nursing mother has already considered this possibility and reassures the physician that she is relaxed and calm. It will require carefully assessing the mother's history to "tease out" the source of stress. This is the time when a home visit by the nurse practitioner from the physician's office or an experienced public health nurse will be valuable. The nurse may observe what is overlooked by the mother: construction of a new building next door, incessant barking from the neighbor's dog, or marital discord. Home observation may lead to the source of the problem.

No Obvious Cause

Even though no obvious cause for failure to thrive is identified, the treatment may have to include establishing a positive attitude. Jelliffe and Jelliffe have often referred to nursing as a "confidence game."[129] Once a mother's breastfeeding goals and intentions are clear, it becomes necessary to share confidence and support and problem solve how to foster those going forward. Quickly recommending to a mother that she stop breastfeeding and switch to formula without additional assistance and support to facilitate breast milk production and delivery does not instill confidence. A physician should prescribe a positive plan for the number and length of feedings, suggest diet and rest for the mother, and set reachable goals for infant growth.

If the let-down reflex is the crux of the problem and simple adjustments have not changed the ejection quality, oxytocin as a nasal spray (Pitocin) can be prescribed (see Chapters 7 and 19). It is available only by prescription and should be used under the physician's guidance because of possible side effects in some women (e.g., headache, vasoconstriction), although it is not dangerous. Oxytocin nasal spray does not affect the milk or the infant. It is contraindicated only in pregnancy or hypersensitivity. A commercial preparation of oxytocin nasal spray is no longer available; it can be prepared by a pharmacist placing Pitocin in a nasal dropper.

Seven mothers whose breastfed infants were contented but failing to grow were given metoclopramide (or chlorpromazine in one) in various dosages.[130] Only one mother thought it was not helpful. The authors did not describe how effective appropriate supportive breastfeeding management was and when the medication was started or how long it was maintained. All the infants gained weight, and breastfeeding was continued for 2 to 12 months.

Other authors have also reported the recovery from lactation failure by mothers taking metoclopramide (10 mg three times per day).[131] Gupta and Gupta reported a 67% success rate in those with no milk and 100% recovery in those with an "inadequate supply."[132] The effect continued after the drug was discontinued. Such a medication is useful only when accompanied by appropriate instructions for proper breastfeeding and assistance in using a breast pump for additional stimulus to increase the supply of milk mechanically. A medication should be prescribed only when routine methods fail. Effect of the drug may dissipate if the infant is still unable to go to the breast. Domperidone (Motilium), a peripheral dopamine antagonist, is known to enhance milk production, although clinical experience in blinded controlled studies is absent. Available internationally but not in the United States, it has to be ordered by prescription. It is reported to modestly enhance milk production with a dosage of 10 to 20 mg orally three to four times per day.[133] Maternal side effects include headaches, dry mouth, gastrointestinal complaints, prolonged QTc, and arrythmias. There is one report of prolonged QTc without clinical symptoms in breastfed infants whose mothers were taking domperidone.[133]

Measurement of prolactin levels is readily available in most laboratories, but the appropriate clinical protocol has not been confirmed by controlled study. Given the information about baseline and response to stimuli (see Chapter 3), it would be advisable to obtain a baseline prolactin level, which should be above normal for the laboratory, and a second value after 10 minutes of breastfeeding. Using a heparin lock with venous line placed well before the baseline specimen is drawn and before feeding ensures the least disturbance to lactation. The prolactin value during feeding should show a significant increase over baseline (usually more than twice baseline).

A group of women diagnosed with lactation insufficiency by history were given thyrotropin-releasing hormone (TRH).[134] Four received 5 mg every 12 hours for 5 days. A consistent 50% increase in prolactin concentrations was seen. Both milk production and let-down were increased. Nine women received 20 mg twice per day, and baseline prolactin was significantly elevated. The women reported subjective and objective increases in breast engorgement and milk let-down, and all returned to full nursing. Two women were given TRH 40 mg daily for 5 days and developed clinical signs of thyrotoxicosis by the seventh day, which disappeared by the tenth day. The investigators had previously given TRH to fully lactating women in a controlled study to demonstrate prolactin response, which occurred within 60 minutes.[134] No change in milk volume or quality in these fully lactating women and no side effects were observed. When Hall and Kay gave TRH 200 mg and followed prolactin and milk production for 6 hours, no dramatic changes in milk production were observed, although the prolactin levels rose.[135] There is no indication that the mothers received more than 1 day's dose. Such an oral TRH product is not clinically available.

A rare infant who does not respond to breastfeeding management adjustment may have a malabsorption or metabolic disease as yet undiagnosed that will not become overt until the child is exposed to formula, cow milk, or solid foods. Infants with a strong family history of cystic fibrosis, milk allergy, or malabsorption should have a careful diagnostic workup before abandoning human milk, which may be the most physiologic feeding available for the infant. Neonatal metabolic screening tests should be repeated.

Dehydration, Hypernatremia, or Hypochloremia

A few cases of severe disease with inadequate breastfeeding have been reported in the literature. These infants were hospitalized because of dehydration and evidence of more severe metabolic disturbance. They illustrate the potential severe outcomes if anticipatory care, early diagnostic assessment, or home management is unsuccessful. The mothers are usually but not always primiparas, new at breastfeeding and child rearing. When the record is reviewed, one often sees that the early danger signs were present at discharge from the hospital. The mother may have a history of difficult delivery or be taking medication for pain that leads to a less vigorous baby and, secondarily, inadequate stimulus for lactation. Supplementary bottles of water or milk were initiated in the hospital instead of directing attention toward the lactation process.[136,137]

As a precautionary measure, a physician should see all breastfeeding dyads promptly in the postpartum period. At this visit, review of the mother's experience and perception of the breastfeeding process and assessment of the infant's weight, feeding history, number of wet diapers, stool pattern, and physical findings should alert the physician to impending difficulties. Observation of the infant at the breast should be part of the assessment. A problem in monitoring breastfed infants is the use of ultra-absorbent diapers, which makes it impossible to detect the number of voidings or volume of urine passed. No specimen can be wrung from the diaper for specific gravity or other analysis. It is recommended that parents of infants younger than 2 months not use ultra-absorbent diapers, especially when the infant is breastfed, until a better monitoring device is developed or until breastfeeding is well established. If, on the other hand, the patient is not seen in the office until there is significant dehydration, it is urgent that laboratory studies, including those for sodium, chloride, potassium, pH, blood urea nitrogen, and hematocrit (bilirubin when indicated), be obtained. An assessment of the degree of dehydration should be made based on skin and tissue turgor and tone and urinary findings.[138,139]

When a breastfed infant has abnormal electrolyte levels, the physician should also obtain levels of sodium, chloride, and potassium from the mother's milk, being certain to sample each breast separately.[136,137] Collecting a few milliliters at the beginning and the end of the feeding and mixing the two samples from a single breast is a good technique. The infant may have occult loss of electrolytes, such as that seen in abnormal renal wasting or retention, cystic fibrosis, hyperaldosteronism, or pseudohyperaldosteronism. The simplest approach is to measure milk electrolytes and infant urine levels to rule out high milk sodium as a cause of the infant's hypernatremia. Weaning milk has elevated sodium, and it occurs when lactation is failing.

In reported cases, infants with hypernatremic failure to thrive are no different at initial presentation from infants with normal sodium levels.[95,136] They may even have an unremarkable neonatal history. At home they develop a poor suck, sleep for long intervals, cry infrequently, and feed infrequently. When observed at the breast, they may be labeled as having a sucking disorder. On examination, however, the lethargy, dehydration, and malnutrition are obvious to a skilled clinician. In the extreme, the infant may have cardiovascular collapse with hypothermia and hypoglycemia. Elevated serum blood urea nitrogen, creatinine, and hematocrit and urinary specific gravity confirm the diagnosis. Hypernatremia has been observed in approximately half of the reported cases of severe dehydration in breastfed infants.[136,138] Although milk sodium levels were not reported in all cases, several cases of elevated milk sodium have been reported. Sodium, chloride, and lactose are the prime constituents that control the osmolarity of the milk. Because the sodium, chloride, and lactose have a reciprocal relationship, inadequate lactose production ultimately results in elevated sodium level (see Chapter 4).[136,139]

Elevated sodium levels in the milk may be a cause or an effect of insufficient milk. When the breast is inadequately stimulated, it begins to involute and produces "weaning milk," which is high in sodium. Milk pumped from non-lactators in the postpartum period has a high sodium content. Maternal sodium intake excesses do not result in elevated sodium levels in the milk.[140] Sodium enters the milk by a controlled mechanism independent of maternal levels in normal women. The milk sodium level is much lower than that of serum sodium, whereas the milk potassium level is much higher than serum levels.

Hypernatremic dehydration is an emergency that requires hospitalization.[95] The mother should room-in if at all possible. Most pediatric units provide this option. It is preferable to maintain lactation in most cases. The treatment of the illness after the dehydration has been treated with intravenous fluids depends on the cause of the hypernatremia. The sodium level of an infant's serum and mother's milk should be followed until normal. Increasing maternal milk output with appropriate lactation counseling, including mechanical pumping between feedings to increase volume, usually normalizes the sodium content. The oral feedings for the infant should be limited to breastfeeding after milk sodium content is normal while the intravenous fluids are tapered. To provide increased caloric resources to the infant and an appropriate sodium load, the Lact-Aid supplementer (see Chapter 19) also may be used to stimulate the breast and to avoid bottle feeding and inadequate intake until the breast increases production.

Chloride deficiency has received attention because of a highly publicized formula-manufacturing error. This syndrome is characterized by failure to thrive with anorexia, hypochloremia, and hypokalemic metabolic alkalosis. Chloride deficiency syndrome has also been reported in an infant whose mother had only 2 mEq/L of chloride in her milk (normal 8 mEq/L).[139] The mother had successfully nourished her previous five infants. The infant had done well until 3 months of age and then had gradually slipped below the 3rd percentile for weight at 6 months. The infant was severely dehydrated and hypotonic with plasma sodium of 123 mEq/L, chloride of 72 mEq/L, potassium of 2.9 mEq/L, and blood pH of 7.61. There were no abnormal urinary losses. When the breastfeeding infant has clinical dehydration, it is important to check not only the sodium but also the chloride content of the infant's serum and urine and the mother's milk.

Human infants younger than 3 weeks of age do not respond to inappropriate solutions by not suckling. This finding is also observed in studies in other species in which pups continue to suck when the solution is unphysiologic. A natural experiment occurred in a newborn nursery and was reported in the literature, when six infants died of hypernatremia after receiving many feedings of formula made from salt rather than sugar.[141] The infants who were younger than 1 week old did not reject the feedings.

Lactation Failure

Occasionally, failure to thrive is actually caused by lactation failure. Historically, sudden complete cessation of lactation was described in the late 1800s after horse-drawn carriage accidents and other great trauma. Advocates of breastfeeding have tended to dismiss this as a possibility and struggle frantically to reverse the situation. Some women who cannot make milk have primary hypoprolactinemia, and others have secondary hypoprolactinemia, as in Sheehan syndrome (see Chapter 15). When reasonable efforts at stimulation are ineffective and the mother is unable to do without the Lact-Aid providing almost a full feeding volume, evaluation of the mother by prolactin level measurement is appropriate.[109,142] Some mothers prefer to discontinue efforts to breastfeed instead of undergoing additional medical evaluation.

If one explores the literature on other mammals, one finds no similar situations in other species. Lactation failure in nursing animals is rare—it is not a trait that is transmitted from generation to generation because the offspring do not survive. Interferences with milk ejection can be identified and treated in some mammals. A syndrome in sows involves agalactia associated with mastitis and metritis.[143] Mammalian lactation failure is attributed to nutritional, pharmacologic, and "emotional stress" causes in animals. Aside from gross dietary deficiency, there is depression or inhibition of the anterior pituitary gland, which is responsible for synthesis in the alveolar cells, and inhibition of transport and discharge of synthesized products from alveolar cells to the lumen. Certain plant alkaloids have been noted in other species to inhibit lactation. Ergot derivatives are best known, but colchicine, vincristine, and vinblastine also inhibit lactation. Some plant lectins such as concanavalin interfere with transport and discharge phases of milk production.

Understanding lactation failure is increasing among clinicians as the diagnostic resources expand.[142] Some herbs may inadvertently suppress lactation. A thorough history of herbal use is always appropriate in any clinical assessment.

MATERNAL AND INFANT OBESITY AND BREASTFEEDING

Obesity Epidemic

There is little doubt that there is an epidemic of being overweight and obese in the world.[144] The WHO has released data estimates through 2016 and noted several disturbing facts: obesity worldwide has tripled since 1975, over 1.9 billion adults (39% of the world's population) were overweight and over 650 million (13%) were obese, 40 million children (younger than 5 years old) were overweight or obese in 2018, and more than 340 million children and adolescents between 5 and 19 years old were overweight or obese in 2016.[145] In the United States, data from the 2013 to 2014 National Health and Nutrition Examination Survey (NHANES) survey of the NCHS are equally dire, with an estimated 70% of adults being overweight (32.5%) or obese (37.7%) and over 9.4% of children 2 to 5 years of age in the United States are obese and over 20.6% of adolescents 12 to 19 years old are obese.[146] Estimates from the WHO, UNICEF, and the World Bank suggest that obesity in children 2 to 4 years old has doubled and increased approximately eight times in the 5- to19-year-

old children and adolescents from 1975 to 2016.[144] These increases are occurring worldwide but to varying degrees in different countries. There are several other facts that make these trends additionally disturbing: (1) a high percentage of children with obesity continue to be obese in adulthood (affected by age of child when first diagnosed with obesity, severity of obesity, and parental obesity); (2) comorbidities associated with obesity in adulthood (hypertension, type 2 diabetes, dyslipidemia, cardiovascular disease, etc.) are being seen more frequently in obese children; (3) the cause of obesity is complex (genetics, environmental, and ecologic) and difficult to pinpoint in an individual; and (4) clinical interventions to prevent or treat obesity are labor and motivationally intense.[147–149]

Definitions and Classifications of Obesity

A practical measure of obesity is BMI.[145] It can be mathematically calculated as follows: BMI = weight (kilograms [kg])/height^2 (meters [m^2]) (kg/m^2). Using a sex-specific chart (Fig. 10.3), the BMI can be determined by plotting for an individual adult the point where the height and the weight intersect. A normal BMI is 18.5 to 24.9, a BMI between 25.0 to 29.9 is considered overweight, obese is a BMI over 30 (obesity class I BMI 30 to 34.9, class II 35.0 to 39.9, class III $\geq$ 40) and underweight is a BMI under 18.5 (Table 10.3). BMI provides a reasonable estimate of adiposity in the pediatric population. BMI may overestimate adiposity in children who are short or have high muscle mass and underestimate adiposity in children with low muscle mass.[150] There are other measures of adiposity, including waist-to-hip ratio for abdominal adiposity and skinfold thickness for generalized adiposity. Because of the difficulty of accurately measuring these or measuring total body fat by various technical procedures (hydrodensity, air displacement plethysmography, computed tomography, or magnetic resonance imaging); BMI is the accepted standard in adults and children. These other measures of adiposity do not currently add anything to understanding the underlying causes of obesity in an individual, nor are they useful to guide prevention or intervention efforts to date (Table 10.4).

Maternal Obesity and Breastfeeding
Obesity Risks in Pregnancy

Maternal obesity is associated with various morbidities both during and after pregnancy that can adversely affect the fetus/infant, including early spontaneous abortion, increased risk for fetal structural anomalies, gestational diabetes, hypertension and preeclampsia, obstructive sleep apnea, gastroesophageal reflex, preterm labor and/or premature birth, dysfunctional labor, operative delivery, postpartum hemorrhage, surgical site infection, thrombotic events, and additional morbidity and mortality.[148] There are numerous national guidelines and medical organization recommendations about the management of obese pregnant women to avoid or diminish such complications.

One of the primary questions about obesity in pregnancy is whether it or any of its associated comorbidities and

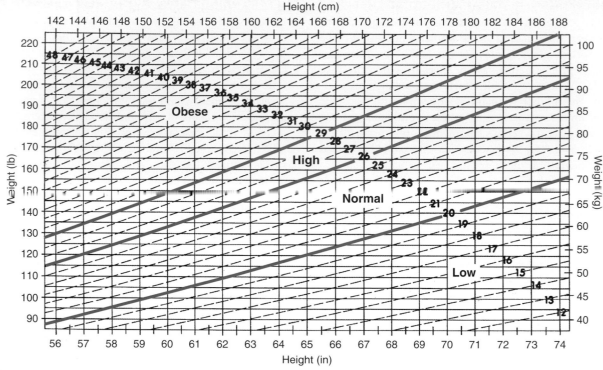

Fig. 10.3 Chart for estimating body mass index (BMI) category and BMI. To find BMI category (e.g., obese), find point where woman's height and weight intersect. To estimate BMI, read *bold number* on the *dashed line* that is closest to the point. (From Subcommittee on Nutrition During Lactation, Committee on Nutritional Status During Pregnancy and Lactation. *Nutrition During Pregnancy and Lactation: An Implementation Guide.* Washington, DC: National Academies Press; 1992.)

variables affect the offspring's risk for obesity, diabetes, or other metabolic abnormalities as a child, adolescent, or adult? A recent investigation of more than 5000 children in The Environmental Determinants of Diabetes in the Young (TEDDY) study reported higher odds of children being overweight at 5 years of age when exposed to maternal gestational

TABLE 10.3   Adult Weight Classification According to Body Mass Index

Relative Weight Classification	Prepregnant BMI (kg/m^2)
Underweight	<18.5
Recommended weight	18.5–24.9
Overweight	25.0–29.9
Obesity	≥30.0
Class I	30.0–34.9
Class II	35.0–39.9
Class III	≥40
Extreme obesity	≥50

Modified from World Health Organization. Obesity and overweight. https://www.who.int/news-room/fact-sheets/detail/obesity-and-overweight. Accessed February 27, 2020; and National Institute of Diabetes and Digestive and Kidney Diseases. Overweight and obesity statistics. https://www.niddk.nih.gov/health-information/health-statistics/overweight-obesity. Accessed February 27, 2020.

diabetes mellitus (odds ratio [OR] 1.48, 95% CI 1.14, 1.92), type 1 diabetes (OR 1.60, 95% CI 1.16, 2.20), and type 2 diabetes (OR 7.39, 95% CI 2.46, 22.23) compared with their unexposed counterparts.[151] Adjustment for BMI and other variables only mildly decreased the odds. The authors reported in the discussion that several meta-analyses suggested an independent effect of exposure to diabetes during pregnancy on childhood adiposity and type 2 diabetes risk. A cohort study in Southern California included 15,710 mother–infant pairs delivered in 2011 to evaluate maternal exposures and childhood overweight status at 2 years of age. Adjusted odds ratios (aORs) demonstrated that maternal prepregnancy obesity (aOR 2.34 95% CI [2.09 to 2.62]) or overweight (1.50 [1.34 to 1.68]) and excessive gestational weight gain (1.23 [1.12 to 1.35]) were associated with an increased risk for the infant being overweight at 2 years of age. In this study, breastfeeding for 6 months or longer was associated with a diminished risk (aOR 0.76 [0.69 to 0.83]) of childhood overweight at 2 years of age.[152] In the prospective cohort study, Programming of Enhanced Adiposity Risk in Childhood-Early Screening (PEACHES), 1671 obese and normal-weight mothers were included to examine late-pregnancy dysglycemia. Late-pregnancy dysglycemia was associated with development of infants who are large for gestational age, greater weight gain during childhood, and higher BMI z-scores at 4 years of age.[153] In a retrospective analysis of maternal risk factor data on 71,892 children born at Kaiser Permanente Southern California hospitals in 2007 to 2011,

TABLE 10.4 Diagnostic Criteria to Classify Obesity in Children by Age

Age	0–2 y	2–5 y	5–18 y
Index	Weight-to-length	BMI*	BMI^
Reference	WHO 2006	WHO 2006	WHO 2007
>85th percentile[†]	At risk for overweight	At risk for overweight	Overweight
>97th percentile[†]	Overweight	Overweight	Obesity
>99th percentile[†]	Obesity	Obesity	Severe Obesity[‡]

*BMI, Body mass index = weight (kg)/height (m^2).

[†]The 85th, 97th, and 99th percentiles approximate z-scores of +1, +2 and +3, respectively.

[‡]A scientific statement from the American Heart Association proposed the 120% above the age and sex 95th percentile of BMI or an absolute BMI ≥ 35 kg/m^2 as an alternative to the 99th percentile. (Kelly AS, Barlow SE, Rao G, et al. Severe obesity in children and adolescents: identification, associated health risks, and treatment approaches—a scientific statement from the American Heart Association. *Circulation.* 2013;128:1689–1712.)

Modified from World Health Organization Multicentre Growth Reference Study Group. WHO child growth standards based on length/height, weight and age. *Acta Paediatr Suppl.* 2006;450:76–85; de Onis M, Onyango AW, Borghi E, et al. Development of a WHO growth reference for school-aged children and adolescents. *Bull WHO.* 2007;85:660–667; and Valerio G, Maffeis C, Saggese G, et al. Diagnosis, treatment and prevention of pediatric obesity: consensus position statement of the Italian Society for Pediatric Endocrinology and Diabetology and the Italian Society of Pediatrics. *Ital J Pediatr.* 2018;44(1):88–109. http://doi:10.1186/s13052-018-0525-6.

one cohort of children was noted to have a high BMI and an increasing BMI trajectory over time.[154] Maternal prepregnancy obesity and overweight was clearly associated with this high-risk group of infants, whereas there was only a moderate association with maternal diabetes and excessive gestational weight gain and a mild association with breastfeeding for months or less.[154] In a separate review, Perng et al.[155] examined developmental overnutrition in mothers before, during, or after pregnancy and its effect on obesity or type 2 diabetes in their offspring. They summarize data supporting that maternal prepregnancy weight and gestational weight gain are associated with their infant's fat mass at birth, at 1 year of age, and in some studies beyond. They specifically point to maternal macronutrient intake during pregnancy and the association of higher energy and carbohydrate and lower protein consumption and elevated infant adiposity. Gestational weight gain and the timing of that weight gain also play a role in offspring adiposity. Maternal gestational weight gain is also correlated with insulin resistance and adipocytokine profiles in their infants with or without obesity.[156,157] Perng et al. and others discuss that these effects may relate to the variable contributions of genetics, shared environment and lifestyle, intrauterine mechanisms, maternal and infant microbiota, and infant feeding across the life span of the mother and infant and may not be readily correlated with single contributing factors.[155,158]

Breastfeeding Barriers or Successes for Overweight Women

Over the last 10 to 15 years, numerous studies have documented that prepregnancy overweight or obesity has been associated with a failure to begin and continue breastfeeding. This is evident worldwide in diverse populations. A large population study reinforces decreased initiation of breastfeeding in obese women with an adjusted odds ratio of 0.84 (95% CI, 0.83 to 0.85) after adjusting for known maternal factors associated with breastfeeding initiation.[159] Race or ethnicity did not affect the magnitude of these findings. There are also systematic reviews and meta-analyses that showed a mixture of results based on race/ethnicity or comorbidities of obesity.[160,161] In a recent systematic review and meta-analysis, higher prepregnancy BMI and gestational weight gain were each associated with being less likely to initiate and more likely to cease breastfeeding earlier.[162] Turcksin et al. raised specific issues such as maternal intent before delivery, initiation, intensity and duration of breastfeeding, and milk supply of obese women and the effect on breastfeeding.[163] Obese women were less likely to intend to breastfeed, were less likely to initiate breastfeeding, and had a "less adequate" milk supply and delayed onset of lactogenesis II compared with normal-weight women. Preusting et al. studied obesity and delayed onset of lactogenesis II in 216 women and found prepregnancy weight and gestational weight gain each were associated with delayed lactogenesis in obese women.[164] In 2019 Huang et al. confirmed in a large study of 3282 women that with higher gestational weight gain throughout pregnancy Chinese women more frequently experienced delayed lactogenesis even after adjustment for various appropriate factors.[165] The question is raised how we can support overweight and obese women to succeed and reach their breastfeeding goals. Chang et al. reviewed potential barriers for these women, including maternal physical barriers (larger breasts, difficulties of positioning while breastfeeding, delayed onset of lactogenesis, impact of cesarean section, perceived insufficient supply of milk), maternal psychologic barriers (low confidence in ability, negative body image, embarrassment at breastfeeding in public, experience of the stigma of obesity) and issues concerning the provision of tailored evidence-based support for obese women who intend to breastfeed.[166] Fair et al.[167] completed a systematic review of interventions for supporting initiation and continuation of breastfeeding among women who are overweight or obese. They concluded there was insufficient evidence for the effectiveness of any physical interventions or various methods of support for initiation or continuation of breastfeeding in this population.[167] There are several reviews of interventions for promoting and supporting breastfeeding in diverse populations of women that emphasize the importance of well-educated professionals and lay persons, with face-to-face contact with mothers using a facilitative, open approach to fully understand individual mothers' needs and open problem solving and support with mothers and families.[168-171] It is important to attend to the potential barriers outlined by Chang et al., to tailor the education and support specifically to the individual mother's needs and for additional study to clarify the most important issues and develop successful interventions for support of overweight and obese women wanting to breastfeed.[166]

Weight Loss During Lactation

It is generally recognized that women who breastfeed return to their prepregnancy weight more quickly and in greater numbers than do bottle-feeding mothers.[102,172] In two separate systematic reviews and analyses the majority of studies showed little or no association between breastfeeding and weight change or change in body composition postpartum.[173,174] Neville et al.[173] reported that of five studies of high methodologic quality in their review, four of the five showed a positive association between breastfeeding and weight change. Additional careful study is needed with controlling for the numerous factors that could contribute to postpartum weight change. When lactation performance was examined, overweight or obese women had less success initiating and continuing breastfeeding than their normal-weight counterparts.[166] The rates of discontinuance of exclusive breastfeeding in overweight and obese women were also higher, even when race or ethnicity, socioeconomic status, and maternal education were controlled, which would affect results examining postpartum weight loss related to breastfeeding. Lovelady,[175] in 2011, reviewed the use of exercise and energy restriction to promote weight loss. Moderate aerobic exercise (45 minutes/day, 5 days a week) improved cardiovascular fitness, plasma lipid levels, and insulin response but did not affect postpartum weight loss. Breast milk composition and volume were not altered. Subsequently she examined overweight women who limited energy intake by 2092 kJ/day and exercised (45 minutes/day, 4 days a week) from weeks 4 to 14 postpartum. Weight loss by control group was less than the diet and exercise group (0.8 kg, standard deviation [SD] 2.3) and 4.8 kg (SD 1.7) without any observed effect on infant growth.[175] In 2012 Bertz et al. examined weight loss, after a 12-week intervention and 9 months after intervention, in overweight and obese lactating Swedish women.[176] Weight loss was noted after the intervention and at 1-year follow-up as −8.3 ± 4.2 and −10.2 ± 5.7 kg, respectively, in the group managed with diet alone compared with −0.8 ± 3.0 and −0.9 ± 6.6 kg in the control group. The exercise alone group lost −2.4 ± 3.2 kg and −2.7 ± 5.9 kg compared with the diet and exercise group at −6.9 ± 3.0 and −7.3 ± 6.3 kg. Additional studies by the same group of the same group of

women demonstrated that the dietary modifications lead to reduced intake of fat and carbohydrates and increased proportions of complex carbohydrates, protein, and fiber by the women, fitting with standard macronutrient intake recommendations in Sweden.[177] These women also had lower total cholesterol, low-density lipoprotein cholesterol, and insulin at the 1-year mark.[178] It is necessary to communicate these results cautiously with appropriate nutritional recommendations such that women can use them without having unrealistic expectations of weight loss. It is important to note that a balanced diet with 500 kcal/day less and 45 minutes a day of exercise 4 to 5 days a week, after breastfeeding is well established at approximately 4 weeks, does not affect milk volume or composition nor infant growth.[175,176]

CHILDHOOD OBESITY AND BREASTFEEDING

Significance of Childhood Obesity

Childhood obesity is a complex disease that is the result of multiple factors. There are single-gene syndromes involving obesity that make up less than 1% of childhood obesity. These single-gene causes of obesity commonly have very early onset of obesity and other syndromic features: short stature, dysmorphic features, or developmental delay (e.g., Prader-Willi, Beckwith-Wiedemann, etc.). Some heritable factor may contribute to obesity in 30% to 40% of persons. Epigenetic factors may also play a role in childhood obesity. Endocrine causes of weight gain are diagnosed in less than 1% of children and adolescents, and they tend to also have poor linear growth and hypogonadism. Possible environmental factors set up equally complex etiologic interactions. They include psychologic or emotional distress affecting adaptive behaviors and eating behaviors (individual, and parental), an "obesogenic environment" (processed foods, sugar-sweetened beverages, fast foods, large portion sizes), and variables affecting decreased activity and caloric expenditure (television, electronic device screen time, etc.). Contributing factors also can be viewed as prenatal (maternal obesity, excessive gestational weight gain, gestational diabetes), perinatal (birth size, antibiotic use, breastfeeding vs. formula feeding), and postnatal (established intestinal microbiota, catch-up growth, maternal/familial/caregiver health beliefs and dietary concerns). There is some evidence for quality and duration of sleep affecting obesity. There is also a proposed association of intestinal microbiota of the infant and dysbiosis leading to metabolic diseases (type 2 diabetes, inflammatory bowel disease) or altered nutrient processing and obesity[149] (Fig. 10.4).

Another concern regarding the increasing prevalence of childhood obesity is that childhood obesity is associated with comorbidities affecting almost every system in the body. These conditions involve the endocrine, gastrointestinal, pulmonary, cardiovascular, musculoskeletal, and dermatologic systems, among others. Many of these comorbidities occur in youth with obesity, including type 2 diabetes mellitus, dyslipidemia, obstructive sleep apnea, and steatohepatitis, although they used to be considered "adult" diseases. The severity of

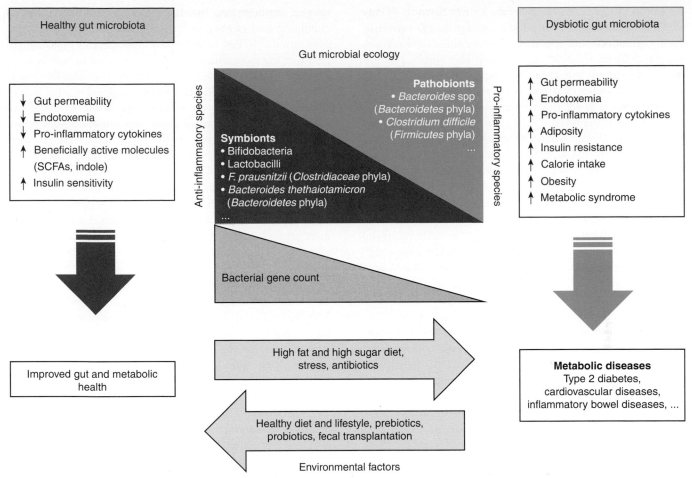

Fig. 10.4 Intestinal microbiota: dysbiosis, obesity, and metabolic disease. *SCFA*, Short-chain fatty acids. (Meldrum DR, Morris MA, Gambone JC. Obesity pandemic: causes, consequences, and solutions—but do we have the will? *Fertil Steril.* 2017;107[4]:833—839, http://doi:10.1016/j.fertnstert.2017.02.104; and Boulangé CL, Neves AL, Chilloux J, et al. Impact of the gut microbiota on inflammation, obesity, and metabolic disease. *Genome Med.* 2016;8[1]:42—55, http://doi:10.1186/s13073-016-0303-2.)

these comorbidities increases with the severity of obesity. There are now medical organizations that recommend classifying obesity in three classes: class I obesity (BMI at or above 95th percentile to less than 120% of the 95th percentile), class II (BMI ≥ 120% to <140% of the 95th percentile, or BMI ≥ 35 kg/m^2), and class III (BMI ≥ 140% of the 95th percentile, or BMI ≥ 40 kg/m^2) to better delineate "degrees" of obesity and to further assess the risk for comorbid conditions. Hypertension, type 2 diabetes mellitus, dyslipidemia, and metabolic syndrome are comorbidities directly associated with obesity and associated with their own health consequences in the short- and long-term health of children and adults.

Effects of Breastfeeding on Overweight and Obesity in Children

A number of reports have proposed that breastfeeding decreases the risk for overweight and obesity in children and adolescents.[179–183] There is biologic plausibility related to mechanisms of how breastfeeding could be protective against obesity. Protein intake and energy metabolism are less in breastfed infants compared with formula-fed infants.[184] There is evidence that lower protein content and energy content as occurs in mature breast milk in comparison to formula are associated with lower fat mass and BMI in infancy and early childhood. There are differences in the hormones in human milk versus formula (specifically adipokines) that affect insulin response, fat deposition, and formation of adipocytes (see Chapter 4 for discussion of adipokines). There may be dietary preferences of infants and children influenced by human milk consumption compared with formula. Theoretical concerns exist regarding dysbiosis of the infant gastrointestinal tract microbiota and the formation of obesity. Despite a degree of biologic plausibility, there is debate about whether breastfeeding does protect against obesity. Various older large trials and systematic reviews suggested a clear relationship between breastfeeding and lower risk for obesity. A study of 32,200 Scottish children showed that the prevalence of obesity was significantly lower in breastfed children, even after adjusting for socioeconomic status, birth weight, and sex. The conclusion was that breastfeeding is associated with a reduction in the risk for childhood obesity.[185] Similar results were reported in a study of over 15,000 adolescents as part of the Growing Up Today Study in the United States.[179] Those who had been breastfed had a lower risk for being overweight during childhood and adolescence. More than 1000 preadolescent children followed in Germany also showed significantly decreased prevalence of being overweight.[186] In reviewing 11 studies of at least 100 participants, Dewey found that 8 showed a lower risk for being overweight in children who had been breastfed.[36] The three studies that did not make that conclusion lacked information on exclusivity and duration. Studies that include children "ever breastfed" dilute the impact of significant breastfeeding. A systematic review of 28 studies involving 298,900 subjects that provided odds ratios from 61 studies published since 1966 demonstrated that breastfeeding protects against obesity. An additional 33 published studies of 12,505 subjects without odds ratios did not change the results.[187] Because obese children have a high risk for becoming obese adults, 9357 German children who were 5 to 6 years old were evaluated for obesity using BMI. After adjusting for confounders, breastfeeding remained a significant protective factor against overweight and obesity.[188]

More recent trials and reviews show mixed results regarding breastfeeding and obesity. Horta and Victora[189] summarized their analysis in a WHO publication in 2013 stating that small-study effect is an issue that tends to overestimate the benefits of breastfeeding. For the larger studies (> 1500 participants) there was a modest protective effect of breastfeeding (aOR = 0.80 [95% CI, 0.80 to 0.91]) but there may be residual confounding related to socioeconomic status. They conclude that their meta-analysis using the "higher quality studies" shows a reduction of approximately 10% in the prevalence of overweight or obesity in children who breastfeed for longer durations. They allow that residual confounding might still explain a large portion of this effect.[189] Oken et al. and The Obesity Society created a position statement in 2017 on breastfeeding and obesity.[190] They raise concerns similar to those of Horta and Victora. They point to a nonobservational randomized intervention by Martin et al.[191] to promote duration and exclusivity of breastfeeding. Even with improved breastfeeding there was no significant improvement in maternal or child weight, adiposity, or blood pressure 11 years after delivery.[191] Oken et al.[190] suggest that randomized controlled trials that compare no breastfeeding with partial or exclusive are neither ethical nor feasible. They propose ongoing mechanistic studies of adiposity, obesity, inflammation, and insulin resistance in pregnant women, lactating women, and their offspring to better understand the issues and possible interventions.[190] Overweight and obesity are more likely the result of multiple contributing and competing factors that may dilute out the potential benefit of breastfeeding in the long term from infancy to adolescence or adulthood. They recommend ongoing support of overweight and obese women (all women) for breastfeeding success and additional support to reduce energy intake and increase expenditure once lactation is established to facilitate achievement of desired postpartum weight loss.

Various researchers and authors point to a plethora of factors that appear to have some relationship with childhood obesity. Monteiro et al. reviewed rapid growth in infancy and childhood and obesity in later life and found a significant association.[192] They noted in the 13 studies of rapid weight gain that the most commonly used definition of rapid weight gain as a z-score change greater than 0.67 in weight-for-age between two ages. Feldman-Winter et al. completed a prospective cohort study on weight gain in the first week of life.[193] Children who gained more than 100 g of weight versus infants who lost weight in the first week of life were 2.3 times (adjusted odds) as likely to be overweight at 2 years of age. They did not find an association between feeding type and BMI at 2 years of age. However, exclusively breastfed children were less likely to gain 100 g or more of weight in the first week of life. Zheng et al. performed a systematic review and meta-analysis of rapid weight gain during infancy and later adiposity.[194] They included 17 studies, all of which used the previous definition of rapid weight gain. They reported that rapid weight gain in infancy was associated with being overweight or obese from childhood to adulthood (pooled OR = 3.66, 95% CI, 2.59 to 5.17). Subgroup analyses showed that rapid weight gain earlier in infancy (birth to 1 year vs. birth to 2 years) was associated with a greater odd of overweight or obesity in later life. Goetz et al. demonstrated from data of 1799 mother–infant pairs in the Infant Feeding Practices Study II, that greater breastfeeding in early infancy is associated with slower weight gain through 7 to 12 months of age in infants with high birth weight.[195] The timing of rapid weight gain in infancy appears important, and interventions to limit rapid weight gain early on are likely to decrease the risk for overweight or obesity in childhood. Given the prevalence of childhood obesity and the potential health consequences, authors are examining possible early risk factors for childhood obesity. Woo Baidal et al. reviewed studies examining risk factors for later obesity in the first 1000 days.[196] Their results showed that higher maternal prepregnancy BMI, prenatal tobacco exposure, maternal excess gestational weight gain, high infant birth weight, and accelerated infant weight gain consistently were associated with later childhood obesity. Fewer studies indicated gestational diabetes, childcare attendance, low socioeconomic status, low strength of maternal-infant relationship, altered infant sleep, inappropriate bottle use, introduction of solid food intake before 4 months of age, and infant antibiotic exposure as risks for childhood obesity.[196] Larqué et al. came up with similar prenatal and postnatal risk factors for childhood obesity.[197] A review by Porter et al. on severe obesity in children younger than 5 years specifically examined "modifiable" risk factors in the early infancy period related to the "obesogenic" environment: consumption of sugar-sweetened beverages and fast foods, low levels of activity (little outdoor play and excess "screen time" with electronic devices), behaviors (low satiety responsiveness, sleeping with a bottle, lack of bedtime rules/structure, and altered sleep), and informal childcare setting.[198] They also included maternal obesity and gestational diabetes as factors that could be important modifiable factors. Breastfeeding duration and exclusivity were not considered in these modifiable or early infancy risk factors by these authors. Pietrobelli et al.[5] take a targeted view of feeding practices in the first 1000 days of life to minimize obesity. Exclusive breastfeeding for 6 months, continued breastfeeding until 1 year, introduction of complementary foods at 4 to 6 months of age, and limiting cow's milk intake are highlighted in the recommended feeding practices.

Comorbidities of Obesity and Breastfeeding

Discussion of the impact of adiposity is rarely undertaken without including a discussion of cholesterol and lipid status, type 2 diabetes, blood pressure, and other measures and risks for cardiovascular health and illness. Previously, energy requirements for infants receiving formula have been overestimated.[13,199] Breastfed infants require and receive 110 kcal/kg per day at 1 month and 70 kcal/kg per day at 4 months and grow appropriately. The low energy intakes are not caused by limitations in maternal milk production as previously assumed but represent physiologically regulated intakes. Breastfed infants deposit less fat than formula-fed infants despite the fact that the two diets appear similar on paper.[200–202] Recommendations for physical activity should fit with dietary recommendations for balanced energy consumption and the types foods consumed (breastmilk, formula, complementary foods) to maintain optimal weight, adiposity, and health.[203]

Lipid Status or Dyslipidemia

Relative to lipid status, there are some older studies on the effect of breastfeeding on plasma cholesterol and weight in young adults as studied longitudinally by Marmot et al. in a sample of people born in 1946.[204] The infant-feeding history was obtained. At age 32, women who had been breastfed had significantly lower mean plasma cholesterol than women who had been bottle fed (Fig. 10.5). The difference for men was smaller, and men who had been breastfed had higher mean weight and skinfold thickness. Multiple studies, both short-

and long-range, with small populations and conflicting results have been reported in humans, although animal studies strongly suggest that species-specific milk reduces the risk for obesity and elevated cholesterol. Indices of fatness and serum cholesterol at age 8 years in relation to feeding and growth during early infancy were reported by Fomon et al. from their detailed longitudinal nutrition project involving 469 children born between 1966 and 1971.[11] In infancy, the formula-fed children had more rapid gains in height and weight, which were attributed to greater food intake. At age 8, there were no differences in indices of fatness related to mode of feeding during infancy and no significant differences in serum cholesterol concentrations. These older studies were also just at the beginning of increasing overweight around the world and children being readily exposed to the obesogenic environment, which is contributing to this increase. In more recent studies there are mixed results on the influence of feeding type on lipid profile in later life. A quantitative review of breastfeeding and blood cholesterol levels in adults (16 years old) by Owen et al. included 17 studies (12,890 breastfed and 4608 formula-fed individuals).[205] The mean total cholesterol was lower in individuals "ever breastfed" versus formula-fed ($p = 0.037$). The difference was larger and more consistent when the analysis used studies (7) of exclusive breastfeeding ($p = 0.005$) compared with studies of nonexclusive breastfeeding (10). Analysis considering potential confounders had minimal effect on the results.[205] Horta et al.[206] performed an updated review and meta-analysis in 2015 with 46 studies. In this review there was no association of total cholesterol level in breastfeeding (−0.01 mmol/L (95% CI, −0.05 to 0.02) versus formula-fed individuals. Serum cholesterol may be too insensitive a quantitation to detect early changes of dyslipidemia or harmful deposition of fat, and it may be necessary to examine lipoprotein classes, apoprotein concentrations, fat deposition, and perhaps insulin and adipokine levels in breastmilk and in infants.

Cardiovascular Disease Risk

Early studies of breastfeeding in infancy were associated with decreased coronary heart disease mortality, but the mechanisms are unclear. In a prospective study of 7276 singleton term infants born between 1991 and 1992 and followed to 7.5 years of age, the systolic and diastolic blood pressures of the breastfed infants were lower compared with those never breastfed (1.2 mm and 0.9 mm, respectively). Even partial breastfeeding had an effect. A further reduction in systolic pressure (0.2 mm) was seen for each 3 months of breastfeeding. Outcome was adjusted for social and economic parameters without significant change in the results.[207] Parikh et al. also examined breastfeeding in infancy in a longitudinal study with adult cardiovascular disease risk factors (BMI, lipid profile, fasting blood glucose, and systolic and diastolic blood pressure).[208] Breastfeeding was not associated with systolic or diastolic blood pressures in the 962 men and women assessed at a mean of 41 years of age. Owen et al. analyzed epidemiologic studies of breastfeeding and cardiovascular risk factors in adult life and reported that long-term observational

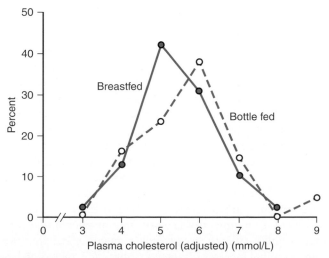

Fig. 10.5 Plasma cholesterol in adults according to type of infant feeding. (From Marmot MG, Page CM, Atkins E, et al. Effect of breastfeeding on plasma cholesterol and weight in young adults, *J Epidemiol Community Health*. 1980;34:164.)

studies suggested that breastfeeding was associated with lower levels of total blood cholesterol and marginally lower adiposity and blood pressure in adult life.[209] They noted that additional control of potential confounding variables and assessment of the duration and exclusivity of breastfeeding needed to be considered. Fewtrell reviewed evidence from randomized trials on breastfeeding and later cardiovascular disease risk.[210] In a trial of preterm infants receiving banked donor breastmilk versus preterm formula, breastfed infants demonstrated significantly lower blood pressure, favorable lipid profile, and less leptin resistance at 13 to 15 years of age. In a cluster controlled trial of breastfeeding promotion in healthy term infants (Promotion of Breast feeding Intervention Trial [PROBIT]) there was no effect of the increased incidence, duration, and exclusivity of breastfeeding in the study on adiposity or blood pressure measured at 6 years of age. Later follow-up of 13,879 breastfeeding mother−infant pairs from the PROBIT study by Martin et al. at 11.5 years of age did not show any effect of breastfeeding on cardiometabolic risk factors, including blood pressure, fasting insulin, glucose, adiponectin, apolipoprotein A1, and the presence of metabolic syndrome.[211] Wong et al. reported a cross-sectional study of 1539 children at 3 to 6 years of age.[212] A "calculated" cardiometabolic risk was associated with increasing breastfeeding duration, but the magnitude of difference in blood pressure was small (1.07 mm Hg (95% CI −2.04, −0.10) comparing breastfeeding for 6 to 12 months with 12 to 24 months. Umer et al. examined longitudinally linked data from three cross-sectional data sets in West Virginia for 11,980 children.[213] Only 43% of mothers self-reported ever breastfeeding (parental recall when children were in the fifth grade), and the adjusted analysis did not show any difference in blood pressure between ever versus never breastfed children. There was a small-magnitude but significant difference in triglyceride level but not in low-density lipoprotein, total cholesterol, or high-density lipoprotein cholesterol. Horta et al. reevaluated breastfeeding and blood pressure in a systematic review and meta-analysis of 43 studies.[206] There was only a small difference in systolic blood pressure (not diastolic) for breastfed children, which was even smaller when controlled for possible confounding socioeconomic and demographic variables. There was also marked heterogeneity among the studies unexplained by study characteristics. In focused systematic reviews by Güngör et al., they concluded that there was insufficient evidence to confirm that blood pressure benefits in children were affected by never versus ever breastfeeding, shorter versus longer duration of breastfeeding, shorter versus longer duration of exclusive breastfeeding, or greater quantities versus less quantities of human milk for mixed-fed infants.[214]

Type 2 Diabetes

Data are conflicting regarding the protective effect of breastfeeding against diabetes in childhood. Two systematic reviews and meta-analyses were published by the same group led by Bernardo Horta. In 2015 they reviewed 11 studies that suggested that breastfeeding lowered the odds ratio for breastfed infants versus formula-fed infants (pooled OR = 0.65, 95% CI 0.49, 0.86).[206] In 2019 another analysis with an additional three studies suggested that breastfeeding protects children from type 2 diabetes. Analysis of each of the three new studies individually supported breastfeeding protection and in the meta-analysis, the pooled odds ratio was 0.67 (95% CI, 0.56 to 0.80) that breastfeeding protects against childhood type 1 diabetes.[215] Güngör et al. also reviewed infant milk-feeding practices and diabetes outcomes in infants in four targeted questions.[216] They reported limited evidence that never versus ever being breastfed is associated with a higher risk for type 1 diabetes; that shorter versus longer duration of exclusive breastfeeding is associated with a higher risk for type 1 diabetes; that the duration of any human milk feeding is not associated with fasting insulin or insulin resistance in childhood or at the transition to adolescence; and that for infants who received some amount of human milk, shorter versus longer duration of any human milk feeding is associated with a higher risk for type 1 diabetes. Otherwise, data were insufficient to determine any relationship among intensity, duration, and amount of human milk for mixed-fed infants, shorter versus longer duration of human milk feeding, and type 2 diabetes, prediabetes, and hemoglobin A1c.[216]

NUTRITIONAL PROGRAMMING

Nutrition in the early stages of growth seems to be essential to glucose and fat metabolism and the potential for obesity or diabetes. The hypothesis of "nutritional programming" states that genetics and the environment in infancy, in particular infant feeding, directly influence the phenotype of the infant with regard to energy metabolism, glucose homeostasis, and fat metabolism.[217] The potential for programming extends from pregnancy (intrauterine milieu) into early feeding. The maternal status during this period influences the environment in which the infant grows, particularly the mother's weight, BMI, glucose metabolism, fat metabolism, energy usage, and nutritional status. Fetal growth is directly affected by the nutrients and hormones provided from the mother. Early in pregnancy this guides cell differentiation and organogenesis. The major period of growth of the fetus occurs in the third trimester and is influenced by glucose homeostasis, insulin, insulin-like growth factor-1 (IGF-1), and the hypothalamic/pituitary axis regulating food intake and metabolism of the mother. During lactation, some of this maternal influence continues through breastfeeding, maternally directed feeding practices (type of food, amount of food, and protein, fat, and energy content of the food provided), and the composition of breast milk or breast milk substitutes. Breast milk provides the macronutrients and micronutrients necessary for human infant growth, and these vary consistently in the amounts from colostrum, transitional milk, and mature milk. Human breast milk contains metabolic hormones (adipokines, see Chapter 4, Table 4.35), including leptin, ghrelin, insulin, adiponectin, obestatin, resistin, apelin, nesfatin, irisin, epidermal growth factor 1 (EGF-1), and platelet-derived growth factor (PDGF). Several groups have reviewed the literature on the hormone content of breast milk to decipher their role in infant growth and nutritional programming.[217–219] Adipokines in breast milk may either pass from maternal serum or be synthesized by mammary epithelial cells. Presumably the adipokine levels in maternal serum and breast milk and in the infant's serum are related, fitting the metabolic status of the mother and the needs of the infant for growth and development. To a degree, the literature regarding breast milk hormone levels and infant growth provides conflicting data.[219] Leptin's activity regulates energy homeostasis and "inhibits" hunger. Even though this should confer an anti-adiposity effect, there is evidence for and against breast milk leptin levels and infant weight gain and adiposity. Ghrelin, known as the "hunger" hormone, acts acutely to stimulate appetite, increase gastric acidity, and improve intestinal motility. Here again data are conflicting regarding serum levels and breast milk levels of ghrelin and satiety and appetite regulation. Adiponectin functions to stimulate hunger and is correlated with fat mass percentage in adults. In infants the data are conflicting regarding breast milk adiponectin levels and the body composition of infants. IGF-1 plays a dominant role in cell proliferation and death and is essential for growth. Data are limited on its levels and infant growth. Insulin directly affects glucose uptake into cells (particularly, muscle, fat, and brain) and is essential for cell growth. Some studies have demonstrated a correlation of breast milk insulin levels and weight-to-length z-scores over the first few months of life, although this is not supported by other studies.[219,220] Further understanding of the role of the specific bioactive factors in human breast milk on infant growth and metabolism will require advanced assessment of the maternal and infant environment and the levels of bioactive factors in mother, breast milk, and the infant along with accurate assessment of desired outcomes in growth and metabolism in infancy, childhood, and later. Research should be expanded to consider "developmental programming" and transgenerational inheritance. This allows that early life environment influences affect not only the mother and the infant but potentially the infant's children by epigenetic effects on the infant's somatic cells, germ-line cells, and the environment generated by the child.[221]

SUMMARY

Optimal growth can be achieved only through the interaction of genetic potential and optimal nutrition at the appropriate times (intrauterine, infancy, childhood, and adolescence) to immediately affect timely active growth and "program" organogenesis and metabolism to optimize future growth and health. Teleologically and as demonstrated in numerous studies, breast milk is the optimal food for infants through the first 6 to 12 months of life combined with culturally, ethnically, and nutritionally appropriate complementary foods from 6 months forward. The WHO growth standards represent appropriate growth references for assessing the optimal growth of breastfeeding infants and children. These standards are appropriate as well, for human variation in growth related to genetics, ethnicity, and culture when breastfeeding and complementary feeding is optimized. It may be useful in the future for individual countries to have their own growth standards to guide national efforts to optimize breastfeeding and use of complementary foods for the specific ethnicities, cultures, and nutritional environments within their country.

Growth faltering in a breastfeeding infant when recognized by comparison of an individual child's growth to the WHO growth standards for breastfeeding infants should be a call for assessment of the situation and intervention to optimize nutrition, allowing the infant to return to appropriate growth. Recognizing that the assessment must include observations for all the potential causes of growth faltering, direct observation of the breastfeeding mother and child is essential to identifying breastfeeding difficulties and potential solutions. When that assessment identifies an infant who is hungry and is not getting adequate nutrition, feeding the baby is the next crucial step. The questions why, what, how much, and how should guide the feeding intervention and ideally generate a plan back to easier breastfeeding and optimal nutrition. Early weight loss in exclusively breastfeeding infants is different from growth faltering in its timing and its assessment using early weight loss nomograms.

Childhood obesity is a complex condition generated through the interaction of genetics and environment. There are numerous potentially contributing factors acting in the prenatal, intrauterine, and postnatal periods. BMI is the accepted practical estimate of adiposity, overweight, and obesity. There remains a tremendous amount to be understood about the various contributing factors, their mechanisms of action and interaction, and possible preventive interventions. At this juncture, a few appropriate recommendations to minimize obesity in infants and children include exclusive breastfeeding from birth to 6 months of age, introduction of appropriate complementary foods at 4 to 6 months of age, continued use of human milk though 12 to 36 months of age, and overall limiting cow's milk intake for any age child.

The Reference list is available at www.expertconsult.com.

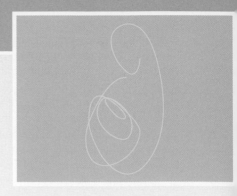

11

Medications, Herbal Preparations, and Natural Products in Breast Milk

Robert M. Lawrence and Ruth A. Lawrence

KEY POINTS

- Medication use during lactation occurs in almost 50% of breastfeeding women. The most common medications reported include oral contraceptives, systemic antibiotics, "cold preparations," analgesics/antipyretics, and nonsteroidal antiinflammatory agents.
- The benefits of continued breastfeeding with maternal medication use almost always outweigh the potential risk to the infant. Every clinical situation is different, based on the specifics for the mother—infant dyad. A careful, informed risk—benefit assessment should be calculated and discussed with the mother to facilitate her informed decision-making. Maintenance of the milk supply should be optimized until a final decision is made.
- Important variables to be considered about a specific medication's use during breastfeeding include route of administration, absorption via that route and orally via

the infant's gastrointestinal tract, half-life, volume of distribution, size of molecule (molecular weight), solubility (in water vs. lipids), dissociation constant (pK_a), and protein binding. Additionally, it is important to know about the specific medication, including its milk-to-plasma ratio, usual maternal plasma levels of the drug, the relative infant dose, and available evidence on the medication's use in lactation and its effects on the breastfeeding infant.

- Given continually changing evidence on medication use and lactation, it is essential that the health care professional review the most recent information on one of the frequently updated online resources before making decisions or recommendations (e.g., LactMed, Infantrisk.com).

As more women breastfeed and breastfeed longer, in keeping with the World Health Organization (WHO) and the American Academy of Pediatrics (AAP) recommendations, questions about the safety of medications during lactation increase, along with estimated use of medications during lactation by 50% of women.[1-3] There are a couple of continually updated information resources on drugs during lactation. One has been developed with advice from an expert panel for the National Library of Medicine called LactMed. It is a peer-reviewed and fully referenced database of possible drugs used during lactation. The data include maternal and infant levels of drugs, possible effects on nurslings and on lactation itself, and a list of alternative drugs. The address is https://www.ncbi.nlm.nih.gov/books/NBK547441/.[4] Another resource is privately managed by Dr. Thomas Hale, PhD, and is available as a book (*Medications and Mothers' Milk*) and as an online resource at http://www.halesmeds.com as well as a website (www.infantrisk.com) and call-line (806-352-2519). Given these resources and the constantly changing available information on medications and lactation, this chapter reports information only on selected medications, herbs and products in breast milk, and how a clinician can utilize the available information on medications and lactation to optimize the health of the mother—infant dyad and facilitate ongoing exclusive breastfeeding. For the most up-to-date information, the previously mentioned resources should be consulted.

MISINTERPRETATION OF DRUG DATA

With the plethora of resources about drugs and chemicals, many of which are available to the layperson and mother herself, there is the risk for an untrained person misinterpreting the data.[5,6] Having said that, there is evidence in the literature that women do engage in a "reiterative, information seeking and analysis process" when faced with a decision about utilizing a complementary medicine product during lactation.[7,8] Even a medical professional untrained in lactation physiology who offers medical advice based on information gleaned from various resources can interfere with safe and appropriate use of a medication for the mother and ongoing breastfeeding. The Pregnancy and Lactation Labeling Rules from the US Food and Drug Administration (FDA), updated in 2014, are intended to provide information (in package labeling) in a narrative summary style, including a "risk summary" (presence of the drug in human milk, effects of the drug on milk production and the breastfed child, a statement on the risk—benefit ratio of use), a section on "clinical considerations" (information on minimizing exposure and monitoring for adverse reactions), and a section on "data" (the published information utilized to formulate the clinical and risk sections).[9] A professional needs to understand not just the plasma and milk levels but also the pharmacology of the drug and physiology of lactation to give helpful instructions that will mitigate the effect of the drug on an infant and avoid discontinuing breastfeeding unnecessarily. LactMed and Hale's online resources give basic instructions on how to use the information contained in their databases.

POSSIBLE RISK OF DRUG APPEARING IN BREAST MILK

Despite the overwhelming advantages of human milk and the advantages of being breastfed, at times, the risk of a maternal medication adversely affecting a nursing infant must be considered. Even when data about the medication, such as the milk-to-plasma ratio, are available, a physician has to consider several factors related to each infant and each situation before deciding if breastfeeding can be initiated or continued.[10] The more complicated a mother's medical problems, the greater the possibility that the infant also has complications of prematurity or illness that will alter its ability to excrete the medication. This situation requires scientific information and experienced clinical judgment to appraise the problems and determine the therapeutic regimen. The clinician must determine the risk—benefit ratio of continued breastfeeding. The data are meager and sometimes conflicting for some drugs, yet maternal medication is the single most common medical problem in managing breastfeeding patients reported to the Breastfeeding and Lactation Center in Rochester, New York.

Risk Categories

The AAP Committee on Drugs published a list of drugs and other chemicals that transfer into human breast milk. The list, which was last updated in 2013, is divided into those that are contraindicated, those that require temporary interruption of breastfeeding, and those that are compatible with breastfeeding.[10] Concern about the issue of drugs in breast milk has spread. That classification is different from the previously used FDA Pregnancy Categories of Risk, which separates medications based on the amount and quality of available studies in pregnant women and animals (A, B, C, D, X) and not on either incidence of reactions or the potential severity of risk.[11] The FDA has new labeling rules for medications, the Pregnancy and Lactation Labeling Rule of 2014.[9] The database and book authored by Dr. Thomas Hale and his team use a lactation risk classification (LRC) based on their assessment of the risk data (L1 = compatible with breastfeeding, L2 = probably compatible, L3 = probably compatible [individualized assessment of the benefits versus risk needed], L4 = possibly hazardous, L5 = hazardous).[12] All of these risk categorization strategies are oversimplifications. The decision about the use of a medication, herb, or product by a lactating woman necessitates an individualized risk—benefit assessment for the mother and the infant based on the available information, with the mother/parents included in that information review and the decision-making.

Extent of Medication Use in Lactation

A study of more than 14,000 pregnant women in 148 hospitals in 22 countries revealed that 79% of women received an average of 3.3 drugs.[10] The drugs most often given were analgesics and anesthetics. Of the 91% of women who initiated breastfeeding, 36% received methylergonovine, and 5% received antibiotics. Another study of 885 women 3 to 5 months postpartum in Oslo showed that breastfeeding women took fewer medications (daily dose/1000 women/day) than nonbreastfeeding women.[13] The most common medication in the latter group was oral contraceptives. Colds, dyspepsia, hemorrhoids, and breast infections were the disorders identified in this study that precipitated the use of albuterol (salbutamol), clemastine fumarate (Tavist), dexchlorpheniramine maleate (cold preparations), phenylpropanolamine hydrochloride (Comtrex, Dimetane), cromolyn sodium, and methotrimeprazine hydrochloride (levomepromazine).

A more recent systematic review of breastfeeding practices and postpartum women's use of medicines included 20 studies (cohort and cross-sectional) from nine countries.[3] The proportion of women using ≥ 1 medicine during lactation ranged from 34% to 100%. The three largest reviews included studies from Sweden ($n = 102,995$), Norway ($n = 106,329$), and Denmark ($n = 15,756$) in which the percentages of medication use were 51%, 57% and 34%, respectively. In the four registered databases, from Norway, Sweden, the Netherlands, and Denmark, the most commonly documented medications were oral contraceptives and systemic antibiotics, whereas in the other studies, analgesics/antipyretics, nonsteroidal antiinflammatory drugs, and antibiotics were the most common (without including iron, vitamins, and minerals). Long-term use of medications for chronic illnesses in Norway, Sweden, and the Netherlands in the first 3 months postpartum included cardiovascular medications, thyroid therapy, antiasthma, antidepressants/antipsychotics, medications for diabetes, and antileptics. In five smaller studies from Brazil and Canada, breastfeeding appeared to be affected by postpartum medication use by the mothers, including noninitiation of breastfeeding or stopping breastfeeding earlier than intended.[3]

Consulting Reliable Information on Humans

No substitute exists for specific knowledge about the individual medications and their use in lactation. It is equally inappropriate to discontinue breastfeeding when it is not medically necessary as it is to continue breastfeeding while taking contraindicated drugs.

Consideration of the pharmacokinetics contributes to the understanding of the potential problems involved. Given the limited data available in humans, some reported data have been extrapolated from experiments performed on cows, goats, and rodents. Bovine experiments have been conducted using continuous infusions, which provide data on the passage of a drug into milk under certain pH and plasma levels. Animal studies are not particularly useful because there is so much variability in the protein and fat composition of different species' milk and the existence of active transport systems in different species. Human pharmacokinetic studies are necessary to quantify the amount of drug that passes to human milk.[14] Medical professionals should not try to "oversimplify" the data but can consult with local pharmacologists knowledgeable in medications and lactation or available hotlines and support groups for assistance. (See Chapter 25 and Appendix G for some of these resources.)

IMPORTANT VARIABLES REGARDING MEDICATIONS IN HUMAN BREAST MILK

Factors that influence the passage of a drug into the milk in humans include the size of the molecule, its solubility in lipids and water, whether it binds to protein, the drug's pH, and diffusion rates. Passive diffusion is the principal factor in the passage of a drug from plasma into milk. The drug may appear in an active form or as an inactive metabolite.

The following outline summarizes these factors:

I. Drugs
    a. Route of administration
       i. Oral
       ii. Intravenous (IV)
       iii. Intramuscular (IM)
       iv. Transdermal drug delivery system (TDDS)
       v. Absorption rate
       vi. Half-life or peak serum time
       vii. Dissociation constant
       viii. Volume of distribution
    b. Size of molecule
    c. Degree of ionization
    d. pH of substrate
       i. Plasma: 7.4
       ii. Milk: 6.8
    e. Solubility
       i. In water
       ii. In lipids
    f. Protein binding more to plasma than to milk protein

INFANT RELATED MEDICATION FACTORS

A most important factor that has received relatively little attention is the infant and how the infant absorbs the medication and is affected by it. Will the infant absorb the chemical from the intestinal tract? If the infant absorbs the chemical, can the infant detoxify and excrete it, or will minimal amounts in the milk accumulate in the infant's system? Is the infant premature, small for gestational age, or high risk because of complications of the pregnancy or delivery? How will these factors affect metabolism or reaction to a medication? Is the drug a material that could be safely given to an infant directly, and at what risk? What dosages and blood levels are safe? Actual data answering these latter two questions are more critical than pharmacokinetic theory. The ultimate question faced by the physician is, "Can this infant be safely exposed to this chemical/medication as it appears in breast milk without a risk that exceeds the benefits of being breastfed?" Almost any drug present in a mother's blood will appear to some degree in her milk.

CHARACTERISTICS OF DRUGS

Protein Binding

Drugs entering the circulation become protein bound or remain free in the circulation. The protein-bound component of the drug serves as an inactive reservoir for the drug that is in equilibrium with the free drug. Most drugs enter the mammary alveolar cells in the unbound form (Fig. 11.1).

At term, plasma proteins may be reduced and the fatty acid and hypoprotein fraction slightly increased in the mother, which results in the displacement of some drugs from plasma proteins. During the early postpartum period, for 5 to 7 weeks, the free fraction of some drugs increases and therefore more readily crosses into milk (e.g., salicylate, phenytoin, diazepam).

Relative Concentration in Plasma Versus Milk

For most drugs, a higher concentration will be found in the plasma than in the milk. Only the small free fraction of a drug can cross the biologic membrane. The total concentration in milk is only minimally influenced by the binding of drugs to milk proteins (milk protein concentration is 0.9% in mature milk). Only those drug molecules that are free in solution can

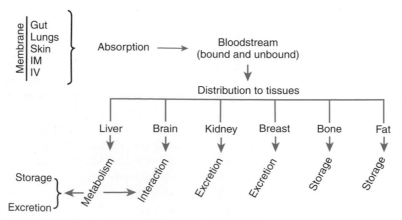

Fig. 11.1 Distribution pathways for drugs once absorbed during lactation. (Modified from Rivera-Calimlim L. The significance of drugs in breast milk. *Clin Perinatol.* 1976;14:51.)

pass through the endothelial pores, either by diffusion or by reverse pinocytosis. *Pinocytosis* is the process whereby drug molecules dissolved in the interstitial fluid attach to receptors located at the surface of the cell membrane. The cell membrane invaginates at the site of the drug attachment, bringing the drug into the cell. The membrane is pinched off, and the drug, surrounded by membrane, remains in the cell. Then the membrane is dissolved, leaving the drug molecule free in the cell.

Reverse pinocytosis is the process by which the apical membrane evaginates after fusion of the intracellular membrane-bound secretion granules with the plasma membrane. The granules include lipids, proteins, lactose, drug molecules, and other cellular constituents. The evagination of the plasma membrane is pinched off and released into the alveolar lumen. Within the extravascular space, the drug may be bound to proteins in the interstitial fluid. Some agents in free solution can pass into the alveolar milk directly by way of the spaces between the mammary alveolar cells. These paracellular areas account for a major portion of the fluid changes across the epithelium. These spaces between adjacent alveolar cells serve to carry water-soluble drugs from the tissue into the milk.

The intercellular junctions are "open" at delivery as lactation is being established and gradually "tighten" over the next few days. The amount of drug passed into milk on day 1 is greater than on day 3 or later. The composition of the milk changes from colostrum to mature milk, altering the amount of protein and fat, which can also influence drug levels in the milk. It is always important to know when plasma and milk samples were measured in relationship to the onset of lactation. Furthermore, some studies have been done on nonlactating women by pumping enough milk to measure the drug. These "weaning samples" do not reflect the normal physiology of lactation and therefore provide only misinformation.

Ionization

Drugs that are nonionized are excreted in the milk in greater amounts than are ionized compounds. Depending on the pH of the solvent and the drug dissociation constant (pK_a), many weak electrolytes are more or less ionized in solution. Blood plasma and interstitial fluid are slightly alkaline (pH 7.4). Drugs that are weak acids are ionized to a greater extent in alkaline solution and are more extensively bound to protein. The amount of drug excreted from plasma (pH 7.4) to milk (pH 6.8 to 7.3, average 7.0) depends on the pH of the compound. Thus a weakly acidic compound has a higher concentration in plasma than in milk. Conversely, weakly alkaline compounds are in equal or higher levels in the milk than in the plasma.

Drug Ionization Changes with the pH

The degree of drug ionization changes with the pH of the plasma and milk. Weak bases become more ionized with decreasing pH; thus the ionized component will increase in milk. Depending on the pH of the solvent and the drug dissociation constant (pK_a), many weak electrolytes are more or less ionized in solution. Blood plasma and interstitial fluid are

TABLE 11.1 Association Between Milk/Plasma (M/P) Ratios and Dissociation Constants (pK_a) of Sulfonamides

Sulfonamide	M/P Ratio	pK_a
Sulfacetamide	0.08	5.4
Sulfadiazine	0.21	6.5
Sulfathiazole	0.43	7.1
Sulfamethazine	0.51	7.4
Sulfapyridine	0.85	8.4
Sulfanilamide	1.00	10.4

Modified from Gaginella TS. Drugs and the nursing mother-infant. *US Pharm*. 1978;3:39.

slightly alkaline (pH 7.4) compared with milk (pH 6.8 to 7.3, average 7.0) The concentration in plasma and milk for the nonionized fraction will be the same, but the total amount of drug in the milk will be greater than in plasma. Drugs that are weak acids are ionized to a greater extent in alkaline solution and are more extensively bound to protein. The amount of drug excreted from plasma to milk depends on the pH of the compound. The amount of drug ionization changes with the pH of the plasma and milk.

The sulfonamides demonstrate the effect of the pK_a on the concentration of drug that reaches the milk. Sulfacetamide, with a low pK_a (5.4), has a low milk-to-plasma (M/P) ratio (0.08), whereas sulfanilamide has a pK_a of 10.4 and an M/P ratio of 1.00 (Table 11.1).

Passage of Molecules Into Milk Depends on Size

The passage of molecules into the milk also depends on the size of the molecule, or the molecular weight (mol wt, in daltons). Water-filled membranous pores permit the movement of molecules of less than 100 mol wt. Because of action similar to the limitation of transport of certain large-molecular-weight chemicals across the placenta, insulin and heparin are not found in human milk either, presumably because of the molecules' large size.

Solubility

The alveolar epithelium of the breast is a lipid barrier that is most permeable in the first few days of lactation when colostrum is being produced. The solubility of a compound in water and in lipid is a determining factor in its transfer. Nonionized drugs, which are lipid soluble, usually dissolve in the lipid phase of the membrane. The solubility is closely linked to the manner in which the drug crosses the membranes (Table 11.2). The membrane of the alveolar epithelial cells is composed of lipoprotein, glycolipid, phospholipid, and free lipids, as described in Chapter 3. The transfer of water-soluble drugs and ions is inhibited by this hydrophobic barrier. Water-soluble materials pass through pores in the

TABLE 11.2 Predicted Distribution Ratios of Drug Concentrations in Milk and Plasma

General Drug Type	Milk/Plasma (M/P) Ratio
Highly lipid-soluble drugs	~1
Highly protein-bound drugs in maternal serum	<1
Small (molecular weight <200) water-soluble drugs	~1
Weak acids	≤1
Weak bases	≥1
Actively transported drugs	>1

Modified from Gaginella TS. Drugs and the nursing mother-infant. *US Pharm.* 1978;3:39.

basement membrane and paracellular spaces. Low lipid solubility of a nonionized compound will diminish its excretion into milk.

Fat solubility. Lipid solubility affects the profile of the drug in the milk and plasma. A drug with high lipid solubility will have parallel elimination curves in the plasma and the milk. A drug with low lipid solubility will clear the plasma at a constant rate, but the clearance curve for the milk will peak lower and later, and the drug will linger in the milk. A prolonged terminal elimination phase may exist when the time between feedings is long.

If the agent is fat soluble, the fat content of the milk may be a significant variable. The fat content at any feeding increases over time; thus the so-called foremilk is low in fat, and the hindmilk is four to five times richer in fat toward the end of a feeding. Even though the total amount of fat will be about the same in each 24-hour period, the total amount of fat in a given feeding is less in the morning, peaks at midday, and drops off in the evening. The coefficient of lipid solubility for a nonionized drug determines both its penetration of the biologic membrane to gain entrance to milk and its concentration in milk fat. Sulfonamides with low fat solubility are in the aqueous and protein fraction of milk, whereas many barbiturates are in the lipid fraction. An inverse relationship exists between a drug's lipid solubility and the amount that appears in the skim fraction. The concentrations in fat differ for each member of the barbital family. Pentobarbital and secobarbital are found in the lipid phase, whereas phenobarbital is found in the aqueous phase.

Half-Life of a Medication

The half-life ($T_{1/2}$) of a medication is the amount of time it takes for half of the drug to be removed from the body by the various metabolic processes and is most often measured as the time it takes for the plasma level to drop by one-half at steady state (plasma half-life). A shorter drug half-life is preferred because there would likely be less exposure of the infant to the drug, and it might be possible to dose the medication to limit the infant's drug exposure in the milk.

Mechanisms of Transport

Drugs pass into milk by simple diffusion, carrier-mediated diffusion, or active transport, as follows:

- Simple diffusion: Concentration gradient decreases
- Carrier-mediated diffusion: Concentration gradient decreases
- Active transport: Concentration gradient increases
- Pinocytosis: Active membrane transport into the cell via receptors
- Reverse pinocytosis: Active membrane transport out of the cell

Nonelectrolytes such as ethanol, urea, and antipyrine enter the milk by diffusion through the lipid membrane barrier and may reach the same concentrations in the milk as in the plasma, regardless of the pH. The main entrance site of molecules is at the basement luminal membrane, where water-soluble materials pass through the alveolar pores. Nonionized drugs cross the membrane more easily than ionized ones because of the structure of the membrane. The nonionized drugs pass through the membrane by diffusion. When simple diffusion takes place, the M/P ratio is 1.0. Passive diffusion provides the same ratio regardless of the plasma concentrations of the drug or the volume of milk secreted. Different M/P ratios depend on the binding to protein and are a measure of the protein-free fraction. The dissimilar ratios for the sulfa drugs (see Table 11.1) partly result from the difference in protein binding and partly from ionization.

Large molecules depend on their lipid solubility and ionization to cross the membrane because they pass in a lipid-soluble, nonionized form. The M/P ratio is determined when equilibrium exists in the amount of nonionized drug in the aqueous phase on both sides of the membrane. When drugs are only partially ionized, the nonionized fraction determines the concentration that crosses the membrane. The drugs for which the nonionized fraction is not very lipid soluble will pass only in a limited degree into breast milk.

Passive drug transport may occur in the form of *facilitated diffusion.* The active compound is transported across the cell membrane by a carrier enzyme or protein. The gradient is toward a lesser or equal concentration in both simple diffusion and facilitated diffusion and is controlled by chemical activity gradients. Facilitated diffusion usually involves water-soluble substance too large to pass through the membrane pores.

Active transport mechanisms provide a process whereby the gradient is "uphill," or higher, in the milk. The process is similar to facilitated diffusion except that metabolic energy is required to overcome the gradient. Examples of substances actively transported include glucose, amino acids, calcium, magnesium, and sodium. Pinocytosis and reverse pinocytosis, as described previously, are involved in the transport of very large molecules and proteins. Chloride ions are secreted into milk via an active apical membrane pump, whereas sodium and potassium diffuse by electrical gradient. Because the level of sodium is kept low, an active return of sodium may occur into the plasma, referred to as a *reverse pump.* Retrograde diffusion, the passage of a drug back into the maternal bloodstream from the milk, is another mechanism influencing the level of drug in the milk. The same variable affecting the drug's diffusion into the milk will affect its passage back into the plasma. Drugs with a shorter half-life will demonstrate greater variations in drug level within the milk as a result of retrograde diffusion.[14]

PHARMACOKINETIC PRINCIPLES

Pharmacokinetic principles relate to the specific variation with time of the drug concentration in the blood or plasma as a result of its absorption, distribution, and elimination. Ultimately, by extrapolation of these factors, one determines the bioavailability of the drug. The most elementary kinetic model is based on the body as a single compartment. Distribution of the drug in the compartment is assumed to be uniform and rapidly equilibrated. In the single-compartment model, the volume of distribution of a drug is considered to be the same as that of the plasma, assuming a rapid uniform distribution.[15]

Volume of Distribution

The volume of distribution (V_d) is calculated as follows:

$$V_d = \frac{\text{Total amount drug in body}}{\text{Concentration of drug in plasma}}$$

The absorption and elimination are considered to be exponential or first-order kinetics. A two-compartment model of drug kinetics considers the phase of decreasing drug concentration as the drug distributes into the tissues. Initially, concentrations fall rapidly as the drug distributes, then first-order elimination follows. When considering the pharmacokinetics of drugs in breast milk, one must also consider that elimination in the breast is by two potential routes: excreted with the milk to the infant and back-diffusion into the plasma to reequilibrate with the falling level in the plasma.

Concentration of Drug in Breast Milk

With access to the volume of distribution of the drug in question, the amount of the dose, and the weight of the mother, the concentration of drug in breast milk may be theoretically calculated as follows:

$$\text{Concentration in breast milk} = \frac{\text{Dose}}{\text{Volume of distribution}}$$

Milk-to-Plasma Ratio

By definition, the M/P ratio is the concentration of a drug in the mother's milk divided by its concentration in the mother's plasma at the same time. A higher M/P ratio indicates that a higher amount of drug will reach the milk for a given concentration. The overall amount of drug reaching the milk is primarily determined by the concentration of the drug in the plasma. If choosing between two drugs with different M/P ratios, then the drug with the lower M/P ratio is less likely to reach the milk than the one with the higher M/P ratio given the same plasma concentrations of the drugs.

Mode of Administration of the Drug

The concentration of the drug in the circulation of the mother depends on the mode of administration: oral, IV, IM, or TDDS. Absorption through the skin, the lungs (inhalants), or vaginally may also need to be considered.

The levels in the blood depend on the route of administration. The curves produced by bolus IV medication peak high and early and taper sharply, thus making avoiding peak plasma levels more feasible. Absorption from IM dosing is less rapid but follows a similar but less sharp curve. Oral dosing depends on other factors, such as whether the medication is taken between or during meals. Depending on the curve of uptake and removal of drug from the plasma, the area under the curve varies. Single doses are simple area-under-the-curve calculations, but calculations for multiple doses or chronic use vary with the steady state of the drug in the body. The mode of administration is important in determining the overall bioavailability of a drug. TDDS patches are constructed to deliver the medication at a constant rate continuously over a period of time.

The TDDS depends on absorption of the drug through the skin at a steady rate; it has become a significant route of administration for certain medications. The delivery rate is determined by diffusion of the drug from the reservoir matrix through the epidermis. This method offers some advantages, including convenience of dosing, reduced dosing frequency, ease of reaching a steady state, increased patient compliance, avoidance of first-pass hepatic biotransformation, avoidance of peaks and valleys in blood levels, and reduction of side effects through heightened selectivity of drug action.[16] The level in the plasma remains constant during the drug's anticipated life span while the patch is in place. The technology is limited to drugs with low molecular weight that are hydrophilic and can diffuse through the stratum corneum. The top molecular weight is 500 daltons. For patient compliance and economics, the patch size is limited to 50 cm in diameter. Occasional patients experience skin irritation. Currently, patches are limited to drugs that are potent in small amounts and highly diffusible through the skin. To maintain a constant rate, a surplus of the drug must be present, often 20 to 30 times the amount that will be absorbed during the time of application. The potential for toxicity is great. If a patch is utilized while lactating, it should be applied and covered so that a nursing infant cannot accidentally get to it. TDDS patches are available for scopolamine, nicotine, clonidine, fentanyl, and other drugs (Table 11.3).

A summary of the steps in the passage of drugs into breast milk follows:

1. Mammary alveolar epithelium represents a lipid barrier with water-filled pores and is most permeable for drugs during the colostral phase of milk secretion (first week postpartum).
2. Drug excretion into milk depends on the drug's degree of ionization, molecular weight, solubility in fat and water, and the relation of the pH of plasma (7.4) to the pH of milk (7.0).
3. Drugs preferably enter mammary cells basally in the nonionized, nonprotein-bound form by diffusion or active transport.

TABLE 11.3   Currently Available Transdermal Patches for Systemic Effects

Generic Drug	Brand Name	Strengths/Release Rate	Application Frequency	Total Drug Content per Patch
Clonidine	Catapres-TTS	0.1, 0.2, 0.3 mg/24 h	7 days	2.5, 5, 7.5 mg
Estradiol	Alora	0.025, 0.05, 0.075, 0.1 mg/24 h	7 days	0.77, 1.5, 2.3, 3.1 mg
	Climara	0.025, 0.0375, 0.05, 0.06, 0.75, 0.1 mg/24 h	7 days	2, 2.85, 3.8, 4.55, 5.7, 7.6 mg
	Estraderm	0.05, 0.1 mg/24 h	3-4 days	4 mg, 8 mg
	Vivelle-Dot	0.025, 0.0375, 0.05, 0.075, 0.1 mg/24 h	0-4 days	0.62/2.7 mg, 0.51/4.8 mg
Estradiol/ Norelgestromin	Ortho Evra	20 mcg/150 mcg/24 h	7 days	0.75 mg/6 mg
Fentanyl	Duragesic	12.5, 25, 50, 100 mcg/h	72 hours	1.25, 2.5, 5, 7.5, 10 mg
Lidocaine	Lidoderm	35 mg/12 h	12 h/day	700 mg
Methylphenidate	Daytrana	10, 15, 20, 30 mg/9 h	9 h/day	27.5, 41, 3, 55, 82.5 mg
Nicotine	Habitrol	7, 14, 21 mg/24 h	16–24 h/day	17.5, 35, 52.5 mg
	NicoDerm CQ	7, 14, 21 mg/24 h	16–24 h/day	36, 78, 114 mg
Nitroglycerin	Nitro-Dur	0.1, 0.2, 0.3, 0.4, 0.6, 0.8 mg/h	12–14 h/day	20, 40, 60, 80, 120, 160 mg
	Minitran	0.1, 0.2, 0.4, 0.6 mg/h	12–14 h/day	Approximately 8.6, 17, 34, 51.4 mg
Oxybutynin	Oxytrol	3.9 mg/24 h	24 h	36 mg
Rotigotine	Neupro	2, 4, 6 mg/24 h	24 h	4.5, 9, 13.5 mg
Scopolamine	Transderm-Scop	1.0 mg/72 h	3 days	1.5 mg
Selegiline	Emsam	6, 9, 12 mg/24 h	24 h	20, 30, 40 mg
Testosterone	Androderm	2.5, 5 mg/24 h	24 h	12.2, 24, 3 mg

4. Water-soluble drugs of less than 200 mol wt pass through water-filled membranous pores.
5. Drugs leave mammary alveolar cells apically by diffusion or active transport.
6. Drugs may enter milk via spaces between mammary alveolar cells.
7. Most ingested drugs appear in milk; drug amounts in milk usually do not exceed 1% of ingested dosage, and levels in the milk are independent of milk volume.
8. Drugs are bound much less to milk proteins than to plasma proteins.
9. The drug-metabolizing capacity of mammary epithelium is not understood.

INFANT-RELATED FACTORS

Absorption from Gastrointestinal Tract

Although concern surrounds the amount of a given agent in the breast milk, of greater importance is the amount absorbed into an infant's bloodstream. No accurate way exists to predict this because numerous factors affect absorption from the gastrointestinal (GI) tract and the metabolic and elimination processes acting on the drug in an infant's bloodstream. The tolerance of the chemical to the pH of the stomach and the enzymatic activity of the intestinal tract are additional significant factors. The volume of milk consumed is a factor as well. Some drugs are not well absorbed with food (see later discussion of food–drug interactions). The oral bioavailability of a compound is a major factor relative to the exposure of an infant to a drug.

Infant's Ability to Detoxify and Excrete Agent

Any drug given to an infant by any route has to be evaluated according to the infant's ability to detoxify or conjugate the chemical in the liver and excrete it in the urine or eliminate it in stool. Some compounds that appear in milk at very low levels are not well excreted by infants and therefore can accumulate in infants' systems to the point of toxicity.

Drugs that depend on the liver for conjugation, such as acetaminophen, are theoretic risks because of the limited reserve of the neonatal hepatic detoxification system. When actual measurements were made of neonates given acetaminophen, they were noted to handle it well because they conjugate it in the sulfhydryl system as an alternative pathway, which is used only to a small extent in adult metabolism of acetaminophen. When a single dose of a drug is given to a mother and the level is measured in her milk and in her infant, it does not give a clear picture of the potential for accumulation in the infant's system. The competition for binding a drug to protein is also important. Some drugs, such as sulfadiazine, compete for binding sites that might normally bind bilirubin in the first week or so of life. This puts an infant in jeopardy of kernicterus at a given bilirubin level because of an increase in the fraction of bilirubin left unbound for lack of binding sites.

The Maturity of Infant in Early Life

The maturity of an infant at birth is an extremely important factor during the first few months of life; thus the gestational age at birth should be established. Clearly, the less mature the infant, the less well tolerated drugs are, not only because of the immaturity of the organ systems but also because of differences in body composition (Fig. 11.2). The less mature an infant, the greater the water content of the body and the proportion of extracellular water. Although the percentage of body weight that is protein is similar for all newborns (i.e., 12%), the absolute amount of protein for binding is less the

smaller an infant is. The amount of body fat is also low, by percentage of body weight and in absolute values. The distribution of highly lipid-soluble drugs therefore will be more apt to deposit in the brain of a 1000-g infant with 3% body fat by weight than in a 3500-g full-term infant with 12% body fat. This may explain the more sedating effect of a drug on the central nervous system (CNS) of a smaller, younger, and less mature infant. The relative lack of plasma protein-binding sites in a small, premature infant compared with a more mature, older infant results in more free (unbound) active drug in circulation. Complications of premature birth, such as acidosis and hypoxia, also contribute to the unavailability of albumin-binding sites and thus result in more unbound drug.

The inability of the liver to metabolize drugs effectively results in the accumulation of some compounds that might be readily cleared by an older infant. At about 42 weeks' conceptual age, an infant's liver is able to metabolize most drugs competently. Renal clearance similarly is less effective with decreasing maturity, which increases the risk for drug accumulation. The need to dose a premature infant less frequently is common to many drugs, such as antibiotics, caffeine, and theophylline, and confirms that a small, premature infant does not clear drugs well.

Metabolic Problems in Early Life

Special problems in neonates, in addition to the presence of jaundice or low serum albumin, may require special consideration. Low Apgar scores at birth, signifying some degree of stress, hypoxia, or acidosis, may alter binding-site availability but may also alter the metabolism and excretion of a drug. Continuing respiratory distress requiring ventilatory support, sepsis, and renal failure demand special consideration when determining if a sick neonate can receive the mother's milk when she is being treated with certain medications. Prescribing for such a mother should be done in consultation with the neonatologist if the woman is providing milk for her infant.

Age

The age of an infant makes a difference in the total volume of milk consumed; in an older child (already taking complementary foods), the child's diet includes other food items so that milk does not compose the total intake. Age can influence the pH of the stomach, the amount of catabolic enzymes in intestinal secretions, and the integrity of the mucosal barrier, thus affecting drug ionization, metabolism, and absorption. Age influences the infant's ability to metabolize drugs more effectively; for example, sulfa drugs can be given to infants after the first month of life, whereas they may cause toxicity in the first month of life. The age of the child also must be taken into consideration with regard to the volume of breast milk ingested per feeding and per day, with a greater volume of milk leading to greater exposure. The usual estimate of intake for an exclusively breastfed infant is 150 mL/kg per day. The agent may appear in low levels in a mother's serum, but mammary blood flow during lactation is 500 mL/min, and a mother produces between 60 and 300 mL of milk per hour. Even an agent that appears in minimal concentrations in the

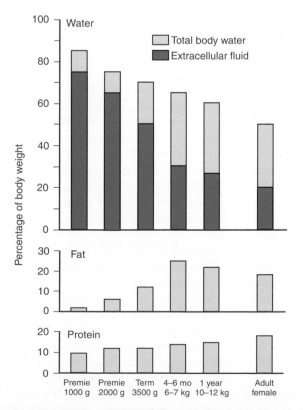

Fig. 11.2 Comparative body composition of infants and adults. (Redrawn from Bechard LJ, Wroe E, Ellisk K. Body composition and growth. In: Duggan C, Watkins JB, Walker WA, eds. *Nutrition in Clinical Practice*. 4th ed. Hamilton, Canada: BC Decker; 2008.)

milk may present a significant problem when one considers that 1000 mL of milk may be consumed in a day by an older infant. Even though the volume is low during the colostral phase of lactation, the breast itself is more permeable to drugs; therefore a higher concentration of drug may enter the colostrum. The immaturity of the infant's developing organs may predispose those organs to greater sensitivity/toxicity to certain medications.

MILK-TO-PLASMA RATIO FOR DRUGS IS USUALLY NOT USEFUL

The M/P ratio for drugs has been measured and reported for many medications. By definition, the M/P ratio is the concentration of the drug in the milk versus the concentration in maternal plasma (serum) at the same time. It presumes that the relationship between the two concentrations remains constant, which, in most cases, it does not. If it were a constant, it would allow the estimation of the amount of drug in the milk from any given plasma level in a mother.

An inaccurate ratio, or one determined under variable circumstances, produces erroneous estimates of the amount of drug in the milk, A pharmacokinetic model is a requisite foundation for studies of drugs in breast milk. A single-point-in-time M/P ratio, or an average ratio calculated with single-dose, area-under-the-curve data, does not work for all drugs. Neither ratio accounts for the importance of time-dependent variations of drug concentration in milk.

The M/P ratio is most valuable if obtained when an infant would be nursed. If the ratio is 1:0, it means only that the levels are equal. If the level is minimal in a mother's plasma because of the large volume of distribution, and if the milk level is also low, the M/P ratio is 1:0. If levels are drawn at the peak plasma level and are equal, the M/P is still 1:0, but the infant receives a large dose. Thus the M/P ratio is valuable only when the time of the measurement is known in relationship to the dosing of the mother. Dose strength, duration of dosing, maternal variation in drug disposition, maternal disease, drug interactions and competition of additional drugs for metabolism or binding sites, and racial variations in drug metabolism all influence the M/P interpretation. The M/P ratio may be greater than 1, which sounds alarming; however, a drug with a large volume of distribution will have low levels in the plasma, leading to a relatively lower amount reaching the milk. The M/P ratio only confirms that the drug gets in the milk; the plasma level of the drug in the mother has to be known at steady state and/or the highest values after intermittent dosing to estimate the likely dose the infant is exposed to.

EVALUATING DRUG DATA

The paucity of carefully controlled studies on large enough samples to validate the results when such a large number of variables are active has been lamented by many authors. Some data collected are not pharmacokinetically sound. A clinician needs to understand these variables, as well as pharmacokinetic principles, to make a reasonable judgment about a given case.

Interethnic and racial differences in drug responsiveness are well recognized. The increased heterogeneity of national populations has brought increased awareness of genetic diversity. Plasma binding, especially with drugs dependent on glycoproteins for binding, often varies greatly between Caucasian and Chinese subjects, for example. Such factors contribute to the differences in drug disposition and pharmacologic response.

It should be theoretically possible to determine how much of a specific drug reaches an infant in the mother's milk by knowing all the properties of the drug, including its volume of distribution, ionization, pK_a, lipid solubility, protein-binding activity, and rate of detoxification in the maternal system. There is enough variation in the levels that reach an infant and in how the infant deals with the agent, however, that makes it necessary to have specific data about a specific drug. Thus specific information about the mother, the infant, the drug, and the clinical scenario should facilitate the identification of relative risks or benefits, leading to an informed decision-making process.

SAFETY FOR INFANT

The first question to ask about infant safety is, "Is this a drug that can be given to the infant directly if necessary?" Antibiotics (e.g., penicillin) that one could give an infant are in this category, whereas an antibiotic such as chloramphenicol, which would not give an infant under ordinary circumstances, should be avoided in a nursing mother. The toxicity of chloramphenicol in an infant is dose related and associated with an unpredictable accumulation of the drug. Also, an idiosyncratic reaction occurs with chloramphenicol, which is unrelated to dose but causes pancytopenia.

If the drug in question can be given to an infant, does the amount in the milk create any risk to the infant? Phenobarbital can be given to infants for various reasons; thus the question is whether enough phenobarbital in the breast milk will reach the infant to cause difficulty. The infant should be watched for symptoms of lethargy or sleepiness, such as a change in feeding or sleeping pattern. If the infant is sleeping long periods and feeding less than usual (specifically, fewer than five or six times per day), the medication may be at fault. Phenobarbital is a significant drug for a mother with seizures; therefore a careful review of the risk—benefit ratio to both mother and infant should be undertaken. Barbiturates vary in their effect in young infants. A newborn does not handle the short-acting barbiturates well because they are dependent on detoxification in the liver, whereas phenobarbital depends more on the kidney for excretion.

If the drug was taken during pregnancy, as for epilepsy, an infant will already have the drug in his or her system via the placenta at a steady state and will have to begin to excrete it on his or her own after delivery.[17] Enzyme induction may have taken place in the neonate, however, because of exposure to the drug in utero; phenobarbital hastens maturation of the fetal liver.[18] Enzyme induction of the hepatic oxygenase system by phenobarbital, phenytoin, primidone, and carbamazepine is well established. Valproate, however, does not induce enzyme activity.

If one can safely give a drug to an infant, administration becomes a question of watching for any symptoms of excessive accumulation. The age of the infant affects the ability to clear the drug.

When the drug in question is one not normally given to an infant at that particular age, weight, or degree of maturity, decision-making is more difficult. Specific information about the amount of the drug that appears in the milk is essential in decision-making. Often, conflicting information is available. Many lists of drug-milk levels have perpetuated the same errors in calculation; thus having more than one reference report the same information may not provide confirmation of its accuracy.

Prolonged Therapeutic Use

If a medication will have to be taken for weeks or months, as with cardiovascular drugs, the drug has a greater potential impact than when taken only for a few days. If the drug exposure has already occurred for 9 months in utero, some think it is less of an issue during lactation; however, the presence of the drug in the milk may compound the problem.

To determine the dose delivered to an infant, the following formula is used:

$$\frac{\text{Dose}}{24 \text{ hours}} = \text{Concentration of drug in milk}$$
$$\times \text{Weight in kg of infant}$$
$$\times \text{Volume of milk per kg}$$
$$\text{ingested in 24 hours}$$

$$\text{Dose}/24 \text{ hours} = C_{\text{milk}} \times \text{Weight} \times \text{Volume}/\text{kg}/24 \text{ hours}$$

The average daily dose the infant receives can also be calculated, as follows:

$$\text{Infant daily dosage} = (\text{Drug concentration in milk})$$
$$\times (\text{Daily volume of milk ingested})$$

There is variability in the daily milk intake for an exclusively breastfed infant because of the age of the child, the child's nutritional needs, and the growth and age of the child.[19] The routinely accepted value for daily milk intake of an exclusively breastfed infant is 150 mL/kg per day, which can be used for estimates.

It has been recommended by Ito and by Hale that the calculation be the relative infant dose (RID), which is the weight-adjusted percentage of the maternal dosage.[12,20] It is commonly calculated as follows:

$$\text{RID} = \frac{\text{Absolute infant dose mg/kg/day}}{\text{Maternal dose mg/kg/day}} \times 100$$

The WHO Working Group on Drugs and Human Lactation and others recommend that the RID be less than 10% of the lower dose of the weight-adjusted maternal or infant dosage. They also state that an RID of greater than 25% is enough to proscribe the use of the medication in a lactating mother. There are no published data to justify these specific cutoff values. There are a number of variables that compound the use of the RID in predicting drug safety in lactating women—for example, a mother's daily dose can vary significantly, the infant's postnatal age will influence the infant's milk intake and the enterohepatic circulation of the drug, the drug's bioavailability in the infant compared with an adult, the existence of active metabolites of a drug, and the fact that the RID may also be reported as a range of percentages. Although there are limitations to the use of RID to predict the safety of medication use during breastfeeding, an appropriately calculated and reported RID can be useful when it is low and is thoughtfully combined with other important drug information for lactating women and infants.

Sensitization

Is sensitization a risk, even in the small dosages of a drug that might pass into the milk? This question arises most frequently with the use of antibiotics, and the use of penicillin is most frequently questioned. Certainly, if a family has a strong history of drug sensitization, it should be considered. In that case, however, it should be questioned for a mother as well. Whether infants are put at risk for developing resistant strains of bacteria in their systems by small amounts of antibiotics in their feedings is a serious question. It is not a question that has been adequately addressed in the literature. It is as pertinent for the dairy and meat industries as for the humans who consume the food products that have a small amount of antibiotics because of administration to livestock.

CORRELATION OF DRUG SAFETY IN PREGNANCY AND LACTATION

Very rarely is valid information on the appearance of a drug in breast milk available on the package insert because pharmaceutical companies usually merely indicate that it should not be taken during pregnancy and lactation. To provide more information, they would have to study it, which they typically choose not to do. Agents that may be safe during pregnancy may not be safe during lactation. During pregnancy, the maternal liver and kidney are serving as detoxification and excretion resources for the fetus via the placenta, whereas during lactation, an infant has to handle the drug totally on his or her own after it has reached his or her circulation. An infant in utero receives a drug in greater quantity via the circulation, whereas a nursing infant receives only what reaches the milk. One should be cautious about translating data pertaining to these two periods back and forth. Drugs that are contraindicated in pregnancy may be acceptable during lactation.

Oral Bioavailability

The dose of a drug delivered via milk to an infant is significantly affected by oral bioavailability, which is the percentage of the drug absorbed into the infant's system via the gut.

Oral bioavailability is the rate and extent to which an active drug is absorbed and enters the general circulation. Absolute oral bioavailability compares the oral route with the IV route. To reach the general circulation, an oral dose must pass through the wall of the gut, liver, or mucosa of the upper respiratory tract.[21] First-pass metabolism or elimination in the tissues of these three organs may reduce a drug's bioavailability. It is possible for a drug to be 100% absorbed and be destroyed or eliminated and have 0% bioavailability because it is so rapidly metabolized.

If a compound is poorly absorbed, it is of less concern than one with 100% bioavailability. Most drugs administered by injection (e.g., insulin, heparin, gentamicin) only are not orally bioavailable.

Food–Drug Interactions

When drugs are taken with meals, numerous opportunities exist for food–drug interactions to occur.[22] Because a breastfed infant receives all maternal medications excreted in the milk "with food," this is an important consideration in the discussion of drugs in milk. The effects of food may reduce GI absorption or irritation. Mechanisms of food–drug interactions can be summarized as follows.[22]

Physiologic
1. Changes in gastric emptying
2. Increased intestinal motility
3. Increased splanchnic blood flow
4. Increased bile, acid, and enzyme secretion
5. Induction and inhibition of drug metabolism
6. Competition in active transport

Physiochemical
7. Food as a mechanical barrier to absorption
8. Altered dissolution of drugs
9. Chelation and adsorption

Pharmacodynamic
10. Altered enzyme activity
11. Changes in homeostasis

Factors Favoring the Safe Maternal Use of a Medication During Lactation

There are a number of factors favoring the maternal use of a medication, drug, or product during lactation once it is clear that that the mother has an appropriate diagnosis and indication for the use of the medication.

1. Pediatric approved use of the medication—The medication is safely used in infants and children with a known dose range.
2. Favorable safety profile—There is a documented side-effect profile from appropriate studies of medication use in children and/or published information regarding the medication's safe use during lactation. Or the agent is listed in the generally recognized as safe (GRAS) listing maintained by the FDA.
3. There is evidence that the medication has little or no effect on the mother's milk supply or breastfeeding.
4. The medication has low or no oral bioavailability

5. Low or very low RID: <10%, <5%, or <1%.
6. The medication has specific characteristics that are likely to lead to a lower amount of the drug in breast milk, such as shorter half-life, high protein binding, and high molecular weight. There are no or limited active metabolites that could add to the amount of active drug in the milk or affect the mother or infant.
7. There is adequate information about the potentially exposed infant, including age, size/weight, and amount of milk ingested daily, and no significant conditions affecting excretion, metabolism, or probable sensitivity to the medication
8. Additional precautions for the use of herbal product include the following: (1) know the chemical substances contained in the herb and their reported effects; (2) consider products from known, reliable sources; (3) use a "pure" form of the herb, not a mixture of herbs; (4) use the lowest dose necessary; and (5) consult a herbalist, lactation consultant, or physician knowledgeable about the herb's use during lactation before use.

Minimizing The Effect of Maternal Medication

If a mother truly needs a specific medication and the hazards to the infant are minimal, the following important adjustments can be made to minimize the effects:

1. Do not use the long-acting form of the drug because the infant may have more difficulty renally excreting such an agent or detoxifying it in the liver. Accumulation of the drug or an active metabolite in the infant is then a genuine concern.
2. Schedule doses so that the smallest possible amount gets into the milk. Check the usual absorption rates and peak blood levels of the drug. Having a mother take the medication immediately after breastfeeding is usually the safest time for the infant with most, but not all, drugs.
3. Watch the infant for any unusual signs or symptoms, such as a change in feeding pattern or sleeping habits, fussiness, or a rash, whenever the mother takes medication.
4. When possible, choose the drug that produces the least amount in the milk (e.g., sulfonamides; see Tables 11.1 and 11.2).

CLASSIFICATION SYSTEMS

The transfer of drugs and other chemicals into human milk also has been detailed in statements by the AAP Committee on Drugs from 1983, with updates through 2013.[10,23]

The list includes only those drugs about which published information is available, and it does not provide the pharmacologic properties of the compounds. The updated 2001 list was divided into the same seven categories as the earlier lists, grouping drugs by their risk factors in relation to breastfeeding. The categories are the following:

1. Cytotoxic drugs that may interfere with cellular metabolism of a nursing infant
2. Drugs of abuse
3. Radioactive compounds that require temporary cessation of breastfeeding

4. Drugs for which the effect on nursing infants is unknown but may be of concern
5. Drugs that have been associated with significant effects on some nursing infants and should be given to nursing mothers with caution
6. Maternal medications usually compatible with breastfeeding
7. Food and environmental agents: effect on breastfeeding

The list of more than 300 items included in the AAP review is not comprehensive or all-inclusive. Further, the committee encourages physicians to report adverse effects in infants consuming the milk of mothers taking specific drugs to the committee at the AAP.[23] The previous category listing from the FDA included succinct categories: Fetal Risk Factors/Pregnancy Categories (A, B, C, D, X).[24] A new rating system was proposed by the FDA in its Pregnancy and Lactation Labeling Rule in 2013, which is more narrative and less "telegraphic."[9] In his book *Medications and Mothers' Milk* and the associated database, Dr. Thomas Hale and his team utilize another LRC based on their assessment of the risk data (L1 = compatible with breastfeeding, L2 = probably compatible, L3 = probably compatible [individualized assessment of the benefits versus risk is appropriate], L4 = possibly hazardous, L5 = hazardous).[12]

Briggs et al., in their classic text *Drugs in Pregnancy and Lactation*, use the AAP classification.[5]

Drugs in Lactation Resources

The Breastfeeding and Human Lactation Study Center at the University of Rochester continually updates its database on drugs, medications, and contaminants in human milk. (See Chapter 25.) More than 4000 references pertain to drugs in the database. In addition, other drugs typically used by women in their childbearing years for which there are no specific milk levels are listed with their oral bioavailability for infants, peak serum time in the mothers, volume of distribution for the drugs, and other pharmacologic information (pH, solubility, protein binding, metabolism) obtained from a host of resources. With this information, a physician should be able to determine relative risk and thus select the best compound and adjust the dose and the time of, and association to, the breastfeeding.

The Breastfeeding and Human Lactation Center is available during limited hours (8 AM to 4 PM EST, Monday to Friday) to address more complex questions (585-275-0088).

LactMed is an extensive database (Drugs and Lactation Database) maintained and updated frequently by the National Library of Medicine and the professional contributors. It can be accessed at http://www.ncbi.nlm.nih.gov/pubmed/30000282.[4]

E-Lactancia is a database resource maintained by the Association for Promotion and Cultural and Scientific Research of Breastfeeding in Spain (http://www.e-lactancia.org).[25]

The Infant Risk Center is a website and call center resource at the University of Texas Tech University Health Science Center connected with Dr. Thomas Hale and his team (available at www.infantrisk.com and 806-352-2519).[26]

Mother to Baby is the database and call center established in 2013 by the Organization of Teratology Information Specialists (OTIS) as the public face for the organization's research and information service to mothers, families, and professionals concerning questions about pregnancy and lactation. OTIS was established in 1987 to connect world-renowned experts in the field of birth defects research to the general public. The Mother to Baby Organization answers questions and concerns related to pregnancy and lactation about the risks of medications, chemicals, herbal products, illicit drugs, diseases, and more via e-mail, telephone, and open chat (https://mothertobaby.org, 866-626-6847).

SPECIFIC DRUG GROUPS

This section will include only selected topics that are of current interest and not specifically addressed by an Academy of Breastfeeding Medicine clinical protocol: 9, Galactogogues; 13, Contraceptives; 15, Analgesia/Anesthesia; 18, Antidepressants in Nursing Mothers; 28, Peripartum Analgesia and Anesthesia; 29, Iron, Zinc, and Vitamin D Supplementation During Breastfeeding; and 31, Radiology and Nuclear Medicine Studies in Lactating Women. Contraceptives are also addressed in Chapter 21, Reproductive Function During Lactation. Many treatment topics (e.g., treatment of migraines, rheumatologic disorders, human immunodeficiency infection) are beyond the scope of this text, and a complete discussion and recommendations will not be addressed. With the available published resources, databases on medications and lactation, websites, and call-lines, it is easier for a practitioner to locate appropriate information about a specific medication and lactation in these other resources. This chapter includes some new tables with specific therapeutic groups of medications, primarily for comparison of the different medications and consideration of medication alternatives.

Analgesics

Analgesia is an essential consideration for the mother in the peripartum and postpartum period through the duration of lactation. Pharmacologic and nonpharmacologic pain relief during labor and the postpartum period can improve overall maternal and infant outcomes by relieving suffering but may have consequences for breastfeeding. The Academy of Breastfeeding Medicine (ABM) has published an evidence-based clinical protocol on peripartum analgesia and anesthesia for the breastfeeding mother.[27] There is a second clinical protocol from the ABM addressing analgesia and anesthesia for the breastfeeding mother outside the immediate postpartum period.[28] Benoit et al. have summarized the evidence for breastfeeding as analgesia for infants.[29] Physicians can familiarize themselves with the guidelines published by the ABM and then refer to the databases, Infantrisk.com and LactMed, to review up-to-date information on specific agents being considered for use in a lactating mother. Refer to Chapter 15, Medical Complications of Mothers, for specific medical conditions.

Anesthesia

The ABM's clinical protocols on anesthesia in the peripartum period and beyond provide appropriate evidence-based guidance on the use of anesthesia for breastfeeding mothers.[27,28] There is a review of obstetrical anesthesia from the anesthesiologist's perspective written by Lim et al. for additional reference.[30]

Antibiotics

Antibiotics are one of the most frequently utilized medications during lactation, along with analgesics and vitamins. The majority of antibiotics have recommended uses in infants and children for their own diagnosed infections and can be safely given to breastfeeding mothers.[31,32] Exposure of infants to antibiotics in any form raises concerns for sensitization, changes in intestinal flora (diarrhea or altered intestinal microbiome), and the development of drug-resistant microorganisms. Data are conflicting concerning early life antibiotic exposure and downstream effects of alteration of the infant's intestinal microbiome (obesity, adiposity, inflammatory bowel disease, autism, or other nervous system effects). Van Wattum et al., in their systematic review, reported on a comparison of the absolute infant dose as a percentage of the therapeutic infant dose for 20 different antibiotics. The absolute infant dose for metronidazole was just over 10% of the therapeutic infant dose, vancomycin and azithromycin were approximately 6%, and the other 17 antibiotics were less than 4%.[32] The low levels of absolute infant dose from breastfeeding are highly unlikely to cause a problem for breastfeeding infants, whether they also are receiving the same antibiotic or not. Specifically, lactating mothers can use the penicillins, cephalosporins, vancomycin, and aminoglycosides without concerns relative to their infants. The notable exceptions to the apparent safety of antibiotics and breastfeeding include sulfonamide exposure in an infant less than 4 weeks of age because of concern for interference with bilirubin binding to albumen, tetracycline-related medications because of teeth staining and abnormal bone growth with prolonged exposure, chloramphenicol in infants related to "gray baby" syndrome or idiosyncratic bone marrow suppression, and erythromycin or azithromycin because of its association with pyloric stenosis when administered to infants in the first 4 to 6 weeks of life. For these antibiotics, a specific risk–benefit assessment should be reviewed with the mother. Chloroquine, gentamicin, streptomycin, and rifampin are reported by the AAP to be safe because they are not excreted in milk.[10]

Fluoroquinolones

Fluoroquinolones had been restricted in pediatric use because of early reports of arthropathy in immature animals and a single report of pseudomembranous colitis in a breastfeeding infant whose mother had self-medicated with ciprofloxacin.[33] More recently, ciprofloxacin has been used in pediatric patients because it is valuable in gram-negative infections and also anthrax. The AAP Committee on Drugs has designated ciprofloxacin to be safe for breastfeeding women, although there are concerns for quinolones' effect on the infant's gut microbiome and development of drug-resistant organisms, as well as diarrhea or candidiasis. Otic or ophthalmic use by the mother is not a concern. Hale has listed ciprofloxacin as L3 (limited data—probably compatible, RID: 2.1% to 6.34%) and recommended avoiding breastfeeding for 3 to 4 hours after a dose to decrease the amount in breast milk. For the other quinolones, Hale has reported gatifloxacin as L3 (no data—probably compatible, RID: unknown), gemifloxacin as L3 (no data—probably compatible, RID: no data), levofloxacin as L2 (limited data—probably compatible, RID: 10.5% to 17.2%), moxifloxacin as L3 (no data—probably compatible, RID: unknown), norfloxacin as L3 (limited data—probably compatible, RID: unknown; little or no drug detected in milk; possibly the best alternative of the quinolones), ofloxacin as L2 (limited data—probably compatible, RID: 3.1%), and trovafloxacin as L4 (limited data—probably hazardous, RID: 4.2%; withdrawn from the US market because of concerns of acute liver failure).[12]

Metronidazole

Metronidazole (Flagyl) does appear in milk at levels approximately equal to those in serum: M/P ratio = 1.15 and RID 12.6% to 13.5%. Metronidazole is directly used in infants and children (dose 15-50 mg PO per kg per day or 22.5-40 mg IV per kg per day). Most researchers consider the risk to an infant insufficient to suggest alternative therapy for the mother. Symptoms in the mother include decreased appetite and vomiting and, occasionally, blood dyscrasia.

One treatment regimen for maternal *Trichomonas vaginalis* is 2 g metronidazole in a single dose. When milk concentrations are measured after a 2-g dose, the highest concentrations are found at 2 and 4 hours postingestion and decline over the next 12 hours to 19.1 mg/mL and to 12.6 mg/mL at 24 hours. The dose to the infant is calculated to be 21.8 mg during the first 24 hours and only 3.5 mg in the second 24 hours.[34] It has been recommended that a single-dose regimen be used in nursing mothers, as well as delaying breastfeeding (3 to 4 hours) after the peak level at 2 hours to decrease the exposure. In another study with mothers receiving 600 mg or 1200 mg orally daily, the average milk metronidazole concentration was 5.7 and 14.4 mg/L, respectively.[35] The authors estimated that the amount metronidazole ingested by an infant would be 3 mg/kg in 500 mL of milk compared with the usual infant dose (15-50 mg PO per kg per day or 22.5-40 mg IV per kg per day). Metronidazole in gel or cream form contains only 0.75% of the medication and is poorly absorbed because the purpose is to work on tissues locally. As a result, maternal plasma levels are 1/50 of levels from comparable oral dosing. Use of the drug in this form would probably result in undetectable amounts in the milk. Metronidazole is often the only drug that works in a serious trichomoniasis, giardiasis, or amebiasis infection when all other treatments have failed.[33] Infant monitoring with maternal use of metronidazole should include observing for vomiting, diarrhea, dry mouth, and a change in the intestinal microbiome.

It is noteworthy that maternal noncompliance with antibiotics was measured by Ito in 203 breastfeeding women who consulted the Motherisk Program for information about antibiotics.[20] Despite reassuring advice, 1 in 5 women either did not initiate therapy or did not continue breastfeeding. This has implications for recurrent infections, drug sensitivity in the infant, and the development of drug resistance based on limited exposure or less-than-appropriate dosing of the antibiotic.

Anticholinergics

Anticholinergic drugs include atropine, scopolamine (hyoscine), and synthetic quaternary ammonium derivatives, some of which are available in over-the-counter medications. Some atropine does enter the milk. There are very limited data on their use during lactation. Infants are particularly sensitive to these drugs; therefore infant monitoring should include drowsiness, insomnia, dry and hot skin, dry mouth, increased heart rate, and constipation or urinary retention. The quaternary anticholinergics, however, should not appear in milk to any degree because, as anions, they do not pass into the relatively acidic milk. Mepenzolate methylbromide (Cantil) does not appear in milk.

Scopolamine is available by dermal patch for motion sickness and causes maternal mucous membrane dryness, which could affect milk production because it restricts the secretions of other secretory glands. Only a small amount appears in milk. The AAP rates it and atropine as category 6, drugs usually compatible with breastfeeding, and Hale ranks atropine as L3 (no data—probably compatible). For the scopolamine patch, which provides a constant level of drug, there are no data on its transfer into breast milk, but it is poorly orally bioavailable. Pressure-point wristbands are reported to be effective for motion sickness in pregnancy and lactation and contain no medication.

Gastrointestinal Medications

Medications for Gastroesophageal Reflux and Heartburn

Oral antacids are appropriate agents for quick-onset treatment of heartburn or gastroesophageal reflux disease (GERD). Antacids are commonly hydroxide salts of aluminum, calcium, or magnesium, alone or in some combination. Although there are few or no data on the concentration of aluminum, calcium, or magnesium in human milk with antacid treatment of lactating women, metals are not well absorbed orally. Antacids are considered acceptable during breastfeeding.[36] Sucralfate in particular is acceptable, given its minimal absorption from the GI tract.[37]

Other ingredients in some antacid products include alginate (a polysaccharide that works as a physical barrier limiting reflux) and simethicone (an antifoaming drug with reportedly minimal GI absorption). These are acceptable during lactation, and simethicone is appropriate for direct use in an infant.

There are a number of histamine H_2-blockers used for the suppression of acid secretion: cimetidine, ranitidine, nizatidine, and famotidine. None of these four is more effective than the others in treating GERD. Famotidine is the preferred medication in this class of medication for use during lactation because it is used directly in infants, has the lowest excretion in milk (RID: 1.9%), and has minimal effects on the P450 cytochrome enzymes. Ranitidine is an alternative choice because relatively low levels of the drug reach the breast milk; it is also used in infants and has less frequent drug interactions through the P450 cytochrome system. Nizatidine is concerning because of animal toxicology studies. Cimetidine causes a dose-related increase in prolactin and is associated with an increased risk of gynecomastia at higher doses (Table 11.4).[38] Cimetidine is actively secreted into human milk (RID: 9.8% to 32.6%, M/P ratio: 4.6 to 11.76) and is reported to have the most drug interactions.[11] Famotidine and ranitidine are probably the best choices for use in lactating mothers.

Proton-pump inhibitors (PPIs) are very effective in acid suppression and include omeprazole, pantoprazole, esomeprazole, lansoprazole, and rabeprazole. The PPIs are safely prescribed in infants despite the fact that they are not approved for use in infants in the United States. Very little omeprazole (RID: 1.1%) or pantoprazole (RID: 1.0%) gets into breast milk, and stomach acid digests PPIs that are not "enterically coated," so the drug that enters the infant's stomach via breast milk is most likely digested and poorly absorbed.[36] Esomeprazole is an isomer of omeprazole and is probably compatible with breastfeeding as well. There are few or no data on lansoprazole and rabeprazole in human milk.[12] PPIs have been reported to raise serum prolactin levels and have been associated with gynecomastia and galactorrhea, which resolve on discontinuation of the drug.

Treatment of Inflammatory Bowel Disease

The treatment of inflammatory bowel disease (IBD) is beyond the scope of this text; however, Witzel has a short review of lactation and biologic immunosuppressive agents.[39] There is a more comprehensive recent consensus report from the Austrian Societies of Gastroenterology and Hepatology and Rheumatology and Rehabilitation that details many of the current immunosuppressive and biologic agents and their usage during pregnancy and lactation.[40] Familiarization of oneself with these two articles and reference to the specific agents in LactMed and Hale's drug database for lactation should facilitate a breastfeeding professional's informed discussion with a breastfeeding mother undergoing treatment for IBD. Given the complexity of the illness and the medication regimens, an individualized risk—benefit assessment is appropriate.

Anticoagulants

There are many new anticoagulants available in several different categories: heparin, low-molecular-weight (LMW) heparin, vitamin K antagonists, direct thrombin inhibitors, direct factor Xa inhibitors, and antiplatelet drugs.[41] Heparin, regular or unfractionated, is a large-molecular-weight molecule that does not pass into breast milk. Because it is not absorbed from the GI tract, its use in the breastfeeding mother is acceptable, although there are no data on heparin levels in human milk.

LMW heparins are glycosaminoglycans consisting of chains of alternating residues of D-glucosamine and uronic acid. Regular or unfractionated heparin is a heterogeneous

TABLE 11.4   Antibiotic Selection for Bacterial Mastitis

Antibiotic	Spectrum	Dose	Safety	Comment
Dicloxacillin	Nonmethicillin-resistant *Staphylococci*	500 mg PO qid	Yes	Highest activity against MSSA
Clindamycin	Penicillin allergic Many CA-MRSA Test susceptibilities	300 mg PO qid	Probably safe	Excreted in milk; active against many strains of CA-MRSA
Erythromycin	Penicillin allergic	500 mg PO qid	Yes	GI intolerance
Azithromycin	Penicillin allergic	500-mg load, then 250 mg/day × 4 days	Probably safe	Limited *Staphylococcus aureus* activity; less GI upset than erythromycin
Trimethoprim Sulfamethoxazole	Some CA-MRSA	One DS tab (160mg/800mg) PO bid	Yes	Less effective when abscess present
Cephalexin	MSSA	500 mg PO qid	Yes	Relatively poor levels in breast tissue

bid, Twice per day; *CA-MRSA*, community-acquired methicillin-resistant *S. aureus*; *GI*, gastrointestinal; *MSSA*, methicillin-susceptible *S. aureus*; *PO*, by mouth; *qid*, four times per day.
From Nathan GG, Uhl K, Kennedy DL. Antibiotic use in pregnancy and lactation: what is and is not known about teratogenic and toxic risks. *Obstet Gynecol.* 2006;107:1120−1138.

mixture of polysaccharide chains ranging from 3000 to 30,000 mol wt. LMW heparin has a mean molecular weight of 5000 daltons (2000 to 8000), with slight variation among brands: ardeparin (Normiflo), dalteparin (Fragmin), enoxaparin (Lovenox), nadroparin (Fraxiparine), reviparin (Clivarine), and tinzaparin (Innohep). Both unfractionated and LMW heparins cause anticoagulation by activating antithrombin. LMW heparins produce a more predictable anticoagulant response because of their better bioavailability, longer half-life, dose-independent clearance, and decreased tendency to bind to plasma proteins and endothelium. They are less likely to interfere with platelets. They are considered safer and more effective in the treatment of venous thromboembolism, can be given subcutaneously without laboratory monitoring, carry less risk for thrombocytopenia and osteoporosis, and can be given at home.[42]

No studies are reported of LMW heparin use in pregnancy or lactation. Because their molecular weights are greater than 1000 and they are charged molecules similar to heparin, it is unlikely that they will pass into breast milk. These LMW compounds are not orally bioavailable and would not be absorbed by an infant. They are considered safe during lactation.

Studies analyzing the milk of mothers using warfarin does not reveal any significant amount of drug in the milk or in their breastfed infants. The infants' prothrombin times remained normal. This was demonstrated by McKenna et al., who followed two breastfed infants whose mothers were anticoagulated before delivery and maintained on warfarin postpartum. They found no immediate or delayed biologic effect on coagulation in 56 and 131 days of follow-up.[43] In a second study of 13 mothers and infants, very low levels of warfarin were detected in milk (<25 ng/mL), and none was detected in the infants.[44] From this, it has been suggested that

warfarin is the drug of choice in lactating mothers who require anticoagulant therapy and want to continue breastfeeding. If surgery is contemplated or unusual trauma occurs, a review of an infant's coagulation status is indicated as a precautionary measure, and 1 mg vitamin K can be given orally or IM if there is concern.

Direct thrombin inhibitors include the injectable medications argatroban, bivalirudin, dabigatran, and desirudin. Bivalirudin and desirudin are large-molecular-weight molecules (too large to be excreted in breast milk) compared with dabigatran and argatroban, which have low molecular weights and probably can reach breast milk. Because there is no information on these medications during breastfeeding, they are proscribed by most authors.

Direct Xa inhibitors include fondaparinux (administered subcutaneously) and the orally bioavailable agents apixaban, edoxaban, and rivaroxaban. One report on rivaroxaban demonstrated a low level of drug in breast milk equivalent to 1.3% of the maternal weight-adjusted dose.[45] No information is available on the other direct Xa inhibitors in human milk, and they are not recommended in breastfeeding women.

Antiplatelet medications include aspirin, an aspirin–dipyridamole combination, and clopidogrel. Clopidogrel irreversibly inhibits platelet aggregation, which could lead to prolonged inhibition of platelet function. High-dose aspirin (as for fever, arthritis, rheumatic heart disease, or arthritis) is not recommended, given the potential side effects at higher doses: fever, metabolic acidosis, thrombocytopenia, tinnitus/ototoxicity, or hemolysis/petechiae. Low-dose aspirin, for its antiplatelet effect, has been proposed as safe during breastfeeding.[46,47]

Low-dose aspirin, warfarin, heparin, and LMW heparins are accepted as compatible with breastfeeding.

Antithyroid Drugs

Iodide (I^-), most often in the form of iodide salts (e.g., NaI, KI, HI, AgI), has been known for generations to pass into the milk in levels higher than in the maternal plasma. It has been reported to cause symptoms in infants when used not only for hyperthyroidism but also in asthma preparations and cough medicines. Iodides have been noted to be goitrogenic and to sensitize the thyroid gland to other drugs, such as lithium, chlorpromazine, and methylxanthines. Iodine is an essential dietary element found in various food sources (e.g., iodized salt, seaweed, yogurt, fish, milk). The Recommended Daily Allowance (RDA) in breastfeeding women is 290 µg/day, per the US Institute of Medicine.[48] Iodine levels in breast milk can exceed the RDA for infants, and the M/P ratio has been reported as up to 26. There are reports of iodine toxicity in the infant associated with lactating mothers consuming seaweed, the use of povidone-iodine vaginal gel, potassium iodide as a medication, and various foods with iodine to excess. Hale recommends limiting the maternal intake to 290 µg/day if breastfeeding.[12]

Propylthiouracil (PTU) has been investigated by several groups, with similar results reported, showing that little of the compound is excreted in the milk (0.025% to 0.077% of total dose) in single-dose studies.[49] An infant who was followed 5 months on maternal doses of 200 to 300 mg PTU daily showed no neonatal thyroid symptoms and normal triiodothyronine (T_3), thyroxine (T_4), and thyroid-stimulating hormone (TSH). The M/P ratio is reported as 0.1, and the RID has been measured as 1.8%.[12] On the strength of these reports, others have proceeded to use PTU and permit breastfeeding. The availability of microdeterminations for T_3, T_4, and TSH levels has improved the quality of monitoring, and all infants receiving PTU via milk should be followed closely.[49] The AAP lists PTU in category 6, compatible with breastfeeding.[10]

Thiouracil is actively transported into the milk and appears in higher concentration in milk than in blood or urine, reported at levels 3 to 12 times higher in milk than in blood. Thiouracil is not used therapeutically because of its excessive toxicity and remains contraindicated during lactation.

Methimazole (Tapazole) is used to suppress the secretion of thyroxine and carbimazole and is a prodrug converted to methimazole. Methimazole does enter breast milk, with an M/P ratio of 1 or above and an estimated RID equal to 2.3%. There are several studies with methimazole or carbimazole demonstrating that methimazole enters the milk, but follow-up of the infants has demonstrated no illness and no alteration in T_3, T_4, or TSH.[50,51] Additional study has demonstrated no evidence of impaired intellectual development or growth in 42 children exposed to methimazole via breastfeeding compared with 40 children without exposure.[52] Propylthiouracil and methimazole can be used during lactation, although some monitoring of infant thyroid function is recommended.

Methylxanthines and Asthma Medications

With an increasing number of women with asthma wanting to breastfeed, a question arises about the impact of methylxanthines and other asthma preparations on human milk.[53]

Methylxanthines (theophylline, caffeine) have also been used in apnea of prematurity. Information has been generated regarding dose, clearance, and toxicity in the neonate.[53,54] In addition, microdeterminations of blood levels of theophylline and caffeine are readily available.

Caffeine

Caffeine occurs naturally in many foods (chocolate) and drinks (coffee, tea, mate). Notably, the $T_{1/2}$ in infants (neonates: $T_{1/2}$ up to 97 hours; 3 to 5 months of age: $T_{1/2} = 14$ hours) is prolonged compared with adults ($T_{1/2} = \sim 4.9$ hours). The amount of caffeine in food products varies significantly, including synthetic caffeine added to soda and energy drinks. It is also added to many over-the-counter pain relievers, weight-loss supplements, and prescription medications and used in products to "counteract drowsiness." Caffeine (or theophylline) is used in premature or low-birth-weight infants to treat apnea of prematurity.[54] The consumption of caffeine is extensive in both adults and children and adolescents. Mitchell et al. estimated in 2014 caffeine consumption at approximately 180 mg/day in more than 85% of US adults.[55] Ahluwalia and Herrick reported data from 1999 to 2011 in the Kanter Worldpanel Beverage Consumption Panel and the National Health and Nutrition Examination Survey (NHANES 2007–2010) showing that approximately 75% of US children (6 to 19 years of age) consume caffeine. Children 2 to 12 years old consume an average of 25 mg/day, and adolescents 12 to 17 years old consume an average of 50 mg/day of caffeine.[56] Around the world, caffeine consumption is reported at even higher daily averages, although there are no reported increases in consumption in the last decade. Given the prevalence and extent of caffeine consumption, it is notable that there is limited published information on the effects of maternal caffeine consumption during lactation.[57] There are some studies on the pharmacokinetics of caffeine and breast milk. Peak levels of caffeine in breast milk occur approximately 60 to 120 minutes after ingestion. The M/P ratio has been calculated as 0.812 based on the area-under-the-curve, and the half-life is 4.6 hours. The reported relative infant dose is highly variable at 6% to 25.9%.[12] The longer $T_{1/2}$ of caffeine in infants could lead to the accumulation of the drug in the infant. Caffeine levels can be measured in clinical situations. Potential effects on infants include agitation, irritability, insomnia, poor sleeping patterns, tachycardia, and tremor, among others. There are some possible nutritional effects of caffeine consumption on human milk, such as decreased iron content.

Although caffeine is not contraindicated during lactation, limiting intake is appropriate with ongoing monitoring of the infant. Various food and health agencies have made recommendations regarding limiting consumption of caffeine in lactating women. The European Food Safety Authority suggests limiting daily consumption in the lactating woman to 200 mg per day. The UK National Health Service recommends restricting intake for breastfeeding women to less than 200 mg per day. There is no clear published evidence for these recommendations related to the health of the mother or infant.[57]

Theophylline

Several studies of theophylline in mothers receiving regular doses have shown that the serum levels are lowest just before the oral dose, and the M/P ratio is 0.60 to 0.73, with milk levels paralleling serum levels.[53,58,59] Infants receive an estimated 1% to 5.9% of the maternal dose. Data on IV and oral medication are similar in terms of the M/P ratio. Maximum exposure was estimated at 7 to 8 mg/24 hours. The $T_{1/2}$ of theophylline in neonates is prolonged compared with older children or adults, suggesting the possibility of accumulation. Theophylline for acute, short-term use in the asthmatic, lactating mother should fit her overall asthma management plan, with monitoring for side effects and theophylline levels in the mother and infant as indicated.[60,61]

The management of asthma has shifted in recent years to asthma control medications, including inhaled medications, inhaled and systemic corticosteroids, long-acting inhaled β-agonists, leukotriene modifiers, mast-cell stabilizers, and combination medications.[60]

Inhaled Medications

Inhalants are unique because they act at the level of the bronchial mucosa and are poorly absorbed. Albuterol (Proventil, Ventolin) is a β_2-adrenergic agonist that is rapidly effective when inhaled, peaking within 30 minutes. The potential for drug levels in the milk is minimal because less than 10% of an inhaled drug is absorbed, but there are few or no published data in lactation. Infant monitoring with maternal use of inhaled albuterol is still appropriate. Formoterol is a long-acting selective β_2 agonist. Extremely low levels in plasma are achieved with twice-daily inhalation, and the very low oral bioavailability should allow this medication to be breastfeeding compatible even though there are no data on formoterol in breast milk. Salmeterol is another long-acting β_2-adrenergic stimulant used for asthma. There are no reports of milk levels in lactating women, although levels measured in animals suggest an M/P ratio of 1. Plasma levels after inhalation are undetectable or very low, suggesting this medication could be breastfeeding compatible with appropriate maternal dosing and infant monitoring.

Inhaled corticosteroids for asthma include fluticasone and mometasone. Again, there is little or no information related to human breast milk. Fluticasone (Flovent inhaled and Flonase nasally) is administered by inhalation, and systemic levels are less than 2% when given nasally and approximately 30% by inhalation. Plasma levels are almost undetectable, and given the usual dosing schedule, no buildup should occur. The very low plasma levels achieved with inhalation and the low oral bioavailability make it probable that these inhaled medications are both compatible with breastfeeding. Additionally, fluticasone has rapid first-pass uptake by the liver, which rapidly eliminates any plasma fluticasone.

Mast-Cell Stabilizers

Cromolyn and nedocromil are mast-cell stabilizers that are used as chronic inhaled medications for asthma. Minimal levels are achieved in the plasma after inhalation, and the <1% oral bioavailability makes it unlikely that an infant would absorb any drug that did reach the breast milk. There are no published data on these medications and breast milk. It is highly likely that both these medications are compatible with breastfeeding.

Leukotriene Modifiers

Montelukast is a leukotriene-receptor inhibitor, and zafirlukast is a receptor antagonist of leukotriene D4; both are administered orally in the long-term treatment of asthma. Montelukast is used in children 2 to 5 years of age. No data are reported on its presence in human milk, although it is secreted in animal milk. Hale reports that montelukast is probably compatible with breastfeeding.[12] Zafirlukast reaches the milk in low concentrations (50 micrograms per liter, with M/P = 0.15). It has very poor oral bioavailability; therefore it is likely compatible with breastfeeding.

Systemic Corticosteroids

Oral prednisone, prednisolone, and methylprednisolone are used for chronic control of asthma, and IV methylprednisolone can be used as acute pulse therapy for severe exacerbations of asthma unresponsive to other therapy (and other acute illnesses, e.g., multiple sclerosis [MS] or acute demyelinating encephalomyelitis [ADEM]). There are limited data on these agents and human breast milk. Small amounts of these medications reach the breast milk, and the reported M/P ratio is 0.25, the $T_{1/2}$ is 2 to 3 hours, and the RID is 1.8% to 5.3%. If possible, high-dose oral or IV steroids and chronic use should be avoided during lactation. Infant monitoring should observe feeding and growth. The mother could reduce the exposure of her infant to high doses (40 mg or more a day) of corticosteroids by waiting to breastfeed for 4 hours after a dose and/or discarding the breast milk for 3 to 6 hours after a very high dose.

DRUGS OF ABUSE AND ALCOHOL

The AAP Committee on Drugs[10] has assigned a special category to drugs of abuse: category 2, which it considers contraindicated during breastfeeding.[9] The list of contraindicated drugs is short: amphetamines, cocaine, heroin, marijuana, and phencyclidine hydrochloride (angel dust, PCP). Various organizations strongly state that these compounds and all other drugs of abuse are hazardous not only to nursing infants but also to the mother's physical and emotional health.[23,28,62] Obviously, maternal use of drugs of abuse is hazardous for bottle-feeding mothers, as well.

There are published resources as well as online resources (LactMed and the Infant Risk Center) that provide direct guidance on breastfeeding and some of the drugs considered in substance use or substance use disorder.[4,21,23,25,26,62] These online resources provide frequently updated information for reference use by health professionals. Only a few topics related to substance use will be considered in this text.

Smoking

The AAP's inclusion of nicotine in category 2 (contraindicated during breastfeeding) was controversial, but it was based on the evidence of nicotine and cotinine (its primary metabolite) in human milk from environmental tobacco smoke exposure and apparent decreases in milk production and poor weight gain early on in the infant.[63] There is certainly a tremendous amount of literature on the negative effects of maternal smoking on pregnancy and the fetus as well as later effects on the child and adult from intrauterine exposure to nicotine/smoking.[64] Analyses of studies on maternal smoking during pregnancy show an increased risk of sudden infant death in infancy. Mothers who quit or reduce their smoking (compared with those who continued smoking) decreased the odds of sudden death in their infants.[65] Asthma, respiratory illnesses, and increased severity of respiratory illness are associated with exposure to second-hand smoke in infants and children.[66-69] In contrast to this, data are clear that children of smoking mothers do better if breastfed in regard to general health, respiratory illness, and risk for sudden infant death syndrome (SIDS).[70,71] Maternal smoking has also been associated with reduced rates and duration of breastfeeding.[72]

The epidemiologic evidence of the impact of maternal smoking on breastfeeding was studied by Amir and Donath.[73] They concluded that psychosocial factors are largely responsible for the lower rates of breastfeeding found in women who smoke compared with those who do not. Fewer smokers intend to breastfeed in the first place. The duration of breastfeeding in smokers is inversely related to the number of cigarettes smoked per day.[74]

Nicotine, cotinine, and other toxicants of tobacco smoking enter the breast milk and can be transferred to the infant. Secondhand smoke also transfers a variety of chemicals directly to the infant through inhaled tobacco smoke. Carbon monoxide is an example of a chemical that can reach an exposed infant directly from heavy smoking by a mother in a confined space. Very little, if any, carbon monoxide would be transferred from the mother in breast milk or orally absorbed by the infant from the milk.[12] Acute changes that occur in relation to smoking and breastfeeding include a change in the taste of the milk, infant tachycardia, and altered sleep-wake patterns.[12,75] The goal of stopping or decreasing smoking during pregnancy and throughout breastfeeding and supporting mothers to successfully breastfeed is an important one for both infant and maternal health.[62,64,72,76] There are now numerous tobacco products used by individuals and mothers that produce plasma levels in the mother and can lead to the transfer of nicotine, cotinine, and tobacco derivatives into various tissues and breast milk.[12,23,64] Nicotine use is more complex than ever previously understood, with a variety of important variables, including the degree of dependence, the rate of nicotine clearance by the individual, the benefits of use to the specific individual, the product or delivery system for nicotine, and the harms of nicotine use and delivery systems.[77] Cigarettes and large cigars tend to have higher mean nicotine concentrations and deliver it to the smoker,

producing higher nicotine plasma levels in shorter amounts of time.[78] A nicotine inhaler delivers less nicotine over a longer period of use than cigarettes or e-cigarettes.[12] E-cigarettes (electronic nicotine delivery systems [ENDS]) can contain varying amounts of nicotine based on the nicotine concentration in the ENDS liquid and the user's puff topology.[79] Smokeless tobacco products (snuff, snus, chewing tobacco) contain variable amounts of nicotine, with differing amounts systemically absorbed. Digard et al. reported that the range of systemic exposure to nicotine was similar for cigarettes and the different smokeless tobacco products.[80] There are also various medications and products in addition to educational and behavioral interventions to promote smoking cessation.[23,64]

Smoking Cessation Products

Bupropion, a norepinephrine-dopamine reuptake inhibitor, and varenicline, a nicotinic-receptor agonist, are agents used to assist in smoking cessation, both of which are not recommended for use during breastfeeding. For bupropion, it seems to be concentrated in breast milk; there are case reports regarding seizures in infants and additional reports of suppressed milk production.[12] There are limited data on varenicline and breastfeeding, but the medication's properties (long $T_{1/2}$, poor protein binding, and LMW) make it likely that it will transfer into human milk.[12] Nicotine replacement therapy with nicotine gum, lozenges, or nicotine patches is described as compatible with breastfeeding, with the intended goal of a lower intake of nicotine via replacement therapy than the mother's usual nicotine consumption in cigarettes, cigars, snuff, chewing tobacco, or e-cigarettes.[23,72] This would lower the amount of nicotine and cotinine in breast milk and diminish the infant's exposure to "smoking" and nicotine. The use of intermittent, short-acting gum or lozenges with refraining from breastfeeding for 2 to 3 hours after use of the gum could further decrease the infant's exposure to nicotine. The use of nicotine patches, in decreasing doses, throughout pregnancy and lactation is another measure to decrease exposure. Diamanti et al. provide a summary of the principles and an approach to smoking cessation in pregnancy for maternity care practitioners. They emphasize the prevalence of women relapsing to smoking in the postpartum period (estimated 47% to 63%) and the importance of both breastfeeding support and smoking cessation support throughout this period to diminish the infant's exposure to secondhand smoke and nicotine and optimize the mother-infant dyad's opportunity to glean the benefits of breastfeeding.[64]

Alcohol

The consumption of alcohol during lactation also deserves careful consideration because of the prevalence of alcohol use worldwide (36% to 83%) and the wide variations in individual intake.[81] The evidence of alcohol's effects on the fetus are well documented but less clear on the breastfeeding infant.[82] Beer and wine are standard beverages in many parts of the world and have been recommended to enhance lactation, especially when a mother is stressed with worldly chores. Some forms of alcohol have also been used as an aperitif to encourage a woman to eat heartily while lactating. The AAP listing is category 6, substances usually compatible with breastfeeding.[10]

Alcohol is one of the most rapidly absorbed compounds. Maximum blood levels are achieved in 15 minutes in adults. Lactating and nonlactating women handle alcohol differently. Lactators tend to peak at lower levels and clear the drug more quickly.[83] The alcohol elimination rate from blood is estimated to be ∼0.015 g alcohol per 100 mL blood per hour. One alcoholic drink equivalent for a "standard drink" (∼12 ounces beer, 1.5 ounces hard liquor, and 5 ounces of wine) equals 14 g of alcohol. Alcohol passes quickly between blood and milk, however, with peak levels in milk at 30 to 60 minutes and at 60 to 90 minutes when taken with food. Studies in men and nonlactating women show an increase in serum prolactin with alcohol.[84–86] This has not been tested in lactators. The impact of alcohol on oxytocin is dose related. No effect is seen on ingesting 0.5 g/kg or less, and varying effects are reported in different women as the dose is increased.[82] At least a partial decrease in milk let-down is seen at 1.0 to 1.5 g/kg, and women have a significant to complete block in milk ejection at 1.5 to 2.0 g/kg.

Although beer and wine have been considered galactagogues, the evidence does not support this. Alcohol is an inhibitor of oxytocin release, thereby inhibiting let-down and milk expression.[87] Alcohol blocks the release of oxytocin rather than blocking the response of the breast.

Many investigations have measured the pharmacologic impact of alcohol consumption.[81,88] Alcohol appears quickly in both foremilk and hindmilk at a level equivalent to, or higher than, corresponding maternal blood samples. The amount of alcohol excreted into milk with doses less than 1 g/kg of absolute alcohol results in minimal exposure of the infant to a very small fraction of the amount of alcohol ingested by the mother and no apparent effect on the infant.[81,85]

Although levels are high in the blood, no acetaldehyde is found in the milk. Levels in milk drop in parallel to those in the blood because alcohol is not stored in the breast. In a study by Lawton, milk levels were very low despite that the participating mothers drank as much as they could as quickly as possible, averaging between 43 and 90 mL of absolute alcohol. Levels were drawn every half hour for 4 hours in this study.[89]

When women served as their own controls in an experiment to observe feeding behavior and the volume of milk consumed by infants with and without maternal alcohol, a significantly increased intensity of odor to their milk was observed, peaking between 30 and 60 minutes after ingestion.[81] The odor paralleled the concentration of alcohol (0 to 32 mg/dL). Infants sucked more frequently but consumed less milk in the presence of alcohol (120.4 ± 9.5 mL vs. 156.4 ± 8.2 mL). When a similar study was done with beer and nonalcoholic beer, the findings were similar: infants sucked less well with the alcoholic beverage. Mothers, however, were unaware of the differences and felt that they had experienced let-down and that their infants had nursed well. This work

has precipitated considerable response because of the belief that a little beer or wine enhances mothers' release of milk.

Although this work suggests that a little alcohol may not enhance the milk volume received by infants, the alcohol was taken in a research setting and consumed in 10 minutes. When the mother takes a little wine socially, it usually creates a different ambiance and may help her relax and improve her ejection reflex. In addition, many women who enjoy sipping an occasional beer or wine may well be discouraged from breastfeeding if they think wine or beer would be forbidden.

An early report by Little et al. regarding the long-term effect of alcohol on nursing infants implied that alcohol causes developmental delay.[90] The drinking would be classified as heavy (2 or more standard drinks a day, $n = 153$) in this group (total $n = 400$), whose infants had slight gross motor delay at 1 year. Furthermore, the infants were subjected to alcohol in utero as well. There were other potential confounders that could have led to this difference. A later study (915 children observed through 18 months of age) by the same authors could not substantiate the original findings.[91] Other longitudinal studies on possible long-term effects of alcohol in breast milk are also affected by confounders, such that clear-cut long-term effects are uncertain.

Infants spent significantly less time sleeping during the 3.5 hours after consuming alcohol-flavored breast milk by bottle (56.8 minutes) compared with plain breast milk by bottle (78.2 minutes). Menella et al. demonstrated in several studies that short-term exposure to small amounts of alcohol in breast milk produces distinctive changes in an infant's sleep–wake pattern, although the long-term consequences of this are uncertain.[86,92]

Recommendations from the AAP, WHO, and ABM advise limiting the infant's exposure to alcohol but do not proscribe it. There is a published nomogram from Motherisk.org using very conservative estimates regarding intake and metabolism that demonstrates estimates of elimination of alcohol by women's body weight. The nomogram provides times after ingesting different amounts of alcohol and using differing maternal weights for when the alcohol should have been cleared from breast milk.[88,93] Use of such a nomogram should allow the health care provider and the mother to reasonably discuss alcohol ingestion and how to diminish the infant's exposure (Table 11.5). This should allow an opportunity to discuss personal, familial, and cultural beliefs and understandings about alcohol use and how to optimize breastfeeding for the individual mother–infant pair.

Marijuana

The potential for the use of marijuana by breastfeeding mothers is a significant concern for several reasons, including increased legalization of its use worldwide; the potency of "available" plant material, which has increased from 4% in 1995 to 12% in 2014; the limited understanding of how much marijuana is transferred from a mother to her infant via breast milk; and the poor understanding of potential health risks to the mother and infant.[94,95] As of 2019, in the United States, 11 states had legalized its use for recreation, and

TABLE 11.5 Estimated Timing Until Clearance of Alcohol From Breast Milk for Women per Body Weight[a]

Mother's Weight, kg (lb)	NUMBER OF DRINKS CONSUMED (HOURS:MINUTES UNTIL CLEARANCE)				
	1	2	3	4	5
40.8 (90)	2:50	5:40	8:30	11:20	14:10
49.9 (110)	2:36	5:12	7:49	10:25	13:01
59 (130)	2:24	4:49	7:13	9:38	12:03
68 (150)	2:14	4:29	6:43	8:58	11:12
79.3 (175)	2:03	4:07	6:11	8:14	10:18
90.7 (200)	1:54	3:49	5:43	7:38	9:32

[a]Assumptions: Metabolism is at a constant rate of 15 mg/dL blood per hour. Women are of average height (1.62 m or 5′4″). One standard drink is 12 oz of 5% alcohol beer, 5 oz of 11% alcohol wine, or 1.5 oz of 40% alcohol liquor. Estimated time begins with first drink.

Adapted from Koren G. Drinking alcohol while breastfeeding. Will it harm my baby? Motherisk Update. *Can Fam Physician.* 2002;48:39.

21 states had broadly legalized medical use.[96] The endocannabinoid system is intimately involved in brain development. Brain development occurring during fetal life and infancy may be affected by marijuana exposure during pregnancy or lactation. Several recent studies and meta-analyses have suggested some apparent effects of marijuana exposure during pregnancy, such as low birth weight or admission to the neonatal intensive care unit (NICU), but cigarette smoking and maternal age were potential confounders.[97−100] Data concerning the effects on the infant of marijuana during breastfeeding are from older studies and present conflicting data regarding development.[101,102] Exposure of infants to secondhand marijuana smoke is associated in one study with a two-times-greater risk of SIDS.[103]

Absorption of cannabinoids after inhalation achieves peak plasma concentrations quickly for both delta-9-tetrahydrocannabinol (THC) and for cannabinol (CBD), equivalent to IV administration. Smoking cannabis does lead to exposure to a variety of toxic pyrolytic substances that does not occur via exposure by other routes. The oral bioavailability of THC is reported as low (10% to 35%), and extensive first-pass metabolism further decreases plasma levels. Oromucosal preparations are rapidly absorbed, reaching levels greater than oral and lower than inhalation intake. Transdermal administration is also limited by the lipophilic nature of THC and CBD. There is some evidence that chronic users achieve higher peak plasma levels than the occasional user.[12] Cannabinoids are quickly distributed to well-perfused organs (brain, heart, liver, lung) and accumulate in adipose tissue. They are metabolized by the cytochrome P450 (CYP 450—isozymes CYP2C9, CYP2C19, and CYP3A4) enzyme system.[104]

There remain significant deficits in our understanding of breastfeeding and marijuana.[105,106] Recent pharmacologic studies on breast milk in lactating mothers are providing some new information. Bertrand et al. studied 54 milk samples from 50 breastfeeding women who reported marijuana use.[107] Δ9-THC was identified in 63% of milk samples, with a median level of 9.47 ng/mL (range 1.01 to 323.0 ng/mL). Five milk samples had measurable levels of 11-hydroxy-Δ-9-tetrahydrocannabinol or cannabidiol. The majority of use was via inhalation, although seven mothers reported marijuana ingestion orally or via the oromucosal route. Variables related to the log value of Δ9-THC in breast milk were time since last use, number of daily uses, and time from sample collection to analysis. Δ9-THC was detectable in breast milk up to 6 days after intake by the mother.[107] Baker et al. measured Δ9-THC levels in breast milk after the inhalation of "standardized" doses of measured cannabis (0.1 g with Δ9-THC content = 23.18%).[108] Breast-milk samples were taken at 20 minutes and 1, 2, and 4 hours after inhalation from eight women 3 to 5 months postpartum who reported "regular" smoking of marijuana of ∼ 0.025 to 1 g/day. A mean concentration−time profile for Δ9-THC was created, and the average Δ9-THC concentration in breast milk was 53.5 ng/mL, with the maximum concentration in milk occurring ∼ 1 hour after inhalation. The authors estimated a relative infant dose as 2.5% (range 0.4% to 8.7%) and an average absolute infant dose of 8 μg/kg per day. Plasma levels of THC have previously been reported to increase quickly even before the end of a smoking session, but distribution into breast milk is slightly slower. The authors propose several important unanswered research questions: What is the plasma level in the breastfeeding infant achieved through breast milk? How do repeated doses affect breast-milk levels? What happens with other cannabis products and breast milk? What are the long-term effects on infants from breast-milk exposure to cannabis?[108]

Given all the remaining uncertainty and needed information about marijuana and breastfeeding, the ABM's caution concerning the use of marijuana and breastfeeding is appropriate. The ABM recommends presenting and discussing the potential benefits of breastfeeding for the mother and infant, along with discussing the potential effects of marijuana exposure, as well as what we do not know. The health care professional should then assist and support mothers in their feeding choice and provide counseling and support to reduce or eliminate marijuana use/exposure during the period of breastfeeding and lactation.[72] Separately, there is a dramatic rise in the use of cannabidiol (CBD) and hemp oils in a variety of topical and ingestible products. CBD oils are derived from *Cannabis sativa* and have low THC amounts.[109] There is even less known about the health-effect benefits of CBD (for pain, sleep, anxiety, postpartum depression, etc.) or its side effects than we know about THC. In the United States, the levels of CBD and the chemical makeup of topical or ingestible products reported to contain CBD are not closely regulated. They can be monitored by the Good Manufacturing Practices of the FDA, and in Europe, Australia, and Canada, they are monitored to meet quality and organic standards.[109] In the study by Bertrand et al. on marijuana use by breastfeeding mothers (primarily smoking), only 5 of 54 maternal milk samples had CBD detected at low levels. These were from stored milk samples, so no additional data were available to calculate CBD pharmacokinetics relative to breast milk.[107] There is no information for CBD's M/P ratio, protein binding, or RID, but CBD is fat soluble and a relatively small molecule, so one could expect to see CBD in human breast milk. There certainly are no controlled studies of the use of CBD in lactating women and infants for any of the reasons it is commonly used (headaches, chronic pain, sleep, anxiety, depression, seizures). A tremendous amount of research needs to be done on cannabidiol before its use should be considered in pregnancy or lactation.[100]

Methadone

Methadone Maintenance and Risks of Breastfeeding

Methadone maintenance treatment for heroin and other addictions has had a significant impact on the recovery of many addicts. When first introduced, it was hoped it would be an ideal treatment for neonatal withdrawal syndrome. It was not. It was also hoped that withdrawal from methadone for an infant born to a woman receiving maintenance therapy would be negligible, but it is not. When pregnant women were maintained on 25 mg/day or less, neonatal withdrawal rarely required treatment. Present regimens during pregnancy typically are for maternal doses of more than 150 mg/day. Neonatal withdrawal from this level is substantial, requiring treatment.

The therapeutic use of methadone in opiate addiction has become a common concern in the childbearing years, especially during pregnancy and lactation. Neonatal abstinence syndrome (NAS) can require 6 to 8 weeks of management and observation for the neonate. The question of breastfeeding is frequently asked.

There are small studies concerning methadone and breast milk. Two women had M/P ratios that remained constant at 0.32 and 0.61, and the infants received a calculated 0.01 to 0.03 mg of methadone per day. Kreek et al. estimated daily infant intake from a mother taking 50 mg daily, assuming consumption of almost a liter of breast milk per day, with a maximum of 0.112 mg/day.[110] Kreek et al. also noted peak levels in the milk at 4 hours after dosing. Pumping and discarding the milk at 3 to 4 hours after dosing has been suggested as a method of reducing exposure. Hale reviews several small studies of maternal methadone maintenance in lactating mothers.[12] There is a lot of variability in the mother's daily dose, as well as in the levels of methadone in plasma and breast milk, in these reported studies. Small amounts of methadone were detected in the infants' plasma, and NAS was not prevented by breastfeeding. There is evidence that the odds ratio for the development of NAS is related to the prescribed maternal methadone dose and that breastfeeding decreases the odds of needing treatment for NAS.[111,112] Review of the literature supports that breastfeeding is beneficial to the infant exposed to methadone or buprenorphine during pregnancy in terms of management of the NAS. Nonpharmacologic support for the mother and infant is essential. An ideal postpartum dosing regimen and pain management for mother or infant remains to be determined.[113]

Neonatal Abstinence Syndrome

NAS describes the potential signs and symptoms in the infant in the early postpartum period, born to a mother treated with or addicted to opioids during pregnancy. Other terms describing the syndrome include *neonatal withdrawal syndrome, neonatal withdrawal,* and *neonatal drug withdrawal syndrome.* In some situations, this includes maternal exposure to nonopioid substances (alcohol, smoking/nicotine, marijuana, amphetamines, selective serotonin-reuptake inhibitors [SSRIs], or serotonin–norepinephrine-reuptake inhibitors [SNRIs], etc.) as well.[114,115] Patrick et al. have reported data on the increasing incidence of NAS in the United States from 1.2 per 1000 hospital births in 2000 to 5.8 per 1000 hospital births in 2012, with the total number of infants diagnosed in 2012 being 21,732.[116] Beyond the potential clinical consequences of maternal opioid use during pregnancy, various infections in the mother associated with use/abuse, fetal effects (growth restriction, abruptio placenta, preterm labor) and certain outcomes in the neonate (low birth weight, preterm delivery, small head circumference, visual disturbances, sleep myoclonus), and interference with appropriate medical care and needed social support can exacerbate the situation for mother and infant.[115] Clinical manifestations of NAS have been extensively described, and there are clinical scoring systems (Finnegan Abstinence Scoring System, Modified Finnegan's Neonatal Abstinence Scoring Tool) to assess and monitor an exposed infant.[114,115] Because NAS occurs in 55% to 94% of exposed newborns and the AAP recommends observation of the exposed infant for 5 to 7 days after birth, before discharge, identification of children at risk in a timely fashion is crucial. Grossman et al. recommend various steps to be taken and to be improved upon: identification of at-risk infants; clarification of pertinent fetal and perinatal factors (including potential exposure to other drugs or toxicants); serial evaluation of neonatal signs and symptoms (standardized, consistent use of a NAS scoring system); nonpharmacologic care (rooming-in, breastfeeding, and breastfeeding support) for every exposed mother–infant pair; standardized treatment protocols; standard pharmacologic management; alternative treatment approaches (outpatient, etc.); and ongoing care and assessment of long-term infant outcomes.[117] The AAP, ABM, and other experts recommend breastfeeding (in the absence of maternal HIV infection) and active supportive care as essential to managing NAS.[72,114,115,117] Initial supportive care for every exposed or at-risk infant includes decreasing exposure to light and noise, minimize handling of the infant, promoting adequate sleep/rest, swaddling and holding the infant when distressed, and adequate nutrition. Pharmacologic treatment is intended to decrease moderate or severe symptomatology (seizures, fever, diminished intake leading to dehydration and excessive weight loss). First-line pharmacotherapy is opioid replacement with oral morphine or methadone solution. Second-line therapy (phenobarbital, clonidine) is indicated if there is an insufficient response to first-line medications. Given issues of safety and lack of efficacy, tincture of opium, paregoric, and diazepam are not recommended for NAS. There is accumulating evidence that breastfeeding infants with NAS when their mothers are on methadone maintenance therapy leads to diminished severity and duration of NAS symptomatology in the infant.[72,115] There is pharmacologic evidence that methadone enters breast milk in low concentrations, and the RID of methadone via breast milk is <3%.[12] Several groups have demonstrated that weaning of pharmacologic therapy of NAS by protocol leads to fewer days of treatment, a shorter length of hospitalization for the infant, and less likelihood of the need for continuing pharmacologic therapy at discharge.[118–120] There is growing evidence that buprenorphine may be a preferred first-line medication for NAS, leading to a shorter course of opioid treatment and length of stay compared with methadone.[121,122] The ABM supports breastfeeding for mothers and infants while mothers remain on methadone maintenance therapy and enhanced support for the mother—infant dyad to diminish barriers to breastfeeding and increase mothers' ability to attain their breastfeeding goals.[72] Researchers continue to explore standardization of NAS treatment and support protocols, how to more effectively support breastfeeding mothers on opioid maintenance therapy, and alternative models of infant care (e.g., "Eat, Sleep, Console Method of Infant Care").[123–126]

HERBS AND HERBAL TEAS

Herbal medicine is the use of plants or plant parts in their natural state without chemical processing. *Natural* is not a synonym for *safe*. Herbs and herbal products are considered dietary supplements; they are not controlled by the FDA, although the FDA has spoken out on the dangers of comfrey and ephedra and other herbal preparations that should be discontinued before surgery (Table 11.6). Herbal products contain many chemicals, some of which may have pharmacologic properties[127,128] (Table 11.7). The major concerns are quality control/standardized processing, cross-contamination, unknown additives, unknown side effects of substances within the herbal product, contamination with heavy metals, and the lack of placebo-controlled studies regarding efficacy and toxicity. Labels in the United States must read, "This product is not intended to diagnose, treat, cure, or prevent any disease." There are several database resources one can consult for information on herbs and herbal preparations, including LactMed, Hale's *Medications and Mothers Milk*, the US Pharmacopeia (USP) Dietary Supplements & Herbal Medicines list (http://www.usp.org/dietary-supplements-herbal-medicines), the Homeopathic Pharmacopoeia of the United States (http://www.hpus.com), and the FDA GRAS list (Table 11.8).

The use of herbs and herbal teas has increased, especially among those interested in natural foods.[129] As is well known to all students of pharmacology, many effective medications originated from these natural products. In the early part of the 20th century, many compounds were being dispensed in their natural form (e.g., foxglove leaves for digitalis). The natural product was unpredictable because one leaf or plant contains more or less active ingredient than another, so careful dose control was impossible, and results were often unpredictable. Much of the interest in herbal teas has evolved as individuals seek a beverage that does not contain caffeine; what they receive is another compound instead, often one more potent and frequently one about which considerably less is known (see Table 11.7). Contamination, adulteration, and misidentification of the products contribute to the problems associated with the use of products that are not regulated by the FDA but can contain various chemicals or active ingredients.[130]

Herbal teas are available that are prepared carefully, using herbs only for essence (e.g., Celestial Seasonings brand tea) and avoiding heavy doses of herbs with active principles. However, the strength of any tea depends on how it is made. An ordinary teabag with hot water run over it will contain little caffeine and theobromine; however, when the tea is steeped for 5 minutes, the potency is increased 10-fold. Some of the preparations are benign or even nutritious, such as rose hips tea, which contains a large amount of vitamin C. Other teas are made from plants known to toxicologists as poisonous. Isolated reports of toxicity from these preparations are appearing in the medical literature; many others probably go undiagnosed and unreported. The use of herbal or "natural" preparations is certainly an important part of a complete and careful medical and dietary history.

Box 11.1 lists herbal teas that are thought to be safe for infants and mothers during lactation when used as flavorings and not in therapeutic doses.

A systematic review of breastfeeding and herbs was conducted by Budzynska et al., who found only 32 studies that met inclusion criteria from 1970 to 2010.[127] Only six were randomized controlled trials, and most were surveys or case reports. Scientific data are rare in the field of herbal consumption.

In edible plants, there may be toxic parts. The potato family is well known for its toxicity in the roots, sprouts, and green coloring. Rhubarb is known for its toxic leaves. Certain mushrooms and some varieties of pea, such as grass pea (*Lathyrus salivus*), have significant toxicity. No systematic reports of data exist for the transmission of such toxins via the milk, although there are now national programs for pharmacovigilance of herbal medicines.[131] The WHO Programme for International Drug Monitoring includes over 150 countries and sets standards for the reporting of data on the safety of medications and chemicals.[132]

In some sense, safety is a matter of dose. In studies of herbs that will safely eliminate the nausea and emesis of pregnancy, ginger and peppermint are reported to be more effective than placebo. Dosing, however, was by capsule of powdered plant (1 g/day) for ginger and oil of peppermint, with no dose provided. It is of concern that ginger in large doses is known as *an emmenagogue*, which is a promoter of menstruation because it increases the blood flow to the uterus and inhibits platelet aggregation and as a galactagogue. In literature reviews, 7% consider peppermint unsafe, and 16% consider ginger unsafe in pregnancy.[133,134] There are limited data for lactation and, in particular, rare data for the use of either of these substances not in combination with other

TABLE 11.6   Clinically Important Effects and Perioperative Concerns of Eight Herbal Medicines and Recommendations for Discontinuation of Use Before Surgery

Herb: Common Name(s)	Relevant Pharmacologic Effects	Perioperative Concerns	Preoperative Discontinuation
Echinacea: purple coneflower root	Activation of cell-mediated immunity	Allergic reactions; decreased effectiveness of immunosuppressants; potential for immunosuppression with long-term use	No data
Ephedra: ma huang	Increased heart rate and blood pressure through direct and indirect sympathomimetic effects	Risk for myocardial ischemia and stroke from tachycardia and hypertension; ventricular arrhythmias with halothane; long-term use depletes endogenous catecholamines and may cause intraoperative hemodynamic instability; life-threatening interaction with monoamine oxidase inhibitors	At least 24 hours before surgery
Garlic: ajo	Inhibition of platelet aggregation (may be irreversible); increased fibrinolysis; equivocal antihypertensive activity	Potential to increase risk for bleeding, especially when combined with other medications that inhibit platelet aggregation	At least 7 days before surgery
Ginkgo: duck foot tree, maidenhair tree, silver apricot	Inhibition of platelet-activating factor	Potential to increase risk for bleeding, especially when combined with other medications that inhibit platelet aggregation	At least 36 hours before surgery
Ginseng: American ginseng, Asian ginseng, Chinese ginseng, Korean ginseng	Lowers blood glucose; inhibition of platelet aggregation (may be irreversible); increased PT and PTT in animals; many other diverse effects	Hypoglycemia; potential to increase risk for bleeding; potential to decrease anticoagulation effect of warfarin	At least 24 hours before surgery
Kava: awa, intoxicating pepper, kawa	Sedation, anxiolysis	Potential to increase sedative effect of anesthetics; potential for addiction, tolerance, and withdrawal after abstinence unstudied	At least 24 hours before surgery
St. John's wort: amber, goatweed, hardhay, hypericum, Klamath weed	Inhibition of neurotransmitter reuptake, monoamine oxidase inhibition	Induction of cytochrome P-450 enzymes, affecting cyclosporine, warfarin, steroids, protease inhibitors, and possibly benzodiazepines, calcium-channel blockers, and many other drugs: decreased serum digoxin levels	At least 5 days before surgery
Valerian: all-heal, garden heliotrope, vandal root	Sedation	Potential to increase sedative effect of anesthetics; benzodiazepine-like acute withdrawal; potential to increase anesthetic requirements with long-term use	No data

PTT, Partial thromboplastin time; *PT*, prothrombin time,
From Ang-Lee MK, Moss J, Yuan CS. Herbal medicines and perioperative care. *JAMA.* 2001;286:213.

substances.[135,136] Any herbal tea consumed in large volumes daily could be a problem, depending on the concentration of individual chemicals within the tea preparation.

Mother's Milk Tea

Mother's milk tea is a blend of plants handed down for many generations as a galactagogue; it contains a mixture of fennel seeds, coriander seeds, chamomile flowers, lemongrass, borage leaves, blessed thistle leaves, star anise, comfrey leaves, and fenugreek seeds (Table 11.9).[137] It is promoted as containing no

caffeine. Although not all the constituents have pharmacologic actions, several do and were used medicinally for centuries. There is one recent randomized, double-blind controlled trial of the safety of Mother's Milk (a registered commercial product with known amounts of specific ingredients). No adverse effects were noted in comparison to a placebo group for healthy, exclusively/fully breastfeeding mothers and their infants.[138] These popular teas have the same potential for problems as do the common popular beverages coffee and cola. The euphoric effects are the most prominent.[129]

TABLE 11.7 Psychoactive Substances Used in Herbal Preparations

Labeled Ingredient	Botanical Source	Active Compound(s)	Suggested Use and Reported Effects
African yohimbe bark; yohimbine	*Corynanthe yohimbe*	Yohimbine	Smoke or tea as stimulant; mild hallucinogen
Broom; scotch broom	*Cytisus* spp.	Cystine	Smoke for relaxation; strong sedative-hypnotic
Buckthorn	*Hiptothae rhamnoides*	Anthraquinones	Tea; cathartic toxin, severe watery diarrhea
Burdock root	*Arctium minus*	Atropine	Tea; anticholinergic blockade, anaphylactic shock
California poppy	*Eschscholtzia californica*	Alkaloids and glucosides	Smoke as marijuana substitute; mild hallucinogen
Catnip	*Nepeta cataria*	Nepetalactone	Smoke or tea as marijuana substitute; mild hallucinogen
Chamomile	*Chamomilla recutita* *Chamaemelum nobile*	Antigens of *Compositae* family	Tea; contact dermatitis (in patients sensitive to ragweed, asters, chrysanthemum)
Cinnamon	*Cinnamomum camphora*	?	Tea; venooclusive disease, hepatic failure, hepatocarcinogen
Comfrey	*Symphytum officinale*	Pyrrolizidine alkaloids	Tea; malignant arrhythmias, cardiac arrest
Foxglove tea	*Digitalis purpurea*	Digitalis	Tea; venooclusive disease, hepatic failure
Gordolobo, groundsel	*Senecio longilobus Senecio vulgaris Senecio spartioides*	Pyrrolizidine alkaloids	Smoke or tea as sedative and marijuana substitute; none
Hops	*Humulus lupulus*	Lupuline	Smoke as marijuana substitute; stimulant
Hydrangea	*Hydrangea paniculata*	Hydrangin, saponin, cyanogens	Tea; PNH-like defect, anticholinergic blockade; CNS intoxication, hallucinations, ataxia, blurred vision
Jimson tea	*Datura stramonium*	Atropine, scopolamine, hyoscyamine, stramonium	Smoke as hallucinogen; strong hallucinogen
Juniper	*Juniperus macropoda*	?	Smoke or tea as marijuana substitute; mild hallucinogen
Kava kava	*Piper methysticum*	Yangonin, pyrones	Smoke, tea, or capsules as stimulant
Kola nut; gotu kola	*Cola* spp.	Caffeine, theobromine, kolanin	Smoke or tea as a marijuana substitute; mild euphoriant
Lobelia	*Lobelia inflata*	Lobeline	Tea as hallucinogen
Mandrake	*Mandragora officinarum*	Scopolamine, hyoscyamine	Tea as stimulant; venooclusive disease
Mate	*Ilex paraguariensis*	Caffeine, pyrrolizidine	Tea as stimulant
Mormon tea	*Ephedra nevadensis*	Ephedrine	Hallucinogen, MAD inhibitor; hallucinogen, CNS intoxicant
Nutmeg	*Myristica fragrans*	Myristin	Hepatic damage
Oleander	*Nerium oleander*	Myristin Cardiac glycosides Digitogenin Nerioside Oleandroside	Malignant arrhythmias, cardiac arrest
Passion flower	*Passiflora incarnata*	Harmine alkaloids	Smoke, tea, or capsules as marijuana substitute; mild stimulant
Periwinkle	*Catharanthus roseus*	Indole alkaloids	Smoke or tea as euphoriant; hallucinogen

(Continued)

TABLE 11.7 Psychoactive Substances Used in Herbal Preparations—cont'd

Labeled Ingredient	Botanical Source	Active Compound(s)	Suggested Use and Reported Effects
Pokeroot, pokeweed	*Phytolacca americana* *Phytolacca decandra*	Saponins Pokeweed mitogen	Gastroenteritis, bloody diarrhea Respiratory depression, mitogenic alterations
Prickly poppy	*Argemona mexicana*	Protopine, berberine, isoquinolines	Smoke as euphoriant; narcotic-analgesic
Sassafras	*Sassafras albidum*	Safrole	Tea or cold beverage; hepatocarcinogen
Senna	*Cassia acutifolia Cassia angustifolia*	Anthraquinones	Tea; cathartic toxin, severe watery diarrhea
Snakeroot	*Rauwolfia serpentina*	Reserpine	Smoke or tea as tobacco substitute; tranquilizer
Thorn apple	*Datura stramonium*	Atropine, scopolamine	Smoke or tea as tobacco substitute or hallucinogen
Tobacco	*Nicotiana* spp.	Nicotine	Smoke as tobacco; strong stimulant
Valerian	*Valeriana officinalis*	Chatinine, valerie, alkaloids	Tea or capsules as tranquilizer
Wild lettuce	*Lactuca sativa*	Lactucarine	Smoke as opium substitute; mild narcotic-analgesic
Woodruff	*Galium odoratum*	Coumarin	Hemorrhagic diathesis, prolonged prothrombin time
Wormwood	*Artemisia absinthium*	Absinthin	Smoke or tea as relaxant; narcotic-analgesic
Yohimbe bark	*Corynanthe yohimbe*	Yohimbine	α_2-Sympathetic (presynaptic) blockade

CNS, Central nervous system; *MAD*, major affective disorder; *PNH*, paroxysmal nocturnal hemoglobinuria.
Modified from Siegel RK. Herbal intoxication: psychoactive effects from herbal cigarettes, tea, and capsules. *JAMA*. 1976;236:473; copyright © 1976, American Medical Association; and Ridker PM. Toxic effects of herbal teas. *Arch Environ Health*. 1987;42:135.

TABLE 11.8 Herbal Medicine and Other Dietary Supplement–Related Sites on the World Wide Web

Organization	Web Address	Site Information
Center for Food Safety and Applied Nutrition, US Food and Drug Administration	https://fda.gov/food/dietary-supplements/dietary-supplement-products-ingredients	Clinicians should use this site to report adverse events associated with herbal medicines and other dietary supplements. Sections also contain safety, industry, and regulatory information.
National Center for Complementary and Alternative Medicine, National Institutes of Health	http://nccam.nih.gov	This site contains fact sheets about alternative therapies, consensus reports, and databases.
Agricultural Research Service, US Department of Agriculture	https://phytochem.nal.usda.gov/phytochem/search	The site contains an extensive phytochemical database with search capabilities.
Quackwatch	http://www.quackwatch.com	Although this site addresses all aspects of health care, there is a considerable amount of information covering complementary and herbal therapies.
National Council Against Health Fraud	http://www.ncahf.org	This site focuses on health fraud and has a position paper on over-the-counter herbal remedies.
HerbMed	https://medlineplus.gov/druginfo/herb_All.html	This site contains information on more than 120 herbal medications, with evidence for activity, warnings, preparations, mixtures, and mechanisms of action. There are short summaries of important research publications with MEDLINE links.
ConsumerLab	http://www.consumerlab.com	This site is maintained by a corporation that conducts independent laboratory investigations of dietary supplements and other health products.

Comfrey and Pyrrolizidine Alkaloids

Considerable concern is mounting over the use of comfrey leaves (*Symphytum officinale*) in the United States. These products have been banned in Canada and Germany. The leaves have been used in teas, salads, and poultices. The use of comfrey has been associated with venoocclusive disease and hepatotoxicity. Comfrey is also rich in hepatotoxic pyrrolizidine alkaloids.[139,140] The highest level of toxin occurs in the roots, which can be obtained in powder form in capsules. Comfrey has been recommended for use to cure various pregnancy, labor, and postpartum symptoms and appears in many home remedy handbooks.[141] It has the greatest potential for toxicity in a fetus and a suckling infant, with fatal fetal venoocclusive disease

reported. It is also known to have carcinogenic properties. All credible references caution against its use topically, orally, or in any form (Table 11.10).[142] Another herb associated with venoocclusive disease and even death is *Senecio longilobus*, commonly known as *thread-leafed groundsel*.[138,139] As with comfrey, it contains hepatotoxic pyrrolizidine alkaloids. Seven cases of hepatitis have been reported resulting from the use of *Teucrium chamaedrys* (germander), a member of the mint family. Botanical identification is essential, as is accurate determination of the chemicals and their concentrations within any prepared product or tea. The label may not be correct or accurate in terms of concentration. Pyrrolizidine alkaloids have also been identified in an herbal tea used in the Southwest that was responsible for the deaths of several children who were given the tea when they were ill. The alkaloid is excreted within 24 hours, but symptoms may not appear for several days or weeks. Death results from liver failure.[143]

Sassafras and Coumarins

Sassafras contains an aromatic oil, safrole, which has been shown to cause cancer in mice; it is therefore no longer permitted as a commercial flavoring, but it appears in herbal teas. It causes CNS symptoms in mice, including ataxia, ptosis, and hypothermia.[144] It is also thought to interfere with the action of other medications. Noted herbalists state that sassafras has no really significant medical or therapeutic use.[141,145]

BOX 11.1 Herbal Teas Considered Safe During Lactation

Tea	Origin/Use
Chicory	Root/caffeine-free coffee substitute
Orange spice	Mixture/flavoring
Peppermint	Leaves/flavoring
Raspberry	Fruit/flavoring
Redbush tea	Leaves, fine twigs/beverage
Rosehips	Fruits/vitamin C

TABLE 11.9 Possible Ingredients and Effects of Mother's Milk Tea

Plant	Constituents	Effects	Toxicity
Fennel seed	Volatile oil, anisic acid	Weak diuretic stimulant	CNS disturbances
Coriander seed	Volatile oil, coriandrol	Increases flow of saliva and gastric juice	CNS disturbances
Chamomile flower	Volatile oil, bitter glycoside	Sudorific, antispasmodic, used to lighten hair	Vomiting, vertigo
Lemongrass	Lemon flavor		
Borage leaf	Volatile oil, tannin, mineral acids	Diuretic, sudorific, euphoric	Possible
Blessed thistle leaf	Volatile oil, bitter principle	Aperitif, galactagogue, diaphoretic	Strongly emetic
Star anise	Volatile oil, anethole, resin, tannin	Stimulant, mild expectorant	
Comfrey leaf (*Symphytum officinale*)	Protein, vitamin B$_{12}$, tannin, allantoin, choline, pyrrolizidine, alkaloids	Used as mucilage to knit bones, weak sedative, demulcent, astringent	Venoocclusive disease Hepatotoxic
Fenugreek seed (Greek hayseed) (coffee substitute and natural dye)	Mucilage, trigonelline, phytosterols, celery flavor	Digestive tonic, galactagogue, uterine stimulant, reduces blood sugar	Hypoglycemia, can induce labor
Other Beverages			
Coffee plant	Volatile oil, caffeine, tannin	Stimulant, diuretic, coloring	Insomnia, restlessness
Blue cohosh	Saponin, glucoside that affects muscles	Oxytocic, potent, acts on voluntary and involuntary muscles	Irritant, causes pain in fingers and toes

CNS, Central nervous system.

TABLE 11.10 Herbal Teas and Their Potential Side Effects

Herb/Parts Used	Common Uses	Method of Application	Side Effects
Aconite (monkshood, wolfsbane)	Aconitine, hypaconitine, aconine, mesaconitine	Tea	Nausea, vomiting, hypersalivation Perioral paresthesia, progressing rapidly to neuromuscular weakness, seizures, coma Cardiac effects: Bradycardia and hypotension (most common), supraventricular or ventricular tachycardia, ventricular fibrillation, asystole
Aloe vera/pure gel from leaves	Burns Constipation Ulcers Canker sores Immunostimulant HIV infection	Gel applied topically or taken internally several times daily Does not standardize	Diarrhea, gastric cramping when taken internally Contact dermatitis from related species *Aloe arborescens*
Chamomile/ flowers	Calming, sedating Aromatherapy Antispasmodic Colic Antiinflammatory Soothe diaper rash Chickenpox, poison ivy	Tea (in infants) or tinctures Essential oil used in aromatherapy or added to bath	Allergic reactions One case of botulism in infant given tea from homegrown plant
Comfrey	Pyrrolizidine Demulcent Sedative Astringent	Tea Poultice Ointment	Hepatic venoocclusive disease marked by severe abdominal pain and vomiting, which may be followed by hepatomegaly and abdominal distention with ascites Hepatic necrosis leading to cirrhosis Not recommended
Echinacea/ leaves, stalks, roots	Immunostimulant Colds, ear and sinus infections HIV infections	Tincture, capsules, or tablets taken internally as immunostimulant Does not standardize	Asthma, atopy, anaphylaxis, immune suppression
Ephedra (ma huang)/ leaves, stalks	Decongestant Asthma, allergy Weight loss "Natural high"	Generally taken internally	Hypertension, tachycardia Toxic psychosis Death Not recommended
Feverfew/fresh or dried leaves	Migraine Prophylaxis Rheumatoid arthritis Insect repellent Menstrual pain	1–3 fresh leaves, 25- to 50-mg capsules, or crushed, dried leaves twice per day to prevent migraine	Allergic reactions Mouth ulcers Rebound headache if discontinued abruptly
Goldenseal/ roots	Diarrhea Antiseptic Antimicrobial for acne, conjunctivitis, eczema, ear infections Possible immunostimulator Antiarrhythmic	1/4 to 1/2 tsp of tincture or 1/2 tsp of fluid extract three or four times per day for diarrhea Can be mixed with 4 oz water or juice	Nausea, vomiting, diarrhea Displaces bilirubin from albumin Not recommended for infants
Pennyroyal	Pulegone	Tea Oil	Hepatoxicity, hepatic failure, nausea, vomiting, abdominal pain Renal failure Delirium, confusion, restlessness, dizziness, seizures, alternating lethargy and agitation Abortion Not recommended

(Continued)

TABLE 11.10   Herbal Teas and Their Potential Side Effects—cont'd

Herb/Parts Used	Common Uses	Method of Application	Side Effects
Tea tree oil/ essential oil from leaves	Minor skin infections Fungicide Acne Vaginitis	Applied topically two to four times per day	Contact dermatitis if applied to broken or irritated skin As little as 10 mL by mouth can affect CNS function and cause muscle weakness Not for internal use

CNS, Central nervous system; *HIV*, human immunodeficiency virus.
Modified from Mack RB. "Something wicked this way comes"—herbs even witches should avoid. *Contemp Pediatr.* 1998;15:49; and O'Hara MA, Kiefer D, Farrell K, et al. A review of 12 commonly used medicinal herbs. *Arch Fam Med.* 1998;7:523.

The oil, along with many other volatile oils, does have mild counterirritant properties on external application. It has a pleasant flavor but many harmful qualities. Although banned by the FDA, sassafras appears in other natural food products.

Licorice

Licorice, the dry root of *Glycyrrhiza glabra*, has been used for medicinal purposes for millennia; stores of licorice were found in the tombs of Egyptian pharaohs, including that of King Tut. Its history is carefully reviewed by Davis and Morris.[146] The active principle is a glycoside of a triterpene called *glycyrrhizic acid*. Licorice continues to be used as a flavoring agent in drinks, drugs, and candies. In addition to its universal role as an expectorant and demulcent and in ointments for various skin disorders, it has been used for peptic ulcers. Its most perplexing properties are those that cause the retention of water, sodium, and chloride and the increased excretion of potassium, mimicking the effects of large doses of desoxycorticosterone. Because licorice is used to flavor chewing tobacco, chewing has been associated with hypertension, sodium retention, and hypokalemia. Licorice derivatives have been found to reroute the metabolism of aldosterone, desoxycorticosterone, and glucocorticoids.[145] Licorice toxicity is well described in the literature.[147] Excessive amounts of licorice should be avoided by lactating women. Its use to lose weight should be discouraged. Some licorice candy contains little or no licorice, and the flavor is provided by anise, which is probably harmless. An occasional stick of licorice candy should not be a risk.[145]

Echinacea

Echinacea (coneflower) is used for the common cold and when "immune system enhancement is desired."[148] A lipophilic fraction of the root and leaves contains the most potent immunostimulating compounds, some yet to be identified. It is used topically to stimulate wound healing and orally to enhance immune response. The public seeks it out for the common cold. No data exist about its entry into milk. It has no known side effects, even when injected in high doses. *Echinacea* preparations tested in clinical trials have varied greatly. There are some data that preparations based on the aerial parts of *E. purpurea* might be effective for the early treatment of colds in adults, but the results are not repeatedly consistent in different studies. Potential beneficial effects of other *Echinacea* preparations and *Echinacea* used for preventative purposes might exist, but they have not been documented in randomized controlled trials.[149]

Taking it for more than 8 weeks has been associated with immunosuppression. It is also important to note that it is a member of the daisy/chrysanthemum family and can cause allergy in those prone to pollen allergies. It has also been reported to have caused asthma, atopy, and anaphylaxis. The use of echinacea during breastfeeding should be undertaken cautiously because of the lack of high-quality human studies on safety. It interferes with immune suppressants and should not be used by patients who have had transplants (see Table 11.10).

Ginkgo biloba

Ginkgo biloba has been known in Chinese medicine since 2800 BC for brain disorders; circulatory problems; and respiratory diseases, including asthma. The *Ginkgo* leaf contains flavonoids (e.g., quercetin, kaempferol, isorhamnetin) and several terpene trilactones (e.g., ginkgolides, bilobalide), as well as numerous minor components. Standardized preparations use measurements based on ginkgo flavone glycoside and terpenoid content. Raw ginkgo seeds contain potentially toxic cyanogenic glycosides, but roasted seeds do not carry the same risk. Ginkgo is commonly used as an antioxidant, as a vasodilator to increase cerebral and peripheral perfusion, and to improve memory. There are no documented uses or safety data in pregnancy. The safety of its use during lactation is unstudied and unknown. It should be avoided, according to Dugoua et al., until some high-quality human studies are reported.[150]

Blue Cohosh

Blue cohosh (*Caulophyllum thalictroides*) root contains N-methylcytosine, with nicotine-like effects. It also contains caulosaponin, a glycoside that constricts coronary vessels and may have oxytocic activity; therefore it has been used to promote labor. Use during lactation has been reported, but data are lacking on efficacy or safety. Various sources recommend it should only be used under medical supervision and not be available over the counter until it is studied thoroughly. One publication from Canada reports that a large percentage of midwives use it in labor in spite of known teratogenic, embryotoxic, and oxytoxic effects.[151]

Chaste Tree

Chaste tree (*Vitex agnus-castus*) was systematically reviewed in the literature in lactation.[152] "Expert opinion" revealed five experts who thought it increased lactation and five who reported that it decreased prolactin and thus milk production.

Chaste tree has some effects on estrogen and progesterone activity. No evidence suggests it passes into milk. Careful blinded controlled studies are needed to determine chaste tree's effect on milk production. Beyond reported expert opinion, there is no indication for the use of chaste tree during lactation.

Ginseng

Ginseng is one of the oldest, most widely recognized, and most documented Oriental herbs. It enjoys a reputation for increasing the capacity for mental work and physical activity and also "antistress" effects. The plant of origin is *Panax schinseng* (Chinese) or *Panax quinquefolius* (American), two species of the *Araliaceae* family. *Panax* is derived from the Greek, meaning "all healing." It has been called an *adaptogen* because it is believed to protect the body against stress and restores homeostasis or provides nonspecific resistance.[153]

The root contains dozens of steroid-like glycosides (ginsenosides), which vary with the species, age, location of growth, and harvest time. It contains sterols, coumarins, flavonoids, and polysaccharides. Although animal studies suggest increased strength and stamina, Engels and Wirth reported that in a carefully blinded and controlled study of 31 healthy men randomized to take 200 mg/day, 400 mg/day, or a placebo, no difference was found in any physiologic or psychologic parameter.[154] They measured oxygen consumption, blood lactic acid, and heart rate while the subjects worked at maximum effort on stationary bikes. It does lower blood sugar and can cause hypoglycemia. It has some effect on coagulation pathways and on platelet coagulability, which may be irreversible (see Table 11.6).

Available products containing ginseng are numerous and variable; more than half are worthless, according to independent studies, and 25% contain no ginseng, which is extremely expensive ($20 per ounce). It is reported to have estrogen-like effects on some women, with mastalgia common with extended use and mammary nodularity also reported. Although animal experimentation has been considerable, no extensive human data, no reliable or standardized preparations, no information on dosage, and no accurate recording of side effects are available. Ginseng is a medical enigma with no proven efficacy for humans, according to Tyler.[148] General side effects include excitement, nervousness, inability to concentrate, hypertension, hypoglycemia, and skin rash. A case of ginseng use during pregnancy and lactation is reported because the infant showed excessive hirsutism and androgen effect, which cleared when breastfeeding was discontinued at 2 weeks of life.[155] Because of the reported breast effects and occasional reports of vaginal bleeding, it is considered problematic during lactation. It should not be used during pregnancy, during lactation, or in children, according to Skidmore-Roth.[129] Panax ginseng should be consumed with caution during lactation based on the absence of studies in humans.[156]

St. John's Wort

St. John's wort is touted in Europe and the United States as an antidepressant and anxiolytic and is now sold in health food stores and supermarkets. It comes from an aggressive perennial weed in meadows and roadsides noted for its spotted leaves, numerous yellow-orange flowers with black spots, and capsular fruit. It contains 10% tannin and hypericin, a reddish dianthrone pigment; other hypericum-like substances (0.2% to 0.5%); and volatile oils. The extract is sold as tablets, capsules, drops, transdermal patches, oils, and teas.

The pharmacology of the extract includes inhibition of the neurotransmitters serotonin, norepinephrine, and dopamine. It also binds to γ-aminobutyric acid receptors in vitro. When the extract is taken orally, hypericin peaks in serum in 5 hours and reaches steady state with continued dosing in 4 days. The half-life in plasma is 25 hours.[157]

Some studies are carefully controlled and include standardized testing of depression and mood before and after 3 to 6 weeks of treatment with St. John's wort versus placebo or versus standard antidepressant medication. In their overview and meta-analysis, Linde et al. conclude that the evidence indicates that extracts of hypericin are more effective than placebo and equally effective as standard antidepressants for mild to moderately severe depressive disorders.[158] Side effects of dry mouth, dizziness, constipation, and confusion occurred in 20% of subjects receiving hypericin and in 53% taking standard antidepressants. The doses, duration, and assessment tools varied widely in these 23 studies and 1757 outpatients. Other systematic reviews report St. John's wort as better than placebo and not different from antidepressant medications for mild to moderate depression, with fewer side effects noted.[159,160]

Adverse effects with chronic high doses (more than 30 mg/day) include photosensitivity; abdominal symptoms; and rarely, tachycardia, tachypnea, fever, and fatigue. Because hypericin inhibits dopamine β-hydroxylase, which leads to increased dopamine, increased prolactin inhibitory factor, and suppression of prolactin, it could decrease lactation. No clinical study has investigated this pharmacologic potential. "Better, longer studies are needed to establish the effectiveness and safety of St. John's for treatment of depression. Twenty-six chemicals have been extracted from St. John's Wort and hypericin may not be the most effective. The active ingredients, potency and purity of preparations sold in the USA are all unknown."[161] It is licensed in Germany but is considered a dietary supplement in the United States and has not been evaluated by the FDA (see Table 11.6).

In a single mother—infant pair, hypericin levels were undetectable in human milk, while hyperforin was excreted into breast milk at low levels and was at the limit of quantification. Neither hypericin nor hyperforin was detected in the infant's plasma.[162] A prospective observational cohort study included 33 breastfeeding dyads compared with 2 matched control groups (101 women matched for clinical condition and 33 women matched for age and parity) that were unmedicated. No difference was found in demographics, symptoms, adverse effects, or milk production between the groups.[163] Lethargy, drowsiness, and colic are infant symptoms reported in case reports with infant exposure to St. John's wort via breast milk. Although the side-effect profile appears favorable, the absence of long-term studies of use during lactation, the multiple components in St. John's wort products, and the limited data on breast-milk levels of the various components in St. John's wort suggest that more study is essential before recommending its use during lactation.

GALACTAGOGUES

A galactagogue is a material or action that stimulates milk production. When trying to increase milk supply, the action of increased draining of the breast (regularly and thoroughly) is the best "galactagogue." When careful lactation management has not produced adequate results, for example, in the case of a mother pumping for her sick, premature infant, various medications and herbs have been recommended. Carefully collected and controlled evidence from randomized, placebo-controlled, appropriately blinded studies is lacking. Even recent systematic reviews and meta-analyses are lacking because the randomized controlled trials to be analyzed are limited in terms of controlled, consistent methodology; small populations studied (n); comparability; and selection of study patients and control groups.[164–168]

Despite the previously mentioned data limitations, the ABM has prepared an outstanding review of galactagogues with appropriate recommendations for approaching the issue of initiating or augmenting milk production and the possible role of galactagogues.[169] The ABM recommends several important principles of problem solving regarding milk production: (1) evaluate the entire feeding process and optimize the nonpharmacologic management of lactation; (2) confirm and objectively measure "low milk supply"; (3) focus on potential interfering factors affecting regular, effective, complete drainage of the breasts or the physiology of milk production; (4) identify the "modifiable factors" and address solutions to those; (5) consider galactagogues with caution, noting drug and herb interactions, an individualized risk–benefit assessment, and informed consent with the mother; and (6) provide close follow-up for the mother–infant pair, monitoring milk production, potential adverse effects of treatment, and potential evolution of the clinical situation. The ABM's review summarizes data on the four dominant galactagogues: domperidone, metoclopramide, fenugreek, and silymarin. Additional resources on specific potential natural or herbal galactagogue agents include LactMed and the FDA's Dietary Supplement Division. A partial list of herbs considered to have galactagogue properties includes fenugreek seed (*Trigonella foenum-graecum*), fennel seed (*Foeniculum vulgare*), anise seed (*Pimpinella anisum*), goat's rue herb (*Galega officinalis*), nettle leaf (*Urtica dioica*), alfalfa herb (*Medicago sativa*), marshmallow root (*Althaea offficinalis*), caraway seed (*Carum carvi*), blessed thistle seed (*Cnicus benedictus*), torbangun herb (*Coleus amboinicus*), shatavari (*Asparagus racemosus*), milk thistle (*Silybum marianum*), and chasteberry (*Vitex agnus-castus*).[127,165]

Metoclopramide

Metoclopramide has been studied in a small series in which mothers took 10 mg three times daily, with an increase in milk supply that, in most cases, dwindled when the drug was tapered after 10 days, which is the recommended limit because of possible maternal side effects. Metoclopramide has been used in infants for reflux; however, when plasma levels were studied, the less mature the infant, the lower the clearance; therefore the drug can accumulate in infants.[170] The FDA has issued a black-box warning for tardive dyskinesia, which can occur even after the drug has been stopped.

It does increase prolactin levels as a dopamine antagonist. Even small doses have a maximum effect on the prolactin levels but less effect on milk production. Kauppila et al. reported on several patients who had high prolactin levels in whom the addition of metoclopramide did not affect the prolactin level or milk production.[171] Other small studies on metoclopramide efficacy demonstrate some variable results. The use of metoclopramide (30 mg/day) for 7 days in 23 women with premature infants did demonstrate an increase in milk production (93 mL/day up to 197 mL/day). In this study, the usual rapid rise in prolactin when milk is expressed seemed to be diminished by metoclopramide.[172] Hansen et al. reported that metoclopramide 30 mg/day did not increase milk production in 28 women with premature infants.[173] Gupta et al. examined the response to metoclopramide in 32 women with low milk supply. In 12 women with "lactation failure," 8 out of 12 had improved milk output within 3 to 4 days of therapy. Overall, 87.5% of the 32 women had increased milk production with metoclopramide dosing 10 mg orally three times daily.[174] In a small study of five women, metoclopramide increased milk production from 150.9 to 276.4 mL/day. Plasma prolactin levels in those women's infants did not show any change.[175] In a more recent randomized controlled trial ($n = 65$) comparing domperidone to metoclopramide in mothers of preterm infants, there was no difference in the response of increased milk production over the mother's own baseline production in either group.[176] Metoclopramide does pass into milk, with a reported M/P ratio range of 0.5 to 4.06 and RID range of 4.7% to 14.3%. Serotonin-like reactions have been reported in women using metoclopramide and a serotonin reuptake inhibitor.[177] Reported side effects for women taking metoclopramide include mood swings, depression, arrhythmias, extrapyramidal signs, headache, itchy skin, and GI complaints. There are no reported pediatric concerns for exposure via milk.[12] A decision to use metoclopramide as a galactagogue should still be made with caution, after a risk–benefit analysis for the mother and infant and perhaps after confirming that the mother has low prolactin levels that could be increased by metoclopramide to then increase milk production.

Domperidone

Domperidone also increases prolactin as a dopamine-receptor blocker. It is used as an antiemetic, for dyspepsia and gastric reflux. It does not enter the brain. When 46 mothers of premature (less than 31 weeks' gestation) babies were given domperidone for lactation failure, levels of nutrients in the milk were compared with controls. By day 14, volume had increased by 267% but only 18.5% in controls. Prolactin increased by 97% versus 17%.

Protein declined by 9.6% in the study group and rose by 3.6% in controls. There was no change in calories, fat, sodium, or phosphate. Carbohydrate and calcium were increased in the study group. Essentially, the milk was not significantly changed except in volume. No adverse effects were reported in the infants or mothers in this study.[178]

A randomized, double-blind, placebo-controlled trial of domperidone's effect on milk production in mothers of premature newborns showed an increase in milk production, 49.5 ± 29.4 mL/day compared with an increase of 8.0 ± 39.5 mL/day in the control group (44.5% increase with the drug and 16.6% with the placebo). The prolactin levels rose significantly with domperidone. A small amount was found in the milk (1.2 µg/L).[179] A multicenter randomized trial, published in 2017, reported on the effects of domperidone on 90 women, their milk production, and their 109 preterm infants. There was an increase of greater than 50% in daily milk volume on day 14 for 77.8% of the women receiving domperidone and only 57.78% of the women receiving placebo for the first 14 days. At 28 days, there was no difference in apparent milk production in the two groups, with the placebo group being given domperidone from days 15 to 28.[180] A review of randomized controlled trials found only a few small studies (four) of high quality and concluded that domperidone produces a greater increase in breast-milk supply than placebo.[167]

A systematic review and meta-analysis that reported on domperidone's effect on milk production in women of preterm infants included five studies ($n = 194$ women). Domperidone compared with placebo increased breast-milk production by approximately 88.3 mL/day (95% confidence interval [CI]: 56.8, 119.8). There were no differences in the two groups regarding maternal adverse events and no apparent episodes of prolonged QTc or cardiac abnormalities.[181] Another systematic review and meta-analysis examined randomized controlled trials of the effect of domperidone on "insufficient" milk production. Five studies were analyzed (239 women included). The reported effect size demonstrated that domperidone administration led to a mean-difference increase in milk production of 93.98 mL/day (95% CI: 71.12, 116.83).[182]

Domperidone has a long history, with many trials for nausea and vomiting and postprandial dyspepsia. It undergoes extensive first-pass hepatic and gut wall metabolism, which results in oral bioavailability of 13% to 17%. After IV administration, the half-life is 7.5 hours, and after oral dosing, the half-life is 14 hours, with time to peak serum levels of 30 to 110 minutes. The volume of distribution is 440. It is metabolized in the liver. Reported adverse effects include arrhythmias, prolonged QTc, extrapyramidal tract effects, and dystonic reactions (more common in children and in patients on antipsychotic medication). Side effects include dry mouth, headache, and abdominal cramps.[12] Galactorrhea is a secondary effect that is not universal. It occurs in both males and females, along with mastalgia and gynecomastia. The augmentation of preexisting lactation in a breast that has been primed by pregnancy appears different. It has been used effectively as an aid to induced or relactation efforts.

Dosage is 10 to 20 mg three to four times per day for 3 to 8 weeks. Some women respond within 24 hours, some take 2 weeks, and some never respond. There are cases of longer-term usage. Withdrawal symptoms of gastric irritability and nausea have been described, and some prescribers recommend tapering the dose. The average milk concentrations with a dosage of 10 mg taken three times per day are 1.2 to 2.6 mcg/L. The total daily dose would be only 180 ng/kg per day. Oral availability is low, 13% to 17%.[178] Domperidone was given to mothers who were pumping for their premature infants and had poor milk production. Two-thirds of the mothers increased their supply at both 30 and 60 mg/day relative to the dose. The amount measured in the milk was low; the mean RID was 0.012% at 30 mg and 0.009% at 60 mg maternal dose per day.[183] No effect on the infants was observed. The AAP rates domperidone a category 6, compatible with lactation.[10] Hale rates it L3, probably compatible, and Schaefer considers it safer than metoclopramide and more effective.[12,184] Because it is banned by the FDA, use in the United States is difficult.[185,186] The recommendations on the use of domperidone from the ABM remain appropriate guides for the clinician: screen mothers for a history of cardiac arrhythmias and the use of other medications associated with prolonged QTc interval, consider obtaining a baseline electrocardiogram (ECG), utilize the medication at the lowest doses for short periods of time, and carefully monitor the response and ongoing breastfeeding care. An informed discussion of the potential risks and benefits of medication use is important and should be documented in the medical record.[169]

Herbs as Galactagogues

Herbs listed as galactagogues are numerous and known by hearsay and historic usage but not by scientific study. Most prominent on the list are fenugreek, fennel, milk thistle (not blessed thistle, which is an entirely different species), lemongrass, goat's rue, and anise. There are several extremely useful recent reviews.[127,165,169,187]

Fenugreek

Fenugreek *(Trigonella foenum graecen)* is a member of the *Leguminosae* family of plants, also called *Fabaceae*, which includes peanuts and chickpeas.[128] Fenugreek is the dried ripe seeds of a small southern European herb known as *Greek hayseed*, which contains 40% mucilage. In addition to being used for poultices and ointments, it is used in teas and syrups and has a faint flavor similar to maple syrup. It is soothing, flavorful, and possibly nutritious. It is available as a spice, flavoring, and tea. It is used as a galactagogue, with use dating back to ancient times. It is generally regarded as safe by the FDA, although it has been noted to cause colic in the infants of mothers using it, similar to that caused by peanuts and chickpeas, and other allergic symptoms in individuals with asthma.[188] It has been noted to lower cholesterol in normal individuals and also to produce hypoglycemia in patients with diabetes. Several cases of mistaken diagnosis of maple syrup urine disease have been published as case reports in which the infant was found to smell of maple syrup. All body fluids smell like maple syrup when an individual receives fenugreek.

In moderate use, fenugreek is considered harmless. As with all things in pregnancy and lactation, moderation is essential. Transport into milk is not documented, but the milk smells like maple syrup, as may the infant. Fenugreek has been touted as a galactagogue, but no scientific reports support or refute this claim. Because it is in the same botanical family as peanuts, soybeans, and chickpeas, a potential for allergy exists. It can interact with anticoagulants and monoamine oxidase (MAO) inhibitors and should not be combined with warfarin (Coumadin) glyburide, or other antidiabetic medications.

The dose is 2 to 3 capsules four times per day, recognizing that varieties differ, and the dose potency will change with variations in plant products. The potential for colic in the infant should be watched for.

Fennel Seed

Fennel seed (*Foeniculum vulgare*) is a common spice with estrogenic properties that has a reputation as a galactagogue but has little supporting evidence.[187]

Milk Thistle

Milk thistle (*Silybum marianum*) also has a reputation as a galactagogue. It is taken as a tea two or three times per day. It is also used as an antispasmodic and has many other uses. Milk thistle is a member of the family *Asteraceae* but should not be confused with blessed thistle, which is *Cnicus benedictus*, an entirely different plant. The active parts of the milk thistle plant are the small hard fruits known as *achenes* (they are not seeds). The leaves have no therapeutic efficacy. The usable material silymarin is an extract of the fruits. It has been credited with inhibiting oxidative damage to liver cells and stimulating the regenerative capacity of liver cells. Micronized silymarin has been studied as a galactagogue in humans because it has been used in cattle. Silymarin is an extract of *S. marianum*, which is the same as milk thistle. Fifty healthy lactating women were given 420 mg/day of silymarin and compared with women who received a placebo. The milk production was increased by 85.9%. Those who received the placebo increased production by 32.1%. No side effects were recorded, and no women dropped out.[189] There is no known toxicity of milk thistle tea. It has been used as a strained tea (simmer 1 tsp crushed fruits in 8 oz water for 10 minutes low dosage).[190]

Lemongrass

Lemongrass (*Cymbopogon citratus*) is used for its dried leaves and oil of citronella. The latter is used as an insect repellent in the United States. It is used for joint pains and GI discomforts. Herbal references do not mention lactation.

Grapefruit Seed

Grapefruit seed extract has been noted in animal experimentation to be an anti-infective, antiviral, antibacterial, and antifungal. Grapefruit itself has been known to contain quinine, especially in the bitter skin and section fibers. Grapefruit seed extract has been recommended as an extract for use by direct application on sore nipples. If it has antiinfectious properties, it should be effective when traumatized nipples have become infected.

Laboratory studies have been reported on the Internet claiming that grapefruit seed extract inactivates herpes simplex (HSV-1), influenza A, and other viruses (see Nutri Team: support@nutriteam.com).

LACTATION SUPPRESSION

Medications that suppress milk production include those that have been used postpartum for women who choose not to breastfeed, such as androgens; estrogens, including those found in low-dose contraceptives; dopaminergic agents, such as bromocriptine or cabergoline, amantadine, and antiparkinsonian drugs; anticholinergics, the smooth muscle relaxants for the GI tract and urinary tract; and some antihistamines and cold preparations. Diuretics also affect milk production. Herbs that are reported to reduce milk supply include sage, peppermint, chasteberry, parsley, and jasmine.[191] The ABM has recently released a protocol on the management of hyperlactation.[192]

Pseudoephedrine

Pseudoephedrine is widely used as a nasal mucous membrane and sinus decongestant. Its effects on milk production were measured by Aljazaf et al., who found it had no effect on breast blood flow or temperature.[193] The mean change in prolactin compared with a placebo was minimal. The milk production, however, was reduced by 24% with a single dose. Little drug was found in the breast milk. This confirms the standard advice that breastfeeding women should not take decongestants and should rely instead on saline nose drops and moisture (vaporizers) for relief of upper respiratory symptoms.

Antiprolactin Medications

Bromocriptine, an antiparkinsonian, synthetic ergot alkaloid that suppresses prolactin secretion, no longer has FDA approval for lactation suppression. A review of adverse effects and bromocriptine in 2015 reported 105 serious adverse effects (cardiovascular, neurologic, and psychiatric) and 2 deaths.[194] Cabergoline, another ergot alkaloid, seems to have fewer side effects than bromocriptine, but both have been associated with postpartum psychosis.[195] There are no large studies of cabergoline's efficacy in stopping lactation, and there is little or no information on its transfer into breast milk or effects on the infant. Cabergoline should be used judiciously for hypergalactia after an appropriate risk–benefit evaluation and with close follow-up during treatment.[191]

Sage

The sage family is a large group of horticulturally important plants consisting of more than 750 species distributed throughout the world. Some are of culinary use and others medicinal. A Central American species is a powerful hallucinogen, traditionally used in religious and ceremonial rites. The best known is *Salvia officinalis*, which has been cultivated for thousands of years. The name *Salvia* is from the Latin word *salvus*, meaning "to be in good health." It is also used as an antiseptic and a gargle and for many other symptoms. It is specifically contraindicated during pregnancy as a suspected abortifacient. Sage has one major physiologic effect: it is antisudorific in cases of excessive sweating, and it is said to reduce lactation. Considering the similarity between sweat glands and alveolar cells of the breast, this cross-relationship is not surprising. No references are found regarding lactation, although there are many references to confirm the antisudorific effect.

The literature supports the use of sage to decrease milk supply, treat engorgement, or hasten weaning.[191] The use of sage as a tea has been recommended to stop hypergalactia. Direct application of sage to the nipples or breast is not recommended unless the goal is to stop lactation.[191]

CARDIOVASCULAR DRUGS AND DIURETICS

The management and treatment of cardiac disease, congestive heart failure, hypertension, and even hypercholesterolemia are incredibly complex. To manage any of these during successful lactation is even more challenging. As outlined in Chapter 15, these chronic conditions can disrupt breast development, lactogenesis, and the composition of milk, not to mention the potential presence of medications to treat these conditions in breast milk and the effects they may have on the infant. A balance must be found between the therapeutic goals of medical treatment and the mother's breastfeeding goals. Risk—benefit information concerning continued breastfeeding and medical therapy must be effectively communicated to facilitate the mother's decision-making for medical therapy with ongoing breastfeeding.

Congestive Heart Failure

Chronic congestive heart failure is usually managed with a combination of medications, most of which are also utilized in the treatment of hypertension. These medications include diuretics, beta-blockers, angiotensin-converting enzyme (ACE) inhibitors, angiotensin II receptor blockers, aldosterone antagonists, and inotropes.[196] See Table 11.11, Ionotropic Agents for Heart Failure, and Table 11.12, Selected Antihypertensive Medications, for a listing of selected cardiac medications from these different classes. These tables (a collation of data from several drug databases) are meant to facilitate comparison of the different agents, including their mechanism of action, compatibility with breastfeeding, important characteristics affecting lactation, ability to enter breast milk (protein binding, M/P ratio, half-life, and RID), and available alternative medications. Three of the inotropes (digoxin, dopamine, and dobutamine) are listed as probably compatible with breastfeeding by Hale.[12]

Digoxin

Digitalis is given to infants but only for significant heart failure. Measurements of digitalis (digoxin) in the milk in mothers maintained on digitalis throughout pregnancy and lactation showed concentrations of 0.825 nmol/L, which was 59% of the maternal plasma level in one study and 75% in another.[5,142] If one calculates the predicted level of digitalis using the higher volume of distribution, 7.5 L/kg, an infant would receive 1.1 ng/mL in the milk of a 60-kg (132-lb) mother receiving a 0.5-mg dose of digoxin. Researchers agree that digoxin levels would be low and the dosage to the infant low, but the long-range effects are not known.[142,197] There is sufficient experience accumulated to date, however, to conclude that mothers taking sustaining doses of digitalis preparations may nurse their infants

without any anticipated harm to the infants. The AAP rates digitalis as category 6, compatible with breastfeeding. Peak plasma levels occur 1.5 to 3 hours after ingestion, so breastfeeding should be avoided during that time to further diminish the infant's exposure to the medication.

Dopamine and Dobutamine

Dopamine is a catecholamine pressor, and dobutamine stimulates beta receptors in the heart. Both are used for congestive heart failure complicated by severe hypotension and shock. Although there is little or no information on their entry into breast milk, the fact that they are destroyed in the GI tract and have very short half-lives (2 minutes) makes it very unlikely that maternal use of either of these medications would affect the infant. Dopamine does inhibit prolactin secretion and could inhibit lactation during its infusion, so dobutamine is likely the preferred choice during lactation.

Peripartum Cardiomyopathy

Peripartum cardiomyopathy as an acute cause of heart failure complicating pregnancy and delivery is discussed in Chapter 15.

Hypertension

Hypertensive disorders associated with pregnancy include gestational hypertension, preeclampsia/eclampsia, chronic hypertension, and underlying hypertension with or without severe exacerbations during pregnancy. Chronic hypertension affects ∼0.9% to 1.5% of pregnancies in the United States, and preeclampsia is estimated to affect 2% to 8% of pregnancies worldwide.[198,199] The effective control of blood pressure in the peripartum period is essential to a safe transition for the mother and the establishment of lactation. The American College of Obstetrics and Gynecology has published protocols for the acute management of hypertension in the perinatal and postpartum period.[198] Many of the antihypertensive agents enter breast milk at low levels and are designated as compatible with breastfeeding. Table 11.12 provides a comparison of medications and alternatives. As a class of agents, the ACE inhibitors are contraindicated during pregnancy, but because of relatively higher protein binding, they are found in low levels in human milk. Benazepril, captopril, and enalapril have some data on their presence in breast milk, have no noted reports of significant effects on breastfeeding infants, and are the preferred ACE inhibitors. The calcium-channel blockers have high protein binding and relatively low levels in breast milk. Nifedipine and verapamil are the preferred calcium-channel blockers because of their relatively shorter half-lives. The angiotensin II receptor antagonists are also contraindicated in pregnancy. They all have very high protein binding, but there is little or no information on their levels in breast milk or observational data on their safe use in breastfeeding. There is a concern regarding diuretics and the potential for reducing the milk supply. There is a history of safe use in lactation of hydralazine and spironolactone, which may be partially explained by their high protein binding and low RID. Clonidine is known to decrease prolactin levels. Nitroprusside, associated with the risk of thiocyanate toxicity, particularly in the fetus and newborn, and nitroglycerin,

TABLE 11.11 Inotropic Agents for Heart Failure

Name	LRC (Hale)	Mechanism of Action	M/P Ratio	PB	RID	Comments	LactMed	Alternative Medications[a]
Digoxin	L2	Na-K pump inhibitor	<0.9	25%	2.7%–2.8%	0.41–0.96 µg/L in BM, no problems noted in BF infants	Given orally, $T_{1/2}$: 36–48 hours Avoid BF for 3 hours after maternal dose (Q 12–Q 24 hours) to decrease exposure	? Another inotrope
Dobutamine	L2	Stimulates beta receptors in heart	?	?	?	Destroyed in the GI tract Given IV, $T_{1/2}$: 2 minutes	No data about transfer into BM, occasionally used IV outpatient	Short $T_{1/2}$ and poor oral bioavailability; unlikely to affect infant
Milrinone	L4	Phosphodiesterase inhibitor	?	70%	?	$T_{1/2}$: 0.8–2.3 hours Short-term IV therapy	Wait 8 hours after a completing infusion before BF	? Another inotrope
Dopamine	L2	Adrenergic and dopaminergic receptor effects	?	?	?	Rapidly destroyed in GI tract Used IV, $T_{1/2}$: 2 minutes Inhibits prolactin secretion—will likely affect lactation	Short $T_{1/2}$ and poor oral bioavailability —unlikely to affect infant	Dobutamine
Norepinephrine	Not listed	Endogenous catecholamine				Poor oral bioavailability and short half-life —any norepinephrine in milk is unlikely to affect the infant		
Levosimendan	Not listed	Calcium sensitizer					Not listed	
Omecamtiv Mecarbil	Not Listed	Affects myosin and actin cross-bridge formation					Not listed	

BF, Breastfed; *BM*, breast milk; *GI*, gastrointestinal; *IV*, intravenous; *LRC*, lactation risk classification; *M/P ratio*, milk-to-plasma ratio; *PB*, protein binding; *RID*, relative infant dose; $T_{1/2}$, drug half-life.

[a]Alternative medications are suggested from Hale TW. *Hale's Medications and Mothers' Milk*. 18th ed. New York: Springer; 2019. Note potential side effects in changing to an alternative medication, and note that the choice of a possible alternative medication is dependent on that medication adequately controlling the seizures specific for that individual.

The LRC (Hale) is as follows:

L2: Probably compatible; studied in a limited number of breastfeeding women without an increase in adverse effects in the infant. L3: Probably compatible; no controlled trials in breastfeeding women; risk of side effects in infants is possible; appropriate to assess the risk–benefit in each situation. L4: Potentially hazardous; there is evidence of risk to a breastfed infant; can be used in mother with appropriate risk–benefit assessment.

Data collated from Hale TW. *Hale's Medications and Mothers' Milk*. 18th ed. New York: Springer; 2019; LactMed. Accessed December 2019.

associated with a risk of methemoglobinemia in children less than 6 months of age, are classified as potentially harmful.

Beta-Blocking Agents

The beta-blockers labetalol and propranolol, which have relatively higher protein binding and lower M/P ratios and lower RDs than atenolol and metoprolol, are the preferred beta-blocking agents.

Propranolol, a beta-adrenergic blocker, is used to treat cardiac arrhythmias, hypertension, migraines, and other illnesses. It was found in the milk of mothers but does not appear to accumulate in infants. Experienced cardiologists have permitted mothers taking propranolol to nurse their infants, without any ill effect observed in the infants. In 1973 Levitan and Manion reported significant quantities of propranolol in breast milk.[200] Propranolol and its major metabolites were measured in milk and found by Smith et al. to provide an infant with a maximum dose of less than 0.1% of the maternal dose or approximately 7 mg/dL.[201] The half-life of elimination from the milk was 3 to 5 hours.[202] Beta-adrenergic blockade effects, including hypoglycemia, have been described in an infant breastfed by a mother taking propranolol. Because the reports

TABLE 11.12   Selected Antihypertensive Medications

Name	Class	LRC (Hale)	M/P Ratio	PB	RID	Concerns	LactMed	Alternative Medications[a]
Captopril	ACE	L2	0.012	30%	0.02%	Contraindicated in pregnancy as a class	Low levels in milk, no noted effects on infant	Enalapril Benazepril Ramipril
Lisinopril	ACE	L3	?	Low	?	Longer $T_{1/2}$,	No information	Enalapril Captopril
Enalapril	ACE	L2	?	60%		active metabolite enalaprilat → poorly absorbed	Low levels in milk, no noted effects on infant	Benazepril Captopril
Benazepril	ACE	L2	0.01	06.7%	?	Benazeprilat active metabolite, poor oral absorption	Low levels in milk, no noted effects on infant	Enalapril Captopril Ramipril
Ramipril	ACE	L3	?	56%	?	Ramiprilat active ingredient	No information	? Another ACE agent
Furosemide	Diur	L3	?	98%	?	Loop diuretic	No information, risk of intense diuresis in infant	? Another diuretic
Hydralazine	Diur	L2	0.4–0.36	87%	1.2%	Long history of use—acceptable in lactation	Limited data, + low levels in milk and infant	? Another diuretic
Hydrochlorothiazide	Diur	L2	0.25	58%	1.68%	Longer $T_{1/2}$, used to suppress postpartum lactation	Low-dose use OK (50–100 mg/day)	Labetalol Nifedipine
Spironolactone	Diur	L3	0.5–0.72	>90%	2.0%–4.3%	K + sparing Aldosterone receptor antagonist, canrenone—major metabolite excreted in BM	Low levels in milk, long history of use—acceptable in lactation	? Another diuretic
Methyldopa	α-ad A	L2	0.19–0.34	Low	0.1%–0.4%	α-adrenergic agonist	Low levels in milk, use OK	?
Prazosin	A-ad block	L3	?	>92%	?		No information	Doxazosin Labetalol
Doxazosin	A-ad block	L3	20	98%	0.58%–0.87%	Limited data, no concerns reported with HM		Propranolol Metoprolol
Nifedipine	CCB	L2	1	>92%		<2% therapeutic infant dose	Rx for nipple vasospasm, low levels in milk	Labetalol
Amlodipine	CCB	L3	?	93%	1.7%–3.1%	Long $T_{1/2}$: 30–50 hours	Found in milk, no effects noted in infants	Nifedipine Labetalol
Nicardipine	CCB	L2	0.25	>95%	<1%		Low levels in milk, use OK	Nifedipine Nimodipine
Nimodipine	CCB	L2	0.06–0.33	95%	<1%	Limited data	Low levels in milk	Verapamil Nifedipine

(Continued)

TABLE 11.12   Selected Antihypertensive Medications—cont'd

Name	Class	LRC (Hale)	M/P Ratio	PB	RID	Concerns	LactMed	Alternative Medications[a]
Verapamil	CCB	L2	0.94	90%	<1%	Variable reports in milk—very low amounts	Low levels in milk, use in infants >2 months of age, use OK	Nifedipine Nimodipine
Atenolol	B-Bl	L3	1.5–6.8	6%–16%	6.6%	Case reports of bradycardia and hypotension	Excreted in BM, use an alternative	Propranolol Metoprolol
Labetalol	B-Bl	L2	0.8–2.6	50%	<3%	Only 1 report of labetalol level in a BF infant	Low levels in milk, caution in preterm infants	Nifedipine Metoprolol
Metoprolol	B-Bl	L2	3.0–3.72	10%	1.4%	Low maternal plasma levels combined with relatively higher M/P ratio limit the amount of drug transferred via BM	Probably safe	Labetalol Propranolol
Propranolol	B-Bl	L2	0.5	90%	0.3%–0.5%	No symptoms reported in BF infants ? Preferred B-Bl	Very low levels in BM, use OK	Metoprolol
Irbesartan	AT-II RA	L3	?	90%	?	Angiotensin II receptor agonist, $T_{1/2}$ is long	Contraindicated in pregnancy, no info—use an alternative	Captopril Enalapril Ramipril
Losartan	AT-II RA	L3	?	99%	?	High PB should reduce its entry into BM	No information—use an alternative	Captopril Enalapril Ramipril
Valsartan	AT-II RA	L3	?	95%	?	Caution with premature infants	No information	Captopril Enalapril Ramipril
Candesartan	AT-II RA	L3	?	>99%	?	Used in children >1 year of age	No information in breastfeeding mothers	Captopril Enalapril Ramipril
Clonidine	Vaso	L3	2	0%–40%	0.9%–7.3%	Decreases prolactin	Central α-agonist	? Alternatives
Nitroprusside	Vaso	L4	?	?	?	$T_{1/2}$: 2 minutes Risk of thiocyanate toxicity	No information on levels in milk, + risk to fetus and newborn	? Alternatives
Nitroglycerin (Nitrates)	Vaso	L4	?	60%	?	Short-acting $T_{1/2}$: 1–4 minutes Children <6 months age: risk methemoglobinemia	Low level in milk, caution with high maternal doses	? Alternatives

α-ad A, Alpha-adrenergic agonist; *A-ad block*, alpha-adrenergic blocker; *ACE*, angiotensin-converting enzyme; *AT-II RA*, angiotensin II receptor antagonist; *B-Bl*, beta-blocker; *BF*, breastfed; *BM*, breast milk; *CCB*, calcium-channel blocker; *Diur*, diuretic; *HM*, human milk; *LRC*, lactation risk classification; *M/P ratio*, milk-to-plasma ratio; *No info*, no or very little information in lactating women; *PB*, protein binding; *RID*, relative infant dose; *Rx*, prescription; $T_{1/2}$, half-life of drug; *Vaso*, vasodilator.

[a]Suggestions for alternative medications are from Hale TW. *Hale's Medications and Mothers' Milk.* 18th ed. New York: Springer; 2019.

The LRC (Hale) is as follows:

L2: Probably compatible; studied in a limited number of breastfeeding women without an increase in adverse effects in the infant. L3: Probably compatible; no controlled trials in breastfeeding women; risk of side effects in infants is possible; appropriate to assess the risk–benefit in each situation. L4: Potentially hazardous; there is evidence of risk to a breastfed infant; can be used in mother with appropriate risk–benefit assessment.

are conflicting, it is appropriate to monitor a breastfed infant carefully when the mother is taking propranolol. Monitoring the plasma levels of the infant may be helpful if there is any concern. Propranolol is a category 6 on AAP scales, considered safe for breastfeeding.

Other beta-blocking agents used to treat hypertension include atenolol (Tenormin), metoprolol tartrate (Lopressor), and nadolol (Corgard, Corzide), which have been evaluated in human milk.[203,204] Metoprolol has a peak level in blood of 713 ng/dL at 1.1 hours and in milk of 4.7 ng/dL at 3.8 hours. The data suggest that metoprolol appears minimally in milk and is probably safe for breastfeeding neonates. Nadolol appears in serum at 77 ng/dL and in milk at 357 ng/dL. Atenolol levels in milk are also higher than levels in the maternal serum. Of this group, metoprolol would be the safest, rated category 6 by the AAP. Serum levels of atenolol in one breastfed infant reached 0.16 mmol/L. It is rated category 5 by the AAP; give with caution. Acebutolol is rated category 6 by the AAP, but the dose must be at or less than 400 mg/day.[205]

Diuretics

Most diuretics are weak acids, and little passes into milk. The use of diuretics, however, requires careful observation because they have the potential for causing diuresis in the neonate, which could be extremely dehydrating.[206] Although diuretics such as furosemide (Lasix) are given to neonates, this is done only when fluid and electrolyte levels can be followed closely. Oral diuretics were used to suppress lactation in a study by Healy in 40 postpartum women who chose not to breastfeed.[207] Bendroflumethiazide (Naturetin) was used, 5 mg twice daily for 5 days. Healy found it more effective than estrogens, with fewer side effects. Milk volume may be reduced by thiazides; therefore they should be used with caution and with monitoring of milk output and infant intake.

Three Diuretics With Bilirubin–Albumin

Complexes. Reports document the interaction of three diuretics with bilirubin–albumin complexes.[208] Chlorothiazide presented the greatest risk for producing free bilirubin, with ethacrynic acid and furosemide producing considerably less. The latter two are clinically effective in lower doses as well. The levels of chlorothiazide and hydrochlorothiazide in milk are less than 100 ng/mL.[209] For most infants, these medications are safe; however, these findings certainly suggest that caution is necessary if an infant is jaundiced or premature and taking diuretics. Furosemide has been shown by several techniques not only to displace bilirubin from albumin in the newborn but also to be slowly excreted by the newborn, with only 84% excreted in 24 hours when given to an infant directly. It is reported, however, that furosemide is not excreted into breast milk and is poorly absorbed orally; thus it would be safe for a lactating mother, although it may suppress milk supply in some women.[12] A mother who is lactating may require substantially less medication, particularly diuretics. Close monitoring of a mother during lactation to try to reduce her medications may provide a therapeutic balance that is good for the mother and safe for the infant. With the short half-life of most diuretics in the adult, dosing can be timed to avoid peak plasma levels during feedings.

Cholesterol-Lowering Drugs

Prevention of cardiovascular disease (CVD) has evolved into a complex set of guidelines using risk assessment and risk categories linked to a series of specific risk-based interventions. The use of lipid-lowering agents is just one of the interventions with the ultimate goal of prevention of CVD, in particular, preventing specific events (myocardial infarction, transient ischemic attacks, stroke, etc.) associated with significant morbidity and mortality.[210] Lifestyle changes, as a first step in CVD prevention, include modifying body weight and physical activity, making choices about nutrition (dietary fat, dietary carbohydrates and fiber, increased fruits and vegetables, increased consumption of fish, and decreased intake of sodium), moderation in alcohol consumption, and decrease in or elimination of smoking. These lifestyle changes will not affect the lipid composition of breast milk and can have other health benefits for the mother. Breastfeeding itself has other benefits on the risk of CVD, including a reduced risk of hypertension, improved blood glucose control, and diminished risk of type 2 diabetes. Lipid-lowering agents include medications with different mechanisms of action, varying degrees of effect on the individual lipids (low-density lipoprotein cholesterol [LDL-C], high-density lipoprotein cholesterol [HDL-C], very low-density lipoprotein [VLDL], cholesterol, triglycerides [TGs]), and very different side-effect profiles. Beyond those considerations, the use of these agents in lactation raises two essential questions: In modifying the mother's plasma lipid profile, how does that change the lipid composition of breast milk? If these medications enter breast milk, how do they affect the infant's plasma lipid profile, nutrition, and growth and development? Cholesterol levels in healthy breastfeeding women are elevated during lactation, which needs to be considered when deciding on the need to lower cholesterol. It has been shown that regardless of dietary intake, mother's milk always contains cholesterol and is remarkably stable at 240 mg/100 g of fat or 9 to 41 mg/dL (average 20 mg/dL). Breastfeeding infants' plasma cholesterol levels are high compared with formula-fed infants who receive no cholesterol in their artificial feeds. There are limited data on the effects of lipid-lowering agents on the breast-milk lipid profile, and to date, these medications have been proscribed during lactation.[211]

Selection of Appropriate Lipid-Lowering Agents

Selecting an appropriate regimen of medications for lipid lowering in an individual is beyond the scope of this chapter. There are online risk calculators from the American Heart Association and the WHO and guidelines available to facilitate this decision-making.[210,212,213] See Tables 11.13, 11.14, and 11.15 for listings of some of these medications and information concerning breast milk and breastfeeding. The tables are meant for comparison, not for recommendation of use. They are a collation of data from Infantrisk.com (LRCs, alternative medications) and LactMed.

TABLE 11.13 Selected Statins for Dyslipidemia

Name	Lactation Risk Category	Effect on Lipids	M/P Ratio	PB	RID	$T_{1/2}$	Comments
Statins: HMG-CoA reductase activity inhibitors, decrease synthesis of cholesterol in liver, increase uptake of LDL-C in hepatocytes							
Atorvastatin	L3	35%–50%	?	98%	?	14 hours	Limited data for BM, likely low BM levels because of poor oral bioavailability and high PB In study of 6 mothers who breastfed 11 infants while on a statin, no long-term effects noted
Fluvastatin	L3	18%–35%	?	>98%	?	1.2 hours	Few or no data
Lovastatin	L3	22%–40%	?	>95%	?	1.1–1.7 hours	Unpublished data says low levels in BM
Pravastatin	L3[a]	20%–25%	?	50%	?	77 hours	Incomplete oral absorption and first-pass effect in liver, BM—estimated 1.4% of maternal weight-adjusted dose
Rosuvastatin	L3[a]	40–55%	?	88%	<1 %	19 hours	Limited data in a breastfeeding woman, BM estimated 1.5% of maternal weight-adjusted dose
Simvastatin	L3	30%–48%	?	95%	?	?	Few or no data
Pitavastatin	? (not listed)					?	

BM, Breast milk; *HMG-CoA*, 3-hydroxy 3-methylglutaryl-coenzyme A; *LDL-C*, low-density lipoprotein cholesterol; *LRC*, lactation risk classification; *M/P ratio*, milk-to-plasma ratio; *PB*, protein binding; *RID*, relative infant dose; $T_{1/2}$, half-life of drug.
[a]Suggestions for alternative medications are from Hale TW. *Hale's Medications and Mothers' Milk.* 18th ed. New York: Springer; 2019.
The LRC (Hale) is as follows:
L2: Probably compatible; studied in a limited number of breastfeeding women without an increase in adverse effects in the infant. L3: Probably compatible; no controlled trials in breastfeeding women; risk of side effects in infants is possible; appropriate to assess the risk—benefit in each situation. L4: Potentially hazardous; there is evidence of risk to a breastfed infant; can be used in mother with appropriate risk—benefit assessment.

The statins remain the first line of therapy in adults who are not pregnant or lactating. As 3-hydroxy 3-methylglutaryl-coenzyme A (HMG-CoA) reductase activity inhibitors, they decrease LDL-C plasma levels. There are scarce or no data on their use in lactation, and decision-making about their use could be based on their pharmacokinetic properties relative to human milk and side-effect profile (myopathy, rhabdomyolysis, hepatocellular damage, proteinuria, and drug—drug interactions with various medications [fibrates, drugs metabolized by CYP3A4]). All the statins are currently classified as LRC L3, but rosuvastatin and pravastatin have been recommended as primary choices during lactation because of the low likelihood of transfer to the infant via breast milk (RID <2%).[214] The bile acid sequestrants (cholestyramine, colestipol, colesevelam) also decrease LDL-C plasma levels and are categorized as LRC L2 because very little medication is absorbed from the GI tract. There are few or no data on their use during lactation, presence in breast milk, and effects on the infant. Ezetimibe and its active metabolite ezetimibe-glucuronide act to decrease the intestinal absorption of dietary or biliary cholesterol from the GI tract and are classified as LRC L3 based on the low likelihood of absorption from the maternal GI tract, despite a lack of data relative to breast milk and breastfeeding. The fibrates (fenofibrate, gemfibrozil) are peroxisome proliferator-activated receptor-alpha (PPAR-α) agonists that decrease TGs and cause a modest increase in HDL-C. They have very high protein binding and are expected to have low breast-milk levels, but there are few or no data on their presence in breast milk, their effect on breast milk, or infant lipid levels. In adults, they are associated with side effects of GI disturbance, myopathy, liver enzyme elevation, and cholelithiasis. The N-3 fatty acids (eicosapentaenoic acid [EPA] and docosahexaenoic acid [DHA]), also classified as LRC L3, are recommended by the AAP and Academy of Nutrition and Dietetics as part of a normal breastfeeding woman's diet, without reference to their potential lipid-lowering effect. There is little or no information regarding their use in lactation for this indication, actual levels achieved in breast milk if supplemented, the lipid profile of milk with supplementation, and their effect on the infant's nutrition and growth and development. Significant clinical research on the use of lipid-lowering agents in lactation is needed before a comprehensive set of recommendations for their use during lactation can be developed.

CENTRAL NERVOUS SYSTEM DRUGS

Anticonvulsants

Protection against seizures during pregnancy is essential to the health of the infant and mother, yet exposure of the fetus to anticonvulsants in utero is associated with an increased

TABLE 11.14 Selected Lipid-Lowering Agents

Name	LRC	Effect on Lipids	M/P Ratio	PB	RID	T$_{1/2}$	Comments[a]
Bile acid sequestrants: Bind bile acids, compensatory increase in LDL receptor activity and decrease in LDL-C (decreases in LDL-C and no effect on HDL-C)							
Cholestyramine	L2	18%–25% decrease	?	?	?	6 minutes?	Not absorbed from the GI tract Lowers mother's lipid level ? Effect on BM LDL-? Alternative
Colestipol	L2	18%–25%	?	?	?	?	? Alternative
Colesevelam	L2	18%–25%	?	?	?	?	0.05% absorption from GI tract Alternative: cholestyramine
Cholesterol-Absorption Inhibitor							
Ezetimibe	L3	Decreases intestinal absorption of dietary and biliary cholesterol Decreases LDL-C 18%–25%	?	90%	?	22 hours	Active metabolite—ezetimibe glucuronide No data relative to BM levels or effect on BM cholesterol or LDL-C levels Alternatives: cholestyramine salts

BM, Breast milk; *GI*, gastrointestinal; *HDL-C*, high-density lipoprotein cholesterol; *LDL*, low-density lipoprotein; *LDL-C*, low-density lipoprotein cholesterol; *LRC*, lactation risk classification; *M/P ratio*, milk-to-plasma ratio; *PB*, protein binding; *RID*, relative infant dose; *T$_{1/2}$*, half-life of drug.

[a]Suggestions for alternative medications are from Hale TW. *Hale's Medications and Mothers' Milk*. 18th ed. New York: Springer; 2019. The LRC (Hale) is as follows:

L2: Probably compatible; studied in a limited number of breastfeeding women without an increase in adverse effects in the infant. L3: Probably compatible; no controlled trials in breastfeeding women; risk of side effects in infants is possible; appropriate to assess the risk–benefit in each situation. L4: Potentially hazardous; there is evidence of risk to a breastfed infant; can be used in mother with appropriate risk–benefit assessment.

risk of congenital malformations, growth restriction, and developmental delay.[215] It has been estimated that about 1.5 million women with epilepsy are of childbearing age in the United States. They give birth to approximately 3 to 5 babies per 1000 infants born each year. The total number of children in the United States exposed in utero to antiepileptic drugs (AEDs) has been estimated to be much greater with prescriptions written for anticonvulsant medications for other indications, including headache, chronic pain, obesity, mood disorders, and other psychiatric diagnoses.[216] The use of anticonvulsants at the time of delivery reportedly increased from 15.7 per 1000 in 2001 in the United States to 21.9 per 1000 deliveries in 2007. Much of the increased use was related to "new" anticonvulsants and their use for other indications beyond seizures.[217] More recently, Meador et al. reported observational data on 351 pregnant women with epilepsy in the United States and their anticonvulsant use.[218] Two hundred and fifty-nine women were on monotherapy (73.8%), 71 (21.9%) were on two or more anticonvulsants, and 15 (4.3%) were on no anticonvulsants. In the women on monotherapy, the most common anticonvulsants were lamotrigine (42%), levetiracetam (37.5%), carbamazepine (5.4%), zonisamide (5.0%), oxcarbazepine (4.6%), and topiramate (3.1%). The benefits of breastfeeding for the infant and mother are significant, well documented, and potentially lifelong. Continued protection of the mother from seizures in the postpregnancy period is important for her health and the care of the infant. The exposure of the infant to anticonvulsants through the ingestion of breast milk still raises concerns regarding the developing brain and the infant's growth and development. A systematic review and network meta-analysis on the safety of antiepileptic drug exposure during pregnancy and breastfeeding wcas conducted by Veroniki et al.[219] Exposure to monotherapy with valproate during pregnancy and breastfeeding was associated with greater odds of cognitive developmental delay. Greater odds of autism were associated with exposure to oxcarbazepine, valproate, lamotrigine, or lamotrigine and valproate together. Valproate and combination drug (valproate + carbamazepine + phenobarbital) exposure were both associated with greater odds of psychomotor delay. This review did not separate the effects of exposure during pregnancy versus breastfeeding and the risk of an adverse outcome.[219] Separately, Meador et al., in a prospective observational multicenter study, assessed 181 children through 6 years of age with exposure to anticonvulsants during pregnancy, comparing breastfed children (42.9% of the total *n*) with ones who did not.[220] There were no apparent adverse outcomes resulting from anticonvulsant exposure via breast milk. The breastfed children demonstrated higher IQs and augmented verbal skills despite continuing exposure to anticonvulsants during breastfeeding (mean 7.2 months).

Maternal Anticonvulsant Therapy

The first decision point for anticonvulsant therapy should be matching the seizure type with an appropriate and effective medication. If the woman has previous experience with a specific agent, then the variables associated with that experience should be reassessed, including efficacy, adherence, tolerance, side effects, and maternal reasons for continuing or discontinuing the medication. Comorbidities are important relative to anticonvulsants, including neurologic conditions, renal and liver dysfunction, behavioral or psychiatric concerns,

TABLE 11.15 Selected Lipid-Lowering Agents

Name	LRC	Effect	M/P Ratio	PB	RID	T$_{1/2}$	Comments[a]
Fibrates: Agonists of peroxisome proliferator-activated receptor-alpha (PPAR-α), decrease triglyceride levels, with modest increases in HDL-C							
Bezafibrate	Not listed		?	?	?	?	No data on BM ? Effect on BM TG or cholesterol levels
Fenofibrate	L3		?	99%	?	20 hours	No data on BM ? Effect on BM TG or cholesterol levels ? Alternative
Gemfibrozil	L3		?	99%	?	1.5 hours	No data on BM ? Effect on BM TG or cholesterol levels ? Alternative
N-3 Fatty Acids: Interact with PPARs and decrease secretion of apoB, decrease TG and VLDL levels							
Eicosapentaenoic acid (EPA)	L3		?	?	?	?	AAP recommends 200–300 mg/day of DHA from dietary sources in mothers No data on supplementation/ treatment doses, except DHA levels can be increased in BM with supplementation No data on effects on lipid composition of BM
Docosahexaenoic acid (DHA)	L3		?	?	?	20 hours	DHA is a common lipid in BM AAP recommends 200–300 mg/day of DHA from dietary sources in mothers No data on effects on lipid composition of BM
Nicotinic acid (Niacin)	?	Reduces TGs and LDL-C and raises HDL-C ? Beneficial effects in clinical trials vs. side effects	?	?	?	?	IOM recommends 13-17 mg/day in lactating women from dietary sources Treatment doses: 100–2000 mg Side effects outweigh benefits Not recommended

AAP, American Academy of Pediatrics; *apoB*, apolipoprotein B; *BM*, breast milk; *HDL-C*, high-density lipoprotein cholesterol; *IOM*, Institute of Medicine; *LDL-C*, low-density lipoprotein cholesterol; *LRC*, lactation risk classification; *M/P ratio*, milk-to-plasma ratio; *PB*, protein binding; *RID*, relative infant dose; *T$_{1/2}$*, half-life of drug; *TG*, triglyceride; *VLDL*, very low-density lipoprotein.
[a]Suggestions for alternative medications are from Hale TW. *Hale's Medications and Mothers' Milk*. 18th ed. New York: Springer; 2019.
The LRC (Hale) is as follows:
L2: Probably compatible; studied in a limited number of breastfeeding women without an increase in adverse effects in the infant. L3: Probably compatible; no controlled trials in breastfeeding women; risk of side effects in infants is possible; appropriate to assess the risk–benefit in each situation. L4: Potentially hazardous; there is evidence of risk to a breastfed infant; can be used in mother with appropriate risk–benefit assessment.
Data collated from Hale TW. *Hale's Medications and Mothers' Milk*. 18th ed. New York: Springer; 2019; LactMed. Accessed December 2019.

and childbearing age and preferences about childbearing and/or contraception. The side-effect profile of the eligible medications is important to review before any decision. Specifically, potential effects on fertility, pregnancy, the fetus (teratogenic or other), and breastfeeding are equally important to consider.[216,221] If the woman is pregnant or pregnancy is possible, then discussion of the use of contraception to prevent/delay pregnancy and supplementation of folic acid and vitamin K during pregnancy are appropriate. An additional important discussion point is that pregnancy can affect blood levels of the medications to different degrees and that monitoring and, potentially, dose adjustment will be essential to effective seizure control.[222] Breastfeeding should be discussed and encouraged. See Box 11.2 and Table 11.16 for comparisons of the individual medications and breast milk and breastfeeding. The table is not meant to guide decision-making for anticonvulsant use in women of

childbearing age; rather, it is for comparison of different agents relative to breast milk and breastfeeding. There are several summaries to guide decision-making for anticonvulsant use in women of childbearing age.[216,221,222] Veiby et al. have published a review of anticonvulsant recommendations for breastfeeding, with "summary" recommendations (safe, moderately safe, possibly hazardous) for specific medications listed.[215] There are some differences in recommendations between Hale, Veiby et al., and LactMed regarding specific anticonvulsants (e.g., Valproate: LRC L4; Veiby et al., safe; and LactMed, monotherapy OK); so before decision-making, review the available databases on anticonvulsant medication use during breastfeeding.

Plasma Levels

When determinations of infant plasma levels are available, it is advisable to check the plasma level after 1 or 2 weeks of

BOX 11.2 Therapeutic Serum Anticonvulsant Levels (mg/L)

Carbamazepine	4–12 mg/L
Ethosuximide	40–80
Felbamate	20–100
Gabapentin	2–20
Lamotrigine	2–20
Phenobarbital	10–20
Phenytoin	10–20
Tiagabine	Not established
Topiramate	Not established
Valproate	50–125
Vigabatrin	Not relevant

nursing to provide an opportunity to evaluate possible accumulation and to check them when mother's daily dose is toward the upper end of the recommended dosing range or the infant is exhibiting concerning signs or symptoms.

PSYCHOTHERAPEUTIC AGENTS

Chapter 15, Medical Complications of Mothers, nicely reviews many of the important considerations related to psychiatric, depression, anxiety, mood, or stress disorders and breastfeeding and lactation. These disorders are common in women of childbearing age and affect 20% to 25% of mothers in the maternal experience during pregnancy and the first year postpartum.[223,224] Medications used in the treatment of psychiatric illness are relatively lipid soluble and able to cross the blood—brain barrier to effectively reach the CNS. There are limited evidence-based data on these medications in breast milk, the potential exposure of the infant via breast milk, medication levels in infants exposed via breast milk, and the safe use of these medications during breastfeeding. There are several comprehensive reviews of the use of antidepressants and other psychiatric medications in breastfeeding.[225–227] The ABM protocol on the use of antidepressants in breastfeeding reinforces screening for depression and psychiatric illness during pregnancy and the postpartum period. It is important to distinguish between primary disease ("postpartum blues," postpartum depression, depression exacerbated during pregnancy or perinatally) and/or comorbid conditions (anxiety, bipolar disease, stress, psychosis, history of traumatic stress or physical or sexual abuse). The protocol provides an outline of considerations and steps in choosing an antidepressant during lactation and is readily applicable to decision-making for other psychiatric medication use as well. Most authors emphasize the importance of the review of previous effective treatment interventions (symptom treatment efficacy, adherence, tolerance, side effects, and reasons for continuation or discontinuation) and open discussion of maternal wishes and concerns regarding treatment. An individual risk—benefit assessment of untreated maternal psychiatric illness, infant health, and the maternal and infant benefits of breastfeeding is essential in each individual situation. Nonpharmacologic therapy plays a crucial role in the management of depression and other psychiatric illnesses, including interpersonal therapy, cognitive—behavioral therapy, and psychodynamic psychotherapy. Extra breastfeeding support, assistance with infant feeding (especially for nighttime feedings), and protection of maternal sleep are important interventions.[225] Given the seriousness of psychiatric illness, the associated symptoms and effects, and the potential for toxicity associated with the psychotherapeutic medications and breastfeeding, it is essential to monitor and reassess the mother's response to therapy, the infant's tolerance of medication exposure via breast milk, and the infant's ongoing growth and development. Reviews and reassessments of up-to-date information on specific psychiatric medication use during lactation that are available through online databases (LactMed, Infantrisk.com) and hotlines (Lactation Study Center, University of Rochester) should be consulted whenever the situation involves psychiatric medications and breastfeeding.

Antidepressants

There are numerous therapeutic agents for depression belonging to a number of different classes of medications: SSRIs, SNRIs, tricyclic antidepressants, MAO inhibitors, miscellaneous medications based on different mechanisms of action, herbal or natural products, and antipsychotics and mood stabilizers.[225,226] See Table 11.17, Selected Antidepressants in Lactation, and Table 11.18, Selected Psychotherapeutic Medications, for collated data on the different medications from several online sources to use for comparison of the different medications.

SSRIs

SSRIs are considered first-line pharmacologic therapy for depression in the peri- and postpartum periods. There are limited long-term data on infant health, growth, and neurobehavioral development with exposure to these agents and even fewer data that separate the effects of the medications only during lactation versus pregnancy and lactation. SSRIs are also used in the treatment of panic attacks, obsessive—compulsive disorder, obesity, substance abuse, sleep disorders, chemotherapy-induced nausea and vomiting, migraine, and appetite suppression. Analyses of the potential risk of autism spectrum disorders with SSRI exposure during pregnancy do not demonstrate statistical significance, with similar results found for SSRI exposure and diminished psychomotor scores in older infants.[228,229] All SSRIs are detected in breast milk at varying levels. Adverse effects noted in infants exposed to SSRIs during breastfeeding include difficulty with sleep, colic, irritability, drowsiness, and poor feeding. Poor neonatal adaptation syndrome (PNAS; also known as *withdrawal syndrome* or *neonatal abstinence syndrome*) with exposure during pregnancy has been observed with SSRIs (and occasionally with SNRIs).[225,230] Continuing maternal medication during breastfeeding may minimize or ease such symptoms in the early postpartum period.[231,232] SSRIs do not seem to affect lactation or milk production. Individual SSRIs

TABLE 11.16 Selected Anticonvulsants

Name	LRC (Hale)	M/P Ratio	PB	RID	LactMed[a]	Veiby et al. (2015)[b]	Comments[c]	Alternative Medications[d]
Carbamazepine	L2	0.69	74%	3.8%–9.5%	BF with carbamazepine monotherapy showed no apparent adverse effects on growth or development	Safe Relatively high PB, M/P <0.7 Serum levels in the infant less than therapeutic and rarely reported side effects	Relatively high BM levels, but BF infants have serum levels < therapeutic range Case reports of liver dysfunction, poor suckling, and poor weight gain	Considered safe ? Alternatives
Clonazepam	L3	0.33	50%–86%	2.8%	Concern of sedation $T_{1/2}$: 18–50 hours	Potentially hazardous Potential for accumulation with long $T_{1/2}$ and reports of sedated breastfed infants	Low incidence of toxicity resulting from drug exposure via BM	Accumulation— potentially hazardous Alternatives: Lorazepam, clobazam
Clobazam	L3	0.13–0.36	80%–90%	4.38%–5.33%	$T_{1/2}$: 36–42 hours Active metabolite → $T_{1/2}$: 71–82 hours	Potentially hazardous, potential for accumulation with long $T_{1/2}$	Short-term use probably compatible with BF	Accumulation— potentially hazardous Alternative: Lorazepam
Diazepam	L3	0.2–2.7	99%	0.88%–7.1%	Active metabolites $T_{1/2}$: 43 hours	Potentially hazardous, potential for accumulation, daily Rx associated with infant sedation	Variable drug levels in BM	Alternative: Lorazepam midazolam
Lorazepam	L3	0.15–0.26	85%–93%	2.6%–2.9%	No active metabolites $T_{1/2}$: 12 hours	Potentially hazardous, potential for accumulation, but lower M/P and shorter $T_{1/2}$ and high PB than other benzodiazepines	Short-term use OK at lowest maternal dose	Accumulation— potentially hazardous Alternatives: Oxazepam, midazolam
Midazolam	L2	0.15	97%	0.63%	$T_{1/2}$: 3 hours Delay BF for 4 hours after maternal dose	Potentially hazardous, shorter $T_{1/2}$, data lacking	Undetectable milk levels after 4 hours	Lorazepam

(Continued)

TABLE 11.16 Selected Anticonvulsants—cont'd

Name	LRC (Hale)	M/P Ratio	PB	RID	LactMed[a]	Veiby et al. (2015)[b]	Comments[c]	Alternative Medications[d]
Ethosuximide	L4	0.94	0%	31%–73% (average = 62%)	+ Transfer via BM No adverse effects reported in breastfed infants	Potentially hazardous, higher RID and higher infant serum levels reported	Often used in combination with other anticonvulsants	More problematic in combination Rx—sedation, hyperexcitability, problems with feeding and weight gain
Felbamate	L4	?	25%	?	Caution—risk for serious side effects	Potentially hazardous, lack of safety data	Minimal data in lactation	Potentially hazardous
Gabapentin	L2	0.7–1.3	<3%	6.6%	Well tolerated by infants	Moderately safe	+ BM levels Infant serum levels 18%–27% of maternal levels	Moderately safe ? Alternatives
Lamotrigine	L2	0.56	55%	9.2%–18.3%	Case report of TTP in an infant	Moderately safe—risk of side effects in the infant	BM levels relatively high	?
Levetiracetam	L2	1	<10%	3.4%–7.2%	Uncommon side effects in exposed infant	Moderately safe	+ Transfer via BM ? Decrease BM production	Alternatives: Gabapentin, Lamotrigine
Oxcarbazepine	L3	0.5	40%	?	No expected symptoms in exposed breastfed infants	Moderately safe	+ Active metabolites	Alternatives: Carbamazepine
Phenobarbital	L4	0.3–0.6%	51%	24%	Lots of variability of levels in BM Infant sedation influences feeding	Potentially hazardous, Long $T_{1/2}$: 96 hours Monitoring for accumulation advisable	Long $T_{1/2}$, relatively low protein binding, risk of accumulation in infant	Caution: Accumulation—watch for drowsiness and poor feeding
Phenytoin	L2	0.18–0.45	89%	0.6%–7.7%	No apparent effect on infant growth or development long term	Safe High PB, low M/P, low serum levels in infants	Low levels in BM, few reports of side effects in infant with combination Rx	Considered safe ? Alternatives
Primidone	L4	0.72	25%	8.4%–8.6%	+ Levels in infants from BF, some sedation	Potentially hazardous, similar to phenobarbital	Metabolized to phenobarbital and other derivatives, exposure to primidone and phenobarbital	Potential to accumulate to high levels in BF infants ? Alternatives

(Continued)

TABLE 11.16 Selected Anticonvulsants—cont'd

Name	LRC (Hale)	M/P Ratio	PB	RID	LactMed[a]	Veiby et al. (2015)[b]	Comments[c]	Alternative Medications[d]
Topiramate	L3	0.86	15%–41%	24.68%–55.65%	No other obvious infant effects, normal development	Moderately safe	Levels in milk—less than therapeutic levels in infants, 1 case report of watery diarrhea	?
Valproate	L4	0.42	94%	0.99%–5.6%	Low levels in infants from BF, no apparent adverse effects on development or growth. Use in mother OK	Safe. High PB, low M/P, low serum levels in infants	1 case report of TTP, low BM levels + developmental benefits of BF > risk from drug exposure	Considered safe, ? Alternatives
Vigabatrin	L3	<1	0	1.5%–2.7%	Limited information in lactation, careful monitoring of the infant is appropriate	Moderately safe	Small amounts in BM, no specific infant concerns except increased brain GABA levels long term	?
Zonisamide	L4	0.7–0.93	40%	28.8%–44.1%	Consider an alternative drug for the mother or limit BM exposure	Possibly hazardous—high levels in neonatal period and potential for accumulation	A sulfonamide. High levels in milk. Long T$_{1/2}$: ~100 hours	Potentially hazardous—little or no toxicity information in infants

BF, Breastfeeding; *BM*, breast milk; *GABA*, gamma-aminobutyric acid; *LRC*, lactation risk classification; *M/P ratio*, milk-to-plasma ratio; *PB*, protein binding; *RID*, relative infant dose; *Rx*, prescription; *T$_{1/2}$*, half-life of drug; *TTP*, thrombotic thrombocytopenic purpura.

[a]Infants exposed to anticonvulsants, as a class of drugs, should be observed for drowsiness, irritability, poor feeding, and weight gain/growth and development.

[b]Data from Veiby G, et al. Epilepsy and recommendations for breastfeeding. *Seizure*. 2015;28:57. doi:10.1016/j.seizure.2015.02.013.

[c]In the question of long-term exposure and the infant's development, t is difficult to distinguish between intrauterine effects and effects from BM exposure.

[d]Alternative medications are suggested from Hale TW. *Hale's Medications and Mothers' Milk*. 18th ed. New York: Springer; 2019. Note potential side effects in changing to an alternative medication. The choice of a possible alternative medication is dependent on that medication adequately controlling the seizures specific for that individual.

The LRC (Hale) is as follows:

L2: Probably compatible; studied in a limited number of breastfeeding women without an increase in adverse effects in the infant. L3: Probably compatible; no controlled trials in breastfeeding women; risk of side effects in infants is possible; appropriate to assess the risk—benefit in each situation. L4: Potentially hazardous; there is evidence of risk to a breastfed infant; can be used in mother with appropriate risk—benefit assessment.

Data collated from Hale TW. *Hale's Medications and Mothers' Milk*. 18th ed. New York: Springer; 2019; LactMed. Accessed December 2019.

are categorized as L2 (probably compatible) by Hale, but sertraline is the most frequently prescribed SSRI, and escitalopram, paroxetine, and fluoxetine are listed as appropriate alternatives.[12] Sertraline and paroxetine have lower levels in human milk and lower reported RIDs (<3%), whereas fluoxetine and citalopram have breast-milk levels that can exceed 10% of the maternal dose. The FDA suggests not using fluoxetine in lactation because of its long half-life ($T_{1/2} = 2$ to 3 days) and that of its active metabolite norfluoxetine ($T_{1/2} = 360$ hours) and potential accumulation.

SNRIs

There are fewer data for SNRIs in breast milk (see Table 11.17). Duloxetine has the lowest breast-milk level and RID compared with desvenlafaxine and venlafaxine, as well as >90% protein binding. Venlafaxine is categorized as L2 (probably compatible) by Hale, and the other two SNRIs are listed as L3 (probably compatible; fewer data for levels in breast milk and possible side effects). These are each associated with isolated reports of PNAS and galactorrhea, and use during breastfeeding should be monitored for infant sedation and weight gain. SSRIs are listed as alternatives to SNRIs by Hale.[12]

Tricyclic Antidepressants

The tricyclic antidepressants include several mediations listed as L2 (probably compatible with lactation) by Hale, although there are limited data on their use.[12] Amitriptyline, clomipramine, desipramine, imipramine, and nortriptyline each have high protein binding and relatively low RIDs. Nortriptyline is the preferred agent in this group for use in lactation, with imipramine being an alternative. Doxepin is listed by Hale as hazardous because of case reports of significant CNS depression in some breastfed infants. There have been reports of galactorrhea and increased prolactin with some of the tricyclic antidepressants.

MAO Inhibitors

There are limited or no data on these MAO inhibitors in breast milk. The need for caution relative to diet and drug interactions when taking an MAO inhibitor is also a concern for lactating mothers. One should consider the alternatives: SSRIs and SNRIs.

Miscellaneous Antidepressants

See Tables 11.17, 11.18, and 11.19. Lithium and quetiapine are used to treat bipolar disorder. There is high variability in lithium levels in breast milk, but the breast-milk levels seem to correlate with maternal plasma levels. Monitoring of levels of lithium in the mother is recommended, as well as in the infant if there are high levels in the mother or suspected symptoms in the infant as a result of toxicity. Hale categorizes lithium as L4 (potentially hazardous) and recommends alternatives: carbamazepine or lamotrigine.[12] There are no reports of significant long-term toxicity in the exposed breastfed infant. Quetiapine has high protein binding, a relatively short half-life, and a low RID. There are no apparent concerns with toxic exposure of the infant, and Hale classifies it as L2

(probably compatible with breastfeeding).[12] Bupropion produces low levels in breast milk, but there are limited data, with individual case reports of seizures in an infant and decreased milk supply in a mother. It is classified as L3 (probably compatible but possible side effects in the exposed infant), and monitoring is recommended for vomiting, diarrhea, jitteriness, and/or sedation. Possible alternatives for bupropion are sertraline and citalopram. Trazadone is considered L2 (probably compatible with breastfeeding) and has high protein binding, a relatively short half-life among psychiatric medications, and an RID of less than 3%. The levels in breast milk are low enough that no adverse effects are expected.

Antipsychotic Medications

Typical antipsychotic medications include the phenothiazines and haloperidol. All of these have been reported to cause galactorrhea and hyperprolactinemia. Most (chlorpromazine, fluphenazine, haloperidol, and perphenazine) are classified as L3 (probably compatible with lactation) but with limited information on their presence in breast milk. They are associated with galactorrhea and hyperprolactinemia. There are no significant side effects reported in exposed breastfed infants, but monitoring is recommended for infant drowsiness and poor feeding. Alternatives include other antipsychotic medications.

The atypical antipsychotic medications include various different medications (see Table 11.19). They are classified as L2 or L3, probably compatible with breastfeeding but with limited available data on their presence in breast milk. There are low amounts of the medications found in breast milk, and thus they are considered relatively safe in lactation, but there are limited long-term data on safety in infants. Olanzapine and risperidone are frequently prescribed. Quetiapine and aripiprazole are recommended alternatives. Risperidone can cause elevated prolactin levels, gynecomastia, and galactorrhea in adults. Monitoring for side effects with the use of antipsychotic medications is recommended, especially if mothers are on more than one psychiatric medication simultaneously.

Other Psychotherapeutic Agents

See Table 11.18, Selected Psychotherapeutic Agents. Mood stabilizers, antianxiety medications, and adjunctive medications (stimulants, e.g., amphetamines) are considered in this group. The mood stabilizers lamotrigine and carbamazepine (also an anticonvulsant medication) each have relatively high breast-milk levels that correlate with maternal serum levels. Although there is little evidence of long-term toxicity or developmental issues, monitoring of infant behavior and growth and development is appropriate. Antianxiety medications include the benzodiazepines and gabapentin. Oxazepam, with high protein binding and relatively short half-life, produces low levels in breast milk. It is not expected to show adverse effects in infants. Lorazepam also has high protein binding, a slightly longer half-life, and an RID of <3%. Short-term lower-dose usage of lorazepam in lactating

TABLE 11.17 Selected Antidepressants in Lactation[a]

Name	LRC (Hale)	M/P Ratio	PB	$T_{1/2}$	RID	LactMed	Comments[b]
Selective Serotonin-Reuptake Inhibitors (SSRIs)							
Citalopram	L2	1.16–3.00	80%	36 hours	3.56%– 5.37%	Low levels in milk Genetic metabolic capacity may affect serum levels in mother and infant	Colic, decreased feeding, somnolence, restlessness Alternatives: Sertraline, escitalopram
Escitalopram	L2	2.2	56%	27–32 hours	5.2%– 7.9%	Low levels in BM A case report of an infant with NEC and one of a seizure in an infant also receiving bupropion	Drug and its metabolite undetectable in most BF infants tested Alternatives: Sertraline, fluoxetine
Fluoxetine	L2	0.286–0.67	94.5%	2–3 days	1.6%– 14.6%	Higher BM levels, long-acting active metabolite, norfluoxetine detectable in BF infant serum	Active metabolite $T_{1/2}$: 360 hours One case of neonatal withdrawal syndrome (NWS) Alternatives: Sertraline, escitalopram
Fluvoxamine	L2	1.34	80%	15.6h	0.3%– 1.4%	Limited data Limited long-term data found no adverse effects Risk of poor neonatal adaptation without BF	Low levels in milk and in infants and no adverse effects Alternatives: Sertraline, escitalopram
Paroxetine	L2	0.056–1.3	95%	21 hours	1.2%– 2.8%	Low levels in BM, not detected in most infants Most authoritative reviewers consider it a preferred antidepressant in lactation	Alternatives: Sertraline
Sertraline	L2	0.89	98%	26 hours	0.4%– 2.2%	Low levels in BM, small amounts ingested by infant Most authoritative reviewers consider it a preferred antidepressant in lactation Mothers may need more support with breastfeeding	Potent inhibitor of 5-HT transporter function in CNS and platelets Very low or undetectable levels of drug in infants Alternatives: Escitalopram, citalopram, fluoxetine
Vilazodone	L3	?	96%– 99%	25 hours	?	No published data Use an alternative	No data on transfer into milk Alternatives: SSRIs, SNRIs
Serotonin–Norepinephrine-Reuptake Inhibitors (SNRIs)							
Duloxetine	L3	0.26–1.29	>90%	12 hours	0.1%– 1.1%	Limited data, low level in milk and in serum of 2 BF infants Galactorrhea reported in women	Very low RID Alternatives: Venlafaxine, sertraline, citalopram
Desvenlafaxine	L3	2.7	30%	11 hours	5.9%– 9.3%	Modest levels excreted in BM, breastfed infants' serum drug levels <10% maternal levels Poor neonatal adaptation syndrome	No reported side effects in infants Alternatives: Sertraline, fluoxetine

(Continued)

TABLE 11.17   Selected Antidepressants in Lactation[a]—cont'd

Name	LRC (Hale)	M/P Ratio	PB	$T_{1/2}$	RID	LactMed	Comments[b]
Venlafaxine	L2	2.75	27%	5 hours	6.8%–8.1%	+ In plasma of most BF infants Monitor for sedation and adequate weight gain Poor neonatal adaptation syndrome	RID higher, no adverse effects Alternatives: Sertraline, fluoxetine
Other							
Bupropion	L3	2.51–8.58	84%	8–24 hours	0.11%–1.99%	Low levels in milk Little reported use Monitor infant for vomiting, diarrhea, jitteriness, sedation	Case reports of decreased milk supply and seizures Alternatives: Sertraline, citalopram
Mirtazapine	L3	0.76	85%	20–40 hours	1.6%–6.3%	Limited info Low levels in milk If used in lactation, monitor infant for behavior and growth	Alternatives: Sertraline, venlafaxine
Trazodone	L2	0.14	85%–95%	4–9 hours	2.8%	Low levels in milk No expected adverse effects	? Alternatives
Tricyclic Antidepressants							
Amitriptyline	L2	1	94.8%	31–46 hours	1.08%–2.8%	Low levels in milk No immediate side effects ? Concern in infants <2 months of age	Very low levels in milk Alternatives: Nortriptyline, SSRIs
Clomipramine	L2	0.84–1.62	96%	19–37 hours	2.8%	Increased prolactin, galactorrhea, withdrawal syndrome reported	Alternatives: Sertraline, paroxetine, fluoxetine
Desipramine	L2	0.4–0.9	82%	7–60 hours	0.3%–0.9%	Milk levels are low, not detected in BF infants, no reported immediate side effects	Few data—undetected in BF infants Alternatives: Amoxapine, imipramine, sertraline
Doxepin	L5	1.08–1.66	80%	15 hours Active metabolite, 31 hours	0.32%–3%	+ Sedating potential, + active metabolite, + infant serum, case reports of adverse effects	2 case reports of serious CNS depression in BF infants Limited data Hazardous
Imipramine	L2	0.5–1.5	90%	8–16 hours	0.1%–4.4%	Low milk levels, not detected in BF infants Active metabolite desipramine	Limited data Alternative: Amoxapine
Nortriptyline	L2	0.87–3.71	92%	16–90 hours	1.7%–3.36%	Authoritative reviewers consider it one of the preferred antidepressants	Rarely detectable in BM or BF infants Alternatives: Imipramine, amitriptyline, SSRIs
Monoamine Oxidase Inhibitors (MAO Inhibitors)							
Selegiline (transdermal)	L4	?	99.5%	10 hours	?	Decreases prolactin	No data in human milk Not recommended in lactation

(Continued)

TABLE 11.17 Selected Antidepressants in Lactation[a]—cont'd

Name	LRC (Hale)	M/P Ratio	PB	T$_{1/2}$	RID	LactMed	Comments[b]
Phenelzine	Not listed					Limited data Galactorrhea Elevated prolactin	Alternatives: Nortriptyline, paroxetine, sertraline
Tranylcypromine	Not listed					Limited data Use an alternative	Alternatives: Nortriptyline, paroxetine, sertraline

BF, Breastfeeding; *BM*, breast milk; *CNS*, central nervous system; *5-HT*, 5-hydroxytryptamine; *LRC*, lactation risk classification; *M/P ratio*, milk-to-plasma ratio; *NEC*, necrotizing enterocolitis; *PB*, protein binding; *RID*, relative infant dose; *T$_{1/2}$*, half-life of drug.

[a]Infants exposed to psychiatric medications, as a broad group, should be observed for drowsiness, irritability, poor feeding, and weight gain/growth and development In the question of long-term exposure and the infant's development, it is difficult to distinguish between intrauterine effects and effects from BM exposure.

[b]Alternative medications are suggested from Hale TW. *Hale's Medications and Mothers' Milk.* 18th ed. New York: Springer; 2019. Note potential side effects in changing to an alternative medication. The choice of a possible alternative medication is dependent on that medication adequately controlling the seizures specific for that individual.

The LRC (Hale) is as follows:

L2: Probably compatible; studied in a limited number of breastfeeding women without an increase in adverse effects in the infant. L3: Probably compatible; no controlled trials in breastfeeding women; risk of side effects in infants is possible; appropriate to assess the risk—benefit in each situation. L4: Potentially hazardous; there is evidence of risk to a breastfed infant; can be used in mother with appropriate risk—benefit assessment.

Data collated from Hale TW. *Hale's Medications and Mothers' Milk.* 18th ed. New York: Springer; 2019; LactMed. Accessed December 2019.

mothers is acceptable, with monitoring of the infant for sedation, sleep disturbance, crying, or irritability. There are case reports of PNAS with the benzodiazepines, which may be ameliorated by breastfeeding in the immediate postpartum period. Stimulants are used as adjunctive medications in treating psychiatric illness and for treatment of attention-deficit/hyperactivity disorder or narcolepsy. Some experts advise against the use of stimulants during lactation, partially because of the limited data on the effects on the infant and partially because of the risk for abuse of these medications. Methylphenidate, with low levels in breast milk, undetectable infant plasma levels, and limited evidence of toxicity in exposed breastfed infants, is classified as L2 (probably compatible with breastfeeding). Dextroamphetamine and lisdexamfetamine are both classified as L3 (probably compatible with breastfeeding), but with even more limited data on breast-milk levels and exposure toxicity through breast-milk exposure.

Psychotherapeutic Medications—Summary

Depression or other psychiatric illness in a pregnant or breastfeeding woman can have significant effects on the health of the mother and the infant. If the symptoms are moderate to severe, they may markedly disrupt routine care of the newborn infant, and the benefits of pharmacologic treatment will outweigh the risks of medication exposure for the mother and infant. Almost all of the psychiatric medications reach the breast milk and can be transferred to the breastfeeding infant. For each mother—infant dyad, an individualized risk—benefit assessment should be performed concerning treatment with medication and subsequent exposure of the mother and infant to one or more medications versus the benefits of breastfeeding and openly discussed with the mother and family. Each mother with depression or psychiatric illness should receive some form of psychotherapy and

additional support for breastfeeding, infant care, and sleep hygiene. Monitoring of the mother's response to medical therapy and the infant's behavior, growth, and development in the face of medication exposure through breast milk is recommended. Long-term follow-up of infant growth and development is crucial, especially when the mother receives more than one psychotherapeutic medication while breastfeeding. Measurement of serum levels of medication does not need to be done routinely, except if there is a clinical indication or suspicion of toxicity. There is the theoretical strategy that infant exposure to maternal medications through breastfeeding can be diminished by administering the mother's medications immediately after breastfeeding or substituting formula for breast milk at different times in the day. There are no controlled trials demonstrating the benefits of this for the mother and infant versus the potential risks.

MIGRAINES AND HEADACHES

Migraines and headaches are both relatively common in women of childbearing age and specifically during pregnancy and postpartum, as discussed in Chapter 15.[233,234] Negro et al. present a systematic review of headaches in pregnancy.[235] The review highlights the four main types of headaches: migraine without aura, migraine with aura, tension-type headache, and cluster headache. It also emphasizes the importance of distinguishing a primary headache disorder from a headache secondary to an underlying cause or illness and outlines "red flags" for headaches and the main causes of secondary headaches in pregnant women. The main causes of secondary headaches and "red flags" for headaches are applicable during lactation as well. Breastfeeding may reduce the occurrence of migraine in the postpartum period but may not affect the overall frequency of headaches in this time period.[236–238]

TABLE 11.18 Selected Psychotherapeutic Medications[a]

Name	LRC (Hale)	M/P Ratio	PB	$T_{1/2}$	RID	LactMed	Comments[b]
Mood Stabilizers							
Lamotrigine	L2	0.56	55%	29 hours	9.2%–18.27%	BM levels relatively high, correlate with maternal plasma levels Case report of TTP in an infant	Monitor for side effects: apnea, rash, drowsiness or poor sucking; measure serum levels if there is a concern ? Alternatives
Valproate	L4	0.42	94%	14 hours	0.99%–5.6%	Low levels in infants from BF, no apparent adverse effects on development or growth Use in mother OK	? Alternatives
Carbamazepine	L2	0.69	74%	18–54 hours	3.8%–5.9%	BF with carbamazepine monotherapy showed no apparent adverse effects on growth or development	Relatively high BM levels, but BF infants have serum levels < therapeutic range Case reports of liver dysfunction, poor suckling, and poor weight gain ? Alternatives
Lithium	L4	0.24–0.66	0%	18–36 hours	0.87%–30%	Highly variable levels in BM Despite this, most reports do not show toxicity or developmental issues	Monitor BF infants and infant levels Alternatives: Carbamazepine, lamotrigine
Antianxiety							
Benzodiazepines							
Alprazolam	L3	0.36	80%	12–15 hours	8.5%	Withdrawal symptoms in infants: Crying, irritability, sedation, sleep disturbances	Alternatives: Lorazepam, midazolam, oxazepam
Chlordiazepoxide	L3	?	96%	6.6–28 hours	?	Limited data in BM Possible accumulation—use an alternative	Alternatives: Lorazepam
Clonazepam	L3	0.33	50%–86%	18–50 hours	2.8%	Concern for sedation, given reports and because accumulation is possible with longer $T_{1/2}$	Low incidence of toxicity resulting from drug exposure via BM Alternatives: Lorazepam
Diazepam	L3	0.2–2.7	99%	43 hours	0.88%–7.1%	Active metabolites $T_{1/2}$: 43 hours Potential for accumulation	Variable drug levels in BM Alternatives: Lorazepam, midazolam
Lorazepam	L3	0.15–0.26	85%–93%	12 hours	2.6%–2.9%	Short-term use or single dose OK at lowest maternal dose	Accumulation—potentially hazardous Alternatives: Oxazepam, midazolam
Oxazepam	L2	0.1–0.33	97%	8 hours	0.28%–1%	Low levels in BM Relatively shorter $T_{1/2}$ Not expected to cause adverse effects in infants	Alternatives: Lorazepam

(Continued)

TABLE 11.18 Selected Psychotherapeutic Medications[a]—cont'd

Name	LRC (Hale)	M/P Ratio	PB	$T_{1/2}$	RID	LactMed	Comments[b]
Gabapentin	L2	0.7–1.3	<3%	5–7 hours	6.6%	Limited data show low levels in BM OK for refractory restless leg syndrome during lactation	Monitor the infant for drowsiness, weight gain, and development, especially in younger, exclusively BF infants or with combinations of anticonvulsant or psychotropic drugs ? Alternatives
Pregabalin	L3	0.34–0.76	Unbound	6 hours	7.18%	Limited data suggest low levels in BM	? Alternatives
Buspirone	L3	?	86%	2–3 hours	?	Limited data—low levels in BM, high PB, relatively low $T_{1/2}$	Alternatives: Lorazepam, oxazepam
Adjunctive Medications: Stimulants							
Amphetamine	Not listed					Contraindicated with abuse No evidence of adverse effects in infants when used at doses for medical reasons Decreases serum prolactin, but milk production not assessed	Some experts advise against any use of stimulants during lactation Alternatives: Dextroamphetamine, lisdexamfetamine, methylphenidate
Dextroamphetamine	L3	2–5.2	16%–20%	9.77–11 hours	2.46%–7.25%	No obvious adverse effects in infants, but long-term development with BF exposure needs study	Alternatives: Methylphenidate, lisdexamfetamine
Lisdexamfetamine	L3	2–5.2	20%	6.8 hours	1.8%–6.2%	Prodrug metabolized to dextroamphetamine Infant plasma levels varied from undetectable to 18 µg/L	Limited data in BM and long-term effects on infants Alternatives: methylphenidate
Methylphenidate	L2	2.8	10%–33%	1.4–4.2 hours	0.2%–0.4%	Limited data shows low levels in BM Not detected in infant's plasma, decreases serum prolactin	? Alternatives

BF, Breastfeeding; *BM*, breast milk; *LRC*, lactation risk classification; *M/P ratio*, milk-to-plasma ratio; *PB*, protein binding; *RID*, relative infant dose; $T_{1/2}$, half-life of drug; *TTP*, thrombotic thrombocytopenic purpura.

[a]Infants exposed to psychiatric medications, as a broad group, should be observed for drowsiness, irritability, poor feeding, and weight gain/growth and development. In the question of long-term exposure and the infant's development, it is difficult to distinguish between intrauterine effects and effects from BM exposure.

[b]Alternative medications are suggested from Hale TW. *Hale's Medications and Mothers' Milk*. 18th ed. New York: Springer; 2019. Note potential side effects in changing to an alternative medication. The choice of a possible alternative medication is dependent on that medication adequately controlling the seizures specific for that individual.

The LRC (Hale) is as follows:

L2: Probably compatible; studied in a limited number of breastfeeding women without an increase in adverse effects in the infant. L3: Probably compatible; no controlled trials in breastfeeding women; risk of side effects in infants is possible; appropriate to assess the risk–benefit in each situation. L4: Potentially hazardous; there is evidence of risk to a breastfed infant; can be used in mother with appropriate risk–benefit assessment.

Data collated from Hale TW. *Hale's Medications and Mothers' Milk*. 18th ed. New York: Springer; 2019; LactMed. Accessed December 2019.

TABLE 11.19 Selected Antipsychotic Medications[a]

Name	LRC (Hale)	M/P Ratio	PB	T {1/2}	RID	LactMed	Comments[b]
Typical Medications							
Chlorpromazine	L3	<0.5	95%	30 hours	0.3%	Identified in BM but not correlated well with maternal dose or serum level ? Infant drowsiness Monitor infant Phenothiazines cause hyperprolactinemia and galactorrhea	Low levels in BM, long $T_{1/2}$, particularly sedating Reports of increased risk of apnea + SIDS Alternatives: Haloperidol, olanzapine, risperidone
Fluphenazine	L3	?	91%–99%	PO 14–16 hours, IM 14 days	?	Phenothiazines cause galactorrhea in 26%–40% of female patients and hyperprolactinemia	Limited data in BM ? Alternatives
Haloperidol	L3	0.58–0.81	92%	12–38 hours	0.2%–12%	Low levels in BM, no adverse effects in infants Galactorrhea, hyperprolactinemia	Increases prolactin in some patients Significant levels in BM Monitor infants Alternatives: Risperidone, olanzapine, aripiprazole
Loxapine	L4	?	?	19 hours	?	Alternatives are preferred	No data in human BM Caution urged Alternatives: olanzapine, risperidone, aripiprazole
Perphenazine	L3	0.7–1.1	?	8–20 hours	0.1%	Limited data show low levels in BM, no adverse effects in infants	Limited data Alternatives: Haloperidol, olanzapine
Trifluoperazine	Not listed					Limited data 1 mcg/L infant plasma level, no observed side effects	Alternatives: Haloperidol, olanzapine
Thiothixene	Not listed					No published data with BM + Hyperprolactinemia, galactorrhea	Alternatives: Haloperidol, olanzapine, risperidone
Thioridazine	L4	?	95%	21–24 hours	?	No published data with BM	No data in BM Alternatives: Haloperidol, olanzapine
Atypical Agents							
Aripiprazole	L3	0.2	99%	75 hours	0.7%–6.44%	Case reports: decreases prolactin, inhibits lactation, hyperprolactinemia and galactorrhea	Limited data show low levels in BM Alternatives: Risperidone, olanzapine, quetiapine, haloperidol
Asenapine	L3	?	95%	24 hours	?	Hyperprolactinemia and galactorrhea reported	No data on levels in BM Alternatives: Risperidone, aripiprazole, quetiapine
Clozapine	L3	2.8–4.3	95%	8–12 hours	1.33%–1.4%	Case reports of sedation and adverse hematologic effects in infants Consider alternatives	Concentrates in BM Alternatives: Haloperidol, olanzapine, quetiapine, risperidone

(Continued)

TABLE 11.19 Selected Antipsychotic Medications[a]—cont'd

Name	LRC (Hale)	M/P Ratio	PB	T {1/2}	RID	LactMed	Comments[b]
Lurasidone	L3	?	99%	18 hours	?	No data, but likely to be low in BM because of high PB and low bioavailability	Alternatives: Quetiapine, risperidone, aripiprazole
Olanzapine	L2	0.38	93%	21–54 hours	0.28%–2.24%	Low levels in BM, undetectable levels in infants. Reports of infant sedation, irritability. Reviews of second-generation antipsychotics state it is a preferred agent	Infant development apparently OK. Alternatives: Risperidone, quetiapine
Paliperidone	L3	?	74%	PO 23 hours, IM 25–49 days	?	Active metabolite of risperidone, but few data on paliperidone during BF. Available only as sustained-release product	Limited data reported, limited long-term data. Reports of hyperprolactinemia, galactorrhea, gynecomastia. Alternatives: Haloperidol, olanzapine
Quetiapine	L2	0.29	83%	6 hours	0.02%–0.1%	Systematic reviews state it is a good choice for second-generation antipsychotics during breastfeeding. Case reports of galactorrhea with minimal effect on prolactin	Low levels in BM. No apparent concerns. Alternatives: Risperidone, olanzapine
Risperidone	L2	0.42	90%	20 hours	2.8%–9.1%	Few published data and little long-term experience. Can cause elevated prolactin serum levels, gynecomastia, and galactorrhea in adults	Low to moderate levels in BM, no detected levels in infant sera, no adverse effects. Alternatives: Quetiapine, haloperidol, olanzapine
Ziprasidone	L2	0.06	99%	7 hours	0.07%–1.2%	Few data—choose alternatives	Couple of case reports: low levels in BM and no adverse effects. Alternatives: Risperidone, olanzapine, haloperidol, quetiapine

BF, Breastfeeding; *BM*, breast milk; *IM*, intramuscular; *LRC*, lactation risk classification; *M/P ratio*, milk-to-plasma ratio; *PB*, protein binding; *PO*, per os; *RID*, relative infant dose; *SIDS*, sudden infant death syndrome; $T_{1/2}$, half-life of drug.

[a]Infants exposed to psychiatric medications, as a broad group, should be observed for drowsiness, irritability, poor feeding, and weight gain/growth and development. In the question of long-term exposure and the infant's development, it is difficult to distinguish between intrauterine effects and effects from BM exposure.

[b]Alternative medications are suggested from Hale TW. *Hale's Medications and Mothers' Milk*. 18th ed. New York: Springer; 2019. Note potential side effects in changing to an alternative medication. The choice of a possible alternative medication is dependent on that medication adequately controlling the seizures specific for that individual.

The LRC (Hale) is as follows:

L2: Probably compatible; studied in a limited number of breastfeeding women without an increase in adverse effects in the infant. L3: Probably compatible; no controlled trials in breastfeeding women; risk of side effects in infants is possible; appropriate to assess the risk–benefit in each situation. L4: Potentially hazardous; there is evidence of risk to a breastfed infant; can be used in mother with appropriate risk–benefit assessment. Data collated from Hale TW. *Hale's Medications and Mothers' Milk*. 18th ed. New York: Springer; 2019; LactMed. Accessed December 2019.

Treatment of Headaches During Lactation

The actual medical decision-making and choice of specific medications for the treatment of acute headaches and prevention of migraines are beyond the scope of this text. It is important to consider all the behavioral and physical therapies available for the treatment and prevention of headaches, including cognitive–behavioral training, biofeedback training, relaxation techniques, acupuncture, cervical manipulation, transcutaneous electrical nerve stimulation, physical therapy, massage, and chiropractic and osteopathic manipulation, for example. These therapies may be beneficial in women based on personal preference, poor tolerance of medications, medical contraindications for medical therapies, planned pregnancy or lactation, or significant stresses and triggers for headaches. There are various reviews available for pharmacologic headache treatment in pregnancy and lactation.[239–242] The American Academy of Neurology and the American Headache Society have published evidence-based guidelines for the treatment and prevention of episodic migraines.[243,244] Hutchinson et al.[245] published a summary of recommendations for common migraine treatments in breastfeeding women. See Table 11.20 for a compilation of data for comparison of the different medications during lactation. Decision-making for lactating women and medical treatment of headaches should be guided by an up-to-date review (LactMed, Infantrisk.com) of the specific medications being considered.

MEDICATIONS FOR AUTOIMMUNE DISORDERS IN LACTATION

There continue to be newly approved disease-modifying agents for the treatment of autoimmune disorders. Although there are data on some of these agents during lactation, there are limited data on the newer agents.[39,246] There are several reviews of biologic immunosuppressants for different conditions in lactation and guidelines published by the British Society for Rheumatology and British Health Professionals in Rheumatology from 2016.[247,248] See Box 11.3 for a listing of some of the available agents. Considering the ongoing approval of new agents and continued need for information on these agents during lactation, practitioners should consult the up-to-date databases (LactMed, Infantrisk.com) for the latest information on specific medications.

PESTICIDES AND POLLUTANTS

Since 1950, human milk has been used as a biomonitoring tool for assessing mothers' and infants' exposures to environmental chemicals. Since that time, a solid database has been created on dichlorodiphenyltrichloroethane (DDT), dioxins, furans, and polychlorinated biphenyls (PCBs) in various geographic areas. Consistency in analytic methods, sampling techniques, postpartum timing, and reporting of chemical concentrations has been lacking. A technical workshop on Human Milk Surveillance and Research on Environmental Chemicals in the United States was held in 2002, and a published report appeared in the *Journal of Toxicology and Environmental Health*.[249] More and more often, human milk is being used as the biologic marker of environmental exposures. The disturbing backlash is that the public interprets this to mean that breast milk is contaminated, and the problem is getting worse. Improving risk communication is equally as important as risk identification.[250] This field of environmental exposure continues to evolve with advancements in hazard identification (identification of all the sources of exposure within an environment over time), dose–response assessment (assessment of risks of specific health outcomes that may occur with a given level of exposure), developmental windows of susceptibility (identifying specific effects resulting from exposure during specific periods of time [e.g., trimesters of pregnancy, first years of life during brain development]), and childhood "origins" of adult disease (early life exposures or triggers that lead to adult disease).[251] Particularly important in hazard identification is the difference in exposure via breast milk or formula and other food sources or local environmental exposure over time. The US Environmental Protection Agency (EPA) reports that more than 40,000 chemicals are available in the United States.[252] LaKind et al., in their review of infant dietary exposures, found data on less than 200 chemicals in the 85 studies they reviewed.[253] There remain significant gaps in knowledge, as well as in terminology and the significance of different exposure terms. The examples include reference dose (RfD), which assumes a threshold response of toxicity with the probability of risk associated with a given level of exposure. This risk can vary significantly based on variables such as the differential toxicity of similar products, age (window of susceptibility), and gender, among others. Tolerable daily intake (TDI) is a measure of subchronic exposure of adult animals to toxins that leads to a specific health outcome. A daily intake that is tolerable for an adult animal may not be so for exposure as a fetus or during breastfeeding. There are reviews that provide fairly comprehensive lists of environmental chemicals/toxins that have been assessed in the human environment, in breast milk, and in formula.[251,254] See Box 11.4, Abbreviated List of Important Environmental Chemical Classes Identified in Breast Milk. A few of these environmental chemicals identified in breast milk are discussed in the following section.

Pesticides and Insecticides

Human milk has been known to contain insecticides. Chlorinated hydrocarbons, such as DDT and its metabolites dieldrin, aldrin, and related compounds, are the best known. The major reason these compounds appear in breast milk is that they are deposited in body lipid stores and move with lipid. A fetus receives the greatest dose in utero, and adult body fat has approximately 30 times the concentration in milk. N, N-diethyl-meta-toluamide (DEET) has been shown to be absorbed through the skin in adult males within 2 hours of application and excreted from the plasma through the urine within 4 hours. A recent review of three WHO/United Nations

TABLE 11.20 Selected Migraine Preventive Therapies[a]

Name	Drug Classification[b]	LRC (Hale)[c]	Evidence-Based Guideline Efficacy[d]	M/P Ratio	PB	T$_{1/2}$	RID	Unique Rx Notes	Comments[e]
Valproate	AE	L4	A	0.42	94%	14 hours	0.99%–5.6%		Long-term effects on IQ from in utero exposure, verbal abilities better if BF
Topiramate	AE	L3	A	0.86	15–41%	21 hours	24.6%–55.6%		Limited data
Metoprolol	BB	L2	A	3.0–3.72	10%	3–7 hours	1.4%		Low levels in BM, monitor exposed infants
Propranolol	BB	L2	A	0.5	90%	3–5 hours	0.3%–0.5%		Low levels, no long-term effects of exposure studied
Timolol	BB	L2	A	0.8	105	4 hours	1.1%		Very low levels, no adverse effects reported in infants
Atenolol	BB	L3	B	1.5–6.8	6%–16%	6–7 hours	6.6%		Alternatives: Propranolol, metoprolol
Nadolol	BB	? Not listed	B		25%	22 hours	?		Higher BM levels than other BB Alternatives: Metoprolol, propranolol
Amitriptyline	AD	L2	B	1	94%	31–46 hours	1.08%–2.8%		Low levels in BM, 1 case report of severe sedation and poor feeding with exposure via BM
Venlafaxine	AD	L2	B	2.75	27%	5 hours	6.8%–8.1%		In utero exposure—poor neonatal adaptation syndrome (withdrawal)
Frovatriptan	Triptans	L3	A	?	15%	26 hours	?		Some transfer into BM expected, but no adequate studies Alternative: Sumatriptan
Naratriptan	Triptans	L3	B	?	29%	6–7 hours	?		No studies in BM or association of adverse effects resulting from BM exposure
Zolmitriptan	Triptans	L3	B	?	25%	3 hours	?		

(Continued)

TABLE 11.20 Selected Migraine Preventive Therapies[a]—cont'd

Name	Drug Classification[b]	LRC (Hale)[c]	Evidence-Based Guideline Efficacy[d]	M/P Ratio	PB	T$_{1/2}$	RID	Unique Rx Notes	Comments[e]
									No studies in BM or association of adverse effects resulting from BM exposure Alternative: Sumatriptan
Fenoprofen	NSAID	? Not listed	B						Limited data in BM BM fenoprofen levels were reportedly 1.6% of those in maternal plasma Alternatives: Other NSAIDs
Ibuprofen	NSAID	L1	B	?	99%	1.8–2.5 hours	0.1%–0.7%		Safe for use in lactation
Ketoprofen	NSAID	? Not listed	B	Calculated average milk concentration of 57 mcg/L (range = 20–177 mcg/L) from 1 study of 61 exposed infants	?	?	0.31%		Fully BF infant would receive an average dosage of 8.5 mcg/kg daily Renal and GI effects in exposed BF infants Alternatives: Ibuprofen
Naproxen	NSAID	L3	B	0.01	99.7%	12–15 hours	3.3%		Very low levels in BM Long T$_{1/2}$—accumulation? Case reports of adverse effects—bleeding, drowsiness, vomiting
Petasites (purified extract of butterbur plant—removes pyrrolizidine alkaloids, keeps active compounds [petasin, isopetasin])	HVM	?	A	?	?	?	?	Trials occurring in pediatrics, not infants	? Data in BM ? Effects on exposed BF infants Effective at decreasing migraine frequency vs. placebo

(Continued)

TABLE 11.20 **Selected Migraine Preventive Therapies[a]—cont'd**

Name	Drug Classification[b]	LRC (Hale)[c]	Evidence-Based Guideline Efficacy[d]	M/P Ratio	PB	$T_{1/2}$	RID	Unique Rx Notes	Comments[e]
Magnesium (Mg^{++})	HVM	L1	B	1.9	30%	?	0.2%	A higher dose for Rx of preeclampsia delayed lactogenesis if continued 6 hours after delivery	Mg concentrated in BM from plasma, oral absorption is very poor, no reported concerns
MIG-99 (feverfew extract; dried leaves of *Tanacetum parthenium*; active ingredients are parthenolides)	HVM	?	B	?	?	?	?	Not recommended in pregnancy—uterine contractions → miscarriage or preterm labor Not recommended in lactation	No data exist on the excretion of any components of feverfew into BM or on the safety and efficacy of feverfew in nursing mothers or infants
Riboflavin (vitamin B$_2$)	HVM	L1	B	?	?	14 hours	?	Equivalent to dietary intake = 32–848 µg/L of BM	High-dose (400 mg/day) used for migraines—no data on this dosage in BM (RDA for all ages = 0.6 mg/1000 kcal) Side effects— diarrhea, polyuria

AD, Antidepressant medication; *AE*, antiepileptic medication; *BF*, Breastfeeding; *BM*, breast milk; *GI*, gastrointestinal; *HVM*, herbs, vitamins, and minerals; *LRC*, lactation risk classification; *M/P ratio*, milk-to-plasma ratio; *NSAID*, nonsteroidal antiinflammatory drug; *PB*, protein binding; *RDA*, Recommended Dietary Allowance; *RID*, relative infant dose; *Rx*, prescription; $T_{1/2}$, half-life of drug.

[a]All the products listed here were reviewed by the American Academy of Neurology and the American Headache Society and listed as either having established efficacy or being probably effective after evidence-based review and categorization. Infants exposed to psychiatric medications, as a broad group, should be observed for drowsiness, irritability, poor feeding, and weight gain/growth and development. In the question of long-term exposure and the infant's development, it is difficult to distinguish between intrauterine effects and effects from BM exposure.

[b]Drug classification: *AE*, antiepileptic medication; *AD*, antidepressant medication; *BB*, beta-blocker; *HVM*, herbs, vitamins, and minerals; *Trip*, triptans; *NSAID*, nonsteroidal antiinflammatory drug.

[c]The LRC (Hale) is as follows: L2: Probably compatible; studied in a limited number of breastfeeding women without an increase in adverse effects in the infant. L3: Probably compatible; no controlled trials in breastfeeding women; risk of side effects in infants is possible; appropriate to assess the risk–benefit in each situation. L4: Potentially hazardous; there is evidence of risk to a breastfed infant; can be used in mother with appropriate risk–benefit assessment.

[d]Evidence-based guidelines efficacy is as follows: Level A—medications with established efficacy (≥2 Class I trials); Level B—medications are probably effective (1 Class I or 2 Class II studies).

[e]Alternative medications are suggested from Hale TW. *Hale's Medications and Mothers' Milk*. 18th ed. New York: Springer; 2019. Note potential side effects in changing to an alternative medication. The choice of a possible alternative medication is dependent on that medication adequately controlling the seizures specific for that individual.

Data collated from Hale TW. *Hale's Medications and Mothers' Milk*. 18th ed. New York: Springer; 2019; LactMed. Accessed December 2019; Silberstein SD, Holland S, Freitag F, et al. Evidence-based guideline update: Pharmacologic treatment for episodic migraine prevention in adults report of the quality standards subcommittee of the American Academy of Neurology and the American Headache Society. *Neurology*. 2012;78:1337. doi:10.1212/WNL.0b013e3'82535d20.

BOX 11.3 Biologic Immunosuppressive Medications During Lactation

Compatible[a]	Not Considered Compatible	Insufficient Data
Adalimumab[a]	Cyclophosphamide	Abatacept
Azathioprine	Methotrexate	Anakinra
Certolizumab[a]	Mycophenolate mofetil	Belimumab
Corticosteroids		Golimumab
Cyclosporin A		Rituximab
Etanercept[a]		Tocilizumab
Hydrochlorothiazide		Ustekinumab
Infliximab[a]		
IVIG		
Sulfasalazine (OK breastfeeding full-term infants)		
Tacrolimus		

IVIG, intravenous immune globulin.

[a]Compatible but with limited data.

From Flint J, Panchal S, Hurrell A, et al. Guidelines BSR and BHPR guideline on prescribing drugs in pregnancy and breastfeeding. Part I: standard and biologic disease modifying anti-rheumatic drugs and corticosteroids on behalf of the BSR and BHPR Standards, Guidelines and Audit Working Group. *Rheumatol.* 2016;55:1693. doi:10.1093/rheumatology/kev404; Flint J, Panchal S, Hurrell A, et al: Guidelines BSR and BHPR guideline on prescribing drugs in pregnancy and breastfeeding. Part II: analgesics and other drugs used in rheumatology practice on behalf of the BSR and BHPR Standards, Guidelines and Audit Working Group. *Rheumatol.* 2016;55:1698. doi:10.1093/rheumatology/kev405; Witzel SJ. Lactation and the use of biologic immunosuppressive medications. *Breastfeed Med.* 2014;9:543. doi:10.1089/bfm.2014.0107.

BOX 11.4 Abbreviated List of Important Environmental Chemical Classes Identified in Breast Milk

Chemical Class	Individual Chemicals
Dioxin/Furans and dioxin-like PCBs	**OCDD** **OCDF**
PCBs	PCBs numbered from PCB-28 "non-sequentially" up through PCB-206
Organochlorine pesticides	Dacthal, DDD, DDE, DDT, endosulfan, HCB, HCH, dieldrin, aldrin, lindane, oxychlordane
Brominated flame retardants	BDEs, HBCDs
Phthalates	MCPP, MECPP, MEHHP, MEOHP
Per- and polyfluoroalkyl substances	PFHxS, PFOA, PFOS, PFOSA, PFNA
Phenols	Benzophenone, BPA, dichlorophenol, triclosan
Parabens	Benzyl-parabens, Butyl-parabens
Perchlorate	
Thiocyanate	
Metals	Lead, arsenic, organic mercury
Volatile organic compounds	Benzene, chloroform, toluene
Organophosphates	
Pyrethroids	Permethrin
Trichloroethylene	
Polycyclic aromatic hydrocarbons	Anthracene, chrysene, fluorene, pyrene
Synthetic musk compounds	AHTN, HHCB, musk ketone, musk xylene

AHTN, Acetyl-hexamethyl-tetrahydronapthalene; *BDE*, brominated diphenyl ether; *BPA*, bisphenol A; *DDD*, dichlorodiphenyldichloroethane; *DDE*, dichlorodiphenyldichloroethylene; *DDT*, dichlorodiphenyltrichloroethane; *HBCD*, hexabromochclododecane; *HCB*, hexachlorobenzene; *HCH*, hexachlorohexane; *HHCB*, hexahydro-hexamethyl-cyclopenta-benzopyran; *MCPP*, mono (3-carboxypropyl) phthalate; *MECPP*, mono (2-ethyl-5-carboxypentyl) phthalate; *MEHHP*, mono (2-ethyl-5-hydroxyhexyl) phthalate; *MEOHP*, mono (2-ethyl-5-oxyhexyl) phthalate; *OCDD*, octachlorodibenzo-p-dioxin; *OCDF*, octachlorodibenzofuran; *PCB*, polychlorinated biphenyl; *PFHxS*, perfluorohexane sulfonic acid; *PFNA*, perfluoro-n-nonanoic acid; *PFOA*, perfluorooctanoic acid; *PFOS*, perfluorooctanesulfonic acid; *PFOSA*, perfluorooctanesulfonamide.

From Lehmann GM, LaKind JS, Davis MH, et al. Environmental Chemicals in Breast Milk and Formula: Exposure and Risk Assessment Implications. *Environ Health Perspect.* 2018;126(9):096001. doi:10.1289/EHP1953.

Environment Programme (UNEP) global surveys of poly-chlorinated dibenzodioxins (PCDDs), polychlorinated diben-zofurans (PCDFs), PCBs, and DDT in human milk was conducted.[255] The levels of PCDDs and PCDFs were the highest in national pooled samples of breast milk (toxic equivalencies [TEQs]; pg/g lipids) for India, some European countries (the Netherlands, Italy, Germany, Spain, Luxembourg, Belgium), and some African countries (Egypt, the Democratic Republic of the Congo, Cote d'Ivoire, Senegal). Indicator PCB levels were noted to be highest in Eastern Europe (Czech Republic, Slovakia, Romania, Ukraine, Croatia, Russia) and Western Europe (Italy, Spain, Germany, the Netherlands, Luxembourg, Sweden, Belgium). However, a downward trend for PCDDs, PCDFs, and PCBs was noted, although the levels were above levels generally considered safe by a variety of toxicity measures (TDI from the WHO, reference dose [RfD] by the EPA, minimum risk level [MRL] from the Agency for Toxic Substances and Disease Registry [ATSDR]). The sum of DDTs was found at the highest levels in less industrialized countries and in countries where spraying to prevent malaria significantly continues (India, Haiti, Mauritius, Mali, Uganda, Sudan, Philippines, Democratic Republic of the Congo).[255]

PCBs in heavily contaminated pregnant Japanese women produced small-for-gestational-age infants who had transient darkening of the skin ("cola babies"). Polybrominated biphenyls (PBBs) are similar compounds associated with heavy exposure to farm animals and contaminated cattle in the lower Michigan peninsula. The women in the United States who have the greatest risk for high exposure to PCBs or PBBs are those who have extensively worked with or eaten the fish caught by sport fishing in contaminated waters.

Studies have refuted earlier observations of concern. No information is available in the United States on the levels of PCDDs or PCDFs in anglers who consume a lot of fish.[256] Persons at high risk are those who live near a waste-disposal site or have been involved in environmental spills. Unless there is heavy exposure, however, no contraindication exists to breastfeeding.

In most cases, the levels of pesticides in human milk have been less than those in cow's milk. The accumulated amounts have not usually exceeded safe allowable limits. In a review of world reports on occurrence and toxicity, Rogan et al. reaffirmed that breastfeeding should be recommended despite the presence of chemical residues.[257] The authors further state that the benefits of breastfeeding outweigh the risks of pollutants. It has been suggested that the body burden at birth can be added to by exposing an infant to small levels in the milk that may indeed exceed the exposure limits allowable for daily intake set by the WHO.[258] Human milk levels are used epidemiologically as markers of human exposure in community exposure because of a close correlation between milk levels and the levels in fat stores.

Chemicals that are lipophilic, biologically stable, nonionized at a physiologic pH, and of low molecular weight transfer easily into maternal milk. Lehmann et al. refer to these compounds as *lipophilic persistent environmental chemicals* (LPECs).[250] Ten to twenty times more of a mother's body burden of persistent organohalogens is transferred via the milk than via the placenta, according to Jensen and Slorach, who published an extensive review of chemical contaminants in human milk.[6] They further caution that the absolute amount transferred depends on the structure of the chemical. PCBs, for instance, are highly chlorinated and transfer more easily than less chlorinated PCBs.

If extractable fat is measured, the levels of persistent organohalogens are about the same in milk, blood, adipose tissue, and muscle. Mobilization from fat stores is greater than that from dietary intake during lactation.[6]

Agent Orange, one of the best known of the dioxins, was identified in Vietnam as a powerful teratogen. Dioxin has been found in human milk from pooled samples from high-risk women with known exposure. No evidence suggests that the population at large is at risk. Women working in dry-cleaning plants, viscose rayon plants, photographic laboratories, and chemical industries where proper precautions are not taken have been noted to absorb tetrachloroethylene, carbon disulfide, and bromides.[259]

Flame retardants, polybrominated diphenyl ethers (PBDEs), are found in upholstery, electronics, automotive interiors, and plastics. Significant increases in PBDEs have been reported in plasma, breast milk, and the environment in the United States. They have been banned in several states because of rising body burdens.[260] Total PBDE concentrations in breast milk are higher in studies reported from North America than either Asia or Europe. The predominant PBDEs in North America are brominated diphenyl ethers (BDEs): BDE-47, BDE-99, BDE-100, and BDE-153. At high levels, PBDEs cause cognitive and behavioral disorders.[261] There are a variety of sources of PBDE exposure (diet, indoor air, and house dust), including in utero exposure. Breast milk seems to contribute to the exposure in infants less than 1 year old.[262] Nevertheless, the risk—benefit ratio for breastfeeding with some exposure to PBDEs is in favor of continued breastfeeding.

Pollutants in Breast Milk Versus Formula

Mother-to-child transfer of essential and toxic elements through breast milk in a mine-waste-polluted area is reported by Castro and colleagues.[263] They reported that lower amounts of toxic elements were ingested by breastfed infants compared with infants who received formula reconstituted with locally contaminated water. Lehmann et al. reviewed environmental chemicals in breast milk and formula. The data were highly variable from substance to substance and country to country. Additional comparisons should be made between powdered formula, concentrated formula, and ready-to-feed formula and the water used to reconstitute powdered formula.[251] Extensive reviews of industrial chemicals and environmental contaminants in human milk are available in Schaefer, Peters, and Miller and Pajewska-Szmyt et al.[264,265]

Heavy Metals

Heavy metals that have been found in milk include lead, mercury, arsenic, cobalt, magnesium, and cadmium, which

TABLE 11.21   Classes and Management of Lead Levels in Blood

Blood Lead Level (mcg/dL)	Class	Management
<10	I	Not considered lead poisoning
10–14	IIA	Many children (or a large proportion of children) with blood lead levels in this range should trigger community-wide childhood lead poisoning prevention activities. Children in this range may need to be rescreened more frequently.
15–19	IIB	Nutritional and educational interventions and more frequent screening; if level persists in this range, environmental investigation and intervention are recommended.
20–44	III	Environmental evaluation and remediation and a medical evaluation; possible pharmacologic treatment of lead poisoning
45–69	IV	Both medical and environmental intervention, including chelation therapy
>69	V	Medical emergency; immediate medical and environmental management

Modified from Centers for Disease Control and Prevention. Blood levels—United States, 1988–1991. *MMWR.* 1994;43:545.

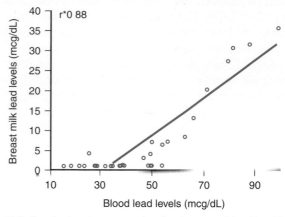

Lead in blood and human milk

Fig. 11.3 Graph showing regression line between blood lead levels and milk lead levels. (From Namihira D, Saldivar L, Pustilnik N, et al. Lead in human blood and milk from nursing women living near a smelter in Mexico City. *J Toxicol Environ Health.* 1993;38:225.)

are also positively correlated with fish consumption.[266] Whenever maternal exposure occurs, a breastfed infant and the milk should be tested. The intake of lead and cadmium by breastfed infants, as reported by the WHO study, is the same as, or somewhat lower than, that of infants fed formula mixed with local water.[267] Levels of these heavy metals in milk, however, are lower than would be predicted from maternal levels.[264] Placental transfer is greater than by breastfeeding.[268] Most common air pollutants are not found in human milk.

Lead

Although the removal of lead from gasoline has been associated with a drop in blood lead levels in children from 15 mg/dL in 1978 to 2 mg/dL in 1999, lead has remained a significant issue because of the number of mothers testing positive for lead on routine screens for lead in the family members of young infants.[269] The release of lead from bone in pregnancy and lactation was studied by Manton et al., who concluded that the entire skeleton undergoes resorption and that blood lead levels of nursing mothers continue to rise, reaching a maximum at 6 to 8 months postpartum.[270] They also noted that lead levels fall from pregnancy to pregnancy, suggesting

that the greatest risk is with the first pregnancy. The Centers for Disease Control and Prevention (CDC) has revised the standards for the treatment of lead intoxication downward (Table 11.21). Meta-analysis reflects a 2.6- to 5.8-point decline in IQ for an increase in lead level from 10 to 20 mg/dL.[269] Blood lead concentrations less than 10 mg/dL are inversely associated with children's IQ scores at 3 to 5 years of age, according to studies by Canfield et al.[271] The first step is always to clean up the environment and identify the source. Lead-abatement resources are available from the US Department of Health. The level of lead in milk depends on its ionization and tight binding to red blood cells. The M/P ratio is 0.2. A blood lead level of 40 mg/dL or less in a nursing mother is considered below the level of transfer through the breast milk (Fig. 11.3). In addition to environmental sources of lead (e.g., old paint, contaminated ground, lead batteries), diet should be reviewed. In some cities, the water supply is a significant source, especially in formula making. Herbs and herbal teas may also be a source. Many traditional and folk remedies contain lead, especially those from China, Mexico, India, and Pakistan. A mother's diet should include extra calcium and iron to reduce the absorption of lead from the diet and mobilization from the bone. Newer lead-removal medications are safer than the traditional British anti-lewisite. Succimer is believed safe during lactation and in infants older than 1 year if milk is pumped and discarded for 5 days.[254]

Arsenic

Arsenic is a heavy metal noted to contaminate some waterways and water supplies. The effects of arsenic exposure on the fetus and in early infancy are still being investigated. It has been suggested that there are critical windows of exposure regarding cognitive development and the potential for early exposure leading to increased mortality in young adults as a result of lung disease.[272,273] Epigenetic effects are a proposed mechanism of action. Arsenic exposure has been evaluated in various parts of the world, including Argentina, Germany, and India. Data are available from these regions on the levels in breast milk and nursing infants. The arsenic level in drinking water in an Argentinean village was 200 mcg/L, the level in maternal blood was 10 mcg/L, and the level in maternal urine was 320 mcg/L. The average amount in the milk was 2.3 mcg/kg. Two infants were tested, and the levels in the urine were 17 and 47 mcg/L, considered very low. In India's West Bengal, an arsenic-affected area, 226 women were tested, some of whom had skin lesions and high levels in their hair.[274] They had arsenic in the breast milk. Most of the arsenic in the milk was inorganic, but the infant levels ranged from 0.3 to 29 mcg/L; those infants who were partially breastfed and formula-fed had levels from 0.4 to 1520 mcg/L. The authors conclude that little arsenic is excreted in breast milk, even when the exposure is high from contaminated water; thus exclusive breastfeeding appears to be protective and safer than formula feeding.[263,275,276]

Mercury

Organic mercury is another heavy metal that is being increasingly identified in food around the world. Fish is a major source, as are herbs and tonics. Levels of mercury in mothers' blood are about three times higher than levels in milk. Two major forms of mercury enter milk. Methylmercury is attached to red blood cells and so has limited access, although it is easily absorbed by infants. Inorganic mercury enters milk easily but is poorly absorbed by infants. When the source of the methylmercury is from breast milk, the developmental scores exceed those of formula-fed infants, suggesting that the advantages of breast-feeding are significant.[266] A similar, more extensive study in the Seychelles Islands of mothers and children followed from birth for 15 years suggests that the value of a fish diet over time and during breastfeeding is significant despite measurable mercury levels.[277] Almost all the infants in the Seychelles were breastfed for at least 6 months and met or exceeded international developmental scores. Acute exposures to methylmercury from industrial or environmental sources should be evaluated on a case-by-case basis, although it appears breastfeeding is safe.

Cadmium

Cadmium is another heavy metal; sources for humans include smoking, lifestyle, diet, and place of residence.[278,279] Around the world, daily intake values range from 10 μg to over 200 μg, and breast-milk levels have been reported as 0.19 to 5.0 μg/L.[265,280] Cadmium enters the body more through the respiratory tract than the GI tract, reaches the blood, and primarily affects the liver and kidneys. Cadmium has been associated with asthma and preterm birth.[265] Ongoing studies are necessary to assess the exposure to cadmium occurring through breast milk versus other environmental sources and other potential health hazards from cadmium exposure.

Well Water

Drinking well water has been a concern because of varying levels of minerals, especially nitrate, contained in drinking water.[281] More than 18% of wells in the state of Iowa are reported to exceed the maximum contaminant level of 45 mg

of nitrate/L or 10 mg NO$_3$/L. Infants younger than 6 months of age are especially susceptible to methemoglobinemia, which can lead to anoxic injury and death. It reportedly occurs at nitrate concentrations greater than 100 mg/L. Although this is a major issue for formula-fed infants, Dusdieker et al. explored the question, "Does increased nitrate ingestion elevate nitrate levels in human milk?"[282] Carefully studying 20 healthy mothers with breastfeeding infants older than 6 months subjected to 47, 168, and 270 mg of nitrate per day, they found that urine spot tests rose from 36 mg on day 1 to 66 mg on day 2 and 84 mg on day 3. Nitrate concentrations in the milk on days 1, 2, and 3 were 4.4, 5.1, and 5.2 mg/L, respectively. The authors concluded that "women who consume water with a nitrate concentration of 100 mg/L or less do not produce milk with elevated nitrate levels."[282] Epidemiologic studies have now demonstrated that nitrates in drinking water leading to higher blood levels are related to other health outcomes, such as adverse reproductive changes, colorectal cancer, bladder and breast cancer, thyroid disease, and neural tube defects.[281] Perfluoroalkyl acids (PFAAs) are synthetic organic chemicals used in industry that are water soluble, persist (not broken down), and accumulate in water and in human tissue. PFAAs can cause toxicity in the liver, endocrine system, and male reproductive system. They also affect the fetus and neonate, which may relate to the accumulated body burden in the pregnant woman.[283,284] Additional ongoing study of drinking water and the various potential contaminants is needed, along with the study of health hazards and the relationship between contaminated drinking water and contaminant levels in human milk.

Chemicals in the Workplace

An increasing number of women return to the workplace after the birth of an infant, and an increasing number are breastfeeding their infants. There is a need for information regarding the transfer of chemicals in the workplace to human milk.

Volatile chemicals in the workplace represent an important but little understood hazard, especially in paint shops, repair shops, garages, and the chemical industry. Fisher et al. developed a physiologically based pharmacokinetic model for lactating women to estimate the amount of chemicals that their nursing infants ingest for a given nursing schedule and maternal occupational exposure.[285] The two major factors are the blood/air partition coefficient, a thermodynamic factor that governs the body burden that may be achieved from inhalation of a chemical, and the pharmacokinetics of the chemical, which determines the length of time a chemical remains in the systemic circulation and is available to transfer into milk. Because milk fat is abundant, preferential uptake of lipophilic chemicals occurs. Of the 19 chemicals simulated in the study, the authors consider bromochloromethane, perchloroethylene, and 1,4-dioxane exposure the highest risk to infants based on EPA guidelines for drinking water (Table 11.22).

Protective gear in the workplace is the most practical way of minimizing exposure to both mothers and infants.

The Occupational Health and Safety Act of the province of Quebec has mandated the establishment and maintenance

TABLE 11.22 Predicted Amount of Chemical Ingested by Nursing Infant (AMILK) During 24-Hour Period and EPA Drinking Water Health Advisory Values

Chemical	Threshold Limit Value (ppm)	AMILK (mg)	EPA Health Advisory Intake (mg/day)[a]
Benzene	10	0.053	0.20[b]
Bromochloromethane	200	2.090	1.00
Carbon tetrachloride	5	0.055	0.07
Chlorobenzene	10	0.229	—
Chloroform	10	0.043	0.1
Methylchloroform	350	3.51	40.0
Diethylether	400	1.49	—
1,4-Dioxane	25	0.559	0.4[b]
Halothane	50	0.232	—
n-Hexane	50	0.052	4.0
Isoflurane	50‡	0.336	—
Methylene chloride	50	0.213	2.0[b]
Methyl ethyl ketone	200	12.08	—
Perchloroethylene	25	1.36	1.0
Styrene	50	0.650	2.0
Trichloroethylene	50	0.496	0.6[c]
1,1,1,2-Tetrachloroethane	100[d]	4.31	0.9
Toluene	50	0.460	2.0
o,p,m-Xylenes	100	6.590	40.0

EPA, US Environmental Protection Agency.

[a]Modified from EPA health advisory values for chronic ingestion of contaminated water by 10-kg (22-lb) children, assuming ingestion of 1 L of water per day. These health advisory concentrations for chemicals in water are thought to be protective of adverse health effects for chronic exposure.

[b]Modified from 10-day health advisory values for ingestion of contaminated water by 10-kg children, assuming ingestion of 1 L of water per day. These health advisory values for contaminated water are thought to be protective of adverse health effects for a 10-day period.

[c]No threshold limit value; concentration value was assigned.

[d]Lifetime health advisory value for ingestion of 2 L water per day in adults.

From Fisher J, Mahle D, Bankston L, et al. Lactation transfer of volatile chemicals in breast milk. *Am Ind Hyg Assoc J.* 1997;58:429.

of a Toxicological Index that provides information on chemical and biologic contaminants potentially present in the workplace.[286] This information can also serve as a basis for the protective reassignment of pregnant or breastfeeding employees. The Infotox database has information about 5500 chemicals. Of the substances in the database, 2.7% (153 of 5736) show evidence of milk transfer and pose relative risks to breastfed infants.[286]

Summary of Toxic Exposures Via Breast Milk

The benefits of breastfeeding for mother and infant outweigh the potential risks of the vast majority of possible toxic exposures that can occur for the infant through breast milk. This is true except in the extreme conditions of documented and measurable toxic exposure of the mother before or during lactation. For each toxic substance, the potential for accumulation of the toxin in the mother and the potential for passing through breast milk to the infant must be assessed on a case-by-case basis. In the interest of informed, shared decision-making, what is known (and unknown) about the exposure, the potential toxicities of the substance, and the degree to which the substance can be transferred from mother to infant through breast milk should be openly discussed with the mother and family. Consulting with a toxicologist and a lactation specialist may be indicated in certain situations.

RADIOACTIVE MATERIALS

Diagnostic Imaging During Lactation

Over the course of lactation, it may be necessary for a lactating woman to undergo diagnostic evaluation for specific health concerns by radiologic imaging or nuclear medicine procedure. With this testing, several questions are raised about the exposure of the mother and the infant (via breast milk) to radiation, either from the radiologic imaging itself or the exposure to a radioactive material or radiopharmaceutical. Questions raised include the following: Should the mother not breastfeed or delay breastfeeding or suspend breastfeeding? Should the breast milk be discarded for a period of time? These questions often cause much angst and disruption of breastfeeding. Various groups (ABM, American College of Obstetrics and Gynecology, American College of Radiology [ACR]) have published guidelines to assist with the answering of these questions.[287-289] Two routes of potential exposure for the breastfeeding infant are considered: radioactive material in the breast milk and radioactive material "concentrated" in the breast tissue. The only agent concentrated in the breast is fludeoxyglucose-F18 (FDG), which is used in performing positron emission tomography (PET) scans.[290] Agencies concerned with radiation exposure include the Nuclear Regulatory Commission (NRC), the International Commission on Radiological Protection (ICRP), and the International Atomic Energy Agency (IAEA). They relatively agree that no interruption of breastfeeding is necessary with radiation doses of less than 100 mrem or 1 mSV. Nevertheless, these agencies have published guidelines that recommend different periods of interruption of breastfeeding based on external radiation or related to free technetium 99m (Tc99m) pertechnetate contained in the contrast media.[289] In particular, the ACR has recognized the need for good information about the administration of contrast medium to nursing mothers. When a conflict of opinion exists, one can refer to the 2018 edition of the ACR *Manual on Contrast Media* (Version 10.3) or the ABM's Protocol on Radiology and Nuclear Medicine Studies in Lactating Women and discuss the particular situation and the mother's breastfeeding goals and preferences with the radiologist.[288,289]

The ACR summarizes a review of the literature, specifically noting that less than 1% of an administered maternal dose of contrast agent is excreted into breast milk and that less than 1% of contrast medium in breast milk ingested by an infant is absorbed from the GI tract.[288]

Breast Imaging

There are no contraindications to performing a mammogram for screening or ongoing evaluation for breast cancer during lactation. To enhance the sensitivity of mammography, nursing or expressing breast milk is encouraged before the procedure to decrease the parenchymal density on imaging. Ultrasound of the breast is another safe adjunctive procedure during lactation. A woman's individual risk of breast cancer should influence ongoing imaging, including magnetic resonance imaging (MRI) for high-risk women in certain situations.[289]

Routine Radiographic Imaging

Radiographic imaging without contrast, often the first step in imaging, includes plain-film radiographs, fluoroscopy, mammography, and computed tomography (CT). The radiation associated with the radiographic procedure does not adversely affect breast milk, nor does any residual radiation enter the breast milk. Breastfeeding can continue on schedule without delay or interruption for such procedures.

CT With Iodinated IV Contrast

The IV contrast currently used for CT is made up of a highly bound iodine substrate. Estimates of the amount of iodinated IV contrast media reaching the breastfed infant via breast milk are less than 0.01% of the dose administered to the mother based on calculations of <0.1% contrast entering the breast milk and <0.1% being absorbed from the infant's gut.[289,291,292] The mother may continue breastfeeding before and after IV iodinated contrast.[288]

Gadolinium-Based IV Contrast

Gadolinium-based IV contrast used for MRI administered to a lactating mother only minimally reaches the breast milk (0.04%), and less than 1% of that amount is absorbed from the infant's gut. The calculated systemic dose reaching the infant is less than 0.0004%.[289] There is good evidence for the safe use of gadolinium-based contrast in the breastfeeding mother–infant dyad.

Nuclear Medicine Imaging

Radioactive agents (radiopharmaceuticals) in various forms are used for imaging of different organs and in different diagnostic situations. The use of Tc99m products for bone scans, renal imaging, and cardiac imaging does not necessitate interruption of breastfeeding because so little of the specific free technetium product enters the breast milk. The exception in

cardiac imaging is a multigated acquisition scan (MUGA) to assess left ventricular ejection fraction. No breastfeeding interruption is needed for in vitro labeling of red blood cells. For in vivo labeling of red blood cells (injection of the Tc-99m pertechnetate into the patient) for the MUGA scan, a 6- to 12-hour interruption of breastfeeding is recommended. If the breast milk is expressed and appropriately stored during a period of 10 physical half-lives (∼60 hours), it can be given to the infant after that.[293] In some situations, an echocardiogram is acceptable, rather than a MUGA scan, for evaluating cardiac function. The same precautions are appropriate for ventilation–perfusion (VP) scans using Tc99m macroaggregated albumin (Tc-99m MAA) as the IV agent. No adjustments are needed for the ventilation agents Tc-99m diethylenetriamine pentaacetate (DTPA) or xenon gas in a VP scan.[293] CT angiography may be the preferred diagnostic testing for pulmonary embolus in the absence of contraindications to iodinated contrast (allergy or renal insufficiency). For PET scans with fludeoxyglucose-F18 (FDG), the FDG does not enter the breast milk, so breast milk can continue to be fed to the infant, but limited contact between the mother and infant is recommended for the 12 hours after FDG administration because it remains in the breast tissue.[289] In general, three different radionuclides might be used for nuclear thyroid imaging: I-131, I-123, and pertechnetate TC-99m. I-123 is preferred over I-131 because less of the radionuclide reaches the thyroid, and its half-life is significantly less (13 hours compared with 8 days). Different resources recommend different periods of breastfeeding interruption for I-123—none up to 3 weeks. One can also express and store the breast milk, testing it for radioactivity until it is gone before using the breast milk for the infant.[289] Tc-99m pertechnetate is the preferred radionuclide in situations when the patient has received thyroid-blocking agents. Different doses of Tc-99m pertechnetate are used in different situations; therefore one could consider expressing the breast milk and appropriately storing it during a period of 10 physical half-lives (∼60 hours) before giving it to the infant.[293]

DERMATOLOGIC MEDICATION

The key issue involved with the dermatologic application of medications is whether they are absorbed through the skin in sufficient quantity to reach the breast milk and affect the infant. A small amount on the skin covering a few square inches may not be a problem from a dose standpoint. Another important issue is the direct application of medication to the nipple and areolar tissue because this area is in the baby's mouth during a feeding. Application to the breast should not be done until after the feeding in any case. It is also possible that the infant could lick the medication from the skin, leading to greater intake than through breast milk. Most prescription dermal medications indicate the percentage of active ingredient absorbed so that the health care provider can determine the risk during lactation. There are various reference sources that can be consulted regarding the safety of dermatologic preparations during lactation.[12,294–296] See Table 11.23 for information about various topical products.

TABLE 11.23 Selected Dermatologic Medications in Lactation

Medication/Product	Medication Class	Concern	Toxicity	Alternatives	Comments
Dosage base/medium for active ingredients					
Ointment (petrolatum)	Dosage form	Paraffins—hydrocarbons accumulate in body fat	?	Do not use on nipples Use a solution > gel > cream	
Solution > gel > cream (degree of "water miscibility" greater to less)	Dosage form	Fewer "inert" ingredients in solutions and slightly more in gels and creams	?	Limit use on nipple or areola if possible Solution > gel > cream	Apply to nipple, areola, or breast after breastfeeding or pumping
Lanolin	Yellow fat from sheep's wool—mixture of fatty acid esters	Pesticide, detergent residues, free alcohols in unpurified form	Wool allergy—avoid in patients with a known allergy to wool	Use highly purified form on the breast	Highly purified modified lanolin—pesticide and detergent residues removed and the natural free alcohols reduced to below 1.5%
Antimicrobial					
Topical iodine, povidone-iodine	Antimicrobial	Increased BM concentration of iodine	Iodine—hypothyroidism	Limit area and time of exposure, do not use on nipple/areola Alternative: chlorhexidine	Avoid vaginal use
Topical antibacterial agents—bacitracin, mupirocin, neomycin, polymyxin	Antibacterial	? Disrupt the infant's GI microbiome	? None	These are poorly absorbable orally	OK on nipples, areola, breast
Clindamycin, erythromycin	Antibacterial	Disrupt microbiome	Potential allergy	Orally absorbable	Used for acne Do not use on breasts, nipples
Metronidazole (topical or vaginal)	Antimicrobial	Absorption through the skin/mucosa Minimal data on use in lactation	? None	Orally absorbable ? Alternatives	<2% reaches maternal plasma levels after topical or vaginal use, so likely low BM levels
Topical antifungal agents—nystatin, amphotericin	Antifungal	No hazard if infants ingest small amounts	? None	Use topically on breast in small amounts Alternatives: another antifungal, or mother takes an oral antifungal — fluconazole (L2), voriconazole (L3)	Nystatin and amphotericin poorly absorbed orally

(Continued)

TABLE 1 | Selected Dermatologic Medications in Lactation—cont'd

Medication/Product	Medication Class	Concern	Toxicity	Alternatives	Comments
Clotrimazole	Antifungal	Clotrimazole, 3%–10% absorption vaginally Miconazole vaginally, <1% absorption Topical, <0.1% absorption	? None	Vaginal and careful topical use is OK	Clotrimazole and miconazole are orally absorbed but metabolized in first pass through liver
Miconazole					
Ketoconazole	Antifungal		Liver toxicity	Do not use on breast OK at other sites or scalp	
Gentian violet (GV)	Antimicrobial	Ulceration of mucous membranes or "tattooing" of skin Allergy Carcinogenic in animals		Topical solution (<0.5%) of GV—OK if used for <7 days Alternatives: Other antifungals for *Candida*	
Insecticides					
Lindane (gamma benzene hexachloride)	Insecticide	Absorbed through skin, reaches plasma and BM	CNS toxicity—lethargy, restlessness, seizures	Do not use during breastfeeding Alternatives: Permethrin products	
Permethrins Pyrethrins	Insecticide	<2% absorption through skin Metabolized rapidly in tissues and serum	None via BM	OK—limited dose and repetition of use during lactation	No observed toxicity in infants of mothers exposed to permethrins
Sulfur 5%–10% in petrolatum base	Insecticide	Absorption	Safe for topical use in infants <2 months old	Do not use on mother's breast (petrolatum base), OK at other sites	
Insect Repellants					
Diethyltoluamide (DEET)	Insect repellant	Little info during BF	?	OK during BF in limited amounts	
Oil of lemon eucalyptus	Insect repellant	Little info during BF	?	OK during BF in limited amounts	
Icaridin	Insect repellant	Little info during BF	?	OK during BF in limited amounts	
Topical corticosteroids					
Low potency	Antiinflammatory	None—low effect and low amounts absorbed	?	Short-term application not likely to lead to high amounts in BM Avoid application to breast and nipples, but low potency and very short exposure is OK	

(Continued)

TABLE 11.23 Selected Dermatologic Medications in Lactation—cont'd

Medication/Product	Medication Class	Concern	Toxicity	Alternatives	Comments
High potency	Antiinflammatory	High effect Absorbed drug can cause systemic effects in mother	Cushingoid changes, electrolyte abnormalities, hypertension, growth affected	Short-term application not likely to lead to high amounts in BM Avoid application to breast and nipples, even with very short exposure	Case reports of toxicity related to prolonged maternal use (6–8 weeks topical exposure of nipples)
Topical Antiinflammatory Drugs					
Tacrolimus, pimecrolimus	Antiinflammatory	Little info during BF	None noted	Poorly absorbed through skin or orally	Poor oral bioavailability
Calcipotriene (synthetic vitamin D₃)	Antipsoriatic, antiinflammatory	Little info during BF	None noted	Solution on scalp even less absorption vs. ointment Avoid nipples/areola	OK on scalp and limited areas of skin
Tazarotene (retinoid for topical use)	Antipsoriatic, antiacne, antiinflammatory	Little info during BF Only 2%–3% of topically applied medication is absorbed	No reports of toxicity	Caution if used on large surface areas of skin Avoid use on breast/nipple	Application to large surface area (>20%) can lead to higher absorption
Miscellaneous					
Coal tar (pyrene metabolites)	Eczema Psoriasis Atopic dermatitis	Absorption by Infant from skin-to-skin or skin-to-mouth contact	?	Avoid application to large areas, and avoid direct contact of infant's skin or mouth with the tar	Caution with vitamins or salicylic acid added
Nitroglycerin (NG)	Anal fissures Raynaud phenomenon of nipples	Concern of nitrates reaching BM vs. infant oral contact with coated nipples	None reported (separately, nitrates cause methemoglobinemia in infants <6 months old)	Use on nipples only in small amounts and after BF	Limited information on NG topical use on nipples with breastfeeding
Hair Products					
Bleaches, dyes, straighteners	Hair treatment/care	Mothers ask about infant exposure with maternal use	None documented in infants related to BM—unlikely to reach BM if maternal plasma levels are low	Avoid direct infant contact with hair products	Limited surface area, relatively low concentrations of various chemicals in hair products, short exposure make systemic levels in mothers unlikely

BF, Breastfeeding; *BM*, breast milk; *CNS*, central nervous system; *GI*, gastrointestinal.
Information collated from Anderson PO. Topical drugs in nursing mothers. *Breastfeed Med.* 2018;13:5. doi:10.1089/bfm.2017.0224; Butler DC, Heller MM, Murase JE. Safety of dermatologic medications in pregnancy and lactation. Part II. Lactation. *J Am Acad Dermatol.* 2014;70:417.e1. doi:10.1016/j.jaad.2013.09.009; Hale TW. *Hale's Medications and Mother's Milk.* 18th ed. New York: Springer; 2019; National Library of Medicine, LactMed (Internet). Drug Levels and Effects Summary of Use During Lactation, 2019. doi:10.10 6/j.foodchem.2007.06.060.

IMMUNIZATIONS

Immunizing Breastfed Infants

Questions often arise about whether breastfed infants should be immunized on a different schedule because of the protective maternal antibodies that might interfere with an infant's response to antigen stimulation.[297] The AAP recommends that all infants should be vaccinated on the regular schedule regardless of the mode of feeding.[298] Vaccinations for diphtheria-pertussis-tetanus are not altered by breastfeeding, and the regular schedule should be followed. Inactivated poliovirus vaccine is the only poliovirus vaccine now used in the United States. There is no evidence for practical interference of breastfeeding with the poliovirus vaccine immunogenicity, and the regular vaccine schedule should be maintained. In areas where rotavirus is endemic, human milk can contain antibodies that could neutralize the live rotavirus vaccine virus. In clinical trials, breastfed and nonbreastfed infants produce comparable antibodies to the rotavirus vaccine. Separately, breastfeeding does decrease the occurrence of rotavirus disease in infants. Measles, mumps, and rubella (MMR) vaccines should be given at the regularly scheduled times because breastfeeding does not interfere with an adequate immune response to the vaccine. There are no data on the combination vaccine MMR and varicella during breastfeeding. A *Haemophilus influenzae* type B (Hib) vaccine is available for infants. The Hib conjugate vaccines should be given at 2 months of age or as soon as possible thereafter, with no modification of the schedule. There have been some variable data on a breastfeeding infant's antibody response to this vaccine, although there is no evidence that breastfeeding reduces the infant's protection from Hib disease. There appears to be an enhanced antibody response to the pneumococcal vaccine in infants who are breastfed for longer than 90 days compared with infants breastfed for less than 90 days.

Immunizing the Nursing Mother

There is no reason for concern about the potential presence of live viruses from vaccines in a mother's milk if she is vaccinated during the postpartum period. Breastfeeding women may follow the same schedule for adults that is followed for other adults for measles, mumps, rubella, tetanus, diphtheria, influenza, *Streptococcus pneumoniae* infection, hepatitis A, hepatitis B, and varicella. When traveling to an endemic area, inactivated poliovirus vaccine can be given to a breastfeeding mother.[297]

Smallpox

Smallpox vaccination is inadvisable for the mother of any infant younger than 1 year of age, nursing or not. The personal contact with the mother's inoculated vaccination site, not the breastfeeding, causes the risk; therefore no advantage exists to weaning if vaccination is necessary. This is consistent with a case of vaccinia virus transmission from a father's smallpox vaccination site to the mother's breast and then from the breast to the infant's mouth, tongue, and cheek. The infant otherwise remained well.[299] This vaccination is not given routinely and is rarely indicated. The CDC advises against vaccination during lactation, and if a mother is vaccinated with an infant younger than 1 year of age, physical contact between the mother and infant (breastfed or nonbreastfed) should be avoided until the vaccination site is fully scabbed over. The CDC also advises against using expressed breast milk in this same time period, although there is insufficient information to support the transmission of vaccinia virus through breast milk itself without evidence of a vaccinia breast lesion.

Yellow Fever Vaccine

Yellow fever vaccine is a live attenuated virus vaccine. There are case reports of encephalitis in breastfed infants whose mother received the vaccine, with confirmation of the vaccine strain of the virus in the infant. Infants ≥ 9 months of age can be vaccinated themselves for travel to endemic areas, but there is an increased risk of encephalitis from the vaccine virus in infants 6 months of age or younger. Avoid vaccinating breastfeeding mothers with infants <9 months old.

Rubella

Following are the considerations with respect to rubella: approximately 85% to 90% of the adult female population is thought to have a high level of naturally acquired immunity, and only 10% to 15% is considered to be susceptible to rubella infection; vaccination of pregnant women is contraindicated under all circumstances because there have been case reports of congenital rubella after rubella vaccination during pregnancy; no woman of childbearing age should be vaccinated without having been first tested for immunity, and if the test is negative, the woman may be vaccinated if there is reasonable assurance that she will not become pregnant for at least 2 months. The rubella virus was found in the milk of 69% of the women immunized with live attenuated rubella (HPV-77 DE5 or RA 27/3 strains).[300] A virus-specific immunoglobulin A antibody response was seen in the milk of all the women. Infectious rubella virus or virus antigen was recovered from the nasopharynx and throat of 56% of the breastfed infants and none of the nonbreastfed infants. No infant had the disease in this study, but 25% of the breastfed group had seroconversion transiently. Although the attenuated virus may appear in the milk, this should not dissuade one from vaccinating a breastfeeding mother at the safest time, which is often immediately postpartum.

Miscellaneous Vaccines[297]

The anthrax vaccine is an inactivated vaccine. There is little or no information on vaccination and breastfeeding. Breastfeeding is not a contraindication to the anthrax vaccine if it is essential to the mother. Cholera is a live attenuated oral vaccine intended for travel to areas with a high risk of cholera. There is no evidence that the cholera vaccine reaches the mother's blood or breast milk; thus it is not considered a risk for the breastfeeding infant. The Japanese encephalitis vaccine is inactivated, so the potential for risk to a breastfeeding infant is very low. The rabies vaccine is an inactivated vaccine, and rabies immune globulins are used after exposure to rabies. There is no evidence that breastfeeding should be discontinued after rabies immune globulin or rabies vaccine is given in a breastfeeding mother. Typhoid exists as both a live attenuated oral vaccine and an injectable inactivated typhoid vaccine. Breastfeeding is not proscribed relative to a mother's immunization with either vaccine.

Rh Immune Globulin

Only rare trace amounts of anti-Rh were present in the colostrum of women given large doses of Rh immune globulin immediately postpartum, and none was found in the mature milk. No adverse response was noted, even with these high dosages. Any Rh antibodies in the mother's milk are thought to be inactivated by the gastric juices. Rh immune globulin or Rh sensitization is not a contraindication to breastfeeding.

SUMMARY OF MEDICATIONS IN BREAST MILK

Many women are exposed to medications over the period of lactation. Although there are questions and concerns raised by these exposures, there is adequate safety information for both the mother and the infant about the use of many medications while breastfeeding. There are excellent resources for medications and lactation in print and online. Careful review of the most current information from one or more of these sources should inform a risk—benefit assessment for the use of a medication during lactation. There are also safer alternative medications and treatments available in many situations, such that in most situations, an appropriate medical regimen can be devised, and breastfeeding can safely continue. Mothers need to receive clear information from the health professional and be supported to make an informed choice for their own medical treatment and continuing breastfeeding to glean the ample benefits of breastfeeding for both the mother and infant. Herbal products should be used with caution during lactation because the purity of the preparations is not routinely regulated, nor are all chemicals within an herbal product named on the labels. The possibility of environmental chemicals or toxins contaminating human milk exists. The levels of such chemicals in human milk are low compared with other sources within the environment. If there is an identified exposure or toxicity in the mother, then her breast milk should be assessed, caution is advised, and clinical observation of the infant should be initiated.

The Reference list is available at www.expertconsult.com.

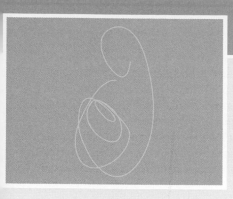

12

Transmission of Infectious Diseases Through Breast Milk and Breastfeeding

Robert M. Lawrence

KEY POINTS

- The basic tenet concerning breastfeeding and infection is that breastfeeding is rarely contraindicated in maternal infection. The few exceptions relate to specific infectious agents with strong evidence of transmission via breast milk and for the development of illness with infection in the infant leading to significant morbidity and mortality.
- The frequency and duration of breastfeeding, along with the "amount" of infectious agent in breast milk, are equivalent to an estimated "dose" of the potential infectious agent and are useful in the estimation of risk of infection.

- Direct contact, contact with body fluids, spread by droplets, and airborne spread are the primary mechanisms of transmission of infectious agents and should be the focus of concern for infectious transmission. Breast milk or breastfeeding is rarely the dominant or a primary mechanism of transmission, the exceptions being cytomegalovirus, human immunodeficiency virus, and human T-cell leukemia virus types I and II.

EVIDENCE FOR TRANSMISSION

A large body of evidence clearly demonstrates the protective effects of breastfeeding and documents the transmission of specific infections to infants through breast milk. The fear and anxiety that arise with the occurrence of any infectious disease are even greater for the breastfeeding mother–infant dyad. Uncertainty and lack of knowledge often lead to proscribing breastfeeding out of fear, which then deprives the infant of the potential protective, nutritional, and emotional benefits of breastfeeding exactly at the time when they are most needed (see the discussion of immunologic benefits of human milk in Chapter 5). Decisions concerning breastfeeding in a mother with an infectious illness should balance the potential benefits of breastfeeding against the known or estimated risk of the infant acquiring a clinically significant infection via breastfeeding and the potential severity of the infection.

Documenting Transmission

Documenting the transmission of infection from mother to infant by breastfeeding requires the demonstration of the infectious agent in the breast milk and a subsequent clinically significant infection in an infant that was caused by a plausible infectious process. The first step is to establish the occurrence of a specific infection (clinically or immunologically evident) in a mother and demonstrate the persistence of the infectious agent, such that it could be transmitted to the infant. Isolation or identification of the infectious agent from the colostrum, the breast milk, or an infectious lesion of the breast is important, but it is not necessarily proof of transmission to an infant. The

identification of the infectious agent simply demonstrates that transmission via breast milk is possible but says nothing about the likelihood or probability of an infection occurring via human breast milk. Other mechanisms of transmission may dominate the natural history of infection by the specific agent (e.g., measles is transmitted predominately via airborne transmission). Demonstration of a clinical or subclinical infection in the infant after exposure to human breast milk is also necessary.

Exclusion of Other Mechanisms of Transmission

Exclusion of other possible mechanisms of transmission (exposure to mother or other persons/animals/environmental sources via airborne, droplet, arthropod, or vector modes of transmission or through direct contact with other infectious fluids) would complete the confirmation of transmission of infection via breastfeeding. It is also essential to exclude prenatal or perinatal transmission of infection to a fetus or infant. Exclusion of all the other possible mechanisms of transmission is very difficult to do.

Epidemiologic Evidence of Transmission

Epidemiologic evidence of transmission can include information from public health surveillance, field investigations, and analytic studies.[1] Descriptive epidemiology may provide information on the chain of infection (agent, reservoir, portal of exit, mode[s] of transmission, portal of entry and susceptible host); disease incidence; and distribution of illness by person, place, and time. Infection via breast milk or breastfeeding can occur by direct contact with an infectious lesion on the mother's breast, the infectious agent persisting in the fluid component of or cells in human milk, or contamination of the milk at the time of expression or during storage and later administration. Analytic epidemiology commonly utilizes an appropriate group for comparison to provide information on rates of infection and calculations of association (e.g., odds ratios or risk ratios). To determine a reasonable estimate of the risk for infection via breast milk, larger analytical epidemiologic studies are needed to compare infection rates in breastfed infants versus formula-fed infants. Other appropriate comparison groups could be breastfeeding mothers with and without the specific infection, or the different timing of maternal infection and the exposure of the infant to a potential pathogen in the colostrum or breast milk. The amount, frequency, and duration of breastfeeding, equivalent to an estimated "dose" of the potential infectious agent, are other important variables to consider in the estimate of risk. (See Chapter 5 regarding additional discussion of "dose" related to breastfeeding.)

These considerations are only some of the variables to consider, in general, to assess the risk for transmission of an infectious agent from mother to infant via breast milk or breastfeeding. Efforts to prove transmission of infection in a specific maternal–infant dyad can be just as difficult and must consider many of the same factors.

This chapter focuses on a discussion of specific, clinically relevant infectious agents and diseases, with reasonable estimates of the risk for infection to infants from breastfeeding. The basic tenet concerning breastfeeding and infection is that breastfeeding is rarely contraindicated in maternal infection. The few exceptions relate to specific infectious agents with strong evidence of transmission and to the association of an infant's illness with significant morbidity and mortality.[2,3]

The risk or benefit of breastfeeding relative to the immunization of a mother or infant is discussed for certain microorganisms. Appendix D addresses precautions and breastfeeding recommendations for maternal infections. Chapter 5 reviews how breastfeeding may protect against infection. Chapter 22 addresses specific concerns relating to banked breast milk and includes standards developed by the Human Milk Banking Association of North America (HMBANA) to guide the appropriate handling of banked human milk relative to possible infectious agents.

INFECTION-CONTROL CONSIDERATIONS

Isolation precautions have undergone some revisions in terminology and conceptualization.[4,5] Understanding that the transmission of microorganisms can occur with a known infection from unrecognized reservoirs or sources of infection, recommendations have been made for standard precautions to be applied to all patients to protect health care workers from potentially infectious body fluids. Additionally, precautions based on the predominant modes of transmission have been recommended to protect against infection through the airborne route, direct contact, or contact with droplets. Although these precautions are intended to be used in clinical situations to protect health care workers, they may be applied in certain situations to the mother–infant dyad to prevent

the transmission of infectious agents from one to the other or to other hospitalized mothers and infants. These precautions are most often useful when a mother and infant are still hospitalized. The use of such precautions within the home is not meant to limit breastfeeding. These precautions are intended to allow breastfeeding in the majority of cases and to facilitate the continuation of breastfeeding with some additional safeguards in certain situations. The guidelines also indicate when to safely use expressed breast milk (see Appendix D).[2]

Standard Precautions

Standard precautions include preventing contact with blood, all body fluids, secretions and excretions, nonintact skin, and mucous membranes by (1) careful handwashing before and after every patient contact; (2) use of gloves when touching body fluids, nonintact skin, mucous membranes, or any items contaminated with body fluids (linens, equipment, devices, etc.); (3) use of nonsterile gowns to prevent contact of clothing with body fluids; (4) use of masks, eye protection, or face shields when splashing with body fluids is possible; and (5) appropriate disposal of these materials. Standard precautions should be applied to all patients regardless of actual or perceived risks. The Centers for Disease Control and Prevention (CDC) does not consider breast milk to be a body fluid with infectious risks, and thus these policies do not apply to breast milk. (See section on misadministration of breast milk later in this chapter as a possible exception to this concept.)

In considering breastfeeding infant–mother dyads and standard precautions, body fluids other than breast milk should be avoided, and only in specified situations should breast milk also be avoided. In general, clothing or a gown for the mother, and bandages if necessary, should prevent direct contact with nonintact skin, potential infectious lesions, or secretions. Avoiding infant contact with maternal mucous membranes requires mothers to be aware of and understand the risks and to make a conscious effort to avoid this type of contact. The use of gloves, gowns, and masks on infants for protection is neither practical nor appropriate. The recommendations concerning the appropriateness of breastfeeding and breast milk are addressed for specific infectious agents throughout this chapter. Human immunodeficiency virus (HIV) infection is an example of one infection that can be prevented using standard precautions, including avoiding breast milk and breastfeeding. The recommendations concerning breastfeeding and HIV and the various variables and considerations involved are discussed later in the chapter.

Airborne Precautions

Airborne precautions are intended to prevent transmission via droplet nuclei (dried respiratory particles smaller than 5 μm that contain microorganisms and can remain suspended in the air for long periods) or dust particles containing microorganisms. Airborne precautions include the use of a private room with negative-air-pressure ventilation and designated respiratory protective devices at all times. In the case of pulmonary tuberculosis (TB), respiratory protective devices (requiring personal fitting and seal testing before use) should be worn.

Airborne precautions are recommended with measles, varicella or disseminated zoster, and TB. Breastfeeding in the presence of these maternal infections is prohibited during the infectious period. This is to protect against airborne transmission of the infection from the mother and to allow the infant to be fed the mother's expressed breast milk by another individual. The exception to allowing breast milk would be local involvement of the breast by varicella-zoster lesions or *Mycobacterium tuberculosis*, such that the milk becomes contaminated by the infectious agent.

Droplet Precautions

Transmission via droplets occurs when an individual produces droplets that travel only a short distance in the air and then contact a new host's eyes, nose, mouth, or skin. The common mechanisms for producing droplets include coughing, sneezing, talking (singing or yelling), suctioning, intubation, nasogastric tube placement, and bronchoscopy. In addition to standard precautions applied to all patients, droplet precautions include the use of a private room (preferred) and a mask if within 3 feet (0.9 m) of the patient. Droplet precautions are recommended for adenovirus, diphtheria, respiratory infections, *Hemophilus influenzae*, *Neisseria meningitidis* or invasive infection, influenza, mumps, mycoplasma, parvovirus, pertussis, plague (pneumonic), and rubella, as well as streptococcal pharyngitis, pneumonia, or scarlet fever. The institution of droplet precautions with a breastfeeding mother who has these infections should be specified for each infection. This may require some period of separation for the infant and mother (for the duration of the illness, for the short term, during treatment of the mother, or for the standard infectious period for that organism) with the use of the mother's fresh expressed breast milk for nutrition in the interim. Prophylactic treatment of the infant and maternal use of a mask during breastfeeding or close contact, combined with meticulous handwashing and the mother's avoidance of touching her mucous membranes, may be adequate and reasonable for certain infections.

Contact Precautions

Contact precautions are meant to prevent the transmission of an infectious agent via direct contact (contact between the body surfaces of one individual and another) and indirect contact (contact of a susceptible host with an object contaminated with microorganisms from another individual). Contact precautions include cohorting or use of a private room, gloves and gowns at all times, and handwashing after removal of gown and gloves. Contact precautions are recommended for a long list of infections, such as diarrhea in diapered or incontinent patients with *Clostridium difficile* infection, *Escherichia coli* O157:H7, *Shigella*, rotavirus, hepatitis A, respiratory illness with parainfluenza virus or respiratory syncytial virus (RSV), multidrug-resistant (MDR) bacteria (e.g., enterococci, staphylococci, gram-negative organisms), enteroviral infections, cutaneous diphtheria, impetigo, herpes simplex virus (HSV) infection, herpes zoster (disseminated or in immunocompromised individuals), pediculosis, scabies, *Staphylococcus aureus* skin

> ### BOX 12.1 Important Points for Infection Control
>
> The Centers for Disease Control and Prevention does not consider breast milk a body fluid with infectious risks.
>
> Infection-control precautions are most useful and applicable within hospitals or health care settings.
>
> These precautions should be utilized to facilitate the continuation of breastfeeding for the individual mother–infant dyad while offering some safeguards to protect against infection transmission via other body fluids, droplets, airborne droplet nuclei, or contact with another infectious source.

infection, viral hemorrhagic fevers (e.g., Ebola, Lassa), conjunctivitis and abscesses, cellulitis, and decubitus that cannot be contained by dressings.[6] For a breastfeeding mother–infant dyad, the implementation of precautions for each of these infections in a mother requires meticulous attention to gowning and handwashing by the mother and a specialized plan for each situation. This is particularly true for uncommon but potentially serious or fatal infections, such as viral hemorrhagic fevers, including Ebola virus disease (EVD), or exposure.

Each of these transmission-based precautions can be used in combination for organisms or illnesses that can be transmitted by more than one route. Within health care settings, they should always be used in conjunction with standard precautions, which are recommended for all patients. The *Red Book: 2018 Report of the Committee on Infectious Diseases* by the American Academy of Pediatrics (AAP)[6] and the CDC website (www.cdc.gov/infectioncontrol/guidelines/index.html) remain excellent resources for infection-control guidelines and recommendations to prevent transmission in specific situations and infections (Box 12.1).

Culturing Breast Milk

The routine culturing of breast milk or the culturing of breast milk to screen for infectious agents is not recommended, except when the milk is intended as donor milk for another mother's child directly or through human milk banks. Most milk banks culture donor milk after pasteurization routinely as quality and safety control. See Chapter 22 for specific bacterial-count standards for raw donor milk and related to pasteurized donor milk. Breastfeeding and the expression or pumping of breast milk (referred to as *expressed breast milk*) for later use are not sterile activities. An emerging practice related to an increase in the use of donor human milk is milk sharing. (This is addressed in the next section and Chapter 22).

Bacterial Isolates From Human Breast Milk

In general, expressed breast milk should not contain large numbers of microorganisms (less than 10^4 for raw milk and less than 10^6 for milk to be pasteurized), nor should it contain large numbers of potential pathogens, such as *S. aureus*, β-hemolytic streptococci, *Pseudomonas* species, *Proteus* species, or *Streptococcus faecalis* or *faecium*. Few studies have examined the "routine" culturing of milk and the significance of specific bacterial colony counts relative to illness in infants.[2] Schanler et al. identified *Staphylococcus epidermidis* as the most frequent bacterial isolate from human breast milk, with a variety of other organisms identified (1963 microbial isolates from 813 milk samples).[7] Other isolates they identified included *Enterococcus faecalis*, *Acinetobacter* sp., *Stenotrophomonas maltophilia*, Coagulase-negative *Staphylococcus*, *S. aureus*, *Pseudomonas* sp., *Klebsiella* sp., and other less common organisms. In this study, initial milk cultures did not predict later milk-culture isolates, and individual milk cultures did not predict subsequent infection in premature infants.[7] Other studies have been primarily concerned with premature or low-birth-weight (LBW) infants who remain hospitalized and are commonly fed via enteral tubes. A study from Canada tested 7610 samples of milk for use in 98 preterm infants.[8] This study also did not identify any adverse events in the infants attributed to organisms growing in the milk samples. A study from Chicago also examined gram-negative bacilli in the milk used for premature infants.[9] Samples were tested before feeding and from the nasogastric tubes during feeding. Milk samples from before feeding were less likely to contain gram-negative bacilli (36%) than milk samples from the nasogastric tubing (60%). Feeding intolerance was observed when there were more than 10^3 colony-forming units per milliliter (CFU/mL), and episodes of sepsis were identified when the bacterial counts in the milk were greater than or equal to 10^6 CFU/mL. Another study from Arkansas focused on the contamination of feeding tubes during the administration of expressed breast milk or formula.[10] Ten infants in the neonatal intensive care unit (NICU) were exposed to greater than 10^5 gram-negative bacteria in their feeding tubes. The three infants who were fed expressed breast milk with contamination at greater than 10^5 organisms remained well, but the seven formula-fed infants with high levels of bacterial contamination in the feeding tubes developed necrotizing enterocolitis. The gram-negative bacteria with high-level contamination in the feeding tubes were either *Enterobacter* or *Klebsiella* in all cases. Many NICUs still consider 10^5 to 10^6 CFU/mL as the significant bacterial count for gram-negative bacilli in breast milk that places premature and LBW infants at greater risk for infection. Even fewer data are available concerning specific bacterial colony counts for gram-positive organisms and the risk to the infant. Generally, less than 10^3 gram-positive organisms per milliliter of milk is considered acceptable, with only case reports and no controlled trials to support this cutoff.

Collection Methods for Culturing Milk

Many small reports comment on the contamination of breast milk with different collection methods. Relative comparisons suggest decreasing contamination of expressed breast milk when collected by the following methods: drip milk, hand-pumped milk, manual expression, modern electric-pumped milk. One group from Malaysia published results showing no difference in contamination between milk collected by electric pump versus manual expression when collected in the hospital. Expressed breast milk collected at home by breast pump had higher rates of contamination with staphylococci and gram-negative bacteria,[11] and in another study, bacterial

contamination of expressed breast milk was more common in samples from home.[12] In a more recent study from Brazil, there was no significant difference in culture results of breast milk collected at home versus at a milk bank.[13] Discussion continues about the need to discard the first few milliliters of milk to lower the bacteria numbers in expressed breast milk, without any evidence to suggest if this is truly necessary.[14,15] No evidence shows that cleansing the breast with anything other than tap water decreases the bacterial counts in cultured expressed breast milk.[16]

Routine Breast-Milk Cultures

Routine breast-milk cultures are not useful in the clinical setting. When the presence of an infectious illness occurs in an infant and breast milk is seriously considered as a possible mechanism of transmission to the infant, culturing breast milk to identify the organism may be warranted and useful. Routine culturing of breast milk from a mother with mastitis or a breast abscess is unlikely to be useful in most situations. With recurrent infection, persistent mastitis, or breast abscess in the mother despite empiric antibiotic therapy, milk cultures with speciation and sensitivity testing of the isolated organisms can guide definitive therapy. Drainage of a breast abscess is often essential for definitive therapy of an abscess. More important than hurrying to culture breast milk is the careful instruction of mothers on the proper technique for collecting expressed breast milk, storing it, and cleaning the collection unit. This reinforcement of proper technique from time to time, especially when a question of contamination arises, is important.

If an infant is directly breastfeeding, collecting milk for culture by manual expression and trying to obtain a "midstream" sample (as is done with "midstream" urine collection for culture) is appropriate. If an infant is being fed expressed breast milk, collecting and culturing the milk at different points during collection (utilizing the same technique the mother uses [manual expression, hand pump, or electric pump]) and administration are appropriate. This can include a sample from immediately after collection, another of stored expressed breast milk, and a sample of milk from the most recent infant feeding at the time the decision to culture is made to identify a point of possible contamination in the handling process. See Box 12.2 for the basic steps in culturing expressed breast milk.

The interpretation of the results of breast-milk cultures can be difficult. When faced with concern for infection via breast milk given to a hospitalized infant, involving a pediatric infectious disease expert, a microbiologist, and a hospital epidemiologist may be appropriate. Additional organism identification is often required, utilizing antibiogram patterns or molecular fingerprinting by various techniques, to correlate a bacterial isolate from breast milk with an isolate causing disease in infant or mother.

Donor Human Milk

The World Health Organization (WHO), the United Nations Children's Fund (UNICEF), and the AAP recommend the

---

BOX 12.2 Culturing Breast Milk

1. Wash hands as per routine.
2. Wash breast with warm tap water and a clean washcloth.
3. Manually express breast milk ("midstream" collection is not required) or attach breast pump flange (previously cleaned as per routine) for collection and collect milk.
4. Place a 3- to 5-mL sample of expressed breast milk in a sterile container with a nonleakable top.
5. Deliver to the laboratory in less than 1 hour or refrigerate at 4°C until delivery. Before sending samples to the viral lab or for nucleic acid/polymerase chain reaction (PCR) testing, confirm that the laboratory will accept and process the sample as requested and that the appropriate collection container and prelaboratory management of the specimen are utilized.
6. Processing of specimens:
   a. Direct examination by Gram stain is not required.
   b. Culture on blood agar (BA) and MacConkey agar (MAC) media as per lab standards.
   c. Quantitate all isolates.
   d. Send separate samples for fungal culture, acid-fast bacilli, and viral culture, as indicated, based on the clinical situation.

Perform routine sensitivity testing on all potential pathogens. (This will require some discussion with the clinician and perhaps a pediatric infectious disease specialist.)

---

use of donor human milk when the infant's own mother's milk is unavailable. The AAP recommends pasteurized donor milk.[3] Possible sources of donor human milk include wet nursing, cross-nursing, milk sharing, and human milk banks. Milk sharing is a more informal process compared with human milk banks, which have guidelines and procedures to maintain the safety and quality of the donated milk. Milk sharing occurs more directly among family and friends or now at greater distances between unknown donors and recipients via the Internet. Human milk banks are either not-for-profit banks (e.g., HMBANA, European Milk Bank Association [EMBA]) or established milk banks in numerous other countries or commercial entities (e.g., Prolacta and Medolac).

Milk Safety

The federal government in the United States does not regulate or oversee milk banking, but the HMBANA and EMBA maintain milk-banking guidelines and procedures for banks within their associations. Prolacta Bioscience, Inc. follows US Food and Drug Administration (FDA) guidelines for both food and pharmaceuticals in the production of its human milk products. Medolac Laboratories does so as well but uses a high-temperature pasteurization process. Donor selection, screening, exclusion, and education; Holder pasteurization (HP) or high-temperature short-time (HTST) pasteurization; and postpasteurization bacterial culture testing are the main components utilized to maintain the safety and quality of donor milk from human milk banks (see Chapter 22).[17]

The proper pasteurization of donor human milk virtually eliminates any infectious risks from donor human milk.

Medolac reports that its process also eliminates *Bacillus cereus* (personal communication with Elena Medo). The risk of drug exposure through donor milk is primarily addressed through donor selection and exclusion. In one study from Spain of donor milk from a nonprofit human milk bank, the breast milk from 36 donors did not contain drugs of abuse, but 50% of them had caffeine detected.[18] In a separate study, 400 milk samples from 63 donors were again tested for drugs and compared with results from the milk bank's required screening questionnaire. No drugs of abuse were identified in any donor milk, nicotine and cotinine were found in one donor's milk who did not report tobacco use, and caffeine was detected in 45% of the donor milk samples. The sensitivity and specificity of the questionnaire to detect caffeine in donor milk were both low; sensitivity was 46%, and specificity was 77%.[19] Prolacta includes donor milk drug testing as part of its screening process.

Milk Sharing

The notable increase in donor human milk sharing via Internet sites has raised concerns about the safety and quality of milk obtained in this manner. Although several of the larger Internet organizations (e.g., Human Milk for Human Babies [HM4HB]. The website for Human Milk for Human Babies is currently under construction as of October 2020, with a statement that it will be reinstated, http://www.hm4hb.net], and Eats on Feets [http://www.eatsonfeets.org] promote the concepts of safe and ethical milk sharing; informed consent; "informal donor screening"; safe collection, storage, shipment, and handling; and home pasteurization, there are many other avenues on the Internet for milk sharing, and the safety of milk sharing via the Internet requires ongoing study.

Two publications by the same group have looked at the process of purchasing human milk on the Internet in terms of the ease and reliability of the process, shipping, costs, delays, the condition of packaging and milk containers, the temperature of the milk samples on arrival, and microbial contamination. Geraghty et al.[20] and Keim et al.[21] reported receiving 50% of the packages on the day after shipment and 37% on the second day after shipment. Nine percent of these shipping boxes were rated as severely damaged, 15% of the milk containers had evidence of leaking milk, and 45% of the milk samples arrived with a surface temperature of the milk >4°C, the recommended refrigerator temperature for the storage of human milk. The surface milk temperature was noted to correlate with the cost of shipping, time in transit, and rating of milk-container condition. The authors also compared the bacteriologic culture results of milk obtained via the Internet and milk obtained from a human milk bank. The Internet samples were colonized with gram-negative bacteria 74% of the time or had colony counts of >10^4 CFU/mL. Compared with samples from a human milk bank, the Internet samples had higher mean total aerobic counts, total gram-negative counts, coliform counts, and *Staphylococcus* sp. counts. Milk bank samples were cytomegalovirus (CMV) DNA positive 5% of the time, with 21% of Internet samples being CMV DNA positive. None of the samples tested positive for HIV ribonucleic acid (RNA).[20,21] Keim and Geraghty and others have also looked at drugs of abuse and cow's milk contamination of human milk purchased from the Internet. Sellers of human milk in these studies reported abstinence from drugs 71% of the time and made no statement about it in 29% of the advertisements. One hundred and two milk samples were tested for 13 groups of drugs of abuse, and none of the samples tested positive. The same 102 samples were tested for bovine DNA, and 10 of the samples contained amounts consistent with at least 10% of the fluid sample being made up of cow's milk.[22,23] Testing for tobacco metabolites and caffeine, the same authors found that 4% of the milk samples contained levels of nicotine or cotinine consistent with active smoking, and 97% of the same samples contained detectable amounts of caffeine.[24] Even though the larger milk-sharing websites recommend guidelines for hygienic collection, appropriate storage, and shipping, the quality and safety of human milk obtained via milk sharing on the Internet fall short of expected standards for donor human milk. Further study is needed with larger numbers of donor human milk samples to provide accurate information on the risk of transmission of infection or contamination with drugs of abuse or cow's milk. This highlights the importance of ethical milk sharing, informed consent, "informal donor screening," and proper and effective home pasteurization of donor human milk by the receiving mother before giving it to an infant.

Collection and use of donor human milk via milk banks are increasing, and human milk-sharing practices in the United States continue to evolve. The Academy of Breastfeeding Medicine (ABM) has published a statement in support of informed and enhanced milk-safety practices for milk sharing.[25] Various studies suggest that milk sharing is a "complex practice," with donors and recipients exchanging roles over time with and without "cross-nursing," and that exchanges were most often face to face or with individuals they knew.[26,27] Participants report milk sharing on the Internet through milk-sharing websites and through their own personal networks. Totally anonymous milk sharing or selling and shipping of breast milk are less commonly reported. Practices of "screening" donors occurred but varied between donor—recipient pairs with greater or less familiarity with the other. Practices for the safe handling and storage of milk are known to most participants, but it is difficult to tell how well they are followed in all situations.[28] Clearly, more study of the safety and quality of donor human milk obtained via the Internet is needed, with a focus on obtaining outcome data on the infants receiving this milk. Additionally, increasing the availability and decreasing the cost of donor human milk from not-for-profit and commercial milk banks while maintaining quality and safety are essential to providing for the needs of an increasing number of infants who have an inadequate supply of their own mother's milk.

MISADMINISTRATION OF BREAST MILK

The misadministration of breast milk, also known as *misappropriation*, *breast-milk exposure*, and *accidental ingestion of breast milk*, among other terms, is a medical-legal issue when it occurs in a hospital. This scenario occurs when one infant receives breast milk from another mother by mistake. This occurrence can be very distressing to the families (recipient patient, recipient parent, and donor mother) and medical staff involved. The actual risk for transmission of an infectious agent to an infant via a single ingestion of expressed breast milk (the most common occurrence) from another mother is exceedingly low. In this scenario, the CDC recommends treating this as an accidental exposure to a body fluid that could be infectious.[29] Bacterial, fungal, or parasitic infection from the single exposure is highly unlikely. The concern is about viral pathogens, known to be bloodborne pathogens that have been identified in breast milk and include but are not limited to hepatitis B virus (HBV), hepatitis C virus (HCV), CMV, West Nile virus (WNV), human T-cell lymphotropic virus types I and II (HTLV-I and HTLV-II), and HIV.

Most hospitals have protocols for managing the situation from both the infection-control/prevention and medical-legal perspectives. These protocols advise informing both families about what occurred, discussing the theoretical risks of harm from the exposure, and reviewing test results and/or recommending testing to determine the infectious status of each mother relative to the mentioned viruses. HCV is not a contraindication to breastfeeding, and WNV infection in lactating women is rare.[30,31] Neither infection has a documented effective form of prevention or acute treatment. Testing either the donor mother or the mother of the recipient infant for these agents is not warranted. Prenatal testing for HIV is more commonplace throughout the world. The incidence of HIV among women of childbearing age is low, although it varies significantly by geographic location, and the hospital- or locale-specific incidence would be important to know to estimate risk. Most women and medical staff are aware that HIV can be transmitted by breastfeeding; therefore breast milk from HIV-positive women is rarely, if ever, stored in hospitals. The risk for transmission of HIV via breastfeeding is a result of the volume of feedings over months (estimated at 400 to 500 feedings in the first 2 months of life) compared with the small "dose of exposure" from one or two "accidental feedings." Transmission of HIV from a single breast-milk exposure has never been documented. Immunologic components in breast milk, along with time and cold-storage temperatures, inactivate the HIV in expressed breast milk. For these reasons, the risk for transmission of HIV via expressed breast milk consumed by another child is thought to be extremely low. HTLV-I/II infection in childbearing women is uncommon, except in certain geographic regions (Japan, Africa, the Caribbean, and South America). Transmission of HTLV via breast milk does occur and, like HIV, appears to be related to the volume and duration of breastfeeding. Limiting the duration of breastfeeding is effective in decreasing transmission.[32,33] Freezing and thawing expressed breast milk decreases the infectivity of HTLV-I.[34] In areas of low prevalence, a positive test in a mother should be suspected to be a false-positive test, and retesting with both antibody and polymerase chain reaction (PCR) testing should be performed. For these reasons, the transmission of HTLV-I/II via accidental expressed breast-milk exposure is thought to be extremely low. Although most women are CMV-positive by childbearing age and CMV transmission occurs via breastfeeding, the risk for CMV disease in a full-term infant is low. Premature or LBW infants are at greater risk for developing disease with CMV infection. Freezing expressed breast milk (at −20°C) for 3 to 5 days significantly decreases the infectivity of CMV. Here again, the risk for CMV transmission from a single accidental exposure to CMV-positive expressed breast milk is extremely low.

Any discussion of theoretical risk should be accompanied by a discussion of possible preventive interventions, such as vaccination or antimicrobial postexposure prophylaxis. If donor mothers are positive for HBV, it is appropriate to give recipient infants hepatitis B virus immunoglobulin (HBIG) and HBV vaccines if they have not already received them. If a donor mother is HIV- or HTLV-I/II-positive, the potential utility of postexposure prophylaxis with antiretroviral medications should be considered on a case-by-case basis. Clinicians participating in these decisions can refer to the AAP *Red Book*[35] or the discussion of pediatric considerations for HIV postexposure prophylaxis offered by Muller and Chadwick.[36] It may also be appropriate to consult a pediatric infectious disease specialist.

Additional important components of the hospital-based protocols for managing accidental expressed breast-milk exposure include ongoing psychosocial support for the families and staff, documentation of medical discussions with the families, investigative steps, consents and interventions, and the demonstration of ongoing infection-control efforts to prevent additional events of misadministration of breast milk.

CLINICAL SYNDROMES AND CONDITIONS

Microorganisms produce a whole spectrum of clinical illnesses or conditions affecting mothers and infants. Many situations carry the risk for transmission of the involved organism from a mother to the infant, or vice versa. In general, however, infants are at greater risk because of such factors as inoculum size and immature immune response. As always, an infection must be accurately diagnosed in a timely manner. Empiric therapy and initial infection-control precautions should begin promptly based on the clinical symptoms and the most likely etiologic agents. When dealing with a maternal infection, clarifying the possible modes of transmission and estimating the relative risk for transmission to the infant are essential first steps to decision-making about isolating a mother from her infant and the appropriateness of continuing breastfeeding or providing expressed breast milk. Breastfeeding is infrequently contraindicated for specific maternal infections.[2] Often, the question of isolation and interruption of breastfeeding arises when symptoms of fever, pain, inflammation, or other manifestations of illness first develop in a mother and the diagnosis is still in doubt. A clinical judgment must be made based on the site of infection, probable organisms involved, possible or actual mechanisms of transmission of these organisms to the infant, estimated virulence of the organism, and likely susceptibility of the infant. In most situations, by the time the illness is clearly recognized or diagnosed in a mother, the infant has already been exposed. Given the dynamic nature of the immunologic benefits of breast milk, the continuation of breastfeeding at the time of diagnosis or illness in a mother can provide the infant protection rather than continued exposure. Stopping breastfeeding is rarely necessary. Many situations associated with maternal fever do not require separation of mother and infant, such as engorgement of the breasts, atelectasis, localized nonsuppurative phlebitis, or urinary tract infections.

Appendix D lists clinical syndromes, conditions, and organisms that require infection-control precautions in hospitals. This appendix also includes short lists of possible etiologic agents for these conditions and appropriate precautions and recommendations concerning breastfeeding for different scenarios or organisms. This chapter considers specific infectious agents and clinical illnesses that are common, clinically significant, or of interest related to breastfeeding or breast milk.

BACTERIAL INFECTIONS

Anthrax

Bacillus anthracis, a gram-positive, spore-forming rod, causes zoonotic disease worldwide. Human infection typically occurs as a result of contact with animals or their products. Three forms of human disease occur: cutaneous anthrax (the most common), inhalation anthrax, and gastrointestinal (GI) anthrax (rare). Person-to-person transmission can occur as a result of discharge from cutaneous lesions, but no evidence of human-to-human transmission of inhalational anthrax is available. No evidence of transmission of anthrax via breast milk exists.[37,38] Standard contact isolation is appropriate for hospitalized patients or patients with draining skin lesions.

The issue of anthrax as a biologic weapon has exaggerated its importance as a cause of human disease. The primary concerns regarding anthrax and breastfeeding are antimicrobial therapy or prophylaxis in breastfeeding mothers and the possibility that the infant and mother were exposed by intentional aerosolization of anthrax spores. The AAP Committee on Infectious Diseases and Disaster Preparedness Advisory Council published recommendations for treatment and prophylaxis in infants, children, and breastfeeding mothers.[39] The recommendations include the use of a range of antibiotics, often in combination, including amoxicillin, ampicillin, chloramphenicol, ciprofloxacin, clindamycin, doxycycline, imipenem, levofloxacin, linezolid, meropenem, moxifloxacin, penicillin, and rifampin. Amoxicillin, ampicillin clindamycin, imipenem, linezolid, meropenem, and penicillin are acceptable for use with breastfeeding.[39] Little information is available on ciprofloxacin, levofloxacin, moxifloxacin, and doxycycline in breast milk for prolonged periods of therapy or prophylaxis (60 days) and possible effects on infants' teeth and bone or cartilage growth during that time period.[40–42] Short-term use is acceptable while breastfeeding for those four drugs, but alternative drugs are preferred for longer-term use in place of chloramphenicol and clindamycin.[43,44] Depending on the clinical situation and sensitivity testing of the identified anthrax strain, specific agents can be chosen to complete the 60-day course of therapy. Guidelines are also given for the use of the adsorbed anthrax vaccine and/or raxibacumab antitoxin, although vaccine use in children is available through an investigational new-drug protocol.[39]

The simultaneous exposure of infant and mother could occur from primary aerosolization or from spores "contaminating" the local environment. In either case, decontamination of the mother–infant dyad's environment should be considered.

Breastfeeding can continue during a mother's therapy for anthrax if she is physically well. Open cutaneous lesions should be carefully covered, and depending on the situation, simultaneous prophylaxis for the infant may be appropriate. If there is no likelihood of contamination of the breast milk from a local skin lesion, breastfeeding or the use of breast milk can continue.

Botulism

Considerable justifiable concern has been expressed because of the reports of sudden infant death from botulism. Infant botulism is distinguished from foodborne botulism from improperly preserved food containing the preformed toxin and from wound botulism caused by spores entering a wound.

Infant Botulism

Infant botulism occurs when the spores of *Clostridium botulinum* germinate and multiply in the gut and produce the botulinal toxin in the GI tract. The toxin binds presynaptically at the neuromuscular junction, preventing acetylcholine release. The clinical picture is a descending, symmetric flaccid paralysis. Not every individual who has *C. botulinum* identified in the stool experiences a clinical illness. The age of infants seems to relate to their susceptibility to illness. The illness is mainly seen in children younger than 12 months of age; the youngest patient described in the literature was 6 days old.[45] Most children become ill between 6 weeks and 6 months of age. The onset of illness seems to occur earlier in formula-fed infants compared with breastfed infants. When a previously healthy infant younger than 6 months of age develops constipation, followed by weakness and difficulty sucking, swallowing, crying, or breathing, botulism is a likely diagnosis. The organisms should be looked for in the stools, and electromyography may or may not be helpful.

In a group reviewed by Arnon et al.,[46] 33 of 50 patients hospitalized in California were still being nursed at the onset of the illness. A beneficial effect of human milk was observed in the difference in the mean age at onset, with breastfed infants being twice as old as formula-fed infants with the disease. The breastfed infants' symptoms were milder. Breastfed infants receiving iron supplements developed the disease earlier than those who were breastfed but not supplemented. Of the cases of sudden infant death from botulism, no infants were breastfed within 10 weeks of death. All were receiving iron-fortified formulas. In most cases, no specific food source

of *C. botulinum* can be identified, but honey is the food most often implicated, and corn syrup has been implicated in infants older than 2 months of age. Honey may contain botulism spores, which can germinate in the infant gut. However, botulin toxin has not been identified in honey. It has been recommended that honey not be given to infants younger than 12 months of age. This includes putting honey on a mother's nipples to initiate an infant's interest in suckling.

Arnon reviewed the first 10 years of infant botulism monitoring worldwide.[47] The disease has been reported in 41 of the 50 states in the United States, and more recently, it has been reported in 26 countries and 5 continents. The United States, Argentina, Australia, Canada, Italy, and Japan reported the largest number of cases from 1976 to 2006.[48] The relationship to breastfeeding and human milk is unclear. In general, the acid stools (pH of 5.1 to 5.4) of human-milk-fed infants encourage *Bifidobacterium* species. Few facultative anaerobic bacteria, or clostridia, existing as spores, are present in breastfed infants. In contrast, formula-fed infants have stool pHs ranging from 5.9 to 8.0, with few bifidobacteria, primarily gram-negative bacteria, especially coliforms and *Bacteroides* species. *C. botulinum* growth and toxin production decrease with declining pH and usually stop below pH 4.6. Breast milk also contains additional protective immunologic components, which purportedly have activity against botulinum toxin.[49]

The relationship between the introduction of solid foods or weaning in both formula-fed and breastfed infants and the onset of botulism remains unclear. For a breastfed infant, the introduction of solid food may cause a major change in the gut, with a rapid rise in the growth of enterobacteria and enterococci, followed by progressive colonization by *Bacteroides* species, clostridia, and anaerobic streptococci. Feeding solids to formula-fed infants minimally changes the gut flora because these organisms already predominate. Although more hospitalized infants have been breastfed, sudden-death victims are younger and have been formula-fed, which supports the concept of immunologic protection in the gut of a breastfed infant.

Much work remains to understand this disease. Clinically, constipation, weakness, and hypotonicity in a previously healthy child constitute botulism until ruled out, especially with recent dietary changes. When the diagnosis of infant botulism is considered, efforts should be made to confirm the diagnosis and Human Botulism Immune Globulin Intravenous (BIG-IV) should be given empirically. Early treatment decreases the length of stay and associated hospital costs.[50]

Currently, no reason exists to suspect breastfeeding as a risk for infant botulism, and some evidence suggests a possible protective effect from breastfeeding. Breastfeeding should continue if botulism is suspected in the mother or infant.[51]

Bacillus cereus

Bacillus cereus is a gram-positive, spore-forming aerobic rod that grows well under anaerobic conditions. It causes at least two kinds of food poisoning: diarrhea and emesis, produced by different toxins. This organism is ubiquitous in the environment, and food-poisoning outbreaks are associated with many types of foods: plant derived, meat, eggs, and dairy.

B. cereus—related disease is not a reportable illness, so the true incidence is unknown. The foods commonly associated with diarrheal disease are meats, soups, vegetables, puddings, sauces, milk, and milk products, and those associated with emetic disease are fried and cooked rice, pasta, pastry, and noodles. The emetic syndrome has a relatively short incubation period, usually less than 6 hours, and lasts 6 to 24 hours, suggesting it is a result of "intoxication" from food containing the emetic toxin cereulide. The infective dose is estimated to be 10^5 to 10^8 cells per g^{-1} of the suspected offending food or toxin present in the suspected food equivalent to 8 to 10 $\mu g k g^{-1}$ body weight (estimated from animal studies). For the diarrhea syndrome, the incubation is approximately 8 to 16 hours, and it lasts from 12 to 24 hours, up to days. The infective dose is 10^5 to 10^8 cells or spores, although there are reports of diarrheal disease with as low as 10^3 *B. cereus* $CFUg^{-1}$ of food. Diarrheal disease is more likely a result of the ingestion of cells or spores that produce one of several enterotoxins during the vegetative phase of growth within the intestine.[52]

Previously, *B. cereus* was noted for being found in dried milk products, including powdered infant formulas. More recently, *B. cereus* has been identified in donor human milk even after Holder pasteurization, which may relate to *Bacillus* spore temperature resistance and the ability to form biofilms.[53,54] A couple of reports contend that human milk could have played a role in *B. cereus* infection in premature infants, even though the strain of *B. cereus* causing disease was not found in milk and contaminated donor human milk was not identified. This has led to new tests to quantify the *Bacillus* toxins by PCR testing or liquid chromatography-tandem mass spectrometry. New techniques for processing donor human milk are being tested, including HTST, high-pressure processing (HPP), ultraviolet irradiation (UV-C), and thermo-ultrasonic processing, with the intent of ensuring the safety and quality of donor human milk.[55] Other processing methods utilizing heat and pressure that eradicate *B. cereus* and other pathogens have been reported.[56]

New research assessing the risk of *B. cereus* infection resulting from pasteurized donor human milk[57,58] and discussion of updated recommendations for quality improvement and processing of human donor milk by milk banks are ongoing.[59,60] With the use of a Monte Carlo simulation, Lewin et al. estimated that the risk of infection from donor human milk to premature infants was very low and that additional precautions in postpasteurization culture testing made little difference in diminishing the apparent risk to exposed infants.[57] To optimize the safety, accessibility, affordability, and quality of donor human milk for neonates, a significant amount of research into *B. cereus* and quality control/improvement is still needed.

Brucellosis

Brucella melitensis has been isolated in the milk of animals. Foods and animals represent the primary sources of infection in humans. Human-to-human transmission is rare, with less than 50 cases reported in the last 49 years, as reported in a recent systematic review.[61] Eleven of those cases were likely via transplacental transmission, and 7 cases were reportedly via breastfeeding based on timing. Only two of the seven cases reported as breastfeeding related were associated with a positive human milk culture. There are no reports of isolation of *Brucella* from human milk on routine culturing.[61] Brucellosis demonstrates a broad spectrum of illness in humans, from subclinical to subacute to chronic illness with nonspecific signs of weakness, fever, malaise, body aches, fatigue, sweats, arthralgia, and lymphadenitis. In areas where the disease is enzootic, childhood illness has been described more frequently. The clinical manifestations in children are similar to those in adults. In infants, the dominant symptoms include respiratory distress, hyperbilirubinemia, fever, hepatomegaly, and arthralgia.[62] Infection can occur during pregnancy, leading to abortion (infrequently), and can produce transplacental spread, causing neonatal infection (rarely). Neonatal brucellosis has been reported rarely, even in endemic areas.[63]

The transmission of *B. melitensis* through breast milk has been implicated in neonatal infection, but the data are circumstantial, at best, for this rare infection in newborns and infants.[64–66]

Separately, *B. melitensis* has been cultured from women with breast lumps and abscesses.[67] Only one of six women described in this report was lactating at the time of diagnosis, and no information about the infant was given. Brucellosis mastitis or abscess should be considered in women presenting with appropriate symptoms and occupational exposure to animals, contact with domestic animals in their environment, or exposure to animal milk or milk products (especially unpasteurized products). The breast inflammation tends to be granulomatous in nature (without caseation). It is often associated with axillary adenopathy, and occasionally, systemic illness in the woman is evident. Brucellosis mastitis or abscess should be treated with surgery or fine-needle aspiration, as indicated, accompanied by 4 to 6 weeks of combination antibiotic therapy with two or three medications. Acceptable medications for treating the mother, while continuing breastfeeding, include gentamicin, streptomycin, trimethoprim-sulfamethoxazole, and rifampin for the longer period of therapy (4 to 6 weeks). Doxycycline should be used with caution in the lactating woman for this longer period.[42]

By the time the diagnosis of *Brucella* mastitis is made, the infant has already been exposed. There is no reason to interrupt breastfeeding or the use of the mother's milk.

Chlamydial Infections

Chlamydial infection is the most frequent sexually transmitted disease (STD) in the United States and is a frequent cause of conjunctivitis and pneumonitis in an infant from perinatal infection. The major determinant of whether chlamydial infection occurs in a newborn is the prevalence rate of chlamydial infection of the cervix.[68] Specific chlamydial immunoglobulin A (IgA) has been found in colostrum and breast milk in a small number of postpartum women who were seropositive for *Chlamydia*. No information is available on the role of milk antibodies in protecting against infection in infants.[69] It is not believed that *Chlamydia* is transmitted via breast milk.

The use of erythromycin or tetracycline to treat mothers and oral erythromycin or azithromycin and ophthalmic preparations of tetracyclines, erythromycin, or sulfonamides to treat suspected infection in infants (with a risk-benefit assessment for the use of the specific antibiotic in the specific infant) is appropriate during continued breastfeeding. Separating infants from mothers with chlamydial infections or stopping breastfeeding is not indicated. The simultaneous treatment of mothers and infants may be appropriate in some situations.

Clostridium difficile

C. difficile is a spore-forming, obligate anaerobic, gram-positive bacillus with Toxins A and B causing intestinal infection. It is acquired via the fecal-oral route from other individuals or the environment. Its increasing incidence in adults and children relates to its relative importance.[70] Infants can readily be colonized (most often asymptomatic carriage), with reported *C. difficile* colonization at approximately 30% to 40% before 1 month of age, 20% to 30% at 1 to 6 months of age, 10% to 20% at 12 months of age, and continuing to decline to about 3 years of age, when the colonization rate approaches the same rate as in adults, 3% to 5%.[71] Various studies show that colonization with *C. difficile* in breastfed infants is almost half of the colonization rate in formula-fed infants.[72–74] Proposed explanations for this include competition with bacteria common in the microbiome in breastfed infants, secretory IgA, and neutralizing antibodies against the *C. difficile* toxins in colostrum. The AAP has advised against routinely testing infants less than 1 year of age because of the high rate of asymptomatic colonization. The AAP recommends testing for alternative etiologies of diarrhea or intestinal disease in children less than 3 years of age.

If a mother is infected with *C. difficile* and hospitalized, standard and contact precautions are likely to be instituted within the hospital. There is no reason to separate the mother and child, except the severity of the mother's illness. Breastfeeding can continue, including during antimicrobial therapy in the mother for *C. difficile*. Vancomycin, rifaximin, and nitazoxanide can be readily utilized in infants, and their very limited absorption from the intestine limits the systemic exposure to the infant. Metronidazole can also be used in the mother or infant with their first episode of *C. difficile* infection, with precaution regarding dosing when the infant is <2 kg in weight and <7 days old.[75] There are limited data on the use of fidaxomicin in infants.[76]

Diphtheria

Corynebacterium diphtheriae causes several forms of clinical disease, including membranous nasopharyngitis, obstructive laryngotracheitis, and cutaneous infection. Complications can include airway obstruction from membrane formation and toxin-mediated central nervous system (CNS) disease or myocarditis. The overall incidence of diphtheria has declined, even though immunization does not prevent infection but does prevent severe disease from toxin production. Fewer than five cases are reported annually in the United States, whereas thousands of cases are reported worldwide (the WHO documented 7097 diphtheria cases reported in 2016), and many more go unreported.[77]

Transmission occurs via droplets or direct contact with contaminated secretions from the nose, throat, eye, or skin. Infection occurs in individuals whether they have been immunized or not, but infection in the nonimmunized is more severe and prolonged. If the skin of the breast is not involved, no risk for transmission exists via breast milk. No toxin-mediated disease from a toxin transmitted through breast milk has been reported in an infant.

Breastfeeding, along with chemoprophylaxis and the immunization of affected infants, is appropriate in the absence of cutaneous breast involvement (see Appendix D).

Gonococcal Infections

Maternal infection with *N. gonorrhoeae* can produce a large spectrum of illness, ranging from uncomplicated vulvovaginitis, proctitis, pharyngitis, and conjunctivitis to more severe and invasive disease, including pelvic inflammatory disease, meningitis, endocarditis, and disseminated gonococcal infection. The risk for transmission from mother to infant occurs mainly during delivery in the passage through the infected birth canal and occasionally from postpartum contact with the mother (or her partner). The risk for transmission from breast milk is negligible, and *N. gonorrhoeae* does not seem to cause local infection of the breasts. Infection in neonates is most often ophthalmia neonatorum and less often a scalp abscess or disseminated infection. Mothers with presumed or documented gonorrhea should be reevaluated for other STDs, especially *Chlamydia trachomatis* and syphilis, because some therapies for gonorrhea are not adequate for either of these infections.

With the definitive identification of gonorrhea in a mother, empiric therapy should begin immediately for the infant. Treatment of the mother with ceftriaxone, cefixime, penicillin, or erythromycin is without significant risk for the infant. Single-dose treatment with spectinomycin, ciprofloxacin, ofloxacin, or azithromycin has not been adequately studied to recommend their use during lactation. Doxycycline use in a nursing mother is not routinely recommended.

Careful preventive therapy for ophthalmia neonatorum should be provided, and close observation of the infant should continue for 2 to 7 days, the usual incubation period. Empiric or definitive therapy against *N. gonorrhoeae* may be necessary, depending on an infant's clinical status, and it should be chosen based on the maternal isolate's sensitivity pattern. The mother should not handle other infants until after 24 hours of adequate therapy. The infant should be separated from the rest of the nursery population, with or without breastfeeding. There is no reason to separate the mother and infant because the infant has already been exposed, and there is no reason to interrupt breastfeeding or hold breast milk.

Hemophilus influenzae

H. influenzae type B can cause severe invasive disease, such as meningitis, sinusitis, pneumonia, epiglottitis, septic arthritis, pericarditis, and bacteremia. Shock can also occur. Because of the increased utilization of the *H. influenzae* type B conjugate vaccines, invasive disease caused by *Hemophilus* has decreased dramatically, with a greater than 95% reduction in the United States. Most invasive disease occurs in children 3 months to 3 years of age. Older children and adults rarely experience severe disease but do serve as sources of infection for young children. Children younger than 3 months of age seem to be protected because of passively acquired antibodies from the mothers, and some additional benefits may be received from breast milk.

Transmission occurs through contact with respiratory secretions, and droplet precautions are protective. No evidence suggests transmission through breast milk or breastfeeding. Evidence supports that breast milk limits the colonization of *H. influenzae* in the throat.[78]

In the rare case of maternal infection, an inadequately immunized infant in a household is an indication to provide rifampin prophylaxis and close observation for all household contacts, including the breastfeeding infant. Breastfeeding or the use of expressed breast milk can continue if the mother is well enough.

Leprosy

Although uncommon in the United States, leprosy occurs throughout the world despite ongoing efforts for eradication with contact testing, postexposure chemoprophylaxis, and ongoing trials of postexposure vaccination with several vaccine formulations. This chronic disease presents with a spectrum of symptoms depending on the tissues involved (typically the skin, peripheral nerves, and mucous membranes of the upper respiratory tract) and the cellular immune response to the causative organism, *Mycobacterium leprae*. Transmission occurs through long-term contact with individuals with untreated or multibacillary (large numbers of organisms in the tissues) disease. Leprosy is believed to be transmitted primarily through the respiratory tract.

Although leprosy can be transmitted to the fetus during pregnancy and young children can manifest with leprosy, there is no evidence of transmission of *M. leprae* via breast milk or breastfeeding. Leprosy is not a contraindication to breastfeeding, according to Jelliffe and Jelliffe.[79] The importance of breastfeeding and the urgency of treatment are recognized by experts who treat infants and mothers early and simultaneously. There are data concerning infants born to mothers with leprosy during pregnancy and the occurrence of smaller placentas and lower birth weights. There is only one long-term study of the growth of children born to mothers with leprosy, which demonstrated slower growth (catch-up by 3.6 years), more childhood infections, and higher infant mortality in comparison to healthy controls.[80] The authors suggested that this could be a result of immunologic factors associated with leprosy, but support of breastfeeding and maternal and infant nutrition during therapy should be included as part of the antimicrobial therapy. Additionally, contact testing within the household and family and postexposure prophylaxis are being studied for their ability to interrupt the cycle of transmission. Breastfeeding and the use of breast milk can continue during maternal therapy and infant prophylaxis. Dapsone, rifampin, and clofazimine are typically and safely used for infant and mother, regardless of the method of feeding (see Appendix D).[81]

Listeriosis

Listeriosis is a relatively uncommon infection that can have a broad range of manifestations. In immunocompetent individuals, including pregnant women, the infection can vary from being asymptomatic to presenting as an influenza-like illness, occasionally with GI symptoms or back pain. Severe disease occurs more frequently in immunodeficient individuals or infants infected in the perinatal period (pneumonia, sepsis, meningitis, and granulomatosis infantisepticum).

Although listeriosis during pregnancy may manifest as mild disease in a mother and is often difficult to recognize and diagnose, it is typically associated with stillbirth, abortion, and premature delivery. Neonatal infection occurs as either early- or late-onset infection from transplacental spread late in pregnancy, ascending infection during labor and delivery, infection during passage through the birth canal, or rarely, during postnatal exposure.

No evidence in the literature suggests that *Listeria* is transmitted through breast milk. There are rare reports of *Listeria* infecting the breast.[82] Treatment of the mother with ampicillin, penicillin, or trimethoprim-sulfamethoxazole is not a contraindication to breastfeeding as long as the mother is well enough. Expressed colostrum or breast milk can also be given if the infant is able to feed orally. The management of lactation and feeding in neonatal listeriosis is conducted supportively, as it is in any situation in which an infant is extremely ill, beginning feeding with expressed breast milk or directly breastfeeding as soon as reasonable.

Meningococcal Infections

N. meningitidis most often causes severe invasive infections, including meningococcemia or meningitis, often associated with fever and a rash and progressing to purpura, disseminated intravascular coagulation, shock, coma, and death.

Transmission occurs via respiratory droplets. Spread can occur from an infected, ill individual or from an asymptomatic carrier. Droplet precautions are recommended until 24 hours after the initiation of effective therapy. Despite the frequent occurrence of bacteremia, no evidence indicates breast involvement or transmission through breast milk.

The risk for transmission of infection from a mother to an infant after birth is from droplet exposure and exists whether the infant is breastfeeding or bottle-feeding. In either case, the exposed infant should receive chemoprophylaxis with rifampin, 10 mg/kg per dose every 12 hours for 2 days (5 mg/kg per dose for infants younger than 1 month of age), or ceftriaxone, 125 mg intramuscularly (IM) once, for children younger than 15 years of age. Close observation of the infant should continue for 7 days, and breastfeeding during and after prophylaxis is appropriate. The severity of maternal illness may prevent breastfeeding, but it can continue if the mother is able.

Pertussis

Respiratory illness caused by *Bordetella pertussis* evolves in three stages: catarrhal (nasal discharge, congestion, increasing cough), paroxysmal (severe paroxysms of cough sometimes ending in an inspiratory whoop, i.e., whooping cough), and convalescent (gradual improvement in symptoms).

Transmission is via respiratory droplets. The greatest risk for transmission occurs in the catarrhal phase, often before the diagnosis of pertussis. The nasopharyngeal culture usually becomes negative after 5 days of antibiotic therapy. Chemoprophylaxis for all household contacts is routinely recommended. No evidence indicates transmission through breast milk, with similar risk to breastfed and bottle-fed infants.

In the case of maternal infection with pertussis, chemoprophylaxis for all household contacts, regardless of age or immunization status, is indicated. In addition to chemoprophylaxis of the infant, close observation and subsequent immunization (in infants older than 6 weeks of age) are appropriate. Prophylaxis for the infant should be azithromycin or erythromycin, although trimethoprim-sulfamethoxazole can be used when the infant is 6 weeks or older. Standard and droplet precautions are recommended for 5 days after the initiation of effective therapy. There are no trials assessing the protection to the infant while utilizing infant prophylaxis and ongoing breastfeeding. Maternal immunization in the third trimester has demonstrated increased passive transfer of antipertussis antibodies to the infant at birth.[83–85] Prenatal maternal immunization is more effective than postnatal immunization at preventing pertussis disease and decreasing the severity of pertussis infection in infants less than 8 weeks of age.[86] Although antipertussis antibodies have been demonstrated in colostrum and breast milk, protection directly from breast milk against pertussis infection in infancy has been difficult to prove.[84] Breastfeeding or the use of mother's milk can continue because exposure has already occurred by the time the diagnosis is made in the mother. There are clear benefits to prenatal maternal immunization, chemoprophylaxis, and immunizing adult caregivers against pertussis in protecting infants.

STAPHYLOCOCCAL INFECTIONS

Staphylococcal infection in neonates can be caused by either *S. aureus* or coagulase-negative staphylococci (most often *S. epidermidis*) and can manifest in a wide range of illnesses. Localized infection can be impetigo, pustulosis in neonates, cellulitis, or wound infection, and invasive or suppurative disease includes sepsis, pneumonia, osteomyelitis, arthritis, and endocarditis. *S. aureus* requires only a small inoculum (10 to 250 organisms) to produce colonization in newborns, most often of the nasal mucosa and umbilicus.[87] By the fifth day of life, 40% to 90% of the infants in the nursery will be colonized with *S. aureus*.[88] The organism is easily transmitted to others from the mother, infant, family, or health care personnel through direct contact. Colonization in the NICU is associated with gestational age and birth weight and not with gender, race, or delivery type.[89]

Outbreaks in nurseries were common in the past. Mothers, infants, health care workers, and even contaminated, unpasteurized, banked breast milk were sources of infection.[90–92] Careful use of antibiotics, changes in nursery layout and procedures, standard precautions, and cohorting as needed decreased the spread of *S. aureus* in nurseries. Currently, the occurrence of methicillin-resistant *S. aureus* (MRSA) is again a common problem, requiring cohorting, occasional epidemiologic investigation, and careful infection-control intervention. There are numerous reports of MRSA outbreaks in NICUs.[93–97] The significance of colonization with *Staphylococcus* and the factors leading to the development of disease in individual patients are not clear. The morbidity and mortality related to *S. aureus* infection in neonates are well described,[98–100] and the management of such outbreaks has been reviewed.[101,102] Little has been written about the role of breastfeeding in colonization with *S. aureus* in NICUs,[93,94] well-baby nurseries, or at home.

Methicillin-Resistant *Staphylococcus aureus*

MRSA is an important pathogen worldwide. Community-acquired MRSA is different from hospital-acquired MRSA. Community-acquired MRSA is usually defined as occurring in an individual without the common predisposing variables associated with hospital-acquired MRSA. Community-acquired MRSA also lacks a multidrug resistance (MDR) phenotype (common with hospital-acquired MRSA) and frequently carries multiple exotoxin virulence factors (e.g., Panton-Valentine leukocidin toxin), as well as the smaller type IV staphylococcal cassette cartridge for the *MecA* gene on a chromosome (hospital-acquired MRSA carries the types I to III staphylococcal cassette cartridge). This is molecularly distinct from the common nosocomial strains of hospital-acquired MRSA. Community-acquired MRSA is most commonly associated with skin and soft tissue infections and necrotizing pneumonia and less frequently associated with endocarditis, bacteremia, necrotizing fasciitis, myositis, osteomyelitis, or parapneumonic effusions. Community-acquired MRSA is so common that it is now being observed in hospital outbreaks.[94,103–105]

Community-acquired MRSA transmission to infants via breast milk has been reported.[93–97] Premature or small-for-gestational-age infants are more susceptible to and at increased risk for significant morbidity and mortality as a result of MRSA, in part because of prolonged hospitalization, multiple courses of antibiotics, invasive procedures and intravenous (IV) lines, their relative immune deficiency related to prematurity and illness, and altered GI tract as a result of different flora and decreased gastric acidity. Therefore colonization with MRSA may pose a greater risk to infants in NICUs in the long run. Full-term infants develop pustulosis, cellulitis, and soft tissue infections, but invasive disease has rarely been reported.[91,106,107] Fortunov et al.[107] from Texas reported 126 infections in term or late-preterm previously well infants, including 43 with pustulosis, 68 with cellulitis or abscesses, and 15 invasive infections. A family history of soft tissue skin infections and male sex were the only variables associated with risk for infection; cesarean delivery, breastfeeding, and circumcision were not.[107] Nguyen et al.[91] reported MRSA infections in a well-infant nursery from California. The 11 cases were all in full-term boys with pustular-vesicular lesions in the groin. The infections were associated with longer length of stay, lidocaine injection use in infants, maternal age older than 30 years, and circumcision. Breastfeeding was not an associated risk factor for MRSA infection.[91] The question of the role of circumcision in MRSA outbreaks was addressed by Van Howe and Robson.[108] They reported that circumcised boys are at greater risk for staphylococcal colonization and infection.[108]

Others report that *S. aureus* carriage in infants (and subsequent infection) is most likely affected by multiple variables, including infant factors (antibiotics, surgical procedures [circumcision being the most common], duration of hospital stay as a newborn), maternal factors (previous colonization, previous antibiotic usage, mode of delivery, length of stay), and environmental factors (MRSA in the family or hospital, nursery stay versus rooming-in, hand hygiene).[98,105,109–113] Gerber et al.[101] from the Chicago area published a consensus statement for the management of MRSA outbreaks in the NICU. The recommendations, which were strongly supported by experimental, clinical, and epidemiologic data, included using a waterless, alcohol-based hand-hygiene product, monitoring and enforcing hand hygiene, placing MRSA-positive infants in contact precautions with cohorting if possible, using gloves and gowns for direct contact and masks for aerosol-generating procedures, cohorting nurses for the care of MRSA-positive infants when possible, periodic screening of infants for MRSA using nares or nasopharyngeal cultures, clarifying the MRSA status of infants being transferred into the NICU, limiting overcrowding, and maintaining ongoing instruction and monitoring of health care workers in their compliance with infection-control and hand-hygiene procedures. The evaluation of the outbreak could include screening of health care workers and environmental surfaces to corroborate epidemiologic data and laboratory molecular analysis of the MRSA strains if indicated epidemiologically. The use of mupirocin or other decolonizing procedures should be determined on an individual basis for each NICU.

S. aureus is the most common cause of mastitis in lactating women.[114–117] Recurrence or persistence of symptoms of mastitis is a well-described occurrence and an important issue in the management of mastitis. Community-acquired MRSA has been associated with mastitis as well[105,116,118] (see Chapter 16 for a complete discussion of mastitis).

Two studies, one from France and one from Brazil, investigated the occurrence of MRSA in expressed breast milk.[119,120] Barbe et al.[119] cultured 9171 expressed breast-milk samples from 378 women and tested 2351 samples before pasteurization and 6820 samples after pasteurization. MRSA and methicillin-susceptible *S. aureus* were identified, respectively, in 8 samples (0.8%) from 3 mothers and 281 samples (19.3%) from 73 mothers, using the tested expressed breast milk before pasteurization. After pasteurization, *S. aureus* was not detected in any of the 6820 samples of expressed breast milk. Colonization of one infant with MRSA was identified, but no

MRSA infections were identified in any of the hospitalized infants in the NICU during the 18 months of the study.[119] Novak et al.[120] identified MRSA in 57 of 500 samples (11%) of expressed fresh-frozen milk from 500 different donors from five Brazilian milk banks. Only 3 of the 57 samples were positive with high-level bacterial counts of MRSA (greater than 10,000 CFU/mL). These were the only samples that would not have been acceptable by bacteriologic criteria according to Brazilian or American criteria for raw milk use. They did not investigate other epidemiologic data to identify possible variables associated with low- or high-level contamination of expressed breast milk with MRSA.[120]

The management of an infant and/or mother with MRSA infection, relative to breastfeeding or the use of breast milk, should be based on the severity of disease and whether the infant is premature, LBW, very low-birth-weight (VLBW), previously ill, or full term.

When full-term infants or their mothers develop mild to moderate infections (impetigo, pustulosis, cellulitis/abscess, mastitis/breast abscess, or soft tissue infection), those infants can continue breastfeeding. An initial evaluation for other evidence of infection should be done in the maternal–infant dyad, the infected child and/or mother should be placed on "commonly" effective therapy for the MRSA infection, and ongoing observation for clinical disease should continue. The mother and infant can "room-in" together in the hospital, if necessary, with standard and contact precautions. Culturing the breast milk is not necessary. Empiric therapy for the infant may be chosen based on medical concerns for the infant and the known sensitivity testing of the MRSA isolate. Appropriate antibiotic choices include short-term use of azithromycin (erythromycin use during infancy [younger than 6 weeks of age] is associated with an increased risk for hypertrophic pyloric stenosis), sulfamethoxazole-trimethoprim (in the absence of G6PD deficiency and older than 30 days of age), clindamycin (short course, 3 to 5 days), and perhaps linezolid for mild to moderate infections.

When infants in NICUs (premature, LBW, VLBW, and/or previously ill) or their mothers have an MRSA infection, those infants should have the breast milk cultured and suspend breastfeeding or receiving breast milk from their mothers until the breast milk is shown to be culture-negative for MRSA. The infant should be treated as indicated for infection or empirically treated if symptomatic (with pending culture results) and closely observed for the development of new signs or symptoms of infection. Pumping to maintain the milk supply and the use of banked breast milk are appropriate. The infant should be placed on contact precautions, in addition to the routine standard precautions. The infant can be cohorted with other MRSA-positive infants, with nursing care cohorted as well. The mother with MRSA infection should be instructed concerning hand hygiene; the careful collection, handling, and storage of breast milk; contact precautions to be used with her infant; and the avoidance of contact with any other infants. The mother can receive several possible antibiotics for MRSA that are compatible with breastfeeding when used for a short period. If the mother remains clinically well, including without evidence of mastitis, but her breast milk is positive for MRSA greater than 10^4 CFU/mL, empiric therapy to diminish or eradicate colonization would be appropriate. Various regimens have been proposed to "eradicate" MRSA colonization, but no single one has been proven to be highly efficacious. These regimens usually include systemic antibiotics with one or two medications (rifampin added as the second medication), as well as nasal mupirocin to the nares twice daily for 1 to 2 weeks with routine hygiene, with or without the usage of hexachlorophene (or similar topical agent or cleanser) for bathing during the 1- to 2-week treatment period. There is no clear information concerning the efficacy of using similar colonization-eradication regimens for other household members or pets in preventing recolonization of the mother or infant. Before reintroducing the use of the mother's breast milk to the infant, at least one negative breast-milk culture should be obtained after the completion of therapy.

The routine screening of breast milk provided by mothers for their infants in NICUs for the presence of MRSA is not indicated in the absence of MRSA illness in the maternal–infant dyad, an MRSA outbreak in NICUs, or a high frequency of MRSA infection in a specific NICU.

Toxin-Mediated *Staphylococcus* Disease

One case of staphylococcal scalded skin syndrome (SSSS) was reported by Katzman and Wald[121] in an infant breastfed by a mother with a lesion on her areola that did not respond to ampicillin therapy for 14 days. Subsequently, the infant developed conjunctivitis with *S. aureus*, which produced an exfoliative toxin, and a confluent erythematous rash without mucous membrane involvement or Nikolsky sign. No attempt to identify the exfoliative toxin in the breast milk was made, and the breast milk was not cultured for *S. aureus*. The child responded to IV therapy with nafcillin. This emphasizes the importance of evaluating the mother and infant at the time of a suspected infection and the need for continued observation of the infant for evidence of a pyogenic infection or toxin-mediated disease, especially with maternal mastitis or breast lesions.

This case also raises the issue of when and how infants and their mothers become colonized with *S. aureus* and what factors lead to infection and illness in each. The concern is that *Staphylococcus* can be easily transmitted through skin-to-skin contact, colonization readily occurs, and potentially serious illness can occur later, long after colonization. In the case of staphylococcal scalded skin syndrome or toxic shock syndrome (TSS), the primary site of infection can be insignificant (e.g., conjunctivitis, infection of a circumcision, or simple pustulosis), but a clinically significant amount of toxin can be produced and lead to serious disease.

TSS can result from *S. aureus* or *Streptococcus pyogenes* infection and probably from a variety of antigens produced by other organisms. TSS-1 has been identified as a "superantigen" that affects the T lymphocytes and other components of the immune response, producing an unregulated and excessive immune response and resulting in an overwhelming systemic clinical response. TSS has been reported in association with vaginal delivery, cesarean delivery, mastitis, and other local infections in mothers. Mortality rates in mothers may be as high as 5%.

The case definition of staphylococcal TSS includes meeting all four major criteria: fever greater than 38.9°C, rash (diffuse macular erythroderma), hypotension, and desquamation (associated with subepidermal separation seen on skin biopsy). The definition also includes the involvement of three or more organ systems (GI, muscular, mucous membrane, renal, hepatic, hematologic, or CNS); negative titers for Rocky Mountain spotted fever, leptospirosis, and rubeola; and lack of isolation of *S. pyogenes* from any source or *S. aureus* from the cerebrospinal fluid (CSF).[122] A similar case definition has been proposed for streptococcal TSS.[123] Aggressive empiric antibiotic therapy against staphylococci and streptococci and careful supportive therapy are essential for decreasing illness and death. Oxacillin, nafcillin, first-generation cephalosporins, clindamycin, erythromycin, and vancomycin are acceptable antibiotics, even for a breastfeeding mother. The severity of illness in the mother may preclude breastfeeding, but it can be reinitiated when the mother is improving and wants to restart. Standard precautions, with breastfeeding, are recommended.

Staphylococcal enterotoxin F has been identified in breast-milk specimens collected on days 5, 8, and 11 from a mother who developed TSS at 22 hours postpartum.[124] *S. aureus* that produced staphylococcal enterotoxin F was isolated from the mother's vagina but not from breast milk. The infant and mother lacked significant levels of antibodies against staphylococcal enterotoxin F in their sera. The infant remained healthy after 60 days of follow-up. Staphylococcal enterotoxin F is pepsin inactivated at pH 4.5 and therefore is probably destroyed in the stomach environment, presenting little or no risk to the breastfeeding infant.[125] Breastfeeding can continue if the mother is able.

Coagulase-Negative *Staphylococcus*

Coagulase-negative staphylococcal infection (*S. epidermidis* is the predominant isolate) produces minimal disease in healthy, full-term infants but is a significant problem in hospitalized or premature infants. Factors associated with increased risk for this infection include prematurity, high colonization rates in specific nurseries, invasive therapies (e.g., IV lines, chest tubes, intubation), and antibiotic use. Illness produced by coagulase-negative staphylococci can be invasive and severe in high-risk neonates but rarely in mothers. There are reports of necrotizing enterocolitis associated with coagulase-negative *Staphylococcus*. At 2 weeks of age, for infants still in the nursery, *S. epidermidis* is a frequent colonizing organism at multiple sites, with colonization rates as high as 75% to 100%. Serious infections with coagulase-negative staphylococci (e.g., abscesses, IV-line infection, bacteremia/sepsis, endocarditis, osteomyelitis) require effective IV therapy. Many strains are resistant to penicillin and the semisynthetic penicillins, so sensitivity testing is essential. Empiric or definitive therapy may require treatment with vancomycin, gentamicin, rifampin, teicoplanin, linezolid, or combinations of these for synergistic activity. Transmission of infection in association with breastfeeding appears to be no more common than with bottle-feeding. As with *S. aureus*, infection control includes contact and standard precautions. Occasionally, during presumed outbreaks, careful epidemiologic surveillance may be required, including cohorting, limiting overcrowding and understaffing, surveillance cultures of infants and nursery personnel, reemphasis on meticulous infection-control techniques for all individuals entering the nursery, and rarely, removal of colonized personnel from direct infant contact.

S. epidermidis is one of the most common organisms identified by molecular studies in human breast milk.[126] It has been identified as part of the fecal microbiota of thriving breast-fed infants.[127] *S. epidermidis* has also been identified in the breast milk of women with clinical evidence of mastitis.[128] Nevertheless, *S. epidermidis* is rarely associated with infection in full-term infants. Conceivably, breast milk for premature infants could be a source of *S. epidermidis* colonization in the NICUs. The benefits of early full human milk feeding potentially outweigh the risk for colonization with *S. epidermidis* via breast milk.[129] Ongoing education and assistance should be provided to mothers about the careful collection, storage, and delivery of human breast milk for their premature infants.[130]

STREPTOCOCCAL INFECTIONS

Group A Streptococcus

S. pyogenes (β-hemolytic group A *Streptococcus* [GAS]) is a common cause of skin and throat infections in children, producing pharyngitis, cellulitis, and impetigo. Illnesses produced by GAS can be classified into three categories: (1) impetigo, cellulitis, or pharyngitis without invasion or complication; (2) severe invasive infection with bacteremia, necrotizing fasciitis, myositis, or systemic illness (e.g., streptococcal TSS); and (3) autoimmune-mediated phenomena, including acute rheumatic fever and acute glomerulonephritis. GAS can also cause puerperal sepsis, endometritis, and neonatal omphalitis. Significant morbidity and mortality rates are associated with invasive GAS infection; the mortality rate is 20% to 50%, with almost half the survivors requiring extensive tissue debridement or amputation.[131] Infants are not at risk for the autoimmune sequelae of GAS (rheumatic fever or poststreptococcal glomerulonephritis). Transmission is through direct contact (rarely indirect contact) and droplet spread. Outbreaks of GAS in the nursery are rare, unlike with staphylococcal infections. Either the mother or infant can be initially colonized with GAS and transmit it to the other.

In the situation of maternal illness (extensive cellulitis, necrotizing fasciitis, myositis, pneumonia, TSS, and mastitis), it is appropriate to continue breastfeeding and use breast milk. The mother can readily receive effective therapy (penicillin, ampicillin, cephalosporins, and erythromycin), the infant can be observed expectantly, and breastfeeding can continue.

Group B Streptococcus

Group B *Streptococcus* (GBS, *Streptococcus agalactiae*) is a significant cause of perinatal bacterial infection. In parturient women, infection can lead to asymptomatic bacteriuria,

urinary tract infection (often associated with premature birth), endometritis, or amnionitis. In infants, infection usually occurs between birth and 3 months of age (1 to 4 cases per 1000 live births). It is routinely classified by the time of onset of illness in the infant: early onset (0 to 7 days, majority less than 24 hours) and late onset (7 to 90 days, generally less than 4 weeks). Infants may develop sepsis, pneumonia, meningitis, osteomyelitis, arthritis, or cellulitis.

Early-Onset GBS Disease

Early-onset GBS disease (EOD) is often fulminant, presenting as sepsis or pneumonia with respiratory failure; three-quarters of neonatal disease is early onset. A recent review showed that the estimated pooled incidence of invasive GBS disease in infants was 0.49 per 1000 live births (95% CI 0.43 to 0.56). The rate was highest in Africa (1.12) and lowest in Asia (0.30). EOD incidence was 0.41 (95% CI 0.36 to 0.47); late-onset disease incidence was 0.26 (95% CI 0.21 to 0.30). The estimated case-fatality rate (CFR) was 8.4% (95% CI 6.6% to 10.2%). Serotype III (61.5%) dominated, with 97% of cases caused by serotypes Ia, Ib, II, III, and V.[132]

Transmission is believed to occur in utero and during delivery. Colonization rates of mothers and infants vary between 5% and 35%. Postpartum transmission is thought to be uncommon, although it has been documented. Risk factors for EOD include delivery before 37 weeks of gestation, rupture of membranes for longer than 18 hours before delivery, intrapartum fever, heavy maternal colonization with GBS, or low concentrations of anti-GBS capsular antibody in maternal sera.[133] The common occurrence of severe GBS disease before 24 hours of age in neonates has led to prevention strategies. Revised guidelines developed by the AAP Committees on Infectious Diseases and on the Fetus and Newborn have tried to combine various variables for increased risk for GBS infection (prenatal colonization with GBS, obstetric and neonatal risk factors for EOD) and provide intrapartum antibiotic prophylaxis (IAP) to those at high risk[133,134] (Fig. 12.1). The utilization of these guidelines, universal culture-based screening, and IAP across the United States have decreased the incidence of EOD by approximately 80% from an estimated 1.4 cases of EOD per 1000 live births in 1990 to 0.28 cases per 1000 live births in 2009.[135] Within the United Kingdom, additional variables and interventions are being identified to further decrease EOD, including giving intrapartum antibiotics to the mother whenever there is prolonged rupture of membranes, regardless of gestational age,[136] and utilizing rapid PCR testing for GBS at presentation for delivery to identify additional infants exposed to GBS and initiate IAP.[137] Researchers in Hong Kong have also noted that the implementation of "universal GBS screening" and improved GBS testing could allow enhanced IAP and decrease EOD in full-term infants.[138] However, there is no clear international consensus, and research is ongoing to develop an optimal evidence-based guideline.[139,140]

Late-Onset Disease GBS

The incidence of late-onset GBS disease (LOD) remains unchanged since 1990 (approximately 0.3 to 0.4 cases per 1000

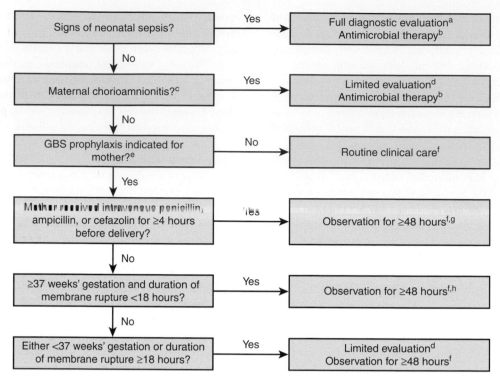

Fig. 12.1 Recommendations for empiric assessment/management of a neonate to prevent early-onset group B streptococcus (GBS) disease. This algorithm is not an exclusive course of management. Variations that incorporate individual circumstances or institutional preferences may be appropriate. (From Committee on Infectious Diseases, American Academy of Pediatrics. Group B streptococcal infections. In: Kimberlin DW, et al. eds. *Red Book: 2018 Report of the Committee on Infectious Diseases.* 31st ed. Itasca, IL: American Academy of Pediatrics; 2018: 762−768, Fig. 3.9, p. 767.)

[a]Full diagnostic evaluation includes complete blood cell (CBC) count with differential, platelets, blood culture, chest radiograph (if respiratory abnormalities are present), and lumbar puncture (if patient stable enough to tolerate procedure and sepsis is suspected).

[b]Antimicrobial therapy should be directed toward the most common causes of neonatal sepsis, including GBS and gram negative pathogens, and should take into account local antimicrobial resistance patterns.

[c]Consultation with obstetric providers is important to determine the level of clinical suspicion of chorioamnionitis.

[d]Limited evaluation includes blood culture (at birth) and CBC count with differential and platelets (at birth and/or at 6-12 hours of life).

[e]GBS prophylaxis indicated if one or more of the following: (1) mother GBS positive at 35−37 weeks gestation; (2) GBS status unknown with one or more intrapartum risk factors, including < 37 weeks gestation, rupture of membranes > or = 18 hours or temperature > or = 100.4°F (38.0° C) or intrapartum nucleic acid amplification test results positive for GBS; (3) GBS bacteriuria during current pregnancy; (4) history of previous infant with GBS disease.

[f]If signs of sepsis develop, a full diagnostic evaluation should be performed and antimicrobial therapy should be initiated.

[g]If > or = 37 weeks gestation, observation may occur at home after 24 hours if other discharge criteria have been met, if there is a knowledgeable observer and ready access to medical care.

[h]Some experts recommend a CBC with differential and platelets at 6 to 12 hours of age.

live births) despite[141] the implementation of screening and guidelines for preventing EOD (GBS Prevention Working Group). LOD is thought to be the result of transmission during delivery or in the postnatal period from maternal, hospital, or community sources. Dillon et al.[142] demonstrated that 10 of 21 infants with late-onset disease were colonized at birth, but the source of colonization was unidentified in the others. Gardner et al.[143] showed that only 4.3% of 46 children who were culture-negative for GBS at discharge from the hospital had acquired GBS by 2 months of age. Anthony et al.[144] noted that many infants are colonized with GBS, but the actual attack rate for GBS disease is low and difficult to predict.

GBS and Breast Milk

Acquisition of GBS through breast milk or breastfeeding was previously believed to be uncommon, but there are more recent reports of GBS transmission via breast milk, and it remains a controversial topic.[145−147] Roca et al. reported from Gambia, in a study of 377 maternal-infant pairs, that maternal colonization was associated with neonatal GBS carriage at 6 days of age. They reported an adjusted odds ratio (aOR) of 3.75 (95% CI, 1.32 to 10.65) for maternal colonization of breast milk and an aOR of 3.42 (95% CI, 1.27 to 9.22) for maternal GBS colonization of the vaginal tract.[148] A number of cases of LOD associated with GBS in maternal milk have been reported.[149−153] Some of the mothers in these reports had bilateral mastitis, at least one had delayed evidence of unilateral mastitis, and the others were asymptomatic. It was not clear when colonization of the infants occurred or when infection or disease began in the infants. The authors discussed the possibility that the infants were originally colonized during delivery, subsequently colonized the mothers' breasts during breastfeeding, and then became reinfected at a later time. Butter and DeMoor[154] showed that infants initially colonized on their heads at birth had GBS cultured from the throat, nose, or umbilicus 8 days later. Whenever they cultured GBS from the nipples of mothers, the authors also found it in the nose or throat of the infants.

Berardi et al.[155] studied GBS colonization prospectively in 160 mother–infant dyads. They noted that few culture-positive women had GBS cultured from their milk through 60 days after hospital discharge. Neonates who were colonized at more than one site (throat, ear, or rectum) were most commonly born to culture-positive carrier mothers who were GBS positive at delivery. One of the three cases of neonatal GBS infection presented as LOD at 35 days of age, and one presented with EOD at birth. The third infant presented with EOD at 20 hours of age and was adequately treated. That same infant was retreated at 18 days of age for a GBS urinary tract infection. They concluded that there was no evidence that mother's milk was the cause of the neonatal infections and that the occurrence of GBS in human milk could have been contamination or colonization from infants who were already heavily colonized with GBS.[141] Filleron et al.[146] reviewed 48 cases in the literature of late-onset neonatal infection (LONI) associated with GBS and breast milk. They noted four cases of LONI that occurred in the absence of maternal GBS detection, in infants born by cesarean section, and with GBS-positive mother's milk as the probable source of infection. Their analysis also demonstrated a high rate of recurrence of LONI; 35% of the 48 neonates had more than one LONI. They concluded,[146] as others have recommended (Berardi et al.,[141] Byrne et al.,[149] Lombard et al.,[156] and Davanzo et al.[157]), that additional attention should be given to the handling and use of raw human milk in "vulnerable" neonates and instances of GBS culture-positive human milk with or without maternal mastitis. Byrne et al.[149] presented a review of GBS disease associated with breastfeeding and made recommendations to decrease the risk for transmission of GBS to infants via breastfeeding or breast milk. Some of their recommendations included confirming appropriate collection and processing procedures for GBS cultures[158] in medical facilities to decrease false-negative cultures; reviewing proper hygiene for pumping, collection, and storage of expressed breast milk with mothers; reviewing the signs and symptoms of mastitis with mothers; and utilizing banked human milk as needed instead of mother's milk.

Proposed Guidance for GBS and Human Milk

Davanzo et al.[157] describe proposed "best-practice guidance" for managing human milk feeding and group B *Streptococcus* in developed countries. This guidance includes the following: (1) Do not routinely perform microbial cultures of breast milk from the mother of the term or preterm infant. (2) Interruption of breastfeeding in most situations of maternal mastitis and healthy full-term infants is unnecessary, but conservative management, including milk removal, supportive measures, and antibiotics for the mother, are appropriate if her symptoms persist or worsen. (3) In the case of mastitis in mothers of preterm infants, drain the affected breast, culture the milk, and treat the mother empirically. If the milk is GBS-positive, then the milk should either be pasteurized before giving it to the premature infant or discarded until there is a subsequent negative culture of the milk. (4) Prevention and management strategies for EOD GBS infection should follow the revised CDC guidelines from 2010 and the more recent recommendations for the prevention of perinatal GBS disease from the AAP's Committee on Infectious Diseases and Committee on Fetus and Newborn (2011)[134] and the *Red Book: 2018 Report of the Committee on Infectious Diseases.*[133] These documents do not recommend routine discontinuation of breastfeeding, discarding breast milk, or pasteurization of breast milk after EOD GBS because there is no evidence that this is protective against LOD GBS. (5) In the situation of LOD GBS disease and a positive breast-milk culture for GBS, treat the mother to eradicate colonization (ampicillin or amoxicillin plus rifampin), pasteurize or discard breast milk until adequate therapy has been given to the mother or there is a negative breast-milk culture, track breast-milk cultures through hospitalization, and consider adding rifampin to the infant's antibiotic treatment to eradicate colonization in the infant, even though the "eradication" of colonization is difficult and inconsistent.

GBS infection in neonates and colonization back and forth between the mother and infant are different from what is seen with other common bacterial pathogens in neonates. The debate continues relative to human breast milk's role in GBS LOD. Even for specific potentially useful interventions (culturing breast milk, stopping use of breast milk, or antibiotics to eradicate colonization), there is insufficient data to establish an evidence-based set of guidelines.[159,160] When a breastfed infant develops GBS LOD, it is appropriate to culture the milk. (See discussion of culturing breast milk earlier in this chapter.) Consider treatment of the mother to prevent reinfection if the milk is culture-positive for GBS (greater than 10^4 CFU/mL), with or without clinical evidence of mastitis in the mother. Withholding the mother's milk until it is confirmed to be culture-negative GBS may be appropriate in certain situations and should be accompanied by providing ongoing support and instruction to the mother concerning pumping and maintaining her milk supply. Serial culturing of expressed breast milk after the treatment of the mother for GBS disease or colonization would be appropriate to ensure the ongoing absence of the pathogen in the expressed breast milk in situations where reinfection as a result of infant susceptibility is high. There are reports of reinfection of the infant from breast milk.[146,156,157,161,162] Eradication of GBS mucosal colonization in the infant or the mother may be difficult. Some authors have recommended the use of rifampin or rifampicin prophylactically in both the mother and infant at the end of treatment to eradicate mucosal colonization.[161,163] (See Chapter 16 for the management of mastitis in the mother.) A mother or infant colonized or infected with GBS should be managed with standard precautions while in the hospital. Ongoing close evaluation of the infant for infection or illness and empiric therapy for GBS in the infant are appropriate until the child has remained well and cultures are subsequently negative at 72 hours. Occasionally, epidemiologic investigation in the hospital will utilize the culturing of medical staff and family members to detect a source of LOD in the nursery. This can be useful when more than one case of LOD is detected with the same serotype. Cohorting in such a situation may be appropriate Selective prophylactic therapy for colonized infants to eradicate colonization may be considered, but unlike GAS or *Staphylococcus* infection, GBS infection in nurseries has not been reported to cause outbreaks. No data support conducting GBS screening on all breastfeeding mothers and their expressed breast milk as a reasonable method for protecting against the spread of GBS infection via expressed breast milk or LOD GBS infection. Selective culturing of expressed breast milk may be appropriate in certain situations.

Tuberculosis

The face of TB is changing throughout the world but is still driven by poverty, HIV coinfection, multidrug-resistant TB (MDR-TB), and migration. In the United States, the incidence of TB rose from 1986 through 1993 and has been declining since then.[164] In 2017 the incidence rate was 2.8 cases per 100,000 population, which represents a decrease of 2.5% from 2016 to 2017. In 2017 the WHO reported an estimated 10 million new cases of TB (133 cases per 100,000 population), which was a 1.8% decline from 2016. The number of deaths resulting from TB also declined by 3.9% from 2016 to 2017, but the case fatality was still 15.7%.[165]

TB During Pregnancy

TB during pregnancy has always been a significant concern for patients and physicians alike.[166] It is now clear that the course and prognosis of TB in pregnancy are less affected by the pregnancy and more determined by HIV coinfection, MDR-TB, the location and extent of disease (as defined primarily by chest radiograph), and the susceptibility of the individual patient. Historically, untreated TB in pregnancy was associated with maternal and infant mortality rates of 30% to 40%.[167] More recent studies have not supported the idea that pregnancy predisposes to worse outcomes of TB.[168] A recent systematic review and meta-analysis also did not show increased maternal mortality compared with pregnant women without TB. There was an increase in maternal and neonatal morbidity, including anemia, cesarean delivery, miscarriage, preterm birth, LBW, acute fetal distress, asphyxia, and perinatal death compared with pregnancies without TB in the mother.[169] Effective therapy is crucial to the clinical outcome in both pregnant and nonpregnant women. TB during pregnancy rarely results in congenital TB, although congenital TB has a mortality rate as high as 50%.[170] A case review and review of the literature from 2011 reported that before 1994, the mortality of congenital TB was 52.6%, and after 1994, the mortality was 33.9%. Data on morbidity in congenital TB was associated with earlier age at the onset of symptoms and the existence of intracranial lesions.[171] Any individual in a high-risk group for TB should be screened with a tuberculin skin test (TST). No contraindication or altered responsiveness to the TST exists during pregnancy or breastfeeding. Interpretation of the TST should follow the most recent guidelines, using different sizes of induration in different-risk populations as cutoffs for a positive test, as proposed by the CDC.[172] Fig. 12.2 outlines the evaluation and treatment of a pregnant woman with a positive TST.[173]

Treatment of active TB should begin as soon as the diagnosis is made, regardless of the fetus's gestational age, because the risk for disease to mother and fetus clearly outweighs the risks of treatment. Isoniazid, rifampin, and ethambutol have been used safely in all three trimesters. Isoniazid and pyridoxine therapy during breastfeeding is safe.[174,175] There is a low risk for hepatotoxicity in the mother during the first 2 to 3 months postpartum.[176,177]

Congenital TB is extremely rare, if one considers that 9 to 10 million new cases of TB occur each year worldwide and that less than 300 cases of congenital TB have been reported in the literature. As with other infectious diseases presenting in the perinatal period, distinguishing congenital infection from perinatal or postnatal TB in infants can be difficult. The Spanish Society for Pediatric Infectious Diseases has published guidelines for the diagnosis of congenital TB.[178]

Postnatal TB infection in infancy typically presents with severe disease and extrapulmonary extension (meningitis; lymphadenopathy; and bone, liver, spleen involvement). Airborne transmission of TB to infants is the major mode of postnatal infection because of close and prolonged exposure in enclosed spaces, especially in their own household, to any adult with infectious pulmonary TB. Potential infectious sources could be the mother or any adult caregiver, such as babysitters, daycare workers, relatives, friends, neighbors, and even health care workers. Mittal et al. recently reviewed the management of the newborn infant exposed to the mother with TB.[179]

TB Exposure for a Neonate or Infant

The suspicion of TB infection or disease in a household with possible exposure of an infant is a highly anxiety-provoking situation (Fig. 12.3). Although protecting an infant from infection is foremost in everyone's mind, separation of the infant from the mother should be avoided when reasonable. Every situation is unique, and the best approach will vary according to the specifics of the case and accepted principles of TB management. The first step in caring for the potentially exposed infant is to determine accurately the true TB status of the suspected case (mother or household contact). This prompt evaluation should include a complete history (previous TB infection or disease; previous or ongoing TB treatment; TST status; symptoms suggestive of active TB; results of most recent chest radiograph, sputum smears, or cultures), physical examination, a TST if indicated, a new chest radiograph, and mycobacterial cultures and smears of any suspected sites of infection. All household contacts should be evaluated promptly, including history and TST, with further evaluation as indicated.[172] Continued risk to the infant can occur from infectious household contacts who have not been effectively evaluated and treated.

When the mother and infant are hospitalized at the initiation of concern for maternal TB, the infant should be

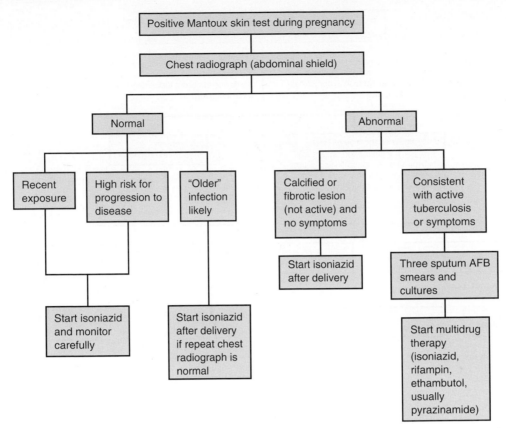

Fig. 12.2 Evaluation and treatment of a pregnant woman with a positive tuberculin skin test. *AFB,* Acid-fast bacilli. (From Starke JR. Tuberculosis, an old disease but a new threat to mother, fetus, and neonate. *Clin Perinatol.* 1997;24:107.)

temporarily separated from the mother or other adult as the suspected source if symptoms suggest active disease or a recent TST documents conversion, and separation should continue until the results of the chest radiograph of the possible source are seen. Because of considerable variability in the course of illness and the concomitant infectious period, debate continues without adequate data about the appropriate period of separation.[180,181] This should be individualized given the specific situation. HIV testing and assessment of the risk for MDR-TB should be done in every case of active TB. Sensitivity testing should be done on every *M. tuberculosis* isolate from a pregnant or lactating woman. Table 12.1 summarizes the management of the newborn infant whose mother (or other household contact) has TB.

Initiation of prophylactic isoniazid therapy in the infant has been demonstrated to be effective in preventing TB infection and disease in the infant. Therefore continued separation of the infant and mother is unnecessary after therapy in both mother and child has begun.[182] The AAP recommends isoniazid (INH) prophylaxis for all infants whose mothers have been diagnosed with active pulmonary TB in the postpartum period. The real risk requiring infant separation is airborne transmission. Separation of the infant from a mother with active pulmonary TB is appropriate, regardless of the method of feeding. However, in many parts of the world, when effective antituberculous therapy in the mother and prophylaxis with isoniazid in the infant have begun, the infant and mother

are not separated.[178] With or without separation, the mother and infant should continue to be closely observed throughout the course of maternal therapy to ensure good compliance with medication by both mother and infant and to identify, early on, any symptoms in the infant suggestive of TB. The mother should be followed to confirm that she is no longer considered infectious, with negative smears and cultures within 2 to 4 weeks of beginning TB therapy.

Tuberculous mastitis occurs rarely in the United States, and it is uncommon even in other parts of the world.[183–192] Tuberculosis mastitis can lead to infection in infants, frequently involving the tonsils. A mother usually has a single breast mass and associated axillary lymph node swelling and infrequently develops a draining sinus. TB of the breast can also present as a painless mass or edema. Involvement of the breast can occur with or without evidence of disease at other sites. Evaluation of the extent of the disease is appropriate, including lesion cultures by needle aspiration, biopsy, or wedge resection and milk cultures. Therapy should be with multiple anti-TB medications, but surgery should supplement this, as needed, to remove extensive necrotic tissue or a persistently draining sinus.[193] Neither breastfeeding nor breast-milk feeding should be done until the lesion is healed, usually after 2 weeks or more of appropriate antituberculous medications. Continued anti-TB therapy for 6 months in the mother and prophylactic isoniazid for the infant for 3 to 6 months is indicated.

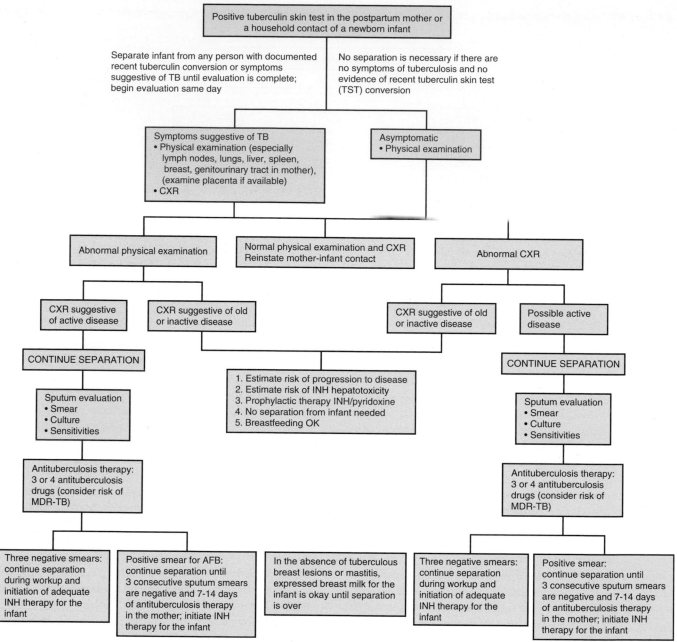

Fig. 12.3 Management of a newborn infant exposed to tuberculin-positive household contact. *CXR*, Chest X-ray film; *INH*, isoniazid; *MDR*, multidrug-resistant; *TB*, tuberculosis.

In the absence of tuberculous breast infection in the mother, the transmission of TB through breast milk has not been documented. Thus, even though temporary separation of the infant and mother may occur pending complete evaluation and initiation of adequate therapy in the mother and prophylactic isoniazid therapy (10 mg/kg per day as a single daily dose) in the infant, breast milk can be expressed and given to the infant during the short separation. Breastfeeding can safely continue when the mother, infant, or both are receiving anti-TB therapy. Anti-TB medications (isoniazid, rifampin, pyrazinamide, aminoglycosides, ethambutol, ethionamide, p-aminosalicylic acid) have been safely used in infancy, and therefore, the presence of these medications in smaller amounts in breast milk is not a contraindication to breastfeeding.

Breastfeeding and Tuberculin Skin Test

Conflicting reports indicate that breastfeeding by TST-positive mothers does influence infants' responses to the bacille Calmette-Guérin vaccine, the TST, and perhaps the *M. tuberculosis* bacillus. Despite efforts to identify either a soluble substance or specific cell fractions (gamma/delta T cells) in colostrum and breast milk that affect infants' immune responsiveness, no unified theory explains the various reported changes, and no evidence has identified a consistent, clinically significant effect.[194–197]

TABLE 12.1 Management of a Newborn Whose Mother (or Other Household Contact) Has Tuberculosis (TB) Infection

Mother–Infant Status	Additional Workup Recommended[a]	Therapy for Mother or Contact	Therapy for Infant	Separation[b]	Breast Milk[c]	Breastfeeding[d]
1. TB infection, no disease[d]	None for mother/contact	Prophylactic[e]	None	No	Yes	Yes
2. TB infection: Abnormal CXR not suggestive of active disease		Decide active vs. inactive disease				
a. Symptoms or physical findings suggestive of active TB	Aerosolized sputum (culture, smears)[f]	Active disease: Empiric[e]	Isoniazid[g]	Yes	Yes	No[h]
		Inactive disease: Prophylactic[e]	None	No	Yes	Yes
b. No symptoms or physical findings suggestive of active TB	Aerosolized sputum in select cases	Prophylactic[e]	None	No	Yes	Yes
3. TB infection: Abnormal CXR suggestive of active disease	Aerosolized sputum (culture, smears)[f]	Empiric therapy[e]	Isoniazid[g]	Yes	Yes	No[h]
4. Active pulmonary TB: Suspected MDR TB	Aerosolized sputum (culture, smears)[f]	Consult TB specialist for best regimen[i]	Consult pediatric TB specialist[i]	Yes	Yes	No
			Consider bacille Calmette-Guérin vaccine			
5. TB disease: Suspected mastitis[j]	Aerosolized sputum (culture, smears)[f]	Empiric[e]	Isoniazid[g]	Yes	No[k]	No
6. TB infection: Status undetermined[l]	Perform/interpret CXR within 24 hours			Yes, until CXR interpreted (see a and b)	Yes	No
a. Abnormal CXR not suggestive of active disease	Proceed as in 2		As in 2	As in 2	As in 2	
b. Abnormal CXR suggestive of active disease	Proceed as in 3		As in 3	As in 3	As in 3	

CXR, Chest x-ray; *MDR,* multidrug resistant.

[a]Further workup should always include the evaluation of the TB status of all other household (or close) contacts by tuberculin skin testing (TST), review of symptoms, physical examination, and CXR. Sputum smears and cultures should be done as indicated.

[b]Separation should occur until interpretation of CXR confirms the absence of active disease, or with active disease, separation should continue until the individual is no longer considered infectious: three negative consecutive sputum smears; adequate ongoing empiric therapy; and decreased fever, cough, and sputum production. *Separation* means movement to a different house or location, not simply separate rooms in a household. The duration of separation should be individualized for each case, in consultation with the TB specialist.

[c]This assumes no evidence of breast involvement, suspected TB mastitis, or lesions (except in status 5, when breast involvement is considered). The risk to the infant is via aerosolized bacteria in the sputum from the lung. Expressed breast milk can be given even if separation of mother and infant is advised.

[d]TST positive, no symptoms or physical findings suggestive of TB, negative CXR.

[e]Prophylactic therapy: isoniazid 10 mg/kg per day, maximum 300 mg for 6 months; pyridoxine 25 to 50 mg/day for 6 months. Empiric therapy: standard three- or four-drug regimens for 2 months, and treatment should continue for total of 6 months with isoniazid and rifampin when the organism is shown to be sensitive. Suspected MDR TB requires consultation with a TB specialist to select the optimum empiric regimen and for ongoing monitoring of therapy and clinical response.

ᶠSensitivity testing should be done on any positive culture.

ᵍIsoniazid 10 mg/kg per day for 3 to 9 months, depending on the mother's or contact's status; repeat TST at 3 months and obtain a normal CXR in the infant before stopping isoniazid. Before beginning therapy, a workup of the infant for congenital or active TB may be appropriate. This workup should be determined based on the clinical status of the infant and the suspected potential risk, and it may include TST after 4 weeks of age, with CXR, complete blood count, and erythrocyte sedimentation rate; liver function tests; cerebrospinal fluid analysis; gastric aspirates; and sonography or computed tomography of the liver, spleen, and chest if congenital TB is suspected.

ʰBreastfeeding is proscribed when the separation of the mother and infant is indicated because of the risk for aerosolized transmission of bacteria. Expressed breast milk given to the infant via bottle is acceptable in the absence of mastitis or breast lesions.

ⁱConsult with a TB specialist about MDR TB. Empiric therapy will be chosen based on the most recent culture sensitivities of the index patient or perhaps the suspected source case, if known, as well as medication toxicities and other factors.

ʲTB mastitis usually involves a single breast, with associated axillary lymph node swelling and, infrequently, a draining sinus tract. It can also present as a painless mass or edema of the breast.

ᵏWith suspected mastitis or breast lesions caused by TB, even breast milk is contraindicated until the lesion or mastitis heals, usually after 2 weeks or more.

ˡPatient has a documented, recent TST conversion but has not been completely evaluated. Evaluation should begin, and CXR should be done and evaluated in less than 24 hours to minimize the separation of this person from the infant. Further workup should proceed as indicated by symptoms, physical findings, and CXR results.

Data from the Committee on Infectious Diseases, American Academy of Pediatrics. *Red Book: Report of the Committee on Infectious Diseases.* 26th ed. Elk Grove Village, IL: American Academy of Pediatrics; 2003.

VIRAL INFECTIONS

Arboviruses

The term *arboviruses* describes a large collection of viruses grouped together because of the common mode of transmission through arthropods. They have now been reclassified into several different families: *Bunyaviridae, Togaviridae, Flaviviridae, Reoviridae,* and others. They include more than 30 human pathogens.

These organisms primarily produce either CNS infections (encephalitis, meningoencephalitis) or undifferentiated illnesses associated with fever and rash, severe hemorrhagic manifestations, and involvement of other organs (hepatitis, myalgia, polyarthritis). Infection with one of these viruses may also be asymptomatic and subclinical, although how often this occurs is uncertain. Some of the notable human pathogens include *Bunyaviridae* (California serogroup viruses), hantavirus, Hantaan virus, phlebovirus (Rift Valley fever), nairovirus (Crimean-Congo hemorrhagic fever), alphavirus (western, eastern, and Venezuelan equine encephalomyelitis viruses, chikungunya virus [CHIKV]), flavivirus (St. Louis encephalitis virus, Japanese encephalitis virus, dengue viruses, yellow fever virus, tick-borne encephalitis viruses, WNV), and orbivirus (Colorado tick fever). Other than for Crimean-Congo hemorrhagic fever and for reported cases of Colorado tick fever associated with transfusion, direct person-to-person spread has rarely been described. Outbreaks in 2005 and 2007 of CHIKV infection on Reunion Island and in India appear to have involved infection in young infants probably secondary to vertical spread from mother to infant transplacentally.[198–200] A few cases of early fetal deaths were associated with infection in pregnant women. The cases of vertical transmission occurred with near-term infection in the mothers, and the infants developed illness within 3 to 7 days of delivery.[198,199] No evidence for transmission via breast milk or breastfeeding is available.

Overall, little evidence indicates that these organisms can be transmitted through breast milk. The exceptions to this include evidence of transmission of three flaviviruses via breast milk: dengue virus, WNV, and yellow fever vaccine virus. Standard precautions are generally sufficient. With any of these infections in a breastfeeding mother, the severity of the illness may determine the mother's ability to continue breastfeeding. Providing the infant with expressed breast milk is acceptable. (See the discussion of dengue virus, WNV, and yellow fever vaccine virus later in this chapter.)

In general, treatment for these illnesses is supportive. However, ribavirin appears to decrease the severity of and mortality from hantavirus pulmonary syndrome, hemorrhagic fever with renal failure, and Crimean-Congo hemorrhagic fever. Ribavirin has been described as teratogenic in various animal species and is contraindicated in pregnant women. No information is available concerning ribavirin in breast milk, with limited information available on the use of IV or oral ribavirin in infants.[201]

Arenaviruses

Arenaviruses are single-stranded RNA viruses that infect rodents and are acquired by humans through the rodents. The six major human pathogens in this group are (1) lymphocytic choriomeningitis virus, (2) Lassa fever virus, (3) Junin virus (Argentine hemorrhagic fever), (4) Machupo virus (Bolivian hemorrhagic fever), (5) Guanarito virus (Venezuelan hemorrhagic fever), and (6) Sabia virus. The geographic distribution of these viruses and the illness they cause are determined by the living range of the host rodent (reservoir).[202] The exact mechanism of transmission to humans is unknown and hotly debated.[203–205] Direct contact and aerosolization of rodent excretions and secretions are probable mechanisms.

Lymphocytic choriomeningitis virus is well recognized in Europe, the Americas, and other areas. Perinatal maternal infection can lead to severe disease in the newborn, but no evidence suggests transmission through breast milk.[206,207] Standard precautions with breastfeeding are appropriate.

Lassa fever (West Africa) and Argentine hemorrhagic fever (Argentine pampas) are usually more severe illnesses, with dramatic bleeding and involvement of other organs, including the brain. These fevers more frequently lead to shock and death than do the forms of hemorrhagic fever caused by the other viruses in this group. Person-to-person spread of Lassa fever virus does occur, including transmission within households.[208] The possibility of persistent virus in human urine, semen, and blood after infection exists for each of the arenaviruses. The possibility of airborne transmission is undecided. Current recommendations by the CDC and others[204,209] are to use contact precautions for the duration of the illness in situations of suspected viral hemorrhagic fever. No substantial information describes the infectivity of various body fluids, including breast milk, for these different viral hemorrhagic fevers. Considering the severity of the illness in mothers and the risk to the infants, it is reasonable to avoid breastfeeding in these situations if alternative forms of infant nutrition can be provided for the short term.

As more information becomes available, reassessment of these recommendations is advisable. A vaccine is in trials in endemic areas for Junin virus and Argentine hemorrhagic fever.[210] Preliminary studies suggest it will be effective, but data are still being accumulated concerning the vaccine's use in children and pregnant or breastfeeding women.

Chikungunya Virus

CHIKV is an alphavirus transmitted most commonly through mosquitoes. Humans are the primary host of the virus during epidemics, but there is limited evidence of transmission from person to person.[211] Bloodborne transmission and intrapartum transmission have been documented. Disease varies from asymptomatic in 10% to 15% of people to symptomatic infection, which most commonly includes fever, polyarthralgia, headache, myalgia, hemorrhage, myelitis, conjunctivitis, nausea/vomiting, and maculopapular rash. Reports from around the world document vertical maternal-fetal transmission, both congenital and perinatal. Data from the epidemic on Reunion Island in 2005 to 2006 show varied results. Lenglet et al. described 160 pregnant women with CHIKV infection during pregnancy. Of these women, 151 had documented infection, 118 did not have viremia at delivery, and none showed congenital disease. Thirty-three mothers were viremic at delivery, and 16 infants demonstrated neonatal chikungunya infection.[212] Fritel et al. compared 658 women infected during pregnancy with 628 uninfected pregnant women in the prolonged epidemic on Reunion Island. Infection was reported to occur in the first trimester for 15% of women, in the second trimester for 59%, and in the third trimester for 26%.[213] There were more frequent hospitalizations in the infected group of women but no reported difference in cesarean deliveries, preterm birth, stillbirths after 22 weeks' gestational age, LBW, or congenital malformations after maternal infection compared with the uninfected women.[213] Separately, Ramful et al. retrospectively described 38 infected neonates from the same epidemic whose mothers presented with evidence of chikungunya infection at delivery or the infant themselves presented with illness within the first days of life. Neonatal symptomatology included pain (in 100% of cases), rash (82%), fever (79%), and peripheral edema (58%). Laboratory abnormalities included elevation of aspartate aminotransferase (77%), thrombocytopenia (76%), decreased prothrombin time (65%), and lymphopenia (47%) of infants. Neonatal

complications included seizures, hemorrhage/hemorrhagic disorders, and cardiac involvement (myocardial hypertrophy, ventricular dysfunction, coronary artery dilatation, and pericarditis). CSF was positive for real-time PCR (RT-PCR) testing in 22 of 24 cases, and magnetic resonance imaging (MRI) results were abnormal in 14 of 25 infants, with white-matter lesions or intraparenchymal hemorrhages noted.[199] Torres et al. reviewed congenital and perinatal complications of chikungunya fever (CHIKF) in Latin America. They described 169 symptomatic infants with CHIKF in four large maternity hospitals in three countries. The reported maternal-to-infant transmission rate ranged from 27.7% to 48.29%. Seventy-nine infected newborns were followed prospectively. The onset of illness was between 3 and 9 days after birth, and the CFR was 5.1% compared with reported CFRs from Reunion Island and Sri Lanka data ranging from 0 to 2.6%.[214] Gérardin et al. reported persistent disabilities in 30% to 45% of the children with apparent clinical CNS involvement.[215]

CHIKV has been detected once in a breastfeeding mother during CHIKV infection, but the infant was not ill and remained PCR and serology negative.[216] There is little other information to suggest CHIKV transmission is common or significant during breastfeeding. The benefits of continuing breastfeeding outweigh the possible protection from stopping breastfeeding with maternal CHIKV infection before delivery or during lactation in most situations.

Cytomegalovirus

CMV is one of the human herpesviruses. Congenital infection of infants, postnatal infection of premature infants, and infection of immune-deficient individuals represent the most serious forms of this infection in children. The gestational age or postconceptual age when the virus infects the fetus or infant, the presence of CMV in the breast milk (virolactia), the infant's immune susceptibility, and the presence or absence of antibodies against CMV provided to the infant by the mother (transplacentally acquired or in colostrum and breast milk)[217] are important determinants of the severity of infection and the likelihood of significant sequelae (congenital infection syndrome, deafness, chorioretinitis, abnormal neurodevelopment, learning disabilities).[218,219] About 1% of all infants are born excreting CMV at birth, and approximately 5% of these congenitally infected infants will demonstrate evidence of infection at birth (approximately 5 symptomatic cases per 10,000 live births). Approximately 15% of infants born after primary infection in a pregnant woman will manifest at least one sequela of prenatal infection.[220]

Various studies have detected that 3% to 28% of pregnant women have CMV in cervical cultures and that 4% to 5% of pregnant women have CMV in their urine.[221,222] Perinatal infection certainly occurs through contact with the virus in these fluids, but it is not usually associated with clinical illness in full-term infants. The lack of illness is thought to result from the transplacental passive transfer of protective antibodies from the mother.

Postnatal infection later in infancy occurs via breastfeeding or contact with infected fluids (e.g., saliva, urine), but again, it rarely causes clinical illness in full-term infants. Seroepidemiologic studies have documented the transmission of infection in infancy, with higher rates of transmission occurring in daycare centers, especially when the prevalence of CMV in the urine and saliva is high.

CMV and Breast Milk

CMV has been identified in the milk of CMV-seropositive women at varying rates (10% to 85%), using viral cultures or CMV DNA PCR.[222–225] CMV is more often identified in the breast milk of seropositive mothers than in vaginal fluids, urine, and saliva. The CMV isolation rate from colostrum is lower than that from mature milk.[222,226] The reason for the large degree of variability in the identification of CMV in breast milk in these studies probably relates to the intermittent nature of the reactivation and excretion of the virus, in addition to the variability, frequency, and duration of sampling of breast milk in the different studies. Some authors have hypothesized that the difference in isolation rates between breast milk and other fluids is caused by viral reactivation in cells (leukocytes or monocytes) in the breast leading to "selective" excretion in breast milk.[223] Vochem et al.[225] reported that the rate of virolactia was greatest at 3 to 4 weeks postpartum, and Yeager et al.[227] reported significant virolactia between 2 and 12 weeks postpartum. Antibodies (e.g., secretory IgA) to CMV are present in breast milk, along with various cytokines and other proteins (e.g., lactoferrin). These may influence the ability of the virus to bind to cells, but they do not completely prevent the transmission of infection.[218,223,228–232]

Several studies have documented increased rates of postnatal CMV infection in breastfed infants (50% to 69%) compared with bottle-fed infants (12% to 27%), observed through the first year of life.[221,224,225,230] In these same studies, full-term infants who acquired CMV infection postnatally were only rarely mildly symptomatic at the time of seroconversion or documented viral excretion. Also, no evidence of late sequelae from CMV was found in these infants.

Postnatal exposure of susceptible infants to CMV, including premature infants without passively acquired maternal antibodies against CMV, infants born to CMV-seronegative mothers, and immunodeficient infants, can cause significant clinical illness (pneumonitis, hepatitis, thrombocytopenia).[233–238] However, the clinical picture varies from asymptomatic to severely ill in various studies. In one study of premature infants followed up to 12 months, Vochem et al.[225] found CMV transmission in 17 of 29 infants (59%) exposed to CMV virolactia and breastfed, as compared with no infants among the 27 exposed to breast milk without CMV. No infant was given CMV-seropositive donor milk or blood. Five of the 12 infants who developed CMV infection after 2 months of age had mild signs of illness, including transient neutropenia, and only one infant had a short increase in episodes of apnea and a period of thrombocytopenia. Five other premature infants with CMV infection before 2 months of age had acute illness, including sepsis-like symptoms, apnea with bradycardia, hepatitis, leukopenia, and prolonged thrombocytopenia.[225] In a prospective study done in the United States, Josephson et al.[239] examined

the role of transfusions and breast milk causing CMV infection in VLBW infants. In the mothers, the seroprevalence of CMV was 76.2% (352/462). In 301 infants receiving 2061 transfusions of CMV-seronegative and leuko-reduced blood, there were no CMV infections linked to transfusion. Postnatal CMV infection had a cumulative incidence at 12 weeks after birth of 6.9% (95% CI, 4.2% to 9.2%), and 5 of 29 CMV-infected infants developed symptomatic disease or died. Twenty-seven of the 29 infants received CMV-positive breast milk. Factors associated with a higher risk of postnatal CMV infection were a higher CMV viral load in the breast milk and a higher number of breast-milk—fed days. This study also demonstrated that the use of CMV-seronegative and leuko-reduced blood products is effective at preventing transfusion-related CMV infection. In a systematic review and meta-analysis, Lanzieri et al.[240] utilized data from 17 studies published between 2001 and 2011. They reported on 299 infants who received untreated breast milk. Of these infants, 19% acquired CMV infection, and 4% developed a sepsis-like syndrome related to CMV infection. Among the 212 infants included who received thawed frozen breast milk (at various temperatures and durations in different studies—18°C to 20°C for over 24 hours or 72 hours), 13% developed CMV infection, and 5% had an associated sepsis-like syndrome. Although the overall rate of CMV infection related to breast milk was slightly lower in the untreated breast-milk group, there was no difference in the occurrence of sepsis-like syndrome in the two groups.

Relative to long-term sequelae related to postnatal CMV infection in VLBW infants, Vollmer et al.[241] followed premature infants with early postnatal CMV infection acquired through breast milk for 2 to 4.5 years to assess neurodevelopment and hearing function. None of the children had sensorineural hearing loss. There was no difference between the 22 CMV-infected children and 22 matched premature control CMV-negative infants in terms of neurologic, speech and language, or motor development.[241] In another small study, Jim et al. did not observe major adverse outcomes in growth, development, or hearing at 24 months of age for 14 infants infected via breast milk compared with 41 control preterm infants.[242] Neuberger et al.[243] examined the symptoms and neonatal outcome of CMV infection transmitted via human milk in premature infants in a case-control fashion; 40 CMV-infected premature infants were compared with 40 CMV-negative matched premature infants. Neutropenia, thrombocytopenia, and cholestasis were associated with CMV infection in these infants. No other serious effects or illnesses were found to be directly associated with the infection, including intraventricular hemorrhage; periventricular leukomalacia; retinopathy of prematurity; necrotizing enterocolitis; bronchopulmonary dysplasia; duration of mechanical ventilation or oxygen therapy; duration of hospital stay; or weight, gestational age, or head circumference at the time of discharge. More recent studies do not further clarify the long-term effects on the neurodevelopmental status of premature or LBW infants with symptomatic postnatal CMV infection.[242,244,245] They present contradictory evidence concerning the occurrence of adverse neurologic outcomes or sensorineural hearing loss in these children.

Exposure of CMV-seronegative, premature, or VLBW infants to CMV-positive milk (donor or natural mother's) should be avoided.[246]

Inactivation of CMV in Human Milk

Various methods of inactivating CMV in breast milk have been reported, including Holder's pasteurization (HP), short-term heat inactivation (5 seconds at 62°C), freezing-thawing (−20°C for 3 days), and brief high temperature (72°C for 10 seconds).[221,227,247,248] Although there is evidence that these procedures and microwave radiation[249] and ultraviolet-C (UV-C) irradiation[250] inactivate CMV, there are mixed results as to whether these treatments effectively decrease the risk of postnatal CMV transmission via breast milk.[251–255] One small prospective study suggests that freezing breast milk at −20°C for 72 hours protects premature infants from CMV infection via breast milk. Sharland et al.[246] reported on 18 premature infants (less than 32 weeks) who were uninfected at birth and exposed to breast milk from their CMV-seropositive mothers. Only 1 of 18 (5%) infants was positive for CMV at 62 days of life, and that infant was clinically asymptomatic. This transmission rate is considerably lower than others reported in the literature. CM-seronegative and leukocyte-depleted blood products were used routinely. Banked breast milk was pasteurized and stored at −20°C for various time periods, and maternal expressed breast milk was frozen at −20°C before use whenever possible. The infants received breast milk for a median of 34 days (range: 11 to 74 days), and they were observed for a median of 67 days (range: 30 to 192 days). Breast-milk samples pre- or postfreezing were not analyzed by PCR or culture for the presence of CMV.[246] Buxmann et al.[233] demonstrated no transmission of CMV in 23 premature infants (≤31 weeks' gestational age) receiving thawed frozen breast milk until 33 weeks (gestational age + postnatal age) born to 19 mothers who were CMV immunoglobulin G (IgG) negative. CMV infection was found in 5 premature infants of 35 infants born to 29 mothers who were CMV-IgG-positive and who provided breast milk for their infants. Three of the five children remained asymptomatic. One child developed a respirator-dependent pneumonia, and the second developed an upper respiratory tract infection and thrombocytopenia in association with the CMV infection.[233] Yasuda et al.[256] reported on 43 preterm infants (median gestational age 31 weeks), demonstrating a peak in CMV DNA copies, detected by RT-PCR assay, in breast milk at 4 to 6 weeks postpartum. Thirty of the 43 infants received CMV-DNA-positive breast milk. Three of the 30 had CMV DNA detected in their sera, but none of the three had symptoms suggestive of CMV infection. Much of the breast milk had been stored at −20°C before feeding, which the authors propose is the probable reason for less transmission in this cohort.[256] Lee et al.[257] reported on the use of maternal milk frozen at −20°C for a minimum of 24 hours before feeding to premature infants in an NICU; 23 infants had CMV-seropositive mothers, and 39 infants had CMV-seronegative mothers. Two infants developed CMV infection, which was symptomatic. They were both fed thawed frozen milk

from CMV-seropositive mothers.[257] Yoo et al. followed 385 extremely LBW infants for evidence of CMV infection. None of 62 infants receiving pasteurized breast milk were infected, whereas 27 of 301 (8%) infants fed thawed frozen breast milk had CMV infection. A lower gestational age and receiving >60% of total oral intake as thawed frozen breast milk in the first 8 weeks of life were associated with CMV infection. Bronchopulmonary dysplasia and an increased number of ventilator days were associated with postnatal CMV infection in this study.[258] Others have reported individual cases of CMV infection in premature infants despite freezing and thawing of breast milk.[259,260] More recent studies, including a prospective cohort study of breast-milk transmission of CMV by Josephson et al.[239] and a systematic review and meta-analysis of breast-milk-acquired CMV infection in VLBW and premature infants by Lanzieri et al.,[240] demonstrate that thawed frozen breast milk provides minimal protection, at best, against breast-milk-acquired CMV infection.[239,240] It is clear that the simple freezing and thawing of breast milk does not completely prevent transmission of CMV to premature and VLBW infants. Eleven of 36 neonatal units in Sweden (27 of which have their own milk banks) freeze maternal milk to reduce the risk for CMV transmission to premature infants.[260]

A prominent group of neonatologists and pediatric infectious disease experts in California, who recognize the significant benefits of providing human milk to premature and LBW infants, recommend screening mothers of premature infants for CMV IgG at delivery and, when an infant's mother is CMV IgG positive at delivery, using either pasteurized banked human milk or frozen and then thawed maternal breast milk for premature infants until they reach the age of 32 weeks.[261] In consideration of the low rates of CMV virolactia in colostrum[224,236] and the predominant occurrence of virolactia between 2 and 12 weeks (peak at 3 to 4 weeks) postpartum,[225,227] they reasonably propose beginning colostrum and breast-milk feedings for all infants until the maternal CMV serologic screening is complete. They recommend close observation and follow-up of premature infants older than 3 weeks of age for signs, symptoms, and laboratory changes of CMV infection until discharge from the hospital or out to 32 weeks postconceptual age.[261] Others are studying different treatments for breast milk to limit or prevent CMV transmission via breast milk while trying to maintain the nutrient and bioactive composition of human milk, including short-term pasteurization (62°C for 5 seconds, high-hydrostatic-pressure and UV-C irradiation).[250,255,262] Additional research and discussion will be necessary to devise guidelines for the use of human milk in premature and VLBW infants to optimize their growth, development, and immune protection while also preventing the risk of acquiring postnatal CMV infection. Our current understanding of the risk of CMV infection via breast milk for premature or LBW infants should be discussed with the mother and parents to facilitate an informed decision.

There has been much discussion of the use of CMV immunoglobulin and/or antiviral medications (acyclovir, ganciclovir, valganciclovir) to treat women during pregnancy to protect against congenital CMV infection. Although these agents have also been used to treat infants with symptomatic congenital CMV and symptomatic acute postnatal CMV infection, they have not been studied as prophylaxis against postnatal CMV infection.

Full-term infants can be safely fed human milk from CMV-seropositive mothers because despite a higher rate of CMV infection than in formula-fed infants observed through the first year of life, infection in this situation is not associated with significant clinical illness or acute or long-term sequelae.

Dengue Disease

Dengue viruses (DENV; serotypes dengue 1 to 4) are flaviviruses associated primarily with febrile illnesses and rash, dengue fever, dengue hemorrhagic fever, and dengue shock syndrome. The mosquitos *Aedes aegypti* and *Aedes albopictus* are the main vector of transmission of dengue virus in countries lying between latitudes 35 degrees north and 35 degrees south. DENV transmission has been documented via blood transfusion, bone marrow transplant, and solid-organ transplant and has the potential for person-to-person transmission because of its hemorrhagic manifestations.[263] DENV in pregnancy manifests a range of fetal/infant illness, from asymptomatic to miscarriage and fetal death.[264–266] Prematurity and LBW were the most frequent adverse outcomes. More than 2.5 billion people live in areas where transmission occurs; DENV infects over 100 million individuals a year and causes approximately 24,000 deaths per year.[267,268] Although dengue hemorrhagic fever and dengue shock syndrome occur frequently in children younger than 1 year of age, they are infrequently described in infants younger than 3 months of age.[269] There are also differences in the clinical and laboratory findings of DENV infection in children as compared with adults.[270] Boussemart et al.[271] reported on two cases of perinatal/prenatal transmission of dengue and discussed eight additional cases in neonates from the literature. Prenatal or intrapartum transmission of the same type of dengue as the mother was confirmed by serology, culture, or PCR. Watanaveeradej et al.[272] presented an additional three cases of dengue infection in infants, documenting normal growth and development at follow-up at 12 months of age. Sirinavin et al.[273] reported on 17 cases in the literature of vertical dengue infection, all presenting at less than 2 weeks of age, but no observations or discussion of breast milk or breastfeeding as a potential source of infection were published.

Phongsamart et al.[274] described three additional cases of DENV infection late in pregnancy, with apparent transmission to two of the three infants and passive acquisition of antibody in the third infant. Arragain et al.[275] reported on vertical DENV transmission in the peripartum period in 10 mother–newborn pairs. DENV RNA was detected at delivery in the sera of all 10 mothers and 9/10 infants. The newborns had prolonged viremia up to 10 to 17 days after disease onset. Separately, DENV RNA was detected in the breast milk of 9/12 mothers tested.[275]

It has been postulated that more severe disease associated with DENV occurs when an individual has specific IgG against the same serotype as the infecting strain in a set concentration, leading to antibody-dependent enhancement of infection. The presence of preexisting dengue serotype-specific IgG in an infant implies either previous primary infection with the same serotype, passive acquisition of IgG from the mother (who had a previous primary infection with the same serotype), or perhaps acquisition of specific IgG from breast milk. Watanaveeradej et al.[272] documented transplacentally transferred antibodies against all four serotypes of DENV in 97% of 2000 cord sera at delivery. Follow-up of 100 infants documented the loss of antibodies to DENV over time, with losses of 3%, 19%, 72%, 99%, and 100% at 2, 4, 6, 9, and 12 months of age, respectively.

No evidence is available in the literature about more severe disease in breastfed infants compared with formula-fed infants. There is one case report of apparent transmission of DENV via breast milk to a 4-day-old infant, however. The mother had clinical illness consistent with DENV disease at delivery, and the infant developed disease on day 4 of life. The mother's blood was positive for DENV by RT-PCR on days 0 to 6 after delivery, and her breast milk was positive on days 2 and 4 after delivery. The infant's blood from days 0 and 2 and the cord blood were repeatedly negative by RT-PCR, but subsequently, the infant's blood was PCR-positive for DENV on days 4 to 13 of life.[276] There is one report of a factor in the lipid portion of breast milk that inhibits DENV, but no evidence for antibody activity against DENV in human breast milk is known.[277] Given the apparent rarity of the transmission of DENV via breast milk, breastfeeding during maternal or infant dengue disease should continue in the majority of situations, as determined by the mother's or infant's severity of illness. A balanced presentation to the mother and family of the apparent low risk of DENV infection via breast milk compared with the known benefits is appropriate.

Epstein–Barr Virus

Epstein–Barr virus (EBV) is a common infection in children, adolescents, and young adults. It is usually asymptomatic, but it most notably causes infectious mononucleosis and has been associated with chronic fatigue syndrome, Burkitt lymphoma, and nasopharyngeal carcinoma. Because EBV is one of the human herpesviruses, concern has been raised about lifelong latent infection, its clear carcinogenic potential, and the potential risk for infection to a fetus and neonate from the mother. Primary EBV infection during pregnancy is unusual because few pregnant women are susceptible.[278,279] Although abortion, premature birth, and congenital infection from EBV are suspected, no distinct group of anomalies is linked to EBV infection in the fetus or neonate. Also, no virologic evidence of EBV as the cause of abnormalities was found in association with suspected EBV infection.

Culturing of EBV from various fluids or sites is difficult. The virus is detected by its capacity to transform B lymphocytes into persistent lymphoblastoid cell lines. PCR and DNA hybridization studies have detected EBV in the cervix and in breast milk. One study, which identified EBV DNA in breast-milk cells in more than 40% of women donating milk to a breast-milk bank, demonstrated that only 17% had antibodies to EBV (only IgG, no IgM).[280] EBV DNA was identified in 33% of 40 human milk samples from normal lactating women in a separate study.[281] However, a study by Kusuhara et al. examining serologic specimens from breastfed and bottle-fed infants showed similar seroprevalence of EBV at 12 to 23 months of age (36/66 [54.5%] and 24/43 [55.8%]) in the breastfed and bottle-fed children, respectively.[282] This suggests that early acquisition of EBV infection in infants is not significantly affected by the consumption of breast milk. Others have identified EBV in breast milk in different situations, such as in T-cell samples of healthy Kenyan children and their mothers' breast milk and saliva or associated with subclinical mastitis and HIV shedding in Zambian women.[283,284] To date, this has not led to a clearer understanding of the significance of EBV in breast milk.

The question of the timing of EBV infection and the subsequent immune response and clinical disease produced requires continued study. Differences exist among the clinical syndromes that manifest at different ages. Infants and young children are most often asymptomatic; have illness not recognized as related to EBV; or have mild episodes of illness, including fever, lymphadenopathy, rhinitis, cough, hepatosplenomegaly, and rash. Adolescents or young adults who experience primary EBV infection more often demonstrate infectious mononucleosis syndrome or are asymptomatic. Chronic fatigue syndrome is more common in adolescents and young adults. Burkitt lymphoma, observed primarily in Africa, and nasopharyngeal carcinoma, seen in southeast Asia, where primary EBV infection usually occurs in young children, are tumors associated with early EBV infection.[285,286] These tumors are related to "chronic" EBV infection and tend to occur in individuals with persistently high antibody titers to EBV viral capsid antigen and early antigen. The questions of why these tumors occur with much greater frequency in these geographic areas and what cofactors (including altered immune response to infection associated with coinfections, immune escape by EBV leading to malignancy, or increased resistance to apoptosis secondary to EBV gene mutations) may contribute to their development remain unanswered.[285,286]

It also remains unknown to what degree breast milk could be a source of early EBV infection compared with other sources of EBV infection in an infant's environment. Researchers from Kenya have reported on the early age of primary EBV infection in infants and associated higher blood EBV viral loads in infancy and the potential contribution to the etiology of endemic Burkitt lymphoma.[287] In a more recent paper, researchers identified that breast milk contains infectious EBV and was associated with mothers infected with *Plasmodium falciparum* malaria at delivery. The mean EBV viral loads in the breast milk of these malaria-infected mothers were the highest at 6 weeks postpartum, declining through 18 weeks postpartum.[288] Similar to the situation of postnatal transmission of CMV in immunocompetent infants, clinically significant illness rarely is associated with primary EBV infection in infants. More data concerning the pathogenesis of EBV-associated tumors should be obtained before proscribing against breastfeeding is warranted, especially in areas where these tumors are common but the protective benefits of breastfeeding are high. In areas where

Burkitt lymphoma and nasopharyngeal carcinoma are uncommon, EBV infection in the mother or infant is certainly not a contraindication to breastfeeding.

Filoviridae

Marburg virus and Ebola virus (EBOV) cause severe and highly fatal hemorrhagic fevers. The illness often presents with non-specific symptoms (conjunctivitis, frontal headache, malaise, myalgia, bradycardia) and progresses, with worsening hemorrhage, to shock and subsequent death in 50% to 90% of patients. Person-to-person transmission through direct contact, droplet spread, or airborne spread are the common modes of transmission. However, the animal reservoir(s) or sources of these viruses in nature for human infection have not been definitively identified. Attack rates in families/households are variable based on age and specific exposures to a corpse and/or fluids, ranging from 8% to 83%.[289,290] No postexposure interventions have proved useful in preventing spread. Monoclonal antibodies, convalescent plasma, and a few antiviral agents continue to undergo testing for possible use against EOV disease in humans.[291]

One report documented the presence of EBOV in numerous body fluids, including breast milk. One acute breast-milk sample on day 7 after the onset of illness in the mother and a "convalescent" breast-milk sample on day 15 from the same woman were positive for EBOV by both culture and PCR testing.[292] In the same study, testing other body fluids in different persons, saliva remained virus-positive for a mean of 16 days after disease onset, urine was positive for a mean of 28 days, and semen was positive for a mean of 43 days after the onset of disease in survivors of Ebola infection. A couple of other case reports document the presence of EBOV in breast milk and possible scenarios consistent with EBOV disease (EVD) in infants associated with breastfeeding.[293] One of the cases showed EBOV in the breast milk of a mother without a reported EBOV-consistent illness.[294] A more recent review acknowledges that transmission of EBOV via human milk has not been confirmed, but the authors go on to support testing of breast milk and avoiding the use of the mother's milk until there are two negative tests obtained 48 hours apart.[295]

There is a single study available concerning the relative risk for transmission of EBOV in breast milk compared with the risk for children less than 2 years of age in a household with a mother who has EVD or does not have EVD.[296] In a review of data from Sierra Leone from an EBOV outbreak in 2015 including 64 children–mother pairs, the adjusted relative risk (aRR) for a child under 2 years of age developing EVD after exposure to a mother with EVD versus a mother who did not have EVD was 7.6 (95% CI 2.0 to 29.1). If the mother died of EVD, the aRR was higher for those infants (aRR 1.5, 95% CI 0.99 to 2.4). Breastfed infants did not have a higher risk of EVD than nonbreastfed infants (aRR 0.75, 95% CI 0.46 to 1.2).[296]

Contact precautions have been recommended for Marburg virus infection and contact and airborne precautions for EBOV infection. The largest epidemic of EVD in West Africa (predominantly Guinea, Liberia, and Sierra Leone), involving over 28,000 cases and over 11,000 deaths, occurred from 2014 to

2016.[297] That outbreak dramatically raised concerns about the transmission of EBOV to family members, close contacts, travelers, and health care personnel. To date, there are no newer publications for this epidemic on transmissibility from different body fluids and particularly from breast milk. A more recent outbreak has been ongoing in the Democratic Republic of the Congo since early 2018, with an estimated 2084 EVD cases (1990 confirmed and 94 probable cases). The highest attack rates reported from this outbreak have been in children aged more than 1 year old and females aged 15 years and older. The overall CFR has been >60%.[298]

The WHO and CDC have developed updated guidance for the use of personal protective equipment for health care workers (https://www.cdc.gov/vhf/ebola/healthcare-us/ppe/index.html). Both guidelines reinforce the high risk of EBOV infection without careful protection against contact with body fluids from a person with EVD. Given the high attack and mortality rates associated with EVD, these precautions should be carefully instituted within health care facilities.

Ebola Virus Disease and Breastfeeding—WHO Guidance

The current breastfeeding recommendations for EVD from the WHO (2014) state:

1. If the breastfed infant of a mother with EVD is asymptomatic, then separate the infant from the mother and offer replacement feeding. The safest replacement feeding for infants less than 6 months old is ready-to-use formula.
2. If the breastfed infant of a mother with EVD has EVD him- or herself or is a suspected Ebola case, continue breastfeeding if the mother is physically able, and if the mother is too ill to breastfeed, then provide replacement feeding. If the mother is well enough to breastfeed, she should be nutritionally, physically, and emotionally supported to do this.
3. Wet nursing or the use of expressed breast milk from another mother in a community where ongoing EVD is occurring is not recommended.
4. If a breastfeeding infant of an EBOV-infected mother has been provided a safe alternative form of nutrition and the infant remains well, then reinitiation of breastfeeding or the use expressed breast milk from that mother should not occur until at least 3 weeks after the mother's recovery (or after two consecutive tests 48 hours apart of mother's milk are negative for EBOV).

At this juncture, the duration for which EBOV persists in breast milk has not been clearly defined.[299]

HEPATITIS IN THE MOTHER

The diagnosis of hepatitis in a pregnant woman or nursing mother causes significant anxiety. The first issue is determining the etiology of the hepatitis, which then allows for an informed discussion of the risk to the fetus or infant. The differential diagnosis of acute hepatitis includes (1) common causes of hepatitis, such as hepatitis A, B, C, and D; (2) uncommon causes of hepatitis, such as hepatitis E and G, CMV,

BOX 12.3 Terminology for Hepatitis	
Hepatitis A Virus (HAV)	
IgM anti-HAV	Immunoglobulin M (IgM) antibody against HAV
HAV RNA	HAV ribonucleic acid
Hepatitis B Virus (HBV)	
HBsAg	Hepatitis B surface antigen
HBeAg	Hepatitis Be antigen
HBcAg	Hepatitis B core antigen
Anti-HBe	Antibody against hepatitis Be antigen
IgM anti-HBcAg	IgM antibody against hepatitis B core antigen
HBV DNA	HBV deoxyribonucleic acid
HBIG	Hepatitis B immunoglobulin
Hepatitis C Virus (HCV)	
Anti-HCV	Antibody against HCV
HCV RNA	HCV ribonucleic acid
Hepatitis D Virus (HDV)	
Anti-HDV	Antibody against HDV
Hepatitis E Virus (HEV)	
HEV RNA	HEV ribonucleic acid
Hepatitis G Virus (HGV)	
HGV RNA	HGV ribonucleic acid
TT Virus (TTV)	
TTV DNA	TT virus deoxyribonucleic acid
Other	
NANBH	Non-A, non-B hepatitis
ISG	Immune serum globulin

echoviruses, enteroviruses, EBV, HSV, rubella, varicella-zoster virus, and yellow fever virus; (3) rare causes of hepatitis, such as EBOV, Junin virus, and Machupo virus (cause hemorrhagic fever), as well as Lassa virus and Marburg virus; and (4) nonviral causes, such as hepatotoxic drugs, alcoholic hepatitis, toxoplasmosis, autoimmune hepatitis, bile duct obstruction, ischemic liver damage, Wilson disease, α_1-antitrypsin deficiency, and metastatic liver disease. The following sections focus on hepatitis viruses A to G. Other infectious agents that can cause hepatitis are considered individually in other sections. Box 12.3 provides hepatitis terminology.

Martin et al.[300] outline a succinct diagnostic approach to patients with acute viral hepatitis and chronic viral hepatitis (Figs. 12.4 and 12.5). The approach involves using the four serologic markers (IgM anti-hepatitis A virus, hepatitis B surface antigen [HBsAg], IgM anti-HBcAg, anti-HCV) as the initial diagnostic tests. Simultaneous consideration of other etiologies of acute liver dysfunction is appropriate depending on a patient's history. If the initial diagnostic tests are all negative, subsequent additional testing for anti-hepatitis D virus (HDV), HCV RNA, hepatitis G virus (HGV) RNA, anti-hepatitis E virus (HEV), or HEV RNA may be necessary. If initial testing reveals positive HBsAg, testing for anti-HDV, HBeAg, and HBV DNA is appropriate. These additional tests are useful in defining the prognosis for a mother and the risk for infection to an infant. During the diagnostic evaluation, it is appropriate to discuss with the mother or parents the

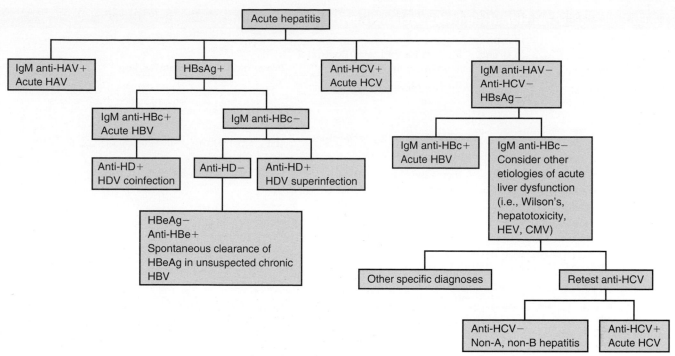

Fig. 12.4 Diagnostic approach to a patient with acute viral hepatitis. See Box 12.3 for definitions of abbreviations. (From Martin P, Friedman L, Dienstag J. Diagnostic approach. In: Zuckerman A, Thomas H, eds. *Viral Hepatitis: Scientific Basis and Clinical Management.* Edinburgh: Churchill Livingstone; 1993.)

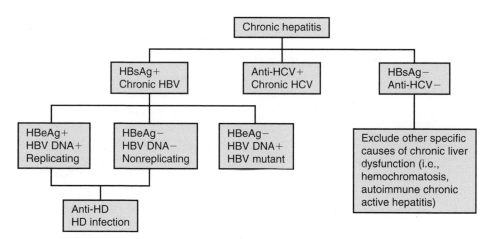

Fig. 12.5 Diagnostic approach to a patient with chronic viral hepatitis. See Box 12.3 for definitions of abbreviations. (From Martin P, Friedman L, Dienstag J. Diagnostic approach. In: Zuckerman A, Thomas H, eds. *Viral Hepatitis: Scientific Basis and Clinical Management.* Edinburgh: Churchill Livingstone; 1993.)

theoretic risk for transmitting infectious agents that cause hepatitis via breastfeeding. The discussion should include an evaluation of the positive and negative effects of suspending or continuing breastfeeding until the exact etiologic diagnosis is determined. The relative risk for the transmission of infection to an infant can be estimated, and specific preventive measures can be provided for the infant (Table 12.2).

Hepatitis A

Hepatitis A virus (HAV) is usually an acute, self-limited infection. The illness is typically mild, and it is generally subclinical in infants. Occasionally, HAV infection is

prolonged or relapsing, extending 3 to 6 months, and rarely, it is fulminant, but HAV infection does not lead to chronic infection. The incidence of prematurity after maternal HAV infection is increased, but no evidence to date indicates obvious birth defects or a congenital syndrome.[301] HAV infection in premature infants may lead to prolonged viral shedding.[302] Transmission is most often person to person (fecal-oral), and transmission in foodborne or waterborne epidemics has been described. Transmission via blood products or transplantation and vertical transmission (mother to infant) are rare. Transmission in daycare settings has been clearly described.

TABLE 12.2   Viral Hepatitis in Association With Breastfeeding[a]

Hepatitis	Virus	Identified in Breast Milk	Factors for Perinatal/Postnatal Transmission	Prevention	Breastfeeding[b]
A	Picornaviridae (RNA)	?	Vertical transmission uncertain or rare	ISG	Limited evidence of transmission via breastfeeding or of serious disease in infants
			HAV in pregnancy associated with premature birth	HAV vaccine	Breastfeeding OK after ISG and vaccine
B	Hepadnaviridae (DNA)	HBsAg	Increased risk for vertical transmission with HBeAg+, in countries where HBV is endemic, or early in maternal infection, before Ab production	HBIG	Low theoretic risk
		HBV DNA		HBV vaccine	Virtually no risk after HBIG and HBV vaccine, breastfeeding OK after HBIG and vaccine
C	Flavivirus (RNA)	HCV RNA detected	Increased risk when mother HIV+ and HCV+ or with increased HCV-RNA titers	None	Positive theoretic risk, inadequate data on relative risk, breastfeeding OK after informed discussion with parents
			Vertical transmission uncommon		
D	Delavirdine (RNA strand, circular)	?	Requires coinfection/superinfection with HBV	None (except to prevent HBV infection, give HBIG/HBV vaccine)	Prevent HBV infection with HBIG and vaccine
			Vertical transmission rare		Breastfeeding OK after HBIG and vaccine
E	Caliciviridae (RNA)	+	Severe disease in pregnant women (20% mortality)	ISG and subunit vaccine being tested	Usually subclinical infection in children, breastfeeding OK
G	Related to calicivirus and flavivirus (RNA)	?	Vertical transmission occurs	None	Inadequate data
TT	TT virus (DNA, circular, single stranded)	TTV DNA detected	Vertical transmission occurs	None	Inadequate data

Ab, Antibody; *HIV*, human immunodeficiency virus.

[a]See Box 12.3 for abbreviations.

[b]With any type of infectious hepatitis, discussion of what is known and not known concerning transmission should be related to the mother/parents, and an informed decision can then be made by the involved adults concerning breastfeeding.

Data from Committee on Infectious Diseases, American Academy of Pediatrics. Hepatitis A–E. In: Kimberlin DW, et al., eds. *Red Book: 2018 Report of the Committee on Infectious Diseases*. 31st ed. Itasca, IL: American Academy of Pediatrics; 2018: 436–437.

Infection with HAV in newborns is uncommon and does not seem to be a significant problem. The usual period of viral shedding and presumed contagiousness lasts 1 to 3 weeks. Acute maternal HAV infection in the last trimester or in the postpartum period could lead to infection in an infant. Symptomatic infection can be prevented by immunoglobulin (Ig) administration, and 80% to 90% of disease can be prevented by Ig administration within 2 weeks of exposure. HAV vaccine can be administered simultaneously with Ig without affecting the seroconversion rate to produce rapid and prolonged HAV serum antibody levels.

The transmission of HAV via breast milk has been implicated in one older case report, and there is a single report of identifying HAV RNA in two of three breast-milk samples from three women with acute HAV infection. The three infants did not have clinical evidence of HAV infection.[303] Because HAV infection in infancy is rare and usually subclinical without chronic disease, and because exposure has already occurred by the time the etiologic diagnosis of hepatitis in a mother is made, no reason exists to interrupt breastfeeding with maternal HAV infection. The exposed infant should receive Ig and/or HAV vaccine per *Red Book* recommendations based on age and time since exposure.[304]

Hepatitis B

HBV infection leads to a broad spectrum of illness, including asymptomatic seroconversion, nonspecific symptoms (fever, malaise, fatigue), clinical hepatitis with or without jaundice, extrahepatic manifestations (arthritis, rash, renal involvement), fulminant hepatitis, and chronic HBV infection. Chronic HBV infection occurs in up to 90% of infants infected via perinatal and vertical transmission and in 30% of children infected between 1 and 5 years of age. Given the increased risk for significant sequelae from chronic infection (chronic active hepatitis, chronic persistent hepatitis, cirrhosis, primary hepatocellular carcinoma), the prevention of HBV infection in infancy is crucial. Transmission of HBV is usually through blood or body fluids (stool, semen, saliva, urine, cervical secretions).[305]

Vertical HBV Transmission

Vertical transmission, either transplacentally or perinatally during delivery, has been well described throughout the world. Vertical transmission rates in areas where HBV is endemic (Taiwan and Japan) are high, whereas transmission to infants from HBV-carrier mothers in other areas where HBV-carrier rates are low is uncommon.[306] The transmission of HBV to infants occurs in up to 50% of infants when the mothers are acutely infected immediately before, during, or soon after pregnancy.[307] There is evidence for the use of antiviral therapy during pregnancy in the situation of chronic hepatitis B infection in the mother to prevent mother-to-child-transmission (MTCT) of hepatitis B. Therapy could include lamivudine, telbivudine, or tenofovir, but there is no standard recommended regimen.[308] Another occasion when antiviral therapy during pregnancy should be considered is with very high hepatitis B viral loads (> 200,000), which increase the risk of MTCT to 25%. Women with "occult" hepatitis B infection may be identified during a pregnancy-associated hepatitis B flare. HBV DNA level, HBeAg level, alanine aminotransferase (ALT) level, and the presence or absence of cirrhosis are some of the other variables utilized to make treatment decisions during pregnancy.[309,310] HBsAg is found in breast milk, but transmission by this route is not well documented. Beasley et al.[311] demonstrated that although breast-milk transmission is possible, seroconversion rates were no different between breastfed and non-breastfed infants in a long-term follow-up study of 147 HBsAg-positive mothers. Hill et al.[312] followed 101 breastfed infants and 268 formula-fed infants born to women who were chronically HBsAg-positive. All infants received HBIG at birth and a full series of the hepatitis B vaccine. None of the breastfed infants and nine of the formula-fed infants were positive for HBsAg after completion of the HBV vaccine series. Breastfeeding occurred for a mean of 4.9 months (range: 2 weeks to 1 year). Transmission, when it does happen, probably occurs during labor and delivery. Another report from China

followed 230 infants born to HBsAg-positive women. The infants received the appropriate dosing and timing of HBIG and the HBV vaccine. At 1 year of age, anti-HB antibodies were present in 90.9% of the breastfed infants and 90.3% of the bottle-fed infants.[313] Risk factors associated with immunoprophylaxis failure against vertical transmission of HBV include HBeAg-seropositive mothers and elevated HBV DNA "viral loads" in the mothers.[314] Zhang et al. also demonstrated, in over 67,000 pregnant women and 1150 HBsAg-positive mothers, that breastfeeding did not increase the risk of HBV MTCT as compared with formula-fed infants.[315] A systematic review and meta-analysis by Shi et al. including 10 controlled clinical trials compared immunized breastfeeding infants with immunized nonbreastfeeding infants, and breastfeeding did not add any additional risk (odds ratio [OR] = 0.98, 95% CI 0.69 to 1.40).[316] In 2018 the AAP Committee on Infectious Diseases stated that "breastfeeding of the infant by an HBsAg-positive mother poses no additional risk for acquisition of HBV infection by the infant with appropriate administration of hepatitis B vaccine and HBIG."[305]

Screening of all pregnant women for HBV infection is an essential first step to preventing vertical transmission. Universal HBV vaccination at birth and during infancy, with the administration of HBIG immediately after birth to infants of HBsAg-positive mothers, prevents HBV transmission in more than 95% of cases. Breastfeeding by HBsAg-positive women is not contraindicated, but the immediate administration of HBIG and the HBV vaccine should occur. Two subsequent doses of the vaccine should be given at appropriate intervals and dosages for the specific HBV vaccine product. This decreases the small theoretic risk for HBV transmission from breastfeeding to almost zero.

When acute peripartum or postpartum hepatitis occurs in a mother and HBV infection is a possibility, with its associated increased risk for transmission to the infant, a discussion with the mother or parents should identify the potential risks and benefits of continuing breastfeeding until the etiology of the hepatitis can be determined. If an appropriate alternative source of nutrition is available for the infant, breast milk should be withheld until the etiology of the hepatitis is identified. HBIG and the HBV vaccine can be administered to the infant who has not already been immunized or has no documented immunity against HBV. If acute HBV infection is documented in a mother, breastfeeding can continue after immunization has begun.

Hepatitis C

Acute infection with HCV can be indistinguishable from hepatitis A or B infection; however, it is typically asymptomatic or mild. HCV infection is the major cause of bloodborne non-A, non-B hepatitis (NANBH). Chronic HCV infection is reported to occur 70% to 85% of the time, regardless of age at the time of infection. The sequelae of chronic HCV infection are similar to those associated with chronic HBV infection.[317]

The rate of perinatal transmission of HCV seems to have been stable in the United States, approximately 5% to 6% over the years 2006 to 2012. The incidence of HCV infection in women of childbearing age has increased dramatically and raises the question of the need for universal screening for HCV during pregnancy.[318,319]

Bortolotti et al.[320] described two groups of children with HCV infection whom they observed for 12 to 48 months. The first group of 14 children, who acquired HCV infection early in life, presumably from their mothers, demonstrated biochemical evidence of liver disease in the first 12 months of life. Two of these children subsequently cleared the viremia and had normal liver function, an additional three children developed normal liver function despite persistent HCV viremia, and the remaining children had persistent viremia and abnormal liver function. The second group of 16 children with chronic HCV infection remained free of clinical symptoms of hepatitis, but 10 (62%) of them had mild alanine-aminotransferase elevations, and 7 of the 16 (44%) who had liver biopsies had histologic evidence of mild to moderate hepatitis.

The two commonly identified mechanisms of transmission of HCV are transfusions of blood or blood products and IV drug use. However, other routes of transmission exist because HCV infection occurs even in the absence of obvious direct contact with significant amounts of blood. Other body fluids contaminated with blood probably serve as sources of infection. Transmission through sexual contact occurs infrequently and probably requires additional contributing factors, such as coinfection with other sexually transmitted agents (especially HIV) or high hepatitis C viral loads in serum and other body fluids. Studies of transmission in households without other risk factors have demonstrated either low rates of transmission or no transmission.

The reported rates of vertical transmission vary widely. In mothers with unknown HIV status or known HIV infection, the rates of vertical transmission were 4% to 100%, whereas the rates varied between 0% and 42% in known HIV-negative mothers.[321] These same studies suggest that maternal coinfection with HIV, HCV genotype, active maternal liver disease, and the serum titer of maternal HCV RNA may be associated with increased rates of vertical transmission.[322–325] The correlation between HCV viremia, the HCV viral load in a mother, and vertical transmission of HCV is well documented.[326–329] Evolution of the HCV during replication with situations of altered maternal cellular immunity (HIV, pregnancy) and "compartmentalization of HCV" in peripheral blood monocytes (PBMCs) may facilitate perinatal transmission of HCV.[330] The clinical significance and risk for liver disease in the infant/child after vertical transmission of HCV are still unknown. The timing of HCV infection in vertical transmission is also unknown. In utero transmission has been suggested by some studies,[331] whereas intrapartum or postpartum transmission was proposed by Ohto et al.[332] when they documented the absence of HCV RNA in the cord blood of neonates who later became HCV-RNA-positive at 1 to 2 months of age. Gibb et al.[333] reported two pieces of data supporting the likelihood of intrapartum transmission as the predominant time of vertical transmission: (1) low sensitivity of PCR for HCV-RNA testing in the first month of life, with a marked increase in sensitivity

after that for diagnosing HCV infection in infants, and (2) a lower transmission risk for elective cesarean delivery (without prolonged rupture of membranes) compared with vaginal or emergency cesarean delivery.[333] Another group, McMenamin et al.,[334] analyzed vertical transmission in 559 mother–infant dyads. The overall vertical transmission rate was 4.1% (18/441), with another 118 infants not tested or lost to follow-up. Comparison of the vertical transmission rate was no different for vaginal delivery or emergency cesarean in labor versus planned cesarean (4.2% vs. 3.0%). This held true even when mothers had HCV RNA detected antenatally (7.2% vs. 5.3%). The authors did not support planned cesarean delivery to decrease vertical transmission of hepatitis C infection. No prospective, controlled trials of cesarean versus vaginal delivery and the occurrence of vertical hepatitis C transmission are available. Even more recent studies report a higher occurrence of MTCT when the mother has uncontrolled HIV coinfection and/or the mother has higher HCV-RNA levels or viral loads (>6 log IU/mL).[325,335–337]

Ongoing challenges to preventing HCV infection include screening during pregnancy; appropriate follow-up and testing of infants born to mothers with HCV; screening higher-risk adolescents and young adults; and further development of safe, effective, direct-acting antiviral (DAA) treatment.[338–340]

The risk for HCV transmission via breast milk is uncertain. Anti-HCV antibody and HCV RNA have been demonstrated in colostrum and breast milk, although the levels of HCV RNA in milk did not correlate with the titers of HCV RNA in serum.[327,341–343] Nevertheless, transmission of HCV via breastfeeding (and not in utero, intrapartum, or from other postpartum sources) has not been proven in the small number of infants carefully studied. Transmission rates in breastfed and nonbreastfed infants appear to be similar, but various important factors have not been controlled, such as HCV-RNA titers in mothers, examination of the milk for HCV RNA, exclusive breastfeeding versus exclusive formula feeding versus partial breastfeeding, and duration of breastfeeding.[322,324,326,332,333,343–345] Zanetti et al.[324] documented the absence of HCV transmission in 94 mother–infant dyads when the mother had only HCV (no HIV) infection and no transmission in 71 mother–infant dyads who breastfed, including 23 infants whose mothers were seropositive for HCV RNA. Eight infants in that study were infected with HCV and their mothers had both HIV and HCV, and 3 of these 8 infants were infected with both HIV and HCV. The HCV-RNA levels were significantly higher in the mothers coinfected with HIV than they were in mothers with HCV alone.

Overall, the risk for HCV infection via breastfeeding is low; the risk for HCV infection appears to be more frequent in association with HIV infection and higher levels of HCV RNA in maternal serum. No effective preventive therapies (Ig or vaccine) exist except direct-acting antiviral chemotherapy to treat HCV-infected women or lower the HCV viral load. The risk for chronic HCV infection and subsequent sequelae with any infection is high. It is therefore appropriate to discuss the theoretic risk for breastfeeding in HCV-positive mothers with the mother or parents and to consider proscribing breast milk when appropriate alternative sources of nutrition are available for the infants. HIV infection is a separate contraindication to breastfeeding. Additional study is necessary to determine the exact role of breastfeeding in the transmission of HCV, including the quantitative measurement of HCV RNA in colostrum and breast milk, the relative risk for HCV transmission in exclusively or partially breastfed infants versus the risk in formula-fed infants, and the effect of duration of breastfeeding on transmission.

The current position of the CDC and the AAP is that no data indicate that HCV is transmitted through breast milk.[346] Therefore breastfeeding by an HCV-positive, HIV-negative mother is not contraindicated. The recommendation does caution about temporarily interrupting breastfeeding to manage bleeding or cracked nipples because of the concern of transmission via blood.

Infants born to HCV-RNA-positive mothers require follow-up through 18 to 36 months of age to determine the infants' HCV status, regardless of the mode of infant feeding. Infants should be tested by anti-HCV antibody at or after 18 months. Testing for HCV-RNA in the first year of life is optional because the ideal time for testing in terms of diagnosis and prognosis is unknown. Repetitive serial testing is not recommended. Children who are anti-HCV positive after 18 months of age should be tested using an HCV-RNA test after 3 years of age to confirm chronic hepatitis C infection.[339]

Hepatitis D

HDV is a defective RNA virus that causes hepatitis only in persons also infected with HBV. The infection occurs as either an acute coinfection of HBV and HDV or a superinfection of HBV carriers. This "double" infection results in more frequent fulminant hepatitis and chronic hepatitis, which can progress to cirrhosis. The virus uses its own HBV RNA (circular, negative-strand RNA) with an antigen, HDAg, surrounded by the surface antigen of HBV, HBsAg. HDV is transmitted in the same way as HBV, especially through the exchange of blood and body fluids. HDV infection is uncommon where the prevalence of HBV is low. In areas where HBV is endemic, the prevalence of HDV is highly variable. HDV is common in tropical Africa and South America, as well as in Greece and Italy, but it is uncommon in the Far East and in Alaskan Inuit despite the endemic occurrence of HBV in these areas.[347]

The transmission of HDV has been reported to occur from household contacts and, rarely, through vertical transmission.[348,349] No data are available on the transmission of HDV by breastfeeding. HDV infection can be prevented by blocking infection with HBV; therefore HBIG and the HBV vaccine are the best protection. In addition to HBIG and HBV vaccine administration to the infant of a mother infected with both HBV and HDV, discussion with the mother or parents should include the theoretic risk for HBV and HDV transmission through breastfeeding. As with HBV, once HBIG and the HBV vaccine have been given to the infant, the risk for HBV or HDV infection from breastfeeding is negligible. Therefore breastfeeding after an informed discussion with the parents is acceptable.

Hepatitis E

HEV is a cause of sporadic and epidemic, enterically transmitted NANBH, which is typically self-limited and without chronic sequelae. HEV is notable for causing a high mortality rate in pregnant women, as well as high neonatal morbidity and mortality when HEV infection occurs in the third trimester.[350] Transmission is primarily via the fecal-oral route, commonly via contaminated water or food. High infection rates have been reported in adolescents and young adults (ages 15 to 40 years). Tomar[351] reported that 70% of cases of HEV infections in the pediatric population in India manifest as acute hepatitis. Maternal-neonatal transmission was documented when the mother developed hepatitis E infection in the third trimester. Although HEV has been demonstrated in breast milk, no transmission via breast milk was confirmed.[352] Five cases of transfusion-associated hepatitis E were reported.[351] In a review by Krain et al.,[353] vertical transmission was noted in reports from India and Ghana in the infants of pregnant women with acute viral hepatitis or fulminant hepatic failure. Chibber et al.[354] reported on the presence of HEV RNA in the colostrum of HEV-infected mothers in significantly lower levels than in maternal serum. They also noted six infants who became infected within 2 weeks postpartum after being anti-HEV antibody and HEV-RNA-negative at birth. Four of these six infants were formula-fed because of severe maternal illness. There was no transmission of HEV in 87 other infants who were exclusively breastfed and born to mothers positive for anti-HEV antibodies or HEV RNA in the third trimester.[354] Other authors report a high rate of severe disease in perinatally infected infants but no evidence of chronic HEV infection after vertical transmission.[355–358] Epidemics are usually related to contamination of water. Person-to-person spread is minimal, even in households and daycare settings.

HEV infection in infancy is rare but does occur after maternal infection in the third trimester of pregnancy.[355,356] Limited available data suggest that transmission of HEV by breastfeeding is rare. There is no evidence of clinically significant postnatal HEV infection or chronic sequelae in association with HEV infection in breastfed infants. Currently, no contraindication exists to breastfeeding with maternal HEV infection. Ig has not been shown to be effective in preventing infection, but there is an HEV vaccine currently under trials.[359]

Hepatitis G

HGV has recently been confirmed as a cause of NANBH distinct from hepatitis viruses A through E. Several closely related genomes of HGV, currently named *GBV-A, -B,* and *-C,* appear to be related to HCV in the groups of pestiviruses and flaviviruses. Epidemiologically, HGV is most often associated with the transfusion of blood, although studies have identified non-transfusion-related cases. HGV genomic RNA has been detected in some patients with acute and chronic hepatitis and a small number of patients with fulminant hepatitis. GBV-C/HGV has also been found in some patients with inflammatory bile duct lesions, but the pathogenicity of this virus is unconfirmed. HGV RNA has been detected in 1% to

3% of healthy blood donors in the United States.[360] Feucht et al.[361] described maternal-to-infant transmission of HGV in three of nine children. Two of the three mothers were coinfected with HIV and the third with HCV. None of these infants developed signs of liver disease. Neither the timing nor the mode of transmission was clarified. Lin et al.[362] reported no HGV transmission in three mother–infant dyads after cesarean delivery and discussed transplacental spread via blood as the most likely mode of HGV infection in vertical transmission. Wejstal et al.[363] reported on perinatal transmission of HGV to 12 of 16 infants born to HGV-viremic mothers, identified by PCR. HGV did not appear to cause clinical hepatitis in these children.[363]

Fischler et al.[364] followed eight children born to HGV-positive mothers and found only one to be infected with HGV. That child remained clinically well, whereas his twin, also born by cesarean delivery and breastfed, remained HGV-negative for 3 years of observation. Five of the other six children were breastfed for variable periods without evidence of HGV infection. Ohto et al.[345] examined HGV mother-to-infant transmission. Of 2979 pregnant Japanese women who were screened, 32 were identified as positive for GBV-C/HGV RNA by PCR; 26 of 34 infants born to the 32 HGV-positive women were shown to be HGV-RNA positive. Reportedly, none of the infants demonstrated a clinical picture of hepatitis, although two infants had persistent mild elevations (less than two times normal) of alanine aminotransferase. The viral load in mothers who transmitted HGV to their infants was significantly higher than it was in non-transmitting mothers. Infants born by elective cesarean delivery had a lower rate of infection (3 in 7) compared with infants born by emergency cesarean delivery (2 of 2) or born vaginally (21 of 25). In this study, HGV infection in breastfed infants was four times more common than it was in formula-fed infants, but this difference was not statistically significant because only four infants were formula-fed. The authors report no correlation between infection rate and duration of breastfeeding. Testing of the infants was not done frequently and early enough routinely through the first year of life to determine the timing of infection in these infants.[345] Schröter et al.[365] reported transmission of HGV to 3 of 15 infants born to HGV-RNA-positive mothers at 1 week of age. None of 15 breast-milk samples was positive for GBV-C/HGV RNA, and all of the children who were initially negative for HGV RNA in serum remained negative at follow-up between 1 and 28 months of age.[365]

The foregoing data suggest that transmission is more likely to be vertical before or at delivery rather than via breastfeeding. The pathogenicity and the possibility of chronic disease as a result of perinatal HGV infection remain uncertain currently. Insufficient data are available to make a policy recommendation concerning breastfeeding by HGV-infected mothers, but it is likely that the benefits of breastfeeding will outweigh the potential risk of HGV infection for the infant in most situations.

Herpes Simplex Virus

HSV types 1 and 2 (HSV-1 and HSV-2) can cause prenatal, perinatal, and postnatal infections in fetuses and infants.

Prenatal infection can lead to abortion, prematurity, or a recognized congenital syndrome. Perinatal infection is the most common form of infection (1 in 2000 to 3000 live births, an estimated 700 to 1500 cases per year in the United States) and is often fatal or severely debilitating.[366] The factors that facilitate intrapartum infection and predict the severity of disease have been extensively investigated. Postnatal infection is uncommon but can occur from a variety of sources, including oral or genital lesions and secretions in mothers or fathers, hospital workers and home caregivers, and breast lesions in breastfeeding mothers. Case reports have documented severe HSV-1 or HSV-2 infections in infants associated with HSV-positive breast lesions in the mothers.[367–370] Cases of infants with HSV gingivostomatitis inoculating the mothers' breasts have also been reported.[368,371]

In the absence of breast lesions, breastfeeding in HSV-seropositive or culture-positive women is reasonable when accompanied by careful handwashing, covering the lesions, and avoiding fondling or kissing with oral lesions until all lesions are crusted. Breastfeeding during maternal therapy with oral or IV acyclovir or valacyclovir can continue safely as well. Inadequate information exists concerning famciclovir, ganciclovir, and foscarnet in breast milk to make a recommendation. Breastfeeding by women with active herpetic lesions on their breasts should be proscribed until the lesions are dried. Treatment of the mothers' breast lesions with topical, oral, and/or IV antiviral preparations may hasten recovery and decrease the length of viral shedding. Maintaining a good supply of mother's breast milk requires a multidisciplinary approach and appropriate support and guidance until full breastfeeding can resume.[372]

Human Herpesvirus 6 and Human Herpesvirus 7

Human herpesvirus 6 (HHV-6) is a cause of exanthema subitum (roseola, roseola infantum) and is associated with febrile seizures. HHV-6 appears to be most similar to CMV based on genetic analysis.[373] No obvious clinical congenital syndrome of HHV-6 infection has been identified, although prenatal infection has been reported,[374,375] and there is one report of a possible adverse effect of congenital HHV-6 infection on neurodevelopment at 12 months of age.[376] Seroepidemiologic studies show that most adults have already been infected by HHV-6. Therefore primary infection during pregnancy is unlikely, but reactivation of latent HHV-6 infection may be more common, and a novel mechanism of vertical transmission through integration of the virus within the germline has been reported.[375] Rare cases of symptomatic HHV-6 prenatal infection have been reported.[377] The significance of reactivation of HHV-6 in a pregnant woman, along with integration of the virus within the germline cells and the production of infection and disease in the fetus and infant, remains to be determined.[378] Primary infection in children occurs most often between 6 and 12 months of age, when maternally acquired passive antibodies against HHV-6 are waning. Febrile illnesses in infants younger than 3 months of age have been described with HHV-6 infection, but infection before 3 months or after 3 years is uncommon.

Various studies involving the serology and restriction enzyme analysis of HHV-6 isolates from mother–infant dyads support the idea that postnatal transmission and perhaps perinatal transmission from the mothers are common sources of infection. One study was unable to detect HHV-6 in breast milk by PCR analysis in 120 samples, although positive control samples seeded with HHV-6-infected cells did test positive.[379]

Given the limited occurrence of clinically significant disease and sequelae of HHV-6 infection in infants and children, the almost-universal acquisition of infection in early childhood (with or without breastfeeding), and the absence of evidence that breast milk is a source of HHV-6 infection, breastfeeding can continue in women known to be seropositive for HHV-6.

Human herpesvirus 7 (HHV-7) is closely related to HHV-6 biologically. Primary infection with HHV-7 occurs most often in childhood, usually later in life than HHV-6 infection. The median age of infection is 26 months, with 75% of children becoming HHV-7 positive by 5 years of age.[380] The seroprevalence of HHV-7 antibodies has been reported to be 80% to 98% in adults, and passive antibodies are present in almost all newborns.[381,382]

Like HHV-6, HHV-7 infection can be associated with acute febrile illness, febrile seizures, and irritability, but in general, it is a milder illness than with HHV-6, with fewer hospitalizations. Virus excretion of HHV-7 occurs in saliva, and PCR testing of blood cells and saliva is frequently positive in individuals with past infection.[383] Congenital infection of HHV-6 was detected via DNA PCR testing in 57 of 5638 of cord-blood samples (1%), but HHV-7 was not detected in any of 2129 cord-blood specimens.[384]

HHV-7 DNA was detected by PCR in 3 of 29 breast-milk mononuclear cell samples from 24 women who were serumpositive for the HHV-7 antibody.[385] In the same study, small differences were seen in the HHV-7 seropositive rates between breastfed infants and bottle-fed infants at 12 months of age (21.7% vs. 20%), at 18 months of age (60% vs. 48.1%), and at 24 months of age (77.3% vs. 58.3%). None of these differences was statistically significant. Given that HHV-6 infection generally occurs earlier than HHV-7 infection in most infants and that HHV-6 is rarely found in breast milk, it seems unlikely that HHV-7 in breast milk is a common source of infection in infants and children. The infrequent occurrence of significant illness with HHV-7 infection, with the absence of sequelae, except in patients who had transplantation or were immunocompromised at older ages, and the common occurrence of infection in childhood suggest that there is no reason to proscribe breastfeeding for HHV-7-positive women.

HUMAN PAPILLOMAVIRUS

Human papillomavirus (HPV) is a DNA virus with at least 100 different types. These viruses cause warts, genital dysplasia, cervical carcinoma, and laryngeal papillomatosis. Types 6 and 11 are most commonly associated with condyloma acuminata, recurrent respiratory papillomatosis, and conjunctival papillomas. High-risk HPV types include 16, 18, 31, 33,

35, 39, 45, 51, 52, 56, 58, 59, 66, and 68. The majority of cervical and anogenital cancers are caused by types 16 and 18.[386] Transmission occurs through direct contact and sexual contact. Laryngeal papillomas are thought to result from acquiring the virus in passage through the birth canal. Infection in pregnant women or during pregnancy does not lead to an increase in abortions or the risk for prematurity, and no evidence indicates intrauterine infection. HPV is one of the most common viruses in adults and one of the most common sexually transmitted infections.

Diagnosis is usually by histologic examination or DNA detection. Spontaneous resolution does occur, but therapy for persistent lesions or growths in anatomically problematic locations is appropriate. Therapy can be topical/local with podophyllum preparations, trichloroacetic acid, imiquimod, green tea extracts (polyphenon E and sinecatechins), cryotherapy, electrocautery, and laser surgery; they should not interfere with breastfeeding.[387] The treatment of recurrent respiratory papillomatosis is surgical or laser treatment with newer adjuvant therapies with intralesional bevacizumab and cidofovir. Rarely, systemic cidofovir has been utilized.[388] Prevention against transmission means limiting direct or sexual contact, but this may not be enough because lesions may not be evident, and transmission may still occur.

Rintala et al.[389] examined the occurrence of HPV DNA in the oral and genital mucosa of infants during the first 3 years of life. HPV DNA was identified in 12% to 21% of the oral scrape samples and in 4% to 15% of the genital scrape samples by PCR. Oral HPV infection was acquired by 42% of children, cleared by 11%, and persisted in 10% of children; 37% of the children were never infected. The authors did not report on breast milk or breastfeeding in that study. Koskimaa et al. studied the association of HPV genotype in the oral mucosa of newborns and their mothers. Oral HPV in newborns was associated with cord blood at delivery (OR = 4.7, 95% CI 1.4 to 15.9) but not at 1 month and with HPV in the placenta (OR = 14.0, 95% CI 3.7 to 52.2).[390] Tuominen et al. examined HPV DNA in breast milk and neonatal oral samples. HPV DNA was detected in 8.6% (3/35) of breast-milk samples and 40% (14/35) infant oral samples.[391] The question of the source(s) of infection in the infant remains undetermined.

The breast is an uncommon site of obvious skin involvement.[392] HPV types 16 and 18 can immortalize normal breast epithelium in vitro.[393] HPV DNA has been detected in breast milk in 10 of 223 (4.5%) milk samples from 223 mothers, collected 3 days postpartum.[394] No attempt was made to correlate the presence of HPV DNA in breast milk with the HPV status of an infant or to assess the viral load of HPV in breast milk or its presence over the course of lactation. Another study found the DNA of cutaneous and mucosal HPV types in 2 of 25 human milk samples and 1 of 10 colostrum samples.[395] Yoshida et al. analyzed 80 maternal milk samples for HPV DNA, and HPV-16 nucleic acid was detected in 2 of 80 samples (2.5%), but there was no evidence of transmission to either of the infants.[396] No reports of HPV lesions of the breast or nipple and documented transmission to an infant secondary to breastfeeding are available.

The questions of viral latency for the various HPV types and the relationship with future cancers and whether the identification of viral sequences correlates with whether the viruses are biologically active remain to be elucidated, especially for human breast milk.[281]

No increased risk for acquiring HPV from breast milk is apparent, and breastfeeding is acceptable. Even in the rare occurrence of an HPV lesion of the nipple or breast, no data suggest that breastfeeding or the use of expressed breast milk is contraindicated.

Measles

Measles is another highly communicable childhood illness that can be more severe in neonates and adults. Measles is an exanthematous febrile illness following a prodrome of malaise, coryza, conjunctivitis, cough, and often Koplik spots in the mouth. The rash usually appears 10 to 14 days after exposure. Complications can include pneumonitis, encephalitis, and bacterial superinfection. With the availability of vaccination, measles in pregnancy is rare (0.4 in 10,000 pregnancies),[397] although respiratory complications (primary viral pneumonitis, secondary bacterial pneumonia), hepatitis, or other secondary bacterial infections often lead to more severe disease in these situations. Despite approximately 85% of children have received one dose of measles vaccine by their first birthday, there were about 89,780 deaths related to measles globally in 2016. There continue to be multistate and multicountry outbreaks yearly.[398]

Prenatal infection with measles may cause premature delivery without disrupting normal uterine development. No specific group of congenital malformations has been described in association with in utero measles infection, although the teratogenic effects of measles infection in pregnant women may rarely manifest in the infants.

Perinatal measles includes transplacental infection when measles occurs in an infant in the first 10 days of life. Infection from extrauterine exposure usually develops after 14 days of life. The severity of illness after the suspected transplacental spread of the virus to an infant varies from mild to severe and does not seem to vary with the antepartum or postpartum onset of rash in the mother. It is uncertain what role maternal antibodies play in the severity of an infant's disease. More severe disease seems to be associated with severe respiratory illness and bacterial infection. Postnatal exposure leading to measles after 14 days of life is generally mild, probably because of passively acquired antibodies from the mother. Severe measles in children younger than 1 year of age may occur because of declining passively acquired antibodies and complications of respiratory illness and rare cases of encephalitis.

Measles virus has not been identified in breast milk, whereas measles-specific antibodies have been documented.[399] A study from a 1970 British cohort study of over 10,000 individuals demonstrated evidence of good protection against measles with measles immunization (OR = 0.14, 95% CI 0.13 to 0.16) and a modest reduction in the risk of measles associated with breastfeeding (OR = 0.69, 95% CI 0.60 to 0.81).[400] A report in 2014 examining measles in pregnancy in France during a resurgence of measles in the community did not demonstrate acquired measles in any of the 13 breastfed infants.[401] Infants exposed to mothers with documented measles while breastfeeding should be given Ig and isolated from the mother until 72 hours after the onset of rash, which is often only a short period after the diagnosis of measles in the mother. The breast milk can be pumped and given to the infant because secretory IgA begins to be secreted in breast milk within 48 hours of the onset of the exanthem in the mother. Table 12.3 summarizes the management of the hospitalized mother and infant with measles exposure or infection.[397] Relative to the measles vaccine or measles, mumps, and rubella (MMR) vaccine during lactation, there is no concern regarding infection of the infant and risk of illness with the attenuated viruses in the vaccine.[402]

Mumps

Mumps is an acute, transient, benign illness with inflammation of the parotid gland and other salivary glands, and it often involves the pancreas, testicles, and meninges. Mumps occurs infrequently in pregnant women (1 to 10 cases in 10,000 pregnancies) and is generally benign. Mumps virus has been isolated from saliva, respiratory secretions, blood, testicular tissue, urine, CSF in cases of meningeal involvement, and breast milk. The period of infectivity is believed to be between 7 days before and 9 days after the onset of parotitis, with the usual incubation period being 14 to 18 days.

Prenatal infection with the mumps virus causes an increase in the number of abortions when infection occurs in the first trimester. A small increase in the number of premature births was noted in one prospective study of maternal mumps infection.[403] No conclusive evidence suggests congenital malformations are associated with prenatal infection, not even with endocardial fibroelastosis, as originally reported in the 1960s.

Perinatal mumps (transplacentally or postnatally acquired) has rarely if ever been documented. Natural mumps virus has been demonstrated to infect the placenta and infect the fetus, and live attenuated vaccine virus has been isolated from the placenta but not from fetal tissue in women vaccinated 10 days before induced abortion. Antibodies to mumps do cross the placenta.

Postnatal mumps in the first year of life is typically benign. No epidemiologic data suggest that mumps infection is more or less common or severe in breastfed infants compared with formula-fed infants. Although mumps virus has been identified in breast milk and mastitis is a rare complication of mumps in mature women, no evidence indicates that breast involvement occurs more frequently in lactating women. If mumps occurs in the mother, breastfeeding can continue because exposure has already occurred throughout the 7 days before the development of symptoms in the mother, and secretory IgA in the milk may help to mitigate the symptoms in the infant.[397]

Parvovirus

Human parvovirus B19 causes a broad range of clinical manifestations, including asymptomatic infection (most frequent manifestation in all ages); erythema infectiosum (fifth disease); arthralgia and arthritis; red blood cell (RBC) aplasia

TABLE 12.3 Guidelines for Preventive Measures After Exposure to Measles in Nursery or Maternity Ward

Type of Exposure or Disease	Measles (Prodrome or Rash) Present[a] Mother	Neonate	Disposition
A. Siblings at home have measles[a] when neonate and mother are ready for discharge from hospital	No	No	1. Neonate: Protective isolation and immunoglobulin (Ig) indicated unless mother has unequivocal history of previous measles or measles vaccination[b] 2. Mother: With history of previous measles or measles vaccination, she may either remain with the neonate or return to older children. Without previous history, she may remain with neonate until the older siblings are no longer infectious, or she may receive Ig prophylactically and return to the older children.
B. Mother has no history of measles or measles vaccination exposure 6 to 15 days antepartum[c]	No	No	1. Exposed mother and infant: Administer Ig to each and send home at the earliest date, unless siblings at home have communicable measles. Test mothers for susceptibility if possible. If susceptible, administer live measles vaccine 8 weeks after Ig. 2. Other mothers and infants: Same approach, unless there is a clear history of previous measles or measles vaccination in the mother. 3. Hospital personnel: Unless there is a clear history of previous measles or measles vaccination, administer IG within 72 hours of exposure. Vaccinate 8 weeks or more later.
C. Onset of maternal measles occurs antepartum or postpartum[d]	Yes	Yes	1. Infected mother and infant: Isolate together until clinically stable, then send home. 2. Other mothers and infants: Same as B-3, except infants should be vaccinated at 15 months of age. 3. Hospital personnel: Same as B-3.
D. Onset of maternal measles occurs antepartum or postpartum[d]	Yes	No	1. Infected mother: Isolate until no longer infectious.[d] 2. Infected mother's infant: Isolate separately from mother. Administer Ig immediately. Send home when the mother is no longer infectious. Alternatively, observe in isolation for 18 days for modified measles,[e] especially if Ig administration was delayed for more than 4 days. 3. Other mothers and infants: Same as C-2. 4. Hospital personnel: Same as B-3.

[a]Catarrhal stage or less than 72 hours after the onset of exanthem.
[b]Vaccination with live attenuated measles virus.
[c]With exposure less than 6 days antepartum, the mother would not be potentially infectious until at least 72 hours postpartum.
[d]Considered infectious from the onset of prodrome until 72 hours after the onset of exanthem.
[e]Incubation period for modified measles may be prolonged beyond the usual 10 to 14 days.
From Gershon AA. Chickenpox, measles and mumps. In: Remington JS, Klein JO, eds. *Infectious Diseases of the Fetus and Newborn Infant.* 4th ed. Philadelphia: WB Saunders; 1995.

(and, less often, decreased white blood cells or platelets); chronic infection in immunodeficient individuals; and rarely, myocarditis, vasculitis, or hemophagocytic syndrome.

Intrauterine vertical transmission can lead to severe anemia and immune-mediated hydrops fetalis, which can be treated, if accurately diagnosed, by intrauterine transfusion. Inflammation of the liver or CNS can be seen in the infant, along with vasculitis. If the child is clinically well at birth, hidden or persistent abnormalities are rarely identified. No evidence indicates that parvovirus B19 causes an identified pattern of birth defects.[404]

Postnatal transmission usually occurs from person to person via contact with respiratory secretions, saliva, and rarely blood or urine. The seroprevalence in children at 5 years of age is approximately 5% to 10%, with the peak age of infection occurring during the school-age years (5% to 40% of children infected), such that about 50% of young adults are seropositive. The majority of infections are asymptomatic or undiagnosed seroconversions.[404] Severe disease, such as prolonged aplastic anemia, occurs in individuals with hemoglobinopathies or abnormal RBC maturation. Attack rates have been estimated to be 17% to 30% in casual contacts and up to 50% among household contacts. In one study of 235 susceptible pregnant women, the annual seroconversion rate was 1.4%.[405]

No reports of transmission to an infant through breastfeeding are available. Excretion in breast milk has not been studied because of limitations in culturing techniques. Rat parvovirus has been demonstrated in rat milk. Immunoglobulin E (IgE) antiparvovirus antibodies have been detected in human breast milk in one study.[406]

The very low seroconversion rate in young children and the absence of chronic or frequent severe disease suggest that the risk for parvovirus infection via breast milk is not significant. The possibility of antibodies against parvovirus or other protective constituents in breast milk has not been systematically studied. Breastfeeding by a mother with parvovirus infection is acceptable.

Polioviruses

Poliovirus infections (types 1, 2, and 3) cause a range of illness, with 90% to 95% being subclinical, 4% to 8% being abortive, and 1% to 2% manifesting as paralytic poliomyelitis. A 1955 review by Bates[407] of 58 cases of poliomyelitis in infants younger than 1 month of age demonstrated paralysis or death in more than 70% and only one child without evidence of even transient paralysis. More than half the cases were ascribed to transmission from the mothers, although no mention was made of breastfeeding. Breastfeeding rates at the time were approximately 25%.

Prenatal infection with polioviruses does cause an increased incidence of abortion. Prematurity and stillbirth apparently occur more frequently in mothers who developed paralytic disease versus inapparent infection.[408] Although individual reports of congenital malformations in association with maternal poliomyelitis exist, no epidemiologic data suggest that polioviruses are teratogenic. Also, no evidence indicates that live attenuated vaccine poliovirus given during pregnancy is associated with congenital malformations.[409,410]

Perinatal infection has been noted in several case reports of infants, infected in utero several days before birth, who had severe disease manifesting with neurologic symptoms (paralysis) but without fever, irritability, or vomiting. Additional case reports of infection acquired postnatally demonstrate illness more consistent with poliomyelitis of childhood. These cases were more severe and involved paralysis, which may represent reporting bias.[409]

No data are available concerning the presence of poliovirus in breast milk, although antibodies to poliovirus types 1, 2, and 3 have been documented.[411] In this era of increasing worldwide poliovirus vaccination, the likelihood of prenatal or perinatal poliovirus infection is decreasing. Maternal susceptibility to poliovirus should be determined before conception, and the poliovirus vaccine should be offered to susceptible women. An analysis of the last great epidemic of poliovirus infection in Italy in 1958 was done using a population-based case-control study.[412] In 114,000 births, 942 infants were reported with paralytic poliomyelitis. A group of matched control subjects was selected from infants admitted to the hospital at the same time. Using the dichotomous variable of never breastfed and partially breastfed, 75 never-breastfed infants were among the cases and 88 among the control group. The authors determined an odds ratio of 4.2, with a 95% confidence interval of 1.4 to 14, demonstrating that the risk for paralytic poliomyelitis was higher in infants never breastfed and lowest among those exclusively breastfed. Because by the time the diagnosis of poliomyelitis is made in a breastfeeding mother the exposure of the infant to poliovirus from maternal secretions has already occurred, and because the breast milk already contains antibodies that may be protective, no reason exists to interrupt breastfeeding. Breastfeeding also does not interfere with successful immunization against poliomyelitis with oral or inactivated poliovirus vaccine.[413]

RETROVIRUSES

Human T-Cell Leukemia Virus Type I

The occurrence of HTLV-I is endemic in parts of southwestern Japan,[414] the Caribbean, South America, and sub-Saharan Africa. HTLV-I is associated with adult T-cell leukemia/lymphoma and a chronic condition with progressive neuropathy. The progressive neuropathy is called *HTLV-I-associated myelopathy* (HAM) or *tropical spastic paraparesis* (TSP)[415] Other illnesses have been reported in association with HTLV-I infection, including dermatitis, uveitis, arthritis, and Sjögren syndrome in adults and infective dermatitis and persistent lymphadenitis in children. Transmission of HTLV-I occurs most often through sexual contact, via blood or blood products, and via breast milk and occurs via the transfer of live infected T lymphocytes. Infrequent transmission does occur in utero or at delivery and with casual or household contact.[415]

Epidemiology HTLV-I

Seroprevalence generally increases with age and varies widely in different regions and in populations of different backgrounds. In some areas of Japan, seropositivity can be as high as 12% to 16%, but in South America, Africa, and some Caribbean countries, the rates are 2% to 6%. In Latin America, seropositive rates can be as high as 10% to 25% among female sex workers or attendees to STD clinics.[416] In blood donors in Europe, the seroprevalence of HTLV-I has been reported at 0.001% to 0.03%. The seroprevalence in pregnant women in endemic areas of Japan is as high as 4% to 5%, and in nonendemic areas, it is as low as 0.1% to 1.0%. HTLV-I is not a major disease in the United States. In studies from Europe, the seroprevalence in pregnant women has been noted to be up to 0.6%. These pregnant women were primarily of African or Caribbean descent.[417]

HTLV-I and Breast Milk

HTLV-I antigen has been identified in the breast milk of HTLV-I-positive mothers.[418] Transmission seems to depend

TABLE 12.4   HTLV-I Transmission Related to the Duration of Breastfeeding

Author (Reference)	Duration (month)	Seroconversion Rate (%)	Number of Children[a]
Takahashi[423]	≤6	4.4	4/90
	≥7	14.4	20/139
	(bottle-fed)	5.7	9/158
Takezaki[32]	≤6	3.9	2/51
	>6	20.3	13/64
Wiktor[33]	<12	9.0	8/86
	≥12	32	19/60

HTLV-I, Human T-cell leukemia virus type I.

[a]Number of children positive for HTLV-I over the number of children examined.

on the transfer of live infected T lymphocytes. Another report shows that basal mammary epithelial cells can be infected with HTLV-I and can transfer infection to peripheral blood monocytes.[419] Human milk from HTLV-I-positive mothers caused infection in marmosets.[420,421] HTLV-I infection clearly occurs via breastfeeding. There are a number of reports documenting an increased rate of transmission of HTLV-I to breastfed infants compared with formula-fed infants and a recent systematic review and meta-analysis of HTLV I and breastfeeding.[422] Boostani et al. utilized seven reports to calculate pooled OR and risk difference (RD), which demonstrated the increased risk of HTLV-I transmission in breastfed infants versus formula-fed infants (OR = 3.48, 95% CI 1.58 to 7.64, RD = 17.1%, 95% CI 7.5% to 26.7%).[422]

Transmission of HTLV-I infection via breastfeeding is also clearly associated with the duration of breastfeeding.[32,33,423,424] It has been postulated that the persistence of passively acquired antibodies against HTLV-I offers some protection through 6 months of life (Table 12.4).

Specific Variables for HTLV-I Transmission

Other factors relating to HTLV-I transmission via breast milk have been proposed. Yoshinaga et al.[425] presented data on the HTLV-I antigen-producing capacity of peripheral blood and breast-milk cells and showed an increased MTCT rate when the mother's blood and breast milk produced large numbers of antigen-producing cells in culture.[425] Hisada et al.[426] reported on 150 mothers and infants in Jamaica, demonstrating that a higher maternal provirus level and a higher HTLV-I antibody titer were independently associated with HTLV-I transmission to the infant. Ureta-Vidal et al.[427] reported an increased seropositivity rate in children of mothers with a high proviral load and elevated maternal HTLV-I antibody titers. Li et al. demonstrated an increased risk of transmission of HTLV-I with increasing provirus load, such that transmission was 4.7/1000 person-months when the provirus load in breast milk was <0.18% and transmission increased to 28.7/1000 person-months when the provirus load was >1.5%.[428] Paiva et al. reported having a previous HTLV-I-infected child as another risk factor for vertical transmission.[429]

Various interventions have been proposed to decrease HTLV-I transmission via breastfeeding. Complete avoidance of breastfeeding was shown to be an effective intervention by Hino et al.[430,431] in a large population of Japanese in Nagasaki. Avoiding breastfeeding led to an 80% decrease in transmission. Breastfeeding for a shorter duration is another effective alternative. Ando et al.[34] showed that freezing and thawing breast milk decreased the infectivity of HTLV-I. Sawada et al.[432] demonstrated, in a rabbit model, that HTLV-I immunoglobulin protected against HTLV-I transmission via milk. It is reasonable to postulate that any measure that would decrease the maternal provirus load or increase the anti-HTLV-I antibodies available to infants might decrease the risk for transmission. The overall prevalence of HTLV-I infection during childhood is unknown because the majority of individuals do not manifest illness until much later in life. The timing of HTLV-I infection in a breastfeeding population has been difficult to assess because of passively acquired antibodies from the mother and issues related to testing. Furnia et al.[433] estimated the time of infection for a cohort of 16 breastfed infants in Jamaica. The estimated median time of infection was 11.9 months, as determined by PCR, compared with the estimated time of infection, based on whole-virus Western blot, of 12.4 months.

In areas where the prevalence of HTLV-I infection (in the United States, Canada, or Europe) is low, the likelihood that a single test for antibodies against HTLV-I would be a false-positive test is high compared with the number of true-positive tests. Repeat testing is warranted in most situations.[434] Quantification of the antibody titer and the proviral load is appropriate in a situation when MTCT is a concern. A greater risk for progression to disease in later life has not been shown for HTLV-I infection through breast milk, but early-life infections are associated with the greatest risk for adult T-cell leukemia.[435]

Recommendations for HTLV-I

The mother and family should be informed about all these issues. If the risk for lack of breast milk is not too great and formula is readily available and culturally acceptable, then the proscription of breastfeeding, or at least a recommendation to limit the duration of breastfeeding to 6 months or less, is appropriate to limit the risk for HTLV-I transmission to the infant. Given the substantial benefits of breastfeeding for the infant and mother, which is especially true in resource-poor countries, there is considerable debate about the cost and benefit of proscribing breastfeeding by HTLV-I mothers in different settings.[436,437] Each individual situation should be evaluated and discussed with the family regarding the potential long-term benefits of not breastfeeding relative to HTLV-I infection versus the potential risks of not breastfeeding.[436–438] Freezing and thawing breast milk before giving it to an infant might be another reasonable intervention to decrease the risk for transmission, although no controlled trials document the efficacy of such an intervention. Neither Ig nor antiviral agents against HTLV-I are currently available.

Human T-Cell Leukemia Virus Type II

HTLV-II is endemic in specific geographic locations, including Africa, the Americas, the Caribbean, and Japan. Transmission is primarily through IV drug use, contaminated blood products, and breastfeeding. Sexual transmission occurs, but its overall contribution to the prevalence of HTLV-II in different populations remains uncertain. Many studies have examined the presence of HTLV-I and HTLV-II in blood products. PCR testing and selective antibody tests suggest that about half of the HTLV seropositivity in blood donors is caused by HTLV-II.

HTLV-II has been associated with two chronic neurologic disorders similar to those caused by HTLV-I, tropical or spastic ataxia.[439] A connection between HTLV-II and glomerulonephritis, myelopathy, arthritis, T-hairy cell leukemia, and large-cell granulocytic leukemia has been reported.

MTCT has been demonstrated in both breastfed and formula-fed infants. It appears that the rate of transmission is greater in breastfed infants.[440–446] HTLV-II has been detected in breast milk.[440] Nyambi et al.[444] reported that HTLV-II transmission did correlate with the duration of breastfeeding. The estimated rate of transmission was 20%. The time to seroconversion (after the initial loss of passively acquired maternal antibodies) for infected infants seemed to range between 1 and 3 years of age.[444] At this time, avoidance of breastfeeding and limiting the duration of breastfeeding are the only two possible interventions with evidence of effectiveness for preventing HTLV-II MTCT.[447]

With the current understanding of retroviruses, it is appropriate in cases of documented HTLV-II maternal infection to recommend avoiding or limiting the duration of breastfeeding and to provide alternative nutrition when financially practical and culturally acceptable. Mothers should have confirmatory testing for HTLV-II and measurement of the proviral load. Infants should be serially tested for antibodies to HTLV-II and have confirmatory testing if seropositive after 12 to 18 months of age. Further investigation into the mechanisms of transmission via breast milk and possible interventions to prevent transmission should occur as they have for HIV-1 and HTLV-I.

Human Immunodeficiency Virus Type 1

Human immunodeficiency virus type 1 (HIV-1) is transmitted through human milk. Refraining from breastfeeding remains a crucial aspect of preventing perinatal HIV infection in the United States and many other resource-rich countries. There are two dilemmas: (1) the use of replacement feeding to prevent MTCT versus breastfeeding in countries where breastfeeding clearly provides infants with significant protection from illness and death as a result of malnutrition or other infections and (2) proscribing breastfeeding for HIV-positive mothers when antiretroviral medications and formula are readily available and depriving infants and mothers of the benefits of breastfeeding. The goals remain the same for the HIV-1-positive woman and the HIV-exposed fetus/infant: prevention of MTCT of HIV; optimization of maternal health; and long-term survival while the exposed infant remains well, with appropriate growth and development, along with HIV-free survival.

Breastfeeding and HIV Transmission

The question of the contribution of breastfeeding in mother-to-child HIV-1 transmission is not a trivial one when one considers the following:

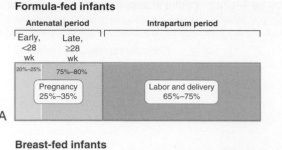

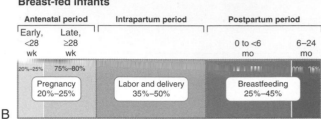

Fig. 12.6 Approximate proportion of human immunodeficiency virus type 1 (HIV-1) transmission (mother-to-child transmission [MTCT]) for an untreated mother and infant, based on gestational period and feeding method. (A) Formula-fed infants. (B) Breast-fed infants. (From Luzuriaga K, Mofenson LM. Challenges in the elimination of pediatric HIV-1 infection. *N Engl J Med.* 2016;374:761–770.)

1. The WHO has estimated that 36.9 million people (estimated range: 31.1 to 43.9) were living with HIV-1 at the end of 2017.[448] There were an estimated 1.6 million new HIV-infected persons 15 years of age or older (down from an estimated 2.8 million in 2000). Despite the actual decline in the annual number of new HIV-infected persons, each week, approximately 7000 women between the ages of 15 and 24 years old become infected with HIV.

2. The WHO estimates that there were 180,000 (110,000 to 260,000) children younger than 14 years old who were newly infected with HIV-1 in 2017. This represents a drop of 35% compared with 2010. Most of the newly infected children are infected via MTCT, and this number has declined as a result of increasing access to and utilization of interventions to prevent MTCT of HIV.

3. The availability of antiretroviral therapy for the prevention of mother-to-child HIV transmission in developing countries has increased to an estimated 80% of the mothers who needed it in 2017 (compared with 59% of all eligible adults receiving antiretroviral therapy).[448]

4. Breastfeeding contributes an estimated 10% to 20% increase in the overall MTCT rates, over and above intrauterine and intrapartum transmission, when no specific interventions to prevent transmission via breastfeeding are utilized. Breastfeeding is responsible for 25% to 45% of all the HIV-infected infants annually[449] (Fig. 12.6).

5. Despite a dramatic increase in the number of people receiving antiretroviral therapy (ART) in developing countries, only 52% of children 0 to 14 years old who were eligible for antiretroviral medications based on current guidelines were receiving them. Without appropriate and timely ART, 50% of HIV-infected infants will die by their second birthday.[448]

Evidence for Mother-to-Child Transmission via Breastfeeding

The evidence of HIV transmission via breastfeeding is irrefutable. Multiple publications summarize the current evidence for HIV transmission via breastfeeding in the literature.[449–455] Primary HIV infection in breastfeeding mothers, with the concomitant high viral load, is associated with a particularly high rate of HIV transmission via breast milk. Palasanthiran et al.[456] estimated that risk at 27%. Large observational studies have demonstrated higher rates of HIV transmission in breastfed infants of mothers with chronic HIV infection compared with formula-fed infants.[457–459] A systematic analysis of published reports estimated the additional risk for perinatal HIV transmission resulting from breastfeeding to be 14% (95% CI 7% to 22%).[460] Other published cohort studies similarly attributed additional risk for HIV transmission resulting from breastfeeding at 4% to 22% over and above the risk from prenatal and intrapartum transmission.[461–463] Laboratory reports and reviews demonstrate the presence of cell-free virus and cell-associated virus in breast milk, as well as various bioactive factors in breast milk and characteristics of the virus that could block or limit infection.[464–472] A dose–response relationship has been observed, correlating the HIV viral load in human milk, as well as a mother's plasma viral load, with an increased transmission risk for the breastfed infant.[473–476]

Many of the potential risk factors associated with human milk transmission of HIV have been described (Box 12.4). The cumulative risk for HIV transmission is higher the longer the duration of breastfeeding.[458,477–480] Maternal characteristics related to the transmission of HIV via human milk include younger maternal age, higher parity, lower $CD4^+$ counts, higher plasma viral loads, and breast abnormalities (mastitis, abscess, or nipple lesions). Characteristics of human milk that relate to a higher risk for transmission include higher viral load in the milk; lower concentrations of antiviral substances (lactoferrin, lysozyme); and lower concentrations of virus-specific cytotoxic T-lymphocytes, levels of various interleukins (interleukin-7 [IL-7], interleukin-15 [IL-15]),[481,482] secretory IgA, and IgM. Mixed breastfeeding is also associated with a higher risk for HIV transmission compared with exclusive breastfeeding.[483–485] The issue becomes how to balance the measurable benefits of breast milk (nutrition and protection against other causes of morbidity and mortality in infancy) against the relative risk for HIV transmission to the infant as a result of breastfeeding (with optimization of other factors to decrease HIV transmission) and how to provide optimal care for each mother–infant dyad within the context of local maternal and child health services. The actual measurable benefits of receiving breast milk versus the relative increased risk for HIV transmission will need to be determined in a prospective fashion in different nations and locales.[454,486–491]

Interventions to Prevent Breastfeeding-Related HIV Transmission

Several potential interventions to prevent breastfeeding transmission of HIV-1 can be utilized depending on the specific situation of the mother and infant. The simplest and most effective is the complete avoidance of human milk. This is a practical solution in places such as the United States, where replacement feeding and other strictly medical interventions are feasible and reasonable and the risk of not providing breast milk to the infant is minimal in the short term. Recommendations proscribing breastfeeding in the setting of an HIV-positive mother within the United States are from the Department of Health and Human Services Panel on Treatment of HIV-Infected Pregnant Women and Prevention of Perinatal Transmission[492] and the AAP Section on Breastfeeding.[3] In resource-poor situations, where the risk for other infections and malnutrition is high without the benefits of breast milk, exclusive breastfeeding is appropriate, with other reasonable and culturally acceptable interventions to decrease HIV transmission via breast milk.[493–496] Recommendations for resource-limited countries are from the WHO.[453,497,498]

Potentially effective interventions include exclusive breastfeeding; avoidance of mixed feeding; utilization of replacement feeding when it is acceptable, feasible, affordable, sustainable, and safe (AFASS) within the woman's community; and education and support to decrease the likelihood of mastitis or nipple lesions.[499] Other crucial issues for the care of HIV-positive women include overcoming inequities of health care and support, diminishing fear of disclosure and stigma, and influencing social circumstances and discrimination.

Other possible interventions include treating a mother with antiretroviral therapy for her own health or prophylactically to decrease the human milk viral load, treating an infant prophylactically for a prolonged period of time to protect against transmission via breastfeeding, treating the milk itself to decrease the viral load (by pasteurization or other methods),[500,501] treating acute conditions in mothers and infants (e.g., mastitis, breast lesions, infant candidiasis), and enhancing an infant's own defenses via vitamins and immunizations. The three options for prevention of MTCT proposed by the WHO are described as Option A, Option B, and Option B + [497,498] (Table 12.5). The use of antiretroviral medications in the mother or the infant to specifically prevent transmission of HIV to the infant via breast milk and breastfeeding should continue through at least 1 week after stopping

---

BOX 12.4 Risk Factors Associated With HIV MTCT Via Breastfeeding

Dose–response relationship between breast-milk HIV viral load and infant infection

Longer duration of breastfeeding (relates to cumulative risk of MTCT)

Mixed feeding (not exclusive breastfeeding)

Early weaning (before 6 months and transition to appropriate complementary foods)

Maternal characteristics: Younger maternal age, higher parity, lower $CD4^+$ lymphocyte counts, higher plasma HIV viral loads, nonadherence to cART

Breast conditions: Mastitis, abscess, nipple lesions

Infant factors: Premature (< 33 weeks' GA), oral lesions, illness

cART, Combined antiretroviral therapy; *GA*, gestational age; *HIV*, human immunodeficiency virus; *MTCT*, mother-to-child transmission.

TABLE 12.5   World Health Organization—Recommended Options for Prevention of HIV MTCT[a]

Options	RECOMMENDATIONS FOR WOMEN	
	Treatment (For CD4 count <350 cells/mm^3)	Prophylaxis (For CD4 counts >35 cells/mm^3)
A	Triple ARVs beginning as soon as possible after diagnosis and continuing for life	Antepartum: AZT starting as early as 14 weeks' gestation (ideally at least 13 weeks before delivery) Intrapartum: At onset of labor, sdNVP and first dose of AZT/3TC Postpartum: Daily AZT/3TC through 7 days postpartum
B	Triple ARVs beginning as soon as possible after diagnosis and continuing for life	Triple ARVs beginning as early as 4 weeks' gestation and continuing through delivery/childbirth and if breastfeeding, continuing postpartum through 1 week after stopping all breastfeeding
B$^+$	Triple ARVs beginning as soon as possible after diagnosis and continuing for life (This should occur regardless of CD4 count in the mother.)	
	RECOMMENDATIONS FOR INFANTS	
A	Daily NVP from birth through 1 week after stopping all breastfeeding (If not breastfeeding or if mother on triple ARVs, continue daily NVP through 4–6 weeks of age.)	
B	Daily NVP or AZT from birth through 4–6 weeks of age regardless of infant feeding method	
B$^+$	Daily NVP or AZT from birth through 4–6 weeks of age regardless of infant feeding method	

3TC, Lamivudine; *ARV*, antiretroviral; *AZT*, azidothymidine; *CD4*, CD4 positive lymphocytes; *HIV*, human immunodeficiency virus; *MTCT*, mother-to-child-transmission; *NVP*, nevirapine; *sdNVP*, single daily dose of NVP; *triple ARV*, one of the current recommended three-drug fully suppressive regimens approved for adults and/or pregnant women; utilization of an individual option by a specific country is dictated by public health considerations and options for that country.
[a]Recommended in WHO 2010 Prevention of MTCT guidelines.
From World Health Organization. Antiretroviral Drugs for Treating Pregnant Women and Preventing HIV Infections in Infants: Recommendations for a Public Health Approach. 2010. http://www.who.int/hiviSBN9789241599818. Accessed July 6, 2019; World Health Organization. Updates on HIV and Infant Feeding: Guideline. 2016. https://www.who.int/maternal_child_adolescent/documents/hiv-infant-feeding-2016/en/.

breastfeeding or stopping the use of mother's milk for that infant. The current recommendations for the duration of breastfeeding by the WHO is at least 12 months and up to 24 months or longer as consistent with local practices, with continued adherence to an effective ART medication regimen.[453] Some of these other interventions may not be feasible in certain settings, such as home pasteurization or maternal ART. Others may not be culturally acceptable, such as treating expressed breast milk before giving it to an infant or even exclusive breastfeeding.

Documented Success of Prevention Options A, B, and B$^+$

Significant data demonstrate the advantage of breastfeeding by HIV-positive mothers for HIV-infected and HIV-exposed infants. The complete avoidance of breastfeeding in certain situations may lead to increased risk for illness and death as a result of other reasons besides HIV transmission.[502,503] A study from Kenya showed improved HIV-1-free survival rates in a formula-fed group of children born to HIV-positive mothers, but the breastfed and formula groups had similar mortality rates (24.4% vs. 20.0%, respectively) and similar incidences of diarrhea and pneumonia in the first 2 years of life.[504] No difference in the two groups was seen in the prevalence of malnutrition, but the breastfed infants had better nutritional status in the first 6 months of life. Arpadi et al.[505] recommend additional nutritional interventions to complement breastfeeding in this population after 6 months of age.

Two reports from Zambia document the benefit of exclusive breastfeeding for decreasing late HIV transmission and the lower mortality at 12 months in infants who had continued breastfeeding rather than discontinued breastfeeding at 4 months of age.[506,507] In Malawi, HIV-infected and HIV-exposed infants who were breastfed (exclusive breastfeeding for 2 months and mixed feeding after that) had lower mortality at 24 months than those who were not breastfed.[508] A report from Botswana examined breastfeeding plus infant zidovudine (ZDV) prophylaxis for 6 months versus formula-feeding plus infant ZDV for 1 month. This study showed a decreased risk for vertical transmission with formula-feeding but also increased cumulative mortality for the HIV-infected infants at 7 months of age who were in the formula-fed group.[509] A study from South Africa examining the use of vitamin A also demonstrated less morbidity in HIV-infected children who were breastfed as compared with those not breastfed.[510] Other abstract reports have shown increased morbidity in HIV-infected children as a result of diarrhea, gastroenteritis, and hospitalization after weaning from breastfeeding.[511–514]

Numerous newer studies[490,515,516] and systematic reviews[454,487,488,491,517] document remarkably improved HIV-free survival out to 6, 12, and 24 months in breastfed infants of mothers receiving combined antiretroviral therapy (cART). These reviews document "pooled" results of HIV-free survival for 89% to 95% of the studied infants with morbidity and mortality from any cause similar to or better than those for formula-fed infants. The recent PROMISE Study provided data on over 2400 mother–child pairs and compared maternal cART with single-daily-dose nevirapine for the child through 18 months. The rates of MTCT were very low, and infant HIV-free survival at 24 months was 97.1% in the maternal ART group compared with 97.7% in the infant NVP group.[516] These successes have led to discussion of what might be the optimal duration of breastfeeding or how to individualize the guidelines to optimize infant HIV-free survival.[490,515]

Reconsidering Breastfeeding and Prevention of MTCT in Resource-Rich Settings

The noted reduction in rates of MTCT across the world and the discussion about the elimination of MTCT as an attainable goal raises the question, Should breastfeeding by effectively treated HIV-positive mothers in high-income settings be reconsidered?[518–521] Waitt et al. point out the different recommendations regarding breastfeeding by HIV-positive women from the European AIDS Clinical Society, the British HIV Association, and the US Panel on the treatment of pregnant women with HIV infection and the prevention of perinatal transmission. They provide an appropriate discussion of the gaps in our knowledge and propose research to provide additional evidence necessary to make an informed choice regarding breastfeeding and HIV.[519] Tuthill et al. report on provider perspectives on infant feeding with HIV in the United States. They note that medical providers are supporting women with HIV infection who are attempting to breastfeed but feel they have inadequate information to optimally do that.[520] Gross et al. present medical evidence on the transmission risks of HIV via breastfeeding and the risks and benefits of breastfeeding and an ethical discussion on breastfeeding and HIV in the United States.[521] They offer recommendations for changing national guidelines utilizing the principles of autonomy, harm reduction, and reduction of health inequities. Kahlert et al. discuss the current estimated risk of HIV MTCT via breastfeeding with maternal suppressive cART compared with the possible benefits of breastfeeding for the mothers and infants in resource-rich settings.[518] For their discussion, they define an "optimal scenario" of regular clinical care for the mother, excellent maternal adherence to the ART regimen, fully suppressed HIV plasma viral load (pVL) to <50 RNA copies/mL on at least two occasions during pregnancy and at delivery, and documentation that the infant has not acquired HIV in utero or in the peripartum period. They note a very low, "unmeasurable" risk in individual situations when the mother is on an effectively suppressive cART but allow that the "prolonged" potential exposure to HIV in human milk over 12 to 24 months of breastfeeding (especially as a result of cell-associated virus) could be significant. The possibility of mastitis in the mother, oral mucosal or gastrointestinal lesions in the infant, or illness in the mother and or infant over the period of breastfeeding could change the risk for an individual infant. Additional risks could include toxicity in the infant as a result of the ART

exposure[522] and immune-response changes in the infant exposed to HIV through breastfeeding. In contrast, they comment on some of the potential benefits from breastfeeding[523,524] and the importance of breast milk containing specific inhibitors of HIV replication; bioactive, antiinflammatory, and antimicrobial factors of acute and long-term benefit to the infant; development of the intestinal microbiota; reduced risk of otitis media, respiratory tract infections, and obesity for the infant; and potential maternal benefits, including uterine involution, lower future risk of breast cancer, and improved glucose homeostasis with diminished risk of type 2 diabetes. The conclusion of Kahlert et al. is that breastfeeding in effectively treated HIV-infected mothers in resource-rich settings is an equipoise proposal. They recommend formally studying this in developed countries and propose how to support HIV-positive women who wish to breastfeed their children.[518]

Exclusive Breastfeeding

Exclusive breastfeeding in most areas of the world is essential to infant health and survival, even in the situation of maternal HIV infection.[483,506,525,526] The duration of exclusive breastfeeding is crucial to decreasing the risk for HIV infection in infants versus the risk for malnutrition and other infections with early weaning. Becquet et al.[527] analyzed data from Cote d'Ivoire for 2001 to 2005; 47% of the HIV-exposed infants were breastfed for a median of 4 months, and 53% were formula-fed and observed for 2 years. No significant difference in the rate of HIV infection was seen in the two groups, and no significant difference between the two groups was seen for morbid events (diarrhea, acute respiratory infections, or malnutrition), hospitalization, or death. The authors attributed these good outcomes to exclusive breastfeeding, effective nutritional counseling and care, access to clean water, and the provision of a safe and continuous supply of breast-milk substitute.[527] Coovadia et al.[525] studied exclusive breastfeeding in the first 6 months of life as an intervention in South Africa. Of the exclusively breastfed infants, 14.1% at 6 weeks of age and 19.5% at 6 months of age were HIV-infected. Breastfed infants who also were fed solids or formula milk were more likely to acquire infection than exclusively breastfed infants. The cumulative mortality at 3 months of age was markedly lower for exclusively breastfed infants (6.1% vs. 15.1%) in the infants receiving mixed feedings.

Early Weaning

Kuhn et al.[528] examined the effects of early, abrupt weaning on HIV-free survival of 958 children in Zambia. Infants were randomly assigned to two different counseling programs that advised either abrupt weaning at 4 months or prolonged breastfeeding (PB). In the weaning intervention group, 69% of mothers stopped breastfeeding by 5 months compared with a median duration of breastfeeding of 16 months in the control group. The study found no significant difference in HIV-free survival at 24 months in the two groups (83.9% vs. 80.7%). Children already infected by 4 months of age had higher mortality if they were assigned to the early-weaning group (73.6% vs. 54.8%). Additional analysis showed that in mothers with less severe HIV disease, early weaning was clearly harmful to the infant.[529] Arpadi et al.[505] studied the growth of HIV-exposed, uninfected children who were exclusively breastfed for 4 months with rapid weaning to replacement foods or exclusively breastfed until 6 months and then continued breastfeeding with complementary foods. Weight-for-age z-scores dropped markedly in both groups from 4 to 15 months of age but less so in the continued-breastfeeding group. Length-for-age z-scores also dropped dramatically but were not influenced by continued breastfeeding. Even in this HIV-exposed, uninfected group of children, additional nutritional interventions are essential to complement breastfeeding beyond 6 months of age.[505]

Human Immunodeficiency Virus and Breastfeeding—Effect on Maternal Health

The potential effect of breastfeeding on the HIV-positive mother needs to be adequately assessed in relation to the mother's health status. From Uganda and Zimbabwe, Mbizvo et al.[530] reported no difference in the number of hospital admissions or mortality between HIV-positive and HIV-negative women during pregnancy. In the 2 years after delivery, the HIV-positive women had higher hospital admission (approximately two times increased risk) and death rates (relative risk greater than 10) than HIV-negative women. Infant feeding status was not reported.[530] Chilongozi et al.[531] reported on 2292 HIV-positive mothers from four sub-Saharan sites followed for 12 months postpartum. Serious adverse events occurred in 166 women (7.2%); 42 deaths occurred in the HIV-positive women, and no deaths occurred in the 331 HIV-negative women. Antiretroviral medications were not available to the women at any of the four sites, and infant feeding was not recorded.

Several studies have examined breastfeeding relative to mothers' health and reported conflicting results. The first study from Kenya demonstrated a significantly higher mortality rate in 425 women randomly assigned to breastfeeding or formula-feeding groups, with 18 deaths in the breastfeeding mothers (18/212) compared with 6 deaths in the formula-feeding group (6/213) in the 2 years after delivery. The hypothesized explanation offered by the authors for this difference was increased metabolic demands, greater weight loss, and nutritional depletion.[532] A second study from South Africa showed an overall lower mortality rate in the two groups, with no significant difference in mortality rate in the 10 months of observation.[526] Kuhn et al.[533] reported no difference in mortality over 12 months after delivery between 653 women randomly assigned to a short breastfeeding group (326 women; 4.93%, 95% CI 2.42 to 7.46) and a long breastfeeding group (327 women; 4.89%, 95% CI 2.38 to 7.40). In a separate analysis, the mortality rates were not associated with prolonged lactation.[533] Walson et al.[534] followed 535 HIV-positive women for 1 to 2 years in Kenya. The mortality risk was 1.9% at 1 year and 4.8% at 2 years of follow-up. Although less than 10% of women reported a hospitalization during the 2 years, they experienced various common infections (pneumonia, diarrhea, TB, malaria, STDs, urinary tract infections,

mastitis). Breastfeeding in these women was a significant cofactor for diarrhea and mastitis but not for pneumonia, TB, hospitalization, or mortality.[534] In 2013 Watts et al. reported on a group of women receiving ART from pregnancy through the postpartum period. In 1285 women, progression to AIDS or a CD4 count <350 cells per microliter was uncommon through 1 year postpartum if the women had CD4 counts over 550 cells per microliter at delivery. Progression to AIDS or a decline to CD4 counts of <350 cells per microliter occurred in over one-third of those with CD4 counts under 550 cells per microliter at delivery. Nine deaths occurred in women with CD4 counts <550 at delivery, and seven deaths occurred in those with CD4 counts >550. They recommended that ART should be continued after delivery or during breastfeeding among women with CD4 counts <550 cells per microliter if follow-up and support for antiretroviral adherence can be maintained.[535] In the IMPAACT PROMISE study (2018), a randomized study of ART strategies for pregnant and postpartum women with high CD4+ T-cell counts, the women were randomized to continue or stop ART in the postpartum period. They were followed for a median of 1.6 years, and progression to AIDS-defining illness or death was rare in both groups. In the group that continued ARV treatment, there were fewer Stage 2 or 3 clinical conditions, and there were few serious clinical events in the breastfeeding women who had high CD4 counts.[536] The majority of the data support HIV-positive women breastfeeding and continuing ART through lactation and "for life" as a means to maintain maternal health and survival. Optimizing the continuum of HIV care, limiting stigma and discrimination, and supporting women in their health choices and ART adherence will be crucial to maternal health and survival.

HIV Child-to-Breastfeeding-Woman Transmission

HIV child-to-breastfeeding-woman transmission (CBWT) has been a theoretical concern since the beginning of the HIV epidemic. There have been rare cases where this has been suspected but not sufficiently investigated to document its occurrence. Little et al. reviewed the topic in 2012, examining a number of published accounts in a systematic review.[537] Two of the studies included in the review, a study from the Russian Federation and one from Libya, examined outbreaks of nosocomial HIV spread in pediatric hospitals. The infants became infected through blood products, unsterilized needles, or injection equipment. The epidemiologic investigations tried to exclude the other possible sources of HIV infection in the women and delineate the character and timing of the exposures of the mothers to their infants. In Russia, 12 mothers of 152 infected infants were documented to be HIV-positive, and the odds of breastfeeding were greater in the HIV-infected group. Infant stomatitis and cracked nipples in the mothers seemed to also correlate, although the duration of breastfeeding did not seem to be a significant factor. In Libya, there were 20 infected mothers associated with 402 children (5.0%) found to be HIV-infected. A sub-study of 118 mother–infant dyads documented HIV infection in 118 infants and 18 mothers while at the same time confirming the

HIV-negative status of the remaining 100 women and all 75 of the fathers tested. Fourteen of the 18 HIV-positive women had no other risk factors identified except breastfeeding their HIV-positive infants. Breastfeeding was an independent predictor of maternal HIV infection. Three other published reports were discussed, documenting the occurrence of CBWT via breastfeeding in Kazakhstan, Kyrgyzstan, and Romania.[537] The authors raise the concern that many parts of the world where wet nursing and cross-nursing are socially acceptable and more common may overlap with higher HIV-prevalence areas and raise the risk of CBWT. They discuss the very high rates of orphanhood in areas with high HIV prevalence and perinatal HIV transmission. They recognize the greater likelihood that female relatives of the orphaned children are wet or cross-nursing without knowing that there is a risk of transmission of HIV to themselves in this practice. The authors conclude that in addition to optimizing the ongoing efforts of HIV-transmission prevention in adults and children, the WHO guidelines on infant feeding should include information about the risks of wet nursing or cross-nursing HIV-infected infants. Women should be counseled about the possibility of CBWT, and the infants and women should be provided HIV testing to offer women the necessary knowledge and information to make informed feeding decisions.[537]

Summary of HIV and Breastfeeding

In summary, the breastfeeding of infants by HIV-positive mothers does lead to an increased risk for HIV infection in the infants. Much remains to be understood about the mechanisms of HIV transmission via breast milk and the action and efficacy of different interventions to prevent such transmission. The complete avoidance of breastfeeding has been a crucial component for the prevention of perinatal HIV infection in the United States and many other countries; however, that premise is being examined, given the continued successes in the prevention of MTCT.[487]

For resource-poor settings, where breastfeeding is the norm and where it provides vital nutritional and infection-protective benefits, management Options A, B, and B+ are the current standard of care, as adopted by specific countries. The WHO, UNICEF, and the Joint United Nations Programme on HIV/AIDS (UNAIDS) created updated recommendations in 2010: *Guidelines on HIV and Infant Feeding 2010: Principles and Recommendations for Infant Feeding in the Context of HIV and a Summary of Evidence* (http://www.who.int/maternal_child_adolescent/documents/9789241599535/en/).[453] There have been subsequent updates to these guidelines.[538,539]

These publications support national authorities deciding on their own country's plan for infant-feeding practice to optimize the health of the mother and infant, to limit the MTCT of HIV, and to accomplish this by incorporating the policy and interventions in the country's maternal and child health services. There are nine key principles proposed to guide national authorities (Box 12.5).

Mothers choosing to breastfeed should receive additional education, support, and medical care to minimize the risk for

> ### BOX 12.5 Nine Key Principles for the Current Guidelines on HIV and Infant Feeding From the WHO
>
> 1. Balance HIV prevention with protection from other causes of child mortality.
> 2. Integrate HIV interventions into maternal and child health services.
> 3. Set national and sub-national recommendations for infant feeding in the context of HIV.
> 4. Provide breastfeeding to infants born to HIV-infected mothers with a greater chance of HIV-free survival even if antiretroviral drugs are not immediately available.
> 5. Inform mothers known to be HIV-infected about infant feeding alternatives.
> 6. Provide services to specifically support mothers to appropriately feed their infants.
> 7. Avoid harm to infant feeding practices in the general population.
> 8. Advise mothers who are HIV uninfected or whose HIV status is unknown about infant feeding alternatives.
> 9. Invest in improvements in infant feeding practices in the context of HIV.
>
> *HIV*, Human immunodeficiency virus; *WHO*, World Health Organization.

From World Health Organization/UNAIDS/UNICEF. Infant Feeding Guidelines. http://www.unicef.org/programme/breastfeeding/feeding.htm. Accessed August 9, 2019.

HIV transmission and to optimize their own health status during and after breastfeeding. Mothers choosing to use replacement feedings should receive parallel education, support, and medical care for themselves and their infants to minimize the effect of the lack of breastfeeding.

Good evidence now shows that antiretroviral prophylactic regimens for mothers or infants, while continuing breastfeeding, do decrease postnatal HIV transmission. Early weaning is associated with increased morbidity and mortality for the infants; therefore the current recommendations are to breastfeed for at least 12 months up to and beyond 24 months. Further carefully controlled research is indicated to adequately assess the overall risks and benefits to infants and breastfeeding mothers with antiretroviral prophylaxis for either or both mothers and infants. Along with this, HIV testing rates must be improved, and access to antenatal care, HIV-prevention services, and HIV medical care for everyone must be increased. The availability and free access to antiretroviral medications must also improve.

The decision about infant feeding for HIV-positive mothers remains a difficult one, but this is slowly improving with increasing options and new evidence. The goals remain 100% prevention of HIV-1 MTCT, optimal maternal health and survival, and optimal infant growth and development with prolonged HIV-free survival. Research continues to be essential to inform future guidelines, including the advisability of recommending or proscribing breastfeeding by HIV-positive women in resource-rich settings.

Resources and guidelines for HIV and breastfeeding.
There are a number of very good references for guidelines for the prevention of HIV MTCT and specifically MTCT via breastfeeding.

The current WHO/UNAIDS/UNICEF infant-feeding guidelines in the context of HIV are summarized at http://www.unicef.org/programme/breastfeeding/feeding.htm (accessed July 8, 2019). Updates are provided in the WHO's 2015 *Guideline on When to Start Antiretroviral Therapy and on Pre-Exposure Prophylaxis for HIV* (https://apps.who.int/iris/bitstream/handle/10665/186275/9789241509565_eng.pdf;jsessionid = 0BC08C7B F59E2A7A0BADDCCF1CD178F0?sequence = 1; accessed July 6, 2019) and the WHO's 2016 *Updates on HIV and Infant Feeding: Guideline* (https://www.who.int/maternal_child_adolescent/documents/hiv-infant-feeding-2016/en/).

The current guidelines for the United States for the management of ART in pregnancy and interventions to diminish HIV MTCT, *Recommendations for the Use of Antiretroviral Drugs in Pregnant Women With HIV Infection and Interventions to Reduce Perinatal HIV Transmission in the United States*, are continually updated by the Panel on Treatment of Pregnant Women With HIV Infection and Prevention of Perinatal Transmission (https://aidsinfo.nih.gov/guidelines; accessed July 8, 2019).

The 2018 guidelines from the British HIV Association8 are available at https://www.bhiva.org/file/WrhwAPoKvRmeV/BHIVA-Pregnancy-guidelines-consultation-draft-final.pdf.

The guidelines from the European AIDS Clinical Society (EACS) are available at http://www.eacsociety.org/files/2018_guidelines-9.1-english.pdf (accessed August 14, 2019).

In 2018 the World Alliance for Breastfeeding Action (WABA) published a comprehensive resource for understanding international policy on HIV and breastfeeding, available at https://waba.org.my/activities/understanding-international-policy-on-hiv-and-breastfeeding-a-comprehensive-resource/ (accessed July 5, 2019).

Human Immunodeficiency Virus Type 2

Human immunodeficiency virus type 2 (HIV-2) is an RNA virus in the nononcogenic, cytopathic lentivirus genus of retroviruses. It is genetically closer to simian immunodeficiency virus than to HIV-1. The clinical disease associated with HIV-2 has similar symptoms to HIV-1 infection, but it progresses to severe immunosuppression at a slower rate.

HIV-2 is endemic in West Africa and parts of the Caribbean and is found infrequently in Europe and North and South America.[540,541] HIV-2 is very uncommon in the United States, with only 166 confirmed cases documented from 1998 and 2009.[542] It is transmitted via sexual contact, blood, or blood products and from mother to child.

Routine testing for HIV-2 is recommended in blood banks. Antibody tests used for HIV-1 are only 50% to 90% sensitive for detecting HIV-2.[543] Specific testing for HIV-2 is appropriate whenever clinically or epidemiologically indicated. Confirmatory HIV-2 testing with nucleic acid testing is appropriate in any low-prevalence area.[544]

Vertical transmission occurs infrequently. Ekpini et al.[463] followed a large cohort of West African mothers and infants:

138 HIV-1-positive women, 132 HIV-2-positive women, 69 women seropositive for both HIV-1 and HIV-2, and 274 HIV-seronegative women. A few cases of perinatal HIV-2 transmission occurred, but no case of late postnatal transmission was observed.[545]

HIV-2 transmission via breast milk is less common than HIV-1 transmission, but data do not support that the risk for transmission is zero. HIV-2 has a 20- to 30-fold lower rate of vertical transmission than HIV-1.[545–547] Mothers who test positive for HIV-2 should be tested for HIV-1, and guidelines for breastfeeding should follow those for HIV-1 until additional information is available.[453] The most current guidelines for management are available through AIDSinfo.[548] The recommendations are based on expert opinion and include maternal therapy during pregnancy with triple ART utilizing medications with documented efficacy against HIV-2, 4 weeks of infant prophylaxis with zidovudine, and no breastfeeding. Follow-up care for the mother and infant and testing should be similar to what is done for HIV-1.[549]

Rabies

The rabies virus produces a severe infection with progressive CNS symptoms (anxiety, seizures, altered mental status) that ultimately proceeds to death; few reports of survival exist. Rabies occurs worldwide, except in Australia, Antarctica, and several island groups. An estimated 60,000 people die from rabies related to dog bites yearly worldwide, and 20 million people receive human rabies vaccine.[550] The elimination of canine rabies in the United States through canine rabies vaccination led to a 10-fold decrease in human rabies cases reported from 1938 through 2018. From 1960 to 2018, there were 125 reported human rabies cases; 89 were US-acquired cases, including 6 organ transplantation cases. Among all US-acquired cases, 62 (70%) were caused by bat rabies virus variants.[551] The rabies virus is endemic in various other animal populations, including raccoons, skunks, foxes, and bats.[552] Since 1960, 36 (28%) US residents have died of rabies acquired from dogs while traveling abroad. Postexposure prophylaxis is given to between 16,000 and 39,000 people annually who encounter potentially rabid animals.[553,554]

Because of aggressive immunization programs, rabies in domesticated dogs and cats in the United States is uncommon.[554] The virus is found in the saliva, tears, and nervous tissue of infected animals. Transmission occurs by bites, licking, or simply contact of oral secretions with mucous membranes or nonintact skin. Many cases of rabies in humans now lack a history of some obvious contact with a rabid animal. This may be a result of the long incubation period (generally 4 to 6 weeks, but up to 1 year, with reports of incubation periods of several years), a lack of symptoms early in an infectious animal, or airborne transmission from bats in enclosed environments (caves, laboratories, houses).

Person-to-person transmission via bites has not been documented, although it has occurred in corneal and other organ transplants.[555,556] Rabies viremia has not been observed in the spread of the virus. No evidence exists indicating transmission through breast milk.

In the case of maternal infection with rabies, many scenarios can occur before the onset of progressive, severe CNS symptoms. The progression and severity of maternal illness can preclude breastfeeding, but separation of an infant from the mother is appropriate regardless of the mother's status and method of infant feeding (especially to avoid contact with saliva and tears).[550] Breastfeeding should not continue when the mother has symptoms of rabies, and the infant should receive postexposure immunization and close observation. An infant may receive expressed breast milk, but the expression must occur without possible contamination with saliva or tears from the mother.

Depending on the scenario, the nature of a mother's illness, the possible exposure of an infant to the same source as the mother, and the exposure of a child to the mother, the postexposure immunization of an infant may be appropriate given the specifics of the situation. There are some data on the safety of the rabies vaccine for the mother and fetus during pregnancy but limited information on its safety during breastfeeding.[557–560] A more common scenario is a mother's apparent exposure to rabies (without exposure for the infant), necessitating the postexposure immunization of the mother with rabies vaccine. In almost all cases, in the absence of maternal illness, breastfeeding can reasonably continue during the mother's four-dose immunization series in 14 days.[561] The CDC and other professional organizations state that breastfeeding is not a contraindication to the rabies vaccine.[562,563] In a rare situation in which apparent exposure of the mother and infant to rabies occurs together, the postexposure treatment of both the mother and infant should be instituted, and breastfeeding can continue. The use of the rabies vaccine for an exposed mother even during breastfeeding is appropriate and should be supported with continued breastfeeding.[560]

Respiratory Syncytial Virus

RSV is a common cause of respiratory illness in children and is relatively common in adults, usually producing a milder upper respiratory tract infection in adults. No evidence indicates that RSV causes intrauterine infection, adversely affects the fetus, or causes abortion or prematurity. RSV does produce infection in neonates, causing asymptomatic infection, afebrile upper respiratory tract infection, bronchiolitis, pneumonia, and apnea. The mortality rate can be high in neonates, especially in premature infants and ill full-term infants, particularly those with preexisting respiratory disease (hyaline membrane disease, bronchopulmonary dysplasia) or cardiac disease associated with pulmonary hypertension.

RSV is believed to be transmitted via droplets or direct contact of the conjunctiva, nasal mucosa, or oropharynx with infected respiratory secretions. Documentation of RSV infection is less commonly made in adults, and spread from a mother or other household contacts probably occurs before a diagnosis can be made. Therefore the risk for RSV transmission from breast milk is probably insignificant compared with transmission via direct or droplet contact in families. In nurseries, however, it is appropriate to make a timely diagnosis of RSV infection in neonates to isolate infants from the others to prevent spread in the nursery. Ribavirin is not recommended for routine use. It is infrequently used in patients with potentially life-threatening RSV infection.[564]

RSV infection should be suspected in any infant with rhinorrhea, nasal congestion, or unexplained apnea, especially in October through March in temperate climates. During this season, prophylaxis against RSV with RSV-specific immunoglobulin IV (RSV-IGIV) for infants at the highest risk for severe disease is appropriate.

Debate surrounds the effect of passively acquired antibodies (in infants from mothers before birth) against RSV on the occurrence and severity of illness in neonates and infants. It appears that a higher level of neutralizing antibody against RSV in neonates decreases the risk for severe RSV disease.[565,566] Some controversy remains concerning the measurable benefit of breastfeeding for preventing serious RSV disease,[567–569] with some studies showing benefit and others no effect. Controlling for possible confounding factors (e.g., smoking, crowded living conditions) in these studies has been difficult. There are well-done studies indicating that breastfeeding, independent of other factors, is protective against hospitalization with RSV or severe RSV disease.[565,568,570–573] Dixon has reviewed the role of human milk in protecting against viral bronchiolitis, proposing a number of potential mechanisms related to human milk immunomodulators.[574] One of the potential mechanisms of protection she describes is the presence of cells in human milk with a specific cytokine profile stimulated in mothers by exposure to RSV.[575] There is certainly more to be learned about the role of human milk in protection against severe bronchiolitis and chronic/recurrent wheezing. At this point, no reason exists to stop breastfeeding because of maternal RSV infection, and a potential exists for benefit from immunomodulatory factors in breast milk against RSV. Infants with RSV infection should breastfeed unless their respiratory status precludes it.

Rotaviruses

Rotavirus infections usually result in diarrhea, accompanied by emesis and low-grade fever. In severe infections, the clinical course can include dehydration, electrolyte abnormalities, and acidosis and can contribute to malnutrition in developing countries. Generally, every child will have at least one episode of rotavirus infection by 5 years of age.[576] In developed countries, rotavirus is often associated with diarrhea requiring hospitalization in children younger than 2 years of age, but it is rarely associated with death. Worldwide, rotavirus is the leading cause of diarrhea-related deaths in children younger than 5 years old. Estimates suggest that in children younger than 5 years old, rotavirus infection leads to more than 100 million occurrences of diarrhea, 2 million hospital admissions, and 500,000 deaths each year.[577] Fecal-oral transmission is the most common route, but fomites and respiratory spread may also occur. Spread of infection occurs most often in homes with young children or in daycare centers and institutions. In hospitalized infants or mothers with rotavirus infection, contact precautions are indicated for the duration of the illness. No evidence indicates prenatal infection from rotavirus, but perinatal or postnatal infection from contact with the mother or others can occur.

Breast Milk and Rotavirus

No case of transmission of rotavirus via breast milk has been documented. Breast milk does contain antibodies to rotavirus for up to 2 years. Human milk mucin has been demonstrated to inhibit rotavirus replication and prevent experimental gastroenteritis.[577] Human milk oligosaccharides (HMOs) have been related to the protective effect of breastfeeding against rotavirus diarrhea.[578] All the mechanisms of rotavirus immunity are not well understood. They are thought to be multifactorial, with cell-mediated immunity limiting the severity and course of infection, whereas humoral immunity protects against subsequent infections. Innate and adaptive responses at the level of the mucosa are probably the most important.[579]

Exclusive breastfeeding may decrease the likelihood of severe rotavirus-related diarrhea by as much as 90%.[580,581] A recent systematic review and meta-analysis demonstrated that exclusive breastfeeding, as reported in six studies, reduced the risk of rotavirus infection in children (OR = 0.62, 95% CI 0.48 to 0.81).[582] Additionally, breastfeeding seems to decrease the severity of rotavirus-induced illness in children younger than 2 years old.[581,583,584] At least one study suggested that this may simply represent the postponement of severe rotavirus infection until an older age.[581] Another study suggested that protection against rotavirus rapidly declines upon discontinuation of breastfeeding.[585] This delay in rotavirus infection until the child is older may be beneficial in that the older child may be able to tolerate the infection or illness with a lower likelihood of becoming dehydrated or malnourished. Continuing breastfeeding during an episode of rotavirus illness, with or without vomiting, is appropriate and often helpful to the infant. No reason to suspend breastfeeding by a mother infected with rotavirus is apparent.

Rotavirus Vaccines and Breastfeeding/Breast Milk

Two rotavirus vaccines (Rotateq and Rotarix) have been licensed for use in more than 90 countries, but fewer than 20 countries have routine immunization programs. Additional types of rotavirus vaccines are undergoing study in various countries, specifically examining the efficacy of the vaccines in low- and medium-income countries.[586] Some of the explanations for the slow global implementation of an effective vaccine include differences in protection with specific vaccines in high-income countries compared with low- or medium-income countries, the unfortunate association with intussusception in the United States, the delayed recognition of the significant rotavirus-related morbidity and mortality, and the cost of the new vaccines. The question of the variable efficacy of the specific rotavirus vaccines in developed and developing countries remains an important one.[587–589] Several trials are examining this issue and attempting to address factors such as transplacentally transferred maternal antibodies, breastfeeding practices (especially immediately before immunization with a live oral rotavirus vaccine),

stomach acid, micronutrient malnutrition, interfering gut flora, and differences in the epidemiology of rotavirus in different locations.[590] Withholding breastfeeding before the administration of oral live-attenuated human rotavirus vaccine has not led to enhanced immune response in infants.[591–593] Evidence indicates that maternal immunization with rotavirus vaccine can increase both the transplacental acquisition of antibodies and secretory IgA in breast milk.[594] Additionally, oral rotavirus vaccines have been able to stimulate a good serologic response in both formula-fed and breastfed infants, although the antigen titers may need to be modified to create an optimal response in all infants.[595] The actual protective effect of these vaccines in different situations and strategies will require measurement in ongoing prospective studies.

Rubella Virus

Congenital rubella infection has been well described, and the contributing variables to infection and severe disease have been elucidated.[596] The primary intervention to prevent congenital rubella has been to establish the existence of maternal immunity to rubella before conception, including immunization with rubella vaccine and reimmunization if indicated. Perinatal infection is not clinically significant. Postnatal infection occurs infrequently in children younger than 1 year of age because of passively acquired maternal antibodies. The predominant age of infection is 5 to 14 years old, and more than half of those with infections are asymptomatic. Postnatal rubella is a self-limited, mild viral infection associated with an evanescent rash, shotty adenopathy, and low-grade transient fever. It most often occurs in the late winter and spring.[597] Infants with congenital infection shed the virus for prolonged periods from various sites and may serve as a source of infection throughout the year. Contact isolation is appropriate for suspected and proven congenital infection for at least 1 year, including exclusion from daycare and avoidance of pregnant women, whereas postnatal rubella infection requires droplet precautions for 7 days after the onset of rash.

Rubella virus has been isolated from breast milk after natural infection (congenital or postnatal) and after immunization with live attenuated vaccine virus. Both IgA antibodies and immunoreactive cells against rubella have been identified in breast milk. Breastfed infants can acquire vaccine-virus infection via milk but are predominately asymptomatic. Because postpartum infection with this virus (natural or vaccine) is not associated with clinically significant illness, no reason exists to prevent breastfeeding after congenital infection, postpartum infection in the mother, or maternal immunization with rubella vaccine.[598]

Severe Acute Respiratory Syndrome

Severe acute respiratory syndrome (SARS) is a term that could be applied to any serious acute respiratory illness caused by or associated with a variety of infectious agents. Since 2003, it has been linked with SARS-associated coronavirus (SARS-CoV). In the global outbreak of 2002 to 2003, more than 8400 probable cases of SARS and more than 800 deaths occurred. Beyond the actual number of affected individuals or its associated mortality rate (approximately 10% mortality overall and closer to 50% mortality in persons older than 65 years of age), the lack of data on this new, unusual illness and the tremendous publicity surrounding it made SARS such a sensation. We now know the cause of this illness, known as the *SARS-CoV*. SARS-CoV was shown to be distantly related to the previously characterized coronavirus groups.[599,600] Despite intense international collaboration to study the illness and the virus, many things are not known, such as the degree of infectiousness, the actual period of transmissibility, all the modes of transmission, how many people have an asymptomatic infection as compared with those with symptoms or severe illnesses, how to make a rapid diagnosis of confirmed cases, and where the virus originated.

SARS in Children

At least 21 cases of probable SARS in children have been described in the literature.[601–604] In general, the illness in children is a mild, nonspecific respiratory illness, but in adolescents and adults, it is more likely to progress to severe respiratory distress. It has been reported that children are less likely to transmit SARS than adults.[602] The overall clinical course, the radiologic evolution, and the histologic findings of this illness are consistent with the host's immune response playing a significant role in disease production.

Five infants were born to mothers with confirmed SARS. The infants were born prematurely (26 to 37 weeks), presumably as a result of maternal illness. Although two of the five infants had serious abdominal illnesses (other coronaviruses have been associated with reported outbreaks of necrotizing enterocolitis), the presence of SARS-CoV could not be demonstrated in any of these infants.[603] No evidence of vertical transmission of SARS is available.

SARS and Infant Feeding

The mode of feeding for any of the reported cases of young children with SARS or the infants born to mothers with SARS was not mentioned. There was no evidence for an increased risk of SARS in formula-fed or breastfed infants.

Middle East Respiratory Syndrome

Since 2012, a second unique coronavirus (CoV) was associated with epidemic SARS: Middle East respiratory syndrome (MERS-CoV), named after the initial outbreak described in Saudi Arabia. Subsequent epidemiologic studies suggest that contact with dromedaries or dromedary products is a source of zoonotic transmission. Unpasteurized camel milk was a common product consumed by MERS cases in one review.[605] This illness has an estimated incubation period of 5 to 14 days and manifests similarly to SARS-CoV, with a variety of extrapulmonary manifestations, and it seems to affect individuals with comorbid conditions.[606] It also appears to be transmitted primarily by respiratory droplets. There is no information on the presence or absence of the MERS-CoV in human milk.

As with other respiratory viruses affecting humans predominantly transmitted by droplets, transmission via breast milk is an insignificant mode of transmission, if it occurs at all. The benefits of breastfeeding being what they are, mothers with SARS or MERS should continue breastfeeding if they are able, or expressed breast milk can be given to an infant until the mother is able to breastfeed.

Smallpox

In this era of worry about biologic terrorism, smallpox is an important concern. The concern for infants (breastfed or formula-fed) is direct contact with mothers or household members with smallpox. Smallpox is highly contagious in the household setting as a result of person-to-person spread via droplet nuclei or aerosolization from the oropharynx and direct contact with the rash. Additional potential exposures for infants include the release of a smallpox aerosol into the environment by terrorists, contact with a smallpox-contaminated space or the clothes of household members exposed to an aerosol, and infection via contact with a mother's or a household member's smallpox vaccination site. These risks are the same for breastfed and formula-fed infants. No evidence for the transmission of the smallpox virus via breast milk exists.

A contact is defined as a person who has been in the same household or had face-to-face contact with a patient with smallpox after the onset of fever. Patients do not transmit infection until after progression from the fever stage to the development of the rash. An exposed contact does not need to be isolated from others during the post-contact observation period (usually 17 days) until that person develops fever. The temperature of the exposed contact should be monitored daily. Personal contact and breastfeeding between mother and infant can continue until the onset of fever, when immediate isolation (at home) should begin. Providing expressed breast milk for the infant of a mother with smallpox should be avoided because of the extensive nature of the smallpox rash and the possibility of contamination (from the rash) of the milk during the expression process. No literature documents transmission of the smallpox virus via expressed breast milk.

Vaccinia—Vaccination

The other issue for breastfeeding infants is the question of maternal vaccination with smallpox in a preexposure-event vaccination program. Children older than 1 year of age can be safely and reasonably vaccinated with smallpox in the face of a probable smallpox exposure. Smallpox vaccination of infants younger than 1 year of age is contraindicated. Breastfeeding is listed as a contraindication to vaccination in the preexposure vaccination program. It is unknown whether the vaccine virus or antibodies are present in breast milk. The risk for infection as a result of contact or aerosolization of virus from a mother's smallpox vaccination site is the same for breastfed and formula-fed infants based on contact or aerosolized transmission. The Advisory Committee on Immunization Practices also does not recommend smallpox vaccination of children younger than 18 years old in a preexposure situation.[607]

Contact Vaccinia

One report documents tertiary-contact vaccinia in a breastfeeding infant.[608] A US military person received a primary smallpox vaccination and developed a local reaction at the inoculation site. Despite reportedly observing appropriate precautions, the individual's wife developed vesicles on both areolae (secondary-contact vaccinia). Subsequently, the breastfeeding infant developed lesions on her philtrum, cheek, and tongue. Both the mother and infant remained well, and the infections resolved without therapy. Culture and PCR testing confirmed vaccinia in both the mother's and the infant's lesions. The breast milk was not tested.[608]

In a review of the literature from 1931 to 1981, Sepkowitz[609] reported on 27 cases of secondary vaccinia in households. The CDC reported 30 suspected cases of secondary/tertiary vaccinia, with 18 of those cases confirmed by culture or PCR. The 30 cases were related to 578,286 vaccinated military personnel. This is an incidence of 5.2 cases per 100,000 vaccinees and 7.4 cases per 100,000 primary vaccinees.[610] In a separate report on the civilian smallpox-prevention vaccination program, 37,802 individuals were vaccinated between January and June 2003, and no cases of contact vaccinia were reported.[611]

The risk for contact vaccinia is low. The risk is from close or intimate contact. In the mentioned case, the risk for the infant was contact with the mother's breasts, the inadvertent site of her contact vaccinia. Breastfed and formula-fed infants are equally at risk from close contact in the household of a smallpox vaccinee or a case of secondary vaccinia, and separation from the individual is appropriate in both situations. If the breast of the nursing mother is not involved, expressed breast milk can be given to the infant.

Monkeypox

Another orthopoxvirus that has emerged as a human pathogen in the past decade is monkeypox. Most commonly it is a zoonotic pathogen, spreading to humans though direct contact with infected animals. There are reports of transmission from person to person, but this seems to be an uncommon event.[612] Similar to smallpox, the likelihood of spread is probably similar for formula-fed or breastfed infants, and as long as the breast of a mother with monkeypox is not involved, then expressed breast milk can be given to the infant.

TT Virus

TT virus (TTV, also known as *Torque teno virus*) is a recently identified virus found in a patient (TT) with posttransfusion hepatitis not associated with the other hepatitis-related viruses, A through G. It has been identified in most human tissues and body fluids, and viral replication has been documented in liver and bone marrow but not peripheral blood mononuclear cells. TTV has been described as an unenveloped, circular, single-stranded DNA virus.[613] This virus is prevalent in healthy individuals, including healthy blood donors, and it has been identified in patients with hepatitis.[614] Its role in liver disease, acute or chronic, remains uncertain. It is also present in persons treated with blood products. TTV has been detected in saliva, throat swabs, semen, vaginal fluid, feces, and breast milk.

TTV in Infants

TTV DNA has been detected in the infants of TTV-positive and TTV-negative mothers. Ohto et al.[615] reported no TTV

DNA was detected in cord blood from 38 infants, and it was detected in only 1 of 14 samples taken at 1 month of age. They noted an increasing prevalence from 6 months (22%) to 2 years (33%), which they ascribed to acquisition via nonparenteral routes. In comparisons of the TTV DNA in TTV-positive mothers and their TTV-positive infants, 6 of 13 showed high-level nucleotide sequence similarity, and 7 of 13 differed by greater than 10%.[615] Tyschik et al. examined the blood and plasma of 100 mother–child pairs by TTV-specific quantitative PCR (qPCR), documenting 84% of the women to be TTV-positive, but TTV was not detected in any cord-blood samples. The TTV load in plasma ranged from 10^3 to 3×10^7 copies/ml.[616] In a separate study of 98 healthy breastfeeding infants from Russia, between the ages of 1 and 12 months, qPCR (test sensitivity ~1000 viral copies per milliliter) analysis of whole-blood samples demonstrated that 67% of the samples were positive for TTV, with a significant positive correlation between age and TTV load ($r = 0.81$, $p < 0.01$).[617] The TTV load demonstrated an increase in number through approximately the first 60 days from initial detection. Breast-milk samples were not tested in this study.

TTV in Breast Milk

Schröter et al.[365] reported on TTV DNA in breast milk examined retrospectively. Notably, TTV DNA was detected in 22 of 23 serum samples of infants at 1 week of age, who were born to 22 women viremic for TTV DNA. Twenty-four women who were negative for TTV DNA gave birth to 24 children who were initially negative for TTV DNA and remained negative throughout the observation period (mean = 7.5 months, range = 1 to 28 months). TTV DNA was detected in 77% of breast-milk samples from TTV-viremic women and in none of the breast-milk samples from TTV-negative women. No clinical or laboratory evidence of hepatitis was found in the 22 children who were observed to be TTV-DNA-positive during the period of the study.[365] Other authors have reported TTV in breast milk, as detected by PCR. They describe the absence of TTV DNA in infants at 5 days and 3 months of age, and 4 of 10 infants were positive for TTV DNA at 6 months of age, suggesting the late acquisition of infection via breastfeeding.[618]

TTV is transmitted in utero infrequently and is found in breast milk.[615] No evidence of clinical hepatitis in infants related to TTV infection and no evidence for a late chronic hepatitis exist. Given the currently available information, no reason to proscribe breastfeeding by TTV-positive mothers is compelling. Certainly, more needs to be understood concerning the chronic nature of this infection and the possible pathogenesis of liver disease.[365]

Mammary Tumor Viruses (Human and Mouse) and Breast Cancer

The worry and discussion about viruses as directly causing breast cancer have continued for decades. Viruses commonly associated with tumorigenesis include bovine leukemia virus (BLV), EBV, HHV-8, HIV, HPV, HTLV-I, mouse mammary tumor virus (MMTV), and human mammary tumor virus (HMTV). The viruses and/or the nucleic acid of BLV and HHV-8 have not been identified in breast milk or breast tissue, whereas the other six have. There has also been the concern that MMTV and HMTV transmitted to infants via breast milk could lead to breast cancer formation later in life. With new technology, including PCR testing, in situ hybridization, immunohistochemistry, and genome sequencing, the questions continue regarding identifying HMTV and MMTV in breast milk and breast tissue and their correlation with breast cancer.

Epidemiology of Breastfeeding and Breast Cancer

Several epidemiologic reviews in the 1970s conveyed disagreement about the protective role of pregnancy and lactation and the development of breast cancer.[619–621] This contrasts with studies after that point in time, which support that lactation decreases the risk of premenopausal breast cancer. Byers et al. (1985) reported a case-control study demonstrating a protective effect of lactation on breast cancer risk in premenopausal women even after correcting for confounding factors.[622] McTiernan and Thomas reported on pre- and postmenopausal women, noting that the risk of breast cancer diminished with increasing lifetime duration of lactation, and this effect persisted even after correcting for other factors.[623] Layde et al. (1989) reported on data from 4599 women with breast cancer and 4536 controls without breast cancer, with their findings strongly supporting parity and duration of breastfeeding as important factors in decreasing the risk of breast cancer after correcting for other variables.[624] Yoo et al. (1992) presented a case-control study from Japan suggesting that lactation had an independent benefit of decreasing the risk of breast cancer in premenopausal women who had ever lactated for 7 to 9 months.[625] Newcomb et al. (1994) reported a decreasing risk of breast cancer in premenopausal women associated with increasing cumulative duration of lactation and younger age at first lactation.[626] Ip et al. (2009) conducted a systematic review and analysis on breastfeeding and maternal and infant health in developed countries for the Agency of Healthcare Research and Quality, and they reported on two previously completed meta-analyses that concluded that there was a reduced risk of breast cancer in women who breastfed their infants.[627] The original meta-analyses were evaluated as fair quality; the first estimated the reduced risk of breast cancer as 4.3% for each year of breastfeeding based on data from 47 studies in 30 countries,[628] and the second study estimated a decrease in breast cancer risk of 28% for 12 or more months of breastfeeding.[629]

Human Mammary Tumor Virus and Mouse Mammary Tumor Virus and Human Milk

MMTV has been shown to produce mammary cancer in mice. HMTV is so named because it has been identified in human breast tissue, but it has also been named *mouse mammary tumor virus-like virus* (MMTV-LV) based on homology with MMTV. It is a single-stranded RNA virus with reverse-transcriptase activity closely related to MMTV. RNA-directed DNA polymerase activity, a reverse transcriptase, has been detected in human breast milk.[630] The search for evidence of a tumor virus either exogenously or endogenously causing breast cancer has been ongoing.

Wang et al. (2003) detected gene sequences homologous to MMTV in human breast cancers.[631] Melana et al. (2007) identified viral particles within human breast cancer cells that had a sequence homology of 95% with the HMTV proviruses as potential etiologic agents in human breast cancer pathogenesis.[632] Nartey et al. (2014) detected HMTV sequences in the breast milk of women who had had a history of breast biopsy for suspicion of cancer, compared with a reference group of women who had not been biopsied. Of the eight women who had breast cancer of the women who underwent biopsy (8/73), only one (1/8) had HMTV sequences detected in her breast milk.[633] HMTV was detected by PCR testing of breast milk in 14 of 65 remaining women in the biopsy group and 7 of 92 women in the reference group (21.54% vs. 7.61%, $p = 0.016$). In a separate study, Nartey et al. (2017) also identified an MMTV-LV in noncancerous breast tissue from 6 of 25 women years before the subsequent development of breast cancer in these same women.[634] MMTV-LV *env* sequences were identified in 9/25 breast cancer samples, 1 to 11 years after the initial noncancerous breast biopsies. Lawson et al. (2018) described the identification of MMTV p14 proteins in 27/50 human breast cancers and PCR detection of MMTV *env* gene sequences in 12/45 human breast cancers. They noted an association between the p14 immunohistochemistry and histology of these human breast cancers and the histologic features found in MMTV-positive mouse mammary tumors. MMTV p14 proteins were also detected in 7/13 benign breast specimens from women who later presented with MMTV-positive breast cancer.[635] Evidence of MMTV-like *env* sequences in breast cancer has been substantiated by several other labs in different parts of the world. The evidence of viral infection in the breast before the development of breast cancer in some studies suggests prior viral infection leading to cancer.[636] Wang et al. (2014) published a meta-analysis of 12 case-control studies of MMTV-LV and the risk of human breast cancer. The analysis demonstrated an increased risk of breast cancer after infection with MMTV-LV based on PCR detection of MMTV-LV DNA in human breast cancer tissue (OR = 15.20; 95% CI 9.98 to 23.13). They also noted that MMTV-LV DNA was identified more commonly in patients with breast cancer from Western countries than Asian patients.[637] Holland and Pogo (2004) enumerate other variables reported in the literature that support causality, including the presence of the entire MMTV in breast cancer tissue, manifested infectivity of breast cancer cells in vitro for normal breast cells, and replication of the virus in vitro from breast cancer cells. They point to the detection of expressed HMTV proteins in breast cancer tissues utilizing MMTV and HMTV antibodies as evidence for horizontal infection before the cancer.[637]

More recently, the debate about MMTV-LV or HMTV as a cause of breast cancer has increased.[638–643] Although various authors agree there are more data than previously, they also name additional points to be explained, such as how MMTV infects human tissue without MMTV receptors and clarification of the source(s) of MMTV infection from the common house mouse (*Mus domesticus*), and correlate this with infectivity and the prevalence of infection and breast cancer. They ask for standardized methodology regarding PCR testing, in situ hybridization, and choice of controls. Particularly important to establish causation would be the characterization of MMTV/HMTV insertion sites in the DNA of human breast cancer cells, explanation of the tumorigenesis mechanisms involved, and the isolation from breast epithelial cells of specific infectious viral particles that could be further studied regarding infectious process and oncogenesis.

Overall, there is good epidemiologic evidence that a longer duration of breastfeeding does decrease the risk of developing breast cancer, and there are insufficient data of a clear causal link between MMTV, MMTV-LV, or HMTV and human breast cancer. Despite the unanswered questions and the need for more research, the presence of these tumor viruses in breast milk is not a reason to stop breastfeeding.

Varicella-Zoster Virus

Varicella-zoster virus (VZV) infection (varicella/chickenpox, zoster/shingles) is one of the most communicable diseases of humans, in a class with measles and smallpox. Transmission is thought to occur via respiratory droplets and virus aerosolized from vesicles. Varicella in pregnancy is a rare event, although disease can be more severe with varicella pneumonia, and it can be fatal.

Congenital Varicella

Congenital VZV infection occurs infrequently, causing abortion, prematurity, and congenital malformations. A syndrome of malformations has been carefully described with congenital VZV infection, typically involving limb deformity, skin scarring, and nerve damage, including to the eye and brain.[644]

Perinatal VZV Infection

Perinatal VZV infection can lead to severe infection in infants if a maternal rash develops 5 days or less before delivery and within 2 days after delivery. Illness in infants usually develops before 10 days of age and is believed to be more severe because of the lack of adequate transfer of antibody from the mother during this period, transplacental spread of virus to the fetus and infant during viremia in the mother, and immature cellular immunity. Varicella in a mother occurring before 5 days before delivery allows for enough formation and transplacental transfer of antibodies to the infant to ameliorate disease, even if the infant is infected with VZV. Mothers who develop varicella rash more than 2 days after delivery are less likely to transplacentally transfer the virus to the infant. Such mothers do pose a risk to their infants from postnatal exposure, which can be diminished by the administration of varicella-zoster Ig to the infant. Postnatal transmission is believed to occur through aerosolized virus from skin lesions or the respiratory tract entering the susceptible infant's respiratory tract. Airborne

precautions are therefore appropriate in the hospital setting. Infants infected with VZV in utero or in the perinatal period (younger than 1 month of age) are more likely to develop zoster (reactivation of latent VZV) during childhood or as young adults. Table 12.6 summarizes the management of varicella in the hospitalized mother or infant.[645]

Postnatal Varicella

Postnatal varicella from nonmaternal exposure can occur, but it is generally mild when it develops after 3 weeks of age or when a mother has passed on antibodies against VZV via the placenta. Severe postnatal varicella does occur in premature infants or infants of varicella-susceptible mothers. When a mother's immune status relative to VZV is uncertain and the measurement of antibodies to VZV in the mother or infant cannot be performed promptly (less than 72 hours), the administration of VZIG[646] or IVIG to the infant exposed to varicella or zoster in the postnatal period is indicated. Ideally, a mother's varicella status should be known before pregnancy, when the varicella virus vaccine could be given if indicated.

VZV and Breast Milk

The VZV has not been cultured from milk, but VZV DNA has been identified in breast milk.[647] Antibodies against VZV have also been found in breast milk.[411] Breast milk from mothers who had received the varicella vaccine in the postpartum period was tested for VZV DNA. Varicella DNA was not detected in any of the 217 breast-milk samples from the 12 women, all of whom seroconverted after vaccination.[648] One case of suspected transfer of VZV to an infant via breastfeeding has been reported, but the virus may have been transmitted by respiratory droplets or exposure to rash before the mother began antiviral therapy.[647]

The isolation of an infant from the mother with varicella and interruption of breastfeeding should occur only while the mother remains clinically infectious, regardless of the method of feeding. As soon as the infant has received the varicella-zoster Ig, expressed breast milk can be given to an infant if no skin lesions involve the breasts. Persons with varicella rash are considered noninfectious when no new vesicles have appeared for 72 hours and all lesions have crusted, usually in 6 to 10 days. Immunocompetent mothers who develop zoster can continue to breastfeed if the lesions do not involve the breast and can be covered because antibodies against VZV are provided to the infant via the placenta and breast milk, and these antibodies will diminish the severity of disease, even if not preventing it. Conservative management in this scenario would include giving an infant varicella-zoster Ig as well (see Table 12.6).

West Nile Virus

WNV disease in the United States is one of the best recent examples of an emerging infectious disease taking on new importance in public awareness about health issues.

WNV Epidemiology

In 2002, 3389 human cases of West Nile infection in the United States were reported to the CDC. Cases were reported

TABLE 12.6 Guidelines for Preventive Measures After Exposure to Chickenpox in the Nursery or Maternity Ward

Type of Exposure or Disease	Chickenpox Lesions Present		Disposition
	Mother	Neonate	
A. Siblings at home have active chickenpox when the neonate and mother are ready for discharge from hospital	No	No	1. Mother: If she has a history of chickenpox, she may return home. Without a history, she should be tested for the varicella-zoster virus antibody titer.[a] If the test is positive, she may return home. If the test is negative, varicella-zoster Ig[b] is administered and she is discharged home. 2. Neonate: May be discharged home with mother if the mother has a history of varicella or is positive for the varicella-zoster virus antibody. If the mother is susceptible, administer varicella-zoster Ig to the infant and discharge home or place in protective isolation.
B. Mother has no history of chickenpox; exposed during period 6–20 days antepartum[c]	No	No	1. Exposed mother and infant: Send home at the earliest date, unless siblings at home have communicable chickenpox.[d] If so, may administer varicella-zoster Ig and discharge home, as above. 2. Other mothers and infants: No special management indicated. 3. Hospital personnel: No precautions indicated if there is a history of previous chickenpox or zoster. In absence of a history, immediate serologic testing is indicated to determine immune status.[a] Nonimmune personnel should be excluded from patient contact until 21 days after an exposure. 4. If the mother develops varicella 1 to 2 days postpartum, the infant should be given varicella-zoster Ig.
C. Onset of maternal chickenpox occurs antepartum[c] or postpartum	Yes	No	1. Infected mother: Isolate until no longer clinically infectious. If seriously ill, treat with acyclovir.[e] 2. Infected mother's infant: Administer varicella-zoster Ig[b] to neonates born to mothers with onset of chickenpox less than 5 days before delivery and isolate separately from mother. Send home with the mother if no lesions develop by the time the mother is noninfectious. 3. Other mothers and infants: Send home at the earliest date. Varicella-zoster Ig may be given to exposed neonates. 4. Hospital personnel: Same as B-3.
D. Onset of maternal chickenpox occurs antepartum[d]			1. Mother: Isolation unnecessary. 2. Infant: Isolate from other infants but not from the mother. 3. Other mothers and infants: Same as C-3 (if exposed). 4. Hospital personnel: Same as B-3 (if exposed).
E. Congenital chickenpox	No	Yes	1. Infected infant and mother: Same as D-1 and D-2. 2. Other mothers and infants: Same as C-3. 3. Hospital personnel: Same as B-3.

Ig, Immunoglobulin.

[a]Send serum to virus diagnostic laboratory for determination of antibodies to varicella-zoster virus by a sensitive technique (e.g., fluorescent antibody to membrane antigen [FAMA], latex agglutination [LA], enzyme-linked immunosorbent assay [ELISA]). Personnel may continue to work for 8 days after exposure, pending serologic results, because they are not potentially infectious during this period. Antibodies to varicella-zoster virus greater than 1:4 are probably indicative of immunity.

[b]Varicella-zoster Ig is available as VariZIG (https://varizig.com/uspage.html or 855-VZV-2466). From Centers for Disease Control and Prevention. Updated Recommendations for Use of VariZIG—United States, 2013. *MMWR, Morb Mortal Wkly Rep*. 2013;62:574–576.

[c]If exposure occurred less than 6 days antepartum, the mother would not be potentially infectious until at least 72 hours postpartum.

[d]Considered noninfectious when no new vesicles have appeared for 72 hours and all lesions have crusted.

[e]The dosage of acyclovir for a pregnant woman is 30 mg/kg per day IV or 80 mg/kg/day PO divided into 4 daily doses for 5–10 days; for a seriously ill infant with varicella, the dosage is 750 to 1500 mg/m² per day IV divided into 3 daily doses every 8 hours.

Adapted from Gershon AA. Chickenpox, measles and mumps. In: Remington JS, et al., eds. *Infectious Diseases of the Fetus and Newborn Infant*. 4th ed. Philadelphia: WB Saunders; 1995.

from 37 states, including 704 cases (21%) of West Nile fever (milder cases), 2354 cases (69%) of West Nile meningoencephalitis, and 201 deaths related to West Nile disease.[649] WNV is endemic in Israel and parts of Africa. Outbreaks have been reported from across the world, including Romania (1996), Russia (1999), Israel (2000), and Canada (2002), as well as the United States (1999 to 2003).[650] WNV is now considered endemic throughout the contiguous United States, with over 16,000 human neuroinvasive disease cases and 1500 deaths reported since 1999. It has been estimated that more than 780,000 illnesses have likely occurred, given how commonly asymptomatic infection occurs.[651] In 2017 there were 2097 reported cases of WNV illness in the United States, including 1425 neuroinvasive disease cases.[652] It is estimated that 150 to 300 asymptomatic cases of West Nile infection occur for every 20 febrile illnesses and for each case of meningoencephalitis associated with WNV. West Nile fever is usually a mild illness of 3 to 6 days' duration. The symptoms are relatively nonspecific, including malaise, nausea, vomiting, headache, myalgia, lymphadenopathy, and rash. West Nile disease is characterized by severe neurologic symptoms (e.g., meningitis, encephalitis, or acute flaccid paralysis and occasionally optic neuritis, cranial nerve abnormalities, and seizures). Children are infrequently sick with WNV infection, and affected infants younger than 1 year of age have rarely been reported.[651] The CFR for 2003 in the United States was approximately 2.5%, but the rate has been reported to be as high as 4% to 18% in hospitalized patients. The CFR for persons older than 70 years of age is considered to be higher, 15% to 29%, as documented among hospitalized patients in outbreaks in Romania and Israel.[651]

WNV Transmission

The primary mechanism of transmission is via a mosquito bite. Mosquitoes from the genus *Culex* are primary vectors. The bird—mosquito—bird cycle serves to maintain and amplify the virus in the environment. Humans and horses are incidental hosts. The pathogenesis of the infection is believed to occur via replication of the virus in the skin and lymph nodes, leading to a primary viremia that seeds secondary sites before a second viremia causes the infection of the CNS and other affected organs.[653,654] Transmission has been reported in rare instances during pregnancy,[655,656] via organ transplant,[657] and percutaneously in laboratory workers.[658]

WNV and Pregnancy

A study of WNV infection in pregnancy documented 4 miscarriages, 2 elective abortions, and 72 live births. Cord-blood samples were tested in 55 infants, and 54 of 55 were negative for anti-WNV IgM. Three infants had WNV infection, which could have been acquired congenitally. Three of seven infants had congenital malformations that might have been caused by maternal WNV infection based on timing in pregnancy, but no evidence of WNV etiology was conclusively demonstrated.[659] WNV transmission occurs via blood and blood-product transfusion,[660] and the incidence has been estimated to be as high as 21 per 10,000 donations during epidemics in specific cities.[661] No evidence of direct person-to-person transmission without the mosquito vector has been found.

WNV and Breastfeeding

One case of possible WNV transmission via breastfeeding has been documented.[658] The mother acquired the virus via packed RBC transfusions after delivery. The second unit of blood she received was associated with other blood products from the same donation causing West Nile infection in another transfusion recipient. Eight days later, the mother had a severe headache and was hospitalized with fever and a CSF pleocytosis on day 12 after delivery. The mother's CSF was positive for WNV-specific IgM antibody. The infant had been breastfed from birth through the second day of hospitalization of the mother. Samples of breast milk were positive for WNV-specific IgG and IgM on day 16 after delivery and positive for WNV-specific IgM on day 24. The same milk was WNV-RNA-positive by PCR testing on day 16 but not on day 24 after delivery. The infant tested positive for WNV-specific IgM in serum at day 25 of age but remained well and without fever. No clear-cut exposure to mosquitoes for the infant was reported. The cord blood and placenta were not available to be tested. IgM antibodies can be found in low concentrations in breast milk, but this is not common or as efficient as the transfer of IgA, secretory IgA, or IgG into breast milk.[31]

A review of WNV illness during breastfeeding identified six occurrences of breastfeeding during maternal WNV illness.[31] Five of the six infants had no illness or detectable antibodies to WNV in their blood. One infant developed a rash and was otherwise well after maternal WNV illness but was not tested for WNV infection. Two infants developed WNV illness while breastfeeding, but no preceding WNV infection was demonstrated in their mothers. Two other breastfeeding infants developed WNV-specific antibodies after their mothers acquired WNV illness in the last week of pregnancy, but congenital infection could not be ruled out. Live virus was not cultured from 45 samples of breast milk from mothers infected with WNV during pregnancy, but WNV RNA was detected in two samples, and 14 samples had IgM antibodies to WNV.[31]

The mentioned data suggest that WNV infection through breastfeeding is rare. To date, evidence of significant disease as a result of WNV infection in young breastfeeding children is lacking. Currently, no reason exists to proscribe breastfeeding in the case of maternal WNV infection if a mother is well enough to breastfeed. As with many other maternal viral illnesses, by the time the diagnosis is made in a mother, the infant may have already been exposed during maternal viremia and possible virolactia. The infant can and should continue to receive breast milk for the potential specific and nonspecific antiviral immunologic benefits.

Yellow Fever Virus

Yellow fever virus is a flavivirus that is transmitted to humans by infected *Aedes* and *Haemogogus* mosquitos in tropical areas of South America and Africa. Large outbreaks occur when mosquitos in a populated area become infected from biting viremic humans infected with yellow fever virus. Transmission from the mosquitos to other humans occurs after an incubation period in the mosquito of 8 days. Direct person-to-person spread has not been reported. Illness resulting from yellow fever virus usually begins after an incubation period of 3 to 6 days, with acute onset of headache, fever, chills, and myalgia. Photophobia, back pain, anorexia, vomiting, and restlessness are other common symptoms. The individual is usually viremic for the first 4 days of illness until the fever and other symptoms diminish. Liver dysfunction and even failure can develop, as can myocardial dysfunction. CNS infection is uncommon, but symptoms can include seizures and coma. Medical care should include intensive supportive care and fluid management.

Yellow Fever Vaccine and Pregnancy

One of 41 infants whose mothers had inadvertently received the yellow fever virus vaccine during pregnancy developed IgM and elevated neutralizing antibodies against the yellow fever virus, without any evidence of illness or abnormalities.[662] A more recent study[663] from Brazil examined inadvertent yellow fever virus immunization during pregnancy during a mass-vaccination campaign in 2000; 480 pregnant women received the yellow fever virus at a mean of 5.7 weeks' gestation, the majority of whom did not know their pregnancy status at the time. Seroconversion occurred in 98.2% of the women after at least 6 weeks after vaccination. Mild postvaccination illness (headache, fever, or myalgia) was reported by 19.6% of the 480 women. The frequency of malformations, miscarriages, stillbirths, and premature deliveries was similar to that found in the general population. At the 12-month follow-up point, 7% of the infants still demonstrated neutralizing antibodies against yellow fever virus, but beyond 12 months, only one child remained seropositive.[663]

Yellow Fever Vaccine and Breastfeeding

Transmission of the yellow fever vaccine virus through breastfeeding was reported from Brazil in 2009.[664] The mother was immunized during a yellow fever epidemic in a nonendemic area in Brazil; 15 days after delivering a healthy female infant (39 weeks' gestational age), the mother received the 17DD yellow fever vaccine, and 5 days later, the mother reported headache, malaise, and low-grade fever that persisted for 2 days. The mother continued breastfeeding and did not seek medical care for herself. At 23 days of age, the infant became irritable, developed a fever, and refused to nurse. The infant developed seizures, and subsequent evaluation of the infant demonstrated an abnormal CSF, and a computed tomography (CT) scan of the brain showed bilateral areas of diffuse low density suggestive of inflammation and consistent with encephalitis. Yellow-fever-specific IgM antibodies were identified in the infant's serum and CSF. Reverse-transcriptase PCR (RT-PCR) testing of the CSF also demonstrated yellow fever virus RNA identical to the 17DD yellow fever vaccine virus. Breast milk and maternal serum were not tested for yellow fever virus.[664] Yellow fever virus, wild or vaccine type, has not been identified in human breast milk, although another flavivirus, WNV, has been detected in milk from a few lactating women with WNV infection.[31] (See the section on WNV.) Neurologic disease

associated with the yellow fever vaccine occurs at different rates in different age groups, including 0.5 to 4.0 cases per 1000 infants younger than 6 months of age.[665] The 17D-derived yellow fever vaccines are contraindicated in infants younger than 6 months of age.

Since 2002, the Advisory Committee on Immunization Practices has recommended, based on theoretical risk, that the yellow fever vaccine should be avoided in nursing mothers, except when exposure in high-risk areas where yellow fever is endemic is likely to occur.[666]

Yellow Fever Virus and Breastfeeding

No case of transmission of yellow fever virus from an infected mother to her infant via breastfeeding or breast milk has been reported. Published information on the severity of yellow fever virus infection in infants younger than 1 year of age, potential protection from passively acquired antibodies, or protection from breast milk is limited. No information on the differential risk for infection in breastfed versus formula-fed infants is available. Given the well-documented method of transmission of yellow fever virus via mosquitos, and the lack of evidence of transmission via breast milk, it makes more sense to protect all infants against mosquito bites than to proscribe breastfeeding, even when the mother is infected with yellow fever virus. Continued breastfeeding or the use of expressed breast milk will depend on a mother's health status and ability to maintain the milk supply while acutely ill. If another source of feeding is readily available, then temporarily discarding expressed breast milk for at least 4 days of acute illness in the mother is a reasonable precaution.

Zika Virus

Zika virus (ZIKV) disease is the newest "emerging infectious disease" to burst onto the scene as a result of the dramatic epidemic across the Americas, the virus's neurotropism, and the clinical picture of congenital Zika syndrome. ZIKV is a flavivirus, as are 52 other viruses, including DENV, St. Louis encephalitis, WNV, and yellow fever virus. Since 2015, when it was first recognized in Brazil related to an excess of neonatal microcephaly cases, there have been millions of infections in the Americas and Caribbean, with ongoing transmission in over 80 other countries.[667] Travel cases have been noted across the United States and the US territories since 2016. Locally transmitted cases of ZIKV illness were reported from Florida and Texas in 2016 as well. The number of cases in the United States appears to be decreasing since 2016:

- 2016: US States = 5168, US Territories = 36,512
- 2017: US States = 452, US Territories = 666
- 2018: US States = 74, US Territories = 148
- 2019 (through May 1, 2020): US States = 22, US Territories = 71[668]

Locally transmitted ZIKV infection in the United States has also dropped off tremendously.[669]

Zika Virus Tracking and Prevention

Clinical case definitions have been created, although they lack sensitivity and specificity.[670,671] The CDC and other global health agencies have issued travel warnings for travel to Latin America, the Caribbean, and specific countries in the Asia-Pacific region and Africa, with targeted warnings for pregnant women and for individuals with concerns for ZIKV sexual transmission during travel. There are ongoing updates available through the CDC Traveler's Health site (https://wwwnc.cdc.gov/travel/page/zika-travel-information). ZIKV disease is a reportable illness, and a US ZIKV Pregnancy Registry was created in 2016 to document and track pregnancy and neonatal outcomes (https://www.cdc.gov/pregnancy/zika/research/registry.html).

Modes of Transmission for ZIKV

There are at least four modes of transmission identified to date: (1) mosquito bites, (2) person-to-person transmission (sexual contact, mother to fetus), (3) blood transfusion, and (4) animal-to-human transmission. Identified animal hosts include monkeys, ducks, goats, cows, horses, bats, rats, rodents, and orangutans.[667,672] Viral detection in human body fluids includes detection in blood, plasma, saliva, urine, semen, vaginal fluid, and breast milk.[667]

ZIKV Clinical Infection

A clinical case definition for congenital and noncongenital ZIKV infection was approved in June 2016 (https://wwwn.cdc.gov/nndss/conditions/zika/case-definition/2016/06/). The salient features of clinical congenital ZIKV disease are congenital microcephaly, intracranial calcifications, structural brain or eye abnormalities, or other congenital CNS-related abnormalities not explained by another etiology. The evaluation of possible congenital ZIKV disease should exclude other possible congenital infections and genetic or teratogenic causes. There should be an epidemiologic link related to maternal illness and travel/exposure. Laboratory criteria can include ZIKV detection by culture, viral antigen, or viral RNA; positive ZIKV IgM of blood, sera, or CSF within 2 days of birth; and serologic exclusion of DENV or other flaviviruses. The clinical features for noncongenital ZIKV disease include a compatible illness with acute onset of fever, maculopapular rash (often with pruritus), arthralgia, conjunctivitis, complications of pregnancy (fetal loss or evidence of possible congenital ZIKV disease), or Guillain–Barré syndrome or other associated neurologic manifestations. The epidemiologic criteria for the case definition are similar to those for congenital infection but include sexual contact with someone with travel to a ZIKV-endemic area. The laboratory criteria are the same. Acute infection is suspected to be asymptomatic in almost 80% of individuals, and most disease is mild. The incubation period is approximately 3 to 14 days.[667] There is limited information on noncongenital infection in children <18 years old. Attack rates are lower, and infection is generally milder in children than adults.[673] The majority of acute ZIKV infections in children are without complications.[674,675] In adults, neurologic complications are the most concerning, encephalopathy, meningoencephalitis, seizures, acute sensory polyneuropathy, myelitis, acute disseminated encephalomyelitis (ADEM), and GBS.[676,677] There are reports of an increased occurrence of

Guillain–Barré syndrome associated with ZIKV infection in adults.[678] Hemorrhagic complications are rare.

Perinatal ZIKV Infection

Perinatal transmission of ZIKV from mother to infant probably occurs, as has been shown with DENV, CHIKV, and WNV. Similarly, it is uncommon, given the very few reports to date. The concern is the neurotropism of ZIKV and the potential for long-term complications in the developing infant. Follow-up on two cases of probable perinatal ZIKV infection did not demonstrate neurodevelopmental abnormalities in either infant.[679]

Congenital ZIKV Infection

Congenital ZIKV syndrome (CZS), a term coined by the CDC, is characterized by severe microcephaly, brain abnormalities, ocular findings, congenital contractures, and neurologic impairment. In 2015, reports of a 20-fold increase in congenital microcephaly in Brazil highlighted the apparent onset of the ZIKV epidemic in the Americas and Caribbean.[680] There is a spectrum of disease affecting the fetus/infant caused by ZIKV infection during pregnancy, and clinical illness in the mother before the 25th week of gestation is the most important factor contributing to the occurrence of CZS.[681] Investigation of the mechanisms of ZIKV neurotropism and the resultant microcephaly, brain abnormalities, and ocular damage are ongoing. Onorati et al. reported data on how ZIKV interferes with phospho-TBK1 localization and mitosis in human neuroepithelial stem cells and radial glia cells.[682] Souza et al. confirmed that ZIKV induced disruption of mitosis and induced apoptosis in human neural progenitor cells.[683] The long-term complications of infants exposed to or infected with ZIKV in utero continue to be explored, especially in the areas of possible treatments to interrupt infection in pregnancy, vaccine prevention, and compassionate clinical management of the affected infants.[673]

ZIKV in Breast Milk

There are at least 10 articles focused on ZIKV and breast milk and breastfeeding; 9 of them report on individual cases, and the 10th is a review article.[684] Nucleic acid/PCR testing of breast milk was positive for ZIKV in 7/10 of the cases reported in the literature. Infective particles of ZIKV were cultured in breast milk from 3/10 of the involved mothers. Breast milk should be considered potentially infectious for the transmission of ZIKV. ZIKV in human milk can be inactivated by prolonged storage or pasteurization.[685] Additional study on efficient ZIKV detection in breast milk, accurate measurement of viral load, and assessment of the persistence and frequency of ZIKV in human milk are needed.

ZIKV and Breastfeeding

Careful analysis of the 10 possible cases of ZIKV infection via breastfeeding suggests that most of the cases reflect no infection in the infant or ZIKV transmission during pregnancy or in the early peripartum period based on the timing of positive laboratory testing in the infants. Most of the children were asymptomatic and have had no evidence of long-term complications.[684] Notably, in one case, the virus identified in the mother and infant revealed 99% identity on genome sequencing, although the timing of the infant's positive urine PCR occurred on day 5 after the onset of maternal illness. This 5-month-old child remained asymptomatic, and the source of infection for the mother and infant could not be definitively identified.[686] Prospective study of breastfeeding infants exposed to ZIKV-positive and ZIKV-negative breast milk is needed to understand the true risk of ZIKV transmission via breast milk.

Given all the data, the WHO recommendation regarding infant feeding in areas of ZIKV transmission remains appropriate: "the benefits of breastfeeding for the infant and mother outweigh any potential risk of Zika virus transmission through breast milk."[687]

SPIROCHETES

Lyme Disease

Lyme disease, as with other human illnesses caused by spirochetes, especially syphilis, is characterized by a protean course and distinct phases (stages) of disease. Lyme borreliosis was described in Europe in the early 20th century. Since the 1970s, tremendous recognition, description, and investigation of Lyme disease have occurred in the United States and Europe. Public concern surrounding this illness is dramatic.

Lyme disease is a multisystem disease characterized by involvement of the skin, heart, joints, and nervous system (peripheral and central). Stages of disease are identified as early localized (erythema migrans, often accompanied by arthralgia, neck stiffness, fever, malaise, and headache), early disseminated (multiple erythema migrans lesions, cranial nerve palsies, meningitis, conjunctivitis, arthralgia, myalgia, headache, fatigue, and, rarely, myocarditis), and late disease (recurrent arthritis, encephalopathy, and neuropathy). The varied manifestations of the disease may relate to the degree of spirochetemia, the extent of dissemination to specific tissues, and the host's immunologic response.[688]

The diagnosis of Lyme disease is often difficult, in part, because of the broad spectrum of presentations, inapparent exposure to the tick, and the lack of adequately standardized serologic tests. Culturing of the spirochete, *Borrelia burgdorferi*, is not readily available. Enzyme-linked immunosorbent assay (ELISA), immunofluorescent assay, and immunoblot assay are the usual tests. PCR detection of spirochetal DNA requires additional testing in clinical situations to clarify and standardize its utility.[689]

Lyme Disease in Pregnancy

Gardner[645] reviewed infection during pregnancy, summarizing a total of 46 adverse outcomes from 161 cases reported in the literature. The adverse outcomes included miscarriage and stillbirth (11% of cases), perinatal death (3%), congenital anomalies (15%), and both early- and late-onset progressive infection in the infants. Silver[690] reviewed 11 published reports and concluded that Lyme disease during pregnancy is uncommon, even

in endemic areas. Although the spirochete can be transmitted transplacentally, a significant immune response in the fetus is often lacking, and the association of Lyme infection with congenital abnormalities is weak at best.[691,692]

In a retrospective review by Lakos and Solymosi, data were reported on 95 women with Lyme borreliosis during pregnancy.[693] They reported on treatment of the mothers and subsequent outcomes. Untreated women had a significantly higher risk of adverse pregnancy outcome (OR = 7.61, $p = 0.004$), with loss of pregnancy and cavernous hemangioma as the most common adverse outcomes. *B. burgdorferi* was not identified in any fetus or infant, and no clear syndrome was associated with Lyme disease in pregnancy. A more inclusive systematic review by Waddell et al. (2018) included 45 relevant studies and 59 cases of reported gestational Lyme disease in the United States. A comparison of the occurrence of adverse birth outcomes in exposed versus unexposed groups in eight studies demonstrated no difference in adverse outcomes. A separate meta-analysis comparing groups of women treated for Lyme disease during pregnancy versus those not treated, in nine studies, showed fewer adverse birth outcomes in the treated groups (11% vs. 50%). The authors concluded that this is indirect evidence of an association of adverse birth outcomes with gestational Lyme disease.[694] In summary, adverse birth outcomes with *B. burgdorferi* infection during pregnancy are uncommon, and the reports present inconsistent evidence for transplacental transmission of *B. burgdorferi*. Treatment of the mother with apparent Lyme disease during pregnancy seems appropriate and relatively safe for the fetus.

Lyme Disease and Breast Milk

Little published information exists on whether *B. burgdorferi* can be transmitted via breast milk. One report showed the detection of *B. burgdorferi* DNA by PCR in the breast milk of two lactating women with untreated erythema migrans, but there was no evidence of Lyme disease or transmission of the spirochete in the one infant followed for 1 year.[695] No attempt to culture the spirochete was made, so it is not possible to determine if the detectable DNA in breast milk was from viable spirochetes or noninfectious fragments. In that same study of 56 women with untreated erythema migrans who had detectable *B. burgdorferi* DNA in the urine, 32 still had detectable DNA in the urine 15 to 30 days after starting treatment, but none had it 6 months after initiating therapy. The lack of adequate information on the transmission of *B. burgdorferi* via breast milk cannot be taken as proof that it is not occurring. If one extrapolates from data on syphilis and the *Treponema pallidum* spirochete, it would be prudent to discuss the lack of information on the transmission of *B. burgdorferi* via breast milk with the mother or parents and to consider withholding breast milk at least until therapy for Lyme disease has begun or has been completed. If the infection occurred during pregnancy and treatment has already been completed, an infant can breastfeed. If infection occurs postpartum or the diagnosis in the mother is made postpartum, infant exposure may have already occurred. Again, discussion with the mother or parents about withholding versus continuing breastfeeding and antibiotic therapy for the mother are appropriate.

After prenatal or postnatal exposure, an infant should be closely observed, and empiric therapy should be considered if the infant develops a rash or symptoms suggestive of Lyme borreliosis. The treatment of mother and infant with ceftriaxone, penicillin, or amoxicillin is acceptable during breastfeeding relative to the infant's exposure to these medications. Doxycycline should not be administered for more than 14 days while continuing breastfeeding because of possible dental staining in the neonate. Continued surveillance for viable organisms in the breast milk and evidence of transmission through breastfeeding is needed.

Syphilis

Syphilis is the classic example of a spirochetal infection that causes multisystem disease in various stages. Both acquired syphilis and congenital syphilis are well-described entities. Acquired syphilis is almost always transmitted through direct sexual contact with open lesions of the skin or mucous membranes of individuals infected with the spirochete *Treponema pallidum*.

Congenital Syphilis

Congenital syphilis occurs by infection across the placenta (placentitis) at any time during the pregnancy or by contact with the spirochete during passage through the birth canal. Any stage of the disease (primary, secondary, tertiary) in a mother can lead to infection of the fetus, but transmission in association with secondary syphilis approaches 100%. Infection with primary syphilis during pregnancy, without treatment, leads to spontaneous abortion, stillbirth, or perinatal death in 40% of cases.[696] Estimated global adverse birth outcomes related to syphilis during pregnancy for 2016 were 143,000 early fetal deaths and stillbirths, 61,000 neonatal deaths, 41,000 preterm or LBW births, and 109,000 infants with symptoms of congenital syphilis.[697] Similar to acquired syphilis, congenital syphilis manifests with moist lesions or secretions from rhinitis (snuffles), condyloma lata, or bullous lesions. These lesions and secretions contain numerous spirochetes and are therefore highly infectious.

The evaluation of an infant with suspected syphilis should be based on the mother's clinical and serologic status, history of adequate therapy in the mother, and the infant's clinical status. Histologic examination of the placenta and umbilical cord, serologic testing of the infant's blood and CSF, complete analysis of the CSF, long-bone and chest radiographs, liver function tests, and a complete blood cell count are all appropriate, given the specific clinical situation. Treatment of the infant should follow recommended protocols for suspected, probable, or proven syphilitic infection.[697]

Postnatal Syphilis in Infants

Postnatal infection of an infant can occur through contact with open, moist lesions of the skin or mucous membranes of the mother or other infected individuals. If the mother or infant has potentially infectious lesions, isolation from each other and from other infants and mothers is recommended. If lesions are on the breasts or nipples, breastfeeding or the use of expressed milk is contraindicated until treatment is complete and the lesions have cleared. Spirochetes are rarely identified in open lesions after more than 24 hours of appropriate treatment. Penicillin remains the best therapy. No evidence indicates that transmission of syphilis via breast milk occurs in the absence of a breast or nipple lesion. When a mother has no suspicious breast lesions, breastfeeding is acceptable if appropriate therapy for suspected or proven syphilis is begun in the mother and infant.

PARASITES

Giardia lamblia

Giardiasis is a localized infection limited to the intestinal tract, causing diarrhea and malabsorption. Immunocompetent individuals show no evidence of invasive infection, and no evidence indicates fetal infection from maternal infection during pregnancy. Giardiasis is rare in children younger than 6 months of age, although neonatal infection from fecal contamination at birth has been described.[698] Human milk has an in vivo protective effect against *Giardia lamblia* infection, as documented by work from central Africa, where the end of breastfeeding heralds the onset of *Giardia* infection.[699] This has been reaffirmed around the world.[700]

The protective effect of breast milk has been identified in the milk of noninfected donors.[701] The antiparasitic effect does not result from specific antibodies but rather from lipase enzymatic activity. The lipase acts in the presence of bile salts to destroy the trophozoites as they emerge from their cysts in the GI tract. Hernell et al.[702] demonstrated that free fatty acids have a marked germicidal effect, which supports the conclusion that lipase activity releasing fatty acids is responsible for killing *G. lamblia*.

G. lamblia has also been reported to appear in the mother's milk, and the parasite has been transmitted to newborns via that route. The exact relationship of breastfeeding to the transmission of *G. lamblia* and the effect on infants continue to be studied, even though symptomatic infection in breastfed infants is rare.[702] One report from the Middle East suggests that even partial breastfeeding is protective against infection with intestinal parasites, including *Cryptosporidium* and *G. lamblia*.[702] A second report from Egypt suggests that breastfeeding has a protective effect against infantile diarrhea caused by intestinal protozoa.[703] The affected organisms included *Cryptosporidium* sp., *Entamoeba histolytica*, *Giardia*, and *Blastocytis*, although the number of infants studied was too small to demonstrate significant protection against each individual protozoon. There remain significant questions about *Giardia*'s role as a commensal or pathogenic organism in children and *Giardia*'s association with acute or chronic diarrhea and poor growth.[704]

Breastfeeding by mothers with giardiasis is a concern mainly because of the medications used for therapy. The safety of the use of metronidazole or tinidazole in infants has not been established, although they have been used in premature neonates and infants.[705,706] There is little information available on quinacrine hydrochloride and furazolidone in breast milk. There is also inadequate information on the use of nitazoxanide during breastfeeding to recommend it.[707] Paromomycin, an orally nonabsorbable aminoglycoside, is a reasonable alternative recommended for the treatment of pregnant women.[708] Breastfeeding by a mother with symptomatic giardiasis is acceptable when consideration is given to the presence of the therapeutic agents in the breast milk.

Hookworm Infection

Hookworm infection, most often caused by *Ancylostoma duodenale* and *Necator americanus*, is common in children younger than the age of 4 years, and there is at least one report on infantile hookworm disease from China.[709] This publication from the Chinese literature reports hundreds of cases of infantile hookworm disease that include the common symptoms of bloody stools, melena, anorexia, listlessness, and edema. Anemia, eosinophilia, and even leukemoid reactions occur as part of the clinical picture in young children. They also note at least 20 cases of hookworm diseases in newborn infants younger than 1 month of age. In the discussion of infantile hookworm infection, they note four routes of infection: direct contact with contaminated soil; "sand-stuffed" diapers; contaminated "washed/wet" diapers; and vertical transmission, transmammary or transplacental. They postulated that infection of infants before 40 to 50 days of age would most likely be due to transplacental transmission, and infection before environmental contact would most likely be due to transmammary transmission. Ample evidence is available in veterinary medicine of transmammary spread of helminths.[710,711] At least two reports suggest the possibility of transmammary transmission of hookworms in humans. Setasuban et al.[712] described the prevalence of *N. americanus* in 128 nursing mothers as 61% and identified *N. americanus* in breast milk in one case. Nwosu[713] documented stool samples positive for hookworms in 33 of 316 neonates (10%) at 4 to 5 weeks of age in southern Nigeria. Most neonatal infections were caused by *A. duodenale*, although *N. americanus* is more prevalent in that area of Nigeria. Examination of colostrum did not demonstrate any hookworm larvae.[713]

Additional epidemiologic work is necessary to determine the potential significance of the transmammary spread of helminths in humans, and more careful examination of breast milk as a source of hookworm infection is required before reasonable recommendations are possible. The probable benefits of breastfeeding in locations where hookworm infections are prevalent outweigh the possible risk of transmammary spread of helminths.

Malaria

Malaria is recognized as a major health problem in many countries. The effect of malaria infection on pregnant and lactating women and thus on the developing fetus, neonate, and growing infant can be significant. The four species of malaria, *Plasmodium vivax*, *Plasmodium ovale*, *Plasmodium malariae*, and *Plasmodium falciparum*, vary in the specific aspects of

the disease they produce. *P. vivax* exists throughout the world, but *P. falciparum* predominates in the tropics and is most problematic in its chloroquine-resistant form. Malaria in the United States is most often seen in individuals traveling from areas where malaria is endemic. The parasite can exist in the blood for weeks, and infection with *P. vivax* and *P. malariae* can lead to relapses years later. Transmission occurs through the bite of the anopheline mosquito and can occur via transfusion of blood products and transplacentally.

Congenital malaria is rare but seems to occur more often with *P. vivax* and *P. falciparum*. It usually presents in the first 7 days of life (range: 1 day to 2 months). It may resemble neonatal sepsis, with fever, anemia, and splenomegaly occurring in the most neonates and hyperbilirubinemia and hepatomegaly in less than half.[714]

Malaria in infants younger than 3 months of age generally manifests with less severe disease and death than it does in older children. Possible explanations include the effect of less exposure to mosquitoes, passive antibody acquired from the mother, and the high level of fetal hemoglobin in infants at this age.[714] The variations in the infection rates in children younger than 3 months of age during the wet and dry seasons support the idea that postnatal infection is more common than congenital infection.

Malaria and Breast Milk

No evidence indicates that malaria is transmitted through breast milk. The greatest risk to infants is exposure to the anopheline mosquito infected with malaria.

The main issues relative to malaria and breastfeeding are how to protect both mothers and infants effectively from mosquitoes and which drugs for treating malaria in mothers are appropriate during lactation. Protection from mosquito bites includes screened-in living areas, mosquito nets while sleeping, protective clothing with or without repellents on the clothes, and community efforts to eradicate the mosquitoes. The CDC provides recommendations for prophylaxis and/or treatment of malaria during breastfeeding.[715,716] Chloroquine, quinine, and tetracycline are acceptable during breastfeeding. Sulfonamides should be avoided in the first month of an infant's life, but pyrimethamine-sulfadoxine (Fansidar) can be used later.[717]

Mefloquine is not approved for infants or pregnant women. However, the milk-to-plasma ratio for mefloquine is less than 0.25, there is a large volume of distribution of the drug, high protein-binding of the drug limits its presence in breast milk, and the relative importance of breastfeeding in areas where malaria is prevalent shifts the risk-to-benefit ratio in favor of treatment with mefloquine. The single dose recommended for treatment or the once-weekly dose for prevention allows for continued breastfeeding with discarding of the milk for short periods after a dose (1 to 6 hours).[718] Maternal plasma levels of primaquine range from 53 to 107 ng/mL, but no information is available on levels in human milk. Primaquine is used in children, and once-daily dosing in the mother would allow for discarding milk with peak levels of the drug. Therefore breastfeeding during maternal malaria, even with treatment or malaria prophylaxis, is appropriate with specific medications.

Strongyloides

Strongyloides stercoralis is a nematode (roundworm) capable of both skin and diffuse organ dissemination. It is found worldwide in tropical and temperate environments. Its true prevalence is probably significantly underestimated because of subclinical infection and the resulting difficulty of diagnosing it. Most infections are asymptomatic, but clinically significant infections in humans can include larval skin invasion, tissue migration, intestinal invasion with abdominal pain and GI symptoms, and a Loeffler-like syndrome resulting from migration to the lungs. Acute infection can cause a cutaneous eruption. In more chronic infection, it is associated with the GI tract and malabsorption, chronic diarrhea, failure to thrive, fever, cachexia, abdominal pain, cramping, and alternating diarrhea and constipation. Hyperinfection and invasive disease are most often evident in the lungs, but *Strongyloides* can include many organs, such as the lymph nodes, skeletal muscle, heart, liver, and brain.[719] There is a syndrome of infantile strongyloidiasis caused by *Strongyloides fuelleborni* affecting the infant in the first months of life, with prolonged diarrhea, abdominal distention, failure to thrive, and malnutrition. Because of the timing, it is suspected that this syndrome appearing in early infancy is a result of vertical transmission. Immune-compromised individuals can develop dissemination of larvae, causing various clinical symptoms. Humans are the principal hosts, but other mammals can serve as reservoirs. Infection via the skin by filariform larvae is the most common form of transmission, and ingestion is an uncommon occurrence.

Strongyloides and Milk

The transmammary transmission of *Strongyloides* species has been described in dogs, ewes, and rats.[710,711] Only one report of transmammary passage of *Strongyloides* larvae in humans is available. In 76 infants younger than 200 days of age, 34% demonstrated the presence of *S. fuelleborni* on stool examination. The clinical significance of this was not elucidated. *Strongyloides* larvae were detected in the human milk of only 1 sample out of 113 samples tested by Brown and Girardeau.[720] Mota-Ferreira et al.[721] identified IgA and IgG antibodies specific against *S. stercoralis* in breast milk by ELISA (IgA in 28.9% and IgG in 25.5% of the samples) and indirect fluorescent antibody test (IFAT; IgA in 42.25% and IgG in 18.9% of the samples, with over 90% concurrence). Given the apparent infrequent evidence of these larvae in human milk and the lack of apparent transmission via breast milk, there is no reason to proscribe breastfeeding in the face of maternal *Strongyloides* infection.

Toxoplasmosis

Toxoplasmosis is one of the most common infections of humans throughout the world. The infective organism, *Toxoplasma gondii*, is ubiquitous in nature. The prevalence of positive serologic test titers increases with age, indicating past exposure and infection. The cat is the definitive host, although infection occurs in most species of warm-blooded animals.

Postnatal infection with toxoplasmosis is usually asymptomatic. Symptomatic infection typically manifests with nonspecific symptoms, including fever, malaise, myalgia, sore throat, lymphadenopathy, rash, hepatosplenomegaly, and occasionally a mononucleosis-like illness. The illness usually resolves without treatment or significant complications.[722]

Congenital infection or infection in an immunodeficient individual can be persistent and severe, causing significant morbidity and even death. Although most infants with congenital infection are asymptomatic at birth, visual abnormalities, learning disabilities, and mental retardation can occur months or years later. The syndrome of congenital toxoplasmosis is clearly defined, with the most severe manifestations involving the CNS, including hydrocephalus, cerebral calcifications, microcephaly, chorioretinitis, seizures, or simply isolated ocular involvement.[773] The risk for fetal infection is related to the timing of primary maternal infection, although transmission can occur with preexisting maternal toxoplasmosis.[724] In the last months of pregnancy, the protozoan is more readily transmitted to the fetus, but the infection is more likely to be subclinical. Early in pregnancy, the transmission to a fetus occurs less frequently, but it more commonly results in severe disease. Treatment of documented congenital infection is currently recommended, although the duration and optimal regimen have not been determined, and the reversal of preexisting sequelae generally does not occur.

The prevention of infection in susceptible pregnant women is possible by avoiding exposure to cat feces or the organism in the soil or water. Pregnant or lactating women should not change cat litter boxes, but if they must, it should be done daily and while wearing gloves. The oocyst is not infective for the first 24 to 48 hours after passage. Mothers can avoid ingestion of the organism by fully cooking meats; carefully washing fruits, vegetables, and food-preparation surfaces; avoiding other high-risk foods; and avoiding increased contact with cat feces.[723]

Toxoplasmosis and Breast Milk

In various animal models, *T. gondii* has been transmitted through the milk to the suckling young. The organism has been isolated from colostrum as well. The newborn animals became asymptomatically infected when nursed by an infected mother whose colostrum contained *T. gondii*. Only one report has identified *T. gondii* in human milk, but there is a question concerning potential contamination of the sample.[724] The possibility of transmission during breastfeeding in humans has been raised in a couple of case reports but has not been proven.[725–727] Breast milk may contain appropriate antibodies against *T. gondii*.

Given the benign nature of postnatal infection in infants, the absence of documented transmission in human breast milk, and the potential protection from antibodies in breast milk, no reason exists to proscribe breastfeeding by a mother known to be infected with toxoplasmosis.

Trichomonas vaginalis

Trichomonas vaginalis is a flagellated protozoan that can produce vaginitis, but it frequently causes asymptomatic infection in both men and women. The parasite is found in 10% to 25% of women in the childbearing years. It is transmitted predominantly by sexual intercourse, but it can be transmitted to the neonate by passage through the birth canal. This parasite often coexists with other STDs, especially gonorrhea.

Infection during pregnancy or while taking oral contraceptives is more difficult to treat. Some evidence suggests that infection with and growth of the parasite are enhanced by estrogens or their effect on the vaginal epithelium. No evidence indicates adverse effects on the fetus in association with maternal infection during pregnancy. Occasionally, female newborns have vaginal discharge during the first weeks of life caused by *T. vaginalis*. This is thought to be influenced by the effect of maternal estrogen on the infant's vaginal epithelium and the acquisition of the organism during passage through the birth canal. The organism does not seem to cause significant disease in a healthy infant.

No documentation exists on the transmission of *T. vaginalis* via breast milk. The difficulty encountered with maternal infection during lactation stems from concerns regarding the use of metronidazole, the drug of choice. There are data on the use of metronidazole in premature infants and neonates, with no difficulty reported. Although topical agents containing povidone-iodine (Betadine) or sodium lauryl sulfate (Trichotine) can be effective when given as douches, creams, or suppositories, metronidazole remains the treatment of choice. The AAP advises using metronidazole only with a physician's direction and considers its effect on a nursing infant unknown but possibly a concern. The potential concerns are metronidazole's disulfiram-like effect in association with alcohol, tumorigenicity in animal studies, and leukopenia and neurologic side effects described in adults.[705] On the other hand, metronidazole is given to neonates and children beyond the neonatal period to treat serious infections with various bacteria or other parasites, such as *E. histolytica*.

The current recommendation for lactating women is to try local treatment first, and if this fails, then try metronidazole. A 2-g single-dose treatment produces peak levels after 1 hour, and discarding expressed breast milk for the next 12 to 24 hours is recommended. If this treatment also fails, a 500 mg of metronidazole twice-daily regimen for 7 days or a 2-g single daily dose of metronidazole or tinidazole for 3 to 7 days is recommended. Some experts recommend discarding of breast milk after the dose and timing of feedings separate from the dose. Infants exposed to metronidazole more frequently demonstrate loose stools; however, diaper rash, feeding difficulty, and *Candida* infection are not more frequent. Tinidazole is an alternative for metronidazole-resistant *Trichomonas*, but less is known about drug levels in breastfed infants of mothers receiving tinidazole.[706]

Trypanosoma cruzi

Chagas disease, caused by the protozoa *Trypanosoma cruzi*, is a major cause of disease in the Americas, and it is endemic in many parts of South America. Pregnant or breastfeeding women can be chronically infected (often asymptomatic) or acutely infected. Infection in pregnancy is associated with an increased risk of preterm birth, LBW, or stillbirth. Women can be chronically infected with relatively low levels of parasitemia, can have a reactivation of an infection (especially in association with HIV coinfection), or can become acutely infected with a high level of parasitemia.

Congenital Chagas Disease

There is a clinical picture of congenital Chagas disease that includes hepatosplenomegaly, myocarditis, anemia, anasarca, and meningoencephalitis in the severest form, but congenital infection is most commonly an asymptomatic infection. A systematic review and meta-analysis reported a prevalence ranging from 0.1% to 8.5% in pregnant women in Brazil, with congenital transmission rates of 0% to 5.2%.[728] In congenital infection, the treatment success is close to 90%. In Spain, a nonendemic country, Ramos et al. reported a seroprevalence rate in pregnant immigrant women from South America of 1.28%, but they were unable to identify a case of congenital Chagas disease in 545 infants.[729] Carlier and Truyens analyzed data on congenital Chagas disease and demonstrated increasing risk of fetal transmission in chronic maternal infection with increasing parasitemia.[730] In another report, Torrico et al. utilized microscopic examination of the buffy-coat layer to estimate parasitemia and demonstrated a significant relationship between the level of parasitemia and mortality and the severity of the clinical picture.[731] In a systematic review, Howard et al. reported transmission rates to fetuses in chronic maternal infection, estimated as 5% in endemic countries and 2.7% in nonendemic countries.[732]

Chagas Disease and Breastfeeding

A recent review of Chagas disease and breastfeeding noted that *T. cruzi* has been identified in the milk of chronically infected mice, but transmission through breast milk has been uncommon, and histologic examination of the breasts did not reveal any parasites.[733] Testing of colostrum and breast milk from women chronically infected with *T. cruzi* did not show evidence of the parasite in the milk.[734] Norman and Lopez-Velez summarized eight reports in the literature of possible transmission of *T. cruzi* via breastfeeding in humans. In the majority of cases, the parasite could not be identified in the human milk, the exact mechanism of transmission could not be effectively pinpointed, and contamination of the breast milk with blood or another mechanism of transmission could not be excluded. They also noted that the "blood-form trypomastigotes," which would be expected to be found in human milk, would potentially have different surface receptors than "infectious metacyclic trypomastigotes" and therefore have altered infectious capability across mucous membranes. They discussed a case of acute Chagas disease with probable parasitemia, noting that in only this one case was *T. cruzi* identified in the breast milk. In that clinical scenario, the infant was not breastfed. In a prospective study of maternal treatment with benznidazole for Chagas disease, pharmacokinetics and breast-milk levels of the drug were assessed. Twelve lactating women were followed for 30 days of treatment and then monthly through 6 months. Five mothers had adverse reactions to the medication, but none of the infants did. The median milk concentration was 3.8 mg/L, and the median "relative dose" of benznidazole received by the infants was 12.3% of the maternal dose per kg. This constitutes limited exposure of the infant to benznidazole through breast milk.[735] Considering the very rare occurrence of possible transmission of *T. cruzi* through human milk, it is not reasonable to proscribe breastfeeding by women with chronic Chagas disease even during treatment with benznidazole. Even in women with acute Chagas and an increased likelihood of a transient parasitemia, by the time the diagnosis is made in the mother, the infant has probably already been exposed. Treating the mother and continuing breastfeeding are appropriate. The medications benznidazole and nifurtimox have been used to treat congenital infection in infants.

Prevention of Vertical Transmission of Chagas Disease

In an effort to limit myocarditis as a result of chronic infection with *T. cruzi* and limit congenital Chagas disease, many authors advocate for screening and treatment of women of reproductive age.[736–738] Other experts recommend screening and treatment of immigrants from Latin America with possible/probable exposure to *T. cruzi*.[739] Alvarez et al. studied 67 women with chronic Chagas disease. The occurrence of congenital Chagas was 16/114 (14%) children born to untreated mothers and 0/42 (0%) children born to mothers treated with benznidazole. In long-term follow-up, 32% of the treated mothers became serologically negative for *T. cruzi*.[736] The CDC, through an investigational new-drug study, treated 369 individuals with *T. cruzi* infection (326 with chronic infection, 4 with new disease, and 35 with reactivated disease) with benznidazole.[737] Moscatelli et al. treated 394 women with a history of chronic Chagas infection; 15 of the women delivered 16 children after treatment with benznidazole, and 13/15 women became PCR-negative for *T. cruzi* at the end of treatment. All the children were full term and of appropriate weight for gestational age and were without any clinical signs of congenital Chagas. They had no laboratory evidence of Chagas infection in the perinatal period and at 8 months of age.[740]

CANDIDA INFECTIONS

The genus *Candida* consists of multiple species. The most common species affecting humans include *Candida albicans*, the dominant agent; *Candida tropicalis, Candida krusei*, and *Candida parapsilosis;* and many other uncommon species. In general, *Candida* exists as a commensal organism colonizing the oropharynx, GI tract, vagina, and skin without causing disease until some change disrupts the balance between the organism and the host. Mild mucocutaneous infection is the most common illness, which can lead to vulvovaginitis, mastitis, or uncommonly, oral mucositis in a mother and thrush (oral candidiasis) and candidal diaper rash in an infant.

Invasive candidal infection occurs infrequently, usually when a person has another illness, impaired resistance to infection (HIV, diabetes mellitus, or neutropenia; decreased cell-mediated immunity in premature infants or LBW or VLBW infants) or disrupted normal mucosal and skin barriers and has received antibiotics or corticosteroids. Invasive disease can occur through local extension, and it may present more often in the genitourinary tract (urethra, bladder, ureters, kidneys), although it usually develops in association with candidemia. The bladder and kidney are more frequently involved, but when dissemination occurs via candidemia, a careful search for other sites of infection should be made (e.g., retina, liver, spleen, lung, meninges).[741]

Transmission usually occurs from healthy individuals colonized with *Candida* through direct contact or contact with their oral or vaginal secretions. Intrauterine infection can occur through ascending infection through the birth canal, but it is rare. This can cause congenital cutaneous candidiasis, usually evident on the first day of life. Most often, an infant is infected in passing through the birth canal and remains colonized. Postnatal transmission can occur through direct contact with caregivers.

The mother and infant serve as an immediate source of recolonization for each other, especially during the direct contact of breastfeeding. For this reason, an infant and breastfeeding mother should be treated simultaneously when treating thrush, vulvovaginitis, diaper candidiasis, mastitis, or mammary candidiasis. Colonization with this organism usually occurs in the absence of any clinical evidence of infection. Simultaneous treatment of the mother–infant dyad should occur even in the absence of any clinical evidence of *Candida* infection or colonization in the apparently uninvolved individual of the breastfeeding dyad.

Candida Infection of the Breast

Considerable discussion of terminology continues with regard to *mammary candidosis* or *candidiasis, mastitis*, and simply *candidal infection of the breast*. The ABM Clinical Protocol 4: Mastitis, last revised in 2014, has a very appropriate discussion and referenced statement regarding mastitis.[742] *Mastitis* means inflammation of the breast, and this inflammation may or may not be related to a microbial infection. The distinction is made between engorgement or blockage or plugging of ducts with redness, pain, and warmth present in a local area of the breast without infection necessarily occurring simultaneously. Additional differentiation is made between mastitis occurring during lactation (lactational or puerperal mastitis) versus at other times in a women's life (nonlactational). Surgeons additionally refer to mastitis or an abscess of the breast as primary, lactational, or postoperative surgical-site infections.[743] Per the ABM protocol, clinical mastitis is present when a local area of the breast is painful, warm, and swollen—often in a "wedge-shape"—with concomitant temperature greater than 101.3°F (38.5°C), chills, and other signs or symptoms of systemic illness. Other publications have considered additional terminology, such as *acute lactational mastitis, subclinical mastitis*, or *subacute mastitis*, without being able to provide clear distinctions in the diagnostic terms based on signs, symptoms, or microbiologic testing with culture or nonculture methods.[744,745] Separately, the term *dysbiosis* has been applied to changes in the human milk microbiome, equating mammary dysbiosis with subacute mastitis or with chronic nipple/breast pain or ductal infection.[746–749] The explanation given for the associated symptoms is that the change in microbial diversity predisposes to an imbalance of the normal milieu and inflammation related to virulence factor(s) and biofilm production by organisms already present in the mammary microbiome.

Candidal infection of the breast is most commonly a local skin infection with superficial signs of inflammation of the nipple and areola consistent with dermatitis or dermatosis. Deeper infection of the breast with candida, ductal candidal infection, and/or nipple or deep breast pain associated with *Candida* continue to be disputed,[750] with various authors demonstrating an association between symptoms and *Candida*[751–754] and other studies that did not demonstrate such an association.[755–758]

Diagnosis of Mammary Candidiasis

The diagnosis of mammary candidiasis is a clinical diagnosis in most situations. Signs or symptoms of mammary candidiasis can include pink to red coloration changes of the nipple and/or areola, a shiny or flaky appearance of the nipple, nipple pain in excess of what is expected by the clinical picture, and "burning nipple pain" or pain extending into the breast.[750,754,759] If the mother or infant has any potentially predisposing factors for *Candida* infection (in addition to compatible symptomatology), such as a documented historical predisposition to *Candida* infections, active *Candida* infection at another site (vagina, perineal area, mouth, diaper region), an immunosuppressive condition, or recent antibiotic or corticosteroid use in mother or child, then the diagnosis of mammary candidiasis should be strongly considered. If there is no response or worsening after the initial management or it is a severe or unusual situation, culturing the nipple, areola, and breast milk for bacteria and fungus, along with sensitivity testing, would be appropriate. Molecular techniques for identification of *Candida* are not routinely available, and measuring 1,3 β-D-glucan, a by-product of *Candida* growth, has not proven useful in making the diagnosis.[756] When treatment is provided for mammary candidiasis, a clinical response to therapy can be useful in confirming the diagnosis. If the clinical situation suggests mastitis, then diagnosis and management should follow the ABM Clinical Protocol 4: Mastitis. Close clinical follow-up with reinforcement of effective milk removal, maintenance of the milk production, and utilization of supportive measures, along with analgesia, are important.

Management of Mammary Candidiasis

No well-controlled clinical trials define the most appropriate or most effective method(s) of treatment for candidal infection in breastfeeding mother—infant dyads. The list of possible treatment products is extensive and includes many anecdotal and empirical regimens. Given the potential for irritation and pain of the nipple and areola, interference with breastfeeding and expression of milk, and potential interference with milk production, management should follow the management of mastitis. Management of irritation of the nipple and areola should be guided by direct feedback from the mother.

Treatment of mild to moderate mammary candidiasis should begin with a topical agent, such as nystatin, clotrimazole, miconazole, econazole, butaconazole, terconazole, or ciclopirox. Treatment should continue for at least 2 weeks, even with obvious improvement in 1 or 2 days. Failures most often result from inadequate therapy involving the frequency of application; careful washing and drying before application; or in the case of diaper candidiasis, decreasing the contact of the skin with moisture. Nystatin oral suspension is less effective for the treatment of oral candidiasis in infants now compared with the past, supposedly as a result of increasing resistance.[760,761] Gentian violet (diluted to a ratio of 0.25% to 1.0%) applied to the breast or painted onto an infant's mouth is again being recommended more frequently. Other topical preparations have been recommended for the mother's breast, including mupirocin; grapefruit seed extract; or mixtures of mupirocin, betamethasone ointments, and miconazole powder. Controlled clinical trials for efficacy and toxicity are not available.

When good adherence to the proposed regimen with topical agents fails, or when the infant or mother are severely affected by pain and decreased breastfeeding, systemic therapy is appropriate. Fluconazole and ketoconazole are the most commonly used systemic agents for oral or diaper candidiasis and vulvovaginitis or mastitis. Fluconazole has a better side-effect profile than ketoconazole, and more data are available concerning its safe use in children younger than 6 months of age and even neonates and premature infants.[762–764] Fluconazole is not currently approved for use in infants younger than 6 months of age. For severe invasive infections in infants, amphotericin B with or without oral flucytosine, IV fluconazole, voriconazole, and echinocandins are reasonable choices in different situations. Other azoles, such as itraconazole or posaconazole, have not been adequately studied in infants to date. Of the echinocandins, micafungin and caspofungin have the most documented experience in infants. Maternal use of fluconazole during breastfeeding is not contraindicated because only a small amount of the medicine, compared with the usual infant dose, reaches the infant through breast milk.[764] Amphotericin or echinocandin therapy in mothers is also not contraindicated because these are both poorly absorbed from the GI tract. Whenever a mother is treated for candidal mastitis or vulvovaginitis, the infant should be treated simultaneously, at least with nystatin oral suspension as the first choice of medication. In the event of severe, invasive candidal infection in the mother or infant, consultation with an infectious disease specialist is appropriate.

Any predisposing risk factors for candidal infection in mothers and infants should be reduced or eliminated to improve the chance of rapid, successful treatment and to decrease the likelihood of chronic or recurrent disease. For mothers, such interventions might include decreasing sugar consumption; stopping antibiotic use as soon as possible; and consuming some form of probiotic bacteria, such as *Lactobacillus acidophilus* (in yogurt, milk, or pill form) to reestablish a normal colonizing bacterial flora. There are individual reports but no systematic reviews or meta-analyses supporting the long-term use of probiotics for vulvovaginitis or mammary candidiasis. For infants, breastfeeding can enhance the growth of specific colonizing bacterial flora, such as *Lactobacillus*, which can successfully limit fungal growth. Breastfeeding and/or breast-milk expression should continue with appropriate support and problem solving with a professional who is knowledgeable about breastfeeding.

SUMMARY

HIV-1, HIV-2, HTLV-I, and HTLV-II are the only infectious diseases that are considered true contraindications to breastfeeding in developed countries. Severe fulminant infections in the mother can be contraindications as well—EVD, Lassa fever, rabies, and so forth. When the primary route of transmission is via direct contact or respiratory droplets/particles, temporary separation of mother and infant may be appropriate (whether the infant is breastfed or formula-fed), but expressed breast milk should be given to the infant for the organism-specific immunologic benefits in the mother's milk. In most instances, by the time a specific diagnosis of infection is made for a mother, the infant has already been exposed to the organism, and providing expressed breast milk to the infant should continue. (Refer to Appendix D for specific exceptions, such as EVD or Lassa fever.) Regarding antimicrobial therapy for mothers and continued breastfeeding, the majority of the antimicrobial medications commonly used in adults can be used to treat the same infection in infants. The additional amount of medication received by infants via breast milk is usually insignificant in comparison to the usual dosing of the medication for infants and children. In almost all instances, an appropriate antimicrobial agent for treating mothers that is also compatible with breastfeeding can be chosen.

Unless there is a documented risk to infants for the transmission of an infectious agent via breast milk that leads to a clinically significant illness, breastfeeding should continue.

The Reference list is available at www.expertconsult.com.

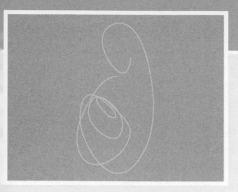

13

Breastfeeding Infants With Problems

Lawrence Noble and Casey Rosen-Carole

KEY POINTS

- Infants with special problems may require procedures, surgeries, or hospitalization to maintain and optimize their health or development. Breastfeeding and breast-milk feeding should be protected throughout these interruptions in an infant's health routine because human milk may offer unique benefits to their health in this period.
- Breastfeeding is the ideal and preferred feeding method for a newborn. Occasionally infant problems interfere with breastfeeding and require the attention of the infant's physician to diagnose and treat the infant's problem and support breastfeeding (e.g., cystic fibrosis).
- Guidelines for preprocedural or preoperative fasting recommend 6, 4, and 1 to 2 hours for solids (and nonhuman milk), breast milk, and clear liquids, respectively. Expressing and storing breast milk in this period of nothing by mouth for the infant will ensure the mother's milk supply is maintained. After minor procedures or surgeries, an infant can return to breastfeeding as soon as the infant is able to feed by mouth.
- Cow's milk protein allergy can occur in exclusively breastfed infants but is less common than in the formula-fed infant. An oral food challenge is usually not necessary or indicated, but having the mother initiate an elimination diet while continuing to breastfeed is often the first intervention.
- Metabolic disorders (galactosemia, phenylketonuria) can interfere with adequate infant feeding. Specialized formulas without the potentially dangerous substrate often supplant breastfeeding. In some instances, some breast milk can be fed in addition to the specialized formula.
- Careful early breastfeeding instruction and hands-on guidance are important, along with ongoing support to assist mothers and parents in identifying the challenges or difficulties of breastfeeding related to infant illness, develop solutions, and optimize infant nutrition despite their illness. (Hypernatremic dehydration is just one example of infant illness that should be preventable by this approach; hyperbilirubinemia should be manageable with continued good breastfeeding, and ankyloglossia is an example of an infant condition that should be managed simultaneously as breastfeeding continues to be facilitated and supported.)
- Breastfeeding has been discouraged in infants with congenital heart disease out of concern for destabilization of the cardiorespiratory system by the act of breastfeeding. Evidence disproves this concern, and breast milk benefits the infant in preventing necrotizing enterocolitis (NEC), improving weight gain, and optimizing long-term health benefits.
- In this era of concern for bedsharing and sudden infant death syndrome (SIDS), bedsharing with breastfeeding (breastsleeping) with an emphasis on safer sleeping and risk minimization with bedsharing are recommended to optimize safe sleeping and successful breastfeeding.

Breastfeeding is a natural behavior for infants and provides the ideal nourishment, but some infants with complicating issues need special assistance or adjustments.[1] Infants with structural abnormalities, metabolic challenges, or neurologic difficulties; stressed infants; and twins and triplets will be discussed in this chapter. Prematurity is discussed in Chapter 14. In this chapter we will briefly review the management of the specific medical conditions and discuss the management of breastfeeding in relation to the medical condition and optimal nutrition.

PROCEDURES AND SURGERY

Infants with special problems may require procedures, surgeries, or hospitalization to maintain and optimize their health or development. Breastfeeding and breast-milk feeding should be protected throughout these interruptions in an infant's routine and may be a solution to the unique problems faced during them.

Procedural Pain Relief

A 2017 systemic review of procedural pain relief for neonates was reported by Benoit et al.[2] Fifteen studies reported on the use of breastfeeding or expressed breast milk in full-term infants, and six reported on preterm infants. Direct breastfeeding was more effective than maternal holding, maternal skin-to-skin contact, topical anesthetics, and music therapy and was as effective or more effective than sweet-tasting solutions in term infants. Expressed breast milk was not consistently found to reduce pain response in full-term or preterm infants. The studies generally had moderate to high risk of bias. The review concluded that there is sufficient evidence to recommend direct breastfeeding for procedural pain management in full-term infants but not expressed breast milk.

A Cochrane systemic review and meta-analysis of procedural pain relief for infants greater than 28 days was published in 2016.[3] Ten studies with a total of 1066 infants were included. All the studies were conducted during early childhood immunization, and all were rated as being at high risk of bias. Breastfeeding reduced behavioral pain responses (cry time and pain scores) during vaccination compared with no treatment, oral water, and other interventions such as cuddling, oral glucose, topical anesthetic, massage, and vapocoolant. Moderate-quality evidence from six studies ($N = 547$ infants) revealed that breastfeeding compared with water or no treatment resulted in a 38-second reduction in cry time (mean difference [MD] $= -38$, 95% confidence interval [CI] -50 to-26; $p < 0.00001$), and moderate-quality evidence from five studies ($N = 310$ infants) disclosed that breastfeeding was associated with a 1.7-point reduction in pain scores (standardized mean difference [SMD] $= -1.7$, 95% CI-2.2 to-1.3).[3]

Preprocedural or Preoperative Fasting

Various societies of anesthesia (American, European, and Scandinavian) have guidelines recommending preoperative fasting for intervals of 6, 4, and 2 hours for solids (and nonhuman milk), breast milk, and clear fluids, respectively.[4–6] The Academy of Breastfeeding Medicine (ABM) supports such recommendations in its Clinical Protocol 25: Recommendations for Preprocedural Fasting for the Breastfed Infant: "NPO" Guidelines.[7] Gastric emptying rates are the primary difference in determining the preprocedural fasting time. The use of clear liquids up to 2 hours, or even 1 hour, before the procedure and nonnutritive sucking on a pacifier or empty breast can be temporary comfort measures.[8] Expressing and storing breast milk during the period of "nothing by mouth" (NPO) is appropriate and will ensure that the mother's milk supply is maintained. For minor procedures under anesthesia, a stable, otherwise-healthy child for which the surgical procedure does not prevent oral intake can resume breastfeeding as soon as the infant is awake.

Surgery or Rehospitalization Beyond Neonatal Period

Anesthesia is a main concern when any patient is scheduled for surgery. Traditionally, a patient has been ordered to have NPO status after midnight or 6 to 8 hours preoperatively. Young infants accustomed to feeding every 4 hours are often frantic when maintained without feeding before going to the operating room. The guidelines, as described previously, are appropriate.

One study reported postdischarge breastfeeding outcomes for a group of infants with complex anomalies that required surgery.[9] One hundred and sixty-five mother—infant pairs cared for in a tertiary care children's hospital and who had

surgery from 2009 to 2012 were included. Of these infants, 60.1% were still receiving human milk at 6 months of age, and 34.5% were still receiving human milk at 12 months of age. Exclusive human milk nutrition continued in 54.3% of infants at 3 months and 35.6% at 6 months. The average duration of ongoing use of human milk was 8 months. Consistent with the required surgery, 30.7% of the infants were still receiving gavage feeding postdischarge. This significant improvement in the level of ongoing use of human milk for infants undergoing surgery was accomplished with an organized lactation program, nursing staff with specific breastfeeding education, and a medical culture that strongly supports breastfeeding and the use of human milk. An infant who requires surgery or rehospitalization can and should be breastfed postoperatively in most cases. The gravity of the surgery and the length of the recovery phase will determine the time necessary for the mother to pump and manually express her milk to maintain her supply. The infant who is hospitalized is already traumatized by the separation, the strange surroundings and contact with multiple unknown persons, and the underlying discomfort of the disease process itself. If the infant is to be fed orally, feeding should be at the breast as often as possible. If the mother can room-in or the hospital has a care-by-parent ward, this works well. If obligations to other family members make it impossible for the mother to stay, she can pump her milk and bring it in fresh day by day or frozen if the time interval between visits is longer than a day. Freezing will destroy the cellular content, but this is not a major problem beyond the immediate neonatal period. The infant should not be subjected to the added trauma of being weaned from the breast when the infant needs the security and intimacy of nursing most, unless weaning is absolutely unavoidable.

The medical professional needs to be aware of these infants and mothers and their special needs for support. An opportunity to discuss the breastfeeding aspect of the infant's management should be offered by the physician. The pediatrician should assume the advocacy role. The parents should not have to fight for the right to maintain breastfeeding. Plans for pumping and saving milk should be discussed and provided. If the infant is recovering in an open ward or a room with other infants and their parents without adequate privacy, a separate room should be provided for the mother to nurse or pump her milk. This room should be clean, neat, adequately illuminated, and equipped with a sink for washing hands. Storerooms, broom closets, bathrooms, and staff dressing rooms are inappropriate. If a mechanical pump is to be used, it should be kept clean and operable with individual tubing and attachments that come in contact with the milk or the breast. If a breast pump is not provided in the pediatric department, it should be available from the newborn unit or neonatal intensive care unit (NICU).

Arrangements for providing sterile containers for collecting milk and storing it are discussed in Chapter 22. Occasionally, a mother may become so concerned about the adequacy of her milk for her infant that she may nurse much too frequently. Her child may need more nonnutritive sucking and holding than usual. A physician should reassure the mother when pointing this out. The father or other parent should also be encouraged to understand all the tubes, bandages, and appliances the infant may have attached. They are important members of the parenting team and should provide some of the soothing and especially the nonnutritive cuddling.

PERINATAL ISSUES

Postmature Infants

Postmature infants are full-grown, mature infants who have stayed in utero beyond the full vigor of the placenta and have begun to lose weight in utero.[10] They are usually "older-looking" and have a wide-eyed countenance. Their skin is dry and peeling, and subcutaneous tissue is diminished; thus the skin appears too large. These infants have lost subcutaneous fat and lack glycogen stores. Initially, they may be hypoglycemic and require early feedings to maintain adequate blood glucose levels. If breastfed, the infants should go to the breast early, taking special care to maintain body temperature, which is labile in postmature infants who lack the insulating fat layer. Blood sugar levels should be followed with a frequency and duration commensurate with the specific risk factors of the individual infant, and monitoring should continue until normal, prefeed blood sugar levels are consistently, successively obtained.[11] Initially, these infants may feed poorly and require considerable prodding to suckle. In extreme cases of hypoglycemia, an intravenous (IV) infusion may be necessary, and management should follow guidelines for any infant who has hypoglycemia that is resistant to routine early feedings. Because the infants lack glycogen stores, hypoglycemia may persist, and glucagon is contraindicated because no glycogen stores are present to be stimulated. Calcium problems, on the other hand, although common in these infants, generally are rare if the infant is adequately breastfed early because of the physiologic calcium—phosphorus ratio in breast milk. After postmature infants begin to feed well, they tend to catch up quickly and adapt well. Problems with hyperbilirubinemia seldom occur because their livers are mature. Postmature infants gain well at the breast once they stabilize.

Fetal Distress, Hypoxia, and Low Apgar Scores

Infants who have been compromised in utero or during delivery because of insufficient placental reserve, cord accidents, or other causes of intrauterine hypoxia have very low Apgar scores at birth and need special treatment.[12] Neonatal asphyxia is a major cause of neonatal mortality worldwide, with an incidence of approximately 0.7 to 1.2 million annually.[13] The incidence of hypoxic-ischemic encephalopathy is 2.5 per 1000 live births, and the proportion of cerebral palsy associated with intrapartum hypoxia-ischemia is 14.5%. Multiple other organs are often involved, including renal (40%), pulmonary (25%), cardiac (30%), and/or gastrointestinal (GI; 30%), and decreases in gastrointestinal blood flow often occur.[14,15] A recent retrospective review of NEC revealed asphyxia to be a major predisposing factor to this

disease process in both term and preterm infants.[16] Therapeutic hypothermia reduces mortality and improves survival with normal neurologic outcome and is now standard treatment.[17] A recent study revealed that celiac and mesenteric artery flow remained low during hypothermia but rose significantly after rewarming (peak systolic velocity in the celiac artery [CA] = 0.63 m/s to 0.77 m/s, $p = 0.004$, and superior mesenteric artery [SMA] = 0.43 m/s to 0.55 m/s, $p = 0.001$).[18] The authors hypothesized that the low GI perfusion during hypothermia may indicate a favorable effect of cooling against reperfusion injury of the GI tract. Enteral feedings are usually withheld during hypothermia, even for mild neonatal encephalopathy.[19]

Colostrum should be expressed and often becomes the first oral feedings, drop by drop. Mothers will need help initiating lactation and understanding the pathophysiology of the infants' disease. These infants often have a poor suck that does not coordinate with the swallow, making nursing at the breast and bottle equally difficult. The mother may need to hold her breast in place and hold the infant's chin as well. These infants are especially susceptible to "nipple confusion" or "nipple preference." That is, the infant seems to prefer feeding via a bottle versus the breast. In the case of a sick infant, this is not likely to be "confusion"; rather, the infant seems to feed "better" via a bottle per the nursing staff or family. In hopes of the infant developing the feeding skills for effectively breastfeeding, a means of sustaining nourishment other than via a bottle should be sought. Cup feeding has been well tolerated using a soft plastic 1-ounce medicine cup. Even infants who will not be breastfed but feed poorly from a bottle for neurologic reasons will do better with a cup.[20–22] Weaning slowly from the IV hyperalimentation fluids while introducing breastfeeding is helpful. Using a dropper and employing the nursing supplementer (feeding tube delivering supplemental feeds directly to the mother's nipple) are options if milk supply from the breasts is low. These infants may continue to feed poorly for neurologic reasons. If the mother is taught to cope with the problem, using specific positions, holds, and supports for the infant, nursing should progress satisfactorily.

Infants can be held in positions that may help an individual baby adapt better. The "football hold" is a popular but poorly named position in which an infant is held close to the mother's body with the feet to her side. The head and face are squarely in front of the breast and steadied by the mother's arm and hand on that side. Cupping the breast and the jaw in one hand facilitates the infant's seal around the breast with the mouth (Fig. 13.1). This position has been called the *dancer hold*.[23] One of the most valuable suggestions is the use of a sling or pleat-seat to hold an infant's body in a flexed position, thus giving the mother both hands free to hold the head and the breast in position for feeding (Fig. 13.2).

Pacing the feedings and pumping after feedings will establish, maintain, or increase a mother's milk supply when the infant is unable to suck vigorously enough. Giving the pumped milk by lactation supplementer, small cup, or dropper ensures proper weight gain in the early weeks.[23] Holding

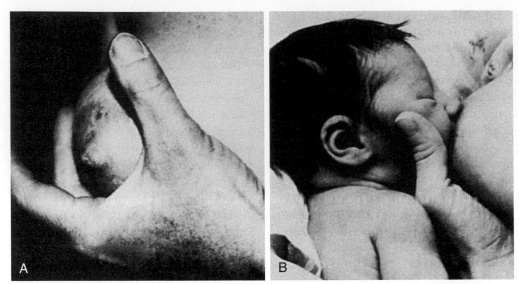

Fig. 13.1 Dancer hold. (A) Hand position of mother. (B) Infant in position at breast with support. (From McBride MC, Danner SC. Sucking disorders in neurologically impaired infants: assessment and facilitation of breastfeeding. *Clin Perinatol.* 1987;14:109.)

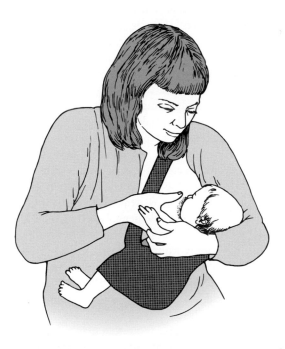

Fig. 13.2 The pleat-seat or sling baby carrier holds the infant in a flexed position that facilitates infant suckling, leaving the mother's hands free to support her breast and the infant. (Redrawn from McBride MC, Danner SC. Sucking disorders in neurologically impaired infants: assessment and facilitation of breastfeeding. *Clin Perinatol.* 1987;14:109.)

an infant in a flexed position that mimics the fetal position relaxes an infant who is hypertonic or arching away from the breast.

In a study of the energetics and mechanics of nutritive sucking in preterm and term neonates, Jain et al.[24] compared 38-gestational-week infants with 35-gestational-week infants and noted that preterm infants used less energy to suck the same volume of milk. The preterm infants took up to 0.5 mL

per suck but generated lower pressures and a lower suck frequency.

Exploring the hypothesis that milk flow achieved during feeding contributes to ventilatory depression during rubber-nipple feeding, Mathew[25] compared nipples with different flow rates. Decreases in minute ventilation and breathing frequency were significantly greater with high-flow nipples, thus confirming that milk flow influences breathing in premature infants who are unable to self-regulate the flow.

Tracings were made from the first oral feeding to time of discharge in term and premature infants. Serial oxygen pressure values showed small undulations across baseline (above and below) while breastfeeding. Substantial dips while bottle-feeding were shown with recovery but not above baseline. The quality and quantity of variation were different in the two modes of sucking (i.e., breast or bottle), with large drops in oxygen saturation occurring during actual sucking of the bottle but only during burping or repositioning while breastfeeding. Meier concludes that the findings do not support the widely held view that breastfeeding is more stressful.[26,27] The comparative data suggest that both the use of a pacifier and bottle-feeding are more stressful than suckling at the breast. For further discussion of the stress of breastfeeding versus bottle-feeding, see Chapter 14 on feeding the 28- to 32-week premature infant. If an infant has significant motor tone disabilities or lacks the usual oral reflexes in response to stimulation of the rooting and sucking reflexes, a neonatal neurologist should assess the infant before any routine exercises are initiated.

It has been suggested that perioral stimulation enhances an immature or neurologically impaired infant's ability to suck and to coordinate suck and swallow.[28] Perioral stimulation, consisting of stimulating the skin overlying the masseter and buccinator muscles by manually applying a quick-touch pressure stimulus lasting 1 second, was studied. This is accomplished by simultaneously squeezing the buccal fat of both cheeks. Suck-monitoring equipment revealed that perioral stimulation increased the sucking rate, suggesting that this may facilitate sucking.[28] Exercising the mouths of infants who already have excessive mouth stimulation may not be appropriate. Many infants in an NICU are being suctioned, tube fed, and orally stimulated for other reasons, which may lead to oral aversion.

Kangaroo care is recommended for full-term infants who are neurologically or metabolically impaired. It involves holding the infant skin to skin inside the parent's shirt. It can stabilize temperature, respirations, and heart rate and be neurologically calming. For a mother who is to breastfeed, it facilitates milk production and helps a mother learn to handle her infant.[29] Kangaroo care is further discussed in Chapter 14.

Galactagogues: Medication-Induced Milk Production When Pumping

Domperidone and metoclopramide are the most commonly used pharmaceutical galactagogues. Both are dopamine antagonists that increase prolactin secretion. A recent meta-analysis reported a significant improvement with the use of domperidone in mothers experiencing insufficient human milk production.[30] Five studies ($N = 239$) showed an increase in the MD of expressed human milk volume in mothers given domperidone of 94 mL/day (95% CI 71.12 to 116.83 mL]; random effect, T^2 0.00, I^2 0%). The use of domperidone in lactation has been the subject of controversy because of the increased risk of ventricular arrhythmia and sudden cardiac death of approximately 4 per 1000 person-years observed among nonlactating adults, including males and females. Numerous studies provide reassuring evidence as to the safety of domperidone use in lactating women. For example, a Canadian population-based cohort study of 320,351 women, of which 45,163 were prescribed domperidone within 6 months postpartum, revealed that no cases of ventricular arrhythmia were identified among those women with no prior history of arrhythmia.[31]

The evidence for metoclopramide is less clear. Brodribb and the ABM protocol team reviewed the use galactagogues for initiating or augmenting maternal milk production in 2018.[32] Although some older trials and observational studies reported increased milk production with metoclopramide, there is concern about the potential for bias in those studies. Five randomized, placebo-controlled blinded trials from 1980 to 2001 did not demonstrate an increase in milk production or duration of breastfeeding with the use of metoclopramide in women diagnosed with poor milk production.

The ABM protocol recommended identifying and correcting any potential cause of low milk production but did not recommend the use of any specific pharmacologic galactagogue for low milk production. Despite the high-quality studies that found domperidone to be useful, they were concerned about rare but significant adverse effects. Since the publication of the ABM protocol, Thomas Hale reported an online survey of self-reported side effects of 1990 mothers, representing 25 countries, who took metoclopramide, domperidone, or both medications to enhance milk production.[33] They found that side effects affected only a small percentage of women who took either medication and that there were fewer side effects with domperidone than metoclopramide. There was no significant difference in cardiac arrhythmias between the two groups. However, there was significantly more depression and tardive dyskinesia symptoms in the metoclopramide group. Of concern, the risk of depression increased by seven times when women took metoclopramide. The authors concluded that recommendations regarding the relative safety of both metoclopramide and domperidone should be reexamined in light of these findings.

Although growth hormone has been observed to enhance milk supply, no recommended protocol exists for its clinical use.[34] In one study, 20 healthy mothers with insufficient milk who delivered between 26 and 34 weeks were given growth hormone, 0.2 international units/kg per day subcutaneously for 7 days. A group of 10 mothers received a placebo. Milk volume increased in the treated mothers. No change was noted in plasma growth hormone levels, but an increase was seen in insulin-like growth factor. No other changes were noted during this short-term therapy.[34]

Other galactagogues are discussed in Chapter 11.

Breastfeeding Twins and Triplets

The medical literature on nursing twins or triplets or multiples in general is limited. Despite this, it is well established that mothers can make enough milk for multiple infants. Many case reports support that a mother can exclusively breastfeed twins and triplets. It has been documented for centuries that an individual mother can provide adequate nourishment for more than one infant. In 17th-century France, wet nurses were allowed to nurse up to six infants at one time. Foundling homes provided wet nurses for every three to six infants.

The key deterrent to nursing twins is not usually the milk supply but time. If a mother can nurse both infants simultaneously, the time factor is reduced (Fig. 13.3). Many strategies have been suggested to achieve this. As the infants become larger and more active, it may be difficult to keep them simultaneously nursing with only two hands to manage infant behavior. However, twins trained from birth to nurse simultaneously will often continue to nurse in a position that allows both to nurse when they are older, even if the other is not nursing at the moment. The first year of life for a parent of a set of twins is an extremely busy one and really requires additional help, particularly if the mother is going to breastfeed. She will need time for adequate rest and nourishment. She often benefits from suggestions from other mothers of twins. The incidence of prematurity with twins is 3 in 10 pregnancies; with triplets, 9 of 10; and with singletons, just 1 in 10. Therefore the challenge of breastfeeding multiples may include some of the challenges of feeding premature infants.

The challenge of breastfeeding twins was investigated through a questionnaire of mothers who were members of the Mothers of Twins Clubs of Southern California, a national organization that offered help and advice to mothers

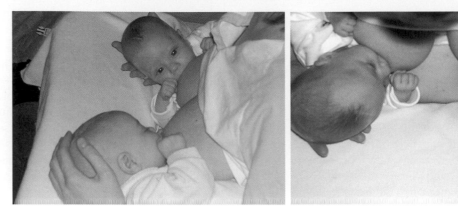

Fig. 13.3 Premature twins nursing simultaneously, resting on a nursing pillow.

of twins in 1975.[35] No other socioeconomic information was available. Of the respondents, 41 mothers (23.7%) breastfed from birth, although 30% of the infants were premature. Of those who did not breastfeed, 9% were told not to do so by their physician, 11% did not think it was possible, and 11% did not think they would have enough milk for two. Of multiparas who had breastfed their first child, an equal number breastfed and bottle-fed. Of the mothers who breastfed, 39 breastfed for more than 1 month, and 12 breastfed for more than 6 months.

In another study from 1986, highlighting the breastfeeding potential of multiples, eight healthy women who were breastfeeding twins and one breastfeeding triplets participated in a study by Saint et al.[36] to determine the yield and nutrient content of their milk at 2, 3, 6, 9, and 12 months postpartum. At 6 months, they fed an average 15 feeds per day. Fully breastfeeding women produced 0.84 to 2.16 kg of milk in 24 hours. Those partially breastfeeding produced 0.420 to 1.392 kg in 24 hours. The mother feeding triplets at 2½ months produced 3.08 kg/day, and the three infants were fed a total of 27 times per day. At 6 months the twins received 64% to 100% of total energy from breastfeeding, and at 12 months, they received 6% to 13%. This further demonstrates that breasts are capable of responding to nutritional demands.

Guidelines for success in breastfeeding twins recommended in 1999 by Hattori and Hattori[37] admit that many obstacles exist but suggest that health care professionals should provide extended support to mothers of multiples to promote successful breastfeeding. The initiation and duration of breast-milk feedings by mothers of multiples compared with mothers of singletons were studied by a mailed questionnaire to 555 women.[38] The 358 mothers who gave birth to twins and multiples in Ohio in 1999 and who answered the questionnaire were older, had higher incomes, were married, and were less likely to return to work by 6 months postpartum. Initiation of breastfeeding was comparable between mothers of multiples and singletons, but mothers of multiples provided milk for a shorter period of time, and mothers of preterm multiples breastfed the shortest period of time. Among mothers who initiated breast-milk feeding, the geometric mean duration of at least some breast-milk feeding

was significantly shorter for preterm multiples than for all other groups: term singletons = 23 weeks, preterm singletons = 19 weeks, term multiples = 24 weeks, and preterm multiples = 12 weeks ($p = 0.002$). At 6 months of age, 31% of preterm singletons were breastfed compared with 16% of preterm multiples.[38] A report in the Cochrane Database in 2017 confirmed the limited published data on breastfeeding for twins and multiples. Of the 10 trials (23 reports), the quality of evidence was mixed, and the risk of bias was high. The authors concluded there was insufficient data to make any reasonable conclusions on specific breastfeeding interventions for twins or multiples.[39] A 2018 study revealed that the main reasons for weaning in the first 6 months cited by mothers of twins were insufficient human milk supply, infants' behavior, and returning to work.[40] On the other hand, books, pamphlets, and websites supply personal stories and advice for mothers, fathers, and families. La Leche League International, Mothers of Twins, pregnancytoday. com, parentingweb.com, multiplebirthsfamilies.com, and others have copious commentaries for mothers. Coping strategies can be helpful. Wisdom from Gromada is shared with mothers in her book *Mothering Multiples, Breastfeeding and Caring for Twins or More.*[41] A case of a mother successfully nursing quadruplets is reported by Berlin.[42] One helpful device is frequently recommended, the "breastfeeding pillow," which is a pillow that wraps around the mother as she sits to nurse. Two infants can be supported by the pillow.

Full-Term Infants With Medical Problems

Infants who have self-limited acute illnesses, such as fever, upper respiratory infection, colds, diarrhea, or contagious diseases such as chickenpox, do best if breastfeeding is maintained. Because of breast milk's low solute load, an infant can be kept well hydrated despite fever or other increased fluid losses. If respiratory symptoms are significant, an infant seems to nurse well at the breast and poorly with a bottle. This observation has been documented many times when nursing mothers have roomed-in with their sick infants in the hospital. The studies of Johnson and Salisbury on the synchrony of respirations in breastfeeding in contrast to the periodic breathing or gasping apnea pattern of the normal bottle-fed infant may well provide the underlying explanation for the phenomenon of an acutely ill infant continuing to nurse at the breast.[43]

In addition to the appropriateness of human milk for a sick infant, nursing and closeness with the mother provide comfort. If an infant is suddenly weaned, psychologic trauma is added to the stress of the illness.[44]

It may be difficult to distinguish the effect of trauma of acute weaning from the symptoms of the primary illness, such as poor feeding or lethargy, if the acutely weaned infant fails to respond to adequate treatment. In this case, returning to breastfeeding may be the treatment because the stress of acute weaning will be removed.

It is not appropriate to give a mother medicine intended to treat the infant, especially antibiotics. This has been tried to the detriment of the child because variable amounts of the drug reach the infant depending on the dose, dosage schedule, and amount of milk consumed. Maternal drugs can produce symptoms in an infant in some cases, and thus maternal history is important in assessing symptoms in a breastfed infant (see Chapter 11).[45]

Buccal Smears in Breastfeeding Infants

Guidelines for buccal smear collection in breastfed infants should be followed when genetic review is indicated. A buccal smear is a noninvasive, fast, and relatively inexpensive diagnostic method for collecting genetic material. It is used for sex determination as well as aneusomy, microdeletion syndromes, and a variety of polymerase chain reaction–based molecular genetic tests. Maternal cells can contaminate smears taken from breastfed infants. The recommendation is to wait at least 1 hour after a feeding. Buccal mucosa should be cleansed thoroughly with a cotton swab applicator. These procedures apply to both neonates and older nursing children.[46]

GASTROINTESTINAL DISEASES

Bouts of diarrhea and intestinal tract disease are less common in breastfed infants than in bottle-fed infants, but when they occur, the infant should be maintained on the breast if possible.[47–48] Human milk is a physiologic solution that normally causes neither dehydration nor hypernatremia. Occasionally, an infant will have diarrhea or an intestinal upset because of something in the mother's diet. It is usually self-limited, and the best treatment is to continue to nurse at the breast. If a mother has been taking a laxative that is absorbed or has been eating laxative foods, such as fruits, in excess, she should adjust her diet. Intractable diarrhea should be evaluated as it would be in any infant. Allergy to mother's milk is extremely rare and would require substantial evidence to support the diagnosis. Allergy to a foreign protein passed into the milk, such as bovine β-globulin, as in cow milk, however, can cause severe allergic symptoms in an infant (see following discussion).

Lactose Intolerance

Suckling milk is the defining characteristic of mammals. Lactose, the major carbohydrate in milk, is hydrolyzed by lactase-phlorizin hydrolase, an enzyme of the small intestine. Lactase plays a critical role in the nutrition of mammalian neonates. Congenital lactase deficiency, present from birth, is extremely rare and is inherited as an autosomal-recessive gene.[49] Most humans (except Northern Europeans) and other adult mammals do not drink milk beyond infancy; it causes indigestion and mild to severe GI symptoms because of an adult's inability to digest lactose. Low lactase levels result from injury or limited genetic expression of lactase. The enzyme hydrolyzes lactose, phlorizin, and glycosyl ceramides. A decline in lactase-specific activity occurs at the time of weaning in most mammalian species. In humans it may occur as early as 3 to 5 years of age; in other species, the elevated juvenile levels of lactase-specific activity persist. The developmental patterns of lactase expression are regulated at the level of gene transcription.[49]

Premature infants and those recovering from severe diarrhea have transient lactose intolerance. The only treatment is a temporary lactose-free diet. Reports of lactose-hydrolyzed human milk suggest that banked human milk can be treated with lactase, which will hydrolyze the lactose (900 enzyme activity units to 200 mL breast milk degraded 82% of the lactose).[50] In one case, the reason for using human milk was that the infant became infection prone when he was weaned from the breast at the time the initial diagnosis was made. That infant showed marked improvement with lactase-treated human milk. In a breastfed infant, lactase deficiency may be manifest by chronic diarrhea and marked failure to thrive.

Cow's Milk Protein Allergy, Food Protein–Induced Allergic Proctocolitis/Non-IgE–Mediated Food Sensitivities, and Food Protein–Induced Enterocolitis Syndrome

Cow's milk protein allergy (CMPA) may be seen in exclusively breastfed infants. Symptoms suggestive of this disorder may be seen in up to 15% of all infants, although the actual incidence is likely closer to 2% to 7.5% in the first year of life. Breastfeeding reduces this incidence to 0.5% to 1.0%.[51] Exclusive breastfeeding may also prevent sensitization to cow's milk protein.[52] CMPA often confused with lactase deficiency (lactose intolerance or cow's milk intolerance) by parents, although it is etiologically distinct and lactose intolerance rarely occurs in infants. CMPA in breastfed infants is generally found to be caused by the passage of bovine β-lactoglobulin. In one study, when mothers ingested cow's milk then breastfed, infants with diagnosed CMPA reacted, but only 63% of their mothers had detectable levels of bovine β-lactoglobulin in their milk.[53] The authors concluded that other proteins may also be responsible for symptoms.

CMPA is currently thought to have two etiologic frameworks: one is immunoglobulin E (IgE) mediated, and the other is non-IgE mediated. IgE-mediated reactions tend to occur within a few hours of ingestion as a type 1 hypersensitivity reaction and include respiratory (wheezing, stridor), dermatologic (hives, atopic dermatitis), allergic (running eyes or nose), and GI symptoms (vomiting and diarrhea). This diagnosis can be made by history, specific IgE blood levels, or skin-prick testing. If the history is clear or symptoms are severe, an oral challenge should be avoided because of the risk.[54]

Non-IgE related reactions are type 4 mediated and generally include reflux, malabsorption, atopic dermatitis, and allergic proctocolitis. This latter results in the characteristic microscopic hematochezia. Symptoms generally present in the first few months of life.[51] Because of the etiology, allergy testing is likely to be inconclusive. Rather, diagnosis is made based on history and elimination diets. A controlled oral food challenge (OFC) with direct medical supervision can help in some situations to confirm or exclude the diagnosis of CMPA.

For exclusively breastfed infants with clinical evidence of allergic colitis, mothers should eliminate all forms of cow's milk protein, including milk products, casein, and whey. The difficulty for mothers in maintaining this diet financially, nutritionally, and psychosocially must be weighed against the potential benefits.[55] Elimination diets with appropriate supplementation of missing nutrients have not been shown to negatively affect infant growth.[56] The ABM has outlined a clinical protocol for a maternal elimination diet in the case of allergic proctocolitis in the exclusively breastfed infant.[57] For supplemented infants, extensively hydrolyzed formula (eHF) or amino acid–based formulas (AAFs) may be used. Some debate exists over whether soy formula should be attempted first, because of its lower cost, increased infant enjoyment, and larger evidence base for growth. However, infants may have cross-reactivity with soy products. Goat, sheep, and other mammal's milk also cross-reacts with CMPA. Studies have shown no increased risk of poor growth from hydrolyzed formulas, and they may result in more rapid resolution of symptoms, particularly if these symptoms are severe.[58] Although allergens likely clear from breast milk within 2 to 7 days, it may take 2 to 4 weeks for inflammation to subside and symptoms to fully resolve.[59] If there is no improvement in symptoms, mothers may consider eliminating other allergens (soy, egg, wheat), seek testing if testing has not yet been done, and reintroduce milk products. An AAF may also be attempted. Very rarely for extremely sick infants, it may be necessary to pause breastfeeding while attempting an AFF, encouraging the mother to pump and store her milk to maintain her supply.

If infants improve with an elimination diet, reintroduction of cow's milk products may be attempted in maternal diets around 9 to 12 months of age, then again periodically if this fails. Most children have outgrown CMPA by school age. If the reaction is IgE mediated or severe, reintroduction should take place under the care of an allergist, or, when unavailable, at the physician's office.

There have been anecdotal reports that severe cases of allergic colitis and also severe GI colic can be alleviated by treating the mother with pancreatic enzymes. These reports noted it was safe for the mother and often showed dramatic improvement for the infant. This treatment is appropriate when eliminating cow protein has not solved the problem.

A formal study of this therapy was reported by Repucci, who described four term infants who were exclusively breastfeeding between 1 and 3 months of age who had a positive family history for atopy.[60] Elimination of bovine protein had not relieved the blood in the stools. Mothers were prescribed pancreatic enzymes (Pancrease MT4 USP units: 4000 units of lipase, 12,000 of amylase, and 12,000 units of protease per capsule), two capsules with each meal and one capsule for snacks. Blood cleared within 2 days. One mother had to increase the dose to three capsules per meal and two with snacks. Mothers experienced no side effects from this therapy.

In severe cases of CMPA, food protein–induced enterocolitis syndrome (FPIES) should be ruled out.[61] This disorder presents somewhat later, between 2 and 7 months of age, and is generally triggered by milk, soy, or grain intolerance.[62] It is characterized by recurrent vomiting, diarrhea, and episodes of pallor and lethargy after ingestion. Acute FPIES may present with hypovolemic shock, hypotension, and hypothermia, whereas chronic FPIES symptoms may be intermittent and cause failure to thrive. Diagnostic criteria are based on history and the outcome of an elimination diet or OFC. Exclusively breastfeeding mothers need extensive dietary counseling for food elimination and milk supply because weaning to solid foods can be very difficult, and even AAFs may not be tolerated by their infants. Time to resolution varies significantly. Close physician counseling and follow-up are recommended. The pathophysiology of FPIES continues to be elusive, with evidence for the stimulation of different components of the immune system. Management involves the treatment of symptoms after an exposure, elimination of suspected food triggers, and ongoing assessment and evaluation using OFCs to identify the resolution of the problem.[61]

Chronic, protracted diarrhea (or enteropathy) includes a variety of abnormalities of the small intestinal mucosa. GI infections are the most common cause of enteropathy. They alter mucosal permeability, antigen penetration in the mucosa, local inflammation, and T-cell activation. Coexisting malnutrition exacerbates the local immune response, alters repair of damaged mucosa, and limits systemic nutritional recovery. Celiac disease and CMPA are other causes of chronic diarrhea. Human milk banks have reported the use of donor human milk in the management of protracted diarrhea. Eleven of 24 children managed by MacFarlane and Miller in a hyperalimentation referral unit recovered when fed banked human milk orally without protracted IV therapy.[63] All the infants had been tried on the available special formulas first. A study of oral rehydration in 26 children younger than the age of 2 years showed that the children who continued to breastfeed while receiving rehydration fluid had fewer stools and recovered more rapidly than those receiving only rehydration fluid.[64] The Pima Infant Feeding Study clearly showed that in less developed and more disadvantaged communities in the United States, exclusive breastfeeding protected against severe diarrhea and other GI disorders.[65]

Celiac Disease

Some chronic diseases are better controlled by keeping an infant on breast milk because symptoms usually become more severe with weaning. If an infant is weaned and does poorly on formula, relactation of the mother should be considered. With the availability of the nursing supplementer, this possibility is no longer remote (see Chapter 19).

Celiac disease or permanent gluten-sensitive enteropathy is an immunologic disease dependent on the exposure to wheat gluten or related proteins in rye and barley.[66]

A case-control study was done on the effect of infant feeding on the development of celiac disease to investigate the association between duration of breastfeeding and age at first gluten introduction into the infant diet and the incidence and age of onset of celiac disease.[67] A significant protective effect on the incidence of celiac disease was related to the duration of breastfeeding after 2 months. It was not related to the age of first gluten in the diet, although the age of first exposure did affect the age of onset of symptoms.[67] The risk for celiac disease was reduced in children younger than 2 years old in a study of 2000 Swedish children if they were still being breastfed when dietary gluten was introduced. The effect was more pronounced if breastfeeding continued after gluten was introduced. The authors conclude that gradual introduction of gluten-containing foods into the diet while breastfeeding reduces the risk for ever getting celiac disease.[66] The declining incidence of celiac disease and transient gluten intolerance has been associated with changing feeding practices, which include later introduction of dietary gluten, the use of gluten-free foods for weaning (rice), and the increased initiation and duration of breastfeeding.[68] The recent US Department of Agriculture (USDA) and US Department of Health and Human Services Pregnancy and Birth to 24 Months Project reviewed nine articles published from January 1980 to March 2016. They concluded, based on limited case-control evidence, that never versus ever being fed human milk is associated with a higher risk of celiac disease. However, concerns about reverse causality precluded a conclusion about the relationship of shorter versus longer duration of any human milk feeding with celiac disease.[69]

A window of opportunity has been suggested to reduce the risk of celiac disease by introducing gluten at specific ages. Two large studies dealt with that hypothesis. The first study, conducted at 20 centers throughout Italy, compared a delayed strategy of the introduction of gluten at 12 months of age to the standard strategy of 6 months of age.[70] The 553 children in this trial were at increased risk for developing celiac disease, with a compatible human leukocyte antigen (HLA) haplotype and a first-degree relative with celiac disease. The cumulative prevalence of celiac disease at age 10 years was 16.8%. This study revealed that although the later introduction of gluten delayed the onset of celiac disease in early childhood, there was no difference between the two groups by the age of 5 or 10 years, suggesting that the age of introduction of gluten had very little impact on the ultimate risk for celiac disease later in childhood.

The second study was a double-blind trial conducted in eight countries on 944 infants with an at-risk HLA haplotype and a first-degree relative with celiac disease who were randomly assigned either 200 mg of vital wheat gluten or placebo

at 4 months of age, and then dietary gluten was introduced to both groups at age 6 months.[71] At 5 years, the cumulative prevalence of celiac disease was 12.1%, and there was no significant difference in the risk of celiac disease when comparing the intervention to the placebo group.

In children at high risk for celiac disease, neither delaying the timing of the introduction of gluten to 12 months or introducing gluten between 4 and 6 months decreased the overall risk of celiac disease, although it may change the timing of onset of the disease.[70,72]

Inflammatory Bowel Disease: Crohn Disease and Ulcerative Colitis

Crohn disease and ulcerative colitis constitute the two major groups of inflammatory bowel disease. Environmental factors, genetic factors, and immune responses are important in the etiology of inflammatory bowel diseases, with resultant excessive and destructive inflammatory reactions of the gut wall. In addition, it is thought that downregulation of the immune responses may allow the damaged mucosa to heal and reset the physiologic functions of the gut back to normal. Because it has been suggested that breast milk is essential for the development of the normal immunologic competence of the intestinal mucosa, investigators have studied the association between breastfeeding and later Crohn disease.

A recent meta-analysis and systemic review have evaluated the risk of inflammatory bowel disease and breastfeeding. A meta-analysis evaluated 35 studies that ran through November 2016 comprising 7536 individuals with Crohn disease, 7353 with ulcerative colitis, and 330,222 controls. They reported that ever breastfeeding was associated with a 29% reduced risk of Crohn disease (odds ratio [OR] 0.71, 95% CI 0.59 to 0.85) and a 22% reduced risk of ulcerative disease (OR 0.78, 95% CI 0.67 to 0.91).[73] Although this inverse association was observed in all ethnicity groups, the magnitude of protection was significantly greater among Asians (OR 0.31, 95% CI 0.20 to 0.48) compared with Caucasians (OR 0.78, 95% CI 0.66 to 0.93; $p = .0001$) in Crohn disease. Breastfeeding duration showed a dose-dependent association, with the strongest decrease in risk when breastfed for at least 12 months for Crohn disease (OR 0.20, 95% CI 0.08 to 0.50) and ulcerative colitis (OR 0.21, 95% CI 0.10 to 0.43) as compared with 3 or 6 months.[73]

The recent USDA systemic review evaluated 17 articles published from January 1980 to March 2016. It concluded, based on limited but consistent case-control evidence, that longer durations of breastfeeding were associated with lower rates of inflammatory bowel disease.[69]

RESPIRATORY ILLNESS AND OTITIS MEDIA

Respiratory Illness

Infants who develop respiratory illnesses should be maintained at the breast as tolerated. The added advantages of antibodies and other antiinfective properties in human milk are valuable to infants over and above the importance of nutritional support during infection.[74,75] The comfort of having the mother nearby is important whenever the infant has a crisis; weaning during illness may be difficult for both the infant and mother.

Wheezing and lower respiratory tract disease and other respiratory illnesses are lower in frequency and duration when the infant is breastfed. The risk of hospitalization for respiratory disease in infants is decreased for breastfed infants.[75] Recovery is accelerated if breastfeeding is maintained. The Millennium Cohort Study, a nationally representative longitudinal study of 18,818 infants in the United Kingdom, revealed that exclusive breastfeeding for 6 months was associated with a decreased risk of lower respiratory tract infections compared with infants who exclusively breastfed for <4 months, stressing the importance of recommending 6 months exclusive breastfeeding.[48] The Environmental Determinants of Diabetes in the Young (TEDDY), a prospective longitudinal study from six centers in the United States and Europe, followed 6861 children between the ages of 3 and 18 months and 5666 children up to the age of 4 years. Breastfeeding was found to be inversely associated with the odds of respiratory infections with fever at 3 to 6 months (any breastfeeding: OR 0.82, 95% CI 0.70 to 0.95, exclusive breastfeeding: OR 0.72, 95% CI 0.60 to 0.8) and with laryngitis and tracheitis at 6 to 18 months (OR 0.79, 95% CI 0.63 to 0.97, $p = 0.03$).[76] The Agency for Health Care Research and Quality (AHRQ) reported a 72% reduction in the risk of hospitalization for respiratory infections in children under a year of age who were exclusively breastfed for at least 4 months.[77]

A meta-analysis of 20 studies on lower respiratory tract infection from respiratory syncytial virus (RSV) revealed that not breastfeeding doubled the incidence (OR 2.24, 95% CI 1.56 to 3.20).[78] It has been estimated that if 90% of US infants were exclusively breastfed for 6 months, this could prevent almost 21,000 hospitalizations and 40 deaths for lower respiratory tract infections in the first year of life.[79] The American Academy of Pediatrics (AAP) Committee on Nutrition and Section of Allergy and Immunology recently concluded that any duration of breastfeeding ≥ 3 to 4 months is protective against wheezing in the first 2 years of life and that longer breastfeeding, as opposed to less breastfeeding, protects against asthma even after 5 years of age.[80] In addition, the USDA Pregnancy and Birth to 24 Months Project recent systematic review concluded, based on moderate, mostly observational evidence, that any breastfeeding is associated with a lower risk of childhood asthma and that longer durations provide more protection.[81]

Young infants who have older siblings may well be exposed to some virulent viruses and bacteria. Developing croup, for instance, may make an infant seriously ill. Hydration can be maintained by frequent, short breastfeeding periods. Studies have shown that respirations are maintained more easily when feeding on human milk than on cow's milk, even from a bottle. Nursing at the breast permits regular respirations, whereas bottle-feeding is associated with a more gasping pattern.[82] Thus breastfed infants should continue to nurse when they are ill. If an infant is hospitalized, every effort should be made to maintain breastfeeding or to provide expressed breast milk if the infant can be fed at all. Staff should provide rooming-in for the mother if a care-by-parent ward is not available.

Colostrum and milk contain large amounts of immunoglobulin A (IgA) antibody, some of which is RSV specific. Breastfed but not bottle-fed infants have IgA in their nasal secretions. Neutralizing inhibitors to RSV have been demonstrated in the whey of most samples of human milk tested.[83] IgG anti-RSV antibodies are present in milk and in reactive T lymphocytes. Breastfeeding-induced resistance to RSV was associated with the presence of interferon and virus-specific lymphocyte transformation activity, suggesting that breastfeeding has unique mechanisms for modulating the immune response of infants to RSV infection.[84] Clinical studies indicating a relative protection from RSV in breastfed infants were clouded by other factors.[85] The populations were unequal because of socioeconomic factors and smoking (i.e., bottle-feeding mothers were in lower socioeconomic groups and smoked more). In general, if breastfed infants become ill, they have less severe illness.[83,85] Although breastfeeding protects, parental smoking and daycare are important negative factors in the incidence of respiratory infection. Respiratory illness in either infant or mother should be treated symptomatically, and breastfeeding should be continued. If the infant has nasal congestion, nasal aspiration and saline nose drops just before a feed are helpful.

Otitis Media

Acute otitis media is a common affliction among young children, with estimates as high as 60% of children experiencing at least 1 episode of acute otitis media (AOM) before 1 year of age and more than 80% by 3 years of age.[86] Beyond the acute illness, AOM can lead to a variety of sequelae, including persistent middle ear effusion, short-term hearing loss, perforation of the eardrum, chronic suppurative otitis media, persistent hearing impairment, and less commonly, mastoiditis, brain abscess, and meningitis.[87] The global incidence of AOM has been estimated at 11% per year, with a peak incidence in the 1- to 4-year age group.[88] There is wide variation in incidence by region and by country. The World Health Organization (WHO) has published data on the occurrence of AOM by region, with sub-Saharan Africa being the highest, followed by southern Asia, South East Asia and the Pacific Islands, and Central America and the Caribbean.[88] Numerous risk factors have been associated with the risk of AOM, including allergy/atopy, upper respiratory tract infection (URTI), snoring, gender (male), attending daycare, multiple children in a household, family history of AOM, patient's previous history of AOM, passive smoking, socioeconomic status, pacifier (or dummy) use, exposure to air pollutants, immunizations (influenza, *Haemophilus influenzae* B, pneumococcal vaccines), obesity, and breastfeeding.[89,90] In different populations and studies, each of these risk factors appeared to be a contributor to the occurrence of otitis media. There is mixed data concerning the contribution or relative effect of these different risk factors, except for passive smoking and breastfeeding.

Otitis media in infants occurs less frequently in breastfed infants because of the infection protection properties of human milk and the protective effect of suckling at the breast. In a prospective birth cohort study, the West Australian Pregnancy Cohort (Raine) Study recruited 2900 mothers through antenatal clinics at the major tertiary obstetric hospital in Perth, Western Australia. A total of 2237 children participated in a 6-year cohort follow-up, and a subset of 1344 children were given ear and hearing assessments. There was a significant, independent association between predominant breastfeeding (OR 1.33, 95% CI 1.04 to 1.69, $p = 0.02$) and otitis media, and breastfeeding duration (OR 1.35, 95% CI 1.08 to 1.68, $p = 0.01$) with otitis media at 3 years of age.[91] The TEDDY Study described earlier reported that breastfeeding was inversely associated with the odds of otitis media at 3 to 6 months (any breastfeeding: OR 0.76, 95% CI 0.62 to 0.94, exclusive breastfeeding: OR 0.64, 95% CI 0.49 to 0.84) and at 6 to 18 months (OR 0.89, 95% CI 0.82 to 0.97, $p = 0.008$). The duration of exclusive breastfeeding was inversely associated with the odds of otitis media up to 48 months of age (OR 0.97, 95% CI 0.95 to 0.99), long after breastfeeding had stopped.[76]

The AHRQ reported that exclusive breastfeeding for 3 to 6 months provided a 50% reduction in otitis media compared with formula-feeding even when controlling for socioeconomic status, parental smoking, and the presence of siblings.[77] A meta-analysis of 24 studies, all from the United States or Europe, revealed that breastfeeding protects against otitis media in the first 2 years of life.[86] Exclusive breastfeeding for the first 6 months was associated with the greatest protection, a 43% reduction in ever having AOM in the first 2 years of life (OR 0.57, 95% CI 0.44 to 0.75), followed by "more versus less" breastfeeding (OR 0.67, 95% CI 0.59 0.76) and "ever versus never" breastfeeding (OR 0.67, 95% CI 0.56 to 0.80), again stressing the importance of recommending 6 months exclusive breastfeeding. The researchers did not report on data showing that breastfeeding offers any protection against AOM beyond 2 years of age.[86] The Italian Society of Pediatrics presents updated guidelines for the management of AOM in children.[90] In those guidelines, the review of the type of feeding as a preventive measure against AOM concludes that breastfeeding is clearly protective. The guidelines state that the heterogeneity of the numerous studies in the review prevents exact statements regarding exclusivity and duration of breastfeeding for protection against AOM. There is biologic plausibility for the protective effect of breastfeeding against AOM based on the multiple immunologic factors in breast milk that can affect mucosal barrier protection, colonization with nonpathogens, and local and systemic immune protection. There is a large amount of clinical and research data demonstrating the protective effect of breastfeeding against AOM. The most benefit from breastfeeding is gained with exclusive breastfeeding and longer duration (at least 6 months in the case of AOM). Discussing and addressing other potential risk factors for AOM is appropriate if there is parental concern or a family history of frequent otitis media.

METABOLIC DISEASE

Galactosemia

Galactosemia, caused by a deficiency of galactose-1-phosphate uridylyltransferase (GALT), is a rare circumstance in which an infant is unable to metabolize galactose and must be placed on a galactose-free diet. The disease can be rapidly fatal in the severe form. The infant may have severe and persistent jaundice, vomiting, diarrhea, electrolyte imbalances, cerebral signs, and weight loss. This is a medical emergency. This does necessitate weaning from the breast to a special formula because human milk, as with all mammalian milks, contains high levels of lactose, which is a disaccharide that splits into glucose and galactose. Until the subtype is discovered, the mother may be encouraged to continue to pump and store milk in case the infant may be partially breastfed. The condition is suspected when reducing substances are found in the urine in the newborn, and the diagnosis is confirmed by measuring the enzyme uridylyltransferase in the red and white blood cells. The several forms can be distinguished by genetic testing. Except for the mild form, the infant must be weaned to a lactose-free diet. An infection with *Escherichia coli* in the newborn period may be the trigger that precipitates serious symptoms associated with this or other metabolic disorders. Galactosemia is screened for in most states in the United States, along with phenylketonuria (PKU) and other metabolic disorders.

When the diagnosis is made, genetic testing should be done. In the more common and milder form of the disease, the Duarte variant (DG), some enzyme is available. A recent study demonstrated that DG, diagnosed on newborn metabolic tests, is not associated with an increased risk of developmental abnormalities and does not benefit from dietary restrictions of galactose. In one study, 350 children between the ages of 6 and 12 in 13 US states were studied, including 206 who had DG and 144 unaffected siblings who served as controls.[92] The children were found to be at no greater risk of long-term developmental abnormalities than their unaffected siblings, regardless of their exposure to milk as infants. Breastfeeding, therefore, should be encouraged with DG.

Although newborns are screened for galactosemia in all 50 US states, screening protocols vary from state to state; some only test for the extreme deficiencies of classic galactosemia, whereas others are designed to detect DG as well. Newborn screening tests for galactosemia look at blood levels of GALT, which helps convert galactose into glucose. Children with GALT enzyme levels of 1% or less are considered to have classic galactosemia, which affects about one out of every 50,000 babies born in the United States. Most babies with DG, which is 10 times more common, have about 25% of the normal level of GALT activity.[93] At present, in most places, the diagnostic evaluation of an abnormal newborn screen for galactosemia can take more than a week for results. The risk of sepsis, hepatic injury, kernicterus, and even death in infants with classic galactosemia leads most providers to respond to an abnormal newborn screening (NBS) result by stopping breastfeeding to use a galactose-free formula. The solution may be to change the NBS by adjusting the cutoff values such that the identification of DG and other benign variants of galactosemia is kept to a minimum. Other solutions would be to change the NBS by adding a screen for the Duarte allele and/or including the several most common classic galactosemia mutations to reduce the number of infants unnecessarily treated. Although the presence of the Duarte allele does not completely eliminate the risk of severe mutations, it would provide reassurance, allowing health care providers to better assess the need to stop breastfeeding without excessive risk to the infant.[94]

With other forms of galactosemia, such as galactokinase (GALK) deficiency or galactose epimerase (GALE) deficiency, the standard treatment is to wean to a lactose-free diet to eliminate complications. Some infants can only be partially breastfed, with some lactose-free formula in addition for necessary calories.[95] A recent review included two infants with GALE who were exclusively breastfed for a mean of 2.5 months. At 7 years of age, their neurologic development was normal, and body length was above the 3rd percentile.[96] An endocrinologist should make the decision for the exact balance of milks. In classic GALT deficiency, breastfeeding is contraindicated.

Inborn Errors of Metabolism

Other metabolic deficiency syndromes may be apparent only as mild failure-to-thrive syndrome until the infant is weaned from the breast and the symptoms become severe. This particularly applies to inborn errors of metabolism caused by an inability to handle one or more of the essential amino acids that are in higher concentration in cow's milk than human milk. Infection is often a complication early in the lives of these infants with inborn errors, most commonly as a result of *E. coli* bacteria. While the acute infection is being treated, the infant may be weaned from the breast, and the metabolic disorder would then become apparent precipitously.

Certain amino acids, including phenylalanine, methionine, leucine, isoleucine, and others associated with metabolic disorders, have significantly lower levels in human milk than in cow's milk. Management of an amino acid metabolic disorder while breastfeeding depends on careful monitoring of blood and urine levels of the specific amino acids involved. Because these are essential amino acids, a certain amount is necessary in the diet of all infants, including those with disease. An appropriate combination of breastfeeding and milk free of the offending amino acid should be developed. The care of such infants should be provided in consultation with a pediatric endocrinologist.

Screening programs that test all newborns have identified many victims early. Almost all NBS programs test for PKU, galactosemia, and hypothyroidism, and increasingly, maple syrup urine disease, homocystinuria, biotinidase deficiency, tyrosinemia, and now cystic fibrosis are included. Most cases can be managed with continued breastfeeding and diet modification. Congenital adrenal hyperplasia requires corticosteroids, but the feeding can be breast milk. If it is the salt-wasting variety, an infant must have added salt.

Phenylketonuria

The most common of the amino acid metabolic disorders is PKU, in which the amino acid phenylalanine (Phe) accumulates as a result of mutations in the liver enzyme phenylalanine hydroxylase. The dietary treatment of PKU is based on the restriction of Phe intake to maintain blood Phe concentrations within the recommended range. Unless the affected child is maintained on a strict low-Phe diet, PKU leads to mental retardation, seizures, behavioral problems, and other neurologic symptoms. In contrast, when identified via newborn screening and if treatment is initiated before 1 month of age, cognitive–neurologic development is preserved.[97] The treatment of PKU involves a lifelong diet low in Phe; frequent monitoring of blood Phe values; and regular consultation with the pediatric metabolic team of physicians, nurses, and dieticians. Normal cognitive development is expected when Phe blood levels are managed and remain within acceptable levels (120 to 360 μmol/L).[98]

Unfortunately, exclusive breastfeeding for the first 6 months of life affects the neurologic development of patients with PKU. Although human milk has less phenylalanine than formula, it still exceeds the tolerance of most infants with PKU. Because breast milk and regular infant formula contain Phe, babies with PKU need to consume a phenylalanine-free infant formula. The standard of care for infants with PKU was immediate discontinuation of breastfeeding with the combination of a standard infant formula and a phenylalanine-free formula. At the time, this was believed to be the only effective way to monitor the infant's intake and allow for precise titration and measurement of Phe to protect the neurologic and cognitive development of the infant. Mothers of infants with PKU titrated Phe-free formula with a standard commercial formula based on Phe levels obtained from infant heel sticks. Breastfeeding is sometimes continued until the diagnosis is confirmed and Phe-free formula is begun. There are reports concerning breastfeeding and PKU that discuss the challenges of doing this and the difficulty of monitoring Phe levels and titrating the amount of Phe-free formula.[99,100]

As soon as the diagnosis is made, an infant should be placed on a low-Phe formula to reduce the levels in the plasma promptly. The mother should pump her breasts to maintain her milk supply. The breastfed infant is offered a small volume of special formula (10 to 30 mL) first and then completes the feeding at the breast. As long as the blood Phe levels can be maintained between 120 and 360 mmol/L, the exact intake need not be measured. Initially, weight checks to ensure adequate growth are essential because poor intake leading to a catabolic state will interfere with control. Because human milk is low in Phe, the offending amino acid, more than half of the diet can be breast milk.

Another protocol for breastfeeding an infant with PKU was studied by van Rijn et al.[101] The feeding schedule was based on alternating breastfeeding and phenylalanine-free formula by bottle. Each child had a separate schedule convenient for the mother–baby dyad, depending on tolerance and age. At the beginning of treatment, the mother breastfed once daily, allowing the infant to feed until satiated, and the mother pumped the rest of the day. Breastfeedings were increased while monitoring phenylalanine plasma levels. Ultimately, breastfeeding and bottle-feeding were alternated and equal. At all feedings, the infant drank until satisfied. The breastfed infants did well on this protocol, and plasma levels were stable. The mean Phe concentration was 170 μmol/L (range 137 to 243 μmol/L) for the breastfed infants and 181 μmol/L (range 114 to 257 μmol/L) for the formula-fed infants; all of the values in each group of infants were within the recommended range. An essential member of the management team is a board-certified licensed lactation consultant to assist the mother in managing her milk supply. It is not known if the type of feeding strategy will affect the duration of breastfeeding in PKU.

A 2018 recent study reviewed 41 infants with PKU, 40 (98%) of whom were breastfed following delivery.[102] After the diagnosis, breastfeeding was continued in 25 (61%) infants. The mean duration of breastfeeding was 7.4 ± 4.0 (1 to 15) months. The serum Phe concentration of breastfed infants (280 ± 163 μmol/L) was significantly lower than that of nonbreastfed infants (490 ± 199 μmol/L, $p < 0.001$), most likely reflecting the lower level of Phe in human milk compared with regular infant formula. Mean monthly weight gain in the first year of life was significantly higher in breastfed patients (493 ± 159 g/month) compared with nonbreastfed patients (399 ± 116 g/month, $p = 0.046$).

Another recent study reviewed early feeding practices in infants with PKU across Europe.[103] Only 42% of centers were likely to have 76% or more of their infants on breastfeeds at the time of diagnosis, and only 26% of centers maintained 76% or more of their infants on breastfeeds after diagnosis. Overall, breastfeeding duration was short, with a mean of 4 weeks in 9%, 5 to 17 weeks in 26%, 18 to 26 weeks in 34%, 27 to 52 weeks in 24%, and >1 year in 6% of centers. For breastfeeding infants, 53% of centers gave premeasured Phe-free infant formula before each breastfeed to satiety, 23% alternated breastfeeds with Phe-free infant formula, 11% gave a premeasured Phe-free infant formula before time-limited breastfeeds, and 6% gave expressed breast-milk feeds followed by Phe-free formula. The authors concluded that controlled prospective studies are needed to assess how different feeding practices influence breastfeeding outcomes to define the optimal infant feeding practices in PKU.

The weaning of this special infant should be similar to that of other infants. Adding solid foods can be initiated at 6 months.[104] The liquid part of the diet continues as before, that is, two feeding components of low-Phe formula and breastfeeding plus solids with little or no Phe (fruits, vegetables, low-protein foods). Rice and wheat contain too much Phe. When the decision is made to wean from the breast, solid foods can be used to replace the Phe in the breast milk as needed. Growth should be followed closely. When weaning is complete, the infant should be given other, less bulky sources of protein free of Phe. This stage will be carefully orchestrated by the endocrinologist and nutritionist. There is one case-control study examining feeding development and progress onto solid foods during weaning for 20 PKU-positive infants

and 20 non-PKU infants.[105] The infants were monitored monthly until 12 months and then again at 15 and 18 months of age. Children with PKU had comparable weaning progression to non-PKU infants, including texture acceptance, infant formula volume, and self-feeding skills. The children with PKU had a longer period of Phe-free infant formula bottle-feeding and parental spoon-feeding than controls. The children with PKU also had fewer meals/snacks per day; more flatulence ($p = 0.0005$), burping ($p = 0.001$), and retching ($p = 0.03$); and less regurgitation ($p = 0.003$). There were negative behaviors associated with Phe-free infant protein-substitute (PS) at ages 10 to 18 months, which overlapped the age of teething. The use of semisolid PS in PKU supported normal weaning development/progression. The authors observed that the parents required additional support to manage the complexity of feeding and to normalize the social interactions in the child's family food environment.[105]

Because infants with PKU are more prone to thrush infection, the mother should be alerted to watch for symptoms in the infant and the onset of sore nipples that could be caused by *Candida albicans*. Treatment is nystatin for both the mother and baby initially. (See discussion in Chapters 15 and 16.)

The other benefits of human milk make the effort to breastfeed valuable for the infant and for the mother, who usually wants to continue to contribute to her infant's nurturing and nourishment. The prognosis for intellectual development is excellent if treatment of PKU is initiated early and the blood levels are maintained at less than 10 mg/dL phenylalanine (120 to 360 mmol/L).

A retrospective study of 26 school-age children who had been breastfed or formula-fed for 20 to 40 days before dietary intervention was conducted by Riva et al.[106] The children who had been breastfed had a 14-point IQ advantage, which persisted at 12.9 points when corrected for maternal social and educational status. The age of treatment onset for PKU was not related to IQ scores. This study strongly supports the belief that breastfeeding in the prediagnostic stage has a positive impact on the long-range neurodevelopmental performance of patients with PKU (Fig. 13.4).

Phe levels in human milk are relatively constant regardless of the mother's diet. Dietary precautions for the mother of a breastfeeding child with PKU are to avoid the artificial

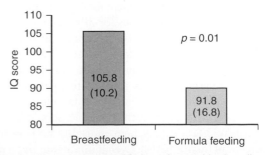

Fig. 13.4 Intelligence quotient (IQ) in patients with phenylketonuria, evaluated by Wechsler Intelligence Scale for Children score, in relation to the type of feeding in the first weeks of life. (From Giovannini M, Verduci E, Salvatici E, et al. Phenylketonuria: dietary and therapeutic challenges, *J Inherit Metab Dis.* 2007;30:1450152.)

sweetener aspartame (NutraSweet), which metabolizes to aspartate and Phe.

Other Metabolic Disorders

Pompe disease (acid maltase deficiency or glycogen storage disease type II) is an inborn error of metabolism caused by a complete or partial deficiency of the enzyme acid α-glucosidase that normally breaks down lysosomal glycogen into glucose. Glycogen accumulates in the tissues, especially muscles. The disease takes various forms. The most severe form, classic infantile-onset Pompe disease (IOPD), typically features dramatic hypertrophic cardiomyopathy at birth, whereas atypical (nonclassical) IOPD can present cardiomyopathy several months later. High-dose (40 mg/kg) enzyme-replacement therapy with recombinant human alglucosidase alpha (GAA; Myozyme) started immediately at newborn screening gives the best outcome.[107] It is safe and reverses cardiomyopathy; improves gross motor outcomes, lingual strength, pulmonary function measures, and biochemical markers; and improves overall survival.[108] Because of the frequency of respiratory infection and difficulty feeding, breastfeeding should be encouraged.

Ornithine transcarbamylase deficiency is a rare, life-threatening genetic disorder. It is one of six urea-cycle disorders named for the specific enzyme deficiency present. Ornithine transcarbamylase deficiency (OTC) is the most common of the urea-cycle disorders. Urea-cycle disorders occur in 1 of 8200 US live births, making these disorders more common in the United States than globally. OTC deficiency occurs more commonly in neonates and early childhood than in adulthood. Males more commonly experience severe symptoms as neonates because the mutation is on the X chromosome. Approximately 10% of female carriers become symptomatic.[109] A lack of enzyme results in excessive and symptomatic accumulation of ammonia in the blood (hyperammonemia). Symptoms vary but can occur within 72 hours of birth and include poor suck, irritability, vomiting, and progressive lethargy followed, if untreated, by hypotonia, seizures, respiratory distress, and coma. Infant-onset disease is more common in males. Treatment includes hydration, arginine, and hemodialysis. Arginine supplementation bypasses the OTC enzyme in the urea cycle, allowing for urea creation and ammonia elimination. Using a combination of sodium benzoate and sodium phenylbutyrate reduces ammonia by using alternative pathways for nitrogen elimination. If ammonia rises above 500 μm/L, the patient should receive urgent hemodialysis. Ammonia levels above 800 μm/L are associated with severe neuralgic damage, limiting treatment options. Once OTC deficiency is suspected, genetic counseling can be helpful for patients and their families. To prevent their condition from deteriorating, patients should limit their protein intake. OTC causes high mortality and morbidity. Fifty percent of infants perish. Even if infants survive a hyperammonemic coma, they will probably face intellectual disabilities if they were in the coma for over 24 hours.[109] Patients diagnosed early and treated emergently have an improved prognosis, as do patients who adhere to low-protein diets and

take medications that bypass the OTC enzyme in the urea cycle. Infants can be breastfed and receive nonprotein caloric supplement. The advantage of human milk is not only dietary but the infection protection and immune-protective qualities. A recent review found that these infants breastfed well.[96] Clinical and biochemical monitoring was performed in at 2- to 4-week intervals, including ammonia and analysis of plasma amino acids. Feeding breast milk was generally uncomplicated in all the patients, without any case of metabolic crisis. An essential amino acid formula is available for those not breastfeeding.

Transient neonatal tyrosinemia, which has been reported to occur in a high percentage (up to 80%) of neonates fed cow's milk, is associated with blood tyrosine levels 10 times those of adults. Wong et al.[110] have associated severe cases with learning disabilities in later years. Tyrosine appears in human milk at low levels. Tyrosinemia type I is an inherited autosomal-recessive trait. Symptoms are caused by the accumulation of tyrosine and its metabolites in the liver. It is treated by dietary control consisting of low protein with limited Phe and tyrosine. Some breastfeeding is possible, combined with protein-free supplements. 2-(2-Nitro-4-trifluoromethyl-benzyl)-1-3-cyclohexanedione reduces the production of toxic metabolites. Liver failure is common. Dietary restrictions are lifelong.

Nutrition management of infants with *organic acidemias* involves limiting the intake of the offending amino acid(s) to the minimum necessary for normal growth and development and suppressing amino acid degradation during catabolic periods by providing alternative fuels, such as glucose. In some disorders, including isovaleric acidemia, specific treatment is included to increase the excretion of toxic metabolites by enhancing the body's capacity to make isovalerylglycine, an acylcarnitine translocase. As more specific amino acid-free formulas are made available, a recipe for combining breastfeeding with the special formula can be engineered to specific infants' needs. The endocrinologist and the nutritionist can provide such a recipe.

A recent study reviewed eight infants with organic acidemias (propionic acidemia [PA; $N = 3$], methylmalonic acidemia [MMA; $N = 2$], malonic acidemia [MA; $N = 1$], and glutaric acidemia type I [GI; $N = 2$]) who breastfed for a mean of 8 months.[96] Five of the eight patients (PA, $N = 3$; GI, $N = 2$; MMA, $N = 1$) received specific amino acid-free formula after the diagnosis was established. In all the patients, the special formula was given mixed with a small amount of expressed breast milk via a standard bottle immediately before breastfeeding. Clinical and biochemical monitoring of the infants was done closely at 2- to 4-week intervals and included ammonia and analysis of urine organic acids and/or plasma amino acids as the metabolic disorders required. Body length was above the 3rd percentile in all the patients except one (G1). Neurologic development was normal in one patient (MA). Five patients had mild to moderate mental retardation (PA, $N = 3$; MMA, $N = 2$), which is consistent with the natural course of the disease.[96]

There are many other variations of these enzyme deficiency diseases. Without treatment, these amino acid enzyme deficiencies lead to deterioration, mental retardation, and often organ failure, especially liver failure. The National Organization for Rare Disorders Inc. (NORD) provides information for professionals, the lay public, and support groups regarding more than 1000 rare diseases. It lobbies for the development of specific treatments (orphan drugs). (Specific treatment information is available at the NORD website, http://www.rarediseases.org.)

Cystic Fibrosis

Cystic fibrosis (CF) is an autosomal-recessive disease caused by mutations in the cystic fibrosis transmembrane conductance regulator (*CFTR*) gene. The CFTR protein is in the epithelia of tissues, including the lungs, sweat glands, pancreas, and GI tract.

Screening tests for CF have been initiated in state-mandated metabolic screening programs for newborns, so a greater number will be identified early. Meconium plugs, especially large plugs and full-blown meconium ileus, have a high correlation with pancreatic enzyme deficiency and CF. As clinicians are alerted to meconium plugs, early tests for CF can be carried out and management adjusted. Breastfeeding is optimal not only for the nutrition but for the presence of enzymes to facilitate digestion and absorption of nutrients. Because infection is a significant morbidity in these children, the infection-protection properties of human milk make a critical impact. A study of infants exclusively breastfed or formula-fed showed that breastfeeding does not compromise growth and is associated with fewer infections and respiratory problems in infants with CF.[111]

The first symptom in infants with CF is often failure to thrive. If an infant is breastfed, the mother may be forced to wean, yet the infant feeds even less well and has no weight gain on formula. Infants do better if placed back on the breast. Pumping to increase the mother's milk supply will help satiate the child's hunger. The use of pancreatic enzymes may be a way to improve tolerance and weight gain in these special breastfed infants rather than weaning to formula.[112] Prescribing pancreatic enzymes for a mother while breastfeeding, as described earlier, is also a consideration.[113]

Breastfeeding is protective for infants with CF. In one study, 146 children (73 males and 73 females) were studied at age 5 to 18 years (mean 10.5 ± 3.9 years).[114] Breastfed compared with formula-fed infants with CF had improved lung function (higher FEV-1, $p = 0.001$) and a reduced incidence of infections in the first 3 years of life ($p = 0.098$) after multivariate analysis. A study of 99 infants with CF revealed that breastfeeding for at least 3 months delayed the first acquisition of *Pseudomonas aeruginosa* to beyond 12 months (4/16, 25% vs. 7/11, 64%, $p = 0.06$).[115] A review of 85 infants with CF and meconium ileus revealed that 31 (37%) had a negative outcome at 12 months, 22 with stunted growth and 9 with chronic *Pseudomonas* infection.[116] Logistic regression showed that the probability of having a negative outcome was decreased if the infant did not have cholestasis (OR 0.125) or did not need intensive care unit (ICU) care (OR 0.141) and increased by not having been breastfed (OR 2.921). The European Society for Clinical Nutrition and Metabolism (ESPEN); the European Society for Paediatric Gastroenterology, Hepatology and Nutrition (ESPGHAN); and the European Society for Cystic Fibrosis (ECFS) have recommended exclusive breastfeeding for infants with CF.[117]

A recent study evaluated a quality improvement project to improve breastfeeding in CF by incorporating international board-certified lactation consultants (IBCLCs) into the initial CF diagnosis visit to support mothers who were breastfeeding at diagnosis.[118] In the preintervention group, only 8/14 (57%) continued to provide breast milk after the first visit, whereas postintervention, 16/17 (94%) mothers continued to do so ($p = 0.03$). The duration of breastfeeding increased to an average of 7.7 months from an average of 6.4 months preintervention ($p = 0.45$). The authors concluded that lactation support to mothers can prolong the duration of breastfeeding in infants with CF.

Alpha₁-Antitrypsin Deficiency

Alpha₁-antitrypsin is a serum protease inhibitor that inactivates a number of proteases. More than 24 genetic variants of this disease are designated B through Z, with the M variant being most common. Children with α_1-antitrypsin deficiency are at increased risk for liver disease, which occurs most often during infancy and often progresses to cirrhosis and death. Udall et al. investigated the relationship between early feedings and the onset of liver disease. Severe liver disease was present in eight (40%) of the formula-fed and one (8%) of the breastfed infants (breastfed for only 5 weeks).[119] Of the 32 infants, 24 were still alive at the end of the study; 12 had been breastfed and 12 formula-fed during their first month of life. All eight of the deceased children had been formula-fed; small-for-gestational-age (SGA) and preterm infants had been excluded from the study so that all infants were equally stable at birth and capable of breastfeeding. A formula-fed infant was seven times more likely to develop liver disease.

With the increasing early diagnosis of α_1-antitrypsin deficiency, encouraging a mother to breastfeed if her infant is affected would appear to have a significant impact on reducing the chance of long-range liver disease in her infant.

Acrodermatitis Enteropathica (Danbolt–Closs Syndrome)

Acrodermatitis enteropathica is a rare and unique disease in which feeding an infant with human milk may be lifesaving. Its onset is as early as 3 weeks.[120] It is inherited as an autosomal-recessive trait and is characterized by a symmetric rash around the mouth, genitalia, and periphery of the extremities. The rash is an acute vesicobullous and eczematous eruption, often secondarily infected with *C. albicans*. It may be seen by the third week of life or not until late in infancy and has been associated with weaning from the breast. Failure to thrive; hair loss; irritability, and chronic, severe, intractable diarrhea are often life threatening. The disease has been associated with extremely low plasma zinc levels. Oral zinc sulfate has produced remission of the syndrome. Zinc deficiency was seen frequently in premature infants on peripheral alimentation until zinc was added to the solution.

Human milk contains less zinc than does bovine milk, with zinc concentrations of both decreasing throughout lactation. Eckert et al. studied the zinc binding in human and cow's milk and noted that the low-molecular-weight binding ligand isolated from human milk may enhance absorption of zinc in these patients.[121] Gel chromatography indicated that most of the zinc in cow's milk was associated with high-molecular-weight fractions, whereas zinc in human milk was associated with low-molecular-weight fractions. The copper—zinc ratio may also be of significance because the ratio is lower in cow's milk. Pabon and Lönnerdal demonstrated in vivo zinc absorption in suckling rat pups dosed with 65Zn-labeled infant diets; the rats were killed, and individual tissues were gamma counted.[122] Lower zinc bioavailability was evident for bovine milk at pH = 4.0 (%65Zn in liver = 18.7 ± 1.4) when compared with whey-predominant infant formula (WPF; 22.8 ± 1.6) or human milk (26.9 ± 0.8). Lowering the pH further decreased zinc bioavailability from human milk, but not from cow's milk or WPF.

The zinc-binding ligand from human milk was further identified as prostaglandin E by chromatography, ultrafiltration, and infrared spectroscopy by Evans and Johnson.[123] Patients also have low arachidonic acid levels. Arachidonic acid is a precursor of prostaglandin. The efficacy of human milk in the treatment of acrodermatitis enteropathica results from the presence of the zinc—prostaglandin complex. The primary deficiency in an infant is an inability to absorb zinc except in this complex form.

The clinical significance of the relationship of human milk to the onset of the disease and its treatment is in successfully developing lactation in the mother of such an infant, rare as the disease may be. Delayed lactation or relactation is possible and should be offered as an option to the mother of such an infant (see Chapter 19).

Several reports of isolated cases of zinc deficiency during breastfeeding have appeared in the literature.[124,125] More recent cases have described zinc deficiency in infants as a result of low concentrations in human milk.[126] In some cases, zinc levels in the milk were low; in others, they were not measured.[127] There are genetic mutations identified as causing an insufficiency of zinc transporter proteins, leading to a deficiency of zinc in human milk.[128] Other authors have described the regulation of iron, zinc, and copper in breast milk and the transport of these minerals across the mammary gland epithelium as poorly understood. Milk values at 9 months postpartum were not associated with maternal mineral status.[129] This suggested an active transport mechanism, according to these investigators.[129] One child had a classic "zinc-deficient" rash that responded to oral zinc therapy. In summary, the three most likely issues related to zinc deficiency in infants are insufficient zinc in their diet, malabsorption of zinc from the GI tract, or defective zinc transportation into milk. In the majority of cases, supplementing the infant with zinc should overcome the deficiency.

The treatment of choice is oral administration of zinc at a dose of 3 mg/kg of elemental zinc.[130] It is usually well tolerated,

safe, inexpensive, effective, and expedient. When zinc deficiency occurs in a breastfed infant, the possibility of zinc deficiency in the milk, although a rare disorder, should be considered.[120] Treating the mother would be the appropriate therapy in such a case.

Premature infants have a negative zinc balance associated with inadequate mineral stores and high requirements associated with rapid growth.[131] Transient zinc deficiency in breastfed infants has been described as manifest by the classic zinc-deficiency rash and was treated by oral zinc to the infant because milk levels are normal in the mother.

NEUROLOGICALLY IMPAIRED INFANTS

In addition to infants who have been neurologically impaired by perinatal hypoxia or asphyxia as demonstrated by low Apgar scores, a rare infant may have an inherited neurologic problem as in a trisomy or a congenital abnormality, such as spina bifida. These infants can be breastfed in most situations, but it requires patience and perseverance. Holding the infant in a flexed position is an essential element of breastfeeding. A sling can work well if muscle tone and posture are part of an infant's difficulties.

Down Syndrome

Down syndrome is one of the more common syndromes, occurring in 1 of 800 to 1000 births. Children with Down syndrome have characteristic phenotypic features and increased risk of congenital diseases and malformations, which may interfere with breastfeeding. These include hypotonia, suction-swallowing disorders, congenital heart disease, macroglossia, gastrointestinal malformations, hypothyroidism, and intrauterine growth restriction or low birth weight. Neonatal illness is common among newborns with Down syndrome, leading to hospital admissions, medical interventions, mother—infant separation, and formula supplementation, all of which limit breastfeeding success. In addition, maternal feelings at the birth of a disabled child, such as stress, frustration, and depression, may also have a negative influence on breastfeeding. However, breastfeeding is important for these infants because of their increased risk of morbidities associated with artificial feeding, such as ear, respiratory, and other infections; malocclusion; and developmental delay.

More than 90% of infants with Down syndrome have hypotonia. Hypotonia is a major feature that, along with a small mouth and a large tongue, makes breastfeeding a challenge. Breastfeeding is challenging, but many can successfully breastfeed at the breast. Sucking behavior with trisomy 21 is less efficient than in normal term infants, with multiple parameters affected, including the pressure, frequency, and duration of sucking and smooth peristaltic tongue movement. Mizuno and Ueda from Japan studied the sucking behavior of 14 infants with Down syndrome at 1, 4, 8, and 12 months of age.[132] Sucking pressure increased significantly from 1 to 4 months and again at 8 and 12 months. Sucking frequency increased from 1 to 4 months; however, sucking duration showed no improvement over time. Sucking efficiency demonstrated a significant stepwise increment throughout the first year. Ultrasound analysis revealed abnormal peristaltic tongue movements at 1 month. Normally, the tongue initially sticks to the palate, shortly after which the posterior portion of the tongue moves downward, releasing the palate. In infants with Down syndrome, the tongue often remains stuck to the palate more than once during the suck cycle. Of note, the mothers reported that feeding difficulties had decreased after 3 or 4 months of age, which is the time when the sucking pressure and frequency had significantly improved. Understanding this time frame allows health professionals to support breastfeeding and assist in maintaining a sufficient milk supply, despite significant difficulties at the beginning.

Breastfeeding is challenging, but many can successfully breastfeed at the breast. There is no evidence that infants with trisomy 21 or other hypotonic infants feed better with the bottle than at the breast and no evidence that these children need to feed from a bottle before attempting to breastfeed. A team of professionals with expertise in assisting infants with special needs to breastfeed should work together to help the mother–infant dyad. The importance of health professionals is highlighted in studies that found that mothers of these children felt they were not given appropriate support for breastfeeding. Instead, they expressed that "health professionals did not encourage breastfeeding and did not pass accurate information, confusing mothers about practices they should have, leaving doubts, discomfort, and a demotivating environment."[133]

In a study of 59 breastfed infants with Down syndrome, Aumonier and Cunningham reported that 31 had no sucking difficulty, 12 were successfully nursing within a week, and 16 required tube feeding initially, which was associated with other medical problems, including low birth weight (LBW), cardiac lesions, and jaundice.[134] Hyperbilirubinemia is common in trisomy and was seen in 49% of the infants in this study. Eighteen babies had multiple medical conditions, and 11 of them sucked poorly. The authors point out that the initial sucking ability of the infants did not appear to be a major cause for nonmaintenance of breastfeeding; 10 of the 13 mothers who discontinued breastfeeding cited insufficient milk as a contributing cause, which might have been prevented by early pumping of the breasts between feedings.[134]

Another review of 73 cases of Down syndrome in Chile revealed that 47% (34/73) of the mothers exclusively breastfed for 6 months, despite the fact that 67% (49/73) of the infants had a disease or malformation that interfered with breastfeeding.[135] Seventy of 73 infants (96%) breastfed (exclusively or not) for at least 1 month, and 71% (52) breastfed for 6 months or more. Among the 39 mothers who did not exclusively breastfeed for 6 months, 25 (64.1%) reported child factors, most commonly poor weight gain and suck-swallow disorder, as reasons for discontinuing. Multivariate analysis revealed that hospitalization during the first 6 months was the most significant factor affecting the cessation of breastfeeding (OR 6.13, 95% CI 1.48 to 25.40). However, other studies show much lower breastfeeding rates, such as a 68% rate of any breastfeeding at birth (compared with a 95% rate in the general population) in a study in Croatia.[136]

To breastfeed successfully, families need to understand that breastfeeding can occur even if the child presents difficulties and has some limitations. Had these mothers received adequate breastfeeding support, they would likely have felt empowered rather than frustrated.

At first, the infant may quickly drift off to sleep at the breast, and weight gain is slow. The mother learns to hold her breast in place because the infant's grasp is not strong enough to overcome gravity. A sling or pillow works to support the infant and free up the mother's hands for additional support. The mother can hold the infant in place and free both the mother's hands to hold both the breast and infant's jaw. This position is referred to as the Dancer hand position or Dancer hold specifically because of the position of the hand which can be helpful for the hypotonic infant in that it supports both the breast and the infant's chin and jaw while the infant is breastfeeding. (For a picture of the Dancer hold, see Fig. 13.1.) The mother supports her breast with the thumb on top and three fingers underneath, while the index finger and thumb form a "U," with the baby's chin resting on the bottom of the "U." This keeps the weight of the breast off the baby's chin and helps him hold his head steady while nursing. Some mothers facilitate milk transfer by using hand compression in conjunction with breastfeeding, and more time may be necessary in the early weeks to complete a feeding. When the suckling is weak initially, the mother should pump between feedings to stimulate the production of milk. If supplements are required, it is best to provide them with a cup or supplemental nursing system. However, the use of a nursing supplementation aid alone may not be as helpful because it works best with an infant who has an effective latch.

Infants with Down syndrome or other genetic trisomies may be difficult to feed because of a variety of contributing factors, such as hypotonia and difficulty with position and/or latch, inadequate sucking force, difficulty with coordinating suck/swallow/breathe, the infant becoming easily fatigued and not completing a feeding session, and so forth. Careful early instruction and hands-on guidance are important, along with ongoing support and instruction to identify challenges or difficulties (see Figs. 13.1 and 13.2).

The initial goals for the mother–infant pair are developing confidence in handling the infant, adjusting to the infant's problem, and dealing with the parental grief and sense of loss—loss of the normal infant who was expected. If the mother has breastfed other children, the emphasis on breastfeeding modifications is more successful, and milk supply usually responds to manual expression and pumping. Initiating sufficient stimulus to the breast to increase milk production is critical in the first few days to induce good prolactin response, especially in primiparas. Renting a hospital-grade breast pump is a good investment, justifiable for reimbursement from health insurance by physician prescription.

With prenatal ultrasound, amniocentesis, and genetic testing or screening in older mothers, the diagnosis is often known before birth so that the family can be prepared. In developing a discharge plan for an infant with Down syndrome, a pediatrician will need to coordinate a team to avoid the fragmented care that develops with a multiple-problem situation, which may require the consultation of a geneticist, genetic counselor, cardiologist, and other medical experts to deal with the infant's problems. Ideally, a pediatrician, family practitioner, or nurse practitioner can provide the additional support and counsel necessary.

The birth of an infant with a major genetic abnormality is a shock, even to the strongest parents. If the mother wants to breastfeed, she should be offered all the encouragement and support necessary. Usually she needs to talk with someone to express her anguish about the infant, not the feeding per se. A sympathetic nurse practitioner or lactation consultant in the pediatric office can be invaluable in providing support and expertise to help with the various management problems. If the mother chooses not to breastfeed, appropriate support can also be provided without disrupting treatment continuity.

It is especially important that these infants be breastfed if possible because they are particularly prone to infection, especially otitis media. Before the advent of antibiotics, they often died of overwhelming infection and rarely survived past 20 years of age. These infants and most other infants with developmental disorders do better with stimulation and affection, so the body contact and communication while at the breast are especially important. Those who have associated cardiac lesions not only can suckle, swallow, and breathe with less effort at the breast but also can receive a fluid more physiologic for their needs. Breastfed or bottle-fed, these infants gain poorly; thus switching to a bottle does not solve the problem. The recommendation that children with Down syndrome receive extra vitamins was tested in a controlled study in children 5 to 13 years of age, and no sustained improvement in the children's appearance, growth, behavior, or development was seen with added vitamins.[137]

Growth charts from birth to 18 years illustrate the deficient growth through the growing periods. In infancy they fall behind, so this observation should not be used to discontinue breastfeeding. Breastfed infants remain healthier. Revised growth charts for infants and children with Down syndrome have been published because these children grow differently, but their growth has improved compared with previous studies.[138] Of note, the growth charts reflect the characteristic short stature, small head circumference, and normal to high relative weight measures (weight for length and body mass index [BMI]) associated with this genetic syndrome. The charts are also published on the Centers for Disease Control and Prevention (CDC) website.[139]

Down syndrome is a lifelong condition. Having a support system is important for a family. Support groups of other families in the community serve as vital peer support.

ENDOCRINE DISEASES

Hypothyroidism

Bode et al. reported that an infant with congenital cretinism was spared the severe effects of the disease because he was breastfed.[140] This was attributed to significant quantities of thyroid hormone in the milk. In a prospective study of 12 cases of hypothyroidism in breastfed infants, however, no protective effect against the disease was found, nor was the onset of the disease delayed. Anthropometric measurements, biochemical values, and psychologic testing at 1 year of age did not differ from those in the 33 bottle-fed hypothyroid infants.[141] Abbassi and Steinour also reported the diagnosis of congenital hypothyroidism in the neonatal period in four breastfed neonates.[142]

Sack et al. measured thyroxine (T_4) concentrations in human milk and found it to be present in significant amounts.[143] Varma et al. studied T_4, triiodothyronine (T_3), and reverse T_3 concentrations in human milk in 77 healthy euthyroid mothers from the day of delivery to 148 days postpartum.[144] From their data, they calculated that if infants received 900 to 1200 mL of milk per day, they would receive 2.1 to 2.6 mg of T_4 per day, based on 238.1 ng/dL of milk after the first week. This amount of T_4 is much less than the recommended dose for the treatment of hypothyroidism (18.8 to 25 mg/day of levo-T_3). T_4 was essentially immeasurable in the milk sampled. In another study, however, comparing 22 breastfed and 25 formula-fed infants who were 2 to 3 weeks old, the levels of T_3 and T_4 were significantly higher in the breastfed infants.[145] No definite relationship between the levels of T_3 and reverse T_3 could be found.

A 6-week-old girl was diagnosed to have congenital hypothyroidism by routine neonatal screening when T_4 was reported at 3 mg/dL (normal is greater than 7 mg/dL).[146] The mother gave a history of multiple applications of povidone-iodine during pregnancy and continuing during lactation. Further testing revealed thyroid-stimulating hormone levels of 0.9 mU/mL (normal 0.8 to 5 μ/mL). Iodine treatment was stopped, and breastfeeding continued while treatment of thyroid replacement was begun. At 1 year, growth and development were normal. It is, therefore, suggested that neonatal screening for thyroid disease may be even more urgent if the clinical symptoms are apt to be masked in a breastfed infant. No contraindication exists to breastfeeding when the infant is hypothyroid, and it would be beneficial.[147] Appropriate therapy should also be instituted promptly. Mandatory screening for hypothyroidism is available to newborns in developed countries. Many infants that screen positive do not have the characteristic signs and symptoms associated with cretinism at birth, but therapy is just as urgent.

Adrenal Hyperplasia

In an analysis of 32 infants with salt-losing congenital adrenal hyperplasia who were in adrenal crisis, 8 had been breastfed, 5 had been breastfed with formula supplements, and 19 had been formula-fed.[148] Infants who were breastfed were admitted to the hospital later than the formula-fed infants, although the breastfed infants had lower serum sodium levels on admission. The breastfed infants did not vomit and remained stable longer, although they had severe failure to thrive.[148] Weaning initiated vomiting and precipitated crises in the breastfed infants. The authors suggest that congenital adrenal hyperplasia should be considered in a breastfed infant with failure to thrive. Electrolytes should be obtained before weaning to make the diagnosis and avoid precipitating a crisis by weaning. Then breastfeeding can continue as treatment is initiated.

Hypernatremic Dehydration Associated With Breastfeeding

The consequences of inadequate intake of breast milk range from hyperbilirubinemia, infant hunger, and low weight gain to life-threatening dehydration and starvation. Neonatal hypernatremic dehydration is a potentially serious condition that can occur in healthy newborns, mainly in association with feeding problems, especially with breastfeeding. It is defined as serum sodium concentrations equal to or greater than 145 mEq/L. It is considered mild when plasma sodium is between 145 and 149 mEq/L and moderate between 150 and 160 mEq/L. Severe forms have been associated with short-, medium-, and long-term complications, especially neurologic problems such as seizures, cerebral edema, or intracranial hemorrhage. It is a rare condition, with an estimated incidence of 20 to 70 per 100,000 births and up to 223 per 100,000 births among primiparous mothers.[149] There has been an apparent increase in the number of reported cases of hypernatremic dehydration in breastfeeding infants. Term breastfed infants with serum sodium levels of 150 mEq/L or higher were found to be 4.1% or 169 of the 4136 term infants hospitalized and reviewed by Unal et al. in the Children's Research Hospital in Ankara, Turkey.[150] These children had lost 15.9% birth weight (range 5.4% to 32.7%). The presenting symptom in 47.3% of cases was hyperbilirubinemia and poor suck in 29.6%. Other complications included acute renal failure in 82.8%, elevated liver enzymes in 20.7%, disseminated intracranial hemorrhage in 3.6%, and thromboses in 1.8%. Ten patients developed seizures, and two died. In another study, 60 term infants less than 28 days old were readmitted to the hospital with dehydration with plasma serum sodium levels greater than 145 mmol/L.[151] The hospital had recently upgraded its newborn discharge policy to include weights by trained midwives at 72 to 96 hours and at 7 to 10 days of age. Voiding, stooling, and breastfeeding were also checked, and infants who lost more than 10% of birth weight were sent to the hospital. The incidence of hypernatremia with plasma serum sodium levels greater than 145 mmol/L was 7.4 and 5.0 per 10,000 live births before and after the new policy, respectively, and the percentages of cases with plasma serum sodium levels greater than 150 mmol/L was 56.5% (before) versus 18.9% (after). It was concluded that weighing and lactation support resulted in less dehydration and less severe hypernatremia and better breastfeeding rates.[151]

Although various factors have been associated with hypernatremic dehydration in neonates as a result of inadequate breastfeeding, the exact pathophysiologic processes leading to its development are not well defined. Insufficient breast-milk intake, infant weight loss, dehydration, free water loss, altered urine output, and ongoing sodium intake are all possible contributing factors.[152] In a systematic review of hypernatremia among breastfeeding infants, significant risk factors included weight loss greater than 10%, cesarean delivery, primiparity, breast anomalies, reported breastfeeding problems, excessive prepregnancy maternal weight, delayed first breastfeeding, lack of previous breastfeeding experience, and low maternal education.[153] To prevent hypernatremia, they recommended daily weights with lactation support during the first 4 to 5 days. Unver Korgali et al. discuss the association of weight loss (percentage loss from birth weight) with sodium value in the dehydrated infants from various reports but only highlight the differing amounts of weight loss implicated in different reports.[154]

A study from Italy prospectively reviewed 53 exclusively breastfed infants admitted to the NICU with a weight loss of ≥ 10% of birth weight.[155] Of these infants, 19 (36%) presented with a serum sodium concentration exceeding 149 mEq/L (range 150 to 160 mEq/L), 42 (79%) had a urea nitrogen greater than 20 mg/dL (range 21 to 56 mg/dL), and 34 (64%) had a metabolic acidosis (range of base excess −5 to −14). The breastfeeding test and volume determination of residual breast milk demonstrated that in 14 (26%), the dehydration was caused by inadequate maternal milk, and in 39 (74%), it was caused by inefficient milk removal because of poor breastfeeding technique. In these 39 neonates, assistance with breastfeeding corrected the problem. In the 14 neonates with inadequate maternal milk supply (3 delivered vaginally and 11 by cesarean section), formula was given. In all neonates, rehydration and increased caloric intake normalized the serum sodium concentration, urea nitrogen, and base excess, and the weight increased.[155]

A study from Turkey reviewed 21 infants admitted to the NICU for hypernatremic dehydration. Infants were monitored by amplitude-integrated electroencephalography (aEEG) and received a neurodevelopmental evaluation at 2 years of age.[156] A statistically significant correlation was found between aEEG abnormalities and serum sodium levels at the time of admission ($p = 0.007$). Neurodevelopmental assessment at a median age of 15 months (9 to 23 months) was available for 17 of the 21 infants. No infant was diagnosed as impaired, and there was no correlation between serum sodium levels on admission and median motor development index (MDI)/psychomotor development index (PDI) scores ($p = 0.286$, $p = 0.904$). The results revealed that hypernatremic dehydration did not adversely affect the long-term outcomes. In a study from Iran, Boskabadi et al. compared the long-term neurodevelopment of 65 healthy breastfed neonates with serum sodium levels <150 mmol/L and 65 breastfed hypernatremic infants with serum sodium levels ≥150 mmol/L (neonatal hypernatremic dehydration [NHD]).[157] The median serum sodium peak value was 158 ± 16 in the cases and 141 ± 9 mmol/L in the control group. Based on Denver II developmental assessment scores, 25% of the infants with NHD had developmental delay at 6 months, 21% at 12 months, 19% at 18 months, and 12% at 24 months, compared with 0.3% in the control group. They found a correlation of poor developmental outcome at 6 months with the degree of hypernatremia ($p = 0.001$).

Early infant weight loss should be evaluated in the context of the clinical status of the infant. Nomograms for newborn weight have been developed using data from more than 160,000 healthy infants from Kaiser Permanente Hospitals in California.[158] Using these nomograms, individual infant weights can be plotted by hours since birth, mode of delivery, and infant feeding type with the use of the Newborn Early Weight Tool (NEWT; https://www.newbornweight.org). Weight loss >75th percentile on NEWT nomograms should prompt a thorough evaluation.[158] Studies have shown that the use of charts for weight loss with standard deviation scores specifically to detect hypernatremic dehydration on days 2, 4, and 7 of life had high sensitivity (97%) and specificity (98.5%).[149,158,159] However, given that the prevalence of NHD is not known in different locations/populations and the fact that we do not know if screening by weight loss to detect hypernatremia will lead to improved outcomes, simply utilizing the degree of weight loss to detect NHD is not yet the evidence-based solution. If the goals are to improve breastfeeding outcomes for healthy infants and detect lactation failure that leads to NHD, then careful serial assessment of breastfeeding (weight loss/gain, latch, milk transfer, number of daily infant voids and stools, breast fullness and let-down, maternal well-being, etc.) with appropriate intervention(s) and support to create breastfeeding success should be the focus.

It is recommended that these dyads be seen by a clinician within 2 days of hospital discharge. Ongoing weight loss should prompt additional assessment, intervention, and close follow-up. Treatment of NHD includes rehydration of the infant, with careful attention to the rate of decline in serum sodium level and skilled, intense establishment of a full milk supply. Follow-up with proper medical care for the infant and the mother—infant dyad by a lactation specialist is essential.

Neonatal Breast Conditions
Neonatal Breasts and Nipple Discharge

A newborn may have swelling of the breasts for the first few days of life, whether male or female; this is unrelated to being breastfed. It is a normal response to falling levels of maternal estrogen at the end of pregnancy, which trigger the release of prolactin from the newborn's pituitary. It is seen in approximately 70% of males and 85% of female neonates.[160] The breast enlargement may considerably vary in size, but the palpable breast tissue usually measures <1.5 cm. If the infant's breast is squeezed, milk can be obtained. This has been called *witch's milk*. These two physiologic phenomena of breast enlargement and milk secretion are usually self-limited but may persist till 2 to 3 months of age.

The constituents of neonatal milk were studied in the milk of 18 normal newborns and infants with sepsis, adrenal hyperplasia, CF, and meconium ileus.[161] Electrolyte values were similar to those in adult women in all infants except one with mastitis, in whom the sodium level was elevated and the potassium decreased. Total protein and lactose were also similar to those in adult women. The fat was different, increasing with postnatal age and being higher in short-chain fatty acids. It was indeed true milk.

The cultural practice of massage of the newborn baby's breasts to express milk is centuries old and persists in some countries. Squeezing the breast to facilitate the discharge may lead to irritation, further enlargement, the persistence of the hypertrophied tissue, or in rare cases, infection (mastitis or abscess). A retrospective analysis of 20 infants (14 girls) with gynecomastia secondary to cultural massage was performed at a tertiary care pediatric hospital in Northwest India.[162] The mean age at presentation was 8 ± 9 months (range 0.25 to 27 months), the average duration of breast manipulation was 39 ± 67 days (range 3 to 270 days), and the mean age at complete resolution was 17 ± 9 months (range 4 to 36 months). The mean palpable breast tissue was 4.4 ± 0.4 cm (range 4 to 6 cm). Galactorrhea was present in 15 (75%) patients. A review of 32 infants with neonatal mastitis in Kashmir, India, revealed that 15 (47%) were secondary to cultural massage.[163]

Bloody discharge from the neonatal breast is extremely rare. Known etiologies are mammary duct ectasia, intraductal papilloma, intraductal cysts, mammary ductal hyperplasia, and gynecomastia, with mammary duct ectasia being the most common. Ultrasound is used to make the diagnosis.[164] Galactorrhea or persistent neonatal milk related to increased prolactin levels has been reported with hyperthyroidism and rarely with neonatal hyperthyroidism.[165] Hyperprolactinemia is more frequent in hyperthyroid females. The serum prolactin level can be increased in hyperthyroidism. In another report, a 21-day-old female infant was seen because of a goiter and galactorrhea.[147] The infant had 50% 24-hour I uptake and elevated prolactin levels, which slowly responded to Lugol solution treatment for hyperthyroidism.

Neonatal Mastitis

Neonatal mastitis occurs infrequently, although it was a common event in the 1940s and 1950s, when staphylococcal disease was rampant in nurseries. A review of 32 infants with neonatal mastitis revealed an age range of 1 to 7 weeks, with a peak incidence for mastitis in the 2nd week and for abscess in the 4th week.[163] The ratio of male:female was 1:2 in the entire group, but there was a greater preponderance of female involvement with increasing age. The babies were generally well, and associated skin pustulosis was common. Cultures revealed *S. aureus* in 18 patients, *E. coli* in 2, and *Klebsiella* in 1 and were sterile in 2 patients. Most strains of *S. aureus* were methicillin sensitive (MSSA; 15), and 3 were resistant but were sensitive to amikacin, ofloxacin, and vancomycin. Treatment with oral antibiotics was not successful. Patients responded well to open drainage via a stab incision, keeping it away from the breast mound. IV antibiotics were prescribed in all patients for 2 to 5 days, followed by oral continuation therapy of 7 to 14 days. The prognosis for cure was excellent. Forty-seven percent were secondary to manipulation of the neonatal breast to express the milk.[163]

HYPERBILIRUBINEMIA AND JAUNDICE

Jaundice in newborns has become a source of considerable misinformation, confusion, and anxiety. From 1994 to 1996, 11.9% of newborns were hospitalized for hyperbilirubinemia; rates rose to 20.0% in 2003 to 2005. The incidence of kernicterus dropped from 5.8 per 100,000 live births in 1988 to 1990 to 1.6 per 100,000 live births in 2003 to 2004 as a result of aggressive preventive measures in these years, according to Burke et al.[166] Current management has further decreased severe pathologic hyperbilirubinemia, defined as total bilirubin of 25.0 to 29.9 mg/dL, from 43 per 100,000 in 2004 to 27 per 100,000 in 2008.[167]

A recent review has highlighted that the burden of severe neonatal jaundice is not evenly distributed and that a heavier burden of disease is born by low-income and middle-income countries.[168] The African region has the highest incidence of severe jaundice per 10,000 live births at 668, followed by Southeast Asia at 251, Eastern Mediterranean at 166, Western Pacific at 9.4, Americas at 4.4, and European regions at 3.7. A meta-analysis concluded that failure to prevent Rh sensitization and manage neonatal hyperbilirubinemia results in over 114,000 avoidable neonatal deaths and 75,000 avoidable cases of kernicterus, mostly in sub-Saharan Africa and South Asia, every year.[169]

More physicians are paying attention to the development of hyperbilirubinemia in newborns. These two factors serve to increase the question of the role of breastfeeding in the development of hyperbilirubinemia. Some of the confusion and inconsistencies associated with the management can be attributed to indecisive terminology. This discussion attempts to clarify the issues and outlines the causes and effects of hyperbilirubinemia.

Why the Concern About Jaundice?

Bilirubin is a cell toxin, as can be demonstrated dramatically by adding a little bilirubin to a tissue culture, which will be quickly destroyed. Excessive bilirubin causes concern because when free, unbound, unconjugated bilirubin is in the system, it can be deposited in various tissues, ultimately causing necrosis of the cells. The brain and brain cells, if destroyed by bilirubin deposits, do not regenerate.[170] The full-blown end result is bilirubin encephalopathy, or kernicterus, which is essentially a pathologic diagnosis that depends on identifying the yellow pigmentation and necrosis in the brain, especially in the basal ganglion, hippocampal cortex, and subthalamic nuclei. At autopsy, 50% of infants with kernicterus also have other lesions caused by bilirubin toxicity. Necrosis of renal tubular cells, intestinal mucosa, or pancreatic cells or associated GI hemorrhage may be seen.

The classic clinical manifestations of bilirubin encephalopathy are characterized by progressive lethargy, rigidity, opisthotonos, high-pitched cry, fever, and convulsions. The mortality rate is 50%. Survivors usually have choreoathetoid cerebral palsy, asymmetric spasticity, paresis of upward gaze, high-frequency deafness, and mental retardation.[171] Premature infants are particularly susceptible to bilirubin-related brain damage and may have kernicterus at autopsy without the typical clinical syndrome. A significant correlation exists between the level of bilirubin and hearing impairment in newborns when other risk factors are present. Classic full-blown kernicterus rarely occurs today, but mild effects on the brain may be manifested clinically in later life in the form of lack of coordination, hypertonicity,

and mental retardation or learning disabilities, symptoms sometimes collectively called *minimal brain damage*.[170] *Bilirubin encephalopathy* is the appropriate term for conditions in which bilirubin is thought to be the cause of brain toxicity.

Recent studies suggest that in the absence of significant comorbidities such as sepsis or Rh hemolytic disease, kernicterus or chronic bilirubin encephalopathy occurs in about 1 in 200,000 live births and only when total serum bilirubin (TSB) levels exceeded 35 mg/dL.[172] As noted earlier, in lower-resource countries, bilirubin encephalopathy and comorbidities are much more common, so kernicterus can and does occur more frequently.[168,169] However, even in high-resource countries, extreme hyperbilirubinemia in apparently healthy infants can cause kernicterus. The US Kernicterus Registry, a database of 125 cases of kernicterus in infants discharged as healthy newborns, reported that a range of bilirubin levels, rather than a specific level, was identified as a threshold for the onset of neurotoxicity in otherwise-healthy term infants.[173] The most frequent clinical factors were late prematurity, undiagnosed hemolytic disease, and genetic abnormalities (such as glucose 6-phosphate dehydrogenase deficiency, congenital spherocytosis, galactosemia, Crigler—Najjar syndrome, and others that were not diagnosed) and concurrent complications of dehydration, sepsis, acidosis, hypoalbuminemia or poor feeding. Case reports of kernicterus were rarely identified in healthy infants when bilirubin levels were <25 mg/dL, and none are reported for bilirubin <20 mg/dL. However, all infants who presented with bilirubin levels >35 mg/dL sustained some degree of chronic sequelae. Vulnerability to chronic sequelae in infants with bilirubin levels between 20 and 35 mg/dL was influenced by postnatal age, rate of bilirubin rise, duration of extreme hyperbilirubinemia, late prematurity (≤37 weeks), gender (male), large for gestational age, dehydration (>15% weight loss over birth weight) and infection that was often associated with genetic abnormalities.[173]

In the US Kernicterus Registry, 98% of 125 infants with kernicterus from 1992 to 2004 were while fully or partially breastfed.[174] Lactation failure was identified in over 90% of infants discharged on exclusive breastfeeding, and there was uniformly suboptimal lactation support, both at the birthing hospital and at follow-up, with a high incidence of excessive weight loss and dehydration. A recent report on 408 infants with extreme neonatal hyperbilirubinemia (bilirubin >450 μmol/L or 26 mg/dL) or kernicterus spectrum disorder in Denmark from 2000 to 2015 revealed that 90% of the infants were exclusively breastfed.[175] These reports highlight that kernicterus has not been eliminated and that appropriate breastfeeding support needs to be part of any prevention initiative.

Mechanism of Bilirubin Production in the Neonate

A normal full-term infant has a hematocrit in utero of 50% to 65%. Because of the low oxygen tension delivered to the fetus via the placenta, the fetus requires more hemoglobin (Hb) to carry the oxygen. As soon as an infant is born and begins to breathe room air, the need is gone. The infant bone marrow does not make more cells, and excess cells are destroyed and not replaced. The life span of a fetal red blood cell (RBC) is 70 to 90 days instead of an adult's 120 days. Normally, when RBCs are destroyed, the released Hb is broken down to heme in the reticuloendothelial system. The reticuloendothelial system cells contain a microsomal enzyme, heme oxygenase, that is capable of oxidizing the α-methene bridge carbon of the heme molecule after the loss of the iron and the globin to form biliverdin, a green pigment. Biliverdin is water soluble and is rapidly degraded to bilirubin. A gram of hemoglobulin will produce 34 mg of bilirubin.

The reticuloendothelial cell releases the bilirubin into the circulation, where it is rapidly bound to albumin. Indirect bilirubin is essentially insoluble (less than 0.01 mg% soluble) and is a yellow pigment. Adult albumin can bind two molecules of bilirubin, the first more tightly than the second. Newborn albumin has reduced molar binding capacities that vary with maturity and other factors, such as pH, infection, and hypoglycemia.

Unconjugated bilirubin is removed from the circulation by the hepatocyte, which converts it, by conjugation of each molecule of bilirubin with two molecules of glucuronic acid, into direct bilirubin. Direct bilirubin is water soluble and is excreted via the bile to the stools. The balance between hepatic-cell uptake of bilirubin and the rate of bilirubin production determines the serum unconjugated bilirubin concentration. Laboratory measurements include both bound and unbound indirect bilirubin. The amount of unconjugated bilirubin that exceeds the binding capacity of an infant's albumin is the unbound unconjugated bilirubin available to deposit in the brain.

Evaluation and Management

Normal full-term newborns have serial bilirubin tests to determine the range of values. The cord bilirubin level may be as high as 2 mg% and rise in the first 72 hours to 5 to 6 mg%, which is barely in the visible range, and gradually taper off, assuming normal adult levels of 1 mg% after 10 days. Less than 50% of normal infants are visibly jaundiced in the first week of life. This would suggest that visible jaundice is idiopathic, not physiologic. The level of bilirubin that is acceptable depends on a number of factors. In some premature infants, even bilirubin levels under 10 mg/dL may be of concern because of the limited albumin-binding sites in premature infants.

Factors that Influence Significance

For a given level of bilirubin, several associated factors may need to be considered. If an infant has acidosis, anoxia, asphyxia, hypothermia, hypoglycemia, or infection, even lower levels of bilirubin may have significant risk for causing deposition of bilirubin in the brain cells. The most important factor is prematurity, which affects liver and brain metabolism and albumin-binding sites. An increased incidence of elevated bilirubin levels occurs in certain races and populations. Asian populations, including Chinese, Japanese, and Korean populations, and

Native Americans may have bilirubin levels averaging 10 to 14 mg%. A higher incidence of autopsy-identified kernicterus also is seen in these populations. Glucose-6-phosphate dehydrogenase deficiency, a genetic disorder, is also common in these groups. Infants who carry the 211 and 388 variants, respectively, in the *UGT1A1* and *OATP2* genes and are breastfed were found to be at high risk of developing severe hyperbilirubinemia, according to Huang et al.,[176] who investigated infants born in Cathay Hospital in Taipei, Taiwan, where glucose-6-phosphate dehydrogenase is prevalent. They also noted that glucose-6-phosphate dehydrogenase is the most common genetic defect and urge more frequent screening. Infants with these genetic variants who were not breastfed had hyperbilirubinemia that was less responsive to phototherapy, thus it is recommended that breastfeeding not be discontinued.[176]

Determination of Cause of Jaundice

Following the chain of events from the destruction of RBCs in newborns through the final excretion of conjugated bilirubin in the stools simplifies understanding the cause of a specific case of jaundice. Causes include (1) increased destruction of RBCs, (2) decreased conjugation in the glucuronidase system, (3) decreased albumin binding, and (4) increased reabsorption from the GI tract and decreased excretion. To be excreted from the body, unconjugated bilirubin has to be conjugated with glucuronic acid in the hepatocyte, which becomes water-soluble bilirubin glucuronide. The enzyme involved is a specific hepatic enzyme isoform (1A1) belonging to the uridine diphosphoglucuronate glucuronosyltransferase (UGT) family of enzymes. Much has been learned about these enzymes and their relationship to bilirubin metabolism.[177] UGTs catalyze the conjugation of not only bilirubin but also steroids, bile acids, drugs, and other xenobiotics. The two separate families of genes, *UGT1* and *UGT2*, have different actions. Gilbert syndrome, an uncommon genetic anemia associated with persistent hyperbilirubinemia in neonates, is associated with a mutation in the coding area of the *UGT1A1* gene. Similar genetic variations are present in Crigler–Najjar syndrome. These genetic variations or ongoing hemolysis are probable causes of persistent hyperbilirubinemia in infants older than 2 months of age.

Ethnic background, risk factors, previous infants with hyperbilirubinemia, and family history of anemia and jaundice are important to correct diagnosis and management, the preservation of breastfeeding, and the safety of the infant.

When albumin binding is altered, the visibility of the jaundice is not affected. The bilirubin level may not be very high, but the substance is not bound to albumin and is available at lower levels to pass into the brain cells.[178] Premature infants have much lower albumin levels and thus have fewer binding sites. Drugs that also bind to albumin (e.g., aspirin, sulfadiazine) compete for the same binding sites. A lower level of bilirubin puts infants who have these medications in their system at risk because the bilirubin is unbound and available to enter tissue cells, including brain cells.

Reabsorption of bilirubin from stool in the GI tract can increase the bilirubin level. This occurs when the conjugated bilirubin that was excreted into the colon and the stool is slow to pass. It is unconjugated by the action of intestinal bacteria and reabsorbed, which happens when stools are decreased or slowed in passage. Poor feedings, pyloric stenosis, and other forms of intestinal obstruction are common causes of this type of jaundice. Some bacteria are more likely than others to unconjugate conjugated bilirubin.

Sepsis, on the other hand, was not found in more than 300 infants readmitted for hyperbilirubinemia while healthy and breastfeeding. Lower total bilirubin and direct bilirubin levels greater than 2.0 mg% in a sick baby have a high correlation with sepsis.

Safe Levels of Bilirubin

Safe levels of bilirubin depend on a number of factors, including acidosis, hypoxia or anoxia, and sepsis. A handy rule of thumb is the correlation of birth weight in a premature infant and the indirect bilirubin level, using a value 2 to 3 mg lower when an infant has multiple problems. The risk for elevated bilirubin is related to the availability of albumin to bind the indirect bilirubin and prevent it from entering the brain cells. The amount of albumin is related to the degree of prematurity, and thus the rule of thumb is based on birth weight and/or gestational age. When an infant is sick, fewer albumin-binding sites are available, and the bilirubin level of concern is even lower.

Any value of 20 mg/dL or greater warrants consideration of aggressive treatment. Jaundice visible when an infant is younger than 24 hours of age is of special concern because it is usually associated with an incompatibility or infection. Rapidly rising bilirubin levels are also of concern, and a 0.5-mg/dL rise per hour is an indication for treatment.

The AAP has published a practice parameter for the management of hyperbilirubinemia in healthy term newborns.[179] Term infants who are visibly jaundiced at or before 24 hours of life are not considered healthy and require a diagnostic workup regardless of feeding method.

The AAP also addresses jaundice associated with breastfeeding in healthy term infants. The AAP discourages the interruption of breastfeeding in healthy term newborns and encourages continued and frequent breastfeeding (at least 8 to 10 times every 24 hours). Supplementing nursing with water or dextrose water does not lower the bilirubin level in jaundiced, healthy, breastfeeding infants.[179] A review of over a million infants born at 116 hospitals before and after universal predischarge bilirubin screening reported that the incidence of infants with total bilirubin levels of 25.0 to 29.9 mg/dL declined from 43 to 27 per 100,000, and the incidence of infants with bilirubin >30.0 mg/dL dropped from 9 to 3 per 100,000.[167]

Early Jaundice While Breastfeeding

Early hyperbilirubinemia while breastfeeding is usually a result of suboptimal intake, often called *breastfeeding jaundice*. It typically occurs on days 3 to 5 after birth and is frequently associated with excess weight loss. Because it is almost always associated with inadequate milk intake rather than breastfeeding per se, "suboptimal intake hyperbilirubinemia" may be a better label.[180] Low milk intake contributes to decreased stool frequency and increased enterohepatic circulation of bilirubin.[181]

Many studies of bilirubin levels in normal newborn nurseries have been conducted that look at the method of feeding.

Unfortunately, few have detailed frequency of feeds, supplementation, and stool pattern. A review summarizing results in 13 studies covering more than 20,000 infants showed a relationship between breastfeeding and jaundice. A pooled analysis of 12 studies showed 514 of 3997 breastfed infants to have TSB levels of 12 mg/dL or higher versus 172 of 4255 bottle-fed infants.[182] In a smaller group of studies, 54 of 2655 breastfed infants had bilirubin levels of 15 mg/dL or greater versus 10 of 3002 bottle-fed infants. Eleven of 13 studies reported that breastfed infants had higher mean bilirubin levels. In a study of more than 12,000 infants, the odds ratio for a breastfed infant having a bilirubin of 10 mg/dL or greater was 1.8 (95% CI 1.6 to 2.0).[183] The odds ratio for a bilirubin of 10 mg/dL or greater for an LBW infant was 3.6 (3.1 to 4.3); for an infant of Asian race, 3.6 (2.5 to 5.0); and with prolonged rupture of membranes, 1.9 (1.6 to 2.4). Exclusively breastfed infants have higher serum bilirubin levels than formula-fed infants because of differences in fluid intake, bilirubin excretion, and increased enterohepatic resorption of bilirubin. In addition, there may also be a genetic predisposition to higher bilirubin levels. Inadequate feeding may increase the bilirubin burden, causing hyperbilirubinemia in neonates who have a polymorphic change in the genes involved in the transport and/or metabolism of bilirubin, such as *UGT1A1*, *SLCO1B1*, and *SLCO1B3* polymorphisms.[184]

Relationship of Bilirubin Level to Passage of Stools

There is 450 mg of bilirubin in the intestinal tract meconium of an average newborn infant. Passing this meconium is critical to avoid the deconjugation and reabsorption of unconjugated bilirubin from the gut into the serum. Failure to pass meconium is correlated with elevated serum bilirubin. The time of first stool is also correlated with the level of serum bilirubin. Bottle-fed infants excrete more stool (82 g) and more bilirubin (23.8 mg) in the first 3 days than breastfed infants, who excreted 58 g of stool and 15.7 mg bilirubin.[185] The serum bilirubin levels were 6.8 mg/dL in bottle-fed and 9.5 mg/dL in breastfed infants on day 3. Furthermore, when the breastfed infants excreted more stools and more bilirubin, they had lower bilirubin levels. This relationship has been confirmed in multiple studies.

Clinical Risk Factors in Hyperbilirubinemia

Clinical examination by visual assessment of jaundice in newborns was not found to be reliable in a study comparing visual estimates with laboratory values by Moyer et al.[186] As stated previously, the current recommendations are for universal predischarge bilirubin screening. Clinical risk factors significantly improve the prediction of hyperbilirubinemia compared with the use of early total bilirubin levels, as reported by Newman et al.[187] based on a study of almost 54,000 infants older than 36-weeks' gestational age and at least 2000 g birth weight. From this group, 207 cases were found with elevated bilirubins drawn before 48-hour discharge. The authors found that the risk index was the best predictor of elevated bilirubin (Table 13.1). Clearly, prematurity carries the greatest risk. The TSB before 48 hours was an accurate predictor of reaching a bilirubin of 20 mg/dL (Fig. 13.5).

When the number of feedings at the breast in the first 3 days of life is related to bilirubin levels, there is a significant

TABLE 13.1   Modified Risk Index for Predicting Hyperbilirubinemia in Infants Who Do Not Have Early Jaundice

Variable	Points
Exclusive breastfeeding at hospital discharge	6
Bruising noted	4
Asian race	4
Cephalohematoma	3
Mother's age ≥25 years	3
Male sex	1
Black race	−2
Gestational age	2 × (40 − gestational age)

Modified from Newman TB, Liljestrand P, Escobar GJ. Combining clinical risk factors with serum bilirubin levels to predict hyperbilirubinemia in newborns. *Arch Pediatr Adolesc Med.* 2005;159:113.

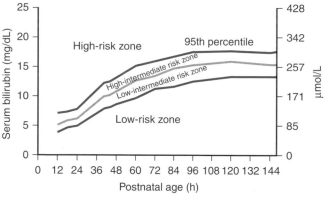

Fig. 13.5 Nomogram for designation of risk in 2840 well newborns of at least 36 weeks' gestational age with a birth weight of 2000 g or greater or of at least 35 weeks' gestational age with a birth weight of 2500 g or greater based on the hour-specific serum bilirubin values. The serum bilirubin level was obtained before discharge, and the zone in which the value fell predicted the likelihood of a subsequent bilirubin level exceeding the 95th percentile (high-risk zone). (From American Academy of Pediatrics Subcommittee on Hyperbilirubinemia. Management of hyperbilirubinemia in the newborn infant 35 or more weeks of gestation. *Pediatrics.* 2004;114:297.)

relationship. The greater the number of breastfeedings, the lower the bilirubin. Infants with more than eight feedings per day were not significantly jaundiced. Water and dextrose supplements were associated with higher bilirubin levels.[188] Sugar-water intake in the first 3 days negatively affects the volume of breast milk available on the fourth day. The infants with high glucose intake have higher bilirubin levels.

Caloric Deprivation and Starvation

Elevated bilirubin does not impede sucking ability. Reduced caloric intake or starvation has been associated with hyperbilirubinemia in adult humans and in many animals. The association between starvation and early neonatal jaundice has been described. Gartner has postulated that starvation may increase bilirubin production, shift bilirubin pools, reduce hepatic bilirubin uptake, diminish hepatic bilirubin conjugation, or increase enteric bilirubin reabsorption.[189] Adequate caloric intake may simply diminish intestinal bilirubin absorption. Infants with intestinal obstruction (pyloric stenosis) at birth or in the early weeks of life are often jaundiced.

Treatment of Early Hyperbilirubinemia

Serum bilirubin levels in newborns and the relationship to breastfeeding were measured, and 8 of 10 infants with serum bilirubin greater than 12.9 mg/dL were breastfed.[178] It is the process of altered nourishment that is the cause of relative starvation. The amount of stress for a mother generated by separation from her infant for phototherapy was measured by urine cortisol levels and compared with levels in mothers who roomed-in with their jaundiced infants during phototherapy. The separated mothers were more stressed and were more likely to discontinue breastfeeding than those who remained with their infants.[190]

In a controlled trial of four interventions, 125 of 1685 infants in the birth cohort whose bilirubin levels reached 17 mg/dL (291 mmol/L) were randomly assigned to treatment. The four interventions were (1) continue breastfeeding and observe; (2) discontinue breastfeeding and substitute formula; (3) discontinue breastfeeding, substitute formula, and use phototherapy; and (4) continue breastfeeding and use phototherapy. The bilirubin reached 20 mg/dL (342 mmol/L) in 24% of group 1, 19% of group 2, 3% of group 3, and 14% of group 4. Phototherapy clearly adds to the decline in bilirubin, and the authors suggest that the parents can be offered the management of their choice.[191] Various groups recommend a blood type and Coombs test as part of the evaluation, and to treat infants with blood type incompatibilities aggressively.

An evaluation of the transcutaneous bilirubinometer demonstrated that it correlated well with TSBs done in the laboratory.[192] The correlation in black infants was not as close, but levels erred on the high side so that underdiagnosing is not a risk. Multiple checks with the meter are easily done to establish trends so that a breastfed infant can be followed closely without painful sticks. Blood levels are essential if phototherapy is needed and after it is initiated.[192]

Hyperbilirubinemia results from unphysiologic management of breastfeeding, expressed largely through insufficient frequency of breastfeeding. To treat the actual cause, that is, failed breastfeeding or inadequate stooling or underfeeding, breastfeeding should be reviewed for frequency, length of suckling, and apparent supply of milk, adjusting the breastfeeding to improve any deficits. If stooling is the problem, an infant should be stimulated to stool. If starvation is the problem, the infant should receive additional calories (formula) while the milk supply is being increased by better breastfeeding techniques. The same would apply to bottle-feeding jaundice (i.e., any infant with idiopathic jaundice who is being bottle-fed and has a bilirubin level greater than 12.9 mg/dL). Stooling, frequency of feeds, and kilocalories would be improved. Box 13.1 provides a management schema for breastfeeding to prevent hyperbilirubinemia. All infants must have the appropriate laboratory studies performed.[193]

BOX 13.1 Breastfeeding Management Outline for Hyperbilirubinemia Prevention

1. Initiate breastfeeding early, ideally within the first hour of life, and encourage frequent breastfeeding on demand. Infants, typically, feed 8 to 12 times a day or more.
2. Ensure that the parents recognize early feeding cues.
3. Promote skin-to-skin contact.
4. Ensure proper latch and milk transfer.
5. Inform caregivers that infants should not be fed water, dextrose water, or formula supplements.
6. Medical supplements should be limited to clinical indications.
7. Monitor infant's weight, voiding, and stooling in association with breastfeeding pattern, recognizing that newborns have a normal weight loss after birth.

BOX 13.2 Key Elements of Hyperbilirubinemia Management

1. Promote and support effective breastfeeding.
2. Establish nursery protocols for the identification and evaluation of hyperbilirubinemia.
3. Identify maternal and infant risk factors for hyperbilirubinemia (see Table 13.2).
4. If infant appears jaundiced in the first 24 hours of life, measure the total serum bilirubin or transcutaneous bilirubin level.
5. Recognize that visual estimation of the degree of jaundice can lead to errors.
6. Interpret all bilirubin levels according to an infant's age according to hours of life (see Fig. 13.5).
7. Recognize that infants born at less than 38 weeks' gestation, particularly those who are breastfed, are at higher risk for developing hyperbilirubinemia and require closer surveillance and monitoring while promoting effective breastfeeding.
8. Screen total serum bilirubin or transcutaneous bilirubin level on all infants before discharge.
9. Provide parents with written and verbal information about newborn jaundice.
10. Provide appropriate follow-up based on the time of discharge and the risk assessment.
11. Treat newborns, when indicated, with phototherapy or exchange transfusion.

TABLE 13.2 Risk Factors for Development of Severe Hyperbilirubinemia in Infants of 35 Weeks' Gestation or Older (in Approximate Order of Importance)

Major Risk Factors

Predischarge TSB or TcB level in the high-risk zone

Jaundice observed in the first 24 hours

Blood group incompatibility with positive direct antiglobulin test, other known hemolytic disease (e.g., glucose-6-phosphate dehydrogenase deficiency), elevated ETCOc

Gestational age 35 to 36 weeks

Previous sibling received phototherapy

Cephalohematoma or significant bruising

Exclusive breastfeeding, particularly if nursing is not going well and weight loss is excessive

East Asian race[a]

Minor Risk Factors

Predischarge TSB or TcB level in the high- or intermediate-risk zone

Gestational age 37 to 38 weeks

Jaundice observed before discharge

Previous sibling with jaundice

Macrosomic infant of a mother with diabetes

Maternal age 25 years or older

Male sex

Decreased Risk

(These factors are associated with decreased risk for significant jaundice, listed in order of decreasing importance.)

TSB or TcB level in the low-risk zone

Gestational age 41 weeks or more

Exclusive bottle-feeding

Black race[a]

Discharge from hospital after 72 hours

ETCOc, End-tidal carbon monoxide corrected for ambient air; *TcB*, transcutaneous bilirubin; *TSB*, total serum bilirubin.
[a]Race as defined by mother's description.
From American Academy of Pediatrics Subcommittee on Hyperbilirubinemia. Management of hyperbilirubinemia in the newborn infant 35 or more weeks of gestation. *Pediatrics.* 2004;114:297.

Key elements of the guidelines for the management of hyperbilirubinemia in newborns by the Subcommittee on Hyperbilirubinemia of the AAP appear in Box 13.2 and Table 13.2. The nomogram for the designation of risk for jaundice is illustrated in Fig. 13.5, and guidelines for the use of phototherapy are illustrated in Fig. 13.6.[179]

When total serum bilirubin levels exceed treatment thresholds, especially when levels are rising rapidly, phototherapy should be started. Phototherapy can be used while continuing full breastfeeding. If intake at the breast is insufficient and supplementation is medically necessary, expressed maternal milk is preferred. The use of pasteurized donor human milk (PDHM) is increasing, despite a lack of data on its benefits on reducing hyperbilirubinemia.[194] Although supplementation with infant formula may decrease the bilirubin level and risk of readmission for phototherapy, it will also interfere with the establishment and continuation of breastfeeding and thus should be used only in extenuating circumstances.[195,196]

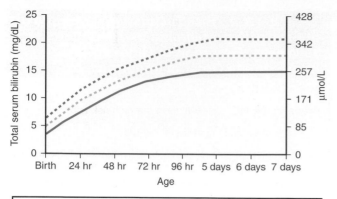

- Use total bilirubin. Do not subtract direct reacting or conjugated bilirubin.
- Risk factors = isoimmune hemolytic dissease, G6PD deficiency, asphyxia, significant lethargy, temperature instability, sepsis, acidosis, or albumin <3.0 g/dL (if measured).
- For well infants 35–37 6/7 wk can adjust TSB levels for intervention around the medium risk line. It is an option to intervene at lower TSB levels for infants closer to 35 wk and at higher TSB levels for those closer to 37 6/7 wk.
- It is an option to provide conventional phototherapy in hospital or at home at TSB levels 2–3 mg/dL (35–50 mmol/L) below those shown but home phototherapy should not be used in any infant with risk factors.

Fig. 13.6 Guidelines for phototherapy in hospitalized infants of at least 35 weeks' gestation. Note: These guidelines are based on limited evidence, and the levels shown are approximations. The guidelines refer to the use of intensive phototherapy, which should be used when the total serum bilirubin exceeds the line indicated for each category. Infants are designated as "higher risk" because of the potential negative effects of the conditions listed on albumin binding of bilirubin, the blood–brain barrier, and the susceptibility of the brain cells to damage by bilirubin. (From American Academy of Pediatrics Subcommittee on Hyperbilirubinemia. Management of hyperbilirubinemia in the newborn infant 35 or more weeks of gestation. *Pediatrics*, 2004;114:297.)

Phototherapy for neonatal jaundice and concerns about insufficient milk can produce anxiety and distress for mothers and can be disruptive to successful breastfeeding.[197] Phototherapy is best done while rooming-in with the mother so that breastfeeding can be continued.[198] Interruption of phototherapy for 30 minutes or longer to permit breastfeeding without eye patches does not alter the effectiveness of phototherapy, and biliblankets can be used while breastfeeding.[199] Infants under phototherapy do not routinely require extra oral or IV fluids. IV fluids are only indicated in cases of infant dehydration, hypernatremia, or inability to ingest adequate milk. Using subthreshold bilirubin levels to initiate phototherapy as a mechanism to prevent readmission is effective but not recommended because this approach increases length of stay and results in many cases of phototherapy that would otherwise not be needed to reduce each case of readmission.[195]

Jaundice in preterm infants at less than 35 weeks' gestation also results from increased bilirubin production, decreased hepatic conjugation in an immature liver, and inadequate excretion via the stool. Hyperbilirubinemia in preterm infants is more prevalent, more severe, and more protracted. The risk

for kernicterus is greater as well. Its management is the purview of a neonatologist.[200] In most cases, if human milk is provided, it is maintained. Maisels et al. add the following recommendations: management and follow-up plans should be based on gestational age, predischarge bilirubins, and risk factors for subsequent hyperbilirubinemia[193] (see Box13.2). The AAP Subcommittee on Hyperbilirubinemia suggests lactation evaluation and support for all breastfeeding mothers.[179] It also recommends that the timing of repeat bilirubin measurements after discharge should depend on age at the time of measurement and on the degree to which the level is above the 95th percentile. Follow-up recommendations can be modified according to the level of risk. Infants should have a predischarge bilirubin, which has been the recommendation to improve the chances of preventing kernicterus. Universal predischarge bilirubin screening using TSB or transcutaneous bilirubin (TcB) measurements, which help to assess the risk of subsequent severe hyperbilirubinemia, is recommended. A more structured approach to management and follow-up according to the predischarge TSB/TcB, gestational age, and other risk factors for hyperbilirubinemia is essential.

Kernicterus in late preterm infants cared for as term healthy infants. Late prematurity (34 6/7 to 36 6/7 weeks' gestational age) has not been recognized as a risk factor for hazardous hyperbilirubinemia by practitioners, according to Bhutani and Johnson, who report cases of acute and chronic posticteric sequelae.[201] Large-for-gestational-age and late preterm infants are disproportionately represented in the group with kernicterus. Unsuccessful and suboptimal lactation experience was the most frequent associated factor. The authors urge attention to early bilirubin values, additional risk factors, and the success of breastfeeding in these infants. These infants require close monitoring by the pediatrician.

Breast-Milk Jaundice

Many breastfed infants have unconjugated hyperbilirubinemia that extends into the second and third week but can continue for as long as 2 to 3 months. At 28 days after birth, 34% of predominantly breastfed infants have TcB levels ≥ 5 mg/dL, 9% have levels ≥ 10 mg/dL, and 1% have levels ≥ 12.9 mg/dL.[178] This cause of prolonged unconjugated hyperbilirubinemia, which can last up to 3 months, is almost always nonpathologic and not associated with direct hyperbilirubinemia or cholestasis. This syndrome has been called *breast-milk jaundice, late-onset jaundice,* and *breast-milk jaundice syndrome.*[189] Breast-milk jaundice should be distinguished from "suboptimal intake jaundice"[180] (Table 13.3). It occurs in less than 1 in 200 births; the numbers are imprecise because not all mothers breastfeed. This syndrome is associated with the milk of a particular mother and will occur with each pregnancy in varying degrees, depending on each infant's ability to conjugate bilirubin (i.e., a premature sibling might be more severely affected).[189] Early-onset jaundice is related to the process of breastfeeding, not the milk itself, and has also been described as "suboptimal intake jaundice."[180] It is essential to rule out other causes of prolonged or excessive jaundice, especially hemolytic disease, hypothyroidism, glucose-6-phosphate

TABLE 13.3 Characteristics Distinguishing Suboptimal Intake Jaundice From Breast-Milk Jaundice

	Typical Time Frame	Weight	Stool Output	Urine Output	Clinical Findings
Suboptimal intake jaundice	Onset 2–5 days of age and usually resolved by 2 weeks	Ongoing weight loss	<5/day with color black, brown, or green	<5/day with uric acid crystals (brick color)	Commonly <38 weeks and rarely ≥40 weeks gestation. May be fussy and difficult to settle between feedings or sleepy and difficult to wake for feeding
Breast-milk jaundice	Onset 2–5 days and may last up to 3 months	Gaining ≥30 g/day[109]	≥8/day with yellow color	≥8/day with yellow or clear color	Waking to feed 8–12 ×/day

From Flaherman VJ, Maisels MJ, Academy of Breastfeeding Medicine. ABM Clinical Protocol #22: guidelines for management of jaundice in the breastfeeding infant 35 weeks or more of gestation—revised 2017. *Breastfeed Med.* 2017;12(5):250–257. https://doi.org/10.1089/bfm.2017.29042.vjf. Epub 2017 Apr 10.

dehydrogenase deficiency, inherited hepatic glucuronyl transferase deficiency (Gilbert syndrome, etc.), and intestinal obstruction. Whenever jaundice in a breastfed newborn is prolonged beyond the third week, it is important to rule out cholestasis by measuring the direct or conjugated bilirubin level and to evaluate for other causes of prolonged indirect hyperbilirubinemia. For indirect hyperbilirubinemia that extends beyond 2 months, conditions such as ongoing undiagnosed hemolysis, Gilbert syndrome, or the very rare Crigler–Najjar syndrome (with an incidence of 1 per million births) should be considered.[180]

The pattern of this jaundice is distinctly different. Normally, idiopathic jaundice peaks on the third day and then begins to drop. Breast-milk jaundice, however, becomes apparent or continues to rise after the third day, and bilirubin levels may peak any time from the 7th to the 10th day, with untreated cases being reported to peak as late as the 15th day. Values have ranged from 10 to 27 mg/dL during this time. No correlation exists with weight loss or gain, and stools are normal.

The syndrome of breast-milk jaundice was attributed by Arias et al. to a substance in the milk of some mothers that inhibits the hepatic enzyme glucuronyl transferase, preventing the conjugation of bilirubin.[202] The substance has been identified as 5β-pregnane-3α,20α-diol, a breakdown product of progesterone and an isomer of pregnanediol that is not usually found in milk but occurs normally in 10% of the lactating population. Although this substance had also been isolated from the milk and serum of mothers whose infants were not jaundiced, this work has not been duplicated. In a definitive study of breast-milk β-glucuronidase, Wilson et al. examined 55 mother–infant pairs.[203] No correlation was found between serum bilirubin levels and breast-milk β-glucuronidase between days 3 and 6 postpartum. The role of lipoprotein lipase and bile salt–stimulated lipase in breast-milk jaundice has also been studied, but again, levels of lipase are not higher in breast-milk jaundice.[204]

Although the undisputed cause of breast-milk jaundice is unresolved, research has focused on numerous factors involved in bilirubin excretion, including increased concentrations of cytokines (including IL-1, IL-10, and TNF-) in human milk; low total antioxidant capacity in human milk; variations in the HO-1 gene promoter; variations in the *UGT1A1* gene; lower serum and milk levels of epidermal growth factor; higher serum alpha-fetoprotein levels; higher cholesterol levels; and lower abundance of *Bifidobacterium adolescentis*, *Bifidobacterium longum*, and *Bifidobacterium bifidum* in human milk and stool.[205–212] The relative contribution of each of these factors, their potential interaction, and their precise mechanism of action remain unknown.

Over time, the jaundice and elevated TSB decline at varying rates to normal adult values even while breastfeeding continues. As in early jaundice associated with breastfeeding, jaundiced infants at 3 weeks do not produce more bilirubin than their unjaundiced breastfed peers or bottle-fed infants.

Diagnosis depends on circumstantial evidence because no easy, rapid laboratory test exists. All other causes, including infection, should be ruled out in the usual manner, and a thorough history should be taken, including medications and family history and ethnic background. If the mother has nursed other infants, were they jaundiced? Usually 70% of the previous children of a given mother whose infant has breast-milk jaundice have been jaundiced. The difference may be related to the greater maturity of the liver of a given infant who then is able to handle the increased demands on the glucuronyl transferase system. Genetic variations in *UGT1A1* and *OATP2* genes may hold answers. To establish the diagnosis firmly, and this is necessary when the bilirubin level is greater than 16 mg/dL for more than 24 hours, a bilirubin reading should be obtained 2 hours after a breastfeeding and then breastfeeding discontinued for at least 12 hours.[187] The infant must be fed fluids and calories. The infant's mother should be assisted in pumping her breasts to maintain her supply. Even more urgent is providing the mother with a sympathetic explanation of the problem and the process. After at least 12 hours without mother's milk, the bilirubin level should be measured. If a significant drop of more than 2 mg/dL occurs, it is diagnostic of breast-milk jaundice. When the level is less than 15 mg/dL, the infant can be put

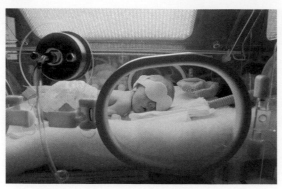

Fig. 13.7 Phototherapy for a premature infant with two overhead banks of lights while lying on a fiber-optic blanket.

back to the breast after the 12-hour "pause." Phototherapy should continue as indicated based on the serum level and assessment of kernicterus risk. Bilirubin levels should be obtained to determine if the bilirubin rises again and, if so, how much. In most cases, in the time not breastfeeding, the infant's body equilibrates the levels sufficiently, so only a slight increase in bilirubin occurs on return to breastfeeding, followed by a slow but steady drop. If that is the case, breastfeeding can continue. The bilirubin level should be checked at 10 to 14 days to be certain the bilirubin is truly clearing.

If the bilirubin has not dropped significantly after 12 hours without breast milk, the time off the breast should be extended to 18 to 24 hours, measuring bilirubin levels every 6 hours. If the bilirubin rises while the infant is off the breast, the cause of jaundice is clearly not the breast milk; breastfeeding should be resumed and other causes for the jaundice reevaluated.

Phototherapy and Breast-Milk Jaundice

If the bilirubin is substantially greater than 20 mg/dL in a full-term infant (or proportionately lower in a preterm infant), it is important to lower the bilirubin promptly; thus phototherapy should be initiated as soon as the blood work is drawn (Fig. 13.7). The relationship to breastfeeding can be established later. Often IV fluids are also necessary.

If one is attempting to establish the diagnosis of breast-milk jaundice, phototherapy should not be used while breast milk is being discontinued. If establishing the diagnosis is not necessary (perhaps because of the same diagnosis in older siblings), phototherapy can be used to bring the values to a more acceptable range (i.e., less than 12 mg/dL). When phototherapy is discontinued, it is most important to establish that no rebound hyperbilirubinemia occurs. In addition, it is important to follow the infant at home after discharge through at least 14 days of life or longer if the values are not less than 12 mg/dL. It should not be assumed that the diagnosis is breast-milk jaundice when breastfeeding has been stopped and phototherapy initiated simultaneously.

Late Diagnosis of Breast-Milk Jaundice

With the frequency of early discharge from the hospital, especially for families enjoying the birthing center concept, breastfed infants are often discharged before jaundice for any

reason has developed. Because breast-milk jaundice is likely to be delayed to the fourth or fifth day, peaking at 10 to 14 days of age, most normal infants are already home. Occasionally, an infant is observed in a pediatrician's office at 10 days of age or older with a bilirubin level greater than 20 mg/dL, often 23 to 25 mg/dL. This necessitates the immediate admission of the infant to the hospital for a complete bilirubin workup. It is important to recognize that other causes of hyperbilirubinemia must be ruled out, including blood type incompatibilities. At this age, it is also necessary to rule out biliary obstruction and hepatitis, which might have a high direct or conjugated bilirubin level.

Phototherapy is used for 4 to 6 hours to establish whether this therapy will be effective in dropping the level sufficiently. When bilirubin is substantially greater than 20 mg/dL and if a possible association with breast milk exists, it is necessary to stop breastfeeding temporarily and start phototherapy immediately on admission while the diagnostic workup is being performed. Otherwise, breastfeeding may continue even though IV fluids may also be necessary.

The AHRQ, through its Evidence-Based Practice Centers, published a report on the management of neonatal hyperbilirubinemia in 2003 after an extensive review of more than 4560 abstracts from which 241 articles were examined and 138 included in the report.[213] In contrast, Chou et al. proposed the management of hyperbilirubinemia using a benchmarking model in a 3-year prospective cohort study.[214] They found associations of high bilirubin with lower gestational age, older mother, and exclusive or partial breastfeeding. The authors recommend assessing breastfeeding and promoting breastfeeding, supplementing if necessary but never with water, in combination with phototherapy as most efficacious.[214] The natural history of jaundice in predominantly breastfed infants is described by Flaherman et al.[180] They measured TcBs in 1044 breastfed infants of at least 35 weeks' gestation and noted that 20% to 30% of predominantly breastfed infants will be jaundiced by transcutaneous measurement at 3 to 4 weeks. Levels of 5 mg/dL or more will be found in 30% to 40%. When drawn, a TcB of zero was highly predictive that the bilirubin was less than 12.9 mg/dL and could be used for screening purposes at 1 month.

Infants discharged early (less than 30 hours of age) were more likely to be rehospitalized for hyperbilirubinemia within 7 days of discharge in a study of 310,000 newborns in the state of Washington when compared with children discharged from 30 to 78 hours after birth. Of the children readmitted, 94% were breastfed.[215] Bilirubin screening at discharge is recommended. Prolonged breast-milk jaundice has not been studied in follow-up when the association of the bilirubin elevation has been made with breast milk. A pediatric practice may see only a few in a lifetime. The safe level for chronic indirect bilirubin has not been established. The Lactation Study Center recommends greater than or equal to 10 mg/dL. Others allow a level of 12 mg/dL. This is accomplished most easily with phototherapy; usually, having an infant sleep under phototherapy 12 hours per day, utilizing home devices such as the "bilirubin blanket," will control the levels. This is not a casual arrangement. The eyes must be protected and the bilirubin monitored. As the liver matures, the problem resolves, and phototherapy can be discontinued. The infant must be under the care of an experienced pediatrician. In some cases, the bilirubin can be controlled with partial breastfeeding with the addition of formula in sufficient amounts to maintain the bilirubin at less than 10 mg/dL. Children with Gilbert syndrome, Crigler—Najjar syndrome, glucose-6-phosphate dehydrogenase, and other genetic variations must be managed individually by a genetic specialist and the pediatrician. These children have chronic hyperbilirubinemia and usually need to sleep under phototherapy.

SUCKLING PROBLEMS RELATED TO ANATOMY AND NEURAL DISORDERS

Most problems with latch-on during breastfeeding can be solved with adjustment of position and approach, but a few cannot because an infant has an anatomic variation of the mouth or a neurodevelopmental problem. A thorough examination is required to evaluate the mouth and cheek for potential associated lesions and syndromes. Premature infants are more often identified with suckling problems as a result of both immaturity and, possibly, the effects of various treatments: suctioning, intubation, feeding tubes, and so forth.[216] They may have a high arched or grooved palate from an endotracheal tube used to ventilate.

There are many variants to normal oral structure, such as high palate, macroglossia, ankyloglossia, cysts on the dental ridge or under the tongue, or clefts.

Primarily Anatomic Feeding Difficulties—The Mouth

High Palate

A number of observations link palatal variation with breastfeeding difficulties (e.g., "bubble palate"). Given how we understand infant suckling, a high-arched palate may contribute low milk transfer by creating a larger intraoral space in which negative pressure must be generated or by limiting the ability of the tongue to compress the nipple against the palate with its peristaltic wave. That high-arched palates and ankyloglossia may coexist could exacerbate this latter mechanical problem.[217,218] One study found an association between 5-year-olds born prematurely and narrow palates, as compared with 5-year-olds who had been born at term.[219] The authors hypothesized that the early introduction of alternative nutritive tools (bottles) and nonnutritive habits (pacifiers) may have contributed to these changes. They also confirmed the previously established link between a lack of breastfeeding and malocclusion.

Marmet and Shell describe a bubble palate as a concavity in the hard palate, usually about {⅜} to {¾} inch (1 to 2 cm) in diameter and {¼} inch (0.5 cm) deep.[220] Only one case report of "bubble palate" exists; from 1997, it describes an infant with bubble palate and failure to thrive and suggests the palate may have contributed to poor milk transfer.[221] Breastfeeding by the

infant improved with repositioning and supplementation with pumped milk. In these reports and anecdotally, it appears that supine positioning with the infant prone ("laid-back" or "Australian hold") may be more comfortable and improve milk transfer (see Fig. 7.4A). This position may encourage the infant's tongue to fall down and forward and keep the nipple deep in the infant's mouth.

Macroglossia. Macroglossia is seen in children born with syndromes such as Beckwith—Wiedemann and congenital hypothyroidism and occasionally is present without an identified cause. The crowding of the oral cavity may represent only part of the reason that macroglossia is associated with feeding difficulties, as not all feeding difficulties resolve after surgery. Prendeville and Sell reported difficulties with "lip seal formation, biting, bolus manipulation and tongue lateralization" in a case series of infants ($N = 25$) under 12 months with Beckwith—Wiedemann and macroglossia.[222] Over 75% of the infants also had aspiration risk. In this series, feeding difficulties in 21 of 25 infants mostly resolved after tongue-reduction surgery, unlike in a prior case series, reported by Style et al., of children aged 9 months to 4 years at repair, where 12 of 47 infants had partial glossectomies and 47% still had significant feeding difficulties after surgery.[223] Although no data exist on breastfeeding with macroglossia, infants are likely to struggle with deep latch and gagging. A laid-back position may be helpful.

Mouth problems. Alveolar lymphangiomas are elevations along the alveolar ridge that are isolated, bluish, firm cysts 3 to 10 mm in diameter. More than one may be present. They may interfere with suckling. They contain no dental tissue and gradually disappear in the first year. Breastfeeding is less influenced than bottle and pacifier sucking.

Ankyloglossia (tongue-tie). Ankyloglossia, or *tongue-tie*, refers to a lingual frenulum that is positioned toward the tip of the tongue or is restricted in function. The frenulum may also be referred to as *shortened, inelastic*, or *thickened*. The true incidence is not known because of differing definitions used in research, but it is probably present in 5% to 10% of newborns; there appears to be a male predominance.[224] Although it may therefore be considered rare, in a thriving practice that sees 40 newborns a month, approximately 2 per month may present with difficulty breastfeeding and ankyloglossia. Additionally, in one study of mothers presenting with nipple pain in Thailand, 23% attributed it to tongue-tie.[225] Either the incidence or diagnosis (or both) of ankyloglossia is increasing in the United States and Canada, most rapidly in the past 6 years, although this varies geographically.[226] This may be a result of the increased rates of breastfeeding or increased awareness by health care providers. Unfortunately, the research has not been done to complete our understanding of tongue-tie, which raises the concern of overdiagnosis and inappropriate management. The "anterior" type (Coryllos types 1 to 3) has been studied, and its prompt diagnosis and management are recommended by the AAP, the National Institute for Health and Care Excellence (UK), and the Canadian Agency for Drugs and Technologies in Health (CADTH).[227–229] There remains some controversy regarding appropriate classification and indications for treatment. In particular, the "posterior" (Coryllos types 3 to 4, submucosal, "short tongue") tongue-tie is an emerging phenomenon because it has been found that these frenula may also benefit from frenotomy. In addition to inadequate research, these types of disagreements are fueled by the division of the mother–infant dyad between pediatrics (which focuses on infant health) and obstetrics (which may treat nipple pain or mastitis), with the lactation consultant, family medicine provider, or breastfeeding medicine provider being more likely to see the whole picture.

Essentially, ankyloglossia affects breastfeeding in two ways: by limiting milk transfer or causing maternal nipple damage. Both of these conditions can lower maternal milk supply, trigger mastitis, or lead to inadequate infant growth. There is emerging evidence that ankyloglossia may also contribute to the pathogenesis of reflux, perhaps through aerophagia or abnormal tongue and esophageal peristalsis.[230] One typical presentation of ankyloglossia will include an infant who is hungry all of the time but rapidly falls asleep while eating and damages maternal nipples. In cases in which there is no nipple damage, we have occasionally seen failure to thrive around 4 to 6 weeks of age. With ankyloglossia, an infant cannot protrude the spread tongue over the gums to latch to the areola, which is essential in maintaining negative pressure and a stretched maternal nipple. There is also abnormal peristalsis. This means that there is a "shallow latch," and the mother's nipple may be caught between the hard palate and a tongue that pistons (drops up and down in the back) instead of waves (peristalses tip to back). Nipples may be creased and cracked as a result. Milk expression is thereby limited, more so if there is a high palate.

On physical exam, there will be difficulty with tongue extension, and there may be a heart-shaped tongue tip when an effort is made to extend it. The infant will have impaired lift, lateralization, cupping, peristalsis, and extension of the tongue. Several groups have worked to develop classifications for ankyloglossia. The Coryllos classification of types 1 to 4 is the most commonly used in practice.[226] However, visual typing is not necessarily associated with functional breastfeeding. The Hazelbaker tool (HATLFF) has an extensive list for visual inspection and physical functioning and has been found to be highly reliable.[231] Unfortunately, this scale may be impractical and requires significant training. Amir et al. found that a shortened version of the function items relying on lift, lateralization, and extension had the highest levels of agreement between scorers.[232] This may be used in clinical settings, with a score of ≤ 4 out of 6 indicating the need for frenotomy.

Alternatively, Walker et al. propose measuring tip-to-frenulum length as a possible indicator of breastfeeding difficulty. In a cohort study, the group measured this length in 100 healthy full-term neonates and compared these findings with scores on the Infant Breastfeeding Assessment Tool (IBFAT) and maternal pain scales (Fig. 1 from this paper)[233] (See Fig. 13.8). The mean tip-to-frenulum length was 9.11 mm, with a standard deviation of 2.65 mm. Tip-to-frenulum length and IBFAT scores were correlated for mothers who had breastfed two or more children. Maternal pain was also correlated with having a visual band and low tip-to-frenulum length, with a 22% increase in the likelihood of pain for each millimeter of decrease in length. Interrater reliability was strong, which suggests that this may be a promising measure for the evaluation of ankyloglossia.

Because of its significant impact on maternal pain and breastfeeding success, all major pediatric organizations agree that a lingual frenulum should be divided if it is interfering with breastfeeding. However, disagreement continues surrounding definitions and indications. There is no evidence that the frenulum will "stretch" over time. However, the natural history of untreated lingual frenula that negatively affect

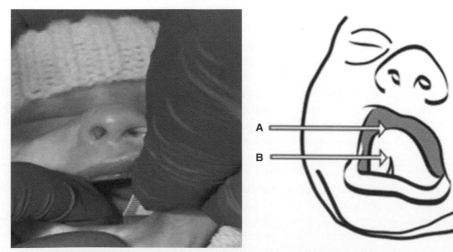

Fig. 13.8 Tip–frenulum measurement. With the infant's tongue retracted superiorly, the distance from the junction of the dorsal papillated and ventral mucosal tongue (A) to the attachment of the lingual frenulum (B) is measured. Color images available online at http://www.liebertpub.com/bfm. (From Walker RD, Messing S, Rosen-Carole C, et al. Defining tip-frenulum length for ankyloglossia and its impact on breastfeeding: a prospective cohort study. *Breastfeed Med.* 2018;13[3]:204–210. https://doi.org/10.1089/bfm.2017.0116. Epub 2018 Mar 20. Right, copyright Ryan Healey.)

breastfeeding has not been studied. In our experience, a lack of treatment rarely results in success.

To evaluate for the need for frenotomy, several tools are available, including the Hazelbaker assessment tool and the abbreviated Hazelbaker; Coryllos typing; and breastfeeding outcome scales, such as the IBFAT, the LATCH score, and the Breastfeeding Self-Efficacy Scale, Short Form (BSES-SF).[224,228,232–235] If the tongue-tie is shown to contribute to the breastfeeding problems, the frenotomy procedure is simple. The cut should be carefully placed to avoid the artery, nerves, salivary ducts, the glossopharyngeal muscle, and other anatomic sites. It has become standard in breastfeeding medicine practices to clip the anterior portion, as well as any posterior portion that may exist, resulting in a diamond-shaped scar under the tongue. The main risk of the procedure is bleeding, although this is more common in cases in which the glossopharyngeal muscle is cut. It is usually relatively bloodless, and the infant can be nursed immediately, now in the correct position. Antibiotic prophylaxis is not indicated for the procedure unless the infant has significant cyanotic cardiac disease or is 6 months or less after cardiac repair. Anesthesia is not recommended because of neurodevelopmental impact, nor is topical benzocaine because of the risk of methemoglobinemia. Clamping the frenulum before clipping had been used in the past to lessen bleeding or direct the scissors but has not been studied and is likely to result in more pain. Observation for bleeding is brief. In the rare case of bleeding beyond 3 minutes, oxymetazoline (Afrin) or silver nitrate may be applied, or a strip of gelatin foam can be used to achieve rapid hemostasis and removed before feeding. Suturing is only required in the case of uncontrollable bleeding.

An alternative to scissors frenotomy is the use of laser, which is increasingly prevalent among pediatric dentists in some countries. There is no comparative data between scissors and laser technique. The laser technique differs from the scissors ("cold") technique in that it vaporizes the tissue, is bloodless, parents are not allowed in the room, and many providers recommend forceful stretches to prevent readherence. It is unclear if the risks of pain to the infant or possibly oral aversion are outweighed by the potential benefit of these exercises because they have not been studied.

There is published work on improvement of breastfeeding after frenotomy for posterior ankyloglossia done by laser[230] and scissors.[236] Ghaheri et al.'s prospective cohort study (N = 237) measured the effect of laser frenotomy on milk transfer, maternal pain, and reflux symptoms at 1 week and 1 month postprocedure. Of subjects, 78% had a posterior tongue-tie, and lingual and labial maxillary frenotomy was done. There was statistically and clinically significant improvement in maternal pain, per the BSES-SF and the Infant Gastroesophageal Reflux Questionnaire, Revised (I-GERQ-R). Breast-milk transfer increased an average of 155%.[230] O'Callahan et al. measured maternal pain and latch difficulties after frenotomy in a retrospective cohort of 157 dyads, 55% of which were classified as posterior, or type 4. There was a 63% improvement in nipple pain and 49%

improvement in latch in the posterior group alone. No group found worsening latch or nipple pain after the procedure.[236]

Ultrasound technologies have allowed the study of suck mechanics before and after frenotomy. Geddes et al. assessed the suck of 24 dyads before and after frenotomy.[237] Milk intake, rate of transfer, maternal pain, and latch improved postfrenotomy. On ultrasound, there was less compression of the nipple tip or base (depending on infant pathology) following the procedure.

After the procedure, some providers recommend mouth exercises, which are meant to help the tongue reestablish its proper use of the eight muscles that make up this remarkable organ. Evidence exists in older children,[238] but as long as it is gentle and does not interfere with feeding, it is conceivable that these exercises may help. Other providers may refer to feeding therapists, craniosacral therapists, and chiropractors to improve tongue function. Although the evidence for all of these is limited, they may be low-risk options and support breastfeeding. Alternatively, they may be costly, increase the risk of exposure to infectious diseases in a high-risk period, or increase parental fatigue and anxiety. Depending on the quality of local resources, these risks should be weighed against potential benefits.

The ABM has a protocol for managing ankyloglossia in breastfeeding, which is in revision. When complete, it will be made available at http://www.abm.com.

Restrictive superior labial frenulum/"lip tie." With the advent of a laser technique for addressing thick superior labial frenula in a bloodless manner, severing lip ties has become increasingly common. There are some case reports on infants who were unable to latch with the upper lip flanged and were associated with maternal pain or infant failure to thrive.

Although the incidence of restrictive labial frenulum is not known, visual anatomy has been recently studied. In a prospective cross-sectional study, 100 infants were examined and photographed.[239] Six experts then assigned grades based on the Kotlow classification scale for upper lip anatomy. All infants were found to have a superior labial frenulum, with 83% being classified as a "grade 2." A thin higher labial frenulum, or "grade 1," has been considered normal and yet was seen in only 6% of subjects. There was very poor interrater reliability for classifying lip tie with the Kotlow classification, which improved when the authors devised their own scale ("Stanford scale"); even then, it remained only 38%.[239]

Clinical opinions have been published regarding classification, diagnosis, and management. Managing an upper lip tie has been part of clinical studies in which tongue-tie was also addressed. Unfortunately, no trials have been completed regarding lip ties alone, or with methodologic rigor, and there remains a significant lack of diagnostic clarity.[240] One case series from 2019 included 22 infants less than 60 days old who underwent an upper lip frenotomy for isolated upper lip tie and breastfeeding problems.[241] Interestingly, cases were not selected by visual appearance but, rather, by restriction on manual eversion and mothers' report of lip eversion during feeding. In this series, 82% of mothers reported improved latch, and 9% reported recurrence after frenotomy performed with fine-tip electrocautery.

When evaluating for ankyloglossia with breastfeeding problems, there exists controversy about whether a frenotomy should be performed for a concurrent low-lying or restrictive upper lip frenulum. Some providers recommend a 1- to 2-week waiting period between a lingual frenotomy and an upper lip evaluation. This may be a result of the relaxing of the compensatory lip-pursing seen with ankyloglossia. That is, many infants' upper lips relax and flange properly after lingual frenotomy alone because the tongue alone can create and maintain negative pressure postfrenotomy. There are some lips for which this is not the case. If a mother has ongoing discomfort or shallow latch after a frenotomy, and a low-lying inflexible maxillary frenulum is observable, it may be indicated to seek treatment. There is insufficient evidence at present to recommend that superior labial frenula of any kind be routinely severed in infants. Also, there are no data to suggest whether such procedures would increase or decrease the risk of future diastema in the upper front teeth or malocclusion.

Buccal frenula/buccal tie/"cheek tie." *Buccal tie* refers to tissue that stretches between the gingiva and the inner cheek. This can be felt by running a finger along the inner cheek between the upper and lower gums. There is no classification scale, known prevalence, or published evidence on the utility of severing such a band to help with breastfeeding. Given the frequency of suck dysfunction without an identifiable cause, it is theoretically possible that managing buccal frenula may be part of the answer. However, at this time, there is no known clinical benefit to a buccal frenotomy, and these should be exceedingly rare to prevent potential negative outcomes.

First-arch disorders: receding chin, choanal atresia, cleft lip and palate. Feeding of any sort may be greatly hindered by abnormalities of the jaw, nose, and mouth. Infants with first-arch abnormalities usually require considerable help in feeding. A receding chin may seem to be a minor problem and require only positioning the jaw forward (Fig. 13.9, recessed chin).[242] It is essential to establish that the jaw is not syndromically dislocated. If choanal atresia is present, because infants are obligatory nose breathers, it may be necessary to insert semipermanent nasal tubes so that the infant can be fed orally until an older age; definitive surgery may be necessary later. Once the

nasal tubes are in place, the infant can be placed at the breast. Feeding by any technique, however, is never easy. A cleft lip or palate may also be present.

Cleft lip and/or palate. Breastfeeding success for infants with cleft lip and/or palate largely depends on the infant's ability to create and maintain negative intraoral pressure to elongate the maternal nipple and hold it in this position (which stimulates let-down and positions the nipple to be expressed with the peristalsis of the infant's tongue)[243] (Table 13.4). It is generally agreed that the ability to generate negative pressure is related to the size and type of cleft.[244] Infants with larger clefts, bilateral clefts, and those including palates will have more difficulty establishing negative intraoral pressure, whereas those with isolated cleft lips will have more success. For instance, one study of 104 infants born at a Baby-Friendly Hospital in the Czech Republic with strong and specific breastfeeding support and neonatal lip repair and 100% breastfeeding initiation rate among subjects found that after surgery, 79% of infants with cleft lip were breastfed, as opposed to only 6% of those with a cleft lip and palate. Of this latter group, 65% continued to be fed expressed breast milk after surgery, thus showing the benefits of active breastfeeding support.[245]

When a cleft is part of a syndrome, other features of the suck/swallow/breathe mechanism may also be impaired.[246] Problems with intraoral muscular movements may be associated with bilateral cleft lip, which causes severe anterior projection of the premaxilla that precludes stabilizing the nipple; with wide palatal clefts, which offer no back guard for tongue movements; and retroplaced tongues that cannot compress the nipple effectively.[243]

Rooming-in after birth and normal newborn care with specialized feeding advice is becoming the standard of care for infants born with cleft lip and/or palate. The pediatric provider, plastic surgeon, and parents should work together as a team from the time of birth to determine a coordinated plan of treatment. The entire cleft lip and/or palate medical team can include many other specialists at different times—a dentist, lactation consultant, occupational therapist, speech therapist, and so forth. Some of the education surrounding options and support may be communicated before birth in the case of a cleft identified by prenatal ultrasound. It is important to make plans for feeding around the surgical plan. Unfortunately, the level of support parents receive to breastfeed or provide breast milk has been historically low and is likely to vary significantly by region.[247] In this study from Kansas, 18% of respondents ($N = 50$) reported being specifically discouraged by their health care team from providing breast milk to their infants with cleft lip and/or palate, whereas only 36% reported being encouraged to do so. Some surgeons have special protocols before and after surgery to ensure optimal healing. Because of these variations, Burca et al. completed a narrative review of the literature in 2016 with the goal of disseminating best practices for support of human milk feeding in the cleft lip/palate population.[248] The authors describe the bedside support needs for parents, including educational needs on the benefits of human milk, assessment of infant's sucking ability, positioning needs, and support

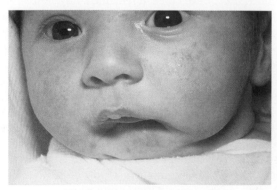

Fig. 13.9 Demonstration of a significantly receding chin. (From Biancuzzo M. *Breastfeeding the Newborn, Clinical Strategies for Nurses.* 2nd ed. St. Louis: Mosby; 2003.)

TABLE 13.4	Assessment of Sucking and Feeding Techniques for Infants With Clefts of Lip and Palate		
Condition	**ASSESSMENT**		**Feeding Techniques**
	Generation of Negative Pressure	**Ability to Make Mechanical Movements**	
Cleft lip and palate	−	±	Breastfeeding is unlikely. Deliver milk into infant's mouth.
Cleft palate only	±	+	Breastfeeding sometimes succeeds. Soft artificial nipples with large openings are effective. Infant may need delivery of milk into the mouth.
Cleft of soft palate	±	+	Breastfeeding or normal bottle-feeding usually works well.
Pierre–Robin syndrome	±	−	Breastfeeding is unlikely. Nipple position is critical. Many infants need delivery of milk into mouth.
Cleft lip only	±	+	Breastfeeding works well. Artificial nipple with large base works well.

+, Present; −, absent; ±, partial.
From Clarren SK, Anderson B, Wolf LS. Feeding infants with cleft lip, cleft palate, or cleft lip and palate. *Cleft Palate J.* 1987;24:244.

for maintenance of milk production. A lactation consultant, specifically a nurse or one well versed in interacting with complex medical teams, should be included to assist the parents in establishing and maintaining a milk supply, an issue perhaps more prevalent in this population than in others.[247]

The ABM has a clinical protocol on best practices to support breastfeeding for infants with cleft lip and palate, which was revised in 2019 and is available online.[244]

Cleft lip. A solitary cleft lip is usually repaired by 3 months of life, with neonatal repair becoming more common. With help, an infant with cleft lip can nurse at the breast if a seal around the areola can be created. Actually, the breast may fill the defect, and suckling may therefore go well. Alternatively, the mother may be able to put her thumb in the cleft to create a seal as she holds the breast to the infant's mouth. Good positioning is therefore critical, and positioning supports such as pillows or slings are helpful. A breast shield may also be tried, and different shapes and flexibilities of these devices exist. In most cases, the mother will need to pump after feedings to establish or maintain a milk supply. In some cases, the mother may have to express or pump milk and offer it by specialized bottle, dropper, or other means if suckling is ineffective. In most cases, the evidence supports immediate resumption of breastfeeding postoperatively.[244]

Cleft palate. The prognosis for successful feeding of an infant with a cleft palate depends on the size and position of the defect (soft palate, hard palate, laterality) as well as any associated lesions and the infant's neurodevelopment.[246] Each child will need their own assessments and unique plan, which may include breastfeeding, nipple shields (regular, cherry-top, or bottle-nipple style), supplemental feeding devices (feeding tubes directed to the maternal nipple), and specialized bottle nipples (Cleft Palate Nurser, Medela Special Needs Feeder/Haberman, Pigeon or Dr. Brown vented bottle). A mother may be able to feed directly from the breast by

holding the breast to her infant's mouth firmly between two fingers, as shown in Figs. 7.5, 13.1, and 13.2. Fig. 13.10 demonstrates angling the nipple toward the area of intact palate; the infant may then be able to milk the areola and nipple with the tongue pressing it against the roof of the mouth, even with the cleft. In this case, the breast must be held in position, just as a bottle must be held throughout the feeding.

If the child is able to gain weight by breastfeeding, with or without assistive devices, this should be encouraged to promote bonding and maternal milk supply. Feeding even once or twice a day at the breast, or for comfort, may theoretically help the infant to learn to feed at the breast after palatal repair. Pre- and postfeed weights may be helpful to determine the amount of milk transfer from the breast, and infants should be carefully watched for fatigue and weight gain. Generally, feedings should be completed within 45 minutes to avoid excess fatigue.

Oral orthopedic devices have been investigated for their use in infants with clefts, to assist with creating negative intraoral pressures to aid nursing, stimulate orofacial and dental development, develop the palatal shelves, prevent tongue distortions, prevent nasal septum irritation, improve phonation, and decrease the number of ear infections. Unfortunately, outcome studies have failed to confirm these theoretical benefits.[249,250] A multicenter randomized controlled trial conducted in the Netherlands with 6 years of follow-up, the DUTCHCLEFT, showed no benefits in the first 6 years of life (including no benefit to maternal satisfaction[251]) and lack of cost-effectiveness.[252] Negative intraoral pressures and improved breastfeeding have also not been demonstrated.[253]

Management and feeding plans continue to vary in the postoperative period. Some centers will use syringe or spoon-feeding for 3 to 5 days after surgery, although this is poorly supported in the literature.[246] The ABM's clinical protocol

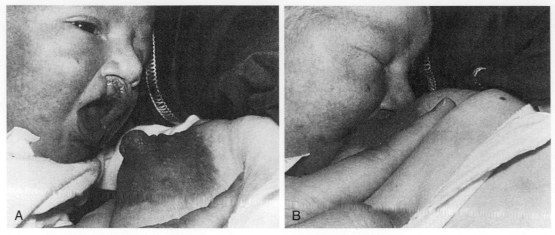

Fig. 13.10 (A) Infant with cleft lip and palate opening wide to latch on for a feeding. (B) Same infant suckling at breast. Defect in lip and palate is comfortably filled by breast tissue. (Photos obtained with assistance of Marie Biancuzzo, RN, MSN.)

states that breastfeeding should be resumed 1 day after surgery.[244] If an infant has been unable to feed at the breast, a family may desire to start breastfeeding after operative repair. Because infants are older at the time of a palate repair (around 12 months), they may need to be "retaught" to feed at the breast, which may or may not be behaviorally appropriate or successful.

Primarily Neurologic Feeding Difficulties
Discoordinated Suck

Although abnormal oral motor patterns are more common in premature infants and those who have been asphyxiated at birth, they may occur in infants without other risk factors as well. Up to 25% to 45% of infants and children with otherwise normal development may have a feeding problem, as compared with 80% of neurodevelopmentally delayed infants and children.[254] These difficulties may include problems along the entire feeding pathway: the suck; the swallowing process, including esophageal action; and the coordination of breathing. Fig. 13.11 by Dr. Chantal Lau outlines where the safety and efficiency of feeds may be interrupted along this pathway, along with some visual signs of the dysfunction.[255] Movements consistent with discoordinated suck include exaggerated tongue thrust, tonic bite, jaw thrust, jaw clenching, pulling away, and lip pursing. Passive signs of dysfunction may include spilling/drooling, reflux, clicking, gagging, aspiration/coughing, and/or oxygen desaturation.[255]

Infants with discoordinated suck should have a full exam to rule out other issues, especially ankyloglossia, which has many overlapping visual signs, and oral thrush, which may cause pain during feeding. Mothers should be evaluated for inverted or flat nipples and low milk supply or difficulty with let-down because these may exacerbate discoordinated suck. Mothers may also have secondary low milk supply as a result of ongoing poor milk transfer.

Treatments for discoordinated suck include encouraging nonnutritive sucking, adding cheek and/or chin support during feeding, or changing feeding positions (laid-back, side-

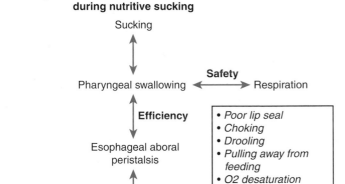

Examples of common "Visual" adverse events during nutritive sucking

Sucking

Pharyngeal swallowing ⟷ **Safety** ⟷ Respiration

Efficiency

Esophageal aboral peristalsis

- *Poor lip seal*
- *Choking*
- *Drooling*
- *Pulling away from feeding*
- *O2 desaturation*
- *Aspiration/penetration*
- *Reflux/vomit*
- *Feeding aversion*

Stomach

Fig. 13.11 Common Adverse events observable during the sucking process. (From Lau C. To individualize the management care of high-risk infants with oral feeding challenges: what do we know? What can we do? *Front Pediatr.* 2020;8:296. Epub 2020 Jun 9. https://doi.org/10.3389/fped.2020.00296.)

lying). Some infants will benefit from cup- or spoon-feeding (Fig. 13.12), and others will benefit from feeding therapy provided by speech—language pathologists or occupational therapists. There are case reports of chiropractors and massage therapists also treating infants with suck difficulties impairing breastfeeding. Hollerman, Nee, and Knapp review potential mechanisms in their case report of an infant whose suck dysfunction improved following chiropractic treatment.[256] For bottle-fed infants, similar supports and positioning may be used, and paced bottle-feeding or altering nipple flow rates may be considered.[256]

Tone abnormalities (hypertonia, hypotonia). Difficulty with latch may also be associated with postural muscle tone abnormalities. Little is known about the effects of hyper- and hypotonia on breastfeeding. However, normal muscle tone and strength throughout breastfeeding, especially alignment

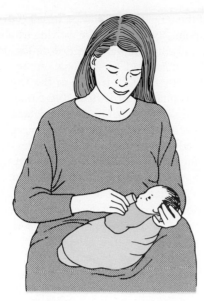

Fig. 13.12 When an infant must be fed but cannot be breastfed (e.g., when mother is ill), the infant can be fed using a small, soft medicine cup. The infant is swaddled and held semiupright, and the liquid is given inside the lower lip.

of the head and neck, are required to form a stable base to anchor the oral and pharyngeal musculature.

Hypertonic infants are usually overflexed or overextended and have hypertonic mouths with tonic bite, jaw thrusting, and clenching. Inducing relaxation with skin-to-skin care, ensuring a calm environment, minimizing handling, and using gentle strokes to calm the infant can be effective. If the infant is extended, flexion may be achieved with a pleat-seat carrier (see Fig. 13.2) or pillows. A flexed position in these infants relaxes the jaw and mouth and allows latching to take place. Finger feeding may help calm or train these infants. If done just before a feed, the infant can be transferred to the breast smoothly.

The ABM has a protocol on best practices for infant feeding with hypotonia.[257] Thomas et al. discuss methods that have been found to be helpful, including skin-to-skin care for state regulation, supportive holds, positioning aids (pillows, slings), "Dancer hold" (see Fig. 13.1), breast compressions during feeds and nipple shields. Mothers' milk supply should be supported with expression because milk transfer is at risk; therefore milk supply may decrease over time.

Oral tactile sensitivity/oral aversion. Infants who have not been able to orally feed after birth as a result of illness or prematurity may develop oral tactile hypersensitivity or even oral aversion. These generally result from repeated negative oral experiences, such as tube placements (e.g., nasogastric, endotracheal), painful procedures, esophagitis, or nausea/vomiting.[258] Signs of oral aversion include turning away from oral stimuli, pursed lips when touched, tongue thrusting (rather than a coordinated suck reflex), and feeding rejection. These infants often lack positive oral experiences, including breastfeeding. They may also have a limited perception of hunger because of their illness or immaturity.

Several interventions have been shown to reduce oral aversion in the ICU setting. Positive oral stimulation without early feeding (e.g., nonnutritive sucking on an expressed breast or pacifier, colostrum care) and offering the normal stimuli of feeding at the same time as a bolus tube feed (sight, smell, position, social interaction, satiety) are preferred methods to help infants transition to oral feeds.[259] Conversely, feeding infants before they demonstrate feeding cues, "urged" or "forced" bottle-feeding, and noxious smells all contribute to worsening.[260] To limit these, feeding by gavage tube at the end of an oral feeding is preferable to "urging" a child to finish a feed at the bottle.

Skin-to-skin care, or kangaroo care, and encouraging feeding experiences at the breast both provide positive experiences that counteract the negative but often necessary procedures infants experience in the intensive care setting. Nonnutritive suckling, licking, or play at an expressed breast can occur as soon as an infant is extubated and stable and has shown safety as early as 28 weeks. This method combines all the normal stimuli of feeding as described previously: positioning and warmth, parental smell and image, taste of the nipple, social interaction with the parent, and satiety from a bolus tube feed that can be given concurrently. It is therefore unsurprising that nonnutritive suckling at the breast lowers stress in preterm infants and their mothers while improving breastfeeding rates.[260] A breastfeeding-only approach has been proposed as a method to improve breastfeeding rates for preterm infants on discharge and throughout the first year of life. This approach includes supplementing infants with cup or tube feeds in addition to early feeding at the breast and avoiding the use of bottles entirely. A Cochrane review from 2016 demonstrated low- to moderate-quality evidence that this approach improves breastfeeding rates and does not prolong hospital length of stay.[261]

In full-term healthy infants, breast aversion may be confused with a strong arching reflex. This is elicited by touching or applying pressure on the back of the head, causing the infant to arch back away from the breast. Positions that require the mother to hold the head (e.g., "football" or "cross-cradle") may trigger this reflex. Patients should be reminded to hold the infant at the base of the skull where it meets the neck, rather than holding the posterior parietal scalp. A laid-back position may also be helpful for infants who have a strong arching reflex because little support for the head is required in this position. Pillows can be used for support of the baby or the mother's arms.

A nursing "strike," when an otherwise healthy infant suddenly and inexplicably refuses to breastfeed, may also be confused with oral aversion. Nursing strikes are covered in Chapters 7 and 9.

Suck dysfunction that is not tongue-tie or lip tie. A small proportion of infants will be evaluated and treated by a multidisciplinary panel of experts from allopathic, complementary, and chiropractic disciplines and still not be able to transfer milk or do so without hurting mothers. These infants represent a conundrum, which in the past would be solved by giving a bottle of formula. However, many mothers remain deeply committed to breastfeeding and will continue to express milk to feed by bottle or express and feed at the breast as well (triple feeding: breastfeed, express, bottle-feed). There is an urgent need for research into the potential causes of these cases.

INTESTINAL TRACT DISORDERS

Tracheoesophageal Fistula and Esophageal Atresia

Esophageal atresia (EA) with or without tracheoesophageal fistula (TEF) is a congenital malformation resulting from abnormal foregut separation. It is uncommon, with estimated prevalence rates for EA/TEF ranging from 1.27 to 4.55 per 10,000 births.[262] There are five generally accepted types of EA/TEF with varying degrees of esophageal atresia and varying position of the fistula. Even with this complexity, the diagnosis is commonly made in the first month of life with cough, choking, cyanosis, difficulty feeding, and/or signs of intestinal obstruction. Suspecting the diagnosis is urgent to make the infant NPO to prevent aspiration, to complete the assessment of the anatomic defects, and to plan the appropriate, timely surgical intervention. If there is aspiration, this complicates the presurgical preparation and can lead to prolonged parenteral nutrition before surgery. Prematurity, LBW, and the presence of additional congenital anomalies are associated with mortality and can complicate the management. Postoperative complications are common despite improvements in intensive care, nutrition, respiratory support, antibiotics, and surgical techniques.[262–264] Establishing effective breastfeeding in the presurgical period with the common presenting symptoms can be difficult. If the mother wants to breastfeed the infant, she should be assisted and supported in expressing or pumping and storing her breast milk (mother's own milk [MOM]) for use either via a gastrostomy tube or when the infant can take oral feedings. Donor human milk is an alternative. Salvatori et al. in Rome reviewed 25 cases of infants with EA whose mothers breastfed after birth, 60% with exclusive human milk feeds, mother's milk, or donor milk.[265] At hospital discharge, 24% were exclusively breastfeeding, 36% were mixed feeding, and 40% were exclusively formula-feeding. At 3 months, 12% were exclusively breastfeeding, 28% were mixed feeding, and 60% were exclusively formula-feeding. The most common reported reason for stopping breastfeeding at 3 months was gastroesophageal reflux disease (GERD).[265] Fiber-optic endoscopic evaluation of swallowing (FEES), which uses a transnasal flexible fiber-optic laryngoscope to visualize the pharynx and larynx during swallowing, has been recommended to evaluate these infants.[266] The procedure is safe, effective, and the only study that can assess swallowing in infants while breastfeeding.[267]

There are no trials comparing breast milk and infant formula in nutritional support of the infant with EA/TEF. The vast majority of reports on the management of EA/TEF do not comment on infant growth or nutritional assessments. Schneider et al. reported on 301 infants with esophageal atresia followed for 1 year in the French National Esophageal Atresia register. Although 219 infants achieved exclusive oral feeding at discharge from the hospital, 15% of those patients were undernourished at that time, and there was no information provided on the use of breast milk versus infant formula.[263] Friedmacher et al. followed up on 109 consecutive patients with EA/TEF born from 1975 to 2011 at a single

center.[262] Of the 92 patients followed up for 3 to 27 years at the last time point, 89 (96.7%) were thriving with normal oral feedings. No information was provided on the use of breast milk or infant formula.[262] Sulkowski et al. reported on 3479 patients with EA/TEF treated in the United States at 43 children's hospitals from 1999 to 2012 based on data from the Pediatric Health Information System database.[268] Thirty-seven percent of the infants were premature, and 83.5% had one or more additional congenital anomalies, with cardiac anomalies being the most common. Within 2 years of the initial diagnosis and management hospitalization, 54.7% were readmitted, 5.2% had a repeat TEF ligation, 11.4% had a repeat operation to reconstruct the esophagus, and 11.7% had a fundoplication. No data were available on enteral feeding and infant nutritional status. The European Society for Pediatric Gastroenterology, Hepatology and Nutrition and North American Society for Pediatric Gastroenterology, Hepatology, and Nutrition (ESPGHAN-NASPGHAN) published guidelines in 2016 for the evaluation and treatment of children with EA/TEF. They analyzed evidence-based data on 36 clinical questions covering the management of EA/TEF, including the issues of abnormal feeding behaviors and the risk of malnutrition.[269] Puntis et al. reported in 1990 on the results of a detailed questionnaire on feeding history and growth for 124 children after EA/TEF repair of 230 families who received the questionnaire.[270] Fifty-eight of 124 infants (46.7%) were breastfed for a median of 3.0 months. There was no comparison of the nutritional status or growth for breastfed and formula-fed infants. There were height and weight measurements for 100 children, of which 19 were stunted based on height-for-weight standard deviation (SD) score, 9 were wasted based on weight-for-height SD score, and 4 were both wasted and stunted. Duerloo et al. reported on 371 consecutive patients treated for EA at a single center without information on enteral feeding. Long term, 7% of the children were at less than the 5th percentile for height and weight.[271] Legrand et al. followed 81 children with type C esophageal atresia for a median 13.3 years, of which 75% had a normal BMI, 16% were obese, and 9% were underweight by BMI.[272]

Given what we already understand about the benefits of breastfeeding or providing human breast milk to infants, the use of MOM or donor human milk for infants with EA/TEF is recommended when enteral feeding or oral feeding is indicated. A lactation consultant and a physician who specializes in breastfeeding should be part of the multidisciplinary team involved in the care of these infants.

Gastroesophageal Reflux and GERD

Gastroesophageal reflux is persistent nonprojectile, postprandial vomiting or regurgitation. Although less common than in bottle-fed infants, esophageal reflux can occur in exclusively breastfed infants. Simple spitting up without discomfort or failure to thrive does not require treatment. However, when reflux is suspected in the etiology of growth delay or causes discomfort, it should be investigated and managed.

GERD is when symptoms or complications occur, including regurgitation, vomiting, poor weight gain, pain, esophagitis, or respiratory problems such as apnea, especially seen in newborns. For breastfed infants with pathologic reflux, crying often begins toward the end of the feeding or after the infant falls asleep and is put down, only to wake up crying inconsolably. Infants may arch their backs, spit up through the nose, or have difficulty settling after a feed. The diagnosis can be confirmed by an esophageal probe test for reflux or by a trial of therapy with omeprazole or ranitidine. On occasion, this type of reflux is a sign of food protein intolerance, and the infant may improve after a maternal elimination diet (see previous discussion). Two cohort studies have seen an association with tongue-tie (see section on ankyloglossia).

Feeding in a sitting position (upright, Dancer hold), or partially laid-back may cause fewer symptoms than football or side-lying positions. Some infants may require frequent breaks to burp, particularly if they frequently lose suction at the breast and thus take in more air. This may be true for infants who "click" when they feed or have on/off behaviors and difficulty staying latched. Although infants who are fed breast milk are less likely to have symptomatic reflux than those fed artificial breast-milk substitutes, bottle-feeding breast milk may also result in more air swallowed during a feed. Parents are advised to keep the infant upright for 30 minutes after a feed, and sleeping in a semiupright position is often palliative.

Pyloric Stenosis

Infantile hypertrophic pyloric stenosis (IHPS) occurs in about 2 to 5 of 1000 live births. A family tendency exists, but the disease is more common in firstborn boys. Usually it occurs between the second and sixth weeks of life, although it can occur any time after birth. Vomiting is characteristic, is intermittent at first, and progresses to include every feeding and is often projectile. These infants are eager feeders and go back for more milk until the weight loss and dehydration make them anxious and irritable.

The risk of pyloric stenosis has reportedly decreased in different reports from the United States, Taiwan, and Nigeria.[273–275] During that time, the incidence of breastfeeding has increased; however, this decline is more likely to be multifactorial. The cause of pyloric stenosis remains elusive, although various factors have been considered (formula-feeding vs. breastfeeding, male gender, exposure to erythromycin [or macrolides], seasons of weather, infectious etiologies, or genetics). Several reviews of the relationship of pyloric stenosis to bottle-feeding (i.e., formula based on bovine milk) have been published. One of the larger studies was from the Danish National Birth Cohort involving 101,000 births from 1996 to 2002.[276] Of that number, 70,000 were singleton births, among which there were 65 infants with the diagnosis of pyloric stenosis requiring surgery. The risk was 4.6 times greater for the formula-fed infants compared with infants not formula-fed in the Danish study.[276] The second study, from Washington State, involved records from January 2003 to December 31, 2009, of 714 infants with a diagnosis of hypertrophic pyloric stenosis.[277] The odds ratio of increased risk

as a result of bottle-feeding was 2.31 (95% CI 1.81 to 2.95). In this study, bottle-feeding versus breastfeeding was "established" at the time of discharge after birth such that the exposure preceded the occurrence of IHPS. The investigators assumed bottle-feeding was equivalent to formula-feeding and did not correct for the potential that infants were fed human milk via bottle or switched from one group to the other after discharge home after birth. The risk remained even with adjustment for other variables (gender, maternal smoking status), although it was modified by maternal age and parity (higher risk with mothers ≥ 35 years old of multiparous. The Danish study noted a six-fold risk of stenosis in never breastfeeding and a five-fold risk of stenosis when switched to formula-feeding from breastfeeding. Male predominance was striking, but the protective factor of breastfeeding was the most consistent finding.[276] Other recent studies report an association between formula-feeding or mixed bottle-feeding with the risk of pyloric stenosis.[278,279] Another large study (case control) including 882 cases of hypertrophic pyloric stenosis and 955 controls demonstrated 1.36-times-greater risk for formula-fed infants versus breastfed infants (relative risk [RR] 1.36, 95% CI 1.18 to 1.57).[280] A meta-analysis from 2017 analyzed 15 studies for perinatal risk factors for IHPS.[281] Being firstborn, cesarean section delivery, preterm birth, and bottle-feeding were associated with IHPS occurrence. Bottle-feeding was the most significant based on odds ratio (OR 2.46, 95% CI 1.76 to 3.43) in this study, although the authors critiqued the included studies for their retrospective nature and poor statistical adjustments in the different studies. They also did not specifically assess how the individual studies defined bottle-feeding (as formula-feeding) or simply bottle-feeding being not breastfeeding. An infectious case of pyloric stenosis in infants seems unlikely based on a few studies including *Helicobacter pylori*, and various viruses (RSV, influenza A and B, adenovirus, metapneumovirus, parainfluenza viruses, rhinovirus and coronavirus [OC43 and 229E]), although large, well-controlled trials have not been performed to look for infectious etiologies.[282,283] The use of macrolide antibiotics in the infant in the first weeks to month(s) of life carries an increased risk of developing infantile hypertrophic pyloric stenosis based on a large cohort study in the United States and two different systematic reviews and meta-analyses of retrospective studies and randomized controlled trials.[284–286] There remains a significant amount of heterogeneity between the various studies included in these reviews. Maternal use of macrolides during breastfeeding, especially in the first 2 weeks after birth, seems to increase the risk of IHPS in the infant, but the risk of IHPS after fetal exposure through maternal ingestion during pregnancy is not as clear.[285,287] A risk–benefit analysis and decision should be discussed concerning the use of a macrolide medication by a breastfeeding mother in the first 2 to 6 weeks after birth. With the 4 to 5 times greater risk in males versus females and an apparent intrafamily association with IHPS, contributing genetic factors have also been examined. Neuronal nitric oxide synthase (nNOS) polymorphisms have not shown a significant association with IHPS. Genome-wide analysis has identified a number of possible loci associated with IHPS. Further investigation of these loci and the significance is indicated.[288,289]

In the investigation of vomiting, it is important to keep in mind that overfeeding can cause spitting and vomiting, even projectile vomiting, but it is not associated with weight loss, decreased urine and stools, and dehydration. Therapy for IHPS consists of pyloromyotomy after correction of the dehydration and associated electrolyte abnormalities. If the procedure is uncomplicated (i.e., intestinal lumen was not entered), the infant can be given enteral feeds on an ad libitum regimen and can go back to the breast in 6 to 8 hours.[290,291] The mother should pump every 3 hours until the infant can be fed. The breastfed infant may be discharged in 24 hours if nursing has gone well. If the duodenum is entered at the time of surgery, gastric decompression and IV fluids may be necessary, and oral feeding may be delayed several days until signs of healing occur. A breastfed infant may resume nursing earlier than a bottle-fed infant returns to formula because of the rapid emptying time of the stomach and the zero curd tension of the breast milk.[290]

Disorders of the Small Intestine

Disorders such as duodenal obstruction, malrotation, jejunal obstruction, and duplications require surgery. Depending on the extent of the lesion, whether the bowel wall is opened, whether bowel segments are removed, and whether associated lesions (e.g., annular pancreas) are present, an infant will need postoperative maintenance on IV fluids and possibly parenteral alimentation. In a study of early postoperative feeding in infants with duodenal atresia ($N = 10$), malrotation ($N = 6$), and jejunal atresia ($N = 1$), enteral feeding was started by postoperative day 2 in 14 cases. Breast milk was the most common nutrient source (numbers and amounts not given). Thirteen infants were discharged (one died of sepsis).[292] A second, larger, more recent retrospective analysis from Baltimore, Maryland, followed 111 infants after gastrointestinal surgery.[293] Intestinal diagnoses included NEC (21), gastroschisis (28), atresia (27), spontaneous intestinal perforation (SIP; 18), and 17 other diagnoses. The majority of infants (77%) were given mother's milk as the first feeding postoperatively. Donor human milk was most frequently utilized after NEC and SIP (11%). Forty-four percent of infants were receiving mother's milk at discharge, and 25% were still receiving it at 1 year of age. Fifty-eight percent of infants had feeding tubes (35% nasogastric, 23% gastric) at discharge. Infants were discharged showing appropriate weight gain, but infants who had NEC or SIP more commonly exhibited growth failure at 3 months, but they were able to grow appropriately at 1 year of age. In a study of human milk versus formula after gastroschisis repair, exclusive human milk feedings led to shorter times to full enteral feeds (5 versus 7 days, $p = 0.03$) and shorter times from initiation of feedings to hospital discharge (7 versus 10 days, $p = 0.01$).[294] A mother who has expressed milk for her sick infant may or may not have ever nursed the infant before surgery, depending on the time of onset of symptoms and their severity. Families should be counseled about the prognosis, and mothers should be encouraged to express milk manually and by pump to provide milk for the infant postoperatively until the time when the infant may be able to feed at the breast. Support for breastfeeding or expressing milk should come from family, the medical team, and especially a lactation consultant to optimize milk production and transfer. Frequently, infants with atresia are also small or premature and have protracted recovery periods because of the removal of a considerable amount of the intestinal tract. If the infant will be breastfed, breast milk can be introduced earlier than formula. Short-gut syndrome requires special management, but human milk is usually tolerated, and donor milk should be obtained if the mother is unable to provide sufficient breast milk. In the study by Varma et al., approximately one-third of infants were still dependent on some form of feeding tube at 1 year postsurgery.[302] There are several areas in which feeding difficulty can arise in these postsurgical infants: feeding intolerance (dysmotility, gastroesophageal reflux, malabsorption, short-gut syndrome, dependency of a feeding tube), diminished milk transfer (insufficient amount for growth; breastfeeding, expressed milk, or use of donor milk), and difficulty with oral feeding (altered muscle tone, delayed development of effective suck-swallow-breathe coordination, feeding aversions). Parenteral nutrition—associated cholestasis (PNAS) and intestinal failure—associated liver disease (IFALD) in infants postgastrointestinal surgery are additional complications related to the prolonged use of parenteral nutrition after intestinal surgery. Various groups have evaluated early postoperative feeding and standardized feeding guidelines in attempts to reduce PNAS and IFALD and improve overall outcomes. Shores et al. demonstrated a decreased incidence of IFALD after initiating a standard regimen for enteral nutrition (beginning volume = 20 mL/kg per day, with daily increases in volume as tolerated).[295] The preguideline cohort ($N = 83$) was historical, and postguideline ($N = 81$) data were collected prospectively. The odds of developing IFALD (moderate to severe) were decreased by 72% (OR 0.28, 95% CI 0.13 to 0.58). Shakeel et al. reviewed postoperative intestinal surgery feeding guidelines and outcomes before and after the initiation of the guidelines.[296] Breast milk was used as the first enteral feeding in 80% of cases in the postguideline cohort and in 65% of cases in the pre-guideline cohort. At discharge, 40% of infants were receiving breast milk postguidelines, 32% were receiving regular formula, 14% were receiving hydrolysate, and 16% were receiving elemental formula. Time to achieving 50% and 100% of calories via enteral feeds also decreased (from 10 to 6 days and 35 to 21 days, respectively).[295] Decreases in the use of parenteral nutrition, length of stay, and central line—associated bloodstream infections also occurred with the standard enteral nutrition guidelines.[296] Otherwise, there is a paucity of data with high-quality prospective studies examining postsurgical outcomes with early enteral feeds or comparing breast milk and (cow-based) formulas. Breast milk (MOM or donor milk) should remain the first choice for feeding infants after GI surgery.[297]

Disorders of the Colon

Disorders of the colon occur more often in full-term infants. Hirschsprung's disease, or congenital aganglionic megacolon, is one of the more common lesions. Passage of meconium is usually delayed; however, only 10% to 15% of all children with delayed passage of meconium have Hirschsprung's disease. Constipation and abdominal distention are the most frequent initial symptoms. They may begin during the first few days of life and gradually progress to include bilious vomiting. The clinical picture may be indistinguishable from meconium ileus, ileal atresia, or large bowel obstruction. In any infant with perforation of the colon, ileum, or appendix, Hirschsprung's disease should be considered. A breastfed infant may have milder symptoms and delayed onset of real distress because of smaller volumes of feeds in the first couple of days, and breast-milk stools are normally loose and seedy and more easily passed. Enterocolitis may occur at any age and is the major cause of death.

No data have been found to distinguish the incidence of this complication in breastfed and bottle-fed infants. The treatment depends on the symptoms, x-ray findings, and biopsy results for the identification of the aganglionic segment. Colostomy is usually done at the time of diagnosis, with definitive surgery later in the first year of life. Feedings can be resumed as soon as the infant is stable, after the colostomy is healing sufficiently to permit bowel activity. Human milk has the same advantages for early postoperative feeding in this disease as well because of its antiinfective properties, antiinflammatory factors/effects, and easy digestibility.[298] The use of human milk could play an important role in enhanced recovery after surgery (ERAS) and immune-nutrition as part of ERAS after colorectal surgery.[298,299]

Meconium plug syndrome and meconium ileus

Meconium plug syndrome and meconium ileus are less common and less severe in breastfed infants who have received a full measure of colostrum, which has a cathartic effect and stimulates the passage of meconium. There are data from one study in Italy that demonstrated an increased risk of a negative outcome for nonbreastfed infants with meconium ileus and cystic fibrosis (OR 2.921).[116] If either disorder is diagnosed, an infant should continue to nurse in addition to any other treatment, which should include an assessment for CF and pancreatic insufficiency. Additional genetic studies may be appropriate for a specific infant and family. One retrospective study in Wisconsin compared growth and pulmonary outcomes through the first 2 years of life for formula-fed and breastfed infants with CF. Breastfeeding was common (51%), but exclusive breastfeeding was less common and short (< 1 month in 53% of the breastfed infants, 1 to 1.9 months in 21%, 2 to 3 months in 17%, and 4 to 9 months in 9%).[111] Infants exclusively breastfed for <2 months did not have difficulty with growth, although exclusive breastfeeding for more than 2 months and pancreatic insufficiency did affect weight z-score growth through 6 months of age. Exclusively breastfed infants had fewer $P.$ $aeruginosa$ infections through 2 years of age than formula-fed infants ($p = 0.003$).

Imperforate anus and other anorectal malformations

Anorectal malformations (ARMs) are another common congenital problem with a spectrum of anatomic presentations.

Individualized treatment is dependent on the specific anatomic defects and potential surgical reconstructions. Cardiac, renal, orthopedic, spinal, sacral, and gynecologic anomalies can be associated with ARMs, and screening for vertebral defects, cardiac, tracheoesophageal fistula, and renal and limb abnormalities (VACTERL) abnormalities is important before surgical intervention. IV fluids, antibiotics, and nasogastric decompression occur in conjunction with the additional evaluation. The type of malformation and sacral and spinal abnormalities will affect bowel motility, anal sensation, and continence. Strictures, insufficient blood supply, wound infection, and dehiscence occur as postoperative complications. There are no studies comparing breast milk to formula in the postoperative period, but the known benefits of breast milk make it the most appropriate first choice for nutrition. Infants may be breastfed as soon as any bowel activity can be permitted, often 2 to 3 days postoperatively.

Gastrointestinal bleeding. The most common cause of vomiting blood or passing blood via the rectum in a breastfed infant is a bleeding nipple in the mother, which may or may not be painful. Any time fresh blood is found in the vomitus or stool of any newborn, the blood should be tested for adult or fetal Hb. If adult Hb, it indicates the source is maternal. This is done by a qualitative test, the Apt test.

Mix RBCs with 2 to 3 mL normal saline solution, and add this mixture to 3 mL of 10% NaOH (0.25 M). Mix gently. Observe for color change. Fetal Hb is stable in alkali and will remain pink, whereas adult Hb turns brown. Use a known adult sample as a color control. If the blood is adult Hb in a breastfed infant, the possibility of a cracked and bleeding nipple should be ruled out by examining the sample of expressed milk for color and guaiac and inspection of the maternal breast (see Chapter 7).

If the blood is fetal Hb, the differential diagnosis for bleeding in any neonate should be followed. Breastfeeding can be maintained unless a lesion requiring surgery is identified. More than 50% of cases of GI bleeding in the neonate go undiagnosed. Anorectal fissure is an uncommon cause in breastfed infants. Allergy to human milk itself has been reported as a cause of intestinal bleeding.[300] The distribution of causes of intestinal bleeding in the neonate, without selection for type of feeding, is as follows: idiopathic, 50%; hemorrhagic disorders, 20%; swallowed maternal blood, 10%; anorectal fissures, 10%; intestinal ischemia, 5%; and colitis, 5%. When the bleeding occurs beyond the newborn period, colitis (see previous discussion in this chapter) becomes a more frequent cause, as does Meckel's diverticulum. Sullivan has reviewed the subject of cow's milk–induced intestinal bleeding in infancy.[300]

Congenital chylothorax

Congenital chylothorax, although uncommon, is the most common cause of pleural effusion in the newborn period. It affects the respiratory, nutritional, and immunologic systems and is potentially life-threatening. Most cases are single abnormalities, but congenital chylothorax may be associated with other anomalies, lymphangiectasia, or neuroblastoma. Management includes mechanical ventilation, transthoracic drainage, surgical drainage, parenteral nutrition, feeding with medium-chain triglyceride formula, close monitoring of absolute lymphocyte count and chest tube output, and administration of octreotide. Parenteral nutrition and mechanical ventilation seem to have improved outcomes. If diagnosed prenatally, transabdominal thoracocentesis can be done and delivery initiated after 32 weeks. The chest can be tapped or put to continuous drainage.

Nutrition most frequently starts with total parenteral nutrition (TPN). Enteral feedings are started as soon as possible (5 to 7 days) using breast milk, medium-chain triglyceride—enriched formula, or regular formula. If the chylothorax worsens, oral feeds are often stopped for another 3 to 7 days and then restarted with a special medium-chain triglyceride-rich formula (e.g., Pregestimil) and later returning to breast milk or regular formula.

In a retrospective study by Al-Tawil et al., 19 infants were reviewed; 18 were followed for 7 years and were successfully managed after 7 weeks with breastfeeding or regular formula.[301] In another study, infants managed with TPN ($N = 9$) recovered more rapidly (mean 10 days) than those treated with medium-chain triglycerides ($N = 8$; mean 23 days). TPN treatment permitted progression to earlier oral feeds and earlier breastfeeding.[302] Iatrogenic chylothorax management is not as simple and may take weeks of TPN and then the use of defatted breast milk. Defatted human milk was used in seven infants with chylous pleural effusion.[303] Mother's milk was placed in a clear 240-mL container and centrifuged at 3000 rotations per minute for 15 minutes at 2°C in a Beckman J2-21 High-Speed Floor Model Centrifuge. The solidified-fat top layer was separated from the liquid portion. The liquid portion was poured into clean cups and frozen for later use. Before and after samples were tested for fat, sodium, potassium, calcium, and zinc. Mean fat removal was 5 g/dL. The infants started on the milk after a month of age for an average of 16 days (7 to 34 days) (Tables 13.5 and 13.6). No reaccumulation of the chylous pleural effusion was observed.[303]

Intensivists and neonatologists have recognized the value of human milk and have reported the practice of defatting human milk for infants with congenital as well as iatrogenic chylothorax.[304] The Children's Hospital of Philadelphia (CHOP) opened a Human Milk Management Center.[304] Skim milk is prepared by their milk technicians utilizing a cold centrifuge (Thermo Fisher Scientific l ST 16). Milk is spun at 4000 rpm for 20 minutes. The center reported on 29 infants with chylothorax over 23 months. Chylothorax was a result of congenital diaphragmatic hernia and congenital cardiac defects that were repaired surgically. Skim milk was used for an average of 16 days (range 1 to 85 days). All milk used had a creamatocrit of less than 1%. The authors concluded that a standard skim milk protocol allowed infants to continue the additional benefits of MOM. Surgical chylothorax in neonates was reviewed from the literature by Costa and Saxena.[303] It was associated with congenital diaphragmatic hernia (CDH; $N = 76$), cardiac malformations ($N = 25$), esophageal atresia ($N = 5$), and one other condition. The use of medium-chain triglycerides was the first treatment in 52 neonates, TPN was used in 51 patients, and 3 patients required no treatment. Octreotide and somatostatin were utilized as the next line of therapy, and 15 patients had 17

TABLE 13.6 Composition of Human Milk Before and After Fat Removal (Mean ± SD)

	Before	After
Fat (g/dL)	5 ± 1	0
Sodium (mEq/L)	40 ± 9	42 ± 9
Potassium (mEq/L)	15 ± 3	14 ± 3
Calcium (mg/dL)	25 ± 4	27 ± 2
Zinc (mcg/dL)	294 ± 135	385 ± 130
Total volume (mL)	100 ± 1	95 ± 1

SD, Standard deviation.
Source of data: Chan GM and Lechtenberg E. The use of fat-free human milk in infants with chylous pleural effusion. *J Perinatol.* 2007;27(7):434—436. https://doi.org/10.1038/sj.jp.7211768. Epub 2007 Jun 7.

TABLE 13.5 Clinical Summary of Infants With Chylothorax

Patient	Gestation (wks)	Birth Weight (g)	Diagnosis	Age FFM Started	Duration of FFM	Supplements Used
1	37	2780	Congenital	5 wks	11 days	Pregestimil
2	31	1681	Congenital	5 mo	34 days	Pregestimil MCT
3	36	2050	Acquired CHD repair	7 wks	14 days	TPN + Intralipid
4	40	3040	Acquired CHD repair	8 mo	21 days	Portagen ProMod
5	39	3430	Acquired CHD repair	2 mo	11 days	MCT glucose polymers
6	33	2750	Congenital	2 mo	7 days	MCT glucose polymers
7	39	3293	Acquired CDH repair	1 mo	14 days	TPN + Intralipid

CDH, Congenital diaphragmatic hernia; *CHD*, congenital heart disorder; *FFM*, fat-free milk; *MCT*, medium-chain triglycerides; *TPN*, total parenteral nutrition.
Source of data: Chan GM and Lechtenberg E. The use of fat-free human milk in infants with chylous pleural effusion. *J Perinatol.* 2007;27(7):434—436. https://doi.org/10.1038/sj.jp.7211768. Epub 2007 Jun 7.

surgeries. Concheiro-Guisan et al. reviewed the literature for the use of defatted human milk in the treatment of congenital chylothorax.[306] They reported only two small controlled trials, one retrospective study, and some laboratory testing data. The data they reported suggest that modified-defatted breast milk does contribute to the resolution of chylothorax in neonates. They described the simple procedure of defatting human milk to a fat concentration of ideally <0.5 g fat per/100 mL (comparable to medium-chain triglyceride—enriched formula). The studies used modified human milk with fat concentrations of <1 g/100 mL. The authors recommend additional clinical trials to establish the duration and level of long-chain triglyceride removal for the effective and safe management of chylothorax (congenital, iatrogenic, and surgical). Fat measurement in the modified milk and fortification of the milk with protein and other nutrients may be necessary to ensure appropriate growth, especially in the premature or sick neonate.

Congenital Dislocation of Hip as a Prototype for Breastfeeding a Child Undergoing Unanticipated Treatments

When procedures or treatments need to be initiated for an infant previously thought to be normal, breastfeeding may not go smoothly. Using congenital dislocation of the hip as a prototype, Elander looked at overall breastfeeding success.[307] Compared with a randomly chosen control group of 113 infants, the 30 study infants who required the von Rosen splint were less successfully fed. However, a higher incidence of cesarean deliveries was seen in the study group (30% vs. 4%). The groups had equal numbers of primiparas (50% vs. 48%). After breastfeeding was established, the long-range success rate was no different. Mothers were pleased to be able to do something special for their splinted children (i.e., breastfeed). This would suggest that special support and guidance regarding breastfeeding issues may be needed, along with details on how to apply the splint and how to cope with the splint while positioning for breastfeeding. Considering this as an example of events or health issues interfering with successful breastfeeding, detailed attention to the basic steps of instruction and support of breastfeeding is indicated. Mothers should be given additional opportunity to review how breastfeeding is going with a lactation consultant, discuss how life and support of the mother and breastfeeding are going at home, and most importantly, discuss any concerns the mother has about breastfeeding and how the maternal-infant dyad is succeeding or having difficulties. The specific issues should be clarified for each infant and mother, potential solutions discussed, breastfeeding goals reviewed, and a plan for ongoing support and follow-up established. Given the variability in health issues, breastfeeding goals, and maternal concerns, this should be a very patient-centered, "personalized," and supportive process.

Congenital Torticollis

Congenital torticollis is another example of a musculoskeletal abnormality that often presents in the neonatal period and can severely affect positioning, latch, and suck for breastfeeding and lead to later complications for the infant. Postural torticollis (positional with "mild" muscle tightness), congenital muscular torticollis (palpable muscle tightness, head tilt, and often restricted movement), and sternocleidomastoid (SCM) tumor or pseudotumor are a rough continuum and constitute important components of severity and prognosis. A detailed classification system and practice guidelines have been established by the Section on Pediatrics of the American Physical Therapy Association.[308] Early diagnosis; screening for other physical abnormalities (facial asymmetry, concomitant spinal and hip asymmetries, SCM tumor and fibrosis, etc.); complete assessment by physical therapy, occupational therapy, and speech therapy; and assessment of the infant feeding plan and process are essential. There is often an intrauterine history of "malposition," breech position, and difficulties with delivery as a result of one of these. The infants are frequently described as "fussy, irritable infants with poor self-calming skills and low tolerance for positional changes and stimulation."[309] Early initiation of therapy along with assessment should include passive stretching, posturing with support to correct position, active rotation exercises, and positioning during feeding. Assistance with positioning, latch, and milk transfer should be initiated as soon as the condition is diagnosed. Personalization of the instruction and support should be fluid, with "trial and error" for the individual mother and infant pair. C. W. Genna, an IBCLC who has investigated breastfeeding infants with congenital torticollis, points out that breast refusal is common, as are feeding difficulties.[310] Wei et al. noted feeding difficulty in 4/170 infants (2.4%).[311] Genna emphasizes a "right-brain approach" to assisting the mother and infant in finding different effective positions that fit for latch and milk transfer and are manageable for the mother and infant. She describes unique positions for breastfeeding the infant with torticollis she has found helpful: torticollis tummy twist, spiderman (hip straddle), belly sit, and arm lie. Images of these positions are presented in a manuscript and on her website (http://cwgenna.com/clinicalcornerpage.html).[310] She recommends close observation of the mother—infant breastfeeding process, including suck and suck-swallow-breathe and milk transfer. Although these recommendations have not been tested in a published clinical trial, Genna reinforces a personalized approach and offers suggestions for parenting practices that soothe and calm the infant (frequent carrying, tummy time on the chest, interactive play to stimulate bilateral active movement, repositioning during sleep) and close collaboration with physical therapy, occupational therapy, and the infant's entire treatment team.

MALFORMATIONS OF CENTRAL NERVOUS SYSTEM

Malformations of the central nervous system (CNS) diagnosed at birth include a broad clinical spectrum from anencephaly and complete craniorachischisis to dermal sinuses. Defects of the spinal column range from complete spinal rachischisis to spina bifida occulta. A mother who had planned to breastfeed an infant with an inoperable condition or for whom breastfeeding is incompatible with life is presented with the additional problem of coping with her desire to nurse her infant. If an infant is to be given normal newborn care and the mother desires to nurse this infant, breastfeeding should be discussed by the pediatrician and parents together. It has been demonstrated that parents grieve more "physiologically" if they have contact with their abnormal infant before the infant's death. This allows the parent to see and potentially understand the actual abnormalities of development rather than what their imagination might create.[312] A professional's personal bias for how to deal with the infant should not overshadow the discussion with the parents. If a mother wants to nurse an infant who has a poor life-expectancy prognosis and the infant is to be fed at all by mouth, the mother and parents should have that choice. This includes infants with trisomy 13 and 18 and congenital Zika microcephaly, among others.[313–315] Breastfeeding can be a concrete action that acknowledges parenthood and the child's life at the same time. It may allow time for attachment/bonding, anticipatory grief, coping, and a recognizable loss and end.[316] Infants with CNS abnormalities requiring surgery in infancy can be breastfed until 4 hours before the procedure and postoperatively as soon as oral intake is permitted.[5] When the GI tract is not involved, breastfeeding can be initiated as early as 4 to 6 hours postoperatively at the surgeon's discretion. The placing of a shunt for hydrocephalus is a simple and common procedure, and breastfeeding is an ideal feeding mode for this infant. There is one report of the successful use of human milk as the first feed in 79.1% of infants with a meningomyelocele and 80.8% being fed at least once at the breast despite also needing bottle-feeding and gavage feeding.[317]

Even without malformations of the CNS, there is evidence that feeding or sucking disorders can be predictive of subsequent neurodevelopment outcomes for children with premature births, cerebral palsy, or neonatal brain injury. Sucking abnormalities may be one of the first signs of neurologic impairment. Abnormal sucking behavior can be the absence of the sucking response; a weak suck; dyscoordination of sucking, swallowing, and breathing; or a mixture of these.[318] Additional assessment of neurologic and feeding status, along with feeding support, including the use of breast milk and breastfeeding, should be done based on the mother's feeding goals. Santoro et al. recommended a multidisciplinary approach for identifying feeding abnormalities in children with cerebral palsy.[319] This should be considered and implemented as soon as cerebral palsy and/or feeding difficulties are detected, even in infancy. In a systematic review, Slattery et al. examined the literature for early sucking and swallowing problems as predictors of neonatal brain injury and neurologic outcomes.[320] They reviewed six studies that reported on assessment of sucking and swallowing problems in neonates with some form of neonatal brain injury and compared subsequent neurodevelopment. Some investigators in these six studies used the Neonatal Oral-Motor Assessment Scale (NOMAS), whereas others used

chart review and feeding observation, imaging, instrumental assessment (fiber-optic endoscopic evaluation of swallowing, videofluoroscopic swallow study, Kron Nutritive Sucking Apparatus), or days to achieve oral feeding. These were prospective and retrospective cohort designs of convenience samples of neonates with a variety of neonatal neurologic insults (hypoxic-ischemic encephalopathy, neonatal arterial ischemic stroke, and mixed neurologic impairments). In this very heterogeneous group of studies without quality statistical measures, five of the six included studies reported a positive association between sucking and feeding problems and later neurodevelopment. A meta-analysis was not deemed reasonable with these studies. None of these studies specifically considered breastfeeding or commented on the use of human milk. Other reviews of infant oral-motor feeding assessment tools have yielded limited data on content validity testing and comprehensive reliability testing for 11 different tools.[321–323] There are two tools applicable to bottle-feeding (Early Feeding Skills Assessment [EFS], NOMAS) and nine tools for breastfeeding (Breastfeeding Evaluation and Education Tool, Systematic Assessment of the Infant at the Breast, Bristol Breastfeeding Assessment Tool [BBAT], IBFAT, LATCH Score for Breastfeeding Assessment, Mother-Baby Assessment [MBA], Mother–Infant Breastfeeding Progress Tool [MIBPT], Potential Early Breastfeeding Problem Tool [PEBT], and the Premature Infant Breastfeeding Behavior Scale [PIBBS]). Each of these tools has limited testing in different populations, term and/or preterm infants, and is intended for slightly different goals. They each assess different items related to actions by the infant in feeding and/or maternal actions during or in response to breastfeeding. None of these tools has been fully validated, tested prospectively in a broad population of infants, or adequately prospectively compared with later neuropsychomotor infant development.

At this time, we are left with a combination of clinician, nursing, and parental reports and a mixture of other tools (ultrasonography, endoscopy, fluoroscopy), along with additional assessment by lactation consultants and physical therapy, occupational therapy, and speech therapy professionals, to guide ongoing discussion about feeding concerns. Nevertheless, when feeding concerns are raised in an infant, it is appropriate to provide early assistance and support for feeding and ongoing assessment for feeding skills development in parallel with neurodevelopment. Future research relating feeding difficulties to later neurodevelopment will require a validated and tested feeding assessment tool to be developed and then tested in prospective controlled clinical trials.

CONGENITAL HEART DISEASE

For many years, parents of infants with congenital heart disease (CHD) were dissuaded from breastfeeding out of concern for a destabilizing effect on the already-fragile cardiorespiratory system. However, the evidence disproves this concern, and breastfeeding plays an important role in the health of infants with CHD, including preventing NEC, improving weight gain, and promoting optimal infant health.[324]

The "Work" of Feeding

For an extubated, stable infant with CHD, there is no medical indication to interrupt the establishment or continuation of breastfeeding unless surgery is imminent. Even infants with cyanotic heart disease, if they can be fed orally, can be breastfed. The "work" required to breastfeed is less than the work required to bottle-feed. Heart and respiratory rates remain stable during feeding at the breast. The misconception that it is more work to breastfeed is incorrect. One small study ($N = 7$ infants) compared oxygen saturation levels (SaO_2) as an indicator of cardiorespiratory effort during breastfeeding versus bottle-feeding.[82] The SaO_2 levels were higher and less variable during breastfeeding than the SaO_2 levels during bottle-feeding in these infants with CHD. In a second study, five small preterm infants were compared, bottle-feeding versus breastfeeding, and functioned as their own controls for 71 feeding sessions. During breastfeeding sessions, the infants became warmer, but there were smaller declines in transcutaneous oxygen pressures compared with bottle-feeding sessions.[26] In two other studies comparing growth patterns of breastfed and bottle-fed infants with cardiac defects, one showed that breastfed infants gained weight more quickly and had shorter hospital stays ($N = 45$ mother–infant dyads), and in the second study ($N = 122$; 81 undergoing heart surgery and 41 undergoing palliative surgery), there were no differences in growth between infants receiving human milk or formula.[325,326] Breastfeeding is less strenuous, as shown in these and other studies.

CHD and Necrotizing Enterocolitis

CHD is known to be a significant risk factor for developing NEC. There are differences in NEC when it occurs in infants with CHD and preterm infants. The pathophysiology of NEC in infants with CHD is likely different than that of NEC in preterm infants, which is thought to result from a mixture of inflammatory and vascular injury involving areas of infarction and necrosis. Cardiac NEC is more of a vascular phenomenon involving mesenteric hypoperfusion from diastolic steal and flow reversal in the abdominal aorta.[327] A recent retrospective case-control study revealed that postnatal age at onset was lower in CHD NEC patients than preterm infants (4 [2 to 24] vs. 11 [4 to 41] days, $p < 0.001$), the lowest pH levels were lower (7.21 [7.01 to 7.47] vs. 7.27 [6.68 to 7.39], $p = 0.02$), and the highest C-reactive protein (CRP) levels were higher (112.5 mg/L [5.0 to 425.0] vs. 66.0 [5.2 to 189.0], $p = 0.05$). The anatomic localization of the disease was also different; the colon was significantly more often involved in CHD NEC than preterm NEC (86% vs. 33%, $p = 0.03$). Mortality caused by NEC was not different (22% vs. 11%, $p = 0.47$).[328] The highest incidence of NEC is in premature infants with CHD because these infants not only have the classic risk factors of preterm babies but also the hemodynamic changes observed in CHD.[329]

A single-center retrospective study at Texas Children's Hospital from 2010 to 2016 found that an exclusive unfortified human milk diet was associated with a significantly lower risk of preoperative NEC (OR 0.17, 95% CI 0.04 to 0.84, $p = 0.03$) in a multivariable regression model controlling for cardiac lesion, race, feeding volume, birth weight, SGA, inotrope use, and prematurity.[330] Therefore exclusive breastfeeding and an exclusive unfortified human milk diet, whether the milk is maternal or donated, is the most significant enteral feeding strategy to decrease the incidence of NEC in infants with CHD.

Breastfeeding Success for Infants with CHD

In a single-center study with 62 mother–infant pairs participating out of 132 eligible pairs, infant feeding data were carefully prospectively collected.[331] The infants were all full term, with a median birth weight of 3.270 kg and with a mixture of congenital cardiac defects. Notable findings regarding the participating mothers included the following: mothers delivering within the institution were more likely to initiate pumping (96%) than those transferred from outside (67%), and mothers pumped an average of five to six times a day, and their daily milk volumes approached 500 mL within the first week of pumping. Relative to the infants, only 13% of all their feeds were via breastfeeding; 63.3% were via bottle, 30.5% were via gavage, and the remainder were mixed. Infants received an average of 53.6% of the daily milk intake as human milk. Comorbidities, hemodynamic instability, periods of being NPO, and the need for additional ventilatory support did interfere with the infants' overall intake. With the majority of infants being discharged by 14 days of age, many were not directly breastfeeding, and there was a need for ongoing instruction and support for breastfeeding and expressing and using expressed breast milk at home to provide human milk to infants after discharge.[331] The use of donor human milk was not discussed in this study.

Breastfed infants enjoy significant health benefits, including those in the cardiovascular system. Given the further demonstrable impact on infant gastrointestinal health in CHD, it is critical that breastfeeding be promoted and supported for families of these infants. They are at higher risk for both complications of not breastfeeding (NEC, neurodevelopmental outcomes) and of breastfeeding not being successful. A coordinated program of support should be implemented, including recommendations by cardiologists, surgeons, critical care physicians, and pediatric providers, with the support of registered nurse–level board-certified lactation consultants to help families through the establishment of breastfeeding and maintenance of milk production during anticipated and unplanned pauses.

SUDDEN INFANT DEATH SYNDROME

SIDS is the sudden, unexplained death of an infant younger than 1 year of age without a known cause after autopsy, review of history, and examination of the death scene. The rate of SIDS in the United States decreased from 130.3 deaths per 100,000 live births in 1990 to 35.4 deaths per 100,000 live births in 2017.[332] Much of the initial decrease in SIDS during the 1990s was secondary to a major public health campaign, started by the AAP in 1992, that focused on decreasing infant sleeping in the prone position, termed *back to sleep*.[333] However, much of the decline in SIDS in the United States since 1999 has been secondary to classifying deaths that previously may have been classified as SIDS as accidental suffocation and strangulation in bed (ASSB) or unknown cause, both of which have increased as the rate of SIDS decreased. The rate of sudden unexpected infant death (SUID), which combines all three classifications (SIDS, ASSB, and unknown cause), has not declined since the 1990s, despite increasing AAP and public health recommendations for supine positioning; use of a firm sleep surface; room-sharing without bedsharing; avoidance of soft bedding and overheating; avoidance of exposure to smoke, alcohol, and illicit drugs; use of a pacifier; and breastfeeding.[334]

A 2017 meta-analysis of eight large international case-control studies, analyzing 2267 SIDS cases and 6837 control infants, confirmed that breastfeeding decreases SIDS.[335] Breastfeeding, however, needs to be continued for at least 2 months to be protective, with greater protection seen with increased duration. Breastfeeding for 2 to 4 months decreased SIDS by 40% (adjusted odds ratio [aOR] 0.60, 95% CI 0.44 to 0.82), breastfeeding for 4 to 6 months decreased SIDS by 60% (aOR 0.40, 95% CI 0.26 to 0.63), and breastfeeding for >6 months decreased SIDS by 64% (aOR 0.36, 95% CI 0.22 to 0.61). Exclusive breastfeeding did not increase the effect. It is, therefore, important that public health messages about SIDS risk reduction emphasize that breastfeeding must continue for at least 2 months to be protective and that longer durations of breastfeeding will result in lower SIDS and lower infant mortality. Because the peak incidence of SIDS occurs between 3 and 6 months, continued exclusive breastfeeding through 6 months will enhance protection during this high-risk period. It has been estimated that optimizing breastfeeding in the United States could prevent 492 infant deaths from SIDS every year.[79]

A 2005 meta-analysis of seven studies revealed that pacifier use has been associated with a reduction in SIDS incidence.[336] In addition, a 2016 Cochrane review found moderate-quality evidence that pacifier use in healthy term infants, started from birth or after lactation is established, did not significantly affect the prevalence or duration of exclusive and partial breastfeeding up to 4 months of age.[337] However, there was insufficient information on the potential harms of pacifiers for infants and mothers. They recommended that mothers who are well motivated to breastfeed should be encouraged to decide on pacifier use based on personal preference. Further research is necessary to assess the effect of pacifiers among women less motivated to breastfeed.

There is growing evidence that more frequent bedsharing increases the duration of breastfeeding and exclusive breastfeeding.[338–340] The AAP Task Force on SIDS, however, campaigns against bedsharing because of the reported risk of suffocation, strangulation, and entrapment that may occur.[334,335] This risk remains controversial because some studies question the conclusion that bedsharing among breastfeeding infants increases the risk of SIDS in the absence of known hazards, such as parental alcohol use, drug use, or

smoking; sleeping in a chair or on a sofa; soft bedding; or a preterm infant.[341,342] Larger well-designed studies are necessary to test the relationship between bedsharing in the breastfeeding infant and infant deaths in the absence of all known hazards.[342] The ABM supports bedsharing and breastfeeding and emphasizes safe-sleeping and risk minimization with bedsharing.[343] The ABM outlines a number of areas for continued research.

ORAL HEALTH

Malocclusion

Three recent meta-analyses have found that breastfeeding decreases malocclusion. A meta-analysis of 41 studies with 27,023 participants revealed that breastfeeding decreased malocclusions (OR 0.34, 95% CI 0.24 to 0.48), exclusively breastfeeding had a greater reduction than nonexclusive (OR 0.54 95% CI 0.38 to 0.77), and longer breastfeeding reduced malocclusions more than shorter breastfeeding (OR 0.40 95% CI 0.29 to 0.54).[344] A meta-analysis of nine studies revealed that nonbreastfeeding increased the risk of posterior crossbite compared with breastfeeding for over 6 months, with an odds ratio of 3.76 (95% CI 2.01 to 7.03), and by an odds ratio of 8.78 (95% CI 1.67 to 46.1) compared with those breastfed for over 12 months.[345] The odds ratio for class II malocclusion was 1.25 (95% CI 1.01 to 1.55), and for nonspaced dentition, it was 1.73 (95% CI 1.35 to 2.22), in children who breastfed for up to 6 months compared with those breastfed for over 6 months. A third meta-analysis of seven studies found that children who had breastfed suboptimally had an increased risk of developing malocclusions and that a strong and significant association existed between a shorter duration of breastfeeding, defined as less than 12 months, and the development of an anterior open bite (RR 3.58, 95% CI 2.55 to 5.03) and a class II canine relationship (RR 1.65 95% CI 1.38 to 1.97).[346]

Oral Health Risk Assessment

Oral health risk assessment has been recommended by the Section on Pediatric Dentistry of the AAP, with the establishment of a dental home by 1 year of age.[347] Although pediatricians have the opportunity to provide early assessment of risk for dental caries and anticipatory guidance to prevent disease, it is also important that children establish a dental home. Recommendations include systematic examination and oral fluoride; elimination of simple sugars in the diet; initiation of oral hygiene early; exclusively breastfeeding infants for 6 months and continued breastfeeding as complementary foods are introduced for 1 year or longer, as mutually desired by mother and infant; weaning the infant from a bottle by 1 year; and not putting an infant to bed with a bottle.[347] The infant is not colonized until the eruption of the primary teeth. Caries are associated with *Streptococcus mutans* and usually occur at the age of 2 years. High caries rates run in families, usually passed from mother to child; 70% of caries occur in

20% of children. Children who sleep with the mother and nurse throughout the night are at higher risk, especially if the mother is prone to caries.

Dental Caries

The development of dental caries occurs in breastfed infants. However, a meta-analysis of seven studies reported that breastfed children had fewer dental caries than bottle-fed children (OR 0.43, 95% CI 0.23 to 0.80).[348] A second meta-analysis of 63 studies revealed that breastfeeding up to 12 months resulted in a reduced risk of caries (OR 0.50, 95% CI 0.25 to 0.99), but children breastfed for >12 months had an increased risk of caries when compared with children breastfed <12 months (OR 1.99, 95% CI 1.35 to 2.95).[349] For children breastfed >12 months, those fed nocturnally or more frequently had a further increased caries risk (OR 7.14, 95% CI 3.14 to 16.23). In addition, a recent oral health study ($n = 1303$) nested in a birth cohort study found that children who were breastfed for ≥ 24 months had a 2.4-times-higher risk of having severe early childhood caries (ECCs; RR 2.4, 95% CI 1.7 to 3.3) than those who were breastfed up to 12 months of age, whereas breastfeeding between 13 and 23 months had no effect on dental caries.[350]

In summary, breastfeeding up to 12 months of age decreases the risk of dental caries by around half, most likely because of its immune-modulating effects and establishment of a protective microbiome, despite the lactose sugar in human milk. In addition, a recent study demonstrated that breastfeeding did not provoke a decrease in biofilm pH and, therefore, should not contribute to ECCs.[351] Breastfeeding at night is a normal feeding pattern, and because breastfeeding for the first 12 months is protective against ECC, advice against nighttime feeding in the first year is not warranted. If infants breastfeed to sleep, the gums and erupting teeth should be wiped to minimize the risk of caries.

Toddlers who breastfeed for more than a year may have increased caries, especially if they suckle at night. Prevention is key. Wiping the gums after night feeds is especially important. Twice-daily brushing with fluoridated toothpaste should be initiated for all toddlers beginning with the eruption of the first tooth (rice grain–sized portion of toothpaste for children <36 months of age and a green pea–sized portion for children ≥ 36 months of age). A physician should be alert to the potential for dental decay when infants nurse frequently, especially through the night. A family history of dental enamel problems is worth investigating.

Some breastfed toddlers develop rampant cavities. The levels of mutans streptococci in saliva and plaque are higher in children with rampant cavities than in control subjects.[352–354] The role of individual bacteria in causing caries seems to be important, although more focus is being placed now on dysbiosis of the oral microbiome and interventions to reestablish oral commensal bacteria and microbiome diversity.[355,356] In addition, infants with rampant cavities often have a strong family history of caries and a cariogenic diet. The most cariogenic solutions are soda, fruit juice, sweetened cow's milk, chocolate milk, and sugar water. If a mother is prone to caries, it increases the risk to the infant, not just because of family history but also because of the shared cariogenic bacteria and diet.

The Reference list is available at www.expertconsult.com.

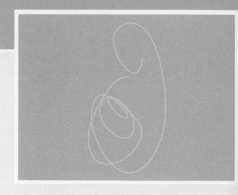

14

Premature Infants and Breastfeeding

Ivan L. Hand and Lawrence Noble

KEY POINTS

- Mother's own milk, appropriately fortified, is the standard for feeding premature infants.
- Provision of mother's own milk for hospitalized premature infants provides short- and long-term health benefits.
- Neonatal providers play an important role supporting lactation in the neonatal intensive care unit with education, milk expression, skin-to-skin care, and breastfeeding.
- Pasteurized human donor milk is recommended instead of formula when mother's own milk is not available or sufficient.
- Promotion of human milk and breastfeeding requires multidisciplinary and system-wide adoption of lactation support practices.

- Reducing disparities in provision of mother's own milk according to demographic and social factors is essential to achieve health equity.
- Before discharge, a plan for feeding at home should be developed with the mother.
- The goal of the discharge feeding plan recommendations for preterm infants is to enable the mother to exclusively breastfeed or provide as much human milk as possible while minimizing nutrient deficits.

BENEFITS OF HUMAN MILK FOR THE PRETERM

The data are overwhelming. Even the most reluctant of neonatologists have accepted the tremendous importance of human milk to all infants from the most immature to term. The American Academy of Pediatrics (AAP) recommends that mother's own milk, fresh or frozen, should be the primary diet for premature infants.[1]

As we shall discuss in this chapter, human milk provides developmental benefits for preterm infants that extend into adolescence. The use of exclusive human milk when paired with standardized feeding guidelines can improve tolerance of feedings and decrease the incidence of necrotizing enterocolitis (NEC). Human milk—fed infants have decreased rates of late-onset sepsis, urinary tract infection, diarrhea, and upper respiratory tract infection. Human milk is also associated with decreases in the incidence and severity of retinopathy of prematurity (ROP), improved neurodevelopmental and visual outcomes, and improved feeding tolerance compared with formula. Improved tolerance allows infants to receive fewer days of parenteral nutrition, significantly decreases morbidity, and decreases length of stay.

Maturation of the gastrointestinal tract is supported by components in human milk resulting in improved motility, smaller gastric residuals, and decreased intestinal permeability. Preterm infants have decreased ability to absorb fats. Enzymes in human milk allow for improved fat absorption and intestinal lipolysis.

Research in the science of nutrition for low-birth-weight (LBW) infants and extremely premature infants has advanced tremendously as the technology to study the important questions has improved. Advances in the field of neonatology have contributed to the survival of increasingly more immature infants. The edge of viability is currently about 22 weeks, and these infants will need to be fed to survive.

One of the key points learned retrospectively about survival, generation after generation, has been the critical impact of fluid and nutrition. For the preterm infant, adequate nutrition and growth are the primary goals during their neonatal intensive care unit (NICU) stay. In the past, the early use of unsupplemented drip milk and some donor milks produced poor growth patterns in preterm infants. Drip milk is low in fat and, therefore, low in calories. The protein levels in donor milk from women late in lactation (i.e., beyond 6 to 8 months, when the protein levels have dropped) parallel a child's decreased biologic needs with the addition of solid foods. These factors contributed to the abandonment of human milk until supplements and fortifiers were developed and studies of the milk of women who had delivered prematurely sparked new investigations.

Policy statements from World Health Organization (WHO), United Nations International Children's Education Fund (UNICEF), AAP, and other international and national organizations confirm the importance of providing a mother's own milk to preterm infants and infants who are small-for-gestational-age (SGA). Standard practice in neonatal units is to promote mother's own milk as the food of choice for all LBW infants.[1]

The absolute standard for evaluating the nutritional outcome of preterm infants remains the intrauterine growth rate. A strategy to minimize mobilization of endogenous nutrient stores is moving from a focus on intrauterine-based, short-term growth and nutrient retention rates to a system that considers long-term growth achievement.[2] For the infant with very low-birth-weight (VLBW), nutritional needs are first met primarily by parenteral nutrition with increasing reliance on the advancement of enteral feeds. The enteral feeding of choice is human milk, preferably mother's own milk or donor human milk if the mother's own milk is not available.[1] The optimal time to initiate oral feedings in the smallest and sickest preterm infants is now thought to be as soon as possible after delivery. Prolonged exclusive parenteral nutrition has been replaced with minimal amounts of oral feedings with parenteral nutrition to preserve and maintain intestinal function. These feeds are known as trophic because they are responsible for the growth of the gastrointestinal tract. Feedings should begin soon after birth once physiologic stability is achieved. Usually this involves stable blood pressure and oxygenation, but many units may have their own criteria for when to initiate oral feeds. It is important to have a standardized feeding protocol in the NICU. This has been shown to reduce the incidence of NEC in the preterm neonate.[3] It is interesting that the specific protocol appears to matter less than that each NICU follow their own protocol and minimize variation.

As nutritional markers shift, a preterm infant's own mother's milk is now recognized, even by the most skeptical clinicians, as the gold standard to prevent short-term morbidities and enhance long-term outcome.[4] With this change comes the recognition that fortified donor milk is clearly superior to artificial feeds.

LBW has been defined by the WHO as a weight at birth of less than 2500 g.[5] Overall, it is estimated that 15% to 20% of all births worldwide are LBW, approximating more than 20 million births per year. LBW infants form a heterogeneous group, some born early, some who are born at term but are SGA, and some both early and small. LBW infants account for 60% to 80% of all neonatal deaths and are at high risk for early growth restriction, infectious disease, developmental delay, and death in infancy and childhood.

GASTROINTESTINAL TRACT DEVELOPMENT

The gastrointestinal tract is one of the first structures defined in the developing embryo. Gut length proceeds rapidly throughout fetal life and for the first years of life. The proton pump is present at 13 weeks' gestation. Intrinsic factor and pepsin are identifiable a few weeks later (Fig. 14.1). Even in premature infants with extremely low-birth-weight (ELBW), the gastric pH can be lowered to below 4.0.[6] Digestive enzymes are capable of intraluminal digestion of fat, protein, and carbohydrates. Although pancreatic lipase and bile salts are minimal in ELBW infants, the introduction of mother's milk will stimulate maturation and provide lipases and other digestive enzymes.

Bile salt—stimulated lipase is a unique component of fresh, unpasteurized breast milk and promotes triglyceride absorption and digestion.[7] The intestinal villi and cellular differentiation occur at about 10 to 12 weeks' gestation and begin a complex interrelationship with developing epithelium and the mesoderm, according to Newell.[8] Lactase and other carbohydrate enzymes begin to appear. Gut motility is thought to appear first as irregular gastrointestinal activity at 23 weeks progressing to organized motility at approximately 28 weeks. Most studies of nutritive sucking and swallowing are done with artificial feeding with a bottle. Suckling at the breast, which begins with peristaltic motion of the tongue and continues down the esophagus, has been initiated by breastfeeding as early as 28 weeks or sooner.

Gastric emptying in premature infants, as measured in most studies, is slow, generating the impression that feedings

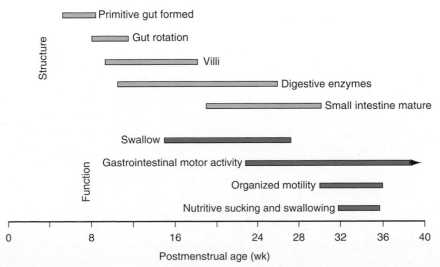

Fig. 14.1 The ontogenic timetable showing structural and functional gastrointestinal development. (Modified from Newell SJ. Enteral feeding of the micropremie. *Clin Perinatol.* 2000;27:221.)

are not tolerated. However, a recent meta-analysis of 66 publications reported no effect of gestational age on the mean gastric emptying time.[9] Gastric emptying is enhanced by human milk and slowed by formula and increased osmolarity (Box 14.1). Half emptying time with human milk is reported to be as rapid as 20 to 40 minutes.[10] Ultrasound studies have assessed small-volume feeds. Some premature infants show delayed antral distention after a nasogastric feeding with emptying that follows a curvilinear pattern after an initial rapid phase.

Maturation of the small intestinal motility, and hence tolerance of feeds, is enhanced by previous exposure of the gut to nutrition. Early feeding precipitates preferential maturation and thus a more mature response to feeds. Total gut transit time in premature infants varies from 1 to 5 days and is more rapid in those who

have received food.[11] In those younger than 28 weeks, it may take as long as 3 days to pass meconium. Breast milk feedings, however, increase motility and stool passage.

When prematurity is complicated by intrauterine growth failure, the resultant cascade of events includes decreased splanchnic circulation and oligohydramnios, poor gut perfusion, decreased growth of the small intestine and pancreas culminating in a fetal echogenic gut, and poor intestinal motility resulting in poor tolerance to milk feeds. It is not uncommon for this to be associated with NEC. These events require careful consideration, including the choice to use mother's milk, especially beginning with colostrum. In a recent study looking at rates of NEC among infants weighing less than 750 g there was no difference in rates of NEC between infants who are appropriate for gestational age (AGA) and SGA infants.[12] This group received colostrum from day 1 and donor milk when mother's own milk was not available, which may have accounted for these results.

Although feeding regimens vary, evidence is strong and consistent that feeding mother's own milk to preterm infants at any gestation is associated with a lower incidence of infections and NEC and improved neurodevelopmental outcome compared with the use of bovine milk products primarily due to the presence of bioactive agents (Fig. 14.2).[4,13] The challenge is to increase the availability of mother's milk and to understand the interactions of bioactive factors to produce these and other clinical benefits (see Fig. 14.2).

GASTROINTESTINAL PRIMING

When feedings are delayed in any newborn, luminal starvation results in epithelial cell atrophy. Lung injury may aggravate this because of multiorgan system dysfunction, increasing the risk for intestinal mucosal injury and associated barrier dysfunction.

BOX 14.1 **Factors Affecting Gastric Emptying**		
Faster Gastric Emptying	**No Effect**	**Slower Gastric Emptying**
Breast milk	Phototherapy	Prematurity
Glucose polymers	Feed temperature	Formula milk
Starch	Nonnutritive sucking	Caloric density
Medium-chain triglycerides		Fatty acids
Prone position		Dextrose concentration
		Long-chain triglycerides
		Osmolality
		Illness

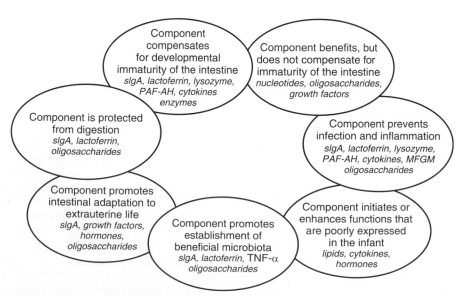

Fig. 14.2 Strategies for beneficial effects of bioactive agents in human milk. Human milk contains bioactive agents with overlapping and synergic effects on intestinal development of neonates. *MFGM*, milk fat globule membrane; *PAF-AH*, platelet-activating factor-acetylhydrolase; *sIgA*, secretory immunoglobulin; *TNF-α*, tumor necrosis factor-α. (Modified from Goldman AS. Modulation of the gastrointestinal tract of infants by human milk: interface and interactions—an evolutionary perspective. *J Nutr.* 2000;130:426S.)

The ultimate injury would be the invasion of bacteria from the gut lumen.[14] Initiating feeds is a delicate balance between insufficient feeds that fail to trigger gut maturation and excessive feeds that overwhelm the digestive capacity. Also, excessive feeds can result in bacterial overgrowth and injury to the brush border.[14] When internal nutrients are absent, the intestinal size and weight are diminished; atrophy of the mucosa, delayed maturation of intestinal enzymes, and increased permeability and bacterial translocation may occur. Intestinal motilities, perfusion, and reactions to the usual gastrointestinal tropic hormones are also affected by lack of nutrients. Trophic hormone levels in the plasma are significantly altered by starvation.

In the words of Lucas,[15] "It is fundamentally unphysiologic to deprive an infant of any gestation of enteral feeding since the deprivation would never normally occur at any stage." This statement is based on the fact that a fetus normally makes sucking motions and swallows amniotic fluid from early gestation. This may even have a trophic effect on the gut. By the third trimester a fetus is swallowing up to 150 mL/kg per day, which provides as much as 3 g/kg per day of protein. The secretion of gastrointestinal hormones is thought to occur in response to the first postdelivery feedings.[15] In animals, after only a few days of deprivation of enteral feeds, atrophic changes take place in the gut.[16] In human infants who have never received enteral feedings, no gut peptide surges occur, not even those of the trophic hormones enteroglucagon, gastrin, and gastric inhibitory polypeptide. These hormones are thought to be key to the activation of the enteroinsular axis[16] (Box 14.2). Clinical trials of early priming in premature infants showed that infants primed in the first few days or first week had better feeding tolerance to advancing feeds and were weaned from parenteral nutrition promptly. It was also associated with lower serum alkaline phosphatase activity and significant stimulation of gastrointestinal hormones such as gastrin. It also resulted in more mature intestinal motility patterns, greater absorption of calcium and phosphorus, increased lactase activity, increased bone mineral content (BMC), and reduced intestinal permeability. Tyson and Kennedy[17] reviewed the studies of early priming and found shorter times to full feeding, fewer days when feedings were held, a shorter duration of hospitalization, and no increase in NEC. Many of the involved infants were at high risk for complications by virtue of their own morbidities, including mechanical ventilation, umbilical catheterization, and patent ductus arteriosus. Schanler and Anderson[18] recommended that ELBW infants who are ill be given small volumes, 10 to 20 mL/kg per day, in the first few days of life to continue for 3 to 7 days before advancing the feeds.[18] Clinical stability is required before advancing the feeds. These volumes are compatible with the volume of mother's milk of a mother of a premature infant (Boxes 14.3 and 14.4). In a meta-analysis by Oddie et al.,[19] consisting of 10 randomized controlled trials (RCTs) with over 3700 infants participating, there was no advantage to slow advancement of enteral feeds (daily increments of 15 to 20 mL/kg compared with 30 to 40 mL/kg infant weight). There was no decrease in the risk for NEC or death, but delays (1 to 5 days) in reaching full feeds and higher rates of invasive infections occurred in the slow advancement group.[19] There have been a number of trials looking at bolus feedings versus continuous feeds. Bolus feeds have been thought to be more physiologic for the infant, resulting in more cyclical hormone surges, and continuous feeds have been described as more appropriate for the extremely preterm infant with better tolerance. All these studies have had issues with blinding and the ideal method of feeding may be infant and unit specific.[20]

Berseth[11] reported that the response of the preterm infant's intestine to entire feedings at different postnatal ages showed significantly more mature motor patterns of the gut and higher plasma concentrations of gastrin and gastric inhibitory peptide. From a management standpoint, early-fed infants were able to tolerate full oral feeds sooner, had fewer

---

BOX 14.2 Biology of the Gut in Infants With Very Low-Birth-Weight

- Swallows amniotic fluid daily, up to 150 mL/kg per day
- Potential for gut atrophy if not fed
- All of gastrointestinal tract is immature
- Enzymes and nutrients in human milk enhance maturation
- Higher total body water, muscle mass, growth accretion rates, and oxygen consumption
- Higher evaporative water loss because of greater surface area
- Prone to hyperglycemia because of poor insulin response
- Lower brown fat reserves and glycogen stores
- Immature thyroid control of metabolic rate

BOX 14.3 Advantages of Gastrointestinal Priming

- Shortened time to regain birth weight
- Improved feeding tolerance
- Reduced duration of parenteral nutrition
- Enhanced enzyme maturation
- Reduced intestinal permeability
- Improved gastrointestinal motility
- Matured hormone responses
- Improved mineral absorption, mineralization
- Lowered incidence of cholestasis
- Reduced duration of phototherapy

BOX 14.4 Advantages of Priming With Mother's Milk

- Earlier use of mother's milk
- Mothers begin milk expression earlier
- Infants receive more mother's milk
- Psychological advantage for mother's safety

Modified with permission from Schanler RJ, Anderson D. The low-birth weight infant in patient care. In: Duggan C, Watkins JB, Walker WA, eds. *Nutrition in Pediatrics*. 4th ed. Hamilton, Ontario, Canada: BC Decker; 2008.

TABLE 14.1   Nutritional Milestones

	Prime Continuous (n = 39)	Prime Bolus (n = 43)	NPO Continuous (n = 44)	NPO Bolus (n = 45)
Duration of parenteral nutrition (days)	34 ± 32[a]	36 ± 32	32 ± 21	32 ± 19
Milk start (days)[b]	6 ± 2	6 ± 3	16 ± 3	16 ± 4
Regain birth weight (days)	12 ± 5	13 ± 5	12 ± 5	13 ± 7
Complete tube-feeding (days),[c] gestation 26–27 wk (days),[d] gestation 28–30 wk (days)	33 ± 19 40 ± 16 30 ± 19	29 ± 19 26 ± 7 31 ± 23	29 ± 9 34 ± 11 27 ± 5	29 ± 9 29 ± 7 30 ± 11
First successful oral feeding (days)	51 ± 19	50 ± 26	49 ± 14	52 ± 18
Full oral feeding (days)	64 ± 20	61 ± 21	64 ± 18	65 ± 20
Duration of hospitalization (days)	91 ± 11	87 ± 45	80 ± 40	81 ± 24

NPO, Nothing by mouth.
[a]Mean ± standard deviation.
[b]Different by study design.
[c]Interaction between gestational age and feeding method, $p = 0.001$.
[d]Continuous versus bolus, $p = 0.001$.
From Schanler RJ, Shulman RN, Lau C, et al. Feeding strategies for premature infants: randomized trial of gastrointestinal priming and tube-feeding method. *Pediatrics*. 1999;103:434.

BOX 14.5   Published and Putative Effects of Early Enteral Intake of Infants Weighing Less Than 1500 Grams

- No change in necrotizing enterocolitis incidence
- Less cholestatic jaundice
- Less osteopenia
- Less physiologic jaundice
- Increased glucose tolerance
- Better weight gain
- Earlier tolerance of full oral nutrient intake
- Increased gut hormones: gastric inhibitory peptide, enteroglucagon, gastrin, motilin, neurotensin
- Induction of digestive enzyme synthesis and release
- Improved antral-duodenal coordination of peristalsis
- Allows gut colonization (vitamin K production) and avoids germ-free gut complications
- Earlier maturation of brush border barrier qualities
- Prevents atrophy and attendant effects of starvation

days of feeding intolerance, and required shorter hospital stays. Studies varied from infants who were fed at younger than 24 hours of age at 1 mL/h to infants who were fed full feeds starting at days 2 to 7 compared with infants on usual delayed protocols. All showed an advantage to early feeds[16] (Table 14.1 and Box 14.5). Early enteral feedings are now being embraced thanks to a number of randomized controlled studies supporting the concept.

Requirements of ELBW infants begin with water, the first great need, followed by energy requirements of 120 kcal/kg per day to meet metabolic and growth rates. Protein is key because ELBW infants miss the last trimester when protein and fat are stored. To stop catabolism and promote protein accretion, Brumberg and LaGamma[14] recommend 3.5 to 4 g/kg per day of protein, presuming a daily loss of 1.1 to 1.5 g/kg of stored protein per day. Protein should start early either orally or by parenteral nutrition.

Human milk is the preferred feeding for all infants, including premature and sick newborns, with rare exception according to the AAP, the WHO, and the National Academy of Medicine (formerly the Institute of Medicine).[1,5,21] For the preterm infant, adequate nutrition and growth are the primary goals during their NICU stay. The goal of postnatal nutrition was proposed to achieve a rate of postnatal growth approximating the intrauterine growth rate of the gestational age–matched fetus.[22] For the VLBW infant, nutritional needs are first met primarily by parenteral nutrition with increasing reliance on the advancement of enteral feeds. The paradigm of extrauterine growth matching intrauterine growth for premature infants based on their gestational age has been called into question.[23,24] The data to support such a paradigm have been called into question based on the measured effects, the period of time postnatally, and potential confounding factors. It has been recommended that new growth standards should be used to assess the postnatal growth of preterm infants based on preterm infants from healthy pregnancies without evidence of intrauterine growth restriction.[25] This standard has been developed and proposed for use by the WHO and the Centers for Disease Control and Prevention (CDC) for use regarding Zika congenital infection and measurement of microcephaly.[24] It is likely that additional data using similar methodology for establishing such a standard will be developed given the primary criticism of such a standard as including too small a cohort of premature infants.

The enteral feeding of choice is human milk, preferably mother's own milk or donor human milk if the mother's own milk is not available.[1] The advantages of human milk feedings include decreased mortality, protection from NEC and sepsis, and improvement in neurodevelopment. Feedings should begin soon after birth, once physiologic stability is achieved. Usually this involves stable blood pressure and oxygenation, but many units may have their own criteria for when to initiate oral feeds. It is important to have a standardized feeding protocol in the NICU. This has been shown to reduce the incidence of NEC in the preterm neonate[3] (Table 14.2). In their review and meta-analysis Patole and de Klerk[3] noted in six studies that the introduction of a standardized feeding regimen (despite it being different from the others) decreased the risk for NEC by 87%. It is interesting that the specific protocol appears to matter less than that each NICU follow its own protocol and minimize variation.

Human milk is better than formula in early feeds in establishing enteral tolerance and discontinuation of parenteral nutrition, in long-term improved neurodevelopmental outcome, and in the psychologic benefit to mothers. Human milk falls short after 4 to 6 weeks in the amount of protein, calcium, and phosphorus, a problem solvable with the use of a human milk fortifier. No substitute has been developed that replaces the many and varied advantages of human milk, however.

COLOSTRUM

The first product produced by the mother is colostrum, which is an important nutrient for the infant and contains many important biofactors. These biofactors are present in the largest amounts in preterm mother's colostrum. Colostrum has the highest amounts of secretory immunoglobulin A (sIgA), lysozyme, lactoferrin, and cytokines. The high immunoglobulin content of colostrum is mainly IgA, but IgM and IgG are also present in significant amounts. The IgA in colostrum binds to potential infectious pathogens and prevents them from adhering to mucosal epithelium in the neonate.[26] Colostrum also provided T and B lymphocytes, which recognize potential antigens. Oral colostrum has been postulated to be a bridge from the protective biofactors found in amniotic fluid to extrauterine life. For these reasons it is important to administer colostrum once it has been obtained. Colostrum is generally produced in very small amounts, and although it can be given by an orogastric tube, the best option may be direct instillation in the oropharynx. This is due to the presence of a significant amount of lymphoid tissue in the oropharynx, critical in the enteromammary pathway.[27] Colostrum should be the first feeding the infant receives.

Most investigators have concluded that minimal enteral feedings with human milk can optimize growth, development, and progress for small premature infants, even if ventilator dependent.[16] In most studies, the incidence of NEC has been similar with and without early feeds.[15] The presence of an umbilical catheter has long been a contraindication to feeding because of the risk for NEC. When Davey et al.[28] investigated this, the incidence of NEC was comparable in infants with and without umbilical catheters.

Other advantages of early feeds include lower serum direct and indirect bilirubin, less apnea and bradycardia, and less need for phototherapy.[29] Benefits from early feeds were measurable with raw maternal milk, pasteurized premature milk, and even to some extent whey-dominant infant formula. Specifically there is evidence of less apnea and bradycardia with early transpyloric tube feedings (Fig. 14.3).

LOW-BIRTH-WEIGHT INFANTS

VLBW refers to an infant weighing less than 1500 g. The birth of an ELBW premature infant, defined as a weight less than 1000 g, is a nutritional emergency. Even with parenteral nutrition from the first day, weight loss exceeds 10% and it usually takes at least 10 days to regain birth weight. The long-term consequences of early nutrition have a great impact on gut development and neurodevelopment and may well reduce the risk for perinatal brain lesions.

With the availability of surfactant for respiratory distress, infants between 500 and 1000 g are surviving in greater numbers. It is evident that the provision of maternal milk also lowers mortality and morbidity in the preterm infant. This includes overall lower rates of bacterial sepsis, NEC, and death.[30] It has been shown that there appears to be a dose response to maternal milk. Infants appear to require more than 50 mL/kg per day of maternal milk to achieve lower rates of sepsis. A similar dose-response relationship between positive blood cultures and cumulative human milk intake had been shown by Schanler et al.[31] This relationship was also seen as a function of human milk intake during the first 2 weeks of life.[32] In this study, there was a 13% decrease in the combined outcome of NEC/death for each 100 mL/kg of ingested human milk. Thus a dose-dependent effect of human milk on mortality was identified. The use of breast milk in the first 10 days of life was shown to decrease combined morbidity and mortality in the first 60 days of life.[33] In this population, minimal enteral feeds were started on the first day within hours after birth. Infants who received greater than 50% of their total enteral intake from mother's milk had a significantly lower combined outcome of sepsis, NEC, or mortality. This protection from NEC, sepsis, and mortality may have to do with the active biologic protection derived from immunoglobulins, lactoferrin, and cytokines. The problems of nutrition, however, pose new challenges to the neonatologist. The feedings appropriate for a 2000-g premature infant vary only in volume and frequency from that for full-term infants in most cases. Feedings for VLBW infants must address the advantages and disadvantages of human milk at this point in their growth curve. The composition of mother's milk varies in some constituents with the degree of prematurity, which is advantageous (Box 14.6).

The advantages of human milk for LBW infants include the physiologic amino acid and fat profile, the digestibility and absorption of these proteins and fats, and the low renal solute load.[34] The presence of active enzymes enhances maturation and supplements the enzyme activity of this underdeveloped gut. The antiinfective properties and living cells protect immature infants from infection and protect against NEC. The psychologic benefit to the mother who can participate in her

TABLE 14.2 Summary of Six Proposed Feeding Regimens for Preterm Infants

Variable	Studies Patole et al.	Kamitsuka et al.	O'Reilly et al.	Premji et al.	Brown et al.	Spritzer et al.
Timing to start feeds	No respiratory assistance or MAP < 10 cm, no PDA or sepsis, no need for cardiovascular support	Day 4, 3, 2 (or longer if needed) for neonates weighing 1250–1500 g (A), 1502–2000 g (B), and 2001–2500 g (C), respectively	1–8 days	Started at day 5 or 6 of life	Feeds delayed for 5–7 days or longer in complicated deliveries with fetal distress	As soon as possible in well neonates. Delayed by 1 wk in presence of ventilation, IUGR, or complicated labor/delivery
Feeding method	Intermittent bolus gavage feeds by nasogastric tube	Intermittent bolus gavage feeds by nasogastric tube	Intermittent bolus gavage feeds by gastric tube	Intermittent bolus gavage feeds by nasogastric tube	Intermittent 3-hourly bolus feeds by nasogastric tube	Not clear
Feeding type	Expressed breast milk (preferred) or 20 kcal/oz formula (later increased to 24 kcal/oz)	Expressed breast milk (preferred) or half-strength formula (later increased to full strength)	Expressed breast milk (preferred) or 20 kcal/oz: iron-fortified formula	Expressed breast milk (preferred) or 24 kcal/oz formula	Sterile water followed by formula (0.45 cal/mL graded up to 0.80 cal/mL)	Dilute formula, graded gradually to full strength
Feed volume start	0.5 mL/h (<28 wk or 1 mL/h (≥28 wk)	Groups A and B: 3 mL 3 hourly Group C: 4 mL 3 hourly	Started as minimal enteral feeds <10–20 mL/kg/day for 3–4 days and then upgraded by 10–20 mL/kg/day	Maximum 24 mL/kg/day. For <750 g: 1 mL/2 h For ≥ 750 to <1000 g: 2 mL/2 h For ≥ 1000 to <1500 g: 1 mL q2h	For <1250 g: 2 mL/2 h For 1250–1500 g: 3 mL/2 h For >1500 g: 4 mL/2 h	20 mL/kg
Increment volume	Start with 0.5 mL/12 h for <28 wk, and 1 mL/12 h for ≥ 28 wk Increase by 1 mL 8 hourly after reaching 100 mL/kg/day (maximum: 24 mL/kg/day)	Not more than 20 mL/kg/day	10–20 mL/kg/day	Maximum: <30 mL/kg/day For <750 g: 1 mL q24h For ≥ 750 to <1000 g: 1 mL q24h For ≥ 1000 to <1500 g: 1 mL q12h	Detailed plan provided for reaching 20 mL/8 h (<1250 g), 25 mL/8 h (1250–1500 g), 29 mL/8 h (>1500 g)	20 mL/kg/day
Total maximum volume	170 mL/kg/day	150 mL/kg/day	150 mL/kg/day or 120 kcal/kg/day	Not clear	See above	Not specified

(Continued)

TABLE 14.2 Summary of Six Proposed Feeding Regimens for Preterm Infants—cont'd

Variable	Studies Patole et al.	Kamitsuka et al.	O'Reilly et al.	Premji et al.	Brown et al.	Spritzer et al.
Minimal enteral feeds (volume and duration)	Not used	Not used	<10–20 mL/kg/day, continued for 3–4 days (breast milk or preterm formula)	Used only for neonates <1 kg at <24 mL/kg/day Start within 48 h of birth and continued for 5–6 days	Not used	Not used
Definition of feed intolerance	Specified	Not specified	Specified	Specified	Not specified Plan of action given for apnea, bradycardia, abdominal distention, gastric retention of formula, occult blood in stools, and for NEC or shock	Not specified
Plan of action for sepsis	Step feeds for 48 h or unit hemodynamic stability	Not specified	Not specified	Not specified	Not specified (see above)	Not specified
Plan of action for PDA and indomethacin	Step feeds until 24 h after completing indomethacin therapy	Not specified	Not specified	Stop feeds during indomethacin therapy	Not specified (see above)	Not specified
Plan of action for "large" gastric aspirates	Step feeds if such aspirates are persistent	Not specified	Stop feeds	Guidelines provided for contacting clinician for decision-making	Step feeds "for a week or two or more till resolution of the problem"	Not specified
Plan of action for bile-stained gastric aspirates	Step feeds if such aspirates are persistent	Not specified	Stop feeds	Guidelines provided for contacting clinician for decision-making	Not specified	Not specified
Policy for umbilical catheters	Catheters were retained as long as they were needed	Not specified	Not specified	Not specified	Not specified	Not specified

IUGR, Intrauterine growth restriction; *MAP*, mean arterial pressure; *NEC*, necrotizing enterocolitis; *PDA*, patent ductus arteriosus.
From Patole SK, de Klerk N. Impact of standardised feeding regimens on incidence of neonatal necrotising enterocolitis: a systematic review and meta-analysis of observational studies. *Arch Dis Child Fetal Neonatal Ed.* 2005;90:F147.

infant's care by providing her milk is a less tangible but no less important advantage.

The disadvantages are the possible gaps in certain nutrients that have been estimated to be required for adequate growth, which include the volume of total protein and macrominerals, especially calcium and phosphorus.[35–37] These disadvantages have been overcome with the use of human milk fortifiers in the preterm population.

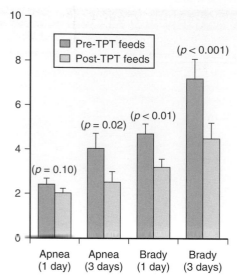

Fig. 14.3 Episodes of apnea and bradycardia before and after initiation of transpyloric tube *(TPT)* feedings especially when limited to human milk. (From Malcolm WF, Smith PB, Mears S, et al. Transpyloric tube feeding in very low birth weight infants with suspected gastroesophageal reflux: impact on apnea and bradycardia. *J Perinatol.* 2009;29:372.)

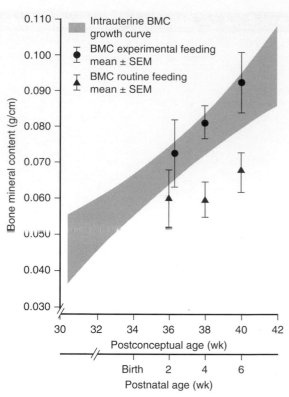

Fig. 14.4 Postnatal bone mineral content *(BMC)* in 33- to 35-week-old appropriate-for-gestational-age or preterm infants compared with intrauterine bone mineralization curve. Regression curve and 95th percentile confidence limits for regression for BMC of infants born at different gestational ages (30 to 42 weeks' gestational age) represent intrauterine bone mineralization curve. Infants fed routine cow milk formula *(solid triangles)* had significantly lower BMC than infants fed standard formula supplemented with calcium and phosphorus *(solid circles)*. In these infants, BMC was not different from intrauterine bone mineralization curve at 4 and 6 weeks' postnatal age. (From Steichen JJ, Gratton TL, Tsang RC. Osteopenia of prematurity: the cause and possible treatment. *J Pediatr.* 1980;96:528.)

BOX 14.6 Milk of Mothers Who Deliver Preterm

Level Increased in Preterm	Level Unchanged in Preterm
Total nitrogen	Volume
Protein nitrogen	Calories
Long-chain fatty acids	Lactose (? less)
Medium-chain fatty acids	Fat (?) by "creamatocrit"
Short-chain fatty acids	Linolenic acid
Sodium	Potassium
Chloride	Calcium
Magnesium (?)	Phosphorus
Iron	Copper
	Zinc
	Osmolality
	Vitamin B_{1-12}

OPTIMAL GROWTH FOR PREMATURE INFANTS

Optimal growth for infants born prematurely is considered to be the growth curve they would have followed had they remained in utero (Fig. 14.4 and Tables 14.3 and 14.4).[37] Achieving this goal using the immature intestinal tract requires that the nutrients be digestible and absorbable and not impose a significant metabolic stress on the other immature organs, especially the kidneys. Although human milk provides the ideal nutrients, it would require an inordinate nonphysiologic volume to achieve adequate amounts of some nutrients without calculated supplementation. To fill these growth needs, one can use an artificial or chemical formula or use human milk as a base, with all its advantages, and add the deficient nutrients to it.

SPECIAL PROPERTIES OF PRETERM MILK

The identification of special quantitative differences in nutrients in the milk of mothers who delivered prematurely created new interest in the use of human milk for premature infants (see Box 14.6). Many investigators have contributed to the pool of knowledge after the initial revelations in 1980 by Atkinson et al.,[38,39] who reported the nitrogen concentration of milk from mothers of premature infants to be greater than that of milk from mothers delivering at term.[40]

The composition of breast milk is highly variable depending on many factors, including gestational and postnatal age. Mature human milk contains about 87% water, 1% protein, 4% fats, and 7% carbohydrate (Table 14.5).[41] Breast milk of mothers who deliver prematurely has higher protein content that generally decreases with advancing gestational age.[42] These differences were maximal in the first few days of life with differences of approximately 35%. Initial mean protein

TABLE 14.3 Estimated Requirements and Advisable Intakes for Protein by Infant's Weight as Derived by Factorial Approach

Birth Weight Range (g)	Tissue Increment (g/day)	Dermal Loss (g/day)	Urine Loss (g/day)	Intestinal Absorption (% intake)	Estimated Requirement (g/day)	ADVISABLE INTAKE		
						g/day	g/kg[a]	g/100 kcal[b]
800–1200	2.32	0.17	0.68	87 g[b]	3.64	4.0	4.0	3.1
1200–1800	3.01	0.25	0.90	87 g	4.78	5.2	3.5	2.7

[a]Assuming body weight of 1000 and 1500 g for 800- to 1200-g infant and 1200- to 1800-g infant, respectively.
[b]Assuming calorie intake of 120 kcal/day.
Modified from Ziegler EE, Biga RL, Fomon SJ. Nutritional requirements of the premature infant. In: Suskind RM, ed. *Textbook of Pediatric Nutrition.* New York, NY: Raven; 1981;29–39.

TABLE 14.4 Accumulation of Various Components During Last Trimester of Pregnancy

Component	ACCUMULATION DURING VARIOUS STAGES OF GESTATION (WK)				
	26–31	31–33	33–35	35–38	38–40
Body weight (g)[a]	500	500	500	500	—
Water (g)	410	350	320	240	220
Fat (g)	25	65	85	175	200
Nitrogen (g)	11	12	12	6	7
Calcium (g)	4	5	5	5	5
Phosphorus (g)	2.2	2.6	2.8	3.0	3.0
Magnesium (mg)	130	110	120	120	80
Sodium (mEq)	35	25	40	40	40
Potassium (mEq)	19	24	26	20	20
Chloride (mEq)	30	24	10	20	10
Iron (mg)	36	60	60	40	20
Copper (mg)	2.1	2.4	2.0	2.0	2.0
Zinc (mg)	9.0	10.0	8.0	7.0	3.0

[a]Body weight of 26-week fetus is 1000 g and of 40-week fetus is 3500 g.
Modified from data of Widdowson from Heird WC, Anderson TL. Nutritional requirements and methods of feeding low birth weight infants. In: Gluck L et al., eds. *Current Problems in Pediatrics.* vol. 7, no. 8, Chicago, IL: Year Book; 1977:1–4.

levels of preterm milk were 2.2 g/dL in a large meta-analysis. Differences were no longer statistically significant by 10 to 12 weeks of life, although in actuality by 5 weeks of age differences in true protein levels were 0.1 to 0.2 g/dL.[41] Growing preterm infants require between 3.5 and 4.5 g/kg of enteral protein, which breast milk alone cannot provide.[43] Fat content was not statistically different between preterm and term milk, initially at a mean of 2.2 g/dL in the preterm milk, although this was 23% higher than in term milk. Fat and energy content also change with time of day and from start to finish of the feed. Lactose in preterm milk averages 6.2 g/dL

and up to 7.05 g/dL at 28 days, peaking at approximately 6 weeks of age (Fig. 14.5).[44]

The macronutrients calcium and phosphorus are slightly higher in preterm milk than term milk (14 to 16 mEq/L vs. 13 to 16 mEq/L calcium and 4.7 to 5.5 m/L vs. 4.0 to 5.1 m/L phosphorus). Neither term nor preterm milk has adequate calcium and phosphorus for the VLBW infant.[45] The preterm infant is missing the third trimester of gestation when accretion rates for calcium and phosphorus are highest and two-thirds of mineral content is acquired. Preterm infants need large amounts of these minerals to achieve adequate extra-uterine growth. Magnesium levels in preterm milk are 28 to 31 mg/L, dropping to 25 mg/L at 28 days, and term milk levels are 25 to 29 mg/L. Zinc levels are higher in preterm milk, beginning at 5.3 mg/L and dropping to 3.9 mg/L, whereas term milk begins at 5.4 mg/L and drops to 2.6 mg/L. Sodium levels in preterm milk are higher (26.6 mEq/L, dropping to 12.6 mEq/L), whereas term milk is 22.3 mEq/L, decreasing to 8.5 mEq/L at 28 days.[45] Chloride has a similar average (preterm 31.6 mEq/L, decreasing to 16.8 mEq/L, and term 26.9 mEq/L, decreasing to 13.1 mEq/L).

Requirements for Growth in Premature Infants
Protein Requirements in Premature Infants
The whey protein in human milk is an advantage for all infants but especially for premature infants. It includes the nine amino acids known to be essential to humans, as well as taurine,[46] glycine, leucine, and cystine, which are considered essential for premature infants. Taurine is not present in cow milk and has to be manufactured and added to formula.[47] The premature infant lacks the necessary enzymes for metabolism and has been noted to accumulate nonphysiologic levels of methionine, tyrosine, phenylalanine, blood urea, and ammonia. The placenta provides about 3.5 to 4.0 g/kg per day of amino acids to the fetus. The placenta is able to optimize the amino acids, however, something that cannot be done with enteral feeds. If energy intake is deficient, protein synthesis can be depressed and protein retention reduced. Greater protein intake is risky if energy intake is limited because the amino acids will be oxidized to ammonia and urea. Preterm infants require 30 to 40 kcal/g of protein provided. LBW infants fed mother's milk exclusively for 2 weeks have been found to have a low protein level. This has led to

TABLE 14.5 **Mean Values for Macronutrients and Energy Content in Human Milk at Different Times During Lactation**

	Protein (g/100 mL)	Lactose/Carbohydrates (g/100 mL)	Fat (g/100 mL)	Energy (kcal/100 mL)
Days 1–3	$n = 163$ 2.57 ± 1.44	$n = 143$ 6.2 ± 0.92	$n = 173$ 2.52 ± 0.98	$n = 143$ 58.8 ± 7.91
Days 4–7	$n = 44$ 2.11 ± 0.44	$n = 87$ 6.17 ± 0.49	$n = 110$ 3.31 ± 1.27	$n = 96$ 67.9 ± 14.1
Week 2	$n = 383$ 1.98 ± 0.68	$n = 389$ 6.72 ± 0.46	$n = 426$ 3.19 ± 1.04	$n = 417$ 691 ± 101
Week 3–4	$n = 528$ 1.6 ± 0.5	$n = 464$ 7.05 ± 0.51	$n = 485$ 3.83 ± 1.01	$n = 481$ 70.87 ± 9.34
Week 5–6	$n = 330$ 1.43 ± 0.25	$n = 354$ 7.14 ± 0.36	$n = 371$ 4.04 ± 0.91	$n = 361$ 73.97 ± 9.1
Week 7–9	$n = 223$ 1.34 ± 0.2	$n = 235$ 7.13 ± 0.38	$n = 236$ 4.21 ± 0.92	$n = 239$ 74.24 ± 8.77
Week 10–12	$n = 120$ 1.26 ± 0.2	$n = 120$ 7.12 ± 0.28	$n = 120$ 4.25 ± 0.91	$n = 120$ 74.53 ± 8.71

From Mimouni FB, Lubetzky R, Yochpaz S, Mandel D. Preterm human milk macronutrient and energy composition. *Clin Perinatol.* 2017;44:165. doi:10.1016/j.clp.2016.11.010.

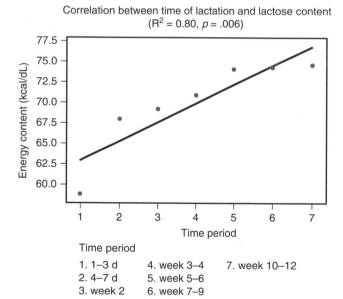

Fig. 14.5 Lactose content correlates with time of lactation. (From Mimouni FB, Lubetzky R, Yochpaz S, Mandel D. Preterm human milk macronutrient and energy composition: a systematic review and meta-analysis. *Clin Perinatol.* 2017;44:165. doi:10.1016/j.clp.2016.11.010.)

the need to supplement human milk when the infant tolerates significant amounts of enteral feeds (120 to 150 mL/kg per day). To achieve adequate weight gain, preterm infants require 3.4 g/kg per day of protein.[48] In most instances, human milk feeding will progress gradually from small trophic feedings designed to stimulate the newborn gut to full enteral nutrition. Fortifiers are added to human milk when infants are typically tolerating a substantial amount of feeds

at about the time when protein levels in their own mother's milk drops from about 2.5 to 1.5 g/dL.[49] Most neonatologists consider fortification at the time when the infants are receiving 80 to 100 mL/kg. Sullivan and Schanler[50] and others have shown that introduction of fortifier in human milk does not increase the risk for adverse events, including NEC. In randomized trials there were no adverse effects of introducing fortifier at 40 mL/kg of feeds compared with 100 mL/kg of feeds.

Protein has been shown to be an important component and necessary for adequate growth.[48,49] In a randomized trial by Brumberg et al.,[51] it was demonstrated that infants fed at equivalent energy levels but higher protein contents had significantly improved weight gain, head circumference, and mid-arm circumferences. Assuming a human milk protein level of 1.5 g/dL, most fortifiers add an additional 1.5 to 2.2 g/dL bringing the total enteral protein intake to 3.5 to 4.5 g/dL when fed at 150 mL/kg. These fortifiers derive their protein from either a bovine source or from pooled human milk. Powdered fortifiers are no longer recommended because of the increased risk for bacterial contamination and sepsis. Exclusive human milk diets including human milk–derived fortifier have been associated with a lower rate of NEC than mixed human milk and bovine-based products.

Fat Requirements in Premature Infants

A diurnal variation in the creamatocrits (see Chapter 22) of expressed breast milk of mothers delivering prematurely was demonstrated in 39 mothers by Lubetzky et al.[52] The creamatocrit was significantly higher in the evening—7.9% ± 2.9% compared with first morning samples, 6.6% ± 2.8% ($p < 0.005$)—regardless of gestational age or birth weight.

The fat content of mother's milk is not affected by fetal growth of the infant. Fifty-six lactating mothers of newborns (26 SGA and 30 AGA) had their creamatocrits measured on the third day postpartum and again at 7 and 14 days.[53] Other parameters (maternal age, body mass index, gestational age, weight gain, or parity) were similar except for birth weight for gestational age (SGA or AGA). Fat content of the milk was not affected by fetal growth status.

The requirement for fat for appropriate growth is based on the essential fatty acid proportion as 3% of total caloric intake. Human milk has high levels of linoleic acid (9% of lipids) and adequately meets this requirement. Human milk fat is more readily absorbed in the presence of milk lipase and other enzymes in human milk. It is reported that infants less than 1500 g absorb 90% of human milk fat and 68% of cow milk formula fats.[54] This phenomenon is due to the fact that human milk has a very special fat globule containing another protein coat and inner lipid core membrane (milk fat globule membrane [MFGM]) (see Chapter 4). The pattern of fatty acids (i.e., high in palmitic 16.0, oleic 18:1, linoleic 18:2 omega-6, and linolenic 18:3 omega-3), their distribution on the triglyceride molecule, and the presence of bile salt—stimulated lipase characterize the lipid system in human milk.[55] Digestion of milk triglycerides requires three gastrointestinal lipases: gastric, pancreatic, and bile salt—stimulated lipase (BSSL). Fat globules are broken down into droplets by gastric lipase, further hydrolyzed by pancreatic lipase, and broken down into free fatty acids and free glycerol by the bile salt lipase.[7] BSSL activity is high in fresh human milk but nearly completely eliminated after Holder pasteurization. High-pressure processing of donor human milk preserves much of the BSSL activity and may be a promising alternative[56] (Fig. 14.6). BSSL is not present in formula, so despite the fact that formula has higher levels of fat, it is not as well absorbed or metabolized.

Fat digestion is efficient in LBW infants who receive their own mother's milk fresh and untreated. Fat absorption is decreased by calcium supplementation, however, and by sterilizing the milk. If human milk is supplemented with lipids, it will change the ratio of vitamin E to polyunsaturated fatty acid (PUFA). It may be necessary to add vitamin E to keep the ratio of vitamin E to PUFA greater than 0.6 (normally the ratio of human milk vitamin E to PUFA is 0.9).[57]

Special attributes of human milk for VLBW infants have been confirmed as investigators inspect the value of adding nutrients to formulas specifically for these infants.[58] In a study of omega-3 fatty acids on retinal function using electroretinograms, human milk was associated with the best function, followed by formula supplemented with omega-3 fatty acids. This supports the concept that omega-3 fatty acids are essential to retinal development.[59]

Although human milk contains 250 mg of calcium and 140 mg/L of phosphorus in readily absorbable form, preterm and term milk do not contain sufficient calcium and phosphorus for bone accretion in LBW infants. Rickets has developed in LBW infants who are not supplemented because the

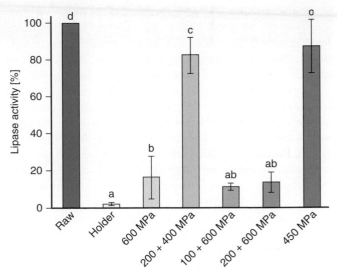

Fig. 14.6 Lipase activity in human milk samples after treatment with different temperatures and pressures (forms of pasteurization). Results are shown as a percent value of (d) raw milk with error bars representing standard deviation (SD). (a) Holder pasteurization was 62.5°C for 30 minutes. For the other test conditions temperature was between 19° and 21°C. Pressure was applied for different periods of time (b) 600 MPa, 10 min; (ab) 100 MPa, 10 min, interval 10 min, 600 MPa, 10 min; (c, light blue bar) 200 MPa, 10 min, interval 10 min, 400 MPa, 10 min; (ab) 200 MPa, 10 min, interval 10 min, 600 MPa, 10 min; and (c, dark blue bar) 450 MPa, 15 min. The pressure generation time was 15 to 25 seconds, and the decompression time was 1 to 4 seconds. *MPa*, Megapascals or 1,000,000 pascals. (From Wesolowska A, Brys J, Barbarska O, et al. Lipid profile, lipase bioactivity, and lipophilic antioxidant content in high pressure processed donor human milk. *Nutrients.* 2019;11:ii:E1972. doi:10.3390/nu11091972.)

requirement for bone growth at this point in the growth curve is high. Calcium and phosphorus fetal accretion increases steadily during the last trimester of pregnancy. Magnesium accretion is unchanged in that period.

Mineral accretion is a complex phenomenon dependent on a number of variables beyond simple levels of calcium, phosphorus, magnesium, and vitamin D.[60] Absorption and retention are altered by the quantities of other minerals and other nutrients, including fat, protein, and carbohydrate. Although the calcium-to-phosphorus ratio in human milk is more physiologic than that of cow milk, the low levels of phosphorus may lead to loss of calcium in the urine if not supplemented.[61]

Even with optimal vitamin D and magnesium, the amount of calcium absorbed from preterm milk is not enough to meet intrauterine accretion rates without supplementation. Because human milk phosphorus levels are low, even with high intestinal absorption and high renal tubular reabsorption, compared with the needs of the premature infant, supplementation is necessary to avoid depletion or deficiency.[62] Intrauterine accretion rates for calcium and phosphorus were achieved when Schanler and Abrams[63] fed human milk supplemented with calcium gluconate and glycerophosphate to VLBW infants. In their study, supplementation with magnesium was not included. The authors concluded that greater intakes of calcium and phosphorus and not improved bioavailability were responsible for the improved net retention. Premature infants who receive only unfortified human milk never achieve intrauterine retention rates of calcium and phophorus.[63] Therefore it is necessary to fortify human milk for premature infants. Vitamin D requirements in this period of high skeletal development depend on maternal vitamin D status because significant correlation exists between maternal serum and preterm infant cord serum 25-hydroxyvitamin D values. Recommendations for vitamin D have changed dramatically. No longer are maternal stores considered adequate. Work by Wagner et al.[64] demonstrated that average women, even with a healthy lifestyle, have low vitamin D levels and thus their infants are relatively deficient at birth, especially infants born prematurely. Mothers of premature infants tend to have lower vitamin D levels than their term counterparts with their preterm newborns showing similar levels of vitamin D insufficiency. The milk was also low in vitamin D. The recommended daily dose of vitamin D for mothers is 1000 units. Obtaining vitamin D blood levels is simple and should be checked early in pregnancy and the dose adjusted. Because infants are no longer exposed to sunlight, dietary sources are crucial. LBW infants quickly become dependent on exogenous vitamin D because fetal storage is minimal. The recommended dietary allowance of 400 units of vitamin D appears to be appropriate for all LBW infants, regardless of feedings, and for term infants. Vitamin D intake of 200 to 400 IU/day for VLBW infants is recommended by the AAP Committee on Nutrition. As the infant grows and weight exceeds 1500 g the dose should be increased to 400 IU/day.[65]

Other vitamin needs of LBW infants depend on body stores, intestinal absorption, bioavailability of the vitamin, and rates of utilization and excretion.[66] Little information suggests that major differences exist in absorption between term and LBW infants, although fat-soluble vitamins depend on bile acids for absorption. (See Chapter 8 for vitamin requirements.) It is recommended that LBW infants receive daily vitamin supplements to address the increased need and borderline levels provided in the volume of human milk they can reasonably consume (Box 14.7).

The mineral supplementation required for LBW infants fed human milk is based on intrauterine accretion rates, which actually may not be achieved (Table 14.6). Not all premature infants fed human milk develop rickets, which occurs infrequently in infants greater than 1500 g. VLBW infants do need supplementation, and cases of rickets are well documented in the literature for this group.[67] Supplements are usually not necessary while an infant is receiving fortified human milk or formula and when an infant reaches 40 weeks' postconceptional age. Hypophosphatemia is a sensitive biochemical indicator of low bone mineralization in VLBW infants fed human milk. Tsang et al.[67] recommend weekly measurements of serum phosphorus for the first month and biweekly until 2000 g or 40 weeks' gestation. A level less than 4 mg/dL phosphorus should be followed by radiographs of the wrists for osteopenia and rickets. Supplementation should be based on an infant's needs. Calcium levels should also be obtained weekly to evaluate levels

BOX 14.7 Vitamin Supplements for Low-Birth-Weight Infants Fed Human Milk

- Vitamin B_{12}: Only if mother's diet deficient
- Folic acid: Human milk usually adequate
- Thiamin (B_1): Borderline
- Riboflavin (B_2): Borderline
- Vitamin B_6: Human milk usually adequate
- Niacin: Human milk usually adequate
- Vitamin A: 1000 to 1500 IU/day
- Vitamin C: If infant receives supplementary protein up to 60 mg/day
- Vitamin D: 400 IU/day
- Vitamin K: All infants should receive 0.5 to 1 mg at birth; recommended 5 mg/kg per day; human milk borderline
- Vitamin E: 25 IU/day for first month, 5 IU/day after first month; human milk adequate

IU, International units.

TABLE 14.6 Required Calcium (Ca), Phosphorus (P), and Magnesium (Mg) Intake to Meet Fetal Accretion Rate at 27 and 30 Weeks[a]

	27 WEEKS			30 WEEKS		
	Ca	P	Mg	Ca	P	Mg
Accretion (mg/kg/day)	121	72	3.37	123	72	3.17
Retention (% intake)	50	89	59	50	89	59
Intake (mg/kg/day)	242	81	5.70	246	81	5.37

[a]Assuming a weight of 1000 g and 1250 g, respectively, in an infant fed human milk.

From Steichen JJ, Krug-Wispe SK, Tsang RC. Breastfeeding the low birth weight preterm infant. *Clin Perinatol.* 1987;14:131.

greater than 11 mg/dL for too much calcium or too little phosphorus.[63] Supplements of calcium and phosphorus are incorporated in available human milk fortifiers and supplements derived from formula (Table 14.7). Now such supplementation is also available from human milk products: Prolacta CR, product of Prolacta (Fig. 14.7, Box 14.8; see Table 14.7), and Medolac.

Trace minerals in general appear in physiologic amounts in human milk and are more bioavailable from human milk than artificial feedings. The minimum daily requirements for LBW infants are based on daily accretion rates as calculated from third-trimester data and calculated obligatory losses.

Zinc is known to be readily available in human milk, although zinc deficiency syndromes from hyperalimentation are well known in the literature and in NICUs. Zinc requirements for the growing preterm infant are 1.4 to 2.5 mg/kg day[69] (are and may be met initially by mother's own milk because the concentration in colostrum starts out very high. Levels quickly fall, however, from 5.4 mg/L in colostrum to 1.1 mg/L by 3 months postpartum. Zinc requirements are met through supplementation with human milk fortifiers of mother's own milk or donor milk.

TABLE 14.7 Nutrient Composition of Selected Fortifiers and Supplements

| | BOVINE-BASED PRODUCTS (PER GRAM OF POWDER) | | | | | | | | | | HUMAN MILK–BASED FORTIFIER (PER VOLUME) | | | |
| | MULTICOMPONENT FORTIFIERS | | | | | PROTEIN SUPPLEMENTS | | | | | | | | |
Fortifier	A	B	C	D	E	F	G	H	I	J	K	L	M	N
Volume (ml)	/	/	/	/	/	/	/	/	/	/	20	30	40	50
Energy (kcal)	4.4 (L)	3.5	3.6	4.9 (L)	3.9 (L)	3.4	3.6	3.6	4	3.7	28	42	56	71
Protein (g)	0.36[PH]	0.25[EH]	0.2[EH]	0.4	0.3	0.82[EH]	0.72[EH]	0.86[W]	0.8[W]	0.9[W]	1.2	1.8	2.4	3
Na (mg)	9.2	8.0	5.4	5.6	4.2	7.8	8.2	2.1	2	0	20	40	42	45
Ca (mg)	18.9	14.9	10	32	33	5.2	12.8	0	4	0	103	106	108	111
P (mg)	11	8.7	7	18	19	5.2	0.73	0	3	0	53.8	54.9	56	57.5
Iron (mg)	0.5	0	0	0.5	0.1	0	0.007	0	0	0	0.1	0.15	0.2	0.25

EH, Extensively hydrolyzed; *HMBF*, human milk–based fortifier; *L*, lipids; *PH*, partially hydrolyzed; *W*, whole protein. *A*, Fortipré, Nestle; *B*, Fortema, Danone; *C*, FM85, Nestle; *D*, Enfamil, Mead Johnson; *E*, Similac, Ross; *F*, Aptamil PS, Danone; *G*, Preemie, Nestle; *H*, Beneprotein, Nestle; *I*, Pro-Mix, Corpak; *J*, Protein instant, Resource; *K*, HMBF + 4, Prolacta; *L*, HMBF + 6, Prolacta; *M*, HMBF + 8, Prolacta; *N*, HMBF + 10, Prolacta.
From Arslanoglu S, Boquien C-Y, King C, et al. Fortification of human milk for preterm infants: update and recommendations of the European Milk Bank Association (EMBA) Working Group on Human Milk Fortification. *Front Pediatr.* 2019;7:76. doi:10.3389/fped.2019.00076.

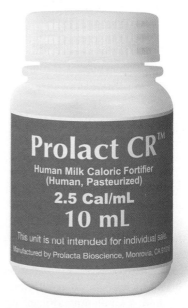

Fig. 14.7 Prolact CR. (Reproduced with permission from Prolacta Bioscience.)

Recommendations have been put forth by various groups/organizations on the recommended amounts of individual daily nutrient intake by premature infants and VLBW infants receiving enteral feedings (Table 14.8).

Preterm infants absorb approximately 50% of copper from fortified human milk and only 27% from formula. To absorb 50 mcg/kg per day the preterm infant is recommended to take in 100 to 230 mcg/kg per day.

Manganese requirements are 1 to 15 mcg/kg per day and are met by the combination of human milk and fortifier. The provision in human milk is 0.35 ng/mL, or 0.5 mg/kg per day, but no information is available recommending supplementation.[35]

The selenium suggested requirement is 5 to 10 mcg/kg per day. Human milk provides 1 to 2 mcg/dL and is stable throughout lactation, so no supplementation has been recommended.[70]

Preterm infants need approximately 30 mcg/kg of iodine to remain sufficient. Maternal breast milk contains about 100 to 150 mcg/L of iodine, and although human milk fortifiers do not contain iodine, there does not appear to be any benefit in iodine supplementation.

Chromium requirements are calculated to be 1.0 to 2.0 mg/kg per day based on an accretion rate of 0.1 to 0.2 mg/kg per day and only 10% absorption. Levels in human milk are reported to be 0.03 mg/dL, which, with 150-mL/kg per day intake, would supply 0.045 mg/kg per day. Supplementation is not usually provided, and absorption in human milk is probably greater than 10%.

Molybdenum levels in human milk are thought to be sufficient to meet LBW accretion rates (1 mg/kg per day).

Iron requirements are a complex issue, and intrauterine accretion rates are not appropriate values on which to base requirements.[71,72] Most of iron accretion, like that of calcium and phosphorus, happens in the third trimester, so preterm infants are at high risk for iron deficiency. Iron stores are partially enlarged by hemoglobin breakdown in early life and blood transfusions, although this is balanced by iatrogenic blood loss through blood sampling in the NICU. Providing iron, however, interferes with the immunologic properties of human milk, especially the bacteriostatic properties of lactoferrin in the gut.

The recommendations for iron supplementation for preterm infants are that supplementation should begin after 2 weeks of age and supply 2 to 3 mg/kg per day of enteral iron. Preterm infants should generally continue these supplements for 6 to 12 months of age.

It is necessary also to ensure adequate vitamin C and vitamin E supplementation (4 to 5 mg/day), even though human milk

---

BOX 14.8 Prolact CR 10 mL Human Milk Caloric Fortifier (Human, Pasteurized)

Product Description

- Prolact CR is pasteurized human milk cream derived from human milk. It is composed of 25% fat and provides 2.5 cal/mL. It contains no added minerals.
- Store at −20°C or colder until ready to thaw for preparation and use.
- Available frozen in 30-mL bottles containing 10 mL of product (four bottles per package).

Intended Use

- Prolact CR is intended for use with mom's own breast milk or donor human milk to achieve a 20 cal/fl oz feeding solution.

Directions for Thawing

Under no circumstances should the product be defrosted or warmed in a microwave.

Remove bottle from the freezer and label with date and time. Thaw product using one of the following methods:

1. Refrigeration: (2° to 8°C) Place unopened bottle in refrigerator. Once thawed, must be administered within 24 hours. Do not refreeze, keep refrigerated.
2. Rapid thawing: Place bottle under lukewarm running water, or place in a water bath. Do not submerge top of bottle. Warm only until product is thawed. Continued warming, or exposure to high temperatures, could result in undesirable changes to the product. Wipe outside of bottle with appropriate disinfectant to reduce the risk for contamination. Once thawed, keep refrigerated, do not refreeze. Product must be administered within 24 hours of thawing.

Ingredients

Human milk cream and human milk ultrafiltration permeate.

Preparation Instructions

Always maintain aseptic technique when preparing and handling human milk products. **Do not add water.**

1. Thaw mom's own or donor milk according to hospital policy.

2. Measure caloric content of mom's own or donor milk.
   a. If using a commercial human milk analyzer, follow the manufacturer's instructions.
   b. If using a creamatocrit, ensure the milk is room temperature and follow the manufacturer's instructions.
3. Thaw Prolact CR according to "Directions for Thawing." Swirl gently before each aliquot.
4. Based on the measured caloric content of mom's own or donor milk, follow the instructions in the following table to formulate 100 mL of human milk plus Prolact CR:

Cal/oz (equivalent to)	Cal/ 100 mL	Mom's Own or Donor Milk Volume	+ Add to Milk
19–20	64–67.9	98 mL milk	2 mL Prolact CR
18–18.9	61–63.9	96 mL milk	4 mL Prolact CR
17–17.9	57–60.9	94 mL milk	6 mL Prolact CR
16–16.9	54–56.9	93 mL milk	7 mL Prolact CR
15–15.9	51–53.9	91 mL milk	9 mL Prolact CR
14–14.9	47–50.9	90 mL milk	10 mL Prolact CR

5. Swirl gently to mix.
6. Once completed, the product is ready for use, *OR*
7. Store bottle in refrigerator (2°C to 8°C). Use within 24 hours after thawing Prolact CR.

For More Information

Visit http://www.prolacta.com or call 1 (888) PROLACT #1 for Customer Service
Manufactured by:
Prolacta Bioscience, Inc.
City of Industry, CA 91746
Reproduced with permission from Prolacta Bioscience.

---

normally contains 5 mg/dL vitamin C and 0.25 mg/dL vitamin E. Vitamin C levels in mother's milk can be increased by dietary increases. However, vitamin C is affected by pasteurization.

The different human milk fortifiers available for use provide different amounts of macronutrients and micronutrients when used to fortify human milk enteral feedings (Table 14.7).

USE OF HUMAN MILK

Human milk provides developmental benefits for preterms that extend into adolescence. The use of exclusive human milk when paired with standardized feeding guidelines can improve tolerance of feedings and decrease the incidence of NEC. Human milk–fed infants have decreased rates of late-onset sepsis, urinary tract infection, diarrhea, and upper respiratory tract infection. The protection against NEC and sepsis appears to be dose dependent. Human milk is also associated with decreases in the incidence and severity of ROP, improved neurodevelopmental and visual outcomes, and improved feeding tolerance compared with formula. Improved tolerance allows infants to receive

fewer days of parenteral nutrition, significantly decreases morbidity, and decreases length of stay.

Human milk contains bioactive factors that benefit growth and development. This includes improved immunity with antibacterial, antiviral, and antiinflammatory effects. A healthy microbiome is promoted by probiotics and the high oligosaccharide content.[73] The oligosaccharides not only have a prebiotic effect but also decrease infections by not allowing pathogenic bacteria and viruses to attach to the intestinal mucosa. This blunts the intestinal inflammatory response to pathogenic bacteria. The gut of the human milk–fed infant is colonized mostly by bifidobacteria and lactobacilli as opposed to the coliforms, enterococci, and *Bacteroides* sp. that colonize formula-fed infants.[74] Abnormal colonization is also promoted by delayed enteral feeding, the use of broad-spectrum antibiotics, and exposure to the pervasive organisms in the NICU milieu. Studies have revealed that preterm infants who develop NEC have an abnormal microbiota 3 weeks before NEC, providing evidence that dysbiosis is a risk factor for NEC.

TABLE 14.8 Recommendations of Nutrient Intake for Fully Enterally Fed Preterm Infants With Very Low-Birth-Weight

Nutrient	Current Recommendation (per kg/day)	Current Recommendation (per 100 kcal)
Fluids	135–200	—
Energy, kcal	110–130 (85–95 IV)	—
Protein, g	3.5–4.5	3.2–4.1
Lipids, g	4.8–6.6	4.4–6
Linoleic acid, mg	385–1540	350–1400
α-Linolenic acid, mg	>55	>50
DHA, mg	(18-) 55–60	(16.4-) 50–55
EPA, mg	<20	<18
ARA, mg	(18-) 35–45	(16.4-) 32–41
Carbohydrate, g	11.6–13.2	10.5–12
Sodium, mg[a]	69–115	63–105
Potassium, mg[b]	78–195	71–177
Chloride, mg	105–177	95–161
Calcium, mg	120–200	109–182
Phosphate, mg	60–140	55–127
Magnesium, mg	8–15	7.3–13.6
Iron, mg	2–3	1.8–2.7
Zinc, mg	1.4–2.5	1.3–2.3
Copper, µg	100–230	90–210
Selenium, µg	5–10	4.5–9
Manganese, µg	1–15	0.9–13.6
Fluoride, µg	1.5–60	1.4–55
Iodine, µg	10–55	9–50
Chromium, ng	30–2250	27–2045
Molybdenum, µg	0.3–5	0.27–4.5
Biotin, ng	1.7–16.5	1.5–15
Vitamin A, µg RE	400–1100	365–1000
Vitamin D, IU	(400–1000 per day, from milk + supplement)	100–350 from milk only
Vitamin E, mg α-TE	2.2–11	2–10
Vitamin K₁, µg	4.4–28	4–25
Nucleotides, mg	NS	NS
Choline, mg	8–55	7.3–50

(*Continued*)

TABLE 14.8 Recommendations of Nutrient Intake for Fully Enterally Fed Preterm Infants With Very Low-Birth-Weight—cont'd

Nutrient	Current Recommendation (per kg/day)	Current Recommendation (per 100 kcal)
Inositol, mg	4.4–53	4–48
Thiamin, µg	140–300	127–273
Riboflavin, µg	200–400	181–364
Niacin, mg	1–5.5	0.9–5
Pantothenic acid, mg	0.5–2.1	0.45–1.9
Pyridoxine, µg	50–300	45–273
Cobalamin, µg	0.1–0.8	0.09–0.73
Folic acid, µg	35–100	32–91
L-Ascorbic acid, mg	20–55	18–50

ARA, Arachidonic acid; *α-TE*, α-tocopherol equivalents; *DHA*, docoshexanoic acid; *EPA*, eicospentaenoic acid; *IV*, intravenous; *RE*, retinol equivalents.
[a]1 mEq Na = 23 mg.
[b]1 mEq K = 39 g.
From Koletzko B, Poindexter B, Uauy R. Recommended nutrient intake levels for stable, fully enterally fed very low birth weight infants. In: Koletzko B, Poindexter B, Uauy R, eds. *Nutritional Care of Preterm Infants: Scientific Basis and Practical Guidelines*. New York, NY: Karger; 2014:297–299.

Maturation of the gastrointestinal tract is supported by components in human milk resulting in improved motility, smaller gastric residuals, and decreased intestinal permeability. Preterm infants have decreased ability to absorb fats. Enzymes in human milk allow for improved fat absorption and intestinal lipolysis.

Important methodologic issues have been raised regarding the quality of research examining associations of breastfeeding and health outcomes among preterm infants in the NICU. Studies are limited by sample size, quality of data sets, and inadequate adjustment for confounders. Measurement of breastfeeding for preterm infants in the NICU is a significant issue, because many studies examine breastfeeding at single time points, when the NICU hospitalization lasts weeks to months, or measure provision of mother's breast milk as "any versus none," which may not accurately represent the "dose" or amount of mother's breast milk an infant received over the course of the hospitalization. As the use of pasteurized human donor milk and human milk fortifiers have increased in the past two decades, studies examining health outcomes vary in their inclusion of these supplements to mother's own breast milk. Practical and ethical issues have precluded prospective randomized interventional trials to examine mother's breast milk versus formula. Thus the majority of published reports are observational cohort studies.

Antiinfective Properties of Breast Milk

Human milk contains bioactive factors that benefit growth and development. This includes improved immunity with antibacterial, antiviral, and antiinflammatory effects. In addition to the microbiome, colonization of the gastrointestinal tract with nonpathogenic organisms and the effect of oligosaccharides blocking attachment of certain pathogenic bacteria and viruses, there are many other proposed antiinfective effects of human breast milk. Antiinfective properties of breast milk also have been related to its components, such as immunoglobulins, lysozyme, lactoferrin, and various cytokines. In response to maternal pathogens, IgA and IgM are produced and secreted into milk. sIgA and IgM are resistant to breakdown in the neonatal gut and protect the newborn with the memory of maternal pathogens.[75] This often has been referred to as the enteromammary pathway.

Lactoferrin

Lactoferrin is a glycoprotein present in significant amounts in colostrum as well as milk with significant antiinfective properties. It is the dominant whey protein in human milk and is critical in protecting the newborn from infection. Lactoferrin levels are sensitive to both freezing and Holder pasteurization, so levels are significantly decreased from levels in fresh mother's milk. Lactoferrin avidly binds iron, which is essential for microbial growth. It also exerts an antimicrobial effect by its interactions with cell membrane surfaces. In addition to its antimicrobial properties, lactoferrin stimulates intestinal growth and proliferation.[76] This may be due to either direct effects on the cell membrane or its ability to remove iron from the environment.[77,78] Lactoferrin has been shown to sequester ferric iron, which is an essential substrate for pathogenic gut bacteria. It also has been postulated to protect the gut by the process of anoikis. This is an apoptotic process that destroys the gut epithelial cells that are infected by bacteria and allows them to be excreted in the stool.[79] Lactoferrin has also been the subject of a number of randomized controls trials among very LBW infants. These trials have shown lactoferrin to reduce the incidence of late-onset sepsis and fungal infections.[80,81] In another trial, bovine lactoferrin was shown to reduce the incidence of combined death or NEC from 10% to 4% in very LBW infants.[82]

Human Milk Oligosaccharides

Human milk oligosaccharides (HMOs) are an important component of human milk and have higher levels in preterm than term milk. These oligosaccharides serve as prebiotics for commensal bacteria in the neonatal intestine and modulate the neonate's immune response. These functions are especially important in the preterm gut, in which gut dysfunction and NEC have the highest incidence.[83] The HMOs have been shown to decrease the inflammatory response of the preterm gut and thus reduce gut injury. The HMOs are a diverse group of monosaccharides and depend on the mother's blood group characteristics for their structure. Interestingly, one particular HMO, disialyllacto-N-tetraose (DSLNT) has been identified to be effective in preventing NEC in neonatal rats. In a study to examine the importance of this HMO, 200 mother–infant pairs were recruited and breast milk composition was analyzed. It was found that infants who developed NEC during their NICU hospitalization received significantly less DSLNT in their milk than those who did not develop NEC.[84] Thus specific HMOs in human milk may serve as biomarkers for NEC risk or as potential therapeutic agents for prevention.

Necrotizing Enterocolitis

One of the most significant morbidities befalling preterm infants is NEC. NEC is a multifactorial disease that includes risk factors such as immaturity, infection, and tissue hypoxia.[85] Because NEC is a multifactorial disease there must be a multipronged attempt to decrease its incidence. This has occurred in neonatal units with evidence of decreasing rates of NEC as reported by the Vermont Oxford Network database. One of the factors associated with NEC is increased intestinal permeability and the breakdown of tight junctions. The metalloproteinases (MMPs) have been shown to be largely responsible for this breakdown. Another factor, tissue inhibitor of metallopeptidase 1 (TIMP-1), inhibits MMP activity and is overexpressed in preterm human milk.[86] Lactoferrin also has been shown experimentally to downregulate inflammation and upregulate cell proliferation and is a key component of human milk.[87] Another factor playing a role are HMOs.[88] These nondigestible carbohydrates serve as prebiotics for commensal bacteria and interact as structural analogs with pathogens and Toll-like receptors to downregulate the inflammatory process. Thus preterm human milk may directly decrease the increased permeability seen in NEC. NEC has been clearly shown to be reduced in human milk feeds compared with formula feedings.[32] Corpeleijn et al.[33] retrospectively analyzed milk intake and morbidity in 349 infants with birth weights below 1500 g. They used the combined outcome of NEC, sepsis, or death and found that any intake of mother's milk in the first 5 days of life was protective. Furthermore they showed that between days 6 and 10 there was a protective effect if the infant ingested more than 50% of their enteral intake as mother's milk.[33] Significant protection against NEC among preterm infants fed human milk versus preterm formula has been published in multiple studies.[30,89–92] A large, multicenter study of more than 1200 ELBW infants (<1000 g) reported a dose-dependent relationship between greater human milk consumption and risk for NEC, in which each 10% increase in the proportion of total intake that was human milk was associated with a 17% risk reduction in NEC (hazard ratio [HR] 0.83 [0.72, 0.96]).[32] A recent meta-analysis reviewed 44 studies and found a clear protection for NEC, with a 4% reduction for any NEC and a 2% reduction for severe NEC. The meta-analysis concluded that any volume of human milk is better than preterm formula and the higher the dose the greater is the protection.[92]

Late-Onset Sepsis

A study examining dose of mother's milk found that 50 mL/kg or more per day of mother's milk was associated with a 31% reduction in incidence of late-onset sepsis.[30] Other studies have shown a significant negative correlation between the number of positive blood cultures and the cumulative intake of human milk throughout NICU hospitalization. Lactoferrin has been shown to inhibit microbial growth and enhance host defense. In a meta-analysis of studies using supplemental enteral lactoferrin it was shown to decrease late-onset sepsis and NEC.[31,94] Because lactoferrin is a significant component of colostrum and human milk, the lower rates of sepsis and NEC in the mother's milk—fed group are not surprising.

Feeding Tolerance

Faster advancement to full enteral feedings (22 days vs. 27 days, $p = 0.01$),[95] was seen in a cohort of VLBW infants fed a high volume of human milk (> 50% intake) versus a lower volume.

In a randomized trial of feeds with an exclusive human milk diet versus preterm formula, infants in the human milk group demonstrated a reduction in parenteral nutrition days (36 vs. 27 days, $p = 0.04$) and rates of surgical NEC ($p = 0.08$) and fewer times that feeds were held,[96] among preterm infants fed human milk versus preterm formula. Although the mechanism is not completely understood, human milk proteins may be more easily digested compared with bovine proteins within the preterm gut, leading to fewer clinical signs of feeding intolerance and subsequent stoppage of feeds.

Brain Growth and Subsequent Intelligence

Observational studies examining the neurodevelopmental outcomes of preterm infants vary in adjustment for important confounders, such as socioeconomic factors that affect both feeding choice and neurodevelopment, age of follow-up, and comparator feeding groups; thus results may not always be clear. One of the classic studies in the field was a carefully controlled, long-range study of preterm infants by Lucas et al.[97,98] over a 10-year period that produced some remarkable results. Mothers who provide their milk have a special desire to be good parents and embrace positive health behaviors, which has been suggested as the real cause of this study's measured differences. Several points deserve attention, however. LBW infants are born at a time of rapid brain growth. In fact, term infants have considerable brain growth in the first year of life, doubling the size of the brain by 1 year of age. Several nutrients in human milk have been associated with brain tissue growth, including taurine, cholesterol, omega-3 fatty acids, and amino sugars in the free and bound forms.[99] Amino sugars such as N-acetylneuraminic acid are important constituents of brain glycoproteins and gangliosides.

The Lucas studies[97,98] included infants weighing less than 1850 g at birth delivered at multiple centers, who were entered in four parallel trials of preterm feedings from 1982 to 1985. Mothers decided whether to provide their milk; the remaining infants were assigned to receive preterm formula. All feedings were by feeding tube the first 4 weeks. At both age 18 months and age 7½ to 8 years, when the children were tested by an examiner blinded to their feeding method, the children who had received their mother's milk scored better. At 18 months, they were more advanced on the Bayley Scales of Infant Development.[98] In a subset of the larger study, comparison groups of infants who received preterm formula were more advanced than infants who received regular formula. At the

second point, 7½ to 8 years of age, using the Wechsler Intelligence Scale for Children, the children who received their mother's milk had an 8.3-point advantage, even after adjustments for mother's education and social class ($p < 0.0001$).[98]

A subset of this large study was reported on infants who had been randomly assigned for 30 days to receive preterm formula, unfortified donor milk, or their mother's milk (with donor milk supplements as necessary).[97] The infants fed donor milk or those whose mothers produced less than 50% of the diet and were supplemented with donor milk were disadvantaged by 0.25 standard deviation (SD) on the developmental scales. This was not pronounced in infants with mental growth restriction. The method of collection of milk from the donors was by drip; that is, the donor fed her baby at the breast and collected milk by drip from the other breast.[97] Drip milk is low in fat and fat-soluble nutrients. Donor milk actively pumped has a higher fat and calorie content. An important feature of these studies was that they focused on the first month of life, a critical time to protect the brain and facilitate its growth.[97,98,100] The infants were all tube fed, thus removing the physical interaction of the breastfeeding mother. Impact of early diet on long-term neurodevelopment continues in multicenter studies on infants fed human milk supplemented with human milk—based supplements. Unfortified human milk has been shown to have measurable impact on neurodevelopment, but investigation of these same parameters comparing fortification of human milk with bovine-based supplements has not shown improvement over unfortified milk. Neurodevelopmental outcomes at 18 months were not affected by bovine fortification.[97,101] Fortification in these previous studies was with a bovine milk—based supplement.

The effect of human milk on cognitive and motor development was compared with the effect of formula in a matched cohort of premature infants. Assessment at 3, 7, and 12 months corrected ages revealed higher motor scores at 3 and 7 months and higher cognitive scores at 12 months when adjusted for maternal vocabulary score on the Peabody Picture Vocabulary Tests. The improved development scores persisted.[102]

In a study of three groups of preterm infants matched for birth weight (mean 1308 g, range 640 to 1780 g), gestational age (mean 30.8 weeks, range 26 to 35 weeks), medical status, birth order, sex, parental age, and educational and socioeconomic level, grouped by (1) more than 75% breast-milk intake, (2) 25% to 75% breast milk, and (3) less than 25% breast milk, the infants in group 1 scored highest, independent of whether mother's milk was given by bottle, tube, or breastfeeding. The more milk the infant received, the greater the score on the Brazelton Neonatal Behavioral Assessment Scale (NBAS). The authors concluded that human milk enhances neurodevelopment quantitatively. The mothers who provided more milk were less depressed and had better interactive affiliative care styles.[103,104]

Some, but not all, studies examining a dose-response between mother's milk consumed and neurodevelopmental outcomes have reported a positive relationship. In a multicenter study of more than 1000 of ELBW infants, each

10 mL/kg of mother's milk consumed was associated with a 0.5-point increase on the Bayley mental developmental index and 0.6-point increase on the Bayley psychomotor developmental index at 18 to 22 months corrected age. This translates to 5 higher points on the Bayley Mental Developmental Index in an infant receiving 110 mL/kg per day of mother's milk during the birth hospitalization.[105]

In another study of preterm infants, 180 preterm infants were followed for 7 years and had magnetic resonance imaging (MRI) performed at term-equivalent age and at 7-year follow-up as well as intelligence quotient (IQ) scores as a function of their breast milk intake.[106] Once again, the more milk the infant received the better was the outcome. For each additional day that breast milk intake was greater than 50% of total enteral intake, IQ was 0.5 points higher and 0.7 points higher per additional 10 mL/kg per day at 7 years of age. This study also demonstrated greater gray matter and hippocampal volumes at term-equivalent age. In another study of preterm infants with follow-up into adolescence, there was a positive correlation between verbal IQ scores, white matter brain volume, and total brain volume as assessed by MRI as a percentage of NICU breast milk intake.[107] Mechanisms that explain the relationship between provision of mother's milk and infant neurodevelopment are likely multifactorial and may include changes in the volume of certain structures in the brain or be a marker mother-infant feeding interaction or attachment, which are associated with better neurodevelopmental outcomes.

Retinopathy of Prematurity

Visual function is improved in premature infants fed human milk.[108] This is thought to be a result of the long-chain polyenic fatty acids and the antioxidant activity of human milk in β-carotene, taurine, and vitamin E.[109] ROP is a disease of the preterm infant associated with extreme prematurity and is a product of oxidative stress on the neonate deficient in antioxidant protection. At this point few interventions have demonstrated success in preventing the development of ROP other than oxygen reduction strategies. Breast milk has the advantage of having many natural antioxidants, such as superoxide dismutase, inositol, vitamin E, and glutathione, and is therefore a good candidate to lower ROP rates. There have been conflicting studies demonstrating that human milk intake may or may not influence development of ROP.[110-112] A recent meta-analysis including several of these studies concluded that ingestion of any amount of human milk in the preterm infant significantly reduces the risk for developing any ROP and the most severe forms of ROP requiring intervention.[108] In a report by Hylander et al.,[113] the diagnosis of ROP was 2.3 times greater in formula-fed infants than in those fed human milk. Few infants fed human milk advanced to severe retinopathy, and none required cryotherapy. Results were similar in fortified and unfortified human milk feeds.

Chronic Lung Disease

Another disease of prematurity is chronic lung disease (CLD). CLD is a multifactorial disease related to ventilator-induced lung injury and oxidative stress. It has been postulated that because human milk contains antioxidants it may help prevent CLD. Although CLD has never been the main outcome of any RCT examining human milk versus formula, recent large observation studies reported a protective effect of human milk against the development of CLD.[90,114] A large multicenter study from the German Neonatal Network studied 1433 infants of gestational age younger than 32 weeks. They found an 11.2% rate of CLD in exclusive breast milk feeders as opposed to a rate of 20.9% in exclusive formula feeders (odds ratio [OR] 2.59).[90] Donor milk also has been associated with some beneficial effects on CLD incidence. Although a meta-analysis of three randomized clinical trials did not show a difference between the use of supplemental donor milk versus formula, there was a reduction in days of mechanical ventilation. When observational studies were included, a reduction in the diagnosis of CLD and days of mechanical ventilation were shown.[115] A recent study reported a dose-dependent relationship between mother's milk and risk for CLD, in which each 10% increase in the proportion of total intake of mother's milk was associated with a 9.5% reduction in odds of CLD (OR 0.905 [0.824, 0.995]).[114] A recent meta-analysis reviewed 17 cohort studies and 5 RCTs involving 8661 preterm infants and concluded that both exclusive human milk and partial human milk feedings are associated with a lower risk for BPD.[116]

GASTROINTESTINAL CHARACTERISTICS OF PREMATURE INFANTS

The anatomic differentiation of the intestinal tract begins before 20 weeks' gestation, but the functional development is limited before 26 weeks.[117] Different parts of the fetal gut develop at different times so that some nutrients are better tolerated than others (Tables 14.9 and 14.10). The concentration of digestive enzymes determines the rate of digestion and absorption, along with the maturity of membrane carriers. The presence of active enzymes in the gut improves the digestion and absorption of human milk. As noted earlier, the gastric emptying time in preterm infants when given human milk is biphasic, with an initial fast phase in which 50% has left the stomach in the first 20 to 25 minutes.[118] In a comparison of breast milk versus formula feeds in a group of preterm infants, the breast milk–fed infants had significantly shorter gastric emptying times ($t_{1/2}$ of 47 minutes) versus formula ($t_{1/2}$ of 65 minutes)[119] (Fig. 14.8).

Our understanding of gut microbiota in the health and growth of premature infants is escalating rapidly partially because of metagenomics technologies that permit the measurement of the entire microbiome, including some microbes not readily culturable at this time. Early gut microbiota plays a major role in intestinal health and disease.[74] The human milk glycans, especially the oligosaccharides and human microbes, are a major component of the immune system by which breastfeeding mothers protect their infants from disease, especially their micropremature infants. The interaction of breast-milk bioactive components (particularly HMOs, lipids, and

TABLE 14.9 Gastrointestinal Tract in Human Fetus

First Appearance of Developmental Markers

Anatomic Part	Developmental Marker	Weeks of Gestation
Esophagus	Superficial glands develop	20
	Squamous cells appear	28
Stomach	Gastric glands form	14
	Pylorus and fundus defined	14
Pancreas	Differentiation of endocrine and exocrine tissue	14
Liver	Lobules form	11
Small intestine	Crypt and villi develop	14
	Lymph nodes appear	14
Colon	Diameter increases	20
	Villi disappear	20
Stomach	Gastric motility and secretion	20
Pancreas	Zymogen (proenzyme) granules	20
Liver	Bile metabolism	11
	Bile secretion	22
Small intestine	Active transport of amino acids	14
	Glucose transport	18
	Fatty acid absorption	24
Enzymes	α-Glucosidases	10
	Dipeptidases	10
	Lactase	10
	Enterokinase	26
Functional ability		
Suckling	Mouthing only	24
Swallowing	Immature suck-swallow	26

Modified from Lebenthal E, Leung Y-K. The impact of development of the gut on infant nutrition. *Pediatr Ann*. 1987;16:215.

TABLE 14.10 Digestion and Absorption in Human Fetus and Neonate

Factors	First Detectable (Weeks of Gestation)	Term Neonate (% of Adult)
Protein		
H^+ (hydrogen ion)	At birth	<30
Pepsin	16	<10
Trypsinogen	20	10–60
Chymotrypsinogen	20	10–60
Procarboxypeptidase	20	10–60
Enterokinase	26	10
Peptidases (brush border and cytosol)	<15	>100
Amino acid transport	?	>100
Macromolecular absorption	?	>100
Fat		
Lingual lipase	30	>100
Pancreatic lipase	20	5–10
Pancreatic colipase	?	?
Bile acids	22	50
Medium-chain triglyceride uptake	?	100
Long-chain triglyceride uptake	?	10–90
Carbohydrate		
α-Amylases		
Pancreatic	22	0
Salivary	16	10
Lactase	10	>100
Sucrase-isomaltase	10	100
Glucoamylase	10	50–100
Monosaccharide absorption	11–19	>100 (?)

From Lebenthal E, Leung Y-K. The impact of development of the gut on infant nutrition. *Pediatr Ann*. 1987;16:215.

fatty acids) and the gastrointestinal tract are known to benefit infant health.[120]

USE OF HUMAN MILK FOR PREMATURE INFANTS

A clear distinction must be made between an infant's own mother's milk and pooled human milk for the feeding of LBW infants. The mother's premature milk has some higher levels of nutrients but never lower levels than term milk. Mothers who donate to milk banks are also feeding their own infants, who may be any age from birth to 6 months or older. Donor milk also must be prepared by sterilization. An infant's own mother's milk may be fed fresh or fresh-frozen and is rarely heat treated. Chapter 22 discusses milk storage and milk banking.

When the volume of milk produced by a mother is not sufficient to meet the infant's needs each day, providing

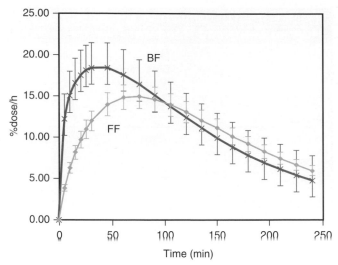

Fig. 14.8 Gastric emptying in formula-fed and breast-fed infants. (Measured with the 13C-octaoic acid breath test). *BF*, Breastfed infants; *FF*, formula-fed infants; mean (standard error of the mean) gastric emptying over time as a percentage of the feeding volume ingested. (From Van Den Driessche M, Peeters K, Marien P, et al. Gastric emptying in formula-fed and breast-fed infants measured with the 13C-octanoic acid breath test. *J Pediatr Gastroenterol Nutr.* 1999;29:46.)

additional nourishment by donor milk is clearly needed. Donor human milk has become increasingly available to mothers of preterm infants. Availability of donor human milk in regional NICUs has increased from below 40% to over 80% in the past few years.[121] Donor human milk has gained acceptance as the feeding of choice for the preterm newborn if mother's own milk is unavailable.[122] The availability of pasteurized donor milk has increased dramatically in the last 4 years, with Human Milk Banking Association of North America (HMBANA) distributing over 5.25 million ounces in 2016 and there now being over 500 milk banks collaborating with HMBANA, the European Milk Bank Association (EMBA), and the International Milk Banking Initiative worldwide. Pasteurized donor human milk is increasingly affordable, especially compared with other nutritional interventions such as parenteral nutrition.[123] In one study from Cincinnati, the provision of human milk for the first 14 days of life was developed as a quality improvement project for the NICU. Over the course of 5 years they were able to go from exclusive human milk feeds in 65% of the infants to 94%.[124] The use of donor milk did not decrease the provision of mother's own milk but decreased the use of formula in the NICU. Because the first 2 weeks of life are critical periods in a preterm infant's life, this was a significant achievement.

A 2001- to 2500-g infant without complications may be weaned from the incubator to an open crib within 24 hours. Although the suck reflex may be poor, the infant usually can be breastfed. The infant is ready to breastfeed even if he or she takes a bottle poorly. If the infant can stimulate the breast briefly and obtain the rich, antibody-containing, cell-filled colostrum, the infant will be protected against infection while

receiving nutrition. Inadequate stimulation of the breast by the infant will require mechanical pumping after the feeding. If the infant cannot suck and must be tube fed, any colostrum the mother can manually express or pump from the breast can be given by gavage tube along with donor milk, or, if human milk is not available, the prescribed formula necessary for nourishment. Chapter 5 reviews the protective value of colostrum to the infant.

Intestinal permeability is another parameter of great importance to LBW infants. The gastrointestinal tract development provides an important barrier to infectious materials and a path for protective and nourishing substances. A precarious balance of intestinal permeability is required to promote infant growth and to avoid severe preterm infant diseases.[125] Decreasing intestinal permeability is associated with gut maturation. In a study of 62 preterm infants (≤32 weeks' gestation), the children were evaluated using enteral lactulose and mannitol administration and urinary measurements at three points in the first month postnatally while assessing their feeding type.[125] Those infants receiving predominantly human milk (more than 75%) had significantly lower intestinal permeability compared with those receiving formula and little or no human milk. The portion of human milk received increased in importance over time, with more than 25% of daily intake as human milk required by 30 days of age to see a significant advantage. Other groups have also documented the decrease in intestinal permeability with ingestion of human milk.[126]

A study in Guatemala that was repeated in the special care nursery of the Rainbow Children's Hospital in Cleveland showed that the infection rate among sick and premature newborns was greatly diminished by providing 15 mL of human colostrum contributed by random donors daily.[127] These findings were especially dramatic in Guatemala, where the mortality rate from infection in the nursery was extremely high. It has been suggested that mixed feedings of an infant's own mother's milk and formula to necessary volume be calculated over a 24-hour period so that the infant receives some mother's milk at each feeding and a supplement of formula, in contrast to alternating feedings or using all mother's milk until it runs out and finishing the day with formula. The reasoning is based on the concept of "inoculating" every feeding with human milk to provide the enzymes and bioactive factors with each feeding. Generous levels of active enzymes in the milk will also assist in the digestion and absorption of the formula. The immunologic properties are less measurable, but the only known interference with function is the addition of iron, which blocks the effectiveness of lactoferrin. Therefore the nutritional and infection-protective properties are also spread throughout each feeding around the clock. Now that donor milk is more readily available, it is recommended to make up the deficit in volume of mother's milk with donor milk.

The quantities of direct-acting antimicrobial factors in human milk vary according to the method of collection, processing, and storage.[128] The ability of donor milk to protect against infection in premature infants is being tested in multiple clinical studies.[93,129]

SUPPLEMENTATION OF MOTHER'S OWN MILK OR POOLED HUMAN MILK

No supplement to human milk is usually needed if the infant weighs more than 1500 g at birth.

The options for supplementing an infant's own mother's milk depend on need for additional volume or for specific nutrients, especially protein, calcium, and phosphorus, based on birth weight and growth rates.[130,131]

The ideal supplementation is one using human milk nutrients and is referred to as *lacto engineering*, in which nutrient concentration is increased by adding specific nutrients derived from human milk. Techniques involve use of donor milk and separating the cream and protein fractions, reducing the lactose content, and heat-treating the product with a high-temperature, short-time (HTST) process of pasteurization. This completely human milk product provides higher protein and energy needs so that weight gains and nitrogen retention are similar to intrauterine rates.

Using a feeding prepared from human milk protein and medium-chain triglyceride supplementation of human milk for VLBW infants was reported by Rönnholm et al.[34] Forty-four infants averaging 30 weeks' gestation with birth weights ranging from 710 to 1510 g were nourished by one of four protocols: plain human milk, human milk and protein, human milk and triglycerides, or human milk and protein and triglycerides. The triglycerides did not influence weight and length, but the two groups receiving added protein gained along a curve comparable with the intrauterine growth for their birth weight, gaining faster from 4 to 6 weeks than the unsupplemented infants. The protein-supplemented groups also grew more in length; however, head circumference growth was similar in all groups.

Total protein is usually calculated by determining the total nitrogen content (Kjeldahl method) and multiplying the number by the protein factor (6.25). Total protein corrected for nonprotein nitrogen, which is high in human milk, is true protein.[132] True milk protein is a heterogeneous mixture of casein and whey proteins. Whey proteins include lactoferrin, immunoglobulin, and lysozyme. True protein minus those more or less indigestible proteins is called *digestible protein*. Analysis of preterm milk by Beijers et al.[132] demonstrated that nonprotein nitrogen was dependent on the degree of prematurity and averaged 20% to 25%, increasing during the time of lactation. Only 30% to 60% of total protein is available for synthesis. However, in absolute amounts over lactation time, it remains stable.

Schanler et al.[133] compared plasma amino acid levels in VLBW infants (mean age 16 days, mean birth weight 1180 g, mean gestation 29 weeks) fed either human milk fortified with human milk or whey-dominant cow milk formula. The infants received continuous enteral infusions of isonitrogenous, isocaloric preparations. Taurine and cystine were significantly higher in the infants fed human milk, and threonine, valine, methionine, and lysine were significantly higher in the infants fed formula. Mother's own milk shows a wide variability in nutrient components when being pumped for a hospitalized premature infant. Nutrient supplementation is necessary

> ### BOX 14.9 Steps to Preserve the Nutrient Value of Mother's Milk
>
> I. Most variable component: Fat
>   A. Lost in collection and storage
>   B. Settles out on standing
>   C. In one report fat content ranged from 2.2 to 4.7 g/dL
>   D. Steps to enhance fat
>   (1) Avoid separation of fat
>   (2) Avoid continuous feeds
>   (3) Use intermittent bolus feeds
>   (4) Orient syringe of milk upward
>   (5) Use short length of tubing
>   (6) Empty syringe completely at end of infusion
>   E. Use hind milk preferentially if volume is adequate
> II. Protein content declines from transitional to mature milk.
> III. Nutrient needs for premature are higher.
> IV. Mineral content has increased bioavailability, but content is lower than needs of premature infants.
> V. Vitamins A and C and riboflavin levels decrease with collection, storage, and delivery.

to maintain adequate growth and good nutritional status. According to Herman and Schanler,[134] extraordinary efforts should be made to use mother's own milk because the advantages of nonnutrient components in human milk are significantly diminished by storage and heat processing. Other groups have reported on the benefit of individualized or targeted fortification of human breast milk and the use of mother's own milk to optimize nutrition and growth for premature infants.[135,136]

The most variable constituent is fat (Box 14.9). Protein does not meet the needs of a small premature infant. Although levels of minerals (calcium and phosphorus) are stable, the needs of VLBW infants require supplementation. Substantial benefits of mother's own milk include reduced infection, enhanced neurodevelopmental outcome, and healthy postnatal growth. The minimum dose of mother's milk when given with various fortifications has been found to be more than 50 mL/kg per day to protect against infection, especially late-onset sepsis.[30] A systematic review looking at multinutrient fortification for human milk involved 14 trials and a total of more than 1000 preterm infants.[137] The data showed improvement in weight gain increments in length, head circumference, and BMC during hospitalization compared with infants receiving unsupplemented milk. There was no evidence of other benefits or harms with supplementation nor an increased risk for NEC.[137] Other studies show neurodevelopmental outcomes were significantly improved with mother's milk. The magnitude of the effect was seen as mother's milk intake increased to 110 mL/kg per day; the developmental scales showed an increase of 5 points, an important gain for these ELBW infants. Preterm infants have lower energy expenditure when they are fed breast milk than when they are fed preterm infant formula.

Preterm infants with birth weight from 750 to 1250 g were randomly assigned to a cream or control group. The cream group received a human milk—derived cream supplement if the energy density of the human milk tested below 20 kcal/oz, measured using a near-infrared human milk analyzer. The control group received their mother's own milk or donor human milk with donor human milk—derived fortifier. Premature infants who received human milk—derived cream as a fortifier had improved weight and length compared with the control group.[138] Cream can be used as an adjunctive supplement to an exclusive human milk—based diet to improve growth rates (see Fig. 14.7).

All preterm infants should receive human milk fortified with protein, minerals, and vitamins when birth weight is less than 1500 g according to the AAP's section on breastfeeding.[1]

ARTIFICIAL FORTIFICATION OF HUMAN MILK

Although breast milk is the ideal food for newborns and the preferred feed for preterm infants, it is not sufficient on its own for the growth of the preterm infant. Preterm breast milk has higher levels of protein for the first few weeks of life but only provides about one-third of the protein and only a fraction of other nutrients needed by the preterm infant. Therefore it must be fortified with protein, minerals, and vitamins to provide optimal nutrient intake for growth.[1] To achieve adequate weight gain preterm infants require 3.4 to 4 g of protein per kilogram per day.[48] In most instances, human milk feeding will progress gradually from small trophic feedings designed to stimulate the newborn gut to full enteral nutrition. Fortifiers are added to human milk when infants are typically tolerating a substantial amount of feeds at about the time when protein levels in their own mother's milk drops from about 2.5 to 1.5 g/dL.[49] Most neonatologists consider fortification at this time when the infants are receiving 80 to 100 mL/kg. The introduction of fortifier in human milk does not increase the risk for adverse events, including NEC. In randomized trials there was no adverse effects of introducing fortifier at 40 mL/kg of feeds compared with 100 mL/kg feeds.[136]

Protein has been shown to be an important component and necessary for adequate growth. In a randomized trial by Brumberg et al.,[51] it was demonstrated that infants fed at equivalent energy levels but higher protein contents had significantly improved weight gain, head circumference, and mid-arm circumferences. Assuming a human milk protein level of 1.5 g/dL, most fortifiers add an additional 1.5 to 2.2 g/dL bringing the total enteral protein intake to 3.5 to 4.5 g/dL when fed at 150 mL/kg. These fortifiers derive their protein from either a bovine source or pooled human milk. Powdered fortifiers are no longer recommended because of the increased risk for bacterial contamination and sepsis. Exclusive human milk diets including human milk—derived fortifier has been associated with a lower rate of NEC than mixed human milk and bovine-based products.

No longer is supplementing an infant's own mother's milk with specially prepared formula supplements necessary. Available commercial preparations for such supplementation were intended to complement human milk and not to be used as an exclusive formula. When multicomponent fortified human milk product for promoting growth in preterm infants was examined in a Cochrane review,[137] the authors found short-term increases in weight gain, linear growth, and head circumference. No effect was seen on serum alkaline phosphatase levels, and the effect on BMC was unclear. Nitrogen retention and blood urea levels were increased. Conclusions about long-term neurodevelopmental and growth outcomes were limited by insufficient data after 1 year. The significance of increased blood urea nitrogen and blood pH levels was unclear. Preparations are different and are used differently (Table 14.11). The powdered supplement is intended to add special nutrients to an adequate volume of mother's own milk (Enfamil human milk fortifier or Similac human milk fortifier), or it can be used to enhance pooled donor human milk. Neither fortifier contains fat. Milk fortification extends the mother's milk and provides additional nitrogen, calcium, phosphorus, and vitamins for an LBW infant. If an infant is fed the mother's milk, pooled donor milk, and a fortifier, the total should meet the infant's daily requirements (Table 14.12). Any addition of artificial formula interferes with the infection protection qualities and other benefits of human milk; therefore use of formula-based supplementation should be avoided unless human milk—based formula is not available. Preventing one case of NEC saves $100,000.

Studies comparing fortified mother's milk with premature infant formulas have shown comparable growth in weight, length, and head circumference. This makes it possible to lose many advantages of a mother's milk while trying to provide the additional nutrients for appropriate accretion rates.[139]

When powdered fortifier was added to a mother's milk, the supplemented infants had significantly greater weight gain, linear growth, and head circumference growth than those not supplemented. The supplemented infants also had higher blood urea nitrogen levels (Table 14.13). The loss of human milk benefits related to fortification/supplementation with bovine milk products is of significant concern.

When a preterm infant's own mother's milk was fortified with protein (0.85 g/dL), calcium (90 mg/dL), and phosphorus (45 mg/dL), the rate of weight gain was greater than that of the unfortified group and comparable with that of the Similac Natural Care formula group.[140–142] Bone mineralization improved during the 6 weeks of the study but did not reach the intrauterine accretion rate of 150 mg/kg per day. A relative phosphorus deficiency occurred in the human milk groups, both with and without supplementation. Fortifying preterm mother's milk permits biochemically adequate growth comparable with that provided by special care formula (Table 14.14).

The effect of calcium supplementation on fatty acid balance studies in LBW infants fed human milk or formula has been shown to be significant. A decrease in total fatty acid absorption both in LBW infants fed their own mother's milk and in formula-fed infants was seen when calcium was added. Fecal output of fat and fatty acid excretion was higher in the formula-fed infants. In mother's milk—fed infants, the total fat absorption and the coefficient of absorption were higher.

TABLE 14.11   Composition of Infant Feeding Using Human Milk With and Without Various Supplements

	PRETERM HUMAN MILK		Similac Natural Care	50:50 MIX SIMILAC NATURAL CARE AND PRETERM HUMAN MILK[a]		Enfamil Human Milk Fortifier (Four Packets)	ENFAMIL HUMAN MILK FORTIFIER (FOUR PACKETS) ADDED TO PRETERM HUMAN MILK[a]	
Weeks postpartum	1	4		1	4		1	4
Kilocalories	67	70	81	72	76	14	81	84
Protein (g)	2.44	1.81	2.1	2.27	1.96	0.7	3.14	2.5
Carbohydrate (g)	6.05	6.95	8.6	7.3	7.8	2.7	8.75	9.65
Fat (g)	3.81	4.00	3.6	3.7	3.8	0.04	3.85	4.04
Vitamin A (IU)[b]	330	230	550	440	390	780	1110	1010
Vitamin E (mg)[b]	0.9	0.25	3	2.0	1.61	3.4	4.3	3.65
Vitamin K (mcg)[b]	NA	1.5	10	NA	5.8	9.1	NA	10.6
Vitamin D (IU)[b]	NA	2.5	120	NA	61	260	NA	262
Thiamin (mcg)	5.4	8.9	200	103	104	187	192	196
Riboflavin (mcg)	36.0	26.6	500	268	263	250	286	277
Niacin (mg)	0.11	0.21	4.0	2.1	2.1	3.1	3.2	3.3
Pyridoxine (mcg)	2.6	6.2	200	101	103	193	196	199
Folate (mcg)	2.1	3.1	30	16.1	16.6	23	25	26
Vitamin B_{12} (mcg)	NA	0.1	0.45	NA	0.27	0.21	NA	0.3
Vitamin C (mg)[b]	7	5	30	19	18	24	31	29
Calcium (mg)	25	22	170	98	96	60	85	82
Phosphorus (mg)	14	14	85	50	50	33	47	47
Magnesium (mg)	3	2.5	10	6.5	6.3	4	7	6.5
Iron (mg)	0.1	0.1	0.3	0.2	0.2	0	0.1	0.1
Sodium (mEq)	2.2	1.3	1.7	2.0	1.5	0.3	2.5	1.6
Potassium (mEq)	1.8	1.7	2.9	2.4	2.3	0.4	2.2	2.1
Chloride (mEq)	2.5	1.6	2.0	2.3	1.8	0.5	3.0	2.1
Zinc (mg)	0.48	0.39	1.2	0.84	0.80	0.31	0.79	0.70
Copper (mg)	0.08	0.06	0.2	0.14	0.13	0.08	0.16	0.14
Manganese (mcg)[b]	NA	0.4	NA	NA	NA	9	NA	9.4
Biotin (mcg)	0.15	0.54	NA	NA	NA	0.8	0.95	1.34
Pantothenic acid (mg)	0.16	0.23	1.5	0.83	0.87	0.79	0.95	1.02
Osmolality (mOsm/kg H_2O)[b]	302	305	300	301	303	+ 60	362	365

IU, International units; *NA*, not available.

[a]Volume 100 mL (1 dL).

[b]Listed values for 1 and 4 weeks reflect reported values for full-term transitional and mature human milk, respectively.

TABLE 14.12 Protein, Calcium, and Sodium Requirements by Growing Premature Infants and Composition of Banked Human Milk

	Protein (g/100 kcal)	Calcium (mg/100 kcal)	Sodium (mEq/100 kcal)
Estimated requirements for hypothetic, growing premature infants[a]	2.54	132[b]	2.3
Composition of banked human milk	1.50	43	0.8

[a]Assumed body weight is 1200 g; weight gain, 20 g/day; energy intake, 120 kcal/kg/day. The basis for estimating requirements is described in the text.
[b]This estimate does not apply to infants fed formulas from which calcium absorption is less than 66% of intake.
From Fomon SJ, Ziegler EE, Vazquez HD. Human milk and the small premature infant. *Am J Dis Child*. 1977;131:463.

TABLE 14.13 Fortified Versus Unfortified Human Milk

Growth	Fortified
13 studies, 596 infants; randomized[a]	
Weight gain	+3.7 g/kg/day
Length	+0.13 cm/wk
Head circumference	+0.12 cm/wk
Bone mineral content	+8.3 mg/cm
Nitrogen balance	+66 mg/kg/day
Blood urea nitrogen	+5.8 mg/dL
Necrotizing enterocolitis	No significant difference
Feeding tolerance	No significant difference

[a]Some comparisons with partial supplements.
From Kuschel CA, Harding JE. Multicomponent fortified human milk for promoting growth in preterm infants. *Cochrane Database Syst Rev*. 2004;(1):CD000343.

Preterm milk with routine multivitamin supplementation (providing 4.1 mg of tocopherol) uniformly resulted in vitamin sufficiency in VLBW infants in a control study by Gross and Gabriel.[143] This was true when they received iron and when they were not iron supplemented. VLBW infants were fed preterm milk, bank milk, or formula, using 2 mg/day of iron. Vitamin E content of preterm milk does not differ significantly from that of term human milk from days 3 to 36.[57]

Jocson et al.[144] studied the effects of nutrient fortification and varying storage conditions on host-defense properties of human milk. Total bacterial colony counts and IgA were not affected by the addition of fortifier.

The effect of powdered human milk fortifiers on the antibacterial actions of human milk were also explored by Chan.[145] Human milk inhibited the growth of *Escherichia coli*, *Staphylococcus aureus*, *Enterobacter sakazakii*, and group B *Streptococcus* when Enfamil and Similac human milk

fortifiers were mixed with human milk, along with medium-chain triglycerides and 1.09 mg ferrous sulfate (in 25 mL milk). The fortifiers containing iron, and the iron alone inhibited the protective effect of human milk against the bacteria. The probable explanation is the interference of iron with the protective action of lactoferrin in human milk. The ferrous iron in the fortifier is changed to a ferric state in human milk, which readily binds with lactoferrin.[146] Based on concerns over the use of powdered milk fortifiers, liquid bovine fortifiers have been developed to avoid the issue of bacterial contamination and low protein supply. These fortifiers were manufactured by two different methods, one was acidified to achieve sterility and the other was heated aseptically. In two randomized trials of the fortifiers the more acidified fortifier had higher rates of metabolic acidosis, lower rates of weight gain, and increased feeding intolerance, thus supporting a greater use of the nonacidified fortifier.[146,147]

Concerns over the nutrient content of supplemented human milk have been expressed by many authors since the early work on premature infants from the Houston group.[61] After noting growth failure in some premature infants, it was discovered that some mother's milk was lower in calories than 20 kcal/oz. This has been reported by Prolacta Biologicals, which tests the protein and caloric content of all donations. This is a major issue for premature infants who have a restricted fluid intake in the early months of life. Preterm infants fed a commercially prepared, bovine-based human milk fortifier receive less protein than they need, according to Arslanoglu et al.[148] They tested the actual nutrient intakes observed in a previously reported study, with assumed nutrient intakes based on the usual assumptions about the composition of human milk. Actual protein intakes were significantly and consistently lower than the levels assumed based on the standard protein content of human milk. Actual intakes of protein by preterm infants fed bovine-fortified human milk were significantly lower, especially after 3 weeks postpartum when the mother's milk no longer had the higher protein content of the milk of a mother who delivers prematurely. Calorie content was not significantly lower (Fig. 14.9).

In a recent update, Arslanoglu et al. and the European Milk Bank Association Working group on Human Milk Fortification[136] discussed the shortfall of standard fortification in the NICU in meeting the nutritional needs of preterm infants. They thought that even though most NICUs use a standard fortification method, a more individualized method using blood urea nitrogen may be a better yet simple choice. (See Box 14.10 for different fortification methods and Table 14.15 for protein and energy requirements, estimated by factorial and empiric methods.)

The AAP Committee on Nutrition has outlined requirements for the premature infant who is less than 27 weeks' gestation and less than 1000 g at birth, regarding calcium and vitamin D. Bone mineral status should be assessed by 4 to 5 weeks after birth. Alkaline phosphatase above 800 to 1000 IU/L or clinical evidence of fractures require radiographic evaluation. A persistent serum phosphorus concentration less than 4 mg/dL should be monitored and supplementation with

TABLE 14.14   Comparison of Selected Fortifiers for Human Milk (Prepared per 100 mL Milk)

Fortifier	PrHM	EHMF	SNC	Eoprotin[a]	S-26/SMA HMF	FM85[b]	SHMF
Energy (kJ) (kcal)	298 (71)	357 (85)	319 (76)	357 (85)	361 (86)	374 (89)	357 (85)
Fat (g)	3.6	3.6[c]	4.0	3.6[c]	3.65	3.6	4.0
Carbohydrate (g)	7.0	9.7	7.8	9.8	9.4	10.6	8.8
Protein (g)	1.8	2.5	2.0	2.6	2.8	2.6	2.8
Calcium (mg)	22	112	97	72	112	73	139
Phosphorus (mg)	14	59	50	48	59	48	81
Magnesium (mg)	2.5	3.5	6.3	5.3	4.0	4.5	9.5
Sodium (mEq)	0.7	1.0	1.1	1.9	1.1	1.9	1.35
Zinc (mcg)	320	1030	760	320[c]	450	320[c]	1320
Copper (mcg)	60	122	1045	60[c]	60[c]	60[c]	230
Vitamins	Yes	Multi[d]	Multi[d]	A, C, E, K	Multi[d]	Multi[d]	Multi[d]

EHMF, Enfamil Human Milk Fortifier (Mead Johnson Nutritionals, Evansville, IN); *HMF,* human milk-fed; *PrHM,* preterm human milk; *S-26/SMA HMF,* SMA Human Milk Fortifier (Wyeth Nutritionals, Philadelphia, PA); *SHMF,* Similac Human Milk Fortifier (Ross Laboratories, Columbus, OH); *SNC,* Similac Natural Care (Ross Laboratories, Columbus, OH) mixed 1:1 (vol:vol) with PrHM. From Schanler RJ. The use of human milk for premature infants. *Pediatr Clin North Am.* 2001;48:207.
[a]Milupa, Friedrichsdorf, Germany.
[b]Nestle, Vevey, Switzerland.
[c]Nutrient not contained in fortifier.
[d]Multivitamins: A, D, E, K, B_1, B_2, B_6, C, B_{12}, niacin, folate, pantothenate, and biotin.

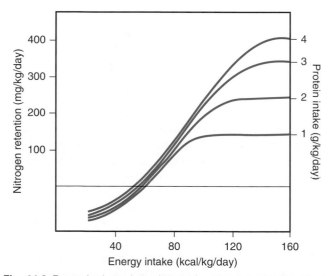

Fig. 14.9 Energy intake and protein retention based on protein intake in low-birth-weight infants. (From Edmond K, Bahl R; World Health Organization. Optimal feeding of low birth-weight infants. Technical Review; 2019. https://www.who.int/nutrition/publications/globaltargets2025_policy brief_lbw/en/. Accessed September 30, 2019.)

phosphorus considered. Postdischarge monitoring is also necessary if exclusively breastfed. When the infant reaches 1500 g, vitamin D intake should be 400 IU/day minimum and up to a maximum of 1000 IU/day. A mineral intake between 100 and 166 mg/kg per day of highly absorbed calcium and 60 to 75 mg/kg per day of phosphorus is recommended to provide appropriate mineralization.[149] Protein requirement is considered

to be a matter of some debate, because human milk protein is readily absorbed and bovine protein is less well absorbed. The revised recommendations for protein appear in Box 14.11. These adjustments were an effort to reduce metabolic stress from protein overload and unbalanced amino acid supply. Human milk has the ideal balance of casein and whey.

FORTIFICATION OF HUMAN MILK WITH HUMAN MILK

The problem of adding nutrients to mothers' milk to meet the increased nutrient needs of premature infants, especially ELBW premature infants, has challenged neonatologists for years. The commercial products developed from a bovine milk base have been widely used and have improved the nutrient intake of these infants. The theoretical concern about the impact of bovine milk on the infection protection properties of human milk has been argued.[150] A minimum of 50 mL/kg per day of the mother's milk is deemed necessary to maintain the protection provided by the mother's milk. A number of investigators have explored the possibility of a fortifier made of human milk, so the feeding would meet needs with entirely human constituents. The antibacterial activity inherent in human milk was inhibited when a bovine-based fortifier containing added iron was mixed with human milk. Chan et al.[151] tested the same antibacterial activity when a newly derived human milk–based product became available (Prolacta Bioscience, Monrovia, CA). Human milk samples from 10 fully lactating mothers were used to test the

BOX 14.10 Recommended Human Milk Fortification Methods for Premature or Very Low-Birth-Weight Infants

Fortification Method	Principle	Advantages Disadvantages
1. Standard (STD) fortification	Fortification method currently in use in most of the neonatal units. A fixed amount of fortifier is added to a fixed volume of human milk according to the manufacturers' instructions.	Practical. But has not solved the problem of protein undernutrition for VLBW infants. Despite STD fortification, many VLBW infants continue to have suboptimal growth.
2. Individualized human milk fortification methods a. Adjustable (ADJ) fortification	Protein adequacy is monitored by BUN twice weekly. Cutoff levels of BUN are 10–16 mg/dL.[a] If the level is <10 mg/dL, extra protein is added to the STD fortification.	Practical, not labor intensive. Does not need expensive devices. Monitors protein intake of each infant. Safeguards also against excessive protein intake. Proven to be effective in optimizing growth and protein intake with a RCT. A real individualization method taking into consideration each infant's protein requirement.
b. Targeted fortification	Macronutrient concentrations in human milk are analyzed and based on the results milk is supplemented with extra protein and/or fat.	All macronutrients can be supplemented. Bedside human milk analyzers are required. May be labor intensive. Supplementation is done according to the population recommendations. Does not take into consideration that each individual infant's requirement may be different.

BUN, Blood urea nitrogen; *RCT*, randomized controlled trial; *VLBW*, very low-birth-weight.

[a] BUN levels of 10–16 mg/dL correspond to BUN concentrations of 21.40–34.24 mg/dL (3.57–5.71 mmol/L).

From Arslanoglu S, Boquien CY, King C, et al. Fortification of human milk for preterm infants: update and recommendations of the European Milk Bank Association (EMBA) Working Group on Human Milk Fortification. *Front Pediatr.* 2019;7:76, 2019. doi:10.3389/fped.2019.00076. eCollection 2019

TABLE 14.15 Protein and Energy Requirements, Estimated by Factorial and Empiric Methods

Body Weight (g)	500–1000	1001–1500	1501–2000
Weight gain of fetus (g/kg/day)	19.0	17.4	16.4
Protein(g/kg/day)	4.0	3.9	3.7
Energy(kcal/kg/day)	106	115	123
Protein/energy(g/100 kcal)	3.8	3.4	3.0

From Arslanoglu S, Boquien CY, King C, et al. Fortification of human milk for preterm infants: update and recommendations of the European Milk Bank Association (EMBA) Working Group on Human Milk Fortification. *Front Pediatr.* 2019;7:76. doi:10.3389/fped.2019.00076. eCollection 2019.

effect on the antimicrobial activity of human milk, milk plus bovine fortifier, and milk plus human milk fortifier against *E. sakazakii, E. coli, Clostridium difficile,* and *Shigella soneii.* Human milk inhibited the growth of all the test organisms. The antibacterial activity was almost completely inhibited by the addition of the bovine-based fortifier. The activity was unaffected by the addition of human milk–based fortifier. Further studies of human milk–based fortifier (H²MF) have been conducted at national and international sites. The fortifier (H²MF) is available from Prolacta Bioscience. Results from University of Florida, Schneider's Children's Hospital, Baylor College of Medicine, and Yale New Haven Medical Center were reported on 207 extremely premature infants whose mothers intended to provide their milk.[50] The infants were randomized to one of three groups: mother's milk plus human milk based fortifier started when the enteral intake was 40 ml/kg per day (HUM40) or human milk based fortifier started when the enteral intake was 100 mL/kg per day (HUM100); the third group received mother's milk plus 100 mL/kg per day of the bovine-based product (Table 14.16). The groups had similar lengths of stay and rates of growth, CLD, and sepsis. However, significantly lower rates of NEC, surgical NEC, and combined deaths were observed with the human milk–based fortifier.[50] More recent additional results are available from other centers completing similar research with human milk diets for premature infants.

BOX 14.11 Protein Recommendations

- Categorized by life stage and gender, because among healthy individuals, these are the two parameters responsible for variations in the body's need for protein.
  - The pediatrics stage has been subdivided into six groupings: *infancy*, 0 to 6 months of age; *infancy*, 7 to 12 months of age; *toddlers*, 1 to 3 years of age; *early childhood*, 4 to 8 years of age; *puberty*, 9 to 13 years of age; and *adolescence*, 14 to 18 years of age.
- Optimal food for full-term infants is human milk.
  - Recommended that it be the sole source of nutrition for infants during the first 6 months of life.
  - On average, infants to 6 months of age consume 0.78 L of milk per day.
- Average value of 11.7 g/L used to calculate adequate intake for protein.
- Nonprotein nitrogen component of human milk contains substantial quantities of taurine, which is virtually absent from cow milk.
- Human milk proteins have a high nutritional quality and are digested and absorbed more efficiently than cow milk proteins.
- Breastfed infants' protein intakes appear to satisfy the infant requirements for maintenance and growth without an amino acid or solute excess.

Data from Rigo J, Senterre J. Nutritional needs of premature infants: current issues. *J Pediatr*. 2006;149:880; Kleinman RE, ed. *Pediatric Nutrition*. 7th ed. Washington, DC: American Academy of Pediatrics; 2013; and World Health Organization. *Protein and Amino Acid Requirements in Human Nutrition*. Geneva, Switzerland: World Health Organization; 2007.

LONG-TERM FOLLOW-UP OF GROWTH PARAMETERS IN INFANTS WITH VERY LOW-BIRTH-WEIGHT

Weight gain and growth in length and head circumference are similar in VLBW infants who are breastfed or given standard formula after discharge. BMC was also followed at 10, 16, and 25 postnatal weeks in those graduates from the NICU who had formerly received fortified human milk. At 16 and 25 weeks, the breastfed infants had lower BMC, ratio of BMC to bone width, and serum phosphorus concentration and higher alkaline phosphate activity than the formula-fed group. These data suggest a need to carefully monitor this select group of VLBW infants for suboptimal bone accretion while receiving their mother's milk. However, human milk—based fortifier should solve this problem.[152]

Reduced bone mineralization is common in preterm infants and has been associated with growth stunting at 18 months of age and dietary insufficiency of calcium and phosphorus. Bishop et al.[153] evaluated 54 children at a mean age of 5 years who were born prematurely and had been part of a longitudinal dietary growth study. The diets included were either banked donor milk or preterm formula as a supplement to the mothers' own milk. Increased human milk intake was strongly associated with better BMC. Those children who had the greater proportion of human milk had greater BMC than children born at term. That is, supplementing with donor milk produced a better outcome at age 5 years than supplementing with infant formula, even though the nutrient content of formula was greater. The later skeletal growth and mineralization of an infant can be calculated and feeding

TABLE 14.16 Use of Human Milk Fortifier Made From Human Milk

	BOV	HUM40	HUM100	*p* Value[a]
N	69	71	67	
Gestation (wk)[b]	27.3 ± 2.0	27.2 ± 2.3	27.2 ± 2.2	NS
Birth weight (g)[b]	922 ± 197	921 ± 188	945 ± 202	NS
MOM consumed, mL (% of enteral intake)[c]	5676 (82%)	4539 (70%)	4048 (73%)	NS
Days of PN[c]	22	20	20	NS
NEC, n (%)	11 (15.9)	5 (7.0)	3 (4.5)	0.05
Surgical NEC, n (%)	8 (11.6)	1 (1.4)	1 (1.5)	0.007
Death, n (%)	5 (7.2)	2 (2.8)	1 (1.5)	NS
Death or NEC, n (%)	14 (20.3)	6 (8.5)	5 (7.5)	0.04

Results: The groups had similar lengths of stay and rates of growth, CLD, and sepsis. Other results are shown. *BOV*, Bovine; *CLD*, central line day; *HUM40*, human milk (mother's milk) plus fortifier (Prolacta Bioscience); *HUM100*, human milk (mother's milk) 100 mL/kg/day; *MOM*, mother's own milk; *NEC*, necrotizing enterocolitis; *PN*, parenteral nutrition.
[a]Chi square, Kruskal-Wallis, log-rank test.
[b]Mean ± SD.
[c]Median.
From Sullivan S, Schanler RJ, Kim JH, Patel AL, Trawöger R, Kiechl-Kohlendorfer U, et al. An exclusively human milkbased diet is associated with a lower rate of necrotizing enterocolitis than a diet of human milk and bovine milkbased products. *J Pediatr*. 2010;156:562. Available from: http://doi:10.1016/j.jpeds.2009.10.040.

adjusted to add necessary mineralization with human milk-based supplements.

Iron status also has been studied in LBW infants at 6 months' chronologic age. The incidence of iron deficiency was 86% in the breastfed group of LBW infants and only 33% in those receiving iron-fortified formula.[154] The breastfed group had significantly lower serum ferritin and hemoglobin values at 4 months of age. Abouelfettoh et al.[59] recommended that these special breastfed infants should receive iron from 2 months of age because they have additional risk for developing iron deficiency above that of full-term infants.

The AAP recommends that infants less than 1500 g birth weight receive 1 mg/kg per day of iron. There were no studies to test this until Taylor and Kennedy[155] compared the effect of 2 mg/kg per day in a multivitamin on the hematocrit at 36 weeks' postmenstrual age. It was concluded that this iron therapy for infants under 1500 g at birth, in addition to dietary intake, did not improve the hematocrit or the number of transfusions required compared with the controls who received no additional iron. A subsequent systematic review and meta-analysis of iron supplementation in preterm and LBW infants showed supplementation resulting in improved iron status and less iron deficiency and anemia. Nevertheless, additional study is needed to fully assess iron overload and short- and long-term health effects.[156]

The feeding of these special VLBW infants after discharge and for the next 6 to 9 months is an important consideration. Breastfeeding with added supplementation has been studied. Some important results came from a randomized, double-blind trial of the effect of supplementary standard formula feedings.[157] Growth and clinical status of infants receiving nutrient-enriched "postdischarge" formula were significantly affected, without vomiting, gas, or stool problems. The group receiving the enriched formula ingested volumes similar to those receiving regular formula.

A large multicenter follow-up study of more than 1000 ELBW infants who had extensive nutritional data collected was reported by Vohr et al.[105] Birth weight, gestational age, intraventricular hemorrhage status, sepsis, bronchopulmonary dysplasia, and hospital stay were similar between those never receiving human milk and those for whom variables of socioeconomic status, race, ethnicity, educational attainment, and parity were adjusted. Effects of human milk intake on mental and motor development were significantly positive. The impact of receiving 110 mL/kg per day of human milk was correlated with a 5-point increase on the Bayley scales. Human milk feedings affect scores even when donor milk is used, compared with term formula.[105]

Infants fed breast milk were found to have faster brainstem maturation, compared with those infants who received formula. This was determined by an analysis of the rate of maturation of the brainstem auditory evoked responses (BAERs). Components of human milk improved cognitive and neurologic outcomes in a series of studies on VLBW infants. Lack of breastfeeding was a major predictor of poor cognitive outcome in very preterm infants, compared with low social status and cerebral lesions by ultrasound.[158]

BOX 14.12 Feeding Schedule for Human Milk in Low-Birth-Weight Infants

1. Use refrigerated milk from the preterm infant's mother when it is available and has been collected within 48 hours of feeding.
2. When fresh milk is not available, use frozen human milk from the infant's mother. This milk should be provided in the sequence that it was collected to provide the greatest nutritional benefit.
3. When the preterm infant is tolerating human milk at greater than 100 mL/kg per day, supplementation using a human milk fortifier is started.
   a. If it requires more than 1 week to reach 100 mL/kg per day intake, fortifier is added even though volume tolerance has not been achieved.
   b. Milk volumes should increase to 150 but not exceed 200 mL/kg per day. Weight gain is optimally 15 g/kg per day and length increment 1 cm/wk. Urinary excretion of calcium should be less than 6 mg/kg per day and phosphorus greater than 4 mg/kg per day.
   c. If weight gain is less than 15 g/kg per day, hind milk is used if mother's milk production exceeds the infant's requirements by 30%.
4. If the mother's milk supply is inadequate to meet her infant's feeding needs, an infant formula designed for preterm feeding is used as described.
5. Fortification of human milk is recommended until the infant is taking all feedings from the breast directly or weighs 1800 to 2000 g, depending on nursery policy on infant discharge weight. During the transition from feeding human milk by gavage or bottle and nipple to feeding at the breast, only those feedings given by gavage or bottle require fortification.
6. Multivitamin supplementation is started once feeding tolerance has been established. This supplementation varies depending on the composition of human milk fortifier.
7. Iron supplementation providing 2 mg/kg per day is started by the time the infant has doubled birth weight.

The association of human milk feedings with a reduction in ROP among VLBW infants compared with formula-fed infants, after adjusting for confounding variables, is significant. It can be considered as an available intervention.

Box 14.12 lists recommendations modified from the work of Schanler and Hurst[159] and Tsang et al.[160]

ANTIMICROBIAL PROPERTIES OF PRETERM BREAST MILK

The infection-protective properties of human milk have been considered a key reason to provide human milk to high-risk infants who are prone to devastating infections such as NEC, sepsis, and meningitis and viral infections such as respiratory syncytial virus and rotavirus. The antimicrobial properties of milk produced by mothers who deliver preterm have been studied by several investigators.

The antiinfective factors in preterm human colostrum ($n = 25$) were studied by Mathur et al.,[161] who compared the colostrum values of a comparable group of 10 full-term postpartum mothers. The mean concentrations of IgA, lysozyme, and lactoferrin were significantly higher than in full-term colostrum. IgG and IgM were similar in both groups. The absolute counts of total cells, macrophages, lymphocytes, and neutrophils were significantly higher in preterm colostrum. The mean percentage of IgA in the premature colostrum was also significantly higher. The degree of prematurity had no effect, although the study group ranged in gestation from 28 to 36 weeks (mean 33 ± 2.1 weeks), compared with the control infants, who were at 38 to 40 weeks (mean 39.1 ± 0.8 weeks). The colostrum of preterm mothers had an even greater potential for preventing infection than term colostrum and are an additional reason to begin early enteral feeds with human colostrum.[162] Table 14.17 lists the specific antiinfective components.

The cells of preterm milk were compared with those of term milk and found to be similar in number and in capacity to phagocytose and kill staphylococci.[162] The ability of the preterm cells to produce interferon on stimulation with mitogens was marginally better than that of term cells. The cells survived 24 hours refrigerated at $4°C$ ($39.2°F$); at 48 hours, cell number, but not function, was reduced. Passing the milk through a feeding tube did not diminish the number or function of the cells. The levels of lactoferrin and lysozyme were greater in preterm milk than in term milk from the 2nd to 12th weeks postpartum.[128]

The predominant form of IgA is sIgA, and values increased from the 6th to 12th weeks in preterm milk. The increase in IgA does not depend on method of collection, rate of flow, or time of day, but the concentration varied inversely with the milk volume. Thus some investigators think that total production of IgA in 24 hours is comparable for the two groups (term and preterm infants).[163] Preterm infants (31 to 36 weeks' gestation) were fed human milk and compared with a matched group of premature infants fed infant formula. The serum levels of IgA at 9 to 13 weeks were higher in the human milk–fed infants.[164] Those infants who received at least 60% of their own mother's milk had higher IgA levels at 3 weeks of age than those receiving less than 30% of the feedings from their mother's milk.

Serum IgG levels were higher in the breast milk group, and serum IgM levels were similar in the two feeding groups. Samples of precolostrum collected from undelivered mothers were assayed and found to contain equal amounts or greater amounts of IgA, IgG, IgM, lactoferrin, and lysozyme than mature colostrum.[165]

When the impact on actual prevention of infection among premature infants is reviewed, significantly less infection is found in infants receiving human milk compared with those receiving formula (9/32 receiving breast milk, 28.1%; 24/38 receiving formula, 63.2%). In this prospective evaluation of the antiinfective property of varying quantities of expressed human milk for high-risk LBW infants, infections were found to be significantly less frequent in the groups that received human milk.[166] This has been documented for decades.

NEC is a major cause of morbidity and death in preterm and other high-risk infants. The absolute cause has eluded neonatologists, although many theories have been put forth and associations suggested (Box 14.13).[167] When researchers investigate its prevention, the role of human milk is prominent.[168] In a large prospective multicenter study of 926 infants, 51 infants (5.5%) developed NEC. The mortality rate was 26% (Fig. 14.10).[169] In exclusively formula-fed infants, the incidence was 6 to 10 times more common than in those

TABLE 14.17 Comparison of Antiinfective Properties in Colostrum of Preterm Versus Term Mothers		
	Preterm Colostrum	Term Colostrum
Total protein (g/L)	0.43 ± 1.3	0.31 ± 0.05
IgA (mg/g protein)	310.5 ± 70	168.2 ± 21
IgG (mg/g protein)	7.6 ± 3.9	8.4 ± 1
IgM (mg/g protein)	39.6 ± 23	36.1 ± 16
Lysozyme (mg/gprotein)	1.5 ± 0.5	1.1 ± 0.3
Lactoferrin (mg/gprotein)	165 ± 37	102 ± 25
Total cells (mL^{-3})	6794 ± 1946	3064 ± 424
Macrophages	4041 ± 1420	1597 ± 303
Lymphocytes	1850 ± 543	954 ± 143
Neutrophils	842 ± 404	512 ± 178

Modified from Mathur NB, Dwarkadas AM, Sharma VK, et al. Antiinfective factors in preterm human colostrum. *Acta Paediatr Scand.* 1990;79:1039.

BOX 14.13 Issues and Risk Factors Associated With Enteral (Oral) Intake and the Causation of Necrotizing Enterocolitis

- Initiation of oral fluids too early
- Excessively rapid increases in volume or concentration of oral fluids
- Nutritional and nonnutritive sucking
- Hyperosmolar fluids
- Formula compared with human breast milk
- Feeding intolerance (cannot advance, residuals)
- Transpyloric compared with gastric gavage
- Bolus compared with continuous gavage
- Malabsorption of carbohydrates (lactose)—low luminal pH and ischemia
- Malabsorption of protein—low luminal pH
- Differences in gut bacterial or viral flora (epidemic necrotizing enterocolitis)
- Labile or inadequate gut blood flow (e.g., diving reflex, apnea, asphyxia)
- Increased work of gut muscle (increased oxygen consumption) because of gut motility

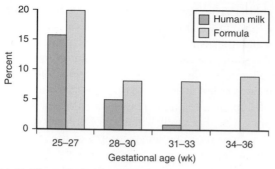

Fig. 14.10 Effect of gestational age and human milk versus formula feeding on necrotizing enterocolitis (NEC). In infants fed formula, incidence of NEC decreases after 27 weeks and then remains the same. In infants fed human milk, incidence of NEC continues to decline. (From Lucas A, Cole TJ. Breast milk and neonatal necrotising enterocolitis. *Lancet.* 1990;336:1519.)

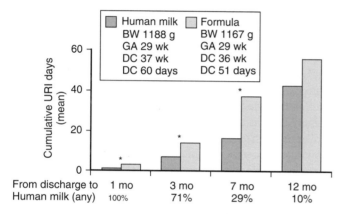

*1 month comparison p<0.025, 3 month p=0.06, 7 month p<0.025, 12 month p=not significant

Fig. 14.11 Effect of human milk on upper respiratory infection symptoms in premature infants during their first year. *BW,* Birth weight; *DC,* discharge; *GA,* gestational age; *URI,* upper respiratory infection. (From Blaymore Bier J-A, Oliver T, Ferguson A, et al. Human milk reduces outpatient upper respiratory symptoms in premature infants during their first year of life. *J Perinatol.* 2002;22:354.)

who received human milk exclusively. In those who received human milk and formula, it was three times more common than in the exclusively breastfed group. Pasteurization did not diminish the effect of human milk in these studies.[170] The comparison was more dramatic at more than 30 weeks' gestation, when formula-fed infants were 20 times more apt to develop NEC than human milk–fed infants. Early enteral feeding did not change the risk in those receiving breast milk, whereas delaying feedings of formula did lower the rate of NEC.[171] In a study of the prevention of NEC in LBW infants, with feedings higher in IgA and IgG, none of the infants in the study group or the breastfeeding comparison group developed NEC. Six cases developed among the 91 infants in the untreated group.[172]

It is notable that human milk also affects the incidence of other infections in the premature infant, including upper respiratory tract infections (Fig. 14.11).

When stool colonization and incidence of sepsis in human milk–fed and formula-fed infants were studied in an intensive care nursery, a protective effect was seen against nosocomial sepsis, which was unrelated to gastrointestinal flora. It was concluded that human milk feeding is associated with a significantly decreased incidence of nosocomially acquired sepsis that cannot be explained by the effect of human milk feeding on the gastrointestinal flora.[129] Various older studies have reported decreased infection in preterm infants with human milk compared with preterm formula. Infants fed predominantly human milk (i.e., more than 50 mL/kg per day) had significantly less late-onset sepsis and NEC and shorter hospital stays compared with those receiving preterm formula. This dose of at least 50 mL/kg per day as protective was confirmed in another study.[30] The greater the dose of human milk, the greater was the effect.[2] A large multicenter study in Norway reported that early feeding of extremely premature infants with human milk and subsequent fortified human milk was associated with significantly less late-onset sepsis and improved survival.[173] A systematic review of human milk for preterm infants and the effect on infection reported that inconsistent definitions of feedings, and infection outcomes, and issues with study design, sample size and potential confounding variables limits the clear conclusion that human milk use prevents infection in preterm or low-birth-weight infants.[174]

Probiotics for the prevention of NEC in preterm infants were subjected to a Cochrane review. Milk feeding and bacterial growth play a role. Dietary supplements containing potentially beneficial bacteria reduce the occurrence of NEC and death in premature infants under 1500 g.[175] However, this review did not find support for probiotics in infants under 1000 g at birth.

The impact of postnatal antibiotics on the preterm intestinal microbiome was studied in a group of premature infants between 24 and 31 weeks' gestation. They received at least 50% or more of breast milk per day and had received only 2 days of antibiotics or 7 days of antibiotics. The results showed that antibiotics disturbed the acquisition of bacteria in the gut.[176]

Dysbiosis in the first week of life is related to later onset of NEC.[177] Neuregulin-4 (NRG4) is an ErbB4-specific ligand that has been shown to help epithelial cells survive. Epithelial cell death is a major pathologic feature of NEC. Studies of ErbB4, which is found in the developing human intestine, as well as NRG4 (its receptor), which is found in human milk, suggest that NRG4-ErbB4 signaling may be a special pathway for therapeutic intervention to prevent NEC.[178] Perhaps this explains the role of human milk.

An exclusively human milk–based diet is associated with a lower rate of NEC than a diet of human milk and bovine milk–based product. This was demonstrated by a multicentered study involving 207 infants.[50] A human milk diet with human milk–based fortification allows the neonatologist to feed premature infants on totally human milk, meeting nutritional needs and preventing NEC.

NEC has historically had a variable rate in nurseries, but the cause has remained elusive. Patel et al.[179] developed an NEC quality improvement initiative when their NEC rates went from

4% in 2005 to 2006 to 10% in 2007 to 2008. A change in feeding protocol had no effect. However, NEC rates did change significantly when nasogastric tube management was redesigned to include more frequent nasogastric tube changes, as well as reeducation of parents about pump cleaning and storage. This project demonstrated the need for ongoing evaluation of routines and protocols.[179]

Changing to an exclusively human milk diet for infants under 33 weeks' gestational age was tested to reduce the incidence of NEC. The diet was limited to the mother's milk and human milk—based fortifier and excluded any trace of bovine protein. It was compared with the incidence of NEC during the years that formula was used, and human milk was fortified with bovine-based supplements. It reduced the incidence of NEC from 3.4% down to 1%.[180]

DONOR MILK

The use of expressed human milk and donor human milk in preterm infants is essential to their short- and long-term health.[181] Given the importance of human milk use for premature infants there should be clear standards for managing and using human milk for these infants.[182] Of particular importance to donor milk use is the effect pasteurization has on human milk cells, microbiome, and bioactive factors and their preservation in biologically active forms to benefit the infant[183] (Tables 14.18 and 14.19). (See Chapter 22 for additional information on handling expressed human milk.) Further investigation into pasteurization techniques is important. HTST techniques appear to protect more infectious protection properties, such as sIgA, than the Holder technique.[184]

TABLE 14.18 Impact of Holder Pasteurization on Human Milk Bioactive Factors

Component	Maintained (>90%)	Maintained (50%–90%)	Maintained (10%–50%)	Abolished (<10%)
Macronutrients	Carbohydrate (lactose, oligosaccharides)	Protein Total fat		
Micronutrients	Calcium	Iron		
	Copper			
	Magnesium			
	Phosphorus			
	Potassium			
	Sodium			
	Zinc			
Vitamins	Vitamin A	Folate		
		Vitamin B$_6$ Vitamin C		
Biologically active (immune)	IL-8, IL-12p70,	IgA, sIgA	CD14 (soluble)	IgM
	IL-13	IgG	IL-2	lymphocytes
	TGF-α	IGF-1, IGF-2	Lactoferrin-iron binding	
		IGF-BP2,3	capacity	
		IFN-γ	lysozyme	
		IL-1β, IL-4, IL-5, IL-10		
		TGF-β		
		Gangliosides		
Biologically active (metabolism)	Epidermal growth factor	Adiponectin	Erythropoietin	Bile salt—dependent lipase
	Heparin-binding growth factor	Amylase Insulin	Hepatocyte growth factor	Lipoprotein lipase

Bioactive components are affected to varying degrees by Holder pasteurization; some components remains intact, and cellular components are completely abolished. *IFN-γ*, Interferon-gamma; *Ig*, immunoglobulin; *IGF*, insulin-like growth factor; *IL*, interleukin; *sIgA*, secretory IgA; *TGF*, transforming growth factor.

From O'Connor D, Ewaschuk J, Unger S. Human milk pasteurization: benefits and risks. *Curr Opin Clin Nutr Metab Care.* 2015;18:269. doi:https://doi.org/10.1097/MCO.0000000000000160.

TABLE 14.19   Effects of Refrigeration Versus Freezing on Pasteurized High-Temperature, Short-Time Milk

Component	Refrigerated	40°C Frozen	Pasteurized HTST
Vitamin C	40%			
Lysozyme	40%	20%	0–65%	20%–40%
Lactoferrin	30%	NC	0–65%	0–85%
Lipase	25%		100%	
Secretory IgA	40%		20–50%	0–20%
Specific IgH	Variable	?		

HTST, High temperature, short time.
Modified with permission from Schanler RJ, Anderson D. The low-birth weight infant in patient care. In: Duggan C, Watkins JB, Walker WA, eds. *Nutrition in Pediatrics.* 4th ed. Hamilton, Ontario, Canada: BC Decker; 2008.

In South Africa, where mothers remain with and help care for their premature babies, a study compared feeding an infant its own mother's milk with feeding pooled pasteurized breast milk. Birth weight was between 1000 and 1500 g. Babies who were not on ventilators began feedings by 96 hours of age. Weight gain was significantly greater using untreated mother's milk, both for regaining birth weight and reaching 1800 g sooner. Both SGA and AGA infants did better on their own mothers' milk. This diet decreased hospital stays and decreased hospital-acquired infection. The authors attribute the advantages to the milk being fed fresh, with early initiation of feeding at the breast, compared with the pooled pasteurized milk.[139]

As much as we would like all mothers to supply their own mothers' milk to nourish their preterm infants there are specific difficulties encountered. Mothers of preterm infants are less likely to initiate milk expression, have delayed lactogenesis stage II, and are less likely to sustain expression than mothers of term infants. This has led to a growing use of donor human milk throughout the world. The use of donor milk has not decreased the amount of breastfeeding; rather it has increased by 10% the number of VLBW infants breastfeeding at hospital discharge.[121] The same study in California NICUs demonstrated a 2.6% reduction in hospital rate of NEC with the introduction of donor milk. In a study of 53 infants randomized to a human milk diet versus a formula diet, Cristofalo et al.[96] found significantly less need for prolonged parenteral nutrition and less NEC in the donor milk—fed group than the formula fed. There was also a trend toward less late-onset sepsis, but it was not significant. Comparing two epochs before and after the introduction of donor breast milk a study of 550 very low-birth-weight neonates showed that after the introduction of donor breast milk the rates of NEC fell significantly, although weight gain and head growth were worse in the donor milk epoch.[185] In a meta-analysis of 12 trials with 1879 infants, donor milk was shown to significantly lower the risk for NEC compared with formula ($p = 0.004$).[186] Formula-fed infants did demonstrate higher rates of weight gain, linear growth, and head circumference, although there was no effect on posthospital growth.

One of the reasons why donor milk does not yield the same strong benefits of mother's own milk relates to the sterilization procedures. There are two currently used methods of pasteurization, the Holder method of 62.5°C for 30 minutes and the HTST method of 72°C for 16 seconds. Pasteurization of donor milk destroys bacteria, viruses, and other pathogens and helps ensure milk safety. The problem is that many of the active bioactive agents are destroyed. All living cells such as lymphocytes and stem cells are killed. In addition, other protective bioactive agents are affected. The Holder method shows a variable loss of sIgA (20% to 50%), IgA (0 to 50%), lactoferrin (0 to 65%), lysozyme (0 to 65%), and lipase (100%). The HTST method better preserves with losses of sIgA (0 to 25%), lactoferrin 0 to 85%), and lysozyme (20% to 40%).[187] Both methods preserve oligosaccharides, vitamins, long-chain PUFAs, and epidermal growth factor.

KANGAROO CARE AND SKIN-TO-SKIN CARE

Kangaroo care and skin-to-skin care are important constituents of the support program for milk production by mothers who are pumping to produce milk, without the benefit of the infant suckling at the breast. The conduction of heat from parent to infant is sufficiently high to compensate for the increase in evaporative and conductive heat loss.

Extensive studies have been carried out to substantiate not only the safety but also the benefits of the skin-to-skin contact for fragile premature infants, including micropremature infants, at 24 weeks' gestation. All the reports recommend initiation directly after birth, even when the infant requires ventilator care. Stability of heart rate, respirations, and oxygen saturation during skin-to-skin care is remarkably calm.[188] This technique was started initially in resource-poor countries but has been so effective in calming stabilizing infants that it has become universal. It is particularly effective when the mother is initiating breastfeeding and pumping to start milk production. The Kangaroo Mother Care (KMC) method is a standardized, protocol-based system for preterm and/or LBW infants. The cardiorespiratory instability seen in separated infants during the first hours is consistent with the mammalian "protest-despair" biology and with a hyperarousal and dissociation response.[189] The aim is to empower the mother (and father, if possible) by gradually transferring the skills and responsibility for becoming the child's primary caregiver. It has been formally organized internationally[190,191] (Boxes 14.14 and 14.15).

Skin to skin has been evaluated by using a number of measurements to demonstrate the physiologic benefits of this close contact with a parent for premature infants. Measurements of salivary cortisol showed that the infant's cortisol reactivity decreased in response to handling. In addition, skin to skin improves the symmetry between the mother's and the infant's salivary cortisol levels.[192] It also helps allay the father's fears of spousal relationship problems, because he feels abandoned when the mother is totally consumed by the infant's needs. Breastfeeding was more common and more exclusive in the skin-to-skin group than in the control group at 1 and 4 months (all 18 dyads vs. 16 of 19).[192]

Kangaroo Care

Kangaroo care was first introduced in 1979 in a hospital in Bogota, Colombia, because of a shortage of incubators, high death rate from infection, and abandonment of premature infants by their mothers. Since that time, many investigators have carefully evaluated kangaroo care and found it to be beneficial to mother and infant.[193] Dressed only in a diaper, an infant is held skin to skin against the mother's chest between her breasts, snug inside the mother's clothing, often for hours. The father can do the same. Many advantages have been noted, including more stable respirations, heart rates, and temperatures. The infants spend less time crying and more time in a quiet, alert state and deep sleep.[194] Some studies suggest better weight gain and earlier discharge.[195] Hurst et al.[196] also reported an increase in milk volume during pumping (Fig. 14.12).

Mothers who give kangaroo care breastfeed longer and more frequently. They also report greater confidence in caring for their fragile infant than those who experience traditional care.[197] NICU nurseries should encourage kangaroo care. All parents should be assisted in providing it whenever they are in the nursery to benefit both the mother and the infant. This skin-to-skin contact enhances milk production, especially when the infant is too immature to suckle.

MILK PRODUCTION BY MOTHERS OF PREMATURE INFANTS

The AAP Committee on Nutrition published a handbook in 2014 that included a section on nutritional needs of LBW

BOX 14.14 Kangaroo Mother Care

There is sufficient evidence to make the following general statements about KMC:

- The kangaroo position provides a neutral thermal environment that provides immature infants with optimal thermal regulation, which is the same or better than provided by an incubator.
- KMC enhances bonding and attachment, universal human needs that apply to all preterm and low-birth-weight infants, their parents, and families.
- Avoiding unwarranted mother-infant separation and initiating the kangaroo position as early as possible helps repair a bonding process that is disrupted by delivering a preterm or ill infant.
- KMC helps reduce maternal postpartum depression symptoms and increases parental sensitivity to infant cues.
- Initiation of KMC as soon as possible is essential for the establishment of breastfeeding and for increasing the duration of exclusive and any breastfeeding.
- KMC has positive effects on infant/parent psychologic development and the development of mutual communication, understanding, and social recognition; reduces parenting stress; and contributes to an optimal family home environment.

KMC, Kangaroo Mother Care.
From Nyqvist KH, Anderson GC, Bergman N, et al. Towards universal Kangaroo Mother Care: recommendations and report from the first European conference and Seventh International Workshop of Kangaroo Mother Care. *Acta Paediatr.* 2010;99:820.

BOX 14.15 Kangaroo Mother Care Principles

The following guiding principles should pervade all components in KMC protocols:

- All intrapartum and postnatal care should adhere to a paradigm of nonseparation of infants and their mothers/families.
- Preterm/low-birth-weight infants should be regarded as extero-gestational fetuses needing skin-to-skin contact to promote maturation.
- KMC should begin as soon as possible after birth and continue as often and for as long as appropriate (depending on circumstances).

KMC, Kangaroo Mother Care.
From Nyqvist KH, Anderson GC, Bergman N, et al. Towards universal Kangaroo Mother Care: recommendations and report from the first European conference and Seventh International Workshop of Kangaroo Mother Care. *Acta Paediatr.* 2010;99:820.

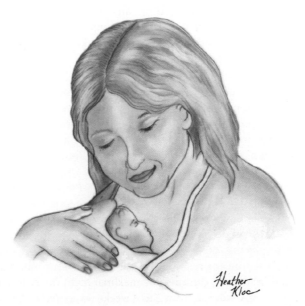

Fig. 14.12 Kangaroo care method.

infants.[198] They suggest that the mother's own milk and new special formulas for those babies who need breast milk substitutes are promising alternatives.

Although human milk is the feeding of choice for preterm as well as term infants there remain several barriers to its implementation. In a CDC PRAMS study, women who delivered infants before 34 weeks were more likely to initiate breastfeeding (OR 2.24) and to breastfeed for longer than 4 weeks (OR 2.58) but less likely to breastfeed beyond 10 weeks compared with term mothers.[199] Thus mothers often find it difficult to meet and maintain their nutritional goals. Some of the barriers the mothers of preterm infants face include separation from their infants, delayed initiation of milk expression, a stressful environment for the mother and baby and a lack of knowledge of the specific benefits mother's own breast milk conveys to the preterm infant. Often the mother of a preterm infant is scared and feels inadequate to help her baby. One way to approach this is to discuss the importance of breast milk to her infant and the mother's ability to give her baby something that no one else can and that is extremely impactful. The presence of lactation specialists in the NICU is also important. Although there are clear recommendations for the presence of lactation consultants on inpatient units, there remains a lack of standards for lactation support in the NICU, and only a limited number of NICUs have dedicated lactation consultants. The presence of an international board-certified lactation consultant or a certified lactation counselor can significantly improve the amount of direct breastfeeding on NICU discharge.[200] A joint effort of the AAP Committee on the Fetus and Newborn and the American College of Obstetricians and Gynecologists Committee on Obstetric Practice states that "human milk has a number of special features that make its use desirable in feeding preterm babies."[201]

The production of milk by a mother who is not actively nursing her infant, as is frequently the case in LBW infants and other neonates in NICUs, is a challenge to the resources of the NICU and the postpartum staff. Insufficient milk production is a common problem that becomes more critical as time passes. As production continues to drop, an infant's needs increase. Evaluation of various protocols has been undertaken by investigators who looked at onset of pumping postpartum, frequency of pumping, and duration in total minutes per day and length of time when no pumping occurred.

Hopkinson et al.[202] enrolled 32 healthy mothers, 19 of whom had no previous breastfeeding experience, into a study protocol. Their infants were 28 to 30 weeks' gestation. All of the mothers initiated pumping between days 2 and 6. The day of initiation was correlated with the volume of milk at 2 weeks, but not at 4 weeks, with mothers who had nursed previously and initiated pumping sooner. Parity, gravidity, age, and previous nursing experience were not correlated with volumes at 2 weeks. Parity and previous nursing experience were associated with milk volume at 4 weeks, with multiparas producing 60% greater volumes. The investigators found no significant relationship between 24-hour milk volume and frequency, duration, or maximal night interval. The change in milk volume from 2 to 4 weeks was correlated with frequency and duration of pumping but not to maximal night

intervals. The range in number of pumpings per day was four to nine. The authors concluded that optimal milk production occurs with at least five expressions per day and pumping durations that exceed 100 min/day.[202]

The frequency of milk expression was evaluated by de Carvalho et al.[127] in a crossover design study of 25 mothers who delivered at 28 to 37 weeks' gestation. Frequent expression of milk was significantly associated with greater milk production (342 ± 229 mL) than with infrequent expression (221 ± 141 mL). They compared three or fewer pumpings per day to four or more. The mean numbers were 2.4 versus 5.7, neither equaling the frequency that a mother would usually feed her infant in the first few weeks.

Minimum frequency and duration figures have been provided. However, it is advisable to increase the frequency of pumping because the need to raise production increases and as the time for discharge and feeding the infant exclusively at the breast approaches. Consideration for increasing nighttime pumpings is also important as discharge approaches. Some mothers experience a dread of the pump when demands are increased for "more milk production." The management of the mother producing milk for her hospitalized infant should be coordinated by a neonatologist and a primary care physician. She should be assisted by a primary care nurse and the unit's lactation coordinator and lactation consultants to maximize support and minimize stress.

Peer counselors have become important members of the lactation support teams in the NICU, as they have been in birth centers and in the community. Peer support was originated by the La Leche League. Anthropologist Dana Raphael coined the expression "a friend from across the street." Health departments and Women, Infants, and Children (WIC) programs have developed peer counselor programs in which women (peers) with breastfeeding experience are trained to provide support and counsel but not practice medicine.[203] Very successful programs have been developed in NICUs. A combination of a lactation consultant and a peer counselor provides the most effective breastfeeding support in the NICU (Fig. 14.13; see Chapter 22).[204]

The NICU at Rush University Medical Center developed a lactation support program that included peer counselors who were former NICU parents.[205] They work directly with NICU mothers and babies, in collaboration with the NICU nurses, to promote successful breastfeeding. The health care providers (n = 17) in a study of university NICUs thought the peer counselors improved the care of the infants by empowering the mothers to provide milk and modeling good infant care for the mothers.

When the physiology of lactation is applied to the practical management of inducing milk supply without the benefit of an infant's participation, it is apparent that mimicking natural breastfeeding is more effective. The breast can be prepared with massage and manual expression. Although some women succeed with manual expression alone, it is rare, and a good pump should be recommended. None of the hand pumps can truly duplicate the milking action of the infant, and all are essentially vacuum extractors. They should be used only as a stopgap measure when

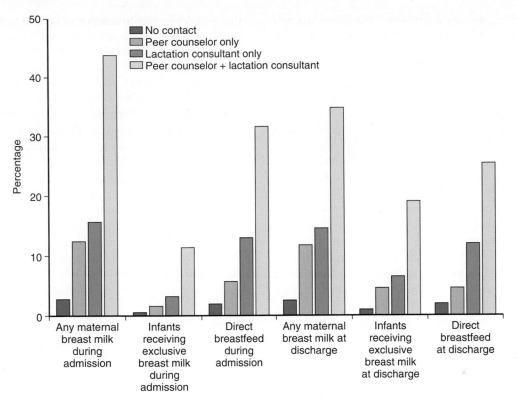

Fig. 14.13 Breastfeeding outcomes during hospital stay by lactation staff type. χ^2 tests for overall differences within each outcome were significant at $p < 0.001$. Breastfeeding outcomes were classified as any maternal breast milk (infant receiving *any* maternal breast milk by direct breastfeeding and/or pumping regardless of supplementation with formula), *exclusive* breast milk (infant receiving exclusive maternal milk by direct breastfeeding and/or pumping without any formula supplementation), and any direct breastfeeding during NICU admission and at discharge (infant fed directly at the breast for at least one feeding with or without subsequent formula supplementation) during neonatal intensive care unit admission and at discharge. Estimates do not include exclusive donor milk. (From Oza-Frank R, Bhatia A, Smith C. Combined peer counselor and lactation consultant support increases breastfeeding in the NICU. *Breastfeed Med.* 2013;8:509.)

the electric pump is unavailable (see Chapter 22). A pump that can be used on both breasts simultaneously saves time and generates higher levels of prolactin.[206] These pumps also generate a greater total milk volume than pumping each breast separately for the same length of time.[206] Subsequent studies have produced variable observations. Groh-Wargo et al.[142] studied 32 women who were randomly assigned to single or double pumping for 6 weeks. No difference was found in prolactin levels or total volume of milk produced by these investigations, although the time-saving effect was considered important.[142]

Jones et al.[207] reported an RCT that was designed to compare methods of milk expression after preterm delivery. It involved 36 women: 19 used simultaneous pumping, and 17 used sequential pumping by random assignment. A crossover design was used to evaluate the effect of breast massage on milk volume and fat content (estimated by creamatocrit). The authors reported that the results were unequivocal, showing that pumping both breasts simultaneously produced more milk—125.1 g with massage and 87.7 g without. This was compared with sequential volumes of 78.7 g with massage and 51.3 g without.

Pumping should be initiated as soon as a mother's condition permits. Offering this opportunity to the mother should be part of the supportive care offered by postpartum staff. All the points of preparation for pumping should be included: comfortable position, tranquil atmosphere, preparation of the breast with gentle stroking and warmth, massage during pumping, confidence, and reassurance from the staff. The obstetrician is in an important position to initiate the offer to pump, because he or she should know whether the mother intends to breastfeed from conversations during the mother's prenatal care. The mother may not know it is appropriate to ask for a pump. Providing knowledgeable, accurate, consistent, and sensitive support should be the rule in every perinatal center, especially for mothers of high-risk infants who choose to breastfeed.[205,206] The opportunity to pump should be offered to all women, regardless of previous feeding choice. Often a mother changes her mind when her infant is at high risk and would receive many additional benefits from her milk.

Providing an appropriate room for pumping after the mother has been discharged is critical to individual success and is an expression of commitment to breastfeeding by the NICU. This room should be clean, bright, and cheerful and accommodate more than one mother and companion at a time, unless several rooms are available. It should have a sink for washing hands and storage for equipment and supplies. A nurse call button or other alarm system is also essential. Additional features are soft music, a telephone, and reading material. The hospital should have a supply of approved electric pumps and individual disposable attachment packets for each mother. A place should be available to store her properly labeled and dated milk in a freezer or refrigerator. Sterile storage containers should be readily available.

A mother should be encouraged to rent a pump for home use and around-the-clock pumping. These are available from medical supply stores, pharmacies, home care services, hospitals, and some lactation consultants. Insurance companies reimburse for the cost of the rental when the milk is prescribed for a high-risk infant. A neonatologist can provide an appropriate letter of support. The hospital support staff who are coordinating the mother's care or the NICU staff should be sure that the mother understands how to use the equipment effectively. Ideally, NICUs have at least one staff member who is a licensed, certified lactation consultant who will coordinate this effort under the direction of the obstetrician, pediatrician, and neonatologist. One lactation consultant per 15 infants in the NICU is ideal. The mother should not be subjected to pressures of pump equipment entrepreneurs and unsolicited advice. The best remedy is for the NICU to provide on-staff, up-to-date experience and support to the mother in her efforts to provide milk and breastfeed her high-risk infant. Box 14.16 outlines key strategies for successful pumping when an infant is unable to suckle the breast. All neonatal nurses should be familiar with the available pumps and their use and be supportive of mothers who are pumping.[207]

Concerns Related to Cytomegalovirus and Human Milk for Premature Infants

Cytomegalovirus (CMV) is a pathogen that can be transmitted to the fetus and newborn in utero, during the perinatal period through direct contact and postnatally by breast milk. Mothers with CMV infection may shed the virus into their milk and risk transmission of the virus to their infants. Transmission of CMV postnatally to term infants has been thought to be inconsequential, but this is not the case for preterm infants. Preterm infants are at highest risk for developing symptomatic disease. In one meta-analysis, 19% of preterm infants acquired CMV infection

---

BOX 14.16 Guidelines for Initiating Milk Supply Without Infant Suckling

1. Begin as soon after delivery as maternal condition permits.
2. Initiate use of electric pump while in hospital.
3. Begin slowly, increasing time over first week.
4. Pump on more regular basis as soon as engorgement is evident.
5. Pump at least five times in 24 hours.
6. Allow a rest period for uninterrupted sleep of at least 6 hours.
7. Pump a total of at least 100 min/day.
8. Use "double" pump to pump both breasts simultaneously, which can cut total time proportionately.
9. Prepare breast with warm soaks, gentle stroking, and light massage to maximize production of milk.
10. Encourage skin-to-skin care (kangaroo care).

---

and about 20% of those developed a CMV-related sepsis-like syndrome.[208] These symptoms can include thrombocytopenia, neutropenia, respiratory distress, and hepatic disease. The AAP recommends considering screening for mothers of infants born at less than 32 weeks. Mothers who are CMV positive may choose to have their breast milk pasteurized before administration to their infant. Pasteurization by either the Holder method or a HTST pasteurization has been shown to inactivate CMV. Of course, pasteurization also has an effect on the components of breast milk. (See discussion under the earlier section on donor milk.) Freezing milk at $-20°C$, which is a routine part of milk storage in the NICU, has been shown to decrease viral titers but does not eliminate the risk for CMV transmission. In a large retrospective cohort study, Weimer et al.[209] described significantly higher rates of failed hearing screens, postnatal age at discharge, biparietal diameter, and lower weight for age in those infants with acquired CMV. This was a retrospective study, however, and there was a very low rate of CMV recognition (0.4%). This could indicate that the majority of preterm infants who developed CMV were unrecognized and asymptomatic. Further prospective studies are needed to clarify the risk for acquired CMV to the preterm infant and whether interventions such as pasteurization or antivirals are indicated (see Chapter 12).

WHO PRODUCES MILK FOR LOW-BIRTH-WEIGHT OR SMALL-FOR-GESTATIONAL-AGE INFANTS?

Nationwide, mothers who give birth to infants who are admitted to special care nurseries are less likely to initiate lactation than mothers of healthy term infants, according to Meier.[47] The profile of mothers who give birth to these high-risk infants includes a higher percentage of low-income, low-education, young mothers, who do not breastfeed in great numbers. Postpartum and NICU staff should work to encourage these women to initiate lactation.

Maternal choice to breastfeed or provide milk for an LBW infant is influenced by many factors beyond those that affect most feeding decisions of normal full-term infants.[210] Lucas et al.[97,100] sought to answer two major questions in a study of 925 mother-infant pairs in five hospitals. Do health care professionals in neonatal units exert a major influence on a mother's feeding preference and availability of her milk for her infant? Are there population differences between mothers who do and do not provide their milk? In these two studies in five centers, the demographic characteristics of the mother were important, not those of the staff. These studies did not look at success rates, however.

Mothers in a study by Verronen[211] had delivered infants at a mean of 31 weeks' gestation; the infants weighed less than 1850 g, with a mean of 1370 g. More educated mothers provided their milk (98%) than uneducated (40%). Factors of higher socioeconomic class, lower parity or fewer living children, being married, and being older than 20 years of age were associated with providing milk. Boys were more apt to receive mother's milk, as shown in other studies. Birth weight and extreme immaturity were not a determinant, nor was transfer of the infant to another center. The Rush Mother's Milk Club, which is a breastfeeding intervention for mothers of VLBW infants in Chicago, was developed and directed by Meier et al.[212,213] In the 52-bed urban NICU, the staff provided facilitated learning. Transportation was provided for mothers from home, as well as a weekly interactive social luncheon. They employ five peer counselors and provide a 24-hour, toll-free pager information line. The peer counselors also contact mothers at home. Low milk supply is aggressively managed with record keeping, encouragement, and counseling. The lactation initiation rate among these predominantly low-income African-American women was 72.9%. Exclusive mother's milk was attained by 57.2% and some mother's milk by 72.5%.[214] Skin-to-skin and kangaroo care are important features of this program and many others.[215]

FEEDING THE NEAR-TERM INFANT (35 TO 37 WEEKS' GESTATION) AT THE BREAST

Near-term infants (i.e., 35 0/7 weeks to 36 6/7 weeks) may be nursed at the breast if otherwise stable. Breastfeeding should be initiated by 1 hour of age if mother and infant are stable. Health care professionals should monitor to ensure that frequent ongoing feedings are occurring "on demand" at least 10 to 12 times a day. Communication among staff and with the parents is key to success. Involvement of lactation-trained staff who are also skilled neonatal nurses mitigates confusion and conflicting messages to the family. Particular care should be given to assist a mother in getting the infant to suckle, especially if the breast and nipples are large or engorged.[216,217] Weight should be followed closely to prevent excessive weight loss. Infants who receive sugar water and formula supplements lose more weight than those who are nursed frequently at the breast without supplementation. If breastfeeding is going well, the infant could be discharged with the mother from the hospital as soon as the infant begins to gain substantially, with close follow-up at home. Poor weight gain, less than 20 g/day, is usually the result of inadequate intake. Average weight gain should be 26 to 31 g/day (see Appendix I, ABM Protocol #10). A mother may need to pump between feedings if the infant does not stimulate the breasts adequately. The milk can be provided by cup or lactation aide device (see Appendix I, ABM Protocol #10 and Fig. 13.12). Difficulties with latch should be investigated with a careful examination of the infant's mouth and the mother's breast and nipples. Before discharge, the physician, as well as the nurse, should observe the dyad.[218] If a mother is a low producer, galactagogues can be considered. (See Chapter 11 and ABM Protocol #9 in Appendix I.) Follow-up should include frequent weighing and growth measurements (length and head circumference should increase approximately 0.5 cm/wk). Home visits or office checks are crucial to monitor progress. An extensive review of practice guidelines for the care of the late preterm infant has been prepared by the National Perinatal Association.[218]

PREMATURE INFANTS OF 28 6/7 WEEKS TO 32 6/7 WEEKS

Infants of gestational age more than 28 weeks but less than 35 weeks are frequently breastfed in NICUs, because the value of human milk has been recognized by most neonatologists.

Feeding at the breast when an infant is less than 1500 g is considered too strenuous by many neonatologists, even though it has been proved that it takes less energy and less impact on vital signs to breastfeed than bottle-feed.[219] When the feeding of infants of less than 1500 g was examined, however, the growth of those fed at the breast was comparable with that of matched control infants fed expressed human milk by bottle.[207] Breastfeeding was started when sucking movements were observed. Initially, they received supplementary human milk by tube plus 800 units of vitamin D and 60 mg of vitamin C daily. Unrestricted visiting of parents to the neonatal unit, an optimistic and knowledgeable attitude of the nursing staff toward breastfeeding, and the avoidance of a bottle for the infants are important to success.[220,221] Encouraging the expression of milk by the mothers early in the postpartum period is essential. The main deterrent to successful breastfeeding was lack of maternal interest and commitment.

Blaymore Bier et al.[102] undertook a clinical study of breastfeeding and bottle-feedings in ELBW infants (birth weight 800 g or less) when they were considered ready to bottle-feed. This was at a mean age of 35 weeks since conception (corrected gestational age). One breastfeeding and one bottle-feeding were monitored each day for 10 days. Prefeeding and postfeeding weights, oxygen saturation, respiratory and heart rates, and axillary temperature were recorded. Higher oxygen saturation and higher temperatures during breastfeeding and less likelihood of desaturation below 90% were noted in the breastfed infants. The weights reflecting intake were higher in the bottle-fed infants. The authors concluded that it was physiologically safe and less stressful for infants to breastfeed. The lower intake requires monitoring, however.[102]

The ontogenic and temporal organization of nonnutritive sucking during active sleep was studied by Hack et al.[222] in preterm infants. One of the six infants studied had recognizable rhythmic sucking bursts at 28 weeks, and all had bursts by 31 to 32 weeks. The number of bursts increased and the interval between bursts decreased as the infants matured, with the earliest indications of intrinsic rhythm beginning at 30 weeks.

Nonnutritive sucking has become a subject of controversy in NICUs. Allowing premature infants to suck on a pacifier during gavage feedings was initially reported to be associated with increased weight gain and shorter hospitalization. When nutrient intake and other parameters were controlled, however, no advantages to nonnutritive sucking were observed in somatic growth, serum proteins, energy absorption, or feeding tolerance, nor was any increase in tropic hormones or growth promoters seen.[221,223,224] Infants have been observed to have transcutaneous oxygen saturation measurements increase by 3% to 4% during nonnutritive sucking.[127] Nonnutritive sucking does not appear to carry risk for infants destined for further bottle-feeding. However, it should be avoided for infants destined to breastfeed, to avoid interference with normal sucking. Unfortunately, most studies have been done with bottles.[225]

Of greater significance is the value of having these infants placed at the "emptied" breast during gavage tube feedings. When Narayanan et al.[226] studied this practice, they found no change in weight gain or length of hospital stay. The practice did, however, result in more successful and longer duration of breastfeeding after discharge. This technique was originally designed in our nursery to improve the mother's milk production and encourage mothers who were becoming discouraged. As the infant matures and begins swallowing with sucking, it becomes unnecessary to **pump** the breast "empty" before presenting it to the infant. This is because any milk provided could be suckled and swallowed. Suckling at the breast initiates a peristaltic action that also triggers swallowing and the physiologic response of the entire gastrointestinal tract (see Chapter 7). Suckling the breast also improves the mother's success when pumping. Readiness to wean from tube feedings to oral feeding is poorly defined and based on observations using a bottle and/or a pacifier. Stable cardiopulmonary status at 33 to 34 weeks is associated with sucking patterns that resemble term infants (i.e., rhythmic alteration of suction and expression and the positive pressure generated by compression). Mature sucking pattern is not necessary for safe, successful feeding at the breast.[227] Infants can feed orally without suction. The undulating motion of the tongue does trigger let-down and the swallowing of fluid. An infant's behavioral state and organization during feeding, the nursery environment (especially light and sound), and a caretaker's approach to oral feeding all affect an infant's performance.[227] This is another point supportive of early breastfeeding. Avoidance of bottles during the establishment of breastfeeding in premature infants has been evaluated in a Cochrane review.[228] Small premature infants begin with tube feedings of their mother's milk. As they mature, breastfeedings are added. But in many nurseries, the bottle with the mother's milk is introduced. Its impact on successful breastfeeding is challenged. Five studies of 543 infants were included in a Cochrane review by Collins et al.[228] Four of the studies substituted cup feeding when mother was not available to breastfeed. The cup feedings increased the probability of successful breastfeeding and continuation of breastfeeding. Cup feedings, however, prolonged hospitalizations by 10 days. Noncompliance was an issue as well. A study in Egypt, after this review, reported 30 cup-fed premature infants compared with 30 bottle-fed infants who were breastfed on discharge because mothers did not provide their milk or breastfeed before discharge. The cup-fed infants breastfed for longer durations and in greater numbers.[60] The crucial role of adequate nutrition in brain growth, especially in the premature infant, is generally acknowledged. Although nutrition may not overcome all the problems of extreme prematurity and its impact on the immature brain, it reduces infections and NEC and has immunomodulatory properties when it includes over 50% human milk. The impact of human milk constituents on the white matter and its development is remarkable. This is being attributed to the gut-immune-brain axis.[193] The nutritional adjustments to use human milk

and human milk supplements are considered safe, are inexpensive, cause few side effects, and are easily implemented.

BREASTFEEDING THE EXTREMELY PREMATURE INFANT

Evaluations of feeding strategies are rarely conducted or published, in spite of rigid protocols in some nurseries. Early initiation of feedings has been thought valuable and safe. In a study of 171 premature infants between 26 and 30 weeks' gestation, Schanler et al.[61] tested the validity of gastrointestinal priming and continuous infusion, versus intermittent bolus tube feeding with human milk or preterm formula. Infants were randomized to four treatment combinations in a balanced two-way design. Investigators compared the presence or absence of gastrointestinal priming for 10 days and continuous infusion versus intermittent bolus tube feeding. Time to full feeding was similar in all groups. Gastrointestinal priming had no adverse effects, improved calcium and phosphorus retention, and shorter intentional transient times. Bolus feeding was associated with less feeding intolerance and greater weight gain than the continuous method. The more human milk fed, the lower was the morbidity rate. The authors concluded that early gastrointestinal priming with human milk and bolus feedings provided the best advantage for premature infants.[61] Very preterm infants, born at 26 to 31 weeks' gestation, have the capacity for the early development of oral motor competence that is sufficient for establishment of full breastfeeding at a low postmenstrual age, according to Nyqvist.[191] Using the Preterm Infant Breastfeeding Behavior Scale (Table 14.20), designed for use by mothers and professionals to observe levels of competence in oral motor behavior during breastfeeding, the author studied 15 infants born at 26 to 31 weeks' gestational age. The author made daily assessments. Semi-demand feeding was used with a prescribed total daily income volume. Breastfeeding was initiated at 29 weeks. Rooting, efficient areolar grasp, and repeated short sucking bursts were noted at 29 weeks. At 31 weeks, long sucking bursts and repeated swallowing were observed. Sucking rates ranged from 5 to 24, with a median of 17. Full breastfeeding was reached between 32 and 38 weeks, with a median of 35 weeks. Weight gain was described as adequate.[191] Alternative techniques were described in a report from a nursery in Brazil, in which they placed infants in groups trying techniques of re-lactation, translactation, and breast-orogastric tubes.[229] They described 432 infants who, at discharge, were breastfeeding 85%, 100%, and 100% in each group, respectively. All attained good weight gain, with only 1.6% feeding-related problems. The definition of re-lactation and translactation resembles other nurseries' use of lactation aide devices for additional nutrition.

Transpyloric tube feeding in VLBW infants with suspected gastroesophageal reflux has been used successfully by Malcolm et al.[29] They described 72 VLBW infants with a median birth weight of 870 g (a range of 365 to 1435 g) and a gestational age of 26 weeks (range 23 to 31 weeks) who received transpyloric

TABLE 14.20 The Preterm Infant Breastfeeding Behavior Scale (PIBBS)

Scale Items	Levels of Competence
Rooting	Did not root
	Showed some rooting behavior (mouth opening, tongue extension, hand-to-mouth/face movements, head turning)
	Showed obvious rooting behavior (simultaneous mouth opening and head turning)
Areolar grasp (how much of the breast was inside the baby's mouth)	None, the mouth only touched the nipple
	Part of the nipple
	The whole nipple, not the areola
	The nipple and some of the areola
Latched on and fixed to the breast	Did not latch on at all so the mother felt it
	Latched on for <1 min
	Latched on for 1–5 min or more, recorded by marking a cross along a line graded 1–15 min
Sucking	No sucking or licking
	Licking and tasting, but no sucking
	Single sucks, occasional short sucking bursts (2–9 sucks)
	Repeated (2 or more consecutive) short sucking bursts, occasional long bursts (10 sucks or more before a pause)
	Repeated long sucking bursts
Longest sucking bursts	Maximum number of consecutive sucks, recorded by marking a cross along a line graded 1–30
Swallowing	Swallowing was not noticed
	Occasional swallowing was noticed

From Nyqvist KH. Early attainment of breastfeeding competence in very preterm infants. *Acta Paediatr.* 2008;97:776–778, Figure 1.

feedings. They observed a reduction in apneic episodes and a decrease in bradycardia. Five infants developed NEC, none of whom were receiving human milk. The authors concluded that transpyloric feedings, when limited to human milk, may safely reduce episodes of apnea and bradycardia in preterm infants suspected of gastroesophageal reflux. They suggest confirmation of this work in other NICUs, with the potential of changing hospital procedures.

SMALL-FOR-GESTATIONAL-AGE INFANTS

Infants who are below the 10th percentile (or 2 SDs) in weight for their gestational age are termed *small for gestational age* (SGA). These infants may also be shorter in length and have smaller heads, depending on when in gestational life the insult to their growth occurred. The more general the growth failure is, the earlier the intrauterine effect appears. For example, rubella in the first trimester causes total growth restriction, whereas hypertension in the mother in the third trimester predominantly affects weight. The more profound the growth restriction is, the more difficult are the nutritional problems.

SGA infants are prone to be hypocalcemic; however, if they can be provided with adequate breast milk early, this complication may be avoided. This is because the calcium-to-phosphorus ratio is more physiologic in human milk than in formula. Other problems, including hypothermia and hypoglycemia, which lead to a vicious circle of acidosis and associated problems, can be triggered by unmonitored exposure of an infant to thermal stress in the first hours of life and failure to identify the hypoglycemia early. Hypoglycemia in an SGA infant cannot be ignored. The potential exists for significant stress to the nervous system, which can result in seizures that require aggressive therapy and a detailed diagnostic workup. SGA infants lack glycogen stores, so they cannot raise their own blood sugar level by mobilizing stores.

Using human α-lactalbumin as a marker protein, Schanler et al.[61] demonstrated that SGA infants with intrauterine growth restriction have delayed postnatal decrease in macromolecular absorption and delayed intestinal maturation, even compared with premature infants of the same weight. Their management demands special care. The enzymes in human milk can facilitate catch-up maturation of the intestinal tract.

Thus perinatal nursery staff may appear to be obstructive to breastfeeding when they hover over this infant or even insist on transfer to the nursery. Initial breastfeeding at delivery is permissible; however, adequate external heat must be provided. Testing the blood glucose should be performed in the delivery room recovery area. The infant should be sent to the nursery if hypoglycemia or hypothermia cannot be controlled. Frequent breastfeeding can be initiated unless the blood glucose level is too low (less than 30 mg/dL) or unresponsive to oral treatment. It may not be possible for even an actively lactating multipara to sustain an SGA infant initially, but the infant should be put to breast at least every 3 hours and given intravenous glucose as well. (See Appendix I, ABM Protocol #1 Hypoglycemia.)

Term SGA infants often have a poor suck and poor coordination with the swallow reflex. They may have considerable mucus, with gagging and spitting. A simple lavage of the stomach with a no. 8 feeding tube (or no. 5 if the infant weighs less than 2600 g) and warmed glucose water usually relieves the gagging. Once this SGA infant begins to eat, he or she will do well and will require sufficient kilocalories to meet the needs of an AGA infant. The mother may need to use a breast pump initially to stimulate lactation and increase the volume she produces.

Children born SGA are at a neurodevelopmental disadvantage. When these infants receive enriched formula, it does improve their growth, but breastfed SGA infants grew best in a series of children followed by Morley et al.[54] Three groups fed regular formula, enriched formula, or breast milk were followed: 147 were randomized to regular formula, 152 received enriched formula, and 175 were in the reference group of breastfeeding. The developmental scores using the Bayley Mental Development Index or the Psychomotor Development Index at 18 months were measured. No difference between formula groups was seen. The breastfeeding infants had significantly higher Psychomotor Development Index scores and a 6-point advantage in the Bayley Mental Development Index. The authors suggested that SGA infants clearly benefited from being breastfed.[54]

TRANSITIONING FROM HOSPITAL TO HOME

The transition from hospital to home is a stressful time for all families, but when an infant is premature and has been in the NICU for days, weeks, or months, transition can be extremely difficult. The stress can be reduced by appropriate discharge planning. The mother should spend as much time as possible with her infant, breastfeeding when present. A lactation consultant or trained staff member should observe these interactions. The presence of sucking and swallowing should be documented. If mothers have received adequate assistance in the days and weeks before discharge, positioning and latch should be perfected by discharge.

The AAP Committee on Fetus and Newborn has delineated the following three physiologic competencies that are recognized as essential before hospital discharge of the preterm infant:

- The ability to maintain body temperature in a home environment
- Sufficiently mature respiratory control
- Oral feeding sufficient to support appropriate growth

Hospitals that have facilities to accommodate care by parent overnight are helpful in the transition. At minimum, parents should be given all the medications and treatments before discharge and be breastfeeding. If a mother's supply is not adequate yet, she should be instructed in the use of the lactation supplementer before discharge, with a plan for the amount and substance to be placed in the supplementer. If she has stored milk available, it can be used. If not, the neonatologist will have to order donor milk. If not, a special care formula or special human milk supplementer, which is designed to be used separately from mixing with mother's milk as a feed, can be used. Mothers should be instructed to continue pumping until the infants are exclusively breastfed and gaining weight adequately. Pumping three to four times per day to completely empty the breasts at home is critical. Preterm infants usually do not completely empty the breasts at first. They lack the suction strength and sustainable effective organization of sucking until they approach 40 weeks' corrected gestational age, according to Meier.[47] To guarantee adequate production and intake, these preterm infants need scheduling to ensure feeding every 3 hours, although feeding on cue is more effective in the long run.

In Sweden, preterm infants who are less than 32 weeks' gestation are fed their mother's milk or, if that is not available, donor milk. Of 36 NICUs in Sweden that responded to a questionnaire on breast milk handling, 27 had their own milk bank.[230] The authors have established national guidelines for the hospital use of human milk. In North America, the Human Milk Banking Association of North America oversees volunteer milk banking (see Chapter 22).

Follow-up after discharge from the NICU is essential and should be involved as the dyad is prepared for discharge. Independent predictors of human milk receipt at NICU discharge were determined by Brownell et al.[231] from analysis of the Vermont Oxford Network clinical data at a Level IV NICU in the inner city. They concluded that a strong NICU lactation program, in combination with a community-based peer counselor program, may increase rates of human milk consumption among VLBW infants of black/Hispanic mothers, as well as those with more complicated courses.

Community-based peer support programs are very helpful in supporting postdischarge mothers to continue to provide their own milk.

Early discharge with tube feeding of preterm infants under close supervision by pediatric nurse practitioners in the Netherlands was done. The effect was an increase in the duration of breastfeeding.[232] The finding continued for 6 months after discharge. This approach needs confirmation but is important.

Not all premature infants will need supplementation at home. Before and after feeding weighing (see Chapter 7) can be done while an infant is still in the hospital to measure the infant's intake at each feeding. Digital scales, accurate to 2 g, are available in hospitals, and home models can be rented. As the preterm infant matures and is approaching discharge from the NICU the ideal discharge plan involves maximizing the intake of human milk.[233] This should be a shared decision with the mother and clinician and focus on a plan that considers the mother's needs as well as the infant's. When an infant is first discharged, it is helpful to both the physician and the parents to know what intake actually is.[152] Some mothers produce large volumes of milk, but the infants do not gain weight. Pumping first to remove the foremilk (and freeze it) and having the infant suckle the hind milk can help this problem. A pediatrician plays a critical role in the success of feeding after discharge. Most infants will have received fortified human milk during the NICU stay. All preterm infants should be discharged on supplemental iron at 2 to 4 mg/kg per day and vitamin D 400 IU/day as recommended by the AAP (AAP Committee on Nutrition: Nutritional Needs of the Preterm Infant, 8th edition).[234] In planning for discharge it is important to closely monitor growth and milk intake both before and after discharge. If the mother has been exclusively breastfeeding the infant before discharge, this should be maintained with close follow-up of growth parameters. If the infant has been receiving fortified breast milk by bottle or cup feeds this should be continued after discharge. The breast milk may be fortified using a powdered preterm discharge formula (22 kcal/30 mL) if milk supply is adequate or supplemented with preterm discharge formula if additional volume is needed. The discharge plan and ongoing nutritional management must be highly individualized, taking into account growth and biochemical parameters, including hemoglobin, alkaline phosphatase, and phosphorus levels. Monitoring of progress and knowledge of the unique concerns in breastfeeding premature infants are key. The Academy of Breastfeeding Medicine Protocol #12 in Appendix I details the steps to follow.

IMPROVING MILK PRODUCTION

The following steps improve milk production:
1. Begin pumping as soon postpartum as possible.
2. Use hospital-grade double (two-breast) pumps.
3. Pump 10 to 15 minutes every 3 hours until more than a few drops are produced (72 hours).
4. When the amount increases, continue to pump for 2 minutes after the last drop is produced (total 20 to 30 minutes).
5. Keep a record of times pumped and volumes produced.
6. Pump at baby's bedside when possible.
7. Start with kangaroo care.
8. Stroke and massage breast during pumping.
9. As soon as infant is able, place at emptied breast to suckle or during gavage feedings.

Pump-dependent mothers are at risk for diminishing milk supply. Mothers of preterm infants can attain and sustain high production levels by combining the use of electrical pumps with manual techniques, including hand expression taught by an experienced nurse. This includes mothers of normal term babies. It is essential for mothers of infants in the NICU. Dr. Morton has developed several videotapes demonstrating these techniques that are excellent for mothers and staff alike.[235] Chapter 11 and Protocol #9 Galactagogues in Appendix I discuss pharmacologic stimulation of milk production.

CONCLUDING RECOMMENDATIONS

Infants who weigh less than 1800 g at birth and have to be gavage fed and infants of any weight who are acutely ill present complex problems. A mother should be instructed to express her milk initially and contribute any colostrum she produces. This can be given by gastric tube spoon or cup. A hospital-grade electric pump is effective in helping a mother increase the volume produced. When an infant is born at 1000 g, requires ventilator support for days, and is not discharged for 8 weeks (Fig. 14.14), it is difficult to maintain a large volume of milk by pumping. It can be done, however, with supportive counseling by staff and the initiation of kangaroo care. Milk volumes usually increase when an infant begins to actually breastfeed, not unlike re-lactation (see Chapter 19) or increasing milk volume in other situations (see Chapter 7).

When nipple feeding is possible, an infant can be put to the breast. It requires less energy to suckle at the breast than to feed from a bottle. The peristaltic motion of the tongue, which is the normal innate suckling mode, initiates the peristaltic motion of the gastrointestinal tract, and triggers the swallow. If no pacifiers or rubber nipples have been given, an infant may be able to suckle at the breast well before reaching 1500 g. Fig. 19.4 illustrates an infant who first nursed at 1100 g. If little or no breastfeeding has been done in the hospital and the mother has been unable to pump enough to sustain the daily needs, an infant may be frustrated at the breast when sent home from the hospital unless intervention is provided.

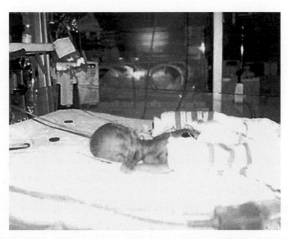

Fig. 14.14 A 1100-g infant shown at 4 hours of life in a busy neonatal intensive care unit. Infants in these situations require early intervention to ensure successful breastfeeding.

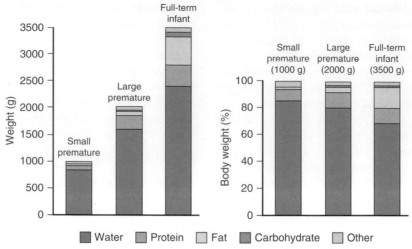

Fig. 14.15 Absolute and relative body composition of infants weighing 1000, 2000, and 3500 g at birth. (From Heird WC, Anderson TL. Nutritional requirements and methods of feeding low birth weight infants. *Curr Probl Pediatr.* 1977;7(8):1–40)

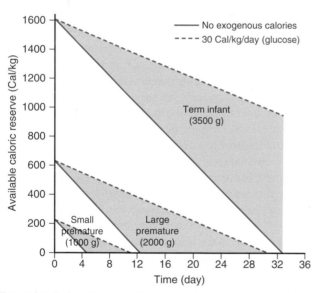

Fig. 14.16 Estimated survival of starved and semistarved infants weighing 1000, 2000, and 3500 g at birth. (From Heird WC, Anderson TL. Nutritional requirements and methods of feeding low-birth-weight infants. In: Gluck L et al., eds. *Curr Probl Pediatr.* vol. 7, no. 8, Chicago, 1977, Year Book.)

TABLE 14.21 **Postdischarge Nutritional Screening Assessment**	
	Action Values
Growth	
Weight gain	<20 g/day
Length growth	<0.5 cm/wk
Head circumference	<0.5 cm/wk
Biochemical Tests	
Phosphorus	<4.5 mg/dL
Alkaline phosphatase	>450 IU/L
Urea nitrogen	<5 mg/dL

IU, International units.
Modified from Hall RT. Nutritional follow-up of the breastfeeding premature infant after hospital discharge. *Pediatr Clin North Am.* 248:435, 2001.

One can see that the reserves of premature infants are limited if one studies the absolute and relative body compositions of infants at birth (Fig. 14.15). If one considers how little time it takes to starve a premature infant compared with a full-term infant, the risks of starving a premature infant while the infant adapts to nursing at the breast are real (Fig. 14.16).[31] The solution to the problem is to provide nourishment while the infant stimulates maternal milk production by suckling at the breast. A piece of equipment called a nursing supplementer provides this setup very effectively (see Fig. 19.1). It was developed to provide nourishment for an adopted infant who is being nursed by a mother who has not been pregnant or has never lactated. It

sustains the infant while the mother's milk supply develops (see Chapter 19). The same effect can be provided for premature or sick infants who have not nursed at the breast since birth and need nourishment while the mother's supply develops, even though she has been pumping.

The infant can continue to gain weight while stimulating the breast if a supplementer is used. The volume required from the nursing supplementer drops continually in a week or so. Occasional infants require the supplementer for a month. The mother should continue to pump after breastfeeding until her volume increases.

The nursing supplementer provides a simple means of ensuring adequate nourishment while adapting to the breast. It is preferable to using supplemental bottles because the infant is not confused by the rubber nipple, which requires a different mechanism of sucking than the human nipple. Furthermore, the suckling of the breast provides the continued stimulus necessary for increasing milk production. Cup feeding is an alternative to the bottle if the infant needs additional nourishment.

The parameters that are to be met before discharge home from the hospital include sustained weight gain, growth in length and head circumference, and stable biochemical parameters (Table 14.21).[236] After discharge from the hospital, these same parameters should be met. If faltering is persistent, fortifying breastfeeding may be indicated. This can be accomplished without interfering with the breastfeeding process again by using a lactation supplementer containing enriched breast milk that had been previously pumped or donor milk, which is preferable to formula.

Posthospitalization breastfeeding patterns of moderately preterm infants (30 to 35 weeks) were studied by Wooldridge and Hall[237] using daily feeding diaries in 55 women for the first month after discharge. Those women who were able to exclusively breastfeed before the end of the first week at home were able to maintain their supply. In general, those women who did not have an adequate supply during the first week were unlikely to achieve it by week 4. The proportion of breastfeeds increased during the 4 weeks of observation, but only 56% achieved exclusive breastfeeds by 4 weeks in this study. Proper preparation before discharge and adequate support at home ensures success.

The Reference list is available at www.expertconsult.com.

15

Medical Complications of Mothers

Alison M. Stuebe

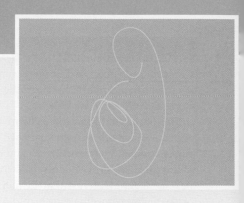

KEY POINTS

- Lactation is a two-person system, and breastfeeding both affects and is affected by the mother's physiology. Both acute maternal health conditions and chronic disorders may have an impact on the mother–baby dyad.
- Often, the mother's acute health condition itself does not affect breastfeeding physiology, but the process of navigating the health care system disrupts lactation. It is the healthcare professional's responsibility to assist her to sustain breastfeeding through the management of the acute condition.
- Any clinician who cares for women of childbearing age cares for women who are lactating must consider both the effects of lactation on maternal health conditions and the

effects of maternal health conditions on lactation. Such care requires consideration of the whole mother–baby dyad, centered on the values and preferences of the lactating woman.
- The distinct individual health conditions affecting mothers must be examined along with any proposed medical management to optimize the initiation and maintenance of lactation and the health of the mother and infant.
- Medication use in the mother should be guided by the medication's safety profile during lactation. Consultation of regularly updated databases of the newest information on the medication's use in lactation is essential to optimal use safely for the mother and infant.

Lactation is a two-person system, and breastfeeding both affects and is affected by the mother's physiology. Understanding these relationships is imperative for clinicians, given that globally more than 70% of women sustain breastfeeding through 1 year after birth, and 45% of women breastfeed for at least 2 years.[1] All clinicians who care for women of childbearing age are thus caring for breastfeeding mother–baby dyads. Moreover, the prevalence of chronic health conditions among childbearing women is increasing (Fig. 15.1).[2] Both acute maternal health conditions and chronic disorders may have an impact on the mother–baby dyad through their effects on fetal development, pregnancy complications, neonatal behavior, and milk production and transfer. Moreover, treatment of maternal conditions can affect lactation through medications that enter milk or through separation of mother and infant for treatment. At the same time, the endocrine and metabolic effects of lactation alter maternal physiology. Breastfeeding duration is associated with long-term differences in women's health outcomes, including lower risk for hypertension, diabetes, cardiovascular disease, and both breast and ovarian cancer.[3] Understanding lactation is thus a fundamental part of understanding women's health.

SHARED DECISION-MAKING

When caring for a breastfeeding woman with acute or chronic health conditions, decisions about risks and benefits of continuing to breastfeed are highly sensitive to the woman's

preferences and values. Similarly, for medication choices for the breastfeeding mother, data are often limited, and different families may make different decisions based on their tolerance for risks for exposure to medications in milk or to disruption of breastfeeding. In their committee opinion on breastfeeding, the American College of Obstetricians and Gynecologists (ACOG) recognizes that each woman "is uniquely qualified to decide whether exclusive breastfeeding, mixed feeding, or formula feeding is optimal for her and her infant."[4] The clinician's role is to ascertain the preferences and values of the mother and her family and share the clinical evidence so that she is able make an informed decision in the context of her life circumstances.

MANAGEMENT OF ACUTE CONDITIONS IN THE BREASTFEEDING MOTHER

Acute maternal health problems can have an impact on the breastfeeding dyad if they interfere with the mother's ability to continue to provide milk, separate mother and child, or require treatment with a medication that is of concern during breastfeeding. Often, the acute condition itself does not affect breastfeeding physiology, but the process of navigating the health care system disrupts lactation. When providing care for women of childbearing age, health care professionals should assess each woman to determine whether she is lactating and assist her to sustain breastfeeding while the acute condition is being addressed.

Diseases	1989–1993		1994–1998		1999–2003		2004–2008		2009–2013	
	n	%	n	%	n	%	n	%	n	%
IDDM and NIDDM	509	0.38	447	0.36	526	0.46	565	0.49	692	0.64
Thyroid disorders	548	0.41	742	0.60	1182	1.03	1781	1.53	2471	2.29
Parathyroid diseases	6	0.00	15	0.01	16	0.01	30	0.03	37	0.03
Cushing syndrome	41	0.03	30	0.02	27	0.02	26	0.02	41	0.04
Polycystic ovary syndrome	94	0.07	171	0.14	511	0.45	1048	0.90	1835	1.70
Polyglandular dysfunction	0	0.00	0	0.00	0	0.00	3	0.00	1	0.00
Polyarthritis nodosa	29	0.02	41	0.03	16	0.01	6	0.01	9	0.01
Rheumatoid arthritis	128	0.10	241	0.19	459	0.40	652	0.56	786	0.73
Systemic lupus erythematosus	27	0.02	47	0.04	75	0.07	73	0.06	78	0.07
Inflammatory bowel disease	401	0.30	623	0.50	792	0.69	1021	0.88	1177	1.09
Epilepsy	666	0.50	768	0.62	891	0.78	1083	0.93	1056	0.98
Multiple sclerosis	53	0.04	98	0.08	168	0.15	218	0.19	277	0.26
Hypertension	183	0.14	220	0.18	417	0.36	601	0.52	740	0.69
Ischemic heart disease	7	0.01	27	0.02	63	0.05	86	0.07	124	0.11
Chronic heart disease	224	0.17	218	0.18	133	0.12	148	0.13	148	0.14
Cardiovascular diseases	80	0.06	98	0.08	143	0.12	217	0.19	240	0.22
Atherosclerosis	2	0.00	13	0.01	22	0.02	35	0.03	30	0.03
Coagulation disorders	26	0.02	37	0.03	105	0.09	428	0.37	793	0.73
Chronic lung disease, including asthma	703	0.53	1182	0.95	2171	1.89	3098	2.67	3443	3.19
HIV	3	0.00	5	0.00	17	0.01	34	0.03	40	0.04
Mood disorders	324	0.24	251	0.20	422	0.37	1158	1.00	2305	2.14
Schizophrenia and other paranoid psychoses	325	0.24	286	0.23	259	0.23	395	0.34	592	0.55
Anxiety and personality disorders	364	0.27	638	0.51	1520	1.33	2537	2.18	3076	2.85
One or more chronic disease	4392	3.28	5698	4.58	9021	7.87	13 191	11.36	16 709	15.49

Fig. 15.1 Prevalence of maternal chronic disease for first pregnancies in Denmark, 1989 to 2013 (N = 42,358). *HIV*, Human immunodeficiency virus; *IDDM*, insulin dependent diabetes mellitus; *NIDDM*, non–insulin dependent diabetes mellitus.

Key Principles

1. *Minimize mother–child separation.* Whenever possible, a mother should be supported to have her nursing child with her when receiving medical care. Breastfeeding dyads should be welcomed in outpatient offices, and emergency and inpatient settings should implement policies to accommodate nursing dyads. Ideally, these accommodations should include single rooms and bassinets for infants, as well as a space for another adult caregiver to room-in and care for the infant.

2. *Support the lactating patient to drain her breasts every 2 to 3 hours or as often as her child is currently nursing.* If the mother is separated from her infant, she should be provided with an electronic breast pump and appropriate supplies. Urgent care centers, emergency departments, surgical centers, and hospitals that care for women of childbearing age should have multiuser breast pumps and supplies available, as well as personnel who are trained to show the lactating patient how to set up the pump to express milk if she is separated from her nursing child.

3. *Select medications with attention to safety profile in lactation.* Most medications enter milk in quantities that are unlikely to affect the health of the infant and are therefore safe to use during lactation. The breast functions differently from the placenta, and drug metabolism in lactation differs from drug metabolism in pregnancy; providers should

therefore resist the assumption that medication safety in pregnancy can be extrapolated to breastfeeding. Detailed information about specific medications is provided in Chapter 11. As studies regarding medication in lactation are ongoing, clinicians should consult regularly updated resources such as the National Library of Medicine LactMed database or the Infant Risk Center.

4. *Drain the breasts just before and after procedures.* Mothers who have received systemic analgesia or anesthesia can resume breastfeeding once they are awake and alert. Draining the breasts before surgery helps maintain milk production and prevents overfilling, reducing the risk for engorgement and mastitis. After surgery, once the woman is alert and awake, medications have redistributed from the plasma compartment and thus from the milk compartment. For healthy term infants, breastfeeding can resume immediately. A brief delay (6 to 12 hours) may be prudent for infants at high risk for apnea, hypotension, or hypotonia;[5] during this time, the mother should be supported to express and discard milk to maintain her supply.

5. *Care plans should address emotional, psychologic, and medical measures to manage the acute illness and support continued lactation.* Well-intentioned individuals may advise the patient and her family that it is "too much" to continue to breastfeed in the setting of an acute medical problem. However, abruptly weaning may complicate

treatment by precipitating engorgement, mastitis, or breast abscess. Moreover, a hasty decision to interrupt a breastfeeding relationship may lead to long-term regret for the mother. Whenever possible, lactation should be sustained so the mother can participate in a decision regarding whether to continue breastfeeding once she has recovered from the acute phase of her illness.

PREGNANCY COMPLICATIONS

Pregnancy complications have an impact on circumstances of birth and early postnatal care. Ideally, spontaneous labor is followed by an uncomplicated vaginal birth of a vigorous term infant who is placed skin to skin undisturbed for the first 90 minutes of life. In reality, induction of labor or surgical birth may be necessary for the well-being of mother and infant. Cesarean birth can interfere with skin-to-skin care and infant-led attachment, although skin-to-skin care in the operating room is becoming more common for healthy, stable mother—infant dyads.[6]

Key Principles

1. *Address the potential effects of pregnancy complications on breastfeeding as part of routine prenatal care.* Obstetric providers should be familiar with the effects of pregnancy complications on infant feeding and should provide tailored anticipatory guidance as part of routine prenatal care.
2. *Communicate maternal risk factors for breastfeeding difficulties to the infant's care team.* Sharing this information will help to facilitate appropriate follow-up of the infant in the early postnatal period.

Hypertensive Disorders of Pregnancy

Hypertensive disorders of pregnancy (HDPs) are associated with fetal growth restriction and indicated preterm birth, both of which can affect early breastfeeding.[7,8] Moreover, women with preeclampsia with severe features are typically treated with intravenous (IV) magnesium for 24 hours after delivery, with side effects of muscle weakness and fatigue that may interfere with rooming-in and caring for a newborn. When postpartum magnesium is planned, consider encouraging a support person to stay with the mother to assist with rooming-in. A published case series describes some of the challenges of establishing breastfeeding among women with HDP,[9] suggesting that they may benefit from additional support to establish and sustain breastfeeding.

A research group in India has reported differences in milk composition among mothers with preeclampsia compared with normal controls;[10,11] the clinical significance of this variation is unknown. Women with HDPs are at increased risk for cardiovascular disease in later life, and breastfeeding is associated with reduced cardiovascular risk.[3] In a small prospective study of women with gestational hypertension, maternal blood pressure at 8 months postpartum was lower among those who had lactated compared with those who had never lactated.[12]

Supporting women with hypertensive disorders to breastfeed may improve long-term maternal health.

Antenatal Corticosteroids

When preterm birth is anticipated, antenatal corticosteroids are recommended to reduce the risks for respiratory distress syndrome and other sequelae of prematurity. A 48-hour course of betamethasone 12 mg q24h $\times$ 2 doses or dexamethasone 6 mg q12h $\times$ 4 doses reduces the risk for perinatal death, neonatal death, respiratory distress syndrome, intraventricular hemorrhage, necrotizing enterocolitis, need for mechanical ventilation, and systemic infections in the first 48 hours of life.[13] Evidence is limited that antenatal corticosteroids may delay onset of lactogenesis II. In an ovine model, antenatal administration of corticosteroids triggered premature lactogenesis II during pregnancy and disrupted milk production after birth.[14] In an observational study of women receiving antenatal corticosteroids for anticipated preterm birth, corticosteroid administration was associated with a transient increase in urinary lactose, indicating premature activation of lactogenesis.[15] Women who delivered at 28 to 34 weeks (N = 37) and had received antenatal corticosteroids 3 to 9 days before birth expressed less milk in the first week than women who received antenatal corticosteroids 0 to 2 days before birth.[16] Women who have recently received antenatal corticosteroids may benefit from additional support to establish lactation.

Operative Birth

Evidence is mixed regarding associations between cesarean birth and breastfeeding outcomes. In a 2012 systematic review of 48 studies enrolling more than 500,000 women in 31 countries,[17] cesarean birth was associated with lower breastfeeding initiation than vaginal birth (odds ratio [OR] 0.57, 95% confidence interval [CI] 0.50 to 0.64). Among studies that distinguished unlabored from in-labor cesarean birth, only unlabored cesarean was associated with lower initiation compared with vaginal birth (unlabored: OR 0.83, 95% CI 0.80 to 0.86; in labor: OR 1.00, 95% CI 0.97 to 1.04). Among women who initiated breastfeeding, cesarean birth was not associated with a difference in any breastfeeding at 6 months (OR 0.95, 95% CI 0.89 to 1.01). A subsequent systematic review of cesarean birth and breastfeeding in China[18] found considerably lower rates of exclusive breastfeeding in the early postpartum period (OR 0.53, 95% CI 0.41 to 0.68) and of any breastfeeding at 4 months (OR 0.61, 95% CI 0.53 to 0.71).

Few studies have tested strategies for enabling women to breastfeed after cesarean birth. Promising strategies include targeted assistance[19] and early skin-to-skin contact in the operating room.[20] A small randomized controlled trial (RCT) found that advising women who birthed by cesarean to pump after at-breast feeding in the first 72 hours postpartum did not improve milk transfer and reduced median duration of breastfeeding among primiparous women (4.2 vs. 9.7 months, $p = 0.18$); routine mechanical expression after cesarean is thus not recommended.

Few studies have evaluated the relationship between operative vaginal delivery and breastfeeding outcomes.[21–23] In a study of 370 births in a Denmark hospital in 1986, infants born by vacuum extraction were more likely to be supplemented with formula than spontaneously born infants, and mothers reported that their milk came in later, but breastfeeding rates were similar through 6 months of life. A 2003 study of 393 women with operative births in the second stage at two teaching hospitals in Bristol, United Kingdom in 1999 to 2000 found similar breastfeeding outcomes among women with cesarean versus operative vaginal births. However, compared with women with a failed instrumental birth, women who underwent cesarean without a trial of instrumental birth were more likely to be breastfeeding at 1 year postpartum (39.8 vs. 29.1%, adjusted OR [aOR] 1.59, 95% CI 1.09 to 2.32). In a Hong Kong study of 8327 births in 1997, instrumental vaginal birth was associated with higher odds of stopped breastfeeding before 1 month compared with spontaneous vaginal birth (OR 1.32, 95% CI 1.04 to 1.68). In a recent RCT[24] of prophylactic antibiotics after operative vaginal birth in which 89% underwent episiotomy, 51% of women were breastfeeding at 6 weeks. Treatment was associated with lower rates of women reporting "perineum ever too painful or uncomfortable to feed baby" (11 vs. 17%, $p < 0.001$). The rate of perineal discomfort in both groups suggests that women with significant perineal lacerations may benefit from help feeding while side-lying.

Intrapartum Analgesia and Anesthesia

The association between intrapartum pain management and breastfeeding outcomes is complicated by multiple factors, including maternal coping and pain tolerance, length and difficulty of labor, and maternal intention to breastfeed.[25] Moreover, RCTs are difficult to conduct given personal preferences among laboring women regarding pain management. A 2016 systematic review identified 23 studies that evaluated epidural anesthesia and breastfeeding outcome: 12 found negative associations, 10 showed no association, and one showed a positive association.[26] The Academy of Breastfeeding Medicine (ABM) recommends that particular care be taken to provide mothers who have received neuraxial anesthesia with good breastfeeding support and close postpartum follow-up.[25]

Parenteral opioids cross the placenta and can depress newborn respiration and neurobehavior. Long-acting opioids with active metabolites, such as meperidine/pethidine, should be avoided.[25] Data on nitric oxide for labor analgesia and breastfeeding outcomes are limited, but the half-life of nitric oxide in the neonate is 3 minutes and extant evidence is reassuring.[27]

Postpartum Hemorrhage

Postpartum hemorrhage is associated with difficulty initiating and sustaining lactation. In a population-based study in Australia of women with a discharge diagnosis code for postpartum hemorrhage (N = 39,787), transfusion was associated with lower rates of any breastfeeding (adjusted relative risk [aRR] 0.91, 99% CI 0.92 to 0.95) and of exclusive breastfeeding (aRR 0.93, 99% CI 0.91 to 0.95) at hospital discharge.[28] Among transfused women, there was a dose-dependent association between lower pretransfusion hemoglobin and lower

breastfeeding rates at discharge.[29] A multicenter longitudinal study of women with a postpartum hemorrhage of greater than 1500 mL found lower rates of full breastfeeding in the first week among women with cesarean or assisted vaginal births or whose first suckling was delayed for longer than 5 hours. Full breastfeeding rates were 63% at 1 week, 58% at 2 months and 45% at 4 months postpartum. In qualitative analyses of women who experienced hemorrhage, the three key themes were (1) difficulty initiating or sustaining breastfeeding, (2) need for education and support, and (3) emotional sequelae. For some women, the trauma of a severe postpartum hemorrhage was compounded by breastfeeding difficulties. One participant wrote, "not being 'mobile' meant the only thing I can do for my new son was to breastfeed, and when that fell over, upset and feelings of uselessness set in. . . . I did begin to develop postnatal depression when I was unable to continue breastfeeding, which I found very difficult and disappointing."[30]

Sheehan Syndrome

Hypotension in the setting of postpartum hemorrhage can cause Sheehan syndrome, an infarction of the anterior pituitary gland, resulting in loss of pituitary function.[31] The expansion of the pituitary because of proliferation of lactotrophs during pregnancy is thought to make it vulnerable to hypoperfusion. Sheehan syndrome is more common in low-resource settings in which women do not have access to modern obstetric care. Along with failure of lactation, acute Sheehan syndrome may manifest with severe hypopituitarism with symptoms of hypotension, hypoglycemia, hyponatremia, shock, headache, visual disturbances, or loss of consciousness. Damage to the posterior pituitary can cause diabetes insipidus. Loss of adrenocorticotropin hormone (ACTH) can be fatal if not treated with glucocorticoids to restore adrenal function.

In other cases, patients may present with a chronic-onset panhypopituitarism or partial hypopituitarism years after the inciting hemorrhage. Symptoms include somnolence, premature aging, mental apathy, physical weakness, nausea, anorexia, anemia, and marked cold sensitivity. Most patients also report a history of being unable to produce milk, with postpartum breast involution and prolonged amenorrhea. This gradual loss of pituitary function may be mediated by pituitary autoantibodies that develop after postpartum pituitary necrosis. In a published case report, a 54-year-old woman presented with a syncopal episode and was found to be in adrenal crisis with panhypopituitarism. Her medical history was significant for postpartum hemorrhage at the birth of her son 19 years ago. Magnetic resonance imaging (MRI) revealed an empty pituitary sella, confirming the diagnosis of Sheehan syndrome.[32]

The three essential diagnostic criteria for Sheehan are (1) typical history of severe postpartum uterine bleeding, particularly at last delivery; (2) at least one pituitary hormone deficiency; and (3) partial or complete empty sella on MRI or computed tomography (CT) in the chronic phase.[31] Suggesting criteria include (1) severe hypotension/shock at index delivery, (2) postpartum amenorrhea, and (3) postpartum agalactia. Laboratory workup includes assessment of pituitary hormones. Findings of hypopituitarism include low serum cortisol with a low or normal ACTH level; low free triiodothyronine (T_3) and free thyroxine (T_4) with low thyroid-stimulating hormone (TSH), low estradiol with a low or normal follicle-stimulating hormone (FSH), and luteinizing hormone (LH) level; low insulin-like growth factor levels; and low baseline prolactin in the setting of agalactia. An ACTH stimulation test may be normal in the early postpartum period before the adrenal cortex has atrophied.

Intensive Care Unit Admission

In surgical and medical intensive care units, mothers are typically separated from their infants and may be intubated and paralyzed. Regular stimulation and draining of the breasts is important to establish lactation, because the critically ill mother may not be able to express milk herself. Clinical staff should assist the critically ill patient to express milk so that once she is awake and alert, she can make a decision about whether to breastfeed.[33]

Retained Placenta

Withdrawal of placental hormones after birth facilitates onset of lactogenesis II, and retained placenta has been described as a cause of delayed lactogenesis. Neifert et al.[34] reported three cases of failed lactogenesis that resolved after emergency curettage with recovery of placental fragments in the setting of delayed postpartum hemorrhage. A 2001 case report describes a woman with two pregnancies and one birth (G2P1) who had previously breastfed without difficulty.[35] At day 9 postpartum, she was producing minimal colostrum. On day 18, her beta human chorionic gonadotropin (hCG) was 225 mIU/mL and she was diagnosed by MRI to have placenta increta. After treatment with methotrexate and an episode of heavy vaginal bleeding, she experienced engorgement. Her hCG at that time was less than 5 mIU/mL. After a period of expressing and discarding her milk to avoid infant exposure to methotrexate, she fully breastfed her infant. Failure of lactation in the setting of abdominal pregnancy with placenta left in situ also has been described, although the authors acknowledge that multiple factors may have contributed.[36] These cases support evaluation for retained placenta in the setting of failed lactogenesis.

Hyperreactio Luteinalis

Hyperreactio luteinalis (HL) manifests with massive cystic enlargement of the ovaries in response to abnormally elevated hCG or ovarian hypersensitivity. HL is more common in the setting of multiple gestations and gestational trophoblastic disease. Theca lutein cysts may be detected incidentally on antenatal ultrasound or at cesarean, or patients may present with abdominal pain or torsion. Women with HL may also present with elevated testosterone or symptoms of virilization. In a literature review, authors identified 52 reports describing 58 pregnancies affected by HL, among whom 30% reported symptoms of maternal virilization.[37]

It has been proposed that elevated testosterone levels after birth may delay onset of lactation. Two case series have reported on lactation outcomes in a total of four women,[38,39] with onset of lactogenesis as serum testosterone fell. In the reported cases, after an initial period of supplementation, three of the four women were able to exclusively breastfeed. Serum testosterone may be helpful in evaluating delayed onset of lactation in women with ovarian cysts.

Postpartum Emergency Visits and Readmissions

In the United States, approximately 2 in 100 women are readmitted within 6 weeks postpartum; the most common indications for readmission are hypertensive disorders, wound infection or breakdown, psychiatric disease, uterine infection, and gallbladder disease.[40] Among publicly insured women in the United States, one in four had at least one emergency room visit in the 6 months postpartum.[41] To ensure that breastfeeding is not disrupted, acute care settings should assess whether patients are lactating and accommodate mother–infant contact and/or access to a breast pump, as detailed earlier in the discussion of acute care.

BREASTFEEDING AND MATERNAL CHRONIC CONDITIONS

Breastfeeding both affects and is affected by maternal health. Providers caring for women of childbearing age need to have a working knowledge of lactation physiology so they can support their patients to nurture their infants and attend to their own health needs.

Key Principles

Maternal health conditions affect breastfeeding through multiple mechanisms (Box 15.1), as follows:
1. *Risk for congenital anomalies.* Fetal anomalies complicate about 3% of live births. Craniofacial anomalies, such as cleft lip and palate, directly interfere with at-breast feeding (see Chapter 13); other anomalies, such as congenital heart defects, may require newborn intensive care or surgical repair in the early days of life, complicating breastfeeding

---

BOX 15.1 Mechanisms Through Which Maternal Health Conditions Affect Breastfeeding

1. Risk for congenital anomalies
2. Fetal growth and risk for preterm delivery
3. Transition to extrauterine life (neonatal physiology) and initiation of lactation (milk synthesis and production)
4. Environment, health, and milk composition
5. Maternal medications, milk synthesis, and the breastfed infant
6. Physiologic demands of breastfeeding and maternal health (effects of breastfeeding on mother's chronic condition)
7. Practical demands of breastfeeding
8. Lactation duration, intensity, and long-term maternal health

initiation. Both maternal chronic diseases and medications are associated with an increased risk for birth defects.

2. *Fetal growth and risk for preterm delivery.* Maternal health conditions can affect the risk for pregnancy complications, fetal growth restriction, and preterm birth. Cardiometabolic diseases, including obesity, hypertension, and diabetes, confer an increased risk for preeclampsia, which may result in indicated preterm or early term birth. As discussed in Chapter 14, prematurity complicates establishment of breastfeeding, particularly if the mother and infant are separated and the infant is admitted to the neonatal intensive care unit (NICU).

3. *Transition to extrauterine life and initiation of lactation.* Maternal disease can have impact on neonatal physiology through effects on placental growth and development and through transplacental transfer of maternal medications, glucose, antibodies, and other bioactive molecules affecting the newborn's transition to extrauterine life. Maternal health conditions can also disrupt the endocrinology of breast development and milk synthesis, resulting in delay of lactogenesis II and reduced or absent milk production.

4. *Environment, health, and milk composition.* Anthropologic studies have found that human milk composition varies depending on characteristics of the maternal environment, and this variation reflects protective adaptations that improve the fitness of the mother–infant dyad.[42,43] Emerging studies have characterized the "omics" of human milk composition and explored variations in milk macronutrients, oligosaccharides, hormones, and microbiome.

5. *Maternal medications, milk synthesis, and the breastfed infant.* When considering the impact of medical management of maternal disease on breastfeeding, it is critical to understand that the pharmacology of medication exposure during pregnancy is different from the pharmacology of medication exposure during lactation. During pregnancy, agents in maternal circulation are transferred via the placenta to the fetal circulation by diffusion or active transport. These medications may affect early breastfeeding through their effects on fetal development and transition to extrauterine life. During breastfeeding, agents may or may not transfer into milk, and any agents ingested by the infant may be digested in the infant gut and may or may not be enterally absorbed. Maternal medications can also affect milk production through effects on blood flow to the breast and through hormonal signals that regulate milk production. Medications and herbal preparations during breastfeeding are discussed in detail in Chapter 11, and the relationship between lactation physiology and reproductive hormones is discussed in Chapter 3.

6. *Physiologic demands of breastfeeding and maternal health.* Both pregnancy and lactation change maternal physiology, and these endocrine and immunologic changes may aggravate or alleviate maternal diseases. Pregnancy downregulates cellular immunity to support tolerance of the fetal allograft, and some autoimmune diseases improve during pregnancy, only to relapse in the postpartum period. Studies of breastfeeding and relapse rates are potentially confounded by maternal disease severity, in that women with more significant disease before pregnancy may be less likely to initiate breastfeeding, because of concerns such as maternal fatigue or infant exposure to maternal medications. The maternal endocrine effects of exclusive breastfeeding, including elevated prolactin and reduced estrogen and progesterone, are distinct from mixed feeding[44] and may have different effects on maternal disease course.

Lactation substantially affects maternal metabolism. Mothers of exclusively breastfeeding infants produce about 700 to 800 g of milk a day, at an energy cost of 597 to 716 kcal (2.5 to 3 MJ) per day (Table 15.1).[45] This metabolic load may be mobilized from fat stores or from dietary intake, depending on the local availability of nutrition to the mother. This significant metabolic load affects and is affected by maternal diseases. Women with health conditions that affect nutrient absorption may have difficulty sustaining sufficient caloric intake and may benefit from consultation with a nutritionist.

TABLE 15.1	**Energy Cost of Milk Production for Exclusive and Partial Breastfeeding**[a]				
Postpartum Period (mo)	0–2	3–5	6–8	9–11	12–23
	Energy cost of milk production (MJ day^{-1})				
Exclusive breastfeeding					
Industrialized countries	2.49	2.75	2.81	3.15	
Developing countries	2.50	2.74	2.72		
Partial breastfeeding					
Industrialized countries	2.24	2.40	2.07	1.53	1.57
Developing countries	2.16	2.32	2.31	2.16	1.92

[a]Energy cost of lactation based on milk production rates from Brown K, Dewey KG, Allen L. *Complementary Feeding of Young Children in Developing Countries: a Review of Current Scientific Knowledge.* Geneva: World Health Organization, 1998., milk energy density of 2.8 kJg^{-1} and energetic efficiency of milk synthesis of 0.80.
From Butte NF, King JC. Energy requirements during pregnancy and lactation. *Public Health Nutr.* 2005;8(7A):1010–1027.

In addition, lactation suppresses the hypothalamic-pituitary-ovarian axis. Prolactin suppresses gonadotropin-releasing hormone (GnRH) and delays return of menses, resulting in lower circulating estrogen and progesterone levels, as discussed in detail in Chapter 3. During lactation, the hypothalamic–pituitary–adrenal (HPA) axis is also suppressed; cortisol levels decrease during breastfeeding episodes,[46–48] and the HPA response to physical stress is diminished in breastfeeding women compared with that in bottle-feeding women.[49] Breastfeeding mothers also demonstrate increased parasympathetic and decreased sympathetic activation, compared with bottle-feeding mothers.[49–52] These changes, in turn, may have an impact on maternal chronic disease trajectories.

Prolactin is secreted from the anterior pituitary and stimulates milk production. Downregulation of dopamine stimulates pulsatile secretion of pituitary prolactin; other triggers for pituitary prolactin include thyrotropin-releasing hormone, estradiol, oxytocin, vasopressin, ghrelin, endogenous opioids, serotonin, and angiotensin II. Prolactin is also produced in the breast, the brain, the decidua, and multiple cell lines, including lymphocytes, skin fibroblasts, and adipose cells.[53] Alternative splicing of prolactin mRNA as well as posttranslational modifications result in multiple prolactin isoforms, which likely mediate its pleiotropic effects. Both B cells and T cells express prolactin and prolactin receptors, such that prolactin participates in both endocrine and paracrine/autocrine regulation of immune function.[54] Higher levels of prolactin are reported in patients with autoimmune diseases[55,56] (discussed in the later section on breastfeeding and autoimmune disease). Prolactin is also implicated in pancreatic beta cell expansion during pregnancy,[57] and higher prolactin levels during pregnancy are associated with improved beta cell function at 3 months postpartum.[58]

7. *Practical demands of breastfeeding.* Exclusive breastfeeding is demanding. In a time use study, Smith and Forrester[59] found that lactating mothers spent about 8.5 hours more per week feeding and caring for infants than nonlactating mothers.[59] This investment of time may be difficult to sustain for women with chronic health conditions. Moreover, nighttime feedings may be especially challenging for women for whom sleep is a medical need, such as women with epilepsy[60] or bipolar disorder.[61] These medically necessary periods of rest can result in breast overfilling and engorgement, and strategies are needed to support draining the breasts with minimal disruption of maternal sleep. The mother and her provider should work together to develop a strategy for both supporting her health and enabling her to breastfeed.[62] Options to consider include the following:

- Before going to sleep, feed and/or express milk to prolong the time until the breasts feel uncomfortably full.
- Express milk and sleep through a nighttime feeding while another caregiver looks after the baby.
- Have another adult caregiver assume responsibility for all aspects of infant care except for feeding. When the

infant cues to feed, the other caregiver can bring the baby to the mother, gently wake her, and assist the baby to nurse while she is side-lying, so that she can continue to rest. When the feeding ends, the other caregiver is responsible for changing, settling, and soothing the baby while the mother goes back to sleep.

- Keep a pump and a cooler at the bedside so that if the mother wakes and feels uncomfortably full, she can express milk to comfort and resume sleep with minimal disruption.

For some women, getting sufficient sleep to prevent complications such as mania, postpartum psychosis, or recurrent seizures may affect milk production. It is imperative for breastfeeding medicine providers to support the whole mother–baby dyad and work with the family to craft a sustainable strategy that takes into account the importance of both human milk and maternal well-being.

8. *Lactation duration, intensity, and long-term maternal health.* In observational studies, longer duration and greater intensity of breastfeeding are associated with substantial differences in women's health across the life span, as detailed in Chapter 6. These findings suggest that enabling women to breastfeed may improve long-term health for women. These population-level differences likely reflect both the effects of breastfeeding on maternal physiology and the extent to which being able to sustain breastfeeding is a marker for maternal health and well-being.[63]

Illustrating the Intersection Between Lactation and Maternal Chronic Conditions: Diabetes

Diabetes is one of the most common chronic diseases among childbearing women, and its multiple effects illustrate the interplay between maternal disease and breastfeeding. About 1% to 2% of pregnancies are complicated by pregestational diabetes,[64] and an additional 6% develop gestational diabetes, defined as glucose intolerance first diagnosed during pregnancy.[65] Here, we use diabetes to illustrate the links between breastfeeding and maternal chronic health conditions.

Effects of Maternal Conditions on Breastfeeding
Fetal Anomalies

Pregestational diabetes is associated with an increased risk for fetal anomalies. This risk is increased in women with poor glucose control before conception, as measured by hemoglobin A1c. Among women with optimal glucose control (hemoglobin A1c < 6.0%), the risk for birth defects is similar to the background rate of 3%. Among women with a hemoglobin A1c greater than 13.9%, the birth defect rate is 20%.[66]

Pregnancy Complications

When maternal glucose is elevated, glucose transfer across the placenta increases, resulting in high fetal glucose levels and increased fetal insulin secretion, as well as accrual of adipose stores in the infant. Excess fetal growth increases risk for shoulder dystocia and traumatic injury during delivery or may necessitate cesarean birth.[64,65] Compared with women without diabetes, women with gestational or pregestational diabetes are more likely to have a preterm birth, to birth by cesarean, and to have an infant admitted to the NICU.[67] These complications and their management can impede establishment of breastfeeding.

Neonatal Physiology

In pregnancies complicated by diabetes, the fetal pancreas compensates for elevated glucose levels by increasing fetal insulin levels. After delivery, this maternal glucose infusion stops, and the insulin secretion continues, resulting in neonatal hypoglycemia. In women with long-standing diabetes and associated vascular disease, poor placental perfusion may result in intrauterine growth restriction and the newborn also may have reduced glycogen and fat stores at birth, further affecting neonatal glucose control. The infant of the diabetic mother requires careful monitoring of glucose levels and frequent opportunities to feed, as recommended in the ABM Clinical Protocol #1: Guidelines for Blood Glucose Monitoring and Treatment of Hypoglycemia in Term and Late-Preterm Neonates, Revised 2014.[68]

Anticipatory guidance and ongoing support for the diabetic mother can prepare her for the baby's transition and reinforce the value of at-breast feeding, hand-expressed colostrum, and skin-to-skin care to maintain normoglycemia. An RCT found that antenatal colostrum expression among women with uncomplicated diabetes modestly increased exclusive breastfeeding rates in the first 24 hours postpartum (69% vs. 60%, aRR 1.15, 95% CI 1.02 to 1.28) without affecting NICU admission rates.[69]

Exposure to maternal diabetes in utero has also been associated with differences in early infant suckling patterns: infants of mothers with gestational diabetes mellitus (GDM) that required insulin (N = 15) had fewer sucks and bursts per 5 minutes than infants of mothers with diet-controlled GDM (N = 31) or normal controls (N = 55).[70] Mothers with diabetes may benefit from targeted lactation support.

Milk Synthesis and Production

Glucose intolerance during pregnancy is associated with delayed onset of lactogenesis II[71,72] and earlier cessation of exclusive[73] and any breastfeeding.[74] Translational research suggests that maternal insulin resistance and reduced milk production may be mediated by changes in lactocyte expression of *PTPRF*, which interferes with *INSR-B*−mediated stimulation of milk synthesis.[75] Interestingly, several commonly used herbal galactagogues, including goat's rue and fenugreek, affect insulin resistance. Insulin resistance has been proposed to mediate associations between maternal obesity and poor lactation outcomes.[76]

Milk Composition

Several authors have reported differences in milk composition between diabetic and nondiabetic mothers, including variation in immune factors,[77,78] proteins,[79] fatty acid

composition,[80] and energy content.[81] The clinical significance of this variation is not known. Differences in human milk composition among women with diabetes may reflect adaptations for the infant who has been exposed to elevated glucose levels in utero.

Pharmacologic Treatment of Diabetes in Breastfeeding

Some women with gestational diabetes can control their glucose with diet, but others require medical therapy, as do most women with pregestational type 2 diabetes and all women with type 1 diabetes. Insulin is the standard treatment for pregestational diabetes. Insulin is a large molecule that would not be expected to enter milk via diffusion. A small study (N = 14) of mothers with type 1 diabetes (N = 4), type 2 diabetes (N = 5), and without diabetes (N = 5) found that insulin was present in milk at similar levels for all three groups. The authors speculate that an active transport mechanism is responsible, and that insulin may play a role in infant gut development. Of note, higher milk insulin levels have been associated with lower infant weight-for-length z-scores at 4 months and 1 year.[82] Insulin is considered to be compatible with breastfeeding (Hale: L1).

Both glyburide and metformin are oral agents that have been used to treat gestational diabetes and pregestational type 2 diabetes. Glyburide stimulates insulin secretion and appears to enter milk in very low levels. It is considered compatible (Hale: L2), although infants should be monitored for signs of hypoglycemia (LactMed). Metformin is a biguanide that reduces insulin resistance. It appears in milk in negligible amounts and is considered safe in lactation (Hale: L1), although caution is suggested for infants who are premature or who have impaired renal function (LactMed). The Endocrine Society recommends that women with overt diabetes continue metformin or glyburide during breastfeeding (strong recommendation, high-quality evidence).[83]

Effects of Medications to Treat Diabetes on Milk Supply

Given the potential role of insulin resistance in low milk production, metformin has been proposed as a galactogogue. Metformin is a derivative of guanidine, one of the metabolically active compounds in *Galega officinalis*, or goat's rue.[84] Goat's rue is so-named because it increases milk production in goats. In an RCT of metformin during pregnancy for women with polycystic ovary syndrome (PCOS), women randomized to metformin had a slightly longer duration of exclusive breastfeeding (4.5 vs. 3.9 months, *p* = 0.08).[85] A pilot study (N = 15) of initiating postpartum metformin for women with insulin resistance and low milk supply found a small increase in milk produced among women in the metformin arm, and a decrease in women in the placebo arm (median change [interquartile range], + 22 [−5 to + 54] mL/24 h versus −58 [−83 to −1] mL/24 h, metformin versus placebo + noncompleters, Wilcoxon rank-sum *p* value = 0.07). These results support the hypothesis that modulating insulin resistance may improve milk supply; however, the increase in production was modest. An ongoing clinical trial of insulin versus metformin + insulin to treat overt diabetes in pregnancy [NCT02932475] is collecting data on breastfeeding outcomes, which may inform future treatment recommendations.

The Effects of Lactation on Maternal Diabetes Management

The energy load of lactation modifies metabolic requirements for women with diabetes. Among a small sample of postpartum women with type 1 diabetes who underwent continuous glucose monitoring, breastfeeding women (N = 8) had slightly higher carbohydrate intake, but similar insulin requirements, to formula-feeding women (N = 8). In the 3 hours after suckling, glucose levels gradually dropped, resulting in hypoglycemia (glucose < 4 mmol/L or 72 mg/dL) in 9.9% of episodes at 2 hours and 13.5% of episodes at 3 hours after suckling. Overall, there was no difference in frequency of hypoglycemia among breastfeeding versus formula-feeding women in this small sample. The authors speculate that women who were breastfeeding increased their carbohydrate intake to compensate for the demands of breastfeeding.

For women with gestational diabetes, breastfeeding during the postpartum oral glucose tolerance test (OGTT) is associated with differences in postload results. In a prospective cohort study of women with GDM who were breastfeeding at their 75-g oral OGTT visit, fasting glucose levels were similar, but 2-hour insulin levels and postload glucose levels were lower (glucose mean adjusted difference: −6.2 mg/dL, 95% CI −11.5 to −1.0), and insulin sensitivity was higher, for women who breastfed during the OGTT than for women who did not in models adjusted for race, parity, age, number of abnormal results for 3-hour prenatal OGTT, amount of formula supplementation (oz/24 h), and fasting period (hours).[86]

Maintenance of Breastfeeding in the Setting of Maternal Disease

Particularly for women requiring insulin, attention to timing and composition of meals is important to maintain euglycemia. In the setting of on-cue feeding of a newborn, mothers need material support to attend to scheduled dosing of insulin and regular meals and snacks with appropriate macronutrient composition.

Long-Term Maternal Health

Longer breastfeeding is associated with a reduced progression of gestational diabetes to type 2 diabetes and reduced risk incident of type 2 diabetes among women who were normoglycemic in pregnancy.[3] These data underscore the importance of enabling women to breastfeed as a strategy to improve women's health. At the same time, preexisting metabolic dysregulation may contribute both to curtailed breastfeeding and long-term metabolic disease risk. In a longitudinal study of women with PCOS, greater change in prolactin from the first trimester through 32 weeks of pregnancy was associated with a more favorable cardiometabolic profile

at 32 weeks. In the same cohort, lack of breast growth during pregnancy was associated with a more adverse metabolic profile at 5 to 11 years postpartum.[87] It may be that adverse lactation outcomes, like adverse pregnancy outcomes, are a window to future maternal health.[63]

ENDOCRINE AND METABOLIC DISORDERS

Breast development, onset of lactation, and maintenance of milk production involve oxytocin and prolactin, cortisol, thyroid hormone, growth hormone, estrogen, and progesterone (see Chapter 3). Endocrine disorders thus affect and are affected by lactation.

Thyroid Disorders

During pregnancy, thyroid binding globulin (TBG) and total T_4 levels increase dramatically, peaking by 16 weeks of pregnancy.[88] After delivery, estrogen, TBG, and total T_4 levels decline.[89] Data are limited on normal thyroid levels in lactation; in a small sample of exclusively breastfeeding women (N = 28), free T_4 levels fell from 2 to 8 weeks postpartum (median values, CI 5% to 95%; 2 weeks: T_4 = 0.97 ng/dL, 0.79 to 1.32; 8 weeks: T_4 = 0.90 ng/dL, 0.67 to 1.18, [paired t test, 2 versus 8 weeks, probability < 0.001]).[90]

Effects of Thyroid Disease on Breastfeeding

Thyroid dysfunction is associated with lactation difficulties and is common in women of childbearing age. In animal models, experimentally induced hyperthyroidism and hypothyroidism disrupt lactation.[88] In a published case report, a 4-month-old exclusively breastfed infant presented with failure to thrive. The mother was found to have Hashimoto thyroiditis. With thyroid replacement, her milk supply increased and infant growth resumed.[91] Hyperthyroidism also appears to adversely after milk production in animal studies. The American Thyroid Association recommends evaluating TSH levels in women experiencing poor lactation of unclear cause. Furthermore, they recommend that breastfeeding women ingest about 250 mcg of dietary iodine daily.[88]

Parathyroid Disorders
Effects of Lactation on Calcium Metabolism

Calcium homeostasis changes during pregnancy and lactation to support the needs of the fetus and neonate.[92,93] During pregnancy, intestinal absorption of calcium doubles, mediated by increased levels of 1,25 dihydroxyvitamin D (calcitriol), prolactin, human placental lactogen, and other factors. By term, the fetus accrues 30 g of calcium, more than 80% of which is transferred in the third trimester. During lactation, women transfer 210 mg/day into breast milk for the neonate (Fig. 15.2). This calcium is primarily obtained from resorption of maternal bone stores, caused by low levels of estrogen and by parathyroid-related peptide (PTHrP) produced in the mammary gland. Indeed, the lactating breast has been described as an accessory parathyroid.[92,93] Increased calcitonin levels in the first 6 weeks of lactation counter the effects of PTHrP, preventing excessive maternal bone loss.

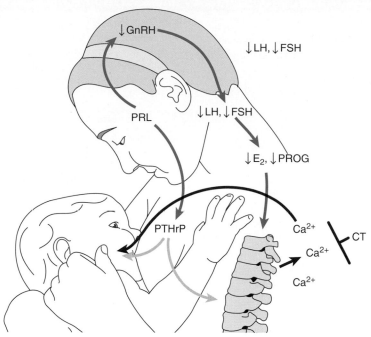

Fig. 15.2 The brain-breast-bone circuit. *CT*, Calcitonin; *E₂*, estradiol; *FSH*, follicle-stimulating hormone; *GnRH*, gonadotropin-releasing hormone; *LH*, luteinizing hormone; *PRL*, prolactin; *PROG*, progesterone; *PTHrP*, parathyroid-related peptide. (From Kovacs CS. Calcium and bone metabolism during pregnancy and lactation. *J Mammary Gland Biol Neoplasia.* 2005;10(2):105–118.)

This transfer of calcium results in a 5% to 10% loss of bone density in the first 2 to 6 months of breastfeeding. Although one longitudinal study found lasting changes in maternal bone microarchitecture,[94] most studies have found that maternal bone density returns within 6 to 12 months of weaning.[95] Of note, a systematic review of 11 studies including 101,726 women found no association between breastfeeding and postmenopausal fracture risk.[3]

Calcium supplementation beyond the recommended daily allowance of 1.2 g/day of calcium is not recommended during pregnancy or lactation, and dietary supplements do not change milk composition or affect maternal bone metabolism. For women with low dietary calcium intake (<600 mg/day), supplementation is recommended by the World Health Organization to reduce risk for HDPs and preterm birth.[96] However, the effects of supplementation on bone health are unclear. In a postnatal follow-up study of Gambian women with low dietary calcium intake (<350 mg/day), those randomized to supplementation with 1500 mg calcium per day had lower bone mass through 12 months postpartum. These differences persisted after weaning.[97] The authors propose that calcium supplementation altered women's ability to conserve calcium in the setting of a low-calcium diet.[98]

Osteoporosis in Pregnancy and Lactation

In the setting of appropriate dietary calcium intake, little bone loss occurs during pregnancy, because fetal demand for calcium is met by increased intestinal absorption. During lactation, however, calcium is mobilized from bone, particularly from the trabecular-rich spine. In case reports of vertebral fractures during lactation,

women have had additional risk factors for low bone mineral density,[93,99] such as treatment with glucocorticoids, hypothalamic amenorrhea, or low dietary calcium intake (Box 15.2). Workup for lactating women with nontraumatic fractures includes bone mineral density assessment by dual-energy x-ray absorptiometry (DXA), assessment for nutritional deficiencies, and assessment of hormones (parathyroid hormone [PTH], PTHrP, TSH, LH, FSH, estradiol, prolactin), biochemistry (electrolytes, estimated glomerular filtration rate [eGFR], ionized calcium, serum phosphate, alkaline phosphatase, 25-hydroxyvitamin D, tissue transglutaminase [TTG]), and hematologic parameter (complete blood count [CBC], erythrocyte sedimentation rate [ESR], serum protein electrophoresis).[100] Recommended treatment for women with low bone mineral density (BMD) and fractures includes a calcium intake of 1200 mg/day and vitamin D supplementation to achieve 25-hydroxyvitamin D levels greater than 50 nmol/L, as well as weight-bearing physical activity. Data are limited on the utility and safety of antiosteoporosis medications in lactation.

Prolactin Disorders

Prolactin is a 23-kDa protein that stimulates milk synthesis by binding the prolactin receptor (see Chapter 3). In addition to its role in lactation, more than 300 functions have been identified for this hormone across multiple species.[101] During pregnancy and lactation, physiologic elevations of circulating prolactin stimulate breast differentiation and milk synthesis. Dysregulation of prolactin can result in hyperprolactinemia, most commonly as a result of pituitary adenomas. In addition, emerging evidence suggests that dysregulation of prolactin signaling may be a cause of failed lactation.

BOX 15.2 Factors Contributing to Pregnancy and Lactation-Related Fractures

Hormonal
Excess PTHrP-mediated bone resorption during pregnancy
Excess PTHrP- and low-estradiol–mediated resorption during lactation
Primary hyperparathyroidism
Hyperthyroidism
Cushing syndrome
Chronic oligoamenorrhea
Hypothalamic amenorrhea
Pituitary disorders leading to sex steroid deficiency
Premature ovarian failure
Prolonged lactation

Nutritional
Low dietary calcium intake
Dairy avoidance
Lactose intolerance
Low vitamin D intake/vitamin D deficiency
Anorexia nervosa

Mechanical
Petite frame
Low body weight
Low peak bone mass
Excess exercise
Increased weight-bearing of pregnancy
Lordotic posture of pregnancy
Bedrest
Carrying child
Prolonged lactation with insufficient skeletal recovery afterward

Pharmacologic
GnRH analog treatment

Depo-Provera
Glucocorticoids
Proton pump inhibitors
Certain antiseizure medications (phenytoin, carbamazepine)
Cancer chemotherapy
Alcohol

Gastrointestinal
Celiac disease
Crohn disease
Cystic fibrosis
Other malabsorptive disorders

Renal
Hypercalciuria/renal calcium leak
Chronic renal insufficiency
Renal tubular acidosis

Primary Disorders of Bone Quality
Osteogenesis imperfecta
Osteopetrosis and other sclerosing bone disorders
LRP5 inactivating mutations

Connective Tissue Disorders
Ehlers-Danlos syndrome
Marfan syndrome

Rheumatologic Disorders
Rheumatoid arthritis
Systemic lupus erythematosus

Other Nonspecified Genetic Disorders
Family history of osteoporosis or skeletal fragility
Idiopathic osteoporosis

From Kovacs CS, Ralston SH. Presentation and management of osteoporosis presenting in association with pregnancy or lactation. *Osteoporos Int.* 2015;26(9):2223–2241.

Types of Prolactin and Implications for Assessment

In addition to the monomeric physiologically active form, prolactin multimers also can be present in the circulation, including dimeric "big prolactin" and multimeric "big-big prolactin" (Fig. 15.3). Of note, commonly available laboratory assays detect both biologically active monomeric prolactin and the inactive multimers.[102,103] When elevated prolactin is detected, particularly in the absence of clinical symptoms, assessment for macroprolactin is recommended.[104]

Hyperprolactinemia

Elevations of prolactin other than during pregnancy and lactation can result in gonadal suppression, infertility, and galactorrhea. Stress, including excessive stress during venipuncture, can elevate serum prolactin levels; however, in the absence of an unusually difficult venipuncture, a single occurrence of elevated prolactin is considered adequate to establish the diagnosis of hyperprolactinemia.[104] The differential diagnosis for hyperprolactinemia includes medication use, renal failure, hypothyroidism, and parasellar tumors (Box 15.3). If medication use is suspected, the Endocrine Society recommends discontinuing the drug of concern for 3 days and

reevaluating prolactin levels. If they remain elevated, pituitary MRI is recommended to assess for a pituitary or hypothalamic mass.

Management of Pituitary Prolactinomas in Pregnancy and Breastfeeding

The Endocrine Society recommends discontinuing dopamine agonist therapy during pregnancy in women with prolactinomas.[104] Serial assessment of visual fields is recommended for women who have macroadenomas and have not undergone surgical resection. Bromocriptine is recommended for women with symptomatic growth of a prolactinoma during pregnancy.

Two case series evaluated outcomes among women with a history of prolactinoma after pregnancy and lactation,[105,106] and neither found an association between breastfeeding duration and risk for recurrence. In a subsequent series, one in four women had spontaneous normalization of prolactin levels after pregnancy.[107] With respect to breastfeeding outcomes, a 1987 case series compared prolactin levels at 4 days postpartum and feeding at 1 month among women with prolactinomas who had been treated with surgery, surgery plus

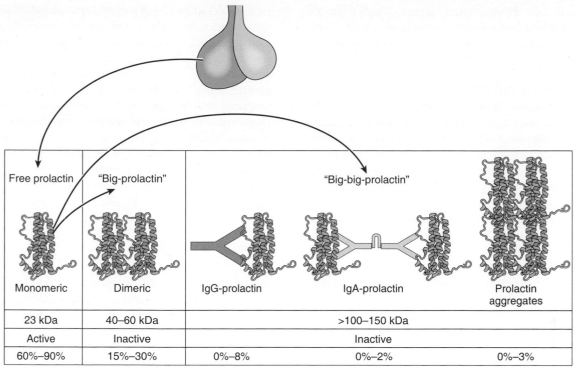

Fig. 15.3 Macroprolactin. *Ig,* Immunoglobulin. (From Lippi G, Plebani M. Macroprolactin: searching for a needle in a haystack? *Clin Chem Lab Med.* 2016;54(4):519–522.)

BOX 15.3 Causes of Hyperprolactinemia

Physiologic

Coitus
Exercise
Lactation
Pregnancy
Sleep
Stress

Pathologic

Hypothalamic-pituitary stalk damage
Granulomas
Infiltrations
Irradiation
Rathke's cyst
Trauma: Pituitary stalk section, suprasellar surgery
Tumors: Craniopharyngioma, germinoma, hypothalamic metastases, meningioma, suprasellar pituitary mass extension
Pituitary
    Acromegaly
    Idiopathic
    Lymphocytic hypophysitis or parasellar mass
    Macroadenoma (compressive)
    Macroprolactinemia
    Plurihormonal adenoma
    Prolactinoma
    Surgery
    Trauma

Systemic disorders
    Chest: Neurogenic chest wall trauma, surgery, herpes zoster
    Chronic renal failure
    Cirrhosis
    Cranial radiation
    Epileptic seizures
    Polycystic ovarian disease
    Pseudocyesis

Pharmacologic

Anesthetics
Anticonvulsant
Antidepressants
Antihistamines (histamine 2)
Antihypertensives
Cholinergic agonist
Drug-induced hypersecretion
Catecholamine depleter
Dopamine receptor blockers
Dopamine synthesis inhibitor
Estrogens: Oral contraceptives, oral contraceptive withdrawal
Neuroleptics/antipsychotics
Neuropeptides
Opiates and opiate antagonists

From Melmed S, Casanueva FF, Hoffman AR, et al. Diagnosis and treatment of hyperprolactinemia: an Endocrine Society clinical practice guideline. *J Clin Endocrinol Metab.* 2011;96(2):273–288.

bromocriptine, or bromocriptine alone. Women in the surgery-only group had lower prolactin levels on day 4 and were less likely to be breastfeeding at 1 month postpartum than women in the bromocriptine-only group.[108]

Prolactin Receptor Variants

The prolactin receptor *PRLR* is a member of the cytokine family of receptors, and emerging research has identified genetic variants in *PRLR* associated with various lactation phenotypes. A 2013 study reported on three sisters, one of whom had persistent galactorrhea after weaning for each of four pregnancies. She and one of her sisters had oligomenorrhea, and the third sister had infertility. All three were found to have a loss-of-function mutation of *PRLR*.[109] Kabayashi et al.[110] reported on a compound heterozygote with inactivating mutations of *PRLR* who was not able to produce milk for either of her two pregnancies. She had been found to have elevated circulating prolactin during a workup for subfertility, before conceiving with intrauterine insemination. Future genotyping studies of *PRLR* may elucidate the mechanisms underlying interindividual differences in milk production.

Polycystic Ovarian Syndrome

PCOS is a common condition that presents with irregular menses, evidence of excess androgens, and polycystic ovaries on ultrasound. Insulin resistance and obesity are also common features of this condition. Several clinical criteria have been proposed for diagnosis; the Rotterdam criteria were endorsed by a 2012 National Institutes of Health Workshop. Two of the following three criteria are required[111]:

- Oligo-ovulation and/or anovulation
- Clinical and/or biochemical signs of hyperandrogenism
- Polycystic ovaries (by ultrasound)

Although PCOS has been proposed as a risk factor for low milk supply in a three-patient case series,[112] both PCOS and milk supply concerns are common. The prevalence of PCOS is estimated at 6% to 10% in the general population,[113] with 45% of women reporting not having enough milk as a reason for weaning.[114] If no association exists between these two conditions, 3% to 5% of mothers would have both PCOS and low milk supply.

Two published studies have quantified the association between PCOS and breastfeeding outcomes. In a case-control study enrolling 135 women, women with PCOS were less likely to initiate breastfeeding (86% vs. 98%), but among women who initiated breastfeeding, women with PCOS were no less likely to be exclusively breastfeeding at 1 month than women without PCOS (87% vs. 91%, $p = 0.56$).[115] In a community-based Australian study enrolling more than 4000 women, 6.5% of women reported having PCOS. After adjusting for body mass index (BMI), PCOS was not associated with breastfeeding outcome but higher BMI was associated with lower breastfeeding initiation and duration.[116]

The elevated androgens characteristic of PCOS have been proposed as a mechanism for reducing milk production, and there is tentative evidence supporting this hypothesis. Among women with PCOS (N = 36), dehydroepiandrosterone sulfate (DHEAS) levels at 32 and 36 weeks were inversely associated

with breastfeeding at 1 month.[115] In a secondary analysis, the same research group reported that higher androgens during pregnancy were associated with reduced breastfeeding duration.[117] However, in a prospective randomized trial of metformin to treat PCOS during pregnancy (N = 186), there was no association between DHEAS or free testosterone index levels in pregnancy and duration of any or exclusive breastfeeding. Treatment with metformin did not affect duration of any or exclusive breastfeeding; however, higher BMI was associated with shorter duration of any breastfeeding.[85] These results suggest that higher BMI, rather than PCOS per se, may be the causal risk factor for earlier cessation of breastfeeding. Women with elevated BMI may benefit from targeted breastfeeding support.

Hypercholesterolemia

Lipid levels increase during pregnancy as part of normal physiology. In women with hypercholesterolemia, these increases are magnified and can result in complications such as acute pancreatitis.[118] Therapeutic apheresis has been proposed as a potential treatment strategy to reduce lipid levels without exposing the fetus or neonatal to statins.[118,119] Statin therapy is not recommended in pregnancy or lactation because of concerns about potential deleterious effects on the fetus and neonate; however, Holmsen et al. propose that the benefits of breastfeeding for mother and infant outweigh the risks of statin therapy.[120]

Data are limited regarding the impact of lipid disorders on milk composition. In a 1985 case report, the authors analyzed milk samples form a lactating patient with type I hyperlipoproteinemia and reported abnormally low concentrations of essential linoleic ($C_{18:2,20:4}$) and arachidonic ($C_{20:4}$) acids.[121] However, in a more recent case report, a mother with homozygous familial hypercholesterolemia breastfed for 2 months while undergoing low density lipoprotein (LDL)-apheresis, and the authors report that "lactation proceeded without complications." At 3 months, the mother weaned and resumed statin therapy.[119]

Inherited Metabolic Diseases

With improved detection and treatment of inherited metabolic disease, more women are conceiving and carrying pregnancies.[122] The physiology of the early postpartum period can aggravate maternal inborn errors of metabolism. For the mother, this is a highly catabolic period, because energy and nutrients are mobilized for milk production (reviewed in reference 123). Moreover, uterine involution mobilizes amino acids, resulting in an increased nitrogen load. This can elevate ammonia levels in women with urea cycle disorders such as ornithine transcarbamylase deficiency.[123,124] Lactation can affect the health of the mother with inherited metabolic disease, and toxic metabolites can accumulate in milk, potentially affecting the infant.

Galactosemia

Galactosemia is an autosomal recessive defect in metabolism of galactose, resulting in toxic accumulation of galactose and its metabolites. Classic galactosemia is the most severe form, affecting 1 in 30,000 to 1 in 60,000 newborns. This disorder is treated with elimination of galactose from the diet. In affected infants, breastfeeding is contraindicated.

Among women with this disorder, premature ovarian failure is common, but some do conceive. During pregnancy, the mammary gland synthesizes lactose, and urinary levels rise approaching delivery. This circulating lactose could adversely affect women with galactosemia. In a 1989 report, a woman with galactosemia initiated breastfeeding and was found to have elevated levels of erythrocyte galactose-1-phosphate. She was treated with bromocriptine and levels dropped dramatically. In a more recent series of five women with classic galactosemia, Schadewaldt et al.[125] found a moderate increase in urinary levels of galactose, galactitol, galactonate, and lactose, with peak values in the first week postpartum, independent of whether the women chose to breastfeed. Three of the five women breastfed without adverse effects on maternal or infant health. In another short report, a woman with galactosemia breastfed two children and experienced a transient increase in galactose-1-phosphate in the early postpartum period.[126]

Two case reports of milk composition in women with galactosemia found normal levels of milk lactose. In one case, a 25-year-old woman exclusively breastfed her infant for 5 months with appropriate growth. Analysis of her milk at 4½ weeks postpartum revealed protein 1.42 g/dL, lactose 7.5 g/dL, fat 4.25 g/dL, and calculated energy content 74 kcal/dL.[127] A second case report has similarly documented normal lactose levels in milk.[128]

Phenylketonuria

Phenylketonuria (PKU) is an autosomal recessive metabolic disorder caused by mutations in hydroxylase (PAH) that result in toxic levels of phenylalanine. Neonatal diagnosis and treatment are necessary to prevent neurotoxicity. Guidelines diverge regarding target levels in adolescence and adulthood, with the European Society for Phenylketonuria and Allied Disorders Treated as Phenylketonuria (ESPKU)[129] recommending goal levels less than 600 μmol/L after age 12, whereas the American College of Medical Genetics (ACMG) recommends a lifelong goal of 120 to 360 μmol/L.[130]

There is consensus that for women of childbearing age who could become pregnant or who are pregnant, target levels of blood phenylalanine should be 120 to 360 μmol/L to minimize toxicity to the fetus. Both the ESPKU and ACMG encourage mothers with PAH deficiency to breastfeed. The ACMG recommends that mothers maintain a phenylalanine (PHE)-restricted diet postpartum for optimal maternal and infant outcomes; recommended intakes during lactation are 700 to 2275 mg/day of phenylalanine and 6000 to 7600 mg/day of tyrosine.[130]

An online survey by the National Society for Phenylketonuria among 300 women with PKU[131] encountered substantial challenges in the postpartum period, including conflicting information on breastfeeding with PKU and difficulty taking in enough calories to sustain breastfeeding while adhering to a PHE-restricted diet. Women with PKU may benefit from antenatal guidance and additional support in the postpartum period to initiate and sustain breastfeeding.

GASTROINTESTINAL DISORDERS

Inflammatory Bowel Disease

Inflammatory bowel disease (IBD) most commonly manifests in individuals of childbearing age, with the highest prevalence in Europe (ulcerative colitis [UC], 505 per 100,000 persons; Crohn disease [CD], 322 per 100,000 persons) and North America (UC, 249 per 100,000 persons; CD, 319 per 100,000 persons).[132] Pregnancy does not affect the course of CD, but UC is more likely to flare.[133] IBD is associated with obstetric complications, including low birthweight and preterm delivery.[134] A 2005 study found higher rates of postpartum IBD flares among women who breastfed, but this was association confounded by medication discontinuation among women who breastfed.[135] Two subsequent studies found no association between breastfeeding and postpartum IBD flare risk.[136,137]

Effect of IBD on Milk Composition

In a study comparing milk composition among women with CD or UC with healthy controls,[138] the authors found lower levels of immunoglobulin A (IgA), lactose, and 2-aminobutyrate in women with IBD, as well as higher levels of inflammatory cytokines. Maternal treatment with 5-aminosalicylic acid versus biologics was also associated with differences in milk composition. The clinical significance of this variation in milk composition is not known.

Medications to treat IBD in lactation

Treatments for IBD include sulfasalazine and mesalamine, corticosteroids, antibiotics, azathioprine/6-mercaptopurine, methotrexate, and biologics. Methotrexate is contraindicated in lactation; data for other agents is generally reassuring at the doses used to treat IBD. In a prospective cohort study of 824 mothers with IBD, 620 breastfed their infants, among whom 412 were treated with thiopurines, biologics, or both.[139] Levels of biologic agents in milk were measured for 72 women and found to be very low (Table 15.2). There were no differences in milestone scores or infection rates among breastfed versus formula-fed infants. A survey of physicians in Canada found widespread variation in knowledge regarding safety of medications to treat IBD in lactating women.[140] Clinicians are encouraged to consult an up-to-date lactation pharmacology resource, such as LactMed, for the most current recommendations.

Bariatric Surgery

Bariatric surgery is common among women of childbearing age. It is suggested to avoid pregnancy for 12 to 24 months after weight loss surgery.[141] After bariatric surgery, the risk for gestational diabetes and preeclampsia appears to be reduced but the risk for growth restriction is increased.[142]

TABLE 15.2   Levels of Inflammatory Bowel Disease Biologics in Human Milk

Drug	Total Patients, n	Total Patients With a Detectable Level, n (%)	Peak (Range) (mcg/mL)	Peak Time Range, hr
Infliximab	29	19 (66.0)	0.74 (0.15–0.74)	24–48
Adalimumab	21	2 (9.5)	0.71 (0.45–0.71)	12–24
Certolizumab	13	3 (23.0)	0.29 (0.27–0.29)	24–48
Golimumab	1	0 (0)	N/A	N/A
Ustekinumab	6	4 (66.7)	1.57 (0.72–1.57)	12–24
Natalizumab	2	1 (50.0)	0.46	24

N/A, Not applicable.
From Matro R, Martin CF, Wolf D, et al. exposure concentrations of infants breastfed by women receiving biologic therapies for inflammatory bowel diseases and effects of breastfeeding on infections and development. *Gastroenterology.* 2018;155(3):696–704.

Effects of Bariatric Surgery on Milk Macronutrient Composition

In a prospective study, researchers collected longitudinal milk samples from normal weight, overweight, and obese women, as well as women who had undergone bariatric surgery, and found similar energy, total fat, total carbohydrates, protein, and vitamin A levels among the four groups.[143] Roux-en-Y gastric bypass surgery can adversely affect maternal absorption of vitamin B_{12}, resulting in B_{12} deficiency in exclusively breastfed infants. Case reports have described failure to thrive, pancytopenia, and developmental delay in vitamin B_{12}—deficient exclusively breastfed infants of mothers who had undergone gastric bypass surgery.[144,145] In one case, neurologic deficits persisted after the pancytopenia resolved.[145] It may be advisable to monitor maternal B_{12} status during lactation, with parenteral supplementation if needed, in mothers who have undergone gastric bypass surgery.

PULMONARY DISORDERS

Asthma

Asthma is the most common respiratory disorder of pregnancy, affecting 2% to 13% of pregnancies worldwide. Adverse pregnancy outcomes associated with maternal asthma include antepartum and postpartum hemorrhage, placenta previa, placental abruption, cesarean delivery, gestational diabetes, HDPs, premature rupture of membranes, stillbirth, intrauterine growth restriction, and cleft lip and palate.[146,147] In epidemiologic studies, breastfeeding is associated with lower risk for asthma in children, although data are mixed.[148] Guidelines regarding lactation in the setting of asthma state that women should be encouraged to breastfeed and asthma treatment medications should be used as in nonlactating women.[149]

Cystic Fibrosis

Cystic fibrosis (CF) is an autosomal recessive genetic disorder of chloride transport that results in a triad of chronic obstructive pulmonary disease, pancreatic exocrine insufficiency, and elevation of sweat sodium and chloride concentrations.[150] Whereas individuals with CF typically died in infancy in the 1950s, median survival in high-income countries is now greater than 40 years. As a result, a growing proportion of women with CF are reaching adulthood and carrying pregnancies. Breastfeeding is encouraged in women with CF, with careful attention to support, nutrition, and hydration.[151] Edenborough et al.[151] note that hands-on support is critical to ensure that the mother is able to continue her treatment regimen while caring for her newborn. Because pancreatic insufficiency affects nutrient absorption in women with CF, support is needed to ensure adequate nutrition to meet the mother's needs and the increased caloric burden of lactation. Fluid intake is particularly important for women with CF, because dehydration can precipitate distal intestinal obstructive syndrome. At least an additional 2 L of fluid intake per day is recommended during lactation. In a 2016 review[152] the majority of medications for CF were found to be compatible with breastfeeding.

AUTOIMMUNE DISORDERS

General Principles

Lactation, Prolactin, and Autoimmune Disorders

Autoimmune diseases disproportionately affect women, and the hormonal changes of pregnancy and lactation affect disease course.[153] Gonadal corticosteroids and prolactin are implicated in the underlying physiology. Prolactin levels are elevated in several autoimmune diseases, including systemic lupus erythematosus (SLE), multiple sclerosis (MS), and systemic sclerosis,[55,56,154] Because T-cell—mediated autoimmune diseases tend to abate during pregnancy and flare after birth, some have theorized that breastfeeding should be discouraged to reduce postpartum relapse.[155] However, the causal relationships among breastfeeding, prolactin, and autoimmune disease are unclear. For example, although MS is associated with increased prolactin levels, and breastfeeding increases prolactin, in observational studies, exclusive breastfeeding is associated with *reduced* risk for MS relapse postpartum.[44,156] Similarly, although prolactin is associated rheumatoid arthritis (RA),[157] longer durations of breastfeeding are associated with reduced risk for developing RA.[158,159]

Transplacental exposure to maternal autoantibodies.
Maternal IgG antibodies cross the placenta during pregnancy, providing short-term passive immune protection for the neonate. In autoimmune diseases, autoantibodies can similarly cross to the fetal circulation and cause transient autoimmune disease in the fetus. Neonatal lupus erythematosus (NLE) is characterized by a transient photosensitive rash, thrombocytopenia, and transaminitis in the setting of maternal anti-Ro/SSA and/or anti-La/SSB antibodies. The most significant manifestation NLE is congenital heart block, which affects approximately 2% of pregnancies in mothers with these antibodies. The recurrence risk for congenital heart block in the setting of these antibodies is 15%.[160]

Other maternal autoimmune conditions mediated by IgG antibodies that can affect the neonate include myasthenia gravis, bullous pemphigoid, and idiopathic thrombocytopenic purpura. Neonates exposed to these antibodies in utero may require monitoring in the NICU; they will thus require additional support to establish breastfeeding.

Medical therapy for autoimmune disorders in lactation.
Many medications used to treat autoimmune disorders are considered compatible with lactation. In 2016 the British Society for Rheumatology and British Health Professionals in Rheumatology issued guidelines on medication use in breastfeeding.[161,162] Disease-modifying agents considered compatible with breastfeeding include corticosteroids, hydrochlorothiazide, azathioprine, cyclosporin A, tacrolimus, intravenous immunoglobulin (IVIG), and, for healthy full-term infants, sulfasalazine. The anti–tumor necrosis factor (TNF) agents infliximab, etanercept, adalimumab, and certolizumab are also considered compatible, although data are limited. There are no data on leflunomide, golimumab, or other biologics, including rituximab, tocilizumab, anakinra, abatacept, belimumab. Drugs not considered compatible include methotrexate, cyclophosphamide, and mycophenolate mofetil. For analgesics and other drugs used in rheumatology practice, the guidelines rated as compatible with breastfeeding acetaminophen, tramadol, amitriptyline, nonsteroidal antiinflammatory drugs (NSAIDs), low-dose aspirin, angiotensin-converting enzyme (ACE) inhibitors, and nifedipine. Caution was advised for fluoxetine, paroxetine, and sertraline, based on limited data, and for codeine. The guideline reported insufficient data regarding gabapentin and venlafaxine and no data for pregabalin, rivaroxaban, dabigatran, bisphosphonates, amlodipine, or the pulmonary vasoconstrictors sildenafil, bosentan, or prostacyclines. Cyclooxygenase 2 (COX-2) inhibitors were rated as not compatible. The American College of Rheumatology recommends the guideline available at https://www.rheumatology.org/Practice-Quality/Clinical-Support/Clinical-Practice-Guidelines/Reproductive-Health-in-Rheumatic-Diseases. The clinician is encouraged to consult LactMed or the Infant Risk Center for the most up-to-date guidance.

Effects of Autoimmune Disorders on Caregiving

Symptoms of autoimmune disorders, including pain, weakness, and limited mobility, can have an impact on caregiving. In a mixed methods study of women with autoimmune rheumatic disorders, women expressed a need for holistic care that accommodated their disease process. For example, one mother with nonspecific inflammatory arthritis could not participate in an infant massage class because the class was on the floor. Another mother struggled to breastfeed through mobility and pain, "but I marched on and then at 6 weeks I dropped the child." Women expressed a need for support from occupational therapists who took into account their role as mothers who had to look after their children.[163]

Systemic Lupus Erythematosus

Few studies have evaluated breastfeeding in women with SLE. In an Argentinian study, women with SLE were less likely to initiate breastfeeding than the general population and they discontinued breastfeeding earlier.[164] Moreover, women with SLE were more likely to report stopping breastfeeding because of a maternal medication, even though half of these women were prescribed medications considered compatible with breastfeeding. In a US study of women with SLE (N = 51), 68% intended to breastfeed, and 49% were breastfeeding at the postpartum rheumatology visit.[165] Prenatal intention was the strongest predictor of breastfeeding outcome.

Effects on Pregnancy

SLE is associated with pregnancy complications, including intrauterine growth restriction, preeclampsia, and preterm birth, each of which can complicate initiation of breastfeeding and require additional support. In addition, In the US study, women with preterm births were less likely to be breastfeeding at follow-up than women with term births (23% vs. 57%, $p = 0.03$).[165]

Effects of Breastfeeding on Disease Course

Given associations between prolactin and disease activity, prolactin inhibitors have been studied as a treatment for SLE. In two unblinded clinical trials conducted in China, postpartum treatment with bromocriptine reduced disease activity and dose of disease-modifying medications.[166,167] Data are limited on associations between breastfeeding and SLE flares in the postpartum period. In the US cohort study, women who were not breastfeeding in follow-up had more SLE symptoms than those who were breastfeeding, indexed by Systemic Lupus Erythematosus Pregnancy Disease Activity Index ($p < 0.05$).

Rheumatoid Arthritis

A case-control study in the early 1990s found that breastfeeding was associated with increased odds of incident RA in the first year postpartum (N = 88 cases, 129 controls).[168] Two subsequent studies found a dose-dependent association between longer lifetime breastfeeding and reduced risk for RA (prospective cohort N = 121,700; nested case-control N = 136 cases, 544 controls).[158,159] These studies have led researchers to explore relationships between circulating prolactin and disease activity, with mixed results.[169] Prolactin is expressed in immune cells in synovial fluid in patients with RA, leading to speculation that autocrine or paracrine prolactin signaling may play a role in pathogenesis of RA.

Anaphylaxis and Breastfeeding

Anaphylaxis associated with breastfeeding has been described in case reports.[170–176]. The first case was reported by Mullins et al.[170] in a patient who had symptoms when achieving letdown with breastfeeding. The first episode occurred at first feeding with the first infant. Although the patient did not react to a skin test with oxytocin, manual expression of the breast precipitated laryngeal edema and hypotension, as did every attempt to breastfeed. Lactation was suppressed by bromocriptine, and there were no recurrences. The patient remained symptom free for 5 years until the birth of her fourth child. At 48 hours postpartum, urticaria, upper airway angioedema, and hypotension occurred within minutes of each breastfeeding. She was again given bromocriptine, lactation ceased, and she was symptom free. Hormonal changes associated with birth, including progesterone withdrawal and associated destabilization of mast cells,[177] has been proposed as an underlying mechanism. Mechanical stimulation of the breast causing degranulation of mast cells may also contribute. Others have suggested that NSAIDs, which are commonly administered in the postpartum period, may contribute.[174] Some women have been able to manage symptoms with a second-generation antihistamine such as cetirizine 10 mg twice daily.[174]

NEUROLOGIC DISORDERS

Multiple Sclerosis

Women with MS have a reduced risk for relapse during pregnancy; however, risk increases in the first 3 months postpartum. Evidence is mixed regarding whether breastfeeding influences risk for relapse of MS in the postpartum period. Although any breastfeeding compared with never breastfeeding is not associated with relapse, exclusive breastfeeding is associated with a reduced risk for relapse.[44,156] This association may be mediated by suppression of estrogen and progesterone, in that relapse rates are similar after introduction of complementary foods.[156] The Association of British Neurologists recommends that women with MS be encouraged to breastfeed. They further suggest that women with MS consider storing extra expressed milk in the freezer in the event of fatigue, relapse-associated disability, or need for treatment that is incompatible with breastfeeding. Because maternal MS is associated with an increased risk for postpartum depression for both parents, additional support from home visiting services is recommended.[178]

Spinal Cord Injury

Data are limited on spinal cord injury (SCI) and breastfeeding. The supraclavicular (C3,C4) and intercostal (T3-T6) nerves provide sensory innervation of the breast, and the sympathetic neurons (T1-T5) provide autonomic innervation. The brachial plexus (C5-T1) provides motor innervation of the upper limbs

to support positioning the infant during feeding. Higher level SCIs would be expected to have a greater adverse impact on breastfeeding. A complication of SCI above T6 is autonomic dysreflexia, which occurs when a strong sensory stimulus triggers vasoconstriction and hypertension as a result of interruption of sympathetic outflows below the level of the SCI.

In a snowball-sample online survey of women with SCI (N = 52),[179] women with high-level SCI (defined as T6 or above) had shorter durations of exclusive breastfeeding than women with low-level SCI (below T6). Women with high-level SCI were less likely to report experiencing the let-down reflex (46.4 vs. 79.2%); of the eight women surveyed with cervical motor-sensory complete injuries, none experienced the letdown reflex. High-level SCI was associated with higher rates of insufficient milk production (77.8 vs. 35.0%, $p = 0.048$). In the survey sample, 38.9% of women with high-level SCI experienced autonomic dysreflexia with breastfeeding, two of whom cited dysreflexia as the primary reason for weaning.

In addition to autonomic dysreflexia, SCI may also affect lactation through interruption of descending reticulospinal autonomic pathways. In a case report of a woman with C4 tetraplegia and right-sided motor function impairment, milk production was markedly reduced in the right breast. With mechanical expression, she produced about 10 mL on the right breast, compared with 60 mL from the left. The authors proposed that loss of sympathetic efferent fibers that modulate myoepithelial cells and blood vessels impeded milk production.[180]

Headaches

Headaches are common among postpartum women; in the Listening to Mothers III study, frequent headaches were a major new problem health problem for 8% of women and a minor problem for 21% of women in the first 2 months postpartum.[181] Evaluation of maternal blood pressure is essential when women present with headache in the early postpartum period to exclude postpartum preeclampsia. Migraine headaches are estimated to affect one in five women over a 3-month period.[182] Evidence suggests that migraines abate to some extent during pregnancy; this is thought to reflect the reduction in hormonal fluctuations during gestation. Postpartum migraine recurrence may be reduced among breastfeeding women;[183,184] however, overall headache prevalence does not appear to vary by infant feeding method.[185] Analgesics that are compatible with breastfeeding include acetaminophen and ibuprofen; aspirin should be used with caution because of the possibility of Reye's syndrome in the infant. Additional safety recommendations for pharmacologic management have been reviewed in detail.[186] Clinicians are encouraged to review LactMed for the most up-to-date information on specific therapies in lactation.

Epilepsy

Epilepsy had a lifetime prevalence of 7.6 per 1000 population (95% CI 6.17 to 9.38), with higher rates in low- and middle-income countries (8.75 per 1000, 95% CI 7.23 to 10.59) than in high-income countries (5.18 per 1000, 95% CI 7.23 to 10.59).[187]

Management of epilepsy among childbearing women is complicated by concerns about teratogenic effects of antiepileptic drugs (AEDs), particularly with valproic acid, phenytoin, topiramate, and phenobarbital.[60] Seizure risk during pregnancy appears to be highest at delivery, including the day before and the day after birth.[188] Importantly, sleep deprivation is a common trigger for seizure, and this medical need for sleep conflicts with the physiology with on-cue exclusive breastfeeding.[60] As for women with psychiatric disorders that are aggravated by sleep deprivation, arranging for another adult caregiver to take responsibility for a period of more than 4 to 6 hours of nighttime care and bringing the infant to the mother to nurse while side-lying may be helpful. To ensure infant safety, it is suggested that mothers should not bathe the baby alone and they may wish to consider feeding in a supine position to minimize infant fall risk. Data on infant exposure to AEDs by breast milk is limited as is evidence-based recommendations, and consultation with LactMed for the most up to date information is recommended.[189] However, in a prospective multicenter study of children exposed to AEDs during pregnancy and lactation,[190] breastfeeding was independently associated with higher IQ at age 6 (+ 4 points, 95% CI 0 to 8, $p = 0.045$).

Restless Leg Syndrome

Restless leg syndrome (RLS), or Willis-Ekbom disease, is common in pregnancy and lactation, affecting one in five women in Western countries.[191] Known exacerbating factors include iron-deficiency, prolonged immobility, and serotonergic antidepressants. Other risk factors include caffeine, tobacco, alcohol, hypoxia, sleep apnea, sleep deprivation, medications such as antiemetics, antipsychotics, and sedating antihistamines. Nonpharmacologic treatments include moderate exercise, yoga, massage, pneumatic compression devices, treating obstructive sleep apnea, and avoiding aggravating factors. If serum ferritin is less than 75 mcg/L, treatment with oral iron is suggested; intravenous iron may be considered for refractory symptoms with serum ferritin less than 30 mcg/L. Other pharmacologic treatments for refractory symptoms include low-dose clonazepam and gabapentin. For women with comorbid depression, bupropion may be preferable to selective serotonin reuptake inhibitors (SSRIs) because SSRIs can aggravate RLS.

RENAL DISORDERS

Data on the effects of renal insufficiency on milk composition are limited to two case reports. One case describes a woman with acute kidney injury secondary to a postpartum hemorrhage.[192] Milk macronutrient composition was similar to that of a sample from a normal control; however, milk levels of creatinine, creatine phosphate, and hippurate were markedly higher. A second case report documents milk composition in a woman undergoing dialysis three times a week for chronic kidney disease (CKD), compared with milk from six healthy control women.[193] Milk urea, creatinine, and uric acid levels decreased from before to after dialysis. Lower phosphate and glucose levels were found in the patient with CKD; however,

total protein, triglyceride, and cholesterol, as well as immunoglobulin levels, were similar. Given the low phosphate levels, the authors recommended monitoring maternal vitamin D levels and supplementing the infant with phosphate. The option of expressing and discarding milk immediately before dialysis was also discussed. There are no reports in the literature regarding effects of lactation on the mother with renal insufficiency; however, it is logical to account for milk production in assessing fluid intake and output.

CARDIAC DISORDERS

Hypertension

Approximately 0.9% to 1.5% of birthing women in the United States have chronic hypertension,[7] which is associated with an increased risk for preterm birth and intrauterine growth restriction, as well as superimposed preeclampsia. During pregnancy, commonly prescribed oral medications include labetalol, nifedipine, and methyldopa. Hydrochlorothiazide is considered a second-line agent. Blood pressures tend to increase in the 1 to 2 weeks after birth, and women are at risk for postpartum preeclampsia. The ACOG states that early ambulatory visits or home blood pressure monitoring may be prudent. A postpartum woman with a headache or visual changes should have her blood pressure evaluated. Prompt control of severe-range blood pressure is essential in the peripartum period, with a goal of treatment within 30 to 60 minutes for blood pressure greater than 160/110 mm Hg that persists for 15 minutes or more. The ACOG has published protocols for acute treatment with intravenous labetalol, intravenous hydralazine, or oral nifedipine.[7]

Most antihypertensive drugs enter milk in low levels and are considered compatible with lactation. Among beta-blockers, labetalol and propranolol have lower milk-to-plasma ratios and are preferred compared with atenolol and metoprolol. Although ACE inhibitors are contraindicated during pregnancy, they are highly protein bound and enter milk at minimal levels and thus are compatible with breastfeeding. There is a theoretical risk for reduced milk supply with diuretics, which should be factored into clinical decision-making.[7]

Peripartum Cardiomyopathy

Peripartum cardiomyopathy complicates 1 in 1000 to 1 in 4000 live births and is characterized by new-onset, non-ischemic cardiomyopathy presenting in late pregnancy or the first few months postpartum.[194]

Diagnostic criteria include the following:
1. Heart failure secondary to left ventricular systolic dysfunction with a left ventricular ejection fraction (LVEF) less than 45%
2. Occurrence toward the end of pregnancy or in the months after delivery (mostly in the month after delivery)
3. No other identifiable cause of heart failure

The cause of peripartum cardiomyopathy (PPCM) is unknown, but an anti-angiogenic 16-kDa subfragment of prolactin may contribute to endothelial damage. In a pilot RCT (N = 20), women with severe PPCM were treated with bromocriptine or placebo. In the bromocriptine group, one woman died, and the nine surviving women recovered to New York Heart Association (NYHA) Class I functional status at 6 months. In the control group, four women died, three recovered to NYHA Class II status, and three remained at Class III status at 6 months postpartum (*p* comparing change in functional class = 0.008). A subsequent RCT enrolled 63 women with LVEF of 35% or less and randomized them to 1 week versus 8 weeks of bromocriptine treatment. Recovery of left ventricular function was similar in the two groups, and there were no deaths or heart transplants in either group.[195] An RCT of 8 weeks of bromocriptine therapy versus guideline-driven medical therapy is underway in Canada (NCT02590601) with an expected completion date of 2023.

The Heart Failure Association of the European Society of Cardiology Study Group on PPCM states that bromocriptine may be considered in patients with PPCM (class IIb recommendation)[196]; however, this drug is considered investigational in the United States.[194] Recommendations similarly vary regarding breastfeeding. The European Society of Cardiology Study Group on Peripartum Cardiomyopathy states that breastfeeding should be encouraged in women with mild cardiac dysfunction, particularly in areas without access to clean water for preparation of formula; in women with severe dysfunction, they recommend treatment with bromocriptine and cessation of breastfeeding.[197] In their guidelines for the management of cardiovascular diseases during pregnancy, the European Society of Cardiology states that bromocriptine may be considered to stop lactation and enhance recovery. They also state that because of the metabolic demands of lactation, preventing lactation may be considered in women with severe heart failure (NYHA III/IV). In contrast, the ACOG states that bromocriptine treatment for PPCM remains investigational and requires further study, and "breastfeeding should not be discouraged in women with peripartum cardiomyopathy because there are no data to suggest it negatively affects maternal cardiac status."[194]

Given conflicting recommendations from different professional societies and the morbidity of PPCM, it is critically important to incorporate the individual woman's preferences and values into decisions about whether to continue breastfeeding or initiate bromocriptine treatment. (See previous discussion of shared decision-making.)

ORGAN TRANSPLANT

Whereas pregnancy after organ transplant was once thought to be unacceptably risky, a growing number of women with transplants are conceiving and carrying pregnancies, albeit with an increased risk for preterm birth or low birthweight.[198] Based on data from the Transplant Pregnancy Registry,[198,199] a growing proportion of women who have undergone transplant are breastfeeding their infants (Fig. 15.4). In a 2014 review, Constantinescu et al.[198] concluded that transplant recipients taking prednisone, azathioprine, cyclosporine, and tacrolimus need not be discouraged from breastfeeding. Data are limited regarding mycophenolic acid products, sirolimus, everolimus, and belatacept.

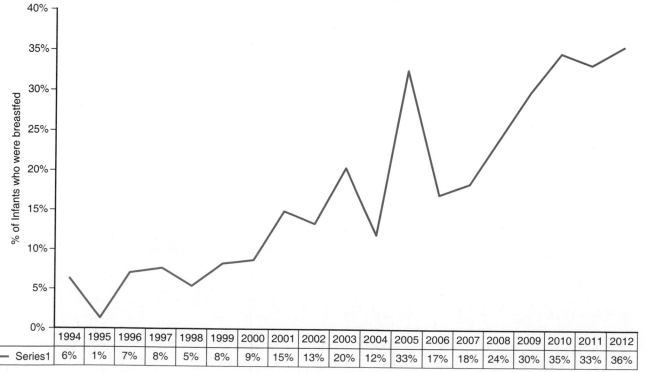

	1994	1995	1996	1997	1998	1999	2000	2001	2002	2003	2004	2005	2006	2007	2008	2009	2010	2011	2012
— Series1	6%	1%	7%	8%	5%	8%	9%	15%	13%	20%	12%	33%	17%	18%	24%	30%	35%	33%	36%

Fig. 15.4 Breastfeeding rates among transplant recipients. (From Constantinescu S, Pai A, Coscia LA, et al. Breast-feeding after transplantation. *Best Pract Res Clin Obstet Gynaecol.* 2014;28(8):1163–1173.)

MUSCULOSKELETAL DISORDERS

Ergonomics of Breastfeeding

In an effort to position and attach the infant or to express milk, nursing mothers may assume positions and postures that result in musculoskeletal discomfort. Moreover, carrying an infant in a car seat or a sling may strain the back, neck, and shoulders. Women who have significant perineal lacerations may find it uncomfortable to sit upright. Hormonal changes of pregnancy continue to affect joint mobility in the early postpartum period, further affecting musculoskeletal health. Attention to appropriate ergonomic positioning can increase maternal comfort (Box 15.4).

Neuropathies Associated With Breastfeeding

A number of neurologic symptoms have been described in association with lactation. During periods of engorgement, pressure on nerves in the axilla, especially from an engorged tail of Spence (see Chapter 2), has caused numbness and tingling down the arms on the flexor surface to the ulnar distribution of the hands, similar to crutch palsy. The numbness and tingling usually abate as soon as the infant nurses and then gradually return as the breast fills again. Symptoms gradually disappear after several weeks, as engorgement resolves.

Tennis Elbow With Hand Pumping

Symptoms similar to those associated with tennis elbow—pain and tingling with flexion of the forearm—have developed in nursing women who are pumping milk with a Kaneson-style cylinder hand pump.[200] Similar symptoms have been experienced by mothers just holding a newborn over time, especially primiparas and especially heavy infants.

Carpal Tunnel Syndrome

Carpal tunnel syndrome (CTS) is common in pregnancy, causing paresthesia of the hands. In a prospective population-based cohort study in the Netherlands, 34% of women reported symptoms of CTS during pregnancy. In the postpartum period, prevalence decreased to 11% at 6 weeks, 6% at 4 months, and 5% at 12 months. Factors associated with persistent postpartum symptoms included earlier onset and greater severity of symptoms in pregnancy and higher depression scores postpartum.[201] This population-based study did not report on associations between CTS and breastfeeding; however, a retrospective mail survey of 27 women with postpartum onset of CTS symptoms found that breastfeeding women reported resolution of symptoms within 1 to 3 weeks of weaning. All were symptom free within a year.[202] The recommended treatment for CTS is conservative, with rest, diuretics, hand splint, and local corticosteroid injection, because it is usually reversible.

PSYCHIATRIC DISORDERS

General Principles

Psychiatric disorders are common in women of childbearing age: 20%[203] to 25%[204] of women will experience an anxiety, mood, substance use, or psychotic disorder during pregnancy or within 12 months of birth. The risk for acute exacerbation is highest in the first month after birth. In a population-based study, the highest rate of both initial psychiatric hospitalization and outpatient psychiatric contact was seen at 10 to 19 days postpartum.[205] Providers caring for breastfeeding dyads should be familiar with symptoms of maternal psychiatric disorders and be prepared to screen and refer or treat women as needed. As many as 80% of women experience the "baby blues," characterized by mild depression and anxiety, mood swings, and tearfulness that peaks at 4 to 5 days and resolves by 10 days postpartum. In contrast, peripartum depression is the onset of symptoms within 12 months of birth that persist for at least 2 weeks.[206] Regardless of how the infant is fed, the mother with psychiatric illness may require additional social and material support for recovery from birth and infant caregiving. For example, for many women with psychiatric disorders, adequate periods of uninterrupted sleep are essential for maternal health.

Effect of Psychiatric Disease on Breastfeeding

It is not uncommon for women to discontinue their psychiatric medication in early pregnancy because of concerns about fetal exposure and potential risk for birth defects. However, the evidence linking most psychiatric medications with fetal anomalies is limited and fraught with confounding. In large studies that have used advanced methods to adjust for confounding, previously described associations between SSRIs and persistent pulmonary hypertension of the newborn were no longer statistically significant.[207,208] Decisions about medical therapy during pregnancy require a thoughtful, shared decision between the patient and her provider, weighing both the risks for fetal exposure and the risks for worsening maternal disease.

Poor neonatal adaptation syndrome has been described among neonates exposed to psychiatric medications in utero, with symptoms including respiratory distress and tremors in

---

BOX 15.4 General Principles of Joint Protection and Proper Body Mechanics

- Avoid using a sustained, tight grasp or pinch, especially if the wrist is bent.
- Avoid static or awkward positions for prolonged periods.
- Minimize repetition.
- Avoid bending, extending, or twisting the wrist during activities.
- Use a power grasp (loose grip, keeping all the fingers together, thumb straight).
- Avoid reaching, grasping, and lifting with the palm down (especially with wrist bent). Rather, support objects from underneath with the palm up (wrist straight).
- Avoid leaning over a work surface or twisting the torso while lifting.

From Roberts D. Preventing musculoskeletal pain in mothers: ergonomic tips for lactation consultants. *Clin Lact*. 2011;2(4):13–20.

the infant.[209] These dyads may benefit from additional support in the first few days of breastfeeding.

In a meta-analysis, women with depression were less likely to initiate breastfeeding.[210] Findings regarding depression and prenatal breastfeeding intention vary.[211-213] Most authors have found that women with antenatal depression symptoms have shorter durations of any[214-217] and exclusive[218-220] breastfeeding, although others have not found an association with continuation through 1 month[221] or 3 months[213] postpartum. Antenatal anxiety also has been linked with reducing breastfeeding intensity and duration.[222]

In clinical practice, breastfeeding difficulties and depression symptoms may manifest together, underscoring the importance of screening women who present with breastfeeding concerns for depression and anxiety symptoms. In a secondary analysis of the US Infant Feeding Practices Study II, women who experienced severe pain with early breastfeeding were more likely to screen positive for depression at 2 months postpartum.[223] In another analysis of the same cohort, women with depression symptoms (Edinburgh Postnatal Depression Scale [EPDS] ≥ 13) were far more likely than women with an EPDS less than 13 to experience early, undesired weaning, 56% vs. 44%) and disrupted lactation (19% vs. 11.3%), defined as unplanned, undesired weaning in the setting of pain, low milk supply, or latch difficulties.[224] The authors of a 2015 systematic review concluded that clinicians need to identify and assist women with depressive symptoms or with early breastfeeding problems "in order to enhance breastfeeding and promote postpartum psychological adjustment."[225] Given these associations, screening for depression is suggested for women presenting with breastfeeding difficulties.

Stress and Lactation

Pain and stress inhibit milk let-down and oxytocin release, as Niles Newton demonstrated in her classic experiment published in 1948. Newton had read that if a cow is stressed while being milked, the cow would make less milk, and she sought to test whether stress might similarly affect breastfeeding mothers. She was nursing her 7-month-old daughter, and she and her husband designed a cross-over design study. Each morning, before the first feed, her baby was weighed, breastfed under various conditions, and weighed again after feeding. In addition to normal feeding, conditions included putting the mother's feet in ice water, asking difficult math questions and administering an electric shock if she gave the wrong answer, and wrapping a piece of gauze around her big toe and pulling until it was painful. When the mother was being stressed, the infant transferred much less milk. During these experiments, she received a dose of either oxytocin or placebo; the oxytocin "rescued" milk transfer. In the paper's discussion, Newton noted:

It is interesting to speculate on the possible application of this knowledge to breast feeding in general. Many mothers are nervous about feeding their first baby; they are upset by the strange hospital surroundings; they are embarrassed by having to expose their breasts among strangers; their nipples are often sore and their breasts engorged. Emotional disturbances, embarrassment, and pain inhibit let-down to the sucking baby, and thus the baby gets little milk.

Research has subsequently demonstrated that acute stress reduces pulsatile oxytocin release during breastfeeding.[226]

Although acute stress reduces milk production, there is also evidence that relaxation may enhance milk flow. In an RCT among NICU mothers, listening to a guided relaxation imagery recording increased milk production.[227] In a study among mothers of healthy term infants in Malaysia,[228] women were randomized to listen to a relaxation therapy audio recording daily while breastfeeding and compared with a control group. The relaxation intervention reduced maternal stress and increased infant milk volume intake and weight gain. These results underscore the importance of providing mothers with both emotional and material support in the months after birth.

The effects of stress on lactation also manifest in studies of local environmental stressors and breastfeeding outcomes. In the UK Millennium Cohort Study, low neighborhood environmental quality was associated with lower initiation and duration of breastfeeding.[229] These effects were buffered among women in the top two income quintiles, whereas among women in the lower quintiles, worse neighborhood quality was associated with lower breastfeeding rates (Fig. 15.5). These results underscore the importance of addressing social determinants of health to enable women to initiate and sustain breastfeeding.

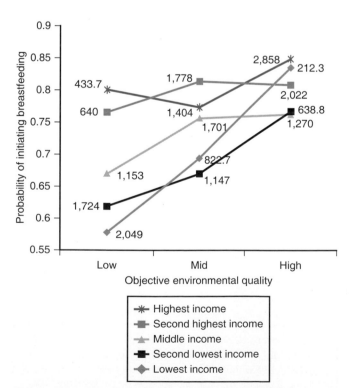

Fig. 15.5 Breastfeeding initiation and neighborhood environmental quality. (From Brown LJ, Sear R. Local environmental quality positively predicts breastfeeding in the UK Millennium Cohort Study. *Evol Med Public Health.* 2017;2017(1):120–135.)

Medication Exposure

Many women with psychiatric disorders require treatment with psychiatric medications: from 2007 to 2010, 14.8% of women of childbearing age were treated with an antidepressant. Use of medications during pregnancy has also increased. From 2001 to 2007, antiepileptic medication use increased from 15.7 to 21.9 per 1000 deliveries[230] and use of atypical antipsychotics increased from 0.33% to 0.82%.[231] Management of the breastfeeding dyad is complicated by limited data on the risks of exposure to psychotropic medications by milk and the benefits of breastfeeding for mother and child.[62]

Data regarding medication exposure by breast milk are limited and primarily comprise case series and small pharmacokinetic studies measuring drug levels in milk. Medications to treat psychiatric disease are typically lipid soluble, to cross the blood-brain barrier, and therefore are also present in milk. Most medications are safe for use in breastfeeding;[232] however, as data continue to emerge, clinicians should consult LactMed for the most up-to-date information on specific agents. To ensure appropriate infant follow-up, the mother's provider should communicate with the infant's provider regarding prescribing and medication changes. As reviewed by Payne,[232] existing data for most antidepressants are reassuring, with the exception of doxepin and monoamine oxidase inhibitors, for which there are little to no data. Among mood stabilizers, infants exposed to lithium should have blood levels monitored. There are limited data on both typical and atypical antipsychotics, and infants should be monitored for extrapyramidal side effects and sedation. Benzodiazepines can cause infant sedation, and shorter acting agents are preferred.

The Effects of Breastfeeding on Psychiatric Disease

Women are often counseled that oxytocin promotes bonding and therefore breastfeeding prevents postpartum depression. In observational studies, women who are exclusively breastfeeding are less likely to have symptoms of depression than women who are mixed feeding or have weaned, but the causal direction of this association is unclear. For some women, breastfeeding may improve mood and prevent depression, but for others, depressive symptoms may derail breastfeeding. In the early days after birth, onset of lactogenesis II is facilitated by falling levels of progesterone. In the brain, progesterone is metabolized into allopregnanolone, a potent agonist of the gamma-aminobutyric acid (GABA) receptor. As progesterone levels fall in the days after birth, allopregnanolone levels also fall, resulting in increased anxiety and irritability known clinically as the baby blues, coinciding with lactogenesis II and engorgement. Interestingly, these symptoms were described together in a 19th-century psychiatric textbook:[233]

About two days after delivery some women become excited, sleepless, and incoherent; they have a flushed face, a rather full pulse and slight elevation of temperature; this is called 'milk fever,' and coincides with the beginning of the flow of milk.

Animal studies have shown that the plasticity of the GABA receptor affects the severity of mood symptoms after birth; mouse dams lacking the delta subunit of the GABA receptor exhibited normal behavior except in the days after birth, when they were unable to care for their pups.[234] Human mothers who are sensitive to fluctuations in progesterone, such as women with premenstrual dysphoric disorder, may experience more severe symptoms after birth and may thus be more vulnerable to postpartum depression.

Oxytocin has been described as the "love hormone," given its important role in maternal behavior in animal studies. However, evidence is emerging that the relationship between oxytocin and maternal behavior is complex. The effects of oxytocin may vary based on life experience; among men who experienced separation from a parent before age 12, administration of oxytocin increased, rather than decreased, cortisol levels.[235] Studies among women with postnatal depression show mixed effects. In a small study of women with postpartum depression, women were administered inhaled oxytocin or placebo and then asked to describe their infants. When given oxytocin, women made more negative initial statements about their infants and were less happy than when given placebo.[236] The same research group found that after receiving nasal oxytocin, women with depression who listened to a recording of an infant crying were more likely to perceive the cry as urgent and to choose a harsh caregiving response than when they received placebo.[237]

Differences in both oxytocin genotype and life experiences may play a role. In the Maternal Adversity, Vulnerability and Neurodevelopment (MAVAN) study, oxytocin genotype modified the relationship between early-life adversity and both depression and breastfeeding outcome.[238] Among women with the OXT rs2740210 CC genotype, low early-life adversity was associated with less depression and slightly shorter breastfeeding duration than the AA/CA genotype. However, in the setting of high early-life adversity, women with the CC genotype breastfed for markedly shorter periods and were considerably more depressed that women with the AA/CA genotype (Fig. 15.6).

In clinical care, these nuances underscore the importance of addressing the mother's experience of infant feeding. For some women, breastfeeding is a source of joy and contentment and for others it is a burden. Indeed, in a cross-sectional study of 217 U.K. women, breastfeeding duration was not associated with postpartum depression symptoms; however, depression scores were higher among women reporting physical difficulty, pain, lack of support, and pressure from others to stop breastfeeding.[239] Women who reported weaning because of inconvenience had lower depression scores. In a longitudinal US study, liking breastfeeding in the first week was associated with longer duration of exclusive breastfeeding and more positive recalled experience of breastfeeding across the entire lactation period.[240] Among women with anxiety, positive emotions during breastfeeding at 2 months was

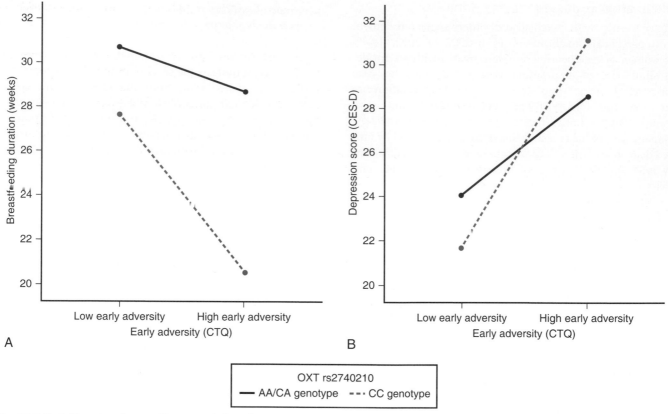

Fig. 15.6 Early-life adversity modifies associations between oxytocin genotype and both (A) breastfeeding duration and (B) depression symptoms. *CES-D*, Center for Epidemiological Studies Depression Scale; *CTQ*, Childhood Trauma Questionnaire. (From Jonas W, Mileva-Seitz V, Girard AW, et al. Genetic variation in oxytocin rs2740210 and early adversity associated with postpartum depression and breastfeeding duration. *Genes Brain Behav.* 2013 Oct;12(7):681–694.)

associated with fewer anxiety symptoms through the first year postpartum.[241]

Bipolar Disorder

The hormonal changes after birth can aggravate bipolar disorder.[242] In a population-based study, women with bipolar disorder were 23 times more likely to be admitted in the 30-day period after birth, compared with the period from 3 to 11 months postpartum.[205] A substantial proportion of women who first present with depression symptoms after birth meet the criteria for bipolar disorder, with rates ranging from 15% to 50%.[243] Distinguishing between unipolar depression and bipolar disorder is important because antidepressants may be ineffective in women with bipolar disorder and can also precipitate mania.

Sleep disruption can trigger manic episodes,[242] and women who have had manic episodes triggered by sleep disruption report higher rates of postpartum psychosis.[244] For the mother with bipolar disorder, sleep is thus a medical need.

Case reports have described manic episodes associated with weaning, suggesting that this may be a higher risk time for women with bipolar disorder.[245] The underlying hormonal mechanisms have not been determined; however, Schmidt et al.[245] speculate that rising dopamine levels may contribute. Suckling stimulates prolactin production by lowering dopamine levels, and when suckling ceases, the resulting rise in dopamine might precipitate manic symptoms. Anticipatory guidance regarding mood symptoms with weaning and close psychiatric follow-up are prudent.

Schizophrenia

Data are limited on breastfeeding outcomes among mothers with schizophrenia. In the World Federation of Societies of Biological Psychiatry (WFSBP) Guidelines for Biological Treatment of Schizophrenia, the authors review the limited data lactation in the setting of schizophrenia. A meta-analysis cited in the WFSBP guideline concluded that quetiapine and olanzapine were acceptable for breastfeeding, and chlorpromazine, haloperidol, risperidone, and zuclopenthixol were possible to use with medical supervision.[246] A thoughtful discussion of risks, benefits, and the family's values and preferences is important to support a shared decision.

Relapse of schizophrenia is common in the postpartum period, and ongoing support is essential.[247] The risk for postpartum psychosis for women with schizophrenia is 25%, and risk factors for psychosis include hormonal shifts, obstetric complications, sleep deprivation, marital discord, and psychosocial stress.[248] Wrap-around services, including home visits, that use a strengths-based approach are recommended. If maternal psychiatric admission is indicated, a mother–baby unit[249] can enable the mother to continue to nurture and care for her baby.

Breastfeeding Among Trauma Survivors

Adverse childhood experiences, such as sexual abuse and physical or emotional abuse or neglect, are common. In a US population-based survey, one in four individuals had experienced three or more adverse childhood experiences.[250] Among women surveyed, 16.3% reported childhood sexual abuse (CSA). The US Centers for Disease Control and Prevention National Intimate Partner and Sexual Violence Survey found that 43.6% of women have experienced contact sexual violence, and 21.3% have experienced completed or attempted rape.[251] The same report found that one in three women have experienced intimate partner violence. Given the high prevalence of traumatic life experiences, there is a growing movement to apply a trauma-informed approach as the standard for maternity care.[252]

Quantifying the relationship between trauma history and breastfeeding is challenging because information on trauma history may not be routinely collected in clinical care, and given the stigma associated with a history of trauma, women may not disclose this information even when asked. One of the first studies to explore childhood sexual trauma and breastfeeding found higher rates of initiation among women with a history of childhood sexual abuse (77% vs. 65%, aOR 2.58, 95% CI 1.14 to 5.85); however, women with a history of CSA who breastfed were less likely to continue through 1 month postpartum (73% vs. 82%, p = not significant).[253] Studies in Norway[254] and Australia[255] found lower rates of breastfeeding continuation among women with a history of childhood sexual abuse. Adverse childhood experiences similarly have been associated with earlier cessation of exclusive breastfeeding.[220,256] The Norway study further evaluated adult emotional, physical, and sexual abuse and found that all were associated with lower rates of breastfeeding beyond 4 months postpartum.[254] These findings are consistent with a cohort study in Tanzania that found women exposed to intimate partner violence were more likely to terminate exclusive breastfeeding before 6 months postpartum.[257]

Women with a history of CSA were more likely to report both mastitis (49.4% vs. 27.6%) and pain (29.4% vs. 18.8%) in a Swiss case-control study.[258] Among women with a history of CSA, 20% reported that breastfeeding triggered memories of CSA and 58% reported dissociative symptoms. These findings are consistent with qualitative findings that loss of control, both during birth and while breastfeeding, can be triggering. Describing breastfeeding, one woman said:[259]

> It's like it's happening again because you are being controlled by another person. And even though I really tried not to feel like that, it happened every single time um that I tried breast feeding. I felt that immense feeling of being controlled by someone else.

The relationship between childhood maltreatment (CMT) and breastfeeding outcome may vary for women who have recovered versus women who have ongoing posttraumatic stress disorder (PTSD). In an observational cohort study, women who had experienced CMT but did not have PTSD, who were classified as CMT-resilient, were twice as likely to be exclusively breastfeeding at 6 weeks postpartum as women who experienced CMT and had PTSD.[260] This distinction between CMT-resilient and PTSD groups may explain findings of a cross-sectional internet survey that found women with a history of CSA who were exclusively breastfeeding reported better mood, sleep, and overall health than women who were mixed feeding or formula feeding.[261] Exclusive breastfeeding may be a marker for CMT resilience, rather than a cause of improved sleep and well-being.

When sexual trauma is disclosed, the obstetric provider can take steps to support women to engage in care and minimize triggers, both during prenatal care and during the birth itself.[262] Therapists have similarly proposed steps to support mothers with a history of sexual abuse who wish to breastfeed:[263]

- In discussing concerns, clinicians should listen carefully, validate the mother's feelings, and explore solutions together.
- When assisting with feeding, ask permission before touching.
- Nighttime feedings may be difficult for the woman with a history of abuse, especially if the abuse occurred at night or in bed. Having another caregiver feed the infant at night, or moving from bed to a comfortable chair, may be helpful.
- The phrase "feed on demand" can be triggering. Consider using different language, such as "feed on cue."

To the extent that overly directive or coercive advice can re-traumatize, clinicians engaging in infant feeding care should take care to apply key principles of trauma-informed care. The six key principles are safety; trustworthiness and transparency; peer support; collaboration and mutuality; empowerment, voice and choice; and cultural, historical, and gender issues.[264]

Substance Use

Substance use is common among women of childbearing age, and although many women are able to cut down or quit during pregnancy, relapse in the postpartum period is common. Tobacco, alcohol, marijuana, and other substances cross the placenta and enter breast milk. Counseling about breastfeeding in the setting of using any of these substances includes sharing information with the patient regarding what is known about the effects of exposure through breast milk, as well as the effects of formula feeding versus breastfeeding. It can be helpful to ask the patient what she has heard about breastfeeding and about breastfeeding in the setting of using a particular substance. Using principles of shared decision-making, explore the patient's preferences and values and support her to make an informed decision. Trauma is common among individuals with use disorder, and the principles of trauma-informed care are important to incorporate into counseling.[265]

Of note, recommendations regarding substance use and breastfeeding often note that effects on maternal judgement or mood may affect this mother's ability to care for the infant.

This is not a concern limited to breastfeeding mothers: regardless of how the infant is fed, substance use can interfere with infant care, and safety plans should address who will care for the infant in the event of recurrent substance use.

The ABM outlines circumstances in which breastfeeding for women with a history of use disorder should be encouraged, carefully considered, and not recommended.[266] These circumstances are summarized in Box 15.5.

Alcohol

Alcohol is a small molecule that freely enters and leaves the milk compartment, and is excreted from the maternal bloodstream through first-order hepatic metabolism. MotherRisk modeled the maternal alcohol clearance and estimated that for a woman of average height, it would take between 1 hour 51 minutes and 2 hours 50 minutes for a single serving of alcohol—340 g (12 oz) of 5% beer, or 141.75 g (5 oz) of 11% wine, or 42.53 g (1.5 oz) of 40% liquor—to clear completely from the mother's bloodstream and from her milk.[267] Because the alcohol leaves the milk compartment as it is metabolized, there is no need to express and discard after a single serving. Women consuming multiple servings may need to express and discard to relieve breast fullness while the alcohol is metabolized.

Tobacco

Because second-hand smoke exposure increases risk for sudden infant death syndrome (SIDS), all members of the infant's household should be counseled to stop smoking. For women who have quit using tobacco during pregnancy, relapse risk should be addressed, because 65% to 80% of women who quit during pregnancy relapse within the first year.[268] According to the American Academy of Pediatrics (AAP), "Maternal smoking is not an absolute contraindication to breastfeeding. . . . Lactating women should be strongly encouraged to stop smoking and to minimize secondhand exposure."[269] In observational studies, maternal smoking while breastfeeding is associated with better infant outcomes than maternal smoking while formula feeding.[270,271] Families should be counseled that there is a markedly increased risk for SIDS for infants who bedshare with parents who smoke compared with infants who sleep in the same room on a separate sleep surface.[272]

Data are limited on nicotine cessation medications in lactation. The AAP considers nicotine replacement in doses equivalent to or less than the amount typically smoked to be compatible with lactation and recommends short-acting formulations, such as gum or lozenges, to minimize exposure.[269]

Opiates

For women who are enrolled in a treatment program to receive maintenance opiate replacement therapy with methadone or buprenorphine, breastfeeding is encouraged.[266,269] In observational studies, breastfed infants born to women treated with opiate replacement therapy have less severe symptoms of neonatal abstinence syndrome than formula-fed infants.[273] However, qualitative data indicate that women on opiate replacement therapy encounter barriers to breastfeeding.[274]

BOX 15.5 Academy of Breastfeeding Medicine Recommendations Regarding Breastfeeding in the Context of Maternal Use Disorder

Encourage women under the following circumstances to breastfeed their infants (III):

- Engaged in substance abuse treatment; provision of maternal consent to discuss progress in treatment and plans for postpartum treatment with substance abuse treatment counselor; counselor recommendation for breastfeeding
- Plans to continue in substance abuse treatment in the postpartum period
- Abstinence from drug use for 90 days before delivery; ability to maintain sobriety demonstrated in an outpatient setting
- Toxicology testing of maternal urine negative at delivery
- Engaged in prenatal care and compliant.

Evaluate carefully women under the following circumstances, and determine appropriate advice for breastfeeding by discussion and coordination among the mother, maternal care providers, and substance abuse treatment providers (III):

- Relapse to illicit substance use or legal substance misuse in the period of 90 to 30 days before delivery
- Concomitant use of other prescription medications deemed to be incompatible with lactation
- Engaged later (after the second trimester) in prenatal care and/or substance abuse treatment
- Attained drug and/or alcohol sobriety only in an inpatient setting
- Lack of appropriate maternal family and community support systems
- Report that they desire to breastfeed their infant to either retain custody or maintain their sobriety in the postpartum period

Counsel women under any of the following circumstances not to breastfeed (III):

- Not engaged in substance abuse treatment or engaged in treatment and failure to provide consent for contact with counselor
- Not engaged in prenatal care
- Positive maternal urine toxicology screen for substances other than marijuana at delivery. Strongly advise mothers to discontinue exposure while breastfeeding and counsel them as to the substance's possible long-term neurobehavioral effects.
- No plans for postpartum substance abuse treatment or pediatric care
- Women relapsing to illicit drug use or legal substance misuse in the 30-day period before delivery
- Any behavioral or other indicators that the woman is actively abusing substances
- Chronic alcohol use.

From Reece-Stremtan S, Marinelli KA. ABM Clinical protocol #21: Guidelines for breastfeeding and substance use or substance use disorder, revised 2015. *Breastfeed Med.* 2015;10(3):135–141.

Marijuana

Second-hand marijuana exposure is associated with an increased risk for SIDS, and all members of the infant's household should be counseled to quit or cut down on use. Similarly, it is recommended that breastfeeding women who are using marijuana cut down or stop using. Existing data on the association between maternal marijuana use during lactation and infant neurodevelopment are limited to two studies published more than three decades ago, as reviewed in an AAP Clinical Report.[275] The authors recommend that women be informed of the potential risks of marijuana exposure during lactation and encouraged to abstain. The ACOG similarly recommends that breastfeeding women be discouraged from using marijuana.[276]

Other Drugs of Abuse

Adverse events have been reported in infants exposed to cocaine, amphetamines, heroin, lysergic acid diethylamide (LSD), and phencyclidine.[269] Women who are actively using these substances should be advised not to breastfeed.

SUMMARY

Globally, more than 90% of women give birth;[277] more than 90% initiate breastfeeding, and half continue to breastfeed for at least 12 months. As a result, any clinician who cares for women of childbearing age cares for women who are lactating and must consider both the effects of lactation on maternal health conditions and the effects of maternal health conditions on lactation. Such care requires consideration of the whole mother—baby dyad, centered on the values and preferences of the lactating woman. By "putting the Mother in Breastfeeding Medicine,"[278] we can address each woman's unique needs and craft sustainable approaches to support the health and well-being of mother and child.

The Reference list is available at www.expertconsult.com.

16

Breast Conditions in the Breastfeeding Mother

Katrina B. Mitchell and Helen M. Johnson

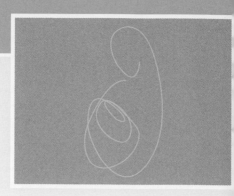

KEY POINTS

- The breast is a complex organ with growth, evolution, and regression over life. Its functional capacity changes dramatically throughout pregnancy and lactation. Many benign and malignant conditions affect the breast in general, and some conditions occur specifically during lactation.
- A careful and complete history, physical examination, and documentation remain essential to understanding, diagnosing, and managing breast disease. A good understanding of the anatomy and physiology of the breast and nipple-areolar complex is essential, including anatomic variations of normal.
- Clinicians caring for breastfeeding mothers should master the management of common lactation-related conditions: plugging, mastitis, galactocele, milk fistula, dermatitis/dermatoses, pain, and hyperlactation. Clinicians also should

be familiar with breast disease that is not related specifically to lactation but can occur in the setting of lactation, such as fibroepithelial tumors, idiopathic granulomatous mastitis, and nipple-areolar complex lesions.
- Breast cancer care can significantly affect lactation, both in patients with prior treatment and those who receive a new diagnosis while lactating. The individual and cumulative effects of breast cancer care, including chemotherapy, surgery, radiation, and endocrine therapy, should be considered in the management of the breastfeeding dyad.
- It is important to understand the surgeries of the breast and nipple-areolar complex and their potential effects on breastfeeding. Patients with a history of breast surgery should receive prenatal counseling and close postpartum support.

Although health care providers should consider the breastfeeding dyad as a unit, certain maternal breast conditions warrant specific evaluation and management. As a foundation for approaching the lactating breast, this chapter begins with a review of the standard breast history and physical exam. It then explores issues affecting the nipple-areolar complex (NAC), as well as inflammatory and obstructive complications, such as mastitis and abscess. Breast masses occurring in the setting of lactation may represent benign or malignant pathology, and this chapter describes appropriate intervention when patients present with a new breast concern during lactation. It outlines how providers can support lactation in patients with a previous or new diagnosis of breast cancer and also reviews common plastic surgery procedures and how they can affect breastfeeding.

BREAST PHYSICAL EXAMINATION

History and Prenatal Counseling

Health care providers should be familiar with the components of a comprehensive examination of the breasts, NAC, and regional lymph node basins. A prenatal breast examination provides an opportunity to evaluate a patient for concerning lesions and begin discussions about breastfeeding. In addition to the physical exam, providers also should inquire

about the patient's previous experience with breastfeeding and any underlying medical conditions that may affect milk production, such as infertility, obesity, and diabetes (see Chapter 15). Surgical and procedural history should be documented (Box 16.1). No history should preclude breastfeeding, but conditions should be identified prenatally, and the patient should be counseled appropriately about potential impacts on breastfeeding.

Prenatal breastfeeding counseling should include anticipatory guidance about normal physiologic breast changes during pregnancy, including growth throughout all trimesters and production of colostrum in late pregnancy. Providers also can address significant breast growth causing pain or lymphedema and recommend targeted interventions such as breast lymphatic massage. Prenatal counseling also affords the opportunity to discuss patient concerns about the potential for breastfeeding challenges resulting from individual anatomy. Providers should reassure patients that breast size is related to the amount of intervening fat in a breast, and smaller breasts do not correlate with a decreased ability to produce milk. However, patients with examination findings consistent with breast hypoplasia (detailed under "Tubular Breast Deformity") should be prepared for potential low milk production. Women with flat or inverted nipples should be reassured that breastfeeding is often successful and that no interventions are advised.

BOX 16.1 Pertinent History Related to Breast Procedures

- Nipple piercing
- Breast biopsy
- Breast cancer surgery
- Operations for benign breast disease
- Chest-wall radiation
- Chest burns and/or skin graft procedures
- Plastic surgical procedures, including the following:
  - Augmentation
  - Reduction, with or without free nipple graft
  - Nipple-inversion correction
  - Gender-affirming top surgery

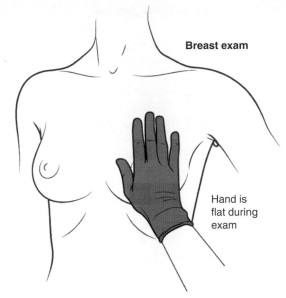

Fig. 16.1 Breast-palpation technique. The provider should use the palm of the hand to palpate the breast during the physical examination because palpation with the fingertips may result in false-positive findings.

Breast Examination

Inspection

The breast examination should begin with inspection. The patient should sit upright with her arms relaxed at her sides. The provider should observe for anatomic variants and symmetry, noting any asymmetries in chest-wall contour, breast size, shape, or protruding masses. The chronicity of any changes should be obtained. The patient should then roll her shoulders forward and raise and lower her arms above her head. This allows for visualization of lower-quadrant lesions and any potential involvement of the pectoralis muscles and/or skin, should a concerning lesion such as breast cancer be present. The provider should observe the skin for scars, edema, erythema, ulceration, skin lesions, and any retraction. The provider should then examine the NAC, assessing for symmetry, retraction, discharge, eczematous changes, and erythema. Montgomery glands, which serve to lubricate the nipple and areola in breastfeeding, likely will be more prominent in pregnant and lactating women than others.

Palpation

After careful inspection, the provider should palpate the breast and regional lymph node basins with the patient in both an upright and supine position. The examiner should use the flat part of the fingers and support the breast with the contralateral hand; because of the nodularity and density of pregnant and lactating breasts, using the fingertips or pinching between two fingers for the examination can produce false-positive findings (Fig. 16.1). The upright position is best for assessing upper-outer-quadrant lesions, and the supine position reveals inframammary-fold lesions and other inferior lesions. The entire breast should be scanned with the flat of the provider's hand in either spiral, radial, concentric circle, or vertical patterns (Fig. 16.2). Palpation of the whole breast should be performed in an overlapping pattern with varying degrees of lighter and deeper pressure applied to survey the entire extent of the parenchyma. The examination should be extended superiorly to the clavicle, inferiorly to the lower rib cage, medially to the sternal border, and lateral to the midaxillary line. Masses, focal pain, and nipple discharge should be assessed.

The bilateral cervical, supraclavicular, and axillary nodes should be palpated. Enlarged axillary lymph nodes often are encountered in breastfeeding, but they should be mobile, soft, and generally <1 cm in size. They may be slightly tender, which is normal in pregnancy and lactation. Any concern for firm or immobile, matted lymph nodes should be further investigated with breast and axillary imaging, usually starting with an ultrasound.

Documentation

If the provider appreciates a concerning finding on the breast, the provider should document this by describing the size of the lesion, whether it is smooth or irregular and mobile or immobile, its location on the breast clockface, and the distance from the nipple. An examination of this documentation would include the following: "1.5 cm × 2.0 cm smooth, rubbery, mobile mass at 12:00, 3 cm from the nipple" (Fig. 16.3). Nipple discharge should be characterized by laterality, number of involved nipple orifices, discharge color, character, presence or absence of blood, and whether it is spontaneous.

Breast Imaging in Lactation

Breast imaging is an extension of the breast physical exam. Acute breastfeeding issues should resolve with proper intervention. Any persistent issue, such as an unrelieved plug, should be referred for breast imaging. Diagnostic imaging generally starts with a breast ultrasound and may or may not require a mammogram. Mammograms do not require interruption of breastfeeding and are safe; a bilateral mammogram results in 3 to 5 milligray (mGy) of radiation to the breasts, the equivalent of background radiation incurred over 2 months.[1] If recommended, breast magnetic resonance imaging (MRI) can also be performed without interruption of breastfeeding.[2]

Palpation patterns

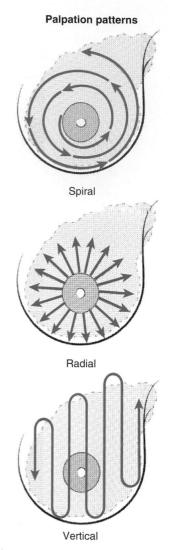

Spiral

Radial

Vertical

Fig. 16.2 Palpation patterns used in breast examination. The provider may palpate the breast in a spiral, radial, or vertical pattern, ensuring overlap in surface area covered and examination of tissues at varying depths.

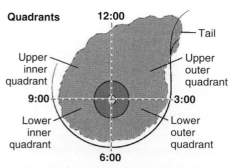

Fig. 16.3 Breast quadrants with superimposed clockface for examination reporting. Uniform documentation of the breast-examination findings includes size, description, location on the clockface, and distance from the nipple.

To reduce density from retained milk, mothers should express milk and drain the breasts fully before any breast-imaging examination.[3] If the radiologist recommends a breast biopsy of a concerning lesion, the mother should understand that this is safe without interruption of breastfeeding and that the incidence of milk fistula is <1.3% within 1 week of procedures.[4] Additionally, it should be noted that routine breast cancer screening in lactation is safe and should be considered in patients with a high-risk family history, a known gene mutation, or who otherwise meet screening guidelines because of age.[5]

ANATOMIC VARIANTS

Congenital variations in breast development may affect lactation.

Poland Syndrome

Poland syndrome is a unilateral anomaly of the pectoralis muscle, breast, NAC, axillary fold, subcutaneous tissue, ribs, and upper limb. Phenotype varies widely, with patients experiencing a spectrum from complete absence of a chest-wall structure to a more mildly asymmetric breast compared with the contralateral side. The thorax, breast, and NAC (TBN) classification helps identify these different phenotypes and the associated degree of hypoplasia. The most common anomaly in women is T1B1N2 (hypoplasia or aplasia of the pectoralis muscle and soft tissue with no rib or sternal defect; breast hypoplasia without aplasia; and NAC hypoplasia and dislocation without the absence of the NAC; Fig. 16.4).[6] Nearly 70% of defects present as right-sided rather than left-sided.[6] Women with asymmetric breasts and/or chest walls should be referred for prenatal counseling and close postpartum support because they may experience challenges with milk production on the affected side. Some of these women also may have undergone previous reconstructive surgery and present with the appearance of a normally developed breast. Therefore the surgical history should always be obtained.

Tubular Breast Deformity

No single definition or terminology exists for the broad category that is variably described as insufficient glandular tissue (IGT), hypoplastic breasts, or tuberous/tubular breast deformity. Many clinicians will utilize the term *IGT* to describe an anatomic phenomenon that includes the following: widely spaced breasts; lack of lower quadrant fullness; a fibrous, inelastic NAC; lack of or minimal breast growth during pregnancy; and lack of or minimal engorgement postpartum. Others will utilize *IGT* to describe breasts that are normal in anatomic appearance but otherwise do not experience normal gestational breast growth or postpartum engorgement and ultimately produce insufficient milk for the infant. It is likely that IGT represents variable clinical scenarios in which embryologic factors result in the development of anatomically abnormal breasts that produce insufficient milk, whereas reproductive and hormonal factors may affect the glandular tissue of anatomically normal-appearing breasts and their ability to produce sufficient milk.

A true tubular or tuberous breast deformity with an anatomically abnormal external appearance has an unknown etiology, although it has been theorized to result from embryologic

Poland syndrome

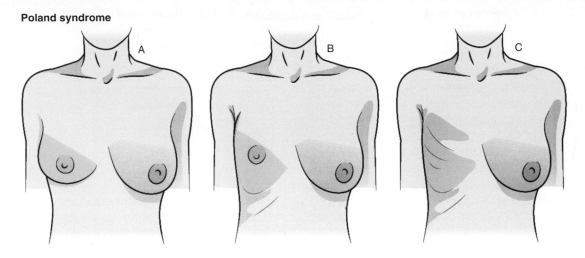

Fig. 16.4 Poland syndrome. Poland syndrome, a unilateral congenital chest wall deformity, presents as a spectrum from mild asymmetry and breast hypoplasia (A) to complete absence of the pectoralis muscle and breast parenchyma (C). The most common presentation includes hypoplasia of the pectoralis muscle, breast, and nipple-areolar complex (B).

failure of thoracic tissue differentiation or fascial maldevelopment. Histologically, these breasts demonstrate marked fibrosis in the glandular tissue and large concentrations of collagen and elastic fibers comprising a constrictive areolar ring.[7] Grossly, the breast resembles a cylindrical shape with an elongated, vertical appearance. Characteristics include parenchymal hypoplasia, superior malposition of the inframammary fold with decreased volume of the inferior breast skin, and herniation of breast glandular tissue through a constricted areolar-nipple complex (ANC) (Fig. 16.5).[8] Grolleau and colleagues developed the most widely accepted classification system, in which type I breasts are hypoplastic in the medial quadrant, type II in the bilateral inferior quadrants, and type III in all four quadrants.[9] As delineated by the classification system, a spectrum of disease exists, and very commonly, patients have asymmetrical breasts.

These patients exhibit variable challenges with breastfeeding. Most have reduced milk production that may improve with each subsequent pregnancy and lactation and may respond to galactagogues.[10] There is no definitive literature or management algorithm, and patients should be counseled during pregnancy and followed closely in the postpartum period. Additionally, many of these patients may have undergone plastic surgery procedures, such as augmentation mammaplasty, before pregnancy. Therefore, as described in the section on plastic surgery, providers should inquire about a patient's reason for undergoing plastic surgery in the past.

Ectodermal Dysplasia

Ectodermal dysplasias are a group of genetic disorders characterized by abnormal embryologic events resulting in malformations of ectodermal appendages, including the sweat glands, hair, nails, and teeth. Phenotype varies considerably and may include breast and/or NAC anomalies. Some individuals have breast hypoplasia, whereas others have amastia—either unilateral or bilateral—and the NAC may be normal, abnormal, or congenitally absent.[11] In a study of 38 women with ectodermal dysplasia, over half reported exceptionally flat nipples, whereas others had inverted nipples, and some had supernumerary nipples.[12] In addition, nearly all women had a paucity or complete lack of Montgomery glands. The majority of participants reported difficulty breastfeeding, and the primary reason for the difficulty was perceived to be flat nipples.[12] Multiple reconstructive surgery options exist for patients with ectodermal dysplasia affecting the breast.[11] However, these procedures are cosmetic in nature and do not improve the underlying developmental disorder affecting the glandular tissue.

Accessory Breast Tissue

Accessory breast tissue presents most commonly in the axilla, although it has been observed in multiple locations throughout the embryologic mammary ridge. It is most common in Native American and Asian populations and has an overall prevalence of approximately 2% to 6%.[13] This tissue can enlarge and become more cosmetically unappealing with each subsequent pregnancy and can also cause pain and chafing with bras. It is frequently engorged postpartum. Nonsteroidal antiinflammatory drugs (NSAIDs) and ice can relieve the pain of engorgement, and the tissue should involute if not stimulated or drained. It is possible for this tissue to develop mastitis and other infectious or inflammatory complications, which should be treated per protocol.[14] Accessory breast tissue can be managed with liposuction and/or surgical resection. However, unless the tissue is causing significant psychological or physical distress, resection should be deferred until childbearing is complete.

Supernumerary Nipples

Like accessory breast tissue, supernumerary nipples can present in any location along the mammary ridge and occur in up to 6% of the population.[15] They may present with a subtle, mole-like appearance or may appear with a full NAC with a

Tubular breast deformity

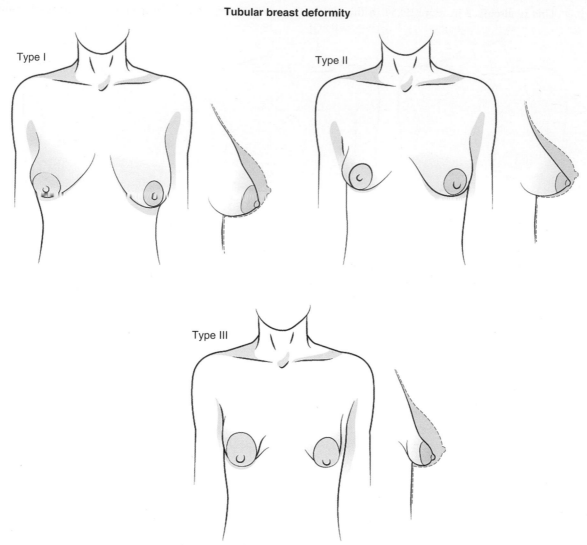

Fig. 16.5 Tubular breast deformity. Tubular breast deformity, a congenital deformity of breast development, presents as a spectrum from more mild hypoplasia and asymmetry to markedly decreased breast-base diameter and a large, fibrotic nipple-areolar complex with a restrictive ring. Hypoplasia may be mild *(left)*, moderate *(right)*, or severe *(bottom)*.

small amount of associated breast parenchyma. *Polythelia* describes an areola with an associated nipple; an isolated areola can present, but a nipple will never exist without an areola. They often enlarge during pregnancy and lactation and will involute if not stimulated. Removal of a small accessory NAC is a minor surgical procedure and may be reasonable to perform before childbearing.

Inverted Nipples

Nipple inversion occurs in approximately 3% to 10% of the population and likely results from congenital connective tissue tethering, failure of the lactiferous sinuses to lengthen, and failure of the complete growth of the mesenchyme. Alternatively, this condition may be acquired after surgery or the development of malignancy or breast infections.[16] Grade I inversions can be manually everted and maintain projection, grade II inversions

return promptly to the inverted position, and grade III inversions are invaginated and difficult to evert. Patients should be reassured that breastfeeding can be successful with flat or inverted nipples, and there are no data to support everting or otherwise "preparing" any nipple while pregnant for breastfeeding.[17,18] In fact, in a small randomized trial, women allocated to breast shells prenatally were less likely to initiate breastfeeding than women in the control group and less likely to be successfully breastfeeding at 6 weeks.[17] Four of the five women allocated to breast shells who decided not to initiate breastfeeding described problems wearing the shells as the reason.

Often, tethering bands may release naturally postpartum with breastfeeding and pumping. However, patient experience is variable, and some of the more tenacious inversions may never release. A history of a surgical procedure to evert the nipple may damage ducts, create scar tissue, and affect breastfeeding. This is discussed in more detail in the plastic surgery section, and it is not recommended that patients undergo this procedure before childbearing.

NIPPLE-AREOLAR COMPLEX

Anatomy

Collecting ducts in the 2-mm size range drain each breast segment and coalesce into 5- to 8-mm subareolar lactiferous sinuses (Fig. 16.6).[19] Most individuals have five to nine nipple orifices.[20] The areola includes sebaceous glands, apocrine glands, and hair follicles, and its pigmentation varies widely. There is minimal subcutaneous fat separating the NAC from the underlying breast parenchyma.[16]

Montgomery glands, also termed *Montgomery tubercles*, are modified sebaceous glands that serve to lubricate the nipple and areola and attract the infant to the breast. They enlarge during pregnancy and lactation.[21] Like other sebaceous glands, they can become obstructed and infected. Treatment involves a focal application of salicylic acid, warm compression, gentle expression, and drainage of any deeper abscess that has developed. If recurrently obstructed, women should avoid excessive use of nipple cream and other lubricants. They also should avoid continually stimulating and expressing the glands because this will potentiate additional drainage and/or hypertrophy and scarring. Aberrant milk drainage through a Montgomery gland is common and also should not be stimulated for similar reasons.

Morphology

Nipple morphology is widely variable with respect to diameter, protrusion, and contour (Fig. 16.7).[22] In the setting of nipple inversion or very small or flat nipples, shaping the NAC to enable a deep latch and milk transfer may be advisable. This can be done by compressing the breast and areola between two fingers with either a C, V, or scissor hold. The

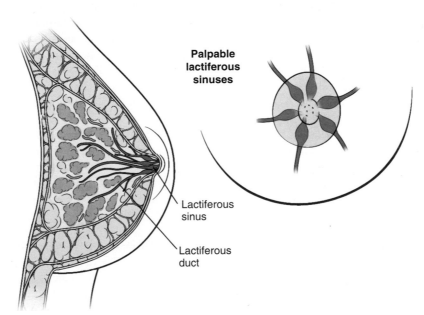

Fig. 16.6 Lactiferous sinuses. Lactiferous sinuses may dilate in the retroareolar region during lactogenesis, presenting as a palpable mass in pregnant or lactating women.

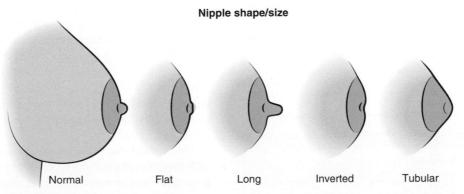

Fig. 16.7 Nipple morphology. Nipples exhibit wide variation in shape, size, and projection and may warrant individual approaches to optimal latch and positioning in each breastfeeding dyad.

laid-back or side-lying positions, particularly in the setting of very large breasts, also may enable a deeper infant latch. Breast shells are not advisable to attempt to evert a nipple because they may promote edema and restrict the pliability of the NAC. Ultimately, latch challenges are usually less related to the size and/or inversion of a nipple and more to the elasticity of the tissue.

Extremely large nipples may present a problem with a small infant or an infant with a small gape. Attempting to feed may result in gagging or inability to latch; in this case, a shield may taper and form the nipple into an acceptable shape and size for the infant. Manual expression and reverse-pressure softening, which soften the areola to make it more pliable before putting the infant to the breast, also may help. In situations of both large and small nipples, limited pre-breastfeeding use of an electric or manual pump may facilitate the infant's latch-on by drawing the nipple into a teat shape. Mothers with extremely large nipples and smaller infants initially may need to pump to maintain their milk production if the baby is not able to latch deeply into the breast parenchyma to transfer milk and/or stimulate maternal production.

Nipple Care

Excessive cleansing, whether prenatally or postpartum, can remove natural oils and predispose the skin to breakdown; patients should not use any drying agents such as antiseptics, alcohol, or saline.[23] Some women may choose to lubricate dry skin with nursing balms. Although this may not cause harm, women should be aware of potentially allergenic ingredients, such as lanolin and coconut, and tailor choice of balm accordingly (Box 16.2).

In the setting of trauma, nipples should be treated with moist, closed wound healing, as detailed later in the chapter. Following known principles of wound care, the nipples should not be soaked in saline, be rubbed with washcloths, undergo rigorous cleaning regimens with alcohol and other irritating drying products, or be "dried out." Gentian violet may produce tissue ulceration, and balms containing multiple products may result in dermatitis from allergens. Topical antifungals and other topical agents can worsen vasospasm. Breast shells designed to evert the nipple are not recommended because of the secondary edema they cause.

It should be noted that many women who exclusively pump without breastfeeding may develop a white crust on their nipples. This may be dried milk or may be related to biofilm production. Researchers have documented the variation in the milk microbiome that occurs with exclusive pumping.[24]

and it is possible that this crust is related to that phenomenon. Although further research is necessary in this area, patients who are asymptomatic, other than noting the appearance of this crust on the nipple, should be counseled that vigorous cleaning and/or attempts to remove this crust may produce nipple trauma and/or infection.

Nipple Shields

A nipple shield is a device made of silicone or latex that is worn over the nipple and areola while an infant is suckling. Shields differ from the shells designed to evert nipples. In addition, they should not be confused with breast-pump flanges. Nipple shields are associated with multiple complications, including mastitis, plugging, and significant reductions in milk production and transfer.[25] Many mothers have difficulty weaning infants off the nipple shield once it has been used regularly.[26]

Given these known complications, the breastfeeding dyad should undergo a thorough evaluation before the introduction of a nipple shield. Often, nipple shields are introduced when a small infant struggles to latch to a larger, pendulous breast. This may instead simply require adjustment of a position that is more amenable to feeding with large breasts, such as the laid-back or side-lying position. Infants also may refuse to latch when the flow of milk is very high; adjusting position also can address this issue without introducing nipple shields. Although nipple shields may be overused, there appear to be instances in which they can be helpful, such as when the infant is not able to latch at all, struggles to maintain a latch, or is causing severe maternal nipple discomfort. These situations may be seen in infant prematurity, tongue restrictions, severe maternal nipple inversions, infant hypotonia, or neurologic delay.

Pain

Up to 96% of mothers report nipple pain while breastfeeding.[27] Nipple pain occurs most commonly in the first week postpartum[27] and generally resolves within 1 to 2 weeks after appropriate intervention.[28] Nipple and breast pain are risk factors for early weaning and therefore warrant prompt attention and close follow-up.[29]

Persistent pain may represent a multitude of different etiologies, and treatment should be tailored to the specific diagnosis[29] (Box 16.3). Overall, suboptimal latch is the most common cause of nipple pain.[28] Other etiologies include trauma, vasospasm, dermatitis, and subacute mastitis, which are discussed individually in this section. It should be noted that because of the complex innervation of the breast and NAC, deeper breast pain may present as NAC pain or may present with concurrent deep breast pain and NAC pain. Similarly, NAC pain resulting from conditions such as vasospasm may radiate posteriorly into the breast (Fig. 16.8).

If a mother has resumed menstruation, she may notice increased sensitivity before her cycle. Mothers who become pregnant while breastfeeding also may experience new nipple and/or breast pain or increased sensitivity.

In the setting of tissue damage, principles of moist, closed wound healing should be followed, as detailed later in this

---

> ## BOX 16.2   Principles for Nipple Balms and Creams
>
> - Avoid petroleum-based ointments.
> - When possible, select single-ingredient agents to reduce the risk of allergic dermatitis.
> - Topical steroid use on the nipple should be time-limited to avoid skin atrophy.

BOX 16.3 Most Common Differential Diagnoses for Nipple and Breast Pain[a]

- Nipple conditions
  - Trauma from suboptimal latch and/or pump trauma
  - Vasospasm
  - Dermatitis
  - Subacute mastitis
  - Nipple bleb
  - Bacterial, fungal, or viral infections
- Breast conditions
  - Engorgement
  - Plugged ducts
  - Mastitis
  - Subacute mastitis
  - Functional/neuropathic pain
  - Musculoskeletal pain
  - Hormonal fluctuations with menstruation or pregnancy
  - Mondor's disease

[a] Because of the rich and complex innervation of the breast, pain originating in the nipple may radiate deep into the breast/chest wall, and the reverse may also be true. For more details about the workup of these differential diagnoses, see the University of North Carolina School of Medicine's nipple/breast pain algorithm: https://www.mombaby.org/wp-content/uploads/2016/04/PainProtocols.v3.pdf.

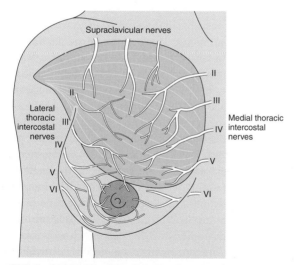

Fig. 16.8 Breast innervation. The breast parenchyma and nipple-areolar complex demonstrate rich, complex innervation patterns that reflect how patients can experience significant pain that radiates throughout the breast during lactation. Innervation largely arises from the medial and lateral branches of the thoracic intercostal nerves, as well as the supraclavicular nerves.

chapter. In brief, the nipples should be moistened with an oil-based lubricating nipple balm and covered with a nonstick dressing, such as hydrogel pads. When selecting a nipple balm, the potential for maternal allergic reactions to components such as lanolin or coconut should be considered. For severe pain in the setting of significant trauma, clinicians may utilize limited topical steroids. However, given the potential for steroids to affect healing, this approach should be individualized and monitored carefully.

Many ineffective and harmful treatments for traumatized nipples exist, and these should be avoided. A Cochrane systematic review concluded that there is insufficient evidence to recommend the "all-purpose nipple ointment" (also known as *APNO* or *triple-nipple cream*) or expressed breast milk for nipple pain in breastfeeding women.[27] Not only are superficial fungal and bacterial infections uncommon in the setting of breastfeeding, but antifungal and antibacterial creams and ointments often contain allergens that may incite dermatitis and worsen vasospasm symptoms. Expression of breast milk followed by air-drying may cause cracking and worsen trauma. Cool, wet tea bags and warm compresses can potentiate skin breakdown. The use of ice theoretically may interfere with the let-down reflex.

When a patient is experiencing significant nipple and/or breast pain, clinicians also may recommend that a patient stop breastfeeding and pump or hand-express instead. This approach should be considered cautiously because pumping can result in additional problems, such as plugging, mastitis, reduction in milk production or stimulation of overproduction, and disinterest of the baby in returning to the breast. If absolutely necessary, hand-expression may represent the most efficacious solution to resting sore nipples.

Overall, we emphasize that the specific etiology of the patient's symptoms should be identified through careful history and examination of the breastfeeding dyad. Once all treatable etiologies have been ruled out, persistent idiopathic pain may require continued support and reexamination of the dyad and continued attention to latch and positioning. As described in the section on mastalgia, patients may benefit from pharmacologic interventions, such as NSAIDs, propranolol, and antidepressants.[29] Persistent pain should be recognized as multifactorial, requiring an integrated treatment approach that addresses not only biological but also psychosocial aspects of pain.[30] Counseling, physiotherapy massage, acupuncture, and other complementary and alternative medicine practices may therefore be helpful.[30]

Trauma

Trauma most commonly results from improper latch, ankyloglossia, unrelieved engorgement, and improperly fitting flanges or pumping on high suction. Providers also should ascertain what interventions patients may have undertaken on their own that could potentiate trauma and/or allergy. This includes soaps, oils, ointments, lubricants, and medications that can cause ulcerations (e.g., gentian violet).

Latch or pump trauma may demonstrate characteristic patterns on the nipple. Scabbing may align with the position causing harm (e.g., horizontally across the nipple for football hold, vertical for cross-cradle or cradle). Cracks at the base of the nipple may result from sucking of the lower lip or biting. Circumferential cracks at the nipple base may occur from pumping with flanges that are either too small or too large or from correctly sized flanges in the setting of excessive suction. When deep fissures have developed, beginning to nurse on the less painful side first may permit the initial let-down to occur with less pain. Then the infant can be put carefully to the affected breast, with attention to using a position that redistributes the pressure of suckling on the nipple.

The normal human wound healing time is 8 to 10 days for reepithelization after traumatic insult.[31] Some patients will question how nipple trauma can heal when an infant continues to stimulate the nipple frequently. The lactating breast and NAC are highly vascular (Fig. 16.9) and therefore heal well, even in the setting of continued breastfeeding. With trauma, patients should apply the principles of wound healing, which include keeping the wound lubricated with an oil-based emollient cream or ointment and keeping it closed or covered with nonstick gauze or hydrogel pads. Wounds with significant exudate and seepage may benefit from polyurethane matrix pads to provide both closed wound healing and absorptive capacity. It is recommended that patients adhere to a regimen both day and night, similar to keeping a burn wound closed at all times, to enable optimal uninterrupted moist wound healing. No drying agents or drying of the nipple should occur. Some wounds respond well to medical-grade honey, which is irradiated and therefore does not pose a risk of botulism to infants who may ingest small amounts. Open wounds should not be closed with suture or surgical glue because they are not clean and therefore at high risk for wound infection. Instead, these wounds should heal following the principles of closure by secondary intention. Additionally, suture material or surgical glue may pose harm to the breastfeeding infant.

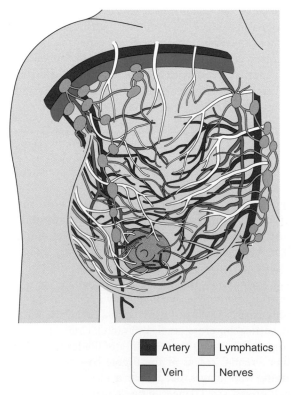

■ Artery	▨ Lymphatics		
■ Vein	□ Nerves		

Fig. 16.9 Vascular and lymphatic systems of the breast. The lactating breast is highly vascular and has a robust lymphatic drainage system. Microvascular injury and edema are common in excessively deep massage.

Vasospasm

Vasospasm is a painful cutaneous vasoconstriction that presents with hardening of the nipple and color changes on a spectrum from white to blue to red. Because of the complex innervation of the breast (see Fig. 16.8), pain can focus in the nipple or radiate deep into the breast and may last for over 30 minutes. Pain is often the worst after the baby unlatches or the mother finishes pumping. It also may present when the mother moves from a warm environment to a cooler environment, such as leaving the shower or pool, going from indoors to outdoors in the winter, or transitioning from warm weather to air conditioning. Alternatively, vasospasm may occur with no apparent trigger.

Nipple vasospasm occurs in approximately one-fifth of breastfeeding women and may be more common in those with a history of Raynaud's phenomenon of the fingers.[32] Secondary vasospasm may occur following trauma to the nipples. Persistent vasospasm can result in a cycle that potentiates trauma as a result of vasoconstriction and inability to heal in the setting of chronic ischemia. Maternal ingestion of vasoconstrictive products, including caffeine, may worsen vasospasm, and nicotine can also contribute to symptoms.[33] Mammary blood vessels are exquisitely sensitive to epinephrine and norepinephrine. Although fewer data exist regarding serotonin and PGF_{20C} as vasoconstrictive agents, it is possible they also may play a role.[34−36]

Treatment of vasospasm involves resolving any underlying persistent trauma, such as improper latch and positioning. As stated earlier, women with larger breasts and/or a history of breast augmentation may benefit from laid-back or side-lying nursing positions to enable deeper latch and reduce trauma from superficial latch. Patients should keep their NACs warm at all times with pads made of wool, fleece, or other insulated fiber. For additional warmth, they may place heating pads or reusable heated products, such as microwaveable rice packs or hand warmers, on top of the pads; these products should not be applied directly to the skin because of the risk of burns. As with healing trauma, these products should be used both night and day. Some women benefit from calcium, magnesium, and fish oil supplements.[32] Women who fail to respond to conservative measures may be recommended to use calcium-channel-blocker agents, such as nifedipine, under the guidance of a medical professional.[33]

Nipple Blebs

Often described as a "white dot" or a "scab," nipple blebs are inflammatory lesions on the surface of the nipple and can cause exquisite pain with latch. They can also cause obstruction of milk flow through the nipple orifice and may present with concurrent acute mastitis. Blebs have no association with candida. Nipple blebs may be solitary and unilateral, or they may present on multiple orifices bilaterally. They generally are 1 mm or less in diameter but at times may grow larger. If repeatedly traumatized with unroofing, they can develop associated reactive tissue and/or scarring and appear larger and more fleshy. Infants may release a superficial bleb while nursing, or more tenacious blebs may persist regardless of interventions. Blebs are often associated with hyperlactation, subacute mastitis/dysbiosis, pumping, and localized plugging.[37]

Despite the morbidity blebs confer to the nursing dyad, little published data exist regarding etiology, prevalence, and management. O'Hara described, in a five-patient cohort, that bleb histology showed signs of inflammation, including histiocytes with foamy cytoplasmic vacuoles and fibrin deposition.[38] This led to the conclusion that mid-potency topical steroids were likely to be helpful in resolving blebs. Other providers have utilized sunflower lecithin by mouth to emulsify milk and treat underlying ductal plugging.[39] If subacute mastitis/dysbiosis and/or hyperlactation is contributing to the development of multiple bilateral blebs, the treatment algorithms for those conditions should be followed. Regardless of additional treatments pursued, topical steroid cream may reduce the tenacity and pain of the bleb. In acutely obstructing situations, health care providers should unroof the bleb using a sterile 18-gauge needle, approaching the nipple parallel to the surface of the bleb. A nipple orifice should never be probed directly with a needle or other traumatic device, and patients should not be encouraged to perform this at home, because continued trauma can potentiate scarring and worsening of symptoms.

It should be noted that blebs are different from the sucking blister that appears early in lactation and results from vigorous suckling, malposition, or high pump suction. This type of blister covers a larger area, appears more vesicular with a thin membrane and underlying fluid, and is not associated with underlying ductal plugging.

Subacute Mastitis

Subacute mastitis, also known as *breast dysbiosis*, represents an imbalance of the breast flora akin to bacterial vaginosis. These patients may present with a history of previously treated recurrent acute mastitis. There may be superimposed hyperlactation and painful nipple blebs, and patients may be exclusively pumping.[37] Patients often describe deep, burning breast pain; feelings of fullness; and painful nipples and latch. A white biofilm may be present on the surface of the nipple. This constellation of signs and symptoms is often misdiagnosed as mammary candidiasis, which is not supported by microbiologic evidence.[40]

Evaluation includes performing a sterile breast-milk culture to tailor the antibiotic choice. Although this culture may often grow a coagulase-negative *Staphylococcus* or *Streptococcus* species, it also may fail to grow any organism.[40] A case series documented that patients can undergo empiric treatment with extended antibiotics that target chronic, intracellular infections, such as azithromycin.[41] In more mild cases, probiotics directed at the breast flora (as described in the section on acute mastitis) may resolve pain; however, no published data on this approach exist. Sunflower lecithin may be used to reduce plugging. Hyperlactation should be addressed and treated.

Dermatitis

Dermatitis of the nipples, areolae, and breasts presents as a red, burning, flaking rash. These skin changes classically start on the areola and may migrate to the nipple, whereas Pagetoid changes present oppositely. Often, patients are misdiagnosed with a "yeast infection" when, in fact, the etiology of their symptoms is dermatitis. Atopic dermatitis is seen in women predisposed to eczema. Irritant contact dermatitis results from topical agents, detergents, clothing, or soaps contacting the skin. Allergic contact dermatitis is a delayed hypersensitivity reaction to an allergen contained in a product used. Common allergens include petroleum, lanolin, coconut, and Bacitracin and the emollients contained in creams, lotions, or ointments. Pump parts, nursing bras, nursing pads (particularly those made of wool, which confer the risk of cross-reaction in women with a lanolin allergy), new detergents or soaps, and nipple shields can also cause allergy. Providers should investigate what an infant may be ingesting that may be allergenic to the mother; this can include antibiotics and complementary foods. Allergens should be eliminated. A short course of moderate-potency steroid rubbed sparingly into the area after each feeding will clear a persistent case in a few days. Rarely, an oral course of corticosteroids may be indicated for women whose symptoms are refractory to a 2-week course of topical steroid therapy.[42] Although limited clinical data are reassuring that oral antihistamines may not affect milk production in most women,[43] providers should exercise caution and advise patients to watch for changes in output, particularly those with lower baseline milk production.[44] Newer, nonsedating antihistamines are preferred because they have little or no anticholinergic activity, and single-agent therapies are preferred to combination drugs.[44]

Bacterial, Fungal, and Viral Infections

Although any concurrent or superimposed superficial skin infection should be considered, this represents a rare scenario in breastfeeding. The lactating breast and NAC are highly vascular and therefore heal well and are unlikely to develop a deep-seated superficial soft tissue infection.

Bacterial

Staphylococcus aureus is the most common cause of soft tissue infections of the NAC or breast skin in lactation.[42] Oral antibiotics appear to more effective than topical antibiotics in relieving symptoms and preventing mastitis, but it is unclear whether this is more attributable to antimicrobial or antiinflammatory properties.[45]

Fungal

The most common superficial fungal infection of the skin of the lactating breast is *Candida* intertrigo, which presents as a pruritic, beefy-red rash with satellite lesions located in the inframammary folds.[46] *Candida* infections of the NAC represent an extremely uncommon clinical scenario, with no scientific data to support this diagnosis.[40] Neither visual assessment of the NAC nor the presence of diaper rash and oral thrush in the infant are sensitive for the diagnosis of nipple or breast fungal infections.[40] In the rare case of culture-proven invasive intraductal *Candida*, both members of the breastfeeding dyad require treatment to clear the infection. Treatment options include topical antifungals, oral fluconazole, and gentian violet. The latter bears risks of skin irritation and ulceration, as well as mucosal irritation in the infant.[42]

Viral

Herpes simplex infection of the NAC presents as a cluster of tender vesicles. The virus can pass between mother and nursling and can be dangerous to neonates with immature immune systems under 3 months of age.[45] If a neonate under the age of 3 months presents with suspected neonatal herpes, the infant should undergo blood and cerebrospinal fluid testing for herpes simplex virus (HSV) polymerase chain reaction (PCR) to confirm the diagnosis and begin empiric treatment with acyclovir until the PCR results are returned.[47] Diagnosis in the mother can be confirmed using a culture, Tzanck smear, serology, or PCR assay.

Mothers with a herpes outbreak undergo treatment with a 5- to 7-day course of acyclovir, which is safe in lactation.[42] If a mother experiences a herpes outbreak on one breast, she can continue to express and discard the milk to maintain milk production.[48] However, she should keep this breast covered until the lesions scab over, and the infant should nurse only from the unaffected breast. There is no recommendation for routine suppression in breastfeeding mothers with a history of herpes simplex virus 1 (HSV-1) to prevent transmission to infants.

The varicella-zoster virus remains dormant in the nerve tissue of individuals with a history of chickenpox. Reactivation of the virus results in herpes zoster, a contagious vesicular rash in a dermatomal distribution. Until lesions are crusted over, women with vesicles on the NAC should avoid breastfeeding from the affected breast.[49] During that time, milk should be expressed to maintain production but is not safe to feed to the infant.

Verruca vulgaris, or viral warts, develop after the human papillomavirus infects epithelial or mucosal cells. Warts less commonly present on the breast and/or NAC than other skin surfaces. However, if a wart develops on the areola, mothers ideally should treat before breastfeeding with topical salicylic acid, cryotherapy, or laser therapy.[50] Very large warts with unusual features may require surgical excision for diagnosis and to rule out malignant transformation.

Nipple Conditions That May Be Related to Atypia and/or Malignancy
Nipple Discharge

Up to 24% of pregnant and lactating women may experience bilateral rusty or bloody discharge that is secondary to physiologic increases in vascularity.[51] This should resolve spontaneously within 1 to 2 weeks of delivery and has been termed *rusty pipe syndrome*.[52] Providers evaluating an infant presenting with bloody emesis should obtain a maternal history of bloody discharge or milk. Persistent unilateral single-duct bloody or clear discharge represents a scenario more concerning for an intraductal lesion such as papilloma or cancer and requires imaging with breast ultrasound and/or mammogram.[5,53] Mothers with hyperlactation or those taking blood-thinning medications may also experience transient bloody

milk. These cases should be evaluated carefully with history and examination and also may warrant imaging. *Serratia marcesans* also has been demonstrated to turn expressed milk pink, and this should be considered.[54]

Nipple Adenoma

Nipple adenoma, also known as *erosive adenomatosis of the nipple* (EAN) or *nipple papillomatosis*, is characterized by nipple nodularity and can progress to erosion. It is more common in middle-aged women and may mimic Paget's disease, although it generally is a benign lesion not associated with atypia.[55] Any nipple disorders not resolving with proper intervention should be referred for further evaluation with a breast surgeon. Biopsy is often performed to confirm diagnosis, and treatment generally consists of excision, which may be able to be deferred if the lesion is not interfering with breastfeeding.

Paget's Disease

Paget's disease presents most commonly in postmenopausal women and comprises 0.5% to 5% of all breast malignancies.[56] The scaling, ulcerating skin changes of Paget's disease represent malignant cells that have migrated from the ducts to surface presentation and are associated with underlying preinvasive or invasive cancer. Pagetoid changes begin on the nipple and migrate to the areola, in contrast to dermatitis. Early Paget's presents with a red, shiny nipple and progresses to a more roughened, flattened nipple with surrounding scaly erythema. Late disease demonstrates complete loss of the nipple and associated ulceration of the skin. Suspected Paget's disease should be referred to a breast surgeon, who will obtain appropriate imaging and undertake treatment that may include surgery and adjuvant therapy.

Miscellaneous
Psoriasis

Psoriasis of the nipple appears as a well-demarcated plaque. Lactation may provoke a psoriatic flare in women with a history of this autoimmune condition, possibly as a result of skin irritation or microtrauma from breastfeeding. Treatment options include topical steroids, ultraviolet phototherapy, immunomodulators, and biologic agents; however, methotrexate is not recommended in lactation.[42]

Dermal Cysts

Sebaceous cysts and epidermal inclusion cysts (EICs) present uncommonly on the breast. These smooth subcutaneous nodules may be difficult to distinguish by physical examination; however, EICs more frequently occur in women with a history of breast procedures or trauma[57] and tend to present in a periareolar location.[58] Nipple-areolar dermal cysts can be repeatedly traumatized by a nursing infant and may become painful. If this occurs, warm compresses and/or antibiotics may be indicated. If diagnosed prenatally, surgical excision under local anesthesia may prevent future trauma, pain, and infection while breastfeeding. Given that cysts are superficial dermal lesions, excision should not affect the underlying ductal tissue or nipple orifices, although attention should be given to careful placement of the incision, closure, and suture type. Nonabsorbable suture produces less tissue reaction and scarring and would be an ideal choice in this circumstance.

Hyperkeratosis

Hyperkeratosis is a thickening of the stratum corneum, the outer layer of skin, and is usually associated with an abnormal quality of keratin. Breastfeeding is possible with hyperkeratosis.[59] To reduce the thickening before breastfeeding, pregnant women should utilize a keratolytic moisturizer (containing urea or lactic acid) or Calcitrene (a synthetic derivative of vitamin D).[60] Laser treatment, cryotherapy, and topical steroids represent alternative treatment strategies.[59]

Leiomyoma

Leiomyoma, a benign tumor comprised of smooth muscle cells, rarely occurs on the breast. When it does present, it most often occurs on the areola because of the presence of smooth muscle fibers. Like other lesions on the NAC, larger leiomyomas may interfere with latch, and treatment is excision. They rarely recur.[61]

Skin Tags (Squamous Papillomas)

Skin tags occurring on the NAC may enlarge with pregnancy and present an issue with postpartum latch. If concerning, they can be excised under local anesthesia during pregnancy. A nonabsorbable suture should be used to reduce tissue reaction and scarring, and a surgical glue may be used for smaller lesions that do not necessitate formal closure with suture.

Lentigo and Seborrheic Keratoses

Lentigo and seborrheic keratosis commonly occur around the NAC and breast and do not present difficulty with breastfeeding unless enlarging in the area where an infant may latch. Any concerning or changing lesions should be referred for dermatologic evaluation.

Hidradenitis Suppurativa

Hidradenitis suppurativa is a chronic inflammatory skin condition of hair-bearing regions of the body. The pathophysiology remains unknown, but it appears to involve obstruction of hair follicles and/or apocrine glands leading to inflammation and secondary infection. It can occur in the axillae, inframammary folds, and periareolar region.[46] Mild cases present as papules, whereas severe cases include nodules, abscesses, fistulae, sinus tracts, and scarring. Treatment includes laser hair removal, antibiotics, corticosteroid injections, and surgical excision.[46] There is no contraindication for breastfeeding with this condition.

OBSTRUCTIVE AND INFLAMMATORY CONDITIONS

Breast engorgement with milk stasis may lead to ductal plugging. If this plugging is unrelieved, noninfectious mastitis may develop. Alternatively, a persistent plug may form a discrete milk-retention cyst, termed *galactocele*. If the obstructed milk remains persistently undrained and bacterial overgrowth results, noninfectious mastitis may progress to infectious mastitis. Severe inflammation and bacterial overgrowth in the setting of mastitis can lead to phlegmon or lactational abscess. This section reviews the spectrum of these obstructive and inflammatory conditions in the lactating breast (Fig. 16.10).

Engorgement

Engorgement is common in the prenatal and early postpartum periods and may occur at other times when regular milk removal is interrupted. Up to 75% of women experience engorgement in the first few weeks after delivery.[62] Engorgement of the breast in the early postpartum period involves three elements: (1) accumulation of milk, (2) hypervascularity and venous congestion, and (3) edema secondary to the swelling and obstruction of drainage of the lymphatic system. Engorgement should be differentiated from gigantomastia of pregnancy, mastitis, and hyperlactation, which are discussed in other sections. It should be noted that engorgement can produce dependent edema and symmetric erythema in the inferior aspects of the breast. Treatment includes frequent and effective removal of breast milk, lymphatic massage (Fig. 16.11), and support of the breasts.[63]

Physiologic engorgement generally peaks on postpartum day 5.[64] Patients should not pump to empty their breasts to relieve engorgement because this may stimulate supraphysiologic milk production and worsen the cycle. Hand-expression or hand-pump use to remove 1 to 2 ounces to relieve pressure may represent the most efficacious management. Although individual success with acupuncture and massage has been reported, no large-scale studies support the use of cabbage-leaf treatment.[62,65] Therapeutic ultrasound may be of use for relieving pain and decreasing inflammation.[66] These supportive interventions are critical because the Infant Feeding Practices Study II demonstrated that 23.9% of mothers who had stopped breastfeeding in less than a month reported feeling too full or engorged.[67]

In addition to breast engorgement, the NAC and accessory breast tissue in the axilla can also become engorged. To improve deep latch and milk transfer in the setting of NAC engorgement, reverse-pressure softening techniques should be applied (Fig. 16.12).[68] Nipple shells, which potentiate obstruction and edema, should be avoided. A supportive bra should be worn to reduce breast and NAC edema.

Hyperlactation

Hyperlactation or "hypergalactia" is the production of milk in excess of what an infant needs and often contributes to engorgement, plugging, and other obstructive and inflammatory breast conditions. Hyperlactation may be iatrogenic or idiopathic. Iatrogenic hyperlactation can be caused by early and excessive pumping, such as can be seen when mothers are separated from their premature infants in the neonatal intensive care unit. It also may be caused by purposeful or inadvertent consumption of galactogogues. When these causes have been ruled out or treated, idiopathic hyperlactation is likely.

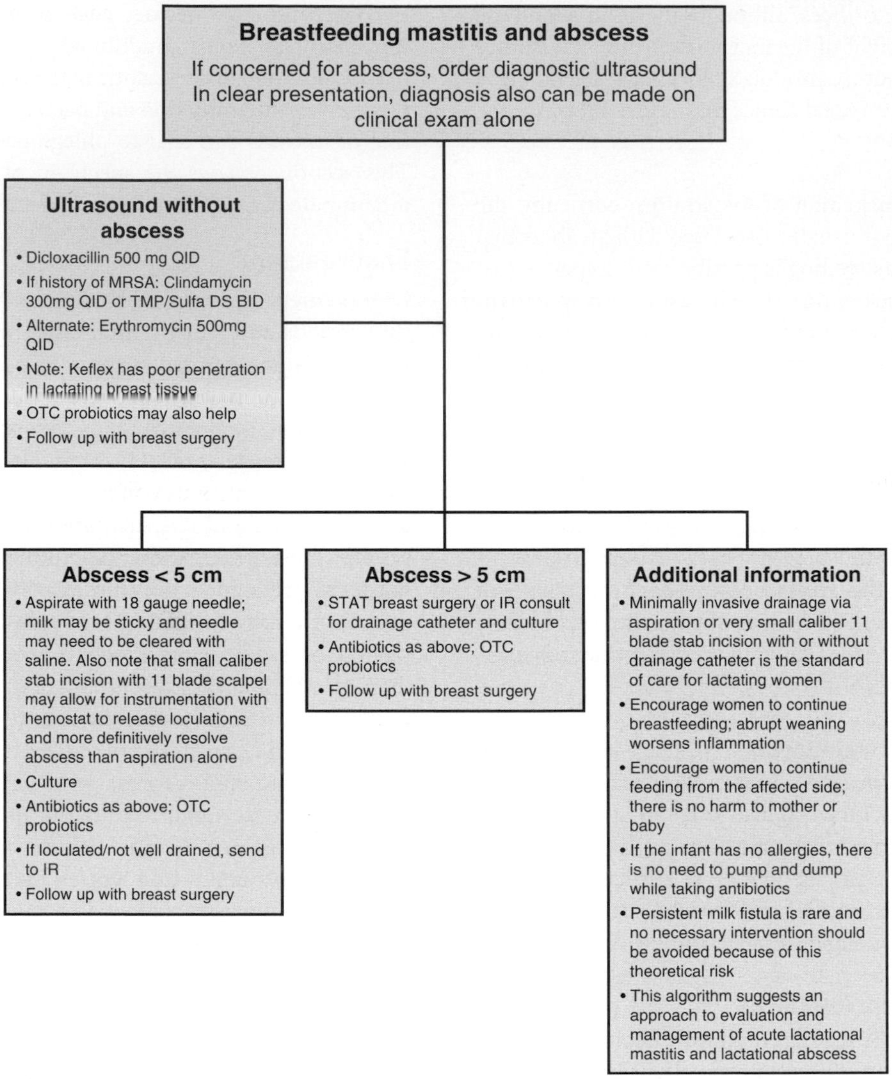

Breastfeeding mastitis and abscess

If concerned for abscess, order diagnostic ultrasound
In clear presentation, diagnosis also can be made on
clinical exam alone

Ultrasound without abscess

• Dicloxacillin 500 mg QID
• If history of MRSA: Clindamycin 300mg QID or TMP/Sulfa DS BID
• Alternate: Erythromycin 500mg QID
• Note: Keflex has poor penetration in lactating breast tissue
• OTC probiotics may also help
• Follow up with breast surgery

Abscess < 5 cm

• Aspirate with 18 gauge needle; milk may be sticky and needle may need to be cleared with saline. Also note that small caliber stab incision with 11 blade scalpel may allow for instrumentation with hemostat to release loculations and more definitively resolve abscess than aspiration alone
• Culture
• Antibiotics as above; OTC probiotics
• If loculated/not well drained, send to IR
• Follow up with breast surgery

Abscess > 5 cm

• STAT breast surgery or IR consult for drainage catheter and culture
• Antibiotics as above; OTC probiotics
• Follow up with breast surgery

Additional information

• Minimally invasive drainage via aspiration or very small caliber 11 blade stab incision with or without drainage catheter is the standard of care for lactating women
• Encourage women to continue breastfeeding; abrupt weaning worsens inflammation
• Encourage women to continue feeding from the affected side; there is no harm to mother or baby
• If the infant has no allergies, there is no need to pump and dump while taking antibiotics
• Persistent milk fistula is rare and no necessary intervention should be avoided because of this theoretical risk
• This algorithm suggests an approach to evaluation and management of acute lactational mastitis and lactational abscess

Fig. 16.10 Sample treatment algorithm for breastfeeding mastitis and abscess. This algorithm suggests an approach to evaluation and management of acute lactational mastitis and lactational abscess. *BID,* Twice daily; *IR,* interventional radiology; *OTC,* over the counter; *QID,* four times daily.

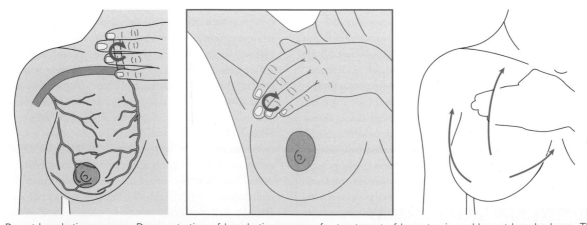

Fig. 16.11 Breast lymphatic massage. Demonstration of lymphatic massage for treatment of breast pain and breast lymphedema. The patient or provider begins with 10 gentle circles at the junction of the internal jugular and subclavian veins. Next, she performs 10 gentle circles in the axillary lymph node region. She then gently sweeps the skin from the nipple-areolar complex to the clavicular and axillary region. This sweeping motion involves very light pressure to lift the skin and allow surface lymphatics to decompress excessive fluid from the breast.

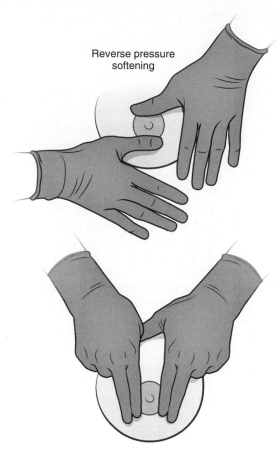

Reverse pressure softening

Fig. 16.12 Reverse-pressure softening. The technique of reverse-pressure softening involves using the fingers to gently compress, in a rotating fashion, all quadrants of the areolar tissue for a minute or two per position. This decreases areolar edema to enable deep, atraumatic infant latch in the setting of engorgement.

Hyperlactation may present with a combination of maternal and infant symptomatology. The breasts may be continuously engorged or painful, and mothers may experience frequent plugging, mastitis, and nipple blebs. Infants may cough, choke, and release the breast when feeding. The presentation may also be more subtle. The infant may not coordinate suck and swallow and may be diagnosed with reflux. Some infants may develop an oral aversion, oral "defensiveness," or sensitive mouth. Because of the large volume of milk, and therefore lactose, some infants develop diarrhea.[69] Because of the fussing, choking, and colicky behavior, pediatricians may diagnose allergy. The mother may be placed on a restricted diet, beginning with dairy products, but the infant usually fails to improve. A situation involving potential hyperlactation well demonstrates the need for careful evaluation of the breastfeeding dyad rather than the mother or infant alone.

Academy of Breastfeeding Medicine (ABM) Protocol 32 summarizes the management of hyperlactation,[70] which begins with eliminating excessive pumping and galactogogues to address any *iatrogenic* component of the presentation. The first intervention with *idiopathic* hyperlactation involves block feeding under close physician supervision. If block feeding does not improve symptoms significantly, the mother can progress to the use of herbal supplements, such as sage, and/

or pharmacologic agents, such as pseudoephedrine. After 6 weeks postpartum, estrogen-containing oral contraceptives can be considered. Extreme cases may require as-needed individual doses of 0.25 to 0.5 mg cabergoline every 3 days.

Plugging

A breast plug represents a focal area of obstructed milk in a specific segment of the breast that follows a ductal distribution. Plugs generally last less than 24 hours and can be quite painful; because it is a localized phenomenon, no systemic symptoms exist as they do with mastitis. Patients with hyperlactation often experience plugging, although patients with average or even low milk supply also may experience plugging. Mothers may report plugging after an infant sleeps longer than usual or when they return to work or school and are separated from the infant for extended periods of time. Other risk factors for plugging include pump usage because pumps do not empty the breast as effectively and dynamically as an infant and may stimulate milk production without adequate removal. Nipple shields may increase plugging because they also may result in inadequate emptying of the breast.[71] Milk rich in fatty acids may be more prone to obstruction. Recurrent plugging also may present in the setting of subacute mastitis/breast dysbiosis, an imbalance of the microbiome that may predispose to plugging as a result of bacterial overgrowth.[37]

If a mother experiences a plug, she should apply moist heat to the area of concern. She should avoid excessive massage because this can traumatize tissue and lead to phlegmon development.[72] Gentle lymphatic massage, as illustrated previously, is helpful in reducing the pain and edema associated with plugs. The mother should breastfeed and minimize unnecessary pumping. Therapeutic ultrasound treatments, which reduce inflammation and edema, have been demonstrated to relieve plugs.[73] Other therapies include prophylaxis with oral sunflower lecithin supplementation and *Phytolacca* (poke root) for acute plug relief. The mechanism of these agents is unknown, although it appears lecithin may emulsify breast milk, and *Phytolacca* likely has antiinflammatory effects. A recanalization manual therapy method that involves techniques of traditional Chinese medicine has been reported to relieve plugged ducts. However, because of the potential for traumatizing the breast, this technique should only be performed by a certified practitioner.[74] Any plug or mass persisting for several days and not resolving with conservative interventions requires referral to a medical provider, who may obtain breast imaging to rule out galactocele and/or other mass. A case of recurrent plugged ducts was reported to be associated with selective immunoglobulin A deficiency.[75]

Mastitis

Mastitis occurs in 3% to 20% of all breastfeeding mothers.[14] Risk factors include primiparity, breast-pump usage, nipple-shield usage, previous history of mastitis, and nipple trauma.[76] Mastitis generally presents with focal breast pain associated with erythema and warmth. Women may or may not feel systemically ill. Systemic signs and symptoms include malaise, myalgias, headache, fatigue, fever, and tachycardia. On physical exam, providers may appreciate erythema and edema in a ductal distribution or retroareolar location. Retroareolar mastitis is common because the coalescence of ducts near the nipple affords the opportunity for milk stasis, bacterial overgrowth, and obstruction. Nipple trauma may be present.

In the early stages of obstruction, mastitis may represent a pure inflammatory phenomenon without superimposed infection. If the obstruction is relieved in a timely fashion, usually within 24 hours, antibiotic therapy may not be required. If the obstruction and inflammation progress, antibiotic therapy is indicated. The antibiotic therapy treats the bacterial overgrowth and helps relieve the obstruction via antiinflammatory effects. Most antibiotics are safe in lactation, and breastfeeding should not be interrupted (Box 16.4). Clinicians can consult online resources such as the National Institute of Health's LactMed database regarding any specific questions related to antibiotics. Breast-milk culture can be utilized in cases of recurrent mastitis or where a resistant organism is suspected. Probiotics directed at the breast flora may reduce the risk of recurrent mastitis; however, current evidence is limited.[77]

Management of mastitis is detailed in ABM Protocol 4.[14] For both noninfectious and infectious mastitis, providers should encourage continued breastfeeding on the affected breast, which will assist in relieving infection, obstruction, and inflammation. Abrupt weaning produces an inflammatory response that will worsen mastitis. Other management strategies include antiinflammatory medications, analgesics, heat or ice packs, lymphatic massage, and therapeutic ultrasound.

Untreated mastitis may progress to abscess formation,[79] and excessive massage in the setting of mastitis may result in lactational phlegmon.[72] Mastitis also can result in reduced milk production and an increase in the sodium content of breast milk as a result of lower volumes, leading the infant to possibly reject the breast. The infant also may reject an engorged and edematous nipple in the setting of retroareolar mastitis. Therefore timely management of mastitis is critical in protecting the breastfeeding dyad relationship.

Abscess

Of women who experience mastitis, 3% to 11% will progress to abscess.[80] Abscesses often occur in the retroareolar location as a result of the convergence of ducts, stasis, bacterial overgrowth, and a decrease in effective milk removal once edema, obstruction, and inflammation develop. If the abscess has progressed to a focal, walled-off, infected fluid collection without surrounding erythema, the patient may not experience any systemic symptoms. On exam, the patient will present with a focal fluctuant, edematous, and erythematous fluid collection. Most often, these are superficial and may drain spontaneously if not promptly treated with controlled drainage. Deeper abscesses are less common but often still present with surface erythema and induration. Ultrasound can help diagnose abscess and differentiate from phlegmon but is not required for diagnosis because clinical signs and symptoms are often characteristic.[72]

Smaller abscesses of less than 5 cm may be amenable to aspiration with an 18-gauge needle, whereas abscesses larger than 5 cm likely will require a small drain placement. These drains can be placed by surgeons or radiologists and are often inserted under ultrasound guidance. Open incision and drainage in the operating room no longer represents the standard of care for treatment of abscesses in lactation.[81] Likewise, surgical packing in the lactating breast should be avoided because this potentiates inflammation, delays healing, and causes pain, and the packing immediately becomes soaked with breast milk. However, a very small stab incision using an 11-blade scalpel produces the same defect as a percutaneous drain and enables the surgeon to break up loculations within an abscess cavity.[72] Fig. 16.13 illustrates the difference between a simple abscess and a loculated abscess containing multiple septated fluid collections. This approach can be easily performed in the clinic setting and may provide more definitive management than aspiration alone, which may require more than one aspiration. Unlike abscesses in other parts of the body, breast milk mixed with purulent fluid can become inspissated and difficult to drain with a needle. It should be noted that no drain in the setting of lactational abscess treatment should be placed on suction because this will promote breast-milk flow through the drain rather than passive removal of purulent fluid. Drains should be placed to gravity alone and removed within 3 to 5 days. As with mastitis, patients should avoid breast-pump usage and should continue breastfeeding from the affected breast. Patients do not need to discard milk. Targeted antibiotic therapy based on culture results is also warranted. Although agents and dosages generally will follow those outlined in Box 16.4, providers may continue a more extended course based on individual patient presentation.

Galactocele

Galactoceles are true milk-retention cysts that develop from unrelieved plugging during lactation or after cessation of

---

BOX 16.4 Recommended Antibiotic Regimens for Acute Infectious Lactational Mastitis

First Line

Dicloxacillin or flucloxacillin 500 mg by mouth four times per day for 10 to 14 days

Methicillin-Resistant *Staphylococcus aureus* Coverage

Refer to institutional/community antibiograms for local resistance patterns

Clindamycin 300 mg by mouth four times per day for 10 to 14 days

Trimethoprim/sulfamethoxazole DS 160mg/800 mg by mouth twice per day for 10 to 14 days; avoid if breastfed infant is full term and <8 days of age or is jaundiced, ill, stressed, premature or G6PD deficient[78]

Alternate Therapy

Erythromycin 250 to 500 mg by mouth four times per day for 10 to 14 days

Consider for history of penicillin hypersensitivity, although resistance is common

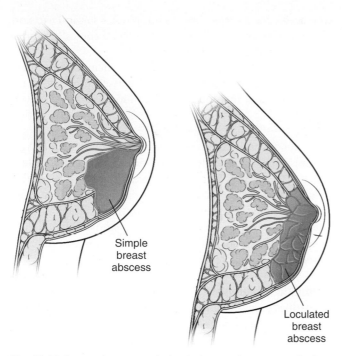

Fig. 16.13 Breast abscesses. A simple breast abscess may be best managed with aspiration alone because a needle can access and empty an entire infected fluid cavity. However, many lactational abscesses become loculated; a very small stab incision may enable access with a small instrument, such as a hemostat, to disrupt septations and more completely drain the complex collection.

breastfeeding. Whereas plugs or early galactoceles may contain more simple milk, more chronic galactoceles ultimately can develop a collection of extremely thick, semisolid material.[82] They can present as a smooth mass or persistent focal swelling. They should be confirmed with ultrasound and/or mammogram. If small, no intervention is required, and they become smaller over the course of lactation. If large and symptomatic, they can be aspirated. It should be noted that they almost always require repeat aspiration and may convert from uninfected to infected galactoceles. A more expeditious approach to management may include drain placement for 3 to 5 days rather than repeated aspiration.[83]

Phlegmon

In contrast to the discrete fluid collections visualized with galactoceles and abscesses, the lactational phlegmon represents a mass with an indistinct fluid collection, surrounding hyperemic parenchyma, and tissue edema.[53] It is often associated with an obstructive, infectious, or inflammatory history, such as plugging or mastitis. Overlying erythema may be present. Often, patients notice an increase in the mass-like area after they have vigorously massaged the breast in an attempt to relieve a plug. Like other phlegmons appearing in the body, such as diverticular and appendiceal, lactational phlegmon may be managed with extended antibiotic therapy of up to 4 weeks.[72] Aspiration or other drainage attempts are not indicated unless the phlegmon converts to an abscess. Therapeutic ultrasound may play a role in decreasing inflammation and

promoting coalescence into a drainable collection. Phlegmons can appear concerning on breast imaging and may be indistinguishable from a concerning mass. Therefore patients may be recommended to undergo biopsy to confirm the diagnosis. Biopsy is not contraindicated, and breastfeeding can continue uninterrupted. Once benign pathology is confirmed, the patient should be followed with interval exams every 3 months with imaging to rule out an occult mass as a lead point for the initial obstruction.

Milk Fistula

Milk fistula, a communication between a lactiferous duct and the skin, is rare. In a large cohort of patients treated in an interventional breastfeeding medicine clinic with core needle biopsies, abscess drainages, NAC procedures, and surgical excisions, the milk-fistula incidence was demonstrated to be 1.3% within 1 week of a procedure, and the overall prevalence was 2.5%.[84] Although incisions on the NAC should be avoided if possible because of potential persistent latch and/or breast-pump trauma that may delay wound healing, no necessary intervention should be delayed in the lactating patient because of the very small risk of milk fistula. Even in the rare cases where a fistula develops, the defect is usually very minor and can be managed well with conservative measures such as keeping the area dry with a breast pad. Given the vascular nature of the lactating breast, most ultimately close within days to weeks of development. Cessation of breastfeeding is neither recommended nor required.[85]

BENIGN BREAST MASSES, BREAST PAIN, AND OTHER CONDITIONS

General Considerations

Breast pain, masses, and other conditions can develop as a direct result of pregnancy and/or lactation. Additional various benign and malignant breast conditions can present in the setting of lactation but are not caused by or related to lactation. Any patients with a concerning breast lesion not resolving with standard interventions should undergo diagnostic breast imaging, starting with a breast ultrasound.[5]

Mastalgia

Breast pain in the nonlactating patient most commonly results from cyclical mastalgia related to hormonal fluctuations with the menstrual cycle.[86] This pain often spontaneously disappears during pregnancy and lactation. Breast and NAC pain in lactation rarely result from hormonal fluctuations and require a thorough workup of this complex issue. Potential etiologies include hyperlactation, engorgement, plugged ducts, vasospasm, subacute mastitis, and dermatitis, as discussed in other sections. As with NAC pain, breast pain may be multifactorial. Persistent idiopathic mastalgia in lactation may benefit from physical therapy interventions, such as therapeutic ultrasound and lymphatic massage; continued attention to breast support and optimal latch/positioning; and consideration of antidepressant medication.[29] Neuropathic pain may improve on a regimen of nonsedating antihistamines and propranolol, based on data from a small case series.[87] Complementary and alternative medicine practices and optimization of psychosocial support may also prove beneficial for persistent mastalgia.[30]

Musculoskeletal chest-wall pain may also refer to the breast. In case series, women with breast pain have responded to physiotherapy.[88,89] The authors recommend evaluating for postural anomalies, such as exaggerated thoracic kyphosis, scapular protraction, or glenohumeral anteriority, as well as circumscribed areas of sharp tenderness along the anterior axillary line close to the border of the breast. Attention to posture and positioning while feeding and carrying the infant may also be helpful.[90]

Breast Conditions Unique to Lactation
Gigantomastia

Gestational gigantomastia has a poorly defined incidence and likely represents a spectrum of excessive breast growth during pregnancy. It may include women who grow multiple cup sizes or those for whom the breast hypertrophy is so significant it can cause mobility impairments. Hormonal factors may play a role in gigantomastia, but the true etiology remains unknown.[91] Extreme cases of enlargement may cause pressure necrosis and tissue loss. Postpartum breastfeeding can be difficult because of the difficulty with latch and milk-transfer issues. It also remains unclear whether the hypertrophy represents true glandular development or intervening stromal edema because patients do not necessarily experience high milk production with this presentation. For more mild cases that demonstrate significant breast growth without concern for necrosis, breast lymphedema and pain can be managed effectively with a supportive bra and lymphatic massage, as described earlier.

Engorgement/Breast Lymphedema/Pain

Outside the presentation of true gigantomastia, patients still may experience breast lymphedema and pain, particularly during periods of early breast growth in the first trimester and in the last trimester nearing childbirth. This discomfort is related to the increasing vascularity of the breast, the development of glandular tissue, and the increasing water content of the breast. Edema tends to present symmetrically in the lower quadrants of the breast and can be mildly erythematous. These cases also can gain significant relief from lymphatic massage and supportive bras. Any asymmetry in presentation warrants referral to a breast surgeon to evaluate for breast masses and/or inflammatory breast cancer.

Lactating Adenoma

Lactating adenomas are benign lesions composed of dense lactational tissue and most commonly occur in the upper-outer quadrant of the breast and the axillary tail tissue. They can present during pregnancy or lactation and likely are related to hormonal stimulation.[92] They may become large; however, most regress as a woman progresses further in the postpartum period and eventually disappear when lactation is complete. They can appear similar to fibroadenoma on breast imaging, as smooth, oval lesions.[92] Diagnosis can be confirmed with a core needle biopsy, but they do not require surgical excision. These masses can be followed with interval clinical examination and imaging to confirm regression.

Other masses specific to lactation include *galactocele*, *phlegmon*, and *abscess*, which are discussed in detail in the "Obstructive and Inflammatory Conditions" section.

Breast Conditions Not Unique to Lactation

Breast conditions that may occur in the lactating patient but are not caused by or related to pregnancy and/or lactation include breast cancer; atypical breast lesions; and benign masses that include but are not limited to fibroepithelial lesions, cysts, lipomas, hamartomas, fat necrosis, and prominent lymph nodes.[53] The management of these lesions is summarized in ABM Protocol 30,[53] and an additional discussion of breast cancer is presented in the next section.

Idiopathic Granulomatous Mastitis

Idiopathic granulomatous mastitis (IGM) is a complex inflammatory disorder affecting the breast of young women in their childbearing years and presents a challenging treatment paradigm. It can result in the development of painful inflammatory masses, abscesses, and fistula formation. It generally self-resolves within 2 to 3 years after presentation but can cause significant distress for patients. Although breastfeeding from the affected breast in the setting of IGM is safe, mothers may report additional pain and difficulty with latch or milk production. IGM traditionally has been treated with oral steroids and/or other immunomodulating medications, such as methotrexate.[93] More recently, intralesional injection of triamcinolone has been documented to improve IGM symptomatology.[94] However, the high local concentration of steroid will be excreted into breast milk and is not safe with breastfeeding from the affected breast.[95] High-dose oral steroids may reduce milk supply,[44] similar to the reported effect of high-dose triamcinolone injections at body sites other than the breast.[96] Methotrexate has a high rate of transfer into milk and is moderately absorbed in the infant's gut; breastfeeding while taking high-dose methotrexate is not recommended, and the lactational safety of lower doses remains controversial.[97] Patients may consider augmenting milk production on the contralateral breast and treating affected-breast symptomatology with intralesional injections rather than systemic steroids or other forms of immunosuppression. If patients prefer to treat their symptoms with systemic therapy, they should be counseled through shared decision-making that they may experience decreased milk production and need to utilize supplementation. Mothers also may elect no treatment during lactation; fluid collections, fistula formation, and other symptomatology can be managed on an as-needed basis.

Dermatitis

Breast dermatitis may occur in the setting of lactation and may be related to an underlying predisposition to eczema and/or reaction to new allergens a mother is exposed to through breastfeeding products and/or her infant. Breast dermatitis management follows the principles of NAC dermatitis management, as outlined previously.

Mondor's Disease

Superficial thrombophlebitis of the anterior chest-wall veins is termed *Mondor's disease*. Women between the ages of 30 and 60 are most commonly affected.[46] The affected vessel, often the lateral thoracic vein, assumes the appearance of a palpable, erythematous, tender "cord." This condition self-resolves in several weeks and may be treated symptomatically with analgesics, moist heat, and ice.

BREAST CANCER AND BREASTFEEDING

Breast cancer care intersects with lactation in multiple situations. These include the following: women who have undergone treatment for breast cancer in the past and later have a child and wish to breastfeed, women who are breastfeeding and receive a breast cancer diagnosis, and women who are diagnosed with breast cancer during pregnancy and wish to breastfeed postpartum.

History of Breast Cancer

Patients with a history of breast cancer at a young age likely will have received multidisciplinary treatments that result in individual and collective effects on subsequent lactation. Chemotherapy may have permanent effects on breast parenchyma and glandular function,[98] but women also have been known to breastfeed successfully after chemotherapy.[99,100] A mastectomy precludes breastfeeding from the absent breast.[101] It should be noted that because of variations in surgical technique, some residual breast parenchyma may hypertrophy during pregnancy and the postpartum period, and some milk may be produced in situations of nipple-sparing mastectomy. However, given that mastectomy is intended to remove >95% of the breast parenchyma, normal lactation should neither be expected nor encouraged from the affected breast. Breastfeeding from the contralateral unaffected breast is safe. With the possible exception of carriers of *BRCA* mutations, bilateral mastectomy confers no survival benefit to patients.[102] Therefore women diagnosed with breast cancer who anticipate childbearing should consider delayed contralateral prophylactic mastectomy to enable breastfeeding from the unaffected breast.

Partial mastectomy ("lumpectomy") removes only the part of the breast affected by cancer. Given that the volume of parenchyma removed is usually small, surgery itself should have a limited effect on future lactational ability unless the nipple or central ducts are removed or are significantly damaged. However, partial mastectomy nearly always requires adjuvant radiation therapy, and radiation will likely significantly affect the future lactational ability of the breast. With radiation, glandular cells undergo apoptosis, the skin becomes fibrotic, and the NAC can lose significant elasticity.[103]

Once initial treatment with chemotherapy, surgery, and radiation is complete, patients with hormone-receptor-positive tumors will be recommended to undergo adjuvant endocrine therapy. Premenopausal women generally receive tamoxifen, which is not recommended in lactation because of the absence of data on transfer into milk and potential negative impact on production.[104] Results are expected in 2020 for the POSITIVE trial (Clinical Trial Registration Number NCT02308085), which is investigating the safety of interruption of endocrine therapy for pregnancy and lactation.[105]

Breast Cancer Diagnosed While Pregnant

Patients diagnosed with breast cancer while pregnant likely will undergo multidisciplinary treatment as described previously. A pregnant patient with a suspicious mass or lesion detected on a screening study should undergo biopsy as indicated. Biopsies are safe, and milk fistula is rare, as described earlier. Patients who begin chemotherapy while pregnant typically have the systemic treatment interrupted at 35 to 37 weeks' gestational age for delivery[106] and likely will be restarted 3 to 4 weeks postpartum. Patients should be counseled about the potential effect of chemotherapy on glandular development during pregnancy.[107] They should also be counseled that breastfeeding during chemotherapy is contraindicated.[97]

In the initial postpartum period, patients can breastfeed their infants and store milk. No data exist to suggests that breastfeeding from an affected breast during this time is harmful to the infant.[108] When they restart chemotherapy, they can choose to wean and utilize donor milk, or they can express milk and discard it until chemotherapy is complete. If they chose the latter approach, they should have a careful discussion with their physicians regarding the risks of mastitis and plugging with pumping, infection in the setting of immunocompromise, decrease in milk production, and anticipated length and type of remaining chemotherapy treatment. Tumors that are HER2-neu amplified will also require monoclonal antibody treatment with trastuzumab and pertuzumab in the postpartum period. There are no data on these agents during lactation;[109] however, like other monoclonal antibodies, they likely are not excreted in milk.

With respect to surgical treatment, unilateral breastfeeding represents a realistic strategy for many patients, regardless of whether surgery is performed during pregnancy or postpartum or whether patients undergo mastectomy or partial mastectomy followed by radiation. The use of technetium for lymph node mapping is likely safe in lactation, but there are no data on blue dyes.[101] If the patient's tumor is hormone-receptor positive, she ultimately will be recommended to start adjuvant endocrine therapy at the completion of other treatments.

Breast Cancer Diagnosed While Lactating

Limited older case reports have described the "milk-refusal sign," in which a mother reports that a baby rejects the breast before her cancer diagnosis.[110–112] Although this may occur in individual cases, mothers should not be falsely reassured if a baby continues to nurse despite the presence of a suspicious mass. Likewise, they should not be concerned that cancer may be present if the baby rejects the breast for a variety of more common reasons. Women should undergo standard, routine diagnostic imaging and biopsy in the setting of clinical concern for malignancy.[113,114]

Diagnostic and screening imaging are safe in lactation, and as described earlier, biopsy is safe, and the risk of milk fistula is very low. Women diagnosed with breast cancer in the postpartum period exhibit a three-fold risk of distant recurrence and death compared with nulliparous controls.[115] These tumors are often high grade, with lymphovascular space invasion,[115] and patients therefore may benefit from neoadjuvant chemotherapy before surgery. As described previously, patients should have a careful discussion with their physicians regarding weaning before chemotherapy or attempting to express and discard milk during their treatment. If patients desire to wean, herbal preparations such as sage and nonprescription medications such as pseudoephedrine may be used to decrease milk volume.[101] In settings of high milk production, 0.25 to 0.5 mg cabergoline dosed every 3 days by mouth may be prescribed by a physician to more rapidly and dramatically decrease volume.[116] Surgery, radiation, and endocrine therapy management proceed as described previously.

PLASTIC SURGERY AND BREASTFEEDING

General Considerations

Discussion with patients regarding prior history of plastic surgery should include background information about why patients elected to undergo a procedure. For example, patients may offer a history of markedly asymmetric breasts, which can be more common in a tubular breast deformity, also known as *IGT*, or hypoplastic breast tissue (see Fig. 16.5). These patients may undergo augmentation and/or mammaplasty and mastopexy. The ultimate cosmetic outcome may not reflect the presence of the previous tubular breast appearance.

Providers should consider that the same volume of breast tissue removed in different individuals may not reflect the composition of the parenchyma removed. For example, a woman could have undergone a breast reduction that removed large amounts of fatty tissue but little glandular tissue, or the opposite may be true. The impact of procedures on the mechanical aspects of breastfeeding also should be considered. For example, very large augmentations may produce difficulty with obtaining a deep latch and may potentiate nipple trauma and pain. Surgical techniques also can influence future lactation, including the technique of parenchymal resection, the location of incisions and type of closure, the types of implants, and varied approaches to NAC procedures. Finally, the time elapsed from surgery should be ascertained, although no studies have proven an association between this and breastfeeding success.[117,118]

Nipple Piercing and Tattooing

Patients with a history of nipple piercings should remove piercings during pregnancy. Breastfeeding generally is uncomplicated after a history of nipple piercing; however, in some cases, patients may develop infection or hematoma at the site of a previous piercing. A small hematoma can be drained for symptomatic relief, and any infection should be treated with antibiotics. On occasion, with very small nipples and very large piercings placed before full nipple development, it is possible that the piercing damages a significant amount of ductal tissue in the nipple and may obstruct milk outflow. Therefore women should be counseled about any potential risk before undergoing this procedure. Tattoos on the breast and NAC do not preclude breastfeeding.

Breast Reductions

The major considerations when counseling a patient with a history of breast reduction (*reduction mammaplasty*, with or without concurrent breast lift, or *mastopexy*) are the choice of surgical pedicle, type of closure, and handling of the NAC. The surgical pedicle represents the area of breast parenchyma that was not resected in the reduction and carries the blood and nerve supply to the NAC. Ideally, this pedicle's connection with the underlying pectoralis muscle and fascia was preserved because connection contributes to nipple vascularity and sensitivity. An intact pedicle also maintains an undisrupted segment of breast lobular and ductal tissue. The most common pedicles are a superior, medial, central, or inferior pedicle (Fig. 16.14). A systematic review of 51 studies evaluating the impact of breast-reduction surgery on breastfeeding concluded that inferior and central pedicles may lead to greater success in breastfeeding and that the amount of parenchyma removed has no appreciable effect.[119] However, variable definitions of breastfeeding success in individual studies limit the interpretation of these data.

Various closure patterns in breast reductions exist, although the most common are the anchor pattern (Wise pattern), circumvertical (lollipop), and circle (periareolar; Fig. 16.15). It should be noted that the pattern of closure noted externally does not correlate with the internal pedicle, volume of tissue resected, or original incisions. Additionally, these closure patterns do not reveal whether the NAC was resected and reattached to the breast using a "free nipple graft" technique or whether the NAC retained its original attachment to the breast and underlying vascular and nerve supply. Data suggest that greater breastfeeding success is tied to the preservation of the column of parenchyma from the NAC to the chest wall rather than partial connection or complete severing and reattachment.[119]

Patients may express remorse regarding a past breast reduction. Providers should validate these emotions but understand that studies document similar breastfeeding rates between unoperated macromastia and patients with a history of breast reduction.[120,121] Macromastia can decrease breast and NAC sensation and present difficulty in obtaining a deep latch and effective milk removal. Further, obesity represents an independent risk factor for poor breastfeeding outcomes,[122,123] and there are no current studies on reductions and lactation control for groups with similar body mass index (BMI). Therefore strong conclusions assessing the potentially independent effects of obesity and macromastia on breastfeeding are difficult to make.

Overall, women commonly cite a lack of support and encouragement as a predominant reason why they did not attempt to breastfeed after a reduction procedure in the past. If women attempted breastfeeding, half of them reported that

Breast pedicles

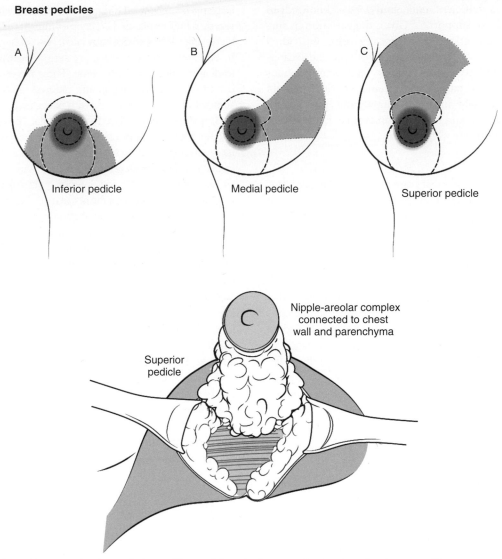

Fig. 16.14 Pedicle-based breast-reduction techniques. The pedicles of a breast reduction describe the area of breast parenchyma that remains connected to the chest wall and nipple-areolar complex during the procedure. The most common pedicles include the inferior (A), medial (B), and superior pedicles (C).

Patterns of closure

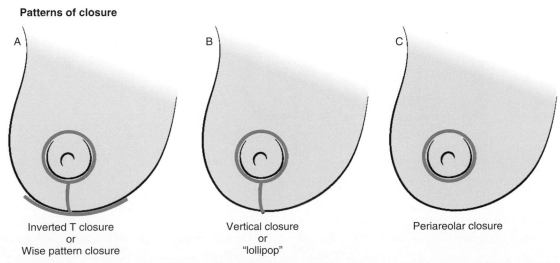

Fig. 16.15 Breast-reduction closure patterns. The external incisions do not provide evidence regarding the type of internal pedicle used during breast-reduction surgery. Common closure patterns include the inverted T or "Wise pattern" closure (A), vertical closure or "lollipop" (B), and periareolar closure (C).

they did not have sufficient milk, and 15% acknowledged reluctance and lack of support.[119] Given the variation in surgical techniques and unknown factors regarding individual ability to hypertrophy remaining glandular tissue and recanalize ducts, few definitive conclusions regarding previous breast reduction and lactation can be made. Providers should support women closely in the prenatal and postpartum period, assist with latch and effective milk transfer, and monitor infants for appropriate weight gain.

Breast Augmentation

Breast augmentation is the most common plastic surgery procedure worldwide.[124] Studies on the impact of augmentation on lactation demonstrate decreased breastfeeding rates, but data quality remains mixed.[124,125] Decreased breastfeeding rates may partially reflect premorbid conditions such as IGT, which prompt women to pursue augmentation, as well as the effects of the procedure itself.

Providers counseling patients who have undergone breast augmentation and subsequently wish to breastfeed should consider several factors regarding the previous procedure, including the following: size of implant, location of implant, location of incisions, and type of implant. These factors may individually and collectively affect lactation. Surgery can affect ducts and glandular tissue. All implants result in the formation of a surrounding reactive capsule, which can undergo capsular contracture, with resulting pain, breast distortion, and loss of elasticity.[126]

The smallest implants generally are 125 mL in size, with the largest silicone implants being 800 mL and the largest saline implants being 960 mL. "Extra-large" implants result from overfilling of saline implants. Larger-size implants likely correlate with increasing challenge with baby latch, positioning, and milk transfer. In addition, they may place pressure on native glandular tissue, leading to attenuation over time. These larger implants may also contribute to nerve traction and reduced sensitivity of the nipple, similar to known phenomena with native macromastia.[127]

Implants may be placed subglandular (posterior to the breast and anterior to the pectoralis muscle, or pre-pectoral); submuscular (posterior to the pectoralis muscle); or "dual plane," where the implant is placed posterior to the muscle, but a portion of the muscle is released to provide inferior pole fullness to the breast (Fig. 16.16). Insertion of submuscular or dual-plane implants may be more likely to disrupt innervation of the NAC.[128] Incisions for the placement of implants include periareolar, inframammary, axillary, and transumbilical. No difference in nipple sensation has been demonstrated to correlate with incision type.[127] Periareolar incisions do not appear to affect breastfeeding rates.[124]

Implants contain either silicone or saline. Silicone levels in the serum and breast milk of women with implants are similar to those without implants,[129] and children of women with silicone implants do not appear to be at increased risk of adverse health outcomes.[130] Patients may report concern with a ruptured implant in the setting of breastfeeding, particularly with extracapsular rupture of silicone implants. Saline poses no risk, and revision/replacement should be deferred until lactation is complete. Deferment of revision of a ruptured silicone implant may also be safe, given exponentially higher silicone levels in cow's milk and formula.[131]

Location of implants

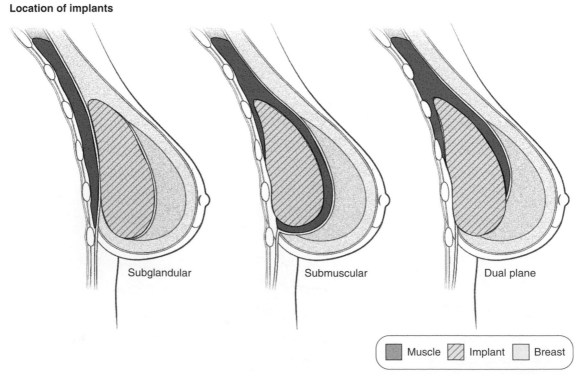

Subglandular   Submuscular   Dual plane

☐ Muscle   ▨ Implant   ☐ Breast

Fig. 16.16 Breast implants. Breast implants may be subglandular, submuscular, or "dual plane." Dual-plane placement involves submuscular placement of the implant with release of the pectoralis muscle inferiorly, such that some implant contacts the breast parenchyma.

If rupture is suspected, breast MRI is the preferred imaging modality for evaluation.[132] Mammogram detects extracapsular rupture but less commonly detects intracapsular rupture.[132] Ultrasound is more operator dependent and has a higher false-negative rate.[132] All these imaging modalities are safe in lactation.

There are no data to support the concern that breastfeeding increases the risk of breast implant infection, even in the setting of rupture. This is likely related to the capsule surrounding the implant as well as the common submuscular implant location.

Overall, patients with a history of breast augmentation, like other plastic surgery procedures, should be counseled in the prenatal period and followed closely postpartum.

Nipple-Areolar Complex Procedures

Nipple Reduction

Countless surgical techniques have been developed to reduce large nipples. These include multiple approaches to flaps that attempt to reduce the outward projection of nipples. A "simplified reduction technique" involves excising the most distal portion of the nipple and placing suture or holding pressure for hemostasis.[133–135] There are limited data regarding lactational outcomes, and we recommend deferment of this elective procedure until breastfeeding is complete.

Nipple Eversion

The etiology of inverted nipples is described in detail earlier in the chapter. Like procedures to reduce nipple size, numerous approaches to nipple eversion have been documented. Many involve division and disruption of the retroareolar ducts and connective tissue and may result in permanent scarring and obstruction of these ducts. Some techniques, such as the "triple flap"[136] or "twist and lock,"[137] involve lengthening parallel to the ducts and external soft tissue flaps to maintain eversion. Nevertheless, no clear demonstration of breastfeeding outcomes has been documented in large studies, and therefore patients should be cautioned against any procedure before childbearing. They also should be counseled that breastfeeding is possible with inverted nipples, and nipples may naturally evert with breastfeeding and pumping.

Gender-Affirming Surgery

Patients who are assigned male at birth (AMAB) or assigned female at birth (AFAB) may undergo gender-affirming "top" surgery and later desire to breastfeed.[138] (see Chapter 20) AMAB patients with a history of augmentation before lactation induction should be counseled similarly to other patients who have undergone augmentation. Because chest-contouring surgeries vary widely based on breast size, BMI, and individual surgical technique,[139] AFAB patients with a history of chest-contouring surgery can experience variable breast hypertrophy and milk production. AFAB patients may have undergone a traditional mastectomy with subsequent free nipple graft or re-creation of the NAC with a tattoo. They also could have undergone a procedure similar to a breast reduction that retains more native breast tissue and NAC attachment to underlying glandular parenchyma. In addition to counseling patients based on needs specific to transgender patients, we recommend prenatal breastfeeding counseling and close postpartum support as would be standard with a history of any previous cosmetic breast surgical procedure.

The Reference list is available at www.expertconsult.com.

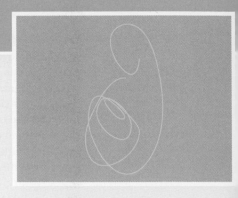

17

Human Milk and Atopic Disease

Robert M. Lawrence and Ruth A. Lawrence

KEY POINTS

- The prevalence of allergy is increasing across the world, and asthma is the most common chronic disease in children.
- The exact role of genetics and epigenetics in the development of allergy are being explored with newer research techniques.
- Exclusive breastfeeding does decrease the occurrence of eczema in the first 2 years of life, and a longer duration of breastfeeding decreases wheezing in the first 2 years of life. A longer duration of breastfeeding protects against asthma even up to 5 years of age.
- Food allergies in breastfeeding infants do occur, although the exact timing and mechanism(s) of sensitization are poorly understood. Maternal elimination diets in pregnancy and/or lactation do not prevent atopic disease, but infant avoidance of foods and maternal elimination diet may be useful in infants with diagnosed food allergies and specifically food protein—induced enterocolitis syndrome.
- An expert panel of the American Academy of Pediatrics now recommends early introduction (4 to 6 months of age) of infant-safe forms of peanuts to decrease the risk for peanut allergy in at-risk infants, including description of risk testing and amount and frequency of peanut allergen.

ATOPIC DISEASE

Atopic disease includes various clinical manifestations of allergy (atopic dermatitis [AD]/eczema, asthma, food allergy, allergic rhinitis) and multiple mechanisms of allergic reaction. The complexity of atopic disease is extended by the differing phenotypes of allergic disease (age of onset, triggers, "target organs/systems," clinical manifestations, severity, response to therapy, and natural history), and the contribution of heredity versus exposure to specific allergens. The several different types of hypersensitivity reactions (type I—immunoglobulin E [IgE] antibody mediated; type II—antibodies mediated; type III—antigen-antibody complex mediated; type IV—activated T-cell and cytokines mediated; and types V and VI—combinations of antibody- and cell-mediated reactions) add to the complexity of atopic disease. Given this complexity and the various mechanisms and clinical manifestations of allergic disease, one should not expect a simple relationship between breastfeeding and atopic disease. Nevertheless, there is accumulating evidence that breastfeeding can offer some protection against the development of specific illnesses, AD, wheezing, and asthma. Equally important is the investigation of the active components of human milk and their contribution to the development of the infant's gastrointestinal tract and immune system and influence on the response to environmental exposures to allergens in infancy.[1] This chapter will attempt to address some of the issues relating breastfeeding to atopic disease (Box 17.1).

Historical Data on Atopic Disease

The association of allergy with cow milk has been documented in the literature for decades.[2–4] The incidence of this allergy in the general population has been noted to increase progressively since the original comments on the subject by Rowe[5] in 1931. The incidence has reportedly increased 10 times in the last 20 + years. This increase has been attributed to increased recognition, increased incidence of exposure to known allergens, and a gradual decrease in infection as a source of morbidity, because the use of antibiotics and immunization revealed an underlying allergic component to chronic symptoms. Glaser[6] attributed the rapid increase in the development of allergic diseases during the 1950s to the abandonment of breastfeeding when safe, pasteurized milk became available. It was noted that 20% of all children had some manifestations of atopic disease by 20 years of age.

Studies of office pediatrics have shown that one-third of the visits are a result of allergy.[7] One-third of all chronic conditions in patients younger than 17 years result from allergy and one-third of lost school days from asthma. In the evaluation of 2000 consecutive, unselected newborns in pediatric practice, 50% had family histories of allergy. Grulee et al.[8] observed, as early as 1934, that eczema was seven times more common in infants fed cow milk than in breastfed infants.

BOX 17.1 Selected Definitions

Allergy:	A hypersensitivity reaction initiated by immunologic mechanisms.
Allergenic foods:	Eight major groups of allergenic foods that account for approximately 90% of all food allergies and must be declared on labels for processed foods in the United States. These include cow milk, eggs, fish, crustacean shellfish, tree nuts, peanuts, wheat, and soybean. More than 170 foods have been described to cause allergic reactions, and additional foods (e.g., sesame) are included in labeling laws in other countries
Atopy:	A personal or familial tendency to produce immunoglobulin E (IgE) antibodies in response to low-dose allergens, confirmed by a positive skin-prick test (SPT) result.
Atopic disease:	A clinical disease characterized by atopy. Atopic disease typically refers to atopic dermatitis, asthma, allergic rhinitis, and food allergy.
Atopic dermatitis (eczema):	A pruritic, chronic, inflammatory skin disease that commonly manifests during early childhood and is often associated with a personal or family history of other atopic diseases.
Asthma:	An allergic-mediated response in the bronchial airways that is verified by the variation in lung function (measured by spirometry), either spontaneously or after pharmacologic bronchodilation.
Food allergy:	An immunologically mediated hypersensitivity reaction to any food, including IgE-mediated and/or non—IgE-mediated allergic reactions.
Allergic rhinitis:	Inflammation of the nasal passages caused by allergic reaction to airborne substances, hypersensitivity reaction initiated by local immunologic mechanisms in the nose.
Hypoallergenic:	Reduced allergenicity or reduced ability to stimulate an IgE response and induce IgE-mediated reactions.
Complementary foods:	Foods and/or beverages (liquids, semisolids, and solids) other than human milk, infant formula, and cow milk (consumed in the first year of life) provided to an infant or young child to provide micronutrients and macronutrients, including energy.
Infants at high risk for developing allergy:	Infants with at least one first-degree relative (parent or sibling) with documented allergic disease.

From Greer FR, Sicherer SH, Burks AW, et al. The effects of early nutritional interventions on the development of atopic disease in infants and children: the role of maternal dietary restriction, breastfeeding, hydrolyzed formulas, and timing of introduction of allergenic complementary foods. *Pediatrics.* 2019;143(4):1—11. http://doi:10.1542/peds.2019-0281.

The incidence of atopic disease (eczema and food allergy) seemed to increase from 1997 to 2011.[9] A 2019 cross-sectional survey of 10 primary care practices in five US states included 652 children; the estimated prevalence of ever having AD was 24% (95% confidence interval [CI] 21 to 28), ranging from 15% among children under the age of 1 to 38% among those aged 4 to 5 years. The occurrence of asthma was higher among AD participants compared with those with no AD, at 12% and 4%, respectively ($p < 0.001$).[10] In industrialized nations, the incidence of AD is reported to have increased two to three times in recent decades. It is estimated to affect 15% to 20% of children and 1% to 3% of adults.[11] AD notably develops early in life; 60% of individuals manifesting symptoms by 1 year of age and 90% by 5 years of age.[12]

Asthma: The Most Common Chronic Disease in Childhood

Asthma is the most common chronic disease of childhood, affecting over 6 million children, according to a Centers for Disease Control and Prevention (CDC) report in 2001.[13,14] These data indicate that, in the United States, people with asthma (over 32 million) collectively have more than 100 million days of restricted activity and 470,000 hospitalizations annually, with more than 5000 deaths annually. Asthma hospitalization rates have been highest among black adults and children, with mortality rates consistently highest among black individuals ages 15 to 24 years. Asthma costs the American public billions of dollars every year. Worldwide, asthma is reported to affect approximately 334 million

people.[15] The prevalence of self-reported asthma in children has continued to increase (10% to 15%) through 2015, with recent declines in admission rates (approximately 2/1000) and mortality rates (<2/1 million) in children.[16] Examining worldwide asthma mortality by country in 5—34 year olds, deaths have declined for 2011—2015 compared to previous years. Most countries exhibit 1—5 asthma deaths per 1 million persons, but large disparities in mortality rates exist between countries.[16] In 2016, asthma in all ages was responsible for 23.7 million Disability Adjusted Life Years (DALYs) worldwide and ranked 28th among the leading causes of burden of disease.[16] Questions remain about the increase in prevalence of asthma and its causes (genetic predisposition, allergens, exposure to smoke and air pollution, antibiotic use, and altered microbiome early in life), although the diminished morbidity and mortality are ascribed to education, treatment programs, and targeted therapies for specific phenotypes and the assessed severity of the disease.[17—20]

Decades of investigation have resulted in conflicting results regarding avoidance of allergenic foods during pregnancy or lactation in prevention of atopic disease. There also have been numerous systematic reviews and meta-analyses trying to resolve the question of prevention and interpret the available data and what it indicates.[21,22] In the past, it was concluded that cow milk should be avoided for at least the first 4 months of life in children at risk for allergy. Maternal avoidance of allergens during pregnancy also produced conflicting results, except for the avoidance of cow milk during pregnancy when there was a family history of atopic disease. Maternal avoidance of cow milk resulted in lower levels of mucosal-specific IgA and a lower incidence of cow milk allergy in the infant.[23] The American Academy of Pediatrics (AAP) had previously recommended that cow milk and dairy products should be avoided in at-risk infants for the first year of life. The AAP and others have declared that soy milk has no role in the prevention of allergy. The AAP is very supportive of breastfeeding for at least 6 months and the delay in starting solids until 6 months. Some mothers with a strong history of atopic disease have attempted strict elimination diets in pregnancy and lactation to avoid sensitization of their infants. It is unclear that such elimination diets are effective. Bone turnover is increased when mothers are on elimination diets that include elimination of cow milk, cow milk products, and eggs, even when they are on supplemental calcium. Mothers who were found to have some bone mobilization for 6 months recovered quickly when breastfeeding was discontinued.[24]

There are new evidence-based guidelines regarding early nutritional interventions for the prevention of atopic disease in infants and children.[22]

NATURAL HISTORY OF FOOD ALLERGY

Similar to the other atopic diseases in children, food allergy prevalence is reportedly increasing and approaching 10% in children.[25] There is concern that the literature presents an imprecise picture, including self-reporting versus confirmatory diagnosis by oral food challenge, use of selected populations in published studies, and selection bias, which would limit the application of results to the larger population.[26] Over 170 foods have been reported as causing allergic reactions, and there are eight major groups of allergenic foods (cow milk, eggs, fish, crustacean shellfish, tree nuts, peanuts, wheat, and soybean), which supposedly account for 90% of all food allergies.[22] The reported increase over time of food allergy could also be secondary to generalized awareness of the condition leading to increased self-reporting.[27]

Salo et al.[28] reported prevalence estimates for sensitization to various foods in 9440 children with serum specific IgEs. In children aged 6 years and older, 44.6% had detectable serum IgEs (sIgEs), whereas 36.2% of children aged 1 to 5 years were sensitized to one or more allergens. In the children aged 1 to 5 years, 6.8% were sensitized to peanut, 21.8% to milk, and 14.2% to egg, and in children aged 6 and over 7.6% were sensitized to peanut, 5.9% to shrimp, 4.8% to milk, and 3.4% to egg. The natural history of food allergy is complicated, requiring information on the onset of clinical allergy and the later persistence or resolution of symptoms with continued exposure. It should also include careful assessment at different time points over the course of the disease by physician-supervised oral food challenge.[25] There are few longitudinal exacting studies that carefully document onset and resolution of allergy symptoms along with careful diagnosis by oral food challenge. Savage and Johns[25] summarized estimates of the age of onset and age of resolution for common food allergens (Table 17.1). In a more recent review led by Savage et al.,[26] specific food allergies were considered to have a high rate of resolution in childhood (milk, >50% resolution by 10 years

TABLE 17.1   Proposed Natural History for Common Food Allergens

Food	Age of Onset	Age of Resolution
Egg	Infant/toddler	Early to late childhood
Milk	Infant/toddler	Early to late childhood
Peanut	Infant/toddler	Early to late childhood—uncommon
	Adulthood	Unknown
Tree nuts	Toddler/early childhood	Early to late childhood—uncommon
	Adulthood	Unknown
Soy	Infant/toddler	Early to late childhood
	Adulthood (rare)	Unknown
Wheat	Infant/toddler	Early to late childhood

From Savage J, Johns CB. Food allergy: epidemiology and natural history. *Immunol Allergy Clin North Am.* 2015;35(1):45–59. http://doi:10.1016/j.iac.2014.09.004.

of age; egg, approximately 50% by 9 years of age; wheat, 50% by 7 years of age; and soy, 45% by 6 years of age), and others more consistently persisted into adolescence or later (peanut 20% resolution by 4 years, and approximately 10% resolution by age 10 for tree nuts, seeds, fish, and shellfish).[26]

The Question of Heredity

Heredity undoubtedly plays a part in the development of allergic disease, an observation first recorded by Maimonides in his Treatise on Asthma in the 12th century. Most studies in the past 60 years have concurred with the concept of a recessive mode of inheritance.[29]

Kern[30] noted that the outstanding etiologic factor in human hypersensitivity is heredity. He stated that few diseases exist in which heredity is so clearly identified and so common.

Hamburger[31] reported that children with two atopic parents had a 47% chance of developing atopic disease. One atopic parent meant a 29% chance of developing atopy, and the risk dropped to 13% with no allergic parent. In a study of asthmatic monozygotic twins, Falliers et al.[32] observed similar serum IgE, blood eosinophil counts, and positive skin tests to allergens in both twins. However, they had dissimilar responses to infection and methacholine. This finding suggests an acquired component to bronchial hyperactivity.

Genetics and Epigenetics of Allergic Disease

New technology is opening the way to studying the genetics and epigenetics of allergic disease. This includes genome-wide association studies, single nucleotide polymorphisms (SNPs), the use of omics (genomics [whole gene sequencing], epigenomics [DNA methylation, histone modification, RNA interference], transcriptomics [microarrays, single-cell RNAseq], and analysis of gene polymorphisms. For asthma, implicated genes include SNPs related to *ADAM33*, *DPP10*, *PHF11*, *GPR*, and *PTGDR* genes and the activation or inhibition of the

Nrf2-mediated antioxidant response in the lung and genetic variants that alter prostaglandins and leukotriene activity related to nonsteroidal antiinflammatory drug–exacerbated respiratory disease (NERD).[33–36] Similarly, for genetic determinants of pediatric food allergy, there are a few implicated genes: *FLG* (filaggrin), *HLA-DR* and *HLA-DQ* (major histocompatibility complex), *IL10* (interleukin [IL] 10), *IL13* (IL 13) and evidence of methylation in genes for the TH1-TH2 pathways (*IL1RL1, IL5RA, STAT4, IL4, CCL18*).[37,38] For AD (eczema), genetic variants of *FLG* and *POSTN* (periostin) may be involved. Obviously the role of the genes related to the innate immune system, skin integrity and immunity, mucosal integrity and mucosal-associated immunity, and antioxidant protection may be important, as are the genetics of T cells (TH2, Treg, and TH1, TH17, and TH22 in the skin) and B cells (IgE- and SIgA-producing cells).

Infants at High Risk for Atopy

To identify infants at high risk for developing atopy, several approaches have been suggested. Cord serum total IgE levels of greater than 100 units/mL are associated with a 5 to 10 times greater risk than lower levels. Eosinophilia and lymphocytes may prove to be markers, but, at present, only the family allergy history and the cord blood IgE have been significantly reliable predictors for recurrent wheezing.[39]

Related to potential environmental risk factors for allergy, several hypotheses have been postulated, including microbial exposure (hygiene), allergen avoidance, dual allergen exposure, nutritional immunomodulation, and a variety of other hypotheses (obesity [chronic inflammatory state]; exposure to processed foods, food additives, and genetically modified foods).[40] In the 1930s, Glaser[41] speculated that if a child was at a high risk for developing allergy, prophylaxis should be able to change the outcome. The original work on prophylaxis was done by Glaser and Johnstone[42] in Rochester, New York and reported in 1953. Only 15% of a group of children whose mothers controlled their own diet in pregnancy and the infants' diets and environments at birth did develop eczema. In contrast, 65% of the sibling controls and 52% of the nonrelated controls who received cow milk developed similar allergic illnesses. Another study was designed and carried out prospectively by Johnstone and Dutton,[43] to investigate dietary prophylaxis of allergic disease. They observed a difference of more than 10 years in the incidence of asthma and perennial allergic rhinitis in those fed soybean milk (18%) and those fed evaporated milk (50%). No infant in this study of 283 children was breastfed, however. A study of 1753 children fed breast milk, soy milk, and cow milk from birth to 6 months of age, who were followed until they were 7 years or older, was published. The children included those with high-risk, low-risk, and no-risk family histories for allergy. No difference in outcome was related to early diet, but a relationship to the family history was seen.[44]

In a prospective study to identify the development of reaginic allergy, infants of allergic parents were placed in a study or control group. The study group followed an allergen-avoidance regimen, including breastfeeding. At 6 months and 1 year, the study infants had less eczema than the control infants, as well as lower serum total IgE levels.[3] The discussion of the efficacy of allergen avoidance, delayed introduction of commonly allergenic foods, and breastfeeding (exclusive and/or longer duration) to avoid food allergens and optimize the intestinal microbiome continue to be debated and studied.

Human Milk Contains Foreign Antigens and Antibodies

Human milk has been analyzed and shown to contain maternal dietary proteins. A small study of 29 women analyzed breast milk by solid-phase radioimmunoassay after the women had ingested either cow milk or a raw egg. Beta-lactoglobulin was detected in breast milk from 10 of 19 women, ovalbumin in 13 of 22 women, and ovomucoid protein in 7 of 9 women. Maximum levels of these foreign proteins in breast milk occurred at approximately 4 to 6 hours after ingestion. There was no evidence of immune complexes in the human milk.[45] Subsequent studies looking for beta-lactoglobulin by an enzyme-linked immunosorbent assay in human milk have also demonstrated its presence at baseline and after a challenge with an oral cow milk load (in 75% of women). In a small percentage of women (15%), no beta-lactoglobulin was detected.[46,47] In a recent study performed with enhanced detection using proteomics, the protein content of human milk was analyzed. Protein detection included 1577 human proteins and 109 nonhuman peptides. Thirty-seven nonhuman peptides were further analyzed, and 9 of these were repeatedly detected in the different human milk samples. These predominant nonhuman proteins were bovine milk products, including casein (α-S1-, α-S2-; beta-, kappa-caseins) and beta-lactoglobulin in quantities of 1 to 10 ng/μL of milk.[48]

Human milk consistently contains antibodies, especially secretory IgA (SIgA), to major food proteins. The levels are influenced by the mother's own external antigen exposure. Savilahti et al.[49] measured IgG subclass antibodies (1 to 4) and IgE to cow milk and hen's egg in 45 infants with documented cow milk allergy based on positive oral challenge testing and skin prick test (SPT) compared with 50 children without cow milk allergy. Infants with cow milk allergy had lower IgG4 levels to alpha-casein, and IgE to beta-lactoglobulin was higher. Infants positive for SPT to egg had elevated levels of sIgG to ovalbumin, beta-lactoglobulin, and alpha-casein and IgA to alpha-casein.[49]

In a study of 500 babies born to families at a high risk for allergies, one group was deliberately not given cow milk and was fed soy milk by random assignment.[50] No benefit resulted from withholding cow milk, but breastfeeding, even for a short period, was clearly associated with a lower incidence of wheezing, prolonged colds, diarrhea, and vomiting. Smoking and environmental molds were also associated with wheezing. Merrett et al.[50] concluded from this that breastfeeding played a significant role in prophylaxis, although this could be explained simply by protection against infection in the respiratory and gastrointestinal tracts.[50]

The effect of breastfeeding on allergic sensitization is proposed to be both direct, through the elimination of nonhuman milk protein as an exposure to antigen, and indirect, by interfering with the absorption of antigen through the intestinal tract.[3]

ENTEROMAMMARY IMMUNE SYSTEM

Maternal antibodies are transferred to breastfed infants as part of what has been called the *enteromammary immune system* (Fig. 17.1).[51] The SIgA antibody present in milk is the result of a mother's enteric immune response to antigens in her gut. SIgA in a mother's milk provides protection against bacterial, viral, and toxic exposures. There are older prospective studies showing that infants at high risk for atopic illness, from a hereditary standpoint, had significantly less disease when breastfed, especially if reared in a protected environment with delayed use of solid foods (Table 17.2).[52] This was compared with children of similar risk fed cow milk and regular solid foods.

Infants with a low incidence of T lymphocytes are at greater risk for developing allergies if fed cow milk rather than breast milk, according to Juto[53] and Juto and Bjorksten.[54] Infants with reduced T-cell fed cow milk also demonstrated higher serum IgE levels and peripheral eosinophil counts. Juto[53] reported that with careful prophylaxis, more than 50% of infants who had both parents with IgE levels greater than 100 mg/mL showed elevated cord and 4-month IgE levels. More than 80% of those infants whose parents had IgE levels less than 100 mg/mL, however, had both low cord blood and low 4-month IgE levels. Such data confirm the genetic effect of both maternal and paternal genes.

Hanson et al.[55] also referred to the enteromammary immune system and the functioning of the breast and infant's intestine as an *immunologic dyad*. Antibodies, lymphocytes, and cytokines in breast milk contribute to the infant's intestinal mucosal barrier, which serves as an enhanced barrier against foreign antigens with less local inflammatory response. At the same time, breast milk constituents facilitate the infant's intestinal and immunologic development. In particular, SIgA, IgG, and IgE are found in human breast milk against cow milk proteins, which may reflect maternal exposures to potential allergens.[1,56-58] Rajani et al.[1] summarize data on immune active factors in human milk and their potential role in the development of atopic disease. Importantly, protein-specific SIgA, cytokines and chemokines are produced by lymphocytes in the breast migrated from the mother's intestine, based on maternal exposure in her intestine (enteromammary system). Various factors in breast milk are considered in their potential role in protection against atopic disease: soluble CD14/LTR, transforming growth factor-β (TGF-β), cytokines (IL-1β, IL-6, IL-10, IL-13), polyunsaturated fatty acids (PUFAs and specifically omega-3 fatty acids and docosahexaenoic [DHA] and eicosapentaenoic acids [EPAs]), and human milk oligosaccharides. Separately the infant's microbiome (intestinal, respiratory tract, and skin) is discussed as influenced by breast milk and its effect on the intestinal milieu and infant's immunologic development during the period of early environmental exposure.[1] The question of how "microbial dysbiosis" in the intestine or the lung might influence the development of atopic disease is an important one to be addressed.[59] The use of "omics" will be important in future studies on the development of atopic disease in infants and the role of breast milk. Type 2 cell-mediated immunity (CMI) (with eosinophils, basophils, mast cells, CD4$^+$ T helper 2 cells, and innate lymphoid cells) contribute directly to chronic allergic diseases (asthma, AD). Along with barrier epithelial cells (ECs) and dendritic cells (DCs) as an early line of defense at mucosal barriers foreign antigens can trigger different responses from the type 2 cell-mediated immunity (CMI), which leads to protection or development of atopic disease. Breast milk plays an important role in barrier function and immunity at mucosal barriers, which certainly plays a role in the development of atopic disease.[60]

PROPHYLAXIS OF ALLERGY

Prophylaxis of Atopic Disease

Efforts to alter the incidence of atopic illness have continued to challenge investigators, who now have access to increased methodologic sophistication. Prevention of IgE-mediated disorders can be directed at the practice of interfering with any of the major forces responsible for the phenotypic expression of atopy.

Review of the plethora of studies directed at measuring the impact of dietary manipulations, including breastfeeding versus not breastfeeding on the incidence of atopic disease demonstrates that retrospective studies show little or no difference in the incidence of asthma and eczema. Prospective studies, however, tend to demonstrate a significant reduction in atopic disease in the treated group.[21,22] In looking at the older data, it is important to recognize that some studies did

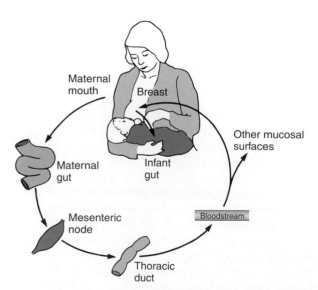

Fig. 17.1 Maternal serum antibodies affect passage of foreign antigens into milk and processing of antigen in infant's intestine. (Redrawn from Kleinman RE. The role of developmental immune mechanisms in intestinal allergy. *Ann Allergy.* 1983;51:222.)

TABLE 17.2 Prevention of Atopy: Prospective Studies

Study	Year Published	No. of Years Followed	No. of Subjects[a]	Type of Milk/Feeding	Impact on Atopy[b]
Johnstone and Dutton	*NEJM* 1966	10	235	Soy, cow	↓ Asthma, rhinitis
Matthew et al.	*Lancet* 1977	1	53 (26)	Breast, soy	↓ Eczema
Chandra	*Acta Pediatr Scand* 1979	>2	134	Breast	↓ Eczema, asthma
Saarinen et al.	*Lancet* 1979	3	(256)	Breast	↓ Eczema, food allergy, asthma
Hamburger	*Excerpta Medica* 1981	1	(300)	Breast	↓ Eczema, asthma
Kaufman and Frick	*Ann Allergy* 1976, *Clin Allergy* 1981	2	(94)	Breast	↓ Asthma
Hide and Guyer	*Arch Dis Child* 1981	1	843 (266)	Breast <6 mo, soy, cow (maternal diet not controlled)	↓ Eczema slight, rhinitis
Gruskay	*Clin Pediatr* 1982	15	908 (328)	Breast 4 mo, soy, cow	↓ Breast symptoms; soy no effect
May et al.	*Acta Paediatr Scand* 1982	1/2	67 normal	Soy, cow, modern formula	↑ Antibodies with no disease symptoms
Businco et al.	*Ann Allergy* 1983	2	(101)	Breast <6 mo; soy, cow	↓ Asthma, eczema
Kajosaari and Saarinen	*Acta Paediatr Scand* 1983	1	(135)	All breast milk <6 mo; half solid foods early	↑ Eczema/food intolerance in those fed solids
Moore et al.	*Arch Dis Child* 1985	1	525	Study—breastfed 3 mo; control —SMA	Not clear: 74% failed to breastfeed or gave cow milk in study group
Zeiger et al.	*J Allergy Clin Immunol* 1989	4	288	Maternal avoidance diet last trimester; controls unrestricted; mother's diet; infants given Nutramigen	↓ Atopy 16% in restricted infants ↑ Atopy in control infants (to 27%) ↓ Urticaria/GI symptoms in restricted group
Sigurs et al.	*Pediatrics* 1992	4	115	All breastfed; 65 mothers restricted diet for first 3 mo of lactation; 50 no restrictions	↓ Atopy/asthma among both groups ↓ Greater among restricted group

GI, Gastrointestinal; *SMA*, formula by Wyeth (no longer available).
[a]Number in study; parentheses indicate number at risk for atopy.
[b]Arrows indicate decrease or increase compared with control group.
Modified from Businco L, Marchetti F, Pellegrini G, Cantani A, Perlini R. Prevention of atopic disease in "at-risk newborns" by prolonged breastfeeding. *Ann Allergy*. 1983;51:296.

not consider the risk for the population developing atopic disease on a hereditary basis. In other studies, breastfeeding may have been carried out for only a few weeks or months. Many of these studies controlled for smoking in the household, and no data were reported on the incidence of respiratory syncytial virus, both potential triggers for wheezing/asthma. In addition, some studies did not control for the breastfeeding mother's diet, the weaning foods, or the use of cow milk products. However, when the long-term effects of breastfeeding, maternal smoking during pregnancy, and recurrent lower respiratory tract infections on asthma in children were

examined, some discordance of results was observed. Breastfeeding for less than 3 months was not an effective intervention as prophylaxis. Breastfeeding reduced the effect of lower respiratory tract infections on episodes of wheezing in infants. Similarly, it reduced the effect of smoking.[39] Asthma in childhood can be prevented by promoting breastfeeding, preventing smoking in pregnancy and infancy, and avoiding recurrent lower respiratory tract infections in early childhood. Recurrent wheezing episodes were evaluated for associated risk factors.[39] Cigarette smoking in the household, heating mode (open stove), and breastfeeding for less than

TABLE 17.3 Relationship of Maternal Total Serum Immunoglobulin E (IgE) Level to Cord and 4-Month Serum IgE Levels in Infants in the Prophylaxis Group

Maternal IgE (U/mL)	CORD IGE (U/ML)		4-MO IGE (U/ML)	
	<0.5, No. (%)	≥0.5, No. (%)	<5.0, No. (%)	≥5.0, No. (%)
≤100	35 (71)	14 (29)	41 (87)	6 (13)
>100	14 (42)	19 (58)	24 (73)	9 (27)
Total	49	33	65	15

$p < 0.01$ by chi-square test for maternal IgE <100 vs. > 100 U/ml for cord IgE with a trend ($p < 0.08$) at 4-month IgE measurement. From Hamburger RN, Heller S, Mellon MH, et al. Current status of the clinical and immunologic consequences of a prototype allergic disease prevention program. *Ann Allergy.* 1983;51:281.

TABLE 17.4 Relationship of Paternal Total Serum Immunoglobulin E (IgE) Level to Cord and 4-Month Serum IgE Levels in Infants in the Prophylaxis Group

Paternal IgE (U/mL)	CORD IGE (U/ML)		4-MO IGE (U/ML)	
	<0.5, No. (%)	≥0.5, No. (%)	<5.0, No. (%)	≥5.0, No. (%)
≤100	29 (63)	17 (37)	40 (83)	8 (17)
>100	10 (56)	8 (44)	14 (82)	3 (18)
Total	39	25	54	11

From Hamburger RN, Heller S, Mellon MH, et al. Current status of the clinical and immunologic consequences of a prototype allergic disease prevention program. *Ann Allergy.* 1983;51:281.

6 months were significantly associated with increased risk for recurrent wheezing.

Hamburger et al.[61] carried out prospective prophylactic studies to include measuring IgE and skin radioallergosorbent tests (RASTs) on mothers, fathers, and infants.[61] They found a significant correlation between maternal IgE and infant IgE and potential allergy in the infants (Tables 17.3 and 17.4). This study was done with controlling the environment and the diet. The process was initiated in pregnancy, to begin by protecting the fetus, and was then continued at birth. Therefore, considerable attention was directed toward breastfeeding in this and other studies.

Longitudinal Studies of Allergy Prophylaxis

In an 18-month study of atopic outcome, atopic mothers (total n = 162 women with respiratory allergy) were randomly allocated to an intervention group or an unrestricted-diet group, and both were compared with nonatopic mothers on unrestricted diets. The intervention was a milk/dairy product–free diet during late pregnancy and lactation. After 7 weeks of the diet, serum beta-lactoglobulin and IgG levels in the mothers were collated to the levels in cord blood. The 163 infants were examined at 12 and 18 months, using a single-blind allergy assessment by a pediatrician. Infants born to nonatopic parents had significantly less allergy than those born to atopic mothers with unrestricted diets.[62] The restricted-diet group of infants had comparable levels to the atopy-free group and had significantly less allergy than the unrestricted-diet group. The nature of the parents' disease and genetic variables probably played a greater role in the occurrence of atopic illness in both groups.

A prospective longitudinal study of 988 healthy infants, from birth to 6 years of age, recorded feeding history, episodes of lower respiratory tract infection in the first 3 years of life, and recurrent episodes of wheezing.[63] Being breastfed was associated with lower rates of recurrent wheeze (3.1% vs. 9.7%, $p < 0.01$) for nonatopic children. The authors concluded that recurrent wheeze at age 6 years is less common among nonatopic children who were breastfed as infants. This effect was independent of whether the child had a wheezing lower respiratory tract illness in the first 6 months of life (Table 17.5). These authors recorded smoking history, but it did not alter the compelling influence of breastfeeding on the outcome.[63]

Another long-term study demonstrated that children who had ever been breastfed had a 50% lower incidence of wheezing than those who had not been breastfed. The effect persisted for the 7 years of the study in nonatopic children.[64] The authors attribute this in part to breastfeeding's protective effect against respiratory illness. They did not distinguish minimal from prolonged breastfeeding. In a 17-year prospective study of 150 healthy children, researchers did consider length of breastfeeding.[65] The three groups had been breastfed less than 1 month or not at all, 1 to 6 months, or more than 6 months. Prolonged breastfeeding was associated with the least eczema at 1 to 3 years, as well as fewer food and respiratory allergies. At age 17 years, the trends continued, leading the authors to conclude that breastfeeding is protective against atopic eczema, food allergy, and respiratory asthma throughout childhood and adolescence (Figs. 17.2 and 17.3).[65]

Systematic Reviews of Maternal Diet as Prophylaxis

A review of five randomized controlled trials (RCTs) or quasi-randomized studies of maternal dietary antigen avoidance in 952 pregnant or lactating women did not demonstrate protection against AD/eczema in the children at 18 months of age.[66] Data were insufficient to analyze allergic rhinitis or urticaria relative to maternal diet antigen avoidance. Two of the included trials focused on antigen avoidance only during lactation in 523 mothers. There was no evidence of a protective effect for AD or the occurrence of positive SPTs to specific allergens (cow milk, egg, peanut) at 1, 2, and 7 years of age in the children. In a larger systematic review of food-based approaches to protection against allergy, 42 studies were included (11 intervention studies, 26 prospective cohort studies, 4 retrospective cohort studies, and 1 case-control study) involving over 40,000 children.[67] In the 7 RCTs the

TABLE 17.5 Odds Ratios and Confidence Intervals for Recurrent Wheeze at Age 6 Years by Logistic Regression

Factor	ODDS RATIO (CONFIDENCE INTERVAL)[a]		
	Total Group ($n = 970$)	Nonatopic Children ($n = 420$)	Atopic Children ($n = 280$)
Not breastfed	1.49 (0.80–2.77)	3.03[b] (1.05–8.69)	1.36 (0.49–3.73)
Maternal education ≤ 12 y	1.48 (0.87–2.53)	1.58 (0.56–4.43)	0.92 (0.36–2.38)
Hispanic	2.48[c] (1.39–4.40)	2.45 (0.82–7.27)	2.50[b] (1.01–6.18)
Maternal hay fever	2.66[d] (1.49–4.72)	2.64 (0.96–7.22)	2.35[b] (1.07–5.16)
Wheezing lower respiratory tract illness in first 6 mo	1.68 (0.88–3.19)	1.86 (0.55–6.25)	2.01 (0.74–5.48)

[a]Excludes children who were missing information for one or more of these factors.
[b]$p < 0.05$.
[c]$p < 0.005$.
[d]$p < 0.0005$.
From Wright AL, Holberg CJ, Taussig LM, et al. Relationship of infant feeding to recurrent wheezing at age 6 years. *Arch Pediatr Adolesc Med.* 1995;49:762.

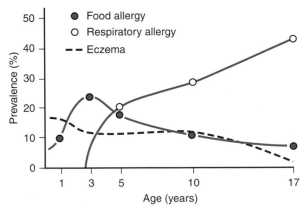

Fig. 17.2 Prevalence of atopic eczema, food allergy, and respiratory allergy in full cohort of initial 236 children during follow-up for 17 years. (Modified from Saarinen UM, Kajossari M. Breastfeeding as prophylaxis against disease: prospective follow-up study until 17 years old. *Lancet.* 1995;346:1065.)

prevalence of eczema and asthma was no different in the infants with mothers participating in antigen avoidance diets for common food allergens. The prospective cohort studies did not show protection from avoidance diets, but mothers who consumed a diet similar to the Mediterranean diet, rich in fruits, vegetables, and fish, with ample in vitamin D, showed greater impact on protection against atopic disorders than those who did not.[67]

RECOMMENDATIONS OF THE COMMITTEE ON NUTRITION AND SECTION ON ALLERGY AND IMMUNOLOGY OF THE AMERICAN ACADEMY OF PEDIATRICS

The incidence of atopic disease in the United States, including asthma, AD, and food allergies, seems to have increased from 1997 to 2011.[9] The literature and the research have been abundant, but evidence is hindered by inadequate or differing study designs. Prevention of disease by dietary restrictions in pregnancy and lactation were reviewed in a clinical report from the AAP in 2008.[21] A revised report was published in 2019, analyzing predominantly RCTs, systematic reviews, meta-analyses, and recommendations from other health groups.[22] The reported recommendations address dietary restrictions for pregnant or lactating women, extent and duration of breastfeeding, hydrolyzed formulas, and the timing of introduction of potentially allergenic foods into the infant's diet. Because of limited data, no recommendations were made regarding the potential role of vitamin D, long-chain PUFAs, and prebiotics and probiotics in protection against atopic disease.

The following are the recommendations from the AAP for nutritional interventions to prevent atopic disease from the 2019 report:

1. "There is lack of evidence to support maternal dietary restrictions either during pregnancy or during lactation to prevent atopic disease. This conclusion is unchanged from the 2008 report.

2. The evidence regarding the role of breastfeeding in the prevention of atopic disease can be summarized as follows:
   A. There is evidence that exclusive breastfeeding for the first 3 to 4 months decreases the cumulative incidence of eczema in the first 2 years of life. This conclusion is unchanged from the 2008 report;
   B. There are no short- or long-term advantages for exclusive breastfeeding beyond 3 to 4 months for prevention of atopic disease. This conclusion is unchanged from the 2008 report;
   C. The evidence now suggests that any duration of breastfeeding beyond 3 to 4 months is protective against wheezing in the first 2 years of life. This

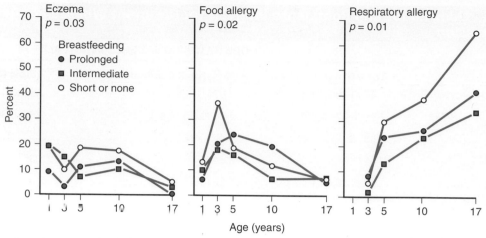

Fig. 17.3 Prevalence of atopic eczema, food allergy, and respiratory allergy in infant feeding groups during follow-up for 17 years. Tests for differences during the appropriate age periods (eczema 1 to 3 years, food allergy 1 to 3 years, respiratory allergy at 5, 10, and 17 years) were done by analysis of variance and covariance with repeated measures. (Modified from Saarinen UM, Kajossari M. Breastfeeding as prophylaxis against disease: prospective follow-up study until 17 years old. *Lancet*. 1995;346:1065.)

effect is irrespective of duration of exclusivity. This conclusion differs slightly from the 2008 report, which stated that exclusive breastfeeding for at least 3 months protects against wheezing early in life;

D. Unlike the 2008 report, there is now some evidence that longer duration of any breastfeeding, as opposed to less breastfeeding, protects against asthma, even after 5 years of age; and

E. Similar to the 2008 report, no conclusions can be made about the role of any duration of breastfeeding in either preventing or delaying the onset of specific food allergies.

3. There is lack of evidence that partially or extensively hydrolyzed formula prevents atopic disease in infants and children, even in those at high risk for allergic disease. This is a change from the 2008 report, in which the AAP concluded that there was modest evidence that hydrolyzed formulas delayed or prevented atopic dermatitis in infants who were formula fed or not exclusively breastfed for 3 to 4 months.

4. The current evidence for the importance of the timing of introduction of allergenic foods and the prevention of atopic disease can be summarized as follows:

A. There is no evidence that delaying the introduction of allergenic foods, including peanuts, eggs, and fish, beyond 4 to 6 months prevents atopic disease. This conclusion has not changed from the 2008 report;

B. There is now evidence that the early introduction of infant-safe forms of peanuts reduces the risk for peanut allergies. Data are less clear for timing of introduction of eggs; and

C. The new recommendations for the prevention of peanut allergy are based largely on the LEAP trial[68] and are endorsed by the AAP.[68] An expert panel has advised peanut introduction as early as 4 to 6 months of age for infants at high risk for peanut

allergy (presence of severe eczema and/or egg allergy). The recommendations contain details of implementation for high-risk infants, including appropriate use of testing (specific IgE measurement, skin-prick test, and oral food challenges) and introduction of peanut containing foods in the health care provider's office versus the home setting, as well as amount and frequency.[69] For infants with mild to moderate eczema, the panel recommended introduction of peanut-containing foods at around 6 months of age, and for infants at low risk for peanut allergy (no eczema or any food allergy), the panel recommended introduction of peanut-containing food when age appropriate and depending on family preferences and cultural practices (ie, after 6 months of age if exclusively breastfeeding).

5. This report describes means to prevent or delay atopic disease through early dietary intervention. For the child who has developed atopic disease, treatment may require specific identification and restriction of causal food proteins; this topic is not addressed in this report."

Other recommendations unchanged from the 2008 report include that solid foods should not be introduced before 4 to 6 months of age and no current evidence is convincing that delaying their introduction beyond this period has a significant protective effect on the development of atopic disease. This is regardless of whether infants are fed cow milk protein formula or human milk. This includes delaying the introduction of foods that are considered highly allergenic, such as fish, eggs, and foods containing peanut protein. For infants older than 4 to 6 months of age, data are insufficient to support a protective effect of any dietary intervention for the development of atopic disease. Additional studies are needed to document the long-term effect of dietary interventions in infancy to prevent atopic disease, especially in children older than 4 years and in adults.[22]

IMMUNOLOGIC ASPECTS OF ALLERGY

A complete discussion of the immunology of allergy and the broad spectrum of clinical atopic diseases is beyond the scope of this text. Much of the original descriptions and concepts of allergy have been modified. Some descriptions of Gell and Coomb's Classification of Hypersensitivity Reactions have been expanded to include types I to VI; type I hypersensitivity reaction—IgE antibody mediated, type II hypersensitivity reaction—antibodies mediated, type III hypersensitivity reaction—antigen-antibody complex mediated, type IV delayed hypersensitivity reaction—activated T-cell and cytokines mediated, type V delayed hypersensitivity reaction—antibody mediated, and type VI delayed hypersensitivity reaction—antibody and cell mediated. However, the terminology of "hypersensitivity reactions" is no longer completely accurate because in some cases the disease process begins with barrier integrity deficits or disruption and the reaction is an inadequate or dysfunctional immune response to foreign antigens. The complexity of atopic diseases has required a distinction of different phenotypes of clinical disease (asthma is being effectively typed based on clinical features, associations and response to treatments), and "endotypes" clarifying the specific pathophysiologic mechanisms causes phenotypes of disease.[18,19] The goal is to improve and guide patient care by determining the underlying mechanisms causing an individual's allergic disease.[70]

Evolving Concepts in Allergic Immunology

It was established that a type 2 immune response is the dominant component in the pathogenesis of eosinophilic asthma (one phenotype of asthma), allergic rhinitis, chronic rhinosinusitis with nasal polyps, eosinophilic esophagitis, and extrinsic AD. The type 2 immune response included TH2 cells, type 2 B cells, group 2 innate lymphoid cells, type 2 macrophages, IL-4 secreting natural killer (NK) cells, IL-4 secreting NK-T cells, basophils, eosinophils and mast cells. Cytokines play a crucial role in the activation and maintenance of the type 2 response with IL-4, IL-5, IL-9, IL-13, and IL-31 produced by immune system cells and cytokines IL-25, IL-33, and thymic stromal lymphopoietin (TSLP) from tissue cells (commonly ECs). The various cells and cytokines have identified roles in the immune response; for example, IL-4 and IL-13 stimulate production of allergen-specific IgE and IL-5 causing eosinophilia. IL-4 and IL-13 also cause tissue migration of eosinophils and TH2 cells and contribute to tight junction maintenance and epithelial barrier integrity. IL-9 and IL-13 contribute to mucus production at mucosal surfaces (Table 17.6).[71] The TH2-type cytokines certainly promote allergic-type airway inflammation that leads to asthma in a large percentage of children. Specific cytokines IL-9, IL-17, and IL-22 mediate airway inflammation dominated by neutrophils. This is different from the allergic type of asthma constituting a different endotype and phenotype of asthma. IL-17 is associated with recruitment of neutrophils, and IL-22 has been described as producing antimicrobial peptide production and affecting mucosal barrier integrity, adding to the local inflammation.[72]

T-regulatory (Treg) and B-regulatory (Breg) cells are involved in tolerance of self-tissues and nonself environmental allergens as well as immune regulation of type 2 inflammation, specifically type 2 innate lymphoid cells. IL-10—secreting Breg cells suppress allergen-specific responses. IL-10, IL-35, and TGF-β are suppressor cytokines adding to immune regulation.

Localized atopic diseases (pruritus, chronic spontaneous urticaria, AD, allergic contact dermatitis) are mediated by a variety of mechanisms that lead to the different clinical manifestations and severity of disease. These pathophysiologic mechanisms demonstrate changes in the systemic immune response related to eosinophils, mast cells, and IgE. Itch, or

TABLE 17.6	Selected Factors in Allergic Mechanisms of Disease		
Factors	**Atopic Diseases**	**Biologic agents**	**Comments**
IL-5/IL5 receptor α	Asthma, CRSwNP, EoE, HES	Benralizumab Mepolizumab Reslizumab	Blood and tissue eosinophils
IL-4Rα subunit	Asthma, AD, CRSwNP	Dupilumab	IL-4
IL-13	Asthma, AD, CRSwNP	Lebrikizumab Tralokinumab	IL-13
IgE receptor cross-linking	Asthma, chronic urticaria, CRSwNP, FA	Ligelizumab Omalizumab	IgE
TSLP	Asthma, CRSwNP, EoE, AD	Tezepelumab	Alarmins—TSLP, IL-33, IL-25
IL-33	Asthma, CRSwNP, EoE, AD	Under development	Alarmins—TSLP, IL-33, IL-25
IL-1 R3, JAK, STAT pathway	Asthma, CRSwNP, EoE, AD	Under development	Other upstream targets

AD, Atopic dermatitis; *CRSwNP*, chronic rhinosinusitis with nasal polyps; *EOE*, eosinophilic esophagitis; *FA*, food allergy; *HES*, hypereosinophilic syndrome; *Ig*, immunoglobulin; *IL*, interleukin; *IL-4Rα*-interleukin-4 receptor alpha chain; *JAK*, Janus-activated kinase; *STAT*, signal transducer and activator of transcription; *TSLP*, thymic stromal lymphopoietin.
From Agache I, Cojanu C, Laculiceanu A, et al. Critical points on the use of biologicals in allergic diseases and asthma. *Allergy Asthma Immunol Res.* 12:24, 2020. http://doi:10.4168/aair.2020.12.1.24.

pruritus, is mediated by various factors, most importantly histamine release, mast cell release of eicosanoids (prostaglandin D2, leukotriene C4, D4, and E4), and activation of specialized sensory neurons that regulate itch, sneeze, cough, and bronchoconstriction.[73] In AD, the issue of a defective skin barrier presumably predisposes to penetration of the barrier by microbes and allergens, leading to subsequent IgE sensitization and type 2 cytokine release and causing local allergic inflammation. A defect in differentiation of keratinocytes may be the original barrier abnormality. Additional downstream barrier dysfunction may be a direct effect of cytokines as well as protein production of periostin and diminished expression of filaggrin, adding to the disruption. "Atopic march" describes the apparent "progression" of disease from AD early in life in an individual to the onset of other allergic diseases (food allergy, asthma, and allergic rhinitis) later on.[74] This fits with the theories of epicutaneous allergen sensitization (through intact or impaired skin barrier) and the dual allergen exposure hypothesis. An initial exposure to environmental food allergens through a disrupted skin barrier leads to sensitization. Protection against the subsequent development of food allergy presumably can occur by immune tolerance as a result of early exposure to food allergens in the intestine. This is partly the theory behind allergen avoidance by exclusion diets and behind the early introduction of highly allergenic foods (peanut, egg, cow milk).

The term *exposome* refers to the entire realm of environmental exposures individuals experience in their life, including in utero, at delivery, while breastfeeding, through the maternal diet, by early-life environment (siblings, pets, farms/farm products, etc.), with antibiotics and other medications, and to their own microbiome. The question with this multitude of exposures is how the individual responds to each potential allergen sequentially and cumulatively. How does predisposition to atopic disease influence the response? There is now evidence that epigenetic changes in response to such challenges also contribute to one's allergic nature.[75] Additional understanding of the molecular mechanisms of these interactions between the environment and the human body is essential.

Microbiome and Allergic Diseases

The human microbiota is made up of multiple local microbiomes (skin, gut, respiratory tract, etc.), each different from the others and interacting differently with the mucosal immune processes and host. Much has been written about the factors influencing the makeup of the microbiomes and their evolution over time and in particular about allergic diseases and the microbiome.[59,76–79] Dysbiosis, or disruption of the microbiome, has been implicated in altering mucosal immunity and local homeostasis. This disruption is associated with allergic sensitization and inflammation and potentially an altered response to allergens.[78] Human milk influences the infant's microbiome by introducing specific bacteria and favoring the growth of certain bacteria through its composition. The intestinal microbiome of the breastfeeding infant has less diversity overall and is dominated by *Lactobacillus, Bifidobacterium,* and Enterobacteriaceae. At cessation of

breastfeeding, more so than with introduction of complementary foods, the intestinal microbiome changes to be dominated by *Clostridium* and *Bacteroides,* becomes more diverse through 2 years of age, and ultimately resembles the adult intestinal microbiome. Human milk oligosaccharides (HMOs) are not digestible by the infant and provide substrate for the intestinal microbiome favoring the growth of specific organisms and additionally support mucosal immunity development and provide antiinflammatory effects. Another important milk component, PUFAs, in particular omega-3 fatty acids (DHA, EPA), have antiinflammatory effects.[80] AD has been described as epidermal barrier dysfunction and chronic recurrent inflammation produced by a decrease in epidermal structural proteins, altered lipid makeup, activated local and systemic inflammation, and diminished microbial diversity of the skin. Increased inflammation, further barrier disruption, and *Staphylococcus aureus* bacterial overgrowth lead to eczematous flares.[81] Mechanistically, the association of the gut microbiome and food allergy appear directly connected via dysbiosis, the intestinal epithelial cell interaction with the microbiome and local barrier, and mucosal immune function development. HMOs and short-chain fatty acids (SCFAs) are implicated in local antiinflammatory effects and oral tolerance. Variation in HMO composition of human milk has been associated with cow milk allergy. Dysbiosis seemingly leads to altered microbial signals favoring the development of type 2 immunity within the intestine.[78] Early-life dysbiosis of the lung and gut microbiomes, within a "window of susceptibility" also have been associated with asthma and allergy. Different studies have described "lower relative abundance" of specific bacterial genera associated with an increased risk for developing asthma later in life. Alternatively, early colonization of the respiratory tract with a variety of respiratory pathogens (*Haemophilus, Moraxella, Streptococcus*) is associated with an increased risk for later asthma. High levels of fecal SCFAs in breastfed infants were associated with protection against asthma.[78]

A number of studies have examined the effect of probiotics in early life on the risk for developing atopic disease later in life. There have been several meta-analyses of studies on the topic. One study including a population of 4031 subjects in 20 cohorts in Europe, Asia, and Australia was reported in a meta-analysis. Studies included 25 double-blind, randomized, and placebo-controlled trials. Probiotics were given prenatally and postnatally (10 studies) and directly to the child (9 studies). Atopic sensitization was measured by positive SPT or elevated serum-specific IgE level to any food or allergen. Asthma was diagnosed by physician or parent. Probiotics did not significantly reduce the prevalence of asthma or wheeze. Introduction of *Lactobacillus acidophilus* as an individual strain was associated with increased atopic sensitization but not a reduction in the actual atopic disease.[82] Two other reviews of allergy and asthma prevention with probiotics also did not find results supporting prevention. The studies were difficult to compare because of sample size, heterogeneity of study design, and variable methods of analyzing gut microbiome.[83,84] A separate systematic review of probiotics for the management of cow milk protein allergy showed that probiotics were associated with more common acquisition of tolerance to cow's milk protein in patients with "confirmed" cow milk protein allergy after 3 years of follow-up when compared with a placebo group. There was no apparent benefit in shortening the occurrence of hematochezia.[85]

There remain significant gaps in our understanding of the microbiome, breast milk, and the immunology of allergy. Ideally, research will continue to focus on the mechanisms of interaction in addition to the epidemiology to guide prevention and therapy of atopic diseases.

COW MILK ALLERGY

Patterns of Clinical Disease Associated With Cow Milk Allergy in Childhood

Cow milk allergy affects 6% to 8% of infants younger than 3 years. Formula-fed or breastfed infants can manifest cow milk protein allergy. Many poorly defined illnesses and pathologic lesions have been associated with the ingestion of milk, making clear diagnosis difficult. Definitions originally proposed by the American Academy of Allergy and Immunology and adapted by Anderson are as follows:[86]

- *Food intolerance* is an adverse reaction to the ingestion of a food related to an enzyme deficiency or metabolic or pharmacologic reaction.
- *Food adverse reaction* with unknown mechanism is an idiosyncrasy; no immunologic mechanism is associated.
- *Food allergy* or *food hypersensitivity* is an adverse reaction to food caused by one or more immune hypersensitivity mechanisms and is not confined to IgE.
- *Food anaphylaxis* reactions are immediate hypersensitivity involving the immunologic activity of IgE homocytotropic antibody and the release of chemical mediators that may be life threatening.
- *Anaphylactoid reaction* to food is an anaphylaxis-like reaction to food as a result of a nonimmune release of chemical mediators.
- *Food toxicity* (poisoning) is toxin from the food itself and not an immune reaction (e.g., scombroid fish poisoning, botulism).
- *Pharmacologic food reaction* is a naturally derived or added chemical that produces a pharmacologic reaction (caffeine in coffee or sodas).

Symptoms associated with food allergy include asthma, eczema, urticaria, and rhinitis, as well as colic and failure to thrive with chronic respiratory and gastrointestinal disease. Skin and the gastrointestinal and respiratory systems are most commonly involved with cow milk protein allergy. Well-defined but uncommon syndromes, including pulmonary hemosiderosis, bronchitis, protein- and iron-losing enteropathy, neonatal thrombocytopenia, and colitis, have been reported to result from cow milk allergy in both breastfed and formula-fed infants.[87] Sleep disturbances have been reported in a series of children evaluated with a prospective double-blind crossover design (Table 17.7).[88]

TABLE 17.7 Clinical Presentations of Cow Milk Protein Allergy

Reaction Type	Presentation
IgE Mediated	
Respiratory	Rhinoconjunctivitis
	Asthma (wheeze, cough)
	Laryngeal edema
	Otitis media with effusion
Cutaneous	Atopic dermatitis
	Urticaria
	Angioedema
	Anaphylaxis
Gastrointestinal	Oral allergy syndrome
	Nausea and vomiting
	Diarrhea
Non–IgE Mediated	
Respiratory	Pulmonary hemosiderosis
Cutaneous	Contact rash
	Atopic dermatitis
Gastrointestinal	Regurgitation
	Vomiting
	Chronic diarrhea
	Protein-losing enteropathy
	Blood in stool
	Colic
	Constipation
	Food refusal
	Food protein–induced enterocolitis syndrome (FPIES)
	Food protein–induced allergic proctocolitis (FPIAP)
	Food protein-induced enteropathy (FPIE)
Mixed Mechanisms	
Cutaneous	Atopic dermatitis
Gastrointestinal	Regurgitation
	Vomiting
	Retrosternal pain
	Food refusal
	Dysphagia
	Food impaction
	Chronic diarrhea

(Continued)

TABLE 17.7 Clinical Presentations of Cow Milk Protein Allergy—cont'd

Reaction Type	Presentation
	Abdominal pain
	Blood in stool
	Protein-losing enteropathy
	Failure to thrive
	Eosinophilic esophagitis
	Eosinophilic gastroenteritis
	Eosinophilic colitis
Other Unclassified (rare)	Arthritis
	Henoch-Schönlein purpura
	Migraine

IgE, Immunoglobulin E.
From Kansu A, Yüce A, Dalgıç B, Şekerel BE, Çullu-Çokuğraş F, Çokuğraş H. Consensus statement on diagnosis, treatment and follow-up of cow's milk protein allergy among infants and children in Turkey Consensus Statement. *Turk J Pediatr.* 2016;58:1–11.

Acute Reactions to Cow Milk in Breastfed Infants

Hippocrates and Gojen described classic cases of milk allergy.[5] External reaction to cow milk was first described in the literature in the 19th century and then by Schloss[89] in 1920 and Tisdale and Erb[90] in 1925. At that time, the reaction was noted to occur during the first feeding of cow milk, which was provided in an effort to wean from the breast at several months of age. The event included sudden crying as if in pain; swelling of the lips, tongue, and throat; stridor; and even generalized urticaria and wheezing lasting for up to an hour.

This type of cow milk allergy is the first of two types described by Gerrard and Shenassa[91] and others. The second type is the well-known reaction to large amounts of cow milk in a cow milk–fed infant and is manifested by vomiting, diarrhea, or colic. This second type is not associated with cow milk–specific IgE antibodies. It usually subsides over time. The acute anaphylactic reactions, however, are associated with alpha-lactalbumin, beta-lactoglobulin, and casein immunity.

Schwartz et al.[92] studied 29 breastfed or soy formula–fed infants who had experienced acute urticarial reactions while being fed cow milk for the first time. One infant had the reaction in the newborn nursery, suggesting in utero sensitization. When charts were carefully reviewed by Schwartz et al., 16 infants were identified as having been given formula in the newborn nursery. Of these, 12 could have been sensitized in utero or through the breast milk. The authors identified elevated serum IgE levels; positive RASTs for alpha-lactalbumin, beta-lactoglobulin, and casein; and recurrent wheezing in 55% of infants (16/29).

In a follow-up study challenging this group of children with whey and casein hydrolysate products, Schwartz et al.[92]

found that 69% had positive SPTs to whey hydrolysate and 38% of SPTs were positive to casein hydrolysate. Children with reactions to cow milk and both hydrolysates had severe reactions, including urticaria, angioedema, and wheezing. Hydrolysates of cow milk protein are not necessarily hypoallergenic. Breastfeeding with small amounts of cow milk proteins in the mother's milk can uncommonly be a risk factor in the development of IgE-mediated cow milk allergy in a susceptible infant. Early exposures may occur in utero, through the breast milk, or with inadvertent feedings of cow milk. Schwartz et al.[93,94] suggest that isolated cow milk not be given to exclusively breastfed infants in the newborn period.

Intrauterine Sensitization

Intrauterine sensitization and allergy in the newborn breastfed infant were described by Matsumura in Japan. Glaser[95] also identified that under certain conditions, an infant with a predisposition for allergy may become actively sensitized in utero because of the mother's consumption of certain foods during pregnancy.[95] For example, Shannon[96] demonstrated the presence of egg antigen in human breast milk in 1922. Infants then responded to reexposure with allergic symptoms on first contact with that same food.[91,97] Kuroume et al.[97] showed that with intrauterine sensitization, hemagglutinating antibody titers against lactalbumin and soybean in the amniotic fluid are high. They suggest that analysis of amniotic fluid could be used to predict future allergy, although this is rarely done. There is a question of whether detection of allergen-specific IgE or IgA in amniotic fluid or cord blood in the infant in the early postnatal period constitutes evidence of sensitization, passive transfer of antibodies from the mother, or actual allergy.[98,99] Most studies do not include testing of cord blood or infant's serum before early feeding to distinguish in utero versus early postnatal sensitization.[100] In utero sensitization to inhaled allergens appears less likely.[101]

FOOD ALLERGY IN BREASTFED INFANTS

Diagnosis of Food Allergy in Breastfed Infants

Various algorithms have been proposed for the diagnosis of food allergy.[102–104] They all begin with a careful history and physical examination to clarify possible triggers and likely pathophysiologic mechanisms (IgE-mediated, non–IgE-mediated, mixed, and other). Targeted SPT and/or allergen-specific IgE testing based on possible food triggers can be performed or an elimination diet initiated for the infant (and for the mother if the infant is breastfeeding). Radioallergoabsorbent sensitivity testing (RAST) is not used commonly when there has been a specific event or illness and there are suspected food triggers. Targeted SPT is very sensitive but less specific. Its negative predictive value is >90%, but a positive test confirms only sensitization to an allergen and does not confirm the diagnosis of food allergy.[102] A positive test for food-specific IgE antibodies has variable predictive value depending on different populations and the specific allergen being tested. Different cutoff points will yield different predictive values for the diagnosis of a food allergy. An oral food challenge is considered the gold standard but is not always readily available.

Oral Challenges for Food-Allergic Disease

Oral food challenges (OFCs) must be physician-supervised for the diagnosis of food-allergic disease to optimize safety. Relative to safety, Lieberman et al.[105] presented a retrospective chart review of OFCs performed at their institution. Of 701 challenges in 521 patients (8 months to 21 years of age) performed on various likely food allergens (milk, egg, peanut, tree nuts, soy, fish, shellfish, sesame, and wheat), there were 132 reactions (18.8%) during the challenges. Cutaneous reactions were most common (75, 56.8%), of which 12 patients with reactions were given epinephrine. The authors reported that OFCs are safe given the need for treatment with epinephrine in only 1.7% of all the OFCs performed.[105] OFC can be done as an open feeding challenge or a blinded, placebo-controlled food challenge.

Elimination Diets for the Breastfeeding Mother

In a technical review, the American Gastroenterological Association comments that breastfeeding is cost effective, but maternally ingested protein can elicit allergic symptoms in infants.[106] Thus, maternal dietary manipulation is required, which should be done to avoid expensive alternative formulas.

When Giovannini et al.[107] studied growth and metabolic parameters of infants fed special formulas for atopy prevention, they noted differences compared with infants who were exclusively breastfed. Lower body mass index values and higher blood urea nitrogen levels were seen at 3 months.[107,108] Plasma aminoacidograms showed higher essential amino acids but lower branched-chain amino acids. Furthermore, the plasma taurine levels were lower in the formula-fed infants, even though the formulas had added taurine. These observations have been confirmed by other investigators, who are most concerned about the elevated threonine levels.[109]

The allergens of specific foods ingested by the mother have been identified in the milk. Cant et al.[110] found 49 eczematous infants who were solely breastfed to be sensitized to cow milk and egg protein; these researchers concluded that infants can be sensitized by foods eaten by the mother. They were able to demonstrate ovalbumin in the breast milk of 14 of 19 mothers who were tested 2 to 4 hours after eating raw egg. This was whether or not their infants had tested positive to egg albumin. Beta-lactoglobulin is often found in human milk, but the amounts vary markedly after maternal cow milk ingestion.[46] Zhu et al.[48] demonstrated by proteomic analysis that bovine milk products are the dominant nonhuman proteins observed in human milk.

Troncone et al.[111] collected samples of breast milk at various times after the mothers were fed 20 g of gluten, after a period of deliberate gluten avoidance. Gliadin was found in 54 of 80 samples; levels peaked at 2 to 4 hours. Gliadin could not be detected in maternal serum. The transfer of gliadin to infants through the milk could be one of the factors producing a protective effect, because breastfeeding is known to decrease the risk for celiac disease.[112]

For each situation a risk-to-benefit analysis for the mother and infant should be done before initiating the elimination diet. This should balance the mother's nutrition status and health with the potential benefit of diminished ongoing sensitization of the infant to various allergens and the potential future tolerance of the offending food(s).

Allergies to Solid Foods

Foods ingested by a mother may present a problem for an allergic child. Nevertheless, food intolerance or adverse reaction to a food are much more common than food allergy or hypersensitivity. The most common problematic allergens have been enumerated previously: milk, egg, peanut, tree nuts, soy, fish, shellfish, sesame, and wheat. Per the recommendations of the Committee on Nutrition and Section on Allergy and Immunology of the AAP, 2019, there is no evidence for prophylactic elimination diets in the breastfeeding mother of an atopic at-risk infant versus an infant who already has a diagnosis of a food allergy.[22]

Allergy to Nuts

The increase in allergies to tree nuts is apparent even in breastfed infants. Peanuts (not tree nuts but legumes) belong to the same family as fenugreek, the ancient herb used as a galactagogue. In many instances, mothers are taking large doses of fenugreek to support or enhance breast-milk production. Although some infants may present symptoms, most commonly colic, with and without diarrheal stools, fussiness, and crying, these are more likely "intolerance" of a medication than evidence of sensitization or allergy to peanuts or other legumes. Stopping the fenugreek improves the symptoms relatively quickly if this is simply intolerance. In a study of peanut allergies in children, 66% were boys and 82% had a first-degree relative with atopy, including 68% with food allergy.[113] Median age of first exposure (known) was 14 months; median age of first reaction was 18 months. Children born before 2000 had the first reaction at 21 months; those born after 2000 had the first reaction at a mean of 14 months. Past recommendations suggested that children not be given peanuts in any form before the age of 3 years and that mothers of allergic children who are breastfeeding avoid peanuts. Allergy to tree nuts has been identified in breastfed infants whose mothers have ingested nuts on more than one occasion. Peanut allergy, in particular, can develop from skin contact and environmental exposure to the nut. There have been a couple of important studies about tolerance and early introduction of potential allergens. The Enquiring About Tolerance (EAT) study team published a randomized trial comparing early introduction (3 months of age) to standard introduction (6 months) of various allergens in exclusively breastfed infants.[114] The prevalence of any food allergy was lower in the early-introduction group versus the standard-introduction group (2.4% vs. 7.3%, $p = 0.01$). The prevalence of peanut allergy was lower in the early-introduction group versus the standard-introduction group (0% vs. 5.5%, $p = 0.009$). The study was not devised to demonstrate the efficacy of early introduction of allergenic foods in the intent-to-treat analysis, and questions were raised about a possible dose-dependent factor in the prevention effect. In a randomized trial from the Learning Early About Peanut Allergy (LEAP) screening study, the prevalence of peanut allergy was significantly lower in two intention-to-treat analyses in the peanut avoidance group versus the consumption group.[115] The enrolled children were considered at high risk for this allergy based on SPT testing and measurement of the wheal size, and the consumption group had modified immune responses to peanuts (SPT, peanut-specific IgE antibody). Based primarily on those studies the current recommendation of the Committee on Nutrition and Section on Allergy and Immunology of the AAP, 2019, is for early introduction of "infant-safe forms" of peanuts as early as 4 to 6 months of age, in children at high risk for peanut allergy.[22] By comparison for children with mild to moderate eczema the recommendation is to introduce peanut containing foods at "around" 6 months of age. For infants at low risk for peanut allergy the recommendation is to begin peanut-containing food at an age-appropriate time depending on family or cultural practices and for exclusively breastfeeding children to start after 6 months of age.

Timing of solid food introduction in relation to AD and atopic sensitization remains a controversial topic. No evidence to date shows that delaying the introduction of solids beyond 6 months is beneficial.[116] The controversy dwells on the 4- to 6-month period. Prescott et al.[117] state that the rising rates of food allergies in early childhood reflect increasing failure of early immune tolerance mechanisms. They are concerned that the practice of delaying complementary foods until 6 months of age may increase, rather than decrease, the risk for immune disorders. They think a critical window exists in development when exposure to these allergens is tolerated. The window may be 4 to 6 months. They concede that favorable microbiome colonization and breastfeeding may promote tolerance. It is agreed that this issue needs study. Breastfed infants are, of course, exposed by breast milk to many flavors and some foods.[117,118] The Australian Society of Clinical Immunology and Allergy states that previous allergy prevention strategies have been ineffective.[119] They admit that more research is needed but recommend starting solids at 4 to 6 months but not beyond 6 months. They do not recommend prophylactic avoidance of known allergens, in spite of family history (egg, peanuts, cow milk, etc.).[119] The most recent recommendations of the Committee on Nutrition and Section on Allergy and Immunology of the AAP, 2019, state that there is no evidence that the delay of introduction of potential allergenic foods beyond 4 to 6 months prevents atopic disease.[22] Specifically concerning breastfeeding: (1) exclusive breastfeeding for the first 3 to 4 months decreases the cumulative incidence of eczema in the first 2 years of life, (2) there is no benefit to exclusive breastfeeding beyond 3 to 4 months for prevention of atopic disease, (3) any duration of breastfeeding beyond 3 to 4 months is protective against wheezing in the first 2 years of life, and (4) a longer duration of breastfeeding as compared with less protects against asthma even up to 5 years of age.

Non—IgE-Mediated Food Protein—Induced Enteropathies

Non—IgE-mediated food protein—induced enteropathies are a loose group of gastrointestinal inflammatory illnesses produced by cell-mediated inflammation. These illnesses occur in breastfed and non-breastfed infants. The list of various clinical entities that are considered in this group includes food protein—induced enterocolitis syndrome (FPIES), food protein—induced allergic proctitis (FPIAP), eosinophilic esophagitis (EE), food protein—induced constipation, food protein—induced gastroesophageal reflux disease (FPI GERD), and food protein—induced enteropathy (FPIE). FPIES is commonly misdiagnosed as sepsis or a surgical abdominal entity.[120,121] The most common triggers are cow milk and soy milk, given directly to the infant or consumed by the breastfeeding mother. There is an increasingly long list of foods associated with FPIES, including legumes, grains, poultry, and almost "any solid food."[122] Rice, a food commonly thought of as "hypoallergenic" and given to highly allergic children, has now been identified as a significant cause of FPIES and hemorrhagic colitis. In one report, 14 children had 26 episodes of colitis, which was likely to be misdiagnosed. Rice caused more severe reactions than cow milk or soy in this report.[123]

Dietary elimination of the trigger food or foods has been the primary management action after stabilization of the patient with FPIES.[120] Routine maternal dietary elimination of potential offending agents for the breastfed maternal—infant dyad is not recommended if the infant has been asymptomatic and is continuing to grow and develop. Current recommendations do include the use of "hypoallergenic" formula in infants who cannot breastfeed or tolerate other formulas and the importance of dietary guidance through the period of introduction of complementary foods. Monitoring growth and development (especially oral sensory feeding behaviors) and recurrence of symptoms is crucial. Reassessment of recurrences of symptoms, apparent tolerance of foods and other possible allergies or food sensitivities is essential to follow-up and management. In the most severe cases of these entities with or without anaphylaxis and with intolerance of extensively hydrolyzed formula, amino acid—based formulas have been recommended. Current recommendations focus on "tolerance induction," which includes oral immunotherapy rather than simply the avoidance of probable allergens.[124]

Allergic proctocolitis in the exclusively breastfed infant has been reviewed by the Academy of Breastfeeding Medicine, and a protocol has been developed.[125] The syndrome of allergic proctocolitis is increasing in the literature, wherein a group of exclusively breastfed infants develop bloody stools and colic but are otherwise well. The protocol describes the events, reviews the literature, and recommends prevention and management of allergic proctocolitis.

1. Early recognition and diagnosis of the acute manifestations should lead to timely management of an urgent situation requiring emergency interventions.

2. Careful history and physical examination guide identification of potential offending foods and co-allergies as well.

3. There is an important differential diagnosis to consider along with the diagnostic criteria for each of the FPIE conditions.[120]

4. An oral food challenge should be considered when there are atypical symptoms or timeline and the food trigger is not identified through careful history. There are proposed criteria for a positive FPIES oral challenge.[126]

5. Dietary management, infant avoidance of trigger foods, and/or maternal elimination diets are the primary long-term interventions. Maternal elimination diets while the mother continues breastfeeding are not recommended if the infant is thriving or asymptomatic. If the infant's food reaction occurs after breastfeeding or there is failure to thrive, hypoalbuminemia, or anemia, the maternal elimination diet is appropriate.

6. Refer mothers for dietary guidance for themselves and at the time of introduction of complementary foods for the infant. The AAP Committee on Nutrition and the World Health Organization have proposed guidance for complementary foods when there is exclusive breastfeeding until 4 to 6 months and continued breastfeeding through the first year of life or longer.[120]

7. Monitoring for normal growth and developmental skill acquisition and additional food reactions should be ongoing. Recommend complementary foods that positively influence the development of age-appropriate eating skills taking into consideration flavors/taste and textures (thin, thick, pureed, soft, hard, etc.).

8. If there is not improvement with avoidance and elimination diets and there is evidence of poor growth or hypoalbuminemia or anemia, hypoallergenic formula may be considered.

9. Referral to pediatric subspecialists may be appropriate if there are ongoing difficulties with diagnosis or management, including referral to an allergist, gastroenterologist, lactation consultant, nutritionist, and developmental team.

10. The development of tolerance to the allergenic foods depends on the specific food and does vary in different countries. The age of tolerance to cow milk varies a lot by country: Korea ± 12 months of age, Israel approximately 3 years, and ± 6.7 years in the United States. Tolerance to soy is often earlier, as is tolerance for grains (oat—median age 4 years, rice—median age 4.7 years).[126]

CELIAC DISEASE

Celiac disease (CD) is not strictly an atopic disorder; rather it is a complex multisystem disorder produced by a complex interaction of genetic and environmental factors and immune dysregulation. It is classically characterized by an enteropathy produced by intestinal exposure to gluten in individuals with a genetic predisposition (commonly identified as genes *HLA-DQ2* and *HLA-DQ8*). Gluten is a water-insoluble protein found in wheat, rye, and barley. The gluten is changed into immunogenic peptides that stimulate innate and adaptive immune-mediated mechanisms leading to inflammation of the intestinal epithelium and lamina propria. The gliadin peptides are deaminated by tissue transglutaminase (TTG) and attach to antigen-presenting cells (APCs). The stimulated APCs lead to a dysregulated immune response with cytotoxic intraepithelial lymphocytes, interleukin 15 production, and B lymphocyte activation. The B lymphocytes produce the celiac disease–specific antibodies (IgA and IgG) against gliadin, endomysium, TTG, and deaminated gliadin peptide, which are used in the serologic diagnosis.[127] The complexity of CD is also related to the various phenotypes of clinical presentation, the epidemiology with worldwide variations, newer non––human leukocyte antigen (non-HLA) genetic susceptibility factors identified by genome-wide associations studies and the still to be determined understanding of its immune dysregulation, multiple modifying environmental factors, and the role of the intestinal microbiome in the development of CD. The phenotype descriptions include CD, CD autoimmunity (persistent TTG antibody and endomysial antibody without documented abnormal intestinal histology on biopsy), nonceliac gluten sensitivity (NCGS, with irritable bowel syndrome symptoms), extraintestinal manifestations (dermatitis herpetiformis, gluten ataxia, and various vitamin and nutritional deficiencies) and asymptomatic/symptomatic, and classic/nonclassic forms of the illness.[128] Diagnosis of CD continues to evolve, using serology, genotyping, histopathology, and gluten challenge as the primary measures.[129]

Numerous studies have been done examining the potential roles of breastfeeding (timing, duration, ± during introduction to gluten), exposure to cow milk, age at gluten introduction, amount of gluten introduction, and their effect on the development of celiac disease. Earlier studies (1980 to 2002) suggested that the duration of breastfeeding played a role in that the risk for CD was higher if breastfeeding was shorter, which was not confirmed with later studies.[130] Similarly, early studies concluded that breastfeeding during the introduction of gluten was protective against the development of CD, which was not demonstrated by subsequent studies. Another systematic review in 2015 and a position paper by the European Society for Pediatric Gastroenterology, Hepatology and Nutrition (ESPGHAN) concluded that breastfeeding or breastfeeding during gluten introduction did not decrease the risk for CD.[131,132] In 2019, one systematic review concluded that case-control evidence suggested that ever receiving human milk versus never receiving it was associated with a lower risk for CD although issues concerning reverse causality prevented any conclusions comparing shorter versus longer durations of breastfeeding being a risk for CD.[133] Popp and Mäki, examining the "changing pattern of childhood celiac disease," concluded that breastfeeding postponed the diagnosis of the disease but did not prevent it. They pointed to genetic risk factors, gluten introduction at an early age (mean of 2 months), gluten intake volume, and the type of cereal used at weaning having clearer effects on the early development of malabsorption or failure to thrive in CD.[134] Despite the many well-established health benefits of breastfeeding; prevention of CD does not appear to be one of those.

SUMMARY

The prevalence of allergy is increasing across the world, and asthma is the most common chronic disease in children. The concepts of the mechanisms of allergy continue to evolve. The exact role of genetics and epigenetics in the development of allergy are being explored with newer research techniques. Increasingly more data are available concerning the prevention of allergy by breastfeeding and the timing of the introduction of foods. Exclusive breastfeeding does decrease the occurrence of eczema in the first 2 years of life, and a longer duration of breastfeeding decreases wheezing in the first 2 years of life. A longer duration of breastfeeding protects against asthma even up to 5 years of age. Food allergies in breastfeeding infants do occur, although the exact timing and mechanism(s) of sensitization are poorly understood. Maternal elimination diets in pregnancy and/or lactation do not prevent atopic disease but may be useful in infants with diagnosed food allergies and FPIES. An expert panel of the AAP now recommends early introduction (4 to 6 months of age) of infant-safe forms of peanuts to decrease the risk for peanut allergy. CD, not an atopic disorder, but rather multisystem manifestations of immune dysregulation, does not seem to be prevented by breastfeeding or the timing of introduction of gluten related to ongoing breastfeeding.

The Reference list is available at www.expertconsult.com.

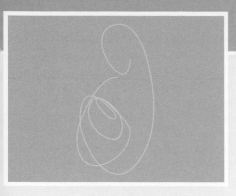

18

Breastfeeding and Return to Work or School

Ruth A. Lawrence

KEY POINTS

- Although it is not easy, mothers need not make any choice between their employment and the optimal nutrition of their infant through breastfeeding.
- As women's role in the workplace continues to assert itself, employers and policy makers must ensure that proper accommodations are available to breastfeeding employees; it is good for business.

- Physicians must advocate for child health and parental well-being by providing sound developmental information, practical advice, and access to appropriate support organizations for employed breastfeeding mothers.

Mothers have always worked. All women work when work is defined as expending energy for a purpose, but not all women are employed when it is defined as earning money for labor. The decision to breastfeed is a very personal one embedded in the context of family, friends, culture, and life. The decision to breastfeed and return to work or education is equally complex with the varied perspectives (personal, social, psychological, emotional, relational, economic, and environmental) on work, life, and balance.

We need to continue to listen to and understand mothers' reasons for breastfeeding, their goals for breastfeeding, and their perception of potential barriers to breastfeeding and engage them in a conversational manner for understanding their reasons for breastfeeding and returning to work or school. This understanding has to be on a familial, communal, social, and generational level but discussed with personal respect, acknowledgment, and empathy for the individual mother's choices. The tremendous variation in types and amount of education and in the myriad job situations, along with the mother's individual reasons for working while pregnant or breastfeeding, make any generalizations about work or return to school and breastfeeding almost irrelevant.

BREASTFEEDING AND EMPLOYMENT

Mothers were the fastest-growing segment of the labor force and the rate of maternal employment outside the home was increasing globally in the early years of this century (2000).[1,2] Reports from 2018 suggest that participation of women in the labor force has been decreasing worldwide from 51.4% in 1990 to 48.5% in 2018 as the participation of men in the workforce has changed from 80% in 1990 to 75% in 2018.[1] In an analysis by the International Labour Organization (ILO), important factors contributing to the differences by gender

included structural barriers, cultural restrictions, increasing number of years that women spend in school, and lack of employment opportunities, especially for young women. There was significant variation in those percentages by country as reflected by a selected sample range of percentage of women participating in the workforce: Yemen 6%, Syria and Algeria 12%, United States 56%, Australia 60%, Lao PDR 77%, and for Madagascar and Rwanda 84%.[3] In many countries throughout the world women account for over 40% of the workforce, including across Europe.[4] Data from the US Department of Labor show that mothers with children under 18 years old are the primary or sole earner in 40% of US households. Nevertheless, women continue to spend more time than men doing "unpaid work," including child care and housework.[5] In the United States, the estimate of time spent in unpaid work was 4 hours and 3 minutes versus 2 hours and 30 minutes for women and men, respectively. In 2017 in the United States mothers with children younger than 3 years of age were 62.3% of the labor force.[6]

Women in general make a huge contribution to national economies and significant contributions to the economic stability of their families. The trend for mothers to work through much of pregnancy has lessened per reports in the United States through 2008.[7] Of women who had a first child in 2006 to 2008, 66% worked during their pregnancy. In that same period approximately 80% of those women worked to within 1 month of delivery of their first child. Similarly, 73% of the women returned to work within 6 months after delivery of a first child occurring in 2005 to 2007.[7] One explanation for this trend is economic, with young households requiring two incomes or the mother is the primary household earner. Another reason is that new mothers are more likely to use paid along with other forms of leave rather than to leave their job.[7] Recognition of women's and mothers' contribution to a growing economy and to a degree an increased understanding of the benefits of breastfeeding to both maternal and infant health has led to an awareness by legislators of the importance of improved working conditions, parental leave, and maternity protection.[8]

Organized Support for Breastfeeding and Return to Work or School

Along with the recognition that mother's return to work is one of the dominant reasons for stopping breastfeeding between 3 and 6 months of age, efforts to counteract this effect have been augmented. This is occurring on the international level (World Health Organization [WHO], United Nations Development Programme [UNDP], United Nations International Children Education Fund [UNICEF], World Alliance for Breastfeeding Action [WABA], La Leche League, ILO) and national level (in individual countries). In the United States, this is being addressed by the efforts of the United States Breastfeeding Committee, the Division of Nutrition Physical Activity and Obesity at the Centers for Disease Control and Prevention (CDC),[9] US Department of Labor, Office of Women's Health of the US Department of Health and Human Services (DHHS), National Conference of State Legislatures (NCSL), Health Resources and Services Administration (HRSA), and the Center for Food Safety and Applied Nutrition of the US Food and Drug Administration (FDA). The efforts of these various organizations range from cataloging the maternity support and paid parental leave laws in individual countries (or states), making recommendations to professionals and businesses about how to support breastfeeding women returning to work and providing guidance to women and families regarding working and breastfeeding and achieving one's breastfeeding goals. The American Academy of Pediatrics (AAP) firmly adheres to the position that breastfeeding ensures the best possible health and the best developmental and psychosocial outcomes for infants.[10] The American Academy of Breastfeeding Medicine (ABM) outlines goals and principles of support for breastfeeding mothers in the workplace or educational settings.[11] Enthusiastic support and involvement of all physicians in the promotion and practice of breastfeeding and continuation as exclusive breastfeeding through 6 months of life are essential to the achievement of optimal infant and child health, growth, and development. The American College of Obstetricians and Gynecologists (ACOG) and the American Academy of Family Practice have made equally strong statements supporting working breastfeeding mothers.[12,13]

Parental Leave Policies Globally

Various international agencies have reported on paid parental leave as it occurs in individual countries around the world. The World Policy Analysis Center reported on the 34 countries in the Organization of Economic Cooperation and Development (OECD), which are predominantly European countries, and developed countries around the world in 2018.[14] Of the 34 OECD countries, 33 have national laws guaranteeing paid leave for mothers of infants and 32 of 34 have legislated paid leave for fathers of infants. The United States is the only country that does not have a nationally regulated policy regarding such paid leave, although various states have passed such legislation.[15] The duration of paid leave for mothers in the OECD countries is guaranteed for at least 14 weeks, and 25 of 34 countries guarantee at least 6 months of paid leave. The 14 weeks fits with the Maternity Protection Convention (2000, no. 183) as the most up-to-date international labor standard on maternity protection produced by the ILO, and 6 months fits with the recommended length for exclusive breastfeeding for all infants.[16] Wage replacement for paid leave is legislated as a maximum rate of two-thirds of one's salary in 31 of 34 OECD countries and a maximum rate of 80% in 25 of 34 countries. The analysis of "Paid Parental Leave" by Raub et al. from the World Policy Analysis Center extensively reviews the connection of paid parental leave with infant health, maternal health, and some aspects of the economic significance of paid parental leave.[14] WABA has a summary document cataloging the nationally mandated maternity protection by country.[17] The list includes all of the world's countries and documents maternity leave and who pays for it, other forms of nationally mandated parental leave, and breastfeeding break legislation. A total of 126 countries have legislation for breastfeeding breaks, the majority of which are intended as paid breaks for a minimum of 60 minutes a day. In the United States, the Patient Protection and Affordable Care Act (ACA) of March 30, 2010 included provisions, specifically Section 4207, amending the Fair Labor Standards Act (FLSA) of 1938, which dictated that employers provide "reasonable break time" for employees to express breast milk for her nursing child for 1 year after birth.[15] There is no required compensation for this break time, but there are stipulations regarding an adequate space for pumping and for the "applicability" of the law under different employment situations. The ACA (2010) also required private health insurance plans to cover breastfeeding support supplies and lactation counseling as a preventive health service. The US Department of Labor Wage and Hour Division developed the Wage and Hour Fact Sheet (no. 73), which is available online.[18] Selected elements of the legal provisions from Fact Sheet no. 73 are outlined in Table 18.1.

All 50 US states now have laws that allow women to breastfeed in any public or private location, and 29 states, the District of Columbia, and Puerto Rico have laws regarding breastfeeding in the workplace. The National Conference of State Legislature supports and tracks much of the ongoing legislation at the state level related to breastfeeding.[15] The obvious goal of all of this legislation is the protection of breastfeeding leading to enabling women to exclusively breastfeed for longer periods and glean the subsequent health benefits related to breastfeeding for both the infant and the mother (Box 18.1).

The Gender Equality and Inequality Indices

The Gender Equality Index (GEI) is a measure used by the UNDP in the Human Development Report to examine the status of gender equality as it influences human development

TABLE 18.1 Select Elements of the Reasonable Break Time for Nursing Mothers Legal Provisions

Elements	Specifics
Time and location of breaks	• Provide a reasonable amount of break time to express milk as frequently as needed by the nursing mother. • A bathroom, even if private, is not a permissible location. • The location must be functional as a space for expressing breast milk. • A temporarily created space is sufficient, provided it is shielded from view and free from any intrusion by coworkers and the public.
Coverage and compensation	• Employers with fewer than 50 employees are not subject to break time requirement if compliance with the provision would impose an undue hardship. • "Undue hardship" is determined by looking at the difficulty or expense of compliance for the employer. • Employers are not required to compensate nursing mothers for breaks taken for the purpose of expressing milk. • If employers already provide compensated breaks and an employee uses such times to express milk, she must be compensated in the same way that other employees are compensated for break times. • The employee must be completely relieved from duty, or else the time must be compensated as work time.
Fair Labor Standards Act prohibitions on retaliation	• It is a violation to discriminate against any employee because such employee has filed any complaint under or related to this act. • Employees are protected regardless of whether the complaint is made orally or in writing.

(Abridged from Fact Sheet no. 73. Washington, DC: Wages and Hours Division, US Department of Labor. Accessed July 9, 2019.)

BOX 18.1 Resources Related to Maternity Protection, Maternity Leave, Paid Parental Leave, and Lactation Accommodations in the Workplace

Academy of Breastfeeding Medicine (ABM). Breastfeeding support for mothers in workplace employment or educational settings: summary statement. Marinelli KA, Moren K, Scott Taylor J; ABM. *Breastfeeding Medicine* 2013;8(1):137–142.

American College of Obstetricians and Gynecologists (ACOG). Employment considerations during pregnancy and the postpartum period. ACOG Comm. Opinion no. 733, April 2018. *Obstetrics & Gynecology* 2018;131(4):e115–e123. ACOG postpartum toolkit: returning to work and paid leave.

Australian Breastfeeding Association (ABA). Breastfeeding friendly workplace toolkits; 2015. https://www.breastfeeding.asn.au/workplace/resources/bfw-toolkits.

Centers for Disease Control and Prevention (CDC). The CDC guide to breastfeeding interventions: support for breastfeeding in the workplace. https://www.cdc.gov/breastfeeding/pdf/breastfeeding_interventions.pdf

Health Resources and Services Administration (HRSA) Maternal and Child Health Bureau (MCHB) DHHS. The business case for breastfeeding: steps for creating a breastfeeding friendly worksite. https://www.womenshealth.gov/files/documents/bcfb_employees-guide-to-breastfeeding-and-working.pdf

International Labour Organization (ILO). Maternity protection resource package. Module 10: Breastfeeding arrangements at work. http://www.ilo.org/publns.

La Leche League International (LLLi). Working and breastfeeding (information for mothers, parents and families). https://www.llli.org/breastfeeding-info/working-and-breastfeeding/.

National Conference of State Legislatures (NCSL). Breastfeeding state laws. http://www.ncsl.org/research/health/breastfeeding-state-laws.aspx

National Partnership for Women and Families. Paid leave. http://www.nationalpartnership.org/our-work/workplace/paid-leave.html.

Office on Women's Health (OWH), US Department of Health and Human Services (DHHS). Breastfeeding and going back to work. https://www.womenshealth.gov/breastfeeding/breastfeeding-home-work-and-public/breastfeeding-and-going-back-work

United States Breastfeeding Committee (USBC). Workplace accommodations to support and protect breastfeeding. http://www.usbreastfeeding.org/p/cm/ld/fid=196

US Department of Labor, Wage and Hour Division. Fact sheet no. 73. Break time for nursing mothers under the FLSA (Fair Labor Standards Act). https://www.dol.gov/whd/regs/compliance/whdfs73.pdf

World Alliance for Breastfeeding Action (WABA). Status of maternity protection by country; 2015. Empower parents, enable breastfeeding: now and for the future. http://www.worldbreastfeedingweek.org.

World Health Organization (WHO). Valuing pregnancy: a matter of legal protection. In: *The World Health Report;* 2005. https://www.who.int/whr/2005/chapter3/en/index5.html.

World Policy Analysis Center. Paid parental leave; 2018. https://www.worldpolicycenter.org/.

in six core domains (power, money, knowledge, work, health, and time).[19] By contrast, the Gender Inequality Index (GII) is used to assess the ongoing inequalities in female reproductive health, education/empowerment, and labor/employment that continue to limit human development on the national, international, and global levels. Another index employed by the UNDP, intimately linked to health, education, and inequality, is the Multidimensional Poverty Index (MPI). MPI is an attempt to understand the "experience of poverty," assessing indicators of nutrition, child mortality, years of schooling, school attendance, cooking fuel, sanitation, drinking water, electricity, housing, and assets. Although none of these indices use breastfeeding rates, and specifically continued exclusive breastfeeding rates after women return to school or work, there is significant discussion of how enabling breastfeeding influences the other measures employed in these indices.[19,20] Additionally, WABA, ILO, WHO, UNICEF, and the UNDP, as well as other global organizations, argue that best practices for human development require a generous, universal, gender-equalitarian, and flexible parental leave policy, financed through social insurance. A more comprehensive parental leave policy (inclusive of mothers and fathers) can lead to improved maternal health throughout pregnancy and delivery and into the postpartum period facilitating exclusive breastfeeding through 6 months or longer.

DEMOGRAPHIC DISPARITIES

Global Disparities

Globally, the largest disparity in the economy or workplace is the difference between the formal economy or employment and the informal economy or employment. Informal employment is a very heterogenous group of employment situations from straightforward self-employment in one's own business, migrant workers, domestic or agricultural workers, or casual or temporary workers to the both visible (push-cart vendors, jitney or cab drivers, daily market vendors, etc., all visible to the passerby) and invisible workers (working in small shops, workshops, and factories or in homes, out of sight).[21] This informal economy is directly linked to the formal economy, each somewhat dependent on the other, but with the informal economy further linked to poverty and inequality as well. Informal employment is in many instances connected to both lower levels of education and higher levels of poor health, morbidity, and mortality. Of the world's workers, 61% are informally employed. Overall, higher rates of men are informally employed; however, in 56% of countries, the rate of informal employment is higher in women, especially in lower income countries. Approximately 90% of employment in Africa is informal, 70% to 80% in eastern and southeastern Asia is informal, and over 60% is informal in northern Africa and the Middle East compared with 54% in Latin America and the Caribbean and 37% in Eastern Europe and Central Asia.[22,23]

Additional barriers to breastfeeding that informal workers may face on return to work after pregnancy include little or no time between delivery and return to work, distance from work and difficult transportation for an infant, dangerous work environment, long working hours, limited or no breaks, and time worked or actual production linked tightly to income. The majority of the interventions to facilitate and sustain breastfeeding on return to work (paid parental leave, legislation for breastfeeding breaks, and interventions in the workplace to increase awareness and acceptance of the benefits of breastfeeding to business) have had an impact only on the formal employment setting. Even though many of the world's leading companies are creating more inclusive and generous parental leave and family-friendly situations and policies, they predominantly affect formal employment.[24] Nevertheless, there are ways to support pregnant women and breastfeeding mothers in informal work settings through adjusting work hours and breaks, assigning different tasks to different individuals, creating informal child-care situations, and making work environments safer for all workers.[20] Guaranteeing breastfeeding protection and support even in informal settings through both legislation and effective interventions is essential to have an impact on the very large numbers of women employed in informal work settings.

Disparities in the United States

The diversity of the US labor force is predicted to continue to increase slowly. Women in low-income jobs are predominantly minorities (black and Hispanic) and return to work earlier and to jobs that do not accommodate breastfeeding.[25] This occurs in both formal employment and informal employment. Some of the barriers in the workplace to returning to work and being able to continue to breastfeed an infant include inflexible schedules, lack of daycare at the site of employment, lack of space for breastfeeding or pumping milk, and lack of understanding and support from employers and colleagues.

There were 131 million working age women (16 years of age or older) in the United States in 2016, representing 51.7% of the total working age population, and 74.4 million were in the labor force. Of that number, 101.4 million were white, 17.4 million were black, 8.1 million Asian, 4.3 million "other," and 20.4 million Hispanic (Fig. 18.1).[26] The percentage of women participating in the workforce approached the percentage of men participating without any consideration for pregnancy or early child care.

The labor force participation rate of mothers in the workforce with children under 18 years of age in 2016 was 70.5%, 75.0% for mothers with children 6 to 17 years of age, 68.6% for mothers with children between 3 and 5 years of age, and 61.8% for mothers with children under 3 (Fig. 18.2).[26] This reinforces what a significant contribution working mothers make to the economy and the importance of protecting maternity, paid parental leave, and accommodations for breastfeeding/pumping in the workplace.

Of employed women, 74.1% worked full time (35 hours or more) and 24.9% worked part time compared with 87.6% and 12.4% of employed men.

Differences in education is a major factor in disparity with the over 64 million women 25 years or older in the labor force; 6.0% had less than a high school diploma, 23.2% had no more than a high school diploma, 16.9% had some college, and 53.8% had a bachelor's degree or higher. The overall women-to-men ratio of earnings is 80.5% (a woman earns approximately $0.80 for each dollar a man earns), with white women only 77.0% and black women 87.3%, Hispanic women 82.3%, and Asian women only 75.9%.[26]

As of 2014 the largest percentage of employed women were in education and health services (36.2%), wholesale and retail trade industry (13.1%), professional and business services (10.5%), and leisure and hospitality services (10.3%).[25]

There are two recent large studies of racial, ethnic, or geographic differences in breastfeeding in the United States.[27,28] McKinney et al.[27] analyzed data from the Community and Child Health Network study with 1636 mother–infant pairs for initiation and duration and demographic variables.[27] Spanish-speaking Hispanic mothers had higher initiation (91%) and longer duration of breastfeeding (mean duration, 17.1 weeks) than English-speaking Hispanic mothers (initiation 90%, mean duration 10.4 weeks) compared with white mothers (initiation 78%, mean duration 16.5 weeks) and black mothers (initiation 61%, mean duration 6.4 weeks). The subsequent analysis demonstrated that demographic factors and formula feeding in hospital explained differences in breastfeeding duration, and demographic factors and family

breastfeeding history accounted for the differences between Hispanic mothers and white or black mothers. In another study using data from the National Immunization Survey (NIS) for children born between 2010 and 2013, Anstey et al. reported significant racial and geographic differences between black and white mother–infant pairs.[28] Breastfeeding initiation rates were lower for black infants than white infants in 23 states, and in 14 of those states in the South and Midwest there were differences of at least 15 percentage points in initiation. There was also a difference of at least 10 percentage points in exclusive breastfeeding through 6 and 12 months (white > black in 12 states at 6 months and white > black in 22 states at 12 months). In a separate analysis using Monte Carlo simulations, Bartick et al.[29] estimated risk for illness for eight pediatric and five maternal illnesses assuming the published causal relationships between breastfeeding and specific illnesses. They created hypothetical cohorts using 2012 breastfeeding rates by race and ethnicity with expected outcomes if 90% of infants met the recommendations for exclusive breastfeeding and recommended duration.[29] Comparing the "hypothetical cohorts," suboptimal breastfeeding would lead to 1.7 times the number of excess cases of otitis media, 3.3 times the cases of necrotizing enterocolitis, and 2.2 times the number of excess child deaths in non-Hispanic blacks compared with a non-Hispanic white population. In a hypothetical Hispanic cohort, there would be 1.4 times the number of gastrointestinal infections and 1.5 the number of excess child deaths compared with a hypothetical non-Hispanic white population. Racial and ethnic disparities in breastfeeding have real and important economic and health consequences.

MATERNAL EMPLOYMENT AFFECTS BREASTFEEDING EXCLUSIVITY AND DURATION

Maternal employment has been cited by many authors as one of the major reasons for the decline in breastfeeding worldwide; however, this may not be universally true. From 1984 through 2002, the Mothers Survey in the United States confirmed that a large percentage of women initiating breastfeeding in the hospital included women who planned to return to full-time employment, the next highest percentage was among women who plan to return to part-time employment, and the lowest percentage of women initiating breastfeeding

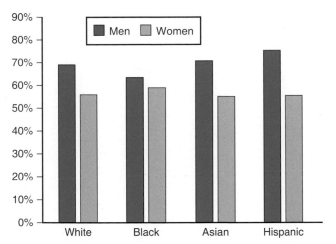

Fig. 18.1 Labor force participation by sex, race, and Hispanic ethnicity, 2016 annual averages. (Data from US Department of Labor, Women's Bureau. Women of working age; 2017. https://www.dol.gov/wb/stats/NEWSTATS/latest.htm#workingwomen. Accessed June 27, 2019.)

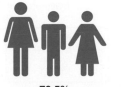

70.5%
with children
under 18 years

75.0%
with children
6 to 17 years

68.9%
with children
3 to 5 years

61.8%
with children
under 3 years

Fig. 18.2 Mothers' participation in the labor force (percentage of total number of women in the workforce). (Data from US Department of Labor, Women's Bureau. Women of working age; 2017. https://www.dol.gov/wb/stats/NEWSTATS/latest.htm#workingwomen. Accessed June 27, 2019.)

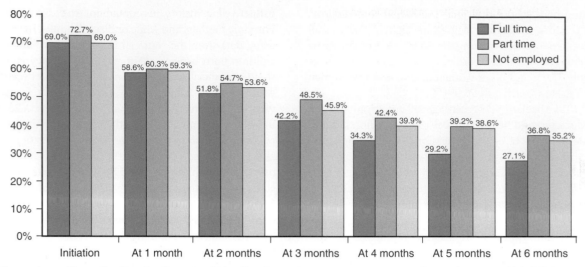

Fig. 18.3 Comparison of breastfeeding duration rates during first 6 months postpartum among mothers who are working full time, working part time, and not employed. (From Ross Products Division, Abbott Laboratories: *Mothers Survey: Updated Breastfeeding Trends Through 2002.* Columbus, OH: Abbott Laboratories; 2002.)

in the hospital was among those who plan to remain at home (see Figure 18.3). In that same review of breastfeeding trends, more women who were employed full time discontinued breastfeeding through the first 6 months compared with those working part time or not working. In 2003 initiation in the hospital was 65.5% among women fully employed, 68.8% among those employed part time, and 64.8% among those not employed. The duration, however, was affected by employment, with 36.6% of those employed part time still breastfeeding at 5 to 6 months, 35.0% of nonemployed women still breastfeeding at that point, and only 26.1% of those employed full time still breastfeeding at 5 to 6 months.[30] Additional data from Listening to Mothers II (2007) and III (2013) from the Reports of National Surveys of Women's Childbearing Experiences reported that of mothers completing the survey 20% exclusively breastfed at 6 months (2007) and 17% exclusively breastfed at 6 months (37% exclusively breastfed at 3 months, 9% at 9 months, and 2% at 12 months) (2013), but did not report data in this report on working status.[31] Reasons given by 8% or more of the mothers for not breastfeeding at the time of follow-up for the survey included trouble getting breastfeeding going well (39%); formula or solid food was more convenient (22%); I fed my baby breast milk as long as I had planned (22%%); my baby stopped nursing, it was the baby's decision (18%); I was working a paying job or attending school and other people were feeding the baby (9%); and I did not have enough support to work through all the challenges (8%). Numerous other studies provide lists of reasons mothers stop breastfeeding in the first year of life. Return to work or school was reported commonly among the reasons along with other significant reasons, including inconvenience or fatigue, concerns about milk supply, medical reasons, lactational factors, psychosocial factors, lifestyle considerations, length of maternity leave, and infant self-weaning (Fig. 18.4).[32–36]

To investigate the effect of maternal postpartum employment on breastfeeding duration in Australia in the first 6 months

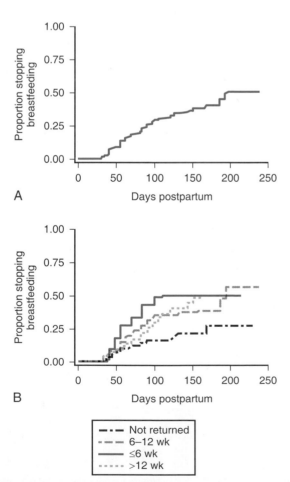

Fig. 18.4 Breastfeeding cessation, Kaplan-Meier failure assessment. **A**, All subjects. **B**, According to length of maternity leave. (From Guendelman S, Kosa JL, Pearl M, et al. Juggling work and breastfeeding: effects of maternity leave and occupational characteristics. *Pediatrics.* 2009;123:e38.)

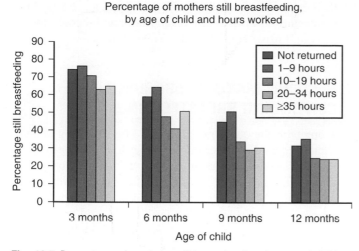

Percentage of mothers still breastfeeding, by age of child and hours worked

Legend:
- Not returned
- 1–9 hours
- 10–19 hours
- 20–34 hours
- ≥35 hours

Fig. 18.5 Percentage of mothers still breastfeeding, by age of child and hours worked. (From Cooklin AR, Donath SM, Amir LH. Maternal employment and breastfeeding: results from the longitudinal study of Australian children. *Acta Paediatr.* 2008;97:620–623.)

after birth in 2008, Cooklin et al.[37] performed a secondary analysis of the Longitudinal Study of Australian Children. Data on 3697 children were completed. Multivariable logistic regression was used to measure the effect of the timing of a mother's return to work and the effect of employment on breastfeeding status. Adjustments were made for maternal age, history of smoking during pregnancy, and socioeconomic status. Breastfeeding rates dropped to 39% at 6 months among employed mothers compared with unemployed mothers at 56%. Full-time employment before 6 months had a major impact; 44% of those who were employed part time were breastfeeding at 6 months. The authors concluded that in spite of controlling for risk factors, employment before 6 months had a negative impact on dedicated breastfeeding (Fig. 18.5).

Effects of Paid Maternity Leave or Workplace Accommodations on Breastfeeding

One modified experimental study documented that access to paid leave, as instituted in California, was associated with increases in the rates of exclusive and overall breastfeeding for 3 to 9 months after birth.[38] The probability of establishing breastfeeding has been associated with a longer maternity leave of 8 weeks of more.[39,40] Additional data reported in 2016, from an analysis of Listening to Mothers III national survey data, noted that only 40% of the women had access to both break time and private spaces at work as stipulated by the breastfeeding workplace accommodation provisions of the ACA. Women who had both private space and adequate break time were 2.3 times (95% confidence interval [CI] 1.03, 4.95) as likely to be exclusively breastfeeding at 6 months.[41] Ogbuanu et al.[40] analyzed data of 6150 mother–infant pairs from the Early Childhood Longitudinal Study–Birth Cohort (ECLS-B) in the United States. Of the study population, 69.4% initiated breastfeeding, although in adjusted analyses neither paid maternity leave nor total time of maternity leave

influenced breastfeeding initiation or duration. When they compared mothers who had returned to work between 1 and 6 weeks postpartum with those who had not returned to work at the 9th-month interview there were greater odds of initiating breastfeeding (odds ratio [OR] 1.46, 95% CI 1.08 to 1.97), continuing any breastfeeding beyond 6 months (OR 1.41, 95% CI 0.87 to 2.27), and continuing predominant breastfeeding longer than 3 months (OR 2.01, 95% CI 1.06 to 3.80) for women who returned to work at the later time. When women returned to work after 13 weeks postpartum the odds ratio of still predominantly breastfeeding after 3 months was 2.54 (95% CI 1.51 to 4.27).[40] In Brazil, Rimes et al.[42] reported on 429 mother–infant pairs, demonstrating that return to work after some maternity leave was associated with a higher adjusted prevalence ratio (APR 1.91, 95% CI 1.32 to 2.78) of exclusive breastfeeding than in mother–infant pairs in whom the mother worked without any maternity leave. In China, a survey of 715 working breastfeeding mothers from a single electronics manufacturing plant demonstrated that higher education level (OR 2.66), lower work load (8 h/day) (OR 2.66), lactation room with dedicated space (OR 2.38), breast pumping breaks (OR 61.6), and encouragement from colleagues (OR 2.78) and supervisors (OR 2.44) to use the breaks were associated with persistent breastfeeding over 6 months after returning to work.[43] A more recent analysis of data from the Listening to Mothers II national survey (2011 to 2012) compared paid maternity leave and maternal and child health.[44] At 21 months postpartum, women who used paid maternity leave compared with taking unpaid or no leave had a 47% decrease in odds of rehospitalization of their infants and a 51% decrease in maternal rehospitalization. Women with paid maternity leave also had 1.8 times the odds of improved stress management and benefits from exercise.

In a review of studies on maternity leave length and workplace breastfeeding policies, Steurer reported on six studies on maternity leave length and eight studies on the effects of workplace breastfeeding policies.[45] She noted the lack of consistency in maternity leave and workplace accommodations by country. Although longer maternity leave had a positive effect on the duration of breastfeeding, she concluded that the optimal duration of maternity leave to achieve the recommended 6 months of exclusive breastfeeding still needs to be determined. Adequate break time for pumping, a private space for pumping, and coworker and supervisor support are each important to foster extending exclusive breastfeeding. It was noted in some of the included studies that some women (especially in lower paying jobs) did not use the policy benefits for fear of consequences at work. Consistent access for all women to multiple breastfeeding accommodations at work and effective enforcement of the policies will be essential to glean the optimal benefits of such policies on breastfeeding exclusivity and duration. The full spectrum of interventions to support breastfeeding should be considered within hospitals, communities, and the workplace to reach the goals of 6 to 12 months of exclusive breastfeeding at home or after returning to work.[46] In another review of the literature Navarro-Rosenblatt and Garmendia (2018)[47] analyzed 21 studies (1996 to 2017) on maternity leave and breastfeeding duration. They reported that women with a maternity leave of 3 months or longer had a 50% likelihood of extending breastfeeding through 3 months than mothers who returned to work before 3 months. Mothers who had 6 months or more of maternity leave had a 30% chance of continuing breastfeeding for 6 months. They also reported on some of the barriers and the importance of providing equal access to the benefits of maternity for all women. In another systematic review of seven studies of paid maternity leave and maternal health outcome, Aitken et al.[48] noted differences between individual-level and policy-level results. The four individual-level studies noted improvements in psychologic stress, depression scores, mental well-being, physical well-being, and reported intimate partner violence with duration of paid leave. The three policy-level comparison studies (from Canada, California, and Norway and Sweden) showed new evidence of an association between maternal health and paid leave. The study from California suggested improved health with 6 weeks of paid leave compared with 12 weeks.[48] A separate systematic review and meta-analysis by McFadden et al.[49] reviewed 73 studies on support for healthy breastfeeding mothers with term infants. "All forms" of additional support for breastfeeding mothers led to a decrease in women stopping exclusive breast by 6 months (relative risk [RR] 0.88, 95% CI 0.85 to 0.92) and at 4 to 6 weeks after delivery (average RR 0.79, 95% CI 0.71 to 0.89). Employment was not a covariable considered in the analysis. The studies were very heterogeneous, as were the analysis by subgroups of covariates (who provided care, type of support, timing of support, and number of postnatal contacts) such that no conclusive comments could be made about the effect of individual factors of support.[49]

Additional interventions to support maternity leave and breastfeeding accommodations in the workplace in all employment and educational settings need to continue to be studied to understand the effects on women's successes with their breastfeeding goals (incidence, duration, satisfaction), their return to work or school, and work and school productivity in "breastfeeding-friendly" environments.

DECISION-MAKING REGARDING CONTINUING BREASTFEEDING

Along with the question, "How can I best feed my infant?" come a myriad of other questions, such as "If I breastfeed, how will I return to work or school?" "If I work, who will care for and feed my child?" "What will the effects of working be on my child?" "What will the effects of working be on me, my spouse, my family, etc.?" "How will I work and breastfeed?" "How can I 'balance'/'juggle' breastfeeding, child care, and family life with work?" And the questions go on. These questions do not come up nor are they answered in a vacuum but rather within the context of the individual mother's life and all that it involves. Nor are these questions answered just once, but they are asked and answered multiple different times, from before pregnancy, during pregnancy before birth, after birth, before returning to work or school, and during the period of working up through weaning. Guides for mothers and families on breastfeeding and returning to work all discuss planning ahead and preparing for return to work while continuing breastfeeding (Box 18.2).

Outcomes for Children of Employed Mothers

Numerous studies since the early 1930s have looked at the effects of maternal employment. Assessment of infant behavior, school achievement and adjustment, children's attitudes, adolescence, and delinquency have been used as outcome measures.[50] Annotated bibliographies covering the range of research on working mothers in areas of medicine, psychology, sociology, and education are available.[51] Four major considerations dealt with commonly in the literature are the variables that facilitate or impede maternal employment, the

---

BOX 18.2 Resources for Parents

Breastfeeding and Employment and Education

American Academy of Pediatrics; Meek JY, ed. *New Mother's Guide to Breastfeeding*. 2nd ed. New York, NY: Bantam Books; 2010.

Australian Breastfeeding Association. Working mothers; 2015. https://www.breastfeeding.asn.au/workplace/working-mothers

Breastfeeding and going back to work. Office of Women's Health, US Department of Health and Human Services. https://www.womenshealth.gov/breastfeeding/breastfeeding-home-work-and-public/breastfeeding-and-going-back-work

Health Resources and Services Administration (HRSA), Maternal and Child Health Bureau (MCHB). The business case for breastfeeding: employees' guide to breastfeeding and working. https://uhs.berkeley.edu/sites/default/files/wellness-womenshealth_breastfeedingandworking.pdf

Huggins K. *The Nursing Mother's Companion*. 6th ed. Cambridge, MA: Harvard Common Press; 2010.

International Labour Organization (ILO). Maternity protection resource package: from aspiration to reality. Module 10: Breastfeeding arrangements at work. http://mprp.itcilo.org/pages/en/modules.html

La Leche League International (LLLi). Working and breastfeeding. https://www.llli.org/breastfeeding-info/working-and-breastfeeding/

Marinelli KA, Moren K, Scott Taylor J; Academy of Breastfeeding Medicine. Breastfeeding support for mothers in workplace employment or educational settings: summary statement. *Breastfeeding Medicine*. 2013;8(1):137−142.

effect of maternal employment on children during the four developmental stages, the effects on the family, and the effects on society in general. Because the literature spans many years, it is reasonable to ask how generalizable past findings are to the current situations for individual working mothers.

It has been emphasized that the presence of a mother in the home does not guarantee high-quality mothering. It also has been shown that well-educated (college) mothers, including those who are employed, spend time with their children at the expense of their own personal needs.[52] Because employed mothers encompass a large group of women with different educational levels, different reasons for working, and different opportunities for employment, it is difficult to generalize about the effects of returning to work or early maternal employment. Literature reviews have emphasized critical factors that are more important than maternal employment, such as good substitute care, maternal role satisfaction, family stability, paternal attitude toward maternal employment, and the quality of the time spent with the children.[53] Despite the abundance of research on school-age children, there is still little reported about preschoolers because no school records or test results are available to use in large-population analysis.

Questions have been raised about the impact of separation of mother and infant and the timing of this separation in early maternal employment.[54] Resumption of full-time employment when the child is younger than 1 year has prompted studies. Using the Ainsworth "strange situation" validated techniques, no relationship between maternal work status and the quality of the infants' attachment to their mothers is reported.[55,56] Early resumption of employment may not impede development of a secure infant-mother attachment. A significantly higher proportion of insecure attachments to fathers in employed-mother families is reported for boys but not for girls. Boys are more insecurely attached than girls in most studies. It is thought that an infant's attachment relationship to mother emerges at approximately 7 months.[57,58] Other studies suggest that maternal employment can have a positive effect on girls but not boys. Whether breastfeeding accounts for some of the variability in these studies is not stated.[59] No study recorded feeding method or considered the impact breastfeeding has on the mother—infant relationship or the infant's development. One of the strategies suggested to address the separation of mother and infant because of early maternal employment is to advocate for infant care centers that provide breastfeeding facilities in the workplace, schools, and other locations serving working women.

A review of the more current literature (last 10 to 15 years) suggests mixed effects of early maternal employment on infant well-being and attachment. A review by Nicol and Hardy[60] that included 13 different studies concluded that there were both positive and negative effects of early maternal employment on child cognition and socioemotional behavior that were often more significantly affected by maternal covariates such as education, socioeconomic status, and job satisfaction. They pointed out that early maternal employment, especially full-time employment, decreased the ability of mothers to breastfeed for a prolonged period and to exclusively breastfeed.[60]

Another recent literature review (2018) extensively examines the psychologic effects of breastfeeding on children and mothers.[61] The authors, Krol and Grossman,[61] provide an extensive review of the effects of breastfeeding on infant cognitive development, brain development, and the social and emotional development of the child. Their analysis concludes that the effects of breastfeeding are generally positive despite a few papers documenting negative effects of breastfeeding on infant development. They propose possible mechanisms of breastfeeding causing positive effects on infant development: long-chain polyunsaturated fatty acids (LC-PUFAs) in human milk contributing to enhanced neuronal growth and repair and myelinization during the crucial window of human brain growth in the first 36 months of life and the positive effects of oxytocin on both maternal and infant attentional responses and response to emotional cues. Several of the studies discussed in this review report on the positive influence of breastfeeding on infant development in the long term into childhood, adolescence, and adulthood. Krol and Grossman[61] do suggest caution regarding the interpretation of the available research and the generalizability of the results related to different definitions of breastfeeding (timing of initiation, exclusivity, and duration), the specificity of the results being attributable to breastfeeding and the limited linking of possible neurobiologic mechanisms of the effects of breast milk and breastfeeding on infant development.

Separately Krol and Grossman[61] discuss the potential effects of genetic predisposition to being affected by breast milk. They quote research by Caspi et al.[62] on the FADS2 genotype and the more efficient processing of LC-PUFAs correlating with the impact of breastfeeding on infant cognitive development. Krol and Grossman[61] also report that a meta-analysis and a case-control study suggest that early initiation of breastfeeding and exclusive breastfeeding for 6 months or more are associated a decreased likelihood of developing autism spectrum disorder (ASD).[63,64] In that discussion they point to another potential genetic predisposition related to CD38 genetic variations, interactive effects of oxytocin and cortisol levels, and the risk for autism in infants.[65–67]

Clearly early maternal employment after childbirth can affect the duration of exclusive or any breastfeeding. Breastfeeding appears to have a positive effect on infant development that can persist beyond infancy. Additional research on the effects of maternal employment and concomitant breastfeeding on infant development should continue with careful attention to contributing factors and potential confounders.

Effects on Mothers of Early Return to School or Work

"Mothering the mother" is a crucial concept in caring for any woman after delivery but even more important for a breastfeeding mother and for one returning to school or work. Of the numerous potential stressors for mothers in the postpartum period, fatigue, adjustment to a new schedule (for baby and mother), and mother's sense of "her daily responsibilities" are three of the most important. The experience of trying to maintain appropriate nourishment, hydration, rest, and self-care can be added burdens for the breastfeeding mother who is trying to feed and care for her newborn on top of her familial and household responsibilities. Returning to work or school can become one more responsibility to be accomplished and balanced with all the mother's other responsibilities.

Psychologic Effects of Breastfeeding on Mothers

Breastfeeding has traditionally been reported to affect mood and stress responsiveness in mothers. Older studies clearly reported reduced anxiety, negative feelings, stress, and depression for breastfeeding mothers compared with formula-feeding mothers.[61] Newer studies have reported on the benefit of breastfeeding on maternal affect and stress related to oxytocin and cortisol levels in breastfeeding mothers.[68] Improved sleeping also has been reported for breastfeeding mothers.[69,70] Breastfeeding and mother–infant attachment have not been found to be directly positively linked.[71] Reports of breastfeeding mothers demonstrating positive mood, less perceived stress, and effective emotional responsiveness are likely to positively affect maternal behavior, but feelings and behaviors have many potential contributors and confounders making it difficult to link them directly to breastfeeding.

Breastfeeding and Postpartum Depression

In the past decade, new studies have demonstrated a link between breastfeeding and less maternal postpartum depression. There have been several prospective studies associating lower depression scores with breastfeeding at 2 to 4 months postpartum and a couple of systematic reviews[72,73] showing higher depression scores leading to decreased breastfeeding (earlier cessation). Higher depression scores at 2 months postpartum were specifically reported as predictive of less breastfeeding at 4 months.[74] It is essential to understand mothers' reasons for stopping breastfeeding while studying postpartum depression and breastfeeding as the reason(s) for stopping may have nothing to do with depression.

There is also the possibility of a "reciprocal relationship" between breastfeeding and maternal depression and the potential that either one may influence the other directly.[74–76] Different studies demonstrate different relationships between maternity leave duration and postpartum depression. Dagher et al.[77] reported that their two-stage least squares analysis demonstrated a U-shaped relationship between depressive symptoms and maternal leave duration (increasing leave associated with decreasing depressive symptoms until 6 months). Kornfeind and Sipsma[78] reported a similarly complex relationship; women with maternity leave of less than 12 weeks were less likely to experience depressive symptoms for each additional week of leave (OR 0.58, 95% CI 0.40 to 0.84), whereas 12 weeks or longer of maternity leave was not associated with postpartum depressive symptoms (OR 0.97, 95% CI 0.73 to 1.29). Chatterji and Markowitz[79] reported data from

the ECLS-B with 14,000 children born in 2001. Mothers who worked before delivery returned to work in the first year postpartum and had less than 12 weeks of leave and less than 8 weeks of paid leave reported increased depressive symptoms.[79] It is difficult to unravel the relationship between breastfeeding and maternal mood and affect. Overall, breastfeeding and depression seem to align with the general positive effects of breastfeeding on maternal mood, affect, and response to stress.

Role of Fathers Regarding Breastfeeding or Return to Work or School

There is increasingly more literature on the role of fathers in pregnancy, childbirth, maternal and newborn health, and breastfeeding.[80–83] This literature includes review of stresses on fathers during pregnancy, the perinatal period and the postpartum period including effects on depression, anxiety and paternal mental health.[84–86] Sihota et al.[83] published a well-organized review of fathers' experiences and perspectives of breastfeeding, including 18 studies in English, with the main focus being fathers of breastfed infants. Fathers generally perceived breastfeeding as optimal nutrition, healthy, and natural and acknowledged other advantages of breastfeeding, including convenience, low cost, freedom from night feedings, and health benefits for the child and breastfeeding partner. Reported paternal concerns from various articles included insufficiency of breast milk, inconvenience compared with formula, and a challenge for the breastfeeding partner. Other important issues for fathers of breastfeeding dyads were noted as father–infant bonding, partner relationships and breastfeeding, breastfeeding in public, and the father's role in the breastfeeding process. One study noted that the fathers had reasonable breastfeeding knowledge and understanding,[87] whereas several others reported limited knowledge about the benefits and the challenges in successful breastfeeding. An important goal for new fathers was reported to be father–infant bonding, which in various studies was perceived to be hindered or limited by breastfeeding and being left out of that process. The authors, deMontigny et al.[82] noted ways fathers proposed to meet the father–infant bonding challenge with breastfeeding by being involved in infant care, including changing diapers, bathing, burping after feeding, cuddling, calming, massaging, singing or playing with the infant, or putting the infant to bed. The concern over how breastfeeding might interfere with their relationship with their partners was commonly expressed and included concerns about intimacy, sleep, a woman's body shape, or increased emotions or conflict during the postpartum period. Fathers' concerns related to breastfeeding in public involved embarrassment, immodesty versus decency, stigma, offending others, other individuals seeing their partner's breasts, and the chance of unpleasant comments made to their partner. Cultural and socioeconomic factors seemed to influence these perceptions, as did the father's overall comfort and acceptance of breastfeeding. The majority of the papers used in this review suggested that fathers thought the decision to breastfeed was the mother's because it involved the partner's body, time, and energy, but they often felt excluded from the decision-making process about breastfeeding and wanted to be involved in that decision. Fathers generally held the perception that their main role was to be supporters and facilitators of the breastfeeding process. This most often meant "practical support" in the form of helping with household chores, caring for older children, providing meals, attending to the comfort of the breastfeeding mother, and recognizing cues from the infant for hunger, fatigue, or need for changing.[88,89] Relative to their role in breastfeeding fathers thought they needed information about breastfeeding that was consistent and specific about "troubleshooting" when difficulties arose, weaning, what to do when breastfeeding was not successful, and how to deal with feelings of exclusion or jealousy.[88–90] Sihota et al.[83] recommended pragmatic education for fathers, with advanced education about troubleshooting common problems or issues, along with practical ways of caring for the infant and supporting their partners. Fathers asked for easier access to targeted information for fathers, use of the term *father* rather than *parent*, and use of images of fathers involved in the care of child and mother during breastfeeding and connection with male peers regarding support for fathers and mentorship.

Breastfeeding Interventions Targeting Fathers

There are at least three systematic reviews in English of breastfeeding interventions directed at fathers. Tadesse et al.[91] reviewed eight articles involving breastfeeding education for fathers in low-and middle-income countries. Each of the educational interventions demonstrated improvement in early initiation, exclusive breastfeeding, or continued breastfeeding when compared with a control group. Mahesh et al.[92] performed an analysis of 8 interventional studies involving 1852 families targeting fathers for breastfeeding promotion. The calculated relative risk of exclusive breastfeeding at 6 months was 2.04 (95% CI 1.58 to 2.65) in the intervention groups. The frequency of "lactation-related problems" (RR 0.24, CI 0.10 to 0.57) and the risk of full-formula feeding (RR 0.69, CI 0.52 to 0.93) were lower in the intervention groups. Abbass-Dick et al.[93] analyzed 12 studies and demonstrated that each study improved at least one specific breastfeeding outcome: duration of breastfeeding in 5 in 9 studies and exclusive breastfeeding up to 24 weeks postpartum in 8 in 10 studies. Six of the studies included demonstrated an increase in paternal breastfeeding support. The authors reported the evidence of beneficial effects when the interventions were face-to-face delivery of breastfeeding information and presented in a "culturally appropriate" manner.

Daycare

Infants in daycare have created special concerns for parents, pediatricians, social scientists, and policy makers. Quality of daycare measures and objective measurable child health and development outcomes other than mortality and infectious diseases have been difficult to construct. Early published information did not discuss the impact of breastfeeding

before or during an infant's involvement with daycare. Haskins and Kotch[94] first reviewed the literature (172 articles) and concluded, "Children in day care, especially those under three years old and sometimes their teachers and household contacts, have higher rates of diarrhea, hepatitis A, meningitis and possibly also otitis media than children not in day care." The data are less clear for respiratory illnesses and cytomegalovirus infection. Parents choosing daycare facilities for their children need to select them with consideration for health and safety. In the United States in 2011, estimates by the US Census Bureau reported 12.5 million children (61% of 20.4 million) under the age of 5 years of age were in regular child-care situations. Approximately 42% were receiving care by a relative, 33% were cared for by a nonrelative, and 18% were in multiple types of daycare situations (overlapping percentages). Fathers made up 17% and grandparents made up 23% of the care by relatives. Almost 38% (7.9 million) of pre-schoolers were not in regular child-care arrangements.[95] In some situations, good daycare facilities may have a very positive influence on the infant's growth and social and cognitive development. Finding affordable child care that the mother/family assesses as safe and nurturing is a tremendous concern in the decision-making for return to work. Finding daycare situations that are also convenient and supportive for breastfeeding and providing breast milk to one's infant is even more challenging.

Concern about infant illness should result in the pediatrician's involvement in ensuring high-quality daycare in the local community. For an infant of an age appropriate for breastfeeding, one possible preventive measure would be to encourage a continuation of breastfeeding or providing breast milk to the infant while in daycare when possible. Furthermore, daycare policy and procedures should encourage and facilitate breastfeeding. Mothers should inquire about daycare centers' policies toward breastfeeding. Physicians who consult for daycare centers should be well informed regarding infection prevention and support of breastfeeding to foster exclusivity and longer duration of breastfeeding as well. Breast milk can safely stand at room temperature for 6 to 8 hours and need not be discarded if the first feeding attempt is incomplete. In contrast, formula must be refrigerated and discarded after the first feeding attempt because it contains no antibodies or infection protection factors. No infant feeding of any kind should be warmed in a microwave oven. Protective gloves are not necessary to feed breast milk. The accidental feeding of a different mother's milk is not cause for alarm, although it should be reported to the families and facility for public health reasons.

The Workplace

Pumping milk at work has been identified as a critical element in the successful return to work for women who work full time outside the home. In a report of over 500 mothers, it was observed that mothers who expressed milk one or more times a day while away were less likely to stop breastfeeding before 6 months. When the problems in the workplace that interfered with pumping and continued lactation were studied by Slusser et al.,[96] it was observed that a mother expressed milk twice a day when the infant is 4 months old and less when the infant is 6 months old. The mothers spent a total of less than an hour a day in the process of pumping, usually divided in two sessions. Pumping facilities at work that are readily accessible are critical for a successful breastfeeding support program.[96]

Although working mothers are common, companies who make working mothers comfortable are still uncommon. Efforts to increase parental leave, even unpaid leave, have not been widely established, although laws requiring minimal parental leave have been passed and apply to both parents. In the interest of equality, institutions have established family leave to provide for a broad spectrum of family health and illness needs consistent with the Family Medical Leave Act (FMLA).

Measuring Breastfeeding Support in the Workplace

Some major companies, however, have been recognized by *Working Mother* magazine's annual survey as making efforts to support mothers in the workplace.[24] The yardstick includes everything from the number of female vice presidents to fair advancement and equal pay for equal work. No company has been nominated solely for its support of breastfeeding. In the top 100 companies, breastfeeding-related accommodations assessed included locked pumping rooms for privacy, breast pumps available, comfortable furniture in the pumping rooms, lactation consultant available 24 hours a day, and encouraging breaks for feeding or pumping. Parental leave and gender-neutral leave policies are other measures considered important measures, as are flextime schedules and child-care options offered and supported by the company. The 2018 report of the eighteenth *Working Mother* magazine's annual survey named Baptist Health South Florida, Bon Secours Virginia Health System, Children's Healthcare of Atlanta, H. Lee Moffitt Cancer Center & Research Institute, and WellStar Health System in the top 100 companies, but only WellStar Health System was in the top 10, even though hospitals should be the model workplace. The top 10 also included pharmaceutical house AbbVie. Hospitals employ a number of professional women in their childbearing years as physicians, nurses, therapists, psychologists, laboratory technicians, and child life specialists, etc. Ideally the health and illness need of children, parents, and families can be better understood by health care professionals such that they could devise model workplaces with regard to physical, mental, and emotional health and well-being. In such a system, appropriate breastfeeding and child-care accommodations would be standard procedure for all employees.

A significant contribution to the workplace could be made by allocating space and providing staff for daycare centers.[97] This would allow mothers to interact with their infants and breastfeed them during the work day. Small experiments of providing daycare in the workplace have shown a decrease in tardiness and absenteeism and a general increase in job satisfaction among employees who are mothers.[98] For hospitals and other businesses in which highly skilled and trained staff require extensive and costly on-the-job training, daycare has been shown to be cost effective for reducing turnover.[11,99]

Physicians who serve as consultants to large and small industries, unions, not-for-profit agencies, and daycare centers are in important positions to influence corporate trends, which are changing slowly. In a study of Women, Infants, and Children (WIC) program employees, it was hypothesized that WIC employees would initiate and continue breastfeeding at significantly higher rates than the national averages because there has been a major breastfeeding campaign at WIC in the past decade.[100] Six Los Angeles WIC agencies participated; 99% of WIC employees began breastfeeding and 68.6% continued to 1 year. Key variables that contributed to the outcome were (1) intention to breastfeed for a year, (2) delayed use of formula, (3) breastfeeding support groups, and (4) availability of pumps at the worksite. Thus it was proved that full-time employment and breastfeeding are compatible if the worksite is appropriate and the environment is supportive.

Other Considerations for Breastfeeding and the Workplace

The Welfare-to-Work program, a central theme of welfare reform, requires recipients to engage in work, even mothers whose newborns are only a few months old, decreasing the incidence of breastfeeding. The negative consequences of these requirements were studied by Haider et al.[101] They indicate that the national breastfeeding rate would have been 5.5% higher at 6 months in 2000 without this mandate. They further suggest that the negative consequences of this policy should be considered because the potential benefits of breastfeeding these at-risk infants are so great.[101] A systematic review and meta-analysis of Welfare-to-Work interventions assessed the physical and mental health of single parents and their children. The analysis showed only moderate- to low-quality evidence and documented very small effects on maternal or child mental and physical health. The magnitude of the effects of Welfare-to-Work programs was assessed as unlikely to have any tangible impact on the participants.[102]

A comparison of maternal absenteeism and infant illness rates among breastfeeding and formula-feeding women showed breastfeeding reduced absenteeism.[37] In two corporations with on-site lactation programs, one had 100 births among 2400 and the second had 30 births among 1200 female employees. Of the 101 mother–infant dyads studied, 59 were breastfed and 42 formula fed. The company provided lactation counseling and pumping and storing facilities. Of the 28% of the infants who had no illnesses, 86% were breastfed and 14% formula fed. Among mothers who were absent because of infant illness, 75% were formula feeding and only 25% were breastfeeding (Fig. 18.6).[98]

In a separate study, questionnaires were sent in late pregnancy and 10 times during the first year after delivery, to clarify mothers' work patterns and breastfeeding practice. Working full time at 3 months decreased breastfeeding duration by 8.6 weeks relative to not working. Part-time work for 4 hours or less per day did not decrease duration of breastfeeding and part-time work more than 4 hours per day decreased breastfeeding duration only slightly. The authors

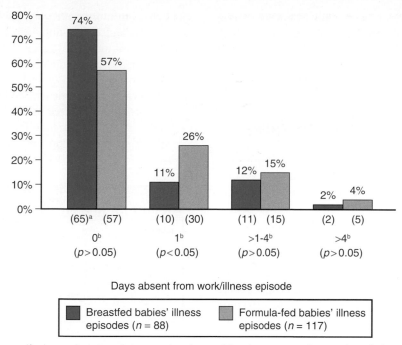

Fig. 18.6 Distribution of illness episodes and maternal absenteeism by nutritional groups. a, the numbers in brackets represent the number of children included in the columns. b, days absent from work/illness episodes. (Modified from Cohen R, Mrtek MB, Mrtek RG. Comparison of maternal absenteeism and infant illness rates among breast-feeding and formula-feeding women in two corporations. *Am J Health Promot.* 1995;10:148.)

concluded that part-time work is actually a good strategy to help mothers combine breastfeeding and work.[103] Planning to return to work before 6 weeks postpartum reduced the likelihood of initiating breastfeeding in this study of more than 10,000 mothers of singleton term infants.

Most of the studies concerning employment and breastfeeding were retrospective, relied on voluntary responses, and did not clearly define breastfeeding in terms of exclusivity or working in terms of part time or full time. A prospective study reported by Kurinij et al.[104] involving more than 1000 women confirmed the reports of others that women with professional occupations breastfeed longer than nonprofessionals and that part-time work is more conducive to longer duration than full-time jobs. Both groups of women found equal satisfaction from breastfeeding. The duration of breastfeeding was evaluated in a separate study in the same two corporations mentioned previously. Cohen et al.[105] reported that of the 187 participants, 75% who returned to work breastfed for 6 months or longer. The average duration for breastfeeding was 8.1 months. These rates, however, were equal to the statistical norms for the region among women not employed outside the home.

The general consensus has been that returning to work diminishes breastfeeding. As the number of women who work outside the home increased and breastfeeding increased in the last decade, the trends have changed. A large study of US mothers found that initiation rates among mothers who were not working after childbirth compared with mothers who were working part time were not different.[30] In 2001 to 2003 it was estimated that 67% of mothers of first children worked during the pregnancy and most of them held full-time jobs.[106]

The Infant Feeding Practice Study II (IFPSII) was conducted by the FDA with the CDC from 2005 to 2007. It was a longitudinal study of women from late pregnancy through the infant's first year of life.[107] Similar to IFPSI conducted in 1992 to 1993, over 1400 mothers were involved. The expected number of hours the mother planned to work was used to categorize each dyad. The actual number of hours worked and baby's age at onset of work were categorized along with demographics, length of maternity leave, past breastfeeding experience, hospital experience, and degree of social support at home. This study showed that compared with not expecting to work, expecting to work less than 35 hours was not positively associated with breastfeeding initiation. Expecting to work full time, however, decreased breastfeeding initiation. Returning to work within 12 weeks regardless of hours worked and returning to work after 12 weeks but working more than 34 hours per week were both associated with shorter breastfeeding. The authors concluded that longer postpartum leave and part-time work promote breastfeeding.[107]

The Early Childhood Longitudinal Study - Birth cohort used a sample of singletons whose mothers had responded to a survey and had worked the 12 months before delivery. The study included 6150 women and classified them by the length of their maternity leave. Almost 70% initiated breastfeeding, which was not influenced by paid maternity leave. Those who returned to work within 1 to 6 weeks were less likely to initiate breastfeeding. Duration of breastfeeding was affected by time of return to work. Those returning to work at or after 13 weeks were more apt to breastfeed for 3 months or longer.[40]

The decision to work or not work is a personal one. Our responsibility is to continue to demonstrate and study the positive effects of paid parental leave on breastfeeding initiation, exclusive breastfeeding, and breastfeeding duration. Along with that we must continue creating breastfeeding interventions and enforce breastfeeding accommodations at work and to foster ongoing breastfeeding successes for all women regardless of their decision to return to work or school.

COUNSELING BREASTFEEDING MOTHERS WHO CHOOSE TO WORK

The AAP periodic survey of members that included questions about breastfeeding was conducted in 1995, 2004, and 2014, and results were compared at the different time points. Pediatricians in 2014 reported they were more likely to recommend exclusive breastfeeding but they were less likely to think that the benefits of breastfeeding outweigh the difficulties or inconveniences and were less confident that mothers can be successful at breastfeeding; younger pediatricians were less confidant than older ones in dealing with breastfeeding problems. Pediatricians with personal experience were much more likely to be supportive. Personal experience seemed to mitigate poor attitudes.[108]

Part of a physician's counseling session before the birth of a baby should include inquiry about a mother's plan to work postpartum. Obstetricians play a crucial role in this period, and the American Academy of Obstetrics and Gynecology have specific statements for obstetricians and counseling women.[109,110] Open discussion about breastfeeding and personal goals for breastfeeding, child-care arrangements, personal support (from spouse/partner, family, friends), available professionals for knowledge and expertise (physicians, nurses, lactation consultants), and general coping skills and resources and plan for back to work (work-life balance, role models, support for working plan [at home, at work]) will be helpful. Most well-educated women who plan to return to a career have thought out the process carefully but may want some reassurance or alternative suggestions. Physicians should know what services are available locally. It may be helpful to have a list of other working mothers who are willing to share experiences and knowledge of resources. It is often helpful for a woman to know another person who has experienced similar career choices. Physicians, however, should not assume that their personal experience should be the model recommended to the patient.

Past experience(s), thoughtful expectations, and reports by other mothers may not fit with an individual woman's experience of caring for a newborn and what it entails. Even pediatricians early in their careers may have an unrealistic view of what to expect.[108] Pediatricians may have to recommend a more realistic view of parenting and after urging the parents to plan carefully and practically for working and parenting make themselves available to problem solve in a timely fashion issues of family life, daycare, work, school, and breastfeeding. A new mother and family need to appreciate that events occur that cannot be totally controlled. Even for a woman who has been an efficient, successful career woman in control of her work situation, an infant with normal needs may be overwhelming at times. Women who have

jobs that are more rigid from the standpoint of work hours, workplace, and expectations will have to consciously address those issues as they arise (Tables 18.2 and 18.3).

Physicians may need to discuss specific issues of child care while a mother is working, such as the following:

1. Child-care arrangements should be sought that permit sufficient time for feeding an infant inexperienced with a bottle and sufficient time for extra cuddling of an infant who is used to a closer relationship with the "feeder." A

TABLE 18.2 Responses for Reasons to Recommend Work

Reason	FREQUENCY	
	No.	%
Economic	1709	25
Never recommend mother work	1566	22
Mother's emotional needs	1220	18
Mother's fulfillment	1059	15
Child is better off without mother	644	9
Reassure mother	270	4
Adequacy of child care	266	4
Child's age	170	2
Mother does important work	64	1
Total	6968	

From Heins M, Stillman P, Sabers D, et al. Attitudes of pediatricians toward maternal employment. *Pediatrics*. 1983;72:283. Copyright © American Academy of Pediatrics, 1983.

TABLE 18.3 Responses for Reasons to Recommend Against Working

Reason	FREQUENCY	
	No.	%
Child's physical health	1724	24
Child's mental health	1445	20
Never recommend against work	1318	18
Inadequate child care	701	10
Child's age	591	8
Mother feels guilty	540	7
No economic need	459	6
Usually say, "Do not work"	72	1
Other	402	6
Total	7252	

From Heins M, Stillman P, Sabers D, et al. Attitudes of pediatricians toward maternal employment. *Pediatrics*.1983;72:286. Copyright © American Academy of Pediatrics, 1983.

child-care specialist should be familiar with the practical issues of breastfeeding and sympathetic to the breastfeeding goals of the mother.

2. The advantages and disadvantages of child care in an infant's home, in a sitter's home, with or without a sitter's children, and with or without other children should be discussed. Is daycare a good arrangement for this family, and what centers take young infants and will work with breastfeeding mothers? Despite lower costs, nursery "warehousing" should be avoided.

3. Are child-care facilities available within the workplace or close to work so that a mother could use breaks to breastfeed?

Plans for feeding an infant while the mother is working depend on the infant's age and feeding pattern. If an infant is totally breastfed and younger than 6 months of age, the mother can breastfeed if she can leave work and go to the infant or if the infant can be brought to the workplace. If a mother cannot leave work to nurse, she may choose to pump her milk at work and save it for the following day. This necessitates having a reasonably sanitary private place to pump and a means of storing the milk until she gets home, either in a refrigerator at work or in a portable refrigerator system. Mothers have used insulated containers with ice, reusable cold packs, or dry ice. If no such arrangement for chilling can be made, the milk can be stored in a sterile container for 8 hours without refrigeration if collected under clean conditions.

Preparation for Breastfeeding and Expressing Breast Milk for the Infant

A woman who is away from her breastfeeding infant past feeding time may need to pump to maintain her milk supply. A mother may also anticipate the infant's needs before she returns to work. She can practice pumping and storing a small amount of her milk daily for several weeks in her home freezer so that a stockpile is available while she is at work (see Chapter 22).

A mother should be instructed to introduce the baby to the bottle and an alternative caregiver before the first day of work. Developing a plan of organization and practicing it before the first day of work will facilitate development of a workable solution. In addition, returning to work part time at first may help minimize the adjustment. In addition, returning to work on a Wednesday or Thursday allows the first week to be a short one.

No evidence indicates that it is necessary to introduce a bottle sooner than 10 days before returning to work. Unless a mother is returning to work immediately after delivery, a bottle should not be introduced before lactation is well established (at least 4 weeks for most primiparas) because it can interfere with a mother's milk-making rhythm. Although some infants readily go back and forth between breast and bottle, there are no readily assessable variables to identify the infant who will develop sucking difficulties and apparent "nipple confusion," ultimately resulting in preference for the bottle if it is introduced too early. Babies given a bottle well before 3 months may easily reject the breast after 3 months.

For the infant who does not accept the bottle gracefully, the following techniques may facilitate the process:

1. Someone other than the mother should give the feeding.
2. The mother should be out of sight and hearing range, preferably out of the building, so the infant does not await her arrival.
3. The infant should be held by the "feeder" in the same position as for breastfeeding, that is, slightly elevated and close to the chest wall at about breast level. The bottle can be slipped down against the caregiver's chest wall.
4. Use a soft nipple and a small bottle at first for easy handling. A clear bottle or plastic cylinder allows a better view of the infant.
5. Create a soothing atmosphere; use a rocking chair, quiet music, and muted light.
6. The initial bottle-feedings, if not all of them, should contain warm mother's milk to reduce the elements of change being introduced.

If the bottle-feedings do not go well and alternative feedings are needed, milk can be provided by medicine cup feeding (see Chapter 14).

If an infant is older than 6 months of age, complementary foods can be part of the solution. The feeding given by the caregiver can be solids by spoon and liquids from a cup so that no breastfeeding is actually missed. A health professional can anticipate these issues and tailor feeding counseling accordingly. Some infants quickly learn the mother's schedule and may adjust their sleep pattern to allow a long stretch while mother is away. This may result in feedings during the night instead, but if the mother is informed of this phenomenon, she may be less anxious if it occurs.

Formula-fed infants have more infections and illnesses, which is another reason to encourage a mother to continue breastfeeding. This is especially important during the first weeks of adjustment to the transient, recurrent separation of mother and infant associated with the mother's return to work.

Resources for Parents

The popular press has been inundated with books on child care and child-rearing, with a significant number on breastfeeding and specifically breastfeeding and employment. These volumes can be extremely helpful to young parents, providing detailed information about how to manage. Many recognize that mothers, fathers, infants, jobs, child-care arrangements, and support resources are all different. A few are dogmatic and single-minded, giving the impression that the author's method is the only recipe for successful lactation. Pediatricians should become familiar with a few of these guidebooks and certainly not recommend any without reading them first. A few of these books have been perceived to produce guilt in a working woman about leaving her infant. Refer to Box 18.2 for a list of practical resources for mothers and parents.

Academy of Breastfeeding Medicine Statement on Breastfeeding Support for Mothers in the Workplace

The ABM published the Breastfeeding Support for Mothers in Workplace Employment or Educational Settings: Summary

Statement. It is an appropriate well-documented resource for additional important accommodations to guide the establishment of a successful lactation program within a work or educational environment.[11]

Surgeon General's Workshop on Breastfeeding and Human Lactation

The Report of the Surgeon General's Workshop on Breastfeeding and Human Lactation,[111] published in 1984, clearly enunciated that strategies need to be developed to reduce the barriers to breastfeeding while employed. All six categories of the report address the issue in some capacity. Twenty-five years later a summit on breastfeeding was convened to review the progress and reset the strategies. The workgroups were the same: work, professional education, public education, health care systems, and support services. The issues were similar, as were the strategies. The urgency of legislative support; workplace support, including daycare; paid maternity leave; child care; alternative work schedules (flextime); and job sharing were on the list for the workgroup on work. The workshop report also states that successful initiation and continuation of breastfeeding will require a broad spectrum of support services involving families, peers, care providers, employers, and community agencies and organizations.[111] The goals remain important ones and the effective collaboration of families, businesses, government agencies, and professional organizations will be needed to accomplish them.

US Breastfeeding Committee Workplace Accommodations to Support and Protect Breastfeeding

The US Breastfeeding Committee has undertaken as a major activity the improvement of the atmosphere for breastfeeding working women. The Committee's policy paper on the subject states the following benefits for employers that adopt a breastfeeding support program:[112]

- Cost savings of $3 per $1 invested in breastfeeding support
- Less illness among the breastfed children of employees
- Reduced absenteeism to care for ill children
- Lower health care costs (an average of $400 per baby in the first year)
- Improved employee productivity
- Higher morale and greater loyalty
- Improved ability to attract and retain valuable employees
- Family-friendly image in the community

Each company or employer should tailor a program to its unique needs. The Committee has suggested that several strategies are feasible, safe, and relatively easy to implement. They include developing a breastfeeding support program, distribution of support policy, consideration of a flexible scheduling option, sufficient break time to feed or pump, and providing useful information. The website also has a very practical list of links for frequently asked questions (FAQs) often asked by parents. The full statement is available at http://www.usbreastfeeding.org.

Breastfeeding Friendly Workplace Kit for Australia

Women in Australia face the same challenges to working while breastfeeding as reported in many other countries.

McIntyre et al.[113] report on a project that promoted balancing breastfeeding and paid work through the development, distribution, promotion, and evaluation of suitable materials to workplaces, employers, and employees. Materials for employees were translated into Arabic, Chinese, Turkish, Spanish, and Vietnamese. In this project targeting employers, women, and workplaces in Australia, 500,000 information kits were distributed with preference for places that had women of childbearing age and women of diverse cultural backgrounds. The project was widely publicized in all media.

The kit contained a poster to display key points and a booklet to provide more detailed information in an easy-to-read format. The contents had been tested in focus groups and evaluated by other key stakeholders, including a working mother and a lactation consultant. The evaluation of the project included a simple survey sent via e-mail or fax to 1571 organizations. Only 202 (12.8%) were returned. Those who responded thought it was excellent, more than half thought it would be useful, and two thirds thought the kit would provide suitable solutions to support balancing breastfeeding and work at their organization. The authors recognize the need for further work to implement the policies and procedures to support breastfeeding in the workplace. A more recent study was conducted to clarify best-practice strategies for breastfeeding support in the Australian workplace.[114] They reported that part-time work and more flexible hours helped mothers breastfeed for longer after returning to work. Mothers who exclusively breastfed for 6 months and returned to work after 7 months reported fewer hospitalizations for their infant. Of women who reported more workplace support for breastfeeding, more were able to exclusively breastfeed for 6 months. The kit disseminated in Australia is now available through the Australian Breastfeeding Association (see Box 18.1).

The Business Case for Breastfeeding

The *Business Case for Breastfeeding*[115] contains the steps for creating a breastfeeding-friendly worksite. This was developed by the US DHHS, Health Resources and Services Administration's Maternal and Child Health Bureau (MCHB). It is a comprehensive resource kit that targets a broad spectrum of individuals and groups involved in supporting breastfeeding women. The kit provides a train-the-trainer approach that results in improving workplace lactation support for employed breastfeeding women. It is intended to provide training for reaching out to local businesses and is working with state breastfeeding coalitions and Healthy Start programs. Healthy Start is a DHHS-funded program providing community-based initiatives to reduce infant mortality rates and to improve the health of women, infants, and children and their families. The training content is based on the MCHB workplace lactation resource kit in a community-based outreach program. Training is targeted at breastfeeding coalitions, Healthy Start Staff, International Board-Certified Lactation Consultants, health care professionals, La Leche League Leaders, and WIC staff. It is a step-by-step program complete with script and slides. The format includes role play. Those who complete the course should be ready to approach employers with why and how to start a program that supports breastfeeding by their employees. A separate section of the kit, "Employees' Guide to Breastfeeding and Working" is specifically for mothers and families and contains anticipatory guidance and practical advice for how to breastfeed and return to work. A printable pamphlet of this guide is available at the Womens Health DHHS site.[116]

Working and Breastfeeding

The international La Leche League has another very practical resource for breastfeeding mothers returning to work. It provides specific steps for planning for the return to work, influencing the breastfeeding-friendly nature of the specific workplace, pumping and storage practices, and links to local laws about breastfeeding and work in the United States, United Kingdom, Australia, and Ireland (See Box 18.2.).

SUMMARY

The benefits of exclusive breastfeeding for 6 months or longer for infant and mother are indisputable. The importance of mothers' education and employment to themselves, their children, their spouse, and their family is equally significant. A judicious and practical merging of breastfeeding and work (or education) to optimize the benefits of breastfeeding and working/education is essential. Further development of best practices supporting mothers in their breastfeeding goals, making breastfeeding-friendly workplaces and child-care environments and collaboratively involving mothers, fathers, families, and communities in these goals are worthy challenges.

The Reference list is available at www.expertconsult.com.

19

Induced Lactation and Relactation (Including Nursing an Adopted Baby) and Cross-Nursing

Ruth A. Lawrence

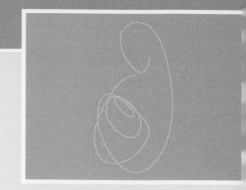

KEY POINTS

- Induced lactation is the process through which a non-puerperal woman is stimulated to breastfeed an infant without a preceding pregnancy. Relactation is when a woman who has given birth but stopped breastfeeding or never initially breastfed is stimulated to lactate.
- Induced lactation and relactation are important processes for assisting women to nourish infants (their own or others) when circumstances have changed and there is an urgent need for ongoing nutrition and nurturing. These situations can arise in the early or late postpartum period,

- as a result of health or social situations for the mother, adoption, and emergencies or disasters that separate infants from their mothers.
- The recommendations for facilitating the processes of induced lactation or relactation have not been studied through rigorous clinical trials but constitute suggestions based on experience or empiric observation. There are a variety of resources, published and online, for assisting and supporting women in their efforts.

Breastfeeding has returned to be the preferred form of nourishment for the infant, and there has been an increased interest in induced lactation. Induced lactation is the process by which a nonpuerperal woman is stimulated to lactate—in other words, breastfeeding without pregnancy. Relactation is the process by which a woman who has given birth but did not initially breastfeed is stimulated to lactate. This may also apply to a mother who may have initially breastfed her infant, weaned the infant, and then chooses to reinstitute lactation. Relactation can also involve a woman who previously breastfed a biologic child, even years before, and now is adopting a newborn. There are no blinded controlled research studies about either induced lactation or relactation. There are occasional observation reports about successes in a small series of dyads. The process has not been confirmed by clinical trials.[1] Otherwise the literature is meager and predominantly in the animal research field.

HISTORICAL PERSPECTIVE

Induced lactation and relactation are not new concepts but rather are well known to history and to other cultures. The motivation historically has been to provide nourishment for an infant whose mother has died in childbirth or is unable to nurse for some reason. A friend or relative would take on the care of the child and with it the responsibility to nourish the infant at the breast because no other alternatives were available.

Relactation has been used in times of disaster or epidemics to provide safe nutrition to weaned or motherless infants.

Numerous historical accounts of induced lactation are recorded in the medical literature and reviewed in the writings of Brown.[2] Mead recorded the occurrence of relactation in her writings about New Guinea in 1935.[3] Other anthropologists have made similar observations in other preindustrialized societies of women who have not recently borne children and, after a few weeks of placing the suckling infant to the breast, produce milk adequate to nourish the infant.[4] Until recently, Western world literature reported the phenomenon as an anecdotal report as part of the discussion of aberrant lactation. In 1971, Cohen reported a patient who had been nursing an adopted child successfully for weeks when first seen in his pediatric office.[5]

Today, the interest in induced lactation in the industrialized world stems from a desire on the part of adopting mothers to nurture an adopted child at the breast even though they were unable to carry the infant in utero. The interest in relactation comes from mothers of sick or premature infants who want to breastfeed their infants after the days and weeks of neonatal intensive care are over. These mothers, although postpartum, have not been lactating.

INDUCED VERSUS INAPPROPRIATE LACTATION

The process of induced lactation is separate from galactorrhea, or inappropriate lactation, which has been described in the medical literature for more than 100 years.[6] Abnormal lactation has been observed in various circumstances in nulliparous and parous women and even in men. There are many eponyms for these conditions, usually based on the name of the physician who first described the syndrome, such as Chiari-Frommel and Ahumada-del Castillo.

Normally in the absence of suckling, lactation ceases 14 to 21 days after delivery. Milk flow that continues 3 to 6 months after abortion or any termination of pregnancy is termed *abnormal* or *inappropriate lactation*, or *galactorrhea*. Galactorrhea also refers to lactation in a woman 3 months after weaning or the secretion of milk in a nulliparous woman in association with hyperprolactinemia and amenorrhea. Although these cases are pathologic in nature and, therefore, different from the groups under discussion, it is noteworthy that some knowledge of the initiation and maintenance of lactation has been gained from the study of these syndromes. A nonpregnant woman who develops spontaneous lactation should be evaluated for hormonal disease. The most common cause is a prolactinoma of the pituitary. Spontaneous lactation should not be ignored. See Chapter 16 Breast Conditions in the Breastfeeding Mother for discussion of nipple discharge and hyperlactation.

ANIMAL STUDIES

Information on the incidence of non-offspring nursing in 100 mammalian species has been assembled by Packer et al.[7] The incidence of non-offspring nursing is increased by captivity. It is more common in species with large litters (polytocous taxa) and differs from that which occurs with single young species (monotocous taxa). In the latter, it is more common for females to continue nursing after they have lost their own young. Among nondomesticated animals, spontaneous lactation has been observed repeatedly only in the dwarf mongoose (*Helogale parvula).*

Lactation has been induced for scientific and commercial purposes in nonpregnant and nonparturient animals by the continual systematic application of a mechanical milking apparatus to the mammary gland of the animal.[8] The response is produced through the release of a mammotropic hormone from the anterior pituitary gland. This effect is abolished if the pituitary stalk is transected. Ruminants respond to the addition of estrogen or estrogen-progesterone combinations, which facilitate mammary growth. Experiments in goats involved applying ointment containing estradiol benzoate to the udders of virgins, which resulted in development of the udder and milk yield almost comparable to that of normal postpartum animals.[9] It was subsequently shown, however, that a combination of estrogen-progesterone not only resulted in better milk yield, but histologically the lobuloalveolar growth was normal, whereas with estrogen alone growth was cystic and irregular. It was also demonstrated that ovariectomized goats could be stimulated to lactate with these two hormones, with resultant normal histology of the udder and good milk production. Initiation of regular milking had a significant impact on production of milk.

Because lactation can be stimulated when the ovaries have been removed but not when the pituitary stalk has been severed, this has significance for understanding some of the postpartum lactation failures in women. Again, in ruminants, growth hormone and thyroid hormone have been shown to increase milk yield, although prolactin does not. This suggests that prolactin is not deficient in ruminants. Because the motivation, goals, and physiologic problems may be slightly different, induced lactation and relactation in women are discussed separately.

INDUCED LACTATION

When a mother chooses to nurse her adopted infant, the goal is usually to achieve a mother–infant relationship that also may have the benefit of some nutrition. In that perspective, success can be evaluated on the basis of whether an infant will suckle the breast and achieve some comfort and security from this opportunity and close relationship with the new mother. As has been well described by Avery,[10] this is nurturing with the emphasis on nurturing, not on "breastfeeding" or nutrition. A mother who is interested in inducing lactation to nurse an adopted infant may need to understand that she may never be able to sustain the infant completely by her milk alone without supplementation. Neither the physician nor the mother should be disappointed. The nurturing goal is still achieved. An adoptive mother induced lactation for premature twins who were exclusively breastfed by 2 months of age. The mother succeeded because of careful planning and support of the health care team.[11]

Preparation of the Breast

Normally the breast is prepared by the proliferation of the ductal and alveolar system throughout pregnancy in anticipation of the time when lactation will begin, when the infant delivers and the placenta is removed.[12] Thus it is appropriate to assume that a period of similar preparation should take place in induced lactation. It has been suggested that a woman should begin systematically to express the breasts manually and stimulate the nipples for up to 2 months before the arrival of the infant, if time permits. A hand pump or other pumping devices can be used, but manual expression may work as well or better. Sometimes some secretion can be produced in this manner if it is carried out systematically on a uniform schedule throughout the day. The schedule should be practical, that is, include times when a mother could take a moment for this activity, such as morning and night plus any times she uses the bathroom or can conveniently handle her breasts.

Hormones and Medications

A more aggressive approach involves hormones and medications. During pregnancy, the breasts are prepared by the hormones generated by the pregnancy, estrogen, progesterone, and human placental lactogen (see Chapter 3, Fig. 3.3).

To mimic this environment, it has been suggested that starting a course of estrogen and progesterone would be appropriate, namely, prescribing oral contraceptive dosing that suppresses ovulation (such as Ortho-Novum). This dosing should be maintained without a pause as it would be during pregnancy.[13] Unfortunately, women who are adopting typically do not have 9 months to prepare, so priming the breasts with hormones may not be possible because the hormones need to be discontinued a month before anticipated lactation.

Concomitant with hormone therapy should be breast stimulation with systematic pumping with a good electric double pump. Timing should begin gradually, 5 minutes three times per day, then 10 minutes three times a day, increasing to a frequency every 4 hours. Pumping about the same time every day is helpful. It usually takes about a month before drops of milk appear. This is a good time to start domperidone (not available in the United States).[14–16] There have been concerns in women taking domperidone about cardiac mortality and prolonged QTc but no such infant mortality resulting from exposure through breast milk. The schedule adopted by Newman[17] in Canada is 10 mg three times per day, increasing during a month's time to 20 mg four times per day. Newman[17] suggests using domperidone from the beginning. Without a placenta, the adoptive mother does not have "prolactin-inhibiting" hormone to block the breast from responding to the prolactin secreted because of the breast stimulation. Health care providers should be able to discuss the use of domperidone and participate in a discussion with the mother about the risks and benefits of its use in induced lactation or relactation.[18,19] When domperidone is initiated, milk should appear in increasing quantities. Many women have achieved success by pumping alone initially and then adding galactagogues.

In other cultures, in which lactation is induced as a survival tactic for the infant, no period of preparation is available. An infant is put to the adoptive mother's breast and allowed to suckle. Emphasis has been placed on herbal teas as galactagogues and good nourishment for the mother, and the infant is also given prechewed food, gruel, or animal milk. Mead attributed much of the success of induced lactation to the ingestion of ample supplies of coconut milk by the new mother.[3] Coconuts are well known in herbal medicine; the oil pressed from ripe fruit is used for wound healing and inflammation reduction.[20] Adoption is not an easy process, and, in fact, it can be quite stressful to become an instant parent. In assisting such a mother, consideration should be given to the infant's age, previous feeding experience, and any medical problems that may exist. Provision for additional nourishment during the process of establishing some milk secretion is most important. Onset of lactation varies from 1 to 6 weeks, averaging about 4 weeks after initiation of stimulation with the appearance of the first drops of milk. When the infant is actually nursing at the breast and being nourished by supplements, milk may appear as early as 1 to 2 weeks.

Some infants are easily confused by switching back and forth between breast and bottle because the sucking technique is slightly different. Other nourishment can be offered by dropper, by small medicine cup, or as solid foods. A unique system is available, however, for providing nourishment for the infant while suckling at the breast. It involves the use of a device to provide a source of nourishment while the infant

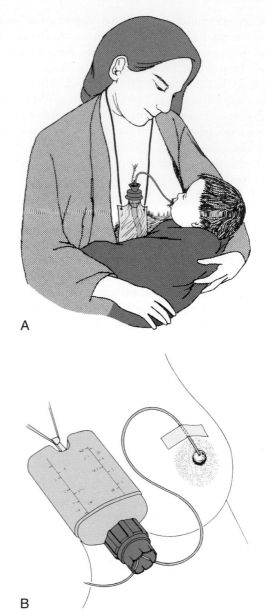

Fig. 19.1 (A) Lact-Aid Nursing Trainer System (Lact-Aid International Inc., Athens, Tennessee). (B) Supplemental Nursing System by Medela (McHenry, Illinois), which provides additional nourishment to infant while suckling at underproducing breast.

suckles at the breast, thus stimulating production. It is further described later in this chapter and is called the *Lact-Aid Nursing Trainer System* (Lact-Aid International Inc., Athens, Tennessee) or *Supplemental Nursing System* (Medela Inc., McHenry, Illinois) (Fig. 19.1).

Other Drug Schedules to Induce Lactation

As described in Chapter 3, estrogen and progesterone stimulate the proliferation of the alveolar and ductal systems. These hormones work in association with an increase in prolactin production. Although the prolactin level is high during pregnancy, milk secretion is inhibited by the presence of the estrogen, progesterone, and placental lactogen, the prolactin-inhibiting hormone. After delivery has occurred and the placenta is removed, these hormone levels fall, and prolactin initiates milk production. Efforts to stimulate this hormonal response have had variable success and are not usually recommended because of the possible effect on an infant through the milk. Women taking oral contraceptives have been noted in some cases to have breast enlargement. In addition, although estrogen and progesterone may enhance proliferation, they may inhibit lactation per se, so they must be discontinued well before lactation is planned to begin.

The dosage of conjugated estrogens recommended by Waletzky and Herman is 2.5 mg twice per day for 14 days beginning on the fourth day of a regular menstrual cycle.[21] Giving 0.35 mg norethindrone once daily for the morning dose of estrogen prevents breakthrough bleeding. Medication is given for 2 weeks and is comparable in dosage to 2 weeks of oral contraceptives. This therapy may be accompanied by some side effects. The regimen should include direct efforts to stimulate lactation by pumping the breasts.

A report from Papua New Guinea, where inducing lactation is critical to adequate infant nutrition, recommends priming the breast tissue of nulliparous women or those who have not lactated with 50 mcg ethinyl estradiol three times per day for a week.[22] Medroxyprogesterone (Depo-Provera) has been used to initiate lactation in nonpuerperal women. A dose of 100 mg is given intramuscularly once, one week before stimulating the breast with massage and pumping. Galactagogues, such as metoclopramide, domperidone, or herbals, can be introduced.[23] (See Chapter 11 for discussion of some galactagogues.) This approach was reported in Papua New Guinea, and success was claimed in 24 of 27 women.[24] When relactation is the goal in women who have previously lactated, pumping and massaging alone are initiated.

Growth hormone and prolactin have considerable genetic similarity, as reflected in some overlap of function.[25] High concentrations of growth hormone can cause lobuloalveolar development and casein expression. Growth hormone may play a role in optimization of milk production during lactation and even an accessory role in the induction of lactogenesis. Both natural and recombinant human growth hormones are potent inductors of milk synthesis in pregnant and lactating rats. This effect is attributed to their effect on the prolactin receptor.[25]

Oxytocin is a critical component in the milk-ejection reflex and may be helpful in the early initiation of ejection. Physiologically, stimulation of the nipple in the lactating woman results in the release of oxytocin by the hypothalamus, which then triggers the release of milk by stimulating the contraction of myoepithelial cells and the ejection of milk (see Chapter 3). The effect of intranasal administration of oxytocin on the let-down reflex in lactating women was well described by Newton and Egli.[26] (Oral administration by tablet is not as effective because oxytocin is destroyed in the stomach; therefore oral administration must be sublingual.) Oxytocin nasal spray has been used in cases of nonpuerperal lactation with some success in enhancing let-down but not necessarily altering the volume produced. The original oxytocin product, Syntonin, is no longer available, but a pharmacist

by prescription can place the intravenous preparation in a dropper bottle or a nasal spray container. The intravenous preparation (10 units/mL) is one-quarter the strength of the old nasal spray (40 units/mL). Therefore the dose needs to be increased four-fold: 4 to 6 drops per dose in one naris and feed the infant or pump immediately. The dose can be repeated. Continued use of oxytocin for weeks has been associated with diminished effect or even suppression of lactation.

In a randomized, double-blind trial of oxytocin nasal spray in mothers expressing breast milk for preterm infants, there were only marginal differences in the pattern of early milk production. The use of oxytocin nasal spray did not significantly improve outcome. Most of the subjects thought they were receiving the real medicine, which demonstrates the power of the placebo effect. All of the mothers had been pregnant, and their breasts had responded to the pregnancy.[27] These data should not be extrapolated without further study to women who had never been pregnant.

The chief benefit of oxytocin is often to break the cycle of failure and instill a feeling of confidence once it has been demonstrated that some secretion can be produced.

Galactagogues

Galactagogues, a substance, product, or medication used to increase milk production, such as metoclopramide, domperidone, or herbals, can be introduced.[23] (See Chapter 11 for additional discussion of some galactagogues.) Chlorpromazine has been observed to act as a galactagogue as well as a tranquilizer when given to patients in large doses (200 mg to 1000 mg). The effect has been observed in both male and female patients in mental institutions. The drug has been reported to increase pituitary prolactin secretion several fold. It acts by the hypothalamus, probably by reducing levels of prolactin inhibitory factor (PIF). Using this information, women well motivated to lactate who have attempted induced lactation by suckling a normal infant have had the process enhanced by small doses of chlorpromazine.

In a program to induce lactation in refugee camps in India and in Vietnam, nonlactating women were given 25 to 100 mg of chlorpromazine three times per day for a week to 10 days while infants were initially put to breast. Brown[28] reports apparent enhancement of lactation with this treatment. Chlorpromazine has the added pharmacologic effect of acting as a tranquilizer. The program of management in these women was supportive in other ways and also included the usual herbal medicines associated with lactation in these Eastern cultures. There was no control group.[28] It is possible that the drug contributed to both the physiologic and the psychologic well-being of the women wanting to lactate. It has been suggested that the desire to lactate is a strong component of success because women whose breasts are frequently stimulated sexually do not begin to lactate.

Theophylline also can increase pituitary prolactin secretions.[29] Therefore both tea and coffee should enhance prolactin secretion and thus lactation. Excessive amounts may inhibit milk let-down, however. (See Tables 19.1 and 19.2 and for other agents that may affect induced lactation.)

TABLE 19.1   Pharmacologic Agents to Induce Lactation: Possibly Effective for Selected Indications

	Domperidone	Fenugreek	Metoclopramide	Silymarin[a]
Chemical class or properties	Dopamine antagonist	A commonly used spice; active constituents are trigonelline, 4-hydroxyisoleucine, and sotolon	Dopamine antagonist	Flavolignans (presumed active ingredient)
Level of evidence	I (one study); other studies have inadequate methodology or excessive dropout rates	II-3 (one study in lactating women—abstract only)	III (mixed results in low-quality studies; effect on overall rate of milk secretion is unclear)	II-I (one study in lactating women)
Suggested dosage	10 mg orally three times per day in the Level I study; higher doses (20 mg orally TID) have been studied in this context	"3 capsules" orally (typically 580–610 mg), three to four times per day; strained tea, 1 cup, three times per day ({1/4} tsp of seeds steeped in 8 oz of water for 10 minutes)	10 mg, orally, three to four times per day; doses of 30–45 mg/day were most effective	Micronized silymarin, 420 mg orally per day; anecdotal; strained tea (simmer 1 tsp of crushed seeds in 8 oz of water for 10 minutes), 2–3 cups/day
Length/duration of therapy	Started between 3 and 4 weeks postpartum and given for 14 days in the Level I study. In various other studies the range was considerable: Domperidone was started between 16 and 17 days postpartum and given for 2–14 days	1 week	7–14 days in various studies	Micronized silymarin was studied for 63 days
Herbal considerations	—	Need reliable source of standard preparation without contaminants	—	Need reliable source of standard preparation without contaminants
Effects on lactation	Increased rate of milk secretion for pump-dependent mothers of premature infants of younger than 31 weeks' gestation in neonatal intensive care unit	Insufficient evidence; likely a significant placebo effect	Possibly increased rate of milk secretion; possible responders vs. nonresponders	Inconclusive
Untoward effects	*Maternal:* Dry mouth, headache (resolved with decreased dosage), and abdominal cramps. Although not reported in studies of lactation, cardiac arrhythmias resulting from prolonged QTc interval are a concern and are occasionally fatal. This may occur with either oral or intravenous administration and particularly with high doses, or concurrent use	Generally well tolerated. Diarrhea (most common), unusual body odor similar to maple syrup, cross-allergy with Asteraceae/Compositae family (ragweed and related plants), peanuts, and Fabaceae family (e.g., chickpeas, soybeans, and green peas—possible anaphylaxis). *Theoretically:* Asthma, bleeding, dizziness, flatulence, hypoglycemia, loss of consciousness,	Reversible CNS effects with short-term use, including sedation, anxiety, depression/anxiety/agitation, motor restlessness, dystonic reactions, extrapyramidal symptoms. Rare reports of tardive dyskinesia (usually irreversible), causing the FDA to place a boxed warning on this drug	Generally well tolerated; occasional mild gastrointestinal side effects; cross-allergy with Asteraceae/Compositae family (ragweed and related plants—possible anaphylaxis)

(Continued)

TABLE 19.1   Pharmacologic Agents to Induce Lactation: Possibly Effective for Selected Indications—cont'd

	Domperidone	Fenugreek	Metoclopramide	Silymarin[a]
	of drugs that inhibit domperidone's metabolism (see Interactions, later). *Neonatal:* Very low levels in milk and no QTc prolongation in premature infants who had ingested breast milk of mothers taking domperidone	skin rash, wheezing, but no reports in lactating women		
Interactions	Increased blood levels of domperidone when combined with some substrates metabolized by CYP3A4 enzyme inhibitors (e.g., fluconazole, grapefruit juice, ketoconazole, macrolide antibiotics)	Hawthorne, hypoglycemics including insulin, antiplatelet drugs, aspirin, heparin, warfarin, feverfew, primrose oil, many other herbal agents	Monoamine oxidase inhibitors, tacrolimus, antihistamines, any drugs with CNS effects (including antidepressants)	Caution with CYP2C9 substrates—may increase levels of the drugs. Possible increased clearance of estrogens (decreased blood levels). Possible increased levels of statins
Comments	In the United States, the FDA has issued an advisory *against* the use of domperidone for lactating women. Do not advise exceeding maximum dosage; no increased efficacy but increased untoward effects. Licensed for use as a drug for gastrointestinal dismotility in some countries (but not in the United States), where for this indication in some regions it is accepted that if no response at the initial dose occurs, dose may be increased. Some areas use as drug of choice when prolactin stimulation is thought to be needed. However, there are no studies of the safety or efficacy of this practice in lactating women	If patient develops diarrhea, reducing the dose is often helpful	Some studies suggest tapering the dose at the end of treatment	No prescription required

CNS, Central nervous system; *CYP*, cytochrome P; *FDA*, US Food and Drug Administration.
[a]Silymarin (micronized silymarin) or *S. marianum* (milk thistle).
Modified from Brodribb W. ABM clinical protocol no. 9: use of galactogogues in initiating or augmenting maternal milk production, second revision 2018. *Breastfeed Med.* 2018;13(5):307–314. doi:10.1089/bfm.2018.29092.wjb.

Because the role of prolactin is the initiation and maintenance of lactation, whereas oxytocin regulates the glandular emptying through the milk-ejection reflex, it is reasonable to speculate that enhancing prolactin release would be productive in inducing lactation. The exact activating mechanism of the neuronal reflex arc from breast to brain has not been deciphered. Secretion of prolactin appears to be influenced, if not controlled, by changes in hypothalamic dopamine turnover. Correspondingly, suckling has been observed to deplete dopamine stores.

TABLE 19.2   Pharmacologic Agents to Induce Lactation: Controversial or Not Recommended, Although Possibly Effective

	Human Growth Hormone	Sulpiride	Thyrotropin-Releasing Hormone
Chemical class or properties	Protein-based polypeptide hormone: stimulates multiple growth, and anabolic and anticatabolic effects	Substituted benzamide (antipsychotic, antidepressant); antagonism of presynaptic inhibitory dopamine receptors	A tripeptide hormone that stimulates the release of TSH and prolactin by the anterior pituitary
Level of evidence	I, II	II-I (only two studies)	I
Suggested dosage	0.2 international units/kg/day, given intramuscularly or subcutaneously	50 mg orally two times per day; do not use higher doses because of sedation of mother and baby	1 mg four times daily by nasal spray
Length/ duration of therapy	7 days, starting 8–18 weeks postpartum	4-day course starting at 3 days postpartum; no evidence to use for a longer course of treatment	10 days
Effects on lactation	Increased milk secretion in a selected population of normally lactating women with no feeding problems and with healthy, thriving infants between 8 and 18 weeks postpartum	Increased milk secretion in a selected population: Primiparous women with total yield of milk not exceeding 50 mL for the first 3 postpartum days	Increased milk secretion in selected population of primiparous women with insufficient milk supply at 5 days postpartum
Untoward effects	None observed in mothers or infants studied to date. *Potentially:* Joint swelling, joint pain, carpal tunnel syndrome, and an increased risk for diabetes or heart disease	Severe drowsiness; extrapyramidal effects same as for metoclopramide (above); weight gain	Elevated TSH and hyperthyroidism
Interactions	Other hormones, including contraceptives, insulin, cortisol, and others	Levodopa, other drugs with CNS effects	Other hormones, including contraceptives, insulin, cortisol, and others
Comments	Insufficient study; not practical— requires injection and is very expensive	Concern about untoward effects	Insufficient study, very expensive, no commercial product available

CNS, Central nervous system; *TSH,* thyroid-stimulating hormone.
Modified from Brodribb W. ABM clinical protocol no. 9: use of galactogogues in initiating or augmenting maternal milk production, second revision 2018. *Breastfeed Med.* 2018;13(5):307–314. doi:10.1089/bfm.2018.29092.wjb.

Investigation of other drugs that are known to stimulate prolactin release has identified some possible therapeutic materials. Kramer reported that metoclopramide induces prolactin release regardless of the route of administration.[22] Prolactin levels are increased three to eight times normal levels within 5 minutes when a 10-mg dose of metoclopramide is given either intravenously or intramuscularly. The effect is achieved within an hour when metoclopramide is given orally. The effect persists for 8 hours. The suggested regimen is 10 mg of metoclopramide, three to four times per day for a week.[30] This is then gradually tapered (see Chapter 11).

Metoclopramide is also used in neonates with esophageal reflux. The side effects are irritability and diarrhea. Rarely, susceptible infants experience dystonic reactions, which have been described in adults. Metoclopramide has also been used in combination with chlorpromazine, 25 mg four times per day, in Papua New Guinea.[22] Metoclopramide has been used to enhance lactation, as well, especially among mothers of premature infants.[28]

The regulation of prolactin secretion in humans has been studied to further the understanding of abnormal lactation and to provide information on the regulation of pituitary function of the brain.[31] It has been shown experimentally that the hypothalamus secretes PIF, which acts on the mammotropin-releasing cells of the pituitary to inhibit release of the hormone prolactin. The hypothalamus can also regulate prolactin secretion by a stimulatory mechanism, the secretion of thyrotropin-releasing hormone (TRH). When human volunteers (nonpregnant, nonlactating) are given infusions of TRH, increases in thyrotropin and prolactin are observed within minutes of injection, with values peaking in 20 minutes. The level of thyroid hormone in the volunteers initially influences the results. Patients with hypothyroidism have been observed to secrete excessive amounts of prolactin, whereas patients with hyperthyroidism are relatively insensitive to TRH. This may explain some of the variable results obtained with prolactin-stimulating drugs used to enhance lactation. Studies using TRH have been done on relactation but not on newly induced lactation. Thyroid activity has not been measured.

TABLE 19.3 Influence of Drugs on Prolactin Secretion

Pharmacologic Agents	Plasma Prolactin Concentration	Mechanism of Drug Action
L-Dopa	Decrease	Increase in hypothalamic dopamine-catecholamine levels, leading to enhanced activity of PIF
Ergot alkaloids (ergocornine, ergocryptine)	Decrease	Direct inhibition of adenohypophyseal prolactin secretion; possible increase of hypothalamic PIF activity (continued PIF function)
TRH (pyroglutamyl histidyl-prolinamide)	Increase	Direct stimulation of adenohypophyseal lactotroph for increased prolactin secretion
Theophylline phenothiazines (chlorpromazine)	Increase	Decreases in hypothalamic dopamine-catecholamine levels, leading to diminution of PIF activity
Metoclopramide	Increase	Inhibition of hypothalamic PIF secretion through dopamine antagonism
Sulpiride	Increase	Increase in hypothalamic prolactin-releasing hormone
Growth hormone	Increase	Causes lobuloalveolar development and casein expression
Recombinant human growth hormones	Increase	Affects prolactin receptors

PIF, Prolactin inhibitory factor; *TRH,* thyrotropin-releasing hormone.
Modified from Vorherr H. Human lactation and breast feeding. In: Larson BL, ed. *Lactation.* New York, NY: Academic Press; 1978.

Table 19.3 summarizes the influence of drugs on prolactin secretion.[29] ABM protocol no. 9 discusses the use of galactagogues and their effects and side effects (see Tables 19.1 and 19.2).[32]

Any pharmacologic regimen to stimulate milk production is most effective if it is initiated after the breast tissue has responded to mechanical stimulation because the hormones that act as the prolactin-stimulating compounds are thought by many to be ineffective in unprimed breast tissue. Jelliffe points out that the most important factor for continued production of milk is not drugs or hormones but "mulging."[33] He explains that *mulging* (stimulation) is a word created by N. W. Pirie to mitigate the confusion between the words *sucking* and *suckling.* The word comes from the Latin *mulgere,* to milk. *Suck,* according to the dictionary, means to draw into the mouth by means of a partial vacuum created by action of the lips and the tongue.[34] *Suckle,* however, refers specifically to the breast and means "to give suck to," as at the breast, or to take nourishment from the breast; thus, by definition, a bottle is not suckled.

Composition of Induced Milk

Concern has been expressed that the composition of the milk produced by stimulation of suckling rather than as a result of pregnancy might differ from "normal human milk."[35] Such induced milk is not different in other species that have been studied extensively, including bovine and rat milk. In developing countries, the fact that the infants showed normal growth and weight gain was taken as evidence that induced milk is adequate.

Kulski et al.[36] reported the analysis of the galactorrheal secretion produced by the breast after hyperstimulation; Table 19.4 lists the comparative analysis of normal breast

TABLE 19.4 Composition of Normal Breast Milk and "Galactorrhea Milk"

Milk Components and Properties	Normal Breast Milk	"Galact-orrhea Milk"	Induced Lactation
Components			
Fat (g/dL)	3.7	3–8	
Lactose (g/dL)	7.0	3–5	5.4
Total protein (g/dL)	1.2	2–7	1.6
Sodium (mg/dL)	15	70	22.0
Potassium (mg/dL)	50	5	19.8
Calcium (mg/dL)	35	38	
Chlorine (mg/dL)	45	50	18.4
Phosphorus (mg/dL)	15	2	
Ash (mg/dL)	20	40–70	
Properties			
Specific gravity	1030–1033	1031	
Milk pH	6.8–7.3	7.3	

From Kulski JK, Hartmann PE, Saint WJ, et al. Changes in the milk composition of non-puerperal women. *Am J Obstet Gynecol.* 1981;139:597 (reprinted with permission from the American College of Obstetricians and Gynecologists).

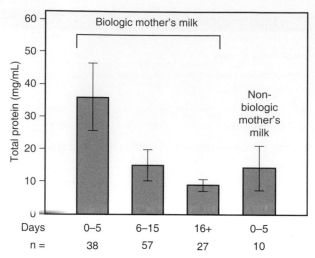

Fig. 19.2 Total protein changes over time: biologic versus non-biologic mother's milk, protein value ± standard deviation. (From Kleinman R, Jacobson L, Hormann E, et al. Protein values of milk samples from mothers without biologic pregnancies. *J Pediatr.* 1980;97:613.)

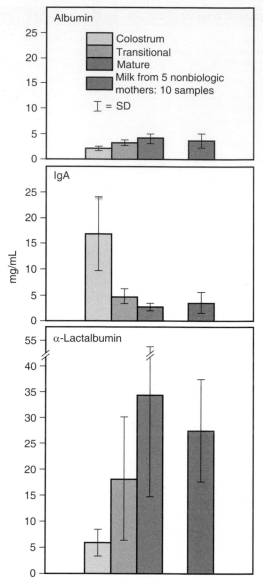

Fig. 19.3 Concentrations of albumin, immunoglobulin A *(IgA)*, and α-lactalbumins: biologic versus nonbiologic mother's milk. *SD,* Standard deviation. (From Kleinman R, Jacobson L, Hormann E, et al. Protein values of milk samples from mothers without biologic pregnancies. *J Pediatr.* 1980;97:614.)

milk with "galactorrhea milk" and milk from induced lactation. The induced lactational milk did not differ from puerperal milk. Brown reported higher values of fat, protein, and lactose in galactorrheal milk.[2] Kleinman et al. reported protein content changes over time and in the milk of biologic and nonbiologic mothers. The volume of secretion was small in these subjects (Figs. 19.2 and 19.3).[37]

The composition of the breast secretion produced by two women who induced lactation artificially by breast hyperstimulation was close to the composition obtained for women with normal lactation, according to Kulski et al. (see Table 19.4).[36] These investigators also examined the milk of a woman in whom lactation had occurred when medicated with a psychotropic drug (haloperidol). She had been pregnant 4 years previously. Her galactorrhea lasted 38 months. Her milk had a composition like that of colostrum for a week but resembled mature milk at 1 month. A woman with hypothyroidism and elevated prolactin and thyroid-stimulating hormone (TSH) had colostrum-like milk for 53 days of sampling. Two women with galactorrhea and amenorrhea associated with pituitary tumor and hyperprolactinemia had transient colostrum-like secretion, which changed to mature-appearing milk.

Protein values of milk samples from five mothers without biologic pregnancies were measured by Kleinman et al.[37] Two of the mothers had nursed previous babies, and three had never been pregnant and had never breastfed. These authors did not distinguish among them. The mean total protein concentration of milk samples from the "nonbiologic" mothers differs from that for "biologic" mothers (see Figs. 19.2 and 19.3). If the goal of induced lactation is nurturing, these differences are clinically less important. However, a clinician needs to keep these values in mind when counseling a mother–infant dyad about induced-lactation nutrition, especially if the infant was premature or small for gestational age. A creamatocrit test for fat and energy content is an appropriate first step (see Chapter 22).

In tandem nursing, when a mother continues to nurse an older child and puts an adopted newborn on the breast simultaneously, the composition of milk will not return to colostrum as it does after a biologic pregnancy.

Lactation has been induced in men, usually when a father tries to replace the mother who has died suddenly. A young married man collected and froze several liters of normal appearing milk over a year's time of taking estrogen and progesterone and using mechanical breast stimulation.

MANAGEMENT OF MOTHER AND INFANT

The collected experiences of counseling women in the Western world who want to induce lactation have resulted in reports on several thousand women. The request for information and advice is increasing and becoming widespread throughout the United States and other Western countries.[35]

Because simple means of supplementing the nutritional needs of an infant are available, counseling should center on the relationship and the nurturing aspects. When the process is undertaken in preindustrialized nations, the antiinfective properties of human milk become important even though total nourishment with human milk may not be possible. One measure of success is having the infant content to nurse at the breast.

A woman should be encouraged to go to a physician's office for a counseling visit before the arrival of the adopted infant to discuss the process of induced lactation. The physician ideally has a lactation-friendly office. There are physicians who specialize in breastfeeding and lactation. They can be located by contacting the Academy of Breastfeeding Medicine (ABM) at 8735 W. Higgins Road, Suite 300, Chicago, IL 60631; (800) 990-4ABM (United States toll free); phone: 847-375-4726; fax: 847-375-4713; email: abm@bfmed.org; website: www.bfmed.org.

A couple who is planning to adopt an infant should have at least one visit with a pediatrician so that parenting can be discussed, just as any couple should do before the birth of a first child. At this visit, while discussing lactation with the couple, it is helpful to explore the motives and general concepts of what is involved. All authors on the subject have pointed out that a husband's interest in, and support of, lactation is critical to success. His participation in the preparation of the breasts may be a means by which the father can share intimately and constructively in the process.

Equally important is to engage the services of a licensed, board-certified lactation consultant (International Board—certified lactation consultant [IBLCL]) who is preferably associated with the physician's office. The lactation consultant will need to spend time in the day-by-day, week-by-week counseling and support of the mother.

Instruction of a mother in preparation of the breasts for suckling is critical in induced lactation, whereas with puerperal lactation it may not be necessary at all. Exercises to stimulate the nipples should be undertaken several times per day and will be most successful if they are scheduled for times when, and situations in which, it is easy, feasible, and readily remembered. A few minutes multiple times per day is more successful and less likely to overemphasize milk versus mothering than rigid excessive exercises once or twice per day. Manual manipulation with gentle traction or horizontal and vertical stretching can be suggested. Avery[10] suggests that a father be encouraged to assist in breast massage and other techniques. She notes that "many adoptive parents felt that this technique (fondling and sucking of the breasts by the husband) added to the mutual sharing in preparation for adoptive nursing similar to the closeness many couples experience in preparing for natural childbirth." Raphael[38] reports that among 40 nursing adoptive mothers, dozens of variations on the theme of preparation were used. A positive attitude seemed to be the only consistent factor.

The need for dietary counseling is obvious. Lip service on behalf of well-balanced nutritious meals is not enough. Discussion should center on the absolute needs in kilocalories, fluids, and nutrients to produce milk (see Chapter 8).

A physician should point out that stimulation of the nipples may cause amenorrhea. Although the variation in menses is not uniform, decreased flow, irregular cycles, and total cessation of menstrual flow are possible. Conversely, the menstrual cycle may be maintained and the flow of milk may seem to vary during menses. Changes in breast size, heaviness, and feeling of fullness should accompany the induced lactation. A woman may have an associated weight gain of 10 to 12 lb (4.5 to 5.4 kg), on average, attributed to the response of the body to developing stores for lactation, just as in pregnancy (i.e., increased fluid retention and appetite increase).[10] The weight gain may be a simple phenomenon of excessive intake. There is no need to gain excessive weight, however, during this experience. Mothers (who may be nutritionally depleted) in non-Western countries who induce lactation are given added diet, nourishment, and herbal teas but do not usually gain weight. Failure to experience change in breast size, menstrual regularity, or weight should not be construed as a failed response as it might be in pregnancy.

Auerbach and Avery[39] reported a retrospective questionnaire study of 240 women: 83 had never been pregnant or lactated, 55 had been pregnant but never lactated, and 102 had breastfed one or more biologic children before the adoptive nursing (lactation). Most respondents used more than one technique to stimulate their nipples. These mothers stated that the most effective method of nipple stimulation was nipple exercises combined with infant suckling. Hand-operated pumps caused soreness and irritation. The nipple exercises included nipple stroking, massaging the breast, and rolling the nipple between thumb and finger.

In this study, infants' willingness to suckle improved over time and was related to the age at which the infant was first put to breast. Infants who were younger than 8 weeks of age had more than a 75% success rate; those older than 8 weeks of age had only 50% success. No infants failed to thrive, but nearly all needed some type of supplementation. Mothers who had nursed a biologic baby before were able to wean from supplementation partially or completely. This group was also more disappointed if they had to supplement.[39]

PROTOCOLS FOR INDUCED LACTATION

The Newman-Goldfarb protocols were developed by Dr. Jack Newman and Ms. Lenore Goldfarb and are on the website Ask Lenore at https://www.asklenore.info/breastfeeding/induced_lactation/gn_protocols.shtml. Also available are protocols for induced lactation with accelerated menopause. The protocols use hormonal stimulus using birth control pills and domperidone initially until the breasts have responded and enlarged; pumping is initiated within 1 month of the beginning of feeding. Various herbs recognized as galactagogues are also added.[33] Domperidone is not available in the United States by Food and Drug Administration mandate.[16] The authors of various protocols for induced lactation point out that starting 9 months before the baby arrives is ideal preparation time. They also provide information for more rapid induction. They do not recommend pumping until the hormone treatment has been effective. They recommend stopping the hormones as pumping is begun. Domperidone is maintained throughout. A woman should always consult her own physician before starting any protocol or trying any medication, hormones, or herbs.

Experience and Expert Opinion

Following personal experience, Bryant prepared a review, "Nursing the Adopted Infant."[40] As a physician she was able to view the issue as a physiologic, pharmacologic, and psychologic challenge.

GUIDELINES FOR INDUCED LACTATION

The following simple guidelines, developed as a result of experiences reported by several authors and many mothers, may be helpful to physicians in counseling mothers to induce lactation:

1. Before arrival of the baby, initiate frequent, brief manual stimulation of nipples and breasts, increasing time gradually to approximately 10 minutes per session. Initiate mechanical pumping stimulus after 2 weeks or so of manual stimulus if time permits. Hand pumps usually cause more soreness. Modern electric pumps with milking action and pressure cycling are most effective. Pumps that can be controlled in cycle frequency and strength are best. Double-sided pumps maximize stimulus and save time.
2. On arrival of the baby, depending on the infant's age, limit sucking to breastfeeding, using a lactation supplementer if necessary.
3. Breastfeed before any other nourishment is provided for a given feeding.
4. Avoid stressing baby with hunger, responding in a timely fashion to early hunger cues.
5. When supplementing, use donor human milk or prepared formula, not cow's milk, with its long stomach-emptying time and potential for allergic response.
6. Avoid rubber nipples and pacifiers to encourage appropriate suckling at breast.
7. Provide other supplements by dropper, spoon, cup, or supplementer.
8. Create a positive atmosphere; "mother the mother."

A trial of oxytocin nasal spray once the infant is established at the breast may facilitate let-down and even encourage prolactin release.

Rigid conformity to a system of feeding may be a symptom of a more serious problem. Women who are rigid and compulsive may have trouble lactating because of the inability to have a good ejection reflex, which can be inhibited by stress and emotional conflict. Mothers who demonstrate an inordinate attention to volume of production of milk more than the value of the relationship may feel as if they have failed.

WHEN ADOPTING MOTHERS ARE A SAME-SEX COUPLE

- As inducing lactation for an adopted infant by same-sex couples has become more common, so has the desire to breastfeed the infant by both women in a lesbian relationship.
- Physiologically inducing lactation is usually possible for both women, although often one is the primary nursing mother. A case is reported by Wilson et al. in which both adopting women and the biologic mother breastfed the infant.[41] Milk induction was stimulated with hormones, domperidone, and scheduled breast pumping. Defining parental roles was complex and maintenance of milk production was difficult.
- Inclusion, open discussion, respect, and consistent lactation support are important when the infant of a same-sex couple has been born to one member of the couple by artificial insemination, and both women plan to breastfeed the baby, one by lactation induction.
- A case is reported as an ethical issue when the physician refuses to assist the patient inducing lactation.[42] The conclusion of the ethics consults was that the physician's objections were unfounded. The value to the infant outweighed any objections. It was thought that the objection showed a troubling unfamiliarity with the clinical facts of lactation and a double standard for treating lesbian, gay, bisexual, transgender, queer, plus (LGBTQ +) patients and heterosexual patients.[42]

RELACTATION OR REINITIATION OF LACTATION

The initiation of lactation and establishing relactation in an outpatient setting with mothers whose infants are younger than 6 weeks old in India is described by Banapurmath et al.; over a thousand mothers were followed with 91.6% succeeding in establishing lactation within 10 days.[43] Proper latch was reported to be essential for success. Focus was on understanding the process, positioning, and building confidence. Medications were not used. Establishing lactation in India for mothers who are adopting babies usually in social crises is challenging. Another report from India was done of 23 mothers, all of whom were given metoclopramide 10 mg twice a day for 15 to 20 days. They put the baby to breast immediately on receipt of the infant.[12] Motivation was critical to success. Lactation has been induced in a primiparous woman with Sheehan syndrome (see Chapter 15), which is usually described as a delivery in which there is excessive loss of blood and maternal shock that also shocks the pituitary. Most of these women develop permanent hypopituitarism. A patient of our Lactation Study center in Rochester, NY suffered such an event. The mother had an emergency hysterectomy. She wished desperately to breastfeed. She was given daily oxytocin by nasal spray and pumped the breasts with increasing frequency. She began producing milk in 2 weeks and fully lactating in 4 weeks. The infant was 36 weeks' gestational age when admitted to the neonatal intensive care unit (NICU). She nursed the infant for a year, although she had hypopituitary function.

Early successful relactation in a case of prolonged lactation failure was reported by Agarwal and Jain.[44] The case was a mother with hemorrhage and shock at delivery. At $3^1/_2$ months the infant was very ill with diarrhea, dehydration, and shock as a result of formula intolerance. The mother induced lactation with the drip and drop method. A tube was used along the breast just beyond the nipple and an assistant presses on the syringe causing milk to drip as the infant suckles, similar to the Lact-Aid device. Supplement was given by cup and spoon until the mother's milk supply was enough to sustain the infant.

Relactation was reported in a series of 15 mothers being managed in a clinic in Davangere, Karnataka, India, who had stopped breastfeeding for 2 weeks or more.[43] The mothers had stopped because they thought they did not have enough milk and began supplementing. The management began immediately with putting the infant to the breast 10 to 12 times per day for at least 10 to 15 minutes on each breast. Key to success was the pouring of milk (formula or donor milk) by spoon or small cup by a helper (a nurse or relative). The amount of milk dripped over the breast was reduced as a mother's supply increased until the process could be stopped. The group of mothers included two with premature infants and two surrogate mothers who had not breastfed for 16 and for 6 years, respectively. Milk appeared at 7 and 8 days of pumping, and exclusive breastfeeding was accomplished in 45 and 40 days, respectively. Follow-up and support were intense. Babies were seen and weighed weekly. Of the 15 mothers, 10 were exclusively breastfed and 5 continued with some supplementation. The authors encourage clinicians to initiate relactation whenever a mother thinks her supply has dwindled.

These protocols have not been tested with placebo-controlled blinded studies but reflect the experience of a number of practitioners.

Nutritional Supplementation

The need to supplement an infant's intake while the milk supply is being developed should be discussed. An older infant who has already been receiving solid foods can be continued on solids by spoon with careful attention to nutritional content so that the diet includes a balance of protein and other nutrients. Supplements with milk or formula should be appropriate to the age of the infant. The infant younger than 12 months should receive infant formula rather than whole milk if donor breast milk is not available. The milk supplements should be full strength, 20 kcal/oz, and provided during the feeding by dropper or supplementer or after the nursing by dropper, spoon, or cup in preference to artificial nipple, which may confuse the infant during adaptation to nursing at the breast.

Postmenopausal Lactation

Women have had infants after menopause thanks to modern fertility techniques and hormone therapy. The question arises as to whether these woman can breastfeed. They will require maintenance hormone therapy paralleling levels in postpartum lactating women. The oxytocin and prolactin should respond with removal of the placenta and suckling of the infant at the breast. Three cases have been reported to the lactation center in which producing milk was successful. No long-term follow-up was available.

A postmenopausal woman may wish to induce lactation. Some of these women are young and had surgical menopause; however, most of them had emergency hysterectomies and still retain their ovaries. The situations are different, and the treatment is different.

In natural menopause, the woman may be on hormone replacement therapy, which should be modified to match pregnancy levels of estrogen and progesterone. A program of regular systematic dual pumping should be initiated with the addition of galactagogues, such as domperidone, after the breast has responded with enlargement, turgescence, and the first drops of milk. The woman who has retained her ovaries can be managed in the same manner as a premenopausal woman.

Support Systems

The process of induced lactation requires considerable commitment and determination.[45] It is far more arduous a task than initiating postpartum lactation, but it is possible and worth the effort, according to the many mothers who have attempted it. The situation is better managed if a doula is available. It is appropriate for a physician to suggest that, in addition to medical support, the mother seek counseling from a licensed, certified lactation consultant experienced in induced lactation. Day-by-day contact for verbal support may be helpful, and these needs may be beyond the scope of a busy office practice unless there is a lactation consultant on staff. A nurse practitioner may be invaluable in this situation, particularly if home visits are made.

Ensuring that the child grows appropriately is the responsibility of a pediatrician; however, this task is best carried out in a nonthreatening way so a mother can concentrate on nurturing and nourishing the infant.[46] Monitoring the usual growth parameters of weight and height and the patterns of voiding and stooling is essential.

Psychological Factors

Although the general process of nipple stimulation, having the infant suckle the breast, and setting the stage for lactation is similar, a woman who has experienced successful lactation previously may have not only the physiologic but also the psychologic edge. As Jelliffe wrote decades ago, "Breastfeeding is a confidence game."[33]

Prospective Study

A prospective study of mothers whose infants were in the NICU in Durham, North Carolina, was reported by Bose et al.[47] The profile of the mothers is listed in Table 19.5. Mothers and babies were admitted to the clinical research unit, where they were assisted with relactating, including help using

TABLE 19.5 Historical and Clinical Data of Mothers in Relactation Study

Case No.	Gestational Age	Time From Delivery to Entry Into Study (Days)	Time From Last Lactation to Entry Into Study (Days)	Postpartum Breast Involution[a]	Time to First Breast Milk (days)	Time to Half Breast Milk Supply[b] (days)	Time to Complete Relactation (days)
1	Term	10	10	None	1	4	8
2	Term	120	120	Incomplete	4	20	28
3[c]	Twins, 31 wk	49	49	Complete	7	28	Never
4	32 wk	70	42	Complete	7	20	Never
5	28 wk	150	135	Complete	9	Never	Never
6	32 wk	30	16	None	4	17	58
7	Term (adopted)	5 yr	5 yr	Complete	21	Never	Never

[a]Mothers were asked if their brassiere size was different from that before this pregnancy.
[b]Estimated on the basis of a decrease in formula intake.
[c]Ceased to suckle her infants after 28 days in the study to return to full-time employment.
From Bose CL, D'Ercole J, Lester AG, et al. Relactation by mothers of sick and premature infants. *Pediatrics*. 1981;67:565.

the Lact-Aid. The infants' nutritional intake was recorded. Mother and infant were discharged when the mother was comfortable with the Lact-Aid and feeding was established (approximately 3 days). Follow-up occurred every week or two. All but one infant were initially reluctant to suckle, but all received their entire nutritional intake at the breast, with or without Lact-Aid, within the first week of the study. Most of the mothers had trouble initiating suckling, with the most significant factor being the length of separation from their infants and not the degree of prematurity, postnatal age, weight, or feeding regimen. Nipple tenderness occurred in all mothers, but it was transient. All the mothers (except number seven, who was an adoptive mother) produced milk in 1 week, with maximum milk production occurring from 8 to 58 days, proportional to the time since delivery.

Although it was done with a small population, this study established some important information. Given appropriate techniques and support, many women appear to be able to relactate and premature infants can learn to breastfeed after initial bottle-feeding.

A retrospective study of relactation was reported by Auerbach and Avery[48] in which 366 women responded with a completed questionnaire of more than 500 contacted from a list of names obtained from manufacturers' lists, magazine ads, and requests to breastfeeding support groups. The bias was in favor of well-educated, affluent women who had probably obtained their lactation goals. The population included those who had untimely weaning (*n* = 174), after delivery of low-birth-weight infants (*n* = 117), and after hospitalization of mother or baby or both (*n* = 75). Three quarters of the study participants rated their experience positively, often stressing the importance of nursing to the mother–infant relationship. Milk production was less often a goal, but when

it was, it was more likely to influence the mother to evaluate her experience negatively and result in difficulty in achieving a total milk supply.[48]

Previous Suckling Experience

An infant's willingness to nurse was related to previous suckling experience, but responses in the first week of effort were not directly correlated with ultimate successful suckling. After 1 month, 50% of mothers were able to discontinue supplementing; however, 24% were never able to eliminate supplements completely. Once established, the nursing patterns were similar to those of ordinary breastfeeding. The authors point out that keeping the baby hungry in the mistaken notion that the infant will nurse more often and for longer periods does not help and may negatively influence outcome. It is of interest that fewer than 10% of respondents thought that they had received helpful advice from health care professionals.[48]

Relactation in mothers of children older than 12 months of age have been reported.[49] Six Australian children 12 to 18 months of age had been weaned by their mothers, with no further stimulus to the breast, and then were reinitiated to breastfeeding. The length of time without breastfeeding ranged from 1 week to 6 months (Table 19.6). All of the children had been actively weaned and initiated the suckling, although the mothers did not forcibly resist. All of the mothers reestablished milk supplies and nursed for 48 months to 5 years.[49]

Tandem Nursing

Tandem nursing an adopted child is a phenomenon in which the adoptive mother is still nursing a biologic child and puts an adopted infant to the breast and intends to nourish the newcomer totally. Usually the older child is a toddler and

TABLE 19.6   Relactation in Mothers of Children Older Than 12 Months of Age

Case No.	Age of Child	Length of Time Off Breast	Methods	Evidence of Presence of Milk	How Long from Relactation to Weaning	Age at Final Weaning
1	48 mo	4 mo	Child suckled from breast Mother relaxed, not anxious over outcome	Child verbally reported presence of milk Mother saw whitish milk	After milk appeared	48 mo
2	12 mo	1 wk	Child took four feeds daily	Milk had not quite dried up	1 yr	2 yr
3	$20\frac{1}{2}$ mo	$2\frac{1}{2}$ mo	Mother gave in to demands of child and suckled her	Mother noticed child's swallowing while breastfeeding	>10 mo	Sometime after $2\frac{1}{2}$ yr
4	2 yr	1 mo	Child suckled from both breasts avidly	Mother saw the milk flow was enough to soak the bed next morning Mother heard swallowing	Approximately 1 yr	>3 yr
5	>3 yr	6 wk	Child suckled from both breasts	Mother saw the milk Mother noticed swallowing	Approximately 2 yr	5 yr
6	Approximately 2 yr	Approximately 6 mo	Mother attached child to breast to demonstrate	Mother began to feel let-down of milk	12 mo	Almost 3 yr

From Phillips N. Relactation in mothers of children over 12 months. *J Trop Pediatr*. 1993;39:45.

feeding only a few times per day or for comfort and receiving the major nourishment from other food and drink. In biologic tandem nursing, the milk returns to colostrum-like constituency with the birth of the new baby; in the absence of a pregnancy, however, the milk volume may increase with increased nipple stimulus while the constituents do not change. Data on milk constituents beyond a year postpartum or in the case of relactation have been noted earlier. In most cases reported anecdotally, the adopted infant is several weeks or months old, so the absence of colostrum is less of a problem. On the other hand, the active state of lactation in terms of immediate availability of milk is an advantage.

An additional concern, as in any situation of tandem nursing, is the development of the younger child. The physician will need to be alert to these issues in counseling the family and ensuring adequate total nutrition for the adopted child.

Eighteen respondents to the survey on adoptive nursing by Auerbach and Avery[39] reported tandem-nursing experiences; 11 of these mothers were able to discontinue supplements totally (two within the first month). Most of the infants were started on solids by $4\frac{1}{2}$ months, which may be the most effective method of supplementing if nutritional value is maintained. For physicians, it is important to be knowledgeable about tandem adoptive nursing and to support the family accordingly.

Drugs to Induce Relactation

Some medications that have been tried in relactation seem to work only when the breast has been primed by mammogenesis, that is, by pregnancy.

Thyrotropin-releasing hormone (TRH) use has been reported by Tyson[50] and Brodribb[32] to induce lactation (see Table 19.2). Each woman in the study was primed with estrogens beforehand. Thyroliberin (also known as TRH) stimulates the pituitary to release both TSH and prolactin. Drugs that produce a decrease in hypothalamic catecholamines, such as phenothiazines, reserpine, meprobamate, amphetamines, and α-methyldopa, cause an increase in prolactin secretion by blocking hypothalamic PIF.

The feasibility of pharmacologically manipulating puerperal lactation was demonstrated by Canales et al.[51] using bromocriptine and thyroliberin sequentially.[51] They suppressed lactation using bromocriptine orally for 8 days in four mothers whose infants were premature or ill and could not be nursed. These mothers did not lactate during this time. On the 8th day, they were given thyroliberin intravenously and then orally daily for 4 days (8th to 12th postpartum days). On the 14th day, they initiated breastfeeding by putting the infants to the breast. Prolactin levels were measured from the day of birth. Levels were depressed by bromocriptine and rose when the thyroliberin was given. The mothers subsequently nursed successfully. Bose et al.[47] also studied thyroliberin and the basal and stimulated serum prolactin concentrations.

Prolactin Concentrations

Prolactin concentrations were measured followed by levels at 15 and 30 minutes after intravenous infusion of 200 mg (range 100 to 500 mg) of thyroliberin. Prolactin levels were also measured before and after suckling at weekly intervals. Serum prolactin levels rose 15 minutes after infusion of thyroliberin or thyrotropin-releasing hormone (TRH) (Table 19.7). The absolute rise in prolactin concentrations did not appear to be related to establishment of milk production. The change over time in the basal prolactin levels was not predictably related to lactation progress.

Lactation can be reestablished with metoclopramide, according to Sousa et al.[52] Metoclopramide is a derivative of procainamide, as is sulpiride (see Chapter 11).

Metoclopramide and sulpiride are potent stimulators of prolactin release.[53] A marked increase in prolactin is seen when metoclopramide is given, as noted previously in this chapter. Sousa et al.[52] used metoclopramide to reestablish lactation in women who had experienced diminished milk supply (Table 19.8). All five mothers experienced increased production of milk when 10 mg was given orally every 8 to

12 hours for 7 to 10 days. No side effects were noted, although this drug is known to cause cardiac arrhythmias and extrapyramidal signs in some adults. No side effects were noted in the infants, but the level of drug was not measured in the milk. The results were encouraging, but further study is needed to determine the minimum dosage necessary to produce the effect and the amount passed into the milk.

In a controlled double-blind study with a placebo, Lewis et al.[54] found no difference in the success rate of induced lactation in 10 patients medicated with 10 mg metoclopramide orally three times daily for 7 days compared with 10 matched patients medicated with lactose capsules. Successful lactation was attributed to the special advice and support provided equally for these women by the nursery staff. Before conducting the study, these authors measured the amount of drug

TABLE 19.7   Basal and Stimulated Serum Prolactin Concentrations (ng/mL)

Case No.	TRH STIMULATION		SUCKLING STIMULATION: PRESUCKLING/POSTSUCKLING					
	Basal	15 min/ 30 min	1st wk[a]	2nd wk	3rd wk	4th–5th wk	6th–7th wk	8th–9th wk
1	179.2	611.1/423.5	136.9/155.4	72.3/123.8	—	—	—	—
2	38.7	80.9/70.3	17.2/119.3	38.6/214.3	16.6/180.6	186.2/244.5	—	—
3	19.9	89.6/77.3	17.9/23.5	—	—	—	—	—
4	9.5	89.9/63.4	12.5/12.7	—	7.0/437.6	5.5/47.3	—	—
5	13.9	40.6/36.3	21.1/58.2	37.8/82.0	38.3/57.7	77.2/98.5	24.6/54.2	—
6	31.7	335.6/274.7	9.5/11.4	—	16.5/18.4	11.8/16.3	7.8/13.3	—
7	43.6[b]	78.8/69.9	8.8/59.6	17.0/77.7	—	—	34.4/147.1	19.2/60.5

[a]Suckling test performed on day 1 or 2 of study.
[b]In this mother, the suckling test was done first, followed 1 h later by thyrotropin-releasing hormone (TRH) infusion; thus 8.8 is the true basal concentration.
From Bose CL, D'Ercole J, Lester AG, et al. Relactation by mothers of sick and premature infants. *Pediatrics.* 1981;67:565.

TABLE 19.8   Data Regarding Mothers Taking Metoclopramide

Case No.	Age of Mother (y)	Age of Infant (mo)	Daily Dose (mg)	Length of Treatment (days)	Side Effects	Results	Education Level of Mother
1	27	2	30	6	None	Increase in milk volume; infant not weaned	University
2	25	10	30	10	None	Same as above	University
3	29	1	20	7	None	Same as above	High school
4	35	3	30	7	None	Same as above	University
5	20	2	20	7	None	Same as above	High school

From Sousa PLR, Barros FC, Pinheiro GNM, et al. Reestablishment of lactation with metoclopramide. *J Trop Pediatr Environ Child Health.* 1975;21:214.

that appeared in the milk of 10 women after a single 10-mg dose of metoclopramide given orally at 7 to 10 days postpartum. The mean 2-hour postdose plasma level was 68.5 ± 29.6 ng/mL. The simultaneous mean concentration in the breast milk was 125.7 ± 41.7 ng/mL. If an infant consumed a liter of milk per day, the dose to the infant would be calculated at 130 mg or 45 mg/kg, a subtherapeutic dose. These data do not address possible accumulation in the infant, however, when multiple doses are given to the mother.

Domperidone has a better track record anecdotally for stimulating lactation but has not been studied in induced lactation or relactation. Herbal agents such as fenugreek have not been studied for this purpose either but could be used as an adjunct to protocol.[55]

SPECIAL DEVICES

Although many mechanical devices have been developed since Roman times to augment lactation and give other feeding opportunities, lactation-supplementing devices provide a unique ability to adequately nourish an infant while the infant is suckling at the inadequately lactating breast (see Fig. 19.1). The suckling stimulates the mother's own supply. On the other hand, the infant continues to suckle the breast because milk is available. The devices have been carefully engineered to provide a source of milk that is obtained by suckling, not by gravity. The capillary tube through which the milk flows can be placed along the human nipple without interfering with suckling. The plastic containers that serve as reservoirs for the supplemental milk are sterilizable or disposable. The milk is naturally warmed by hanging the bag beside the mother's breast, as shown in Fig. 19.1.

Gradual weaning from the supplementer can be provided by putting increasingly less in the container each day. Thus the infant can obtain milk from the breast in increasing amounts because the nipple stimulation affects milk production.

An increasing number of mothers want to nurse their sick premature infants; however, it is often not possible for the infant to breastfeed for weeks. Meanwhile, the mother may pump but only obtain minimal volume. When the infant is finally ready for discharge from the hospital, it is mandatory that the baby continue to receive reliable nourishment every day. Starving the infant into submission is inappropriate and dangerous. A lactation supplementer is an excellent alternative for providing adequate nourishment and continuing stimulating suckling at the breast to increase milk production.

For years, mothers of premature and sick infants have been assisted in breastfeeding their infants in preparation for discharge from the hospital and during the early weeks at home by using dropper feeding, complementary feeds by bottle after each breastfeeding, or solids. The success rate was low and the aggravation for the mother often insurmountable.

Weaning From the Device

Weaning from the supplementation device is usually not a problem for most of the infants. It was a problem, however, for an occasional mother who could not nurse without the supplementer even though it contained less than an ounce of formula per feeding and the breast was supplying the rest. Because the mother may use this as a "crutch," careful anticipatory counseling should address this issue.

Use of a supplementation device should be started with a full understanding of its role in nourishment of infants and with a plan for weaning from it that begins the first day. Weaning should be appropriate to an infant's age and nutritional needs. The nourishment provided should be donor human milk or regular-strength formula, 20 kcal/oz, and not just water, sugar water, or diluted formula. Starvation, even for a day or so in a premature infant, can compromise growth, especially of the brain. An infant who has been in the intensive care nursery is in special jeopardy.

Several alternative devices have been suggested by professionals interested in the transient supplementation of lactation while a mother increased her milk supply for her full-term baby. Usually in these situations, lactation failure has been the result of inadequate initial advice. The devices are rigged from readily available feeding tubes and syringes but lack the special engineering and safety features of the supplementer. Special precautions are advised when employing such handmade equipment to avoid milk aspiration by the infant, which is the chief hazard. Because they will allow milk to flow without sucking, they do not stimulate the infant to suck. Other devices, such as hand pumps and a variety of electric pumps, which are useful in initiating relactation or induced lactation and in puerperal nursing, are illustrated in Chapter 22.

RELACTATION DURING DISASTERS

Relactation has assumed new significance as the plans for disaster preparedness are reviewed. World attention has been drawn to major disasters, hurricanes, earthquakes, tsunamis, tornadoes, and fires that leave infants without their mothers to nurse them (see Chapter 23). Such disasters have allowed people to recognize the value and safety of human milk and breastfeeding when simple things such as clean water, sanitation, heat, and light are not available. Brown recounts the experience of 100,000 orphans in the city of Saigon during a disaster, many of whom were newborns who ended up breastfeeding.[2] In times of disaster, surrogate mothers were housed in orphanages, fed well, and received a daily dose of chlorpromazine for a week. Many women were able to nourish two babies.

The need to relactate exists in a number of circumstances, including the following:
1. A sick or premature infant cannot be fed initially, or at all, until several weeks or months old (Fig. 19.4).
2. An infant is weaned prematurely because of illness in the infant or in the mother.
3. An infant who was not previously breastfed develops an allergy or food intolerance.
4. A mother who has lactated weeks, months, or years earlier wants to nurse an adopted infant.
5. A mother who is nursing a biologic child wants to nurse an adopted child (without benefit of pregnancy).

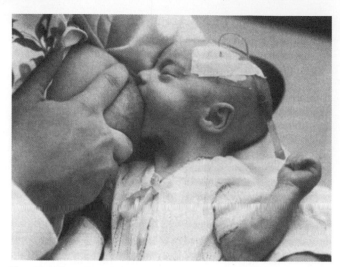

Fig. 19.4 Premature infant at breast: infant weighed 1300 g at time of photograph.

6. A town or village is in a time of crisis in the area and infants need clean, safe food.

Historical reviews provide many examples of infants suckled in times of crisis by women who have not lactated for years. The process of reestablishing lactation under these circumstances is generally easier than that of nonpuerperal lactation. Investigations have shown that a breast that has been previously primed by pregnancy to respond to prolactin will produce milk more readily but the majority of women can succeed at relactating.[2,24,28,48]

WET NURSING, CROSS-NURSING, CO-FEEDING, OR MILK SHARING

Although feeding an infant by one who is not the mother is an established means of sustaining life, it has been uncommon in Western cultures. There are no medical contraindications provided the nursing woman is in good health, was infection free, and was taking no medications. The threat of human immunodeficiency virus (HIV) infection has reinforced the need for assessing the risk-to-benefit ratio in a given situation of one woman providing breast milk for another woman's child. In special cases, surrogate nursing would be acceptable by individual arrangement, with HIV testing in both mother and infant. The chief obstacles have been psychologic or social. Women who are trying to develop a supply of milk when their own infants cannot nurse because of prematurity or illness would be benefited by having a vigorous, normal suckling infant nurse at their breasts.

In contemporary society, the term *cross-nursing* has replaced *wet nursing* to disassociate the phenomenon from negative historical connotations.[56] In reviewing mothers' experiences of sharing breastfeeding or breast milk, Thorley[1] offered a new term to replace *cross-nursing: co-feeding.* She points out that wet nursing initially was an occupation and

was done for hire and did not include any reciprocity. When sisters or friends nurse each other's infants, reciprocity exists. The term *co-feeding* is thought to suggest sharing. The term *milk siblingship* has been proposed to suggest the bond between children breastfed by the same woman. In cross-nursing the mother continues to breastfeed her own child in addition to the child she takes for a feeding or two per day. The circumstances described in the report by Krantz and Kupper[56] usually involve babysitting arrangements, which may be daily and formal or random and informal. They interviewed three women involved in a mutual agreement for babysitting purposes. The mothers were married and well-educated. The babies were girls and 4 months old. The mothers reported no physical effects on the babies. The behavioral reactions of the babies were being disturbed and "looking puzzled" if the surrogate mother spoke. Some difficulty was noticed in let-down, and all three mothers noted a difference in the way each baby suckled.

Another purpose of cross-nursing is for maternal benefit, wherein an experienced, vigorous infant is nursed by a woman whose own baby is unable to give proper stimulus to milk production. This has been done by private arrangement and has not caused any known problems. Usually the normal newborn is younger than 2 months. Cross-nursing also has been used to stimulate lactation in adoptive nursing. In this situation, the infants are exchanged to stimulate the adoptive mother's breasts and also to show the adopted infant that milk comes from breasts and how to suckle at the breast.

Cross-nursing had been used in NICUs by mothers to encourage their own milk production. It is usually a private arrangement between mothers who have babies to nourish. A mother of an immature infant who could not be put to the breast sought out a friend who was actively feeding a full-term infant and borrowed the infant to stimulate her production. An infant who needs to learn how to suckle correctly after weeks of bottle-feeding or no feeding may benefit from being nursed by a fully lactating woman. The best pump is always a suckling infant.

The hazards to cross-nursing are undocumented but worthy of consideration. The physical problems are the potential for infection, either of mother or of baby; interruption of milk supply for the mother's own baby; and the difference in composition of milk if babies are of different chronologic or conceptual ages. The psychologic hazards could include failure of mother let-down, refusal of infant to nurse (which does occur when infants are introduced to the practice after 4 months of age), and negative impact on siblings and the household environment. The long-range effects are not documented.

Reasonable caution is certainly appropriate, taking care to ensure that the cross-nursing mother is healthy and well-nourished without any general or local infection, not taking any medications, and not smoking. The infants probably should be close in age to the mother's own baby and also free of infection, including thrush. If this were a commercial venture in a public daycare setting, regulations of certification and screening for tuberculosis, syphilis, hepatitis, cytomegalovirus, herpesvirus, HIV, and other infectious agents would be in order. Documents of liability might be required with signed consent forms. Mothers' experiences of sharing breastfeeding or breast milk were reviewed in Australia from 1978 to 2008 by Thorley.[1] The objective of the study was to explore the mothers' experiences when they shared breastfeeding, why it was done, and the process used. The most common reason to participate was to provide human milk for their babies, exclusively, including whenever they were separated from their infants or temporarily unable to feed the infants themselves. Most of the respondents to the survey were selective about with whom they would share. They otherwise found positive response from friends and health care professionals, although they noted a change in attitude in the 30 years.

Various cultural "rules" exist for milk-sharing. In Chinese, Japanese, and Thai families, milk can be shared only for infants of the same sex. Moslem tradition is strict in its ban on marriage between children who had the same wet nurse. In some cultures, breast milk is a conduit of ancestral power. Sharing is restricted to the same clan or lineage.

Informal milk sharing is a more recent terminology that describes various situations (not directly nursing) of sharing of breast milk by donor mothers with infants of other mothers without using milk banks. The exchange of breast milk occurs between relatives, friends, connections made specifically for exchange, connections made through websites, and now more directly person to person over the Internet. The responsibility for safe milk exchange is born by the donor and the parents of the infant to receive the milk. The ABM has issued a position statement on informal breast milk sharing to provide guidance to health care providers about the safe sharing of breast milk for the term healthy infant.[57] The statement emphasizes a "mother-to-mother" screening process regarding the donor mother's health, any medication use, most recent prenatal and postnatal infectious screening tests (HIV, hepatitis B or C virus, human T-cell leukemia virus type 1) or risk for such infections, and social practices of the donor mother related to marijuana, alcohol, smoking, or illegal drug use. The statement also provides guidelines for "home pasteurization" of donated breast milk using the flash heating method.

Perhaps as breastfeeding knowledge and understanding reach a greater number of professionals and women, such opportunities may be more common. At present, it is significant to recognize cross-nursing as a viable option, as long as appropriate infection precautions are taken, or safe informal milk sharing can be practiced by using the ABM's recommendations for appropriate use of shared breast milk. A hospital or a physician should not be the agent of arrangement or exchange.

SUMMARY

Relactation or induced lactation may be practiced in a variety of situations to provide breast milk to an infant in need. Careful medical management of an adopted infant who is breastfed is important. Many times the prenatal care of this infant as a fetus in utero and the biologic mother has not been optimal. Any failure in growth should be identified quickly so that appropriate supplementation can be provided. In cases of relactation to provide for sick or premature infants, close follow-up is mandatory. A child who does not have a powerful suck may appear to be content yet be underfed.

Relactation and induced lactation are special events requiring the positive support of medical personnel.[46] A physician can serve as a well-informed stable resource in a process that will require considerable effort and commitment by the participants and will go better if there is an experienced licensed IBLCL available as a supporter. A pediatrician is responsible for monitoring adequate growth, nutrition, adjustment, and development of the child.

Mother-Initiated Preparation
1. Nipple stimulation: Hand massage and nipple exercise, hand pump, electric "milkers"
2. Diet supplementation: Fluids and calories, especially protein
3. Reading, learning, and communicating with others with similar experience

Physician-Initiated Preparation
1. Knowledgeable, sympathetic support
2. Preparatory hormones and lactagogues to promote mammogenesis for prescription
3. Induction of let-down: Oxytocin nasal drops to initiate or enhance let-down
4. Counseling about breast preparation and diet supplementation in the context of total care of the mother and the infant
5. Appropriate use of pumping milk extraction devices and of lactation-supplementing devices

The Reference list is available at www.expertconsult.com.

20

Chestfeeding and Lactation Care for LGBTQ + Families (Lesbian, Gay, Bisexual, Transgender, Queer, Plus)

Casey Rosen-Carole and Katherine Blumoff Greenberg

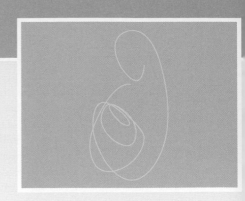

KEY POINTS

- LGBTQ + families may have unique experiences in providing human milk for their infants.
- LGBTQ + individuals may face particular barriers related to their ability to provide human milk for their infants related to discriminatory policies, restricted donor milk regulations, or anatomic/functional limitations.
- Appropriate care for LGBTQ + families includes the use of both respectful and affirming language and background

knowledge of the physiologic impacts of any past or current treatments on milk production.
- As with all families, lactation providers should be careful to provide appropriate information, while not making assumptions or judging parental decisions.

Social science evidence clearly shows that the children of LGBTQ + families thrive on par with children living in different-sex families.[1] Assessments of well-being span cognitive and psychological development, mental health, and adolescent risk-taking behavior, among others.[2] In the United States, where there exist policies related to nondiscrimination, 35% of US LGBTQ + families have children.[3] Internationally, many countries have LGBTQ + -inclusive social norms and policies; however, there are still countries where "homosexual activity" continues to be illegal[4] and many others where same-sex couple adoption is highly restricted. LGBTQ + couples in these countries may have significantly less access to family building opportunities. Box 20.1 lists organizations that provide guidance and information on gender-affirming care.

Family development in LGBTQ + couples may take many forms and can include adoption and assisted reproductive

technologies. The infant children of LGBTQ + families may be at risk for health disparities from birth in the form of reduced access to human milk.[5] Children raised in LGBTQ + families thrive on par with children raised in heterosexual, cisgender families.[2,6] However, given the range of anatomy and fertility that may exist within LGBTQ + families, they may be unable to offer a parent's human milk to their children. Because current donor milk policies prioritize medically high-risk infants, babies in LGBTQ + families may also lack access to donor milk (see Chapter 22 for information on expanding donor milk availability). It is therefore critical for providers to both understand how to support and counsel families about their options with respect to lactation and to compassionately approach any constraints they may face.

Providers should not assume that all parents will desire to lactate because they have the anatomy or hormones to do so.

BOX 20.1 Groups and Organizations That Support Gender-Affirming Care

- *Equaldex:* The Collaborative LGBT Rights Knowledge Base. Includes maps and lists of laws applying to LGBT persons around the world. Access at: http://www.equaldex.com.
- *Transcend Legal:* Medical organization statements. List of medical and nursing groups along with their statements of nondiscrimination and the promotion of safe and affirming care for gender nonconforming patients. Access at: https://transcendlegal.org/medical-organization-statements.
- *World Professional Association for Transgender Health:* International, interdisciplinary, professional association devoted to understanding and treatment of gender identity disorders. Access at: http://www.wpath.org.
- *UCSF Transgender Care.* Website for the Transgender Care Clinic at University of California San Francisco. Includes evidence, terminology, environment guidance and clinical guidance for appropriate care. Access at: https://transcare.ucsf.edu/.
- *National LGBT Health Education Center.* A program of the Fenway Institute. Their mission is to advance health equity for LGBTQIA + people, address and eliminate health disparities, and optimize access to cost-effective health care for the LGBTQIA + community. They provide distance learning, videos, and printed educational health materials. Access at: https://www.lgbthealtheducation.org/publication/lgbt-glossary/.

As with any family, human milk feeding may not be a parental goal; in LGBTQ+ families, specifically, parents may be taking turns gestating, birthing, and lactating or may have histories of medical treatment that will make lactating, breastfeeding, or chestfeeding uncomfortable or impossible. As with all families, lactation providers should be careful to provide appropriate information while not making assumptions or judging parental decisions.[5,7,8,9]

The Academy of Breastfeeding Medicine (ABM) has a protocol for the care of lactating patients who identify as LGBTQ+, which is available on their website.[10] To best care for patients, it is important to understand some basic terminology used within the LGBTQ+ community. Box 20.2 is a list of definitions helpful in this context.

CREATING A RESPECTFUL HEALTH CARE ENVIRONMENT

There are many opportunities for health care systems, hospitals, and clinics to provide affirming care to LGBTQ+ individuals. Increasing the amount of LGTBQ+ training for health care providers and building inclusive systems and documentation can minimize provider and staff mistakes surrounding an individual's gender or sexual orientation. Examples of inclusive practices include updated intake forms with more options for affirmed gender, affirmed pronouns, and partnership status; single-stall, all-gender restrooms; and gestation and lactation spaces that include all parents, not just those identified as mothers. Coupling training and inclusive practices with displaying signs or statements of inclusivity is a subtle but impactful way to welcome individuals with diverse genders, sexual orientations, and families.[11,12] Patient confidentiality is another cornerstone to LGBTQ+ care, because many patients may not be "out" to all of their health care providers,[13] and even a patient's family and friends may not be aware of the patient's gender identity and/or sexual orientation. This information is privileged within provider-patient relationships, and it is critical that providers ask patients about when, how, and why they might disclose their gender and sexuality. Although not a comprehensive list, other considerations include the following:

- An individual's appearance may not match gender identity. Do not assume that a female-appearing individual identifies as female or is interested in breast/chestfeeding.[14]
- Ensure that people are addressed by their affirmed names and pronouns. To know the patient's preference, one needs to ask. For example: "I'd like to address you respectfully, what name and pronouns should I use?"
- Names and pronouns are but one aspect of a parent's experience, and patients may also use different terms for parenting (mom/mama/mum, dad/father, parent, etc.) and lactation (chestfeeding, lactation, breastfeeding, etc.). We recommend ensuring that patients have the opportunity to identify at the beginning of a patient care visit which words they would like to use.
- Calling a patient by a name, pronoun, or parenting term other than the patient's affirmed name/pronoun,

is generally referred to as *misgendering* and is hurtful to the patient. If intentional, misgendering damages the patient-provider relationship; if unintentional, it is an opportunity for providers to acknowledge the mistake, correct it, and continue with the visit using affirming language.[15] Acknowledging the mistake and apologizing is key, but prolonged attention on the mistake may take the focus off of providing appropriate and affirming health care.

PHYSIOLOGY OF LACTATION IN SPECIAL CIRCUMSTANCES

Because of the development of mammary tissue and its hormone responsiveness in critical windows, timing of gender-affirming treatments or practices (e.g., chest binding) may or may not affect the ability to lactate. Following are some examples of hormonal treatments, surgeries, and practices and how they may affect lactation. Because of a dearth of clinical studies on LGBTQ+ human milk feeding, many of these effects are theoretical.

Transmen (Assigned Female at Birth, Affirmed Male)
Chest Binding
Transmen may have bound their mammary tissue with tight clothes or special binders during or after puberty. Though this is unlikely to affect the hormonal axis, it may lead to compression atrophy of the mammary tissue. Studies on breast augmentation show that over time, compression of the mammary tissue can lead to atrophy.[16] Chest binding may provide more, or less, pressure than implants for augmentation, and the distribution is likely to be different. Nevertheless, if a person binds mammary tissue and then desires to lactate, the tissue may be less able to generate a milk supply.

Masculinizing Chest Surgery (Also Known as "Top" Surgery)
Transmen may have undergone surgery of the mammary tissue. This surgery is different from a mastectomy, in that not all breast tissue is removed. Rather, the goal is to create a male-appearing chest contour. It is therefore possible that lactating mammary tissue remains. Depending on surgical technique, the nipple may or may not be fully removed during the procedure. If a nipple is fully removed, reanastomosis of the ducts may be anecdotally reported but is likely uncommon. Pregnant patients who have had this type of surgery should be counseled on engorgement management and pain relief in the postpartum period. If the nipple and areola remain attached to a pedicle of mammary tissue during surgery, ductal structures may be less damaged, and it may be easier to lactate. Studies on breast reduction have shown that preservation of the subareolar mammary parenchyma results in the highest rates of successful breastfeeding.[20] These approaches

BOX 20.2 Definitions Related to LGBTQ + Health[10]

Definitions: Several sources have defined terms related to LGBTQ + health. Here, we reference the University of California San Francisco Transgender Care & Treatment Guidelines[17] and the National LGBT Health Education Center's glossary of terms.[18] However, it is important to note that terminology is fluid and community-specific. In countries speaking languages other than English, these terms may have adaptations or may be irrelevant entirely. Consulting with members of LGBTQ + advocacy communities in such areas, where possible, may be helpful to ensure that language is respectful and inclusive.

- *LGTBQ + :* A term for people who identify as lesbian (L), gay (G), bisexual (B), transgender (T), queer (Q) or questioning (Q) and people with other diversities in sexual orientation and gender identity (+). There are a variety of these terms internationally with their own acronyms. This term is meant to be inclusive.
  - *Lesbian* (adj., noun): A sexual orientation that describes a woman who is emotionally and sexually attracted to other women.
  - *Gay* (adj.): A sexual orientation that describes a person who is emotionally and sexually attracted to people of their own gender. It can be used regardless of gender identity, but is more commonly used to describe men.
  - *Bisexual* (adj.): A sexual orientation that describes a person who is emotionally and sexually attracted to people of their own gender and people of other genders.
  - *Transgender* (adj.): Describes a person whose gender identity and assigned sex at birth do not correspond. Also used as an umbrella term to include gender identities outside of male and female. Sometimes abbreviated as trans.
  - *Queer* (adj.): An umbrella term used by some to describe people whose sexual orientation or gender identity are outside of societal norms. Some people view the term queer as more fluid and inclusive than traditional categories for sexual orientation and gender identity. Because of its history as a derogatory term, the term queer is not embraced or used by all members of the LGBT community.
  - *Questioning* (adj.): Describes individuals who are unsure about or are exploring their own sexual orientation and/or gender identity.
  - *" + "/Plus:* The plus sign represents the ever-growing list of terms people use to describe their sexual orientation or gender identity. There are many different variations of the LGBTQ + acronym, and the " + " acknowledges that it is not possible to list every term people currently use.
- *Affirming care:* Refers to care that supports a patient's gender identity and must include inclusive terminology, practices, insurance coverage, and knowledgeable providers.
- *Affirmed pronouns and name:* Pronouns and name that are chosen by the individual and therefore best represent the person's gender identity. People in the LGBTQ + community may have changed their name and gender, informally or legally, to those that affirm their true gender identity.
- *Assigned Female at Birth, Assigned Male at Birth:* These terms refer to gender assignment at birth medically and socially, generally based on genital anatomy. These terms may be abbreviated (AFAB, AMAB) to communicate birth anatomy in medical documentation.
- *Cisgender:* Someone whose gender identity aligns with the gender assigned to them at birth. For example, someone who was assigned female at birth who identifies as a woman.
- *Chestfeeding:* A term used by many masculine-identified trans people to describe the act of feeding their baby from their chest, regardless of whether they have had chest/top surgery (to alter or remove mammary tissue).[19]
- *Co-lactation:* When more than one parent breastfeeds/chestfeeds their child.
- *Gender-affirming surgery:* Surgeries specific to transgender people include feminizing and masculinizing procedures that align secondary sexual characteristics with a person's gender identity. These may include facial, voice, genital, and hair removal/addition procedures.
- *Gender-expansive, genderqueer, nonbinary:* All different terms for a broad category of gender identities in which the individual identifies outside of a binary concept of gender (binary meaning "male" and "female"). This can mean identifying as both feminine and masculine or as neither.
- *Gender identity:* Persons' innate sense of their own gender. It does not necessarily correspond to anatomy, sex assigned at birth, or how someone expresses self. Examples include but are not limited to cis woman, cis man, trans man, trans woman, nonbinary, gender expansive, and gender fluid. Not the same as sexual orientation (see later).
- *Gender incongruence, formerly "gender dysphoria" or "gender identity disorder":* Incongruence between an individual's experienced or expressed gender and assigned sex.* Dysphoria refers particularly to suffering as a consequence of this incongruence.
- *Heteronormative/cisnormative:* The assumption and/or preference of individuals and institutions that everyone is heterosexual and cisgender. This leads to invisibility and stigmatization of people in the LGBTQ + community.
- *Transition:* The process and time during which persons assume their affirmed gender expression, which may or may not include legal, medical, or surgical components.
- *Sexual orientation:* The aspect of someone's identity, which refers to the gender(s) of the people to whom they are attracted. Examples include but are not limited to homosexual, lesbian, gay, heterosexual, bisexual, asexual, and pansexual.

*World Health Organization. *International Classification of Diseases.* 11th ed. Geneva, Switzerland: WHO; 2018.

should be discussed with patients during a lactation consultation, and a clear history obtained because the scars may look identical.

Testosterone Therapy

Hormone therapy may be used to masculinize features for transmen. It may be started as early as the late teenage years and has been shown to interrupt mammary gland development.[21] For some patients using testosterone after completing female puberty, this may result in a smaller chest, though for others the difference in the mammary gland may not be grossly obvious. It is possible that this type of therapy inhibits anatomic lactocyte development. It may also interrupt the hypothalamic-pituitary axis of milk production and let-down because this axis is influenced by gonadal hormones, though this is incompletely understood.[22]

"Chestfeeding"

The term *chestfeeding* originated in the transmale lactating community as a term that encompasses both gender-affirmed language and the embodied experience of feeding an infant from one's own body. Transmen may or may not have dysphoric feelings toward their chests; if they do have chest dysphoria or have experienced trauma, abuse, or overt discrimination related to their chest, the word "breast" may raise negative emotions. Some in the lactation community have pushed back against this term, as possibly marginalizing an experience long thought to be quintessentially female. However, one must consider the difficulties encountered by lactating transmen along with any histories of gender dysphoria. Furthermore, using a patient's own language concerning their body is widely considered the foundation of respectful provider—patient interactions. Therefore one also should not assume that because a person identifies as "trans" that the person would prefer the term "chestfeeding" over "breastfeeding." As discussed earlier, patients should be asked about their preferred terms, and those terms should be used. Finally, any handouts, videos, or applications (apps) used should be reviewed before being suggested, because many contain gendered language along with highly gendered assumptions about lactation, families, and children.

Transwomen (Assigned Male at Birth, Affirmed Female)
Gender-Affirming Mammoplasty

Transwomen may have undergone augmentation mammoplasty. If this is the case, implants are most often subpectoral, and incisions are most often inferior to the breast. This means that the nipple may not be divided from any ductal tissue, as in masculinizing chest surgery. However, the visual appearance may mask low volumes of mammary tissue or provide uncomfortable pressure during engorgement if mammary tissue is present. Patients with breast augmentation should be counseled to express milk or feed an infant more often in the postpartum period (10 to 12 times per day rather than 6 to 8 times per day), to prevent downregulation of milk supply, uncomfortable engorgement, or mastitis.

Feminizing Therapy

Breasts with physiologic mammary tissue may develop over the course of time during treatment with estrogen and progesterone. Androgen-blocking medication, often spironolactone, is typically used for those who have not had orchiectomy as a part of their surgical transition. This mammary tissue has been shown on case report and in anecdotal reports to be capable of making human milk (see later).

Induced Lactation: Case Report

One published report exists of a transwoman who presented with anatomically typical breasts after treatment with estrogen, progesterone, and spironolactone for 6 years.[23] Over the course of 3 months, she induced lactation by a progressive increase in her estrogen and progesterone dosages, then a withdrawal period combined with domperidone (a dopamine-blocking galactogogue) and pumping. She exclusively breastfed for 3 months. Other providers and patients have induced lactation with/as transwomen, but these cases remain anecdotal. See Chapter 19 for more discussion of induced lactation.

TWO OR MORE LACTATING PARENTS AND CO-LACTATION

Although two or more parents who are able to lactate may see the benefit of sharing the work and bonding of infant feeding, because the physiology of lactation requires frequent breast emptying without prolonged pauses (see Chapter 3 on feedback inhibition of lactation), sharing lactation requires planning and careful consideration. In fact, some parents have reported that having two parents maintain lactation while attending to other children, housework, and employment was overwhelming.

For families who desire to co-lactate, a few considerations should be discussed. First, both milk supplies must be maintained. This means all lactating parents must express milk approximately 8 times per day, whether with a child or a breast pump. To avoid dropping prolactin levels, no break longer than 6 hours should be taken between sessions. Generally, at least one parent in these cases is inducing lactation (see Chapter 19). If this is done before birth, a plan for the birth hospitalization should be considered. For some hospitals, prenatal infectious disease laboratory tests will be required of any individual other than the birth parent providing human milk, unless it is pasteurized processed donor milk. A parent inducing lactation may require extra assistance from lactation consultants, including a supplemental nursing system, nipple shield, or flange fit for adequate pumping. If this is the case, choosing a delivery hospital should include these postpartum considerations. Given that the gestational parent is most likely to make colostrum, it is conceivable that some benefit accrues to having this parent provide milk until lactogenesis 2, if desired. In addition, another person breastfeeding in the first 72 hours may risk interrupting the gestational parent's milk supply by limiting stimulation, emptying, or skin-to-skin contact. However, if the gestational parent can pump, the risk may be mitigated by the extra bonding and stimulation experienced by the other lactating parent.

SURROGACY AND ADOPTION

Same-sex couples may be up to four times as likely to build families through adoption as their opposite-gender peers.[5] In the case of adoption, induced lactation may or may not be possible. If lactation is physiologically possible, patients can be counseled according to their anatomy, hormone status, and time to potential adoption. If it is not possible, parents may still wish to provide their children with human milk. In this case, banked donor milk may be a viable option, though in many countries the cost is prohibitive. If banked milk is not available or is not affordable, some families will turn to informal milk donation. The ABM has a position statement on informal milk donation and summarizes the risks, benefits, and considerations involved. In sum, human milk should not be purchased informally, because this increases the possibility of contamination and/or improper handling. When sharing, an open relationship is ideal, with sharing of medical records and infectious disease/prenatal laboratory test results when possible. Proper handling should be ensured, and pasteurization may be considered. A position statement on informal milk sharing was released by the ABM in 2017 and can be found online.[24]

In the case of surrogacy, and sometimes in adoption, the gestational carrier or birth parent may be willing to provide colostrum or human milk for a time. If there are no contraindications, this milk should be encouraged and can be given by supplemental nursing system at the breast/chest by the surrogate or adoptive parents, if desired. In the case of induced lactation, even when successful, colostrum production has not been seen. Rather, the inducing parent makes mature milk. Therefore colostrum provided in this way is likely an incremental benefit to the newborn. In the case of induced lactation for an adopted infant or an infant born by surrogacy, birth hospitals may require infectious disease/prenatal laboratory test results of any parent providing human milk or breast/chest feeding.

FACTORS COMMON TO ALL OF THESE CASES

LGBTQ + parents who desire to breastfeed, chestfeed, or lactate require routine and robust lactation support, as is the standard of care for any parents. In addition, they should have access to advanced lactation support provided by breastfeeding medicine providers and board-certified lactation consultants. They may desire to use supplemental nursing systems or galactogogues to promote infant time at the breast and milk supply. For further reading, Chapter 19 discusses induced lactation and cross-nursing and Chapter 11 covers galactogogues, as does Appendix I (ABM Protocol #9).

The Reference list is available at www.expertconsult.com.

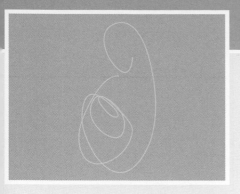

21

Reproductive Function During Lactation

Alison M. Stuebe and Melissa J. Chen

KEY POINTS

- Optimal birth spacing is essential to the health of mothers and children. The suppression of ovulation contributes to birth spacing.
- Return of menses and fecundity are affected by lactation (exclusivity and duration) and maternal energy balance. At the molecular level, there is evidence that the neuropeptide kisspeptin plays a role in lactation-associated fertility suppression through prolactin receptors and sensory input from suckling. Ovulation suppression also occurs at the level of the ovary and pituitary.
- Lactation Amenorrhea Method (LAM) is included in the Medical Eligibility Criteria for Contraception guidance for both the World Health Organization and Centers for Disease Control and Prevention as a highly effective, temporary method of contraception.
- Highly effective methods of contraception include permanent surgical methods and long-acting, reversible methods (implants, intrauterine devices). Moderately effective methods include hormonal methods (injectable, pill, patch, ring)

and the diaphragm. Less effective methods include male and female condoms, withdrawal, the sponge, fertility awareness—based methods, and spermicide.

- The risks and benefits of hormonal contraception during lactation are controversial with concern for the effects on the mother or the infant. Separate from potential breastfeeding concerns, combined hormonal contraceptives are generally avoided because of the increased risks for venous thromboembolism associated with both estrogen-containing methods and the early postpartum state. Overall, the majority of evidence does not demonstrate adverse effects of progestin-only contraception on breastfeeding or infant outcomes.
- The reproductive justice framework focuses on protecting the rights of women to not have a child, to have a child, and to parent children in safe and healthy environments. Women should be provided breastfeeding and reproductive information in a patient-centered fashion to facilitate their autonomous and informed decision-making.

Optimal birth spacing contributes to health and well-being for mothers and children. Lactation suppresses ovulation and delays the return of menses after pregnancy. In natural fertility populations, this suppression of ovulation contributes to birth spacing, with periods of amenorrhea lasting for as long as 2 to 3 years.[1] However, in industrial societies, ovulation resumes earlier, with 20% of breastfeeding women in a US study ovulating by 12 weeks postpartum.[2] Optimal birth spacing thus requires that clinicians and couples understand when lactation provides protection against pregnancy and when additional methods are necessary to prevent conception.

LACTATION AND FERTILITY

Strategies for Mammalian Reproduction and Birth Spacing

In mammalian physiology, lactation follows pregnancy, and provision of species-specific milk is an essential part of neonatal development. However, reproductive strategies vary widely. Life history theory proposes that unfavorable conditions favor a "fast" strategy, with early sexual maturity and

frequent, short pregnancies with many small offspring. Under more favorable conditions, "slow" strategies predominate, with later sexual maturity, longer pregnancies, larger offspring, and greater investment after birth through prolonged lactation and parenting (Fig. 21.1).[3]

While the offspring is suckling and dependent on its mother for care, fertility is suppressed, so that the mother has sufficient energy and time to care for the juvenile. Weaning occurs once the juvenile is able to survive independently; with cessation of lactation, fertility returns and the mother is able to conceive again (Fig. 21.2A). Primates as a group follow a slower life history pattern than many other mammals, with one or two offspring per pregnancy and a prolonged period of maternal care. Compared with nonhuman primates, humans mature later, which reduces the number of years they are able to reproduce; to compensate, anthropologist Daniel Sellen notes that humans have adapted their child-rearing strategy to allow shorter intervals between births.[4,5] Indeed, humans are the only primates who are able to conceive before the older sibling is able to forage for himself or herself; we rely on other caregivers and grandparents to assist with juveniles and provide transitional foods after weaning (see Fig. 21.2B). When resources are constrained,

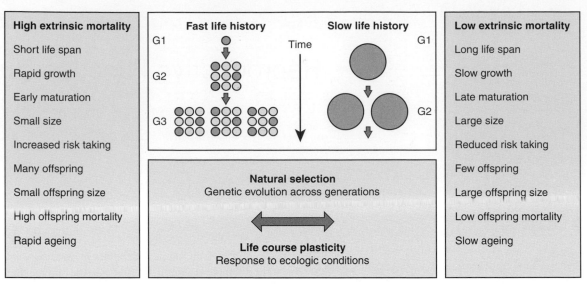

Fig. 21.1 Life history theory. Fast life histories are favored in environments with high mortality risk, whereas slow life histories can evolve when mortality risk reduces. These strategies might evolve under natural selection, but physiology can also respond to cues during the life course through plasticity. The size of the *circles* is proportional to adult body size, and *filled circles* indicate individuals that survive to reproduce. *G1*, First generation; *G2*, second generation; *G3*, third generation. (From Wells JCK, Nesse RM, Sear R, et al. Evolutionary public health: introducing the concept. *Lancet.* 2017;390[10093]:500–509.)

humans may introduce supplemental feeds from birth, with adverse consequences for mother and child (see Fig. 21.2C).

Normal interpregnancy intervals in natural fertility populations appear to have been between 2 and 3 years. In the !Kung hunter-gatherers, breastfeeding occurs continuously through age 2 to 3, with children continuing to sleep near their mothers and nurse at night for years.[1] Sellen notes that foragers, who are able to carry their children with them, tend to wean later than subsistence farmers and herders, whose work requires separation from their infants.[4]

With the introduction of breast-milk substitutes, it became possible to separate mother from infant at birth, allowing resumption of ovulation and pregnancy to follow almost immediately and markedly shortening interbirth intervals. However, rapid repeat pregnancies are associated with risks. In observational studies, interpregnancy intervals less than 18 months are associated with increased risks to the mother, the older child, and the next baby. A variety of mechanisms have been proposed to explain these associations.[6] A major objective of postpartum contraceptive counseling is to share with families the rationale for delaying the next pregnancy and assist them in selecting an appropriate contraceptive strategy.

Factors Affecting Return of Fecundity

Ovulation and return of menses occur earlier in women who do not breastfeed or breastfeed less intensively. A study in US women showed that the average time to first ovulation was 45 ± 3.8 (range 25 to 72) days in nonlactating women compared with 189 ± 14.7 (range 34 to 256) days for lactating women, as determined by urinary pregnanediol-3a-glucuronide, a progesterone metabolite[2] (Fig. 21.3). Among lactating women, frequency and duration of suckling were inversely correlated with return of ovulation. These findings were confirmed in a study of lactation among women in Manila and Baltimore.[7] A larger number of feeds per day, longer durations of feeding, and a greater percentage of feeds that were breast milk were all associated with a lower proportion of women ovulating (Fig. 21.4).

Return of fecundity also varies with maternal energy balance. Lactation imposes a substantial metabolic load on the mother, estimated at 597 to 716 kcal (2.5 to 3 MJ) per day.[8] Valeggia and Ellison[9] propose that the lactating mother cannot "afford" to ovulate unless she has access to sufficient nutrition to sustain herself, her infant, and another pregnancy. These authors studied return of ovulation among well-nourished Toba women in Argentina and found that positive energy balance, indexed by rising C-peptide levels and increasing body mass index (BMI) (Fig. 21.5), precedes return of menses, which occurred at a mean of 10.2 ± 4.3 months postpartum.[9–12] In a study in Sri Lanka, higher BMI was associated with earlier return of menses, providing further support for the importance of energy balance in duration of amenorrhea.[13]

A large international study (N = 4118 mother-infant pairs) by the World Health Organization (WHO) Task Force on Methods for the Natural Regulation of Fertility quantified non–feeding-related and feeding-related characteristics associated with time to return of menses.[14] Lower maternal BMI, a higher number of prior live births and more episodes of infant illness were associated later return of menses. Infant factors independently associated with longer amenorrhea included shorter time between birth and first breastfeed, later introduction of regular supplementation, longer total duration of breastfeeding in 24 hours and greater percentage of feeds that were breast milk. For women who were fully breastfeeding and whose menses had not returned, the 6-month pregnancy rate was 1.0% (95% confidence interval [CI] 0 to 2.1) and the 12-month pregnancy rate was 6.9% (95% CI 2.0 to 11.8).[15]

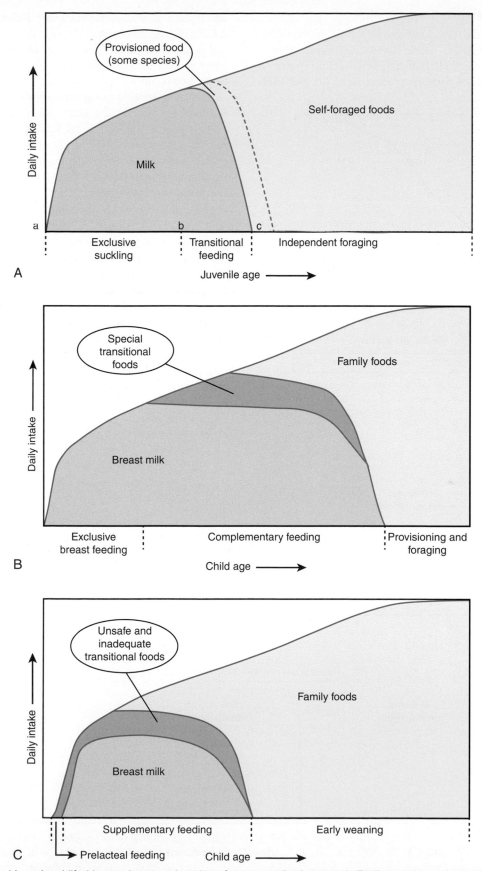

Fig. 21.2 (A) Key nutrition-related life history phases and markers for a generalized mammal. (B) Key nutrition-related life history phases and markers for humans, optimal for infants and young children. (C) Commonly observed pattern of infant and young child feeding, not optimal for child outcomes. Whereas most mammals rely on an exclusive breast milk diet for a prolonged period, followed by a brief period of provisioned foods for some species (A), humans rely on a combination of transitional foods and mother's milk for a prolonged period (B). In the setting of constraints that disrupt exclusive breastfeeding, humans supplement from birth, adversely affecting the health of mother and child (C). (From Sellen DW. Evolution of infant and young child feeding: implications for contemporary public health. *Annu Rev Nutr.* 2007;27:123–148.)

Physiology of Fertility Suppression

Ovulatory cycles require the coordinated activity of gonadotropin-releasing hormone (GnRH), follicle-stimulating hormone (FSH), and luteinizing hormone (LH). Pulsatile release of GnRH from the hypothalamus stimulates pituitary production of LH and FSH, which promote maturation of ovarian follicles, ovulation, and production of progesterone from the ovarian corpus luteum. Estrogen and progesterone in turn stimulate proliferation and secretory differentiation of the endometrium to support a pregnancy, should fertilization occur.

Lactation appears to suppress ovulation through multiple mechanisms. Emerging evidence suggests that the neuropeptide kisspeptin, encoded by the *Kiss1* gene, may play a central role in lactation-associated fertility suppression, both through prolactin receptors on kisspeptin neurons and through sensory input from suckling.[16–21] Moreover, kisspeptin neurons are modulated by nutritional status, and food restriction during lactation in rodents downregulates Kiss1 mRNA expression and delays return of fertility.[22,23] Although animal studies demonstrate lactation-related differences in kisspeptin expression, a small study in women with lactational amenorrhea did not find differences in plasma kisspeptin levels compared with normally cycling women.[24]

Lactation may also suppress ovulation at the level of the pituitary and the ovary. In a longitudinal study of women with lactation amenorrhea, follicular growth was observed, but levels of estradiol and both inhibin A and B were much lower than during ovulatory cycles.[25] Although circulating levels of FSH were similar during lactational amenorrhea and ovulatory cycles, the isoforms of FSH during lactational amenorrhea were more acidic, reflecting posttranslational modifications that may reduce the bioactivity of circulating FSH.[26]

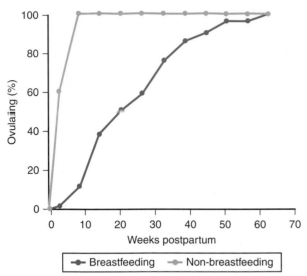

Fig. 21.3 Proportion of ovulation by time postpartum for breastfeeding compared with non-breastfeeding women. (From Campbell OM, Gray RH. Characteristics and determinants of postpartum ovarian function in women in the United States. *Am J Obstet Gynecol.* 1993;169 [1]:55–60.)

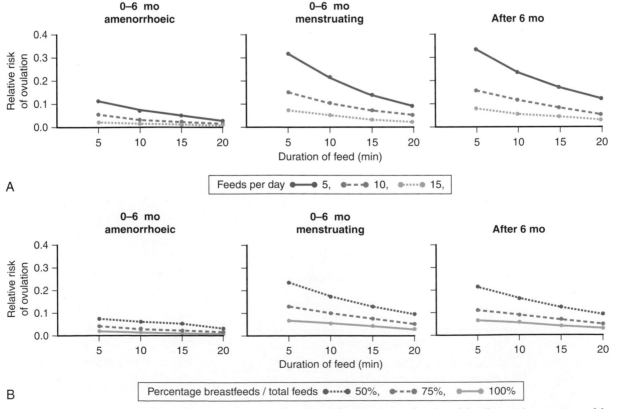

Fig. 21.4 Relative risk of ovulation by 6 months postpartum as a function of feeds per day, duration of feeding, and percentage of feeds that were breast milk. (From Gray RH, Campbell OM, Apelo R, et al. Risk of ovulation during lactation. *Lancet.* 1990;335[8680]:25–29.)

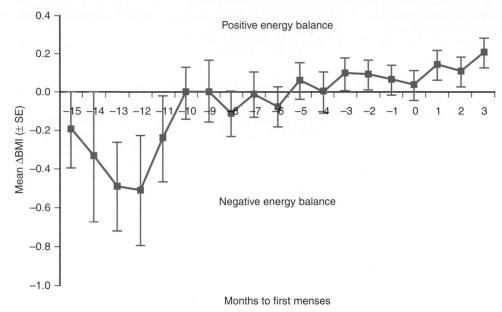

Fig. 21.5 Body mass index increases immediately before return of ovulation, indicating positive energy balance. *BMI*, Body mass index; *SE*, standard error. (From Valeggia C, Ellison PT. Lactational amenorrhoea in well-nourished Toba women of Formosa, Argentina. *J Biosoc Sci.* 2004;36[5]:573–595.)

THE LACTATIONAL AMENORRHEA METHOD

The Lactational Amenorrhea Method (LAM) specifies conditions under which lactation provides effective protection from pregnancy (Fig. 21.6). The Bellagio Consensus Conference on breastfeeding as a family planning method established that a mother who is fully or nearly fully breastfeeding her infant and remains amenorrheic will have more than 98% protection from pregnancy in the first 6 months postpartum.[27] The consensus proposed two strategies for breastfeeding as a contraceptive method.

Breastfeeding can be used as a birth spacing method in its own right, especially when there are no alternatives available or if a couple chooses not to use other family planning methods, or it can be used as a means to delay the introduction of other family planning methods. Where there are problems with family planning availability, acceptability or continuation (especially during breastfeeding) the use of the natural infertility of breastfeeding followed by the use of another family planning method, rather than the simultaneous employment of both, may serve to maximize the interbirth interval.

The LAM was codified as a method of family planning the following year at an international conference at Georgetown University.[28]

In a multisite clinical trial conducted at 11 sites in 10 countries, the 6-month efficacy of LAM with correct use was found to be 98.5% (standard error [SE] 0.7).[29] At 6 months, 72.4% of women remained amenorrheic, and at 12 months, 42.1% remained amenorrheic (Fig. 21.7). Women were counseled to introduce another method of contraception once LAM criteria were no longer met; the mean duration of reliance on LAM was more than 5 months across all sites (Fig. 21.8). Study participants were highly satisfied with LAM as a

contraceptive method, with 84.1% being "very satisfied" and 86.9% reporting "no problems" with the method.[30]

LAM is included in the Medical Eligibility Criteria for Contraception guidance for both the WHO and Centers for Disease Control and Prevention (CDC) as "a highly effective, temporary method of contraception."[31,32] Interestingly, in a systematic review comparing outcomes among women who received instruction in LAM versus women who were fully breastfeeding without formal LAM training, authors did not find differences in return of menses or protection from pregnancy.[33] Patient recall of LAM criteria was not high. Among women in low- and middle-income countries who participated in the USAID Demographic and Health Surveys, only 26% of women who said they were using LAM for contraception met correct practice criteria (Table 21.1), and among women who met LAM criteria, only 6.8% described themselves as LAM users.[34] These results suggest that existing counseling on LAM is not sufficient to ensure that couples understand how to use this method reliably. Implementation efforts can improve outcomes; in a project in Jordan, knowledge of LAM criteria, especially regarding the reduction in protection after 6 months postpartum, increased the proportion of women who transitioned to a modern contraceptive method.[35]

Transitioning From the Lactation Amenorrhea Method to Other Contraceptive Methods

LAM is a highly effective, temporary method of contraception, and couples who wish to avoid pregnancy will require another method once LAM criteria are no longer met. It is therefore imperative to counsel women on options for preventing pregnancy after LAM and ensure that they know how and where to access other methods once they are no longer protected by LAM.

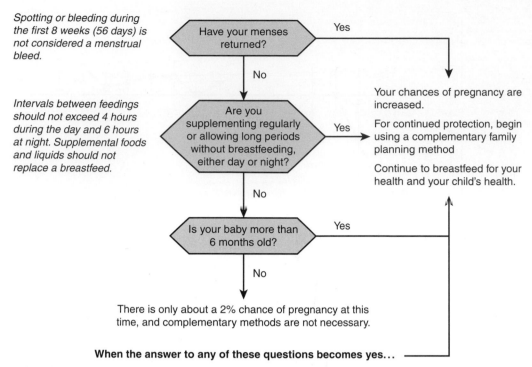

Spotting or bleeding during the first 8 weeks (56 days) is not considered a menstrual bleed.

Intervals between feedings should not exceed 4 hours during the day and 6 hours at night. Supplemental foods and liquids should not replace a breastfeed.

Have your menses returned?

Yes

Your chances of pregnancy are increased.

For continued protection, begin using a complementary family planning method

Continue to breastfeed for your health and your child's health.

No

Are you supplementing regularly or allowing long periods without breastfeeding, either day or night?

Yes

No

Is your baby more than 6 months old?

Yes

No

There is only about a 2% chance of pregnancy at this time, and complementary methods are not necessary.

When the answer to any of these questions becomes yes...

Fig. 21.6 The Lactational Amenorrhea Method.

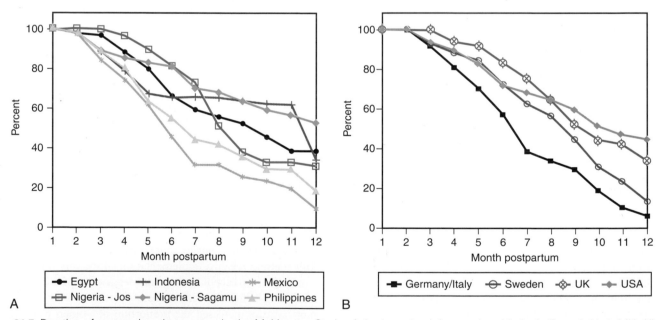

Fig. 21.7 Duration of amenorrhea, by country, in the Multicenter Study of the Lactational Amenorrhea Method. (From Labbok MH, Hight-Laukaran V, Peterson AE, et al. Multicenter study of the Lactational Amenorrhea Method [LAM], I: efficacy, duration, and implications for clinical application. *Contraception.* 1997;55[6]:327–336.)

A randomized controlled trial (RCT) in Egypt tested instruction of LAM alone compared with instruction in LAM and provision of a packet of levonorgestrel 1.5-mg emergency contraception pills as a strategy to prevent undesired pregnancy.[36,37] Women were instructed to return to the clinic to initiate another method when LAM criteria were no longer met; women in the

LAM plus emergency contraceptive (EC) group were instructed to use the pill packet in the case of sexual intercourse after LAM criteria were no longer met and if they had not yet initiated another method. Rates of unprotected intercourse after LAM expiration were similar (LAM-only 71.6 vs. LAM + EC 73.5, $p = 0.22$); however, 46.6% of women in the LAM + EC

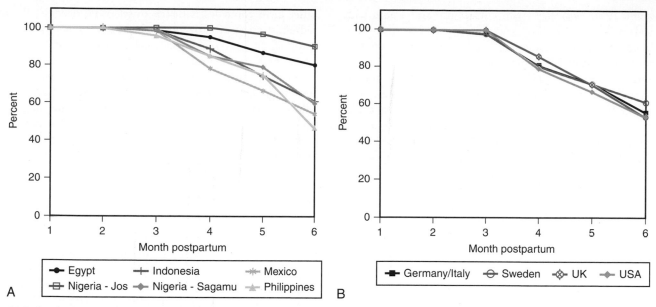

Fig. 21.8 Continuation of the Lactational Amenorrhea Method through 6 months postpartum, by country, in the Multicenter Study of the Lactational Amenorrhea Method. (From Labbok MH, Hight-Laukaran V, Peterson AE, et al. Multicenter study of the Lactational Amenorrhea Method [LAM], I: efficacy, duration, and implications for clinical application. *Contraception.* 1997;55[6]:327–336.)

TABLE 21.1 Self-Reported Lactation Amenorrhea Method (LAM) Users Who Did Not Meet Correct Practice Criteria, by Type of Disqualification Percentage of Respondents Who Self-Reported as LAM Users but Did Not Meet Correct-Practice Criteria, by Type of Disqualification, 39 DHS Surveys, 1998–2011

	Mean of Survey-Specific Percentages
Gave birth 6 + months ago	82.8
Menstrual period returned	23.8
Gave liquid other than water	71.2
Gave food	69.7
Gave food or liquid other than water	91.9

DHS, Demographic and Health Survey.
Notes: These data are drawn from 39 DHS surveys in which the denominator exceeded 30. The mean number of women analyzed in each survey is 102. Correct-practice criteria are based on definition 1, which consists of those (1) who gave birth less than 6 months ago, (2) whose menstruation had not returned, (3) who did not use any other modern contraceptive methods, and (4) whose infant had been either exclusively breastfed or breastfed and given water but given no other liquid or semisolid or solid food.
From Fabic MS, Choi Y. Assessing the quality of data regarding use of the lactational amenorrhea method. *Stud Fam Plann.* 2013;44 (2):205–221.

group used the emergency contraceptive pills. Women in the LAM + EC group were more likely to initiate a regular contraceptive method (LAM + EC 77.4%, LAM only 47.6%,

$p = 0.001$) and were less likely to become pregnant within 6 months (0.4% vs. 5.3%, $p = 0.0001$). These results underscore the importance of providing specific, actionable guidance for how to avoid pregnancy when LAM criteria are no longer met.

Transitioning From the Lactation Amenorrhea Method to Fertility-Awareness Methods

Use of fertility-awareness methods during the transition from LAM is challenging because cycles may be irregular or anovulatory and cervical mucus and temperature monitoring may be less reliable. In a multisite study of the symptothermal method among lactating women in the United Kingdom, Canada, and Australia, serial urine samples were collected from 42 days postpartum to identify fertile and infertile periods.[38] An integrated set of rules for cervical mucus and temperature charting to identify fertile periods had a positive predictive value of 21%, a specificity of 51%, and a negative predictive value of greater than 94%. In theory, this method would be highly effective at preventing pregnancy, but would require abstinence on 50% of days.

The Standard Days Method has been studied for women with regular cycles lasting 26 to 32 days. Couples are advised to avoid intercourse or use a barrier method on cycle days 8 to 19. With correct use, the cumulative probability of pregnancy is 4.8% over 13 cycles, and 12.0% with typical use.[39] To develop a calendar-based method for breastfeeding women, data from the multisite symptothermal method study were used to develop a Bridge strategy. In this method, after the first menses, women were presumed to be fertile from day 11 until the next menses. For subsequent cycles, the fertile period is 8 to 24 days. Once cycles become regular, lasting 26 to 32 days, the Standard Days Method can be used.[40] In an efficacy study of the Bridge in Guatemala and Peru, the 6-month cumulative pregnancy rate was 3.7% with correct use and 11.8% with typical use.[41]

In addition to symptothermal or calendar-based methods, a pilot study evaluated home-based monitoring of urinary estrone-3-glucuronide and urinary LH with coaching by a web-based tool during breastfeeding; the unintended pregnancy rate was 2 per 100 with correct use and 8 per 100 with actual use at 12 months postpartum.[42] The authors note that the cost of the home monitor (USD $150 to $200) and test strips ($15 to 30 per month) may be a barrier to widespread implementation.

Research Gaps in Lactation Amenorrhea Method Implementation

Among lactating mothers in the United States, 85% report incorporating milk expression and 25% regularly express milk.[43] Given the changes in feeding practices, new definitions for "breastfeeding" have been proposed.[44] "Breast-milk feeding" refers to the provision of mother's milk to the infant, and "breastfeeding" indicates feeding at the breast. Although milk expression may be useful in meeting an infant's nutritional needs, less is known about the effects that milk expression has on lactational infertility. A Chilean study found that working mothers who were using hand expression experienced a 5.2% pregnancy rate at 6 months.[45] However, it is unclear whether the women who became pregnant were actually still meeting criteria for LAM. Furthermore, the majority of US women use electric pumping instead of hand expression as a method to express milk, which has been shown to yield higher volumes of milk and stimulate higher prolactin responses than hand or manual expression.[43,46] Therefore the question remains whether a lactating mother who is expressing milk through electric pumping to exclusively feed her child has the same degree of nipple stimulation to inhibit ovulation, and, ultimately, the same contraceptive efficacy when using LAM compared with fully breastfeeding women. Determining whether pumping can provide the same contraceptive efficacy is an issue that is relevant to mothers who wish to use LAM for contraception.

SAFETY AND EFFICACY OF OTHER CONTRACEPTIVE METHODS DURING LACTATION

Although LAM is highly effective, it is temporary, and in settings in which supplementation is common, many women resume ovulating before another pregnancy is desired. The CDC and WHO rate family planning methods by their effectiveness with typical use (Fig. 21.9). Highly effective methods of contraception include permanent and long-acting, reversible methods. Moderately effective methods include hormonal methods (injectable, pill, patch, ring) and the diaphragm; less effective methods include male and female condoms, withdrawal, the sponge, fertility-awareness—based methods, and spermicide.

The risks and benefits of hormonal methods during lactation are controversial. Because withdrawal of progesterone

after birth coincides with the onset of lactogenesis II, early administration of exogenous progestins could disrupt milk production.[47] A secondary analysis of one RCT reported lower breastfeeding rates at 6 months in women allocated to immediate postpartum levonorgestrel intrauterine system versus placement at 6 to 8 weeks.[48] A published case report documented weight loss in an exclusively breastfeeding infant after placement of an etonogestrel-releasing contraceptive implant.[49] In an anonymous, Internet-based survey of postpartum women, 15% of respondents who had started hormonal contraception within 12 weeks after delivery reported new or additional concerns about their milk supply after contraception initiation.[50]

Given these concerns, several randomized trials have been conducted to assess the impact of early initiation of hormonal contraception on lactation. Studies evaluating immediate postpartum implant initiation did not demonstrate any differences in outcomes such as time to lactogenesis II, exclusive breastfeeding through 6 months postpartum, and infant weight.[51-54] Similarly, a randomized trial demonstrated that breastfeeding outcomes with a postplacental levonorgestrel intrauterine device (IUD) was noninferior compared with delayed levonorgestrel IUD.[55]

In addition to the potential effect of hormonal contraception on milk supply, concerns have been expressed regarding hormonal exposure to the infant through breast milk in the early neonatal period, when, in animal models, progesterone receptors are expressed in the developing brain and may play an important role in central nervous system development.[56-59] Although the clinical relevance of progestin exposure through breast milk is not known, a systematic review did not find evidence of adverse effects of progestin-only contraception on infant growth and development.[60] Overall, the majority of evidence does not demonstrate adverse effects of progestin-only contraception on breastfeeding or infant outcomes. However, most sample sizes were small and thus underpowered to detect small but potentially clinically relevant effects. Further, the trials only included participants who delivered term, healthy infants and excluded those who might experience breastfeeding difficulty, such as women who delivered prematurely or had a multiple-gestation pregnancy. These limitations in evidence should be considered in the context of a woman's desire to breastfeed, potential for breastfeeding difficulty, and risk for unplanned pregnancy.

Combined estrogen and progestin contraceptives have traditionally been thought to pose a greater risk to the lactating mother-infant dyad than progestin-only methods. This literature is complicated by studies of higher dose formulations in the early years of combined oral contraception. A 2016 review found some evidence of adverse effects on breastfeeding with initiation less than 6 weeks' postpartum, but not for after 6 weeks postpartum.[61] Aside from potential breastfeeding concerns, combined hormonal contraceptives are generally avoided because of the increased risks for venous thromboembolism associated with both estrogen-containing methods and the early postpartum state.

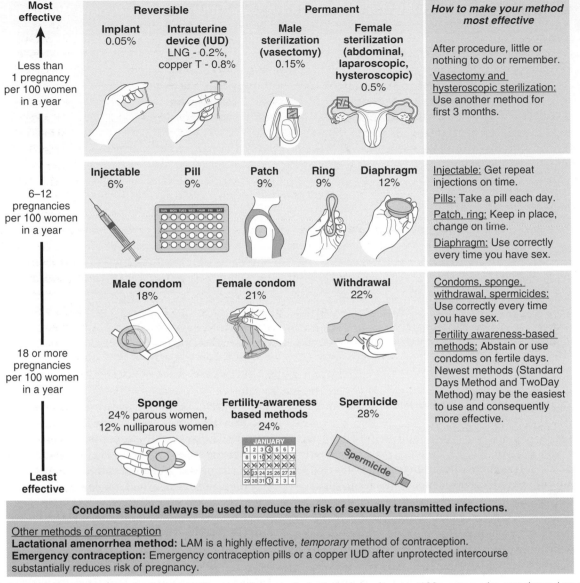

Fig. 21.9 Effectiveness of family planning methods. The percentages indicate the number in every 100 women who experienced an unintended pregnancy within the first year of typical use of each contraceptive method. (From Curtis KM, Tepper NK, Jatlaoui TC, et al. US medical eligibility criteria for contraceptive use, 2016. *MMWR Recomm Rep.* 2016;65[No. RR-3]:1–104.)

Both the WHO and the CDC rate the safety of contraceptive methods on a 4-level scale:

1. A condition for which there is no restriction for the use of the contraceptive method.
2. A condition for which the advantages of using the method generally outweigh the theoretical or proven risks.
3. A condition for which the theoretical or proven risks usually outweigh the advantages of using the method.
4. A condition that represents an unacceptable health risk if the contraceptive method is used.

In their most recent guidance, the WHO and the CDC reached different conclusions regarding timing of initiation and type of hormonal contraception during breastfeeding (Table 21.2), with the CDC considering earlier initiation of hormonal methods to be safer compared with the WHO.

PATIENT-CENTERED COUNSELING ON SEXUALITY, BIRTH SPACING, AND CONTRACEPTION

Breastfeeding and Sexuality

The time to resumption of sexual activity varies widely among couples. Women are routinely counseled to defer intercourse until 6 weeks postpartum, but there are no data supporting this recommendation. The risk for bleeding or infection is minimal after 2 weeks, and guidelines recommend that women resume intercourse when it is comfortable and desired, once the perineum has healed and bleeding has decreased.[62] In one cohort, more than half of women had resumed sexual intercourse by 6 weeks postpartum, and 90% resume by 12 weeks postpartum.[63] Another study found that 43% of women had resumed intercourse by 6 weeks, and 81% had resumed by 12 weeks; the only

TABLE 21.2   Medical Eligibility for Contraceptive Use Among Breastfeeding Women, by Time Since Delivery

	COMBINED HORMONAL CONTRACEPTIVES (PILLS, PATCH, RING, INJECTABLE)		PROGESTIN ONLY, OTHER THAN INJECTABLE (PILLS, LNG, ETG IUS ETG, LNG-IUS OR IMPLANT)		INJECTABLE (DMPA/NET-EN)	
	WHO	CDC	WHO	CDC	WHO	CDC
<21 days	4	4	2	2	3	2
21 to <30 days	4	3	2	2	3	2
30 to 42 days	4	3/2[a]	2	1	3	1
42 days to 6 months	3	2	1	1	1	1
>6 months	2	2	1	1	1	1

CDC, Centers for Disease Control and Prevention; DMPA, depot medroxyprogesterone acetate; ETG, etonogestrel; LNG, levonorgestrel; LNG-IUS, levonorgestrel intrauterine system; NET-EN, norethisterone enantate; WHO, World Health Organization.
1, A condition for which there is no restriction for the use of the contraceptive method; 2, a condition for which the advantages of using the method generally outweigh the theoretical or proven risks; 3, a condition for which the theoretical or proven risks usually outweigh the advantages of using the method; 4, a condition that represents an unacceptable health risk if the contraceptive method is used.
[a]CDC rates CHC at 30–42 days as 3 for women with risk factors for deep venous thrombosis, 2 for women without risk factors.
From World Health Organization. Medical eligibility criteria for contraceptive use. Geneva, Switzerland: World Health Organization; 2015; and Curtis KM, Tepper NK, Jatlaoui TC, et al. US Medical Eligibility Criteria for Contraceptive Use, 2016. MMWR Recomm Rep 2016;65(No. RR-3):1–104.

clinical factor associated with initiation before 6 weeks was use of contraception before 6 weeks.[64]

Data indicate that women receive little information on postpartum sexuality. In the US Listening to Mothers III study, only 30% of women who attended a postpartum visit received enough information about changes in sexual response and feelings, even though many women reported painful intercourse (27%) and lack of sexual desire (43%).[65] The association between breastfeeding and sexual desire appears to vary among women: in a study of predominantly white primiparous women in Minnesota, 42.4% reported a decreased interest in sex postpartum, 48.9% reported no change, and 8.7% reported an increase.[66] Compared with before breastfeeding, 45.2% reported about the same level of arousal, 41.4% reported less arousal, and 13.4% reported more arousal than during pregnancy. In written comments, 15 women described reasons for decreased interest in sex, including weight gain and body image issue ($N = 8$), sore or uncomfortable breasts ($N = 6$), perineal pain with intercourse ($N = 6$), leaking breast milk ($N = 6$), contraception issues ($N = 4$), and constant physical contact with the baby ($N = 2$).

Because lactation reduces circulating estrogen levels, vaginal dryness and pain with intercourse are more common among mothers who are breastfeeding and amenorrheic. In a US study, one third of women reported pain with intercourse at 6 and 12 weeks, and pain was more common among women who were breastfeeding at 12 weeks (relative risk [RR] 3.36, 95% CI 1.77 to 6.37).[67] Signorello et al.[68] similarly found that concurrent breastfeeding was associated with more pain at first postpartum intercourse and at 3 and 6 months postpartum. Women with vaginal dryness should be encouraged to use lubrication.

In a review on postpartum sexuality, Leeman and Rogers[63] note that lactation is associated with increased nipple sensitivity, which may make sexual stimulation uncomfortable or may increase erotic responses. They suggest encouraging couples to talk openly and address these issues. Oxytocin release with orgasm can cause milk let down; women who are concerned about leaking milk may wish to wear a bra.

Patient-Centered Counseling

In the setting of conflicting evidence and recommendations regarding hormonal contraception in lactation, a shared decision-making approach is essential. For some women, reliable prevention of pregnancy may be the highest priority, whereas others might want to avoid even a theoretical possibility of disrupting lactation. Clinicians can use open-ended questions to explore each individual woman's preferences, desires for future childbearing, and desires for breastfeeding (Box 21.1). This approach is consistent with guidance from the American College of Obstetricians and Gynecologists.

Women considering immediate postpartum progestin-only contraception should be counseled about the theoretical risk for reduced duration of breastfeeding and about the preponderance of evidence that has not shown a negative effect on actual breastfeeding outcomes. Obstetric care providers should discuss any concerns within the context of each woman's desire to breastfeed and her risk for unplanned pregnancy, so that she can make an autonomous and informed decision.[69]

Clinicians also should be mindful of the history of coercive contraceptive counseling, particularly among marginalized populations. The concept of stratified reproduction refers to policies and practices that celebrate the reproduction of

BOX 21.1 Questions for Counseling on Breastfeeding and the Use of Hormonal Contraception

Breastfeeding
- What have you heard about breastfeeding? What have you heard about the benefits of breastfeeding?
- What are your goals for breastfeeding?
- Ideally, for how long would you like to continue breast-feeding?
- How is breastfeeding viewed by your community and/or family?
- What could make it harder for you to breastfeed?

Birth Spacing/Contraception
- Are you interested in having another baby after this one? (If yes) When might you want to have another baby?
- How important is it to avoid another pregnancy right now?
- Do you know how long is recommended to wait after giving birth to try and get pregnant again?
- How would you feel if you were to get pregnant sooner than the current recommendation?
- How would your family and/or community react to your pregnancy?
- What contraceptives worked well for you in the past? Do you have any preferences or concerns about contraception?
- What is important to you in a contraceptive method?
- What have you heard about getting pregnant while breast-feeding? What have you heard about breastfeeding and contraception?

Sexuality
- Are you sexually active with men?
- How soon after birth do you think you and your partner will want to resume intercourse?
- What questions do you have about resuming intercourse after giving birth?

Breastfeeding and Hormonal Contraception
Most studies indicate that hormonal contraception does not affect a woman's ability to breastfeed, but more research is needed, and some specialists worry about an effect of contraception on milk production. How do you think you would feel if your contraception made breastfeeding more challenging?

Follow-Up Questions and Phrases
- Tell me more about _____.
- It sounds like ___ (being able to breastfeed for a year, not getting pregnant, etc.) is really important to you. What do you think this means for ___? (using contraception, breastfeeding, etc.)
- Based on what you've told me, it sounds like you might ____.

From Bryant AG, Lyerly AD, DeVane-Johnson S, et al. Hormonal contraception, breastfeeding, and bedside advocacy: the case for patient-centered care. *Contraception.* 2019;99(2):73–76.

privileged women while decrying the reproduction of marginalized women. In the US context, Harris and Wolfe write:[70]

"Throughout the US history, the fertility and childbearing of poor women and women of color were not valued equally to those of affluent white women. This is evident in a range of practices and policies, including black women's treatment during slavery, removal of Native children to off-reservation boarding schools, and coercive sterilizations of poor white women and women of color. Thus reproductive experiences throughout US history were stratified. This ideology of stratified reproduction persists today in social welfare programs, drug policy, and programs promoting long-acting reversible contraception".[70]

Campaigns to increase uptake of contraceptive methods must be undertaken with a clear understanding that preventing pregnancy is not a cure-all for poverty. The reproductive justice framework asserts that "individual choices have only been as capacious and empowering as the resources any woman can turn to in her community."[71] Reproductive justice focuses on protection of three core rights:
1. The right not to have a child
2. The right to have a child
3. The right to parent children in safe and healthy environments

Clinicians can help advance reproductive justice by ensuring that each family understands the relationship between breastfeeding and fertility, sexuality, and birth spacing and by supporting each woman's values and preferences.

The Reference list is available at www.expertconsult.com.

22

The Collection and Storage of Human Milk and Human Milk Banking

Lawrence Noble and Anita Noble

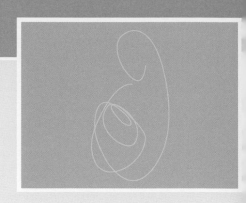

KEY POINTS

- Electric pumps are not necessarily more effective than manual pumps or hand expression.
- Pumped milk volume can be increased with low cost interventions such as listening to music, relaxation, warming or massaging the breast, frequent pumping and starting to pump sooner after birth.
- Milk can be stored at room temperature for 4 hours, but under optimal conditions for 6 to 8 hours. Milk kept with ice packs in a small cooler can be stored for 24 hours. Fresh, refrigerated, milk can be used for 96 hours (4 days). Milk can be frozen for 9 months, but under optimal freezer conditions for 12 months.
- Breastfeeding outcomes are influenced by length of maternity leave and workplace conditions' time and place for pumping.

- The optimal nutrition for feeding preterm infants is mothers' milk, which reduces necrotizing enterocolitis (NEC), late-onset sepsis, chronic lung disease, retinopathy of prematurity, and improves neurodevelopment. Pasteurized donor human milk is the recommended nutrition for VLBW infants when mother's milk is not available, as it decreases NEC, but has no effect on other outcomes.
- Health care providers should assist mothers and families who are considering informal milk sharing by advising recipients on risks and benefits, including the need to evaluate for donor's illnesses, social practices and medications.
- Parents' acceptance of donor human milk may depend on a cultural component such as religion, country of origin, age, parity, breastfeeding experience, and level of education.

The Baby-Friendly Hospital Initiative's revised Ten Steps to Successful Breastfeeding include steps toward health care professionals possessing the knowledge, competence, and skills pertaining to human milk expression.[1] Human milk expression is accomplished either by hand expression or with a pump that is either manual or electric. Human milk is collected and stored for the infant for several reasons. For the premature infant, human milk expression allows the mother to stimulate milk production and provide optimal nutrition even before the infant is able to feed directly at the breast. For infants who are breastfeeding directly from the breast, human milk expression may be used to maintain lactation, increase the milk supply, or make human milk available when the mother and infant are temporarily separated, for example, because of maternal employment. Human milk expression is also a means for mothers to donate their human milk to infants other than their own in need of human milk, such as premature infants in the neonatal intensive care unit (NICU) or informal milk sharing for healthy term infants.

PREVALENCE OF HUMAN MILK EXPRESSION

A review regarding the prevalence of human milk expression found that expressing milk is extremely common and that exclusive breastfeeding at the breast is actually quite rare, at least in the developed world.[2] A 2017 study on 100 postpartum women revealed that 98% stated that they would use a breast pump to express milk for their baby, with most of this subset (69%) intending to start within weeks of delivery.[3] Over a quarter of the participants (29%) had already initiated pumping or intended to start within the subsequent few days. Primiparous women were more likely to report having already started pumping at the time of the interview. For all the postpartum women, the most common reason for pumping was to maintain their milk supply. Women who started pumping while in the hospital also noted that they pumped to increase their milk supply and overcome latch difficulties.

The prevalence of feeding healthy term infants exclusive pumped human milk, without breastfeeding, has also increased. In a study of 2450 women in Hong Kong, the rate of exclusive expressed breast milk feeding in the first 6 months in two cohorts increased from 5.1% to 8.0% in 2006 to 2007 to 18.0% to 19.8% in 2011 to 2012.[4] Factors associated with a higher rate of exclusive expressed human milk feeding included supplementation with infant formula, lack of previous human milk feeding experience, having a planned cesarean section delivery and postpartum return to work. In different locales, the prevalence of human milk expression can vary, as do the reasons for expression and storage of human milk.[5] In a report from Australia of 1003 postpartum women and at 6 months postpartum, 83% (754/911) of the women had a breast pump and 40% (288/715) were expressing at least occasionally. The most common reported reasons for any expressing in the first 6 months postpartum were "to be able to go out and leave the baby" (35%, 268/772), milk supply "not enough" (27%, 207/772), having "too much" milk (19%, 147/772), and, less commonly, returning to work (10%, 80/772).

TECHNIQUES FOR HUMAN MILK COLLECTION

The revised World Health Organization's (WHO's) Ten Steps, Step 5 includes teaching mothers how to collect their human milk in case they are separated from their infant or unable to initiate breastfeeding after birth.[6] Health care professionals should possess the knowledge pertaining to the skills needed to collect human milk.[7] Whether collecting for a mother's own infant or as a donor, it is of prime importance to maintain cleanliness and minimize microbial contamination in the process of collection. Since the era of COVID-19, concern regarding microbial contamination of expressed milk has increased, including bacteria, fungi, and/or viruses from respiratory secretions or other sources.[8] (Heat treatment of the expressed milk before use as is routinely done by milk banks effectively eliminates the vast majority of microorganisms from donor milk.) Primary prevention involves that the mother should be instructed to, preferably, wash her hands with soap and water for 20 seconds and dry her hands with a clean towel before handling the equipment or pumping. If soap and water are not available, an alcohol-based hand sanitizer with 60% alcohol should be used. In the past, mothers have been advised to clean their breasts, but this is not necessary. In a study of human milk expression from mothers of preterm infants, Haiden et al.[9] measured bacterial counts in 1466 expressed human milk samples from women following one of two infection control regimens. The standard regimen used an alcohol-based sanitizer for washing hands before expressing breast milk, whereas the strict regimen comprised a 10-step process, which included additional hand hygiene steps and cleaned the breast using sterile water and an alcohol-based skin sanitizer. They found no significant differences between the standard (11.9% [94/788]) and strict (12.1% [82/678]) regimens ($p = 0.92$). Significantly more samples were contaminated, however, when expressed at home than in the hospital (standard regimen home/hospital: 17.9% vs. 6.1%, $p < 0.001$; strict regimen home/hospital: 19.6% vs. 3.4%; $p < 0.001$). They concluded that attempts to improve personal hygiene during milk collection seem to be of limited value, but good hygiene of collection and storage equipment is likely to be the most important way to ensure the microbiologic quality of expressed human milk, but cleaning of the breast before expression is not necessary.[9] Pumped milk for home or hospitalized infants does not routinely need to be cultured.

Mothers can choose to collect their milk several ways: hand expression, manual pump, or electric pumps intended for single or multiple users.

Hand Expression

Hand expression is a means of removing human milk manually from the breast. There are several benefits for hand expression: no equipment or apparatus needs to be bought or acquired, allowing it to be a method that is affordable by all. Many mothers are able to remove more human milk from the breast by hand expression than by using a pump, and it is always available as a method for human milk collection even in places without electricity or during a disaster. Handwashing before hand expression remains an important step. In addition, hand expression before pumping can soften engorged breasts, making pumping easier. There is no evidence that hand-expressed milk is higher in fat than pumped milk.[10,11] However, hand expression used in conjunction with a pump increases milk production, fat content, and caloric content of the milk (62.5 g/L vs. 25 to 45 g/L; 26.4 calories/oz vs. 20 calories/oz) more than the pump alone.[12,13]

Techniques for hand expression starts with handwashing and preparation of a clean container to collect the human milk. This can be a spoon, cup, collection bag, or a bottle that is suitable for human milk collection. Leaning forward, not lying down, while expressing will use gravity to help the milk flow. The mother can promote milk flow by one or all of the following: making circular movements on the breasts; shaking the breasts with her hands or using something soft, such as a soft towel; or breast massage recommended from the outer areas toward the nipple.

Dr. Jane Morton from the Stanford School of Medicine has a technique of hand expression in which the mother places the thumb and forefinger approximately 1 to 2 inches from the areola, presses in toward the chest wall, and then brings the two fingers together compressing the breast[14] (see Appendix E, Manual Expression of Human Milk). Hand expression also can be used at the start of a breastfeeding session so that the flow of human milk may encourage the baby to taste and smell the milk even before starting to suck.

Another hand expression technique called Therapeutic Breast Massage in Lactation (TBML), uses techniques developed in Russia for the purposes of relieving engorgement, plugged ducts, and mastitis.[15,16] TBML includes gentle breast massage facilitated by rolling the breasts between both hands or kneading the breasts with one or both hands. When needed to relieve engorgement, massaging toward the axillae can facilitate reverse-pressure softening by promoting lymphatic drainage. Hand expression in the TBML method has the mother place two fingers opposite each other near the areola and then bringing the fingers together while compressing behind the nipple. Mothers are instructed to adjust their fingers to areas where milk removal is achieved.

Drip Milk

Drip milk is the milk that drips spontaneously from the contralateral breast during the suckling of an infant. Collection of dripped milk uses the concept that stimulation to one breast will cause a milk ejection reflex by which milk also will be ejected from the second breast.

Traditionally the milk was collected with shells or "nesty cups," which are placed inside the brassiere to collect milk;

the milk was found to have lower caloric value, lower fat, and a much higher incidence of contamination.[17] In recent years, several companies have reintroduced devices to collect dripped milk either in the form of shells or soft silicone containers that are easy to clean or sterilize and stay on the breast by suction created by squeezing the container. The newer devices have a soft flange that can adhere to the breast, allowing the mother to collect drip milk in a "no-hands" manner. (See "drip milk collector" in Table 22.1.) Studies are necessary to determine if these newer devices are safer.

Pumped Milk

The use of breast pumps has been associated in some studies with mastitis, possibly because of nipple damage, because cracked or sore nipples have been associated with mastitis in multiple studies.[18,19] A case-control study of risk factors for infectious mastitis in Spanish breastfeeding women with 368 women with mastitis and 148 controls revealed that breast pumps were associated with almost three times the incidence of mastitis (adjusted odds ratio [aOR] 2.78, 95% confidence interval [CI] 1.68 to 4.58) even after controlling for other contributing factors.[20] In their study, Cullinane et al.[18] reported 20% (70/346) of participants developed mastitis. Women had an increased risk for developing mastitis if they reported nipple damage (incidence rate ratio [IRR] 2.17, 95% CI 1.21, 3.91), oversupply of breast milk (IRR 2.60, 95% CI 1.58, 4.29), nipple shield use (IRR 2.93, 95% CI 1.72, 5.01), or expressing several times a day (IRR 1.04, 95% CI 1.01, 2.68). The presence of *Staphylococcus aureus* on the nipple (IRR 1.72, 95% CI 1.04, 2.85) or in milk (IRR 1.78, 95% CI 1.08, 2.92) also increased the

TABLE 22.1	**Manual Pumping Devices**	
Hand Pump	**Advantages**	**Disadvantages**
Bicycle horn	Inexpensive Portable 	Difficult to clean Bulb retains bacteria Works as vacuum No instructions Can cause trauma Not appropriate for donor milk Milk washes back over nipple Requires constant emptying Not recommended
Plain suction pump	Inexpensive 	Difficult to clean Bulb harbors bacteria even when boiled
Handle pump	Pliable flange Can feed baby from collecting container Works well for less experienced mother with good let- down No milk contacts mechanism 	

(Continued)

TABLE 22.1 Manual Pumping Devices—cont'd

Hand Pump	Advantages	Disadvantages
Cylindric		
Two all-plastic cylindric tubes fit inside one another to create vacuum; inner tube has flange at top and rubber or nylon gasket	Less expensive than electric Portable Can feed baby from collecting container Easily cleaned and sterilized	Requires some dexterity Works as vacuum with some rhythm Rigid flange Can achieve >220 mm Hg of pressure Must follow instructions

Drip Milk Collector		
Passive Breast milk collector	Allows every drop of milk that is leaking to be collected in a passive system when breastfeeding from the other breast or pumping with a single-sided pump	Not intended for use to collect large volumes of milk

risk for developing mastitis.[18] The Academy of Breastfeeding Medicine (ABM) recommends a number of actions to prevent mastitis (effective milk removal, effective management of fullness or engorgement, prompt attention to signs of milk stasis, timely attention to other signs of breastfeeding difficulty, rest, and good hygiene), including effective milk removal from the breast by hand expression and/or pumping.[21]

Manual Pumps

The advantages of manual breast pumps are that they can be used everywhere, with no need for electricity or batteries. This may be important in a disaster. In addition, there is the lower cost compared with electric pumps. Most manual pumps are single sided. Mothers should handle the manual pump with clean hands and assemble the parts as directed by the manufacturer[22] (see Table 22.1 and Figs. 22.1 and 22.2).

As with all pumps, the flange to the manual pump should fit the mother's nipple and areola and not be too tight or too loose to avoid nipple trauma. Manual breast pumps are designed for one user only (single use) and should never be rented or shared for safety reasons. The main parts to a manual pump are the flange, pump, and milk container. The manual pumps vary in the way the human milk is pumped. The lever manual pump is squeezed by a hand lever. Another type uses a smaller cylindrical tube that fits into a larger cylindrical tube and also creates a vacuum so that human milk can be pumped from the breast. The third type, the bicycle horn manual pump, consists of a hollow rubber bulb attached to a flange. Its use has been discouraged as the rubber bulb is difficult to clean and dry and may retain milk and bacteria. In addition, the suction generated by such pumps is not consistent and so may damage breast tissue and cause mastitis.

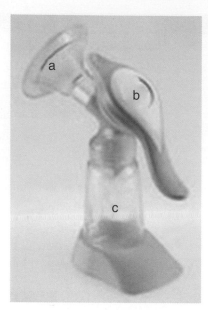

Fig. 22.1 There are three basic components to a breast pump: breast shield, pump, and milk container. (a) The breast shield is a flange that is placed over the nipple and areola. (b) The pump uses negative pressure to express milk and is connected to the breast shield with plastic tubing. (c) The milk container is attached to the breast shield and collects the milk. (From US Food and Drug Administration. Types of breast pumps; 2018. https://www.fda.gov/medical-devices/breast-pumps/types-breast-pumps. Accessed December 26, 2019.)

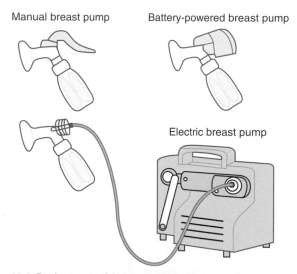

Manual breast pump   Battery-powered breast pump

Electric breast pump

Fig. 22.2 Basic types of breast pumps. (From US Food and Drug Administration. Types of breast pumps; 2018. https://www.fda.gov/medical-devices/breast-pumps/types-breast-pumps. Accessed December 26, 2019.)

These devices may not be enough for a woman trying to build up a supply when the infant cannot stimulate the breast directly (see Table 22.1).

Electrical Pumps

Electrical pumps are used by many to increase the milk supply when it is low or provide human milk at times of separation, for example, when the infant has an extended stay in the NICU or the mother is at work. Although not shown to be superior in the

Cochrane review, many recommend double electric breast pumps at home and in the hospital.[11] (See Fig. 22.2 and US Food and Drug Administration [FDA] website https://www.fda.gov/medical-devices/consumer-products/breast-pumps). Mothers should be instructed in navigating common issues faced while pumping, such as suction strength, pain with pumping, and proper flange fit. Electric pump parts should be checked for cleanliness. Problems of contamination are a significant issue with old models, because they may not protect against milk backing up into the motor or tubing, normally thought to be free of milk. Care must be taken to check each machine and follow the directions for its proper use.

Multiple use electric pumps have been referred to as *hospital grade*; however, this is a misnomer because there are no FDA criteria for "hospital grade" pumps.[23] The FDA does recognize "multiple use" pumps, which refers to pumps with which human milk does not touch any part of the pump except for the kit (not the pump itself). These are safer to use by different mothers each with their own collection kit, which they maintain (see the Centers for Disease Control and Prevention [CDC] website https://www.cdc.gov/healthywater/pdf/hygiene/breast-pump-fact-sheet-p.pdf on How to Keep Your Breast Pump Kit Clean: The Essentials).[24] There does not seem to be a difference in milk contamination whether the milk is pumped or hand expressed, as long as the hands and pump parts are cleaned adequately.[25] In a study of human milk expression from mothers of infants with very low birthweight (VLBW), Boo et al.[26] reported that there was no significant difference in bacterial contamination whether the milk was expressed by hand or pump when the milk was collected in the hospital. However, when breast milk was expressed at home, the rates of bacterial contamination by staphylococci ($p = 0.003$) and gram-negative bacilli ($p = 0.002$) were significantly higher in the breast pump group than the manual group. They concluded that the difference was not considered to be due to method of human milk expression but rather to poor cleaning of the pump at home. Before use, the pump should be inspected for whether the pump kit or tubing has become moldy or soiled during storage. Moldy tubing should be discarded and replaced immediately. If using a shared pump, one should clean pump dials, power switch, and countertop with disinfectant wipe. There is no need to discard the first few drops of milk while initiating milk expression, because there is no increased risk for contamination.[9,25] A 2017 CDC *Morbidity and Mortality Weekly Report* article described an incident with a preterm infant who developed meningitis after being infected with *Cronobacter sakazakii* from expressed maternal milk.[27] *C. sakazakii* was cultured from the valves of the breast pump kit of the mother. The mother reported soaking the breast pump collection kit from her personal breast pump in soapy water for around 5 hours without scrubbing or sanitizing. She then washed and air-dried the kit and placed it in a plastic zip-top bag. At the hospital, she also pumped with the hospital pump. The collection kit from the hospital breast pump was washed and thoroughly air-dried. The mother did not report symptoms or signs of mastitis. The infant had meningitis, resulting in spastic cerebral palsy and global developmental delay, requiring a ventriculoperitoneal shunt and a gastrostomy feeding tube.

Cleaning and Care for Pump Parts

After pumping, pump parts, known as *the kit*, should be dismantled, scrubbed, rinsed, and air-dried by hand or by dishwasher. Because of the risk for *C. sakazakii* infection, the CDC has recently updated its guidelines for infants younger than 3 months old, preterm infants, or immunocompromised infants, suggesting that pump parts should be sanitized at least once daily, using steam, boiling water, or a dishwasher with a sanitize setting.[24] A recent randomized study of steam decontamination after washing the pump collection kit in women pumping to donate to a milk bank revealed that decontamination with steam resulted in a lower proportion of discarded samples (1.3% vs. 18.5%, $p < 0.001$) and of samples contaminated with Enterobacteriaceae (1.3% vs. 22.8%, $p < 0.001$) and *Candida* sp. (1.3% vs. 14.1%, $p < 0.05$) compared with samples collected with a breast pump kit that was only washed.[28] The CDC recommends that mothers positive for COVID-19 who choose to express and provide their breast milk for the baby employ measures to prevent contamination (i.e., wear a mask for breastfeeding or pumping, wash hands and breasts).[8] In the hospital, multiuse pumps should not be used but rather a breast pump should be designated for each mother. The mother should be instructed to wash her hands before touching the pump or any of its parts. After use, the entire pump and all parts should be cleaned according to the manufacturer's recommendations.[24]

Types of Mechanical and Electric Pumps

Most portable electric pumps have a battery mode for use while traveling. Fully battery-operated pumps are available, and many have rechargeable batteries. These small pumps work for some fully lactating women and for those who have no trouble with volume. Battery-operated pumps may supply dual equipment resembling a double pumping system; however, some have been reported to work sequentially instead of simultaneously. New wearable breast pumps are battery operated, portable, convenient and offer either upright or full mobility, depending on the model. The wearable pump is placed in the bra and may or may not have additional parts, depending on the type.

Small, purse-size electric pumps may be effective for the fully lactating woman (Fig. 22.3). They have an advantage over a manually powered hand pump in that the electric power frees one hand for the mother to stroke the breast and encourage let-down. If flow is going well, the hand is free to perform other tasks, such as read, hold a telephone, or write, not an insignificant advantage for a busy, working, breastfeeding woman.

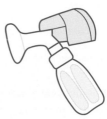

Fig. 22.3 Purse-sized electric pump. This type of breast pump is serviceable for women who are fully lactating.

Small, purse-size electric pumps may come equipped with single and double pumping collection kits. Double pumping allows the mother to pump both breasts at the same time, thereby lessening the total time spent pumping. Some small electric models have a small hole in the flange base that must be closed with a finger to develop the suction, as in many hospital suctioning devices. This also gives the mother control over the pressure. By rhythmically opening and closing the hole with the finger, the operator can simulate a milking action that is effective in extracting milk. Some, but not all, have multiple flange size options or serve as a double pump to express milk from both breasts simultaneously.

Full-size electric pumps may be more efficient because the motor applies the mechanical effort. The mother can concentrate on applying the cup to her breast, massaging the breast, and relaxing so that adequate let-down can take place. They are designed to cycle pressure instead of maintaining constant negative pressure, decreasing the likelihood of causing petechiae or internal trauma to the breast. The ultimate effect of pressure also depends on the length of time the pressure is applied. Tissue cannot withstand sustained high pressure. Pressure sustained for 2 seconds or at a rate of 30 pumps per minute is considered maximum time or minimum rate.[29] Negative pressures should have a governing mechanism to avoid excessive pressures. Mean sucking pressures of most normal full-term infants range from -50 to -155 mm Hg/in^2, with a maximum of -220 mm Hg/in^2. Manufacturers recommend about 200 mm Hg/in^2 to initiate flow in most women. An older study by Johnson[30] of more than 1000 patients at the University of Texas, using a variety of pumps, confirmed some facts about pumps. The amount of negative pressure possible and the control mechanisms were recorded (Table 22.2).

An increasing number of pumps on the market have similar designs, but each has its special nuances. A standard electric pump capable of cycling pressures to 220 mm Hg (2.5 to 8.5 psi/Hg) is usually required to stimulate production de novo (i.e., when an infant is unavailable to suckle directly, such as a small premature infant on a ventilator in the NICU). Breast pumps have been identified repeatedly for years as the source of infection.[31] Improvement in design, with a safety trap between the collecting vessel and the machine to prevent milk getting into the mechanism, is important. In addition, all equipment that comes in contact with milk or the breast should be sterilizable or disposable. The well-designed electric pump properly used is the best system for stimulating lactation and increasing volume for hospitalized infants.

Although attention is usually given to the pressure mechanisms, the cup or flange that is applied to the breast is equally important. The diameter and depth of the flare are fixed for the hand pumps, but a choice is offered for the standard electric pumps (Fig. 22.4). The nipple should have room to be drawn out, and the flange should be adequate to transmit pressure or milking action to the collecting ampullae under the areola. Finding the proper size for a breast flange is based on the diameter of the nipple, not the areola (the softer pigmented skin around the nipple). When the tunnel of the flange is placed on the breast, it should only have a few millimeters (3 to 5 mm) of

TABLE 22.2 **Expression and Pumping Methods**

Type	Action	Equipment	Availability
Hand expression	Hand action stimulates milk ejection reflex and compresses milk ducts	None	Universal
Hot jar (base cooled with cold cloth)	Cooling creates a vacuum so that the milk flows from breast (higher pressure) to the jar (lower pressure); suction pressure may be difficult to control	Suitable glass jar, hot water, cold water, cloth	Widespread
Manual pump: Compressing a bulb, pulling on two connected cylinders, or squeezing and releasing a handle	Negative pressure created by hand; arm action of the pump causes milk to flow from breast to pump; suction pressure may be difficult to control; some brands designed to reduce arm/hand fatigue; some work on a "draw and hold" principle rather than an even in-out action	Pump Cleaning supplies Most pumps have at least three parts One-handed pumps available and two pumps can be used for double pumping	Depends on market demand/distribution
Battery pump: Power provided by battery, manner of creating pressure may vary	Negative pressure at pump causes milk to flow from breast to pump; adjustable suction pressure and cycling time in some brands; some work on a "draw and hold" principle rather than even in-out action	Pump Batteries: New batteries may be needed after 2–4 hours use; some have AC adapters available Cleaning supplies Most pumps have at least four parts Most are hand-held so weight of pump plus milk may be a concern	Depends on market demand/distribution
Small pump: Electric, diaphragm	Negative pressure created by pump action of the pump causes milk to flow from breast to pump; adjustable suction pressure and cycling time in some brands	Pump Electricity supply Cleaning supplies Most pumps have many parts Two collection sets can be used for double pumping for most brands	Depends on market demand/distribution
Large electric: Piston pump, rotary vane pump, diaphragm pump; power may be provided by car battery or by foot treadle	Negative pressure created by action of the pump causes milk to flow from breast to pump; suction pressure may be difficult to control; some brands designed to reduce arm/hand fatigue; some work on a "draw and hold" principle rather than an even in-out action	Electricity supply or other power source Cleaning supplies Most pumps have 10 or more parts Two collection sets can be used	Depends on market demand/distribution; larger pumps generally purchased by hospitals or rental companies for loan to mothers

Note: Some brands of pump have a flexible breast cup that compresses the breast, and some have a choice of sizes of breast cup. Multiuser pumps require high-quality cleaning procedures and frequent servicing.
There is no one type of pump that is suitable for all mothers and all circumstances. To obtain quantities of milk by any method requires an effective milk ejection reflex.
From Becker GE, Smith HA, Cooney F. Methods of milk expression for lactating women. *Cochrane Database Syst Rev.* 2016;9:CD006170.

space around the nipple. The tunnel of the flange fits over the nipple and forms a seal around the areola. The pumping action mimics the nipple stimulation of a baby nursing. Vacuum is created by the pump, and the nipple is gently pulled into the flange tunnel. A good fit allows the nipple to move freely and comfortably within the shaft of the flange, minimizing friction points. The areola is gently compressed, allowing for rhythmic expression of milk. A woman's breasts may be different sizes

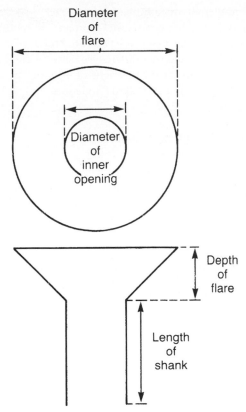

Fig. 22.4 Measurement of nipple cups. (From Johnson CA. An evaluation of breast pumps currently available on the American market. *Clin Pediatr [Phila]*. 1983;22:40.)

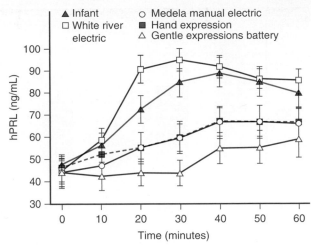

Fig. 22.5 Mean human serum prolactin (hPRL) levels for each of five expression methods. Data given as mean ± standard error of the mean (SEM). (Modified from Zinaman MJ, Hughes V, Queenan JT, et al. Acute prolactin, oxytocin responses and milk yield to infant suckling and artificial methods of expression in lactating women. *Pediatrics*. 1992;89:437.)

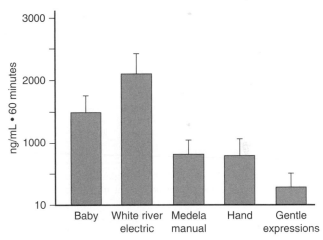

Fig. 22.6 Serum prolactin results, with breast stimulation calculated as mean net area under curves for each of five methods. Data given as mean ± standard error of the mean (SEM). (Modified from Zinaman MJ, Hughes V, Queenan JT, et al. Acute prolactin, oxytocin responses and milk yield to infant suckling and artificial methods of expression in lactating women. *Pediatrics*. 1992;89:437.)

and may require two different flange sizes. The hand pumps are too small; however, bigger is not always better. A mother may find that the smaller model of the two offered may be more physiologically suited to her anatomy. This feature does not correlate directly with overall size of the breast. The average flange size is 24 mm but typically ranges from 21 to 27 mm; however, some women may need 30 or 36 mm (see Fig. 22.4).[30] Silicone funnels adapt well to all sizes and shapes because of their flexibility. A study regarding the type of pump, hand and electric, shows the difference in effect on prolactin production and milk volumes obtained (Figs. 22.5 to 22.7 and Table 22.3).[32] The universal availability of a double collecting system, so both breasts are "pumped" simultaneously, greatly enhances production and saves time. Table 22.2 provides data on expression and pump methods of different types of pumps.

Pump Pressures and Cycles and Efficacy

To test the effect of breast pumps on milk ejection, an electric pump was programmed to cycle 45 to 125 times per minute with vacuums between 45 and 273 mm Hg by the research laboratories of Dr. Peter Hartman. The time it took for milk to be ejected was determined by ultrasound of the opposite breast measuring the dilation of lactiferous ducts in response to a pattern of 45 cycles per minute was 147 ± 13 seconds. For patterns that more closely resemble the sucking frequency of an infant when it first attaches to the breast, milk ejection occurred between 136 ± 12 and 104 ± 10 seconds. This compares with ejection time when the infant suckles at 56 ± 4 seconds. The applied vacuum affected the

volume of milk that was removed up to 50 to 70 seconds after initiation of milk ejection, but not the time of ejection.[33]

When this same research group investigated means of assessing milk injection and breast milk flow, they measured milk flow rates while the mother pumped milk with an electric pump at different settings. They determined the milk duct diameter by ultrasound in the other breast simultaneously. They reported a direct relationship between increases in duct diameter and increases in milk flow rates.[34]

Breast pump efficiency was studied by another group working with Dr. Hartmann, using a procedure for objective determination of breast pump efficiency by measuring milk removal from one breast in a 5-minute period in 30 women using an electric breast pump. They compared these data

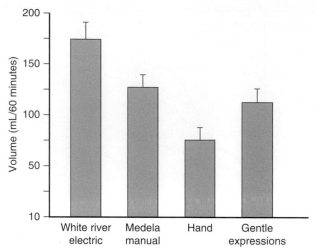

Fig. 22.7 Mean milk volumes obtained with breast stimulation for four of the five expression methods (infant not included). Data given as mean ± standard error of the mean (SEM). (Modified from Zinaman MJ, Hughes V, Queenan JT, et al. Acute prolactin, oxytocin responses and milk yield to infant suckling and artificial methods of expression in lactating women. *Pediatrics.* 1992;89:437.)

TABLE 22.3 Oxytocin Results[a]

Method	Mean Net AUC	SEM
Infant	224.7	75.4
White River Electric	174.1	41.3
Medela Manual	218.5	157.5
Hand expression	140.5	66.5
Gentle Expressions Battery	186.7	67.6

AUC, Area under the curve; *SEM*, standard error of the mean.
[a]Levels of plasma oxytocin with breast stimulation calculated as mean net AUC for each of the five methods for the 60-minute sampling session. No significant differences were noted.
From Zinaman M, Hughes V, Queenan JT, et al. Acute prolactin, oxytocin responses and milk yield to infant suckling and artificial methods of expression in lactating women. *Pediatrics.* 1992;89:437.

with breastfeeding characteristics. They determined each woman's breastfeeding characteristics by collecting milk samples before and after each feed from each breast, by either manual breast pump or hand expression, by test weighing the infant, measuring degree of fullness, and direct measurement of breast volume, techniques standardized in their laboratory. The authors concluded that pump efficiency can be measured if maternal characteristics and the amount of milk in the breast available to be expressed are known. The proportion of available milk expressed varied greatly among mothers.[35]

Investigators in this same laboratory looked at the impact of vacuum on volume of milk expressed. They looked at 23 mothers (two were expressing milk only and not feeding the infant) who expressed their milk for 15 minutes. The pumps were set at their own maximum comfort levels and then at lesser vacuum levels. The mother's maximum comfort level produced more milk than at lesser pressures. Milk flow was greatest at the onset, and cream level was highest at the end of

the 15 minutes at maximum comfort level.[36] Milk output from the right and left breasts was compared in mothers who were exclusively pumping and had not fed their infants at the breast. It was reported that differences between right and left breasts are common, with the right often more productive. The difference was not related to handedness but was consistent through the day and over time.[29]

Consumer Information Resources

Obviously, numerous websites and blogs provide information for mothers and families concerning the choice of a breast pump and their recommendations. We do not recommend any specific breast pumps in this text. A noncommercial resource of information is the FDA's website with helpful information for consumers buying breast pumps, available at https://www.fda.gov/consumers/consumer-updates/what-know-when-buying-or-using-breast-pump. Breast pump recalls by the FDA can be found at https://www.fda.gov/medical-devices/medical-device-safety/medical-device-recalls. Another presumably noncommercial source of information is the Consumer Reports website, Breast Pump Buying Guide, 2016, which has reasonable information for the consumer: https://www.consumerreports.org/cro/breast-pumps/buying-guide/index.htm.

Recommendations of Breast Pumps

In the past, recommendations of breast pumps to individual women tended to be "one size fits all" despite the fact that women and infants are each different and the reasons for expressing/pumping human milk are also different.[37] A tremendous amount of research (as noted earlier) has ensued concerning human milk expression by negative pressure (vacuum, suction) and positive pressure (expression) using newer technology of ultrasound, computerized tomography assessment of breast fullness, and increasingly accurate weighing scales to measure milk transfer (volumes and ejection and flow rates). A couple of reviews of milk expression have proposed that the mechanism of human milk expression should be specific to the individual circumstances of the mother–infant dyad (breastfeeding [exclusively, partially]), milk expression for specific reasons (effective emptying, stimulate transition to lactogenesis II, storage for later use, or to increase milk production, etc.) and the health or illness of the mother and infant.[11,38] What has evolved is that expression or pumping to remove human milk from the breast should be in synchrony with the infant's removal of milk by breastfeeding. One large group in Dr. Peter Hartmann's laboratory in Australia has focused on the anatomy and physiology of milk removal,[33–36] and a second group led by Drs. Paula Meier and Janet Engstrom in Chicago, Illinois, has focused on the functional use of breast pumps based on the "breastfeeding infant as the gold standard," the stage of lactation, the degree of breast pump dependency, and the characteristics of different pumps.[29,37] Meier et al.[37] eloquently examined the evidence regarding human milk transfer during breastfeeding and hand expression versus breast pump. They summarized the importance breast pump suction patterns, the use of percent of available milk removed as a measure of effective milk removal and measurement of pump efficiency as the number of milliliters of human milk removed per unit of time.[37] They also summarized the characteristics of commonly used breast pumps (manual, battery-operated, mini-electric; double electric, and multiuse electric) and their recommendations for pump use based on the phase of lactation and the degree of breast pump dependency.[37] They predominately recommend a multi-use electric pump for partial or complete breast pump dependency regardless of the phase of lactation (initiation, coming to volume or maintenance) and potentially a personal-use electric pump during the maintenance phase of well-established lactation depending on the mother-infant dyad specifics. Manual, mini-electric, or personal-use electric pumps are recommended as appropriate for dyads only minimally pump dependent during the phases of coming to volume and maintenance of lactation. Another publication provides discussion of the functioning of breast pumps and considerations for choosing among the different types.[39]

Clearly, other factors such as sizing and temperature of the breast shields, vacuum pressures and time since last milk removal impact milk removal, and comfort and convenience of pump usage. Other important pump characteristics of modern breast pumps are valued by mothers, including cost, ease of use, simplicity versus complexity, portability, quietness, and facility of use at work or at home.

EVALUATION OF MILK EXPRESSION METHODS

In the latest Cochrane review by Becker et al.,[11] human milk expression methods were evaluated. The review included 41 trials, including 2293 participants, with 22 trials involving 1339 participants contributing data for analysis. The review also included a review of 11 trials of different pumps: hand, manual, and electric. The authors also cautioned readers that 16 of 30 trials received support from pump manufacturers, so that bias may be a factor. This current Cochrane review's primary outcomes were maternal satisfaction/acceptability, lack of contamination of milk, and level of breast or nipple pain/damage. The only acceptable study in the category of maternal satisfaction and acceptability revealed mothers reported that they were more likely not to want anyone to see them when they used an electric pump compared with hand expression (N = 68, mean difference [MD] 0.70, 95% CI 0.15 to 1.25; $p = 0.01$). The studies reviewed could not elicit a preferred pump type. In regard to the outcome of milk contamination, no clinically significant differences were found when comparing any pump to hand expression (N = 28, $p = 0.51$), manual pump to hand expression (N = 142, $p = 0.30$), a large electric pump compared with hand expression (N = 123, $p = 0.61$), or the large electric pump compared with a manual pump (N = 41, $p = 0.59$). The final primary outcome, maternal breast or nipple pain/damage, was evaluated on 68 subjects. Large electric pumps were compared with hand expression and found similar results for sore nipples with both the manual and large electric pump (7%). Engorgement was reported in 4% and 6%, respectively, with the manual and electric pumps. Although no nipple damage was reported in the hand expression group, one case was reported in both the manual and large electric pump groups.[11]

Secondary outcomes included the quantity of milk expressed, milk volume, and nutrient quality. The authors reported that relaxation, massage, music, warmth, initiation, and duration of pumping and correct breast shield sizes contributed to the increased quantity of milk expressed. This is in contrast to other interventions such as sequential versus simultaneous pumping from both breasts that did not result in different milk amounts. The Cochrane review reported differences in nutrient quality among hand expression, large manual pumps, and manual pumps: hand expression and large electric pumps provided better nutrient quality, with higher protein, compared with a manual pump. Hand expression yielded higher sodium and lower potassium than the manual or large electric pump. Breast massage combined with pump use yielded higher fat content in the milk, although no difference was found in the caloric content.

Becker et al.[11] concluded that there is no preferred type of pump, and no difference was found regarding milk contamination between methods or breast/nipple soreness of mothers. Mothers did report approval for relaxation and support interventions. Low-cost interventions, including initiation of milk expression sooner after birth when not feeding at the breast, relaxation, massage, warming the breasts, hand expression, and lower cost pumps, may be as effective, or more effective, than large electric pumps for some outcomes.[11]

However, in a recent study, breastfeeding women were recruited to participate in a study to measure physical changes of the breast with a variety of human milk transfer modalities under close observation.[40] In this small study of 46 lactating women, Francis and Dickton[40] compared the physical changes of the breast after four different types of human milk transfer sessions: direct breastfeeding, hand expression (Jane Morton's method), and by two different popular electric pumps. The study design was a randomized crossover. Inclusion criteria included women who read and spoke English, did not use breast pumps on a regular basis, had breastfeeding infants between 2 and 3 months of age with reported normal growth, and had no history of breast damage. Before and after testing of a 15-minute human milk transfer session included precise measurements obtained for nipple length, diameter, pain, erythema, or swelling to the breast tissue, including the nipple or areola. Breastfeeding and hand expression did not cause any significant changes. The two electric pumps, however, caused significant changes in nipple length and diameter ($p < 0.003$) and increased pain and visible changes to the breast tissue. Pain was associated with visible changes. Limitations of the study included the use of a convenience sample in which many of the participants had received lactation guidance from an international board-certified lactation consultant early in their lactation, which may have improved their baseline breastfeeding experience, that each human milk transfer type was 15 minutes, and that the authors observed and measured each method of milk transfer only once, leaving the effect of repeated pumping episodes unknown. All women received a proper-sized flange for the electric pump at the beginning of the human milk transfer session; however, the authors noted that use of a different size flange during the session may have occurred. The authors concluded that although the use of the pumps was correct and done under the supervision of lactation-experienced professionals, many of the participants still reported pain with erythema and/or swelling evident for 20 minutes or more after the use of pumps. They recommended that health care professionals should evaluate those starting to use a pump. They recommended further research to evaluate the long-term consequences to women who experience untoward physical changes from breast pumps, especially with long-term pump use.

PUMPING IN THE NEONATAL INTENSIVE CARE UNIT

Part of the management of a sick infant is to be sure that the mother's milk production is also progressing. Most hospitals provide a lactation consultant for lactating women with babies in the NICU or have trained the unit's nursing staff to provide assistance. NICUs should have pumping resources available next to the infant's isolette to decrease separation between mother and baby. NICUs should also provide a room with electric pumps for the mothers of infants in the NICU. These are key resources for any NICU because appropriate nourishment is key for the survival of infants in NICUs.

In the hospital, as with all special equipment, it is advisable to select the best equipment to fill the needs of that hospital, and then purchase more of the same model so that staff can learn how to use one model properly and can instruct the patient. Similarly, the equipment should be checked on a routine basis, cleaned, and bacteriologically tested. Breast pump collection kits can be cleaned for the same patient but not for a second patient because the collection kits are meant for a single user. Lactation staff within the hospital should review technique with mothers during their infant's hospitalization.

STORAGE CONTAINERS

Just like breast pump collection kits, the containers for human milk storage must be completely dismantled, washed in hot soapy water, and rinsed or washed in a dishwasher and always should be thoroughly air-dried or dried with paper towels after each use. If soap is not available, boiling water is preferable. Chemical disinfection is not considered the best mode of disinfection, because the chemicals can be easily deactivated, thereby endangering infants to preventable risks for inadequately cleaned containers and residual chemical disinfectant.[7,25] They do not need to be sterilized. The CDC suggests, however, that for infants younger than 3 months, preterm infants, or immunocompromised infants, pump parts should be sanitized at least once daily, using steam, boiling water, or a dishwasher with a sanitize setting.[24]

Chang et al.[41] reported a significant reduction in percent of fat (0.27 to 0.30 g/dL) and an increase in total protein

(0.04 to 0.06 g/dL) and carbohydrate concentrations (0.06 to 0.1 g/dL) following the storage, freezing, and thawing of milk. However, there were no statistical differences in fat, protein, carbohydrate, and energy with either glass or polyethylene, polypropylene, polycarbonate, or polyethersulfone bottles or bags.[41] Garza et al. reported that Pyrex and polypropylene containers were found not to interact with water-soluble and fat-soluble nutrients such as vitamin A, zinc, iron, copper, sodium, and protein nitrogen.[42] Pyrex and polypropylene containers appear to have similar effects on the concentration of immunoglobulin A (IgA) and white blood cells; however, polyethylene containers decreased IgA 60%.[43] Steel containers are associated with a marked decline in cell count and cell viability.[44,45]

Garza et al. reported that polyethylene bags leaked more easily, were harder for mothers to fill without contamination, and were difficult to handle in the nursery.[42] However, a more recent study found no difference between contamination and fat loss when comparing hard polypropylene containers and soft polyethylene bags.[46] It is important that if bags are used, they be sturdy, sealed well, and handled and stored carefully.

Containers made with bisphenol A (BPA), which is found in several plastic containers, including baby bottles, should be avoided because of growing evidence of its effects as an endocrine disruptor increasing the risk for multiple cancers, especially breast cancer.[47] In addition, containers containing bisphenol S, a bisphenol A alternative, should be avoided.[48] Hospital plastic specimen storage containers used for urine or other bodily fluids also should not be used because there is insufficient evidence regarding their chemical safety and effects on infants' health.[49] Only food-grade plastic containers should be used.[49]

HUMAN MILK STORAGE RECOMMENDATIONS

A summary of recommendations for human milk storage at home and in the hospital for full term and premature infants can be found in Table 22.4. These recommendations are based on the studies which are explained in this section. Although it is clear that human milk may be stored safely at room temperature (16° to 29°C [60° to 85°F), studies suggest different optimal times. Ajusi et al.[50] studied freshly expressed human milk kept at room temperature for 8 hours and found that bacterial colony counts were consistently low. Eteng et al.[51] reported significant decreases in protein, lactose, and pH and increased microbial content on storage at 29°C for 6 and 24 hours, compared with storage for 3 hours. Hamosh et al.[52] found that significant differences in pH occurred at all temperatures at 24 hours, proteolysis was minimal at 15° and 25°C, but became apparent at 38°C at 24 hours and lipolysis was marked at 24 hours at all temperatures. Bacterial growth was minimal at 15°C at 24 hours, low at 25°C at 8 hours, and higher at 38°C by 4 hours. The authors concluded that storage of human milk is safe at 15°C for 24 hours (storage with ice

TABLE 22.4 Maximum Human Milk Storage Recommendations

Environment	Maximal Temperature	Freshly Expressed Mother's Milk	Thawed Previously Frozen Mother's Milk	Thawed Frozen Pasteurized Donor Milk[a]
Room temperature	77 °F/25°C	4 h Under optimal conditions 6–8 h	4 h	4 h
Small cooler with ice packs	59 °F/15°C	24 h	24 h	
Refrigerator	40 °F/4°C	96 h	48 h	48 h Never refreeze thawed milk
Freezer	0 °F/−18°C	9 mo Optimal 12 mo acceptable	Never refreeze thawed milk	

[a]Keep frozen for 6–8 months, varies by milk bank, check the expiration date on the container.

packs in a small cooler), 25°C for 4 hours and should not be stored at 38°C. Handa et al. studied thawed and warmed milk maintained at room temperature in a NICU and reported small, but significant differences in milk pH, bacterial colony counts, and free fatty acid (FFA) concentrations.[53] They concluded that because the increased bacterial counts were not greater than baseline and there were no untoward effects that the milk was safe. Our recommendation is that milk can be stored at room temperature for 4 hours, as long as the temperature does not exceed 32° C (85°F). Freshly expressed human milk expressed under optimal very clean conditions can be left at lower room temperatures for 6 to 8 hours.[54–56] Milk stored with ice packs in a small cooler (15°C) can be stored for 24 hours.

Slutzah et al.[57] studied freshly expressed human milk samples brought to a NICU and stored in a refrigerator at 4°C over 96 hours. There were no significant changes for osmolality, total and gram-negative bacterial colony counts or concentrations of secretory immunoglobulin A (sIgA), lactoferrin, and fat. Gram-positive colony counts (2.9 to 1.6×10^5 colony-forming units (CFU)/mL), pH (7.21 to 6.68), white blood cell counts (2.31 to 1.85×10^6 cells/mL), and total protein (17.5 to 16.7 g/L) declined, and FFA concentrations increased (0.35 to 1.28 g/L) as storage duration increased, $p < 0.001$. This suggests that refrigeration (at appropriate temperatures) of fresh human milk is safe for 96 hours.[57]

Vickers et al.[58] studied pasteurized donor milk and found no evidence of microbial growth at 0 to 9 days after thawing of the milk samples. A recent study reported that both unfortified and fortified pasteurized donor milk remained largely free of bacterial growth for up to 96 hours of refrigerated storage in NICU settings.[59] The same group found refrigerated storage for up to 96 hours had no impact on the total protein, lysozyme activity, and IgA activity in fortified Holder-pasteurized donor human milk.[60] However, they did find that acidic fortifiers significantly lowered the lysozyme and IgA activity in Holder-pasteurized donor human milk.

Human milk should be refrigerated or frozen within 4 hours of pumping. Milk may be refrigerated for up to 4 days before freezing, but preferably right after pumping. If there is still room for more milk in the container after one pumping session, more milk may be added before freezing. Fresh milk may be added to frozen milk by chilling fresh milk in the refrigerator for 30 minutes and then pouring chilled fresh milk on top of the frozen milk. However, warm milk should not be added to frozen, because it may thaw the frozen milk. Mothers should be advised to never refreeze human milk once it has thawed. If the baby did not finish the pumped milk intended for the present feed, the milk should only be used within 2 hours afterward.

Fresh, refrigerated, unsterilized mother's milk can be used for 96 hours (4 days) after collection. If the milk is to be used fresh-chilled, it should be refrigerated at home and brought in promptly for use within 96 hours. If it is to be frozen, this should be done immediately at −18°C (0 °F) (standard home freezer) or in the top of a refrigerator freezer. The milk stored in the latter should be frozen within 24 hours if it is to be stored any length of time. A recent study by Ahrabi et al.[61] found that freezer storage of human milk for 9 months at −20°C is associated with decreasing pH and bacterial counts, but preserves key macronutrients and immunoactive components, with or without prior refrigeration for 72 hours. They concluded that freezer storage of human milk is safe for up to 9 months for both freshly expressed and refrigerated milk. Therefore we recommend that optimally mothers' milk can be frozen for 9 months, but it is acceptable to freeze for 12 months. Do not store human milk in the door of the refrigerator or freezer. This will help protect the breast milk from temperature changes from the door opening and closing. Freezing guidelines for pasteurized donor human milk vary by milk bank; check the expiration date of the milk. In addition, the CDC now has a downloadable handout on human milk storage and preparation and a magnet that can be downloaded and printed through a printing service. It is available at https://www.cdc.gov/breastfeeding/recommendations/handling_breastmilk.htm.

In the hospital or at a donor human milk bank, all samples should be labeled with the name of donor, date, and time of collection. Barcoding is the most accurate method. Centralized human milk handling and barcode scanning improved safety and reduced human milk administration errors at the Childrens' Hospital of Orange County.[62] During the first 6 months of human milk bar code scanning, 55 attempts to feed the wrong human milk to the wrong patient and

127 attempts to feed expired human milk were prevented and errors were reduced to zero. A Quality Improvement initiative using barcoding decreased errors from 97.1 per 1000 bottles to 10.8.[63] Specifically, the number of expired milk error scans declined from 84.0 per 1000 bottles to 8.9. The number of preparation errors (4.8 per 1000 bottles to 2.2) and wrong-milk-to-wrong-infant errors scanned (8.3 per 1000 bottles to 2.0) also declined. Milk should be stored in the freezer in such a way that the oldest milk is used first, and all milk of a mother is kept together and used only for the infant of that mother.

RISK OF HUMAN MILK EXPRESSION ON BREASTFEEDING

Several studies have assessed human milk pumping and its effect on the duration of lactation. Yourkavitch et al.[64] examined breast milk feedings and exclusive breast milk feeding of 2595 women (1624 and 971, respectively) in mothers who were both working and not working. Using the Infant Feeding Practices Survey II (IFPS II), mothers were followed from 2 to 12 months after birth. Mothers self-defined themselves as regular and nonregular pumpers. The authors found that regular pumpers were more likely to terminate breast milk feeding and exclusive breast milk feeding earlier than nonregular pumpers or mothers who did not pump. The weighted hazard ratio for time to breast milk feeding and exclusive breast milk feeding termination of regular pumpers compared with nonregular/nonpumpers was 1.62 (95% CI 1.47 to 1.78) and 1.14 (95% CI 1.03 to 1.25), respectively. Further analysis found that nonworking regular pumpers were more likely than nonregular/nonpumpers to stop breast milk feeding. However, there was no effect of pumping among working women. The authors recommend that early, regular pumpers might benefit from tailored support to maintain breast milk feeding.[64]

Felice's qualitative study on 20 mothers from the IFPS II[65] revealed mothers' reasons for pumping, which may be for nonelective (i.e., breastfeeding issues such as separation from the baby for reasons such as employment and problems with the latch) and elective (i.e., giving another caregiver the feeding as a bonding measure). Pumping for nonelective reasons yielded higher pumping frequency, formula use, and breastfeeding termination.

In another study, Felice et al.[66] used the IFPS II cohort and reported findings on 1116 mothers who were breastfeeding and pumping. Results revealed that pumping for nonelective reasons was associated with termination of feeding at the breast (hazard ratio [HR] 2.07, 95% CI 1.77 to 2.42) and were less likely to provide any human milk feeds or exclusive human milk feeds (HR 1.12, 95% CI 1.05 to 1.21; and HR 1.14, 95% CI 1.09 to 1.20, respectively). The likelihood of higher pumpers to terminate was reported to have a 2.6- and 1.7-fold higher hazard at 3 and 6 months after birth, respectively. The authors concluded that higher pumping and nonelective reasons were associated with shorter durations for

human milk feedings. Mothers who report feeding at breast issues or employment may represent a risk group for decreased human milk feeding duration. The findings suggest that it is not pumps or pumping that obstructs human milk goals, rather the nonelective reason necessitating pumping; therefore interventions should be incorporated to promote feeding at the breast.[66]

RISKS OF FEEDING PUMPED MILK ON INFANT HEALTH

Recent data from the Canadian CHILD birth cohort revealed that feeding human milk from a bottle does not have all of the same health benefits as breastfeeding.[67] Feeding human milk from a bottle increased body mass index at 1 year and asthma at 3 years and was associated with a less beneficial microbiota at 3 to 4 months, with increased potential pathogens and decreased bifidobacteria, compared with direct breastfeeding.[68,69] Although we recognize that most US mothers will feed their infants expressed human milk from a bottle, the data suggest that they should direct breastfeed as much and as long as possible.

CULTURAL ASPECTS CONCERNING HUMAN MILK COLLECTION

Paid Leave and Employment

Worldwide provisions vary for maternity and paternity leave, which can influence breastfeeding practices especially when the parent has very limited time to establish lactation before returning to work. This is multifactorial from international, national, local, and individual situations, including residency status in a country, socioeconomic level, education, profession, etc.[70] According to the Organisation for Economic Co-operation and Development (OECD), for its 36 member countries the average government-mandated paid maternity leave was 18.1 weeks, with the highest in Bulgaria (58.6 weeks) and the lowest in the United States (0.0 weeks).[71] Most of the countries mandated 12 to 18 weeks leave (24/36 countries). Only 13 of 36 countries paid 100% of the prepregnancy salary, 16 of 36 paid 50% to 94%, and 7 countries paid less than 50% of the woman's prepregnancy salary (Fig. 22.8 and Table 22.5).

Navarro-Rosenblatt and Garmendia,[72] in their literature review of 21 studies on maternity leave and its impact on breastfeeding, concluded that increased maternity leave was associated with increased breastfeeding. Studies that reported maternity leave of more than 3 months had three times the likelihood of maintaining breastfeeding at 3 months after birth compared with returning to work within 3 months after birth. Women who had maternity leave of 6 months were 50% more likely to maintain their breastfeeding until the sixth month after birth. In contrast, women who had to return to work before the third month after delivery showed, on average, a 20% to 40% greater likelihood of discontinuing

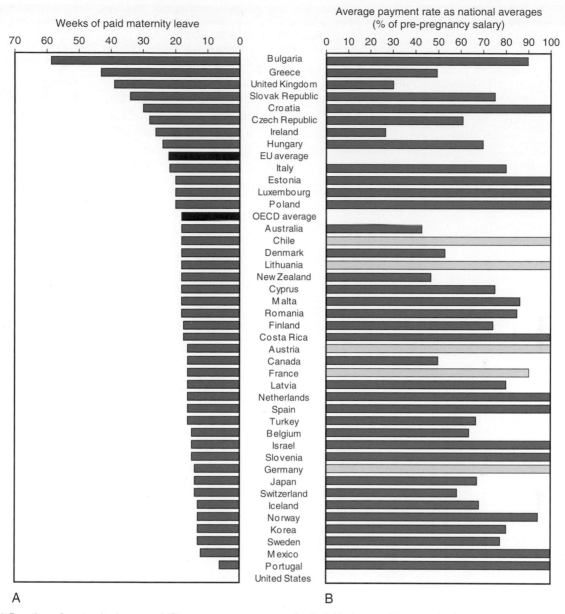

Fig. 22.8 (A) Duration of maternity leave and (B) average payment rate for individuals on paid maternity leave as national averages in 2018. Black bars represent averages of multiple countries, not individual countries. Dark blue bars represent gross pay. Light blue bars represent net pay. From The Organisation for Economic Co-operation and Development. OECD Family Database. Paid maternity leave; 2019. https://www.oecd.org/els/soc/PF2_1_Parental_leave_systems.pdf. Accessed March 2, 2020.)

breastfeeding before 6 months. The authors concluded that socioeconomic status also played a role for black women, women in less privileged positions, and women with less education, who had decreased breastfeeding duration. A limitation of this review is that it did not separate paid versus unpaid leave. A cross-sectional study from Brazil showed a significant association between paid maternity leave and exclusive breastfeeding of infants under 6 months of age.[73] Mothers without maternity leave had lower rates of exclusive breastfeeding (27%) than mothers with unpaid maternity leave (49%, $p = 0.003$) and mothers with paid maternity leave (70%, $p < 0.001$). Conversely, longer paid maternity leave was associated with increased exclusive breastfeeding with an increase of 50% longer duration and 30% any breastfeeding in

countries that have extended maternity leave of 3 and 6 months, respectively.[74–76]

The United Nations International Children's Education Fund's (UNICEF's) breastfeeding and family-friendly policy provides an evidence brief with their findings and recommendations for national policy and legislation to promote and support breastfeeding, suggested time for paid leave in the government and private sector, services that are needed to be in place in the private sector and ideas for collaborations between the government and private sector.[77]

For many employees who are separated from their infants, expressing human milk is a means of providing the optimal nutrition even when separated. The WHO and UNICEF initiated a call to action in which governments, donors, and

TABLE 22.5   Summary of Paid Maternity Leave Entitlements by Country, 2018 (Weeks)

	PAID MATERNITY LEAVE			PAID PARENTAL AND HOME CARE LEAVE AVAILABLE TO MOTHERS			TOTAL PAID LEAVE AVAILABLE TO MOTHERS		
	Length (wk)	Average Payment Rate (%)	Full-Rate Equivalent (wk)	Length (wk)	Average Payment Rate (%)	Full-Rate Equivalent (wk)	Length (wk)	Average Payment Rate (%)	Full-Rate Equivalent (wk)
	(1)	(2)	(3)	(4)	(5)	(6)	(7) = (1) + (4)	(8)	(9)
Australia	18.0	42.9	7.7	0.0	0.0	0.0	18.0	42.9	7.7
Austria	16.0	100.0	16.0	44.0	75.8	33.4	60.0	82.3	49.4
Belgium	15.0	63.7	9.6	17.3	20.3	3.5	32.3	40.4	13.1
Canada	16.0	493	8.0	35.0	53.2	18.6	51.0	52.1	26.6
Chile	18.0	100.0	18.0	12.0	100.0	12.0	30.0	100.0	30.0
Czech Republic	28.0	61.0	17.1	35.3	84.5	29.8	63.3	74.1	46.9
Denmark	18.0	53.0	9.5	32.0	53.0	17.0	50.0	53.0	26.5
Estonia	20.0	100.0	20.0	146.0	44.1	64.4	166.0	50.8	84.4
Finland	17.5	74.4	13.0	143.5	19.1	27.4	161.0	25.1	40.4
France	16.0	90.4	14.5	26.0	13.7	3.6	42.0	42 9	18.0
Germany	14.0	100.0	14.0	44.0	65.0	28.6	58.0	73.4	42.6
Greece	43.0	495	21.3	0.0	0.0	0.0	43.0	49.5	21.3
Hungary	24.0	70.0	16.8	136.0	37.8	51.4	160.0	42.6	68.2
Iceland	13.0	68.2	8.9	13.0	68.2	8.9	26.0	68.2	17.7
Ireland	26.0	26.7	6.9	0.0	0.0	0.0	26.0	26.7	6.9
Israel	15.0	100.0	15.0	0.0	0.0	0.0	15.0	100.0	15.0
Italy	21.7	800	17.4	26.0	30.0	7.8	47.7	52.7	25.2
Japan	14.0	67.0	9.4	44.0	59.9	26.4	58.0	61.6	35.8
Korea	12.9	80.2	10.3	52.0	28.5	14.8	649	388	25.1
Latvia	16.0	80.0	12.8	78.0	49.8	38.8	94.0	54.9	51.6
Lithuania	18.0	100.0	18.0	44.0	100.0	44.0	62.0	100.0	62.0
Luxembourg	20.0	100.0	20.0	17.3	67.2	11.6	37.3	84.8	31.6
Mexico	12.0	100.0	12.0	0.0	0.0	0.0	12.0	100.0	12.0
Netherlands	16.0	100.0	16.0	0.0	0.0	0.0	16.0	100.0	16.0
New Zealand	18.0	465	8.4	0.0	0.0	0.0	18.0	468	8.4
Norway	13.0	94.2	12 2	78.0	39.4	30.8	91.0	473	43.0
Poland	20.0	100.0	20.0	32.0	67.5	21.6	52.0	80.0	41.6
Portugal	6.0	100.0	6.0	24.1	59.6	14.4	30.1	67.7	20.4
Slovak Republic	34.0	75.0	25.5	130.0	21.2	27.6	164.0	32.4	53.1
Slovenia	15.0	100.0	15.0	37.1	90.0	33.4	52.1	92.9	48.4
Spain	16.0	100.0	16.0	0.0	0.0	0.0	16.0	100.0	16.0
Sweden	12.9	77.6	10.0	42.9	57.4	24.6	55.7	62.1	34.6

(Continued)

TABLE 22.5 Summary of Paid Maternity Leave Entitlements by Country, 2018 (Weeks)— cont'd

	PAID MATERNITY LEAVE			PAID PARENTAL AND HOME CARE LEAVE AVAILABLE TO MOTHERS			TOTAL PAID LEAVE AVAILABLE TO MOTHERS		
	Length (wk)	Average Payment Rate (%)	Full-Rate Equivalent (wk)	Length (wk)	Average Payment Rate (%)	Full-Rate Equivalent (wk)	Length (wk)	Average Payment Rate (%)	Full-Rate Equivalent (wk)
							(7) = (1) + (4)		
	(1)	(2)	(3)	(4)	(5)	(6)	(7)	(8)	(9)
Switzerland	14.0	58.4	8 2	0.0	0.0	0.0	14.0	58.4	8.2
Turkey	16.0	66.7	10.7	0.0	0.0	0.0	16.0	66.7	10.7
United Kingdom	39.0	30.1	11.7	0.0	0.0	0.0	39.0	30.1	11.7
United States	0.0	0.0	0.0	0.0	0.0	0.0	0.0	0.0	0.0
OECD average	18.1	—	—	35.8	—	—	53.9	—	—
Costa Rica	17.3	100.0	17.3	0.0	0.0	0.0	17.3	100.0	17.3
Bulgaria	58.6	90.0	52.7	51.9	32.8	17.0	110.4	63.1	69.7
Croatia	30.0	100.0	30.0	26.0	42.1	10.9	56.0	73.1	40.9
Cyprus	18.0	75.1	13.5	0.0	0.0	0.0	18.0	75.1	13.5
Matta	18.0	86.3	15.5	0.0	0.0	0.0	180	863	15.5
Romana	18.0	85.0	15.3	90.7	85.0	77.1	108.7	—	—
EU average	22.1	—	—	43.7	—	—	65.8	—	—

EU, European Union; *OECD*, Organisation for Economic Co-operation and Development.

From Organisation for Economic Co-operation and Development. Family database: summary of paid leave and entitlements available to mothers; 2019. https://www.oecd.org/els/soc/PF2_1_Parental_leave_systems.pdf.

developing partners enact better workplace breastfeeding policies.[78,79] There are a variety of resources for pregnant and breastfeeding women and families regarding workplace policies, allowances, legislation, and continued breastfeeding while working. In England, the National Health Service (NHS) provides a pamphlet with provisions stated for expressing human milk in the workplace.[80] Breastfeeding women are supposed to write a letter to their employer informing their employer that they are breastfeeding. Additionally, the Health and Safety Executive includes the risk assessment that the employer must perform to prepare a safe environment for the pregnant or breastfeeding women and the facilities needed for pregnant and breastfeeding women to rest.[81] The bathroom is not considered an acceptable place for expressing human milk. Although not legally obligated, suggestions include providing a clean, healthy environment for the employee to express and store human milk.

Historically, expressing and storing human milk in the workplace has been a challenge, whether by not being provided sufficient time to express human milk or being relegated to express in a bathroom or storage closet, for example. Even now, there is no universal mandate for adequate provisions in all workplaces. Since 2010, US federal laws mandate that provisions be made for expressing human milk while at work.[82] These laws apply for all employees working for employers covered by the Fair Labor Standards Act. Under the Patient Protection and Affordable Care Act, a provision states that "reasonable time breaks" be provided to express human milk for those with a child (until the child reaches 1 year of age). The employer must provide a space where milk expression can be done and states that a bathroom is not an acceptable option.[82] A designated room should, ideally, be provided; however, if there is no designated room for expressing human milk, another area, which is available when needed and out of view to others with no accessibility by coworkers or the public, may be used. The federal law applies in businesses that employ 50 or more people.

HISTORICAL PERSPECTIVE HUMAN MILK SHARING AND BANKING

The origin of human milk banking can be traced to wetnursing, in which children were breastfed by friends, relatives, or strangers. In the Old Testament (Exodus 2:7), the Pharaoh's daughter sought a wet-nurse for the baby Moses (approximately

1530 BC). The Babylonian Code of Hammurabi (roughly 1800 BC) contains rules governing wet-nursing.[83] By the 11th century, the royalty of Europe almost exclusively used wet-nurses. By the 18th century, wet-nursing in France crossed class lines, as economic conditions forced the urban working class to place their babies with rural families for up to 4 years.[84] Workers' wages were so low during this era and rents so high that even mothers with infants had to work. A high death rate was common among these babies, probably as a result of nutrition, neglect, and infection. One typical father reported that only 3 of his 13 wet-nursed children survived more than a few years.[85] In other Western European countries, wet-nursing was not as common as in France, but it was a significant cultural practice. In England, wealthy married women customarily hired wet-nurses whereas working-class mothers breastfed their own babies. Wet-nurses were also commonly employed in the United States, whereas in the South white slaveholders used enslaved black women as wet-nurses, resulting in their inability to nurse their own children.[86]

During the 19th century, there was a decline in wet-nursing and other non-breastfeeding alternative feeding methods (animal milks by various feeding devices and later bottles and teats [nipples]) began to replace the use of human milk. There was no safe way to store milk of any species and no human milk banks existed.[84] As improvements in infant bottles and nipples occurred (more easily cleanable), simple pasteurization techniques became available and formulas based on milk from other species increased in popularity, the pool of human milk diminished. Wet-nurses were increasingly difficult to locate and often were not safe sources because of wet-nurse lifestyle, risk for infections, and poor nutrition. It already had been clearly demonstrated in the early 20th century that infants who did not receive their mother's milk had six times the risk for dying in the first year of life (see Chapter 1).

The impetus behind milk banks at the turn of the 20th century was actually the medical profession's desire to remove the control of infant feeding from wet-nurses and separate the product (human milk) from the producer. Pediatricians, anxious to improve the prognosis for infants deprived of their own mother's milk for medical and social reasons, developed a means of storing human milk for general use for sick infants. The first milk bank was opened in Vienna in 1900. In the United States, the first milk bank was established 10 years later at the Massachusetts Infant Asylum, where wet-nurses had been the only sources of human milk.[87] In 1919 a human milk bank was founded in Magdeburg, Germany by Dr. Marie-Elise Kayser. In 1934 she wrote the guidelines that were used throughout Europe for the creation and operation of milk banks.[88]

Early attempts at providing donor milk depended on casual screening of donors for tuberculosis, syphilis, and various acute contagious diseases.[89] There was little research investigating human milk, but the dairy industry was rigorous in its attempt to store and market bovine and other mammalian milks. This technology was applied on a small scale, but other human milk banks appeared after Denny and Talbot created

the one in Boston. The American Academy of Pediatrics (AAP) established its first formal guidelines for human milk banks in 1943.[90,91] Similar guidelines were provided in other countries. After World War II, milk banks were mandated on both sides of the Berlin Wall. In 1959 the Federal Republic of Germany (West Germany) had 24 milk banks and the German Democratic Republic had 62.[88] The numbers of milk banks in Germany gradually decreased from then.

As technology advanced in newborn care and in infant nutrition, science replaced nature. The interest in human milk faded and with it the call for banked human milk, in the 1960s and into the 1970s. Experience in Rochester with short-gut syndrome and malabsorption syndromes, however, resulted in the development of a registry of lactating women who donated fresh milk when needed. A milk bank was developed, with donors providing frozen milk on a regular basis. By 1975, five large commercial milk banks were operating in Britain. Milk banks also were opened across the United States. The system thrived with the establishment, in 1985, of the Human Milk Banking Association of North America (HMBANA). The association not only facilitated communications among banks but also began to investigate processes, develop uniform policies, and, most importantly, provide professional and public education.[92]

The threat of human immunodeficiency virus (HIV) and hepatitis, the return of tuberculosis, and drug abuse have cast a long shadow on milk banks in the United States. This resulted in the closure of all but seven milk banks in North America and five in the United States in the 1990s. In Europe, milk banking has been key in the nourishment of premature and other high-risk infants. The Sorrento Maternity Hospital has supplied 50,000 L of milk from 10,000 donors in 40 years and provided 700 L a year both locally and across Britain in the 1990s.[93] In 1994 the remaining 18 milk banks in unified Germany supplied about 15,000 L.

Many developing countries, especially in Central and South America, are establishing milk banks as part of national efforts to promote breastfeeding.[94] Studies done in nurseries in Guatemala have shown a marked decrease in mortality and morbidity rates by providing every infant with human milk, especially colostrum.[95] UNICEF has encouraged and supported such efforts.[96,97]

Regulations pertaining to milk banks donations vary by locale. A resurgence of milk banks in the United States has occurred in the last 20 years, stimulated in part by the recognition of the value of human milk for premature and especially infants with VLBW by neonatologists.

INFORMAL MILK SHARING

Informal human milk sharing is becoming increasingly common for healthy infants as families' desire to feed their infants with human milk increases. A recent study has reported that 52% of US lactating women have considered donating to another mother, 12% have provided milk, 21% have considered receiving milk, 7% have received milk, and 1.3% have purchased or sold milk.[98]

Informal human milk sharing is facilitated by donors who are lactating women with surplus milk after feeding their own infant, have milk they cannot provide to their infant because of infant illness (e.g., galactosemia), or who have experienced perinatal loss. Mothers become milk donors because they value the relationship and friendship with the milk sharing partner, which develops because giving and receiving milk is so personal and requires trust, because they see donating as a gift, and because of their high valuation of human milk.[99] They decide to share informally and not to a milk bank for several reasons: their belief in the value of human milk, unexpected versus a planned donation, their lack of information about milk banks, and their desire to directly help and connect with the recipient mother.[100] An online survey of US milk sharing practices has revealed that donors had a long breastfeeding history with a mean lifetime lactation of 26 months and mean longest duration of breastfeeding for a single child of 18 months; 93% were exclusively breastfeeding their current infant for 6 months.[100] They donated milk to a mean three recipients and have donated a mean 1357 oz of milk.

Recipient mothers are motivated by the health benefits and their preference for human milk, but also report the stress of securing adequate milk and their fear of running out of milk.[101] These mothers had received a mean 2834 oz of milk from a mean 8 donors; 50% received milk from multiple sources, including family, friends, and local and online donors.[100,102] There is a concern of mood disorders in the recipient mothers because of their lactation difficulties and from social stigma when they tell others that they are providing shared milk to their infant, which others may perceive as a dangerous practice.[103] Spousal support for milk sharing and the ability to screen donors are associated with positive emotional response.

One major reason for informal milk sharing is low milk supply. A recent anonymous internet-based survey of breastfeeding mothers with low milk supply revealed that 29% reported receiving human milk from an informal milk sharing source for their infants.[104] Users of informal milk sharing were significantly more likely to provide human milk at 6 months (59.3% vs. 39.6%, $p = 0.001$) and be satisfied with their supplementation choice ($p < 0.001$) compared with nonusers.

The 2017 ABM position statement regarding informal milk sharing advises physicians and other health care providers to assist mothers and families who are considering informal milk sharing to make informed choices about the risks and benefits by advising recipients on medical screening of donors for illnesses and medications that are contraindicated.[105] Donors should have no medical illness in which breastfeeding is contraindicated, nor should they be on any medication or herbal preparation that is incompatible with breastfeeding. This will usually require a review of the donor's medical history, including, where possible, a review of her prenatal infectious screening tests and a review of her social practices (Table 22.6). The recipient should review the donor mother's prenatal infectious screening tests, which should be negative for HIV, hepatitis B virus, and, if performed, human T-cell leukemia virus (HTLV-1). The donor should not be using illegal drugs or marijuana; tobacco products, including cigarettes, nicotine gum, patch, or e-cigarettes; or alcohol: more than 1.5 oz liquor, 12 oz beer, 5 oz wine, or 10 oz wine coolers daily. In addition, she should not be at risk for HIV or have had a sexual partner who is at risk for HIV within past 12 months.

Health care providers should discourage the use of informal milk sharing from anonymous donors. Because donors need to be screened, informal milk sharing is safest if the donor and recipient mother can directly meet and least safe if done by the internet, especially if the milk is sold. Milk obtained from the internet should be discouraged because donors are unknown to the recipient and difficult to screen and donor milk may be adulterated or arrive fully thawed, spoiled, and/or contaminated. Milk sold on the internet should be strongly discouraged because donors may not be fully transparent regarding their health histories, medications, and social practices, thereby increasing the risk to the recipient infant. Studies of milk samples purchased on the internet have revealed high

---

TABLE 22.6 Recommended Medical Screening of Potential Milk Donors for Informal Milk Sharing

1. Mother-to-mother screening process through face-to-face and/or telephone interview/conversation. Donor mothers should be:
   - In good health
   - Only on medications or herbal preparations that are compatible with breastfeeding. It is recommended that LactMed and "Medications and Mother's Milk" by Dr. Thomas Hale be used for decisions on whether medications are compatible with breastfeeding.
2. Review the donor mother's prenatal and (if performed) regular postnatal infectious screening tests. The donor mother should be negative for:
   - HIV
   - Hepatitis B virus
   - HTLV-1 (in high prevalence areas)
3. Social practices. A woman is not a suitable breast milk donor if she:
   - uses illegal drugs or marijuana (any)
   - smokes or uses tobacco products including nicotine gum, patch, e-cigarettes,
   - consumes alcohol daily >1.5 ounces (44 mL) of hard liquor/spirits 12 ounces (355 mL) of beer 5 ounces (148 mL) of wine 10 ounces (296 mL) of wine coolers with ETOH
   - Is at risk for HIV or has had a sexual partner within past 12 months who is at risk for HIV

contamination with bacteria and, in some cases, pathogenic bacteria[106] and evidence that the milk was contaminated with cow's milk[107] or with tobacco and caffeine.[108] The authors also reported poor collection, storage, and shipping practices. On the other hand, milk donated and not sold for peer-to-peer sharing or to milk banks has been found to be safe, with no evidence of higher bacteria levels or water dilution, no difference in macronutrients or in antimicrobials,[109] and no evidence of drugs of abuse.[110]

Wet-nursing (as discussed earlier in this chapter) is directly breastfeeding a non-biologic child, and another mode of informal milk sharing that continues to be practiced in many cultures. Whether it occurs within families, or between friends, wet-nurses are directly breastfeeding other women's infants to provide them with breast milk and require screening. In some countries, wet-nursing of infants orphaned at birth is very important for survival. In Nigeria, only 31% of infants orphaned at birth survived to age 5 years without wet-nursing, which is most successful if done by the maternal aunt or grandmother.[111]

Health care providers can advise those mothers who want to further reduce the risk for infections to perform home pasteurization of donated milk before giving it to her infant. The mother needs to be informed that pasteurization can significantly decrease some of the beneficial components of human milk.[112]

HUMAN MILK BANKING

The optimal nutrition for feeding preterm infants with VLBW is the infant's mothers' milk. This human milk contains macronutrients, micronutrients, and biologic components, such as immunoglobulins, cytokines, growth factors, hormones, antimicrobial agents, probiotics, immune cells, stem cells, and prebiotics, such as oligosaccharides. The infant's mother's milk confers a multitude of health benefits for VLBW infants, including reduction of necrotizing enterocolitis (NEC), late-onset sepsis, chronic lung disease, retinopathy of prematurity, and improved neurodevelopment. It is important to encourage and assist mothers to hand express or pump to provide their own milk whenever possible.

Pasteurized donor human milk is recommended for VLBW infants when the mother's own milk is not available or is contraindicated.[113] The process of pasteurization, however, destroys cells, such as neutrophils, stem cells, and probiotic bacteria. Bioactive components of human milk, including lactoferrin and immunoglobulins, are substantially decreased by pasteurization, but there is much less effect on macronutrients or micronutrients, including vitamins. A 2019 Cochrane meta-analysis of 12 trials of 1879 preterm infants fed formula compared with pasteurized donor human milk showed that formula had nearly twice the risk for developing NEC (relative risk [RR] 1.87, 95% CI 1.23 to 2.85), but had no difference in other outcomes, such as all-cause mortality, long-term growth, or neurodevelopment.[114]

The number of human milk banks in the United States is increasing. Currently, there are 26 donor milk banks in the United States and 3 in Canada that are part of the Human Milk Banking Association of North America (HMBANA); 6 others are developing milk banks (http://www.hmbana.org) (Fig. 22.9). In addition, several commercial (for-profit) human milk banks collect, pasteurize, and distribute donor

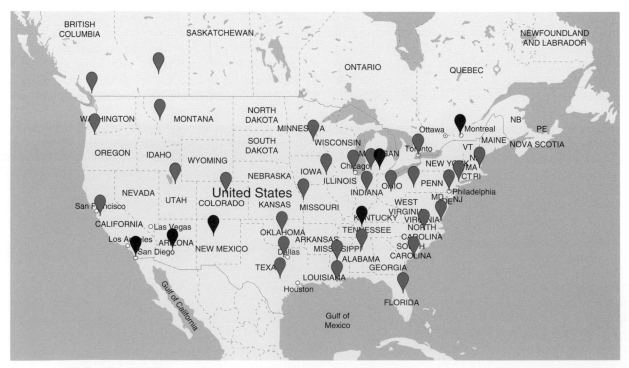

Fig. 22.9 Human Milk Banking Association of North America (HMBANA) milk bank locations in the United States and Canada. *Blue markers* represent established milk banks; *black markers* represent banks in development. (Data from Association of Milk Banking. Find a milk bank. https://www.hmbana.org/find-a-milk-bank/overview.html. Accessed May 5, 2020.)

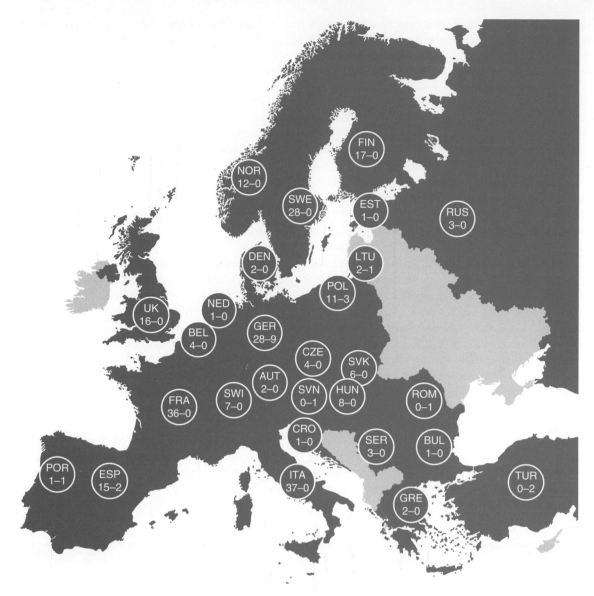

Fig. 22.10 Map of active and planned milk banks in the European Milk Bank Association. (From European Milk Bank Association, Milan, Italy. https://europeanmilkbanking.com/map/. Accessed February 2, 2020.)

human milk but are not part of HMBANA. The European Milk Bank Association (EMBA) lists 239 active milk banks throughout Europe and 15 planned banks on its website (Fig. 22.10).[115] Brazil lists on its website the most milk banks for any country, numbering 224 milk banks.[116]

Safety of Banked Human Milk

Human milk is a biological product; therefore whether from an infant's own mother or a donor mother, there will always be concerns about contamination. Possible contaminants are infectious agents, including both bacteria and viruses, and contamination with other substances, such as medications, drugs, or herbs.

HMBANA has established policies for donor human milk collection, as do commercial human milk banks. Guidelines address three layers of protection from transmission of infections. First, donors are screened for medical and lifestyle risk

factors and serum is screened for HIV, HTLV, syphilis, and hepatitis B and C. Then, milk is pasteurized, a process that kills HIV, cytomegalovirus (CMV), and other viruses and bacteria. Finally, no milk is dispensed after pasteurization until a culture is negative for bacteriologic growth. Prolacta, a commercial human milk bank, has additional tests for drug testing and DNA matching. HMBANA has developed guidelines for expressing, storing, and handling of human milk.[117]

Heat Treatment of Donor Human Milk

Several methods may be used to pasteurize donor human milk. The Holder pasteurization method uses heating at 62.5°C for 30 minutes and is the primary method used by HMBANA milk banks. One commercial milk bank, Medolac Laboratories, uses retort processing,[118] which heats milk to 121°C for 5 minutes, at 15 lb/in² above atmospheric pressure, to produce donor milk with a shelf life of 3 years without refrigeration. Recent studies have reported that shelf-stable milk loses more bioactive factors than milk that has undergone Holder pasteurization.[119] When human milk was pasteurized at 73°C (163 °F) for 30 minutes, minimal immunoglobulins A and G (IgA, IgG), lactoferrin, lysozyme, and C3 complement remained. When the temperature was kept at 62.5°C (144.5 °F) for 30 minutes (Holder pasteurization), there was a loss of 23.7% of the lysozyme, 56.8% of the lactoferrin, and 34% of the IgG, but no loss of IgA, according to work done by Evans et al.[120] Similar studies of heat treatments of graded severity were carried out by Ford et al.[121] The findings were similar. Pasteurization at 62°C for 30 minutes (Holder pasteurization) reduced IgA by 20% and destroyed IgM and lactoferrin. Lysozyme was stable at 62.5°C but destroyed at 100°C, as were lactoperoxidase and the ability to bind folic acid against bacterial uptake.[122] Growth of *Escherichia coli* increased when introduced into heated milk. Vitamin B_{12}—binding capacity declined progressively with increasing temperature of the heat treatment.[123]

The effects of the Holder pasteurization on antiinfective agents were reviewed by Orloff et al.,[124] who concluded that high temperatures destroyed much of the bacteriostatic effect of human milk, thus decreasing the benefit to infants. These data raise the question of whether any heat treatment might not increase the risk for enteric infection in infants. The alterations of the lymphocyte and antibody content after processing were of concern. Significant changes with heat, including a decrease in total lymphocyte count and in specific antibody titer to *E. coli*, are noted.

Welsh and May[125] discussed antiinfective properties of breast milk and provided two tables to demonstrate the stability of the antibacterial and antiviral properties of human milk (Tables 22.7 and 22.8).

Low-temperature short-time pasteurization of human milk was reported by Wills et al.[126] using the Oxford human milk pasteurizer. Heating at 56°C for 15 minutes destroyed more than 99% of the inoculated organisms, which included *E. coli*, *S. aureus*, and group B beta-hemolytic streptococci. The remaining activity of antimicrobial proteins after different time/temperature treatments is shown in Table 22.9.

Bacteriologic screening of donor human milk before and after Holder pasteurization was done at the Mother's Milk Bank at Austin, Texas. A total of 810 samples from 219 certified donors were used to create 303 pools of pasteurized donor milk. Forty-four pools of preterm donor milk were also studied. Of individual donor milk samples, 78% had some bacteria on routine cultures. After Holder pasteurization, 93% of the pooled milk samples had no growth on routine cultures. All donor milk with any detectable bacterial growth after pasteurization was discarded or used for research purposes. Holder pasteurization was considered by the authors to be an effective means to remove detectable bacteria from samples. They recommended routine bacteriologic surveillance of donor milk after pasteurization to detect heat treatment failures or contamination during or after the treatment process.[127]

High-temperature short-time (HTST) pasteurization is a method used in the commercial dairy industry. It requires establishing 72°C (87 °F) for 15 seconds, which involves greater technical skill than the Holder pasteurization. The investigators report that HTST is effective in the elimination of bacteria and important pathogenic viruses. A time of 16 seconds is recommended rather than the original 15 seconds. Subsequently, they demonstrated that HTST preserves the nutrients in human milk. HTST treatment (72 °F or 87°C

TABLE 22.7 Antibacterial Factors in Breast Milk

Factor	Shown In Vitro To Be Active Against	Effect of Heat
Bifid[a] growth factor	Enterobacteriaceae, enteric pathogens	Stable to boiling
Secretory IgA	*Escherichia coli*, *E. coli* enterotoxin, *Clostridium tetani*, *Corynebacterium diphtheriae*, *Streptococcus pneumoniae*, *Salmonella*, *Shigella*	Stable at 56°C for 30 min Some loss (0–30%) at 62.5°C for 30 min Destroyed by boiling
C1–C9	Effect unknown	Destroyed by heating at 56°C for 30 min
Lactoferrin	*E. coli*, *Candida albicans*	Destroys approximately two thirds at 62.5°C for 30 min
Lactoperoxidase	*Streptococcus*, *Pseudomonas*, *E. coli*, *Salmonella typhimurium*	Unknown, presumably destroyed by boiling
Lysozyme	*E. coli*, *Salmonella*, *Micrococcus lysodeikticus*	Stable at 62.5°C for 30 min Activity decreased by 97% by boiling for 15 min
Lipids (fatty acids)	*Staphylococcus aureus*	Stable to boiling
Milk cells	Phagocytosis: *E. coli*, *C. albicans* Sensitized lymphocytes: *E. coli*	Destroyed at 62.5°C for 30 min

[a]Lactobacillus bifidus/Bifidobacterium bifidum.
From Welsh LK, May JT. Anti-infective properties of breast milk. *J Pediatr.* 1979;93:1.

TABLE 22.8 Antiviral Factors in Breast Milk

Factor	Shown In Vitro To Be Active Against	Effect of Heat
Secretory IgA	Poliovirus types 1, 2, 3 Coxsackie-virus types A9, B3, B5 Echo virus types 6, 9 Semliki Forest virus Ross River virus Rotavirus	Stable at 56°C for 30 min Some loss (0–30%) at 62.5°C for 30 min Destroyed by boiling
Lipids (unsaturated fatty acids and monoglycerides)	Herpes simplex Semliki Forest virus Influenza Dengue virus Ross River virus Murine leukemia virus Japanese B encephalitis virus Human immunodeficiency virus	Stable at boiling for 30 min
Nonimmunoglobulin macromolecules	Herpes simplex Vesicular stomatitis virus Rotavirus	Stable at 56°C for 30 min Destroyed by 60°C Destroyed by boiling for 30 min Unknown
Milk cells	Induced interferon activity against Sendai virus Sensitized lymphocytes? Phagocytosis?	Destroyed at 62.5°C for 30 min

From Welsh LK, May JT. Anti-infective properties of breast milk. *J Pediatr.* 1979;93:1.

TABLE 22.9 Remaining Activity of Antimicrobial Proteins After Heat Treatment of Human Milk

Temperature / Time	IgA (%)	Lactoferrin (%)	Lysozyme (%)
62.5°C for 30 min	67	27	67
62.5°C for 5 min	77	59	96
56°C for 15 min	90	91	106

IgA, Immunoglobulin A.
From Wills ME, Han VEM, Harris DA, Baum JD. Short-time low-temperature pasteurization of human milk. *Early Hum Dev.* 1982;7(1):71–80.

up to 16 seconds) of human milk inoculated with endogenous bacteria and CMV rendered the milk bacteria free in 5 seconds and CMV free in 15 seconds.[128] Folic acid and vitamins B_1, B_2, B_6, and C were not affected. Bile salt–stimulated lipase was inactivated by these conditions. Lactoferrin and IgA and sIgA antibody activity were stable at 72°C (162 °F) for 15 seconds. Lysozyme concentration and enzymatic activity were increased, suggesting that lysozyme may be sequestered in the milk.

The HTST technique was thoroughly studied by Terpstra et al.[129] to determine its effect on the bioburden of human milk. HTST was effective in eliminating all bacteria and lipid-enveloped viruses, as well as at least one nonlipid envelope virus from spiked samples. Furthermore, Welsh and May[125] and Goldblum et al.[128] demonstrated that HTST preserved sIgA, IgA, and lactoferrin, proteins important to immune defenses and folic acid; vitamins B_1, B_2, B_6, and C levels in human milk were not affected (Tables 22.10 and 22.11). These authors suggested HTST is the method of choice for milk banks.

The effect of temperature on transforming growth factor-α (TGF)-α and TGF-β2 of human milk concentrations during pasteurization (at temperatures commonly used by donor milk banks) slightly decreased TGF-α concentrations, but not milk TGF-β2. There was little difference when temperature was increased to 71°C.[130]

In the United States and Canada, most donor milk is distributed by established milk banks to NICUs using shipping guidelines established by the milk banks. Receiving hospitals receive guidance related to temperature and other storage conditions for the milk, and these may be subject to state and local regulations. Hospitals that use frozen donor human milk must have properly regulated freezers and other methods for handling and tracking donor milk.

The AAP Policy Statement regarding the use and safety of donor human milk concluded that "families and caregivers may be reassured that, at the time of this publication, there are no reported cases of pasteurized donor human milk causing an infection with hepatitis viruses or HIV and that the

TABLE 22.10 Effect of High-Temperature Short-Time (HTST) Pasteurization on Selected Vitamins in Human Milk

	Time (s)							
	0		**1**		**3**		**15**	
	$P = V \times I$	n	$P = V \times I$	n	$P = V \times I$	n	$P = V \times I$	n
Vitamin B$_1$ (mcg/mL)	0.104 ± 0.013	9						
72°C			0.098 ± 0.005	3	0.091 ± 0.008	3	0.088 ± 0.009	3
87°C			0.084 ± 0.011[a]	3	0.095 ± 0.027	3	ND	
Vitamin B$_2$ (mcg/mL)	0.724 ± 0.132	9						
72°C			0.75 ± 0.08	3	0.70 ± 0.09	3	0.56 ± 0.07	3
87°C			0.66 ± 0.13[b]	3	0.72 ± 0.22	3	ND	3
Vitamin B$_6$ (mcg/mL)	0.237 ± 0.081	9						
72°C			0.27 ± 0.05	3	0.26 ± 0.025	3	0.22 ± 0.012	3
87°C			0.25 ± 0.07	3	0.26 ± 0.02	3	ND	
Folic acid (mcg/mL)	0.106 ± 0.020	9						
72°C			0.089 ± 0.005[c]	3[a]	0.065 ± 0.018	3	0.101 ± 0.012	3
87°C			0.088 ± 0.008	3	0.080 ± 0.023	3	ND	
Vitamin C (mcg/mL)	9.2 ± 2.4	9						
72°C			11.2 ± 1.2	3	21.5 ± 3.0[a]	3	8.7 ± 1.7	3
87°C			16.0 ± 4.9[a]	3	22.5 ± 13.3	3	ND	

ND, not done. *s*, second(s).
[a] $p < 0.07$.
[b] $p < 0.001$.
[c] $p < 0.04$.
From Goldblum RM, Dill CW, Albrecht TB, et al. Rapid high-temperature treatment of human milk. *J Pediatr*. 1984;104:380.

likelihood of this type of infection occurring in a neonate given donor human milk is extremely small."[113]

Noninfectious Contaminants

With regard to noninfectious contaminants, the safety of donated milk was evaluated by Bloom[110] in a study of milk samples donated to Prolacta, a for-profit milk bank. DNA fingerprinting of donations revealed only 2 nonmatched donations in 13,491 samples. Both of the nonmatched donations, however, were determined to be a mix-up of human milk stored in hospital NICUs. There is always the theoretical risk for a donor mixing her collections with cow milk. Bloom's study revealed that only 2 samples in almost 5000 that had evidence of "other protein source." Drug screening of 12,400 milk samples revealed 2 samples with oxycodone/oxymorphone and 40 samples with cotinine, a metabolite of nicotine used as a biomarker for exposure to tobacco.[110]

DONOR HUMAN MILK

The 2019 Cochrane meta-analysis of 12 trials of 1879 preterm infants fed formula compared with pasteurized donor human milk found that formula-fed infants had higher in-hospital rates of weight gain (mean difference [MD] 2.51, 95% confidence interval [CI] 1.93 to 3.08 g/kg per day), linear growth (MD 1.21, 95% CI 0.77 to 1.65 mm/wk), and head growth (MD 0.85, 95% CI 0.47 to 1.23 mm/wk), but no effect on long-term growth or neurodevelopment.[114] A 2019 study by McGee et al.[131] randomized infants to fortified donor milk or formula as a supplement when mother's milk was unavailable and evaluated growth at 5.5 years of age. Substantial differences were not found for body composition outcomes between these groups at 5.5 years of age, although the use of greater amounts of mother's own milk during hospitalization was associated with a greater height z score in participants at 5.5 years of age. The authors concluded that using fortified donor human milk does not pose long-term metabolic or growth risks relative to preterm formula.

Indications for Donor Human Milk

A goal of providing donor human milk to supplement the mother's milk for all preterm infants may be ideal; however, at the present time, there are limitations because of supply and cost concerns. The AAP policy pertaining to donor human milk for the high-risk infant states that priority should be given to providing donor human milk to infants less than 1500 g.[113] Relatively few data are available on whether this would include infants who are small for gestational age, such

TABLE 22.11   **Effect of High-Temperature Short-Time (HTST) Pasteurization on Immunologic Proteins in Human Milk**

	Time (s)							
	0		**1**		**3**		**15**	
	P = V × I	**n**	**P = V × I**	**n**	**P = V × I**	**n**	**P = V × I**	**n**
Lactoferrin (mg/mL)	0.67 ± 0.10	8						
72°C			0.95 ± 0.21	2	0.58 ± 0.2	3	0.83 ± 0.05	3
87°C			0.50 ± 0.02	3	0.50 ± 0.2	3	0.47 ± 0.17	2
Lysozyme (mcg/mL)	15.0 ± 8.7	8						
72°C			86.0 ± 3.5[a]	2	78.0 ± 16.0	3[b]	59.0 ± 7.0[a]	3
87°C			86.0 ± 9.1[a]	3	59.0 ± 9.0	3[b]	36.0 ± 7.7	2
Total IgA (mg/mL)	0.37 ± 0.08	8						
72°C			0.37 ± 0.07	2	0.25 ± 0.06	3	0.3 ± 0.04	3
87°C			0.06 ± 0.04[a]	3	0.04 ± 0.02	3[b]	0.05 ± 0.03	2
sIgA Ab (reciprocal titer)	10.0 ± 4.8	7						
72°C			10.2 ± 12.4	2	10.6 ± 4.8	2	15.0 ± 3.5	3
87°C			<1	3	<1	2	<1	2

n, Number of experiments; *sIgA*, secretory immunoglobulin A.

[a]$p < 0.01$.

[b]$p < 0.05$.

From Goldblum RM, Dill CW, Albrecht TB, et al. Rapid high-temperature treatment of human milk. *J Pediatr.* 1984;104:380.

as those who are older than 32 to 33 weeks' postmenstrual age at birth who also weigh less than 1500 g; but, in general, the primary guide for use is birthweight, not gestational age, in prioritizing donor milk use.

There are no clear guidelines for discontinuing the use of donor human milk in an infant less than 1500 g birthweight when the mother's milk volume is not adequate, but most centers discontinue at a range of 32 to 36 weeks' postmenstrual age, because this range covers the highest risk period for NEC. Further research is needed to clarify the optimal timing of discontinuing donor human milk.

Fewer data are available regarding the use of donor human milk in other high-risk infants, including infants with abdominal wall defects, such as gastroschisis or omphalocele, and other conditions, such as congenital heart disease. Nonetheless, some infants with these conditions or other neonatal disorders may benefit from donor human milk because of either a direct effect on intestinal growth or improved feeding tolerance.

Donor Milk From a Milk Bank

The following scenarios are common reasons for obtaining donor milk from a bank.

1. An infant is at risk for infection or NEC. Fresh colostrum is held to be especially protective and may be collected from low-risk, carefully screened mothers who are not breastfeeding their own infants.
2. An infant has a gastrointestinal anomaly or other reasons for intestinal tract surgery, especially short-gut syndrome.
3. A physician thinks an infant would benefit from the nourishment in human milk because of prematurity, especially if the infant weighs less than 1500 g.
4. A mother is temporarily unable to nourish her own breastfed infant completely. It may be that the mother's supply is inadequate when she first puts the infant to the breast after weeks of pumping or when the mother has been ill or hospitalized. Usually these infants are already at home.
5. Donor milk is an excellent transition from parenteral nutrition when mother's milk is not available. It allows earlier weaning from parenteral solution—earlier than when formula is known to be tolerated.
6. Metabolic disorders, especially amino acid disorders, respond well because of the physiologic profile of human milk (decreased casein, tyrosine, and phenylalanine). In addition, human milk is protective against infection, which may be a serious complication of these disorders.
7. An older infant or child has unique feeding difficulties, usually characterized by an inability to tolerate any oral nourishment except human milk (e.g., a child dying of HIV infection).

Qualifications of Donors

A mother who is willing to donate milk should be healthy and fulfill the following qualifications:

1. Normal pregnancy and delivery
2. Serologically negative for syphilis, hepatitis B surface antigen, CMV, and HIV

BOX 22.1 Donor Screening Procedures

1. Donors answer questions on a verbal health history screening form. Primary health care providers for the prospective donor and her infant are asked for verification of health.
2. Donors are tested serologically for:
   a. HIV-1 and HIV-2
   b. HTLV-1 and HTLV-2
   c. Hepatitis B
   d. Hepatitis C
   e. Syphilis
3. Repeat donors are treated as new donors with each pregnancy.
4. Milk banks will cover the cost of the serologic screening if the tests are done by the milk bank.
   Reasons for excluding a donor:
- Receipt of a blood transfusion or blood products within last 12 months
- Receipt of an organ or tissue transplant within last 12 months
- Regular use of more than 2 oz of hard liquor or its equivalent in a 24-hour period
- Regular use of over-the-counter medications or systemic prescriptions (replacement hormones and some birth control hormones acceptable)
- Use of megadose vitamins or pharmacologically active herbal preparations
- Total vegetarians (vegans) who do not supplement their diet with vitamins
- Use of illegal drugs
- Use of tobacco products
- Silicone breast implants
- History of hepatitis, systemic disorders of any kind, or chronic infections (e.g., HIV, HTLV, TB)

HIV, Human immunodeficiency virus; *HTLV,* human T-cell leukemia virus; *TB,* tuberculosis.

3. No infection, acute or chronic (i.e., not at high risk)
4. Not taking medications, smoking, or using excessive alcohol
5. Capable of carrying out sterile technique
6. If donating for other infants, own child is healthy and without jaundice
   See Box 22.1 for recommended donor screening procedures.

Discarding milk during maternal illness is the most difficult regulation to which a mother must adhere. The desire to contribute may overshadow the mother's understanding of the risk it poses for an infant who is not her own receiving such milk. The amount of protein has been noted to be lower after 6 months of lactation in some women; thus after 6 months or, at most, 8 months postpartum it is advisable to evaluate a given mother's contributions to confirm that protein and caloric content is sufficient.

Standards for Pasteurization of Donor Milk

Milk suitable for pasteurization should meet the following minimum standards:
1. A total aerobic count that does not exceed 1×10^6 CFU/mL.

2. *S. aureus* that does not exceed 1×10^3 CFU/mL; risk for feeding heat-treated enterotoxins when *S. aureus* exceeds 1×10^6 CFU/mL.
3. Presence of organisms defined as being of fecal origin does not exceed 1×10^4 CFU/mL.
4. Presence of organisms not part of normal flora does not exceed 1×10^7 CFU/mL.
5. Presence of no unusual organisms such as *Pseudomonas aeruginosa,* spore-bearing aerobes, or spore-bearing anaerobes.[92]

Pasteurization by Holder Method

Recommended pasteurization of human milk for banks, according to HMBANA guidelines, follows these steps[92,132]:
1. All containers shall be tightly closed with new caps to prevent contamination of milk during heat treatment.
2. Heat processing.
   a. Aliquots of milk shall be processed by completely submerging the containers in a well-agitated or shaking water bath preheated to a minimum of 63°C.
   b. A control bottle, containing the same amount of milk or water as the most filled container of milk in the batch, shall be fitted with a calibrated thermometer to register milk temperature during heat processing. The control bottle should follow the same process as the rest of the batch at all times.
   c. The thermometer shall be positioned such that approximately 25% of the milk volume is below the measuring point of the thermometer.
   d. The monitored aliquot shall be placed into the water bath after all other aliquots and shall be positioned centrally among the treated aliquots.
   e. After the temperature of the monitored control bottle has reached a minimum of 62.5°C, the heat treatment shall continue for 30 minutes. Milk shall not reach a core temperature higher than 63°C.

Viruses in Mother's Own Milk and Donor Human Milk

CMV is a ubiquitous double-stranded DNA virus, and 60% to 70% of American women are infected with CMV before pregnancy.[133] Most CMV IgG—positive women shed the virus in breast milk during lactation. In a study of postpartum women, CMV was recovered from the genital tract in 10%, from the urine in 7%, from the saliva in 2%, but from the breast milk in 30%.[134] The dilemma of CMV is a significant one for preterm infants, but not term infants. Mother's own milk is the primary source of CMV transmission among term newborns, and nearly all term infants who acquire CMV during breastfeeding are infected without signs of illness. In contrast, VLBW infants are at risk for disease. A 2013 meta-analysis determined that rates of postnatally acquired CMV infection from mother's milk in VLBW infants was 19% for asymptomatic CMV infection and 4% for CMV sepsis-like syndrome.[135] Manifestations of infection include apnea, pneumonitis, leukopenia, thrombocytopenia, hepatitis, cholestasis, and colitis.[136] VLBW infants fed mother's own milk who present with evidence of late-onset sepsis should be tested for CMV. Freezing mothers' milk has been shown to reduce, but not eliminate, the viral load of CMV in mother's own milk and is associated with loss of bioactive components.[137] In addition, freezing has not decreased the incidence of CMV sepsis-like syndrome.[137] Further studies are needed to determine the relative impact of breast milk—acquired CMV infection given the many benefits of mother's own milk among VLBW infants. At this time, mothers who are seropositive may be permitted to provide raw milk for their own infants. It is destroyed by Holder's pasteurization at 62.5°C after 30 minutes. Donor milk should be accepted only from CMV-negative mothers.

Hepatitis virus also passes into milk, and donors should therefore be screened and be seronegative. The question of having seropositive women feed their own infants is discussed in Chapter 12.

HIV has been identified in human milk.[138,139] Human milk banks require that donors be HIV negative. The viruses associated with HIV and HTLV were incubated at temperatures from 37° to 60°C, and the virus titer was determined over time by a microculture infectivity assay. It required 32 minutes at 60°C to reduce the virus titer.[140] Using the HMBANA standard of Holder pasteurization with 62.5°C for 30 minutes totally destroyed the viruses. No virus could be recovered after the process, even with repeated subculturing. Human milk contains one or more components that inactivate HIV-1, but that are not toxic for the cells in which the virus replicates.[124] These components are under continued study and are probably lipids/fatty acids.

The bottom line is that are no reported cases of pasteurized donor human milk from an approved milk bank causing an infection with hepatitis viruses or HIV and that the likelihood of this type of infection occurring in a neonate given donor human milk is extremely small.[113]

In response to the COVID-19 pandemic of 2020 caused by the novel coronavirus (severe acute respiratory syndrome [SARS]-CoV-2), questions have arisen as to the safety of breast milk.[8] In a small study of 6 mothers with COVID-19, breast milk samples were collected and tested after the first lactation.[141] Samples were tested for COVID-19 using quantitative real-time polymerase chain reaction (qRT-PCR), with results demonstrating that all tests were negative. A slightly larger study of 19 mothers did not find SARS-CoV-2 in breast milk, as did other smaller studies.[142–156] This is similar to past reports on SARS in which the virus did not seem to be vertically transmitted, although breast milk samples were rarely tested or analyzed.[147,148] A review of SARS-CoV-2 and human milk analyzed data from 14 studies and 48 milk samples from 33 mothers showed evidence of SARS-CoV-2 viral RNA by PCR in one sample and another sample with SARS-CoV-2—specific IgG in human milk. The authors noted that none of the PCR testing methods had been standardized for use on human milk.[149] Of note, breast milk of a pregnant woman who contracted a severe case of SARS in the second trimester was negative by SARS PCR but did contain antibodies to SARS at 130 days after the infection onset.[150] Since that review by Lackey et al.[149] there have been at least three published case reports

that identified COVID-19 in breast milk samples.[151–153] The infants were all clinically well. Of note, a recent report found sIgA antibodies against SARS-CoV-2 in the breast milk from 80% of mothers previously infected with COVID-19.[154]

The CDC concluded that the limited data available suggest that breast milk is not likely to be a source of transmission and supports breastfeeding and the use of breast milk from COVID-19—positive mothers.[8] The AAP guidance states that before breastfeeding or pumping milk the COVID-19 positive mothers should wear a mask and clean their hands and breasts and any pump parts, bottles, and artificial nipples.[155] Pasteurized donor human milk has remained safe during the epidemic, and evidence shows that the virus is inactivated by the HMBANA standard of Holder pasteurization.[156] The limited data available do not suggest that breast milk is a common source of SARS-CoV-2 infection in neonates or infants nor that infants who are infected in the first month of life are at risk for severe SARS-CoV-2 disease.[157] Breastfeeding should be initiated and continued depending on the mother's health relative to SARS-CoV-2 infection in the mother. Appropriate management of respiratory secretions by the mother during breastfeeding or milk expression is appropriate. There is no concern that donor human milk, treated by standard pasteurization would be a source of SARS-CoV-2 infection of the infant fed donor human milk. There remains a tremendous amount about SARS-CoV-2 and human milk to be studied.

Lyophilization and Freezing

Lyophilization is the creation of a stable preparation of a biologic substance by rapid freezing and dehydration (freeze drying) of the frozen product under high-vacuum freeze drying. The technique involved freezing to −23°C (−9°F) and thawing at 1, 2, 3, and 4 weeks. This technique is being used to store the human milk fortifier produced by Prolacta Biologics (Monrovia, California). The impact of lyophilization was similar to that of heating, showing a decrease in total lymphocyte count, immunoglobulin concentration, and a specific antibody titer to E. coli. Freezing specimens up to 4 weeks showed no change in IgA or E. coli antibody titer, although the lymphocyte count was decreased. Although cells were present after freezing, they showed no viability when tested with the trypan blue stain exclusion method.

The storage of human milk at 4°C (39°F) for 48 hours caused a decrease in the concentration of milk macrophages and neutrophils, but not of the lymphocytes, which also maintained their activity, according to Pittard and Bill.[158] The loss of cells may be desirable if the graft-versus-host reaction in a premature infant, who is possibly immunodeficient, is of concern.

Evans et al.[120] reported their results with 3-month storage at −20°C and with freeze drying and reconstitution (lyophilization). They found no significant change in lactoferrin, lysozyme, IgA, IgG, and C3 after 3-month freezing, but a small loss of IgG after lyophilization (Table 22.12).

Nutritional Consequences

Initially, the focus in processing donor human milk was the effect on its unique antiinfective properties,[159,160] but attention

TABLE 22.12   Effect of Deep Freezing (3 Months) at −20°C and Lyophilization of Human Milk Proteins (mg/dL Milk)

	Raw Milk (Mean ± SE)	DEEP-FROZEN MILK			LYOPHILIZED MILK		
		Mean ± SE	Mean as % Raw	p	Mean ± SE	Mean as % Raw	p
α₁-Antitrypsin (16 samples)	2.38 ± 0.3	1.98 ± 0.2	83.2	<0.05	2.22 ± 0.3	93.3	>0.1
IgA (8 samples)	9.55 ± 0.84	9.25 ± 0.83	96.9	>0.1	9.33 ± 0.74	97.7	>0.1
IgG (16 samples)	0.42 ± 0.05	0.42 ± 0.04	100	>0.1	0.33 ± 0.04	78.6	<0.05
Lactoferrin (11 samples)	332 ± 71.7	338 ± 57.4	102	>0.1	363 ± 79	109.3	>0.1
Lysozymes (11 samples)	5.1 ± 1.20	4.0 ± 0.07	90.2	>0.1	4.8 ± 1.19	94.1	>0.1
C3 (16 samples)	1.35 ± 0.13	1.26 ± 0.11	93.3	>0.1	1.27 ± 0.13	94.1	>0.1

Ig, Immunoglobulin; *SE,* standard error.
From Evans TJ, Ryley HC, Neale LM, et al. Effect of storage and heat on antimicrobial proteins in human milk. *Arch Dis Child.* 1978;53:239.

has been given to the nutritional consequences as well.[161] Storage for 24 hours did not affect vitamin A, zinc, iron, copper, sodium, or protein nitrogen concentrations at 37°C.[162,163] Ascorbic acid levels decreased greatly when stored at 37° and 4°C at 24 and 48 hours. (They remained stable for 4 hours.) Other investigators have found that ascorbic acid levels drop 40% with heating.[42,161]

Levels of unsaturated fatty acids apparently are also affected by heating and cold storage, but the data need clarification.[164] It is anticipated that heating or freezing and thawing are capable of damaging membranes surrounding milk fat globules.[165] The fat globule could then undergo fragmentation and allow greater access of milk lipases to triglycerides. The percentages of polyunsaturated fatty acids linoleic acid (C18:2) and linolenate (C18:3) decreased after both heating and freezing, but monounsaturated and saturated fatty acids were unaffected.[166] When milk is stored at −11°C for 48 hours, release of fatty acids progresses over time with an increase in the proportion of free C18:2, C20:4, and other long-chain polyenic acids. No measurable lipolysis occurred when milk was stored at −70°C. The higher the temperature and the longer the time, the greater is the accumulation of FFAs.[167] Other investigators have confirmed this, concluding that the lipoprotein lipase and bile salt−stimulated lipase remain fully active at −20°C, but not −70°C, with or without the presence of serum. Berkow et al.[168] therefore recommend that milk be stored at −70°C. Other enzymes were not affected by freezing and storing except lactoperoxidase, which lost activity.

A 2019 study revealed that long-term storage of milk at −80°C is associated with better fat and energy preservation compared with storage at −20°C.[169] Milk at −80°C was compared with paired samples stored at −20°C for each time point, and fat and energy content were consistently higher ($p < 0.05$). Milk stored at −20°C for 24 weeks lost significantly more fat (0.3 g/100 mL [7.9%], $p = 0.001$) and energy (2.3 kcal/100 mL [3.3%], $p = 0.03$) than milk stored at −20°C for 4 weeks. Fat and protein declined less, but also significantly in the −80°C group (by 0.14 g/100 mL [3%], $p = 0.009$, and 0.06 g/100 mL [6.4%], $p = 0.02$, respectively) (Fig. 22.11).

Because the nourishment of low-birth-weight (LBW) infants has been the purpose of many human milk banks, the ability of preterm infants to use treated bank human milk is relevant. Holder pasteurization at 62.5°C for 30 minutes was reported not to influence nitrogen absorption or retention in LBW infants.[160] When raw, pasteurized, and boiled human milks were fed to VLBW (less than 1.3 kg) preterm infants in three separate consecutive weeks, fat absorption was reduced by one third in the heat-treated group. There was a reduction in the amount of nitrogen retained in the heat-treated group, as well, although the absorption was unaffected. The absorption and retention of calcium, phosphorus, and sodium were unaffected by heating or freezing. The mean weight gain was one-third greater when the infants were fed raw human milk.[162]

Pasteurization decreased vitamin B₁ (thiamine) by approximately 50% and folate-binding capacity by 10% (Table 22.13).[122] Sterilization (100°C for 20 minutes), on the other hand, had similar effects on vitamin B₁₂ binding and completely inactivated folate binding.[122] Vitamins A, D, E, B₂, and B₆, choline, niacin, and pantothenic acid were barely affected by pasteurization, whereas thiamine was reduced up to 25%, biotin up to 10%, and vitamin C up to 35%.[170] Quick freezing and frozen storage do not significantly affect levels of biotin, niacin, folic acid, vitamin E, and the fat-soluble vitamins. Photooxidation and absorption by the container or tubing are always a consideration. Vitamin C is reduced by both of these processes.[171]

Analysis
Infrared Spectroscopy

On December 21, 2018, the FDA approved the Miris Human Milk Analyzer (Uppsala, Sweden), an infrared spectroscopy system to analyze samples of human milk and provide a quantitative measurement of fat, protein, and total carbohydrate content and calculations of the total solids and energy content contained in the milk.[172] The device provides results within minutes using only a small sample of milk and allows clinicians to provide individualized fortification to both mothers' milk and donor milk for preterm babies. The FDA reviewed data on 112 samples of

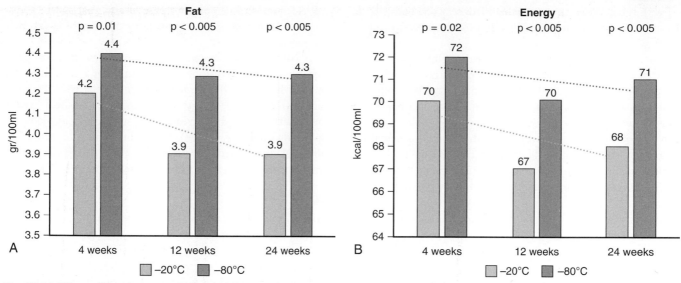

Fig. 22.11 Effect of freezing temperature and time on fat and energy content of human milk. (A) Mean human milk fat content. (B) Mean human energy content. At different freezing temperatures (*gray*, −20°C; *black*, −80°C). Different durations of storage are listed (4, 12, and 24 weeks). (From Orbach R, Mandel D, Mangel L, et al. The effect of deep freezing on human milk macronutrients content. *Breastfeeding Med.* 2019;14[3]:172−176. http://doi:10.1089/bfm/2018.0226.)

TABLE 22.13 Thermal Destruction of Milk Components (Follows First-Order Reaction Kinetics)

	D Value[a] at 60°C (s)	Z Value[b] (°C)
Immunoglobulin A	4.9×10^4	5.5
Lactoferrin	2.4×10^3	4.7
Thiamine	7.7×10^5	28.4
Folic acid	1.9×10^4	6.4

[a]90% degradation at 60°C in seconds.
[b]Temperature change to alter degradation rate by a factor of 10.
Modified from Morgan JN, Toledo RT, Eitenmiller RR, et al. Thermal destruction of immunoglobulin A, lactoferrin, thiamin, and folic acid in human milk. *J Food Sci.* 1986;51:348.

human milk tested in the machine and compared with the expected true values obtained by independent methods; the systems provided similar results for each test.

Creamatocrit

Testing milk for protein, fat, and carbohydrate has not been done by most banks. However, Lucas et al.[173] suggested a quick method of analysis. It involves standard hematocrit microtubes and a centrifuge. The percentage of cream, or "creamatocrit," is read from the capillary tube. Fat and energy content have a linear relationship, as follows:

$$\text{Fat}\left(\frac{g}{L}\right) = \frac{\text{Creamatocrit[\%]} - 0.59}{0.146}$$

$$\text{kcal/L} = 290 + (66.8 \times \text{Creamatocrit[\%]})$$

Accuracy is within 10%.

The Research Institute for Health Sciences provides the following formula for calculating the fat and energy content of milk, using the measurement of the creamatocrit (%)[174]:

$$\text{Fat}\left(\frac{g}{L}\right) = (6.24 \times \text{Creamatocrit[\%]}) - 3.08$$

$$[r = 0.98, 95\% \text{ confidence limit} = \pm 4.39 \text{ g/L}]$$

$$\text{kcal/dL} = (5.57 \times \text{Creamatocrit[\%]}) + 45.13$$

$$[r = 0.92, 95\% \text{ confidence limit} = \pm 12.61 \text{ kcal/dL}]$$

Studies done comparing energy value calculated by creamatocrit with energy value from percentage of carbon, as measured by Manchester bomb calorimeter using pooled pasteurized milk samples, were somewhat inaccurate compared with data obtained by creamatocrit on fresh or fresh-frozen samples.[165]

The methodology was validated with further analysis by Lemons et al.,[175] who repeated the studies and confirmed actual measurements of total fat and caloric content. Because the protein and lactose content remains relatively constant over time, the variation in fat content is the primary constituent affecting caloric value of the milk. Neither freezing for up to 2 months, nor pasteurization, affected the creamatocrit. There was no evidence of fat globule degradation during storage that affected the test.

Special cautions while performing this simple test should include the following:

- Use a representative, well-mixed sample.
- Complete a sample of pumping from at least one breast; do not take just a spot sample.
- Use a well-mixed 24-hour sample.

- Use a tube at least three-fourths filled; seal one end.
- Centrifuge for 15 minutes in a standard table-top centrifuge.

The Creamatocrit Plus (EKF Diagnostics, Elkhart, Indiana) has been evaluated by Meier et al.[176] The device is a special centrifuge that spins and calculates the creamatocrit. It automatically calculates the fat and calorie content. This device has been in use in research and in NICUs. Its accuracy was compared with that of the standard laboratory centrifuge with a hematocrit reader, and the standard laboratory centrifuge with digital calipers, using 36 milk specimens from 12 women. The results varied less than 1% from each other. Laboratory measurements for lipids and calories were confirmatory.[177] NICUs that use mother's milk can easily check the content of a mother's milk with this device.

A 2017 study compared gravimetric, esterified fatty acid (EFA) and creamatocrit measurement of human milk fat.[178] The gravimetric method is considered the gold standard for measuring the fat content of human milk. However, it is labor intensive and requires large volumes of human milk. Other methods, such as creamatocrit and EFA, have been used widely in fat analysis. Comparison of the three methods was conducted with human milk of varying fat content. Correlations among these methods were high ($r(2) = 0.99$). Statistical differences ($p < 0.001$) were observed in the overall fat measurements and within each group (low-, medium-, and high-fat milk) using the three methods. Overall, stronger correlation with lower mean (4.73 g/L) and percentage differences (5.16%) was observed with the creamatocrit than the EFA method when compared with the gravimetric method.[177] Furthermore, the ease of operation and real-time analysis make the creamatocrit method preferable.

Ultrasonic Homogenization

Pooling specimens of human milk may not result in a milk of uniform fat content after storage. The separation of fat during processing, storage, and administration by continuous nasogastric infusion, whether by gravity flow or continuous mechanical pump, results in significant loss of fat and variation in the milk received (47.4% of fat with slow infusion and 16.8% with fast infusion).

Homogenization by ultrasonic treatment was studied by Martinez et al.,[178] who found that changes in fat concentration during infusion and loss of fat during administration, caused by the fat sticking to the container and tubes, were eliminated. Furthermore, the fat-soluble vitamins are preserved. Because 31% of iron, 15% of copper, 12% of zinc, 10% of calcium, and 2% of magnesium sulfate are in the fat fraction of both human and cow milk, preserving the fat is essential to maximizing nutrient intake from human milk, especially in compromised infants. Tube feedings have been noted to reduce vitamins B_2, B_6, A, and C in human milk. Ultrasonic homogenization was accomplished in this study by subjecting the milk to treatment in a Tekmar Sonic Disruptor TSD-P 250 (Tekmar Co., Cincinnati, Ohio). The homogenization time (2, 4, or 8 minutes) is a function of the volume of milk and intensity of vibration. The procedure should be done with milk in an ice bath. It has not been tested

to determine the amount of lipase, if any, that survives pasteurization and would be capable of digesting the fat after homogenizing.

A 2017 study evaluated the effect of ultrasonic homogenization of pasteurized donor human milk on gastric digestion in eight hospitalized tube-fed preterm infants who served as their own control.[179] Homogenization increased the degree of lipolysis ($p < 0.01$) by increasing the surface area available for lipase adsorption ($p < 0.01$). Thus homogenization could be a potential strategy to improve fat absorption and thus growth and development in infants fed with donor human milk.

Microwave Effects

Milk should be thawed in the refrigerator, and each bottle should be used completely within 24 hours. Defrosting in the microwave oven may lead to separation of layers and decreased vitamin C content. The greatest danger of microwaving is that the milk heats and the container does not, so that an infant could be burned or the milk significantly overheated.

The effects of microwave radiation on human milk have been much debated. The only nutritional effect identified has been the lowering of the vitamin C level. Lysozyme activity, total IgA, and specific IgA to *E. coli* serotypes 01, 04, and 06 were tested in 22 freshly frozen milk samples before and after heating for 30 seconds at low-power and high-power settings of the microwave oven, leading to decreasing antiinfective factors with increasing power (temperature)[180] (Table 22.14). Additional samples were tested at low (20° to 25°C), medium (60° to 70°C), and high (98°C or higher) microwave powers, before the addition of *E. coli* suspension. Microwaving at high temperatures (72° to 98°C) greatly decreased all the tested antiinfective factors (Table 22.15). *E. coli* growth in milk after heat treatment at 98°C or higher was 18 times that of untreated thawed human milk. Low temperatures did not affect total IgA or specific IgA to *E. coli* serotypes 01 and 04 or specific IgA to *E. coli* serotype 06, but even at only 20° to 25°C, the growth of *E. coli* was five times that of the untreated thawed milk.[179] In experimental laboratories, the microwaves are carefully controlled. In the home, they vary tremendously. Ovesen et al.[181] admitted that the temperature had to stay under 60° C (140°F). Above that, antibodies were decreased and at 77°C (170°F), they were totally destroyed. Vitamins B_1 and E were apparently stable, but they did not test for vitamin C. It is very clear that IgA, sIgA, and lysozyme were affected by microwaving at 14° to 25°C (i.e., lower temperatures). Time is important because even at 30% power the temperature will increase over time.

Microwaving clearly interferes with the antiinfective properties of human milk—the higher the temperature (because of higher power), the greater the effect (see Table 22.14)—and is not appropriate for heating human milk.[180]

Specialty Milks

New technologies offer the potential for providing specialty milks. Simple homogenization would preserve the fat, as noted. However, because of the presence of active enzymes,

TABLE 22.14   Impact of Microwaving on Antiinfective Factors in Human Milk[a]

	No.	Control	Low Microwave	High Microwave
Lysozyme activity (mcg/mL)	22	23.7 ± 4.0	19.2 ± 3.4	0.9 ± 0.72
			$p < 0.005$	$p < 0.0005$
Total IgA (mg/dL)	22	73.3 ± 16.1	48.9 ± 15.8	1.55 ± 1.54
			NS[b]	$p < 0.0005$
Antigen-Specific Antibody to *Escherichia coli* Serotype				
01	22	100%	91 ± 9.2^c	24.9 ± 10.0^c
04	22	100%	90.3 ± 6.5^c	12.3 ± 3.7^c
06	22	100%	79.8 ± 5.7^c	17.1 ± 3.6^c
			$p < 0.005$	$p < 0.0005$

IgA, Immunoglobulin A.
[a]Results are mean ± standard error of the mean. All significant differences were also confirmed by the Fisher protected least significant difference test.
[b]Not significant.
[c]Percentage of control.
From Quan R, Yang C, Rubinstein S, et al. Effects of microwave radiation on anti-infective factors in human milk. *Pediatrics*. 1992;89:667.

TABLE 22.15   Impact of Microwaving on *Escherichia coli* Growth in Human Milk at 3.5 Hours[a]

	No.	Colony Count
Control	10	$8.4 \pm 2.7 \times 10^7$
Low microwave (20°–25°C)	10	$43.9 \pm 11.4 \times 10^{7b}$
Medium microwave (60°–70°C)	10	$90.1 \pm 24.1 \times 10^{7c}$
High microwave (72°–98°C)	10	$152 \pm 43 \times 10^{7c}$

[a]Results are mean ± standard error of the mean. All significant differences were also confirmed by the Fisher protected least significant difference test.
[b]$p = 0.005$ compared with control.
[c]$p = 0.001$ compared with control.
From Quan R, Yang C, Rubinstein S, et al. Effects of microwave radiation on anti-infective factors in human milk. *Pediatrics*. 1992;89:667.

once the fat membrane is ruptured by homogenization, the milk should be used promptly to prevent excessive fat breakdown. Lyophilization, or freeze drying, is an opportunity to concentrate the nutrients without increasing the volume. Adding a freeze-dried aliquot to liquid human milk is preferable to using the commercial bovine-based products. Such a human milk product is available from Prolacta. In Denmark, infrared analysis of milk donations is used to provide high-protein or high-fat pools of milk. In Canada and the United States, some banks identify donors with dairy-free diets for specific infants with bovine protein allergies.[91,182,183] Gluten-free milk from mothers on gluten-free diets is available. Fat-free milk that does not need pasteurization can be prepared from a mother's own milk by NICU staff for an infant with chylothorax. It is described in Chapter 14.

Sour Milk After Storage

For decades, women have reported to the Lactation Study Center that their fresh-frozen breast milk smells sour and even rancid. Although a slightly soapy odor had sometimes been noted, it had never been reported to be harmful or to be rejected by the infant. This soapy smell has been attributed to a change in the lipid structure associated with the freeze-thaw effects of the self-defrost cycle in the freezer-refrigerator.

The cases reported to the Lactation Study Center, however, have suggested true lipid breakdown is associated with the rancid smell. Speculation first suggested that some women have more lipase activity than others, leading to increased lipid breakdown, as noted in the study of lipase and hyperbilirubinemia. Some mothers reported that their milk began to smell as soon as it cooled, whether refrigerated or frozen. Others have noted that their stockpile of milk, meticulously stored in anticipation of returning to work, was rancid and rejected by their infants when thawed months later. When these mothers heated their milk to a scald (not boiling) immediately after collection and then quickly cooled and froze it, the effect was not apparent, and their infants accepted the heat-treated milk. That process, it was speculated, inactivated the lipase and halted the process of fat digestion. On the other hand, scalding rancid milk will not improve the flavor or smell. Scalding does not work for all mothers. A few mothers have noted improvement when they lowered the pressure and speed of the pump. This is also noted in the bovine literature.

In the over four decades since the first thoughts about sour milk were published, many women have experienced the devastation of discovering they had stored quarts and quarts of sour milk. Some women found scalding helped prevent souring. But no studies were done predominately because no investigator could accumulate enough samples to study lipase levels. This problem was solved thanks to the wise thinking of the Medolac Bank leadership. Medolac had received thousands of donor milk samples and, in the screening process, identified some that were sour. They separated the sour milk samples out, kept them frozen, and shared them with the Lactation Study Center at the University of Rochester. Analysis of lipase activity, fatty acids, and pH were done. The samples had already been cultured at Medolac, and no samples had excessive growth or any species except skin flora. Cultures were unremarkable.

Lipase levels were compared with levels in known normal milk samples. Lipase in the sour milk was half that of the normal samples, not increased. Lactic acid was increased, and lactate was low or unmeasurable, similar to the normal samples. This was reported during discussions at the ABM meetings in Los Angeles, California, in October 2015. Further studies are under way at the Lactation Study Center. The cause of the souring of human milk is still unconfirmed.

A 2019 study confirmed that the rancid smell was not due to lipase.[184] Frozen milk previously refused by the mother's own infant was collected from 16 mothers at five different time points when available (postpartum days 30, 60, 90, 120, and 150). The lipase activity for all samples was at or below literature values for mature human milk and lower compared with control milk ($p < 0.001$). Macronutrient composition was not different from that in control values and did not change significantly over 150 days ($p < 0.005$). The pH for all postpartum time groups was lower ($p < 0.02$) in refused milk and was inversely associated with lipase activity and FFA. FFA and bacterial counts were not different from those in control samples. The authors concluded that infant refusal of previously frozen milk was not due to endogenous lipase activity and that the milk is suitable for donation to human milk banks.

FINANCIAL ASPECTS OF BANKING

A major limitation in the use of pasteurized donor human milk is the cost to hospitals or families. Reimbursement for pasteurized donor human milk is variable across states and often among sources of insurance coverage. The AAP Policy on Donor Human Milk states that "the use of donor human milk in appropriate high-risk infants should not be limited by an individual's ability to pay.[113] Policies are needed to provide high-risk infants access to donor human milk on the basis of documented medical necessity, not financial status." As of 2018, only six states in the United States provided Medicaid coverage for donor milk reimbursement[185] and an estimated 50% of families who have a premature baby in the United States are recipients of Medicaid funding.[185] The national preterm birth rate of 10% raises the question that finances could dictate who will receive human donor milk.[186]

All human milk banks, even nonprofits and those in which human milk is donated, charge hospital and private recipients the costs of processing, labor, equipment, and supplies. In the HMBANA milk banks, the charge is not for the human milk itself, because all of the milk is donated. The cost of donor milk varies but is generally estimated as $3 to $5 per ounce, which includes both direct costs, such as screening of donors and processing and pasteurizing of human milk, and indirect costs, such as research and infrastructure.[187] A 2018 single-center study calculated a mean number of days that an infant received pasteurized donor human milk to be 23 days (range 1 to 134 days), and the mean volume consumed daily was 195 mL (range 6 to 1335 mL).[188] Estimating a cost of US $4.50 per oz, the authors calculated the average cost of pasteurized donor human milk per day was only US $29.19 (range US $0.90 to $200.23).

For-profit companies such as Prolacta and Medolac have patents to protect their human milk products that come from mothers who donate their milk. Another ethical issue that has been raised pertains to their policy to compensate mothers for their milk donations. In 2015 the Detroit-based Black Mothers' Breastfeeding Association raised concerns against Medolac's monetary compensation that could lead to situations in which low-income mothers would be enticed to donate human milk at the expense of their own child. The company defended their practice of milk donation compensation stating that it potentially allowed mothers to prolong their maternity leave. Women who donate to Medolac are compensated, approximately US $600 to $800 per month, an amount that could be the deciding factor for mothers to donate. Additionally, Prolacta provides cost benefit analysis and guidance regarding insurance reimbursement on the purchase of Prolacta's donor milk by hospitals.[189]

The costs of purchasing pasteurized donor human milk must be compared with the costs of not purchasing it. A 2017 systematic review evaluated the cost of donor milk, the cost of treating NEC, and the cost-effectiveness of exclusive donor milk to reduce the short-term treatment costs of NEC.[190] Seven studies with donor milk costs and 17 with NEC treatment costs were included. The mean cost for the four US studies was $14 per 100 mL, which is a cost of just under $300 per VLBW infant or around $1500 for an infant with a birth-weight of 500 to 1250 g fed exclusive donor milk. Estimates of the increased length of stay associated with NEC were approximately 18 days for medical NEC and 50 days for surgical NEC. The authors concluded that donor milk provides short-term cost savings by reducing the incidence of NEC.

Costs of NEC and the cost-effectiveness of exclusively human milk–based products, including donor milk as a supplement to mothers' milk, when necessary, and human milk–based fortifier, in feeding extremely premature infants were determined by Ganapathy et al.[191] The cost of patients without NEC averaged $74,000, and with NEC $236,000. The cost of bovine fortifier was $1.30 per packet, the cost of human milk fortifier was $6.25 per milliliter, and donor human milk was $3 per ounce. The calculated saving per infant given human milk was over $8000 because of the lower length of stay and costs of hospitalization. The cost analysis ignored the benefit of avoiding the lifelong burden of NEC. Two 2019 studies, one from the United States[192] and one from Germany,[193] confirmed that an exclusive human milk diet for VLBW infants is cost effective.

The neonatal period, the first 28 days of life, is the time when a child is most vulnerable and at most at risk for dying.[194] In 2018 the global neonatal mortality rate was 18 deaths per 1000 live births. Most of these deaths are preventable. In 2018 worldwide, a reported 2.5 million children died in the first month of life, which is approximately 7000 deaths every day, with a third not surviving the first day. Approximately 15 million babies are born prematurely, with more each year. Cost-effective interventions have the potential to decrease the related morbidity and mortality. The Every Newborn Action Plan considers breastfeeding a key component of essential newborn care, together with other interventions such as hygienic care, thermal control, and newborn resuscitation (if required). Only 44% of newborns worldwide are breastfed within the first hour of life, only 40% of infants are exclusively breastfed for 6 months, and fewer than two in three infants over the age of 1 year are breastfed.[195]

On a global level, the leading cause of death among children under the age of 5 years is preterm birth complications, with approximately 1 million deaths in 2015.[196] Reports note that approximately 40% of infants in a NICU setting do not receive their mother's milk for the first hours or days or longer.[197] Interventions are needed to increase human milk intake by direct breastfeeding, pumped milk, Kangaroo Mother Care, and pasteurized donor human milk, when needed.[197] Infrastructure and equipment on a global level are needed for pasteurizing, screening, and storing human milk for later use. This can be achieved with innovations to lower costs that enable low-resource settings to achieve the same safety and quality as high-resource settings.

CULTURAL ISSUES PERTAINING TO MILK SHARING

Parents' cultural beliefs, attitudes, and practices should be explored before using donor milk. This is because culture plays a role in the beliefs, attitudes, and practices concerning the use of donor human milk. Several studies have revealed that the parents' acceptance of donor human milk may depend on a cultural component such as religion, country of origin, age, parity, breastfeeding experience, and level of education.[198–202]

A small study of 174 postpartum inner city New York women compared the attitudes for those whose infants were receiving care in the NICU or regular nursery.[198] Results revealed that women with post–high school education believed that donor milk was beneficial. US-born mothers had knowledge of donor milk when compared with foreign-born mothers; however, that did not correspond to believing that donor milk was better to use than formula. Banked donor milk was more apt to be accepted rather than informal milk sharing from a friend or relative by mothers whose babies were in the NICU than those in the regular nursery. The authors recommended that educational interventions to increase awareness and knowledge of donor milk banks become a public health initiative to increase acceptance.

Informal and formal milk sharing may not be acceptable for all families because of religious considerations. For example,

Islam has a concept called *milk kinship*, whose origin is derived from a passage in the *Qur'an*: "Prohibited to you (for marriage) are your milk mothers who nursed you and your sisters through nursing" (*Qur'an*: Surat al-Nisa 04:23) and refers to situations in which an infant receives breast milk from someone other than the mother.[202] In practice, milk kinship means that a wet-nurse, her family members (maternal and paternal), and all those that she breastfed become "milk siblings" and are forbidden to marry. Implications of milk kinship are that donor breast milk by informal or formal sharing may not be acceptable to those following Islamic law because of concerns that "milk siblings" will marry.

Because of the issue of milk kinship, an acceptable means of sharing human milk has been sought. Several initiatives have been reported, such as those in Malaysia,[203] Kuwait,[205] and Turkey.[202] Approximately 20 years ago, in Kuwait, a milk sharing program was introduced in which mothers were able to share their human milk in a culturally acceptable manner.[204] Likewise, in Malaysia, a study was conducted on 48 infants who were hospitalized (42 in the NICU and 6 on the pediatric unit).[203] Mothers of infants hospitalized in the NICU or pediatric units who were in need of human milk were introduced and given time to speak with healthy mothers in the rooming-in unit who had enough milk to donate and expressed a desire for donated human milk. This was undertaken to ensure that future milk kinship would not occur, because the women would know which mother had donated her milk to which infant. Written informed consent was obtained. Conditions for using donated human milk were that the donator was negative for HIV and syphilis. The donated milk was frozen for 72 hours at $-20°C$. The donated human milk was unpasteurized, frozen-thawed. The authors reported that this endeavor of using donated human milk was an alternative to human milk donor banks.

Turkey was the first Muslim country to establish a human milk bank; however, it closed while in the pilot stage because of religious concerns.[202] In a recent study, the beliefs and practices of 435 Turkish mothers was examined in a descriptive, cross-sectional, web-based study. Results revealed that 85% of the respondents would not share milk, whereas 50% used formula and only 11% and 4% were donors or recipients, respectively. Although the overwhelming majority of mothers were not comfortable donating or receiving shared milk, 77% of the mothers thought it necessary to establish a human milk bank in Turkey.

In a scholarly explanation of milk kinship and acceptable ways to provide human donor milk to those infants in need, Ghaly[205] provided a detailed analysis pertaining to the complex issues regarding Islamic concept of milk kinship. The author presented the religious guidelines (fatwa) of the Egyptian born scholar, Yūsuf al-Qaradāwī's 1983 religious law ruling that establishing human milk banks and using the human milk from these banks is acceptable. This ruling was ultimately accepted in 2004 by the European Council of Fatwa and Research, based in Dublin, Ireland for Muslims living in non-Muslim countries.[206]

At the present time, there are no known Western-style milk banks in the Muslim world. Several health care professionals and scholars have proposed possible solutions to make milk banking permissible in Muslim countries. In a commentary published in the *Journal of Paediatrics and International Child Health*,[207] the authors, Alnakshabandi and Fiester, suggested a voluntary database that they entitled the Conditional Identified Milk Banking System (CIMBS), in which donors' and recipients' identities are accessible in a voluntary registry and milk pooling would be limited to three donors. Khalil et al.[199] proposed a different solution of establishing milk banks in which there would be a single known donor and recipient or more than three unknown donors. These proposals seem to be culturally competent approaches that may be feasible in Muslim countries in which families can preserve their beliefs and practice regarding milk kinship while providing donor human milk to infants when needed.

Breastfeeding for the first 2 years of life is recommended by Jewish Law (*Talmud* Ketubot 60 A). Eidelman[208] writes that the *Talmud* gives allowances to breastfeeding mothers with laws endorsing food and employment conditions that promote the quantity and quality of breast milk. He concludes that because the *Talmud* explicitly focuses on the positive values of human milk and breastfeeding it is understandable that Jewish women may have a deep religious and cultural commitment to breastfeeding.

Informal and formal milk sharing are permissible in Judaism, and the Old Testament attests that women in Biblical times shared their milk (Exodus 2:9). For many Jewish women, milk sharing is considered a religious imperative because it is a means of assisting others *(chesed)* and saving a life *(pikuach nefesh)*. The *Talmud* statement that "he who saves a life, saves the whole world" (Sanhedrin 37 A) can be applied to donor human milk. A recent qualitative study of 14 ultra-Orthodox women reported that these mothers commonly engaged in milk sharing to support hospitalized at-risk infants.[209] Jewish law includes keeping dietary requirements known as *kosher*, which includes special restrictions. For that reason, women in the ultra-Orthodox Jewish community may request that donor human milk be obtained from donors who observe Jewish dietary laws.[210]

Health care professionals should possess cultural knowledge about the reasons that families may not use human banked milk as an option. Parents may be hesitant to discuss cultural issues with health care professionals. Cultural beliefs and practices pertaining to donor human milk can influence health care decisions. Health care professionals can discuss possible options so that parents can make informed decisions.

The Reference list is available at www.expertconsult.com.

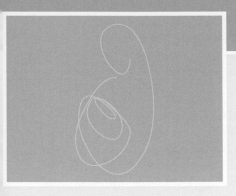

23

Infant Feeding After a Disaster

Cindy Calderon-Rodriguez and Lawrence Noble

KEY POINTS

- The care and feeding of infants and young children after any disaster is an important priority, because they are vulnerable as a result of their total dependence on adults for survival. Breastfeeding is the recommended way to feed all infants, and after a disaster it is often the safest way available.
- Even with maternal dehydration, malnutrition, or limited food intake, mothers' milk will provide proper nutrition in the initial phase of recovery until further aid arrives. Human breast milk contributes bioactive factors that are both nutritive and protective against diarrhea and respiratory illnesses and supports the infant's developing immune system.
- Challenges and circumstances after a disaster will vary according to the type of disaster and the degree of preparedness to deal with them. Under inadequate hygienic

conditions and limited clean water and food supplies, the use of formula may increase infants' risk for illness as a result of contamination. Breastfeeding mothers have the safest method to provide for infant nutrition, and the most beneficial aid is providing direct support, nutrition, and clean water to mothers to continue breastfeeding.
- To mitigate infant morbidity and mortality in disasters, it is necessary to include breastfeeding support and safe infant feeding strategies in preparedness plans. This should include keeping the family together (at least mothers and infants), creating safe environments for breastfeeding and infant feeding, providing education and support for pregnant and breastfeeding women, and arranging for ongoing assessment of infant and child hydration and nutritional status.

BENEFITS OF BREASTFEEDING AFTER A DISASTER

Among the many priorities to address in a disaster scenario are the care and feeding of infants and young children, vulnerable because of their total dependence on adults for survival. When a disaster strikes, caretakers and parents will be expected to be feeding infants younger than 6 months one of three options: exclusive breastfeeding, breastfeeding combined with baby formula, or exclusive baby formula.[1] Infants older than 6 months would also be receiving complementary foods. Under normal living conditions, breastfeeding is the recommended way to feed an infant, and after a disaster becomes the safest way available, even in infants older than 6 months, until supplemental food is available.[1–8] Breastfeeding has the advantages of providing nutrients required for growth and being ready to feed, at the adequate temperature, and without the need of supplies or clean water. It also has the additional benefits of providing warmth and comfort to the infant and the mother in the mist of the chaos after a disaster.[1,4,7] Even with maternal dehydration, malnutrition, or limited food intake, mother's milk will provide proper nutrition in the initial phase of recovery until further aid arrives.[1,3–5,8,9] Not only does it provide needed nutrients, it

also provides immunoglobulin A, many bioactive factors, and live cells with protective immunologic properties contributing to protect the gastrointestinal tract against infectious diseases that cause diarrhea, a protective benefit for the immature immunologic system and gastrointestinal tract of the infant and against respiratory illnesses.[1,3–5,7,10–12] Infants are at a higher risk for both during a disaster because of poor hygienic and adverse environmental conditions and increased risk for contamination in overcrowded living conditions in shelters.[4,6] Given the stressful circumstance encountered in such disaster situations, mothers may require additional support to establish successful exclusive breastfeeding in disaster situations because of unexpected changes in their living circumstances and to overcome emerging challenges and barriers.

PREVIOUS EXPERIENCES FEEDING INFANTS

Challenges and circumstances after a disaster will vary according to the type of disaster and the degree of preparedness to deal with it. A family with an infant who are fleeing a war scene will face different challenges and needs than a family fleeing a life-threatening forest fire, or a family sheltering from a hurricane; however, they all will have the common need of protecting their infant and procuring safe feedings.[4,13] Various authors have categorized different types of disasters into large categories: natural disasters and "human-made" disasters; and further subdivided human-made disasters into technologic and industrial, terrorism, and complex (meaning conflicts or wars).[4,13] Natural disasters can include hurricanes or cyclones, tornadoes, floods, avalanches, mud slides, tsunamis, hailstorms, droughts, forest fires, earthquakes, and epidemics. Terrorism or various forms of violence as disasters include bombs or explosions, release of chemical materials, biologic agents, radioactive agents, and intentional fires. What is important is the disruption of life, safety, food supply, and risks to health that occur with any of these disasters and how to respond to them given the available or unavailable resources.[4,13]

Earthquake: Indonesia, 2006

Previous disasters have provided opportunities to better understand the emerging needs of infants and how to improve disaster plan preparation, as well as prioritizing breastfeeding and safe infant feeding. In 2006 a severe earthquake struck Indonesia, causing the estimated death of about 6000 lives, 60,000 injured people, and hundreds of thousands displaced from their homes. Data obtained in a survey in the recovery phase after the disaster suggested a significant increase in the prevalence of diarrhea in infants after an earthquake (29%) compared with 1% to 7% before the earthquake with the prevalence twice among those who received donations of infant formula (25.4%) compared with those who did not (11.5%).[14] The authors associated this rise to the changing feeding practices and artificial feeding in conditions of poor sanitation and hygiene after the disaster. They also observed a protective effect of breastfeeding, with decreased incidence of diarrhea among these infants.[15]

Earthquake: Haiti, 2010

In 2010 Haiti suffered a major earthquake, measuring 7.3 on the Richter scale, that killed over 220,000 people, injured 300,000, and caused the displacement of 1.5 million. The local and international nongovernmental organizations (NGOs), established baby tents in shelter camps, offering infant nutrition counseling throughout the areas affected by the earthquake, with the main purpose to promote and sustain optimal infant feeding practices while reducing the health risks associated with unsafe infant feeding practices in the emerging precarious conditions.[16] Baby tents offered safe private havens for mothers to receive breastfeeding support by trained counsellors and their own peers.[16] These tents were instrumental in implementing and sustaining breastfeeding in the population and safe infant feeding practices. Volunteers providing support described how besides technical support to establish effective breastfeeding, they had to provide education to counter the cultural belief that breast milk is spoiled after a mother suffers an emotional shock such as an earthquake.[17] Other challenges to establish breastfeeding are low prevalence of breastfeeding before the disaster, the health care provider's lack of skills in providing support, and mother's confidence

in breastfeeding undermined by the indiscriminate distribution of formula.[6,10,12] The baby tents in Haiti were able to overcome these challenges and helped promote breastfeeding and safe infant feeding.[16]

Hurricane: Puerto Rico, 2017

In September 2017, Puerto Rico was hit by two major hurricanes, Irma and Maria, that caused the destruction of the electrical grid and communications network, disruption in the water supply, and damage to homes and infrastructures. People who lost their homes were sheltered in government-run facilities or in relatives' homes. Because of the severe damage, rebuilding the infrastructure and electrical grid took a prolonged time, forcing many families to survive with no electricity, tap water, and limited access to basic supplies. Promoting breastfeeding and safe infant feeding became a priority of the local government and local and international NGOs that provided aid. In the recovery phase, obstetricians handed out water filters to pregnant and postpartum women to provide a safe source of drinking water for mothers and to promote breastfeeding. This was a collaborative effort between the Puerto Rico District of the American College of Obstetricians and Gynecologists (ACOG); the American Academy of Pediatrics (AAP) Puerto Rico Chapter; the Women, Infants, and Children (WIC) program; and the Puerto Rico Department of Health denominated the "Water for Milk" initiative.[18] A group of lactation consultants created *Alimentacion Segura Infantil* (Safe Infant Feeding) and with the support of Save the Children visited communities training leaders on safe infant feeding practices and providing breastfeeding and relactation support to mothers.[19] A similar initiative was accomplished by the Liga de la Leche under the sponsor of the International Medical Corps. A total of 150 women successfully relactated under the guidance of the Puerto Rico Chapter of La Leche League International when most of the island lost electricity and had trouble accessing tap water and other basic needs for months. The success of these women demonstrates how providing support and motivation to mothers may help them achieve relactation. A campaign promoting breastfeeding was sponsored by the local health department through radio and local newspaper, the only means of mass communication for months. Lessons learned were incorporated by the Puerto Rico Department of Health in the updated policy statement, *Alimentacion infantil segura en emergencias* (Safe Infant Feeding in Emergency), to improve preparedness and response plan (2019).[20]

CHALLENGES IN FEEDING INFANT FORMULA AFTER DISASTERS

Depending on the specifics of the disaster and its interference with the mother's ability to provide appropriate nutritional food for her infant (see Table 23.1), various infant feeding options include continued breastfeeding with guidance and support, relactation to breastfeeding if the mother had stopped before or during the disaster, pasteurized donor human milk (if available and safe), informal donor milk (from women volunteering to directly feed another woman's infant or providing expressed milk to the mother for use for her infant), and, finally, when no other options are available and safe, providing mothers and infants with ready-to-use standard formula. For any of these options, health authorities should make public health recommendations specifically related to the ongoing circumstances and lactation consultants can provide specific information, guidance, and support for continued breastfeeding, relactation, and use of pasteurized donor human milk or informal donor human milk.

Although the recommended alternative from breastfeeding in normal living conditions is infant formula until the age of 12 months, safely feeding formula may be a challenge because of multiple adverse conditions after a disaster.

Concentrated powder baby formula requires a safe source of clean water, which may not be readily available after a disaster, to prepare the formula, and to clean the bottles and nipples. If the use of formula is necessary, ready-to-feed formula is recommended over concentrated powder.[1,5,6,10] Therefore caretakers who use formula should adopt additional precautions to ensure safe infant feeding or modify their infant feeding practices.

A clean space dedicated to formula preparation, decreasing the risk for contamination, also will be indicated.[3] Formula also requires specific recommended temperatures for storing and transporting, to avoid spoiling, which under the circumstances after a disaster may not be easily achieved. A surplus of powdered and ready-to-feed baby formula may accumulate from well-intentioned recovery aid efforts that, if not properly

TABLE 23.1 Consequences of Specific Challenges After Various Disasters.

Challenges After a Disaster	Consequences for the Population	Consequences for Pregnant Women, Mothers, Infants, and Young Children
Loss of home	Dependence on the conditions and supplies of shelter, either official shelter or at relative's home. Overcrowding in shelters with increased risk for transmissible diseases and deterioration of sanitary conditions (shared bathrooms, limited source of water and cleaning products). Exposure to extreme temperatures, cold or hot.	Separation of infant or young child from mother. Higher risk for transmissible diseases in infants (vulnerable because of immature intestinal and immune system). Lack of privacy for breastfeeding mothers. Lack of clean area specifically assigned for formula preparation. In infants and young children evaporation loss is higher when skin is wet or cold, and they are less able to cope with temperature problems, with higher risk for hypothermia.
Damage to water supply or water treatment plant	Lack of a source of tap water. Risk for dehydration. Risk for contaminated water supply. Dependence on bottled water or oasis.	Risk for dehydration in breastfeeding mother, maternal dehydration (>10%) likely affecting milk production. Lack of a safe source of water to prepare formula. Increased risk for diarrhea in infants because of contaminated water with a higher risk for dehydration from vomiting and diarrhea after exposure to contamination.
Damage to electrical grid	No electricity to preserve perishable food, cook, or boil water. Limited services in hospitals, primary care practices and immunization clinics because of lack of electricity and structural damage. Loss of vaccines as a result of prolonged electrical and refrigeration failure. Short supply of gasoline and diesel because of increased demand to operate equipment with electric power generators.	Limited resources to boil water to prepare formula. Increased risk for transmissible diseases prevented by vaccines.
Damage to communication grid and internet	Lack of communication with agency and organizations that provide aid. Lack of communication with family members. No digital access to obtain cash, use credit cards or ATM to pay for food and services.	Mothers unable to purchase formula or obtain formula.
Damage or blockage of roads and bridges	Transportation routes for distribution of food, water, and aid blocked, increasing food shortage. Isolation of populations.	Food and water shortage for pregnant women, mothers, infants, and young children. Formula shortage.

(Continued)

TABLE 23.1   Consequences of Specific Challenges After Various Disasters.—cont'd

Challenges After a Disaster	Consequences for the Population	Consequences for Pregnant Women, Mothers, Infants, and Young Children
Damage to ports (airport, seaport, river port)	Limited arrival of food, water, and aid.	Food and water shortage for pregnant women, mothers, infants, and young children. Formula shortage.
Damage to health care services	Limited medical supplies and medicines because of interruption in distribution of supplies. Limited number of pharmacies and primary care services because of damage to structures or lack of electricity. Overcrowding in hospitals and emergency rooms because of limited availability of urgency medical services.	Limited access for sick pregnant women, mothers, infants and young children, increasing infant mortality and morbidity risk.
Environmental issues	Poor air quality because of debris in air and smoke. Poor air quality, increased risk for accidental poisoning with electric power generator emissions. Garbage piles in communities (debris and human activity) with increased transmission of disease by vectors (rats, roaches, flies, etc.). Toxins or radioactive elements leaked into the environment.	Increased risk for health complications for vulnerable populations, pregnant women, mothers, infants, and young children. Infants and young children because of higher minute respiratory volume have increased risk from exposure to inhaled agents. Infants and young children have a higher body surface area with an increased risk for skin exposure. Skin is thinner and more susceptible to injury from burns, chemicals, and absorbable toxins. Nuclear fallout and heavier gases settle lower to the ground, where children breathe, affecting children more severely. Increased risk for thyroid cancer from radiation exposure.
Malnutrition	Food shortage as a result of food contamination or interruption in distribution. Lack of cash to purchase food. Isolated community.	Food and water shortage for pregnant women, mothers, infants, and young children. Formula shortage. Separation of breastfeeding mother and infant.
Psychological	Posttraumatic stress.	Infants and young children at risk for posttraumatic stress and separation anxiety. Pregnant women and postpartum mothers at risk for maternal depression.

ATM, Automated teller machine.
Adapted, in part, from Berman S, ed. *Pediatric Education in Disasters Manual.* American Academy of Pediatrics; 2009.

managed, may become spoiled. Under the stressful situations after a disaster, mothers may be physically and emotionally drained and confused. If breastfeeding is not adequately supported, they may resort to infant formula, which may be readily available. In the presence of formula that is not distributed in a targeted manner to infants who will require it, mothers may choose to feed their children formula instead of breastfeeding. Readily available formula may undermine breastfeeding mothers' confidence in their capacity to feed their infant, because of their lack of confidence in producing enough milk, or cultural beliefs related to poor quality of their milk because of stress.[2,4,6,9,16] It may also incorrectly influence mothers to think that formula is a better alternative than breastfeeding. Another consequence is that mothers may combine breastfeeding with formula, resulting in a dwindling breast-milk supply.[4] If the amount of formula provided to the disaster area declines, these infants will be in danger of developing malnutrition. Under inadequate hygienic conditions, the use of formula

may increase their infants' risk for illness from contamination.[3,4] Therefore breastfeeding support and encouragement are even more critical in these disaster situations. Breastfeeding mothers have the safest method to provide for infant nutrition, and the most beneficial aid is providing direct support, nutrition, and clean water to mothers to continue breastfeeding.

PREPAREDNESS PLANS TO SUPPORT BREASTFEEDING AND SAFE INFANT FEEDING AFTER A DISASTER

To mitigate infant morbidity and mortality in disasters, it is necessary to include breastfeeding support and safe infant feeding strategies in preparedness plans. Health care professionals have a leading role in their communities to identify emerging needs and advocate for implementation of strategies to ensure the safest and most effective way to feed infants.[21,22] Proposing strategies in emergency response and preparedness plans serve to guide emergency relief agencies, organizations, shelters, and hospitals for a better response. The following are strategies to be considered when developing and adopting protocols to address challenges faced in feeding infants after a disaster (Box 23.1 and Box 23.2):

- Strategies to *determine the population to be served* in shelters, including a census of infants and children by age groups (younger than 2 months, 2 to 6 months, 6 to 12 months, 12 to 24 months, older than 24 months), pregnant women, and breastfeeding women and determining their feeding needs.[2,3,10] This allows the identification of mothers who will require support to sustain breastfeeding and of infants who will require an alternative safe feeding method if mothers are not breastfeeding or absent. By conducting a careful evaluation of infant and young child feeding requirements, the unnecessary offering of formula to breastfeeding mothers may be avoided. Breastfeeding women and pregnant women

---

BOX 23.2 Challenges to Implementing a Safe Infant Feeding Plan

- Lack of knowledge and policies on supporting breastfeeding and safe infant feeding by agencies and nongovernmental organizations that coordinate and provide aid after disasters.
- Lack of training on supporting breastfeeding and safe infant feeding methodology for administrators, staff, and volunteers in shelters.
- Lack of strategies to incorporate volunteers with knowledge and skills to provide support for breastfeeding and safe infant feeding in shelters and/or aid teams.
- Acceptance and untargeted distribution of unsolicited breast-milk substitute.
- Low prevalence of breastfeeding in affected population before disaster.
- Myths and cultural beliefs: Mother's milk is spoiled due to stress; hungry mothers do not produce enough milk.

BOX 23.1 Disaster Preparedness Planning

Strategies for Safe Infant Feeding

- Determine the population census and type and amount of food required to be served in shelters.
- Prevent the separation of mothers and infants during evacuation transport and sheltering.
- Establish a monitoring/tracking and reunification plan for those who do become separated.
- Create specific areas designated for pregnant women and breastfeeding mothers.
- Provide education and counseling to pregnant women and breastfeeding mothers on arrival at the shelter.
- Promote exclusive breastfeeding.
- Include breastfeeding support specialists in the aid community to help support breastfeeding, teach and supervise relactation and hand milk extraction techniques if necessary.
- Support the successful initiation and establishment of exclusive breastfeeding by mothers of newborns before discharge from birthing hospitals.
- Provide feeding options for orphaned infants, infants who are separated from their mothers, and/or whose mothers cannot lactate. Refer to the American Academy of Pediatrics algorithm.
- Implement safe formula feeding if formula is to be used.
- Prefer ready-to-feed formula over concentrated formula.
- Implement procedures for the preparation of formula in a clean, sanitary, and uncontaminated area assigned for this purpose and used only if bottled or boiled water is available.
- Procedures to ensure the safe storage, feeding, and distribution of purchased and donated infant formula for infants who, despite best efforts, will need formula.
- Facilitate procedures to sanitize hands before preparing formula, feeding infants, extracting milk manually, or using breast pumps.
- Implement trainings for emergency relief agencies (all staff and volunteer workers) to ensure adequate implementation of strategies that appropriately support and protect breastfeeding.

---

should be included on the priority list for clean water and food.[1,7,11,14] If there is a shortage of safe, complementary foods for infants older than 6 months of age, mothers can be assured that their milk can contribute significant nutrition in the absence of other foods for the first year after birth and beyond.[1,23]

- Strategies to *keep families together* and prevent separation of mothers and infants during evacuation transport and sheltering, as well as a monitoring and tracking and reunification plan for those who do become separated during an emergency.[6,7,10,21] Reunification as soon as possible helps decrease families' anxiety.
- Specific areas designated for pregnant women and breastfeeding mothers: create a haven, providing security, counseling, clean water, food, and a *safe environment for breastfeeding* or expressing milk, including providing a private area or a way to breastfeed discreetly if the mother desires it.[3,5,11,12]
- Strategies to *provide education and counseling to pregnant women and breastfeeding mothers* on arrival at a shelter regarding the importance of breastfeeding their infants, and assurance and further support to sustain and increase their milk supply.[1,5-7] Mothers should be assured that stress does not cause their milk supply to dry up and that even malnourished women can breastfeed successfully. Breastfeeding mothers should be encouraged to exclusively breastfeed as much as possible and taught that optimal human milk supply is maintained by infant demand, and further supported by appropriate nutrition and hydration for the mother.[6,7,14]
- Breastfeeding support should include *assessment of the lactating infant's hydration and nutritional status.*[1] Those who give birth during a disaster period should be advised of the life-saving importance of breastfeeding and should be supported in initiating and continuing exclusive

breastfeeding. Mothers who previously breastfed may be able to reestablish milk production.[1,5] This would require breast stimulation by the child suckling at the breast while continuing to feed the infant from a wet nurse, donated human milk, or available formula while establishing the production of breast milk. Even women who previously did not breastfeed may try establishing breastfeeding with appropriate stimulation and by following relactation strategies.[1,2,5] Highly motivated mothers with support of knowledgeable professionals may establish adequate milk production and wean from formula.

- Strategies to *include breastfeeding support specialists* in the aid community to help address the difficulties that may arise for mothers to sustain breastfeeding after a disaster and teach mothers relactation skills and milk extraction techniques if necessary.[5–8,12] Maintaining good attachment and positioning during suckling are necessary to successfully initiate and sustain breastfeeding and may require the support of a person who is knowledgeable in the correct technique for breastfeeding (attachment and position).[3,4]
- Strategies to *educate mothers on how to express milk by hand*, in case mother and infant are separated and breast pumps are not available, so as to not interrupt milk production, avoid mastitis, and serve as a human milk donor to other babies until they are reunited with their own, if determined to be the best action.[1,5]
- Strategies to support the successful initiation and establishment of exclusive breastfeeding by mothers of newborns before discharge from birthing hospitals.[1,8,12] The implementation of the recommended Baby Friendly Steps has demonstrated an increase to the prevalence of breastfeeding on discharge.[5,24] After a disaster, hospitals contribute in the recovery phases by complying with these recommendations and including in their preparedness plan strategies to support breastfeeding.
- Strategies for *optimal feeding options for orphaned infants*, infants who are separated from their mothers and/or whose mothers cannot lactate.[1,5,6,8,14] When a mother's own milk is not available, the next best option is the use of pasteurized donor human milk, which may not be feasible in the early recovery phase if no refrigeration is available to transport and store it. Another option is termed *"informal" human milk donation*—that is, wet nursing, delivered by direct breastfeeding, or feeding babies expressed human milk from volunteers, delivered immediately by using disposable cups or clean bottles and nipples.[1,5,8,10] If informal human milk donation is used, the parent or person responsible for the baby must be informed of the risks and benefits of feeding unpasteurized human milk to babies, such as the possibility of transferring disease from the donor through contaminated milk, even if the risk is minimal. "In populations where there is a high prevalence of human immunodeficiency virus (HIV) infection, the risk to infants of being infected with HIV through breastfeeding should be carefully weighed against the risk of their becoming seriously ill or dying from other causes if they are not breastfed" (cited from the World Health Organization "Guiding principles for feeding infants and young children," 2004).[5] The benefit of informal human milk donation over formula is that it may be readily available; it does not require mixing with water, which may be unsanitary; and it provides nutritional and immunologic protective factors, which are so important to the infant during a disaster. The use of cups for infant feeding requires trained personnel to teach caretakers the proper technique.[2,5]

- Strategies to implement *safe formula feeding*. If there is a need to feed an infant formula, the on-site health care professionals should recommend ready-to-feed formula.[1,3,7] The preparation of concentrated or powdered formula should be done in a clean, sanitary, and uncontaminated area assigned for this purpose and used only if bottled or boiled water is available.[3] Water that has been treated with iodine or chlorine tablets should be avoided, except as a last resort, because of the risk for errors in the concentrations of these substances in the water when these methods of disinfection are used.[25] Bottles and nipples used for feeding also must be clean.
- Strategies to ensure the *safe storage, feeding, and distribution of purchased and donated infant formula* for infants who, despite best efforts, will need formula.[5,6] Acquisition and distribution must consider the special dietary needs for certain formulas for those babies who are formula fed, for example, those who will require soy-based formula. Ready-to-feed formulas should be chosen over other formulas that require preparation requiring access to bottled or clean water supply to mix into the formula before feeding.[1] Formula feeding, besides clean storage containers, bottles, and nipples, will also require cleaning supplies: water, soap, brushes, clean surface, and access to bleach or heat to sanitize feeding utensils. It will also require a space that is not a bathroom to prepare, store, and clean items, which may be a challenge in a shelter situation. In circumstances where there is limited access to clean water, bottles and nipples can be hard to clean effectively; therefore disposable cups ought to be made available. Emergency relief volunteers should be trained on how to safely cup feed infants.[10]
- Strategies to include *clean containers, bottles, and bottle nipples* in the list of supplies for immediate infant feeding available to store pumped human milk.[12] The use of breastfeeding supplementary feeding devices and breast pumps should be considered only when their use is vital and where it is possible to clean them adequately. If human milk is to be pumped for storage, adequate refrigeration must be available.
- Strategies to *implement hand sanitizing* before preparing formula, feeding infants, pumping milk manually, or using breast pumps. Hand washing with water and soap is the recommended practice, but in the absence of clean water, hand sanitizing may be accomplished by using an alcohol-based hand sanitizer that contains at least 60% alcohol.[25]
- Training for emergency relief agencies (all staff and volunteer workers) to ensure adequate implementation of

strategies that appropriately support and protect breast-feeding.[6,7,10] Trainings should consider including provision of emotional support to pregnant or breastfeeding mothers, fathers, and other family members, so that they understand why it is critical for mothers to continue breastfeeding, remain hydrated, and receive appropriate nutrition and support. Staff and volunteers' cultural expectations and personal experiences may represent barriers to understanding and implementing breastfeeding support and need to be addressed.[3,5,6,10]

In overcrowded conditions, the risk for contagious disease spreading is higher. Prioritizing lactating women and children in vaccination campaigns may help minimize infection risk. Lactating women should be immunized as recommended for adults and adolescents to protect against measles, mumps, rubella, tetanus, diphtheria, pertussis, influenza, *Streptococcus pneumoniae, Neisseria meningitis,* hepatitis A, hepatitis B, varicella, and polio.[1] It is highly recommended that mothers are vaccinated for influenza to protect their infants, who may not be vaccinated until reaching 6 months of age. Antibiotics and other medications can be given to lactating women during a disaster, because they are usually compatible with breastfeeding.

Infant feeding practices and resources should be assessed, coordinated, and monitored throughout the disaster. Families affected by the disaster who are not in a shelter (e.g., at home) also benefit by support efforts to sustain breastfeeding.

These strategies should be developed, trained, and practiced before a disaster by all personnel and volunteers (Table 23.2).[26] Recruiting volunteers from the community in the development of preparedness plans and providing aid should be considered to maximize the implementation of the recovery plan when disaster strikes.

BREASTFEEDING AND RADIATION EXPOSURE

In situations in which there is contamination with ionizing radiation and radionuclides, such as after a nuclear accident, questions arise pertaining to the safety of breast milk in contaminated mothers and of the proper management and treatment of mothers and infants. A leak or explosion at a nuclear reactor site may cause radioactive materials to be released into the air causing contamination of soil, food, and water.[27] External contamination of clothes and skin and internal contamination by inhalation of contaminated air with volatile radionuclides or contaminated dust or particles may occur to exposed populations.[27] The effects of radiation on exposed persons will depend on the amount of radiation absorbed by the body (the dose), the type of radiation, and how and for how long the person was exposed.[28] Exposure to high doses of radiation increases the risk for developing cancer later in life. Children are at a higher risk because of their accelerated organ and tissue growth and longer life span.[22] Previous nuclear accidents, Chernobyl (1986) and Fukushima (2011), released radioactive iodine (RAI) and radioactive cesium

(RAC).[28,29] RAI is rapidly taken up into the thyroid gland, increasing the risk for thyroid cancer.[30] Epidemiologic studies of the effects of the Chernobyl accident report that there was a 30−60 fold increase in thyroid cancer in children over the expected rate; who were 0−4 years of age when exposed to the radiation.[30,31] Children are particularly vulnerable because they have higher minute ventilation than adults and are therefore at a greater risk for breathing in more of the aerosolized particles.[28] Nursing mothers who are near the affected area may be exposed to internal contamination, and radioactive material can be passed to babies through their breast milk.[28,32] RAI is actively transferred into mammalian milk, both human and bovine, contaminating these sources of nutrition. If contaminated water is used to mix formula for babies, it serves as another source that can cause or lead to internal radiation exposure. Treatment with potassium iodine (KI) accumulates in the thyroid and blocks the RAI absorption for the next 24 hours.[31] It does not block RAI from entering the body and cannot reverse the effects caused by RAI once the thyroid is damaged.[27] It does not protect other parts of the body from RAI, nor does it protect the body from other radioactive elements. The protective effect of KI is most effective displacing the absorption of RAI when administered in the first 4 hours after exposure but will also depend on how fast it is absorbed and distributed in the blood to the thyroid.[27] Because all infants have the highest risk for getting thyroid cancer after being exposed to RAI, the Centers for Disease Control and Prevention recommends that all infants should receive a single dose of KI, including breastfed infants.[33] Administering more than 1 dose of KI to newborns younger than 1 month old increases their risk for developing hypothyroidism; therefore other protective measures should be used.[31] Breastfeeding women should also take only 1 dose of KI if they have been internally contaminated with (or are likely to be internally contaminated with) RAI. They should be prioritized to receive other protective action measures. KI is available in two forms (KI), tablets (130 and 65 mg) and liquid (65 mg of KI/mL) (Table 23.3).

Higher doses of KI, or more doses than recommended, may not offer additional protection and may represent a risk for severe illness or death. KI should be taken only on the advice of public health or emergency management officials, closely their recommendations.[34] The AAP 2018 Policy Statement recommends that local governments have available stockpiles that can be readily distributed immediately after exposure, increasing its effectiveness in the first 4-hour window.[28]

Relevant to breastfeeding mothers, the AAP recommends that mothers who are temporarily exposed to nonlethal levels of RAI should continue to breastfeed if appropriate doses of KI are given to her and the infant within 4 hours of the contamination.[28] The levels of radiation exposure, availability of KI treatment, and availability of human milk substitutes may determine recommendations for decisions related to continuing breastfeeding.[29] If local water supplies are contaminated, formula and cow milk also may be unsafe; therefore ready-to-feed formula may be an option, if available. Infants' thyroid function should be monitored, and if hypothyroidism

TABLE 23.2 Resources for the Development of a Safe Infant Feeding Plan

Carolina Global Breastfeeding Institute (CGBI): Resources for lactation and infant feeding in emergencies https://sph.unc.edu/cgbi/cgbi-resources-l-i-f-e-support-basic-kit	Links to additional resources to develop a safe infant feeding plan, including posters to support strategies for implementation
Infant Feeding in Emergencies (multilingual), La Leche League International https://www.llli.org/breastfeeding-info/infant-feeding-emergencies-multilingual/	Links to resources for infant feeding in emergencies (multilingual)
Operational Guidance on Infant Feeding in Emergencies (OG-IFE) version 3.0 (Oct 2017) Interagency Working Group on Infant and Young Child Feeding in Emergencies IFE Core Group; co-led by the Emergency Nutrition Network (ENN) and UNICEF, eight languages https://www.ennonline.net//resources/operationalguidancev32017	Recommendations to develop a safe infant feeding plan after a disaster, available in eight languages
Emergency Health and Nutrition, IYCF-E Toolkit: Rapid start-up resources for emergency nutrition personnel. This IYCF-E Toolkit was made possible by a grant from the USAID Technical and Operational Performance Support (TOPS) program in addition to Save the Children's Innovation, Development, Evaluation and Action (IDEA) Fund https://sites.google.com/site/stcehn/documents	Document available on Google drive for download. Recommendations for developing and implementing a safe infant feeding plan
Pediatric Education in Disasters Manual https://www.aap.org/en-us/advocacy-and-policy/aap-health-initiatives/Children-and-Disasters/Documents/peds-full-eng_2012.pdf	Training modules on disasters, Section V on feeding programs in disaster situations
Disaster Planning: Infant and Child Feeding, Center for Disease Control and Prevention (CDC) https://www.cdc.gov/nccdphp/dnpao/features/disasters-infant-feeding/index.html	Information and recommendations on safe infant feeding and links to resources to develop safe infant feeding plan
Infant Feeding During Disasters, Office of Human Services, Emergency Preparedness and Response (OHSEPR), Administration for Children and Families, US Department of Health and Human Services https://www.acf.hhs.gov/ohsepr/resource/infant-feeding-during-disasters	Information and advice for safe infant feeding
Infant and Young Child Feeding in Emergencies, United States Breastfeeding Committee http://www.usbreastfeeding.org/emergencies	Information and links to resources for safe infant feeding
Infant Feeding in Emergencies Module 1 For emergency relief staff Authors: World Health Organization (WHO), United Nations International Children Education Fund (UNICEF), Linkages Project, International Baby Foods Network (IBFAN), Emergency Nutrition Network (ENN) https://www.who.int/nutrition/publications/emergencies/ife_module1/en/ Infant Feeding in Emergencies Module 2 Version 1.1 For health and nutrition workers in emergency situations for training, practice, and reference Authors: ENN, IBFAN-GIFA, Foundation Terre des hommes, CARE USA, Action Contre la Faim, UNICEF, United Nations High Commissioner for Refugees (UNHCR), WHO, World Food Programme (WFP), Linkages Project https://www.who.int/nutrition/publications/emergencies/ife_module2/en/	Training modules on safe infant feeding from the WHO

TABLE 23.3	Potassium Iodide Dosing to Block Radioiodine Accumulation With Exposure
Age	**Dose**
FDA Dose Recommendation for Internal Contamination With RAI	
Newborns up to 1 month	16 mg PO single dose
Infants and children older than 1 month to 3 years	32 mg PO single dose
Older than 3 years to 12 years	65 mg PO single dose
12 years to 18 years (<150 lb)	65 mg PO single dose
Adult dose (including breastfeeding women and adolescents older than 12 years who weigh >150 lb)	130 mg PO single dose

FDA, US Food and Drug Administration; *PO*, orally; *RAI*, radioactive iodine.
Modified from US Department of Health and Human Services, US Food and Drug Administration, Center for Drug Evaluation and Research. Guidance: potassium iodide as a thyroid blocking agent in radiation emergencies; 2001. https://www.fda.gov/drugs/bioterrorism-and-drug-preparedness/radiation-emergencies, https://www.fda.gov/media/72510/download.

develops, thyroid hormone therapy should be instituted. Infants and mothers should have priority for evacuation and food supply.[1,28,34] If KI is not available, nursing mothers should consider temporarily stopping breastfeeding and switching either to stored breast milk (that was pumped before the exposure) or formula if safe formula is available. Formula supplementation should be provided as a temporary solution until KI becomes available or until public health authorities declare breastfeeding safe again. The outside of containers of formula and feeding supplies should be cleaned with a damp cloth or clean towel. Nursing mothers who temporarily discontinue breastfeeding are recommended to pump and discard it to maintain their milk production and avoid mastitis until it is safe to restart breastfeeding.[1] If no other source of food is available, the mother should continue to breastfeed after taking the precautions to wash the nipple and breast thoroughly with soap and warm water and gently wipe around and away from the infant's mouth.[28]

Medical treatments, such as Prussian blue and diethylenetriamine pentaacetate (DTPA), limit or eliminate internal contamination with other radionuclides.[28] Prussian blue reduces the time that RAC and thallium stay in the body, by trapping it in the intestines and passing it out in the feces. DTPA binds to radioactive plutonium, americium, and curium, decreasing the amount of time these radioactive isotopes are in the body. These treatments cannot prevent radioactive isotopes from entering the body but by early administration may help decrease damaging effects on the body. They may be administered to all infants and children younger than 12 years of age and breastfeeding women, following the recommended doses and the recommended treatment for the specific radionuclides targeted.[28] These medications have specific radionuclide targets with minimal or no effect on others.

During the 2011 earthquake and tsunami in Japan, there was damage to the nuclear reactors in Fukushima, resulting in a radionuclide spill. Concerns were raised related to maternal contamination with RAI and therefore infant contamination by breast milk. Dr. Ruth Lawrence was interviewed, and her opinion summarizes the recommendations previously discussed. She expressed that "It's better to breastfeed unless there's absolute proof that it's dangerous," emphasizing that the many benefits of breastfeeding—hydration, nutrition, and protection against infection and disease—become even more important after a disaster. "You have to look at the alternatives, too," she added. The water used to mix formula may have been the original source of the mother's contamination. To stop breastfeeding in that case would not only deprive the baby of all the considerable benefits of nursing but would still allow radiation to concentrate in the child. Nursing mothers who are taking KI to prevent a buildup of iodine-131 should not stop breastfeeding while taking the pills, because the benefits of the medicine are safely passed to the infant through the breast milk. "You have to look at the risk-to-benefit ratio," she explained. "It's not that nursing under these conditions is completely safe—but it is likely the best response to a bad situation."[35]

When deciding the best actions to implement after a disaster to deliver aid, two major principles should guide the decisions: Do the least harm and deliver the aid after assessing the needs of the affected population. Assuming what the population needs without proper evaluation and without including the voices of the affected communities may entail incurring the mistake of providing unnecessary aid or causing further harm.

The Reference list is available at www.expertconsult.com.

24

Establishing a Breastfeeding Medicine Practice or Academic Department

Casey Rosen-Carole

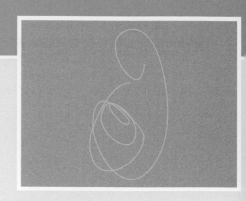

KEY POINTS

- Breastfeeding is unique in medicine as a process that occurs at the juncture of (at least) two interdependent physiologies, those of the lactating parent and of the child. Although much can be known about lactation by all types of providers, expert breastfeeding medicine providers have a role in treating complex problems facing lactating families.
- There are increasing numbers of breastfeeding medicine clinics and programs at academic institutions. These programs vary widely in funding, billing, sponsoring department, and involvement with lactation consultants.
- Some features common to building these programs include choosing a model type, business plan considerations, access, liability issues, and integration with community agencies and lactation consultants.

Practices that serve the medical needs of breastfeeding families are on the rise. At first, these practices were led by visionary physicians who noticed that the physiology and pathology of breastfeeding parents and infants were not being addressed by the medical field.[1] Parents and lactation consultants have long thought this to be true, and studies continue to document not only the poor support families receive from the health care system, but also the devastation brought on by policies and procedures that directly interfere with lactation.

A combination of factors has led to an expansion of both clinical sites devoted to serving breastfeeding and academic programs that also expand education and research surrounding lactation. These include rising breastfeeding rates, increasing percentages of women in medical fields, increasing complexity of pregnant patients and newborns, improved interdisciplinary support of patients, increasingly empowered medical students, and increased public health focus on breastfeeding as a human right. One survey of members of the Academy of Breastfeeding Medicine (ABM) and the American Academy of Pediatrics identified 32 academic breastfeeding medicine programs across 7 countries (25 of the 32 were in the United States); 75% of these were housed in pediatrics units.[2]

Given the fact that this is a relatively new and expanding phenomenon, there is also a need for guidance surrounding the development of breastfeeding medicine practices and academic departments. Although significant differences exist around the world with respect to paying for health care, certain commonalities will be discussed here, to the extent possible.

WHO IS A BREASTFEEDING MEDICINE PROVIDER?

Breastfeeding medicine providers may be initially trained in a variety of fields, but generally have the knowledge and expertise to address common and uncommon breastfeeding problems. There have been breastfeeding practices established by advanced-practice professionals (nurse practitioners, physician assistants), midwives, and physicians. Physicians may come from obstetrics and gynecology, pediatrics, family medicine, preventive medicine, surgery, or other fields. The ABM is a "worldwide organization of medical doctors dedicated to the promotion, protection, and support of breastfeeding," and is developing a standard canon of knowledge to which an expert in breastfeeding may be held. In the absence of clear guidelines, a breastfeeding medicine provider should be up to date with standard breastfeeding knowledge and practices, have advanced knowledge of the anatomy and physiology of lactation and suck, and have extensive experience managing complex breastfeeding difficulties.

CHOOSING A MODEL TYPE

Good medical care surrounding breastfeeding can be provided in many ways. The type used in a particular community should take into account (1) what is feasible and sustainable; (2) the primary needs of the community, as identified by community activists and services, parents, lactation consultants, broad types of medical providers, students, and employees; (3) who the local champions are; (4) where the money is or should come from (business analysts, marketing directors, and office managers may have important input about the types of successful programs in a particular area); and (5) what already exists for parents and babies in the communities served. These factors may help determine which would be the most streamlined approach and where the barriers are likely to arise.

Needs Assessment

Given that those who control budgets are unlikely to be familiar with breastfeeding medicine programs, formal or informal needs assessment data are often useful in bringing attention to the needs of the community. A brief analysis may include strengths, weaknesses, opportunities, and threats/barriers (SWOT) analysis for such a program.[3] This may include data that are already available surrounding rates of disease, economic variables, marginalized communities, or access concerns. They should also include information about numbers of births and other important pregnancy variables such as maternal and infant mortality rates, maternal complications rates, and an estimate of the numbers of families who struggle with breastfeeding in a community. Standard numbers used may include the fact that worldwide 80% to 90% of women have reported at least one problem with breastfeeding[4,5] or that over 40% of women do not meet their breastfeeding goals.[6,7] If a neonatal intensive care unit (NICU) is part of the plan, data surrounding mother's own milk use, donor milk use, costs of donor milk programs (if any), rates of necrotizing enterocolitis and bronchopulmonary dysplasia, length of stay, and breast milk/breastfeeding on discharge are numbers that are likely to exist. When considering an academic program, it is critical to break these numbers out by race or geography to ensure that marginalized populations are served equally. Tools to help guide needs assessments are widely available; an example is a free community needs assessment workbook by the Centers for Disease Control and Prevention. Global and local data on breastfeeding outcomes tend to be available from local health authorities. References useful for a needs assessment or business plan for the creation of a breastfeeding medicine practice or department are readily available on the web.

Types of Models

Different types of models may be used based on the needs of the community and the SWOT analysis, including the following:

- A primary care physician with advanced training in breastfeeding who blocks time for breastfeeding/lactation medicine visits
- A breastfeeding medicine provider embedded in a primary care practice or obstetric/midwifery practice
- A stand-alone breastfeeding medicine clinic
- A university-supported or academic breastfeeding medicine clinic

Types of Providers

Each type may include a variety of providers to meet the needs of the community, including a primary provider, such as a physician, midwife, or advanced care practitioner (nurse practitioner, physician's assistant, etc.), and lactation consultants, lactation counselors, social workers/postpartum therapists, and occupational or feeding therapists. In some communities, home visitors, grant-supported trained counselors, peer counselors, doulas, massage therapists, chiropractors, acupuncturists, craniosacral providers, herbalists, or practitioners of traditional medicines may be part of a lactation community. Inclusion of these types of providers may enrich the tapestry of support for breastfeeding families. Getting paid for these types of providers will vary based on geography. There is one report of a "trifecta" model, in which good outcomes were seen with a provider, lactation consultant, and social worker who saw each dyad at each visit.[8] Other models have successfully included health care providers trained as lactation counselors.[9] Finally, many currently used models with two lactation consultants and one provider working a half day together, referring to a variety of other specialists as needed. For management of ankyloglossia, one report included an otolaryngologist working with a speech language pathologist, although breastfeeding outcomes were not reported.[10]

Because the skills and credentialing for breastfeeding medicine providers is in development, and there exist many certification pathways for the other lactation supports, it is important to ensure that each provider has adequate training and safe practice to care for patients.[11] Specifically, lactation consultants should have their international board certification (IBCLC). For academic programs with NICU or complex care, nurses with advanced training (e.g., registered nurses) with an IBCLC should be strongly considered. Physicians should have, or be working toward, their Fellowship in the Academy of Breastfeeding Medicine (FABM) designation.

BUSINESS PLAN

A business plan, if required, will need to consider spending and revenue. It has been our experience that within 1 to 2 years, a breastfeeding medicine practice that is adequately reimbursed can be cost neutral to positive. Spending may include salaries of providers and support persons; rent for space; supplies needed; any office supplies, scheduling, and record-keeping costs; liability, malpractice, license, and insurance costs; and marketing needs (for events, flyers, advertising, and giveaways). Revenue considerations may include estimated patient volume, time to achieve that volume, predicted reimbursement, procedures billed, any supplies sales, and which department(s) or program(s) will cover costs. Programs that are supported between departments may be able to come to scale more quickly, because two budgets are being used. Proposed departments include pediatrics, neonatology, obstetrics, midwifery, general pediatrics, public health, family medicine, and preventive health.

Supplies Needed

Table 24.1 includes supplies useful to have when establishing a practice for the care of advanced problems with breastfeeding. Table 24.2 highlights needs specific to in-office frenotomy procedures.

TABLE 24.1	**Specific Supplies Useful in Establishing a Breastfeeding Medicine Practice**
One Time	**Recurring**
• Couch or bench	• Nipple shields in different sizes
• Foot stool	• Pump kits (including flanges, attachments, bottles, tubing)
• Medical-grade infant scale	• Flanges in different sizes (to attach to pump parts for fittings)
• Pillows: Breastfeeding specific or general, pillowcases	• Supplemental nursing systems or KITS (5-French feeding tubes, 30- to 60-mL syringes, paper tape)
• Towels, sheets, and gowns (will need laundering)	• Breast pads
	• Gloves
	• Tongue depressors
	• Q-tips
	• Disposable breast pads
	• Gel pads, nipple creams, as desired
	• Measuring tapes for babies

TABLE 24.2	**Supplies Needed to Perform Scissors Frenotomy in a Breastfeeding Medicine Practice**
One Time Recurring, Sterilization/ Cleaning Costs	**Recurring**
• Headlamp	• Sweet-Ease
• Blunt-tip tape scissors (to cut the ruler)	• 3-mL syringe
• Probe and groove director, sterile (these are also available as disposable)	• Disposable sterile ruler, 6 inch (with millimeter marks)
• Curved iris scissors or straight, as desired, sterile (these are also available as disposable)	• Emergency kit:
	• Silver nitrate sticks
	• Neo-Synephrine spray
	• Gauze, sterile
	• Q tips

Billing Considerations

In areas in which billing takes place, several barriers have been encountered by those starting practices, including the following:

1. A primary care physician cannot bill as a specialist without a separate tax identification number (ID) in the United States. Therefore a first step in creating an independent practice will be determine under which tax ID billing should be done. If between departments, the nonprimary department's tax ID may be used (e.g., an obstetrician and gynecologist with a secondary appointment in pediatrics could use a pediatrics tax ID). Alternatively, a new tax ID could be created.

2. Breastfeeding medicine providers at academic programs almost universally described not being reimbursed for their services.[2] Although this model may persist with adequate passion and support, it is unlikely to be sustainable or lead to growth. Breastfeeding medicine is a medical service with a specific area of expertise and should be reimbursed as such.

3. Insurers should be notified that a visit for a breastfeeding dyad (or triad, or more) is reimbursed as a visit for the parent/mother and a visit for the infant/child. This means there are at least two different notes, two physical examinations, and two separate plans. When these criteria are met, reimbursement has proceeded successfully with

insurers, although negotiation may be required at the local level.

DOCUMENTATION TO SUPPORT SOUND CLINICAL PRACTICE, FOR BILLING, AND TO LIMIT LIABILITY

Documentation

To clearly communicate maternal/infant medical concerns and interventions, notes should be comprehensive and in both the child/children and the lactating parent's medical chart. This will also support billing, if applicable. Some payors may require different notes in each chart. In addition, privacy considerations may mandate that consent is obtained to share visit information with other care providers, or that some information is limited when sharing consult notes. In these cases, in general, the history of present illness, birth history, and assessments will be similar if not the same. Other parts, including a review of systems, the medical history, physical examinations, and plan will vary. In general, we recommend collecting and documenting the following information:

• History:
  • Lactating parent/mother's history of present illness, review of systems, current depression, medical history,

surgical history, family history of breastfeeding, breast changes in pregnancy, parental leave, family support, and social history, including smoking and tobacco smoke exposure

- Infant/child review of systems, medical history, surgical history, family history of tongue tie or speech delay, and social history, including sleep location
- Latch assessment, weights before and after feeds
- Infant/child physical examination, including tongue assessment using standardized tools (e.g., Hazelbaker, Coryllos),[12] neck assessment, skin assessment for jaundice, other assessments as indicated
- Parent/maternal physical examination, including breasts, nipples, axillae, and other assessments as indicated
- Any procedures done, including pump fitting, frenotomy, supplemental nursing system, or hand expression for breast-milk culture
- Assessment and plan

Because breastfeeding medicine providers care for both parents and children, and training and certification of said providers is unclear, legal liability may be a concern. To date, there has been one breastfeeding medicine case in which the provider was sued. In this case, a woman who developed breast cancer years after being seen for breast pain while breastfeeding brought suit against the breastfeeding medicine clinic. This case was presented by the provider and lawyer at one of the annual meetings of the ABM International Conference. The clear documentation of clinical examination findings and follow-up was considered essential in clearing the physician in the case of wrongdoing and is an important point to consider when considering one's own legal liability.

In our experience, the highest acuity settings for breastfeeding medicine providers, and those in which providers should demonstrate excellent documentation include infants with failure to thrive, parent refusal to supplement, infant fever, maternal use of medications or drugs that may affect the infant and any counseling done, any testing or signs of retained placenta, sequelae of maternal hemorrhage, breast masses, and mastitis management with abscess.

To mitigate risk, providers may consider the following:

1. Clear documentation of all clinical work in parents and children's charts is essential. For instance, even if a pediatric provider cares for an infant and diagnoses thrush, then also treats the mother for painful nipples, this encounter and any physical examination findings should be documented in the mother's chart as well as the child's. This should occur regardless of primary patient being billed and is true in the converse setting as well (i.e., primarily maternal issue, documentation in the infant's chart).
2. Clear communication with the primary care provider is sound clinical practice and may decrease liability. As in the case described previously, any maternal physical findings or treatments should be communicated with the mother's primary care or obstetric provider(s).
3. Follow-up plans are also essential to appropriate care, but should be clearly documented, with the burden of responsibility clearly stated. That is, if a patient should call if pain persists, this should be stated. Conversely, if a provider will follow up with a patient to determine improvement or discuss laboratory test results, this, too, should be clear.
4. Considering privacy is important when sharing notes between parent and infant charts. For instance, in a clinical situation with two mothers (one inducing lactation, another birthing the baby) and an infant, there may be three or more providers caring for these patients, and clinicians should be careful that parents have agreed that visit information can be shared. In addition, providers can consider removing some information from parent and/or child charts before sending, depending on clarity and local laws (see earlier discussion on documentation).
5. Providers should ensure their notes meet standards of compliance and privacy and should consider sharing examples of notes with their legal office. Ensuring that these departments understand the unique scenarios that develop in breastfeeding medicine may help if a clinical situation is later questioned.

COMMUNITY INTEGRATION, ACCESS, AND FOLLOW-UP

Community Integration and Noncompetition With Other Providers

To provide the best care, breastfeeding medicine providers should meet and work with others involved in lactation in their community. Given the novelty of the field and historically low breastfeeding rates, there is rarely an abundance of support. Therefore creating local support networks is likely to be helpful to patients. In some communities, lactation consultants may be the only other providers of care. In other areas, midwives, other medical providers, occupational therapists, social workers, body workers, chiropractors, and doulas may support breastfeeding mothers. Lactation consultants or other supports may or may not have experience with breastfeeding medicine or may be concerned about competition. Meeting, establishing fair referral practices, and helping to support their missions will be helpful in creating collaboration. Regular meetings on topics that have historically caused dissent can be helpful and may prevent parents from receiving conflicting information. Such topics are likely to differ geographically, but in our area have included ankyloglossia diagnosis and management, contraception and milk supply, informal milk sharing, nicotine replacement products, postoperative pain control and breastfeeding, diversity and equity in support services, and breast abscess management.

Ensuring Access to Care

In many communities internationally, persons with lower incomes or less access to health care are least likely to receive appropriate medical care and have lowest breastfeeding rates. For example, in the United States, it has been shown that women who identify as African American or black have lower rates of breastfeeding and live in communities with less support. This has also been seen in many other analyses, such as India, where those in the rural south have been found to have less prenatal care and lower breastfeeding rates,[13] and Ethiopia.[14]

Breastfeeding medicine providers can be leaders in supporting breastfeeding parents and should be attentive to issues of inequity in medical care. Some considerations when building a practice will therefore include the following:

- *Geography and transportation:* Is the clinic site accessible to those with lower incomes? If not, how might services extend to such communities? (e.g., telemedicine, satellite office days in other practices, telephone consulting services, medical transportation assistance, etc.)
- *Race, ethnicity, and inequity:* Providers should consider which groups tend to be left out of breastfeeding conversations and support in the provider's area and strive to improve their access to care. Who are the leaders in those communities and what ideas do they have to improve care? (e.g., helping to train lactation consultants of color, considering offering services at community centers, specialized support groups, ensuring marketing materials are representative of the communities they intend to serve, etc.)
- *Affordability:* Providers should consider which payment options may be offered and whether reduced rates, sliding-fee scales, or free drop-in groups may be offered.
- *LGBTQI + services:* With improved access to fertility options and adoption, families identifying as gender expansive or LGBTQI + (lesbian, gay, bisexual, transgender, queer, questioning, intersex) will require increased access to lactation care. International standards for such care are being developed (see Chapter 20). Providers should ensure their office is a welcoming atmosphere with well-trained staff and gender-inclusive language.

Triage and After-Hours Care

Access to care includes how to offer advice and care when the office may be closed. Breastfeeding medicine services are likely to be offered by a small group of providers and lactation consultants, and staffing may not be adequate to provide after-hours access to care or weekend care. Despite this, families will use the clinic as a primary site for concerns over infant feeding and breast care, some of which may be urgent. Therefore considering how evenings, weekends, and holidays may be covered is of crucial importance. Some ideas include the following:

- Sharing an after-hours call center with an obstetrics and gynecologic or pediatric practice, which can triage basic problems, or connect patients with their primary provider in the case of an urgent medical situation or emergency
- Working with in-hospital lactation consultants to check messages on weekends
- Creating an on-call system with providers and lactation consultants, using expanded staff as needed
- Training triage centers or secretaries in basic breastfeeding triage and ensuring access to triage supports (books, materials), such that urgent issues are not inappropriately deferred.

INPATIENT ROUNDING AND SUPPORT

Although it can be initially unclear to those in traditional medical fields how breastfeeding medicine providers can support the inpatient service, hospital lactation consultants may quickly realize the value of collaboration with breastfeeding medicine providers. Opportunities for clinical work, quality improvement, research, and medical education can be found across departments.

Medical Direction

An academic hospital may consider appointing a medical director to coordinate these services, a growing trend. A review of academic programs in 2017 found that of the 32 medical directors of lactation in academic programs, 75% of programs were created in the preceding 10 years and 34% in the preceding 2 years.[2] Given that care of lactating persons necessarily spans at least two departments, it may be useful to appoint breastfeeding medicine providers between several, including obstetrics, pediatrics, family medicine, and/or preventive medicine. This distributes staffing costs, leverages resources, minimizes risk for lost revenue, and facilitates inclusion of breastfeeding priorities into departmental projects.

Support of Lactation Consultants

Direct support of hospital/network lactation consultants should form the bedrock of any successful breastfeeding medicine program. With adequate staffing, lactation-specific leadership, and educational support, lactation consultants can be the first experts to be involved in advanced breastfeeding problems. For example, a breastfeeding family whose infant is readmitted for failure to thrive should be provided with a thorough lactation consult, including a review of medications, pump practices, physical assessments, and a plan for immediate and long-term breastfeeding support of the parents while the infant is evaluated and managed. The breastfeeding medicine provider may be called if there are concerns for infant oral anatomy, maternal milk production, etc., which require diagnosis and treatment. Using this model, clear scope of practice should be determined by the team, with frequent communication about cases and procedures to best assist lactating families.

Unfortunately, many lactation departments are underfunded, to the detriment of both normal deliveries and more complex neonatal intensive care or readmission cases. Although no current guidelines exist, we suggest using the 2010 United States Lactation Consultants Association (USLCA) recommendations and the full-time equivalents (FTE) calculations provided by Mannel and Mannel[15,16] (e.g., 1 FTE for 783 deliveries; 1 FTE per 235 infant admits to NICU; 1 FTE per 1292 outpatient dyads; 1 FTE per 818 outpatient follow-up NICU). Essentially, lactation coverage should be ensured in the hospital setting 7-days per week, all days of the year, and on multiple shifts. All shifts may need to be covered if bedside nursing care is not adequate because of competing priorities or training.

Although lactation consultants are rarely licensed, they often function at a nursing level, and their certification maintenance requires provider-level continuing education. We therefore also suggest that programs provide stipends and opportunities for continuing education, along with requirements for certification, professional growth, and peer review.

Where Do Breastfeeding Medicine Providers Consult?

Breastfeeding medicine consults can inform a wide range of clinical scenarios on inpatient services, including:

- *Birth centers/normal deliveries:* Early diagnosis and management of ankyloglossia, delayed lactogenesis 2, mammary hypoplasia, maternal medication use, maternal substance use/abuse
- *Neonatal intensive care units:* Prenatal consultations on medications, anatomy, breastfeeding a high-risk or premature infant, postpartum early identification and management of low milk supply, breast-milk contaminants, ankyloglossia versus premature suck, rapid management of maternal infections such as candida nipple infections and mastitis
- *Inpatient pediatrics:* Failure to thrive assessments (ankyloglossia, maternal milk supply), maternal medication review, parental substance abuse
- *Inpatient obstetric/medicine:* Mastitis and sepsis, pumping protocols for comatose patients, pain management considerations with breastfeeding
- *Emergency departments:* Mastitis management with or without abscess, medication reviews
- *Surgical/imaging:* Medications, anesthesia, pumping in the operating rooms

What Else Can Breastfeeding Medicine Providers Do for Hospitals?

Breastfeeding medicine providers will also be able to consult on and create a wide range of quality improvement projects, including disseminating best practices for infant and child feeding (e.g., Baby Friendly Hospital Initiative, hand expression, and colostrum care), management of specific conditions (e.g., cleft lip/palate, parental substance abuse), and parent–patient relations. They can also promote and support employee lactation, ensuring policies are in line with best practices and any legal requirements, advocating for lactating employees with human resources and space planning, and building lactation support programs for employees returning from parental leave.

SUMMARY

Breastfeeding medicine practices serve as centers for breastfeeding and lactation knowledge and function to serve all breastfeeding infants, women, and families in support of breastfeeding. Beyond that they should provide "specialty care" for complex and difficult health situations during lactation and breastfeeding. They should also optimize access to breastfeeding knowledge and care in a truly equitable manner. Within the broader medical profession, the practice and the lactation specialists should provide ongoing education for the next generations of lactation specialists, especially clinical experience in breastfeeding medicine, and potentially even serve as a center for lactation and breastfeeding research.

To achieve these goals, the establishment of a breastfeeding practice or academic department should be built on an open needs assessment within the medical and broader community, collaborating directly with both those communities to foster an open and equitable collaboration. In this way, the model of practice can be chosen and developed to fit the specific needs and goals understood through the needs assessment.

The Reference list is available at www.expertconsult.com.

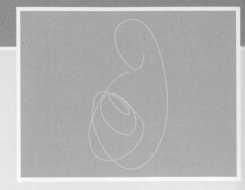

25

Breastfeeding Support Groups and Community Resources

Ruth A. Lawrence

KEY POINTS

- Breastfeeding success requires support for the mother from individuals, groups, and organizations.
- Peer breastfeeding support is important in any of its forms—personal, group, and professional (e.g., lactation consultants).

- The needs of breastfeeding mothers and their families call for the continued growth and development of governmental and nongovernmental organizations for the protection, promotion, and support of breastfeeding.

SUPPORT FOR BREASTFEEDING

The transition into motherhood, through pregnancy, childbirth, breastfeeding, and on to the extended period of child-rearing is a challenging metamorphosis. In traditional societies, the mother has most often been supported, instructed, and cared for through this transition by the women of her extended family and her community. The African proverb "it takes a village to raise a child" also can be applied to breastfeeding; it takes a community to breastfeed a child. That is to say, the new mother and family need information, instruction, advice, encouragement, and support to successfully breastfeed an infant. The question is, what form does that support take? It can come directly from sisters, mothers, mothers-in-law, aunts, friends, neighbors, doulas, lactation consultants, and other medical professionals. Sometimes, in the absence of access to those one-on-one relationships, there is a need to get additional support from breastfeeding support groups and community resources for infant feeding and child-rearing. This chapter focuses on the development and the nature of such support groups and resources for breastfeeding. Appendix G provides a list of various groups and organizations that promote and support breastfeeding.

HISTORICAL PERSPECTIVE

Rites of passage were described by the French author Van Gennep[1] as the ceremonies and rituals that mark special changes in people's lives. The list includes marriage, motherhood, birth, death, circumcision, pubescence, graduation, ordination, retirement, etc. In present day cultures, the recognition of these transitions takes many forms. In some situations, educational, physical, psychological, and emotional support exists for the period of change and adjustment. The support needed and desired by the mother and family continues to evolve for

pregnancy, childbirth, and lactation. Anthropologist Dana Raphael emphasized in her writing and lecturing that the most critical rite of passage in a woman's life is when she becomes a mother. Raphael further distinguished this period of transition with the term *matrescence*, "to emphasize the mother and to focus on her new life-style."[2] Traditional cultures herald a mother giving birth, whereas current cultures tend to "announce" the birth of an infant. The former highlights the mother, the latter the infant. Matrescence is a time of caring for and supporting the mother as she adds new responsibilities and roles to her life. This includes instructing, advising, and supporting the mother in breastfeeding through the entire period of lactation, 6 to 12 months and longer. Over time, various factors in our societies and culture diminished the occurrence of breastfeeding along with the support for breastfeeding. Mothers increasingly were working outside the home, which led to the need for child care outside the family and different methods of infant feeding. Paralleling this was an emphasis on the "science" of infant care and feeding. Various infantformulas and foods were developed and touted as "medically approved." Adding to the momentum of the bottle-feeding trend that began in the 1920s, manufacturers were able to mass produce an inexpensive container and rubber nipple with which to feed infants inexpensively. Pediatrics evolved as a new specialty to guard the health of children. The focus was on measuring and calculating calories and nutrition and growth. Physicians seemed more secure when they could prescribe a measure of nutrition as they might measure formula. The science and technology of the infant food industry was a continuing influence on the nutritional thinking of both medical and lay groups.

Need for New Forms of Breastfeeding Support

Breastfeeding was never totally abandoned. The perception that formula was "as good as breast milk" increased, and the knowledge about breastfeeding and support for breastfeeding within the community and the medical profession diminished. Nevertheless, there were always groups of women who prepared themselves for childbirth and read and researched feeding and nutrition and chose to breastfeed.

In the mid-1940s, Dr. Edith Jackson began the Rooming-In Project at Yale University in New Haven, Connecticut. Families in New Haven who sought "childbirth without fear" and an opportunity to room-in with their infants usually chose to breastfeed. In the rooming-in unit, breastfeeding was often "contagious" because one mother successfully nursing would encourage others to try. Hospital stays averaged 5 to 7 days, during which time a mother-infant couple was cared for as a pair. More than 70% of the patients left this hospital breastfeeding. The national average of breastfeeding initiation at that time (1945 to 1955) was less than 25%.

Students and staff who were exposed to the philosophy of this unit went to many parts of the country, taking with them tremendous commitment to prepared childbirth and nurturing through breastfeeding. The classic article on the management of breastfeeding by Barnes et al.[3] was published as a result of counseling hundreds of nursing mothers. The students of Dr. Jackson inoculated many hundreds of hospitals and communities with a zeal for breastfeeding.

DEVELOPMENT OF MOTHER SUPPORT GROUPS

The need remained for mothers and nuclear families to have access to information, support, and conversation about healthy infants, mothering, and breastfeeding.

La Leche League

The La Leche League, developed by a group of seven mothers to meet these needs, was established in Franklin Park, Illinois, in 1957. The original intent was to provide other nursing mothers with information, encouragement, and moral support. Thousands of local chapters and a network of 32,000 state and regional coordinators synchronized their activities with the headquarters in Schaumburg, Illinois. La Leche League International's (LLLI's) 4000 groups are now in 66 countries, including the United States, Canada, parts of Europe, New Zealand, Africa, and other parts of the world.

An excellent publication, *The Womanly Art of Breastfeeding*,[4] was first published in 1958 (8th edition and update in 2007) by the original group of mothers involved in the La Leche League. La Leche League continues to provide information and updated publications about common questions that arise during lactation. Local groups offer classes for preparing mothers to breastfeed. They help with suggestions about the nitty-gritty details of preparation, nutrition, clothing, and mothering in general. They also provide every mother with a telephone counselor. To be qualified to serve as a counselor to another mother, a member must demonstrate knowledge and expertise in breastfeeding and an understanding of how to counsel and render support. "Telephone mothers" do not give medical advice and are instructed to tell a troubled mother to call her own physician for such advice.

Interested local physicians provide medical expertise for the group when a medical opinion is appropriate. The league provides support for mothers to reduce the time the physician needs to spend counseling on the nonmedical aspects of lactation. Most information needed by new mothers is not medical.

Doulas

In the 1960s in the United States, along with the "natural childbirth" movement, came the concept of another woman supporting the pregnant woman through the process of pregnancy, childbirth, and the postpartum period. Dana Raphael used the term *doula* to describe such an assistant in an anthropologic study and popularized that term in her book, *The Tender Gift: Breastfeeding*. A doula is described as a professional person trained to provide physical, emotional, and informational support to a mother throughout her transition into motherhood. There are various international programs to train doulas. Research supports the concept that personal, continuous physical and emotional support in addition to regular nursing care is associated with better childbirth outcomes.[5-7] Additional data demonstrate the benefits of doulas into the postpartum period and specifically for increasing duration and exclusivity of breastfeeding in black and Hispanic mothers.[8] Other forms of breastfeeding support in addition to La Leche League are available. Similar programs have been developed as needed to provide support based on local and cultural practices of breastfeeding and infant nutrition in more than 70 other countries. Examples of such programs include the Ammehjelpen International Group in Norway, the Australian Breastfeeding Association, and in the United Kingdom the National Childbirth Trust.

The Breastfeeding Association of South Africa is an example of a nongovernmental, nonprofit, voluntary organization. It was founded in 1978 by South Africans for the express needs of South African women. Their particular issues and solutions are well described by Bergh.[9]

Individual Groups and Special Needs

Support groups for all of life's events, especially those covering health and specific illnesses, have become commonplace. Pregnancy and prenatal classes have evolved to provide mothers and fathers with information and support through pregnancy and childbirth. In the broader field of perinatal care, groups are available for infertile couples; couples who are expecting; those who have experienced pregnancy loss, loss of a premature infant, or loss of a term baby; those who had a cesarean delivery; and so on.

Adolescents are an example of a subset of women who need special support to improve the outcome of their pregnancies, to encourage them to breastfeed, and to establish the special relationship with, and commitment to, their infants. A study done in the Breastfeeding Educated and Supported Teen Club in Melbourne, Florida, looked at the impact of specific breastfeeding education provided by a lactation consultant in group classes. Teens were randomly assigned to the program or as a control; ethnicity and age were not significant factors. Of the 43 adolescents in the education group, 28 (65%) initiated breastfeeding, but of the 48 control subjects without education, only 7 (14.6%) initiated breastfeeding ($p < 0.001$). The authors concluded that targeted education makes a difference in adolescents initiating breastfeeding.[10]

A similar study was performed involving low-income women using a community-based program. It examined interventions in a hospital, a home visit, and telephone support system provided by a community health nurse and a peer counselor for 6 months. After random assignment, those receiving the interventions breastfed longer. The infants in the intervention group had fewer sick visits and use of medications than the group with "standard care." The cost of the program per mother was $301, which was offset by the savings on the cost of formula and health care.[11]

In another study, adult women without a personal breastfeeding support system at home were randomized to receive or not receive support. The support group received assistance and support in the hospital and at home from a practicing midwife in the community. The midwife made daily visits to the hospital. After discharge, she telephoned within 72 hours and then weekly for 4 weeks. At home the participants had access to the midwife by phone and pager. One home visit was made the first week and then as necessary. In the supported group, 26 of 26 were still breastfeeding at 1 month, but only 17 of 25 (68%) in the unsupported group were breastfeeding, proving that intensive professional support works. The costs of the program were not provided.[12]

There are numerous other examples of effective breastfeeding support in many forms.[13] Active individualized support outreach clearly affects the duration of breastfeeding and ultimately saves health care dollars.

Peer Support Groups

There are many forms of support that have been successfully provided to breastfeeding mothers. The Centers for Disease Control and Prevention (CDC) has published a guide to various strategies for support, including maternity care practices, professional education, access to professional support, support in the workplace, breastfeeding education, and information and social marketing that positively influence breastfeeding.[13] Systematic reviews of peer support programs have found them to be effective in increasing breastfeeding.[14–16] Significant increases in initiation, duration, and exclusivity were observed among women who received support from a peer or other lay person providing the counseling. Often peer support, added to other components of breastfeeding support, leads to increased maternal satisfaction and trust in the education and care provided.

Resources

As different forms of breastfeeding support were identified to be effective there was a need to make the support readily available to all mothers. Many hospitals started to provide training in preparation for childbirth. Part of those programs were about the new infant and how to plan for neonatal care. These programs often serve as the initial stimulus to consider breastfeeding. Often such programs are given by hospital-based lactation consultants.

When a large health maintenance organization looked at 5213 new mothers enrolled in a commercial managed care plan by telephone survey at 4 to 6 months postpartum, 75% had breastfed for some time. Of these, 75% breastfed for more than 6 weeks. Breastfeeding for more than 6 weeks was associated with level of education, employment status (part-time, 84%), and adequacy of postpartum information. The authors of the report concluded that health plans and employers should consider promoting breastfeeding.[17]

Because hospitals have become competitive and are marketing their services, many are developing birthing centers and are trying to capture the attention of the childbearing public with special services. These services often include classes on child-rearing, including breastfeeding. Physicians should investigate the programs and printed materials distributed by the hospitals where their patients deliver. Pediatricians can assist mothers and families in coping with the flood of patient information from conflicting sources by being familiar with the different materials and being able to competently answer parental questions. This is especially helpful if the patients give birth at more than one hospital or more than one lay advocacy group is active in the community. Hospital procedures and policies can influence the success or failure of breastfeeding mothers.[18] Pediatricians should be aware of the policies at the hospital(s) with which they are associated and support those policies that effectively support breastfeeding.

Trusted Information and Trusted Sources

In a couple of decades, we have gone from a paucity of support groups and resource literature to an overwhelming flood. The flow is greatest over the Internet. Health care books and childbearing and family-rearing advice books are cascading off the presses, written by everyone from qualified experts to poorly informed freelance writers. Some are written by health care professionals who have personal and professional experience in childbearing. Websites, blogs, Twitter, Facebook, etc., send an avalanche of information with the smallest question or search. Physicians should be familiar with a few good references/websites for parents, provide a list of references/websites for patients to access and be ready to review the sources of information their patients are using. Along with that, physicians should openly demonstrate respect for their patients' concerns and questions, legitimize their search for information and dilemmas with inconsistent information, and support their ongoing decision-making and choices regarding infant feeding and breastfeeding.

Community Resources

Within the communities where families live are many community resources of breastfeeding information and support. The Young Women's Christian Association (YWCA) in most communities may also provide preparation for childbirth. Its classes usually provide programming that appeals to young and unwed women, a group in need of services rarely provided by other sources.

The Visiting Nurses Association and the public health nurses on the staff of the local county health department are special resources particularly skilled at counseling new mothers with their infants. They can provide valuable information to the physician who is working with an infant who fails to thrive at the breast by witnessing the breastfeeding scene at home. As discharge from the hospital occurs earlier and earlier, pediatricians should consider employing nurse practitioners who are prepared to make house calls immediately after birth.

Many other organizations, local and national in scope, have the perinatal period and the family as their focus. Many of these are also interested in promoting breastfeeding as part of their overall goals. In the United States, the United States Breastfeeding Committee maintains a directory of state/territory, cultural, and local/community organizations that support breastfeeding in all 50 states.[19] A number of these organizations provide breastfeeding support for specified cultural and community groups.

The Women Infants Children (WIC) program was permanently established in 1974 to support and safeguard the health of women, infants, and children (younger than 5 years old) who are at risk for nutritional deficiency. This is a national program available "locally" in all 50 states, including 34 Indian Tribal Organizations, and territories. WIC is administered by 90 state agencies, with services provided at a variety of community clinic locations, including county health departments, hospitals, schools, and Indian Health Service facilities. WIC has a breastfeeding support program linked to its nutritional services.[20] WIC also partners with local community organizations to develop local breastfeeding support programs.

GOVERNMENT ORGANIZATIONS

The United States government has taken an active interest in the promotion of breastfeeding.

United States Department of Health and Human Services

The breastfeeding goals for national health prepared by the US Department of Health and Human Services, Healthy People 2010 and 2020, have evolved as progress continues. Adjusted new goals for breastfeeding in 2020 include 81.9% of infants ever being breastfed, 60% of children still being breastfed at 6 months of age, 25.5% still being exclusively breastfed at 6 months of age, and 34.1% of children still being breastfed at 1 year of age.[21] These adjustments were made because of progress and expectations that these goals could be met. Various national organizations collaborate to achieve these breastfeeding goals, and these goals serve as national guideposts.

Office of the Surgeon General

The US Office of the Surgeon General conducted a national workshop on breastfeeding and human lactation in Rochester, New York, in June 1984 to develop recommendations for national policy. A publication from the workshop was available

from the US Government Printing Office in Washington, DC.[22] A follow-up workshop was held in Washington, DC in 1985, gathering the representatives of the major official national organizations for obstetrics, pediatrics, and family physicians, including the credentialing organizations for physicians, nurses, nurse midwives, and dietitians. The organizations responded to a request for each to approve a model statement in support of breastfeeding. This was accomplished by January 1987. The organizations prepared a review of curriculum within their disciplines to ensure adequate education, training, and accreditation regarding human lactation and breastfeeding for their members. Although improvements have been made and certifying examinations have incorporated questions about breastfeeding and human lactation, curriculum development in most institutions has lagged. Available curricula to solve this problem have been developed by the American Academy of Pediatrics (AAP), American College of Obstetricians and Gynecologists (ACOG), and Wellstart.

C. Everett Koop, US Surgeon General in the 1980s, maintained his commitment to breastfeeding. Twenty-five years to the day later, June 9, 2009, the Academy of Breastfeeding Medicine (ABM) convened the first summit on breastfeeding in Washington, DC. Dr. Koop opened the meeting with a televised message, the same message he concluded with in 1984.[23] The summit was directed at a different audience, not at breastfeeding advocates and supporters but the US government, its many agencies, and the health care and insurance industries. The purpose was to educate the participants on the value of breastfeeding and the necessity to support breastfeeding, including reimbursement for services provided to patients in hospitals and at home. Progress has been made. The CDC, the Office of Women's Health (OWH), and the Surgeon General took up the cause and have participated in collecting data and changing programs. In 2011 the sitting Surgeon General, Regina M. Benjamin, MD, issued the first "call to action" charge for governmental and societal support of breastfeeding.[24] Annual summits were convened, continuing to involve the government agencies, the health care industry, and insurance providers. Ten summits have been convened through 2018.[25] The ABM organized these summits with generous grant support from the W.K. Kellogg Foundation from the very first summit. The W.K. Kellogg Foundation has not only funded the summits but also has dedicated its grant resources to breastfeeding issues across the country. It now supports over 100 programs large and small. Nothing has done more to facilitate the progress of breastfeeding in the United States than the commitment of the W.K. Kellogg Foundation.

During these 10 years of summits, progress has occurred broadly across disciplines and across culture. Progress has occurred among minority groups who have formed their own organizations for breastfeeding support such as Mocha Mothers, Black Mothers' Breastfeeding Association, and Reaching Our Sisters Everywhere (ROSE) among others. Although there remain disparities in breastfeeding,[26,27] there are also documented effective interventions and ongoing initiatives.[28,29]

Through the efforts of the W.K. Kellogg Foundation and the office of the Surgeon General collaborating with other US organizations the WIC program has changed its policy to encourage breastfeeding and support breastfeeding mothers. There is a toolkit to guide employers and employees on creating support for breastfeeding mothers at work available through the Office on Women's Health.[30,31] The National Conference of State Legislatures (NCSL) maintains a listing and tracks state laws that promote and protect breastfeeding across the 50 states.[32]

US Department of Agriculture

The US Department of Agriculture's (USDA's) WIC nutrition services provides supplemental nutrition and counseling to more than 50% of US families with young children. There are large differences in rates of breastfeeding among the different racial groups in WIC. A study of services in North Carolina confirmed the racial/ethnic disparities in breastfeeding rates.[33]

The differences in availability of support services were also associated with racial/ethnic composition of the catchment area. These observations of disparity among services at WIC were also reported in an analysis of data from the Early Childhood Longitudinal Study, Birth Cohort. Breastfeeding duration was a result of cultural trends, not WIC programming. Multiple studies have done analysis outcomes at WIC sites. When the barriers to reaching the national goals for breastfeeding among the WIC population were counted, they were (1) lack of support in and outside the hospital, (2) returning to work, (3) practical issues, (4) WIC-related issues, and (5) social and cultural barriers.[34] Issues affecting breastfeeding included young age, non-Hispanic ethnicity, obesity, and depression.

Solutions that worked for local WIC programs have been peer counselors, breast pump programs, and discontinuing free formula at the hospital and by the WIC program. The major obstacle to WIC program success is budgetary. Nationally, WIC spends 25 times more money on formula than on breastfeeding initiatives.[35] The new food packages, however, implemented in the fall of 2009, have improved breastfeeding outcomes in Los Angeles County, where exclusive breastfeeding rates at 3 and 6 months have doubled.[36]

Issues of rural health have begun to include those surrounding birth and the infant's welfare. Programs are being developed to increase breastfeeding among rural women. Although the incidence of breastfeeding has increased among well-educated, self-motivated, middle-class Americans, the number of impoverished, less well-educated women who breastfeed remains small. Progress is being made, community by community, by dedicated health care workers, dietitians, and WIC staff. Health professionals often serve as a catalyst in developing such programs but should always be ready to serve as knowledgeable, supportive consultants to the efforts of groups of mothers and members of the community.[37]

The USDA's breastfeeding program, through the WIC's Nutrition Program, has launched a major effort to increase breastfeeding initiation and duration throughout the 50 states.

One of the programs, Best Start, included social marketing research, a media campaign, a staff support kit, a breastfeeding resource guide, a training conference, and continuing education and technical assistance. WIC has been made a permanent national health and nutrition program, and breastfeeding has been written into the legislation. The program even mandates that every WIC agency must have accommodations for employees who are breastfeeding their infants to pump and store their milk.[38]

Office of Women's Health

The OWH invested time, talent, and resources in the issues of maternal health overall. Out of those efforts and collaboration with other governmental groups came specific initiatives to support breastfeeding and foster breastfeeding support for working women embedded within their broad programs for women's health (general wellness, specific illnesses and conditions, reproductive health, and patient information). The OWH program for breastfeeding support includes a guide to breastfeeding, practical online information for making the decision to breastfeed, learning to breastfeed, breastfeeding challenges, pumping and storing breast milk, breastfeeding resources, and breastfeeding at home and at work. The Business Case for Breastfeeding resource maintained by OWH is an internationally recognized toolkit for employees and employers to enhance breastfeeding support for working women.[39]

Centers for Disease Control and Prevention

The CDC has a comprehensive program for supporting breastfeeding within the United States that has evolved over decades.[40] They assess, monitor, and publicize breastfeeding rates within the United States by the Breastfeeding Report Card, which is updated frequently.[41] It is shared nationally and with all 50 states as a "motivator" for ongoing breastfeeding support efforts at multiple levels nationally. It has developed an evidence-based Guide to Strategies to Support Breastfeeding Mothers and Babies, which continues to evolve.[13] It has a publication on how Hospital Actions Affect Breastfeeding for hospitals and for individuals to inform them about the important influence hospitals have on breastfeeding initiation and continuation. The publication about hospitals and breastfeeding includes the Ten Steps to Successful Breastfeeding for Baby Friendly Hospitals.[42] The CDC has also participated in the Best Fed Beginnings program and reported on the successes for improving minority breastfeeding rates in the United States.[43]

LactMed Database in the National Library of Medicine

LactMed was created by the National Library of Medicine within the National Institutes of Health (NIH), US Department of Health and Human Services.[44] This database contains information on drugs and other chemicals that might be contained in breast milk as a result of maternal exposure. It provides information on the levels of such substances in breast milk and infant blood and discusses potential adverse effects in the nursing infant based on data from the scientific literature and peer review of the presented information. Suggested therapeutic alternatives to medications are presented as well if available and appropriate. In addition to the website an application and a widget are available.

Health Resources and Services Administration, Maternal and Child Health Bureau

The Maternal and Child Health Bureau of the Health Resources and Services Administration supports over 50 million women, including half of pregnant women and one third of the infants and children younger than 5 years old in the United States. The Bureau's programs for supporting breastfeeding are located within the Title V Maternal and Child Health Block Grants (state and federal collaborative programs to support breastfeeding), Women's Preventive Services (for lactation support and publicizing the known benefits of lactation on women's health), the Healthy Start Program for healthy pregnancies and breastfeeding counselors, and the Children's Healthy Weight Collaborative Improvement and Innovation Network promoting evidence-informed practices for breastfeeding, nutrition and exercise.[45]

NONGOVERNMENTAL ORGANIZATIONS

United States Breastfeeding Committee

To fulfill a mandate of the Innocenti Declaration (1990),[46] that each country should have a national breastfeeding committee, a group of interested breastfeeding supporters and advocates met in Florida in January 1996. The National Alliance of Breastfeeding Advocacy (NABA) and the Healthy Children Project convened the first National Breastfeeding Leadership Roundtable (NBLR). This small group of breastfeeding advocates met to discuss the need for coordination of breastfeeding activities in the United States. Working on the international model created by other signers of the Innocenti Declaration, this group worked to establish a multisectoral, national breastfeeding committee composed of representatives from relevant government departments, nongovernmental organizations, and health professional associations in every country.

The NBLR proposed four major goals: (1) to support ongoing breastfeeding projects in the United States; (2) to develop a strategic plan for breastfeeding in the United States; (3) to reorganize the National Breastfeeding Leadership Roundtable into the US Breastfeeding Committee (USBC), and (4) to incorporate the organization of the USBC and its leadership. The organization continued to meet twice a year and in January 1998 voted to declare itself, with the encouragement of Assistant Surgeon General Audrey Nora, MD, the USBC.

The USBC is a collaborative partnership of organizations not under governmental control. The mission of the committee is to protect, promote, and support breastfeeding in the United States. The USBC exists to ensure the rightful place of

breastfeeding in society. Major organizations that are members include but are not limited to the ACOG, the AAP, the American Academy of Family Practice, the LLLI, the International Lactation Consultant Association (ILCA), Wellstart, and the NABA. The NIH, Maternal and Child Health Bureau of the Health Resources Division of the US Department of Health and Human Services, Women's Health, the US Food and Drug Administration (FDA), and the CDC also participated. After more than 10 years of developing its organizational skills and attracting more than 30 organizational members, the USBC has assumed a vital role in the United States' national breastfeeding activity and agenda. It has organized coalitions in all states, has hosted coalition meetings to train state representatives, and provided a forum for sharing strategies among the members. USBC is an organization of organizations, not individuals. An important effort has been to create federal legislation to support breastfeeding women. The USBC's understanding of the barriers that employment creates for working breastfeeding mothers was a major catalyst for the development of the national program, the Business Case for Breastfeeding.[31] The interdisciplinary nature of its membership and its collaborative approach are part of what has made the USBC so successful in its mission to promote, protect, and support breastfeeding in the United States.

Best Start: The Concept of Social Marketing

Using the concept of social marketing, Bryant et al.[47] designed an approach to promoting breastfeeding that used the counseling strategies, educational materials, policies, and community-based activities that formed the Best Start Program. Social marketing "combines the principles of commercial marketing with health education to promote a socially beneficial idea, practice or product."[9] Typically a well-articulated program involves a combination of mass media, print materials, personal counseling, and community-based activities and services.

From these findings, a multifaceted breastfeeding promotion campaign was designed for new mothers, family members, health professionals, and the community at large. The Best Start Program proved to be extremely successful and has been replicated by others successfully using strategies developed in social marketing and segmentation modeling for health communication.[48] Best Start developed the multimedia program, Loving Support Makes Breastfeeding Work. This program was the substance of the WIC National Breastfeeding Promotion Project launched in April 1997.[47,49] Best Start has turned the program over to WIC for its continuation.

Wellstart International

A program to extend the scope of breastfeeding promotion was launched by Wellstart International in a cooperative agreement with the US Agency for International Development (AID). Wellstart International, a private nonprofit organization headquartered in San Diego, grew out of clinical and teaching experiences at the University of California, San Diego Medical

Center in the late 1970s.[50] In 1983, in response to a clear need to improve the breastfeeding knowledge of health professionals, a Lactation Management Education program was initiated with funding from AID. Almost 400 participants of the Lactation Management Education program now form a global network of Wellstart Associates in 28 countries.

In late 1991, Wellstart joined in a cooperative agreement with AID to expand and diversify its global breastfeeding promotion activities.[50] The Expanded Promotion of Breastfeeding program can be implemented in any country, with cultural and local adaptation. Wellstart continues to provide educational information for the training of physicians, nurses, and dietitians. Wellstart was active in global events as well.[51] These activities included the development of the "Ten Steps" for hospital care of the mother—baby dyad, the Innocenti Declarations of 1990 and 2005, the formation of the World Alliance for Breastfeeding Advocates (WABA), and the initiation of World Breastfeeding Week and the Baby Friendly Hospital Initiative (BFHI).

Baby Friendly Hospital Initiative

The Baby Friendly Hospital Initiative was originally designed to rid hospitals of their dependence on artificial infant formulas and encourage the support of breastfeeding in these facilities. It is now intended to be a comprehensive program for hospitals to present a supportive atmosphere with trained and knowledgeable staff. The Ten Steps describe the essentials of the program. In 2009 the BFHI materials were revised by the World Health Organization. The program was expanded to integrate BFHI with the Global Strategy for Infant and Young Child Feeding. This revision included the expectation that staff be trained to provide support and education for mothers who were not breastfeeding. The 2009 update also included a review of labor and delivery practices. Step 4 has been extensively revised to promote skin-to-skin contact and the process of the infant finding the breast and latching on immediately after delivery. BFHI expects that every infant will spend up to an hour accomplishing the first feeding while skin-to-skin with the mother. Worldwide achievement of Baby Friendly Hospitals accreditation has been extensive. In the United States progress has been slow.

Breastfeeding and Human Lactation Study Center

The Lactation Study Center of the University of Rochester School of Medicine and Dentistry in New York encourages and promotes human lactation and breastfeeding through physician education and support. The goal is to provide information that will help practitioners encourage and support breastfeeding for all patients. Information is available to the health care professional by telephone. Originally federally funded and established at the request of the Office of the Surgeon General in 1984, the center now depends on private grants and donations from users. The drug information line operates Monday through Friday from 9 AM to 4 PM Eastern Standard Time. Physician consultation is available by call back.

LACTATION CONSULTANTS

For years, many medical and nursing professionals have served as lactation consultants ready to respond to any colleague's request for knowledge and expertise. With the increasing international movement to embrace breastfeeding, however, a new type of lactation consultant has evolved from the vast pool of women who have served in local mother-to-mother programs to help others breastfeed. The health care professional needs to ensure that the lactation resources available in the community are truly of professional quality and background and that the individuals have obtained proper education, training, preparation, certification, and licensure. Counseling on any topic is a special skill requiring more than personal experience with the situation.

International Board of Lactation Consultant Examiners

The International Board of Lactation Consultant Examiners (IBLCE) was developed as a separate organization by the LLLI to credential individuals who want to counsel about breastfeeding.[52] Those who successfully complete the IBLCE certification process, which includes a written examination, are entitled to use the designation IBCLC (International Board Certified Lactation Consultant) after their names. The IBLCE has defined lactation consultants as "allied health care providers who possess the necessary skills, knowledge, and attitudes to facilitate breastfeeding." These lactation consultants perform as employees in some situations and as independent contractors in states where the medical practice act allows such activity. A lactation consultant should have professional liability insurance coverage and a license to practice in the health field in the state. Nurses, midwives, nurse practitioners, dietitians, and physicians are commonly certified as IBCLCs.

International Lactation Consultants Association

The International Lactation Consultants Association (ILCA) constitutes an association of individuals who support lactation/breastfeeding, but not all members are certified lactation consultants.

The ILCA describes "A lactation consultant as a health care professional whose scope of practice is focused on providing education and management to prevent and solve breastfeeding problems and encourage a social environment that effectively supports the breastfeeding mother—infant dyad." The ILCA published Standards of Practice for Lactation Consultants, which is available in print and at the website http://www.ILCA.org.

Lactation Specialist as a Member of Health Care Team

Modern medicine has developed a team approach to the management of many patient populations, such as elderly or handicapped persons.[53] A team approach also is used in the management of many categories of diseases, such as cancer and diabetes. A health care team provides medical service for the family during the perinatal period. This team includes an obstetrician and a pediatrician or a family physician; nurse midwives; nurses working in prenatal care, obstetrics, neonatal care, and public health; social workers; and dietitians. When a problem develops the team can expand to include maternal-fetal medicine specialists, perinatologists, neonatologists, and the skilled team from the perinatal center. These team members are well-educated and extensively trained professionals. Together they have lowered the morbidity and mortality rates of childbirth. The long-range prognosis for the intact survival of infants has been significantly improved.

The need for information, education, and support of the breastfeeding mother and nuclear family continues. This support can come from many sources, but increasingly it is coming from the health care team. The result is a medically successful birth and a team of professionals to support the mother, father, and family and assist in their ongoing development into capable, informed parents. Ideally, education and support that begins during pregnancy continues in the postpartum period and is maintained as needed as the child grows and the family develops.

Lactation specialists become an important addition to the health care team, replacing individuals in the traditional family support system, with their expertise in the knowledge, practice, and support of breastfeeding. Specialists not only must know their role as counselors interacting with the family, but also must understand how they interact with other members of the health care team. The professional team members are beginning to understand the importance of lactation specialists and how to work most effectively with them. Some physicians, however, provide a nurse practitioner, whose role is to fill that gap between medical care and family support. The nurse practitioner is usually skilled in well-baby care, especially breastfeeding, and in the era of early postpartum discharge home, may make house calls within 48 hours of arrival home.[54]

Lactation consultants quickly earn the respect of health care teams when they communicate openly with them, support mothers in a positive manner, and encourage a relationship of mutual trust and respect between the mothers and the teams.[53]

PEER COUNSELING

Peer counseling is part of a system developed by health care providers and health educators to change personal health behavior.[55] It is an adaptation of a cultural technique that has been used for generations wherein the family provides a personal advocate/assistant to help the individual carry out good health practices. In lay midwifery, for example, members of the group attend women throughout pregnancy, delivery, and the postpartum period. The key requirements are that the peer counselor is a member of the same sociocultural group as the recipient, is selected for leadership qualities and experience, and is trained in the necessary knowledge and skill for mastery of the health behavior.

Public health programs have used peer counselors to encourage women to seek prenatal or well-child care for their children. Other programs have provided peer counselors for individuals with hypertension, diabetes, or other chronic diseases to help the patient access health care and carry out behaviors and instructions for treatment. This concept has been applied to the WIC program.[27,55] This system of support has been expanded to many parts of the country.

The most successful programs involve the peer counselor in multiple health issues so that the relationship between counselor and client continues. These peer programs are integrated with efforts to improve health habits in general and especially those associated with childbearing. The best programs train community counselors to support women through pregnancy, delivery, and early child-rearing, of which breastfeeding is a part. This type of program encourages the development of a relationship that can last several years.

Because the lowest incidence and duration of breastfeeding in the United States are among low-income women and among black mothers, a peer-support program among these clients has the highest probability of success.[26,27] Using the same model for training candidates that has been developed for other health projects has facilitated initiating the program. The local WIC program or health department is ideal for undertaking a peer-support program because the permanent, full-time staff are knowledgeable about nutrition and lactation and can provide continuity when peer counselors leave the program and new ones need training. This stability is essential to developing some consistency and permanency for the system. The WIC program supports women from early pregnancy through postpartum and early infancy periods.

Given that a peer counselor is an individual from the social or cultural community who is selected because of good health behaviors and an innate ability to help others and gain respect; a peer counselor for breastfeeding is a respected member of the community or neighborhood, is of the same or similar ethnic background and of similar educational and economic level, and has breastfed one or more children. Examples of success of peer counseling for breastfeeding include the La Leche League and peer counseling among well-educated, white, middle-class American women; a WIC program of peer counseling for a mixed population of women in Minnesota; first-time mothers in Toronto initiating breastfeeding; and low- and middle-income countries.[56–59] Peer support programs have been effective in Canada and Britain.[59,60] Systematic reviews and meta-analyses also document the benefits of peer counseling on breastfeeding successes.[61,62]

Some physician practices have employed (yes, peer counselors should be trained and paid) peer counselors successfully to take some of the roles of health care professionals who lack the time to relate on an even plane with a client of different educational or socioeconomic status. Well-established peer-counseling programs have even inspired the counselors to obtain further training as nurses' aides, licensed practical nurses, or registered nurses.

Who Shall Counsel?

Among those working closely with people in critical life situations, some people make good counselors and some equally knowledgeable people are not appropriate as counselors and should have other jobs in the organization.[53]

Counseling is a profession, and professional counselors are carefully screened, educated, and trained. Therefore individuals who help mothers breastfeed should be screened, educated, and trained as well. They should have the following special abilities:

- To listen
- To avoid judgment
- To understand other lifestyles
- To admit when they do not know something
- To seek appropriate help from professionals
- To recognize incompatibility in a given relationship

In the past few decades, peer counseling has become widespread and has been successful, not only with breastfeeding and childbirth, but also with chronic diseases such as cystic fibrosis and with devastating illnesses such as cancer. The first fact that all of these groups had to acknowledge is that experience does not make one qualified to counsel others in similar situations.

A candidate must first put personal experiences into perspective and understand the motivation for seeking this counseling role. Counseling is an opportunity to help by listening, and being a sympathetic listener is the most important quality. This is not a time to talk about the counselor's pregnancies. The counselor cannot have a personal agenda and press personal views or lifestyle choices on a mother being counseled, nor should counseling be used as a personal platform to promote organizational biases.

A counselor must understand that assuming a place on a health care team demands time and effort. One must be available at the convenience and need of a client, even when this is inconvenient to the counselor.

Learning to Help Mothers

The suggestions to guide a counselor in training must be general guidelines about attitude. The emphasis is on listening, encouraging a mother to talk, and ultimately helping her to solve her own problem by understanding it. Professional counselors are trained using didactic sessions, role-play, and supervisory sessions until skills are developed. Continued reinforcement of philosophy and techniques forms the basis of growth and improvement. A lay counselor should attend counselor-training sessions provided by the parent organization and work closely with the supervisor. Sharing counseling situations with others with more experience will give further insight. Returning to reference materials again and again will bring to light new thoughts that have been read before but not truly assimilated initially because of lack of experience.[54]

A peer counselor does not provide medical advice but can encourage a mother to contact her physician. When an infant is doing poorly or is sick, the pediatrician should be consulted promptly. The rare condition of failure to thrive while breastfeeding is increasing in frequency, paralleling the increased incidence of breastfeeding. It has serious health implications for infants and for the continuation of breastfeeding unless treatment is initiated promptly by the physician. A counselor must be able to recognize when a situation is beyond her skills and understand that a physician is powerless to help if not consulted. When an infant's problem is identified and it is prudent to continue breastfeeding, a counselor can be an invaluable asset in supporting and reassuring the mother.

Maternal problems such as mastitis should respond well if treated early, but recurrent mastitis may develop when home remedies are substituted for proper treatment. The role of a counselor in such situations is significant. Encouraging a mother to seek medical care promptly is most important. Reinforcing medical advice will further enhance its effectiveness. For example, if rest is prescribed, a counselor can help a mother understand how critical rest is to recovery and then help her determine how she is going to cope at home with family responsibilities and a newborn and still be able to rest.

The role of a counselor is support of a mother. A counselor should work in concert with the medical health care team as a team player, not as a competitor or an adversary, but as a facilitator. The mission of the team is successful lactation, a satisfying mothering experience, and a healthy infant. The health care team will continue to be responsible for a family long after lactation has been discontinued. The confidence and trust developed between the health team and family will be critical to lasting success. The counselor should be remembered as a gentle facilitator and a caring support person who was present and supportive through the rite of passage of matrescence.

A physician working with a lactation counselor or consultant needs to recognize this specialist's skills and limitations. As in other, similar situations, the physician is the leader of the health care team and carries the ultimate responsibility for education about, promotion of, and support of breastfeeding.

SUMMARY

Support for breastfeeding mothers is crucial to their success in reaching their breastfeeding goals. That support should be available and accessible for all mothers in forms that are most appropriate for them, their families, and their children. The evolution of breastfeeding support should continue along with careful assessment of its effectiveness as well as its cost-effectiveness as a public health intervention. Many examples of breastfeeding support and organizations that contribute to breastfeeding support and promotion are listed in Appendix G for your reference. As someone interested in breastfeeding, please join and support one or more.

The Reference list is available at www.expertconsult.com.

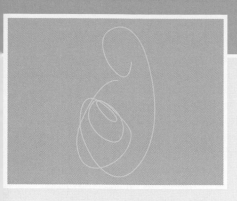

26

Educating and Training Medical Professionals

Casey Rosen-Carole

KEY POINTS

- Untrained health professionals contribute to poor breast-feeding outcomes the world over. Training the health care work force, especially providers, is an important component of any breastfeeding initiative.
- Because of the lack of training, personal experiences influence a provider's guidance about breastfeeding, leading to care that is not evidence-based.
- Many studies have shown that adequate training of health care providers improves knowledge and confidence of providers, and positively affects breastfeeding duration and exclusivity of patients.

- Successful training programs involve at least some in-person or practical components. A combined program, including some online and some in-person training, may provide health care systems with flexibility and lower costs of training while leveraging important in-person skills-based teaching.
- Including breastfeeding and lactation on medical and nursing examinations is a crucial component in ensuring that curricula adequately prepare their students to manage breastfeeding dyads.

Inadequate education of health professionals surrounding normal breast physiology, infant suck, and breastfeeding has been widely recognized as a substantial barrier to improving breastfeeding rates. For example, when a physician recommends excessive or inappropriate supplementation with formula to a mother with breastfeeding difficulties, the breastfeeding relationship often ends. Or, when a health professional fails to notify a woman that breast surgeries carry risks to breastfeeding, she may be disappointed and confused when breastfeeding does not proceed as expected. On the other hand, a health care professional who is well-educated in breastfeeding may be the strongest, or only, support a woman has in her breastfeeding journey.

PROVIDER EDUCATION ON BREASTFEEDING IN THE TWENTIETH CENTURY

Influence of Government and Health Authorities

Action on the part of health authorities to promote, protect, and support breastfeeding was a necessary component in promoting breastfeeding education for health care providers. In some countries, such action preceded public efforts to regain breastfeeding for mothers and infants. For example, Brazil's National Breastfeeding Program (PNBF) began in 1981 in response to declining breastfeeding rates after rapid urbanization. The program created policy-level changes, including a provider education requirement following the Baby Friendly

Hospital Initiative (BFHI)[1] guidelines. Brazil now has some of the highest breastfeeding rates in the world. In contrast, in the US government efforts began well *after* rates increased through grass-roots efforts of women and groups such as La Leche League, founded in 1956.[2]

In 1979 a joint meeting was held by the World Health Organization and United Nations International Children's Emergency Fund (UNICEF) on Infant and Young Child Feeding. One of the central themes discussed was the education and training of health care professionals.[3] The 1984 Surgeon General's Workshop on Breastfeeding and Human Lactation was the first US national meeting to focus exclusively on breastfeeding, and it outlined six major areas of need, one of which was the education of health care professionals. Since that time, all major health care organizations have agreed that educational institutions should be held accountable for professional training and that such accountability is essential to training professionals who are able to effectively support breastfeeding. Nevertheless, it has been an ongoing struggle to instantiate. Although many professional organizations describe requisite breastfeeding knowledge and skills for their fields, there are no consistent standards in medical education on breastfeeding and human lactation, except in midwifery.[4] In other words, it remains unclear how and when providers should obtain this necessary information. It should also come as no surprise that women who are cared for by midwives have the highest rates of breastfeeding initiation and duration.[5,6]

Providers Who Breastfeed

Many physicians rely on experience with their own children in providing breastfeeding support.[7] These providers acknowledge that their medical training on breastfeeding is inadequate. It has been shown that personal experiences influence the type and quality of advice that is given. For instance, if providers had a negative experience, they may be more likely to recommend formula during the return to work period. Unfortunately, it is common for health care workers to have challenging breastfeeding experiences; this is especially true for physicians. One study of health care workers in Nigeria found knowledge, support, and practice of exclusive breastfeeding to be suboptimal. In this study, exclusive breastfeeding was more common among nonphysicians who had good knowledge of the benefits.[8]

A provider's own breastfeeding experience may be most at risk during the years of intensive training, because of the high workload, stress, and long hours. For instance, the American Academy of Pediatrics (AAP) Section on Medical Students, Residents, and Fellowship Trainees found that 75% to 92% of resident physicians encounter difficulties with breastfeeding and about one third do not meet their breastfeeding goals.[9,10] Negative emotions in such studies are common and are reported to affect clinical interactions with patients. Residents reported feeling "frustrated," "depressed," and "devastated."[11]

In one study in Lebanon, medical trainees were found to have low breastfeeding knowledge and self-efficacy, with a poor professional network of support.[12] In response to similar findings in the United States, in 2009 a group of physician mothers started their own grassroots support group, Dr. MILK (Mothers Interested in Lactation Knowledge),[13] and have since leveraged social media to support each other in their particular struggles to breastfeed while carrying on a professional career. This Facebook group has been used by over 20,000 physician mothers for this purpose and continues to grow.

Inadequate Training

In medical education, at least, information on breastfeeding tends to be left for the clinical years, during which time a student may or may not have adequate exposure, depending on patient census or teacher preference.[14] Thereafter, learning is relegated to optional continuing education courses. Because few board questions address breastfeeding management problems, few providers will seek out this education on their own. The AAP developed an online curriculum that has been shown to improve breastfeeding outcomes of patients when cared for by trained pediatricians.[15] Unfortunately, it continues to be implemented only if passion of the local teaching staff exists. No central unified program has been developed to change the curriculum at the seats of learning: medical and nursing schools.

Changing Attitudes?

There is evidence that training on breastfeeding across physician disciplines continues to be limited. However, some evidence from the United States shows that knowledge and attitudes of

providers have changed in the past few decades. One study in a county in New York of 164 prenatal care providers found improvements in support for breastfeeding since 1993, but no change in the amount of education received: only half of respondents had received any breastfeeding education, and more found such education inadequate (54% vs. 19%, $p < 0.001$) as compared with 20 years prior. Unsurprisingly, midwives reported the highest rates of knowledge, confidence, and support. In contrast, in Nevada, a survey of 889 professionals found little change among physicians in the past 10 years, but highest knowledge and attitude scores were found amongst nurses.[16] In fact, in a national review of pediatricians' recommendations about breastfeeding, younger pediatricians were less confident than older pediatricians in managing breastfeeding problems.[17]

Providers Left Out of Decision-Making

Because of the inability of untrained physicians and providers to adequately support breastfeeding, many families seek help elsewhere. There exists, in some communities, robust lay support in the form of extended family, mother groups, lactation groups, La Leche League groups, doulas, peer counselors, mother-to-mother informal milk sharing, and home visiting programs. For management of suck dysfunction and ankyloglossia, dentists, speech language pathologists, occupational therapists, chiropractors and massage therapists may also be assisting families. Such a rich tapestry of supports has the potential to broaden and deepen our knowledge of appropriate breastfeeding support, if coordinated and collegial. Unfortunately, providers without breastfeeding education are likely left out of these discussions. In areas that lack these other supports, it is possible families will have no support at all.

PRINCIPLES OF EDUCATING PROVIDERS

Faculty Leadership and Board Questions

It has long been a concern that medical or nursing students educated on lactation exclusively by lay providers may fail to understand the impact of lactation on their own scope of practice. In contrast, professional curricula have been developed and instantiated by passionate faculty leaders. Unfortunately, such a reliance on individual passion may or may not lead to sustainable change. Rather, to provide future generations with adequate knowledge, board certification examinations must test learners on breastfeeding knowledge suitable to their field (s). In response, schools will ensure their curricular adequacy. Additionally, robust breastfeeding support at affiliated training centers at the nursing, lactation consultant, and provider levels is critical to expose learners to appropriate care and offer opportunities for hands-on learning. It is no longer acceptable for academic centers to lack evidence-based breastfeeding support for patients and learners, from a clinical or educational standpoint.

Interprofessional Education

Interprofessional education refers to the education and training of health care providers in groups combining professions usually taught in silo: medical, nursing, dental, etc. It has been shown that educating in this manner can improve provider and patient satisfaction,[18] and it is gradually becoming incorporated into medical professional education. In breastfeeding education, it may help to emphasize the importance of the topic to learners and allow for an enriched understanding of scope of practice. Various groups of providers can learn ownership of their field's management and support skills, while gaining knowledge of other fields' contributions.

Motivational Interviewing

Patient-centered communication has been shown to promote behavior change and has been widely implemented in graduate medical education.[19] Several feasibility studies using motivational interviewing for breastfeeding have demonstrated a high patient and provider acceptance rate and cost-effectiveness. A small randomized controlled trial in the United States demonstrated improvement in breastfeeding duration after a motivational interviewing-based intervention.[20] Because this technique has its origins in Euro-American psychology, its applicability in cultures that deemphasize patient participation in health care decision making must not be assumed. Indeed, using motivational interviewing in some circumstances may increase anxiety. A systematic review in Canada sought to determine its applicability in other ethnicities and cultures.[21] This review noted particular challenges in Chinese patients, and the need for cultural acknowledgment as part of counseling.

Trauma-Informed Care

Traumatic events affect health care by altering a patient's response thresholds in light of prior vulnerability. That is, a patient's behavior may be unpredictable based on the known medical history, if that history does not include facts related to prior trauma (such as ACES screening for Adverse Childhood Events Screening). A health care worker may therefore inadvertently worsen a patient's condition by disregarding potential triggers or responding inappropriately to patient defensiveness, aggressiveness or silence. The occurrence of posttraumatic stress disorder after birth has been long neglected, but has now been shown to occur in 3.3% to 18.5% of postpartum patients, depending on background risks.[22] Acknowledging the globally estimated 35% of women who experience rape or intimate partner physical or sexual violence in their lifetimes,[23] breastfeeding women are, therefore, likely to have had experiences of trauma. Breastfeeding itself carries significant stressors in terms of autonomy risk, pain, vulnerability concerns, and effort.[24]

Trauma-informed care refers to delivery systems that recognize the role of trauma in lifelong health and seek to provide care that traumatized patients experience as safe. The education of health care providers on breastfeeding should therefore include the tenets of trauma-informed care: screening for prior traumatic events (e.g., with ACES), minimizing distress and maximizing autonomy, and developing trusting relationships with patients.[25] Other considerations may include listening to birth stories and validating feelings and screening for depression in postpartum patients.

SUGGESTED LEARNING OBJECTIVES BY DISCIPLINE

Suggested Curriculum for Medical Students

By the end of medical school, medical students should have a basic understanding of the histology, anatomy, physiology, pathology, pharmacology, public health, and clinical issues surrounding breastfeeding; be able to understand the relevance of this knowledge to clinical scenarios; and begin to apply this knowledge in clinical decision making. Appendix J serves as a guide to facilitate the inclusion of these items into medical education. A recent review of an undergraduate medical curriculum in the United States listed 12 comprehensive knowledge-based and 12 practice-based competencies that all medical students should acquire in breastfeeding education (Boxes 26.1 and 26.2).[26] The authors then performed a survey of over 600 students to determine whether the curricular objectives were met; unfortunately, significant deficits were found. Although this situation is far from unique, having published guidelines for medical student education may begin to pave the way toward increased curricular exposure.

Physician Trainees, Residents, and Continuing Education

Educational objectives and skills for physicians with respect to breastfeeding have been developed by the Academy of Breastfeeding Medicine (ABM). The ABM recommends high-quality breastfeeding education throughout the continuum of medical education and training. This document, "Educational Objectives and Skills for the Physician with Respect to Breastfeeding," is available on the ABM website and is presented in Appendix I.[27]

A few important points should be mentioned with respect to individual fields. All family medicine, pediatric, and obstetric providers should have a comprehensive understanding of the field, regardless of subspecialty. Primary care providers should gain additional skills in counseling, latch assistance, and management of lactation disorders. Internal medicine physicians (internists), though not directly involved in birth and postpartum periods, may be involved in preconception, breast disorders, medication and lactation concerns, and management of endocrinologic impacts on lactation. They should therefore have a strong understanding of the physiology of lactation and medication impacts on lactation and human milk. Surgeons may be asked about the impacts of surgeries on breastfeeding goals, and therefore should understand how their surgical techniques (in both children and lactating parents) affect lactation (see Chapter 16 on breast disorders and surgeries). Radiologists and anesthesiologists are frequently asked about the impacts of various medications, contrast agents, and procedures on lactation and the breastfed infant and should know that most medications and contrast agents are safe for breastfeeding, along with recognized resources for specific cases (see Chapter 12 on medications).

BOX 26.1 **Twelve Knowledge-Based Competencies in Breastfeeding Care for Undergraduate Medical Education**

1. Understand the 10 steps to successful breastfeeding (WHO/UNICEF)
2. Understand the impact of pregnancy, birth, and other health care practices on breastfeeding outcomes
3. Know basic anatomy (including normal anatomy and abnormal pathologic conditions) and physiology of the breast (including hormones of lactation and milk production and secretion)
4. Describe physiology of lactation-related fertility suppression
5. Compare latch (attachment) and suckling dynamics of breastfeeding and bottle-feeding mechanics
6. Understand the role of breastfeeding and human milk in maintaining health and preventing disease (including the biochemical and immunologic properties of human milk)
7. Understand the importance of exclusive breastfeeding and its correlation with optimal health outcomes
8. Understand the role of behavioral, cultural, social, and environmental factors in infant feeding decisions and practices (ethnicity, maternal education, socioeconomic status)
9. Know the evidence-based contraindications to breastfeeding
10. Know the potential adverse outcomes for infants, mothers, societies who do not breastfeed
11. Know the potential problems associated with the use of infant formula
12. Know of the existence and intent of the international code of marketing of breast-milk substitutes

NOTE: The knowledge-based competencies should be introduced during the preclinical years (M1 and M2) and then reinforced in clinical practice during the clinical years (M3 and M4). *UNICEF,* United Nations International Children's Emergency Fund; *WHO,* World Health Organization.
From Gary AJ, Birmingham EE, Jones LB. Improving breastfeeding medicine in undergraduate medical education: a student survey and extensive curriculum review with suggestions for improvement. *Educ Health (Abingdon).* 2017;30:163. Modified from "core competencies in breastfeeding care for all health professionals" and "educational objectives and skills for the physician with respect to breastfeeding."

BOX 26.2 **Twelve Skill-Based Competencies in Breastfeeding Care for Undergraduate Medical Education**

1. Obtain a detailed breastfeeding history and perform a breastfeeding-related breast examination
2. Recognize the effects of labor and delivery interventions on the initiation of breastfeeding
3. Describe the impact of intrapartum and immediate postpartum procedures and medications on lactation (and recommend medications and treatment options that are compatible with breastfeeding)
4. Facilitate and assist with the first feeding immediately after delivery
5. Recognize and correct attachment and effective suckling at the breast
6. Counsel mothers about establishing and maintaining milk supply during separation from their infants (because of illness, return to work, etc.)
7. Provide anticipatory guidance for breastfeeding mothers and children
8. Discuss family planning options for the breastfeeding woman
9. Discuss causes, prevention, and management of common breastfeeding problems (i.e., sore nipples, low milk supply, poor weight gain, jaundice)
10. Describe appropriate timing, introduction, and selection of complementary foods
11. Understand normal growth patterns for breastfed babies
12. Know the indications for referral to lactation services and know the resources available to assist mother seeking breastfeeding and lactation information or services

NOTE: The skill-based competencies should be taught and practiced during the clinical years (M3 and M4), with particular focus during the pediatrics clerkship, obstetrics and gynecology clerkship, and family medicine clerkship.
From Gary AJ, Birmingham EE, Jones LB. Improving breastfeeding medicine in undergraduate medical education: a student survey and extensive curriculum review with suggestions for improvement. *Educ Health (Abingdon).* 2017;30:163. Modified from "core competencies in breastfeeding care for all health professionals" and "educational objectives and skills for the physician with respect to breastfeeding."

Overall, even untrained providers may be supportive of breastfeeding when they understand its importance and know the local and online resources to assist with finding information when they are unsure.

Nursing

By the end of nursing school, nurses should have a basic understanding of clinical and public health issues surrounding breastfeeding. They should also have practical bedside skills supporting breastfeeding families, using best practices with clear evidence. The Registered Nurses Association of Ontario, Canada (RNAO) has developed a best practice guideline aimed at promoting evidence-based nursing

care for breastfeeding persons and children, now in its 3rd edition. It can be purchased and is also free for download.[28] It recommends education for bedside care (assessment and intervention) and at organizational and policy levels. It is an excellent document for learners and teachers alike.

Other Provider Types

As we have already discussed, midwifery training is strong in breastfeeding education. Other provider types, including nurse practitioners, physician's assistants, home health workers, etc., must create and maintain competencies for breastfeeding based on their own scope of practice. These must be comprehensive and applied to all learners in the program, regardless of final career choice.

FORMATS

Various methods have been used to train providers in basic breastfeeding knowledge and management, including recorded, text-based, and in-person, both optional and required.

When choosing a format for breastfeeding education, it is important to consider the needs of the learners and where they practice. For instance, although online education has a significant reach, it is less likely to change practice. On the other hand, though an in-person lesson may show significant changes in knowledge and practice, it may rely on a teaching staff of variable quality or geographic scope. Following are some considerations and examples of the success of different formats.

In Person

Strengths	Weaknesses
• Expert teachers impassion learners and model appropriate care • Group education motivates behavior change • Formative assessments can be used to adjust content based on the needs of the group • Offers opportunities for methods targeted at different types of learners • Hands-on learning promotes retention • Has been shown to change knowledge, attitudes, and practice, including patient outcomes	• Uses most time and resources • Needs motivated leadership at both the school administration and expertise levels • Variable expertise and delivery of teachers • Content may vary between teachers or sessions • Unlikely to cover a wide geographic area

Hillenbrand and Larsen[29] published the results of a 4-day multimodal educational program on the knowledge, confidence, and behaviors of pediatric resident physicians. The program consisted of lectures on statistics, recommendations, physiology, and barriers, as well as role-playing and group practice on breastfeeding basics and management of common problems. Interestingly, the intervention concluded with a panel of breastfeeding mothers discussing their lactation problems, needs, and sources of support. Residents who attended the training were evaluated by pretest and posttest, and their behaviors in the clinical setting were measured before and after the curriculum. The

investigators telephoned the mothers after the clinic visit to gain insight into their experiences. Accurate breastfeeding management increased from 22% to 65% after the training. The resident physicians especially improved in assessment of problems.[29]

Online

Strengths	Weaknesses
• Easily disseminated across large groups • Improves standardization of content across teachers and learning sessions • Offers flexibility for content delivery by popular self-paced online learning • Has been shown to change knowledge and attitudes	• High resource needs for building, maintaining, and supervising effective online teaching • Formative assessment is less likely to result in adjustments to online content (though this is possible with good design) • Less likely to change learners' practice • May generate less commitment than in-person expert exposure

Given the facility of disseminating standardized content and the relative ease of use of online education, these methods have been proposed for breastfeeding education of health care professionals. Some have shown promise in targeting knowledge and attitudes. However, online education in the health professions has a smaller impact on change in practice and professional environment. For example, an intervention was designed by collaboration among the Italian National Institute of Health, UNICEF, and the Local Health Authority of Milan.[30] The training comprised two e-books, four mandatory case studies, and four optional learning activities. A total of 15,004 participants completed the course and were evaluated with a posttest. Significant changes in attitudes and knowledge were noted, although only minor changes were seen in practice, most notably in using evidence-based resources for medication compatibility with lactation. This training was well received by participants, who had a high rate of satisfaction. This is similar to findings of other studies of online lactation education.[31]

Effective online education should not be approached as a video-recorded lecture. It is important for teachers to understand the needs of online learners and adaptations in educational scholarship in the past decade to meet these needs. As with the earlier example, opportunities for activities are critical to gain formative assessments, enable learners with different learning styles, and ensure engagement with the content material. Activities that enrich online teaching include group discussions, collaborative projects, reflections, and hands-on exercises.

Combined

Strengths	Weaknesses
• Leverages strengths of in-person and online teaching • Takes slightly less time to complete • Online component expands geographic reach	• Medium resource needs for building, maintaining, and supervising effective online components • Medium resource needs for in-person content • Continues to rely on variable expertise of in-person teachers

Blended curricula, "flipped classrooms," and learning collaboratives are all examples of combined in-person and online education that have been used to advance breastfeeding knowledge. For example, the US nonprofit the National Institute for Children's Health Quality (NICHQ) led quality improvement initiatives in New York State and Texas that involved local teams, statewide webinar collaboratives, and in-person meetings.[32] Both of these showed improvements in breastfeeding care (e.g., increased rates of rooming-in), and larger structural change (e.g., Baby Friendly Hospital designations).

SPECIFIC CURRICULA

Given the rapidly expanding world of both free and paid content for breastfeeding education, this section will focus on a few well-known or innovative examples of lessons.

The American Academy of Pediatrics Section on Breastfeeding Residency Curriculum

The AAP developed and tested an 8- to 19-hour residency curriculum on breastfeeding directed at all residents and tested in university hospitals with obstetrics, pediatrics, and family medicine residency programs.[15] There are three major sections to the program: advocacy, clinical management, and delivering culturally competent breastfeeding care. The program is organized to be delivered flexibly over a 1-year period and is organized to meet the core competencies of the Accreditation Council for Graduate Medical Education. Lessons include prepared presentations and clinical case studies. The evaluation tools are designed to facilitate review and tracking by a residency director. In a multisite trial with controls, sites with trained residents showed improvement in resident knowledge and practice, as well as improved exclusive breastfeeding rates of infants out to 6 months at trained sites (odds ratio [OR] 4.1, 95% confidence interval [CI] 1.8 to 9.7) (see Table 26.1).[15] This breastfeeding residency curriculum has its own website and is available for downloading.[33]

WEPNKAB

Creating postgraduate educational opportunities is one of the major goals of the ABM, an international organization of physicians, dentists, and trainees founded in 1994. The ABM holds an annual meeting with plenary sessions, workshops, and submitted papers and posters on the wide range of topics involving breastfeeding and human lactation. The first day's program—What Every Physician Needs to Know About

TABLE 26.1	Impact of Curriculum on Breastfeeding Initiation and Continuation			
Type of Feeding	**Pretest**	**Posttest**	**Change**	**Significance**
Breastfeeding Rates at Initiation Before and After Implementation (% Infants)				
Intervention Sites				
Exclusive breastfeeding	15.5	23.1	+7.45	0.002
Overall breastfeeding	76.0	80.7	+4.74	0.071
Control Sites				
Exclusive breastfeeding	27.5	30.5	+3.00	0.239
Overall breastfeeding	64.8	66.6	+1.86	0.500
Breastfeeding Rates at 6 Months Before and After Implementation (% Infants)				
Intervention Sites				
Exclusive breastfeeding	2.3	9.0	+6.7	0.001
Overall breastfeeding	25.3	28.7	+3.3	0.291
Control Sites				
Exclusive breastfeeding	11.6	6.2	−5.4	0.002
Overall breastfeeding	26.9	25.3	−1.6	0.574

From Feldman-Winter L, Barone L, Milcareck KB, et al. Residency curriculum improves breastfeeding care. *Pediatrics.* 2010;126:289–297. http://doi.org/10.1542/peds.2009-3250.

Breastfeeding (WEPNKAB)—is presented by a team of experts at every annual meeting. It is a comprehensive review of breastfeeding physiology, pathology, clinical scenarios, and policies. It has been recorded on video and is also available from the ABM on its website.

Online Learning Resources
Wellstart Program
Wellstart International[34] was founded in 1985 and developed a multidisciplinary approach to breastfeeding education that trained health profession teams, who then became experts in their own community. They were widely hailed as successful, although the training no longer takes place. Their "Lactation Management Self-Study Modules, Level 1," 4th edition, most recently updated in 2014,[35] remains a comprehensive text-based review of foundational breastfeeding knowledge. It includes a pretest and posttest and can be incorporated into other curricula.

The Normal Pregnancy Virtual Patient Program developed at Harvard University included a largely text-based online education module on breastfeeding with some photos and videos. In one review of the complete module, the program was shown to enhance student behavior in medical management and counseling skills.[36]

Bella Breastfeeding is available for free from OPENPediatrics through a grant from the W.K. Kellogg Foundation. It was launched in 2018 and includes 3 hours of educational videos in 15 short learning modules, each with a several-question pretest and posttest.[37] A certificate of completion is available to meet BFHI provider education requirements.

Best Start Canada
A training guide for health care professionals was prepared by Best Start[38] by Health Nexus, a nonprofit funded by the government of Ontario, Canada. Best Start itself is an early child development resource center. Its breastfeeding education training includes seven online modules on the basics of breastfeeding support and includes a completion certificate. It is available for free by registering for an account. The work is audiovisual, with some interactive prompts.

Postgraduate Learning Opportunities for Nurses and Lactation Consultants
Numerous programs across the United States are geared toward nurses and often are provided by nurses. Many of these focus on curricula designed to assist the participant in passing the certifying examination provided by the International Board of Lactation Consultant Examiners. Postgraduate teaching for lactation consultants is provided by the International Lactation Consultants Association and by independent professional groups. These are often rich resources; given gaps in health care education, they also present information that will be new to many health professionals.

Lactation Education Resources. Lactation Education Resources (LER) is an online provider of paid educational content for lactation consultants and health professionals.[39] It was originally formed in 1997 by Vergie Hughes, RN, MS, IBCLC, as a continuation of the National Capital Lactation Center and the Lactation Consultant Training Program developed at Georgetown University Medical Center and canceled in that year. Courses are exclusively online and include an India-specific course and courses to meet the BFHI education requirements. LER provides contact hours for nurses, dietitians and midwives, in addition to lactation consultants. They also offer guidance on how to obtain the International Board Certified Lactation Consultant (IBCLC) certification.

GOLD learning. GOLD is another purveyor of paid online content in maternal child health.[40] The ABM, IABLE (see later), and several lactation consultant and midwifery organizations are partners and share content for the online courses. GOLD provides live-streamed and recorded conferences and offers contact hours for nurses, dietitians, midwives, and physicians, in addition to lactation consultants.

ORGANIZATIONS DEVOTED TO PROVIDER EDUCATION

Various professional organizations have created special interest groups to support professional engagement with breastfeeding. Many have a mission to promote professional education. In addition, these organizations have increased their programming about human lactation at their annual and regional meetings for all attendees. In the following section we offer some of the larger breastfeeding-specific groups and their initiatives.

Academy of Breastfeeding Medicine
The ABM provides WEPNKAB (see earlier) at its yearly and regional conferences.

Institute for the Advancement of Breastfeeding and Lactation Education
The Institute for the Advancement of Breastfeeding and Lactation Education (IABLE) is a nonprofit organization dedicated to educating providers to support knowledgeable medical systems and communities. The group offers conferences in the United States, online resources, and publications.[41]

International Society for Research in Human Milk and Lactation
The International Society for Research in Human Milk and Lactation (ISRHML)[42] is an organization of investigators who meet annually in conjunction with the Federation of American Societies for Experimental Biology and biannually independently to discuss current knowledge of laboratory and clinical research. Membership is limited to qualified investigators in the field.

American Academy of Pediatrics
The AAP has established the Section on Breastfeeding, which is responsible for a position paper updated every 5 years.[43] The section has also produced several publications, including

The Breastfeeding Handbook for Physicians, 2nd edition, edited by Richard Schanler, MD, which is available online.[44]

Milk Club

The Milk Club meets in conjunction with the American Pediatric Society, Society for Pediatric Research, and Academic Pediatric Association. Their mission is to bring new science in the field to the attention of all investigators. The format is usually a symposium with discussion and a poster session at the Pediatric Academic Society annual meeting.

National Association of Podiatrio Nuroo Practitioners

The National Association of Pediatric Nurse Practitioners (NAPNAP), in the United States, has a breastfeeding education special interest group. In their position statement on breastfeeding, they encourage pediatric providers to "Serve as an educational resource for other health care professionals, employers, and the general public regarding breastfeeding."

SUMMARY

Breastfeeding and human lactation education must be integrated into all health care provider education. Given the evidence surrounding breastfeeding physiology, pathology, and appropriate support, it is no longer acceptable for providers to put their patients' health at risk through their own ignorance. Nor is it acceptable for professional schools to rely on the passion of a few faculty members to create site-specific content. Each discipline should develop their own breastfeeding competencies and educate and evaluate their learners' achievements therein.

The Reference list is available at www.expertconsult.com.

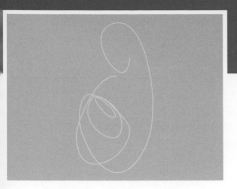

Appendices

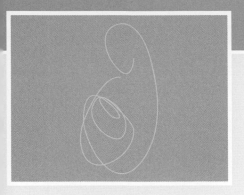

Composition of Human Milk

Ruth A. Lawrence

TABLE A.1 Composition of Human Colostrum and Mature Breast Milk

Constituent (per 100 mL)	Colostrum 1–5 Days	Mature Milk >30 Days
Energy (kcal)	58	70
Total solids (g)	12.8	12.0
Lactose (g)	5.3	7.3
Total nitrogen (mg)	360	171
Protein nitrogen (mg)	313	129
Nonprotein nitrogen (mg)	47	42
Total protein (g)	2.3	0.9
Casein (mg)	140	187
Alpha-lactalbumin (mg)	218	161
Lactoferrin (mg)	330	167
Immunoglobulin A (mg)	364	142
Amino Acids (Total)		
Alanine (mg)	—	52
Arginine (mg)	126	49
Aspartate (mg)	—	110
Cystine (mg)	—	25
Glutamate (mg)	—	196
Glycine (mg)	—	27
Histidine (mg)	57	31
Isoleucine (mg)	121	67
Leucine (mg)	221	110
Lysine (mg)	163	79
Methionine (mg)	33	19
Phenylalanine (mg)	105	44
Proline (mg)	—	89
Serine (mg)	—	54
Threonine (mg)	148	58
Tryptophan (mg)	52	25
Tyrosine (mg)	—	38
Valine (mg)	169	90
Taurine (free) (mg)	—	8
Urea (mg)	10	30
Creatine (mg)	—	3.3
Total fat (g)	2.9	4.2
Fatty Acids (% Total Fat)		
12:0 lauric	1.8	5.8
14:0 myristic	3.8	8.6
16:0 palmitic	26.2	21.0
18:0 stearic	8.8	8.0
18:1 oleic	36.6	35.5
18:2, n-6 linoleic	6.8	7.2
18:3, n-3 linolenic	—	1.0

(Continued)

TABLE A.1   Composition of Human Colostrum and Mature Breast Milk—cont'd

Constituent (per 100 mL)	Colostrum 1–5 Days	Mature Milk >30 Days
C_{20} and C_{22} polyunsaturated	10.2	2.9
Cholesterol (mg)	27	16
Vitamins		
Fat Soluble		
Vitamin A (retinol equivalents) (mcg)	89	67
Beta-carotene (mcg)	112	23
Vitamin D (mcg)	—	0.05
Vitamin E (total tocopherols) (mcg)	1280	315
Vitamin K (mcg)	0.23	0.21
Water Soluble		
Thiamin (mcg)	15	21
Riboflavin (mcg)	25	35
Niacin (mcg)	75	150
Folic acid (mcg)	—	8.5
Vitamin B_6 (mcg)	12	93
Biotin (mcg)	0.1	0.6
Pantothenic acid (mcg)	183	180
Vitamin B_{12} (ng)	200	26
Ascorbic acid (mg)	4.4	4.0
Minerals		
Calcium (mg)	23	28
Magnesium (mg)	3.4	3.0
Sodium (mg)	48	18
Potassium (mg)	74	58
Chlorine (mg)	91	42
Phosphorus (mg)	14	15
Sulfur (mg)	22	14
Trace Elements		
Chromium (ng)	—	50
Cobalt (mcg)	—	1
Copper (mcg)	46	25
Fluorine (mcg)	—	16
Iodine (mcg)	12	11
Iron (mcg)	45	40
Manganese (mcg)	—	0.6 ±
Nickel (mcg)	—	2
Selenium (mcg)	—	2.0
Zinc (mcg)	540	120

Data from multiple references (see Chapter 4). Figures have been averaged.

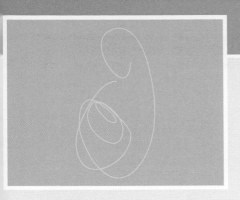

Normal Serum Values for Breastfed Infants

Ruth A. Lawrence

TABLE B.1 Serum Chemical Values of Normal Breastfed Infants[a]

Concentration/100 mL of Serum	AGE 28 DAYS			AGE 56 DAYS			AGE 84 DAYS			AGE 112 DAYS		
	N	Mean	SD	N	Mean	SD	N	Mean	SD	N	Mean	SD
Males												
Total protein (g)	22	5.87	0.50	36	5.96	0.42	29	6.16	0.57	51	6.29	0.51
Albumin (g)	22	4.02	0.35	36	4.14	0.34	29	4.27	0.39	51	4.38	0.40
Globulins (g)												
α_1	22	0.14	0.03	36	0.17	0.03	29	0.18	0.03	51	0.17	0.04
α_2	22	0.53	0.10	36	0.60	0.11	29	0.74	0.14	51	0.81	0.19
β	22	0.61	0.11	36	0.67	0.13	29	0.69	0.20	51	0.67	0.11
γ	22	0.57	0.14	36	0.38	0.09	29	0.28	0.08	51	0.26	0.10
Cholesterol (mg)	21	139	31	32	153	34	25	133	32	47	145	26
Triglycerides (mg)	18	122	36	32	106	57	25	170	76	46	148	57
Urea nitrogen (mg)	43	8.5	3.2	49	6.6	2.1	47	7.0	2.7	51	7.3	4.2
Calcium (mg)	41	10.2	0.8	47	10.3	1.0	42	10.4	0.8	48	10.3	0.8
Phosphorus (mg)	43	6.6	0.7	49	6.4	0.7	47	6.2	0.5	49	6.2	0.7
Alkaline phosphatase[b]	31	**22**	6	40	**21**	7	35	21	8	44	18	7
Magnesium (mg)	40	2.0	0.2	47	2.1	0.2	45		0.2	50	2.2	0.2
Females												
Total protein (g)	18	6.04	0.40	27	5.86	0.44	21	6.21	0.57	42	6.31	0.62
Albumin (g)	18	4.07	0.27	27	4.03	0.35	21	4.29	0.37	42	4.36	0.42
Globulins (g)												
α_1	18	0.15	0.02	27	0.17	0.04	21	0.17	0.03	42	**0.19**	0.04
α_2	18	0.55	0.07	27	0.65	0.12	21	0.74	0.18	42	0.78	0.17
β	18	0.70	0.18	27	0.63	0.11	21	0.71	0.13	42	0.67	0.16
γ	18	0.57	0.10	27	0.38	0.10	21	0.30	0.06	42	**0.31**	0.10
Cholesterol (mg)	13	**180**	35	25	157	37	20	**155**	29	40	**165**	36
Triglycerides (mg)	9	**157**	43	24	112	53	18	195	56	38	**170**	52
Urea nitrogen (mg)	37	8.3	2.3	33	6.4	2.2	40	6.4	2.2	42	6.6	3.5
Calcium (mg)	37	10.3	0.8	33	10.3	0.8	40	10.3	0.8	42	10.7	0.7
Phosphorus (mg)	39	6.9	0.8	33	6.4	0.8	40	6.1	0.7	42	6.1	0.7
Alkaline phosphatase[b]	31	19	5	28	17	5	32	17	5	36	17	5
Magnesium (mg)	39	2.0	0.4	32	2.0	0.2	40	2.1	0.2	41	2.1	0.3

[a]Bold figures indicate that value is greater than the corresponding value for infants of the opposite sex and that the difference is statistically significant at the 95% level of confidence.

[b]King-Armstrong units.

From Fomon SJ, Filer LJ, Thomas LN, et al: Growth and serum chemical values of normal breastfed infants. *Acta Paediatr Scand Suppl.* 1970;202:1.

TABLE B.2	**Leptin Levels in Infants**			
	Leptin (ng mL^{-1})	In (Leptin) (ng mL^{-1})	In (Leptin)/Weight (ng mL^{-1} per kg)	In (Leptin)/BMI (ng m^2 mL^{-1} per kg)
Total ($n = 35$)	7.35 ± 6.87	1.19 ± 0.89	0.21 ± 0.20	0.08 ± 0.06
M ($n = 18$)	6.92 ± 5.72	0.96 ± 1.01	0.13 ± 0.22	0.05 ± 0.07
F ($n = 17$)	7.79 ± 8.02	1.43 ± 0.73	0.29 ± 0.17	0.1 ± 0.05
BF ($n = 13$) (7 M, 6 F)	8.04 ± 5.01	1.62 ± 0.73[a]	0.30 ± 0.13[a]	0.11 ± 0.05[a]
FF ($n = 22$) (11 M, 11 F)	6.93 ± 7.91	0.94 ± 0.95[a]	0.16 ± 0.20[a]	0.06 ± 0.07[a]

[a]$p < 0.05$.

NOTE: Data are mean ± SD. *BF*, Breastfed; *BMI*, body mass index; *F*, female; *FF*, formula fed; *M*, male. From Savino F, Costamagna M, Prino A, et al. Leptin levels in term breastfed (BF) and formula-fed (FF) infants. *Acta Paediatr.* 2002;91:897.

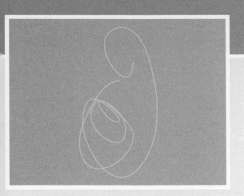

Herbals and Natural Products

Ruth A. Lawrence

TABLE C.1   Herbals and Natural Products: Issues Related to Human Milk

Herb Common Name/Rating[a]	Synonyms	Active Ingredient	Uses	Present in Milk	Safety/Efficacy
Aloe vera AAP — H L3 W —	*Aloe barbadensis, A. capensis, vera*	Polysaccharide, glucomannan	Wound healing and small burns	Unknown, probably none when applied to skin	Orally is a strong purgative; oral dosing not recommended during lactation. Dermal use ok.[1,2]
Asparagus	Wild asparagus root	*Asparagus racemosus*		Unknown (for Asparagus) from LactMed reference	Nourishing herb; used in those debilitated or galactagogue (1 g powdered root per day in milk or juice).[3]
Blessed thistle AAP — H L3 W —		Many chemicals and volatile oils	Gastrointestinal symptoms	Unknown	This is not a galactagogue. It is a different plant from milk thistle. No known toxicity.[1] Many uses.
Borage AAP — H L5 W —	*Borage officinalis*	Pyrrolizidine alkaloid	Pain therapy		Contraindicated in pregnancy and lactation.[4]
Botulism AAP — H L3 W —	Toxin				In natural cases of botulism toxin does not get into the milk. Pharmaceutical product Botox treatment unlikely to reach milk.[5]
Cannabis AAP 2 H L5 W —	Marijuana	Δ9-Tetrahydrocannabinol (THC)	Sedative, hallucinogen	Yes	Remains in infant's system for weeks, especially in fat.[1,6,7]
Capsaicin AAP — H L3 W —	Cayenne peppers (Capsicum)	Capsaicin	Topical anesthesia	Unknown	Available as a cream, lotion, or oral tablets. Used where vasodilation or warmth is needed. Can cause burning, stinging. Do not use on breasts.[2,8]
Chamomile AAP — H L3 W —	*Matricaria recutita,* Aster, Aceae family	Terpenoids (coumarins), flower heads	Antiinflammatory, carminative, antiseptic, sedative (all unproved)	Unknown	Potential for allergic reaction. Animal studies question safety in pregnancy and lactation.[6,10]
Cohosh (black) AAP — H L4 W —	*Cimicifuga racemosa,* black cohosh, black snakeroot, found in Lydia Pinkham's compound	Estrogenic compounds, tannins, terpenoids, use roots and rhizome	Dysmenorrhea, dyspepsia, rheumatism, menopause	Unknown	May cause hypotension; could decrease milk production? Efficacy and safety in lactation.[4]

Herb (AAP/H/W)	Scientific name / Synonyms	Parts / Active ingredients	Uses	In milk	Comments / Safety
Cohosh (blue) AAP – H L5 W –	*Caulophyllum*, blue cohosh, squaw root	Roots and rhizome, methylcytosine, caulosaponin	Uterine stimulant, emmenagogue, increased blood pressure, similar to nicotine, induces labor		Safety of concern, can constrict coronary vessels; leaves and seeds are known to be toxic. Can induce labor.[4]
Comfrey FDA banned AAP – H L5 W –	*Symphytum officinale*	Roots, rhizome, and leaves; allantoin; hepatotoxic; pyrrolizidine alkaloids	"Wonder drug," heals wounds, used as poultice, used as tea	Yes	Venoocclusive disease causing hepatic failure. Banned in many countries; unsafe.[1,12–16]
Echinacea AAP – H L3 W –	*Echinacea angustifolia*, coneflower	Whole plant, flowers, dried roots	Immunostimulant, antiinfective, tested for upper respiratory tract infections	Unknown	Has been studied; effective in short courses, not continual use. No known toxicity; probably safe during lactation.[2,17,18]
Evening primrose AAP – H L3 W –	*Oenothera biennis*	Biennis, oil from seeds, cis-gamma-linoleic acid (GLA), a precursor of prostaglandin E_1, essential fatty acids (EFA)	Lower cholesterol, lower blood pressure, lower dysmenorrhea, mastalgia, eczema	Yes	Efficacy: Conflicting reports. Safety: ± probably in small amounts. Supplements increase EFA in milk[19], increase bleeding time.[20] Do not use with phenol thiazines.
Fennel AAP – H L4 W –	*Foeniculum vulgare*	Dried ripe fruit, volatile oil, transanethole estrogenic effect	Carminative, loosen phlegm, galactagogue, increase libido	Probable	Volatile oil can be toxic; use only fruits (seeds). Because of estrogenic effect, its reputation as a galactagogue is questioned.[1,4,7]
Fenugreek AAP – H L3 W –	*Trigonella foenumgraecum*, Greek hayseed	Dried ripe seeds, diosgenin, and alkaloids smell like maple syrup	Hypoglycemia, galactagogue, anticoagulant, see text	Probable / Unknown	Risk: Cross allergy to chrysanthemum family. Probably in milk; infants smell of maple syrup. No studies of efficacy.[4,7,21–25]
Feverfew (not rated by AAP, Hale)	*Tanacetum parthenium, Chrysanthemum parthenium*, Family: Asteraceae, Bachelor's button	Leaves, parthenolide = active ingredient extracted from the leaves	Associated with migraines. Menstrual irregularity antiinflammatory	Unknown	Enhances effect of warfarin contraindicated during pregnancy. Value as galactagogue undocumented; decreases platelet aggregation.[4,7]
Garlic (supplement form) AAP – H L3 W –	Lily family: *Allium sativum*, poor man's treacle, clove garlic, common garlic, allium, stinking rose	Alliin, ajoenes	Has over 100 different uses, some contradictory, both high and low blood pressure, antibacterial, antithrombotic, lower cholesterol	Yes	Can cause colic in breastfed infants. Can enhance warfarin. Not tolerated by some infants.[25,26]

(Continued)

Herb Common Name/Rating[a]	Synonyms	Active Ingredient	Uses	Present in Milk	Safety/Efficacy
Ginkgo AAP – H L3 W –	*Ginkgo biloba*	Flavones and glycosides, seeds, ginkgotoxin, ginkgo biloba extract (GBE), leaves for tea	Herbal antioxidant, used as an herbal supplement and for many conditions	Unknown	There are no well controlled studies of its efficacy against various conditions. Conflicting reports of safety. Not recommended in lactation.[25] Enhances the effect of warfarin. Can cause bleeding even alone.
Ginseng AAP – H L3 W –	Panax ginseng (*P. quinquefolius*), Asian ginseng	Root and extracts	Panacea, cure-all, adaptogen, strengthening, increasing mental capacity	Unknown	A lot has been written, with considerable conflict of opinion. Ginseng abuse syndrome; research done mostly by manufacturers. Safety: Not for long-term use; efficacy questionable.[27–29] Not recommended in lactation.[25] Reduces effect of warfarin.
Grapefruit seed extract AAP – H – W –		Flavonols	Antimicrobial inhibits intestinal cytochrome 450. Used topically on breasts for candida or orally (250 mg a day)	No data	Noted to have antiviral, antibacterial, and antifungal effects. Grapefruit is known to contain quinine, especially in the bitter skin and section fibers. Recommended as an extract for use by direct application on sore nipples. If it has antiinfectious properties, it should be effective when traumatized nipples have become infected.[25]
Grape seed AAP – H – W –	*Vitis vinifera* Grape seed extract	Proanthocyanidin, resveratrol	Used as a supplement and in treatment of circulatory problems	No data	Antioxidant, anticancer agent for varicose veins, circulatory problems. May increase risk for bleeding.
Herbal teas	Tablets, powders, tea leaves	May include germander, comfrey, mistletoe, skull cap, pennyroyal, all of which are toxic. **Always check constituents.**			Many cause hepatotoxicity and/or venous occlusive disease. Many associated with hemorrhagic disease.[10,20] See Chapter 11, Box 11.1, Tables 11.9 and 11.10.
Kava AAP – H L5 W –	*Piper methysticum*, Kew, tonga	Roots/rhizomes, dihydropyrones with central nervous system activity, kavapyrones	Inebriation, muscle relaxants, antianxiety, antistress alternative to benzodiazepams	Unknown	Unsafe in pregnancy and lactation. Numbs the mouth; nauseating. Causes yellow discoloration of the skin, hair, nails.[1,2] The FDA has issued a safety alert about kava and liver toxicity.

Herb / Rating	Scientific name / preparation	Constituents	Uses	Lactation	Comments
Licorice root AAP – H L3 W –	Glycyrrhiza glabra family	Glycyrrhizin acid rhizomes and roots	Laxative effects and symptoms of acid reflux or gastritis, hypokalemia	Glycyrrhizin has been measured in the breastmilk in a few reports.	Known for 4000 years; large doses: weakness, edema, weight loss, hypertension, hypokalemia, and confusion. Consumption should be avoided in pregnancy and lactation.[25,30]
Milk thistle (holy thistle) (not blessed thistle) AAP – H L3 W –	Silybum marianum, St. Mary's thistle, Silymarin is a standardized preparation extracted from the fruits (seeds) of milk thistle.	Fruits, flavolignans, inhibits oxidative damage to cells	Protective effect, concentrates in the liver	Unknown	Purported galactagogue. Only one study, no randomized or well controlled reported a positive effect as a galactagogue. Problem: can cause allergy; low oral bioavailability. Probably safe.[1,35]
Raspberry root AAP – H – W –	Rubus idaeus leaves	Reportedly promotes urinary tract health, fight morning sickness, ease labor	No proven effective treatments. Used as a dietary supplement	There are polyphenols from raspberry leaves detectable in breastmilk.	Limited safety data in pregnancy and lactation - caution.[31]
Sage AAP – H L4 W –	Salvia officinalis	Fresh leaves and fresh flowering aerial parts, dried leaves, and oils prepared as extracts and teas	Loss of appetite, inflammation of mouth and pharynx, excessive perspiration	Unknown	Contraindicated in pregnancy. Suppresses lactation. Okay as a flavoring.[5]
St. John's wort AAP – H L2 W –	Hypericum perforatum Hyperforin Flavonolignans seeds	Naphthodianthrones, phloroglucinols, hypercin, hyperforin Antioxidant	Depression	Hypericin not detected and hyperforin detected in small amounts	Can cause photosensitivity. Risk for self-medication for a serious psychiatric problem. Can reduce the effect of warfarin, induce cytochrome P450 enzyme system.[32–34]
Valerian root AAP – H L3 W –	Valeriana officinalis, all-heal, Amantilla, setwell, setewale, capon's tail, heliotrope, vandal root	Liquid, tablets, tea, volatile oil	Nervousness and insomnia	Unknown	Not recommended in lactation. Used as a sedative, hypnotic.[36] Generally regarded as safe in foods by the FDA.

AAP, American Academy of Pediatrics; *FDA*, US Food and Drug Administration.

[a]Ratings for each drug represent three classification systems: American Academy of Pediatrics (AAP), Hale (H), and Weiner (W). See text for a complete listing of categories in each system. A dash indicates that the drug is not listed in that system.

The Reference list is available at www.expertconsult.com.

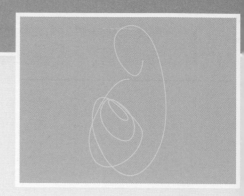

D APPENDIX

Precautions and Breastfeeding Recommendations for Selected Maternal Infections

Robert M. Lawrence

TABLE D.1 Precautions and Breastfeeding Recommendations for Selected Maternal Infections[a]

Organism, Syndrome, or Condition[b,c]	Empiric Precautions[d]	Breastfeeding Acceptable[e]	Compatibility of Medications With Breastfeeding[f]
Adenoviruses			
Conjunctivitis	Contact		
Upper/lower respiratory infections	Droplet	Yes[g]	
Gastroenteritis	Standard		
Amebiasis			
Entamoeba histolytica			
Intestinal	Standard	Yes	Iodoquinol, paromomycin, metronidazole, tinidazole
Extraintestinal	Standard	Yes	
Anaplasmosis	Standard No human to human transmission documented	Yes	Doxycycline, rifampin
Anthrax			
Bacillus anthracis (cutaneous, inhalation, gastrointestinal)	Standard, add contact precautions for draining cutaneous lesions	Yes, if cutaneous lesion is not on the breast and can be covered	Ciprofloxacin
Arboviruses			
Arthropod-borne infections, meningoencephalitis, hemorrhagic fevers, hepatitis	Standard	Yes[h]	
California encephalitis	Standard	Yes	
Colorado tick fever	Standard	Yes	
Dengue fever	Standard	Yes	
Eastern equine encephalitis	Standard	Yes	
Japanese encephalitis	Standard	Yes	
St. Louis encephalitis	Standard	Yes	
West Nile virus	Standard	Yes[h]	
Yellow fever	Standard	Yes	
Yellow fever vaccine virus	Standard	No[h]	
Arcanobacterium haemolyticum			
Pharyngitis, skin infections	Standard	Yes	Erythromycin, azithromycin clindamycin, cefuroxime, tetracycline

(Continued)

TABLE D.1   Precautions and Breastfeeding Recommendations for Selected Maternal Infections[a]—cont'd

Organism, Syndrome, or Condition[b,c]	Empiric Precautions[d]	Breastfeeding Acceptable[e]	Compatibility of Medications With Breastfeeding[f]
Ascaris lumbricoides Gastrointestinal infections, pneumonitis	Standard	Yes	Pyrantel pamoate, mebendazole, albendazole, piperazine
Aspergillosis Bronchopulmonary, sinus, or invasive infections	Standard	Yes	Amphotericin B, flucytosine, rifampin
Astroviruses Gastroenteritis	Standard, but contact for incontinent individuals	Yes	
Babesiosis			
Babesia microti Subacute/chronic febrile illness	Standard	Yes	Clindamycin + quinine, atovaquone + azithromycin
Bacillus cereus (toxin-mediated disease)	Standard	Yes—breastfeeding No—contaminated powdered formula No—contaminated donor milk	Vancomycin—only for invasive infection
Blastocystis hominis Gastrointestinal infection	Standard	Yes	Metronidazole, nitazoxanide, trimethoprim-sulfamethoxazole (TMP-SMX)
Blastomycosis			
Blastomyces dermatitidis Pulmonary, cutaneous, or invasive infection	Standard	Yes	Amphotericin B, fluconazole, itraconazole
Borrelia			
Relapsing fever *Borrelia hermsii*	Standard (tick-borne)	Yes	Penicillin, erythromycin, tetracycline
Borrelia recurrentis	Contact (louse-borne)	Yes	
Borrelia turicatae	Standard (tick-borne)	Yes	Doxycycline
Botulism			
Clostridium botulinum Hypotonia, progressive weakness, toxin-mediated paralysis	Standard	Yes	Antibiotics not indicated
Breast abscess (see Mastitis) *Staphylococcus aureus* Enterobacteriaceae *Streptococcus pyogenes*	Contact (24 h)	Yes (after 24 h if no drainage into breast milk; discard breast milk for first 24 h after surgery)	First-generation cephalosporin, amoxicillin/clavulanate, ampicillin/sulbactam
Brucellosis Febrile illness with variable manifestations	Standard	Yes (after 48 h of therapy in mother; discard breast milk for 48 h)	Doxycycline, TMP-SMX, rifampin, gentamicin, streptomycin, tetracycline

(Continued)

TABLE D.1   Precautions and Breastfeeding Recommendations for Selected Maternal Infections[a]—cont'd

Organism, Syndrome, or Condition[b,c]	Empiric Precautions[d]	Breastfeeding Acceptable[e]	Compatibility of Medications With Breastfeeding[f]
Brucella abortus *Brucella melitensis* *Brucella suis*	Contact (for draining wounds)	Yes	
Caliciviruses Gastroenteritis	Standard, but contact for incontinent individuals	Yes	
Campylobacter Gastrointestinal infection *Campylobacter fetus* *Campylobacter jejuni*	Standard, but contact for incontinent individuals	Yes	Erythromycin, azithromycin, ciprofloxacin
Candidiasis Mucocutaneous infection, vulvovaginitis, invasive infections *Candida albicans* *Candida krusei* *Candida tropicalis*	Standard	Yes (therapy for the infant simultaneous with mother's therapy)[h]	Topical agents, fluconazole, ketoconazole, itraconazole, amphotericin B, flucytosine
Cat-scratch disease Skin infection, regional lymphadenitis, and rarely, invasive infection *Bartonella henselae*	Standard	Yes	Azithromycin, TMP-SMX, rifampin, ciprofloxacin, gentamicin, doxycycline, erythromycin
Chikungunya virus	Standard	Yes—breastfeeding, no virus identified in breast milk	
Chlamydia *Chlamydophila pneumoniae*	Standard	Yes	Tetracycline, doxycycline, erythromycin, azithromycin
Pharyngitis, pneumonia *Chlamydophila psittaci* Psittacosis, pneumonia, rarely invasive infection	Standard	Yes	Tetracycline, doxycycline, erythromycin, azithromycin,
Chlamydia trachomatis Urethritis, vaginitis, endometritis, salpingitis, lymphogranuloma venereum, conjunctivitis, pneumonia	Standard	Yes (consider treating the infant simultaneously)	Erythromycin, azithromycin, doxycycline, sulfonamide, levofloxacin, ofloxacin
Clostridia			
Clostridium botulinum Toxin-mediated paralysis	Standard	Yes	Antibiotic therapy not indicated
Clostridium difficile Antimicrobial-associated diarrhea, pseudomembranous colitis	Contact	Yes	Metronidazole, vancomycin, fidaxomicin
Clostridium perfringens Food poisoning, wound infection, gas gangrene, myonecrosis	Standard	Yes	

(Continued)

TABLE D.1   Precautions and Breastfeeding Recommendations for Selected Maternal Infections[a]—cont'd

Organism, Syndrome, or Condition[b,c]	Empiric Precautions[d]	Breastfeeding Acceptable[e]	Compatibility of Medications With Breastfeeding[f]
Coccidioides immitis			
Pulmonary, invasive infections rarely, extrapulmonary	Standard, but contact for draining lesions	Yes	Amphotericin B, fluconazole, itraconazole
Conjunctivitis			
Adenovirus	Contact	Yes	
Chlamydia trachomatis	Standard	Yes	Tetracycline, doxycycline, erythromycin
Neisseria gonorrhoeae	Standard	Yes[i]	Penicillin, ceftriaxone
Coronavirus (HCoV) (also SARS, MERS, epidemic disease)	Standard, SARS, MERS → Airborne, droplet, contact	Yes	
Cryptococcus neoformans			
Meningitis, pneumonia	Standard	Yes	Amphotericin B, flucytosine, fluconazole
Cryptosporidiosis			
Cryptosporidium parvum			
Diarrhea	Contact	Yes	Nitazoxanide, paromomycin, azithromycin
Cytomegalovirus (CMV)			
Asymptomatic infection	Standard	Yes (for full-term infants)	
Infectious mononucleosis	Standard	No (for premature or immunodeficient infants, do not give expressed breast milk)[h]	
Dengue fever			
Acute febrile illness, hemorrhagic fever	Standard	Yes	
Diphtheria			
Corynebacterium diphtheriae			
Membranous nasopharyngitis	Droplet (DI)	Yes (with infant receiving chemoprophylaxis-P)	Erythromycin, penicillin
Obstructive laryngotracheitis	Droplet (DI)		
Cutaneous infection, toxin-mediated myocarditis, or neurologic disease	Contact (cover lesions)	No (only if skin lesion involves breast)	
Diarrhea			
Campylobacter fetus	Standard	Yes	Azithromycin
Campylobacter jejuni	Standard + Contact for infants	Yes	Erythromycin, ciprofloxacin
Escherichia coli (O157:H7)	Contact	Yes	None indicated
Giardia lamblia	Standard	Yes	Metronidazole, tinidazole, nitazoxanide
Rotavirus	Contact	Yes	
Salmonella enteritidis	Standard	Yes	
Shigella boydii	Contact	Yes	Ciprofloxacin, ceftriaxone, TMP-SMX
Shigella dysenteriae	Contact	Yes	Ciprofloxacin, ceftriaxone, TMP-SMX
Shigella flexneri	Contact	Yes	Ciprofloxacin, ceftriaxone, TMP-SMX

(Continued)

TABLE D.1   Precautions and Breastfeeding Recommendations for Selected Maternal Infections[a]—cont'd

Organism, Syndrome, or Condition[b,c]	Empiric Precautions[d]	Breastfeeding Acceptable[e]	Compatibility of Medications With Breastfeeding[f]
Shigella sonnei	Contact	Yes	Ciprofloxacin, ceftriaxone, TMP-SMX
Vibrio cholerae	Standard	Yes	Doxycycline, azithromycin, tetracycline, ciprofloxacin, furazolidone
Vibrio parahaemolyticus	Standard	Yes	None
Yersinia enterocolitica	Standard + Contact for incontinent persons	Yes	For sepsis or invasive disease—ciprofloxacin, norfloxacin, ceftriaxone, TMP-SMX, doxycycline
Yersinia pseudotuberculosis	Standard	Yes	
Ebola virus	Contact, droplet, and airborne	No (and do not give expressed breast milk) (see text Chapter 12)	
Ehrlichiosis	Standard, no evidence of person-to-person transmission	Yes	Doxycycline, rifampin
Encephalitis			
Enteroviruses	Standard	Yes	
Lyme disease *(Borrelia burgdorferi)*	Standard	Yes	Ceftriaxone, doxycycline, amoxicillin
Rabies	Standard	No (BM +) Return to BF/BM after infant has received RIG and rabies vaccine series	Rabies immune globulin (RIG), rabies vaccine
Endometritis, pelvic inflammatory disease			
Anaerobic organisms	Standard	Yes	Clindamycin, metronidazole, cefoxitin, cefmetazole
Chlamydia trachomatis	Standard	Yes	Erythromycin, azithromycin, tetracycline, levofloxacin
Enterobacteriaceae	Standard	Yes	Ampicillin, aminoglycosides, cephalosporins
Group B streptococci	Standard	Yes[h] (after 24 h of therapy for mother, breast milk is permissible with observation of infant) No[h] (if infant is sick with suspected or proven group B streptococcal infection and the breast milk is being cultured to identify a source of infection; permissible if breast milk is culture negative) (see Chapter 12 text for additional discussion)	Penicillin, cephalosporin, macrolides
Mycoplasma hominis	Standard	Yes	Clindamycin, tetracycline
Neisseria gonorrhoeae	Standard	Yes[i]	Ceftriaxone, spectinomycin, doxycycline, azithromycin
Ureaplasma urealyticum	Standard	Yes	Erythromycin, azithromycin, clarithromycin, tetracycline

(Continued)

TABLE D.1   Precautions and Breastfeeding Recommendations for Selected Maternal Infections[a]—cont'd

Organism, Syndrome, or Condition[b,c]	Empiric Precautions[d]	Breastfeeding Acceptable[e]	Compatibility of Medications With Breastfeeding[f]
Enteroviruses			
Myocarditis: respiratory, gastrointestinal, skin, central nervous system, and eye infections	*Adults:* Standard *Children:* Contact		
Coxsackievirus		Yes	
Echovirus		Yes	
Polioviruses		Yes	
Epstein–Barr virus			
Infectious mononucleosis, broad range of infections	Standard	Yes	
Erythema infectiosum			
Parvovirus B19	Standard	Yes (no infectious risk after the appearance of the rash in immune-competent individuals)	
Flaviviruses			
Dengue	Standard	Yes[h]	
Powassan		Rare transmission through breast milk, benefits > > > risk	
St. Louis encephalitis			
Japanese encephalitis			
Tickborne encephalitis			
West Nile virus			
Yellow fever virus			
Zika virus			
Febrile illness ±	Standard	Yes[h]	
Rash			
Neuroinvasive			
Hemorrhagic fever, congenital infection			
Food poisoning			
Bacillus cereus			
Toxin mediated	Standard	Yes	
Invasive infection			
Clostridium perfringens			
Toxin mediated	Standard	Yes	
Escherichia coli			
Enterohemorrhagic (O157:H7)	Contact	Yes	
Hepatitis A	Standard	Yes (immune serum globulin and hepatitis A vaccine for the infant)	
Norwalk virus	Standard	Yes	
Salmonella enteritidis	Standard	Yes	
Shigella	Contact	Yes	Ciprofloxacin, TMP-SMX
Staphylococcus aureus			
Enterotoxin	Standard	Yes	
Gastroenteritis (see Diarrhea or Food Poisoning)			
Giardiasis			
Giardia lamblia	Standard, no contact with incontinent individuals	Yes	Metronidazole, tinidazole, nitazoxanide

(Continued)

TABLE D.1   Precautions and Breastfeeding Recommendations for Selected Maternal Infections[a]—cont'd

Organism, Syndrome, or Condition[b,c]	Empiric Precautions[d]	Breastfeeding Acceptable[e]	Compatibility of Medications With Breastfeeding[f]
Gonorrhea			
Genital, pharyngeal, conjunctival, or disseminated infection			
Neisseria gonorrhoeae	Standard	Yes[i]	Ceftriaxone, azithromycin, erythromycin, doxycycline
Haemophilus influenzae			
Meningitis, epiglottitis, pneumonia, cellulitis, sinusitis, bacteremia	Droplet	Yes (24 h after initiating therapy in mother; breast milk[b]; P[h] if infant has not been fully immunized, observation)	Cefotaxime, ceftriaxone, ampicillin
Hantavirus			
Pulmonary syndrome, hemorrhagic fever with renal syndrome	Standard	Yes	Intravenous ribavirin is investigational
Hemorrhagic fevers			
African hemorrhagic fever			
Ebola virus	Contact	No (no expressed breast milk)	
Marburg virus	Contact	No (no expressed breast milk)	
Dengue virus (1—4)	Standard	Yes (breast milk +)	
Hantavirus	Standard	Yes (breast milk +)	
Lassa fever	Contact	No (no expressed breast milk)	Intravenous ribavirin?
Yellow fever	Standard	Yes[h] (breast milk +)	Vaccine
Yellow fever vaccine virus immunization in mother[h]	Standard	No[h]	
Hepatitis[h]			
A Acute only	Standard, but contact for incontinent individuals	Yes (after immune serum globulin [ISG] and vaccine)	
B Chronic hepatitis, cirrhosis, hepatocellular carcinoma	Standard	Yes (after hepatitis B immunoglobulin [HBIG] and vaccine)	
C Chronic hepatitis, cirrhosis, hepatocellular carcinoma	Standard	Yes	
D Associated with hepatitis B	Standard	Yes (after HBIG and vaccine)	
E Severe disease in pregnant women	Standard	Yes	
G	Standard	Inadequate data	
Herpesviruses			
Cytomegalovirus (CMV)	Standard	Yes for full-term infants	Ganciclovir, valganciclovir, foscarnet
Asymptomatic, infectious mononucleosis-like syndrome: severe disease in the immunodeficient person		No for premature or immunodeficient infants (infant of CMV-negative mother should not receive milk from CMV-positive mothers)	
Epstein—Barr virus			
Asymptomatic, infectious mononucleosis, associated with chronic fatigue syndrome, African Burkitt lymphoma, and nasopharyngeal carcinoma	Standard	Yes	

(Continued)

TABLE D.1   Precautions and Breastfeeding Recommendations for Selected Maternal Infections[a]—cont'd

Organism, Syndrome, or Condition[b,c]	Empiric Precautions[d]	Breastfeeding Acceptable[e]	Compatibility of Medications With Breastfeeding[f]
Herpes simplex			
Types 1, 2 (HSV$_{1,2}$)			
Mucocutaneous	Contact	Yes (in the absence of breast lesions)	Acyclovir, valacyclovir, famciclovir
Neonatal	Contact		
Encephalitis	Standard		
Varicella-zoster virus[h]			
Varicella	Airborne	No (breast milk + is permissible in absence of lesions on the breast.) Give VariZIG for the exposed infant.	Acyclovir, valacyclovir, famciclovir
Zoster	Standard in normal patient		
	Airborne/contact in immunocompromised individuals	No, VariZIG for the exposed infant, especially less than 1 month of age[h]	
Human herpesvirus 6 (HHV-6)			
Roseola (exanthema subitum, sixth disease), acute febrile illness	Standard	Yes	
Histoplasmosis			
Acute pulmonary disease, disseminated	Standard	Yes	Amphotericin B, itraconazole, fluconazole
Human immunodeficiency viruses (HIV)[h]			
HIV-1	Standard	Yes/no[h]	Limited information on antiretrovirals in breast milk[h] Antiretroviral medications for the mother and/or infant through period of lactation
HIV-2	Standard	Yes/no[h]	
Human T-cell leukemia viruses (HTLV)			
HTLV1			
T-cell leukemia/lymphoma, myelopathy, dermatitis, adenitis, Sjögren's syndrome	Standard	No[h]	
HTLV-II			
Myelopathy, arthritis, glomerulonephritis	Standard	No[h]	
Impetigo	Contact	Yes	Oxacillin, dicloxacillin, erythromycin, first-generation cephalosporins
Infectious mononucleosis (see CMV, EBV)			
Influenza	Droplet	Yes	Oseltamivir, zanamivir, amantadine, rimantadine
Junin virus			
Argentine hemorrhagic fever	Contact	No (do not give expressed breast milk)	

(Continued)

TABLE D.1   Precautions and Breastfeeding Recommendations for Selected Maternal Infections[a]—cont'd

Organism, Syndrome, or Condition[b,c]	Empiric Precautions[d]	Breastfeeding Acceptable[e]	Compatibility of Medications With Breastfeeding[f]
Lassa fever	Contact	No (do not give expressed breast milk)	Intravenous ribavirin
Legionnaires' disease			
Legionella pneumophila	Standard	Yes	Azithromycin, erythromycin, levofloxacin
Pneumonia ± gastrointestinal, central nervous system, or renal involvement			
Leprosy			
Mycobacterium leprae	Standard	Yes	Dapsone, rifampin, clofazimine
Chronic disease of skin, peripheral nerves, and respiratory mucosa			
Leptospirosis			
Abrupt febrile illness, often biphasic, with multiple organ involvement			
Leptospira interrogans	Standard	Yes (no mother-infant contact except for breastfeeding)	Penicillin, cefotaxime, ceftriaxone
Leptospira icterohaemorrhagiae			
Leptospira canicola			
Listeria monocytogenes	Standard	Yes	Ampicillin, penicillin, TMP-SMX
In adults: nonspecific febrile illness; in neonates: meningitis, pneumonia, sepsis, granulomatosis infantisepticum			
Lyme disease			
Borrelia burgdorferi			
Multistaged illness of skin, joint, and peripheral or central nervous system	Standard	Yes, with informed discussion[h]	Ceftriaxone, ampicillin, doxycycline
Lymphocytic choriomeningitis			
Aseptic meningitis to severe encephalitis, with variable presentation of other symptoms	Standard	Yes	
Malaria	Standard	Yes	Pyrimethamine-sulfadoxine, chloroquine, quinidine, quinine, tetracycline, mefloquine
Marburg virus			
Hemorrhagic fever	Contact	No (no expressed breast milk)	
Mastitis			
Candida albicans	Standard	Yes, with simultaneous treatment of the infant[h]	Nystatin, ketoconazole, fluconazole
Enterobacteriaceae	Standard	Yes	First-generation cephalosporin,
Staphylococcus aureus	Contact	Yes[h] (after 24 h of therapy, during which milk must be discarded) (If infant becomes ill during	Dicloxacillin, oxacillin, erythromycin

(Continued)

TABLE D.1 Precautions and Breastfeeding Recommendations for Selected Maternal Infections[a]—cont'd

Organism, Syndrome, or Condition[b,c]	Empiric Precautions[d]	Breastfeeding Acceptable[e]	Compatibility of Medications With Breastfeeding[f]
		evaluation and treatment of mother, infant should be treated for presumed staphylococcal infection, and breast milk should be withheld until proven to be culture negative.)	
Group A *Streptococcus*	Contact	Yes[h] (after 24 h of therapy, during which milk must be discarded) (If infant becomes ill during evaluation and treatment of mother, infant should be treated for presumed streptococcal infection, and breast milk should be withheld until proven to be culturally negative.)	Ampicillin, third-generation cephalosporin
Group B *Streptococcus*	[h]	Yes[h] (after 24 h of therapy for the mother, breast milk is permissible with observation of the infant) No[h] (If infant is sick with suspected or proven group B streptococcal infection and the breast milk is being cultured to identify a source of infection; BM is permissible if breast milk is culture negative.)	Penicillin, cephalosporin, macrolides
Mycobacterium tuberculosis	Standard (if mother has pulmonary involvement, then airborne precautions as well)	No[h] (breastfeeding for 2 weeks of maternal therapy, consider prophylactic INH for infant [see Fig. 12.3 and Table 12.1], breast milk permissible with INH)	Isoniazid (INH), rifampin, ethambutol, pyrazinamide ethionamide
Measles			
Febrile illness with coryza, conjunctivitis, cough, and an erythematous maculopapular rash	Airborne	Yes (after 72 h of rash in mother and after infant receives ISG, expressed breast milk is permissible)	Ribavirin is experimental
Meningitis			
Aseptic meningitis (nonbacterial, viral meningitis)	Standard	Yes	
Fungal meningitis	Standard	Yes	Amphotericin, itraconazole, flucytosine
Haemophilus influenzae	Droplet (for first 24 h of appropriate therapy and carrier eradication with ceftriaxone or rifampin)	Yes (after 24 h of maternal therapy, with the infant receiving prophylaxis, prophylactic antibiotics begin infant vaccination; expressed breast milk is permissible)	Ceftriaxone, ampicillin, chloramphenicol, rifampin
Neisseria meningitidis	Droplet (24 h of appropriate therapy and carrier eradication with ceftriaxone or rifampin)	Yes (after 24 h of maternal therapy, with the infant receiving prophylaxis, prophylactic antibiotics expressed breast milk is permissible)	Ceftriaxone, penicillin, chloramphenicol
Streptococcus pneumoniae	Standard	Yes	Ceftriaxone, penicillin, vancomycin
Mumps	Droplet	Yes	

(Continued)

TABLE D.1   Precautions and Breastfeeding Recommendations for Selected Maternal Infections[a]—cont'd

Organism, Syndrome, or Condition[b,c]	Empiric Precautions[d]	Breastfeeding Acceptable[e]	Compatibility of Medications With Breastfeeding[f]
Mycobacterium tuberculosis[h]	Standard and airborne	Yes	Antituberculosis medications are acceptable during breastfeeding (see Chapter 12, section on Tuberculosis and *Red Book*, 31st edition)
Mycoplasma pneumoniae Bronchitis, pneumonia, pharyngitis, otitis media, and a broad range of unusual manifestations, including central nervous system, cardiac, skin, muscle, and joint involvement	Droplet	Yes	Erythromycin, clarithromycin, azithromycin, tetracycline
Neisseria meningitidis Meningitis, meningococcemia	Droplet (for 24 h of appropriate therapy and carrier eradication with ceftriaxone or rifampin)	Yes (after 24 h of appropriate therapy, and with prophylaxis for the infant)	Penicillin, ceftriaxone, chloramphenicol, rifampin
Norwalk agent Gastroenteritis	Standard	Yes	
Papillomaviruses Skin or mucous membrane warts, laryngeal papillomas	Standard	Yes (in the absence of breast or nipple involvement)	
Parainfluenza viruses Laryngotracheobronchitis, upper and lower respiratory infections	Standard (contact for infants and children)	Yes	
Parvovirus B19 Erythema infectiosum, fifth disease, aplastic crisis, arthritis	Standard Droplet for mothers with aplastic crisis or immunodeficient and prolonged illness	Yes (no infectious risk after the appearance of the rash in immune-competent individuals) No (for aplastic crisis or infection in individuals with hemoglobinopathy or immune deficiency infection for the duration of the illness [DI])[d]	
Pelvic inflammatory disease (see Endometritis)			
Pertussis Whooping cough, pneumonia, bronchitis, encephalitis *Bordetella parapertussis* and *Bordetella pertussis*	Droplet (for 5 days of appropriate therapy)	Yes (after 5 days of appropriate therapy and chemoprophylaxis for the infant, expressed breast milk is permissible) If no appropriate Rx is given, then 3 weeks of droplet precautions	Erythromycin, clarithromycin, TMP-SMX
Pneumocystis jiroveci pneumonia (previously *Pneumocystis carinii* pneumonitis)	Standard	Yes, but suspect HIV infection if mother develops symptoms and reassess breastfeeding with HIV infection in mind	Pentamidine, TMP-SMX, atovaquone, prednisone

(Continued)

TABLE D.1   Precautions and Breastfeeding Recommendations for Selected Maternal Infections[a]—cont'd

Organism, Syndrome, or Condition[b,c]	Empiric Precautions[d]	Breastfeeding Acceptable[e]	Compatibility of Medications With Breastfeeding[f]
Pneumonia (see specific causative agents)			
Poliomyelitis	Standard	Yes	
Rabies			
Severe, progressive central nervous system infection, generally fatal	Standard	No[h] (when mother is clinically sick) Yes[h] (BM +) (during postexposure immunization of mother without symptoms; yes if both mother and infant are receiving postexposure RIG and immunization)	Rabies immune globulin (RIG), rabies vaccine
Rat-bite fever			
Spirillum minus	Standard	Yes	Tetracycline, chloramphenicol, streptomycin
Streptobacillus moniliformis	Standard	Yes	Penicillin
Relapsing fever			
Borrelia recurrentis	Standard (tick-borne)	Yes	Tetracycline, doxycycline, TMP-SMX, streptomycin, rifampin
	Contact if louse infested	Yes with simultaneous treatment of mother and infant for body lice	Topical Pediculicides are OK Ivermectin (oral or topical)
Respiratory syncytial virus			
Upper respiratory infection, pneumonia, bronchiolitis	Contact	Yes	Ribavirin
Retroviruses			
(See Human immunodeficiency viruses 1, 2 and Human T-cell leukemia viruses I, II)			
Rickettsial diseases			
Fever, rash, vasculitis; arthropod, louse-borne			
Ehrlichiosis, leukopenia	Standard	Yes	Doxycycline, tetracycline
Ehrlichia chaffeensis			
Q fever			
Coxiella burnetii			
Pneumonia, hepatosplenomegaly, endocarditis	Standard	Yes	Doxycycline, tetracycline, TMP-SMX
Rickettsial pox			
Rickettsia akari			
Scab or eschar, rash, regional lymphadenopathy, self-limited	Standard	Yes	Doxycycline, tetracycline, fluoroquinolones
Rocky Mountain spotted fever			
Rickettsia rickettsii	Standard	Yes	Doxycycline
Typhus (flea-borne)			
Rickettsia typhi	Standard	Yes	Doxycycline, fluoroquinolones
Typhus (louse-borne)			
Rickettsia prowazekii	Standard	Yes	Doxycycline (in epidemic situations a single dose may be adequate), chloramphenicol

(*Continued*)

TABLE D.1   Precautions and Breastfeeding Recommendations for Selected Maternal Infections[a]—cont'd

Organism, Syndrome, or Condition[b,c]	Empiric Precautions[d]	Breastfeeding Acceptable[e]	Compatibility of Medications With Breastfeeding[f]
Rotavirus Diarrhea, vomiting, "winter vomiting disease"	Contact	Yes	
Rubella virus Self-limited, mild exanthem with fever: congenital rubella syndrome	Contact	Yes	
Salmonella (see Diarrhea/gastroenteritis)			
SARS-associated coronavirus, severe acute respiratory syndrome	Droplet	Yes	
***Shigella* (see Diarrhea)**			
Smallpox Variola virus (variola major)	Contact, airborne	No (no expressed breast milk)	
Vaccinia virus (smallpox vaccine) secondary contact infection	Contact	Yes, except if breast involved with lesions	
Staphylococcus aureus Cellulitis, abscess	Contact	Yes	Oxacillin, dicloxacillin, first-generation cephalosporins, erythromycin, vancomycin
Enterocolitis, diarrhea	Standard	Yes	
Scalded-skin syndrome	Contact	Yes (after 24 h of effective therapy; discard breast milk for 24 h)	
Toxic shock syndrome	Standard	Yes[h]	
Methicillin-resistant *S. aureus* (MRSA)	Contact	Yes[h] (after 24 h of therapy, during which milk must be discarded) (If infant becomes ill during evaluation and treatment of mother, infant should be treated for presumed MRSA infection, and breast milk should be withheld until proven to be culture negative.)	Vancomycin, TMP-SMX, clindamycin, linezolid
Staphylococcus epidermidis Opportunistic infections	Standard	Yes	Oxacillin, dicloxacillin, vancomycin
Streptococcus Group A: Cellulitis, pharyngitis, pneumonia, myositis/fasciitis, scarlet fever	Standard	Yes (24 h after beginning appropriate therapy; discard breast milk for 24 h)	Penicillin, erythromycin, cephalosporin
	Contact (for extensive skin infection unable to be covered until after 24 h of therapy)	Yes (24 h after beginning appropriate therapy; discard breast milk for 24 h)	
Group B: Urinary tract infection, endometritis, mastitis; infants: sepsis, pneumonia, meningitis, osteomyelitis, arthritis	Standard	Yes[h] (after 24 h of therapy, during which milk must be discarded) (If infant becomes ill during evaluation and treatment of mother, infant should be treated for presumed streptococcal	Penicillin, ampicillin, third-generation cephalosporin

(Continued)

TABLE D.1   Precautions and Breastfeeding Recommendations for Selected Maternal Infections[a]—cont'd

Organism, Syndrome, or Condition[b,c]	Empiric Precautions[d]	Breastfeeding Acceptable[e]	Compatibility of Medications With Breastfeeding[f]
		infection, and breast milk should be withheld until proven to be culture negative.)	
Streptococcus pneumoniae Pneumonia, occult bacteremia, otitis media, sinusitis	Standard	Yes	Penicillin, ceftriaxone, vancomycin, cefotaxime, rifampin
Strongyloidiasis *Strongyloides stercoralis*	Standard	Yes	Ivermectin, Albendazole
Syphilis **Treponema pallidum** Multisystem, multistage infection with widely varying presentations, congenital infection	Standard	Yes (after 24 h of effective therapy; discard breast milk for 24 h)	Penicillin, doxycycline, tetracycline
Open skin lesions of breast or nipples	Contact	No, until 24 h of effective therapy in mother if open skin lesions involve breasts	Penicillin, doxycycline, tetracycline
Tetanus Exotoxin-mediated severe muscular spasms *Clostridium tetani*	Standard	Yes (age-appropriate vaccination of the child, no tetanus immunoglobulin [TIG] necessary for infant)	Penicillin, metronidazole
Tinea capitis *Microsporum audouinii*	Standard	Yes	Griseofulvin, terbinafine, selenium sulfide shampoo, prednisone
Microsporum canis *Trichophyton tonsurans*			
Tinea corporis, cruris, pedis *Epidermophyton floccosum*	Standard	Yes	Topical agents
Trichophyton canis *Trichophyton rubrum*			
Tinea versicolor *Malassezia furfur*	Standard	Yes	Topical agents, ketoconazole, itraconazole
Toxoplasmosis *Toxoplasma gondii*	Standard	Yes	Pyrimethamine, sulfadiazine, TMP-SMX, dapsone, atovaquone, clindamycin
Asymptomatic or mononucleosis-like illness with lymphadenopathy, ocular symptoms; congenital infection			
Toxic shock (see *S. aureus, Streptococcus* [group A])			

(Continued)

TABLE D.1   Precautions and Breastfeeding Recommendations for Selected Maternal Infections[a]—cont'd

Organism, Syndrome, or Condition[b,c]	Empiric Precautions[d]	Breastfeeding Acceptable[e]	Compatibility of Medications With Breastfeeding[f]
Toxin-mediated illness (see specific agents)			
Bacillus cereus			
Botulism			
Food poisoning			
Staphylococcal scalded-skin syndrome (SSSS)			
Trichinosis			
Trichinella spiralis			
Asymptomatic, or may cause myalgia, periorbital edema, myocardial failure, CNS involvement, or pneumonitis	Standard	Yes	Albendazole, mebendazole, thiabendazole, prednisone
Trichomonas vaginalis			
Vaginitis, urethritis, or asymptomatic infections	Standard	Yes	Metronidazole, tinidazole
Trypanosomiasis			
Trypanosoma brucei			
"Sleeping sickness"; tsetse fly vector (African)	Standard	No	Suramin, pentamidine, eflornithine, melarsoprol
Trypanosoma cruzi			
Chagas disease (American)	Standard	Yes[h]	Nifurtimox, benznidazole
TT virus			
Hepatitis	Standard	Yes	
Tuberculosis (see *Mycobacterium* in this Appendix; see Chapter 12, Figures 12.2 and 12.3 and Table 12.1; see *Red Book*, 31st edition)			
Tularemia			
Francisella tularensis			
Acute febrile illness with various syndromes; oculoglandular, ulceroglandular, glandular, oropharyngeal, typhoidal, pneumonia	Standard	Yes	Streptomycin, gentamicin, doxycycline, ciprofloxacin
Ureaplasma urealyticum			
Nongonococcal urethritis (NGU), endometritis, pelvic inflammatory disease	Standard	Yes	Doxycycline, erythromycin, azithromycin, clarithromycin, ciprofloxacin
Urinary tract infection			
Group B streptococcus (see *Streptococcus* [group B])	Standard	Yes	Ampicillin, aminoglycosides, cephalosporin
Enterobacteriaceae	Standard	Yes	Ampicillin, cephalosporins, fluoroquinolones
Staphylococcus saprophyticus	Standard	Yes	Vancomycin, clindamycin + rifampin
Vaginitis			
Bacterial	Standard	Yes	Metronidazole, clindamycin
Candida albicans (see Candidiasis)			
Varicella-zoster virus (see Herpesviruses)			

(Continued)

TABLE D.1   Precautions and Breastfeeding Recommendations for Selected Maternal Infections[a]—cont'd

Organism, Syndrome, or Condition[b,c]	Empiric Precautions[d]	Breastfeeding Acceptable[e]	Compatibility of Medications With Breastfeeding[f]
West Nile virus	Standard	Yes[h]	
Asymptomatic, fever, meningoencephalitis			
Whooping cough			
Bordetella parapertussis and *Bordetella pertussis*: see also Adenovirus, *Chlamydia* (*Chlamydia pneumoniae*, *Chlamydia trachomatis*), *Mycoplasma pneumoniae* as other agents may mimic the clinical picture of whooping cough	Droplet (for 5 days of appropriate therapy and chemoprophylaxis for infant)	Yes, after 5 days of appropriate therapy, breast milk + , P[h]	Erythromycin, clarithromycin, TMP-SMX
Yellow fever			
Yellow fever virus	Standard	Yes[h]	
Yellow fever vaccine virus	Standard	No[h]	Avoid yellow fever vaccine virus immunization during lactation if possible[h]
Yersinia enterocolitica			
Diarrhea, pseudoappendicitis, focal infections, and bacteremia	Contact precautions for incontinent individuals	Yes	Cefotaxime, aminoglycosides, TMP-SMX, fluoroquinolones
Yersinia pseudotuberculosis			
Fever, rash, abdominal symptoms	Standard	Yes	TMP-SMX
Zika virus	Standard	Yes[h]	

BF, Breastfeeding; *BM*, breastmilk; *DI*, duration of illness; *HCoV*, human coronavirus; *INH*, isoniazid; *MERS*, Middle Eastern respiratory syndrome; SARS, severe acute respiratory syndrome; TMP/SMX, trimethoprim/sulfamethoxazole.

[a]To ensure that appropriate empiric precautions are always implemented, hospitals must have systems in place to routinely evaluate patients according to these criteria as part of their preadmission and admission care.

[b]Patients with the syndromes or conditions listed may present with atypical signs and symptoms (e.g., pertussis in neonates and adults may not have paroxysmal or severe cough). A clinician's index of suspicion should be guided by the prevalence of specific conditions in the community and clinical judgment.

[c]The organisms listed are not intended to represent the complete, or even most likely diagnoses, but rather possible etiologic agents that may require additional precautions, beyond *standard precautions*, until they can be excluded.

[d]These are the usual precautions (Standard, Airborne, Contact, and Droplet) outlined in the text, as proposed by the Centers for Disease Control and Prevention. Symbols for duration of precautions: *24 hours*, 24 hours of antibiotic therapy; *CN*, until off antibiotics and culture negative; *DI*, duration of the illness; *PI*, period of infectivity.

[e]*Yes* means that if, in a hospitalized mother and infant, the proposed precautions are followed, breastfeeding is acceptable and may be beneficial to the infant. Any infant breastfeeding during a maternal infection should be observed closely for signs or symptoms of illness. *BM* + , Expressed breastmilk is OK to give the infant even if breastfeeding is not OK.

[f]See Chapter 11 on medications in breast milk, in this book, and refer to LactMed at http://toxnet.nlm.nih.gov/newtoxnet/lactmed.htm.

[g]Adenovirus types 4 and 7 have been known to cause severe respiratory disease in premature infants or individuals with immunodeficiency or underlying respiratory disease. In certain situations, feeding of expressed breast milk to an infant may not be advisable.

[h]See text for more complete explanation. *P*, Prophylactic antibiotics for the infant. See the 2018 Report of the Committee on Infectious Diseases, *Red Book*, 31st edition, for current recommendations on the specific antibiotics for the specific condition.

[i]Breastfeed immediately if mother receives ceftriaxone intramuscularly or intravenously. Breastfeed after 24-hour antibiotic therapy for other treatment regiments, with feeding expressed breast milk for the first 24 hours.

Modified from Garner JS. Hospital Infection Control Practices Advisory Committee guidelines for isolation precautions in hospitals. *Infect Control Hosp Epidemiol.* 1996;17:53.

E APPENDIX

Manual Expression of Breast Milk

Casey Rosen-Carole

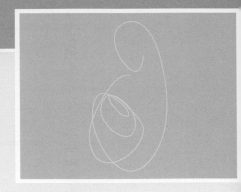

A health care professional should be familiar with the technique of manual expression and be able to correct improper technique. Ideally this technique is taught to mothers in the prenatal period or soon after birth, before discharge from the hospital in the case of a hospital birth. It should be demonstrated by postpartum nursing staff, lactation consultants, or birth attendants, and women should be given the opportunity to practice with assistance.

Reasons to express breast milk include the following:

1. To initiate flow and assist an infant to grasp the breast properly
2. To encourage production of milk early in lactation when an infant is premature or ill
3. To relieve engorgement
4. To remove milk when it is not possible to nurse an infant at a given feeding
5. To pump and save milk for feeding an infant at another time
6. To contribute to a milk bank
7. To pump and discard milk while temporarily on a specific medication

As opposed to a pump, hand expression has a low cost and may be more hygienic in certain circumstances. It may also promote self-efficacy, particularly when used to express colostrum before lactogenesis II. Manual expression also may be used to initiate flow before applying a pump or at the end of pumping to ensure drainage.

PROCEDURE

Step 1—Preparation, Hygiene, Containers, and Position: Hands should be washed and a clean container obtained. For colostrum, a spoon or syringe is often adequate. After lactogenesis II, a large bowl may be used to catch errant sprays, and milk can then be poured into a storage container. The mother should find a comfortable clean location and be as relaxed as possible.

Step 2—Facilitating Letdown, Reminders of Infant, Breast Massage, and Heat: Whether planning to manually express or mechanically pump, preparing the breast for ejecting the milk facilitates the process. The release of oxytocin and the ejection reflex are stimulated by external stimuli: a baby's cry, a picture of the baby, or gentle handling of the breast. Prolactin release and milk production are stimulated by "sucking" stimulation.

The breast can be gently stroked from periphery to areola and gently massaged. One should avoid roughly rubbing the hand across skin and irritating tissues; this should not be painful or leave marks. A warm washcloth, heat pack, or soaking in warm water are also helpful in initiating flow through the ducts. Gentle fingertip massage around all quadrants should follow and be repeated several times during extended mechanical pumping. A good example of therapeutic breast massage and hand expression is studied and taught by Dr. Ann Witt and Maya Bolman, IBCLC,[1,2] and can be viewed for free online.

Step 3—Positioning Hands on the Breast (the C-hold near, but not on, the areola): Usually placing the fingers below and thumb on top is natural for most women (Fig. E.1). One hand placed above and one hand placed below the areola may be easier when the hand is small compared with breast size. The target area is beyond the ampullae, which are the collecting areas of the main ducts that radiate out from the nipple to the areola. The ampullae are approximately 3 cm from the nipple base and are generally, but may not be, at the edge of the areola. Compressing at the areola, however, may cause pain and should be avoided. The hand should be pressed toward the chest wall, and then the thumb and fingers compressed together (Fig. E.2). Continue to compress the breast while moving the hand away from the chest wall in a "milking" action toward the nipple (Fig. E.3). The fingers should roll, rather than rub, toward the areola (pulling, squeezing, or rubbing motions should be avoided). This motion should be performed in a repeated rhythmic manner at a comfortable rate. The hand should be rotated around the breast to massage and stroke all quadrants, including the periphery and the axillae. Dr. Jane Morton, a breastfeeding advocate and expert clinician, suggests the terms "Press, Compress, Release" to teach parents this technique.[3] Her video series on hand expression is evidence-based, widely used, and available for free online.[4]

Of note, every mother develops her own natural pattern, so rigid adherence to methods may be counterproductive. Effectiveness is measured by the comfortable release of milk.

Total emptying of the breast will generally require 20 to 30 minutes of manual expression. If engorgement or mastitis is present, warm compresses, hot showers, or suspending the breast in a bowl of warm water may help. Leaning over and gently shaking the breast may help stimulate flow. Manual expression while leaning over may help empty the lower quadrants.

The Reference list is available at www.expertconsult.com.

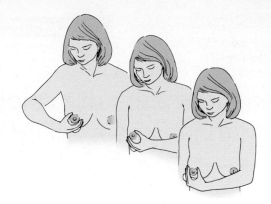

Fig. E.1

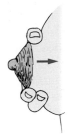

Fig. E.2

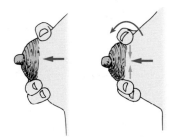

Fig. E.3

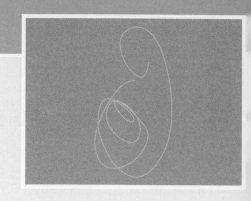

Measurements of Weight Loss and Growth in Breastfed Infants

Casey Rosen-Carole

WEIGHT LOSS IN THE FIRST DAYS OF LIFE: THE NEWBORN WEIGHT TOOL

The Newborn Weight Tool (NEWT) tool was developed from 2014 to 2016 as a collaboration across several academic medical centers in the United States led by Drs. Ian Paul and Valerie Flaherman and statistician Eric Schaefer. Data extraction of 161,471 singleton infants was used to create nomograms for infant weight loss in the first 72 to 96 hours of life depending on feeding and delivery type[1] (Fig. F.1). The online calculator[2] will plot a neonate's weight loss percentile and trajectory and identifies infants at high risk if they exceed the 75th percentile of weight loss or increase in weight loss percentiles, rather than decrease, after the first 24 hours. There is now a calculator for the first 30 days of life as well.

STANDARDS FOR GROWTH UNTIL AGE 5: WORLD HEALTH ORGANIZATION

Growth standards for breastfed infants and children were developed by the WHO from 1997 to 2003, after a large prospective trial of healthy children 0 to 59 months in 6 countries.[3] Participating children were breastfed according to WHO recommendations. These curves therefore represent longitudinal growth and growth velocity in appropriately fed, thriving children. They are available for free online[4] and are included here (Figs. F.2 through F.9).

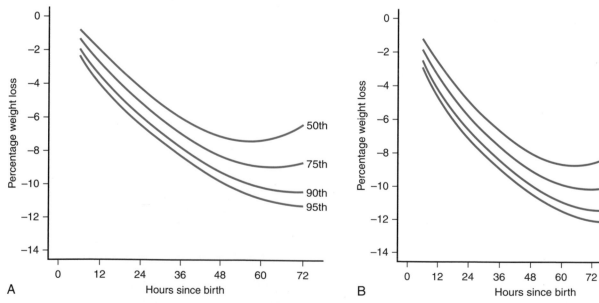

Fig. F.1 (A) Estimated percentile curves of percent weight loss by time after birth for vaginal deliveries. (B) Estimated percentile curves of percent weight loss by time after birth for cesarean deliveries. (From Flaherman VJ, Schaefer EW, Kuzniewicz MW, et al. Early weight loss nomograms for exclusively breastfed newborns. *Pediatrics.* 2015;135[1]:e16–23. doi:10.1542/peds.2014–1532.)

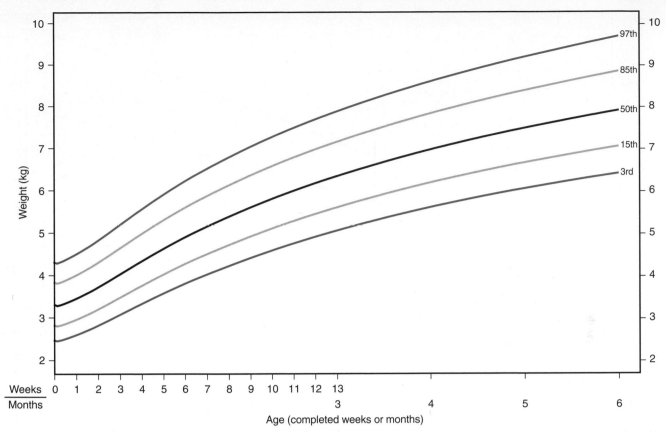

Fig. F.2 Weight-for-age in BOYS 0 to 6 months. Graph lines represent the 3rd to the 97th percentiles. (From World Health Organization. World Health Organization growth standards. Geneva, Switzerland.)

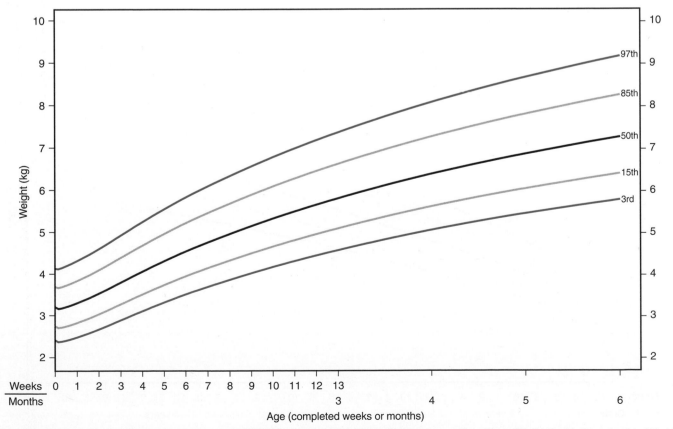

Fig. F.3 Weight-for-age in GIRLS 0 to 6 months. Graph lines represent the 3rd to the 97th percentiles. (From World Health Organization. World Health Organization growth standards. Geneva, Switzerland.)

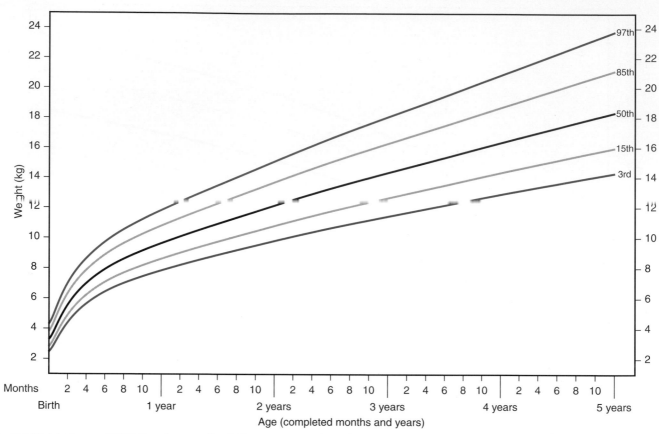

Fig. F.4 Weight-for-age BOYS 0 to 5 years. Graph lines represent the 3rd to the 97th percentiles. (From World Health Organization. World Health Organization growth standards. Geneva, Switzerland.)

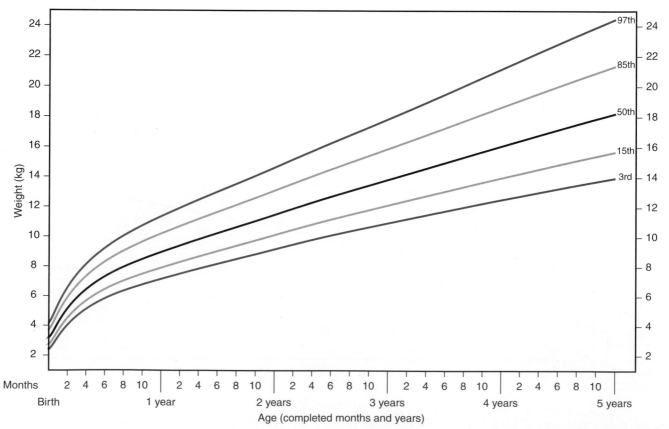

Fig. F.5 Weight-for-age GIRLS 0 to 5 years. Graph lines represent the 3rd to the 97th percentiles. (From World Health Organization. World Health Organization growth standards. Geneva, Switzerland.)

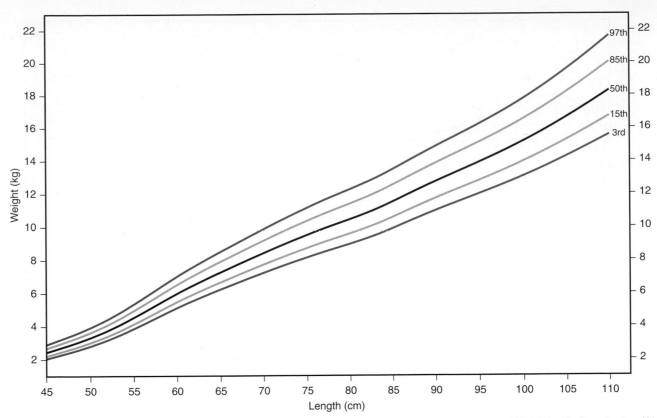

Fig. F.6 Weight-for-length BOYS 0 to 2 years. Graph lines represent the 3rd to the 97th percentiles. (From World Health Organization. World Health Organization growth standards. Geneva, Switzerland.)

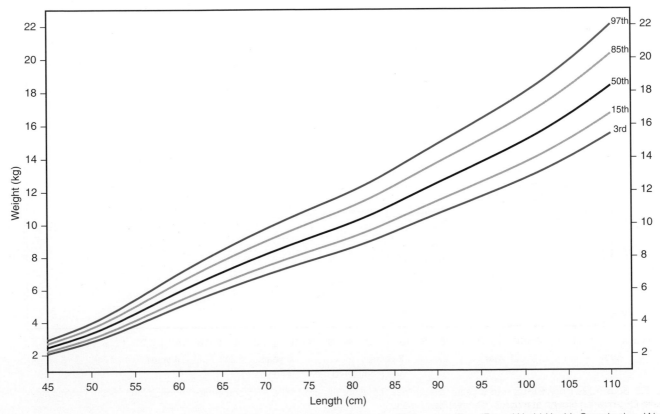

Fig. F.7 Weight-for-length GIRLS 0 to 2 years. Graph lines represent the 3rd to the 97th percentiles. (From World Health Organization. World Health Organization growth standards. Geneva, Switzerland.)

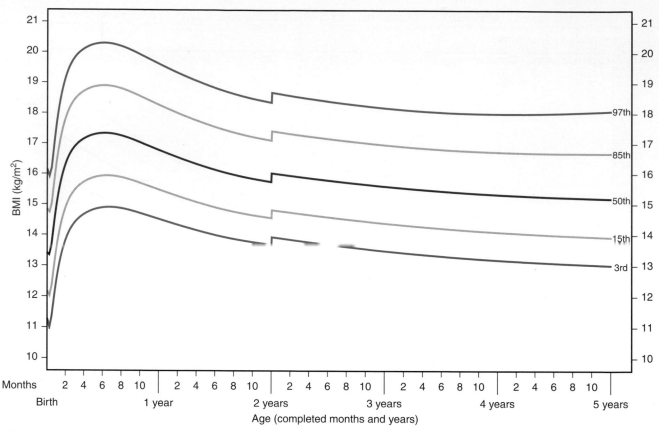

Fig. F.8 Body mass index BOYS 0 to 5 years. Graph lines represent the 3rd to the 97th percentiles. (From World Health Organization. World Health Organization growth standards. Geneva, Switzerland.)

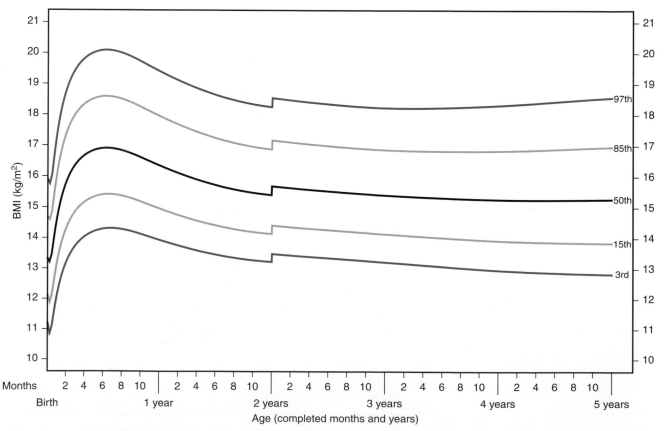

Fig. F.9 Body mass index GIRLS 0 to 5 years. Graph lines represent the 3rd to the 97th percentiles. (From World Health Organization. World Health Organization growth standards. Geneva, Switzerland.)

The Reference list is available at www.expertconsult.com.

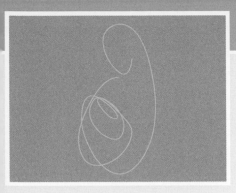
Organizations Supporting Breastfeeding and Promoting Lactation Knowledge

Robert M. Lawrence

GOVERNMENT AGENCIES

Food and Nutrition Information Center
National Agricultural Library, USA-ARS
10301 Baltimore Avenue, Room 108
Beltsville, MD 20705-2350
Phone: 301-504-5414
Fax: 301-504-6409
E-mail: ndlinfo@ars.usda.gov
Website: http://ndb.nal.usda.gov

This center provides information on human nutrition, nutrition education, food service management, consumer education, and food technology and functions as a resource library loaning books, journal articles, and audiovisual materials for nutrition and breastfeeding.

Office of the Assistant Secretary for Health, Office of the Secretary
US Department of Health and Human Services
1101 Wootton Parkway, Suite LL100
Rockville, MD 20852
Phone: 240-453-8280
Fax: 240-453-8281
E-mail: info@nhic.org
Website: http://www.health.gov/NHIC/
    This office supports three websites:
    Healthy People healthypeople@hhs.gov
    Healthfinder.gov healthfinder@hhs.gov
    National Health Information Center nhic@hhs.gov

These sites help consumers answer questions and locate health information at these different sites/databases. Health questions can be referred to appropriate health agencies that, in turn, respond directly to inquirers.

Office of Women's Health (OWH)
Office of the Assistant Secretary for Health at the US Department of Health and Human Services
200 Independence Avenue, SW

Washington, DC 20201
Phone: 800-994-9662
Website: http://www.womenshealth.gov

This office supports programs and activities for women's health, including a focus on breastfeeding. There is a broad range of informational materials concerning women's health available through the site. There are focused materials specifically for breastfeeding: The Business Case for Breastfeeding and "Your Guide to Breastfeeding."

National Information Center on Health Services Research and Health Care Technology (NICHSR)
National Institute of Health/US National Library of Medicine
8600 Rockville Pike
Bethesda, MD 20894
Phone: 888-346-3656 or 301-594-5983
Website: www.nlm.nih.gov/hsrph.html

This website maintains a search program for accessing health information contained anywhere in the National Library of Medicine and the National Institute of Health. NICHSR ONESearch at https://hsric.nlm.nih.gov/hsric_public.

Agency for Healthcare Research and Quality (AHRQ)
US Department of Health and Human Services
5600 Fishers Lane
Rockville MD, 20857
Phone: 301-427-1364
Website: http://www.ahrq.gov

This agency works to produce evidence to affect health care, making it safer, of higher quality, and more equitable, affordable, and accessible. They foster collaboration between research entities and clinical practice through the production of clinical practice guidelines, share research tools and data, evaluate programs for quality and patient safety, and produce evidence-based reports. It creates, catalogs, and makes available materials to teach and train health care professionals and institutions to improve care for patients.

US Food and Drug Administration (FDA)
10903 New Hampshire Avenue
Silver Spring, MD 20993
Phone: 888-463-6332
Website: http://www.fda.gov

This agency regulates the safe use and availability of food and medications within the United States. It is a resource of information and guidance for consumers, patients, health professionals, scientists, and industry. It provides information on the requirements for labeling of prescription drugs and biologic products for use during pregnancy and lactation. It maintains information on safety of product use during lactation and the use of donor human milk.

Centers for Disease Control and Prevention (CDC)
National Center for Chronic Disease Prevention and Health
    Promotion
Division of Nutrition, Physical Activity and Obesity
1600 Clifton Road
Atlanta, GA 30333
Phone: 800-232-4636
Website: http://www.cdc.gov/breastfeeding

The division of Nutrition, Physical Activity, and Obesity maintains and analyzes data on all aspects of health related to those issues but has a focus on breastfeeding for health promotion. It conducts national surveys to assess breastfeeding data for the United States and produces a yearly "Breastfeeding Report Card, United States." It supports a national "Call to Action" for breastfeeding, and the Healthy People 2020 Objectives focused on breastfeeding and newborn health. It provides information for consumers and health care professionals on numerous aspects of breastfeeding and lactation.

World Health Organization (WHO)
Publications Center (US location)
5 Sand Creek Road
Albany, NY 12205-1400
Phone: 518-436-9686
Fax: 518-436-7433
Website: http://www.who.int/nutrition
E-mail: QCORP@compuserve.com

The WHO maintains a large database for numerous health care issues and breastfeeding comes under its focus on maternal, infant, and child nutrition (Department of Nutrition for Health and Development). Publications available include a statement on infant and young child feeding, a breastfeeding guide for use by community health workers, and a study on patterns of breastfeeding, among other focused publications.

The Global Breastfeeding Collective
WHO and UNICEF (US location)
125 Maiden Lane
New York, NY 10038
Phone: 212-686-5522
Website: http://www.unicef.org/nutrition/index_98470.html

This organization, led by the WHO and UNICEF, is a partnership with 20 international agencies to increase investment in breastfeeding worldwide. The WHO and UNICEF collaborate to develop evidence-informed guidance and policies, support adoption of guidance and actions to improve health, and monitor implementation of policy and programs with resultant outcomes for nutrition and breastfeeding. The Global Breastfeeding Collective partners include 1000 Days, Academy of Breastfeeding Medicine, Action Against Hunger, Alive and Thrive, Bill and Melinda Gates Foundation, CARE, Carolina Global Breastfeeding Institute, Center for Women's Health and Wellness, Centers for Disease Control and Prevention, Concern Worldwide, Helen Keller International, International Baby Food Action Network, International Lactation Consultant Association, La Leche League International, New Partnership for Africa's Development, Nutritional International, PATH (formerly known as Program for Appropriate Technology in Health), Save the Children, UNICEF, United States Agency for International Development, WHO, World Alliance for Breastfeeding Action, World Bank, and World Vision International.

PRIVATE EDUCATIONAL AND SUPPORT ORGANIZATIONS

Health Education Associates (HEA)
327 Quaker Meeting House Road
East Sandwich, MA 02537-1300
Phone: 888-888-8077 (toll-free), 508-888-8044
Fax: 508-888-8050
E-mail: info@healthed.cc
Website: https://healthed.com

Health Education Associates, an independent health publishing company, make inexpensive pamphlets and other materials available as teaching aids on breastfeeding. They sponsor training programs for breastfeeding counseling and promotion techniques.

**Institute for the Advancement of Breastfeeding & Lactation
    Education (IABLE)**
Website: https://lacted.org

This is a nonprofit organization supporting breastfeeding education with handouts, courses, and conferences and developing and sustaining breastfeeding support systems and communities. They are associated with The Milk Mob and with GOLD Learning Online Continuing Education to accomplish their goals.

International Childbirth Education Association (ICEA)
110 Horizon Drive, Suite 210

Raleigh, NC 27615
Phone: 919-674-4183
Fax: 919-459-2075
E-mail: info@icea.org
Website: http://www.icea.org

The association's *Bookmarks* catalog has a large selection of books and inexpensive pamphlets on breastfeeding, childbirth, and parenting. It publishes *ICEA News*, with news about childbirth, prenatal, and parenting issues, and *ICEA Review*, which provides in-depth reviews of current perinatal issues. It also has a resource committee on breastfeeding.

International Lactation Consultant Association (ILCA)
2501 Aerial Center Parkway, Suite 103
Morrisville, NC 27560
Phone: 919-861-5577
Fax: 919-459-2075
E-mail: info@ilca.org
Website: http://www.ilca.org

The International Lactation Consultant Association (ILCA) provides many services, including newsletters, the *Journal of Human Lactation* and annual conferences.

La Leche League International, Inc. (LLLI)
110 Horizon Drive, Suite 210
Raleigh, NC 27615, USA
Phone: 919-459-2167; 1-800-LaLeche
Fax: 919-459-2075
E-mail: info@llli.org
Website: http://www.llli.org

La Leche's publications catalog includes a large variety and broad scope of materials for mothers and health professionals to use in promoting and supporting breastfeeding. There is also a directory of league area coordinators by state and foreign country. The coordinators can give information about local support groups.

United States Breastfeeding Committee (USBC)
4044 N Lincoln Avenue, No. 288
Chicago IL 60618
Phone: 773-359-1549
Fax: 773-313-3498
Website: http://www.usbreastfeeding.org

This is a coalition of over 50 organizations collaborating to improve policies and practices to support breastfeeding within the United States. It works on strategic planning for breastfeeding and legislation in the United States and hosts the National Breastfeeding Coalitions Conference, yearly. It is a resource for breastfeeding publications and position statements. It connects people with the resources provided by the various collaborating breastfeeding organizations through "Breastfeeding Frequently Asked Questions" on the website.

Baby Friendly, USA
Corporate Headquarters
125 Wolf Road, Suite 402
Albany, NY 12205
Phone: 518-621-7982
Fax: 518-621-7983
E-mail: info@babyfriendlyusa.org
Website: http://www.babyfriendlyusa.org

This organization is the originator of the Baby Friendly Hospital Initiative (BFHI), including guidelines and evaluation criteria. BFHI was adapted by the WHO and UNICEF for use worldwide. The Baby Friendly organization continues to work for the dissemination of lactation information and hospital and community support of breastfeeding.

WABA Secretariat: World Alliance for Breastfeeding Action
PO Box 1200
10850 Penang
Malaysia
Phone: 604-658-4816
Fax: 604-657-2655
E-mail: waba@waba.org.my
Website: http://www.waba.org.my

The World Alliance for Breastfeeding Action (WABA) is a network of organizations and individuals dedicated to protecting, promoting, and supporting breastfeeding as a right of all children and women. It also provides publications on breastfeeding and infant feeding with a focus on knowledge, advocacy, and lactation management.

OTHER INTERNATIONAL BREASTFEEDING SUPPORT ORGANIZATIONS

Australian Breastfeeding Association (ABA)
PO Box 4000
Glen Iris, Victoria 3146
Australia
Phone: 03-9885-0855, or from outside Australia + 61-3-98850855
Fax: 03-9885-0866, or from outside Australia + 61-3-98850866
E-mail: info@breastfeeding.asn.au
Website: http://www.breastfeeding.asn.au

This is a national association with some support from the Australian government. It focuses on providing consumers and professionals with lactation information. It also supports a breastfeeding phone helpline: 800-686-268 (800-mum-2-mum).

Baby Milk Action Group
34 Trumpington Street
Cambridge CB2 1QY

United Kingdom
Phone: 01223 464420 (UK); + 44 1223 464420 (international)
Website: http://www.babymilkaction.org

This group is part of a global network, International Baby Food Action Network (IBFAN), whose mission is to protect infants receiving breast milk or formula from adverse outcomes. It focuses on stopping misleading marketing by formula companies and pushes for companies to comply with the CODE requirements for product labeling.

Center for Science in the Public Interest (CSPI)
1220 L Street NW, Suite 300
Washington, DC 20005
Phone: 202-332-9110
Fax: 202-265-4954
E-mail: cspi@cspinet.org
Website: http://www.cspinet.org

This is an independent science-based consumer advocacy group that focuses on nutrition information for consumers, including eating healthy, protecting one's health, what individuals can do, and actions that support good nutrition.

National Childbirth Trust (NCT)
Brunel House, 11 The Promenade, Clifton
Down, Bristol, United Kingdom BS8 3NG
Phone: + 44 300 330 0700
E-mail: enquiries@nct.org.uk
Website: http://www.nct.org.uk/

This group focuses on supporting parents through the first 1000 days of an infant's life through building community and society initiatives. They conceived and developed the First 1000 Days program of support for parents and infants. They provide information and courses for parents and professionals that focus on the important issues for infants and parents in the first 1000 days of the infant's life. They also sponsor a support line for parents that includes practical and emotional support with feeding the infant. (Helpline: 0300 330 0700)

International Society for Research in Human Milk and Lactation (ISRHML)
5841 Cedar Lake Road, Suite 204
Minneapolis, MN 55416
E-mail: info@isrhml.com
Website: https://www.isrhml.com

This is a nonprofit organization committed to research and the dissemination of scientific findings in human milk and lactation.

ORGANIZATIONS FOR PHYSICIANS

Academy of Breastfeeding Medicine (ABM)
8735 West Higgins Road, Suite 300

Chicago, IL 60631
Phone: 800-990-4ABM (toll-free); 847-375-4726
Fax: 847-375-4713, attn: ABM
E-mail: ABM@bfmed.org
Website: http://www.bfmed.org

The Academy of Breastfeeding Medicine is a worldwide organization of physicians dedicated to the promotion, protection, and support of breastfeeding and human lactation. Its mission is to unite into one association of members of the various medical specialties with this common purpose. The academy's goals include physician education, expansion of knowledge in both breastfeeding science and human lactation, facilitation of optimal breastfeeding practices, and encouragement of the exchange of information among breastfeeding supportive organizations.

American Academy of Family Physicians (AAFP)
11400 Tomahawk Creek Parkway
Leawood, KS 66211-2680
Phone: 800-274-2237 or 913-906-6000
Fax: 913-906-9075
Website: http://www.aafp.org

This academy provides member services for education and resources concerning breastfeeding support and practice and lactation knowledge.

American Academy of Pediatrics (AAP)
National Headquarters
345 Park Boulevard
Itasca, IL 60143
Phone: 800-433-9016
Fax: 847-434-8000
E-mail: csc@aap.org
Website: http://www.aap.org

This academy is the largest organization for pediatricians in the United States that supports parents and professionals through development of evidence-based guidelines and policy statements. It participates in research, clinical support, quality improvement, journals and publications, and education and certification of pediatricians. It has a specific section on breastfeeding that formulates policy, develops educational resources for consumers and physicians on breastfeeding and lactation, works on advocacy and changing policies related to breastfeeding in the United States, and has a curriculum on breastfeeding for physicians in training.

American College of Obstetricians and Gynecologists (ACOG)
409 12th Street SW
Washington, DC 20024-2188
Mailing address: PO Box 96920
Washington, DC 20024-9998
Phone: 800-673-8444; 202-638-5577
Website: https://acog.org

This group provides services for over 58,000 members. It maintains resources for education and practical management of breastfeeding, including a "toolkit," a conversation guide, coding for billing for lactation management, informational resources, patient education pamphlets, and infographics.

Dr. MILK: Mothers Interested in Lactation Knowledge

E-mail: admin@drmilk.org
Website: https://drmilk.org

This is a group of and for doctor mothers interested in lactation knowledge. It provides evidence-based support and education for physician women to reach their breastfeeding goals and apply that knowledge to their medical practice. This is an online/Facebook maintained group.

DIRECT ACCESS LACTATION INFORMATION SOURCES

Breastfeeding and Human Lactation Center

Lactation Study Center: Encouraging and Promoting Breastfeeding
Phone (Warmline): 585-276-MILK or 585-276-6455 8 AM to 5 PM EST
Website: https://www.urmc.rochester.edu/breastfeeding.aspx

The Lactation Study Center at the University of Rochester Medical Center encourages and promotes human lactation and breastfeeding through physician education and support. The goal is to provide the information that will help practitioners encourage and support breastfeeding for all patients. The study center maintains a phone information center operated by specialists in lactation and networked databases, including a bibliography database, searchable by keyword, subject, medications, biochemicals, and health conditions of the mother or infant.

LactaMap

Family Larsson-Rosenquist Foundation and University of Western Australian

Family Larsson-Rosenquist Foundation
Rheinstrasse 1, 8500
Frauenfeld, Switzerland
Phone: +41-41-510-05-10
Website: https://www.lactamap.com/home

This is an online lactation care support system to assist medical practitioners in answering lactation questions to ensure consistent, high-quality, practical information for breastfeeding mothers and their infants. The system was developed by the University of Western Australia's International Breastfeeding Centre and was opened in March 2019.

Infant Risk Center

Infant Risk Center at Texas Tech University Health Sciences Center

Phone: Hotline: 806-352-2519
Website: http://www.infantrisk.com

This hotline was established specifically to answer questions about over-the-counter or prescription medications while pregnant or nursing. It is co-located at Texas Tech's research center for medication safety during pregnancy and lactation. They are a resource for ongoing pharmacologic research and information related to lactation.

National Breastfeeding Helpline

Association of Breastfeeding Mothers and The Breastfeeding Network
Phone: Helpline in United Kingdom: 0300 100 0212
Website: http://nationalbreastfeedinghelpline.org.uk

This is a helpline partially funded by Public Health England and the Scottish Government. Breastfeeding mothers can get direct assistance from women who have breastfed and as volunteers who are trained by the Association of Breastfeeding Mothers (http://www.abm.me.uk) and The Breastfeeding Network (http://www.breastfeedingnetwork.org.uk).

LactMed (TOXNET Database)

US National Library of Medicine (National Institutes of Health [NIH] and Department of Health and Human Services [DHHS])
8600 Rockville Pike
Bethesda, MD 20894
Phone: 301-594-5983 or 1-888-346-3656
Fax: 301-480-3537
E-mail: tehip@teh.nlm.nih.gov
Website: http://www.toxnet.nlm.nih.gov/newtoxnet/lactmed.htm

This a database and resource maintained by the US government through TOXNET as part of the National Library of Medicine, NIH, and DHHS. It is searchable for drugs or other chemicals to which breastfeeding mothers may be exposed. It provides pharmacokinetic information about the drugs, maternal and infant exposure, drug levels in breast milk and infant blood, and management after exposure along with suggested therapeutic alternatives for specific health conditions. LactMed can be accessed, free of charge, via NCBI's Bookshelf. https://www.ncbi.nlm.nih.gov/books/NBK501922 Alternatively, the dataset can be downloaded from National Library of Medicine's Data Distribution site. https://www.nlm.nih.gov/databases/download/data_distrib_main.html

National Breastfeeding Helpline (USBC and Office of Women's Health)

4044 North Lincoln Avenue, No. 288
Chicago, IL 60618
Phone: 773-359-1549
OMH Helpline: 800-994-9662 (9 AM to 6 PM EST, Mon.–Fri.)
Fax: 773-313-3498

E-mail: office@usbreastfeeding.org
Website: http://www.usbreastfeeding.org

This is a helpline maintained within the Office of Women's Health and supported by the US Breastfeeding Committee.

PUBLIC AND PRIVATE HUMAN MILK BANKS/LABORATORIES

Medolac Laboratories
Phone: 866-599-7740
Fax: 866-239-3654
Website: http://www.medolac.com

This is a public benefit corporation founded to provide human donor milk safely and at a reasonable cost to any infant who needs it. The bank/laboratory formulates human milk to create products with appropriate nutrient levels for preterm infants. They do research on shelf life, safety, nutritional content, and the benefits of specially formulated milk for premature infants.

Prolacta Bioscience Inc.
1800 Highland Avenue
Duarte, CA 91010
Phone: 888-776-5228
Website: http://www.prolacta.com

This is a private company that produces human milk—based nutritional products. It maintains milk banks to supply the production of human milk—based products. It is involved in scientific research on human milk, safety and quality of human milk—based products, and the nutritional benefits of their use in premature infants and other infants at risk.

Human Milk Bank Association of North America (HMBANA)
4455 Camp Bowie Boulevard, Suite 114-88
Fort Worth, TX 76107
Phone: 817-810-9984
Website: http://www.hmbana.org

This is the ongoing collaboration of the 28 milk banks in North America whose focus is to provide pasteurized human donor milk in hospitals, homes, and childcare settings to infants with significant medical needs. The association also prints guidelines for establishing and operating a donor human milk bank and best practices for expressing, storing, and handling human milk.

European Milk Bank Association (EMBA)
c/o Biomedia
Via Libero Temolo, 4
20126 Milano, Italy

Phone: +39 (0)2 454 98282 ext. 230
Fax: +39 (0)2 454 98199
E-mail: embamembership@biomedia.net
Website: https://europeanmilkbanking.com

This association fosters collaboration of over 200 active milk banks in over 20 countries. It is a resource for women looking to donate or have their infants receive donor human milk. They have a yearly meeting for milk bank members and other interested persons.

INFORMATION ABOUT EXAMINATION AND CERTIFICATION

International Board of Lactation Consultant Examiners (IBLCE)
10301 Democracy Lane Suite 400
Fairfax, VA 22030
Phone: 703-560-7330
Fax: 703-560-7332
E-mail: exam@iblce.org or international@iblce.org
Website: http://www.iblce.org

This group provides information regarding eligibility to become a lactation consultant and for the examination for certification as a lactation consultant. It also makes available other educational material on breastfeeding and lactation.

Academy of Breastfeeding Medicine
140 Huguenot Street, 3rd Floor
New Rochelle, NY 10801
Phone: 800-990-4ABM (toll-free); 914-740-2115
Fax: 914-740-2101, attn: ABM
E-mail: ABM@bfmed.org
Website: http://www.bfmed.org

This academy provides information for physicians, to become a physician specialist in lactation (Faculty of the Academy of Breastfeeding Medicine [FABM]) through membership in the academy. Its goals include physician education, expansion of knowledge in both breastfeeding science and human lactation, dissemination of optimal breastfeeding practices and protocols, and encouragement of the exchange of information among breastfeeding supportive organizations.

Academy of Lactation Policy and Practice (ALPP)
PO Box 1288
Forestdale, MA 02644
Phone: 508-833-1500
Fax: 508-833-6070
Website: http://www.alpp.org

This group provides for certification of lactation counselors and maintains policy and requirements for their training based on the WHO/UNICEF Breastfeeding Counseling Training Course, a code of ethics for lactation counselors, and examinations for certification. There is a Candidate Handbook available, a list of training partners and a course pathway for becoming a lactation counselor.

The Center for Breastfeeding
327 Quaker Meeting House Road
East Sandwich, MA 02537
Phone: 508-888-8044
Fax: 508-888-8050
Website: http://www.centerforbreastfeeding.org

This group organizes and produces training for certified lactation counselors as designated by the ALPP. They are part of the Healthy Children Project, a nonprofit research and educational institution to improve child health outcomes.

FOUNDATIONS SUPPORTING BREASTFEEDING AND LACTATION RESEARCH AND KNOWLEDGE

Family Larsson-Rosenquist Foundation
Rheinstrasse 1
8500 Frauenfeld, Switzerland

Phone: +41 41 510 05 10
E-mail: info@larsson-rosenquist.org
Website: http://www.larsson-rosenquist.org

This independent charitable organization has as its primary focus promoting and supporting breastfeeding and breast milk. It does this through supporting research and education on breastfeeding, specifically the University of Western Australia's LactaResearch Group (https://research-impact.uwa.edu.au) and LactaMap (http://www.lactamap.com).

W.K. Kellogg Foundation
1 Michigan Avenue
East Battle Creek, MI 49017
Phone: 269-968-1611
Fax: 269-968-0413
Website: http://www.wkkf.org

This foundation supports research and community interventions that focus on the health and welfare of children, working families, and the establishment of equitable communities. The foundation has a long history of supporting breastfeeding research and initiatives in the United States.

H APPENDIX

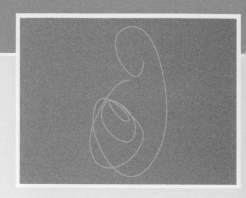

Breastfeeding Health Supervision

Alison M. Stuebe

GLOSSARY

Asbill's sign Pink, lacy capillary pattern.

Crisco Regular shortening used in cooking, used as barrier for sensitive skin and dermatitis.

Medical grade honey Irradiated honey to facilitate wound healing.

Shower sign Cold air hitting breasts when getting out of shower is painful, pain in frozen food section of grocery store or when opening the freezer.

Towel sign Touch of a towel or dress is excruciating.

Yeast screen Highly sensitive microbiology assay for yeast; order to rule out ductal candida.

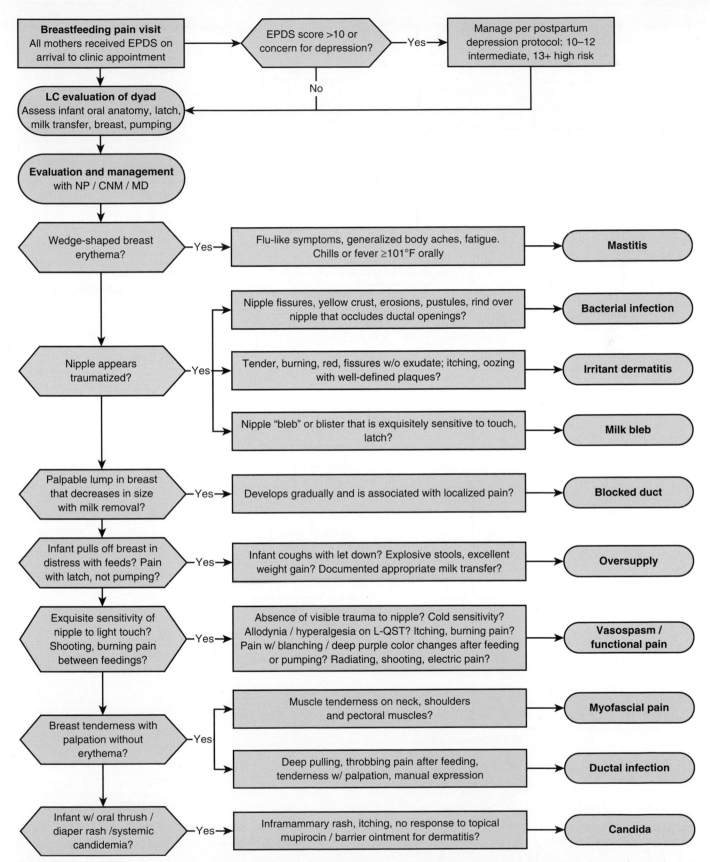

Fig. H.1 Breastfeeding pain visit. *CNM*, Clinical nurse midwife; *EPDS*, Edinburgh Postpartum Depression Screen; *LC*, lactation consultant; *L-QST*, laboratory quantitative sensory testing; *MD*, medical doctor; *NP*, nurse practitioner. (Courtesy Alison Stuebe, MD, Department of Obstetrics and Gynecology, University of North Carolina School of Medicine, Chapel Hill, North Carolina.) (Last updated June 2018.)

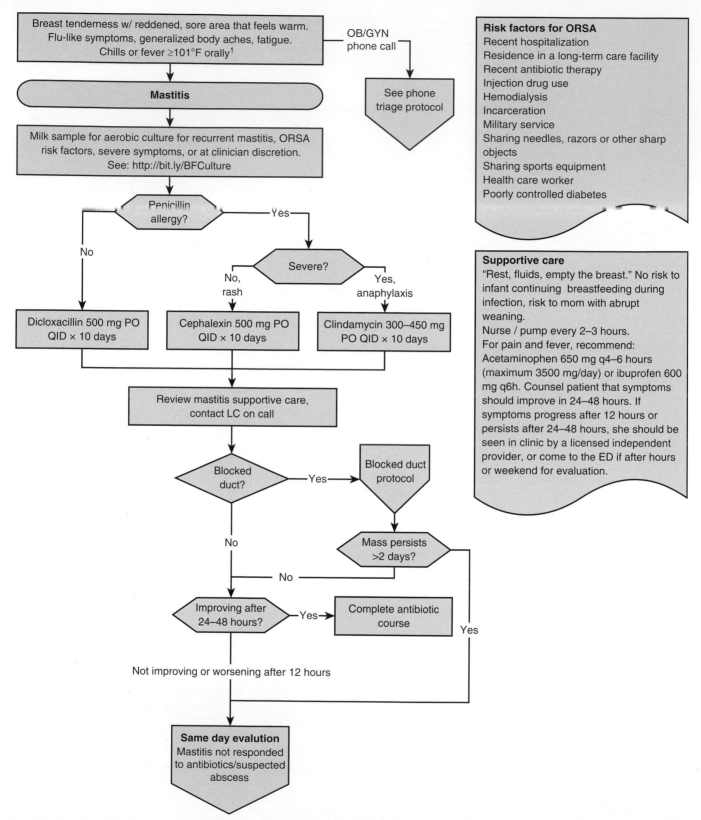

Fig. H.2 Mastitis. *ED*, Emergency department; *LC*, Lactation consultant, *OB/GYN*, obstetrician/gynecologist; *ORSA*, oxacillin-resistant *Staphylococcus aureus*.[1] (Courtesy Alison Stuebe, MD, Department of Obstetrics and Gynecology, University of North Carolina School of Medicine, Chapel Hill, North Carolina.) (Last updated June 2018.)

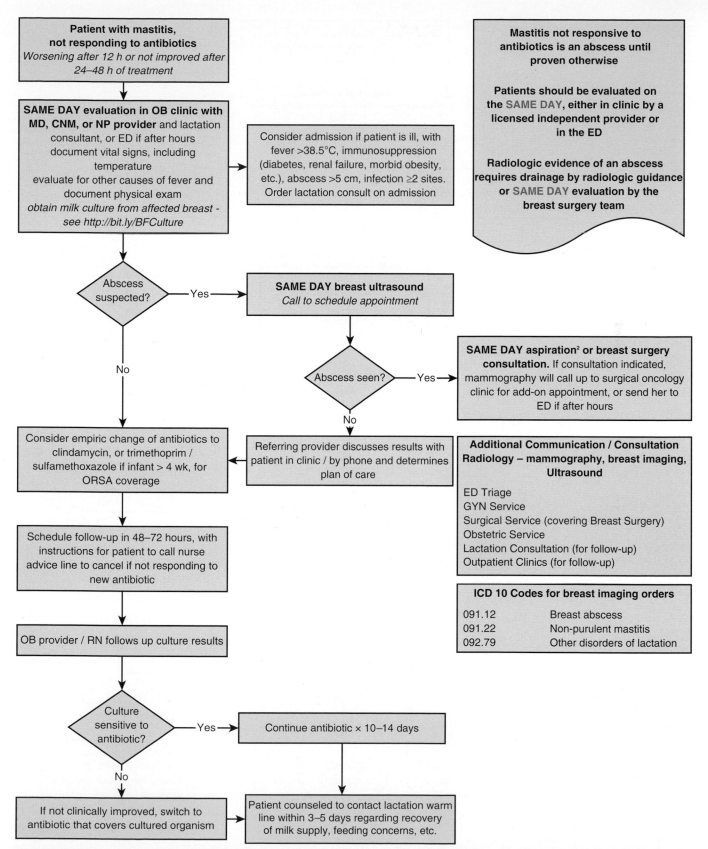

Fig. H.3 Mastitis not responding to antibiotics/suspected abscess. *CNM*, Clinical nurse midwife; *ED*, emergency department; *LC*, lactation consultant; *MD*, medical doctor; *NP*, nurse practitioner; *OB*, obstetric; *RN*, registered nurse.[2] (Courtesy Alison Stuebe, MD, Department of Obstetrics and Gynecology, University of North Carolina School of Medicine, Chapel Hill, North Carolina.) (Last updated June 2018.)

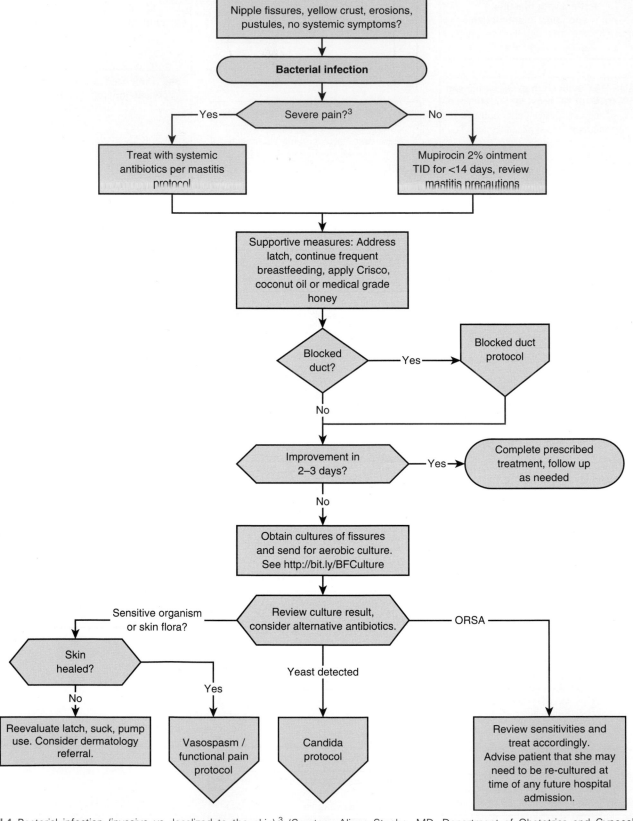

Fig. H.4 Bacterial infection (invasive vs. localized to the skin).[3] (Courtesy Alison Stuebe, MD, Department of Obstetrics and Gynecology, University of North Carolina School of Medicine, Chapel Hill, North Carolina. (Last updated June 2018.)

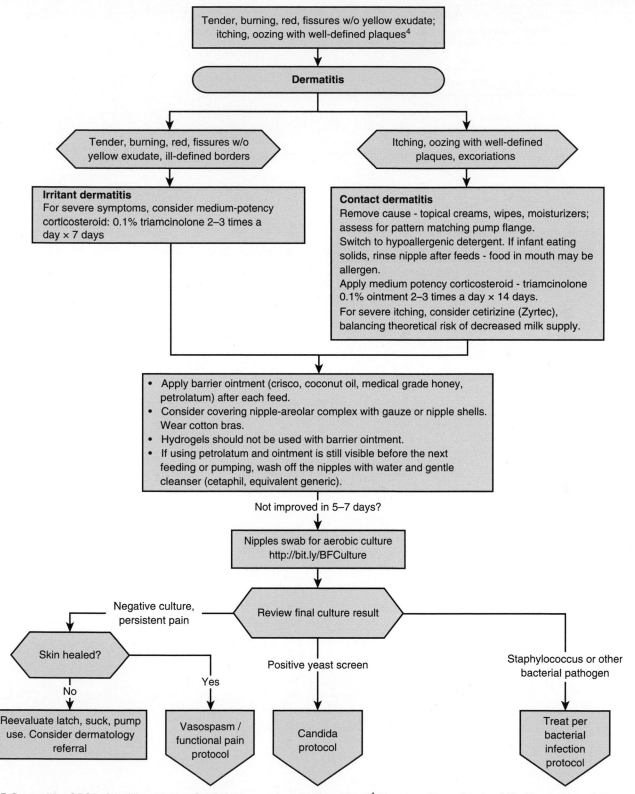

Fig. H.5 Dermatitis. *ORSA*, Oxacillin-resistant *Staphylococcus aureus; w/o*, without.[4] (Courtesy Alison Stuebe, MD, Department of Obstetrics and Gynecology, University of North Carolina School of Medicine, Chapel Hill, North Carolina.) (Last updated June 2018.)

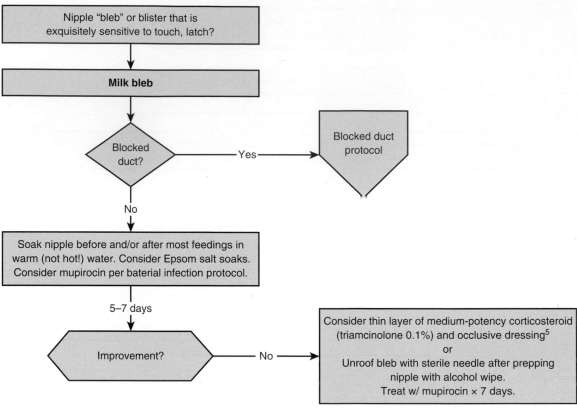

Fig. H.6 Milk bleb.[5] (Courtesy Alison Stuebe, MD, Department of Obstetrics and Gynecology, University of North Carolina School of Medicine, Chapel Hill, North Carolina.) (Last updated June 2018.)

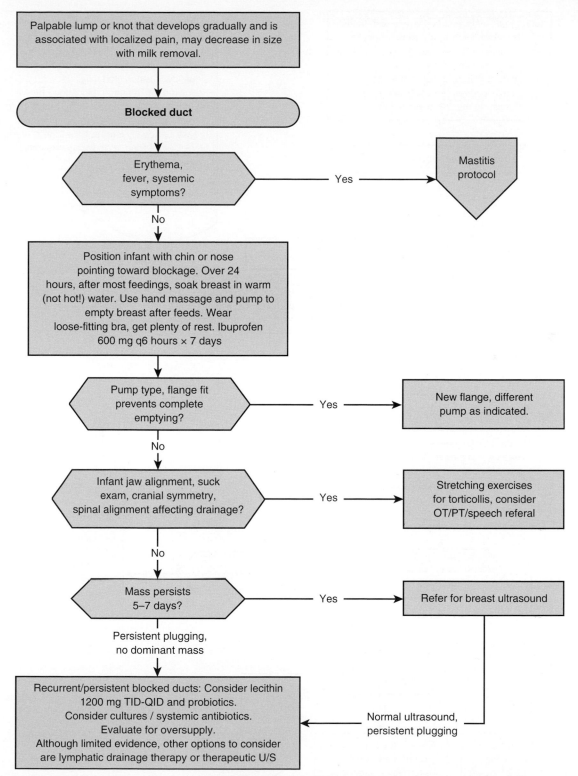

Fig. H.7 Blocked duct. *OT*, Occupational therapy; *PT*, physical therapy; *US*, ultrasound. (Courtesy Alison Stuebe, MD, Department of Obstetrics and Gynecology, University of North Carolina School of Medicine, Chapel Hill, North Carolina.) (Last updated June 2018.)

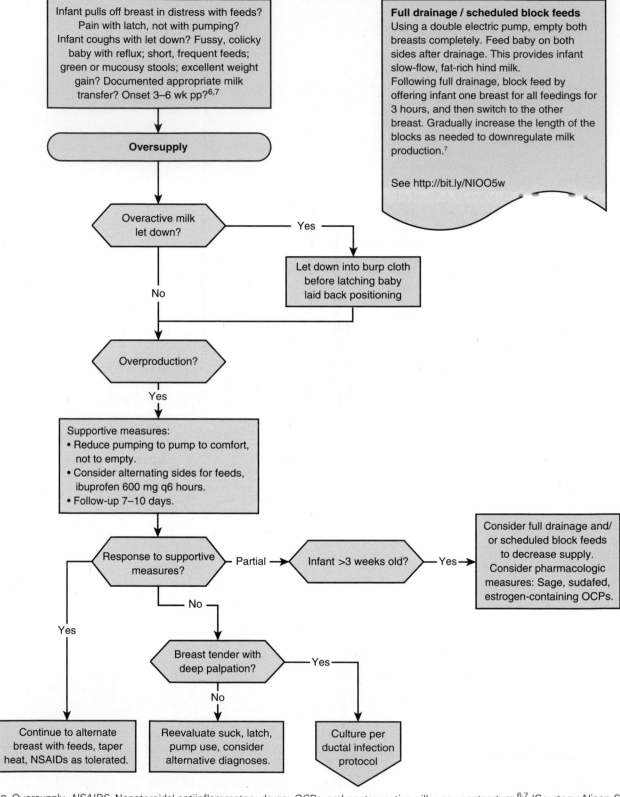

Fig. H.8 Oversupply. *NSAIDS,* Nonsteroidal antiinflammatory drugs; *OCPs,* oral contraceptive pills; *pp,*; postpartum.[6,7] (Courtesy Alison Stuebe, MD, Department of Obstetrics and Gynecology, University of North Carolina School of Medicine, Chapel Hill, North Carolina.) (Last updated June 2018.)

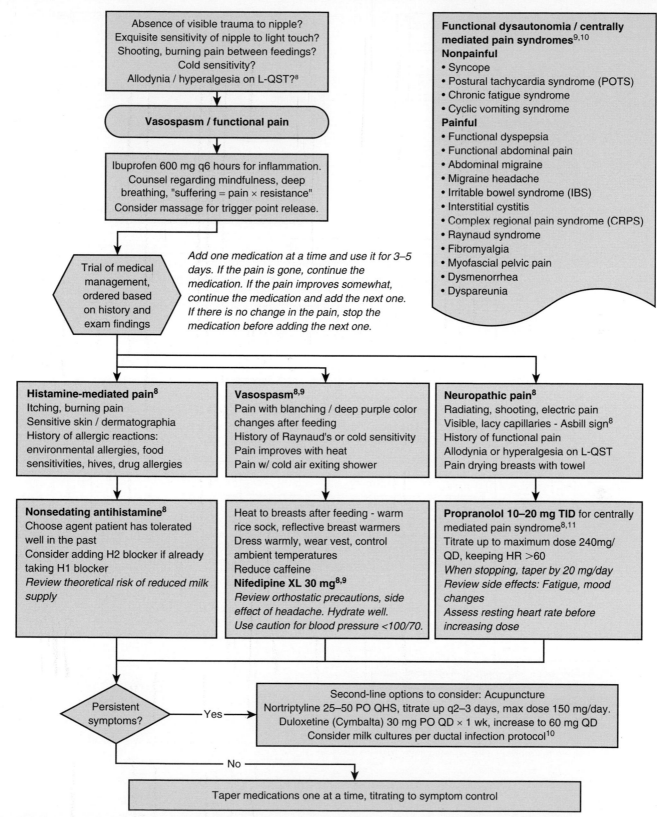

Fig. H.9 Vasospasm/functional pain. *Asbill's sign,* Pink lacy capillary pattern on skin; *H1,* histamine 1; *HR,* heart rate; *L-QST,* laboratory quantitative sensory testing; *PO,* orally; *QST,* quantitative sensory testing.[8–11] (Courtesy Alison Stuebe, MD, Department of Obstetrics and Gynecology, University of North Carolina School of Medicine, Chapel Hill, North Carolina.) (Last updated June 2018.)

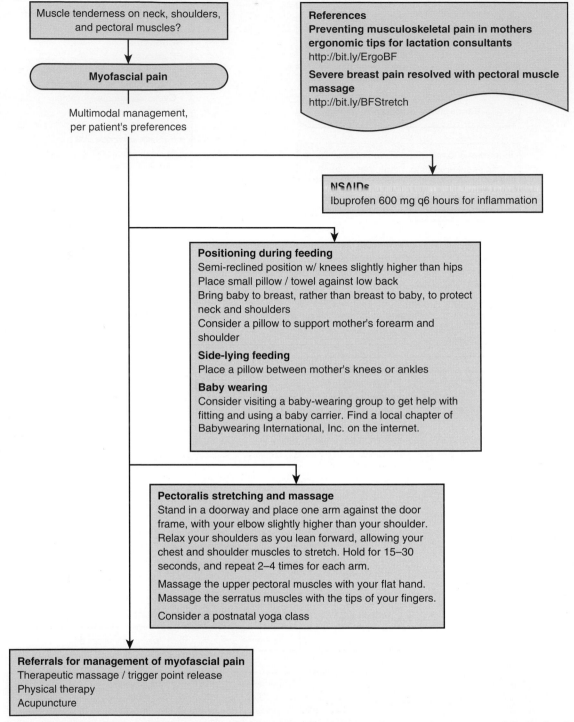

Fig. H.10 Myofascial pain. (Courtesy Alison Stuebe, MD, Department of Obstetrics and Gynecology, University of North Carolina School of Medicine, Chapel Hill, North Carolina.) (Last updated June 2018.)

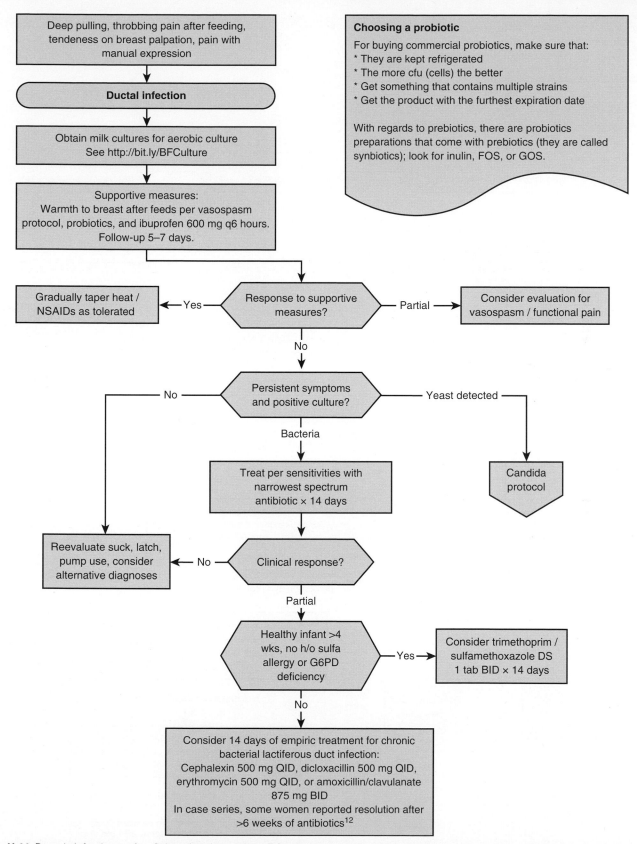

Fig. H.11 Ductal infection. *cfu*, Colony-forming units; *DS*, double-strength; *FOS*, fructooligosaccharides; *G6PD*, glucose-6-phosphate dehydrogenase; *GOS*, galactooligosaccharides; *h/o*, history of; *NSAIDs*, nonsteroidal antiinflammatory drugs.[12] (Courtesy Alison Stuebe, MD, Department of Obstetrics and Gynecology, University of North Carolina School of Medicine, Chapel Hill, North Carolina.) (Last updated June 2018.)

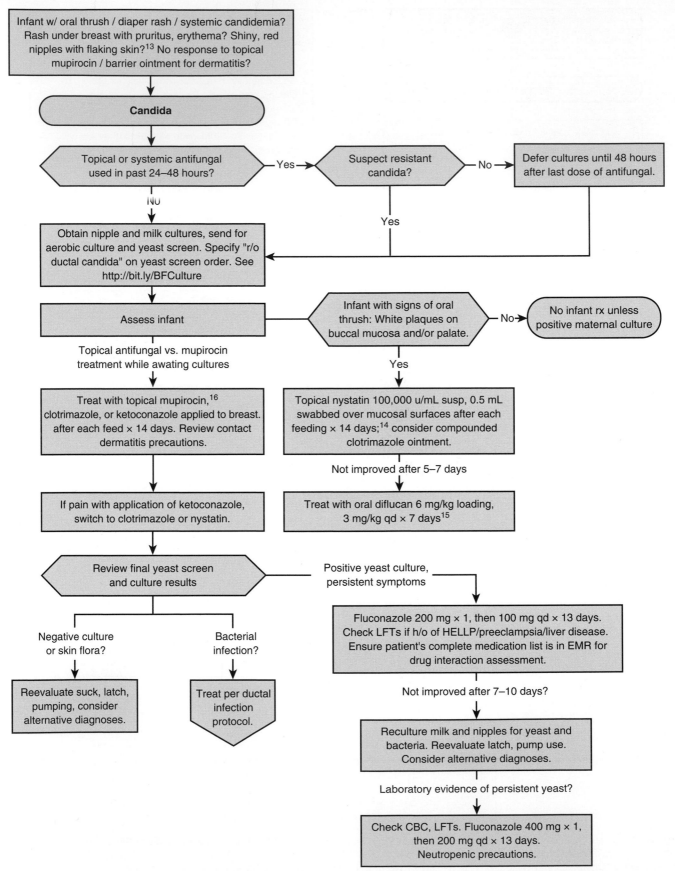

Fig. H.12 Candida. *CBC*, Complete blood count; *EMR*, electronic medical record; *HELLP*, hemolysis, elevated liver enzymes, low platelet count; *h/o*, history of; *LFTs*, liver function tests; *r/o*, rule out; *Rx*, treatment; *susp*, suspension.[13–16] (Courtesy Alison Stuebe, MD, Department of Obstetrics and Gynecology, University of North Carolina School of Medicine, Chapel Hill, North Carolina.) (Last updated June 2018.)

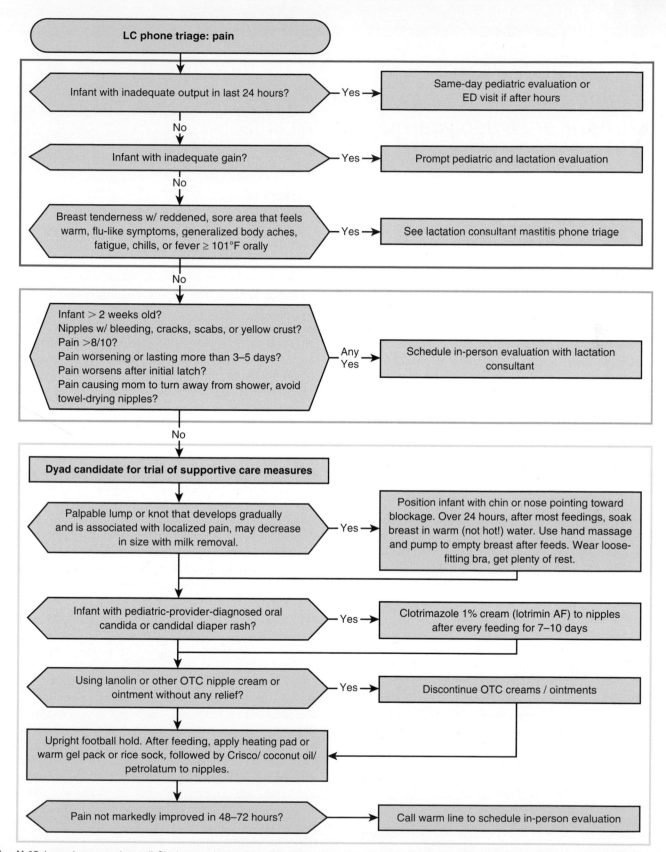

Fig. H.13 Lactation consultant *(LC)* phone triage: pain. *ED*, Emergency department; *OTC*, over-the-counter. (Courtesy Alison Stuebe, MD, Department of Obstetrics and Gynecology, University of North Carolina School of Medicine, Chapel Hill, North Carolina. (Last updated June 2018.)

The Reference list is available at www.expertconsult.com.

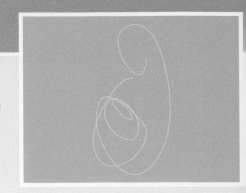

ABM Clinical Protocol #1
Guidelines for Blood Glucose Monitoring and Treatment of Hypoglycemia in Term and Late-Preterm Neonates, Revised 2014*

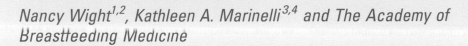

Nancy Wight[1,2], Kathleen A. Marinelli[3,4] and The Academy of Breastfeeding Medicine

ABSTRACT

A central goal of The Academy of Breastfeeding Medicine is the development of clinical protocols for managing common medical problems that may impact breastfeeding success. These protocols serve only as guidelines for the care of breastfeeding mothers and infants and do not delineate an exclusive course of treatment or serve as standards of medical care. Variations in treatment may be appropriate according to the needs of an individual patient.

PURPOSE

To provide guidance in the first hours/days of life to:

- Prevent clinically significant hypoglycemia in infants
- Appropriately monitor blood glucose levels in at-risk term and late-preterm infants
- Manage documented hypoglycemia in infants
- Establish and preserve maternal milk supply during medically necessary supplementation for hypoglycemia or during separation of mother and baby

BACKGROUND

Physiology

The term "hypoglycemia" refers to a low blood glucose concentration. Clinically significant neonatal hypoglycemia reflects an imbalance between the supply and utilization of glucose and alternative fuels and may result from several disturbed regulatory mechanisms.[1] Transient hypoglycemia in the first hours after birth is common, occurring in almost all mammalian newborns. In healthy, term human infants, even if early enteral feeding is withheld, this phenomenon is self-limited, without clinical signs, and considered to be part of adaptation to postnatal life, as glucose levels spontaneously rise within the first 24 hours after birth (for some, it is even longer but still physiological).[2–6] Most neonates compensate for this "physiological" low blood glucose with endogenous fuel production through gluconeogenesis, glycogenolysis, and ketogenesis, collectively called "counter-regulation." Even in those situations where low blood glucose concentrations do develop secondary to prolonged intervals ($>$ 8 hours) between breastfeeding, a marked ketogenic response occurs. The enhanced capability of the neonatal brain to utilize ketone bodies provides glucose-sparing fuel to the brain, protecting neurological function.[3,7–9] The compensatory provision of alternate fuels constitutes a normal adaptive response to transiently low nutrient intake during the establishment of breastfeeding,[3,10] resulting in most breastfed infants tolerating lower plasma glucose levels without any significant clinical manifestations or sequelae.[10]

No studies have shown that treating transiently low blood glucose levels results in better short-term or long-term outcomes compared with no treatment, and in fact there is no evidence at all that hypoglycemic infants with no clinical signs benefit from treatment.[11,12] Increases in neurodevelopmental abnormalities have been found in infants who have hypoglycemia associated with abnormal clinical signs, especially those with severe, persistent hyperinsulinemic hypoglycemia.[11–16] Rozance and Hay[17] have delineated the conditions that should be present before considering that long-term neurologic impairment might be related to neonatal hypoglycemia. Transient, single, brief periods of hypoglycemia are unlikely to cause permanent neurologic damage.[18–21] Therefore, the monitoring of blood glucose concentrations in healthy, term, appropriately grown neonates is unnecessary and potentially harmful to parental well-being and the successful establishment of breastfeeding.[18–23]

---

* Courtesy of the Academy of Breastfeeding Medicine. Please go to https://www.bfmed.org/protocols for complete protocols, translations, and the most up-to-date information (protocols are updated every 5–7 years).

[1] San Diego Neonatology, Inc., San Diego, California.

[2] Sharp HealthCare Lactation Services, Sharp Mary Birch Hospital for Women and Newborns, San Diego, California.

[3] Division of Neonatology and The Connecticut Human Milk Research Center, Connecticut Children's Medical Center, Hartford, Connecticut.

[4] University of Connecticut School of Medicine, Farmington, Connecticut.

Definition of hypoglycemia

The definition of hypoglycemia in the newborn infant has remained controversial because of a lack of significant correlation among plasma glucose concentration, clinical signs, and long-term sequelae.[10,24,25] An expert panel convened in 2008 by the U.S. National Institutes of Health concluded that there has been no substantial evidence-based progress in defining what constitutes clinically important neonatal hypoglycemia, particularly regarding how it relates to brain injury.[26] Multiple reviews have concluded that there is no specific plasma or blood glucose concentration or duration of low blood glucose level that can be linked to either clinical signs or permanent neurologic injury.[17,25,27] In addition, blood glucose test results vary enormously with the source of the blood sample, the assay method, and whether whole blood, plasma, or serum glucose concentration is determined. Plasma or serum glucose concentrations are 10–15% higher than in whole blood.[28,29]

Breastfed, formula-fed, and mixed-fed infants follow the same pattern of glucose values, with an initial fall in glucose level over the first 2 hours of life, followed by a gradual rise in glucose level over the next 96 hours, whether fed or not.[2,5,6] Artificially fed infants tend to have slightly higher levels of glucose and lower levels of ketone bodies than breastfed infants.[3,5,18,30–32]

The incidence of "hypoglycemia" varies with the definition.[33,34] Many authors have suggested numeric definitions of hypoglycemia, usually between 30 and 50 mg/dL (1.7–2.8 mmol/L) and varying by postnatal age.[2,5,18,24,26,33,35–38] There is no scientific justification for the value of < 47 mg/dL (2.6 mmol/L) that has been adopted by some clinicians.[10,25–27,39] Cornblath et al.[10] summarized the problem as follows:

> *Significant hypoglycemia is not and cannot be defined as a single number that can be applied universally to every individual patient. Rather, it is characterized by a value(s) that is unique to each individual and varies with both their state of physiologic maturity and the influence of pathology.*

A meta-analysis of studies published from 1986 to 1994 looked at low plasma glucose thresholds in term healthy newborns who were mostly mixed fed (breastfed and formula-fed) or formula-fed. It presented statistical ranges of low thresholds for plasma glucose level based on hours after birth in healthy term infants (Table 1).[40] The authors specifically noted that given the known lower plasma glucose levels in healthy term breastfed infants as compared with formula-fed infants, the low thresholds for exclusively breastfed infants might even be lower. Table 1 gives recommendations for this timed threshold approach.

This information is translated into guidelines for clinical intervention by the operational treatment guidance of Cornblath et al.[10] As they stated, an operational threshold is that concentration of plasma or whole blood glucose at which clinicians should consider intervention, based on the evidence currently available in the literature (Table 2). It needs to be underscored that the therapeutic objective (45 mg/dL [2.5 mmol/L]) is different from the operational threshold for intervention (36 mg/dL [2.0 mmol/L]), which is different from the population low thresholds in normal babies with no clinical signs or risk factors who do not need to be treated (Table 1). The higher therapeutic goal was

TABLE 1   Population Low Thresholds: Plasma Glucose Level[40]

Hour(s) after birth	≤5th percentile plasma glucose level
1–2 (nadir)	28 mg/dL (1.6 mmol/L)
3–47	40 mg/dL (2.2/mmol/L)
48–72	48 mg/dL (2.7 mmol/L)

TABLE 2   Operational Thresholds for Treatment of Plasma Glucose Levels[10]

Infant	Plan/PGL	Treatment
Infant with clinical signs	If <45 mg/dL (2.5 mmol/L)	Clinical interventions to increase blood glucose concentration
Infants with risk factors[a]	Initiate glucose monitoring as soon as possible after birth, within 2–3 hours after birth and before feeding, or at any time there are abnormal signs.	Clinical interventions to increase blood glucose concentration: at very low glucose concentration (20–25 mg/dL, 1.1–1.4 mmol/L), intravenous glucose infusion to raise plasma glucose levels to >45 mg/dL (2.5 mmol/L) is indicated.
	If plasma glucose concentration is <36 mg/dL (2.0 mmol/L), close surveillance should be maintained. Intervention is recommended if plasma glucose remains below this level, does not increase after a feed, or if abnormal clinical signs develop.	

PGL, plasma glucose level.
[a]See Table 3.

TABLE 3   At-Risk Infants for Whom Routine Monitoring of Blood Glucose Is Indicated

Small for gestational age: <10th percentile for weight commonly cited in the United States; <2nd percentile cited in the United Kingdom as above this considered small normal[a]
Babies with clinically evident wasting of fat and muscle bulk
LGA: >90th percentile for weight and macrosomic appearance[b]
Discordant twin: weight 10% < larger twin All infants of diabetic mothers, especially if poorly controlled
Low birth weight (<2,500 g)
Prematurity (<35 weeks, or late preterm infants with clinical signs or extremely poor feeding)
Perinatal stress: severe acidosis or hypoxia-ischemia
Cold stress
Polycythemia (venous Hct > 70%)/hyperviscosity
Erythroblastosis fetalis
Beckwith–Wiedemann's syndrome
Microphallus or midline defect
Suspected infection
Respiratory distress
Known or suspected inborn errors of metabolism or endocrine disorders
Maternal drug treatment (e.g., terbutaline, beta-blockers, oral hypoglycemics)
Infants displaying signs associated with hypoglycemia (see Table 4)

Hct, hematocrit.
[a]As per Dr. Jane Hawdon (personal communication).
[b]Unnecessary to screen all large for gestational age (LGA) babies. Glucose monitoring is recommended for infants from maternal populations who were unscreened for diabetes during the pregnancy where LGA may represent undiagnosed and untreated maternal diabetes.

chosen to include a significant margin of safety in the absence of data evaluating the correlation between glucose levels in this range and long-term outcome in full-term infants.[10]

Given this information, it is clear that routine monitoring of blood glucose in healthy term infants is not only unnecessary, but is instead potentially harmful to the establishment of a healthy mother–infant relationship and successful breastfeeding patterns.[1,20,22,23,41,42] This recommendation has been supported by the World Health Organization,[18] the American Academy of Pediatrics,[1,41] the U.S. National Institutes of Health,[26] and the National Childbirth Trust of the United Kingdom.[43] These organizations all conclude that (1) early and exclusive breastfeeding is safe to meet the nutritional needs of healthy term infants and that (2) healthy term infants do not develop clinically significant hypoglycemia simply as a result of a time-limited duration of underfeeding.

Testing methods

Bedside glucose reagent test strips are inexpensive and practical but are not reliable, with significant variance from true blood glucose levels, especially at low glucose concentrations.[22,38,44–46] Bedside glucose tests may be used for screening, but laboratory levels sent STAT (immediate determination, without delay) (e.g., glucose oxidase, hexokinase, or dehydrogenase

method) must confirm results before a diagnosis of hypoglycemia can be made, especially in infants with no clinical signs.[1,18,22] Other bedside rapid measurement methods such as reflectance colorimetry and electrode methods may be more accurate.[47–50] Continuous subcutaneous glucose monitoring, as is used in diabetic patients, has been used experimentally in neonates with good correlation with laboratory glucose values but is not currently recommended for screening.[51,52]

Risk factors for hypoglycemia

Neonates at increased risk for developing neonatal hypoglycemia should be routinely monitored for blood glucose levels irrespective of the mode of feeding. At-risk neonates fall into two main categories:

1. Excess utilization of glucose, which includes the hyperinsulinemic states
2. Inadequate production or substrate delivery[32,53,54]

Infant risk factors for hypoglycemia are listed in Table 3.[3,10,18,19,21,30,32,34,53–56]

Clinical manifestations of hypoglycemia

The clinical manifestations of hypoglycemia are nonspecific, occurring with various other neonatal problems. Even in the presence of an arbitrary low glucose level, the physician must

TABLE 4   Clinical Manifestations of Possible Hypoglycemia

Irritability, tremors, jitteriness
Exaggerated Moro reflex
High-pitched cry
Seizures or myoclonic jerks
Lethargy, listlessness, limpness, hypotonia
Coma
Cyanosis
Apnea or irregular breathing
Tachypnea Hypothermia; temperature instability
Vasomotor instability
Poor suck or refusal to feed

assess the general status of the infant by observation and physical examination to rule out other disease entities and processes that may need additional laboratory evaluation and treatment. Some common clinical signs are listed in Table 4.

A recent study found that of the[23] maternal/infant risk factors and infant signs/symptoms studied, only jitteriness and tachypnea were statistically significant at predicting low blood glucose—not even maternal diabetes![57] A diagnosis of hypoglycemia also requires that signs abate after normoglycemia is restored (the exception being if brain injury has already been sustained).

GENERAL MANAGEMENT RECOMMENDATIONS (TABLE 5)

Any approach to management needs to account for the overall metabolic and physiologic status of the infant and should not unnecessarily disrupt the mother—infant relationship and breastfeeding.[1,21] Because severe, prolonged hypoglycemia with clinical signs may result in neurologic injury,[11,14,15,58] immediate intervention is needed for infants with clinical signs. Several authors have suggested algorithms for screening and treatment.[1,17,26,27,59] (Quality of evidence [levels of evidence I, II-1, II-2, II-3, and III] is based on the U.S. Preventive Services Task Force Appendix A Task Force Ratings[60] and is noted in parentheses.)

Initial management

Early and exclusive breastfeeding meets the nutritional and metabolic needs of healthy, term newborn infants. Healthy term infants do not develop clinically significant hypoglycemia simply as a result of time-limited underfeeding.[18,19,21] (III)

1. Healthy, appropriate weight for gestational age, term infants should initiate breastfeeding within 30—60 minutes of life and continue breastfeeding on cue, with the recognition that that crying is a very late sign of hunger.[41,61,62] (III)

2. Initiation and establishment of breastfeeding, and reduction of hypoglycemia risk, are facilitated by skin-to-skin contact between the mother and her infant immediately after birth for at least the first hour of life and continuing as much as possible. Such practices will maintain normal infant body temperature and reduce energy expenditure (thus enabling maintenance of normal blood glucose) while stimulating suckling and milk production.[31,41] (II-2, III)

3. Feedings should be frequent, at least 10—12 times per 24 hours in the first few days after birth.[41] (III) However, it is not unusual for term infants to feed immediately after birth and then sleep quite a long time (up to 8—12 hours) before they become more active and begin to suckle with increasing frequency. They mount protective metabolic responses throughout this time so it is not necessary to try to force-feed them. However, an unusually, excessively drowsy baby must undergo clinical evaluation.

4. Routine supplementation of healthy term infants with water, glucose water, or formula is unnecessary and may interfere with the establishment of normal breastfeeding and normal metabolic compensatory mechanisms.[3,30,41,43] (II-2, III)

Blood glucose screening

Glucose screening should be performed only on at-risk infants and those with clinical signs compatible with hypoglycemia. Early breastfeeding is not precluded just because the infant meets the criteria for glucose monitoring.

1. At-risk infants should be screened for hypoglycemia with a frequency and duration related to the specific risk factors of the individual infant.[1,19] (III) Monitoring should begin no later than 2 hours of age for infants in risk categories.[1] Hawdon[63] recommended blood glucose monitoring should commence before the second feeding (i.e., not so soon after birth that the physiologic fall in blood glucose level causes confusion and overtreatment). (III)

TABLE 5   General Management Recommendations for All Term Infants

A. Early and exclusive breastfeeding meets the nutritional and metabolic needs of healthy, term newborn infants.
   1. Routine supplementation is unnecessary.
   2. Initiate breastfeeding within 30–60 minutes of life and continue on demand.
   3. Facilitate skin-to-skin contact of mother and infant.
   4. Feedings should be frequent, 10–12 times per 24 hours in the first few days after birth.

B. Glucose screening is performed only on at-risk infants or infants with clinical signs.
   1. Routine monitoring of blood glucose in all term newborns is unnecessary and may be harmful.
   2. At-risk infants should be screened for hypoglycemia with a frequency and duration related to the specific risk factors of the individual infant.
   3. Monitoring continues until normal, prefeed levels are consistently obtained.
   4. Bedside glucose screening tests must be confirmed by formal laboratory testing

TABLE 6   Management of Documented Hypoglycemia

A. Infant with no clinical signs
   1. Continue breastfeeding (approximately every 1–2 hours) or feed 1–5 mL/kg of expressed breastmilk or substitute nutrition.
   2. Recheck blood glucose concentration before subsequent feedings until the value is acceptable and stable.
   3. Avoid forced feedings (see above).
   4. If the glucose level remains low despite feedings, begin intravenous glucose therapy.
   5. Breastfeeding may continue during intravenous glucose therapy.
   6. Carefully document response to treatment.

B. Infant with clinical signs or plasma glucose levels <20–25 mg/dL (<1.1–1.4 mmol/L)
   1. Initiate intravenous 10% glucose solution with a minibolus.
   2. Do not rely on oral or intragastric feeding to correct extreme or clinically significant hypoglycemia.
   3. The glucose concentration in infants who have had clinical signs should be maintained at >45 mg/dL (>2.5 mmol/L).
   4. Adjust intravenous rate by blood glucose concentration.
   5. Encourage frequent breastfeeding.
   6. Monitor glucose concentrations before feedings while weaning off the intravenous treatment until values stabilize off intravenous fluids.
   7. Carefully document response to treatment.

2. Monitoring should continue until acceptable, prefeed levels are consistently obtained, meaning until the infant has had at least two consecutive satisfactory measurements.[63] A reasonable (although arbitrary) goal is to maintain plasma glucose concentrations between 40 and 50 mg/dL (between 2.2 and 2.8 mmol/L)1 or >45 mg/dL (2.5 mmol/L).[10] (III)

3. Bedside glucose screening tests must be confirmed by formal laboratory testing, although treatment should begin immediately in infants with clinical signs.
   Table 5 summarizes these recommendations.

MANAGEMENT OF DOCUMENTED HYPOGLYCEMIA (TABLE 6)

Infant with no clinical signs (absence of clinical signs can only be determined by careful clinical review)

1. Continue breastfeeding (approximately every 1–2 hours) or feed 1–3 mL/kg (up to 5 mL/kg)[18] of expressed breastmilk or substitute nutrition (pasteurized donor human milk, elemental formulas, partially hydrolyzed formulas, or routine formulas). Glucose water is not suitable because of insufficient energy and lack of protein. Recent reports of mothers with diabetes expressing and freezing colostrum prenatally (beginning at[34–36] weeks of gestation) to have it available after birth to avoid artificial feedings should their infant become hypoglycemic are mixed in terms of association with earlier births, and currently this procedure is not widely recommended.[64–68] (III)

2. Recheck blood glucose concentration before susequent feedings until the value is acceptable and stable (usually >40 mg/dL [2.2 mmol/L]). If staff is unavailable to check blood glucose and an infant has no clinical signs, breastfeeding should *never* be unnecessarily delayed while waiting for the blood glucose level to be checked.

3. If the infant is simply worn out and not otherwise ill, nasogastric feeds of human milk can be initiated, watching carefully for signs of intolerance or evidence of significant underlying illness. If the neonate is too ill to suck or enteral feedings are not tolerated, avoid forced

oral feedings (e.g., nasogastric tube) and instead begin intravenous (IV) therapy (see below). Such an infant is not normal and requires a careful examination and evaluation in addition to more intensive therapy. Term babies should not be given nasogastric feedings. They are much more likely to fight and aspirate.

4. If the glucose level remains low despite feedings, begin IV glucose therapy and adjust the IV rate by blood glucose concentration. Avoid bolus doses of glucose unless blood glucose is unrecordable or there are severe clinical signs (e.g., seizures or coma). If a bolus dose is given, use 2 mL/kg of glucose in 10% dextrose preparation.

5. Breastfeeding should continue during IV glucose therapy when the infant is interested and will suckle. Gradually wean from the IV glucose as the serum glucose level normalizes and feedings increase.

6. Carefully document physical examination, screening values, laboratory confirmation, treatment, and changes in clinical condition (i.e., response to treatment).

7. The infant should not be discharged until reasonable levels of blood glucose are maintained through a fast of 3−4 hours. Monitoring must be recommended if there are adverse changes in feeding.

Infants with clinical signs or with plasma glucose levels <20−25 mg/dL (<1.1−1.4 mmol/L)

1. Initiate IV 10% glucose solution with a bolus of 2 mL/kg and continuous IV treatment at 5−8 mg/kg/minute.

2. Do not rely on oral or intragastric feeding to correct extreme or symptomatic hypoglycemia. Such an infant most likely has an underlying condition and, in addition to IV glucose therapy, requires an immediate and careful examination and evaluation.

3. The glucose concentration in infants with clinical signs should be maintained at >45 mg/dL (>2.5 mmol/L).

4. Adjust the IV rate by blood glucose concentration.

5. Encourage frequent breastfeeding after initiation of IV therapy.

6. Monitor glucose concentrations before feedings while gradually weaning from the IV solution, until values are stabilized off IV fluids.

7. Carefully document physical examination, screening values, laboratory confirmation, treatment, and changes in clinical condition (i.e., response to treatment).

SUPPORTING THE MOTHER

Giving birth to an infant who develops hypoglycemia is of concern to both the mother and family and thus may jeopardize the establishment of breastfeeding. Mothers should be explicitly reassured that there is nothing wrong with their milk and that supplementation is usually temporary. Having the mother hand-express or pump milk that is then fed to her infant can overcome feelings of maternal inadequacy as well as help establish a full milk supply. It is important for the mother to provide stimulation to the breasts by manual or mechanical expression with appropriate frequency (at least eight times in 24 hours) until her baby is latching and suckling well to protect her milk supply. Keeping the infant at breast or returning the infant to the breast as soon as possible is important. Skin-to-skin care is easily accomplished with an IV line in place and may lessen the trauma of intervention, while also providing physiologic thermoregulation, thus contributing to metabolic homeostasis.

RECOMMENDATIONS FOR FUTURE RESEARCH

1. Well-planned, well-controlled studies are needed that look at plasma glucose concentrations, clinical signs, and long-term sequelae to determine what levels of blood glucose are the minimum safe levels.

2. The development and implementation of more reliable bedside testing methods would increase the efficiency of diagnosis and treatment of significant glucose abnormalities.

3. Studies to determine a clearer understanding of the role of other glucose-sparing fuels and the methods to measure them in a clinically meaningful way and time frame are required to aid in understanding which babies are truly at risk of neurologic sequelae and thus must be treated.

4. For those infants who do become hypoglycemic, research into how much enteral glucose, and in what form, is necessary to raise blood glucose to acceptable levels is important for clinical management.

5. Randomized controlled studies of prenatal colostrum expression and storage for mothers with infants at risk of hypoglycemia are important to determine if this is a practical and safe treatment modality.

SUMMARY

Healthy term infants are programmed to make the transition from their intrauterine constant flow of nutrients to their extrauterine intermittent nutrient intake without the need for metabolic monitoring or interference with the natural breastfeeding process. Homeostatic mechanisms ensure adequate energy substrate is provided to the brain and other organs, even when feedings are delayed. The normal pattern of early, frequent, and exclusive breastfeeding meets the needs of healthy term infants.

Routine screening and supplementation are not necessary and may harm the normal establishment of breastfeeding. Current evidence does not support a specific blood concentration of glucose that correlates with signs or that can predict permanent neurologic damage in any given infant. At-risk infants should be screened, followed up as needed, and treated with supplementation or IV glucose if there are clinical signs or suggested thresholds are reached. Bedside screening is helpful, but not always accurate, and should be confirmed with laboratory glucose measurement. A single low glucose value is not associated with long-term neurological abnormalities, provided the treating clinician can be assured that the baby was entirely well up until the time of the low value. Hypoglycemic encephalopathy and poor long-term outcome are extremely unlikely in infants with no clinical signs and are more likely in infants who manifest clinical signs and/or with persistent or repeated episodes of severe hypoglycemia.

ACKNOWLEDGMENTS

This work was supported in part by a grant from the Maternal and Child Health Bureau, U.S. Department of Health and Human Services.

REFERENCES

1. Adamkin DH. Committee on Fetus and Newborn. Postnatal glucose homeostasis in late-preterm and term infants. *Pediatrics.* 2011;127:575–579.

2. Srinivasan G, Pildes RS, Cattamanchi G, et al. Plasma glucose values in normal neonates: A new look. *J Pediatr.* 1986;109:114–117.

3. Hawdon JM, Ward Platt MP, Aynsley-Green A. Patterns of metabolic adaptation for preterm and term infants in the first neonatal week. *Arch Dis Child.* 1992;67(4 Spec No):357–365.

4. Cornblath M, Reisner SH. Blood glucose in the neonate and its clinical significance. *N Engl J Med.* 1965;273:378–381.

5. Heck LJ, Erenberg A. Serum glucose levels in term neonates during the first 48 hours of life. *J Pediatr.* 1987;110:119–122.

6. Hoseth E, Joergensen A, Ebbesen F, et al. Blood glucose levels in a population of healthy, breast fed, term infants of appropriate size for gestational age. *Arch Dis Child Fetal Neonatal Ed.* 2000;83:F117–F119.

7. Lucas A, Boyes S, Bloom SR, et al. Metabolic and endocrine responses to a milk feed in six-day-old term infants: Differences between breast and cow's milk formula feeding. *Acta Paediatr Scand.* 1981;70:195–200.

8. Edmond J, Auestad N, Robbins RA, et al. Ketone body metabolism in the neonate: Development and the effect of diet. *Fed Proc.* 1985;44:2359–2364.

9. Yager JY, Heitjan DF, Towfighi J, Vannucci RC. Effect of insulin-induced and fasting hypoglycemia on perinatal hypoxic-ischemic brain damage. *Pediatr Res.* 1992;31:138–142.

10. Cornblath M, Hawdon JM, Williams AF, et al. Controversies regarding definition of neonatal hypoglycemia: Suggested operational thresholds. *Pediatrics.* 2000;105:1141–1145.

11. Boluyt N, van Kempen A, Offringa M. Neurodevelopment after neonatal hypoglycemia: A systematic review and design of an optimal future study. *Pediatrics.* 2006;117:2231–2243.

12. Koivisto M, Blanco-Sequeiros M, Krause U. Neonatal symptomatic and asymptomatic hypoglycemia: A follow-up study of 151 children. *Dev Med Child Neurol.* 1972;14:603–614.

13. Kinnala A, Rikalainen H, Lapinleimu H, et al. Cerebral magnetic resonance imaging and ultrasonography findings after neonatal hypoglycemia. *Pediatrics.* 1999;103:724–729.

14. Dalgic N, Ergenekon E, Soysal S, et al. Transient neonatal hypoglycemia—Long-term effects on neurodevelopmental outcome. *J Pediatr Endocrinol Metab.* 2002;15:319–324.

15. Burns C, Rutherford M, Boardman J, et al. Patterns of cerebral injury and neurodevelopmental outcomes after symptomatic neonatal hypoglycemia. *Pediatrics.* 2008;122:65–74.

16. Menni F, deLonlay P, Sevin C, et al. Neurologic outcomes of 90 neonates and infants with persistent hyperinsulinemic hypoglycemia. *Pediatrics.* 2001;107:476–479.

17. Rozance PJ, Hay WW Jr. Describing hypoglycemia—Definition or operational threshold? *Early Hum Dev.* 2010;86:275–280.

18. Williams AF. *Hypoglycemia of the Newborn: Review of the Literature.* Geneva: World Health Organization; 1997.

19. Eidelman AI. Hypoglycemia and the breastfed neonate. *Pediatr Clin North Am.* 2001;48:377–387.

20. Hawdon JM, Ward Platt MP, Aynsley-Green A. Prevention and management of neonatal hypoglycemia. *Arch Dis Child Fetal Neonatal Ed.* 1994;70:F60–F64. discussion F65.

21. Wight N. Hypoglycemia in breastfed neonates. *Breastfeed Med.* 2006;1:253–262.

22. Hawdon JM, Platt MP, Aynsley-Green A. Neonatal hypoglycemia—Blood glucose monitoring and baby feeding. *Midwifery.* 1993;9:3–6.

23. Hawdon J. Neonatal hypoglycemia: The consequences of admission to the special care nursery. *Child Health.* 1993;(Feb) 48–51.

24. Kalhan S, Peter-Wohl S. Hypoglycemia: What is it for the neonate? *Am J Perinatol.* 2000;17:11–18.

25. Sinclair JC. Approaches to the definition of neonatal hypoglycemia. *Acta Paediatr Jpn.* 1997;39(Suppl 1): S17–S20.

26. Hay WW, Raju T, Higgens R, et al. Knowledge gaps and research needs for understanding and treating neonatal hypoglycemia: Workshop report from Eunice Kennedy Shriver National Institute of Child Health and Human Development. *J Pediatr.* 2009;155:612–617.

27. Rozance PJ, Hay WW. Hypoglycemia in newborn infants: Features associated with adverse outcomes. *Biol Neonate.* 2006;90:74–86.

28. Aynsley-Green A. Glucose: A fuel for thought! *J Paediatr Child Health.* 1991;27:21–30.

29. Cornblath M, Schwartz R. Hypoglycemia in the neonate. *J Pediatr Endocrinol.* 1993;6:113–129.

30. Swenne I, Ewald U, Gustafsson J, et al. Inter-relationship between serum concentrations of glucose, glucagon and insulin during the first two days of life in healthy newborns. *Acta Paediatr.* 1994;83:915–919.

31. Durand R, Hodges S, LaRock S, et al. The effect of skin-to-skin breast-feeding in the immediate recovery period on newborn thermoregulation and blood glucose values. *Neonatal Intensive Care.* 1997;10:23–29.

32. Cornblath M, Ichord R. Hypoglycemia in the neonate. *Semin Perinatol.* 2000;24:136–149.

33. Sexson WR. Incidence of neonatal hypoglycemia: A matter of definition. *J Pediatr.* 1984;105:149–150.

34. Harris DL, Weston PJ, Harding JE. Incidence of neonatal hypoglycemia in babies identified as at risk. *J Pediatr.* 2012;161:787–791.

35. Cole MD, Peevy K. Hypoglycemia in normal neonates appropriate for gestational age. *J Perinatol.* 1994;14:118–120.

36. Stanley CA, Baker L. The causes of neonatal hypoglycemia. *N Engl J Med.* 1999;340:1200–1201.

37. Schwartz RP. Neonatal hypoglycemia: How low is too low? *J Pediatr.* 1997;131:171–173.

38. Alkalay A, Klein A, Nagel R, et al. Neonatal nonpersistent hypoglycemia. *Neonatal Intensive Care.* 2001;14:25−34.

39. McGowan JE. Commentary: Neonatal hypoglycemia—Fifty years later, the questions remain the same. *Neoreviews.* 2004;5:e363−e364.

40. Alkalay AL, Sarnat HB, Flores-Sarnat L, et al. Population meta-analysis of low plasma glucose thresholds in full-term normal newborns. *Am J Perinatol.* 2006;23:115−119.

41. Section on Breastfeeding. Breastfeeding and the use of human milk. *Pediatrics.* 2012;129:e827−e841.

42. Haninger NC, Farley CL. Screening for hypoglycemia in healthy term neonates: Effects on breastfeeding. *J Midwifery Womens Health.* 2001;46:292−301.

43. National Childbirth Trust, United Kingdom. Hypoglycemia of the newborn: Guidelines for the appropriate blood glucose screening of breast-fed and bottle-fed babies in the UK. *Midwives.* 1997;110:248−249.

44. Ho HT, Yeung WK, Young BW. Evaluation of "point of care" devices in the measurement of low blood glucose in neonatal practice. *Arch Dis Child Fetal Neonatal Ed.* 2004;89:F356−F359.

45. Altimier L, Roberts W. One Touch II hospital system for neonates: Correlation with serum glucose values. *Neonatal Netw.* 1996;15(2):15−18.

46. Hussain K, Sharief N. The inaccuracy of venous and capillary blood glucose measurement using reagent strips in the newborn period and the effect of haematocrit. *Early Hum Dev.* 2000;57:111−121.

47. Ellis M, Manandhar DS, Manandhar N, et al. Comparison of two cotside methods for the detection of hypoglycemia among neonates in Nepal. *Arch Dis Child Fetal Neonatal Ed.* 1996;75:F122−F125.

48. Dahlberg M, Whitelaw A. Evaluation of HemoCue blood glucose analyzer for the instant diagnosis of hypoglycemia in newborns. *Scand J Clin Lab Invest.* 1997;57:719−724.

49. Sharief N, Hussein K. Comparison of two methods of measurement of whole blood glucose in the neonatal period. *Acta Paediatr.* 1997;86:1246−1252.

50. Schlebusch H, Niesen M, Sorger M, et al. Blood glucose determinations in newborns: Four instruments compared. *Pediatr Pathol Lab Med.* 1998;18:41−48.

51. Harris D, Weston P, Williams C, et al. Cot-side electroencephalography monitoring is not clinically useful in the detection of mild neonatal hypoglycemia. *J Pediatr.* 2011;159:755−760.

52. Harris D, Battin M, Weston P, et al. Continuous glucose monitoring in newborn babies at risk of hypoglycemia. *J Pediatr.* 2010;157:198−202.

53. de Lonlay P, Giurgea I, Touati G, et al. Neonatal hypoglycemia: Aetiologies. *Semin Neonatol.* 2004;9:49−58.

54. Cowett RM, Loughead JL. Neonatal glucose metabolism: Differential diagnoses, evaluation, and treatment of hypoglycemia. *Neonatal Netw.* 2002;21:9−19.

55. Sunehag AL, Haymond MW. Glucose extremes in newborn infants. *Clin Perinatol.* 2002;29:245−260.

56. Kalhan S, Parmimi P. Gluconeogenesis in the fetus and neonate. *Semin Perinatol.* 2000;24:94−106.

57. Hoops D, Roberts P, VanWinkle E, et al. Should routine peripheral blood glucose testing be done for all newborns at birth? *MCN.* 2010;35:264−270.

58. Yager J. Hypoglycemic injury to the immature brain. *Clin Perinatol.* 2002;29:651−674.

59. Jain A, Aggarwal R, Jeeva Sankar M, et al. Hypoglycemia in the newborn. *Indian J Pediatr.* 2010;77:1137−1142.

60. Appendix A Task Force Ratings. Guide to Clinical Preventive Services: Report of the U.S. Preventive Services Task Force, 2nd edition. www.ncbi.nlm.nih.gov/books/NBK15430 (accessed March 28, 2014).

61. American Academy of Pediatrics, American College of Obstetricians and Gynecologists. *Guidelines for Perinatal Care.* 6th ed. Elk Grove Village, IL: American Academy of Pediatrics; 2008.

62. World Health Organization, UNICEF. *Protecting, Promoting and Supporting Breast-Feeding: The Special Role of Maternity Services, A Joint WHO/UNICEF Statement.* Geneva: World Health Organization; 1989.

63. Hawdon JM. Neonatal hypoglycemia: Are evidence-based clinical guidelines achievable? *Neoreviews.* 2014;15:e91−e98.

64. Cox SG. Expressing and storing colostrum antenatally for use in the newborn period. *Breastfeed Rev.* 2006;14:11−16.

65. Forster DA, McEgan K, Ford R, et al. Diabetes and antenatal milk expressing: A pilot project to inform the development of a randomised controlled trial. *Midwifery.* 2011;27:209−214.

66. Soltani H, Scott AM. Antenatal breast expression in women with diabetes: Outcomes from a retrospective cohort study. *Int Breastfeed J.* 2012;7:18.

67. Chapman T, Pincombe J, Harris M. Antenatal breast expression: A critical review of the literature. *Midwifery.* 2013;29:203−210.

68. Chapman T, Pincombe J, Harris M, et al. Antenatal breast expression: Exploration and extent of teaching practices amongst International Board Certified Lactation Consultant midwives across Australia. *Women Birth.* 2013;26:41−48.

ABM protocols expire 5 years from the date of publication. Evidence-based revisions are made within 5 years or sooner if there are significant changes in the evidence.

The Academy of Breastfeeding Medicine Protocol Committee
Kathleen A. Marinelli, MD, FABM, Chairperson
Maya Bunik, MD, MSPH, FABM, Co-Chairperson
Larry Noble MD, FABM, Translations Chairperson
Nancy Brent, MD
Amy E. Grawey, MD
Alison V. Holmes, MD, MPH, FABM
Ruth A. Lawrence, MD, FABM
Tomoko Seo, MD, FABM
Julie Scott Taylor, MD, MSc, FABM
For correspondence: abm@bfmed.org

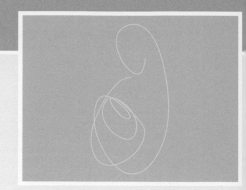

ABM Clinical Protocol #2
Guidelines for Hospital Discharge of the Breastfeeding Term Newborn and Mother: "The Going Home Protocol," Revised 2014*

Amy Evans[1,2], Kathleen A. Marinelli[3,4], Julie Scott Taylor[5] and The Academy of Breastfeeding Medicine

ABSTRACT

A central goal of The Academy of Breastfeeding Medicine is the development of clinical protocols for managing common medical problems that may impact breastfeeding success. These protocols serve only as guidelines for the care of breastfeeding mothers and infants and do not delineate an exclusive course of treatment or serve as standards of medical care. Variations in treatment may be appropriate according to the needs of an individual patient.

BACKGROUND

The ultimate success of breastfeeding is measured in part by both the duration of and the exclusivity of breastfeeding. Anticipatory attention to the needs of the mother and infant at the time of discharge from the hospital is crucial to ensure successful, long-term breastfeeding. The following principles and practices are recommended for consideration prior to sending a mother and her full-term infant home.

Clinical Guidelines

1. A health professional trained in formal assessment of breastfeeding should perform and document an assessment of breastfeeding effectiveness at least once during the last 8 hours preceding discharge of the mother and infant. Similar assessments should have been performed during the hospitalization, preferably at least once every 8–12 hours. In countries such as Japan, where the hospital stay may last up to a week, assessment should continue until breastfeeding is successfully established and then may decrease in frequency. These should include evaluation of positioning, latch, milk transfer, clinical jaundice, stool color and transition, stool and urine output, and notation of uric acid crystals if present. Infant's weight and percentage weight loss should be assessed but do not need to be checked frequently. For example, in Australia, infants are weighed at birth and at discharge or on Day 3 of life, whichever comes first. All concerns raised by the mother such as nipple pain, inability to hand express, perception of inadequate supply, and any perceived need to supplement must also be addressed.[1–7] (I; II-3; III) (Quality of evidence [levels of evidence I, II-1, II-2, II-3, and III] for each recommendation as defined in the U.S. Preventive Services Task Force Appendix A Task Force Ratings[8] is noted in parentheses.) It is important to ask detailed questions—many mothers may not bring up these concerns if not directly questioned.

2. Prior to discharge, anticipation of breastfeeding problems should be assessed based on maternal and/or infant risk factors (Tables 1 and 2). (III)

   All problems with breastfeeding, whether observed by hospital staff or raised by the mother, should be attended to and documented in the medical record prior to discharge of the mother and infant. This includes prompt recognition and treatment plans for possible ankyloglossia, which can affect latch, lactogenesis, and future breastfeeding.[9,10] (An updated clinical protocol is in development.) (I) A plan of action that includes follow-up of the problem after discharge must be in place.[11–14] (II-3) If the mother's and infant's caregivers are not the same person, there needs to be coordinated communication of any issues between the obstetric and pediatric providers for optimal follow-up care (see Guideline #10).

* Courtesy of the Academy of Breastfeeding Medicine. Please go to https://www.bfmed.org/protocols for complete protocols, translations, and the most up-to-date information (protocols are updated every 5–7 years).
[1] University of California San Francisco—Fresno, Fresno, California.
[2] Center for Breastfeeding Medicine and Mother's Resource Center at Community Regional Medical Center, Fresno, California.
[3] Division of Neonatology and Connecticut Human Milk Research Center, Connecticut Children's Medical Center, Hartford, Connecticut.
[4] University of Connecticut School of Medicine, Farmington, Connecticut.
[5] Alpert Medical School of Brown University, Providence, Rhode Island.

TABLE 1 Maternal Risk Factors for Lactation Problems

Factors

History/social
- Primiparity
- Intention to both breastfeed and bottle or formula feed at less than 6 weeks
- Intention to use pacifiers/dummies and/or artificial nipples/teats at less than 6 weeks
- Early intention/necessity to return to school or work
- History of previous breastfeeding problems or breastfed infant with slow weight gain
- History of infertility
- Conception by assisted reproductive technology
- Significant medical problems (e.g., untreated hypothyroidism, diabetes, cystic fibrosis, polycystic ovaries)
- Extremes of maternal age (e.g., adolescent mother or older than 40 years)
- Psychosocial problems (e.g., depression, anxiety, lack of social support for breastfeeding)
- Prolonged labor
- Long induction or augmentation of labor
- Use of medications during labor (benzodiazepines, morphine, or others that can cause drowsiness in the newborn)
- Peripartum complications (e.g., postpartum hemorrhage, hypertension, infection)
- Intended use of hormonal contraceptives before breastfeeding is well established (6 weeks)
- Perceived inadequate milk supply
- Maternal medication use (inappropriate advice about compatibility with breastfeeding is common)

Anatomic/physiologic
- Lack of noticeable breast enlargement during puberty or pregnancy
- Flat, inverted, or very large nipples
- Variation in breast appearance (marked asymmetry, hypoplastic, tubular)
- Any previous breast surgery, including cosmetic procedures (important to ask—not always obvious on exam)
- Previous breast abscess
- Maternal obesity (body mass index ≥ 30 kg/m^2)
- Extremely or persistently sore nipples
- Failure of "secretory activation" lactogenesis II. (Milk did not noticeably "come in" by 72 hours postpartum. This may be difficult to evaluate if mother and infant are discharged from the hospital in the first 24–48 hours postpartum.)
- Mother unable to hand-express colostrum
- Need for breastfeeding aids or appliances (such as nipple shields, breast pumps, or supplemental nursing systems) at the time of hospital discharge

Adapted with permission from Neifert[51,p.285] and the *Breastfeeding Handbook for Physicians*.[2,p.90] (III)

TABLE 2 Infant Risk Factors for Lactation Problems

Factors

Medical/anatomic/physiologic
- Low birth weight or premature (<37 weeks)
- Multiples
- Difficulty in latching on to one or both breasts
- Ineffective or unsustained suckling
- Oral anatomic abnormalities (e.g., cleft lip/palate, macroglossia, micrognathia, tight frenulum/ankyloglossia with trained medical assessment)
- Medical problems (e.g., hypoglycemia, infection, jaundice, respiratory distress)
- Neurologic problems (e.g., genetic syndromes, hypertonia, hypotonia)
- Persistently sleepy infant
- Excessive infant weight loss (> 7–10% of birth weight in the first 48 hours)

Environmental
- Mother–infant separation
- Breast pump dependency
- Formula supplementation
- Effective breastfeeding not established by hospital discharge
- Discharge from the hospital at < 48 hours of age[50]
- Early pacifier use

Adapted with permission from Neifert[51,p.285] and the *Breastfeeding Handbook for Physicians*.[2,p.90] (III)

3. Physicians, midwives, nurses, and all other staff should encourage the mother to breastfeed exclusively for the first 6 months of the infant's life and to continue breastfeeding through at least the first year and preferably to 2 years of life and beyond.[3,15,16] (III) This is the recommendation of the World Health Organization, as well as organizations from many individual countries such as the National Health and Medical Research Council in Australia.[17] The Joint Commission, an organization that accredits hospitals and health care institutions in the United States and globally, is now mandating documentation of exclusive breastfeeding rates as part of its accreditation process for hospitals and birthing centers in the United States. The U.S. Centers for Disease Control and Prevention has similar recommendations.[14,18-21] (III) The addition of appropriate complementary food should occur at 6 months of life.[22] (I) Mothers benefit from education about the rationale for and practical advice on exclusive breastfeeding. The medical, psychosocial, and societal benefits for both mother and infant and why artificial milk supplementation is discouraged should be emphasized. Such education is a standard component of anticipatory guidance that addresses individual beliefs and practices in a culturally sensitive manner.[23-25] Special counseling is needed for those mothers planning to return to outside employment or school (see Guideline #7).[26] (II-2)

4. Families will benefit from appropriate, noncommercial educational materials on breastfeeding (as well as on other aspects of child health care).[27] (I) Discharge packs containing infant formula, pacifiers, commercial advertising materials specifically referring to infant formula and foods, and any materials not appropriate for a breastfeeding mother and infant should not be distributed. These products may encourage poor breastfeeding practices, which may lead to premature weaning.[27]

5. Breastfeeding mothers and appropriate others (fathers, partners, grandmothers, support persons, etc.) will benefit from simplified anticipatory guidance prior to discharge regarding key issues in the immediate future. (I) Care must be given not to overload mothers. Specific information should be provided in written form to all parents regarding:
   a. prevention and management of engorgement
   b. interpretation of infant cues and feeding "on cue"
   c. indicators of adequate intake (evacuation of all meconium stools, three to four stools per day by Day 4, transitioning to yellow bowel movements by Day 5, at least five to six urinations per day by Day 5, and regaining birth weight by Day 10-14 at the latest)
   d. signs of excessive jaundice[4,28] (III)
   e. sleep patterns of newborns, including safe cosleeping practices[29] (III)
   f. maternal medication, cigarette, and alcohol use
   g. individual feeding patterns, including normality of evening cluster feedings

   h. regarding the use of pacifiers (in communities where the use of sanitary pacifiers is commonly recommended to prevent sudden infant death syndrome [SIDS]), discouraging their use until breastfeeding is well established, at least 3-4 weeks. (These recommendations are in accordance with the U.S.-based American Academy of Pediatrics recommendations for the use of pacifiers as a possible prevention of SIDS. Breastfeeding, in itself, is thought to be preventative for SIDS. The Japanese Ministry of Health, Labour and Welfare supports breastfeeding, no smoking, and back sleeping but does not encourage pacifier use.)[30-34] (I)
   i. follow-up and contact information

6. Every breastfeeding mother should receive instruction on the technique of expressing milk by hand (whether or not she uses a pump) so she is able to alleviate engorgement, increase her milk supply, maintain her milk supply, and obtain milk for feeding to the infant should she and the infant be separated or if the infant is unable to feed directly from the breast.[35-37] (II-1)

7. Every breastfeeding mother should be provided with the names and phone numbers of individuals and medical services that can provide advice, counseling, and health assessments related to breastfeeding, ideally on a 24-hour-a-day basis.[1,3] (I)

8. Every breastfeeding mother should be provided with lists of various local peer support groups and services (e.g., mother-to-mother support groups such as La Leche League, Australian Breastfeeding Association, hospital/clinic-based support groups, governmental supported groups [e.g., Special Supplemental Nutrition Program for Women, Infants, and Children (WIC) in the United States] with phone numbers, contact names, and addresses. (II-1; III) Mothers should be encouraged to contact and consider joining one of these groups.[38-44] (II-3; III)

9. If a mother is planning on returning to school or outside employment soon after delivery, she may benefit from additional information.[36,37] (II-1) This should include the need for ongoing social support, possible milk supply issues, expressing and storing milk away from home, the possibility of direct nursing breaks with the infant, and information about any relevant regional and/or national laws regarding accommodations for breastfeeding and milk expression in the workplace. It is prudent to provide her with this information in written form, so that she has resources when the time comes for her to prepare for return to school or work.

10. In countries where hospital discharge is common within 72 hours after birth, appointments for the infant and mother where breastfeeding can be viewed should be made prior to discharge for an office or home visit within 3-5 days of age by a physician, midwife, or a physician-supervised breastfeeding-trained healthcare provider. All infants should be seen within 48-72 hours after discharge; infants discharged before 48 hours of age should be seen within 24-48 hours after discharge.[1,3] (III)

In countries where discharge is 5−7 days after birth, the infant can be seen several times by the physician prior to discharge. In Japan, where this is the case, the next routine visit is recommended at 2 weeks unless there is a problem. Based on the mother's choice, her postpartum visit can be scheduled before discharge, or she can be given the information to make the appointment herself once she is settled at home. In many countries this appointment will be with the obstetrician, family physician, or midwife who participated in the birth of her infant. In other countries such as Australia, if she gave birth in a public hospital, it will be with her general practitioner or family practitioner, who did not attend her birth.

11. Additional visits for the mother and the infant are recommended even if discharge occurs at later than 5 days of age, until all clinical issues such as adequate stool and urine output, jaundice, and the infant attaining birth weight by 10−14 days of age are resolved.

An infant who is not back to birth weight by the first 10 days of life, but who has demonstrated a steady, appropriate weight gain for several days, is likely fine. This baby needs continued close follow-up but may not need intervention.

Any baby exhibiting a weight loss approaching 7% of birth weight by 5−6 days of life needs to be closely monitored until weight gain is well established. Should 7% or more weight loss be noted after 5−6 days of life, even more concern and careful follow-up must be pursued. These infants require careful assessment. By 4−6 days infants should be gaining weight daily, which makes their percentage weight loss actually more significant when that lack of daily weight gain is taken into account. In addition to attention to these issues, infants with any of these concerns must be specifically evaluated for problems with breastfeeding and milk transfer.[1−7] (III)

12. If the mother is medically ready for hospital discharge but the infant is not, every effort should be made to allow the mother to remain in the hospital either as a patient or as a "mother-in-residence" with access to the infant to support exclusive breastfeeding. Maintenance of a 24-hour rooming-in relationship with the infant is optimal during the infant's extended stay.[19,20,43] (II-1)

13. If the mother is discharged from the hospital before the infant is discharged (as in the case of a sick infant), the mother should be encouraged to spend as much time as possible with the infant, to practice skin-to-skin technique and kangaroo care with her infant whenever possible, and to continue regular breastfeeding.[45−49] (I; II-2) During periods when the mother is not in the hospital, she should be taught to express and store her milk and to bring it to the hospital for the infant. At the least she should demonstrate successful expression of her milk before hospital discharge. If she has problems with her milk supply, early referral to a lactation consultant and/or a physician skilled in breastfeeding management and medicine is indicated. (III) Milk may be expressed at home and brought in to the hospital for use by the baby. Some countries discourage this practice, but there is no evidence to contradict this recommendation and much evidence to support the use of mother's milk for these fragile infants.[3]

SUGGESTIONS FOR FUTURE RESEARCH

Although the majority of the clinical recommendations in this policy are firmly evidence-based, areas for future study remain. We know that in some areas of the world, initiation rates are high in the hospital but fall precipitously after hospital discharge. Once mothers and infants receive the best evidence-based information and assistance possible in hospital, what best practices need to be established to ensure that the process of "going home" is a smooth one? What culturally appropriate safety nets of support, help, and advice need to be readily and easily available to them, regardless of where they live and their socioeconomic or educational level? There is much work that can be done in this area to develop and test model policies and plans in action that could then be replicated in similar areas to determine best practices to support exclusive breastfeeding.

A Cochrane Review was done in 2002[50] looking at the effect of "early discharge" (less than 48−72 hours) on maternal/infant outcomes, including breastfeeding out to 6 months. The results were equivocal, with no differences in sample and control groups, but there was no standardization of definitions or any attempt to quantify teaching in hospital and follow-up on "going home." This is an area ripe for examination as we try to discern when a dyad is ready for discharge home.[5] Finally, if future research deliberately uses the same primary and secondary outcome measures currently described in the literature, then meta-analysis of these data will become possible.[49]

ACKNOWLEDGMENTS

This work was supported in part by a grant from the Maternal and Child Health Bureau, U.S. Department of Health and Human Services.

REFERENCES

1. Langan RC. Discharge procedures for healthy newborns. *Am Fam Physician*. 2006;73:849−852.
2. Schanler RJ, Krebs N, Mass S, eds. *Breastfeeding Handbook for Physicians*. 2nd ed. Elk Grove Village, IL: American Academy of Pediatrics and American College of Obstetrics and Gynecologists; 2014.
3. American Academy of Pediatrics, Section on Breastfeeding. Policy statement: Breastfeeding and the use of human milk. *Pediatrics*. 2012;129:e327−e341.
4. Gartner L. ABM Clinical Protocol #22: Guidelines for management of jaundice in the breastfeeding infant equal or greater than 35 weeks gestation. *Breastfeed Med*. 2010;5:87−93.

5. American College of Obstetricians and Gynecologists. Committee Opinion No. 570. Breastfeeding in underserved women: Increasing initiation and continuation of breastfeeding. *Obstet Gynecol.* 2013;122:323–428.

6. Academy of Breastfeeding Medicine Board of Directors. Position on breastfeeding. *Breastfeed Med.* 2008;3:269–270.

7. Lawrence RA, Lawrence RM. Breastfeeding: A Guide for the Medical Professional. 7th ed. Philadelphia: Saunders; 2010.

8. Appendix A Task Force Ratings. Guide to Clinical Preventive Services: Report of the U.S. Preventive Services Task Force. 2nd edition. www.ncbi.nlm.nih.gov/books/NBK15430 (accessed December 15, 2013).

9. Buryk M, Bloom D, Shope T. Efficacy of neonatal release of ankyloglossia: A randomized trial. *Pediatrics.* 2011;128:280–288.

10. Ballard J, Academy of Breastfeeding Medicine Protocol Committee. Clinical protocol #11: Guidelines for the evaluation and management of neonatal ankyloglossia and its complications in the breastfeeding dyad, 2004 [Members Only page]. http://www.bfmed.org/Media/Files/Protocols/ankyloglossia.pdf (accessed December 19, 2013).

11. Yanicki S, Hasselback P, Sandilands M, et al. The safety of Canadian early discharge guidelines. *Can J Public Health.* 2002;93:26–30.

12. Ahluwalia IB, Morrow B, Hsia J. Why do women stop breastfeeding? Findings from the Pregnancy Risk Assessment and Monitoring System. *Pediatrics.* 2005;116:1408–1412.

13. Britton JR, Baker A, Spino C, et al. Postpartum discharge preferences of pediatricians: Results from a national survey. *Pediatrics.* 2002;110:53–60.

14. Centers for Disease Control and Prevention (CDC). Vital signs: Hospital practices to support breastfeeding, United States, 2007 and 2009. *MMWR Morb Mortal Wkly Rep.* 2011;60:1020–1025.

15. American Academy of Family Physicians. Breastfeeding Policy Statement, 2013. www.aafp.org/about/policies/all/breastfeeding.html (accessed December 13, 2013).

16. James DC, Dobson B, American Dietetic Association. Position of the American Dietetic Association: Promoting and supporting breastfeeding. *J Am Diet Assoc.* 2005;105:810–818.

17. National Health and Medical Research Council. *Infant Feeding Guidelines.* Canberra: National Health and Medical Research Council; 2012.

18. World Health Organization, United Nations Children's Fund. Protecting, promoting and supporting breastfeeding: The special role of maternity services (a joint WHO/UNICEF statement). *Int J Gynaecol Obstet.* 1990;31:171–183.

19. U.S. Department of Health and Human Services. *The Surgeon General's Call to Action to Support Breastfeeding.* Washington, DC: Office of the Surgeon General, U.S. Department of Health and Human Services; 2011.

20. Joint Commission Perinatal Core Measures. http://manual.jointcommission.org/releases/TJC2013A/PerinatalCare.html (accessed December 13, 2013).

21. World Health Organization. The Optimal Duration of Exclusive Breastfeeding: Report of an Expert Consultation. March 2001. www.who.int/nutrition/publications/optimal_duration_of_exc_bfeeding_report_eng.pdf (accessed December 13, 2013).

22. Kramer MS, Kakuma R. Optimal duration of exclusive breastfeeding. *Cochrane Database Syst Rev.* 2002;(1)CD003517.

23. Setrakian HU, Rosenman MB, Szucs K. Breastfeeding and the Baháʼí faith. *Breastfeed Med.* 2011;6:221–225.

24. Centers for Disease Control and Prevention. Racial and ethnic differences in breastfeeding initiation and duration, by state—National Immunization Survey, United States, 2004–2008. *MMWR Morb Mortal Wkly Rep.* 2010;59:327–334.

25. Segawe M. Buddhism and breastfeeding. *Breastfeed Med.* 2008;3:124–128.

26. Guendelman S, Kosa JL, Pearl M, et al. Juggling work and breastfeeding: Effect of maternity leave and occupational characteristics. *Pediatrics.* 2009;123:e38–e46.

27. Sadacharan R, Grossman X, Matlak S, et al. Hospital discharge bags and breastfeeding at 6 months: Data from the Infant Feeding Practices Study II. *J Hum Lact.* 2013 Dec 4; [Epub ahead of print]. Available from: https://doi.org/10.1177/0890334413513653. http://jhl.sagepub.com/content/early/2013/11/25/0890334413513653.full.pdf + html (accessed December 19, 2013).

28. American Academy of Pediatrics Subcommittee on Hyperbilirubinemia. Management of hyperbilirubinemia in the newborn infant 35 or more weeks of gestation. *Pediatrics.* 2004;114:297–316.

29. Academy of Breastfeeding Medicine Protocol Committee. ABM clinical protocol #6: Guideline on co-sleeping and breastfeeding. Revision, March, 2008. *Breastfeed Med.* 2008;3:38–43.

30. Kramer MS, Barr RG, Dagenais S, et al. Pacifier use, early weaning, and cry/fuss behavior. *JAMA.* 2001;286:322–326.

31. Task Force on Sudden Infant Death Syndrome. SIDS and other sleep related infant deaths: Expansion of recommendations for a safe infant sleeping environment. *Pediatrics.* 2011;128:1030–1039.

32. Task Force on Sudden Infant Death Syndrome. Technical report: SIDS and other sleep related infant deaths: Expansion of recommendations for a safe infant sleep environment. *Pediatrics.* 2011;128:e1341–e1367.

33. Blair PS, Sidebotham P, Evason-Coombe C, et al. Hazardous cosleeping environments and risk factors amenable to change: Case control study of SIDS in South West England. *BMJ.* 2009;339:b3666.

34. Hauck FR, Thompson JM, Tanabe KO, et al. Breastfeeding and reduced risk of sudden infant death syndrome: A meta-analysis. *Pediatrics.* 2011;128:1–8.

35. Eglash A, Academy of Breastfeeding Medicine Protocol Committee. ABM clinical protocol #8: Human milk storage information for home use for full-term infants (original protocol March 2004; revision #1 March 2010). *Breastfeed Med.* 2010;5:127–130.

36. Eldridge S, Croker A. Breastfeeding friendly workplace accreditation. Creating supportive workplaces for breastfeeding women. *Breastfeed Rev.* 2005;13:17–22.

37. Health Resources and Services Administration. The Business Case for Breastfeeding. Steps for Creating a Breastfeeding Friendly Worksite: Bottom Line Benefits. 2008. http://mchb.hrsa.gov/pregnancyandbeyond/breastfeeding/ (accessed December 13, 2013).

38. Phillip BL. Every call is an opportunity. Supporting breastfeeding mothers over the telephone. *Pediatr Clin North Am.* 2001;48:525–532.

39. Anderson AK, Damio G, Young S, et al. A randomized trial assessing the efficacy of peer counseling on exclusive breastfeeding in a predominantly Latina low-income community. *Arch Pediatr Adolesc Med.* 2005;159:836–841.

40. Graffy J, Taylor J. What information, advice, and support do women want with breastfeeding? *Birth.* 2005;32:179—186.

41. Bronner Y, Barber T, Vogelhut J, et al. Breastfeeding peer counseling: Results from the national WIC survey. *J Hum Lact.* 2001;17:119—168.

42. Bronner Y, Barber T, Davis S. Breastfeeding peer counseling: Policy implications. *J Hum Lact.* 2001;17:105—109.

43. Mickens AD, Modeste N, Montgomery S, et al. Peer support and breastfeeding intentions: Among black WIC participants. *J Hum Lact.* 2009;25:157—162.

44. Gross SM, Resnik AK, Nanda JP, et al. Early postpartum: A critical period in setting the path for breastfeeding success. *Breastfeed Med.* 2011;6:407—412.

45. DiGirolamo AM, Grummer-Strawn LM, Fein SB. Effect of maternity-care practices on breastfeeding. *Pediatrics.* 2008;122 (Suppl 2):S43—S49.

46. Browne JV. Early relationship environments: Physiology of skin-to-skin contact for parents and their preterm infants. *Clin Perinatol.* 2004;31:287—298.

47. Carfoot S, Williamson PR, Dickson R. A systematic review of randomized controlled trials evaluating the effect of mother/baby skin-to-skin care on successful breastfeeding. *Midwifery.* 2003;19:148—155.

48. Kirsten GF, Bergman NJ, Hann FM. Kangaroo mother care in the nursery. *Pediatr Clin North Am.* 2001;48:443—452.

49. Moore ER, Anderson GC, Bergman NJ. Early skin-to-skin contact for mothers and their healthy newborn infants. *Cochrane Database Syst Rev.* 2011;(3)CD003519.

50. Brown S, Small R, Argus B, et al. Early postnatal discharge from hospital for healthy mothers and term infants. *Cochrane Database Syst Rev.* 2002;(3)CD002958.

51. Neifert MR. Prevention of breastfeeding tragedies. *Pediatr Clin North Am.* 2001;48:273—297.

ABM protocols expire 5 years from the date of publication. Evidence-based revisions are made within 5 years or sooner if there are significant changes in the evidence.

Academy of Breastfeeding Medicine Protocol Committee
Kathleen A. Marinelli, MD, FABM, Chairperson
Maya Bunik, MD, MSPH, FABM, Co-Chairperson
Larry Noble, MD, FABM, Translations Chairperson
Nancy Brent, MD
Amy E. Grawey, MD
Alison V. Holmes, MD, MPH, FABM
Ruth A. Lawrence, MD, FABM
Tomoko Seo, MD, FABM
Julie Scott Taylor, MD, MSc, FABM
For correspondence: abm@bfmed.org

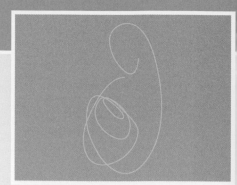

ABM Clinical Protocol #3
*Supplementary Feedings in the Healthy Term Breastfed Neonate, Revised 2017**

Ann Kellams[1], Cadey Harrel[2], Stephanie Omage[3], Carrie Gregory[5], Casey Rosen-Carole[4,5] and the Academy of Breastfeeding Medicine

ABSTRACT

A central goal of The Academy of Breastfeeding Medicine is the development of clinical protocols for managing common medical problems that may impact breastfeeding success. These protocols serve only as guidelines for the care of breastfeeding mothers and infants and do not delineate an exclusive course of treatment or serve as standards of medical care. Variations in treatment may be appropriate according to the needs of an individual patient.

DEFINITIONS USED IN THIS PROTOCOL

- *Exclusive breastfeeding*: Feeding only breastmilk (at the breast or own mothers' expressed breast milk), no food or water except vitamins, minerals, and medications.
- *Supplementary feedings*: Additional fluids provided to a breastfed infant before 6 months (recommended duration of exclusive breastfeeding). These fluids may include donor human milk, infant formula, or other breast milk substitutes (e.g., glucose water).
- *Complementary feedings*: Solid or semisolid foods provided to an infant in addition to breastfeeding when breast milk alone is no longer sufficient to meet nutritional needs.

* Courtesy of the Academy of Breastfeeding Medicine. Please go to https://www.bfmed.org/protocols for complete protocols, translations, and the most up-to-date information (protocols are updated every 5—7 years).

[1] Department of Pediatrics, University of Virginia, Charlottesville, Virginia.

[2] Department of Family & Community Medicine, University of Arizona College of Medicine and Family Medicine Residency, Tucson, Arizona.

[3] Discipline of General Practice, The University of Queensland, Brisbane, Australia.

[4] Department of Pediatrics, University of Rochester, Rochester, New York.

[5] Department of OBGYN, University of Rochester, Rochester, New York.

- *Term infant*: In this protocol "term infant" also includes early-term infants (gestational age 37—38 6/7 weeks).

BACKGROUND

Given early opportunities to breastfeed, breastfeeding assistance, and instruction the vast majority of mothers and infants will successfully establish breastfeeding. Although some infants may not successfully latch and feed well during the first day (24 hours), most will successfully breastfeed with time, appropriate evaluation and support, with minimal intervention. Exclusive breastfeeding for the first 6 months is associated with the greatest protection against major health problems for both mothers and infants.[1-3] Unfortunately, infant formula supplementation of healthy neonates in hospital is commonplace,[4,5] despite widespread recommendations to the contrary.[6-8] Early supplementation with infant formula is associated with decreased exclusive breastfeeding rates in the first 6 months and an overall shorter duration of breastfeeding.[9,10] Therefore, hospitals, healthcare facilities, and community organizations that promote breastfeeding are integral in improving the exclusivity and duration of breastfeeding.[10] One way of achieving this is by following The Ten Steps to Successful Breastfeeding (the basis for the Baby-Friendly Hospital Initiative), both in the hospital and community.

Newborn physiology

Small quantities of colostrum are appropriate for the size of a newborn's stomach,[11-13] prevent hypoglycemia in a healthy, term, appropriate for gestational age infant,[14,15] and are easy for an infant to manage as he/she learns to coordinate sucking, swallowing, and breathing. Healthy term infants also have sufficient body water to meet their metabolic needs, even in hot climates.[16-18] Fluid necessary to replace insensible fluid loss is adequately provided by breast milk alone.[7,18] Newborns lose weight because of physiologic diuresis of extracellular fluid following transition from intrauterine to extrauterine life and the passage of meconium. In a prospective cohort of mothers in a U.S. Baby-Friendly designated hospital with optimal support of infant feeding, the mean weight loss of exclusively breastfed infants was 5.5%; notably, greater than 20% of healthy breastfed infants lost more than 7% of their birthweight.[19] A study of over 160,000 healthy breastfed infants resulted in the creation of hour-specific nomograms for infant weight loss for exclusively breastfed newborns that showed differentially increased weight loss in those born by cesarean section than by vaginal birth. In this study, almost 5% of vaginally born infants and >10% of those born by cesarean section had lost ≥ 10% of their birth weight by 48 hours after birth. By 72 hours, >25% of infants born by cesarean section had lost ≥ 10% of their birth weight.[20] Breastfed infants regain birth weight at an average of 8.3 days (95% confidence interval: 7.7—8.9 days) with 97.5% having regained their birth weight by 21 days.[21] Infants should be followed closely to identify those who lie outside the predicted pattern, but the majority of those breastfed infants will not require supplementation. It should also be noted that excess newborn weight loss is correlated with positive maternal intrapartum fluid balance (received through intravenous fluids) and may not be directly indicative of breastfeeding success or failure.[22,23]

Early management of the new breastfeeding mother

Some breastfeeding mothers question the adequacy of colostrum feedings and perceive that they have an insufficient milk supply.[24,25] These women may receive conflicting advice about the need for supplementation and would benefit from reassurance, assistance with breastfeeding technique, and education about the normal physiology of breastfeeding and infant behavior. Inappropriate supplementation may undermine a mother's confidence in her ability to meet her infant's nutritional needs[26] and give inappropriate messages that may result in supplementation of breastfed infants at home.[27] Introduction of infant formula or other supplements may decrease the feeding frequency of the infant, thereby decreasing the amount of breast stimulation a mother receives, which results in a reduction of milk supply.[28]

Postpartum mothers with low confidence levels are very vulnerable to external influences, such as advice to offer breastfeeding infants supplementation of glucose water or infant formula. Well-meaning healthcare professionals may recommend supplementation as a means of protecting mothers from fatigue or distress, although this can conflict with their role in promoting breastfeeding.[29–31] Several sociodemographic factors are associated with formula supplementation in the hospital, and vary geographically. It is important to recognize and address these factors in a culturally sensitive manner. Inappropriate reasons for supplementation and associated risks are multiple (Appendix 1 Table A1).

There are common clinical situations where evaluation and breastfeeding management may be necessary, but SUPPLEMENTATION IS NOT INDICATED, including:

1. The healthy, term, appropriate for gestational age infant when the infant is feeding well, urinating and stooling adequately, weight loss is in the expected range, and bilirubin levels are not of concern (depending on gestational age, time since birth, and any risk factors).[32]
   - Newborns are normally sleepy after an initial alert period after birth (∼2 hours). They then have variable sleep—wake cycles, with an additional one or two wakeful periods in the next 10 hours whether fed or not.[33]
   - Careful attention to an infant's early feeding cues, keeping the infant safely skin-to-skin with mother when she is awake, gently rousing the infant to attempt frequent breastfeeds, and teaching the mother hand expression of drops of colostrum,[34] may be more appropriate than automatic supplementation after 6, 8, 12, or even 24 hours.
   - Increased skin-on-skin time can encourage more frequent feeding.
2. Ten percent weight loss is not an automatic marker for the need for supplementation, but is an indicator for infant evaluation.
   - The infant who is fussy at night or constantly feeding for several hours
   - Cluster feeding (several short feeds close together) is normal newborn behavior, but should warrant a feeding evaluation to observe the infant's behavior at the breast[35] and the comfort of the mother to ensure that the infant is latched deeply and effectively.
   - Some fussy infants are in pain that should be addressed.
3. The tired or sleeping mother
   - Some fatigue is normal for new mothers. However, rooming out for maternal fatigue does not improve mothers' sleep time[36] and has been shown to reduce breastfeeding exclusivity.[37] Extreme fatigue should be evaluated for the safety of mother and baby to avoid falls and suffocation.[38]
   - Breastfeeding management that optimizes the infant feeding at the breast may make for a more satisfied infant AND allow the mother to get more rest.

The following guidelines address strategies to prevent the need for supplementation (also see Appendix 2) as well as indications for and methods of supplementation for the healthy, term (37- to 42-week), breastfed infant. Indications for supplementation in term, healthy infants are few.[7,39] Table 1 lists possible indications for the administration of supplemental feeds. In each case, the medical provider must decide if the clinical benefits outweigh the potential negative consequences of such feedings.

RECOMMENDATIONS

Step 1. Prevent the need for supplementation

1. There is mixed, but mainly positive, evidence about the role of antenatal education and in-hospital support on the rates of exclusive breastfeeding.[40–42] (I) (Quality of evidence

TABLE 1   Possible Indications for Supplementation in Healthy, Term Infants (37–41 6/7 Weeks Gestational Age)

1. Infant indications

  a. Asymptomatic hypoglycemia, documented by laboratory blood glucose measurement (not bedside screening methods) that is unresponsive to appropriate frequent breastfeeding. Note that 40% dextrose gel applied to the side of the infant's cheek is effective in increasing blood glucose levels in this scenario and improves the rate of exclusive breastfeeding after discharge with no evidence of adverse effects.[78] Symptomatic infants or infants with glucose <1.4 mmol/L (<25 mg/dL) in the first 4 hours or <2.0 mmol/L (<35 mg/dL) after 4 hours should be treated with intravenous glucose.[15] Breastfeeding should continue during intravenous glucose therapy.

  b. Signs or symptoms that may indicate inadequate milk intake:

  i. Clinical or laboratory evidence of significant dehydration (e.g., high sodium, poor feeding, lethargy, etc.) that is not improved after skilled assessment and proper management of breastfeeding.[79]

  ii. Weight loss of ≥8–10% (day 5 [120 hours] or later), or weight loss greater than 75th percentile for age.

   1. Although weight loss in the range of 8–10% may be within normal limits if all else is going well and the physical examination is normal, it is an indication for careful assessment and possible breastfeeding assistance. Weight loss in excess of this may be an indication of inadequate milk transfer or low milk production, but a thorough evaluation is required before automatically ordering supplementation.[19,20,80]

   2. Weight loss nomograms for healthy newborns by hour of age can be found at: www.newbornweight.org[20,80]

  iii. Delayed bowel movements, fewer than four stools on day 4 of life, or continued meconium stools on day 5 (120 hours).[48,80]

   1. Elimination patterns for newborns for urine and stool should be tracked at least through to the onset of secretory activation. Even though there is a wide variation between infants, the patterns may be useful in determining adequacy of breastfeeding.[81,82] II-2. Newborns with more bowel movements during the first 5 days following birth have less initial weight loss, earlier the transition to yellow stools, and earlier return to birth weight.[83]

  c. Hyperbilirubinemia (see ABM Clinical Protocol #22: Guidelines for Management of Jaundice)

  i. Suboptimal intake jaundice of the newborn associated with poor breast milk intake despite appropriate intervention. This characteristically begins at 2–5 days and is marked by ongoing weight loss, limited stooling and voiding with uric acid crystals.

  ii. Breast milk jaundice when levels reach 340–425 μmol/L (20–25 mg/dL) in an otherwise thriving infant and where a diagnostic and/or therapeutic interruption of breastfeeding may be under consideration. First line diagnostic management should include laboratory evaluation, instead of interruption of breastfeeding.

  d. Macronutrient supplementation is indicated, such as for the rare infant with inborn errors of metabolism.

2. Maternal indications

  a. Delayed secretory activation (day 3–5 or later [72–120 hours] and inadequate intake by the infant).[80]

  b. Primary glandular insufficiency (less than 5% of women—primary lactation failure), as evidenced by abnormal breast shape, poor breast growth during pregnancy, or minimal indications of secretory activation.[84,85]

  c. Breast pathology or prior breast surgery resulting in poor milk production.[84]

  d. Temporary cessation of breastfeeding due to certain medications (e.g., chemotherapy) or temporary separation of mother and baby without expressed breast milk available.

  e. Intolerable pain during feedings unrelieved by interventions.

[levels of evidence I, II-1, II-2, II-3, and III] is based on the U.S. Preventive Services[43] Task Force Appendix A Task Force Ratings and is noted in parentheses.)

2. All staff who care for postpartum women should be able to assist and assess breastfeeding infants, especially when other staff with expertise are not available.

3. Both mothers and healthcare professionals should be aware of the risks of unnecessary supplementation.

4. Healthy infants should be placed skin-to-skin with the mother, if she is awake and alert, immediately after birth to facilitate breastfeeding.[7,44] (I) The delay in time between birth and initiation of the first breastfeed is a strong predictor of infant formula use and may affect future milk supply.[10,45,46] (II-3, II-2, II-3)

5. It is ideal to have the mother and infant room-in 24 hours per day to respond to infant feeding cues, enhance opportunities for breastfeeding, and hence secretory activation (lactogenesis II).[7,39,47,48] (III)

6. If mother–infant separation is unavoidable, milk supply is not well established, or milk transfer is inadequate, the mother needs instruction and encouragement to express her milk by hand or pump to stimulate milk production and provide expressed milk for the infant.[7,39,48,49] (I, III) This process should begin within 1 hour of birth.[45] (II-2)

Step 2. Address early indicators of the possible need for supplementation

1. The infant's medical providers should be notified if the infant or mother meets any criteria for supplementation, as listed in Table 1.

2. All infants must be formally evaluated for position, latch, and milk transfer before the provision of supplemental feedings. This evaluation should be undertaken by a healthcare provider with expertise in breastfeeding management, when available.[7,48]

Step 3. Determine whether supplementation is required and supplement with care

1. The status of the infant requiring supplementation should be determined and any decisions made on a case-by-case basis (guidelines in Table 1).
2. Hospitals should strongly consider formulating and instituting policies to require a medical provider's order when supplements are medically indicated and informed consent of the mother when supplements are not medically indicated. It is the responsibility of the healthcare provider to fully inform parents of the benefits and risks of supplementation, document parental decisions, and support the parents after they have made a decision.[50,51] (III)
3. All supplemental feedings should be documented, including the content, volume, method, and medical indication or reason.
4. When supplementary feeding is medically necessary, the primary goals are to feed the infant and to optimize the maternal milk supply while determining the cause of low milk supply, poor feeding, or inadequate milk transfer. Supplementation should be performed in ways that help preserve breastfeeding such as limiting the volume to what is necessary for the normal newborn physiology, avoiding teats/artificial nipples,[52] (I) stimulating the mother's breasts with hand expression or pumping, and for the infant to continue to practice at the breast.
5. Optimally, mothers need to express milk frequently, usually once for each time the infant receives a supplement, or at least 8 times in 24 hours if the infant is not feeding at the breast. Breasts should be fully drained each time.[53] (II-2) Maternal breast engorgement should be avoided as it will further compromise the milk supply and may lead to other complications.[54] (III)
6. Criteria for stopping supplementation should be considered from the time of the decision to supplement and should be discussed with the parents. Stopping supplementation can be a source of anxiety for parents and providers. Underlying factors should be addressed and mothers should be assisted with their milk supply, latch, and comfort with assessing the signs that their infant is adequately fed. It is important to closely follow up mother and infant.
7. When the decision to supplement is not medically indicated (Table 1), discussions with the mother should be documented by the nursing and/or medical staff followed by full support of her informed decision.

CHOICE OF SUPPLEMENT

1. Expressed breast milk from the infant's mother is the first choice for extra feeding for the breastfed infant.[7,55] (III) Hand expression may elicit larger volumes than a breast pump in the first few days following birth and may increase overall milk supply.[56] Breast massage and/or compression along with expressing with a mechanical pump may also increase available milk.[57] (II-3)
2. If the volume of the mother's own colostrum/milk does not meet her infant's feeding requirements and supplementation is required, donor human milk is preferable to other supplements.[55]
3. When donor human milk is not available or appropriate, protein hydrolysate formulas may be preferable to standard infant formula as they avoid exposure to intact cow's milk proteins and reduce bilirubin levels more rapidly,[58] (II-2) although recent data are less supportive of its role in preventing allergic disease.[59] (I) The use of this type of formula may also convey the psychological message that the supplement is a temporary therapy, not a permanent inclusion of artificial feedings.
4. Supplementation with glucose water is not appropriate because it does not provide sufficient nutrition, does not reduce serum bilirubin,[60,61] and might cause hyponatremia.
5. The potential risks and benefits of other supplemental fluids, such as cow's milk formulas, soy formulas, or protein hydrolysate formulas, must be considered along with the available resources of the family, the infant's age, the amounts needed, and the potential impact on the establishment of breastfeeding.

VOLUME OF SUPPLEMENTAL FEEDING

1. Several studies give us an idea of intakes at the breast over time. In most studies, the range of intake is wide, while formula-fed infants usually take in larger volumes than breastfed infants.[62–66] (II-3)
2. Infants fed infant formula ad libitum commonly have much higher intakes than breastfed infants.[65,66] (II-3) Acknowledging that ad libitum breastfeeding emulates evolutionary feeding and considering recent data on obesity in formula-fed infants, it appears that formula-fed infants may be overfed.
3. As there is no definitive research available, the amount of supplement given should reflect the normal amounts of colostrum available, the size of the infant's stomach (which changes over time), and the age and size of the infant. Intake on day 2 postbirth is generally higher than day 1 in relation to infant's demand.[65]
4. Based on the limited research available, suggested intakes for healthy, term infants are given in Table 2, although feedings should be based on infant cues.

TABLE 2	Average Reported Intakes of Colostrum by Healthy, Term Breastfed Infants
Time (hours)	Intake (mL/feed)
First 24	2–10
24–48	5–15
48–72	15–30
72–96	30–60

METHODS OF PROVIDING SUPPLEMENTARY FEEDINGS

1. When supplementary feedings are needed, there are a number of delivery methods from which to choose: a supplemental nursing device at the breast, cup feeding, spoon or dropper feeding, finger-feeding, syringe feeding, or bottle feeding.[67] (III)

2. An optimal supplemental feeding device has not yet been identified, and may vary from one infant to another. No method is without potential risk or benefit.[68]

3. When selecting an alternative feeding method, clinicians should consider several criteria:
   a. cost and availability
   b. ease of use and cleaning
   c. stress to the infant
   d. whether adequate milk volume can be fed in 20–30 minutes
   e. whether anticipated use is short- or long-term
   f. maternal preference
   g. expertise of healthcare staff
   h. whether the method enhances development of breastfeeding skills.

4. There is no evidence that any of these methods are unsafe or that one is necessarily better than the other. There is some evidence that avoiding teats/artificial nipples for supplementation may help the infant return to exclusive breastfeeding[20,52,69] (I); however, when hygiene is suboptimal, cup feeding is the recommended choice.[55] Cup feeding also allows infants to control feeding pace[68] (II-2). Cup feeding has been shown safe for both term and preterm infants and may help preserve breastfeeding duration among those who require multiple supplemental feedings.[52,70–72] (II-2, I, I, I, II-2)

5. If bottles are being used, pacing the feed may be beneficial, especially for preterm infants.[73] (III)

6. Supplemental nursing systems have the advantages of supplying a supplement while simultaneously stimulating the breast to produce more milk, reinforcing the infant's feeding at the breast, enabling the mother to have a breastfeeding experience, and encouraging skin-to-skin. However, mothers may find the systems awkward to use, difficult to clean, relatively expensive, requiring moderately complex learning, and the infant must be able to latch effectively.[67] A simpler version, supplementing with a dropper, syringe, or feeding tube attached to the breast while the infant is feeding at breast, may be effective.

7. Bottle feeding is the most commonly used method of supplementation in more affluent regions of the world, but concerns have been raised because of distinct differences in tongue and jaw movements, and faster flow may result in higher (and unnecessary) volumes of feeds.[67] Some experts have recommended a teat/ nipple with a wide base and slow flow to try to mimic breast-feeding and to avoid nipple confusion or preference,[68,74] (II-2), but little research has been done evaluating outcomes with different teats/nipples.

RESEARCH NEEDS

Research is necessary to establish evidence-based guidelines on appropriate supplementation volumes for specific conditions and whether this varies for colostrum versus infant formula.

Specific questions include the following:
1. Should the volume be independent of infant weight or a per kilogram volume? Should supplementation make up for cumulative losses?
2. Should feeding intervals or quantities be different for different types of delivery of supplementation (e.g., bottles, cup feeding)?
3. Are some methods (type and delivery mechanism) best for infants with certain conditions, ages, and available resources? Which methods interfere least with establishing direct breastfeeding?

NOTES

This protocol addresses the healthy, term newborn. For information regarding appropriate feeding and supplementation for the late preterm infant (35–37 weeks), see "ABM Protocol #10: Breastfeeding the Late Preterm Infant"[75] and "Care and Management of the Late Preterm Infant Toolkit."[76] The World Health Organization broadened the annex of the "Global Criteria for the Baby Friendly Hospital Initiative: Acceptable Medical Reasons for Supplementation."[77] to include acceptable reasons for use of breast milk substitutes in all infants. The handout (#4.5) is available at: www.who.int/nutrition/topics/BFHI_Revised_Section_4.pdf

APPENDIX 1

TABLE A1   Inappropriate Reasons for Supplementation in the Context of a Healthy Newborn and Mother, Responses, and Risks

Concerns/inappropriate reasons	Responses	Risks of supplementation
There is "no milk,"[5] belief that colostrum is insufficient until the milk "comes in"	Mother and family should be educated about the benefits of colostrum including dispelling myths about the yellow color. Small amounts of colostrum are normal, physiologic, and appropriate for the term, healthy newborn	Can alter infant bowel flora and microbiome.[86,87] Potentially sensitizes the infant to foreign proteins.[88,89] Increases the risk of diarrhea and other infections, especially where hygiene is poor.[3] Potentially disrupts the "supply-demand" cycle, leading to inadequate milk supply and long-term supplementation.
Supplementation is needed to prevent weight loss and dehydration in the postnatal period[5]	A certain amount of weight loss is normal in the first week of life and is due to diuresis of extracellular fluid and passage of meconium.	Supplementation in the first few days may interfere with the normal frequency of breastfeeding. Supplementation with water or glucose water, increases the risk of jaundice,[90] excessive weight loss,[91] and longer hospital stays.[92]
Infant could become hypoglycemic	Healthy, full-term infants do not develop symptomatic hypoglycemia as a result of suboptimal breastfeeding.[15]	Same risks as for weight loss/dehydration
Breastfeeding is related to jaundice in the postnatal period	The more frequent the breastfeeding, the lower the bilirubin level.[93,94] Bilirubin is a potent antioxidant[95] and jaundice is normal in the newborn. Colostrum acts as a natural laxative helping to eliminate meconium that contains bilirubin	Same risks as for weight loss/dehydration
Lack of time for counseling mother about exclusive breastfeeding when mothers request a supplement	Train all staff in how to assist mothers with breastfeeding. Mothers may benefit from education about artificial feeds and/or how supplements may adversely affect subsequent breastfeeding.[29] Time spent by healthcare professionals listening to and talking with mothers is at least as important as other more active interventions (which may be viewed more as "real work" to them).[29]	If the supplement is infant formula, which is slow to empty from the stomach[96] and often fed in larger amounts,[66] the infant will breastfeed less frequently. Depending on the method of supplementation,[52,74] or the number of supplements[97] an infant may have difficulty returning to the breast. Feeds given before secretory activation and copious breast milk production (as opposed to supplementation) may be associated with delayed initiation of breastfeeding and negatively associated with exclusivity and duration of breastfeeding.[98]
Medications may be contraindicated with breastfeeding	Accurate references are available to providers (e.g., Medications and Mothers' Milk 2017,[99] LactMed on Toxnet website[15]) For most medical conditions, medication safe for breastfeeding mothers and babies is available	Risk of decreasing breastfeeding duration or exclusivity.[9,10]

(Continued)

TABLE A1   Inappropriate Reasons for Supplementation in the Context of a Healthy Newborn and Mother, Responses, and Risks—cont'd

Concerns/inappropriate reasons	Responses	Risks of supplementation
Mother is too malnourished or sick to breastfeed or eats an inappropriate diet.	Even malnourished mothers can breastfeed. Breast milk quality and quantity is only affected in extreme circumstances. Supplements are better given to the mother (with continued breastfeeding) than the infant	Risk of decreasing breastfeeding duration or exclusivity.
Supplementation will quiet a fussy or unsettled infant[5]	Infants can be unsettled for many reasons. They may wish to cluster feed or simply need additional skin-to-skin time or holding.[67] Filling (and often overfilling) the stomach with a supplement may make the infant sleep longer,[96] missing important opportunities to breastfeed, and demonstrating to the mother a short-term solution which may generate long-term health risks. Teaching other soothing techniques to new mothers such as breastfeeding, swaddling (but not if prone or side lying),[100] swaying, singing, encouraging father or other relatives to assist. Caution should be taken to not ignore early feeding cues.[101] Ensure comfortable, effective latch to maximize signal to mother's body and intake for the infant	Risk of decreasing breastfeeding duration or exclusivity. Maternal engorgement due to decreased frequency of breastfeeding in the immediate postpartum period.[54]
Concern about the cause of frequent feeding and cluster feeding and other changes in infant behaviour	Periods when infants demand to breastfeed more are sometimes interpreted by mothers as insufficient milk. This may happen in later weeks but also in the second or third night (48–72 hours) postbirth. Changes in stooling patterns that often occur after 6–8 weeks of age can also be misinterpreted as insufficient milk. Anticipatory guidance for normal infant development and behavior is helpful.	Risk of decreasing breastfeeding duration or exclusivity.
Mothers need to rest or sleep	Postpartum mothers are restless when separated from their infants and actually get less rest.[29] Mothers lose the opportunity to learn their infants' normal behavior and early feeding cues.[48] Infants are at highest risk for receiving a supplement between 7 p.m. and 9 a.m.[102]	Risk of decreasing breastfeeding duration or exclusivity.
Sore nipples will improve if mother takes a break from breastfeeding[5]	Sore nipples are not a function of length of time breastfeeding. Position, latch, and sometimes individual anatomic variation (e.g., ankyloglossia) are more important.[103] There is no evidence that limiting time at the breast will prevent sore nipples. The nipple should not be rubbed or compressed during breastfeeding even if the feedings are frequent or "clustered."[104]	Problem with latch not addressed. Risk of decreasing breastfeeding duration or cessation of breastfeeding. Risk of breast engorgement.

APPENDIX A2: Sample Maternity Care Infant Nutrition Algorithm

Step 1: Prenatally and on admission to hospital

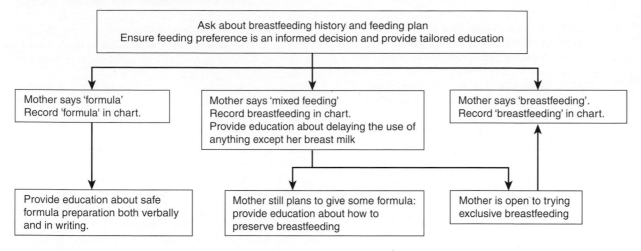

Step 2: When a mother or the family requests formula supplementation

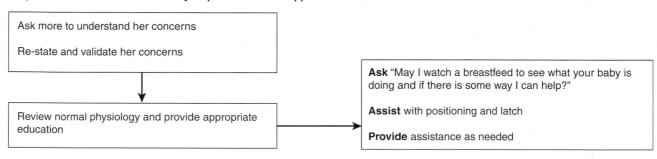

Step 3: Determine medical necessity for and decide on supplementation

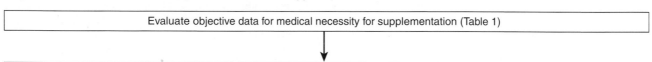

If 'YES' to any of these indications for supplementation:
Consider the need for supplementation with donor human milk (if available) or infant formula and discuss with appropriate hospital staff
Teach the mother how best to preserve breastfeeding by keeping the infant skin-to-skin while she is awake, continuing to put the infant to the breast with every feeding cue, using breast compression during a breastfeed, hand expressing after each breastfeed and expressing (hand or pump) for 10-15 minutes every time the infant receives supplementation to encourage milk production.
Always use mother's own expressed breast milk first and then limited amounts of donor human milk or infant formula.

If 'NO' to all these questions:
Probably no medical need for supplementation at this time
Provide reassurance to the family based on objective data and normal physiology
Evaluate at least every 12 hours for changes in clinical status

If 'NO' to these questions but parents still prefer to offer infant formula:
Educate parents on the potential risks of supplementation including, early cessation of exclusive and any breastfeeding, different sucking mechanisms with breast and other methods of supplementation, issues with milk production and potential risk of cows milk allergy.

REFERENCES

1. Kramer MS, Kakuma R. Optimal duration of exclusive breast-feeding. *Cochrane Database Syst Rev.* 2012;CD003517. Available from: https://doi.org/10.1002/14651858.CD003517.pub2.

2. Smith HA, Becker GE. Early additional food and fluids for healthy breastfed full-term infants. *Cochrane Database Syst Rev.* 2016;CD006462. Available from: https://doi.org/10.1002/14651858.CD006462.pub4.

3. Victora CG, Bahl R, Barros AJD, et al. Breastfeeding in the 21st century: Epidemiology, mechanisms, and lifelong effect. *Lancet.* 2016;387:475−490.

4. Biro MA, Sutherland GA, Yelland JS, et al. In-hospital formula supplementation of breastfed babies: A population-based survey. *Birth.* 2011;38:302−310.

5. Boban M, Zakarija-Grkovic I. In-hospital formula supplementation of healthy newborns: Practices, reasons and their medical justification. *Breastfeed Med.* 2016;11:448−454.

6. World Health Organization. *The Optimal Duration of Exclusive Breastfeeding: A Systematic Review.* Geneva: WHO; 2002.

7. American Academy of Pediatrics Section on Breastfeeding. Breastfeeding and the use of human milk. *Pediatrics.* 2012;129:827−841.

8. National Health and Medical Research Council. *Infant Feeding Guidelines.* Canberra: National Health and Medical Research Council; 2012.

9. Dabritz HA, Hinton BG, Babb J. Maternal hospital experiences associated with breastfeeding at 6 months in a northern California county. *J Hum Lact.* 2010;26:274−285.

10. Perrine CG, Scanlon KS, Li R, et al. Baby-Friendly hospital practices and meeting exclusive breastfeeding intention. *Pediatrics.* 2012;130:54−60.

11. Naveed M, Manjunath CS, Sreenivas V. An autopsy study of relationship between perinatal stomach capacity and birth weight. *Indian J Gastroenterol.* 1992;11:156−158.

12. Zangen S, Di Lorenzo C, Zangen T, et al. Rapid maturation of gastric relaxation in newborn infants. *Pediatr Res.* 2001;50:629−632.

13. Scammon R, Doyle L. Observations on the capacity of the stomach in the first ten days of postnatal life. *Am J Dis Child.* 1920;20:516−538.

14. Wight NE. Hypoglycemia in breastfed neonates. *Breastfeed Med.* 2006;1:253−262.

15. Wight N, Marinelli KA. ABM clinical protocol #1: Guidelines for blood glucose monitoring and treatment of hypoglycemia in term and late-preterm neonates, Revised 2014. *Breastfeed Med.* 2014;9:173−179.

16. Cohen RJ, Brown KH, Rivera LL, et al. Exclusively breastfed, low birthweight term infants do not need supplemental water. *Acta Paediatr.* 2000;89:550−552.

17. Marchini G, Stock S. Thirst and vasopressin secretion counteract dehydration in newborn infants. *J Pediatr.* 1997;130:736−739.

18. Sachdev HP, Krishna J, Puri RK. Do exclusively breast fed infants need fluid supplementation? *Indian Pediatr.* 1992;29:535−540.

19. Grossman X, Chaudhuri JH, Feldman-Winter L, et al. Neonatal weight loss at a US Baby-Friendly Hospital. *J Acad Nutr Diet.* 2012;112:410−413.

20. Flaherman VJ, Schaefer EW, Kuzniewicz MW, et al. Early weight loss nomograms for exclusively breastfed newborns. *Pediatrics.* 2015;135:e16−e23.

21. Macdonald PD, Ross SR, Grant L, et al. Neonatal weight loss in breast and formula fed infants. *Arch Dis Child.* 2003;88:F472−F476.

22. Noel-Weiss J, Woodend A, Peterson W, et al. An observational study of associations among maternal fluids during parturition, neonatal output, and breastfed newborn weight loss. *Int Breastfeed J.* 2011;6:9.

23. Chantry C, Nommsen-Rivers L, Peerson J, et al. Excess weight loss in first-born breastfed newborns relates to maternal intrapartum fluid balance. *Pediatrics.* 2011;127:171−179.

24. Gatti L. Maternal perceptions of insufficient milk supply in breastfeeding. *J Nurs Scholarsh.* 2008;40:355−363.

25. Robert E, Coppieters Y, Swennen B, et al. The reasons for early weaning, perceived insufficient breast milk, and maternal dissatisfaction: Comparative studies in two Belgian regions. *Int Sch Res Notices.* 2014;2014:678564.

26. Blyth R, Creedy DK, Dennis C-L, et al. Effect of maternal confidence on breastfeeding duration: An application of breastfeeding self-efficacy theory. *Birth.* 2002;29:278−284.

27. Reif M, Essock-Vitale S. Hospital influences on early infant-feeding practices. *Pediatrics.* 1985;76:872−879.

28. Crowley WR. Neuroendocrine regulation of lactation and milk production. *Evaluation.* 2015;5:255−291.

29. Cloherty M, Alexander J, Holloway I. Supplementing breastfed babies in the UK to protect their mothers from tiredness or distress. *Midwifery.* 2004;20:194−204.

30. Kurinij N, Shiono PH. Early formula supplementation of breast-feeding. *Pediatrics.* 1991;88:745−750.

31. Akuse RM, Obinya EA. Why healthcare workers give prelacteal feeds. *Eur J Clin Nutr.* 2002;56:729−734.

32. American Academy of Pediatrics Subcommittee on Hyperbilirubinemia. Management of hyperbilirubinemia in the newborn infant 35 or more weeks of gestation. *Pediatrics.* 2004;114:297−316.

33. Emde RN, Swedberg J, Suzuki B. Human wakefulness and biological rhythms after birth. *Arch Gen Psychiatry.* 1975;32:780−783.

34. Flaherman VJ, Gay B, Scott C, et al. Randomised trial comparing hand expression with breast pumping for mothers of term newborns feeding poorly. *Arch Dis Child.* 2012;97:F18−F23.

35. Berens P, Eglash A, Malloy M, et al. ABM Clinical Protocol #26: Persistent pain with breastfeeding. *Breastfeed Med.* 2016;11:46−53.

36. Waldenström U, Swenson A. Rooming-in at night in the postpartum ward. *Midwifery.* 1991;7:82−89.

37. Jaafar SH, Ho JJ, Lee KS. Rooming-in for new mother and infant versus separate care for increasing the duration of breastfeeding. *Cochrane Database Syst Rev.* 2016;CD006641. Available from: https://doi.org/10.1002/14651858.CD006641.pub3.

38. Feldman-Winter L, Goldsmith JP. Safe sleep and skin-to-skin care in the neonatal period for healthy term newborns. *Pediatrics.* 2016;138:e20161889.

39. World Health Organization. *Evidence for the Ten Steps to Successful Breastfeeding.* Geneva: WHO; 1998.

40. Su L-L, Chong Y-S, Chan Y-H, et al. Antenatal education and postnatal support strategies for improving rates of exclusive

breast feeding: Randomised controlled trial. *BMJ.* 2007;335:596.

41. Lumbiganon P, Martis R, Laopaiboon M, et al. Antenatal breastfeeding education for increasing breastfeeding duration. *Cochrane Database Syst Rev.* 2016;CD006425. Available from: https://doi.org/10.1002/14651858.CD006425.pub4.

42. Balogun OO, O'Sullivan EJ, McFadden A, et al. Interventions for promoting the initiation of breastfeeding. *Cochrane Database Syst Rev.* 2016;11:CD001688.

43. Guide to Clinical Preventive Services, 2nd ed., Report of the U.S. Preventive Services Task Force. US Preventive Services Task Force Washington (DC). US Department of Health and Human Services. 1996. Available at www.ncbi.nlm.nih.gov/books/NBK15430 (accessed January 4, 2016).

44. Moore ER, Bergman N, Anderson GC, et al. Early skin-to-skin contact for mothers and their healthy newborn infants. *Cochrane Database Syst Rev.* 2016;11:CD003519.

45. Parker LA, Sullivan S, Krueger C, et al. Association of timing of initiation of breastmilk expression on milk volume and timing of lactogenesis stage II among mothers of very low-birth-weight infants. *Breastfeed Med.* 2015;10:84−91.

46. Parry JE, Ip DKM, Chau PYK, et al. Predictors and consequences of in-hospital formula supplementation for healthy breastfeeding newborns. *J Hum Lact.* 2013;29:527−536.

47. Pang WW, Hartmann PE. Initiation of human lactation: Secretory differentiation and secretory activation. *J Mammary Gland Biol Neoplasia.* 2007;12:211−221.

48. Spangler A, Flory J, Wambach K, et al. Clinical Guidelines for the Establishment of Exclusive Breastfeeding: International Lactation Consultant Association; 2014.

49. Becker GE, Smith HA, Cooney F. Methods of milk expression for lactating women. *Cochrane Database Syst Rev.* 2016; CD006170. Available from: https://doi.org/10.1002/14651858.CD006170.pub5 [Epub ahead of print].

50. Academy of Breastfeeding Medicine Protocol Committee. ABM Clinical Protocol #7: Model breastfeeding policy (Revision 2010). *Breastfeed Med.* 2010;(5)173−177.

51. Hawke BA, Dennison BA, Hisgen S. Improving hospital breastfeeding policies in New York State: Development of the model hospital breastfeeding policy. *Breastfeed Med.* 2013;8:3−7.

52. Howard CR, Howard FM, Lanphear B, et al. Randomized clinical trial of pacifier use and bottle-feeding or cupfeeding and their effect on breastfeeding. *Pediatrics.* 2003;111:511−518.

53. Hill PD, Aldag JC, Chatterton RT. Initiation and frequency of pumping and milk production in mothers of non-nursing pre-term infants. *J Hum Lact.* 2001;17:9−13.

54. Berens P, Brodribb W. ABM Clinical Protocol #20: Engorgement, Revised 2016. *Breastfeed Med.* 2016;11:159−163.

55. World Health Organization. *Global Strategy for Infant and Young Child Feeding.* Geneva: WHO; 2003.

56. Morton J, Hall JY, Wong RJ, et al. Combining hand techniques with electric pumping increases milk production in mothers of preterm infants. *J Perinatol.* 2009;29:757−764.

57. Morton J, et al. *Breast massage maximizes milk volumes of pump-dependent mothers [abstract 7720.9]. Pediatric Academic Societies Scientific Program.* Toronto: Pediatric Academic Societies; 2007.

58. Gourley GR, Li Z, Kreamer BL, et al. A controlled, randomized, double-blind trial of prophylaxis against jaundice among breastfed newborns. *Pediatrics.* 2005;116:385−391.

59. Boyle RJ, Ierodiakonou D, Khan T, et al. Hydrolysed formula and risk of allergic or autoimmune disease: Systematic review and meta-analysis. *BMJ.* 2016;352:i974.

60. de Carvalho M, Hall M, Harvey D. Effects of water supplementation on physiological jaundice in breast-fed babies. *Arch Dis Child.* 1981;56:568−569.

61. Nicoll A, Ginsburg R, Tripp JH. Supplementary feeding and jaundice in newborns. *Acta Paediatr Scand.* 1982;71:759−761.

62. Saint L, Smith M, Hartmann PE. The yield and nutrient content of colostrum and milk of women from giving birth to 1 month post-partum. *Br J Nutr.* 1984;52:87−95.

63. Casey CE, Neifert MR, Seacat JM, et al. Nutrient intake by breast-fed infants during the first five days after birth. *Am J Dis Child.* 1986;140:933−936.

64. Evans K, Evans R, Royal R, et al. Effect of caesarean section on breast milk transfer to the normal term newborn over the first week of life. *Arch Dis Child.* 2003;88:F380−F382.

65. Dollberg S, Lahav S, Mimouni FB. A comparison of intakes of breast-fed and formula-fed infants during the first two days of life. *J Am Coll Nutr.* 2001;20:209−211.

66. Davila-Grijalva H, Troya AH, Kring E, et al. How much do formula-fed infants take in the first 2 days? *Clin Pediatr (Phila).* 2017;56:46−48.

67. Wight NE. Management of common breastfeeding issues. *Pediatr Clin North Am.* 2001;48:321−344.

68. Cloherty M, Alexander J, Holloway I, et al. The cup-versus-bottle debate: A theme from an ethnographic study of the supplementation of breastfed infants in hospital in the United kingdom. *J Hum Lact.* 2005;21:151−162.

69. Flint A, New K, Davies MW. Cup feeding versus other forms of supplemental enteral feeding for newborn infants unable to fully breastfeed. *Cochrane Database Syst Rev.* 2016;CD005092. Available from: https://doi.org/10.1002/14651858.CD005092.pub3.

70. Howard CR, de Blieck EA, ten Hoopen CB, et al. Physiologic stability of newborns during cup- and bottle-feeding. *Pediatrics.* 1999;104(Pt 2):1204−1207.

71. Malhotra N, Vishwambaran L, Sundaram KR, et al. A controlled trial of alternative methods of oral feeding in neonates. *Early Hum Dev.* 1999;54:29−38.

72. Marinelli KA, Burke GS, Dodd VL. A comparison of the safety of cupfeedings and bottlefeedings in premature infants whose mothers intend to breastfeed. *J Perinatol.* 2001;21:350−355.

73. Kassing D. Bottle-feeding as a tool to reinforce breastfeeding. *J Hum Lact.* 2002;18:56−60.

74. Neifert M, Lawrence R, Seacat J. Nipple confusion: Towards a formal definition. *J Pediatr.* 1995;126:S125−S129.

75. Boies E, Vaucher Y. ABM Clinical Protocol #10: Breastfeeding the late preterm (34−36 6/7 weeks of gestation) and early term infants (37−38 6/7 weeks of gestation), second revision 2016. *Breastfeed Med.* 2016;11:494−500.

76. California Perinatal Quality Care Collaborative. Care and management of the late preterm infants toolkit. 2013. Available at http://www.cpqcc.org/sites/default/files/LatePretermInfantToolkitFINAL2-13.pdf (accessed August 25, 2016).

77. UNICEF/WHO. Baby Friendly Hospital Initiative, revised, updated and expanded for integrated care, Section 4, Hospital Self-Appraisal and Monitoring. 2006. Available at

www.who.int/nutrition/topics/BFHI_Revised_Section_4.pdf (accessed November 21, 2016).

78. Weston P, Harris D, Battin M, et al. Oral dextrose gel for the treatment of hypoglycaemia in newborn infants. *Cochrane Database Syst Rev.* 2016;CD011027. Available from: https://doi.org/10.1002/14651858.CD011027.pub2.

79. Boskabadi H, Maamouri G, Ebrahimi M, et al. Neonatal hypernatremia and dehydration in infants receiving inadequate breastfeeding. *Asia Pac J Clin Nutr.* 2010;19:301−307.

80. Neifert MR. Prevention of breastfeeding tragedies. *Pediatr Clin North Am.* 2001;48:273−297.

81. Nommsen-Rivers LA, Heinig MJ, Cohen RJ, et al. Newborn wet and soiled diaper counts and timing of onset of lactation as indicators of breastfeeding inadequacy. *J Hum Lact.* 2008;24:27−33.

82. Thuiler D. Challenging expected patterns of weight loss in full-term breastfeeding neonates born by Cesarean. *J Obstet Gynecol Neonatal Nurs.* 2017;46:18−28.

83. Shrago LC, Reifsnider E, Insel K. The Neonatal Bowel Output Study: Indicators of adequate breast milk intake in neonates. *Pediatr Nurs.* 2006;32:195−201.

84. Neifert MR, DeMarzo S, Seacat JM, et al. The influence of breast surgery, breast appearance, and pregnancy-induced breast changes on lactation sufficiency as measured by infant weight gain. *Birth.* 1990;17:31−38.

85. Huggins K, Petok E, Mireles O. Markers of lactation insufficiency: A study of 34 mothers. In: Auerbach K, ed. *Current Issues in Clinical Lactation.* Sudbury: Jones & Bartlett; 2000:27−35.

86. Bullen CL, Tearle PV, Stewart MG. The effect of "humanized" milks and supplemented breast feeding on the faecal flora of infants. *J Med Microbiol.* 1977;10:403−413.

87. Goldsmith F, O'Sullivan A, Smilowitz JT, et al. Lactation and intestinal microbiota: How early diet shapes the infant gut. *J Mammary Gland Biol Neoplasia.* 2015;20:149−158.

88. Liao S-L, Lai S-H, Yeh K-W, et al. Exclusive breastfeeding is associated with reduced cow's milk sensitization in early childhood. *Pediatr Allergy Immunol.* 2014;25:456−461.

89. Saarinen K, Juntunen-Backman K, Järvenpää A, et al. Supplementary feeding in maternity hospitals and the risk of cow's milk allergy: A prospective study of 6209 infants. *J Allergy Clin Immunol.* 1999;104:457−461.

90. De Carvalho M, Hall M, Harvey D. Effects of water supplementation on physiological jaundice in breastfed babies. *Arch Dis Child.* 1981;56:568−569.

91. Glover J, Sandilands M. Supplementation of breastfeeding infants and weight loss in hospital. *J Hum Lact.* 1990;6:163−166.

92. Martens P, Phillips S, Cheang M, et al. How baby-friendly are Manitoba hospitals? The Provincial Infant Feeding Study. Breastfeeding Promotion Steering Committee of Manitoba. *Can J Public Health.* 2009;91:51−57.

93. De Carvalho M, Klaus MH, Merkatz RB. Frequency of breast-feeding and serum bilirubin concentration. *Am J Dis Child.* 1982;136:737−738.

94. Yamauchi Y, Yamanouchi I. Breast-feeding frequency during the first 24 hours after birth in full-term neonates. *Pediatrics.* 1990;86:171−175.

95. Kumar A, Pant P, Basu S, et al. Oxidative stress in neonatal hyperbilirubinemia. *J Trop Pediatr.* 2007;53:69−71.

96. Van Den Driessche M, Peeters K, Marien P, et al. Gastric emptying in formula-fed and breast-fed infants measured with the 13C-octanoic acid breath test. *J Pediatr Gastroenterol Nutr.* 1999;29:46−51.

97. Matheny RJ, Birch LL, Picciano MF. Control of intake by human-milk-fed infants: Relationships between feeding size and interval. *Dev Psychobiol.* 1990;23:511−518.

98. Pérez-Escamilla R, Segura-Millán S, Canahuati J, et al. Prelacteal feeds are negatively associated with breastfeeding outcomes in Honduras. *J Nutr.* 1996;126:2765−2773.

99. Hale T, Rowe H. *Medications and Mother's Milk.* 17th ed. New York: Springer Publishing Company; 2017.

100. Pease AS, Fleming PJ, Hauck FR, et al. Swaddling and the risk of Sudden Infant Death Syndrome: A meta-analysis. *Pediatrics.* 2016;137:e20153275.

101. Bystrova K, Matthiesen A, Widstrom A, et al. The effect of Russian Maternity Home routines on breastfeeding and neonatal weight loss with special reference to swaddling. *Early Hum Dev.* 2007;83:29−39.

102. Gagnon A, Leduc G, Waghorn K, et al. In-hospital formula supplementation of healthy breastfeeding newborns. *J Hum Lact.* 2005;21:397−405.

103. Slaven S, Harvey D. Unlimited suckling time improves breastfeeding. *Lancet.* 1981;1:392−393.

104. Geddes DT, Langton DB, Gollow I, et al. Frenulotomy for breastfeeding infants with ankyloglossia: Effect on milk removal and sucking mechanism as imaged by ultrasound. *Pediatrics.* 2008;122:e188−e194.

ABM protocols expire 5 years from the date of publication.

Content of this protocol is up-to-date at the time of publication. Evidence based revisions are made within 5 years or sooner if there are significant changes in the evidence.

The 2009 edition of this protocol was authored by Nancy E. Wight and Robert Cordes.

The Academy of Breastfeeding Medicine Protocol Committee:
Wendy Brodribb, MBBS, PhD, FABM, Chairperson
Larry Noble, MD, FABM, Translations Chairperson
Nancy Brent, MD
Maya Bunik, MD, MSPH, FABM
Cadey Harrel, MD
Ruth A. Lawrence, MD, FABM
Kathleen A. Marinelli, MD, FABM
Sarah Reece-Stremtan, MD
Casey Rosen-Carole, MD, MPH, MSEd
Tomoko Seo, MD, FABM
Rose St. Fleur, MD
Michal Young, MD
For correspondence: abm@bfmed.org

ABM Clinical Protocol #4
Mastitis, Revised March 2014

Lisa H. Amir[1,2] and
The Academy of Breastfeeding Medicine Protocol Committee

ABSTRACT

A central goal of The Academy of Breastfeeding Medicine is the development of clinical protocols for managing common medical problems that may impact breastfeeding success. These protocols serve only as guidelines for the care of breastfeeding mothers and infants and do not delineate an exclusive course of treatment or serve as standards of medical care. Variations in treatment may be appropriate according to the needs of an individual patient.

INTRODUCTION

Mastitis is a common condition in lactating women; estimates from prospective studies range from 3% to 20%, depending on the definition and length of postpartum follow-up.[1–3] The majority of cases occur in the first 6 weeks, but mastitis can occur at any time during lactation. There have been few research trials in this area.

Quality of evidence (levels of evidence I, II-1, II-2, II-3, and III) for each recommendation as defined in the U.S. Preventive Services Task Force Appendix A Task Force Ratings[4] is noted in parentheses in this document.

DEFINITION AND DIAGNOSIS

The usual clinical definition of mastitis is a tender, hot, swollen, wedge-shaped area of breast associated with temperature of 38.5°C (101.3°F) or greater, chills, flu-like aching, and systemic illness.[5] However, mastitis literally means, and is defined herein, as an inflammation of the breast; this inflammation may or may not involve a bacterial infection.[6,7] Redness, pain, and heat may all be present when an area of the breast is engorged or "blocked"/"plugged," but an infection is not necessarily present. There appears to be a continuum from engorgement to noninfective mastitis to infective mastitis to breast abscess.[7] (II-2)

PREDISPOSING FACTORS

The following factors may predispose a lactating woman to the development of mastitis.[7,8] Other than the fact that these are factors that result in milk stasis, the evidence for these associations is generally inconclusive (II-2):

- Damaged nipple, especially if colonized with *Staphylococcus aureus*
- Infrequent feedings or scheduled frequency or duration of feedings
- Missed feedings
- Poor attachment or weak or uncoordinated suckling leading to inefficient removal of milk
- Illness in mother or baby
- Oversupply of milk
- Rapid weaning
- Pressure on the breast (e.g., tight bra, car seatbelt)
- White spot on the nipple or a blocked nipple pore or duct: milk blister or "bleb" (a localized inflammatory response)[9]
- Maternal stress and fatigue

INVESTIGATIONS

Laboratory investigations and other diagnostic procedures are not routinely needed or performed for mastitis. The World Health Organization publication on mastitis suggests that breastmilk culture and sensitivity testing "should be undertaken if

- there is no response to antibiotics within 2 days
- the mastitis recurs
- it is hospital-acquired mastitis
- the patient is allergic to usual therapeutic antibiotics or
- in severe or unusual cases."[7] (II-2)

Breastmilk culture may be obtained by collecting a hand-expressed midstream clean-catch sample into a sterile urine container (i.e., a small quantity of the initially expressed milk is discarded to avoid contamination of the sample with skin flora, and subsequent milk is expressed into the sterile container, taking care not to touch the inside of the container). Cleansing the nipple prior to collection may further reduce skin contamination and minimize false-positive culture

* Courtesy of the Academy of Breastfeeding Medicine. Please go to https://www.bfmed.org/protocols for complete protocols, translations, and the most up-to-date information (protocols are updated every 5–7 years).
[1] Judith Lumley Centre (formerly Mother & Child Health Research), La Trobe University, Melbourne, Australia.
[2] Royal Women's Hospital, Melbourne, Australia.

results. Greater symptomatology has been associated with higher bacterial counts and/or pathogenic bacteria.[10] (III)

MANAGEMENT

Effective milk removal

Because milk stasis is often the initiating factor in mastitis, the most important management step is frequent and effective milk removal:

- Mothers should be encouraged to breastfeed more frequently, starting on the affected breast.
- If pain interferes with the let-down, feeding may begin on the unaffected breast, switching to the affected breast as soon as let-down is achieved.
- Positioning the infant at the breast with the chin or nose pointing to the blockage will help drain the affected area.
- Massaging the breast during the feed with an edible oil or nontoxic lubricant on the fingers may also be helpful to facilitate milk removal. Massage, by the mother or a helper, should be directed from the blocked area moving toward the nipple.
- After the feeding, expressing milk by hand or pump may augment milk drainage and hasten resolution of the problem.[11] (III)

An alternate approach for a swollen breast is fluid mobilization, which aims to promote fluid drainage toward the axillary lymph nodes.[12] The mother reclines, and gentle hand motions start stroking the skin surface from the areola to the axilla.[12] (III)

There is no evidence of risk to the healthy, term infant of continuing breastfeeding from a mother with mastitis.[7] Women who are unable to continue breastfeeding should express the milk from breast by hand or pump, as sudden cessation of breastfeeding leads to a greater risk of abscess development than continuing to feed.[11] (III)

Supportive measures

Rest, adequate fluids, and nutrition are important measures. Practical help at home may be necessary for the mother to obtain adequate rest. Application of heat—for example, a shower or a hot pack—to the breast just prior to feeding may help with the let-down and milk flow. After a feeding or after milk is expressed from the breasts, cold packs can be applied to the breast in order to reduce pain and edema.

Although most women with mastitis can be managed as outpatients, hospital admission should be considered for women who are ill, require intravenous antibiotics, and/or do not have supportive care at home. Rooming-in of the infant with the mother is mandatory so that breastfeeding can continue. In some hospitals, rooming-in may require hospital admission of the infant.

Pharmacologic management

Although lactating women are often reluctant to take medications, women with mastitis should be encouraged to take appropriate medications as indicated.

Analgesia

Analgesia may help with the let-down reflex and should be encouraged. An anti-inflammatory agent such as ibuprofen may be more effective in reducing the inflammatory symptoms than a simple analgesic like paracetamol/acetaminophen. Ibuprofen is not detected in breastmilk following doses up to 1.6 g/day and is regarded as compatible with breastfeeding.[13] (III)

Antibiotics

If symptoms of mastitis are mild and have been present for less than 24 hours, conservative management (effective milk removal and supportive measures) may be sufficient. If symptoms are not improving within 12–24 hours or if the woman is acutely ill, antibiotics should be started.[7] Worldwide, the most common pathogen in infective mastitis is penicillin-resistant S. aureus.[14,15] Less commonly, the organism is a Streptococcus or Escherichia coli.[11] The preferred antibiotics are usually penicillinase-resistant penicillins, 5 such as dicloxacillin or flucloxacillin 500 mg by mouth four times per day,[16] or as recommended by local antibiotic sensitivities. (III) First-generation cephalosporins are also generally acceptable as first-line treatment, but may be less preferred because of their broader spectrum of coverage. (III)

Cephalexin is usually safe in women with suspected penicillin allergy, but clindamycin is suggested for cases of severe penicillin hypersensitivity.[16] (III) Dicloxacillin appears to have a lower rate of adverse hepatic events than flucloxacillin.[17] Many authorities recommend a 10–14-day course of antibiotics[18,19]; however this recommendation has not been subjected to controlled trials. (III)

S. aureus resistant to penicillinase-resistant penicillins (methicillin-resistant S. aureus [MRSA], also referred to as oxacillin-resistant S. aureus) has been increasingly isolated in cases of mastitis and breast abscesses.[20–22] (II-2) Clinicians should be aware of the likelihood of this occurring in their community and should order a breastmilk culture and assay of antibiotic sensitivities when mastitis is not improving 48 hours after starting first-line treatment. Local resistance patterns for MRSA should be considered when choosing an antibiotic for such unresponsive cases while culture results are pending. MRSA may be a community-acquired organism and has been reported to be a frequent pathogen in cases of breast abscess in some communities, particularly in the United States and Taiwan.[21,23,24] (I, II-2) At this time, MRSA occurrence is low in other countries, such as the United Kingdom.[25] (I) Most strains of methicillin-resistant staphylococci are susceptible to vancomycin or trimethoprim/sulfamethoxazole but may not be susceptible to rifampin.[26] Of note is that MRSA should be presumed to be resistant to treatment with macrolides and quinolones, regardless of susceptibility testing results.[27] (III)

As with other uses of antibiotics, repeated courses place women at increased risk for breast and vaginal Candida infections.[28,29]

FOLLOW-UP

Clinical response to the above management is typically rapid and dramatic. If the symptoms of mastitis fail to resolve within several days of appropriate management, including antibiotics, a wider differential diagnosis should be considered. Further investigations may be required to confirm resistant bacteria, abscess formation, an underlying mass, or inflammatory or ductal carcinoma. More than two or three recurrences in the same location also warrant evaluation to rule out an underlying mass or other abnormality.

COMPLICATIONS

Early cessation of breastfeeding

Mastitis may produce overwhelming acute symptoms that prompt women to consider cessation of breastfeeding. Effective milk removal, however, is the most important part of treatment.[7] Acute cessation of breastfeeding may actually exacerbate the mastitis and increase the risk of abscess formation; therefore, effective treatment and support from healthcare providers and family are important at this time. Mothers may need reassurance that the antibiotics they are taking are safe to use during breastfeeding.

Abscess

If a well-defined area of the breast remains hard, red, and tender despite appropriate management, then an abscess should be suspected. This occurs in about 3% of women with mastitis.[30] (II-2) The initial systemic symptoms and fever may have resolved. A diagnostic breast ultrasound will identify a collection of fluid. The collection can often be drained by needle aspiration, which itself can be diagnostic as well as therapeutic. Serial needle aspirations may be required.[31–33] (III) Ultrasound guidance for needle aspiration may be necessary in some cases. Fluid or pus aspirated should be sent for culture. Consideration of resistant organisms should also be given depending on the incidence of resistant organisms in that particular environment. Surgical drainage may be necessary if the abscess is very large or if there are multiple abscesses. After surgical drainage, breastfeeding on the affected breast should continue, even if a drain is present, with the proviso that the infant's mouth does not come into direct contact with purulent drainage or infected tissue. A course of antibiotics should follow drainage of the abscess. (III)

Photographs of breast abscesses and percutaneous aspiration can be found in a 2013 review by Kataria et al.[34]

Candida *infection*

Candida infection has been associated with burning nipple pain or radiating breast pain symptoms.[18] Diagnosis is difficult, as the nipples and breasts may look normal on examination, and milk culture may not be reliable. Careful evaluation for other etiologies of breast pain should be undertaken with particular attention to proper latch and ruling out Raynaud's/vasospasm and local nipple trauma. When wound cultures are obtained from nipple fissures, they most commonly grow *S. aureus.*[35–37] (I)

A recent investigation of women with these typical symptoms, using breastmilk cultures after cleansing the nipples, found that none of the[35] cultures from the control group of women grew *Candida*, whereas only one of[29] in the symptomatic group grew the organism.[38] (I) There was also no significant difference in the measurement of a by-product of *Candida* growth [(1,3)b-d-glucan] between groups.[38] Yet, evidence is conflicting as another recent study on milk culture found that 30% of symptomatic mothers were positive for *Candida*, whereas 8% of women in the asymptomatic group grew the organism.[39] (I)

Women with burning nipple and breast pain may also be more likely to test positive for *Candida* on nipple swab by polymerase chain reaction.[40] Using molecular techniques as well as standard culture, a large cohort study of women followed up for 8 weeks postpartum found that burning nipple pain with breast pain was associated with *Candida* species, but not with *S. aureus.*[41] (II-2)

Further research in this area is required. Until then, a trial of antifungal medications, either with or without culture, is the current expert consensus recommendation. (III)

PREVENTION (III)[8]

Effective management of breast fullness and Engorgement

- Mothers should be helped to improve infants' attachment to the breast.
- Feeds should not be restricted.
- Mothers should be taught to hand-express when the breasts are too full for the infant to attach or the infant does not relieve breast fullness. A breast pump may also be used, if available, for these purposes, but all mothers should be able to manually express as the need for its use may arise unexpectedly.

Prompt attention to any signs of milk stasis

- Mothers should be taught to check their breasts for lumps, pain, or redness.
- If the mother notices any signs of milk stasis, she needs to rest, increase the frequency of breastfeeding, apply heat to the breast prior to feedings, and massage any lumpy areas as described in the section Effective milk removal.
- Mothers should contact their healthcare provider if symptoms are not improving within 24 hours.

Prompt attention to other difficulties with breastfeeding

Skilled help is needed for mothers with damaged nipples or an unsettled discontent infant or those who believe that they have an insufficient milk supply.

Rest

As fatigue is often a precursor to mastitis, healthcare providers should encourage breastfeeding mothers to obtain adequate rest. It may also be helpful for healthcare providers to remind family members that breastfeeding mothers may need more help and encourage mothers to ask for help as necessary.

Good hygiene

Because *S. aureus* is a common commensal organism often present in hospitals and communities, the importance of good hand hygiene should not be overlooked.[14,42] It is important for hospital staff, new mothers, and their families to practice good hand hygiene. Breast pump equipment may also be a source of contamination and should be washed thoroughly with soap and hot water after use.

RECOMMENDATIONS FOR FUTURE RESEARCH

There are several aspects of prevention, diagnosis, and treatment of mastitis that require research. First, a consensus on a definition of mastitis is vital.[43] We need to know when antibiotics are needed, which are the most appropriate antibiotics, and the optimal duration of treatment. The role of probiotics in prevention and treatment needs to be determined. Finally, the role of massage to prevent and treat breast engorgement and infection needs to be clarified.

ACKNOWLEDGMENTS

This work was supported in part by a grant from the Maternal and Child Health Bureau, U.S. Department of Health and Human Services.

REFERENCES

1. Waldenström U, Aarts C. Duration of breastfeeding and breastfeeding problems in relation to length of postpartum stay: A longitudinal cohort study of a national Swedish sample. *Acta Paediatr.* 2004;93:669–676.
2. Foxman B, D'Arcy H, Gillespie B, et al. Lactation mastitis: Occurrence and medical management among 946 breastfeeding women in the United States. *Am J Epidemiol.* 2002;155:103–114.
3. Amir LH, Forster DA, Lumley J, et al. A descriptive study of mastitis in Australian breastfeeding women: Incidence and determinants. *BMC Public Health.* 2007;7:62.
4. Appendix A Task Force Ratings. Guide to Clinical Preventive Services: Report of the U.S. Preventive Services Task Force, 2nd edition. www.ncbi.nlm.nih.gov/books/NBK15430 (accessed May 7, 2014).
5. Lawrence RA. The puerperium, breastfeeding, and breast milk. *Curr Opin Obstet Gynecol.* 1990;2:23–30.
6. Inch S, Renfrew MJ. Common breastfeeding problems. In: Chalmers I, Enkin M, Keirse M, eds. *Effective Care in Pregnancy and Childbirth.* Oxford, United Kingdom: Oxford University Press; 1989:1375–1389.
7. World Health Organization. Publication number WHO/FCH/CAH/00.13 *Mastitis: Causes and Management.* Geneva: World Health Organization; 2000.
8. Walker M. *Mastitis in lactating women. Lactation Consultant Series Two.* Schaumburg, IL: La Leche League International; 2004.
9. O'Hara M-A. Bleb histology reveals inflammatory infiltrate that regresses with topical steroids; a case series [platform abstract]. *Breastfeed Med.* 2012;7(Suppl 1). S-2.
10. Matheson I, Aursnes I, Horgen M, et al. Bacteriological findings and clinical symptoms in relation to clinical outcome in puerperal mastitis. *Acta Obstet Gynecol Scand.* 1988;67:723–726.
11. Thomsen AC, Espersen T, Maigaard S. Course and treatment of milk stasis, noninfectious inflammation of the breast, and infectious mastitis in nursing women. *Am J Obstet Gynecol.* 1984;149:492–495.
12. Bolman M, Saju L, Oganesyan K, et al. Recapturing the art of therapeutic breast massage during breastfeeding. *J Hum Lact.* 2013;29:328–331.
13. Sachs HC, Committee on Drugs. The transfer of drugs and therapeutics into human breast milk: An update on selected topics. *Pediatrics.* 2013;132:e796–e809.
14. Amir LH, Garland SM, Lumley J. A case-control study of mastitis: Nasal carriage of *Staphylococcus aureus*. *BMC Fam Pract.* 2006;7:57.
15. Kvist LJ, Larsson BW, Hall-Lord ML, et al. The role of bacteria in lactational mastitis and some considerations of the use of antibiotic treatment. *Int Breastfeed J.* 2008;3:6.
16. Antibiotic Expert Group. *Therapeutic Guidelines: Antibiotic.* Melbourne: Therapeutic Guidelines Ltd.; 2010.
17. Olsson R, Wiholm BE, Sand C, et al. Liver damage from flucloxacillin, cloxacillin and dicloxacillin. *J Hepatol.* 1992;15:154–161.
18. Lawrence RA, Lawrence RM. *Breastfeeding: A Guide for the Medical Profession.* 7th edition St. Louis: Mosby; 2011.
19. Neifert MR. Clinical aspects of lactation: Promoting breastfeeding success. *Clin Perinatol.* 1999;26:281–306.
20. Perez A, Orta L, Padilla E, et al. CA-MRSA puerperal mastitis and breast abscess: A potential problem emerging in Europe with many unanswered questions. *J Matern Fetal Neonatal Med.* 2013;26:949–951.
21. Branch-Elliman W, Golen TH, Gold HS, et al. Risk factors for *Staphylococcus aureus* postpartum breast abscess. *Clin Infect Dis.* 2012;54:71–77.
22. Stafford I, Hernandez J, Laibl V, et al. Community-acquired methicillin-resistant *Staphylococcus aureus* among patients with puerperal mastitis requiring hospitalization. *Obstet Gynecol.* 2008;112:533–537.
23. Berens P, Swaim L, Peterson B. Incidence of methicillin-resistant *Staphylococcus aureus* in postpartum breast abscesses. *Breastfeed Med.* 2010;5:113–115.
24. Chen CY, Anderson BO, Lo SS, et al. Methicillin-resistant *Staphylococcus aureus* infections may not impede the success of ultrasound-guided drainage of puerperal breast abscesses. *J Am Coll Surg.* 2010;210:148–154.
25. Dabbas N, Chand M, Pallett A, et al. Have the organisms that cause breast abscess changed with time?—Implications for appropriate antibiotic usage in primary and secondary care. *Breast J.* 2010;16:412–415.
26. Johnson MD, Decker CF. Antimicrobial agents in treatment of MRSA infections. *Dis Mon.* 2008;54:793–800.

27. Rodvold KA, McConeghy KW. Methicillin-resistant *Staphylococcus aureus* therapy: Past, present, and future. *Clin Infect Dis.* 2014;58(Suppl 1):S20–S27.

28. Dinsmoor MJ, Viloria R, Lief L, et al. Use of intrapartum antibiotics and the incidence of postnatal maternal and neonatal yeast infections. *Obstet Gynecol.* 2005;106: 19–22.

29. Pirotta MV, Gunn JM, Chondros P. "Not thrush again!" Women's experience of post-antibiotic vulvovaginitis. *Med J Aust.* 2003;179:43–46.

30. Amir LH, Forster D, McLachlan H, et al. Incidence of breast abscess in lactating women: Report from an Australian cohort. *BJOG.* 2004;111:1378–1381.

31. Dixon JM. Repeated aspiration of breast abscesses in lactating women. *BMJ.* 1988;297:1517–1518.

32. Ulitzsch D, Nyman MKG, Carlson RA. Breast abscess in lactating women: US-guided treatment. *Radiology.* 2004;232:904–909.

33. Christensen AF, Al-Suliman N, Nielson KR, et al. Ultrasound-guided drainage of breast abscesses: Results in 151 patients. *Br J Radiol.* 2005;78:186–188.

34. Kataria K, Srivastava A, Dhar A. Management of lactational mastitis and breast abscesses: review of current knowledge and practice. *Indian J Surg.* 2013;75:430–435.

35. Livingstone V, Stringer LJ. The treatment of *Staphylococcus aureus* infected sore nipples: A randomized comparative study. *J Hum Lact.* 1999;15:241–246.

36. Amir LH, Garland SM, Dennerstein L, et al. *Candida albicans*: Is it associated with nipple pain in lactating women? *Gynecol Obstet Invest.* 1996;41:30–34.

37. Saenz RB. Bacterial pathogens isolated from nipple wounds: A four-year prospective study. *Breastfeed Med.* 2007;2:190.

38. Hale TW, Bateman TL, Finkelman MA, et al. The absence of *Candida albicans* in milk samples of women with clinical symptoms of ductal candidiasis. *Breastfeed Med.* 2009;4:57–61.

39. Andrews JI, Fleener DK, Messer SA, et al. The yeast connection: Is *Candida* linked to breastfeeding associated pain? *Am J Obstet Gynecol.* 2007;197. 424.e1–e4.

40. Panjaitan M, Amir LH, Costa A-M, et al. Polymerase chain reaction in detection of *Candida albicans* for confirmation of clinical diagnosis of nipple thrush. *Breastfeed Med.* 2008;3:185–187.

41. Amir LH, Donath SM, Garland SM, et al. Does *Candida* and/ or *Staphylococcus* play a role in nipple and breast pain in lactation? A cohort study in Melbourne, Australia. *BMJ Open.* 2013;3:e002351.

42. Collignon PJ, Grayson ML, Johnson PDR. Methicillin-resistant *Staphylococcus aureus* in hospitals: Time for a culture change. *Med J Aust.* 2007;187:4–5.

43. Kvist LJ. Toward a clarification of the concept mastitis as used in empirical studies of breast inflammation during lactation. *J Hum Lact.* 2010;26:53–59.

ABM protocols expire 5 years from the date of publication. Evidence-based revisions are made within 5 years or sooner if there are significant changes in the evidence.

The Academy of Breastfeeding Medicine Protocol Committee
Kathleen A. Marinelli, MD, FABM, Chairperson
Maya Bunik, MD, MSPH, FABM, Co-Chairperson
Larry Noble, MD, FABM, Translations Chairperson
Nancy Brent, MD
Amy E. Grawey, MD
Alison V. Holmes, MD, MPH, FABM
Ruth A. Lawrence, MD, FABM
Tomoko Seo, MD, FABM
For correspondence: abm@bfmed.org

ABM Clinical Protocol #5
Peripartum Breastfeeding Management for the Healthy Mother and Infant at Term, Revision 2013*

Allison V. Holmes[1], Angela Yerdon McLeod[2] and Maya Bunik[3]

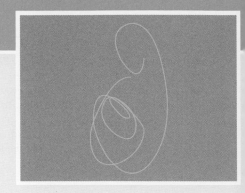

ABSTRACT

A central goal of The Academy of Breastfeeding Medicine is the development of clinical protocols for managing common medical problems that may impact breastfeeding success. These protocols serve only as guidelines for the care of breastfeeding mothers and infants and do not delineate an exclusive course of treatment or serve as standards of medical care. Variations in treatment may be appropriate according to the needs of an individual patient.

BACKGROUND

HOSPITAL POLICIES AND ROUTINES greatly influence breastfeeding success.[1–10] The Baby-Friendly Hospital Initiative (BFHI) has defined the Ten Steps to Successful Breastfeeding, and 20 years of research has now verified that "the achievement of BFHI certification leads to substantially improved breastfeeding outcomes, especially increases in breastfeeding initiation and exclusivity."[1]

The peripartum hospital experience should include adequate support, instruction, and care to ensure the successful initiation of breastfeeding. Such management is part of a continuum of care and education that begins during the prenatal period, promotes breastfeeding as the optimal method of infant feeding, and includes information about maternal and infant benefits. The following principles and practices are recommended for care in the peripartum hospital setting.

---

* Courtesy of the Academy of Breastfeeding Medicine. Please go to https://www.bfmed.org/protocols for complete protocols, translations, and the most up-to-date information (protocols are updated every 5–7 years).

[1] Department of Pediatrics and of Community and Family Medicine, Geisel School of Medicine, Dartmouth, New Hampshire.

[2] Family Medicine, Concord, New Hampshire.

[3] Department of Pediatrics, University of Colorado, Aurora, Colorado.

RECOMMENDATIONS

Quality of evidence (levels of evidence I, II-1, II-2, II-3, and III) for each recommendation as defined in the U.S. Preventive Services Task Force Appendix A Task Force Ratings"[11] is noted in parentheses.

PRENATAL

1. All pregnant women must receive education about the benefits and management of breastfeeding to allow an informed decision about infant feeding.[5–10] An evidence-based review of practices that improve the duration or initiation of breastfeeding found that "prenatal combined with postnatal interventions are more effective than usual care in prolonging the duration of breastfeeding…."[12] Information and advice from a health professional early in pregnancy are also supported by the American College of Obstetricians and Gynecologists and the American Academy of Family Physicians in their policy statements, which read "Advice and encouragement of the obstetrician-gynecologist are critical in making the decision to breastfeed"[6] and "Family-centered care (the belief that health care staff and the family are partners, working together to best meet the needs of the patient) allows support of breastfeeding practices throughout the lifecycle to all family members."[9] (I, II-1, II-2, II-3, III)

2. Prenatal education should include information about the benefits to mother and baby of exclusive breastfeeding initiated in the first hour after birth.[5] Educational materials produced by formula manufacturers are inappropriate sources of information about infant feeding.[13,14] (I, III)

3. Maternity care includes an assessment of any medical or physical conditions that could affect a mother's ability to breastfeed her infant. In some cases, it may be helpful to obtain a prenatal consultation with the infant's physician or a lactation consultant or specialist and to develop a plan of follow-up to be instituted at the time of delivery.[6–8] Women will benefit from moderated group discussions, group prenatal visits, systematic case management, or referral to a lay support organization prior to delivery.[6–8,12] There is also good evidence that peer counseling promotes

the initiation and maintenance of breastfeeding.[15,16] (I, II-3, III)

LABOR AND DELIVERY

1. Women will benefit from the continuous presence of a close companion (e.g., doula, spouse/partner, or family member) throughout labor and delivery. The presence of a doula is known to enhance breastfeeding initiation and duration.[17] Many risk factors are associated with early cessation of breastfeeding, including the mean length of labor, the need for surgical intervention, and the use of pain-reducing interventions such as epidurals and other medications. These risks may be reduced by the presence of a doula.[18-20] (I, II-2, III)

2. Intrapartum analgesia may also have an impact on breastfeeding, and consideration needs to be given to the type and dose of analgesia.[6,21-23] Epidural analgesia, intramuscular opioids, exogenous oxytocin, and ergometrine have all been associated with lower rates of breastfeeding initiation.[24] (I, II-2, III)

IMMEDIATE POSTPARTUM

1. The healthy newborn should be given directly to the mother for skin-to-skin contact until after the first feeding. The infant may be dried and assigned Apgar scores, and the initial physical assessment may be performed as the infant is placed with the mother. Such physical contact provides the infant with optimal physiologic stability, warmth, and opportunities for the first feeding.[10,25-29] Extensive early skin-to-skin contact likely increases the duration of any and exclusive breastfeeding.[27-35] Delaying procedures such as weighing, measuring, administering eye prophylaxis as well as vitamin K, up to 6 hours after birth, and the initial bath enhances early parent–infant interaction.[10,36] Infants are to be put close to the breast, as soon after birth as is feasible for both mother and infant, to allow for a latch and feeding, ideally within an hour of birth.[28,31-35] This practice is to be initiated in the delivery, operating, or recovery room, and every mother should be instructed in proper breastfeeding technique.[5,10,31,37-41] (I, II-2, II-3, III)

2. Mother–baby rooming-in on a 24-hour basis enhances opportunities for bonding and for optimal breastfeeding initiation. Whenever possible, mothers and infants are to remain together during the hospital stay.[10,30,35,42-45] To avoid unnecessary separation, infant assessments in the immediate postpartum time period and thereafter are ideally performed in the mother's room. Evidence suggests that mothers get the same amount and quality of sleep whether infants room-in or are sent back to the nursery at night.[42-44] (II-1, II-2, II-3, III)

3. Education about the benefits of 24-hour rooming-in encourages parents to use it as the standard mode of hospital care for their families. At the same time, from a staffing standpoint, nursing personnel should arrange for time to be available to assess and document the status of the infant and infant feeding while the baby is in the family's room.[5,10,41,45,46] (I, II-3, III)

4. Women may need help from healthcare providers to ensure that they are able to position and attach their babies at the breast. Those delivered by cesarean section may need additional help from nursing staff to attain comfortable positioning. A trained observer should assess and document the effectiveness of breastfeeding at least once every[8-12] hours after delivery until mother and infant are discharged. In countries where the delivery hospital stay may last up to a week, then assessment should continue until breastfeeding is successfully established.[1,10] Peripartum care of the dyad should address and document infant positioning, latch, milk transfer, baby's weight, clinical jaundice, and any problems raised by the mother, such as nipple pain or the perception of an inadequate breastmilk supply. Formal inpatient lactation instruction programs need to be assessed carefully for effectiveness and best practices.[38-41] Some infants are sleepy in the first 24 hours after birth. By the second day, infants who are breastfeeding well will feed on demand. Feedings usually range from eight to 12 times or more in 24 hours, with a minimum of eight feedings every 24 hours. Limiting the time that an infant is at the breast is not necessary and may even be harmful to the establishment of a good milk supply. Infants usually fall asleep or release the breast spontaneously when satiated. (I, II-2, II-3, III)

5. Supplemental feeding should not be given to breastfed infants unless there is a medical indication.[10,13,47-49] Supplementation can inhibit or delay the establishment of maternal milk supply and have adverse effects on breastfeeding (e.g., delayed lactogenesis, maternal engorgement). Supplements may alter infant bowel flora, sensitize the infant to allergens (depending on the content of the feeding and method used), interfere with maternal–infant bonding, and interfere with infant weight gain.[14,47-49] There is no role for the routine supplementation of nondehydrated infants with water or dextrose water; in fact, this practice could contribute to hyperbilirubinemia.[50] Before any supplementary feedings are begun, it is important that a formal evaluation of each mother–baby dyad, including a direct observation of breastfeeding, is completed by a provider trained in lactation.[14] (I, II-2, III)

6. Pacifiers in the neonatal period should be used with caution. Some earlier research showed that pacifier use in the neonatal period was detrimental to exclusive and overall breastfeeding,[51,52] while a recent Cochrane review found that pacifier use in healthy term breastfeeding infants, started at birth or after lactation was established, did not significantly affect the prevalence or duration of exclusive and partial breastfeeding up to 4 months of age.[53] Other recent studies suggest that the relationship among pacifiers, breastfeeding, and supplementation is more complex that previously realized.[54] (I)

7. In general, acute infectious diseases, undiagnosed fever, and common postpartum infections in the mother are not a contraindication to breastfeeding, if such diseases can be readily controlled and treated. Infants should not be breastfed in the case of untreated active tuberculosis, or herpes simplex when there are breast lesions.[55–57] In the case of maternal human immunodeficiency virus the World Health Organization recommends that "national authorities in each country decide which infant feeding practice, i.e. breastfeeding with an antiretroviral intervention to reduce transmission or avoidance of all breastfeeding, should be promoted and supported by their Maternal and Child Health services."[55] Infectious peripartum varicella may require separation of the mother and newborn, limiting direct breastfeeding, but expressed milk can be used.[10] Beyond infectious diseases, the listing of all contraindications is beyond the scope of this document, but reliable sources of information are readily available and include information about medications and radioactive compounds.[56–63] (III)

8. All breastfed infants should be seen by a healthcare provider at 3–5 days of life or within 48–72 hours of discharge to evaluate the infant's well-being and the successful establishment of breastfeeding.[10,64–66] Depending on the length of hospitalization or country of origin, these postpartum practices may vary. For example, in Japan and Australia the mother and infant stay for 4–5 days in the hospital, and in the United Kingdom mothers are home-visited by nurse midwives for about 10 days. (I, III) Peer-to-peer support should also be offered and has been proven to be helpful in promoting breastfeeding success.[16,46] (I, I-2)

PROBLEMS AND COMPLICATIONS

1. Mother–baby dyads at risk for breastfeeding problems benefit from early identification and assistance. Consultation with an expert in lactation management may be helpful in situations including but not limited to the following:
   (a) Maternal request/anxiety
   (b) Previous negative breastfeeding experience
   (c) Mother has flat/inverted nipples.
   (d) Mother has history of breast surgery.
   (e) Multiple births (twins, triplets, higher-order pregnancies)
   (f) Infant is early term (37–38 6/7 weeks of gestation) or premature (< 37 weeks).
   (g) Infant has congenital anomaly, neurological impairment, or other medical condition that affects the infant's ability to breastfeed.
   (h) Maternal or infant medical condition for which breastfeeding must be temporarily postponed or for which milk expression is required
   (i) Documentation, after the first few feedings, that there is difficulty in establishing breastfeeding (e.g., poor latch-on, sleepy baby, etc.)
   (j) Hyperbilirubinemia

2. Discharge of mothers and babies from the hospital at less than 48 hours mandates that risks to successful breastfeeding be identified in a timely manner so that the time spent in the hospital is used to maximal benefit.[64] Recommendations for close follow-up are particularly important for dyads with early discharge.

3. If a neonate needs to be transferred to an intermediate or intensive care area, steps must be taken to maintain maternal lactation. When possible, transport of the mother to the intermediate or intensive care nursery to continue breastfeeding is optimal. If breastfeeding is not possible, arrangements should be made to continue human milk feeding for the neonate. Mothers must be shown how to maintain lactation through both manual and mechanical expression.[5,10] There is evidence that there may be greater maternal milk production with the use of electric breast pumps compared with manual expression alone.[67,68] A combination of manual and mechanical expression (hands-on pumping)[69] may yield optimal milk production. (I, I-2, III)

4. If an infant is not feeding at the breast consistently and effectively at the time of hospital discharge, the mother must be shown how to maintain lactation through both manual and mechanical expression and demonstrate proficiency in emptying her breasts before she is released home.[67,68] The possible need for supplemental feedings for the infant must be addressed, with consideration given to the choice of supplement to be used and the method of feeding. Any and all breastmilk the mother can express should be used, and it should only be supplemented further if maternal supply is inadequate. Cup feeding may help preserve breastfeeding duration among those who require multiple supplemental feedings because of the concerns regarding nipple confusion or bottle preference.[52] The mother–infant dyad will need referral to a lactation professional for continued assistance and support.

RECOMMENDATIONS FOR FUTURE RESEARCH

1. Controversy remains as to the effects of labor medications on breastfeeding outcomes. More studies are needed to evaluate the effects of the various labor medications available on both short- and long-term breastfeeding outcomes.

2. Despite evidence that delaying postpartum interventions to the newborn is associated with improved breastfeeding outcomes, many hospital policies still dictate immediate weighing, measuring, administering eye prophylaxis and vitamin K, and an early initial bath, all of which interfere with early and continued skin-to-skin and breastfeeding initiation. Large implementation and/or multicenter trials may be needed to ultimately influence changes in hospital policies if these findings persist.

3. The relationship between pacifiers and breastfeeding is more complex than previously realized. More research is needed to assess the effect of pacifiers on short-term breastfeeding difficulties and long-term effect on breastfeeding duration.

4. As more hospitals adopt the Ten Steps and are certified as Baby-Friendly Hospitals, we need to continue to collect data concerning which specific peripartum practices are most important in achieving desirable breastfeeding outcomes.

ACKNOWLEDGMENTS

This work was supported in part by a grant from the Maternal and Child Health Bureau, U.S. Department of Health and Human Services.

REFERENCES

1. Holmes AV. Establishing successful breastfeeding in the newborn period. *Pediatr Clin North Am.* 2013;60:147–168.

2. UNICEF Breastfeeding Initiatives Exchange. The Baby Friendly Hospital Initiative. www.unicef.org/programme/breastfeeding/baby.htm (accessed October 31, 2013).

3. Kramer MS, Chalmers B, Hodnett ED, et al. Promotion of breastfeeding intervention trial (PROBIT): A cluster-randomized trial in the Republic of Belarus. *JAMA.* 2001;285:413–420.

4. Martens PJ. What do Kramer's Baby-Friendly Hospital Initiative PROBIT studies tell us? A review of a decade of research. *J Hum Lact.* 2012;28:335–342.

5. World Health Organization, UNICEF, Wellstart International. Baby-Friendly Hospital Initiative. Revised, Updated and Expanded for Integrated Care. 2009. www.unicef.org/nutrition/files/BFHI_2009_s1.pdf (accessed October 31, 2013).

6. American College of Obstetricians and Gynecologists Women's Health Care Physicians, Committee on Health Care for Underserved Women. Committee Opinion No. 570: Breastfeeding in underserved women: Increasing initiation and continuation of breastfeeding. *Obstet Gynecol.* 2013;122:423–428.

7. Rotundo G. Centering pregnancy: The benefits of group prenatal care. *Nurs Womens Health.* 2011;15:508–517.

8. Caine VA, Smith M, Beasley Y, et al. The impact of prenatal education on behavioral changes toward breast feeding and smoking cessation in a healthy start population. *J Natl Med Assoc.* 2012;104:258–264.

9. American Academy of Family Physicians. Family Physicians Supporting Breastfeeding, Position Paper. www.aafp.org/about/policies/all/breastfeeding-support.html (accessed October 31, 2013).

10. Section on Breastfeeding. Breastfeeding and the use of human milk. *Pediatrics.* 2012;129:e827–e841.

11. Appendix A Task Force Ratings. Guide to Clinical Preventive Services: Report of the U.S. Preventive Services Task Force. 2nd edition. www.ncbi.nlm.nih.gov/books/NBK15430 (accessed October 31, 2013).

12. Chung M, Raman G, Trikalinos T, et al. Interventions in primary care to promote breastfeeding: An evidence review for the U.S. Preventive Services Task Force. *Ann Intern Med.* 2008;149:565–582.

13. Howard CR, Howard FM, Lawrence RA, et al. The effect on breastfeeding of physicians' office-based prenatal formula advertising. *Obstet Gynecol.* 2000;95:296–303.

14. Academy of Breastfeeding Medicine Protocol Committee. ABM clinical protocol #3: Hospital guidelines for the use of supplementary feedings in the healthy term breastfed neonate, revised 2009. *Breastfeed Med.* 2009;4:175–182. Erratum in: *Breastfeed Med* 2011;6:159.

15. Chapman DJ, Morel K, Anderson AK, et al. Review: Breastfeeding peer counseling: From efficacy through scaleup. *J Hum Lact.* 2010;26:314–332.

16. Sudfeld CR, Fawzi WW, Lahariya C. Peer support and exclusive breastfeeding duration in low and middle-income countries: A systematic review and meta-analysis. *PLoS One.* 2012;7:e45143.

17. Kozhimannil KB, Attanasio LB, Hardeman RR, et al. Doula care supports near-universal breastfeeding initiation among diverse, low-income women. *J Midwifery Womens Health.* 2013;58:378–382.

18. Hodnett E, Gates S, Hofmeyr G, et al. Continuous support for women during childbirth. *Cochrane Database Syst Rev.* 2013;7: CD003766.

19. Nommsen-Rivers LA, Mastergeorge AM, Hansen RL, et al. Doula care, early breastfeeding outcomes, and breastfeeding status at 6 weeks postpartum among low-income primiparae. *J Obstet Gynecol Neonatal Nurs.* 2009;38:157–173.

20. Mottl-Santiago J, Walker C, Ewan J, et al. A hospital-based doula program and childbirth outcomes in an urban, multicultural setting. *Matern Child Health J.* 2008;12:372–377.

21. Beilin Y, Bodian CA, Weiser J, et al. Effect of labor epidural analgesia with and without fentanyl on infant breastfeeding. A prospective, randomized, double-blind study. *Anesthesiology.* 2005;103:1211–1217.

22. Gizzo S, DiGangi S, Saccardi C, et al. Epidural analgesia during labor: Impact on delivery outcome, neonatal wellbeing, and early breastfeeding. *Breastfeed Med.* 2012;7: 262–268.

23. Montgomery A, Hale TW. Academy of Breastfeeding Medicine. ABM clinical protocol #15: Analgesia and anesthesia for the breastfeeding mother, revised 2012. *Breastfeed Med.* 2012;7:547–553.

24. Jordan S, Emery S, Watkins A, et al. Associations of drugs routinely given in labour with breastfeeding at 48 hours: Analysis of the Cardiff Births Survey. *BJOG.* 2009;116: 1622–1629.

25. Christensson K, Siles C, Moreno L, et al. Temperature, metabolic adaptation and crying in healthy full term newborns cared for skin-to-skin or in a cot. *Acta Paediatr.* 1992;81:488–493.

26. Marin-Gabriel MA, Llana-Martin I, Lopez-Escobar A, et al. Randomized controlled trial of early skin-to-skin contact: Effects on the mother and the newborn. *Acta Paediatr.* 2010;99:1630–1634.

27. Mikiel-Kostyra K, Mazur J, Boøtruszko I, et al. Effect of early skin-to-skin contact after delivery on duration of breastfeeding: A prospective cohort study. *Acta Paediatr.* 2002;91:1301–1306.

28. Moore ER, Anderson GC, Bergman N, et al. Early skin-to-skin contact for mothers and their healthy newborn infants. *Cochrane Database Syst Rev.* 2012;5:CD003519.

29. Bramson L, Lee JW, Moore E, et al. Effect of early skin-to-skin mother-infant contact during the first 3 hours following birth

on exclusive breastfeeding during the maternity hospital stay. *J Hum Lact.* 2010;26:130–137.

30. Bystrova K, Widstrom AM, Matthiesen AS, et al. Early lactation performance in primiparous and multiparous women in relation to different maternity home practices. A randomized trial in St. Petersburg. *Int Breastfeed J.* 2007;2:9.

31. Hung KJ, Berg O. Early skin-to-skin after Cesarean to improve breastfeeding. *Am J Matern Child Nurs.* 2011;36:318–324. quiz 325–326.

32. DiGirolamo AM, Grummer-Strawn LM, Heim SB. Effect of maternity-care practices on breastfeeding. *Pediatrics.* 2008;122 (Suppl 2):S43–S49.

33. Mahmood I, Jamal M, Khan J. Effect of mother-infant early skin to skin contact on breastfeeding status: A randomized controlled trial. *J Coll Physicians Surgeons Pakistan.* 2011;21:601–605.

34. Thukral A, Sankar MJ, Agarwal R, et al. Early skin-to-skin contact and breast-feeding behavior in term neonates: A randomized controlled trial. *Neonatology.* 2012;102:114–119.

35. Murray EK, Ricketts S, Dellaport J. Hospital practices that increase breastfeeding duration: Results from a population-based study. *Birth.* 2007;34:202–211.

36. Preer G, Pisegna JM, Cook JT, et al. Delaying the bath and in-hospital breastfeeding rates. *Breastfeed Med.* 2013;8:485–490.

37. Righard L, Alade MO. Effect of delivery room routines on success of first breast-feed. *Lancet.* 1990;336:1105–1107.

38. Righard L, Alade MO. Sucking technique and its effect on success of breastfeeding. *Birth.* 1992;19:185–189.

39. Cordova do Espirito Santo L, Dias de Oliveira L, Justo, Giugliani ER. Factors associated with low incidence of exclusive breastfeeding for the first 6 months. *Birth.* 2007;34:212–219.

40. Henderson A, Stamp G, Pincombe J. Postpartum positioning and attachment education for increasing breastfeeding: A randomized trial. *Birth.* 2001;28:236–242.

41. Kervin BE, Kemp L, Pulver LJ. Types and timing of breastfeeding support and its impact on mothers' behaviours. *J Paediatr Child Health.* 2010;46:85–91.

42. Keefe MR. The impact of infant rooming-in on maternal sleep at night. *J Obstet Gynecol Neonat Nurs.* 1988;17:122–126.

43. Waldenstrom U, Swenson A. Rooming-in at night in the postpartum ward. *Midwifery.* 1991;7:82–89.

44. Ball HL, Ward-Platt MP, Heslop E, et al. Randomised trial of infant sleep location on the postnatal ward. *Arch Dis Child.* 2006;91:1005–1010.

45. Perez-Escamilla R, Pollitt E, Lonnerdal B, et al. Infant feeding policies in maternity wards and their effect on breastfeeding success: An analytical overview. *Am J Public Health.* 1994;84:89–97.

46. Renfrew MJ, McCormick FM, Quinn WA, et al. Support for healthy breastfeeding mothers with healthy term babies. *Cochrane Database Syst Rev.* 2012;5:CD001141.

47. Bystrova K, Matthiesen AS, Widström AM, et al. The effect of Russian maternity home routines on breastfeeding and neonatal weight loss with special reference to swaddling. *Early Hum Dev.* 2007;83:29–39.

48. Blomquist HK, Jonsbo F, Serenius F, et al. Supplementary feeding in the maternity ward shortens the duration of breast feeding. *Acta Paediatr.* 1994;83:1122–1126.

49. Perrine CG, Scanlon KS, Li R, et al. Baby-Friendly Hospital practices and meeting exclusive breastfeeding intention. *Pediatrics.* 2012;130:54–60.

50. American Academy of Pediatrics Subcommittee on Hyperbilirubinemia. Management of hyperbilirubinemia in the newborn infant 35 or more weeks of gestation. *Pediatrics.* 2004;114:297–316.

51. O'Connor NR, Tanabe KO, Siadaty MS, et al. Pacifiers and breastfeeding: A systematic review. *Arch Pediatr Adolesc Med.* 2009;163:378–382.

52. Howard CR, Howard FM, Lanphear B, et al. Randomized clinical trial of pacifier use and bottle-feeding or cup feeding and their effect on breastfeeding. *Pediatrics.* 2003;111:511–518.

53. Jaafar SH, Jahanfar S, Angolkar M, et al. Effect of restricted pacifier use in breastfeeding term infants for increasing duration of breastfeeding. *Cochrane Database Syst Rev.* 2012;7: CD007202.

54. Kair LR, Kenron D, Etheredge K, et al. Pacifier restriction and exclusive breastfeeding. *Pediatrics.* 2013;131:e1101–e1107.

55. www.who.int/maternal_child_adolescent/documents/ 9789241599535/en/ (accessed October 30, 2013).

56. Lawrence RM. Circumstances when breastfeeding is contraindicated. *Pediatr Clin North Am.* 2013;60:295–318.

57. Lawrence RA, Lawrence RM. *Breastfeeding: A Guide for the Medical Profession.* 7th ed. Philadelphia: Elsevier/Mosby; 2011.

58. Sachs HC. Committee on Drugs. The transfer of drugs and therapeutics into human breast milk: An update on selected topics. *Pediatrics.* 2013;132:e796–e809.

59. Toxnet: Toxicology Data Network. Drugs and Lactation Database (LactMed). http://toxnet.nlm.nih.gov/cgi-bin/sis/htmlgen?LACT (accessed October 31, 2013).

60. Hale TW. *Medications and Mothers' Milk.* 15th ed. Amarillo, TX: Pharmasoft; 2012.

61. Webb JA, Thomsen HS, Morcos SK, et al. The use of iodinated and gadolinium contrast media during pregnancy and lactation. *Eur Radiol.* 2005;15:1234–1240.

62. Chen MM, Coakley FV, Kaimal A, et al. Guidelines for computed tomography and magnetic resonance imaging use during pregnancy and lactation. *Obstet Gynecol.* 2008;112:333–340.

63. American Thyroid Association Taskforce on Radioiodine Safety, Sisson JC, Freitas J, et al. Radiation safety in the treatment of patients with thyroid diseases by radioiodine 131I: Practice recommendations of the American Thyroid Association. *Thyroid.* 2011;21:335–346.

64. Academy of Breastfeeding Medicine Clinical Protocol Committee. ABM clinical protocol #2 (2007 revision): Guidelines for hospital discharge of the breastfeeding term newborn and mother: "the going home protocol". *Breastfeed Med.* 2007;2:158–165.

65. Labarere J, Gelbert-Baudino N, Ayral AS. Efficacy of breastfeeding support provided by trained clinicians during an early routine, preventive visit: A prospective, randomized, open trial of 226 mother-infant pairs. *Pediatrics.* 2005;115:e139–e146.

66. American Academy of Pediatrics Committee on the Fetus and Newborn. Hospital stay for healthy term newborns. *Pediatrics.* 2010;125:405–409.

67. Becker GE, Cooney F, Smith HA. Methods of milk expression for lactating women. *Cochrane Database Syst Rev.* 2011;12: CD006170.

68. Flaherman VJ, Gay B, Scott C, et al. Randomized trial comparing hand expression with breast pumping for mothers of term newborns feeding poorly. *Arch Dis Child Fetal Neonatal Ed.* 2012;97:F18–F23.

69. Morton J, Hall JY, Wong RJ, et al. Combining hand techniques with electric pumping increases milk production in mothers of preterm infants. *J Perinatol.* 2009;29:757–764.

ABM protocols expire 5 years from the date of publication. Evidence-based revisions are made within 5 years or sooner if there are significant changes in the evidence.

The Academy of Breastfeeding Medicine Protocol Committee
Kathleen A. Marinelli, MD, FABM, Chairperson
Maya Bunik, MD, MSPH, FABM, Co-Chairperson
Larry Noble, MD, FABM, Translations Chairperson
Nancy Brent, MD
Amy E. Grawey, MD
Alison V. Holmes, MD, MPH, FABM
Ruth A. Lawrence, MD, FABM
Tomoko Seo, MD, FABM
Julie Scott Taylor, MD, MSc, FABM
For correspondence: abm@bfmed.org

Bedsharing and Breastfeeding
The Academy of Breastfeeding Medicine Protocol #6, Revision 2019*

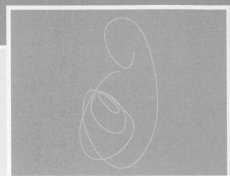

Peter S. Blair[1], Helen L. Ball[2], James J. McKenna[3,4], Lori Feldman-Winter[5], Kathleen A. Marinelli[6,7], Melissa C. Bartick[8] and the Academy of Breastfeeding Medicine*

ABSTRACT

A central goal of the Academy of Breastfeeding Medicine is the development of clinical protocols for managing common medical problems that may impact breastfeeding success. These protocols serve only as guidelines for the care of breastfeeding mothers and infants and do not delineate an exclusive course of treatment or serve as standards of medical care. Variations in treatment may be appropriate according to the needs of an individual patient.

PURPOSE

Bedsharing promotes breastfeeding initiation,[1] duration,[2–7] and exclusivity.[7,8] Medical and public health organizations in some countries recommend against bedsharing, citing concerns over increased risk of sleep-related infant death.[9,10]

[1] Centre for Academic Child Health, University of Bristol, Bristol, United Kingdom

[2] Infancy and Sleep Centre, Department of Anthropology, Durham University, Durham, United Kingdom

[3] Department of Anthropology, Santa Clara University, Santa Clara, California

[4] Mother-Baby Sleep Lab, Department of Anthropology, University of Notre Dame, South Bend, Indiana

[5] Department of Pediatrics, Division of Adolescent Medicine, Cooper Medical School of Rowan University, Camden, New Jersey

[6] Department of Pediatrics, University of Connecticut School of Medicine, Farmington, Connecticut

[7] Connecticut Children's Medical Center, Division of Neonatology, Hartford, Connecticut

[8] Department of Medicine, Cambridge Health Alliance and Harvard Medical School, Cambridge Massachusetts

* Courtesy of the Academy of Breastfeeding Medicine. Please go to https://www.bfmed.org/protocols for complete protocols, translations, and the most up-to-date information (protocols are updated every 5–7 years).

However, bedsharing may only be a risk in hazardous circumstances as demonstrated by epidemiological study (Table 1).[11] We aim to clarify the currently available evidence regarding the benefits and risks of bedsharing, and offer evidence-based recommendations that promote infant and maternal health through increased breastfeeding duration.[12] The recommendations in this protocol apply to mother–infant dyads who have initiated breastfeeding and are in home settings, and are not intended for use in hospitals or birth centers.

SUMMARY AND RECOMMENDATIONS

Summary

Levels of evidence (1–5) from the Oxford Centre for Evidence Based Medicine[13] are listed in parentheses, and are based on the citations are described below in the supporting material. See the supporting material for the ways in which we define "bedsharing," "SIDS," and "separate sleep" for purposes of this protocol. "Breastsleeping" is defined there as well.

Overall, the research conducted to date on bedsharing and breastfeeding indicates that nighttime proximity facilitates breastfeeding duration and exclusivity (levels 2–3).[2,4,14] Discussions about safe bedsharing should be incorporated into guidelines for pregnancy and postnatal care.[15–19] Existing evidence does not support the conclusion that bedsharing among breastfeeding infants (i.e., breastsleeping) causes sudden infant death syndrome (SIDS) in the absence of known hazards (level 3) (see Table 1).[11] Larger studies with appropriate controls are needed to understand the relationship between bedsharing and infant deaths in the absence of known hazards at different ages. Not all hazards are individually modifiable after birth (e.g., prematurity). Accidental suffocation death is extremely rare among bedsharing breastfeeding infants in the absence of hazardous circumstances (levels 2–3),[20] and must be weighed against the consequences of separate sleep. There are consequences to breastfeeding with separate sleep (even with room-sharing)

TABLE 1 Hazardous Risk Factors or Circumstances During Bedsharing
These are factors that increase the risk of SIDS and fatal sleeping accidents, either alone or when combined with bedsharing.[11,26,41,42] • Sharing a sofa with a sleeping adult ("sofa-sharing") • Infant sleeping next to an adult who is impaired by alcohol[a] or drugs • Infant sleeping next to an adult who smokes • Sleeping in the prone position • Never initiating breastfeeding • Sharing a chair with a sleeping adult • Sleeping on soft bedding • Being born preterm or of low birth weight

[a]Amounts of alcohol causing impairment are discussed in the text. SIDS, sudden infant death syndrome. knowledge, beliefs, and preferences and acknowledge the known benefits as well as the risks (level 5).[23,24]

TABLE 2 Elements of Safe Bedsharing Advice, *in Order of Importance*
1. Never sleep with infants on a sofa, armchair, or unsuitable surface, including a pillow (level 3).[11] 2. Place infants to sleep away from any person impaired by alcohol or drugs (level 3).[11] 3. Place infants supine for sleep (level 3)[11] (level 4)[43] (level 5).[44] 4. Place infants to sleep away from secondhand smoke and away from a caregiver who routinely smokes (level 1)[28] and clothing or objects that smell of smoke (thirdhand smoke) (level 5).[45] (In cases where the mother smokes, this will not be possible). 5. The bed should be away from walls and furniture to prevent wedging of the infant's head or body (level 1).[46] 6. The bed's surface should be firm, just as with a crib (level 3),[41] without thick covers (e.g., duvets, doonas), pillows, or other objects that could cause accidental head covering and asphyxiation. 7. The infant should not be left alone on an adult bed (level 1).[47] 8. Adoption of the C-position ("cuddle curl"), with the infant's head across from the adult's breast, adult's legs and arm(s) curled around the infant, infant on their back, away from the pillow, is the optimal safe sleeping position (Fig. 1) (level 4).[48,49] 9. There is insufficient evidence to make recommendations on multiple bedsharers or the position of the infant in bed with respect to both parents in the absence of hazardous circumstances.[50,51] Each locality should consider the cultural circumstances unique to its situation with respect to sleep conditions.

that include the risk of early weaning, the risk of compromise to milk supply from less frequent nighttime breastfeeding, and unintentional bedsharing (levels 1–3).[5,21,22] Recommendations concerning bedsharing must take into account the mother's

Recommendations

All families should be counseled about safe sleep. Table 2 summarizes safe sleep advice in order of importance based on the strength of the evidence. In addition, we recommend the following:

1. Discussion with open-ended questions from health care providers concerning bedsharing safety should happen with *all* parents, as bedsharing is likely to happen whether intended or not (level 4).[25] These discussions should take place early in the perinatal course and continuously throughout infancy, and include as many caregivers as possible. Open-ended questions that have been found to be successful in opening conversations include:
   a. "What are your plans for where your baby will sleep?"
   b. "What does that sleep area look like?"
   c. "Does your baby ever end up in bed with you?"

2. Screen families at increased risk of infant death with bedsharing: infants who were born preterm (level 2)[26] (level 3),[27] exposed to tobacco antenatally (level 1)[28] (level 4)[29] (level 5),[30] live with smokers (level 1)[28] (level 3)[11] (level 4),[31,32] and those who live with people who consume alcohol (level 3)[11] or drugs and, therefore, might be in charge of an infant and could fall asleep with the infant.

3. Information and counseling about safe bedsharing should be provided even to those parents for whom bedsharing should be discouraged (those with hazardous conditions or circumstances), as one must assume that parents may bedshare anyway, even if unintentionally (level 1).[33] See Table 3 for risk minimization strategies.
   a. These discussions can include how to make sleep areas as safe as possible, and can reflect how to minimize hazardous circumstances, even if they are not eliminated (See Table 2).
   b. For instance, if a parent who smokes is bedsharing, breastfeeding, sleep positioning, sleep surface, bedding, and where infant naps when alone can all be discussed.

TABLE 3   Risk Minimization Strategies for Families in Which Bedsharing is High Risk

Increased promotion and support of breastfeeding (level 1)[12,42,52] (level 3).[52]

Referral for smoking cessation and alcohol and/or drug treatment (level 1)[28] (level 3).[11]

Enhanced repeated multimodal messaging regarding risks of sofa-sharing, bedsharing where hazardous factors are present, including sleeping next to an impaired adult and smoke avoidance. Text messaging and e-mail, including use of video and social media may be helpful if available to parents (level 2).[34,53,54]

Sidecars or in-bed devices (e.g., Pēpi-Pod®; *wahakura*) can be considered (level 2).[1,55]

Emphasize room-sharing where and when bedsharing cannot be done safely.

Take into account the importance of the partner and other support persons' involvement in the infants' sleep time activities.

Conversations when a family is bedsharing should be nonjudgmental and acknowledge context

- Ending stigma around bedsharing and educating all parents about safe bedsharing have the potential to reduce infant deaths. Bedsharing evolved from innate human biological and behavioral mechanisms. It is not a singular, discrete, or coherent practice, but is composed of a diverse range of behaviors, some of which may carry risks, making it particularly important to discuss bedsharing safety.

- Discussing the concept of breastsleeping with breastfeeding parents allows a way to discuss safe bedsharing in this context. Using the theory of planned behavior, counseling about safe breastsleeping is most likely to be effective if it is consistent with both social norms and attitudes (level 2).[34]

- Scripting tools are important resources.[35,36] Beginning with an open-ended inquiry helps to identify an understanding of patients' and families' lived experiences. It is critical to recognize that evidence-based medicine integrates "compassionate use of individual patients' predicaments, rights, and preferences" (level 5).[23] Nonjudgmental counseling helps to build trusting patient–professional relationships for both disclosure and effective counseling (level 5).[10]

Public policy recommendations

Structural societal interventions are essential interventions regardless of counseling on sleeping arrangements. As many parents will have limited contact with the health care system,[33] advocating for structural changes is critical. Policymakers should address the following strategies that may lower infant mortality:

1. Increasing tobacco prices, a strategy associated with an immediate marked decrease in infant mortality in Europe (level 5).[37]

2. Ending racial bias in the health care system that undermines breastfeeding and leads to poor maternal and infant outcomes (level 2)[38,39] (level 3).[40]

3. Advocating for the allocation of research funding and resources focusing on the risk factors for sleep-related infant death commensurate with the evidence-based level of risk.

EVIDENCE BASE AND SUPPORTING MATERIAL

Definitions

SIDS is defined as the sudden death of an infant that is unexplained after a case review and/or autopsy and death scene investigation have been performed. SIDS has a specific code, R95, under the *International Classification of Diseases, 10th Revision (ICD-10)*.[56] The code for "other ill-defined and unspecified causes of death" (R99) is used when the cause of death is unknown or there is inadequate evidence to classify as SIDS, as when SIDS is suspected but a full investigation has not been performed. Accidental suffocation or strangulation in bed (ASSB, W75) is coded when the death was due to asphyxia, strangulation, or suffocation, in a bed, crib, sofa, or armchair.

Sudden unexpected infant death (SUID), also known as sudden unexpected death in infancy (SUDI), is an overarching term for all unexpected deaths, both those that remain unexplained (coded as R95 or R99) and those in which a full causal explanation is eventually found.

Proxy measure for SIDS: For any international comparisons for the purpose of this protocol, we use a proxy measure for SIDS by adding deaths assigned to these three codes together (R95 + R99 + W75) as a composite measure of unexplained SUDI (or SUID).[57] This is due to our recognition of the diagnostic shift pointed out by Taylor et al.[58] and Shapiro-Mendoza et al.[59] over the past decade in which some pathologists and medical examiners seem reluctant to use SIDS (R95) because the diagnosis requires the exclusion of any other cause of death. Therefore, the use of codes R99 or W75 is preferred, despite incomplete or minimal evidence that overlaying (accidental smothering) may be the causal factor. Diagnostic shift toward ASSB (W75) is more common in the United States than in the United Kingdom.[60]

Bedsharing is defined as an infant sharing an adult bed with an adult for sleep, and for this protocol we are defining this as with the infant sleeping next to a caregiver, most often the mother. The bed may consist of a mattress or futon with varying levels of firmness depending on the filling.

Cosleeping is a term that may include both sleeping on a shared surface and sleeping in proximity, but not necessarily on a shared sleep surface. For clarity, "cosleeping" is not used in this protocol.

Separate versus solitary sleep: We refer to "separate sleep" as room-sharing without bedsharing, whereas "solitary sleep" refers to sleeping in a separate room from parents.

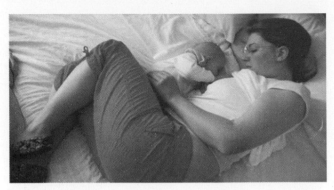

Fig. 1 C-position or "Cuddle curl." Breastsleeping mothers adopt a characteristic position (Protective C or Cuddle Curl) in which they make a safe space for their baby to sleep with their bodies. Mother's arm is above the baby's head preventing him/her moving up the bed into the pillows, and her knees are tucked under his/her feet to prevent him/her moving down the bed. Baby is positioned flat on his/her back on the flat mattress for sleep, and next to the mother's breasts for easy feeding. © Baby Sleep Information Source, licensed for use under Creative Commons, 2016. Color images are available online.

History, context, and anthropology of infant sleep location

Human milk, lower in solute compared with milk of other species (e.g., bovine),[61] is digested very quickly. The rapidly growing infant breastfeeds at least 8–12 times in 24 hours.[62] Frequent feeding is difficult if the infant is not in close contact with his or her breastfeeding mother day and night.[1,8] Parent–infant bedsharing with breastfeeding constitutes the human evolutionary norm as demonstrated in anthropological research.[63–67]

In industrialized countries until the early 20th century, most infants were bedsharing and breastfeeding.[68] After that time, solitary sleep developed as an ideal among the middle classes, reinforced by the growing trends of artificial feeding and medicalization of childbirth, separating infants from mothers.[65,68] Sleep training also became increasingly popular in some industrialized societies.[68] Human milk substitutes (e.g., infant formula) helped this trend, as infants who receive them tend to feed less frequently[69] and may sleep more deeply than breastfed infants.[70]

Concerns about infant sleep duration and location did not appear until after the late 19th and early 20th centuries in industrialized countries,[68] indicating that infant sleep research has taken place within an historical context in which feeding of human milk substitutes and solitary sleep promotion were normative. Although parents and caregivers in the majority of cultures sleep in proximity to their infants, organizations in some countries, including the United States, Canada, and Germany, recommend that even breastfeeding mothers should never share a sleep surface with their infants.[10,71–73]

The concept of "breastsleeping" was proposed to describe a biologically based model of sustained contact between the mother and infant, starting immediately after birth, in which sleeping and breastfeeding are inextricably combined, assuming no hazardous risk factors.[15,64] Described in cultures around the world, the breastsleeping mother and infant feed frequently during the night while lying in bed together, and by morning, the mother may not recall how many times she fed or for how long.[74] The breastsleeping concept acknowledges the critical role that immediate and sustained maternal contact plays in helping establish optimal breastfeeding[63,75,76]; and recognizes that the behavior and physiology of breastsleeping dyads may be different from that of bedsharing nonbreastfeeding dyads, signifying that the safety assessments for bedsharing with breastfeeding versus feeding human milk substitutes likely require different approaches.[4,21,77,78]

When breastfeeding mothers sleep with their infants, they protect them from potential physiological stressors including airway covering and overheating by their characteristic sleep position (curled around their infants, making a constrained sleep space with their bodies), known as the C-position[48] or "cuddle curl"[49] (Fig. 1). Their continued vigilance through microarousals prompts regular infant arousals throughout the night.[21,78–80] In two small video studies, mothers who had never breastfed were observed to exhibit these protective behaviors less frequently.[78,81]

Compared with breastfeeding infants who sleep alone, breastsleeping infants spend less time in stages 3–4 (deep) sleep, and more time in stages 1–2 (lighter) sleep, facilitating rapid infant awakening and termination of apneas. Additional time nurturing through breastsleeping, as compared with less time nurturing when sleeping separately, may affect epigenetic responses to stress in the infant through the possible influence of maternal care on infant regulatory responses.[82]

Despite decades of advice to avoid mother–infant sleep contact, researchers report that on any given night, 20–25% of U.S. and U.K. infants <3 months of age share a bed with a parent for sleep at least some of the nights,[83,84] and >40% of infants in Western* societies, in general, do so at some point in the first 3 months.[83,85–91] These proportions may be underreported due to the stigma associated with bedsharing, especially in the United States. Parents express various reasons for sleeping with their infant, including deeply rooted cultural or religious beliefs and parenting philosophies, physiological links between lactation and nighttime breastfeeding, and a biological compulsion that drives the urge for close contact.[25,89,92–94] They explain that sleeping with their infant makes nighttime care easier, helps them monitor their infant, provides comfort, and still allows them to sleep.[8,25,95] Sometimes parents report having nowhere else to put their infant at night, or that they have fallen asleep with their infant unintentionally.[25,89,96] Others report bedsharing in response to either the mother or her infant being deaf, to keep infants safe from environmental harms (i.e., vermin, gunfire, and earthquakes) and to protect them from SIDS.[97–99]

Breastfeeding mothers comprise the largest group of bedsharers.[92] Sleep contact between mother and infant facilitates

---

* We understand "Western" as an ideological construct, not a geographic one.

nighttime breastfeeding, with multiple studies demonstrating that bedsharing is associated with more frequent nighttime feeds (promoting milk production), and more months of breastfeeding[2,4,14,90] (Fig. 2). Those women with the strongest prenatal intention to breastfeed are more likely to bedshare,[4] whereas breastfeeding women who did not initially intend to bedshare often end up doing so.[8,100] Although bedsharing breastfeeding mothers wake frequently to feed, they are awake for shorter periods and fall back to sleep more rapidly.[79] Thus they achieve greater sleep duration[101] than nonbedsharing mothers.[14] Bedsharing is a strategy used by breastfeeding mothers to reduce physical and social costs, for example, sleep disruption.[102] One observational study has shown that,

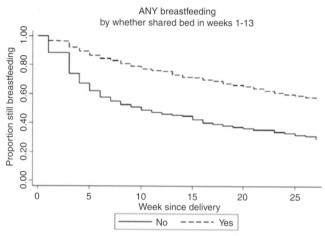

ANY breastfeeding
by whether shared bed in weeks 1-13

Fig. 2 Bedsharing is strongly associated with breastfeeding continuation. *Source:* Ball et al., 2016.

compared with mothers who room-shared without bedsharing, mothers who bedshared were more likely to report exclusive breastfeeding (adjusted odds ratio [OR]: 2.46; 95% confidence interval [CI]: 1.76—3.45) or partial breastfeeding (adjusted OR: 1.75; 95% CI: 1.33—2.31).[7,103] Therefore, advice to avoid bedsharing has the potential to undermine breastfeeding goals,[3,8,104,105] and may increase risk of sleeping in unsafe environments such as sofas.[106]

Although mothers and infants can sleep apart and still breastfeed exclusively, doing so results in fewer sessions of breastfeeding per night: bedsharers have double or triple the number of breastfeeding sessions and total amount of breastfeeding time compared with solitary sleepers.[6] Fewer than half as many feedings occurred for mothers whose infants slept alone in a bedside bassinet (Fig. 3a) in the postnatal ward compared with a sidecar (Fig. 3b) or with bedsharing in a randomized trial examining breastfeeding initiation.[1] In one study among a population with low breastfeeding rates, advice to room-share without bedsharing achieved a similar duration of "any" breastfeeding, but not exclusive breastfeeding.[22]

Bedsharing and SIDS: epidemiological/observational evidence

Feeding of human milk substitutes (formula) is associated with a markedly increased risk of SIDS.[42] This may be due to lower infant arousal thresholds and increased infection risks compared with breastfeeding dyads.[52] In addition, videographic studies show that breastsleeping infants consistently sleep with their heads well below pillows as they are positioned near their mother's breasts,[21,78,81] which might lower

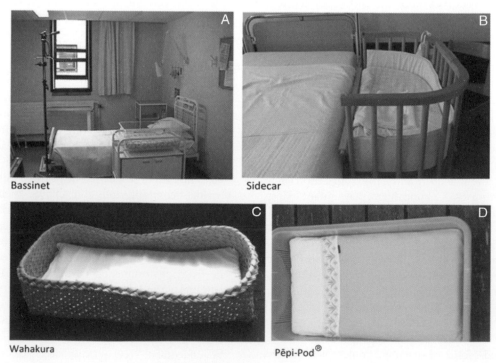

Bassinet   Sidecar

Wahakura   Pēpi-Pod®

Fig. 3 Bassinet, sidecar, *wahakura*, and Pēpi-Pod®. **(a)** bassinet, **(b)** sidecar, **(c)** *wahakura*, **(d)** Pēpi-Pod.

suffocation risk, in contrast to infants who are fed human milk substitutes, who have been noted to be placed intentionally on or around pillows. Videographic data show that breastsleeping infants rarely sleep prone.[21,81] Hauck et al. made the case that breastfeeding is causally associated with a reduction in SIDS based on biologic plausibility, consistency of findings, strength of association (which has since gotten stronger[42]), timing of association, and dose–response effect, and is not merely a marker for other protective factors including absence of tobacco smoke or sociodemographic factors.[52] The protective mechanism is unknown. However, it is likely to be a combination of maternal behavioral factors, immunological and nutritional properties of human milk, and the physiological influence of sucking on arousal.

Approximately half of SIDS cases occur when infants are sleeping alongside an adult as shown in recent observational case–control studies, with the remainder of deaths occurring among infants who sleep alone in a cot/crib.[9,11] In a longitudinal study in England of 300 consecutive SIDS deaths for a 20-year period, the total number of bedsharing SIDS deaths decreased by half after the "Back to Sleep" campaign.[107] However, in this cohort there was a sevenfold reduction in deaths that occurred in the crib/cot, which suggests that placing infants prone to sleep was far more common among those infants sleeping alone than among bedsharing infants.[11,107] This trend also resulted in a higher proportion of deaths that occurred among bedsharing infants, despite a numerical decrease in bedsharing deaths, because of the lower number of overall deaths. This statistical rise in the proportion of bedsharing deaths led policymakers in some countries to recommend against bedsharing, including the American Academy of Pediatrics, beginning with its 2005 statement.[10,108] In a meta-analysis of 11 SIDS case–control studies published in 2012, there was a pooled threefold risk associated with bedsharing, although this did not reach significance in older infants (> 12 weeks) or those not exposed to tobacco smoke, and the risk was only significant for unintentional bedsharers, not routine bedsharers. In addition, breastfeeding was not included in the analysis.[109]

The interaction between infants bedsharing next to mothers who smoked, as a risk for SIDS, first identified in the New Zealand Cot Death Study in 1993,[31] was more than fourfold (OR: 4.55 [95% CI: 2.63–7.88]) compared with no risk among infants sleeping next to nonsmoking mothers (OR: 0.98 [95% CI: 0.44–2.18]) in this case–control study.[32] Antenatal smoke exposure is not merely a marker for socioeconomic status as it is associated with reduced infant arousal, and with pathologic findings in the brains of exposed infants.[29,30]

A combined analysis of 400 SIDS infants and 1,386 controls from two English studies demonstrated an 18-fold increase in SIDS deaths if either an infant slept with an adult on a sofa or slept next to an adult who drank >2 U of alcohol within a 24-hour period (2 U equals 1 pint or large can of beer [440 mL], 1 glass of wine [175 mL], or 2 shots of spirits [50 mL]), with a 4-fold risk with bedsharing if parents smoked.[11] In the absence of hazards, there was no risk of SIDS with bedsharing compared with nonbedsharers (room-sharing or solitary sleeping) (OR: 1.08 [95% CI: 0.58–2.01]). When the data were divided into younger (<3 months) or older infants, an increased but not statistically significant risk in the younger infants (OR: 1.6 [95% CI: 0.96–2.7]) and a significant protective effect for nonhazardous bedsharing among the older infants (OR: 0.08 [95% CI: 0.01–0.52]) were apparent. Further study with larger number of infants would be needed to properly assess any differential effect by infant age or impact of other factors such as parental drug use, infant sleep positioning, or room-sharing.

In contrast, in a similar combined analysis, a fivefold increased risk was associated with younger infants bedsharing in nonhazardous circumstances.[9] However, the reference group for this study was female breastfed infants placed on their backs next to the beds of nonsmoking parents in the absence of any other risk factors. This magnified the risk difference and renders this explanation not generalizable and difficult to interpret, because both protective factors (detailed in the reference group) and potential risk factors (bedsharing) are being quantified at the same time.

Limited data exist on the risk of bedsharing with caregivers other than the mother. A single study from inner city Chicago in the United States found an increased death risk with multiple bedsharers (other children alone or other children with one or both parents) and nonparent bedsharers,[50] but a causal relationship is unclear. In a Scottish study, a markedly increased risk of death was found if the infant was sleeping between two parents,[51] but this study did not account for alcohol and/or drug use, which is notable as the United Kingdom has a high prevalence of heavy episodic drinking (27.1% among those aged 15 years and older) compared with other industrialized countries.[110]

SIDS epidemiology

SIDS is most common among low-income[46,107] and some marginalized communities in wealthy countries, with the world's highest prevalence of SIDS occurring among U.S. American Indians/Alaskan Natives (combined) and non-Hispanic blacks, New Zealand Māori, Australian Aboriginal and Torres Strait Islander peoples, and indigenous Canadians.[33] Bedsharing is often common and culturally valued in these marginalized communities. However, there are also many populations with high bedsharing rates that have low rates of SIDS,[33,111] including Swedes,[33] U.S. Asians, and U.S. Hispanics (Fig. 4). These conflicting observations may be explained by the presence or absence of a variety of attendant hazardous risk factors.[33] The overlap of many of the hazardous circumstances with conditions of poverty, structural racism, and legacies of historical trauma must be noted, including antenatal smoking, alcohol use, preterm birth, poor prenatal care, and lack of breastfeeding (feeding human milk substitutes). In the United States, fewer than half of the mothers of infants who died of SIDS received timely prenatal care,[33] which has been demonstrated as associated with SIDS elsewhere.[112,113] Structural racism also plays a role. For example, African American infants are more likely to be given human milk substitutes in the hospital without a medical indication,[38,39] undermining breastfeeding. Racial discrimination of Māori and Australian Indigenous peoples and other minorities by health professionals and society is associated with a wide range of negative health outcomes in New Zealand and Australia.[40,114]

Risk minimization policies and strategies

Various policies have been adopted to advise parents about bedsharing over the past decade. Countries including the United States, Canada, and Germany[73] have opted to advise against bedsharing. The conclusion of a 2014 review of all international case–control studies for 20 years by the independent U.K. body, the National Institute for Health and Care Excellence, was that bedsharing in itself is not causal for SIDS, and that parents should be informed of the specific hazards associated with this practice.[115] In contrast to the countries advising against all bedsharing, countries such as the United Kingdom and Australia[116] acknowledge that

bedsharing occurs both intentionally and unintentionally and is often linked to breastfeeding. Thus, they advise health practitioners to openly discuss the particular circumstances when it would be risky to bedshare.

Although the United Kingdom and Australian approach lacks the simplicity of the predominant U.S. approach, it is more closely aligned to the evidence, which acknowledges that bedsharing is widespread and may be culturally valued. This strategy allows the issue to be discussed without judgment, and for specific hazardous situations to be emphasized.[48,117,118] The U.S. policy, while calling for nonjudgmental conversations with families about sleep practices, includes the recommendation to room-share without bedsharing. This is a clear direct message to the public that may appear easy to convey to policymakers. A disadvantage of this direct approach, as evidenced by the antibedsharing rhetoric in some campaigns, is the stigmatization that can prohibit honest discussion among parents and health professionals and offend bereaved parents who have lost an infant while bedsharing. Despite campaigns to decrease bedsharing, reported bedsharing has increased in the United States in recent years, especially among black and Hispanic communities.[87,91] In one trial using enhanced messaging with high-risk families to avoid bedsharing,[119] bedsharing was no different than in the control group, and in both arms of the study, bedsharing increased over the first 6 months. Breastfeeding did not decrease, presumably because bedsharing was unaffected.[22] Taking into account diagnostic shift, the proxy SIDS rate (R95 + R99 + W75) in the United States with the strict "no bedsharing" policy appears to be almost unchanged (Fig. 5). In the United Kingdom, where parents are educated about safe bedsharing, the proxy SIDS rate has fallen over the past 10 years (Fig. 6). It is noted, however, that many different factors other than bedsharing may feed into these recent trends.

Risk minimization strategies include the recognition of the role of breastfeeding in SIDS prevention, the potential risk of bedsharing in the context of hazardous circumstances, and

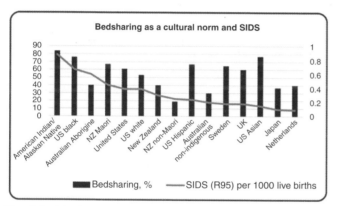

Fig. 4 Bedsharing (any) as a cultural norm and SIDS. *Source:* Taken from data from Bartick and Tomori, 2019. Most SIDS data are 2014. Australia groups are 2008–2012, Japan is 2015, The Netherlands and Sweden are 2013. Aborigine here refers to both Australian Aborigines and Torres Strait Islanders (combined). SIDS, sudden infant death syndrome.

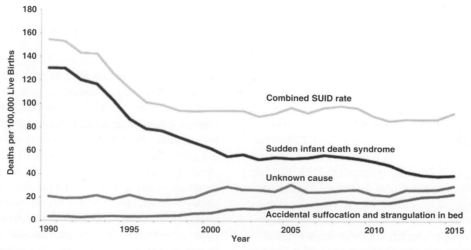

Fig. 5 U.S. trends in SIDS and SUID (1990–2015). *Source:* Centers for Disease Control and Prevention/National Center for Health Statistics (CDC/NCHS), National Vital Statistics System, Compressed Mortality File. SUID, sudden unexpected infant death.

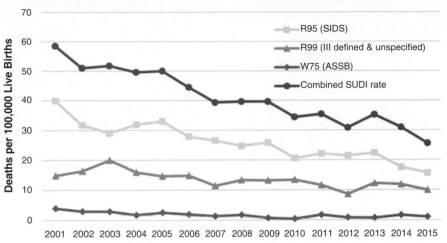

Fig. 6 England and Wales trends in SIDS and SUID (2000–2015). *Source*: Office for National Statistics, England and Wales. SUDI, sudden unexpected death in infancy.

taking into account the importance of the partner and other support persons' involvement in sleep time activities (See Table 3).

Effectiveness of safe sleep interventions

A review of safe sleep interventions shows that most (primarily U.S.-based) one-on-one interventions are unsuccessful, including those addressing smoke exposure and sleep location.[120] One observational U.S. study showed that exclusively breastfeeding women were far less likely to adhere to advice not to bedshare than other women (65% versus 30.5%).[103] There has been some success reaching parents with text messages and e-mail with video, social networks, or other media,[34,53,54,121] but this requires mobile phone and internet access. A simplistic "ABC-Alone, Back, Crib" approach is often rejected by families and caregivers, and has not been shown to decrease sleep-related deaths, leading to the adoption of a conversational approach,[35] which includes exploring patients' needs and perceptions and making informed decisions.[118] Annual U.S. surveys between 1993 and 2010 revealed that bedsharing rates among black and Hispanic families has continually increased, despite nearly half of U.S. nighttime caregivers discussing bedsharing with a physician.[91]

New Zealand, whose Māori population until recently had the highest SIDS rate in the world, driven by high rates of smoking combined with bedsharing,[58] has seen reductions in infant death rates after a novel intervention.[122] It targets high-risk families with provision of the *wahakura* (Fig. 3c), a woven flax bassinet-like structure based on Māori traditions developed for this purpose, used on the bed, to create a separate sleeping space, and the Pēpi-Pod (Fig. 3d), a polypropylene box (food-grade plastic) of similar proportions.[123] Parents also receive one-on-one advice that promotes "Safe Sleep." Importantly, the *wahakura* has the enhanced appeal of reclaiming a traditional Māori infant care practice that supports the highly valued proximity of mother and infant.[124] The high Māori SIDS rate dropped dramatically between 2009 and 2012, especially in targeted areas.[122] Interestingly,

the *wahakura* did not decrease unsafe sleep behaviors compared with a bedside bassinet, but was associated with markedly increased breastfeeding rates at 6 months (*wahakura*: 22.5% versus bassinet 10.7%, $p = 0.04$).[55]

Future areas of research

- How can death investigation techniques be improved to determine whether the death of an infant can be fully explained by asphyxia?
- Is there a significant risk from bedsharing in the absence of all hazardous circumstances?
- Is there a relationship between bedsharing risk and infant age and mode of feeding (adjusting for all hazardous circumstances) (breastfeeding, expressed milk feeding, donor milk feeding, and human milk substitutes)?
- What is the best advice for a safe sleep environment for nonbreastfeeding infants?
- How do multiple bedsharers in the absence of hazardous risks, including bedsharing of twins, impact the safety of the infant? Does the location of the infant in the bed, for example, between the parents or on the edge of the bed next to the mother, make a difference for safety?
- Are in-bed devices and sidecars safe and efficacious, especially for infants in high-risk situations, and if safe, what are their effects on breastfeeding?
- Can the C-position ("cuddle curl") be adopted by nonbreastfeeding bedsharers and is it effective in reducing SIDS?
- Is providing supportive information to parents on "breastsleeping," as defined in this protocol as a separate category of bedsharing, protective or risky to provide these parents with better specific guidance?
- Is there autopsy evidence of the effect of feeding human milk substitutes that can establish a causal link between feeding human milk substitutes and SIDS?
- Do the risks of death from SIDS due to early weaning and potentially related to the lack of safe bedsharing

outweigh the risk of death from SIDS from bedsharing in nonhazardous circumstances? There are many confounders and this will be difficult to study.

- To what extent does maternal obesity modify the risks and benefits of bedsharing?[125,126]

DISCLOSURE STATEMENT

JJM serves as safety consultant for the Arms Reach cosleeper for which he is paid a small honorarium but no royalties. No other competing financial interests exist. PSB serves as the chair of the International Society for the Study and Prevention of Perinatal and Infant Death (ISPID) and is a scientific advisor to UNICEF UK, neither of which are funded positions. HLB is scientific advisor to Lullaby Trust and chair of the Lullaby Trust Scientific Committee, board member of ISPID, and member of editorial review board for Journal of Human Lactation, which are all unfunded positions. As part of her academic role, she is co-founder and co-director of Basis, the Baby Sleep Information Source (www.BasisOnline.org.uk). JJM serves as psychological advisor to Fit Pregnancy magazine, an unpaid respondent for the website Kids in the House, KidsintheHouse.com, and a board member of Speaking of Kids; LFW works as a consultant and physician lead for Communities and Hospitals Advancing Maternity Practices (CHAMPS), Boston Medical Center, Boston, Massachusetts, and as a consultant to National Institute for Children's Health Quality (NICHQ)-National Action Partnership to Promote Safe Sleep Improvement and Innovation Network(NAPPSS-IIN). She is chair of the Section on Breastfeeding for the American Academy of Pediatrics (AAP) and also serves on the AAP Task Force on SIDS. KAM serves on the clinical advisory board of the US Baby-Friendly Hospital Initiative and is associate editor of the Journal of Human Lactation; MCB has received funding from the W.K. Kellogg Foundation for research in breastfeeding and economics and co-leads the Massachusetts Baby-Friendly Collaborative. LFW and MCB serve on the board of the Academy of Breastfeeding Medicine.

FUNDING INFORMATION

This work was unfunded.

REFERENCES

1. Ball HL, Ward-Platt MP, Heslop E, et al. Randomised trial of infant sleep location on the postnatal ward. *Arch Dis Child.* 2006;91:1005−1010.
2. Huang Y, Hauck FR, Signore C, et al. Influence of bedsharing activity on breastfeeding duration among US mothers. *JAMA Pediatr.* 2013;167:1038−1044.
3. Blair PS, Heron J, Fleming PJ. Relationship between bedsharing and breastfeeding: Longitudinal, population-based analysis. *Pediatrics.* 2010;126:e1119−1126.
4. Ball HL, Howel D, Bryant A, et al. Bed-sharing by breastfeeding mothers: Who bed-shares and what is the relationship with breastfeeding duration? *Acta Paediatr.* 2016;105: 628−634.
5. Ball HL. Night-time infant care: Cultural practice, evolution, and infant development. In: Liamputtong P, ed. *Childrearing and Infant Care Issues: A Cross-Cultural Perspective.* Melbourne, Australia: Nova Science; 2006.
6. McKenna J, Mosko S, Richard C. Bedsharing promotes breastfeeding. *Pediatrics.* 1997;100:214−219.
7. Moon RY. Task Force on Sudden Infant Death Syndrome. SIDS and other sleep-related infant deaths: Evidence base for 2016 updated recommendations for a safe infant sleeping environment. *Pediatrics.* 2016;138:e20162940.
8. Ball HL. Breastfeeding, bedsharing, and infant sleep. *Birth.* 2003;30:181−188.
9. Carpenter R, McGarvey C, Mitchell EA, et al. Bed sharing when parents do not smoke: Is there a risk of SIDS? An individual level analysis of five major case−control studies. *BMJ Open.* 2013;3:e002299.
10. Task Force on Sudden Infant Death Syndrome. SIDS and other sleep-related infant deaths: Updated 2016 recommendations for a safe infant sleeping environment. *Pediatrics.* 2016;138:e20162938.
11. Blair PS, Sidebotham P, Pease A, et al. Bed-sharing in the absence of hazardous circumstances: Is there a risk of sudden infant death syndrome? An analysis from two case−control studies conducted in the UK. *PLoS One.* 2014;9:e107799.
12. Victora CG, Bahl R, Barros AJ, et al. Breastfeeding in the 21st century: Epidemiology, mechanisms, and lifelong effect. *Lancet.* 2016;387:475−490.
13. Howick J, Chalmers I, Glasziou P, et al. *The Oxford 2011 Levels of Evidence.* UK: Oxford; 2011.
14. Bovbjerg ML, Hill JA, Uphoff AE, et al. Women who bedshare more frequently at 14 weeks postpartum subsequently report longer durations of breastfeeding. *J Midwifery Womens Health.* 2018;63:418−424.
15. Feldman-Winter L, Goldsmith JP, et al. Safe sleep and skin-to-skin care in the neonatal period for healthy term newborns. *Pediatrics.* 2016;138:e20161889.
16. Lullaby Trust, Baby Sleep Info Source (Basis), Public Health England, UNICEF UK Baby-Friendly Hospital Initiative. Safer sleep for babies: A guide for parents. London, 2019. https://www.unicef.org.uk/babyfriendly/wpcontent/uploads/sites/2/2018/08/Caring-for-your-baby-atnight-web.pdf
17. Crenshaw JT. Healthy Birth Practice #6: Keep mother and baby together: It's best for mother, baby, and breastfeeding. *J Perinatal Edu.* 2014;23:211−217.
18. Drever-Smith C, Bogossian F, New K. Co-sleeping and bed sharing in postnatal maternity units: A review of the literature and critique of clinical practice guidelines. *Int J Childbirth.* 2013;3:13−27.
19. Fetherston CM, Leach JS. Analysis of the ethical issues in the breastfeeding and bedsharing debate. *Breastfeeding Rev.* 2012;20:7−17.
20. Bajanowski T, Vege A, Byard RW, et al. Sudden infant death syndrome (SIDS)—standardised investigations and classification: Recommendations. *Forensic Sci Int.* 2007;165:129−143.
21. Baddock SA, Purnell MT, Blair PS, et al. The influence of bedsharing on infant physiology, breastfeeding and behaviour: A systematic review. *Sleep Med Rev.* 2019;43:106−117.
22. Moon RY, Mathews A, Joyner BL, et al. Impact of a randomized controlled trial to reduce bedsharing on breastfeeding rates and duration for African-American infants. *J Community Health.* 2017;42:707−715.
23. Sackett DL, Rosenberg WM, Gray JA, et al. Evidence based medicine: What it is and what it isn't. *BMJ.* 1996;312:71−72.

24. Jack E, Maskrey N, Byng R. SHERPA: A new model for clinical decision making in patients with multimorbidity. *Lancet.* 2018;392:1397–1399.

25. Ball HL. Reasons to bed-share: Why parents sleep with their infants. *J Reprod Infant Physiol.* 2002;20:207–221.

26. Ostfeld BM, Schwartz-Soicher O, Reichman NE, et al. Prematurity and sudden unexpected infant deaths in the United States. *Pediatrics.* 2017;140:e20163334.

27. Malloy MH, Hoffman HJ. Prematurity, sudden infant death syndrome, and age of death. *Pediatrics.* 1995;96(3 Pt. 1):464–471.

28. Zhang K, Wang X. Maternal smoking and increased risk of sudden infant death syndrome: A meta-analysis. *Leg Med (Tokyo).* 2013;15:115–121.

29. Lavezzi AM, Mecchia D, Matturri L. Neuropathology of the area postrema in sudden intrauterine and infant death syndromes related to tobacco smoke exposure. *Auton Neurosci.* 2012;166:29–34.

30. Kinney HC, Thach BT. The sudden infant death syndrome. *N Engl J Med.* 2009;361:795–805.

31. Scragg R, Mitchell EA, Taylor BJ, et al. Bed sharing, smoking, and alcohol in the sudden infant death syndrome. New Zealand Cot Death Study Group. *BMJ.* 1993;307:1312–1318.

32. Mitchell EA, Thompson JM, Zuccollo J, et al. The combination of bed sharing and maternal smoking leads to a greatly increased risk of sudden unexpected death in infancy: The New Zealand SUDI Nationwide Case Control Study. *N Z Med J.* 2017;130:52–64.

33. Bartick M, Tomori C. Sudden infant death and social justice: A syndemics approach. *Matern Child Nutr.* 2019;15:e12652.

34. Moon RY, Corwin MJ, Kerr S, et al. Mediators of improved adherence to infant safe sleep using a mobile health intervention. *Pediatrics.* 2019;143:e20182799.

35. Bronheim S. *Building on Campaigns with Conversations: An Individualized Approach to Helping Families Embrace Safe Sleep and Breastfeeding.* Washington, DC: National Center for Education in Maternal and Child Health; 2017.

36. UNICEF UK Baby-Friendly Hospital Initiative. *Co sleeping and SIDS: A Guide for Health Professionals.* London: UNICEF UK; 2019.

37. Filippidis FT, Laverty AA, Hone T, et al. Association of cigarette price differentials with infant mortality in 23 European Union countries. *JAMA Pediatr.* 2017;171:1100–1106.

38. Lind JN, Perrine CG, Li R, et al. Racial disparities in access to maternity care practices that support breastfeeding—United States, 2011. *MMWR Morb Mortal Wkly Rep.* 2014;63:725–728.

39. McKinney CO, Hahn-Holbrook J, Chase-Lansdale PL, et al. Racial and ethnic differences in breastfeeding. *Pediatrics.* 2016;138:e20152388.

40. Harris R, Cormack D, Tobias M, et al. The pervasive effects of racism: Experiences of racial discrimination in New Zealand over time and associations with multiple health domains. *Soc Sci Med.* 2012;74:408–415.

41. Kemp JS, Nelson VE, Thach BT. Physical properties of bedding that may increase risk of sudden infant death syndrome in prone-sleeping infants. *Pediatr Res.* 1994;36(1 Pt. 1):7–11.

42. Thompson JMD, Tanabe K, Moon RY, et al. Duration of breastfeeding and risk of SIDS: An individual participant data meta-analysis. *Pediatrics.* 2017;140:e20171324.

43. Li DK, Petitti DB, Willinger M, et al. Infant sleeping position and the risk of sudden infant death syndrome in California, 1997–2000. *Am J Epidemiol.* 2003;157:446–455.

44. Tuladhar R, Harding R, Cranage SM, et al. Effects of sleep position, sleep state and age on heart rate responses following provoked arousal in term infants. *Early Hum Dev.* 2003;71:157–169.

45. Torres LH, Balestrin NT, Spelta LEW, et al. Exposure to tobacco smoke during the early postnatal period modifies receptors and enzymes of the endocannabinoid system in the brainstem and striatum in mice. *Toxicol Lett.* 2019;302:35–41.

46. Erck Lambert AB, Parks SE, Cottengim C, et al. Sleep related infant suffocation deaths attributable to soft bedding, overlay, and wedging. *Pediatrics.* 2019;143:e20183408.

47. Lagon E, Moon RY, Colvin JD. Characteristics of infant deaths during sleep while under nonparental supervision. *J Pediatr.* 2018;197. 57.e36–62.e36.

48. UNICEF UK Baby-Friendly Hospital Initiative. *Caring for Your Baby at Night.* London: UNICEF UK; 2016.

49. Weissinger D, West D, Smith LJ, et al. *Sweet Sleep: Night time and Naptime Strategies for the Breastfeeding Family.* New York: Ballantine Books; 2014.

50. Hauck FR, Herman SM, Donovan M, et al. Sleep environment and the risk of sudden infant death syndrome in an urban population: The Chicago Infant Mortality Study. *Pediatrics.* 2003;111(5 Pt. 2):1207–1214.

51. Tappin D, Ecob R, Brooke H. Bedsharing, roomsharing, and sudden infant death syndrome in Scotland: A case–control study. *J Pediatr.* 2005;147:32–37.

52. Hauck FR, Thompson JM, Tanabe KO, et al. Breastfeeding and reduced risk of sudden infant death syndrome: A meta-analysis. *Pediatrics.* 2011;128:103–110.

53. Kellams A, Parker MG, Geller NL, et al. TodaysBaby Quality Improvement: Safe Sleep Teaching and Role Modeling in 8 US Maternity Units. *Pediatrics.* 2017;140:e20171816.

54. Moon RY, Hauck FR, Kellams AL, et al. Comparison of text messages versus e-mail when communicating and querying with mothers about safe infant sleep. *Acad Pediatr.* 2017;17:871–878.

55. Baddock SA, Tipene-Leach D, Williams SM, et al. Wahakura versus bassinet for safe infant sleep: A randomized trial. *Pediatrics.* 2017;139:e20160162.

56. World Health Organization. *ICD-10, International Statistical Classification of Diseases and Related Health Problems-10th Revision.* 5th edition Geneva, Switzerland: WHO; 2018.

57. Goldstein RD, Blair PS, Sens MA, et al. Inconsistent classification of unexplained sudden deaths in infants and children hinders surveillance, prevention and research: Recommendations from The 3rd International Congress on Sudden Infant and Child Death. *Forensic Sci Med Pathol.* 2019;4:622–628.

58. Taylor BJ, Garstang J, Engelberts A, et al. International comparison of sudden unexpected death in infancy rates using a newly proposed set of cause-of-death codes. *Arch Dis Child.* 2015;100:1018–1023.

59 Shapiro-Mendoza CK, Parks SE, Brustrom J, et al. Variations in cause-of-death determination for sudden unexpected infant deaths. *Pediatrics.* 2017;140:e20170087.

60. Marinelli KA, Ball HL, McKenna JJ, et al. An integrated analysis of maternal-infant sleep, breastfeeding, and sudden infant death syndrome: Research supporting a balanced discourse. *J Hum Lact.* 2019;35:510–520.

61. Hernell O. Human milk vs. cow's milk and the evolution of infant formulas. *Nestle Nutr Workshop Ser Pediatr Program.* 2011;67:17–28.

62. Casiday RE, Wright CM, Panter-Brick C, et al. Do early infant feeding patterns relate to breast-feeding continuation and weight gain? Data from a longitudinal cohort study. *Eur J Clin Nutr.* 2004;58:1290—1296.

63. Ball HL. Evolution-informed maternal-infant health. *Nat Ecol Evol.* 2017;1:73.

64. McKenna JJ, Gettler LT. There is no such thing as infant sleep, there is no such thing as breastfeeding, there is only breast-sleeping. *Acta Paediatr.* 2015;105:17—21.

65. Ball HL. Evolutionary paediatrics: A case study in applying Darwinian medicine. In: Elton S, O'Higgins P, eds. *Medicine and Evolution: Current Applications, Future Prospects.* Vol. 48. Boca Raton, FL: Taylor & Francis; 2008:127—152.

66. McKenna JJ, Ball HL, Gettler JT. Mother-infant co sleeping, breastfeeding and sudden infant death syndrome: What biological anthropology has discovered about normal infant sleep and pediatric sleep medicine. *Am J Phys Anthropol.* 2007; (Suppl. 45)133—161.

67. Trevathan WR, Rosenberg KR. Human evolution and the helpless infant. In: Trevathan WR, ed. *Costly and Cute: Helpless Infants and Human Evolution.* Albuquerque: University of New Mexico Press; 2015:1—28.

68. Stearns PN, Rowland P, Giarnella L. Children's sleep: Sketching historical change. *J Soc Hist.* 1996;30:345—366.

69. Centers for Disease Control and Prevention. *Infant Feeding Practices Study II, Chapter 3, Infant Feeding.* Atlanta, GA: CDC,; 2008.

70. Kahn A, Groswasser J, Franco P, et al. Factors influencing the determination of arousal thresholds in infants—A review. *Sleep Med.* 2000;1:273—278.

71. Canadian Paediatric Society, Canadian Foundation for the Study of Infant Deaths, Canadian Institute of Child Health, Health Canada, Public Health Agency of Canada. *Joint Statement on Safe Sleep: Preventing Sudden Infant Deaths in Canada.* Ottawa, Canada: Canadian Paediatric Society; 2018.

72. European Foundation for the Care of Newborn Infants. *Safe Sleep.* Munich, Germany: EFCNI,; 2018.

73. Kindergesundheit-info.de [Childhealth-info]. Ein schmerzliches Thema: Der Plötzliche Kindstod. Bundeszentrale für gesundheitliche Aufklärung. [A Painful Topic: Sudden Infant Death Syndrome. Federal Center for Health Education]. Published 2019. Available at https://www.kindergesundheit-info.de/themen/risiken-vorbeugen/ploetzlicher-kindstod-sids/sids (accessed September 13, 2019).

74. Tomori C. Breastsleeping in four cultures: Comparative analysis of a biocultural body technique. In: Abington NY, ed. *Breastfeeding: New Anthropological Approaches, Tomori C, Palmquist AE, Quinn E.* Routledge; 2017:55—68.

75. Ball HL, Russell CK. Nighttime nurturing: An evolutionary perspective on breastfeeding and sleep. In: Narvaez D, Panksepp J, Schore A, Gleason T, eds. *Evolution, Early Experience and Human Development: From Research to Practice and Policy.* Oxford: Oxford University Press; 2012:241—261.

76. Ball HL, Klingaman K. Breastfeeding and mother-infant sleep proximity: Implications for infant care. In: Trevathan WR, McKenna JJ, eds. *Evolutionary Medicine and Health: New Perspectives.* New York: Oxford University Press; 2008:226—241.

77. Mobbs EJ, Mobbs GA, Mobbs AE. Imprinting, latchment and displacement: A mini review of early instinctual behaviour in newborn infants influencing breastfeeding success. *Acta Paediatr.* 2016;105:24—30.

78. Ball HL. Parent-infant bed-sharing behavior: Effects of feeding type and presence of father. *Hum Nat.* 2006;17:301—318.

79. Mosko S, Richard C, McKenna J. Maternal sleep and arousals during bedsharing with infants. *Sleep.* 1997;20:142—150.

80. Mosko S, Richard C, McKenna J. Infant arousals during mother-infant bed sharing: Implications for infant sleep and sudden infant death syndrome research. *Pediatrics.* 1997;100:841—849.

81. Volpe LE, Ball HL, McKenna JJ. Nighttime parenting strategies and sleep-related risks to infants. *Soc Sci Med.* 2013;79:92—100.

82. Lester BM, Conradt E, LaGasse LL, et al. Epigenetic programming by maternal behavior in the human infant. *Pediatrics.* 2018;142:e20180194.

83. Blair PS, Ball HL. The prevalence and characteristics associated with parent-infant bed-sharing in England. *Arch Dis Child.* 2004;89:1106—1110.

84. McCoy RC, Hunt CE, Lesko SM, et al. Frequency of bed sharing and its relationship to breastfeeding. *J Dev Behav Pediatr.* 2004;25:141—149.

85. Gibson E, Dembofsky CA, Rubin S, et al. Infant sleep position practices 2 years into the "back to sleep" campaign. *Clin Pediatr (Phila).* 2000;39:285—289.

86. Rigda RS, McMillen IC, Buckley P. Bed sharing patterns in a cohort of Australian infants during the first six months after birth. *J Paediatr Child Health.* 2000;36:117—121.

87. Bombard JM, Kortsmit K, Warner L, et al. Vital Signs: Trends and disparities in infant safe sleep practices United States, 2009-2015. *MMWR Morb Mortal Wkly Rep.* 2018;67:39—46.

88. Hauck FR, Tanabe KO. International trends in sudden infant death syndrome: Stabilization of rates requires further action. *Pediatrics.* 2008;122:660—666.

89. Ateah CA, Hamelin KJ. Maternal bedsharing practices, experiences, and awareness of risks. *J Obstet Gynecol Neonatal Nurs.* 2008;37:274—281.

90. Santos IS, Mota DM, Matijasevich A, et al. Bed-sharing at 3 months and breast-feeding at 1 year in southern Brazil. *J Pediatr.* 2009;155:505—509.

91. Colson ER, Willinger M, Rybin D, et al. Trends and factors associated with infant bed sharing, 1993-2010: The National Infant Sleep Position Study. *JAMA Pediatr.* 2013;167:1032—1037.

92. Salm Ward TC. Reasons for mother-infant bed-sharing: A systematic narrative synthesis of the literature and implications for future research. *Matern Child Health J.* 2015;19:675—690.

93. Crane D, Ball HL. A qualitative study in parental perceptions and understanding of SIDS-reduction guidance in a UK bi-cultural urban community. *BMC Pediatr.* 2016;16:23.

94. Culver ED. Exploring bed-sharing mothers' motives and decision-making for getting through the night intact: A grounded theory. *J Midwifery Womens Health.* 2009;54:423.

95. Rudzik AEF, Ball HL. Exploring maternal perceptions of infant sleep and feeding method among mothers in the United Kingdom: A qualitative focus group study. *Matern Child Health J.* 2016;20:33—40.

96. Volpe LE, Ball HL. Infant sleep-related deaths: Why do parents take risks? *Arch Dis Child.* 2015;100:603—604.

97. Joyner BL, Oden RP, Ajao TI, et al. Where should my baby sleep: A qualitative study of African American infant sleep location decisions. *J Natl Med Assoc.* 2010;102:881—889.

98. Chianese J, Ploof D, Trovato C, et al. Inner-city caregivers' perspectives on bed sharing with their infants. *Acad Pediatr.* 2009;9:26—32.

99. McKenna JJ, Volpe LE. Sleeping with baby: An internet based sampling of parental experiences, choices, perceptions, and interpretations in a Western industrialized context. *Infant Child Dev.* 2007;16:359—385.

100. Tomori C. *Nighttime Breastfeeding: An American Cultural Dilemma*. New York: Berghahn Books; 2014.

101. Quillin SI, Glenn LL. Interaction between feeding method and co-sleeping on maternal-newborn sleep. *J Obstet Gynecol Neonatal Nurs*. 2004;33:580—588.

102. Tully KP, Ball HL. Trade-offs underlying maternal breastfeeding decisions: A conceptual model. *Matern Child Nutr*. 2013;9:90—98.

103. Smith LA, Geller NL, Kellams AL, et al. Infant sleep location and breastfeeding practices in the United States, 2011—2014. *Acad Pediatr*. 2016;16:540—549.

104. Bartick M, Tomori C, Ball HL. Babies in boxes and the missing links on safe sleep: Human evolution and cultural revolution. *Matern Child Nutr*. 2018;14:e12544.

105. Bartick M, Smith LJ. Speaking out on safe sleep: Evidence-based infant sleep recommendations. *Breastfeed Med*. 2014;9:417—422.

106. Kendall-Tackett K, Cong Z, et al. Mother-infant sleep locations and night time feeding behavior: U.S. data from the survey of mothers' sleep and fatigue. *Clin Lact*. 2010;1(Fall).

107. Blair PS, Sidebotham P, Berry PJ, et al. Major epidemiological changes in sudden infant death syndrome: A 20-year population-based study in the UK. *Lancet*. 2006;367:314—319.

108. American Academy of Pediatrics Task Force on Sudden Infant Death Syndrome. The changing concept of sudden infant death syndrome: Diagnostic coding shifts, controversies regarding the sleeping environment, and new variables to consider in reducing risk. *Pediatrics*. 2005;116:1245—1255.

109. Vennemann MM, Hense HW, Bajanowski T, et al. Bed sharing and the risk of sudden infant death syndrome: Can we resolve the debate? *J Pediatr*. 2012;160. 44.e42—48.e42.

110. World Health Organization. *Global Status Report on Alcohol and Health 2014*. Geneva, Switzerland: WHO; 2014.

111. McKenna JJ, McDade T. Why babies should never sleep alone: A review of the co-sleeping controversy in relation to SIDS, bedsharing and breast feeding. *Paediatr Respir Rev*. 2005;6:134—152.

112. Kohlendorfer U, Haberlandt E, Kiechl S, et al. Pre- and postnatal medical care and risk of sudden infant death syndrome. *Acta Paediatr*. 1997;86:600—603.

113. Mitchell EA, Scragg R, Stewart AW, et al. Results from the first year of the New Zealand cot death study. *N Z Med J*. 1991;104:71—76.

114. Shepherd CCJ, Li J, Cooper MN, Hopkins KD, et al. The impact of racial discrimination on the health of Australian Indigenous children aged 5—10 years: Analysis of national longitudinal data. *Int J Equity Health*. 2017;16:116.

115. NICE (National Institute for Health Care Excellence). *Appendix A CG37: Summary of New Evidence from Surveillance, Post-natal Care Up to 8 Weeks After Birth*. London: NICE; 2015.

116. Red Nose National Scientific Advisory Group. Information statement: Sharing a sleep surface with a baby. Published 2018. Available at https://rednose.org.au/article/sharing-asleep-surface-with-a-baby (accessed September 13, 2019).

117. Ball HL. The Atlantic Divide: Contrasting U.K. and U.S. recommendations on cosleeping and bed-sharing. *J Hum Lact*. 2017;33:765—769.

118. Young J, Shipstone R. Shared sleeping surfaces and dangerous sleeping environments. In: Duncan JR, Byard JR, eds. *SUDS Sudden Infant and Early Childhood Death: The Past, the Present and the Future*. Adelaide, Australia: University of Adelaide Press; 2018.

119. Moon RY, Mathews A, Joyner BL, et al. Health messaging and African-American infant sleep location: A randomized controlled trial. *J Community Health*. 2017;42:1—9.

120. Salm Ward TC, Balfour GM. Infant safe sleep interventions, 1990—2015: A review. *J Community Health*. 2016;41:180—196.

121. Moon RY, Mathews A, Oden R, et al. A qualitative analysis of how mothers' social networks are established and used to make infant care decisions. *Clin Pediatr (Phila)*. 2019;58:985—992.

122. Mitchell EA, Cowan S, Tipene-Leach D. The recent fall in postperinatal mortality in New Zealand and the Safe Sleep programme. *Acta Paediatr*. 2016;105:1312—1320.

123. Abel S, Tipene-Leach D. SUDI prevention: A review of Maori safe sleep innovations for infants. *N Z Med J*. 2013;126:86—94.

124. Abel S, Stockdalc-Frost A, Rolls R, et al. The wahakura: A qualitative study of the flax bassinet as a sleep location for New Zealand Maori infants. *N Z Med J*. 2015;128:12—19.

125. Mitchell EA, Thompson JMD. Who cosleeps? Does high maternal body weight and duvet use increase the risk of sudden infant death syndrome when bedsharing? *Paediatr Child Health*. 2006;11:14A—15A.

126. Carroll-Pankhurst C, Mortimer Jr. EA. Sudden infant death syndrome, bedsharing, parental weight, and age at death. *Pediatrics*. 2001;107:530—536.

ABM protocols expire 5 years from the date of publication. Content of this protocol is up-to-date at the time of publication. Evidence-based revisions are made within 5 years or sooner if there are significant changes in the evidence.

Peter S. Blair, PhD
Helen L. Ball, PhD
James J. McKenna, PhD
Lori Feldman-Winter, MD, MPH
Kathleen A. Marinelli, MD, FABM
Melissa C. Bartick, MD, FABM
The Academy of Breastfeeding Medicine Protocol Committee Members 2020:
Michal Young, MD, FABM, Chairperson
Larry Noble, MD, FABM, Translations Chairperson
Sarah Calhoun, MD
Megan Elliott-Rudder, MD
Laura Rachael Kair, MD, FABM
Susan Lappin, MD
Ilse Larson, MD
Ruth A. Lawrence, MD, FABM
Yvonne Lefort, MD, FABM
Nicole Marshall, MD, MCR
Katrina Mitchell, MD, FABM
Catherine Murak, MD
Eliza Myers, MD
Sarah Reece-Stremtan, MD
Casey Rosen-Carole, MD, MPH, MSEd
Susan Rothenberg, MD, FABM
Tricia Schmidt, MD
Tomoko Seo, MD, FABM
Natasha Sriraman, MD
Elizabeth K. Stehel, MD
Adora Wonodi, MD
Nancy Wight, MD
For correspondence: abm@bfmed.org

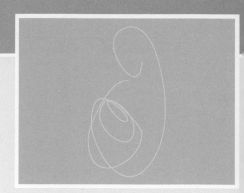

I APPENDIX

ABM Clinical Protocol #7
Model Maternity Policy Supportive of Breastfeeding*

Maria-Teresa Hernández-Aguilar[1,2], Melissa Bartick[3,4], Paula Schreck[5], Cadey Harrel[6] and The Academy of Breastfeeding Medicine

ABSTRACT

A central goal of The Academy of Breastfeeding Medicine is the development of clinical protocols for managing common medical problems that may impact breastfeeding success. These protocols serve only as guidelines for the care of breastfeeding mothers and infants and do not delineate an exclusive course of treatment or serve as standards of medical care. Variations in treatment may be appropriate according to the needs of an individual patient.

BACKGROUND

BREASTFEEDING IS THE BIOLOGICAL NORM and early weaning carries considerable maternal[1–5] (1),[6] and infant health[2,7–14] (1) risks, and considerable social costs worldwide[2,15] (1).[6,16] The care that mother and infant receive in the first postpartum days will influence their future breastfeeding success[17] (2),[18,19] health, and lives[15] (1).[16] To improve this care globally, the World Health Organization (WHO) and the United Nations International Children's Emergency Fund (UNICEF) launched the Baby-Friendly Hospital Initiative (BFHI) in 1991, which has since been revised twice.[20,21] After 27 years, it has been implemented globally[22]; significantly improved infant health[23–25] (1); and increased initiation, duration, and exclusivity of breastfeeding[1,24–27] (1). The BFHI is considered the gold standard of evidence-based policy for maternity facilities[28] that has been endorsed by different international organizations.[28–30] However, breastfeeding disparities associated with social and structural determinants of health are still widespread[8,15,31,32] (1).[33] These result in unequal rates of morbidity and mortality,[33,34] and health injustice for women and children[2,7,35,36] (1).[33] But, inequities may be reduced by implementing evidence-based maternity practices to support breastfeeding such as, BFHI[2] (1), one-to-one continuous support during labor and birth, culturally sensitive care[37] (M) or peer support[38] (1) among others.[33,39]

PURPOSE

Perinatal care practices influence delivery method, affect breastfeeding and maternal and infant health[40–44] (1)[45] (2)[46] (H)[47,48] and impact mother's satisfaction[49] (H). Thus, breastfeeding policies cannot be isolated from policies of maternity care as a whole. The purpose of this Protocol is to offer a "Model Maternity Policy Supportive of Breastfeeding," which includes an "Infant Feeding Policy." The term "Infant Feeding Policy" rather than "Breastfeeding Policy" is used as a step forward recognizing breastfeeding as the norm; it is inclusive (ensuring adequate support for parents feeding with supplements, exclusively with breast milk substitutes, exclusively with expressed breast milk, or chestfeeding in transgender individuals). It is also the language used in the updated 2018 WHO Ten Steps[21] (Table 1).

We have only included statements that are based on evidence or global recommendations in this document, which is intended to be a model for facilities seeking to implement high-quality perinatal care. It will need to be adapted to each specific institution, for example by including the name of the institution, and the date of revision, and follow each facility's institutional process for approval and implementation. We are aware that some of the recommendations listed here may need to be adapted to the specific situations of each country (e.g., a country lacking midwives may have other type of providers attending normal deliveries).

* Courtesy of the Academy of Breastfeeding Medicine. Please go to https://www.bfmed.org/protocols for complete protocols, translations, and the most up-to-date information (protocols are updated every 5–7 years).

[1] Breastfeeding Clinical Unit Dr. Peset, University Hospital Dr. Peset, National Health Service, Valencia, Spain.

[2] National Coordinator of Spain Baby-Friendly Initiative (IHAN-Espana Iniciativa para la Humanización de la Asistencia al Nacimiento y la Lactancia), Madrid, Spain.

[3] Department of Medicine, Cambridge Health Alliance, Cambridge, Massachusetts.

[4] Harvard Medical School, Boston, Massachusetts.

[5] Department of Pediatrics, Ascension St. John, Detroit, Michigan.

[6] Department of Family Medicine, University of Arizona, Tucson, Arizona.

TABLE 1   Ten Steps to Successful Breastfeeding (Revised 2018)

Critical management procedures	Step 1. Policies
	1a. Comply fully with the International Code of Marketing of Breast-milk Substitutes and relevant World Health Assembly resolutions.
	1b. Have a written infant feeding policy that is routinely communicated to staff and parents.
	1c. Establish ongoing monitoring and data-management systems.
	Step 2. Ensure that staff has sufficient knowledge, competence and skills to support breastfeeding.
Key clinical practices	Step 3. Discuss the importance and management of breastfeeding with pregnant women and their families.
	Step 4. Facilitate immediate and uninterrupted skin-to-skin contact and support mothers to initiate breastfeeding as soon as possible after birth.
	Step 5. Support mothers to initiate and maintain breastfeeding and manage common difficulties.
	Step 6. Do not provide breastfed newborns any food or fluids other than breast milk, unless medically indicated.
	Step 7. Enable mothers and their infants to remain together and to practice rooming-in 24 hours a day.
	Step 8. Support mothers to recognize and respond to their infants' cues for feeding.
	Step 9. Counsel mothers on the use and risks of feeding bottles, teats and pacifiers.
	Step 10. Coordinate discharge so that parents and their infants have timely access to ongoing support and care.

Adapted from The Ten Steps, WHO-UNICEF.[21]

This protocol includes all the elements covered by the BFHI "Global Criteria,"[21] because the BFHI is, at present, the best model with proven efficacy. Some countries' national Baby-Friendly accreditation standards may be more or less stringent than Global Criteria and those described herein. Thus, this model policy may require minor changes to conform to specific country requirements. This protocol will not address some specific requirements related to neonatal units, for which thorough recommendations have been published.[50,51]

ABOUT THE 2018 POLICY PROTOCOL

This comprehensive protocol encompasses contents of many other ABM Protocols: #1 (Guideline for Hypoglycemia),[52] #2 "(Going Home),[53] #3 (Supplementary Feedings in the Full-Term Neonate),[54] #5 (Peripartum Breastfeeding Management),[48] #8 (Milk Storage Information for Home Use for Full-Term Neonates),[55] #10 (Breastfeeding the Late Preterm and Early Term Infant),[56] #14 (Breastfeeding-friendly Physician's Office),[57] #19 (Breastfeeding Promotion in the Prenatal Setting),[58] #21 (Guidelines for Breastfeeding and Substance Use or Substance Use Disorder),[59] #26 (Persistent Pain with Breastfeeding),[60] and 28# (Peripartum Analgesia for the Breastfeeding Mother).[61]

A thorough scientific literature review (including recent statements/guidelines[21,50,51,62–66] was conducted in PubMed and LILACS. The search included documents in English, Spanish, French, and Portuguese published between 2011 and 2018. More than 1,000 abstracts were reviewed, those of low quality were discarded and a final total of 302 articles were analyzed in full. Quantitative evidence was rated according to the 2011 Oxford Center for Evidence-Based Medicine criteria: Levels of evidence are graded from (1) to (5) according to this criteria.[67] Qualitative evidence was graded using GRADECERQual: H (HIGH), M (MODERATE), L (LOW), VL (VERY LOW).[68] All citations grouped before a given level of evidence share that level of evidence. Expert or international guidelines, including ABM protocols, are not assigned levels of evidence, and certain research studies do not fall into the level of evidence categories.

We acknowledge that partners of birthing individuals may be of any gender. Also, although the vast majority of birthing individuals are women, we acknowledge that transgender men and nonbinary-gendered individuals may also give birth and many may want to breastfeed or feed at the chest (chestfeed). Some transgender female to male individuals who have undergone surgery to remove all or some of the breast parenchyma to achieve a flat chest wall may report variable experiences with milk production. They may wish to feed at the chest through supplemental devices or breastfeed, or conversely, some transgender parents may feel uncomfortable with the idea of breastfeeding or chestfeeding[69] (M)[70] (VL). Throughout this document, we may refer interchangeably to "mothers," "birthing individuals," or "parents."

We recognize that adopted newborns and their adoptive parents[71] (5), and infants born to surrogate mothers and their nonpuerperal mothers/parents[72] (5) equally need to bond and have the right for help with infant feeding (breastfeeding if chosen) and therefore are included in the words "mothers," "parents," and "infants."

Hereafter, the term "formula" refers to any kind of infant formula or breast milk substitute, including follow-up or any kind of "special formula."

RECOMMENDATIONS

Model maternity policy supportive of breastfeeding

Policy

1. This institution promotes breastfeeding considering that it is the biological norm for the human mother and

infant (dyad)and that artificial feeding and early weaning carries considerable maternal and infant health risks[1–5,7–14] (1).[6]

2. This institution recognizes the BFHI as the best and most efficacious intervention improving institutional maternity care with a significant positive effect on the incidence and duration of breastfeeding[24–27] (1) and infant health[23] (1).[62]

3. This document constitutes the Maternity Policy of this institution and includes an Infant Feeding Policy supportive of breastfeeding (or a dedicated Breastfeeding Policy). This policy is mandatory for all staff and nonabiding activities must be justified and written in the mother's and/or infant's clinical record.[21] This Policy:

   A. Addresses institutional responsibilities with respect to complying with the International Code of Marketing of Breast Milk Substitutes and subsequent resolutions of the World Health Assembly (The Code)[65,66] guaranteeing staff clinical competency and skills to promote, protect, and support breastfeeding, and monitoring its implementation.

   B. Addresses staff responsibilities (the implementation of key clinical practices) to ensure best maternal and infant care and adequately support best infant feeding practices.

   C. Addresses the need for all protocols and standards related to breastfeeding and infant feeding used in the maternity facility to be in line with WHO recommendations (i.e., BFHI standards) and current evidence-based guidelines and protocols.[21,63]

   D. Promotes skin-to-skin contact (SSC) immediately after birth and active support of breastfeeding, as part of the delivery of essential quality care during labor and delivery and childbirth quality care.[73]

   E. Ensures respectful, nondiscriminatory care practiced with cultural humility[74] for all parents and newborns, including adopted infants.[21,63,73]

   F. Guarantees that care and support for mothers and families is timely, appropriate and, sensitive to their needs,[21,62,63] honors privacy and informed choice,[57,63] and secures coordination among providers.[63]

4. To guarantee implementation of this policy:

   A. An Infant Feeding/Breastfeeding Committee whose primary focus is breastfeeding will be established to monitor and oversee the implementation of this Policy[75] (1). This committee is at the level of other Hospital Quality improvement committees and clinical practices.[21]

   B. The policy must be multidisciplinary and culturally appropriate and be composed of representatives of decision makers in the areas of maternal and newborn health, quality assurance and management, providers/physicians, nurses, midwives, lactation specialists, other appropriate staff, and parents. An elected breastfeeding coordinator and a secretary will chair and respond to the board.[21]

   C. Committee members will meet at least every 6 months for monitoring purposes. They will assess implementation of the policy and determine how often to assess institutional compliance with the policy. Committee members will define actions needed to remain compliant with the policy.[21]

   D. A mechanism for data collection directed to routinely track breastfeeding and mother–infant care indicators and policy implementation will be in place to continually monitor and improve quality of perinatal care.[21] Incorporation of breastfeeding indicators into the facility quality-improvement monitoring system is mandated.

   - Early initiation of breastfeeding and exclusive breastfeeding are considered sentinel indicators and must be routinely tracked.[21,63]
   - Other indicators may be added whenever considered necessary by the Infant Feeding/Breastfeeding committee.

   E. All staff will receive appropriate orientation to this Policy in the first weeks after hiring and periodically afterward.[21]

   F. A user-friendly summary of the policy will be made easily available to parents. There are clear written accountability mechanisms to redress comments, compliments, or complaints on the Policy compliance and there is a comment mechanism easily accessible to mothers and families whose content is periodically revised.[63]

5. This institution facilitates breastfeeding to their employees, allows for breastfeeding breaks, and has suitable areas available where staff (including residents)[76] (3) may breastfeed, express, and store their milk in appropriate conditions[77] (1)[78] (3).

6. This institution abides by The Code and related World Health Assembly resolutions[21,66] because noncompliance is a major undermining factor for breastfeeding[79–82] (1)[83] (M)[84] (3).

   A. This institution does not promote formula (nor related products covered in the Code). Direct contact of employees, manufacturers, or distributors of these products ("The Industry") with the public is not allowed inside premises[79] (1)[83] (M).[21,63,66]

   B. Gifts of any kind (including nonscientific literature, materials, equipment or money for staff, and materials, samples, coupons, or gift packs for mothers/families), any display (including posters or placards) or educational material with brand logos, and any educational or other type of events supported or paid by "The Industry" and directed to the staff, pregnant women, mothers, or families, are prohibited[63,84] (3).[66]

   C. Any product under the Code that may be needed by the institution (formula, teats, bottles, or pacifiers and others) will be bought at fair market value[80] (1).[66]

   D. Health care providers will receive training on the Code to avoid conflicts of interest and to avoid giving conflicting advice to mothers[81,85] (1)[83] (M).

   E. No promotional messages of industry foods or products, will be allowed in education materials aimed at mothers or families.[21]

F. This institution ensures that safe preparation and feeding of infant formula, and safe handling of bottles and teats, are demonstrated to birthing individuals and significant others only when needed (clinical indication for supplementation, breastfeeding contraindicated (Table 2), or not possible) or, after an informed choice made by parents (after a full explanation of the risks of breast milk substitutes).[21,63,179] This institution does not give group instruction on formula use and, the risks of not breastfeeding are fully explained to mothers who choose not to breastfeed.[21]

Staff training

7. This institution ensures that all staff caring for mothers and infants have the knowledge and skills needed for appropriate mother—infant care and breastfeeding management[86,87] (1)[17] (2) (Table 3).[21] A designated staff member coordinates staff training activity and keeps training records[75] (1).
   A. Health staff's knowledge and skills, about breast-feeding management[88,89] (1), mother infant care, interpersonal communications, and counseling[90] (2),[63] shall be assessed at hiring and periodically.
   B. The BFHI Breastfeeding education and skills standards will be the minimum required for all staff.[21]

TABLE 2   Potential Contraindications to Breastfeeding

Mother's conditions

Ebola Virus	Suspected (until ruled out) or confirmed maternal Ebola virus.
Herpes virus	Mothers with active herpetic lesions on the breast(s) should not breastfeed from the affected breast, but may breastfeed from the unaffected breast. Milk can be pumped from the affected breast, as there is no concern of hematologic transmission through the milk itself. However, milk can become contaminated via the breast pump, and thus should any part of the breast pump come in contact with herpetic lesions, that milk should be discarded. In this case, expression with discarding of milk should be encouraged to maintain milk supply until breastfeeding is resumed.
HIV	Maternal Human Immunodeficiency Virus infection is a contraindication in locations where artificial feeding is acceptable, feasible, affordable, sustainable, and safe. Check with local authorities as recommendations from individual countries may vary (for example, the US government stated that breastfeeding is not recommended for women living with HIV in the US, as of 2018, but offers guidance and counseling for those who wish to breastfeed).
HLTV I and II	Mothers with human T-cell lymphotropic virus type I or type II Current use of illicit drugs (e.g., cocaine, heroin, phencyclidine) as determined on a case-by-case basis by the infant's health care provider.
Varicella	If there is onset of Varicella within 5 days before or up to 48 hours after delivery, separation of the mother and infant with feeding of expressed milk until mother is no longer contagious is recommended, with administration of Varicella-Zoster Immune Globulin to the infant as soon as possible. Avoid close contact with skin lesions. (For older infants, separation of the mother and infant is not recommended, as the mother was contagious prior to the appearance of skin lesions and thus the infant was already exposed.) Expert consultation is advised.
Brucella	Untreated maternal brucellosis.
Tuberculosis	Mothers with active, untreated pulmonary tuberculosis (until no longer contagious: 15 days of treatment), should not breastfeed but infant can be given mother's own expressed milk.However, unless the diagnosis has been made in the 15 days pre-delivery, the infant will have been exposed by the time of the diagnosis, and must receive prophylaxis with isoniazid. There might thus be no reason to separate them, if the infant is already being treated. Expert consultation is advised.
Medications	Treatment with some medications such as chemotherapy, temporary or permanent cessation of breastfeeding may be advised. Check with LactMed, InfantRisk.com, or e-lactancia, Lactation Study or other local available accurate resources.
Illicit drugs	Current use of illicit drugs (e.g., cocaine, heroin, phencyclidine) as determined on a case-by-case basis by the infant's health care provider.

Infant's conditions

Inborn errors of metabolism	Galactosemia (except for Duarte variant, in which partial breastfeeding is possible).
	Congenital lactase deficiency.
	Some inborn errors of metabolism may require supplementation (phenylketonuria, maple syrup disease).

Sources: (ABM Protocols),[59,60] (official recommendations),[172,179,180] (web pages),[169–171] and (5).[181–184] Numbers in parentheses refer to Levels of Evidence (LOE) assigned, according to the OCEBM[67] (as in the rest of the text).

TABLE 3   List of Abilities to Be Assessed Among Staff Working with Mother and Infants in Maternity Facilities

1. How to use listening and learning skills to counsel a mother and use skills for building confidence and giving support to counsel a mother.
2. How to counsel a pregnant woman about breastfeeding.
3. How to explain to a mother about the optimal pattern of breastfeeding.
4. How to counsel a mother about benefits of breastfeeding to her own health.
5. How to help a mother to initiate breastfeeding within the first hour after birth.
6. How to adequately assess a breastfeed.
7. How to efficiently help a mother to position herself and her infant for breastfeeding and achieve a proper attachment of the infant.
8. How to help a mother to express her breast milk and to cup feed her infant.
9. How to help mothers with most frequent breastfeeding issues:
   a. mother who thinks she does not have enough milk;
   b. mother with an infant who cries frequently;
   c. mother whose infant is refusing to breastfeed;
   d. mother who has flat or inverted nipples;
   e. mother with engorged breasts;
   f. mother with sore or cracked nipples;
   g. mother with mastitis;
   h. mother breastfeeding a low-birth-weight or sick infant, using a supplemental tube at the breast or other devices, if indicated.
10. How to implement the Code in the health facility.

Source: World Health Organization-UNICEF.[21]

Whenever previous training does not meet the requirements, additional training will be required and breastfeeding and lactation management, and competencies will be verified within 6 months of hire, but ideally within 2 months of hire.

C. In-service training and periodic updates[75,87,91,92] (1)[62] with the appropriate content and duration to ensure compliance with BFHI Guidance[87,93] (1) and this policy, will be provided as needed.[21]

D. Supportive supervision[94] (2) will ensure that care is offered according to this Policy[63] and that correct, current, and consistent information is provided to all parents.[63]

Antenatal

8. Mothers will be empowered to have the birth experience most conducive to breastfeeding. A detailed breastfeeding history, including breastfeeding desired objectives, will be part of the prenatal history in the clinical record[95] (1).[58]

9. This facility ensures that all pregnant mothers attending prenatal care in this facility will be offered personalized antenatal breastfeeding support and education[75,87,96] (1)[41] (2) tailored to their concerns and needs. It will work with related facilities providing prenatal care to ensure that all mothers receive the information they need.

   A. Sessions will start early in the first or second antenatal visit to avoid lack of information to women who may deliver prematurely.[21]

   B. One-on-one and/or small group sessions will be delivered[97] (1) and partners and family will be encouraged to participate[98,99] (1).[58]

C. Midwives[100] (1)[101] (1) and other health care providers with lactation specialization[102] (1) will be the preferred staff providing this antenatal education.

10. The education provided at each visit will be documented in the woman's clinical history and all women will be provided a schedule with the information that will be offered (Table 4).[21] The curriculum taught to pregnant women includes essential information pertinent to breastfeeding and is shared with nearby organizations that offer antenatal education to families in the community.

11. Special consideration will be given to behavioral and psychoeducational approaches[58] to increase selfconfidence[103] (3) and empowerment techniques, including gender equity.

12. Education will be tailored to mothers' personal determinants (background, ethnicity, culture, socioeconomic)[58] and the special needs of women at risk of low breastfeeding: adolescents[104] (1), obese[105] (1), disenfranchised[102] (1),[106] (M) or disadvantaged groups[87,96] (1),[107] (2),[108] (M). mHealth (the use of mobile and wireless devices for health services) training will be offered if deemed necessary for families with difficult access to the institution[109] (1).[21]

Labor and delivery care

13. Physiological labor and birth will be promoted[49] (H) and harmful practices and unnecessary outdated interventions will be avoided.[63,73]

   A. All practices and interventions during labor, childbirth, and the early postnatal period in this institution conform to a written, up-to-date guidance that minimize the risk of cesarean delivery and instrumental vaginal delivery.[73] Both have been associated with

TABLE 4   Topics To Be Covered In Antenatal Education, Model Schedule

Visit date (weeks gestation)	Topics	Staff signature
Gest. week:__Visit #:__	1. The right to receive respectful maternity care — which refers to care organized for and provided to all women in a manner that maintains their dignity, privacy and confidentiality, ensures freedom from harm and mistreatment, and enables informed choice and continuous support during labour and childbirth.	
Gest. week:__Visit #:__	2. Non-pharmacologic pain relief methods during labor and the influence of delivery methods on breastfeeding success	
Gest. week:__Visit #:__	3. Global recommendations and importance of breastfeeding the importance of exclusive breastfeeding for the first 6 months, the risks of giving breast milk substitutes, and the importance of continuing breastfeeding after 6 months with appropriate complementary foods, for the first two years or beyond	
Gest. week:__Visit #:__	4. The importance of immediate and sustained skin-to-skin contact after birth	
Gest. week:__Visit #:__	5. The importance of early initiation of breastfeeding and rooming in on a 24-hour basis	
Gest. week:__Visit #:__	6. The basics of milk supply and demand, to ensure the infant's adequate nourishment.	
Gest. week:__Visit #:__	7. The basics of good positioning and attachment and recognition of feeding cues	
Gest. week:__Visit #:__	8. Management of most common initial challenges such as pain, cluster feeding, sleepy newborns, latching issues, engorgement and practice of safe sleep	

Depending on each institution's and/or BFHI national country requirements, topics and antenatal information may be needed to be covered at a certain time point (e.g., Baby-Friendly USA requires topics to be covered before 28 weeks). Visit #, visit number; Gest. week:, Gestational week at which the visit should take place.

Sources: (numbers in parentheses refer to the LOE assigned according to OCEBM[67]: (1),[40,44,186,187] (2),[43,107,188–190] (5),[189,190] (guidelines or protocols are not rated).[21,28,62,63,73]

adverse mother—child health outcomes[44,96,110] (1)[42] (2) and adverse breastfeeding outcomes[111,112] (1)[43] (2).

B. Patient-centered[47] sensitive and supportive care shall be offered.[63,73] The benefits, risks, and possible complications of interventions, such as pain control measures, route and type of narcotic analgesia, planned Cesarean delivery, and induced delivery, will be discussed.[73] Birthing individuals' informed choices will be respected[40,43,44] (1)[49] (H).

C. Mothers will be encouraged to choose the companion(s) of their choice during labor.[48,63,73]

D. Women with low-risk pregnancies who have the expectation of a normal delivery should be offered the option of a Midwife-Led Continuity of Care model service,[113] with one-on-one support being offered whenever possible[38,114,115] (1)[49] (H). (This recommendation applies only to settings with well-functioning midwifery programs).[63]

E. A trained birth companion or doula, will be allowed following the mother's wishes and the country/institution policies[38] (1).[48]

F. Nonpharmacological measures will be favored for uncomplicated cephalic deliveries. Medication, timing, and route of narcotic analgesia will be carefully chosen and discussed with the mother[113] (1)[61] to minimize risks for the dyad's health and breastfeeding[40] (1).

Postnatal care

14. Immediately after vaginal and Cesarean births, SSC will be offered and encouraged for all mothers and newborns

without complications[115,116] (1), regardless of feeding choice, and including late preterm (LPT) infants (34–36 6/7 weeks gestation)[56] and low birth weight (LBW) (between 1,200 and 2,500 g),[117] whenever stability of mother/infant allows.[117,118]

A. All well and alert newborns will be placed prone on mother's bare chest, naked, immediately after birth[119] (2). They will then be thoroughly dried (except hands), a diaper placed (if mother desires), and cover provided with a warm blanket to contain mother's heat[120] (5). Dyad and partner will be allowed to bond while being carefully observed. Infants should be left to experience the nine phases of newborn behavior that occur naturally when an infant is placed skin-to-skin at birth[121] (2), such as smelling, licking, resting, and crawling toward the nipple before latching spontaneously[121] (2)[122] (4)[123] (5).[28,117]

B. SSC will not be interrupted for at least 2 hours1[15,116,124,125] (1)[126] (2)[127] (5) (Table 4) or until first breastfeed, unless required for justified medical reasons. If a delay or interruption of initial SSC has been necessary, staff will ensure that mother and infant receive SSC as soon as clinically possible[127] (5).[21,28,48,62,128] Time of initiation and end of SSC shall be documented in the medical record.

C. The room temperature in the birthing environment will be set at or above 25°C (77°F) and free of draughts.[63] Staff will avoid bright lights and loud noises to help the infants unfold their innate reflexes.[28,63]

D. Needed measures will be in place to facilitate immediate (or as soon as possible) SSC after a Cesarean delivery, ideally in the operating room or the recovery area[115,125] (1)[126] (2). Use of transparent surgical drapes will be favored attending to the mother's wishes to provide a positive experience for the mother.

E. Continuous supervision (intervening only if needed) and safe positioning to minimize the risk of Sudden Unexpected Postnatal Collapse with directions for staff and the mother's companions to monitor the mother and infant are included in skin-to-skin procedures protocol. A protocol with recommendations on safe sleep and SSC in the neonatal period based on evidence[127] (5) will guide staff practice.

F. Apgar scores will be performed with the infant skin-to-skin[127] (5). Oral, nasal, or tracheal suction will not be done for babies who start to breathe on their own even when meconium is present in the amniotic fluid.[117]

G. Umbilical cord clamping will be delayed in both preterm and term infants[129] (1)[117,130] except when mother or infant are unstable[131] (1)[117] or if harvesting of cord blood is desired.[132]

H. The infant's anthropometric measurements,[133] (3) intramuscular vitamin K administration,[134,135] ophthalmic prophylaxis,[136] and hepatitis B vaccine administration[137] will be delayed at least after the first hours of uninterrupted mother–infant contact or first breastfeeding.[48,63]

I. Bathing will be delayed for at least 24 hours.[73]

J. Immediate SSC with father or partner will be offered only if mother is not available[126] (2).[50]

K. All parents (with preference time for the mother) will be encouraged to have their newborns SSC during their stay in the postpartum unit[127] (5).

15. All mothers and all newborns able to breastfeed (including LBW and preterm infants) shall be supported to breastfeed as soon as possible within the first hour of birth[125,138,139] (1).[56,62,118]

A. Help will be offered to facilitate the infant's first latch, if the infant does not latch spontaneously in the first hour or at the request of the mother[115] (1).[48,118]

B. Preterm infants, and early term babies will be offered special help to ensure latch and adequate transfer of milk[140] (1).[56] Close observation needed by preterm and LBW infants for the first 12–24 hours will be offered during skin-to-skin care, Kangaroo care,[141] (1) breastfeeding, and rooming-in.[56,117] Mothers will be encouraged to breastfeed on demand as soon as the infant's condition permits.[21]

16. Every mother shall be offered as much help as needed with breastfeeding. The staff will ensure that the mother is able to position and attach her infant at the breast. At-risk mothers (complicated and Cesarean deliveries, obese, adolescents, patients with tobacco use, lack of partner support, intimate partner violence) will have tailored extra help.[21,48]

A. Trained staff will observe carefully the first breastfeeding sessions, looking for signs of effective latch, position, and effective feeding. If everything goes well they will not intervene. If improvement is needed, the mother will first be gently shown how to improve the latch and positioning herself, and avoid having the staff do it for her.[28]

B. Trained staff will observe and document at least one feed every shift until discharge and, with each staff contact with the mother whenever possible. Positioning, latch, milk transfer, infant's output frequency and characteristics, jaundice and infant's weight, and any feeding problem will be recorded in the clinical history.[48]

C. Maternal semirecumbent position (biologic nurturing) will be encouraged in the early postpartum period,[122] (4) but each mother will be empowered to find her own most comfortable position.

D. Mothers and partners will be enabled to recognize hunger cues, signs of good positioning and effective latching, to identify suckling, swallowing, and milk transfer and, to optimize milk production.[21,48]

E. The staff will address any breastfeeding problem (nipple pain, latch difficulties, insufficient milk supply)[48] and referral will be made to a lactation specialist whenever needed. Management of most common breastfeeding difficulties will be discussed with every breastfeeding parent before discharge (Tables 3 and 5).[21]

17. All mothers will be taught breast massage and breast milk hand-expression techniques during their stay[142] (1)[143] (2) and, if desired they will be taught how to use a breast pump. Mothers and families will be taught that obtaining only a few milliliters is frequent during the first episodes of milk expression, and does not signify low milk production.

A. Breast massage and hand expression shall be taught early whenever:
   - Newborns are not able to get colostrum through latch alone.
   - Preterm, early term, and any infant are not latching effectively in the first 24 hours[143] (2).
   - Newborns are at risk of hypoglycemia (diabetic mothers, undernourished infants), to supplement with colostrum on the first feeds after breastfeeding.
   - The infant cannot breastfeed directly (e.g., preterm or sick infants).
   - Mother–infant separation is unavoidable.
   - Mother is at risk for delayed lactogenesis II (Table 6).

B. Whenever separation lasts more than a few days mothers will be advised to use a double set-up electric breast pump, at least eight times per day, combined with hand expression[144] (3) (which has proven useful in mothers of preterm infants), and breast massage and hand expression will also be taught early.

TABLE 5   List of Essential Issues That Every New Breastfeeding Mother (and Family) Should Know and/or Demonstrate (to Be Verified with Mothers Before Discharge)

1. The importance of breastfeeding exclusively and mother/parent infant eye-to-eye and body contact while feeding.
2. Feeding cues and signs of an adequate latch, swallowing, milk transfer and infant satisfaction and how to recognize all of them.
3. The average feeding frequency (8–12 times per 24 hours) with some infants needing more frequent feedings.
4. How to breastfeed in a comfortable position without pain.
5. Infants should be fed in response to feeding cues, offered both breasts per feeding and fed and until they seem satisfied.
6. How to ensure and enhance milk production and let down.
   a. Why and how to hand express colostrum/breastmilk.
   b. Mothers who need to pump must know how to correctly use and care for their breast pump.
7. The effects of pacifiers and artificial teats on breastfeeding and why to avoid them until lactation is established.
8. Not all medications nor mother's illnesses contraindicate breastfeeding.
   a. Accurate information resources: www.e-lactancia.org and www.mommymeds.com are user-friendly resources for parents.
   b. Reasons for a breastfeeding mother to avoid tobacco, alcohol and other drugs.
9. Safe sleeping instructions (how to make co-sleeping safer), particularly avoiding sofas and tobacco.
10. Recognize signs of undernourishment or dehydration in the infant and warning signs for calling a health professional.
    a. <u>Infant</u>: usually not waking for more than 4 hours or, always awake or, never seeming satisfied or, more than 12 feeds per day, or no signs of swallowing with at least every 3–4 sucks, too few wet/heavy or soiled diapers per day, fever.
    b. <u>Mother</u>: persistent painful latch or, breast lumps, breast pain, fever, doubts with milk production, aversion to the child, profound sadness and any doubt with breastfeeding self-efficacy.

Adapted from WHO-UNICEF[21] with additions from the following sources: (numbers in parentheses refer to the LOE assigned according to OCEBM[67]): (web pages),[172,192] (5),[191] (4),[185] (1).[192]

TABLE 6   Risk Factors for Delayed or Failed Lactogenesis II or Low Milk Supply

Maternal factors	Infant factors
Age over 30, Primiparity.	Early term birth (37–39 weeks).
Breast problems: Insufficient glandular tissue, flat or inverted nipples tissue, history of breast surgery.	Infant Apgar <8.
Delivery problems: Cesarean delivery (especially if unplanned), complicated delivery, significant hemorrhage, prolonged labor, preterm delivery (<37 weeks), retained placenta.	High birth weight >3600 g.
Postpartum depression.	Low birth weight (<2500 g).
Metabolic problems: Diabetes (gestational, types 1 or 2), hypertension, preeclampsia, polycystic ovary syndrome, obesity (pre-pregnancy BMI >30), high cortisol levels, hypothyroidism, extreme tiredness, fatigue or stress.	Poor or painful latch / restricted feedings.
Previous low supply.	Prelacteal feeds.
Tobacco use and some drugs and medications may cause low milk supply.	Prematurity (<37 weeks).

Delayed Lactogenesis II is defined as little or no maternal perception of breast fullness or leaking at least 72 hours post-birth.
Sources: This table has been constructed with information from references (numbers in parentheses refer to the LOE assigned according to OCEBM[67]): (1),[141,193] (5).[194]

C. Mothers identified prenatally or soon after delivery, as at risk of delayed lactogenesis II (Table 6), will be assigned to special help as deemed appropriate. A feeding plan and close follow-up of the infant (for adequate hydration and nutrition besides help with expression) will be offered. At discharge, continuum of care will be ensured with a feeding plan and close follow-up.[48]

D. Enough staffing time will be allocated to ensure that adequate supervision and help is possible for all new mothers and infants.[21,48]

E. Painful procedures, such as Immunizations, vitamin K administration, or heel pricks shall be done while breastfeeding as it is the best method to soothe pain in the neonate[145] (2).

18. Individualized appropriate care for each mother of preterm or LBW infants will be offered, both for attending to the infant needs as well as family centered care and continuity of care.[50,51]

A. Preterm infants may be able to root, latch, and suck from 27 weeks; however, ineffective breastfeeding is likely.[21] Preterm and early term infants will be offered special help to ensure adequate latch and milk transfer[140] (1).[56]

B. Every effort will be made for LBW (including Very Low Birth Weight) infants, to be fed their mother's own milk or, if that is unavailable, pasteurized donor human milk.[117,128] Mothers of preterm and LBW infants will be helped to start expressing as soon as possible, preferably within 1 hour of birth[146] (3),[21,63] (if no SSC has been possible)[147] (3) but at least in the first 6 hours[146] (3).[56]

C. Mothers will be supported and encouraged to express their breasts at least five times per day aiming to eight sessions per day, and at least one night session in 24 hours, to ensure an adequate milk supply. Space to pump milk near their infants in the neonatal ward will be made available and privacy may be provided with screens upon request. Guidance will be offered on breast massage, hand expression, usage of an electric breast pump (double set-up if feasible)[148] (2). Encouragement to pump immediately after SSC[149] (2) and hand expression accompanied by pumping at least eight times[56] will be offered to increase milk supply whenever needed[144] (3).

D. For infants <2,000 g, Kangaroo mother care will be instituted as soon as possible after birth for infants and as close to continuously as possible,[63,117] and will be facilitated to all mothers once the infant is stable[141,150] (1)[151] (5). Unlimited access to the neonatal ward for mothers and partners[141,152] (1) is guaranteed. For that purpose, mothers will be provided with clothing and adequate space to sit–lay in a semireclined position and enabled to hold their infants prone and naked between their breasts. Staff will facilitate feedings whenever infant shows early feeding cues.

E. When going home, written and spoken instructions for proper storage and labeling of breast milk will be provided for all mothers who are separated from their infants.[55] Mothers will be encouraged to continue pumping and whenever possible, the institution will facilitate the provision of breast pumps.

19. Breastfeeding mothers will be encouraged to exclusively breastfeed (feeding only breast milk, no other liquids or solids except for vitamins/medications) unless supplements (water, glucose solutions, formula, or other liquid) are medically indicated (ABM Protocol #3).[54] Supplements will not be offered to newborns unless medically indicated or by the mother's documented and informed request.[21,62] If supplements are needed:

A. Preferred order will be: colostrum/mother's own milk, pasteurized donor human milk,[21,62] ready-mixed formula, and powdered or concentrated formula mixed with clean water. On the first 1–2 days of life, term infants do not need more than 2–15 mL per feeding.[48]

B. Mothers will be encouraged to express colostrum or milk directly into the infant's mouth or to feed by

alternative methods other than bottle/artificial teats (a cup, finger, syringe, paladai, or a spoon are preferred).[54] Supplementing through tubing at chest may help stimulate the mother's breast while feeding the infant[153] (1).

C. Supplements will not be given without a medical order,[21] including by mother's request. Orders given for medical indications will require daily review and renewal. Medical indications for supplementation, type of supplement, times, amount, method of feeding the supplement, and instructions given to mothers regarding supplementation will be documented in the clinical record of mother/infant.[21,54]

D. Mothers who ask for supplementation when not medically indicated will have their reasons listened to and explored. A careful assessment of breastfeeding will be offered and the risks of supplementing will be discussed with mothers and relatives.[54]

E. Safe preparation, feeding, handling, and storage of breast milk substitutes will be individually taught to families who do not breastfeed or need supplements, at discharge,[21] and written instructions will be given if appropriate.

20. In this institution, we recognize and facilitate the need for all mothers and healthy term babies to remain together 24 hours per day (rooming-in) for their mutual well-being, regardless of parent's feeding choice, or delivery method)[154] (1).[63,117] Unless legally mandated, this facility does not have a dedicated nursery space for healthy term newborns (although eliminating the nursery is not a requirement of BFHI). Should this institution maintain a nursery, the infants therein would not be visible to passersby, thereby deflecting interest, and neither normalize separation nor appear to endorse or encourage its use.

A. Rooming-in is facilitated for all newborns[155] (2),[21] including LPT infants[140] (1)[56] or LBW >1,750 g who meet specific medical and safety criteria[156] (2). Maternity beds with sidecar basinets will be facilitated for hospital use[157,158] (2).

B. Separation of mothers and infants will occur only for justified clinical reasons. Documentation of interruption of rooming-in with reason for interruption, location of infant during interruption, and time parameters for interruption is required[154] (1)[56] from staff. Rooming-in will be reinstated as soon as the reason ceases. Whenever a mother must be separated from her infant the staff will support the mother to begin expressing her milk as soon as possible and at least within the first 6 hours of separation.[21] Whenever parents request their infant be kept apart from them, their reasons for such care will be explored and the importance of rooming-in for the infant's health and wellbeing will be explained[154] (1). The education will be documented. If the infant is separated either for medical reasons or parental choice, the nurse caring for the infant will be responsible for bringing the infant to the mother as soon as the infant displays feeding cues, to support exclusive breastfeeding.

C. All routine procedures, assessments, newborn screens, cardiac screens, immunizations, hearing screens, and routine laboratory draws shall be performed at the mother's bedside.[48,63] Routine blood glucose monitoring of term healthy infants is not indicated.[52,73] Newborn bathing is not necessary in most cases, but if desired, parents will perform it whenever possible, with assistance of staff.[48,73]

D. Infants who need intravenous antibiotics or phototherapy, but are otherwise healthy and stable, will be allowed to remain with the mother[125] (1).[56]

E. Safe rooming-in practices training to prevent infant falls and suffocation incidents, will be regularly offered to families, including information about high-risk hours (early morning) and risk factors (exhausted parents), particularly advice to feed the infant in an adult bed at night or when tired, instead of on a sofa or recliner.[159] Increased surveillance will be offered to mother–infant dyads that have been identified at higher risk[127] (5).[56]

21. Hospital staff will ensure that all mothers, regardless of delivery method or feeding choice, know how to respond to their infant cues for feeding, closeness, and comfort. Scheduled feeding of stable newborns is not recommended.[21,30,73]

A. No restrictions will be placed on the frequency or length of feeding (crying is a late feeding cue).[21]

B. Mothers will be taught that:
- Infants need at least breastfeed eight times per day, and, many need more frequent feedings.
- It is important to offer both breasts at each feeding, but if the infant gets satiated only with one breast, the opposite side should be offered at the next feed.
- Cluster feedings (several feeds close together) are common in the first 24–36 hours and may stimulate breast milk production. They are not a sign of insufficient milk neither is supplementation required.[30] Later, they may signal insufficient milk transfer[160] (5).

C. While rooming in, parents of LBW, preterm or early term newborns, and newborns who are losing excess weight, will be instructed to feed the infant at early feeding cues and awaken them if necessary, so that the infant receives at least 8 feeds per 24 hours.[56] Whenever separation occurs, staff will bring infants to mothers for feeding, every time staff notice feeding cues.[21]

22. Pacifiers, artificial nipples, or teats will not *routinely* be used nor routinely offered to healthy-term breastfeeding infants[161,162] (1)[155,163] (2)[164,165] (3).[54]

A. If a mother requests that her infant be given a bottle or teat, staff will explore reasons for the request, address concerns, and educate on the risks

of their use, with emphasis on the effects on suckling. Breastfeeding will be assessed to rule out breastfeeding difficulties[165] (3).[21]

B. Staff will not routinely give pacifiers to breastfeeding infants. If a mother requests a pacifier, the staff will explore the reasons for the request, address the mother's concerns, and educate her on potential problems with pacifier use and the education will be documented. Informed mother decisions on teats or pacifier use will be honored and documented in the medical record.[54]

C. Preterm or sick infants in the Neonatal Intensive Care or Special Care Unit may have pacifiers indicated for non-nutritive sucking.[21,50,163]

D. Nipple shields (or bottle nipples) will be only used on recommendation by a lactation specialist and after other attempts to correct the difficulty have failed[166] (1)[167] (2).[50]

E. Breastfeeding will be the preferred soothing method for any breastfed infant undergoing a painful procedure[145] (2). Pacifiers will be given for pain soothing during a procedure, only if breastfeeding is not possible and will be discarded after the procedure.

23. This institution will use evidence-based sources for medication safe use with lactating mothers, such as LactMed,[168] InfantRisk,[169] the Lactation Study Center,[170] or APILAM webpage: www.e-lactancia.org.[171] Pharmacological inhibition of lactation will not be offered routinely to inhibit lactation.[172,173] Nonpharmacological measures, such as ice and mild analgesics to alleviate discomfort, breast expression to comfort, and breast support to avoid engorgement, will be advised[174] (1).[172] In birthing individuals, where inhibition of lactation may be necessary for medical or psychological reasons, and after the birthing individual has made an informed decision[173] (5), lisuride and cabergoline may be used[175] (1).

Continuum of care/going home

24. This institution offers coordinated care with clear, accurate information exchange between relevant health and social care professionals[63] for all mothers, infants, and family.

A. Before discharge, the health care team will ensure that there is effective breastfeeding that breastfeeding mothers are able to efficiently breastfeed their infants and that continuity of care is guaranteed, either by follow-up visits (including home visits) or by arranging qualified primary care providers and/or lactation specialists visits and/or support groups or peer counseling contacts[1,21,28,62,176] (1).

B. If the infant is still not latching or feeding well at the time of discharge, an individualized feeding plan will be devised and depending on the dyad's clinical situation and resources, the infant's discharge may be delayed.[53,54] A healthy infant will not be discharged without his mother if she needs to stay for any clinical reason, unless staying together is impossible (e.g., mother in the medical intensive care unit).

C. Education written material on breastfeeding will be facilitated and discussed with mothers and partners[177] (2) as appropriate, but will not be substituted for person-centered, proactive personal support[178] (1)[46] (H). Efforts will be made to include family in educational activities. Before leaving the hospital, staff will make sure that birthing individuals have certain knowledge and skills (Table 4).

25. This institution collaborates with community-based programs to coordinate breastfeeding messages and offer continuity of care.

A. Before discharge, contacts with local support groups or other breastfeeding support community resources will be provided for all dyads[1] (1).

B. A visit with a health care provider will be secured for every mother—infant dyad to assess the mother and infant's general well-being, feeding situation, presence of infant jaundice, 2—4 days after birth and again in the next week.[21]

C. Whenever needed, a visit for specifically following up on feeding issues will be arranged. Home visits may be planned or arranged as they have demonstrated importance to extend breastfeeding duration[1] (1).

APPLICATION

All birthing individuals.

OTHER RELATED ABM PROTOCOLS

Protocols #1, #2, #3, #5, #8, #10, #14, #19, #21, #26, #28.

RESEARCH NEEDS

While researching for evidence to build this protocol, certain issues have arisen as lacking enough or at all evidence, such as effective strategies to increase implementation of BFHI practices in the hospital setting or best ways to monitor staff adherence to a hospital's breastfeeding policy. There is need for controlled studies of prenatal and early hand expression in mothers of term infants at risk for delayed lactogenesis II; and its effect on the timing of lactogenesis II, milk volume, and duration of breastfeeding should be better determined. On-demand feeding, best positions for breastfeeding, SSC with nonfather parents and other relatives (if mother is not available), best treatment to inhibit lactation when needed and, transgender parents' chest-feeding experiences and how to support them, are other issues where adequate research or any research at all is lacking.

REFERENCES

1. Feltner C, Palmieri Weber R, Stuebe AM, et al. *Breastfeeding Programs and Policies, Breastfeeding Uptake, and Maternal Health Outcomes in Developed Countries.* Rockville, MD: Agency for Healthcare Research and Quality; 2018 .

2. Victora CG, Bahl R, Barros AJ, et al. Breastfeeding in the 21st century: Epidemiology, mechanisms, and lifelong effect. *Lancet.* 2016;387:475—490.

3. Chowdhury R, Sinha B, Sankar MJ, et al. Breastfeeding and maternal health outcomes: A systematic review and meta-analysis. *Acta Paediatr.* 2015;104:96—113.

4. Merritt MA, Riboli E, Murphy N, et al. Reproductive factors and risk of mortality in the European Prospective Investigation into Cancer and Nutrition; a cohort study. *BMC Med.* 2015;13:252.

5. Nguyen B, Jin K, Ding D. Breastfeeding and maternal cardiovascular risk factors and outcomes: A systematic review. *PLoS One.* 2017;12:e0187923.

6. Bartick MC, Schwarz EB, Green BD, et al. Suboptimal breastfeeding in the United States: Maternal and pediatric health outcomes and costs. *Matern Child Nutr.* 2017;13:3—6. Erratum in *Matern Child Nutr* 2017.

7. Sankar MJ, Sinha B, Chowdhury R, et al. Optimal breastfeeding practices and infant and child mortality: A systematic review and meta-analysis. *Acta Paediatr.* 2015;104(Suppl 467):3—13.

8. Cleminson J, Oddie S, Renfrew MJ, et al. Being baby friendly: Evidence-based breastfeeding support. *Arch Dis Child Fetal Neonatal Ed.* 2015;100:F173—F178.

9. Bowatte G, Tham R, Allen KJ, et al. Breastfeeding and childhood acute otitis media: A systematic review and meta-analysis. *Acta Paediatr.* 2015;104(Suppl 467): 85—95.

10. Giugliani ER, Horta BL, Loret de Mola C, et al. Effect of breastfeeding promotion interventions on child growth: A systematic review and meta-analysis. *Acta Paediatr.* 2015;104 (Suppl 467):20—29.

11. Horta BL, Loret de Mola C, Victora CG. Long-term consequences of breastfeeding on cholesterol, obesity, systolic blood pressure and type 2 diabetes: A systematic review and meta-analysis. *Acta Paediatr.* 2015;104(Suppl 467):30—37.

12. Horta BL, Loret de Mola C, Victora CG. Breastfeeding and intelligence: A systematic review and meta-analysis. *Acta Paediatr.* 2015;104(Suppl 467):14—19.

13. Horta BL, de Sousa BA, de Mola CL. Breastfeeding and neurodevelopmental outcomes. *Curr Opin Clin Nutr Metab Care.* 2018;21:174—178.

14. Lodge CJ, Tan DJ, Lau M, et al. Breastfeeding and asthma and allergies: A systematic review and meta-analysis. *Acta Paediatr.* 2015;104(Suppl 467):38—53.

15. Rollins NC, Bhandari N, Hajeebhoy N, et al. Why invest, and what it will take to improve breastfeeding practices? *Lancet.* 2016;387:491—504.

16. Hansen K. Breastfeeding: A smart investment in people and in economies. *Lancet.* 2016;387:416.

17. Babakazo P, Donnen P, Akilimali P, et al. Predictors of discontinuing exclusive breastfeeding before six months among mothers in Kinshasa: A prospective study. *Int Breastfeed J.* 2015;10:19.

18. Graham W, Woodd S, Byass P, et al. Diversity and divergence: The dynamic burden of poor maternal health. *Lancet.* 2016;388:2164—2175.

19. McDougall L, Campbell OMR, Graham W. *Maternal Health. An Executive Summary for the Lancet's Series.* London: The Lancet Maternal Health Series; 2016.

20. World Health Organization. *Baby-Friendly Hospital Initiative: Revised, Updated and Expanded for Integrated Care.* Geneva: World Health Organization; 2009.

21. World Health Organization-UNICEF. *Implementation Guidance: Protecting, Promoting, and Supporting Breastfeeding in Facilities Providing Maternity and Newborn Services: The Revised Baby-Friendly Hospital Initiative.* Geneva: World Health Organization; 2018.

22. World Health Organization. *National Implementation of the Baby-Friendly Hospital Initiative 2017.* Geneva: World Health Organization; 2017.

23. Martens PJ. What do Kramer's Baby-Friendly Hospital Initiative PROBIT studies tell us? A review of a decade of research. *J Hum Lact.* 2012;28:335−342.

24. Perez-Escamilla R, Martinez JL, Segura-Perez S. Impact of the Baby-Friendly Hospital Initiative on breastfeeding and child health outcomes: A systematic review. *Matern Child Nutr.* 2016;12:402−417.

25. Meek JY, Noble L. Implementation of the ten steps to successful breastfeeding saves lives. *JAMA Pediatr.* 2016;170:925−926.

26. Spaeth A, Zemp E, Merten S, et al. Baby-friendly hospital designation has a sustained impact on continued breastfeeding. *Matern Child Nutr.* 2018;14.

27. Vieira TO, Vieira GO, de Oliveira NF, et al. Duration of exclusive breastfeeding in a Brazilian population: New determinants in a cohort study. *BMC Pregnancy Childbirth.* 2014;14:175.

28. EU Project on Promotion of Breastfeeding in Europe. *Protection, promotion and support of breastfeeding in Europe: Blueprint for action (revised 2008).* Luxembourg: European Commission, Directorate Public Health and Risk Assessment; 2008.

29. US Department of Health and Human Services. *The Surgeon General's Call to Action to Support Breastfeeding.* Washington, DC: US Department of Health and Human Services, Office of the Surgeon General; 2011.

30. Perinatal Services BC. *Breastfeeding Healthy Term Infants.* Vancouver, BC: Perinatal Services BC; 2015.

31. Renfrew MJ, Pokhrel S, Quigley M, et al. *Preventing Disease and Saving Resources: The Potential Contribution of Increasing Breastfeeding Rates in the UK.* London: UNICEF UK; 2012.

32. Jones KM, Power ML, Queenan JT, et al. Racial and ethnic disparities in breastfeeding. *Breastfeed Med.* 2015;10:186−196.

33. UNICEF. *World Health Organization. Capture the moment: Early initiation of breastfeeding: The best start for every newborn.* New York: UNICEF; 2018.

34. Bartick MC, Jegier BJ, Green BD, et al. Disparities in breastfeeding: Impact on maternal and child health outcomes and costs. *J Pediatr.* 2017;181(49−55):e46.

35. Sacker A, Kelly Y, Iacovou M, et al. Breast feeding and intergenerational social mobility: What are the mechanisms? *Arch Dis Child.* 2013;98:666−671.

36. Victora CG, Requejo J, Boerma T, et al. Countdown to 2030 for reproductive, maternal, newborn, child, and adolescent health and nutrition. *Lancet Glob Health.* 2016;4:e775−e776.

37. Condon LJ, Salmon D. 'You likes your way, we got our own way': Gypsies and Travellers' views on infant feeding and health professional support. *Health Expect.* 2015;18:784−795.

38. Bohren MA, Hofmeyr GJ, Sakala C, et al. Continuous support for women during childbirth. *Cochrane Database Syst Rev.* 2017;7:CD003766.

39. Centers for Disease Control and Prevention. Breastfeeding Among U.S. Children Born 2002−2014, CDC National Immunization Survey. 2017. Available at https://www.cdc.gov/breastfeeding/data/nis_data/results.html (accessed March 3, 2018).

40. French CA, Cong X, Chung KS. Labor epidural analgesia and breastfeeding: A systematic review. *J Hum Lact.* 2016;32:507−520.

41. Carvalho ML, Boccolini CS, Oliveira MI, et al. The Baby Friendly Hospital Initiative and breastfeeding at birth in Brazil: A cross sectional study. *Reprod Health.* 2016;13(Suppl 3):119.

42. Black L, Hulsey T, Lee K, et al. Incremental hospital costs associated with comorbidities of prematurity. *Manag Care.* 2015;24:54−60.

43. Hobbs AJ, Mannion CA, McDonald SW, et al. The impact of caesarean section on breastfeeding initiation, duration and difficulties in the first four months postpartum. *BMC Pregnancy Childbirth.* 2016;16:90.

44. Hofmeyr GJ, Barrett JF, Crowther CA. Planned caesarean section for women with a twin pregnancy. *Cochrane Database Syst Rev.* 2015;CD006553.

45. Cabrera-Rubio R, Mira-Pascual L, Mira A, et al. Impact of mode of delivery on the milk microbiota composition of healthy women. *J Dev Orig Health Dis.* 2016;7:54−60.

46. Sudhinaraset M, Afulani P, Diamond-Smith N, et al. Advancing a conceptual model to improve maternal health quality: The person-centered care framework for reproductive health equity. *Gates Open Res.* 2017;1:1.

47. World Health Assembly. *Framework on Integrated People Centered Health Services.* Geneva: World Health Organization; 2016.

48. Holmes AV, McLeod AY, Bunik M. ABM clinical protocol #5: Peripartum breastfeeding management for the healthy mother and infant at term, revision 2013. *Breastfeed Med.* 2013;8:469−473.

49. Downe S, Finlayson K, Oladapo O, et al. What matters to women during childbirth: A systematic qualitative review. *PLoS One.* 2018;13:e0194906.

50. Nyqvist KH, Maastrup R, Hansen MN, et al. *Neo-BFHI: The Baby-Friendly Hospital Initiative for neonatal wards. Core document with recommended standards and criteria.* Raleigh, NC: International Lactation Consultant Association; 2015.

51. International Lactation Consultant Association. *Neo-BFHI Package.* Raleigh, NC: ILCA; 2018.

52. Wight N, Marinelli KA. Academy of Breastfeeding M.ABM clinical protocol #1: Guidelines for blood glucose monitoring and treatment of hypoglycemia in term and late-preterm neonates, revised 2014. *Breastfeed Med.* 2014;9:173−179.

53. Evans A, Marinelli KA, Taylor JS. Academy of Breastfeeding Medicine. ABM clinical protocol #2: Guidelines for hospital discharge of the breastfeeding term newborn and mother: "The going home protocol. *Breastfeed Med.* 2014;9:3−8.

54. Kellams A, Harrel C, Omage S, et al. ABM clinical protocol #3: Supplementary feedings in the healthy term breastfed neonate, revised 2017. *Breastfeed Med.* 2017;12:188−198.

55. Eglash A, Simon L. Academy of Breastfeeding M. ABM clinical protocol #8: Human milk storage information for home

use for full-term infants, revised 2017. *Breastfeed Med.* 2017;12:390–395.

56. Boies EG, Vaucher YE. ABM Clinical Protocol #10: Breastfeeding the late preterm (34–36 6/7 weeks of gestation) and early term infants (37–38 6/7 weeks of gestation), second revision 2016. *Breastfeed Med.* 2016;11:494–500.

57. Grawey AE, Marinelli KA, Holmes AV. Academy of Breastfeeding M. ABM clinical protocol #14: Breastfeeding friendly physician's office: Optimizing care for infants and children, revised 2013. *Breastfeed Med.* 2013;8:237–242.

58. Rosen-Carole C, Hartman S. Academy of Breastfeeding M. ABM clinical protocol #19: Breastfeeding promotion in the prenatal setting, revision 2015. *Breastfeed Med.* 2015;10:451–457.

59. Reece-Stremtan S, Marinelli KA. ABM clinical protocol #21: Guidelines for breastfeeding and substance use or substance use disorder, revised 2015. *Breastfeed Med.* 2015;10:135–141.

60. Berens P, Eglash A, Malloy M, et al. ABM clinical protocol #26: Persistent pain with breastfeeding. *Breastfeed Med.* 2016;11:46–53.

61. Martin E, Vickers B, Landau R, et al. ABM clinical protocol #28, peripartum analgesia and anesthesia for the breastfeeding mother. *Breastfeed Med.* 2018;13:164–171.

62. World Health Organization. *Guideline: Protecting, Promoting and Supporting Breastfeeding in Facilities Providing Maternity and Newborn Services.* Geneva: World Health Organization; 2017.

63. World Health Organization. *Standards for Improving Quality of Maternal and Newborn Care in Health Facilities.* Geneva: World Health Organization; 2016.

64. Spangler A, Wambach K. *Clinical Guidelines for the Establishment of Exclusive Breastfeeding.* Raleigh, NC: International Lactation Consultant Association; 2014.

65. World Health Organization. *The International Code of Marketing of Breast-Milk Substitutes, 2017 Update, Frequently Asked Questions.* Geneva: World Health Organization; 2017.

66. World Health Organization. Code and subsequent resolutions. 2016. www.who.int/nutrition/netcode/resolutions/en (accessed July 17, 2018).

67. Howick J, Chalmers I, Glasziou P, OCEBM Levels of Evidence Working Group. The Oxford 2011 Levels of Evidence. 2011. www.cebm.net/index.aspex?o = 5653 (accessed July 9, 2018).

68. Lewin S, Bohren M, Rashidian A, et al. Applying GRADECERQual to qualitative evidence synthesis findings-paper 2: How to make an overall CERQual assessment of confidence and create a summary of qualitative findings table. *Implement Sci.* 2018;13(Suppl 1):10.

69. MacDonald T, Noel-Weiss J, West D, et al. Transmasculine individuals' experiences with lactation, chestfeeding, and gender identity: A qualitative study. *BMC Pregnancy Childbirth.* 2016;16:106.

70. Reisman T, Goldstein Z. Case report: Induced lactation in a transgender woman. *Transgend Health.* 2018;3:24–26.

71. Fontenot HB. Transition and adaptation to adoptive motherhood. *J Obstet Gynecol Neonatal Nurs.* 2007;36:175–182.

72. Farhadi R, Philip RK. Induction of lactation in the biological mother after gestational surrogacy of twins: A novel approach and review of literature. *Breastfeed Med.* 2017;12:373–376.

73. World Health Organization. *WHO Recommendations: Intrapartum Care for a Positive Childbirth Experience.* Geneva: World Health Organization; 2018.

74. Tervalon M, Murray-Garcia J. Cultural humility versus cultural competence: A critical distinction in defining physician training outcomes in multicultural education. *J Health Care Poor Underserved.* 1998;9:117–125.

75. Li CM, Li R, Ashley CG, et al. Associations of hospital staff training and policies with early breastfeeding practices. *J Hum Lact.* 2014;30:88–96.

76. Orth TA, Drachman D, Habak P. Breastfeeding in obstetrics residency: Exploring maternal and colleague resident perspectives. *Breastfeed Med.* 2013;8:394–400.

77. Sattari M, Levine D, Serwint JR. Physician mothers. An unlikely high risk group-call for action. *Breastfeed Med.* 2010;5:35–39.

78. Sattari M, Serwint JR, Shuster JJ, et al. Infant-feeding intentions and practices of internal medicine physicians. *Breastfeed Med.* 2016;11:173–179.

79. Piwoz EG, Huffman SL. The impact of marketing of breast-milk substitutes on WHO-recommended breastfeeding practices. *Food Nutr Bull.* 2015;36:373–386.

80. Tarrant M, Lok KY, Fong DY, et al. Effect of a hospital policy of not accepting free infant formula on in-hospital formula supplementation rates and breast-feeding duration. *Public Health Nutr.* 2015;18:2689–2699.

81. Barennes H, Empis G, Quang TD, et al. Breast-milk substitutes: A new old-threat for breastfeeding policy in developing countries. A case study in a traditionally high breastfeeding country. *PLoS One.* 2012;7:e30634.

82. Barennes H, Slesak G, Goyet S, et al. Enforcing the international code of marketing of breast-milk substitutes for better promotion of exclusive breastfeeding: Can lessons be learned? *J Hum Lact.* 2016;32:20–27.

83. Parry K, Taylor E, Hall-Dardess P, et al. Understanding women's interpretations of infant formula advertising. *Birth.* 2013;40:115–124.

84. Feldman-Winter L, Grossman X, Palaniappan A, et al. Removal of industry-sponsored formula sample packs from the hospital: Does it make a difference? *J Hum Lact.* 2012;28:380–388.

85. McFadden A, Gavine A, Renfrew MJ, et al. Support for healthy breastfeeding mothers with healthy term babies. *Cochrane Database Syst Rev.* 2017;2:CD001141.

86. de Jesus PC, de Oliveira MI, Fonseca SC. Impact of health professional training in breastfeeding on their knowledge, skills, and hospital practices: A systematic review. *J Pediatr (Rio J).* 2016;92:436–450.

87. Balogun OO, Kobayashi S, Anigo KM, et al. Factors influencing exclusive breastfeeding in early infancy: A prospective study in North Central Nigeria. *Matern Child Health J.* 2016;20:363–375.

88. Beake S, Pellowe C, Dykes F, et al. A systematic review of structured compared with non-structured breastfeeding programmes to support the initiation and duration of exclusive and any breastfeeding in acute and primary health care settings. *Matern Child Nutr.* 2012;8:141–161.

89. Britton C, McCormick FM, Renfrew MJ, et al. Support for breastfeeding mothers. *Cochrane Database Syst Rev.* 2007; CD001141.

90. Coutinho SB, Lira PI, Lima MC, et al. Promotion of exclusive breast-feeding at scale within routine health services: Impact

of breast-feeding counselling training for community health workers in Recife, Brazil. *Public Health Nutr.* 2014;17:948–955.

91. Gavine A, MacGillivray S, Renfrew MJ, et al. Education and training of healthcare staff in the knowledge, attitudes and skills needed to work effectively with breastfeeding women: A systematic review. *Int Breastfeed J.* 2016;12:6.

92. Sinha B, Chowdhury R, Sankar MJ, et al. Interventions to improve breastfeeding outcomes: A systematic review and meta-analysis. *Acta Paediatr.* 2015;104(Suppl 467):114–134.

93. Spiby H, McCormick F, Wallace L, et al. A systematic review of education and evidence-based practice interventions with health professionals and breast feeding counsellors on duration of breast feeding. *Midwifery.* 2009;25:50–61.

94. Ekström AC, Thorstensson S. Nurses and midwives professional support increases with improved attitudes—Design and effects of a longitudinal randomized controlled process-oriented intervention. *BMC Pregnancy Childbirth.* 2015;15:275.

95. Kraft JM, Wilkins KG, Morales GJ, et al. An evidence review of gender-integrated interventions in reproductive and maternal-child health. *J Health Commun.* 2014;19(Suppl 1):122–141.

96. Esteves TM, Daumas RP, Oliveira MI, et al. Factors associated to breastfeeding in the first hour of life: Systematic review. *Rev Saude Publica.* 2014;48:697–708.

97. Nguyen PH, Kim SS, Sanghvi T, et al. Integrating nutrition interventions into an existing maternal, neonatal, and child health program increased maternal dietary diversity, micronutrient intake, and exclusive breastfeeding practices in Bangladesh: Results of a cluster-randomized program evaluation. *J Nutr.* 2017;147:2326–2337.

98. Tadesse K, Zelenko O, Mulugeta A, et al. Effectiveness of breastfeeding interventions delivered to fathers in low and middle-income countries: A systematic review. *Matern Child Nutr.* 2018;14:e12612.

99. Wouk K, Tully KP, Labbok MH. Systematic review of evidence for Baby-Friendly Hospital Initiative step 3. *J Hum Lact.* 2017;33:50–82.

100. Balyakina E, Fulda KG, Franks SF, et al. Association between healthcare provider type and intent to breastfeed among expectant mothers. *Matern Child Health J.* 2016;20:993–1000.

101. Costanian C, Macpherson AK, Tamim H. Inadequate prenatal care use and breastfeeding practices in Canada: A national survey of women. *BMC Pregnancy Childbirth.* 2016;16:100.

102. Wouk K, Lara-Cinisomo S, Stuebe AM, et al. Clinical interventions to promote breastfeeding by Latinas: A meta-analysis. *Pediatrics.* 2016;137.

103. Liu L, Zhu J, Yang J, et al. The effect of a perinatal breastfeeding support program on breastfeeding outcomes in primiparous mothers. *West J Nurs Res.* 2017;39:906–923.

104. Leclair E, Robert N, Sprague AE, et al. Factors associated with breastfeeding initiation in adolescent pregnancies: A cohort study. *J Pediatr Adolesc Gynecol.* 2015;28:516–521.

105. Bever Babendure J, Reifsnider E, Mendias E, et al. Reduced breastfeeding rates among obese mothers: A review of contributing factors, clinical considerations and future directions. *Int Breastfeed J.* 2015;10:21.

106. Johnson AM, Kirk R, Rooks AJ, et al. Enhancing breastfeeding through healthcare support: Results from a focus group study of African American mothers. *Matern Child Health J.* 2016;20(Suppl 1):92–102.

107. Khan AI, Kabir I, Eneroth H, et al. Effect of a randomised exclusive breastfeeding counselling intervention nested into the MINIMat prenatal nutrition trial in Bangladesh. *Acta Paediatr.* 2017;106:49–54.

108. Behera D, Anil, Kumar K. Predictors of exclusive breastfeeding intention among rural pregnant women in India: A study using theory of planned behaviour. *Rural Remote Health.* 2015;15:3405.

109. Lee SH, Nurmatov UB, Nwaru BI, et al. Effectiveness of mHealth interventions for maternal, newborn and child health in low- and middle-income countries: Systematic review and meta-analysis. *J Glob Health.* 2016;6:010401.

110. Keag OE, Norman JE, Stock SJ. Long-term risks and benefits associated with cesarean delivery for mother, baby, and subsequent pregnancies: Systematic review and meta-analysis. *PLoS Med.* 2018;15:e1002494.

111. Prior E, Santhakumaran S, Gale C, et al. Breastfeeding after cesarean delivery: A systematic review and meta-analysis of world literature. *Am J Clin Nutr.* 2012;95:1113–1135.

112. Chien LY, Tai CJ. Effect of delivery method and timing of breastfeeding initiation on breastfeeding outcomes in Taiwan. *Birth.* 2007;34:123–130.

113. Sandall J, Soltani H, Gates S, et al. Midwife-led continuity models versus other models of care for childbearing women. *Cochrane Database Syst Rev.* 2016;4:CD004667.

114. Fortier JH, Godwin M. Doula support compared with standard care: Meta-analysis of the effects on the rate of medical interventions during labour for low-risk women delivering at term. *Can Fam Physician.* 2015;61:e284–e292.

115. Beake S, Bick D, Narracott C, et al. Interventions for women who have a Caesarean birth to increase uptake and duration of breastfeeding: A systematic review. *Matern Child Nutr.* 2017;13.

116. Cleveland L, Hill CM, Pulse WS, et al. Systematic review of skin-to-skin care for full-term, healthy newborns. *J Obstet Gynecol Neonatal Nurs.* 2017;46:857–869.

117. World Health Organization. *WHO Recommendations on Newborn Health.* Geneva: World Health Organization; 2017.

118. Work Group of Clinical Practice Guide on Breastfeeding. *Clinical Practice Guide on Breastfeeding.* San Sebastián, Spain: Ministry of Social Services and Equality, Basque Government; 2017.

119. Dumas L, Lepage M, Bystrova K, et al. Influence of skin-to-skin contact and rooming-in on early mother-infant interaction: A randomized controlled trial. *Clin Nurs Res.* 2013;22:310–336.

120. Righard L. The baby is breastfeeding—Not the mother. *Birth.* 2008;35:1–2.

121. Widström AM, Lilja G, Aaltomaa-Michalias P, et al. Newborn behaviour to locate the breast when skin-to-skin: A possible method for enabling early self-regulation. *Acta Paediatr.* 2011;100:79–85.

122. Colson SD, Meek JH, Hawdon JM. Optimal positions for the release of primitive neonatal reflexes stimulating breastfeeding. *Early Hum Dev.* 2008;84:441–449.

123. Brimdyr K, Cadwell K, Stevens J, et al. An implementation algorithm to improve skin-to-skin practice in the first hour after birth. *Matern Child Nutr.* 2018;14:e12571.

124. Stevens J, Schmied V, Burns E, et al. Immediate or early skin-to-skin contact after a Caesarean section: A review of the literature. *Matern Child Nutr.* 2014;10:456–473.

125. Moore ER, Bergman N, Anderson GC, et al. Early skin-to-skin contact for mothers and their healthy newborn infants. *Cochrane Database Syst Rev.* 2016;11:CD003519.

126. Guala A, Boscardini L, Visentin R, et al. Skin-to-skin contact in cesarean birth and duration of breastfeeding: A cohort study. *Scientific World Journal.* 2017;2017:1940756.

127. Feldman-Winter L, Goldsmith JP. Committee on Fetus and Newborn, Task Force on Sudden Infant Death Syndrome. Safe sleep and skin-to-skin care in the neonatal period for healthy term newborns. *Pediatrics.* 2016;138. pii:e20161889.

128. Pallás Alonso CR, Rodriguez López J,. *Comité de Estándares de Sociedad Española de Neonatología. [Factors associated with the safety of early skin-to-skin contact after delivery]. An Pediatr (Barc).* 80. 2014203−205.

129. Rabe H, Reynolds G, Diaz-Rossello J. A systematic review and meta-analysis of a brief delay in clamping the umbilical cord of preterm infants. *Neonatology.* 2008;93:138−144.

130. World Health Organization. *Delayed Umbilical Cord Clamping for Improved Maternal and Infant Health and Nutrition Outcomes.* Geneva: World Health Organization; 2014.

131. Garofalo M, Abenhaim HA. Early versus delayed cord clamping in term and preterm births: A review. *J Obstet Gynaecol Can.* 2012;34:525−531.

132. American College of Obstetricians and Gynecologists. ACOG committee opinion No. 648: Umbilical cord blood banking. *Obstet Gynecol.* 2015;126:e127−e129.

133. Flaherman VJ, Schaefer EW, Kuzniewicz MW, et al. Early weight loss nomograms for exclusively breastfed newborns. *Pediatrics.* 2015;135:e16−e23.

134. McMillan D, Canadian Paediatric Society Fetus and Newborn Committee. Position statement: Routine administration of vitamin K to newborns. 2018. Available at https://www.cps.ca/en/documents/position/administrationvitamin-K-newborns (accessed June 16, 2018).

135. World Health Organization. *Recommendations for Management of Common Childhood Conditions: Newborn Conditions, Dysentery, Pneumonia, Oxygen Use and Delivery, Common Causes of Fever, Severe Acute Malnutrition and Supportive Care.* Geneva: World Health Organization; 2012.

136. U.S. Preventive Services Task Force. Clinical Summary: Ocular Prophylaxis for Gonoccocal Ophthalmia Neonatorum. 2011. Available at https://www.uspreventiveservicestaskforce.org/Page/Document/ClinicalSummaryFinal/ocularprophylaxis-for-gonococcal-ophthalmia-neonatorum-preventive-medication (accessed June 20, 2018).

137. AAP Committee on Infectious Diseases, AAP Committee on Fetus Newborn. Elimination of perinatal hepatitis B: Providing the first vaccine dose within 24 hours of birth. *Pediatrics.* 2017;140. pii:e20171870.

138. Neovita Study Group. Timing of initiation, patterns of breastfeeding, and infant survival: Prospective analysis of pooled data from three randomised trials. *Lancet Glob Health.* 2016;4:e266−e275.

139. Smith ER, Hurt L, Chowdhury R, et al. Delayed breastfeeding initiation and infant survival: A systematic review and meta-analysis. *PLoS One.* 2017;12:e0180722.

140. Goyal NK, Attanasio LB, Kozhimannil KB. Hospital care and early breastfeeding outcomes among late preterm, early-term, and term infants. *Birth.* 2014;41:330−338.

141. Conde-Agudelo A, Diaz-Rossello JL. Kangaroo mothercare to reduce morbidity and mortality in low birthweight infants. *Cochrane Database Syst Rev.* 2016;.

142. Johns HM, Forster DA, Amir LH, et al. Prevalence and outcomes of breast milk expressing in women with healthy term infants: A systematic review. *BMC Pregnancy Childbirth.* 2013;13:212.

143. Flaherman VJ, Gay B, Scott C, et al. Randomised trial comparing hand expression with breast pumping for mothers of term newborns feeding poorly. *Arch Dis Child Fetal Neonatal Ed.* 2012;97:F18−F23.

144. Morton J, Wong RJ, Hall JY, et al. Combining hand techniques with electric pumping increases the caloric content of milk in mothers of preterm infants. *J Perinatol.* 2012;32:791−796.

145. Soltani S, Zohoori D, Adineh M. Comparison the effectiveness of breastfeeding, oral 25% dextrose, kangaroo-mother care method, and EMLA cream on pain score level following heal pick sampling in newborns: A randomized clinical trial. *Electron Physician.* 2018;10:6741−6748.

146. Parker LA, Sullivan S, Krueger C, et al. Association of timing of initiation of breastmilk expression on milk volume and timing of lactogenesis stage II among mothers of very low-birth-weight infants. *Breastfeed Med.* 2015;10:84−91.

147. Spatz DL, Froh EB, Schwarz J, et al. Pump early, pump often: A continuous quality improvement project. *J Perinat Educ.* 2015;24:160−170.

148. Fewtrell MS, Kennedy K, Ahluwalia JS, et al. Predictors of expressed breast milk volume in mothers expressing milk for their preterm infant. *Arch Dis Child Fetal Neonatal Ed.* 2016;. pii:fetalneonatal-2015-308321.

149. Acuña-Muga J, Ureta-Velasco N, de la Cruz-Bértolo J, et al. Volume of milk obtained in relation to location and circumstances of expression in mothers of very low birth weight infants. *J Hum Lact.* 2014;30:41−46.

150. Puthussery S, Chutiyami M, Tseng PC, et al. Effectiveness of early intervention programs for parents of preterm infants: A meta-review of systematic reviews. *BMC Pediatr.* 2018;18:223.

151. Charpak N, Ruiz JG. Latin American clinical epidemiology network series—Paper 9: The kangaroo mother care method: From scientific evidence generated in Colombia to worldwide practice. *J Clin Epidemiol.* 2017;86:125−128.

152. Chan GJ, Labar AS, Wall S, et al. Kangaroo mother care: a systematic review of barriers and enablers. *Bull World Health Organ.* 2016;94:130−141J.

153. Collins CT, Gillis J, McPhee AJ, et al. Avoidance of bottles during the establishment of breast feeds in preterm infants. *Cochrane Database Syst Rev.* 2016;9:CD005252.

154. Jaafar SH, Ho JJ, Lee KS. Rooming-in for new mother and infant versus separate care for increasing the duration of breastfeeding. *Cochrane Database Syst Rev.* 2016; CD006641.

155. Colombo L, Crippa BL, Consonni D, et al. Breastfeeding determinants in healthy term newborns. *Nutrients.* 2018;10.

156. De Carvalho Guerra Abecasis F, Gomes A. Rooming-in for preterm infants: How far should we go? Five-year experience at a tertiary hospital. *Acta Paediatr.* 2006;95:1567−1570.

157. Ball HL, Ward-Platt MP, Heslop E, et al. Randomised trial of infant sleep location on the postnatal ward. *Arch Dis Child.* 2006;91:1005−1010.

158. Tully KP, Ball HL. Postnatal unit bassinet types when rooming-in after cesarean birth: Implications for breastfeeding and infant safety. *J Hum Lact.* 2012;28:495−505.

159. Task Force On Sudden Infant Death Syndrome. SIDS and other sleep-related infant deaths: Updated 2016 recommendations for a safe infant sleeping environment. *Pediatrics.* 2016;138. pii:e20162940.

160. Douglas P, Geddes D. Practice-based interpretation of ultrasound studies leads the way to more effective clinical support and less pharmaceutical and surgical intervention for breastfeeding infants. *Midwifery.* 2018;58:145−155.

161. Jaafar SH, Ho JJ, Jahanfar S, et al. Effect of restricted pacifier use in breastfeeding term infants for increasing duration of breastfeeding. *Cochrane Database Syst Rev.* 2016; CD007202.

162. Buccini GDS, Perez-Escamilla R, Paulino LM, et al. Pacifier use and interruption of exclusive breastfeeding: Systematic review and meta-analysis. *Matern Child Nutr.* 2017;13.

163. Kair LR, Kenron D, Etheredge K, et al. Pacifier restriction and exclusive breastfeeding. *Pediatrics.* 2013;131: e1101−e1107.

164. Lindau JF, Mastroeni S, Gaddini A, et al. Determinants of exclusive breastfeeding cessation: Identifying an "at risk population" for special support. *Eur J Pediatr.* 2015;174:533−540.

165. Kair LR, Colaizy TT. Association between in-hospital pacifier use and breastfeeding continuation and exclusivity: Neonatal intensive care unit admission as a possible effect modifier. *Breastfeed Med.* 2017;12:12−19.

166. Chow S, Chow R, Popovic M, et al. The use of nipple shields: A review. *Front Public Health.* 2015;3:236.

167. Ekström A, Abrahamsson H, Eriksson RM, et al. Women's use of nipple shields: Their influence on breastfeeding duration after a process-oriented education for health professionals. *Breastfeed Med.* 2014;9:458−466.

168. U.S. National Library of Medicine. LactMed: A ToxNet Database. 2018. Available at https://www.toxnet.nlm.nih.gov/newtoxnet/lactmed.htm (accessed June 28, 2018).

169. Infant Risk Center. InfantRisk. 2018. Available at www.infantrisk.com (accessed August 7, 2018).

170. University of Rochester Medical Center, Golisano Children's Hospital. Human Lactation Center. 2018. Available at https://www.urmc.rochester.edu/childrens-hospital/neonatology/lactation.aspx (accessed September 4, 2018).

171. e-lactancia.org. *Is it compatible with breastfeeding?* Valencia, Spain: Association for Promotion and cultural and scientific Research into Breastfeeding (APILAM); 2018 (accessed August 4, 2018).

172. European Medicines Agency. *CMDh Endorses Restrictive Use of Bromocriptine for Stopping Breast Milk Production.* London: European Medicines Agency of the European Union; 2014.

173. Marcellin L, Chantry AA. *[Breast-feeding (part II): Lactation inhibition—Guidelines for clinical practice].* J Gynecol Obstet Biol Reprod (Paris). 2015;44:1080−1083.

174. Spitz AM, Lee NC, Peterson HB. Treatment for lactation suppression: Little progression in one hundred years. *Am J Obstet Gynecol.* 1998;179 (6, Part 1):1485−1490.

175. Oladapo OT, Fawole B. Treatments for suppression of lactation. *Cochrane Database Syst Rev.* 2012;CD005937.

176. Sudfeld CR, Fawzi WW, Lahariya C. Peer support and exclusive breastfeeding duration in low and middle-income countries: A systematic review and meta-analysis. *PLoS One.* 2012;7:e45143.

177. Abbass-Dick J, Stern SB, Nelson LE, et al. Coparenting breastfeeding support and exclusive breastfeeding: A randomized controlled trial. *Pediatrics.* 2015;135: 102−110.

178. Renfrew MJ, McCormick FM, Wade A, et al. Support for healthy breastfeeding mothers with healthy term babies. *Cochrane Database Syst Rev.* 2012;CD001141.

179. Centers for Disease Control and Prevention. Contraindications to Breastfeeding or Feeding Expressed Breast Milk to Infants. 2018. Available at https://www.cdc.gov/breastfeeding/breastfeeding-special-circumstances/Contraindications-to-breastfeeding.html (accessed June 28, 2018).

180. UNICEF. WHO/UNAIDS/UNICEF Infant feeding guidelines. Available at https://www.unicef.org/programme/breastfeeding/feeding.htm (accessed June 28, 2018).

181. Amiri M, Diekmann L, von Kockritz-Blickwede M, et al. The diverse forms of lactose intolerance and the putative linkage to several cancers. *Nutrients.* 2015;7:7209−7230.

182. Kimberlin DW, Brady MT, Long SS, Jackson MA. *Red Book: 2018 Report on the Committee on Infectious Disease.* 31st Edition Itasca, IL: American Academy of Pediatrics; 2018.

183. Centers for Disease Control and Prevention. Updated recommendations for use of VariZIG—United States, 2013. *MMWR Morb Mortal Wkly Rep.* 2013;62:574−576.

184. U.S. Department of Health and Human Services. Guidance for Counseling and Managing Women Living with HIV in the United States Who Desire to Breastfeeding. 2018. Available at https://aidsinfo.nih.gov/guidelines/html/3/perinatal/513/counseling-and-management-ofwomen-living-with-hiv-who-breastfeed (accessed September 17, 2018).

185. Blair PS, Sidebotham P, Pease A, et al. Bed-sharing in the absence of hazardous circumstances: Is there a risk of sudden infant death syndrome? An analysis from two case-control studies conducted in the UK. *PLoS One.* 2014;9: e107799.

186. Thompson JMD, Tanabe K, Moon RY, et al. Duration of breastfeeding and risk of SIDS: An individual participant data meta-analysis. *Pediatrics.* 2017;140.

187. Ball HL, Howel D, Bryant A, et al. Bed-sharing by breastfeeding mothers: Who bed-shares and what is the relationship with breastfeeding duration? *Acta Paediatr.* 2016;105:628−634.

188. Ball HL. The Atlantic divide: Contrasting U.K. and U.S. recommendations on cosleeping and bed-sharing. *J Hum Lact.* 2017;33:765−769.

189. Bartick M, Tomori C. Sudden infant death and social justice: A syndemics approach. *Matern Child Nutr.* 2018; e12652.

190. Centers for Disease Control and Prevention. How to keep your breast pump kit clean: The essentials. 2017. Available at https://www.cdc.gov/healthywater/hygiene/healthychildcare/infantfeeding/breastpump.html (accessed August 2, 2018).

191. Infant Risk Center. MommyMeds. 2018. Available at mommymeds.com (accessed August 7, 2018).

192. De Bortoli J, Amir LH. Is onset of lactation delayed in women with diabetes in pregnancy? A systematic review. *Diabet Med.* 2016;33:17—24.

193. Nommsen-Rivers LA. Does insulin explain the relation between maternal obesity and poor lactation outcomes? An overview of the literature. *Adv Nutr.* 2016;7:407—414.

194. Riddle SW, Nommsen-Rivers LA. Low milk supply and the pediatrician. *Curr Opin Pediatr.* 2017;29:249—256.

ABM protocols expire 5 years from the date of publication.

Content of this protocol is up-to-date at the time of publication. Evidence-based revisions are made within five years or sooner if there are significant changes in the evidence.

The previous version of this protocol was authored by Barbara L. Philipp.

Maria-Teresa Hernández-Aguilar, MD, MPH, PhD lead author
Melissa Bartick, MD, MSc, FABM

Paula Schreck, MD
Cadey Harrel, MD
The Academy of Breastfeeding Medicine Protocol Committee:
Michal Young, MD, FABM, Chairperson
Larry Noble, MD, FABM, Translations Chairperson
Sarah Calhoun, MD
Sarah Dodd, MD
Megan Elliott-Rudder, MD
Susan Lappin, MD
Ilse Larson, MD
Ruth A. Lawrence, MD, FABM
Kathleen A. Marinelli, MD, FABM
Nicole Marshall, MD
Katrina Mitchell, MD
Sarah Reece-Stremtan, MD
Casey Rosen-Carole, MD, MPH, MSEd
Susan Rothenberg, MD
Tomoko Seo, MD, FABM
Adora Wonodi, MD
For correspondence: abm@bfmed.org

ABM Clinical Protocol #8
*Human Milk Storage Information for Home Use for Full-Term Infants, Revised 2017**

Anne Eglash[1], Liliana Simon[2] and The Academy of Breastfeeding Medicine

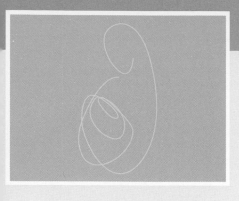

ABSTRACT

A central goal of The Academy of Breastfeeding Medicine is the development of clinical protocols, free from commercial interest or influence, for managing common medical problems that may impact breastfeeding success. These protocols serve only as guidelines for the care of breastfeeding mothers and infants and do not delineate an exclusive course of treatment or serve as standards of medical care. Variations in treatment may be appropriate according to the needs of an individual patient.

BACKGROUND

BREASTFEEDING MOTHERS MAY ENCOUNTER unforeseen reasons for separation from their infants, but more often women express and store milk for planned events, lifestyle flexibility, and returning to work. Knowledge of appropriate human milk handling and storage is essential for breastfeeding success in these situations. One study indicated that although most women store their milk as recommended, ~12% heated their milk in a microwave, and 17% rinsed bottle nipples/teats with only water before reuse,[1] which may reduce the milk's biological properties and increase risk of contamination, respectively. Another study showed that neonatal nurses' knowledge and practice of breast milk collection and storage were adequate, however, there was inadequacy related to discarding, storing, and thawing breast milk.[2]

Human milk is a fresh, living food with many antioxidant, antibacterial, prebiotic, probiotic, and immune-boosting properties in addition to nutrients. Although some of these nutrients and health properties change with storage, there is good evidence that human milk storage can be safe, allowing provision of optimal nutrition to the child when breastfeeding or immediately expressed milk is not available. When direct breastfeeding is not possible, stored human milk maintains unique qualities, such that it continues to be the gold standard for infant feeding.

PREPARATION FOR HUMAN MILK STORAGE

1. Washing: Women should wash their hands with soap and water, or a waterless hand cleanser if their hands don't appear dirty, before milk expression. Unclean hands may transmit viruses and bacteria, some of which can cause illness. Studies show that human milk containing fewer bacteria at the time of expression develops less bacterial growth during storage and has higher protein levels compared to milk that has an abundance of bacteria.[3–5] Additional hand hygiene and cleaning of the breasts before expression are not necessary.[6] (IIB) (Quality of evidence [levels of evidence IA, IB, IIA, IIB, III, and IV] is based on levels of evidence used for the National Guidelines Clearing House[7] and is noted in parentheses.)

2. Hand or Pump: Milk expression can be achieved by hand or by a pump. As long as the appropriate steps are taken for hand cleansing and cleaning of pump parts as per the pump manufacturer's instructions, there does not seem to be a difference in milk contamination with pumping versus hand expression.[8,9] (IIB, IV) There is no need to discard the first few drops of milk with initiating milk expression. This milk is not more likely to be contaminated than milk that is subsequently expressed.[7] One study found that milk expressed at home appears to have more bacterial contamination than milk expressed at the hospital, possibly related to equipment at home or transport, not related to personal hygiene.[6] (IIB)

3. Storage Container Choice: Several studies have been done to evaluate a range of available storage containers. There is a significant reduction in percent of fat and an increase in total protein and carbohydrate concentrations with

* Courtesy of the Academy of Breastfeeding Medicine. Please go to https://www.bfmed.org/protocols for complete protocols, translations, and the most up-to-date information (protocols are updated every 5–7 years).

[1] Department of Family and Community Medicine, University of Wisconsin School of Medicine and Public Health, Madison, Wisconsin.

[2] Department of Pediatrics, Pediatric Critical Care, University of Maryland School of Medicine, Baltimore, Maryland.

either glass or polyethylene, polypropylene, polycarbonate, or polyethersulfone bottles or bags.[10] Glass and polypropylene containers appear similar in their effects on adherence of lipid-soluble nutrients to the container surface,[11] the concentration of immuno-globulin A(IgA), and the numbers of viable white blood cells in the stored milk.[12] Use of polyethylene containers was associated with a marked drop (60%) of IgA[12] and milk's bactericidal effect when compared to Pyrex, a type of tempered glass.[13] Steel containers were associated with a marked decline in cell count and cell viability when compared to polyethylene[14] and glass.[15] (IIB)

There has been concern about possible contamination of milk stored in polypropylene bags because of the risk of contamination by puncturing the plastic.[16] (IV) However, one study showed no difference between contamination and fat loss when comparing hard and soft polypropylene containers.[17] Therefore, plastic bags used for human milk storage should be sturdy, sealed well, and stored in an area of the freezer where damage to the bag would be minimized. (IIB) Containers made with bisphenol A, which is found in several plastic containers including baby bottles, should be avoided based on strong evidence of its adverse effects as an endocrine disruptor.[18] There should be caution about the use of bottles with bisphenol S, a bisphenol A alternative, as it may also have deleterious effects, although this is not well established in the literature.

Human milk should not be stored in hospital plastic specimen storage containers such as those used for urine or other bodily fluids because there is insufficient evidence regarding their chemical safety and effects on infants' health;[19] only food grade plastic containers should be used for human milk storage. (IV)

4. Care of Containers: Containers for human milk storage and breast pump milk collection kits must be completely dismantled, washed in hot soapy water and rinsed or washed in a dishwasher,[8] and should always be thoroughly air dried or dried with paper towels.[20] They do not need to be sterilized. If soap is not available, then boiling water is preferable. (IIB) Chemical disinfection is not ideal, as the disinfectant can be easily deactivated and could expose infant to unnecessary risk of both inadequately clean containers and residual chemical disinfectant.[20] (IV)

STORAGE OF HUMAN MILK

1. Freshly expressed human milk may be stored safely at room temperature (10−29°C, 50−85°F) for some period of time. Studies suggest different optimal times for room temperature storage because conditions vary greatly in the cleanliness of milk expression technique and the room temperature. Warmer ambient temperatures are associated with faster growing bacterial counts in stored milk. For room temperatures ranging from 27°C to 32°C (29°C = 85°F), 4 hours may be a reasonable limit.[5,21,22] For very clean expressed milk with very low bacterial counts, 6−8 hours at lower room temperatures may be reasonable, but it is best to chill or refrigerate as soon as possible if the milk will not be used during that time.[4,23−25] (IIB)

2. Ice packs: Very few studies have evaluated milk storage safety at 15°C (59°F), which would be equivalent to an ice pack in a small cooler. Hamosh et al.[21] suggested that human milk is safe at 15°C for 24 hours, based on minimal bacterial growth noted in the samples from their study. (IIB)

3. Refrigeration: Several studies have demonstrated the safety of refrigerating human milk (4°C, 39.2°F), either by evaluating the bactericidal capacity of stored milk as a marker for milk quality or by measuring bacterial growth in the stored milk samples. Bactericidal capacity of stored refrigerated human milk declines significantly by 48−72 hours.[26−28] However, studies of expressed human milk with little contamination at the time of expression demonstrate safe, low levels of bacteria growth in milk at 72 hours[24] and even after 4−8 days of refrigeration.[3,4,29]

Few studies have been done on the change in milk composition during refrigerator storage. One study found that lipid composition and lipase activity remained stable up to 96 hours in the refrigerator.[30] Lactoferrin levels are stable in the refrigerator for 4−5 days.[31,32] Many immunologic factors in colostrum such as IgA, cytokines, and growth factors are not diminished with refrigeration for 48 hours.[33] (IIB)

4. Freezing expressed human milk (−4°C to −20°C = 24.8°F to −4°F) has been demonstrated to be safe for at least 3 months. Evidence indicates that thawed human milk, previously frozen for at least 6 weeks at −20°C (−4°F), has the same bacterial viability and diversity as it did when it was freshly expressed.[34] The basic principles of freezing dictate that frozen foods at −18°C (0°F) are safe indefinitely from bacterial contamination, although enzymatic processes inherent in food could persist, with possible changes in milk quality.[35]

Fat, protein, and calories decrease in human milk when frozen for 90 days compared to fresh human milk.[36] Frozen human milk has a significant increase in acidity by 3 months, likely due to ongoing lipase activity, that increases free fatty acids in the milk.[37] Based on a few studies with very small samples sizes, vitamin E appears stable in frozen milk over time, and vitamin C levels decrease significantly after 1−5 months of storage.[38,39] There is a paucity of research on how freezer storage affects nearly all vitamins and minerals in human milk.[38−40]

Bioactive factors in human milk variably diminish with freezing. Lactoferrin levels and bioactivity are significantly lower in human milk frozen at −20°C for 3 months.[13,31,32] However, several cytokines, IgA and growth factors from colostrum are stable for at least 6

TABLE 1   Milk Storage Guidelines

Location of storage	Temperature	Maximum recommended storage duration
Room temperature	16–29°C (60–85°F)	4 hours optimal
		6–8 hours acceptable under very clean conditions
Refrigerator	~4°C (39.2°F)	4 days optimal
		5–8 days under very clean conditions
Freezer	<−4°C (24.8°F)	6 months optimal
		12 months acceptable

months at −20°C (−4°F).[10,33] One trial evaluating milk frozen for 9 months found a progressive decline in pH and in bacterial counts, and increases in nonesterified fatty acids. Other macronutrients, osmolality, and immunoactive proteins remained unchanged in this study after 9 months.[41] Frozen human milk should be stored in the back of the freezer to prevent intermittent rewarming due to freezer door opening, and should be kept away from the walls of self-defrosting freezers. All containers with human milk should be well sealed to prevent contamination. (IIB)

5. Smell of stored milk: Refrigerated and frozen human milk may have an odor different from fresh milk due to lipase-mediated triglyceride breakdown, releasing fatty acids. The odor likely comes from oxidation of these fatty acids.[42,43] This lipolysis process has antimicrobial effects preventing the growth of microorganisms in thawed refrigerated milk.[44] There is no evidence to suggest that infants often reject human milk due to this odor. Many foods that humans eat, such as eggs, cheese, and fish, have an unpleasant odor that does not affect taste. One study demonstrated that freezing human milk to −80°C (−112°F) leads to less change in smell as compared to conventional freezing to −19°C.[43] Heating milk to above 40°C to deactivate lipase is not advised because this may destroy many of the immunologically active factors in human milk. (IIB)

6. Expansion while freezing: When filling a container with human milk, space should be left at the top to allow for expansion with freezing. All stored containers of human milk should be labeled with the date of milk expression and the name of the child if the milk will be used in a child-care setting. It is typical for infants in daycare to take 60–120 mL (2–4 ounces) of human milk at one feeding. Therefore, storing human milk in a variety of small increments such as 15–60 mL is a convenient way to prevent waste of thawed human milk.

7. Mixing milk: Freshly expressed warm milk should not be added to already cooled or frozen milk, to prevent rewarming of the already stored milk. It is best to cool down the newly expressed milk first before adding it to older stored milk.

A summary of milk storage guidelines is given in Table 1.

USING STORED HUMAN MILK

1. Cleaning of feeding devices: Containers and feeding devices used to feed the infant should be cleaned with soap and water and air dried or dried with a paper towel before/after every use. They do not need to be sterilized for a healthy infant. (IIB)

2. Using fresh milk first: Fresh milk is of higher quality than frozen milk. Fresh milk contains current maternal secretory IgA antibodies that may be relevant to the dyad's recent infectious exposures.[45] Freshly expressed milk is highest in antioxidants, vitamins, protein, fat, and probiotic bacteria compared to refrigerated or frozen milk.[27,36,38,39] Fresh human milk also has the greatest immunologic activity compared to refrigerated or frozen milk.[10,31,46] (IB)

3. Thawing frozen milk: There are several ways to thaw frozen human milk: by either placing the container in the refrigerator overnight; by running it under warm water; by setting it in a container of warm water; or by using a waterless warmer. Slow thawing in the refrigerator causes less fat loss than thawing in warm water.[47] (IIB)

4. Warming human milk: Most infants drink milk cool, at room temperature, or warmed; infants may demonstrate a preference. Warming thawed human milk to body temperature is best done over a period of 20 minutes in lukewarm water (at most 40°C). Even warming the milk just to 37°C brings the fat to its melting point, promoting changes from solid fat, which is present at 4°C refrigerator temperature, to liquid or oil fat. Oil fat appears to adhere to the side of the container at 37°C more than it does at 4°C, therefore lowering the fat content of the milk. One study compared tepid water warming at 37°C and waterless warming and found there was no difference between them in regards to changes in fat, protein, lactoferrin, and secretory IgA.[44]

   Milk placed in hot water bath (80°C, which is not uncommon in the real setting) creates islets of high temperature milk due to lack of stirring.[48] Overheating during the warming process causes denaturation and inactivation of milk's bioactive proteins and decreased fat content. (IIB)

5. Microwaving: Studies done on defrosting human milk in a microwave demonstrate that controlling the

temperature in a microwave is difficult, causing the milk to heat unevenly.[49] Although microwaving milk decreases bacteria in the milk much like pasteurization does, it also significantly decreases the activity of immunologic factors, which may reduce its overall health properties for the infant.[50,51] (IIB)

6. Using thawed milk: Once frozen milk is brought to room temperature, its ability to inhibit bacterial growth is lessened, especially by 24 hours after thawing.[52] Previously frozen human milk that has been thawed for 24 hours should not be left out at room temperature for more than 2 hours.[44] (IIB)

7. Refreezing: There is little information on refreezing thawed human milk. Bacterial growth and loss of antibacterial activity in thawed milk will vary depending on the technique of milk thawing, duration of the thaw, and the amount of bacteria in the milk at the time of expression. At this time no recommendations can be made on the refreezing of thawed human milk.

8. Using previously fed milk: Once an infant begins drinking expressed human milk, some bacterial contamination occurs in the milk from the infant's mouth. The length of time the milk can be kept at room temperature once the infant has partially fed from the cup or bottle would theoretically depend on the initial bacterial load in the milk, how long the milk has been thawed, and the ambient temperature. There has been insufficient research done to provide recommendations in this regard. However, based on related evidence thus far, it seems reasonable to discard the remaining milk within 1–2 hours after the infant is finished feeding. (IV) To avoid wasting or discarding unfed milk, mothers may consider storing milk in a variety of increments such as 15, 30, or 60 mL.

9. Handling: Expressed human milk does not require special handling (such as universal precautions), as is required for other bodily fluids such as blood. It can be stored in a workplace refrigerator where other workers store food, although it should be labeled with name and date.[53] (IV) Mothers may prefer to store their milk in a personal freezer pack or cooler, separate from communal refrigerator areas.

10. Infections: Uncontaminated human milk naturally contains nonpathogenic bacteria[54,55] that are important in establishing the neonatal intestinal flora. These bacteria are probiotics—they create conditions in the intestine that are unfavorable to the growth of pathogenic organisms.[55] If a mother has breast or nipple pain from a bacterial or yeast infection, there is no evidence that her stored expressed milk needs to be discarded. Human milk that appears stringy, foul, or purulent should, however, be discarded and not be fed to the infant. (IV)

AREAS FOR FUTURE RESEARCH

The evidence for some aspects of human milk storage is lacking. Many studies are older, and because of differences in methodology, are difficult to compare. The studies vary in many respects, such as technique of milk collection, cleanliness and types of containers, duration of storage, method of thawing and warming milk, temperature and type of storage unit, and culture techniques of milk samples. Large high-quality studies evaluating human milk storage in a variety of circumstances over a longer duration of time are needed. Standards for evaluating milk quality, such as culture techniques, need to be established. Although it is ideal to have a universal international guideline for human milk storage, it may be impossible for one guideline to represent unusual or limited circumstances in some cultures

Human milk naturally has both prebiotic and probiotic activity that is essential in establishing the infant gut microbiome. Human milk's prebiotic components are nondigestible factors such as oligosaccharides that promote the growth of beneficial microorganisms in the intestines. Human milk's probiotic components are commensal organisms. Because of the impact of refrigeration, freezing, thawing, and warming on the bactericidal activity of human milk, feeding an infant stored human milk may have different consequences on infant intestinal health compared to breastfeeding, and this should be investigated further. Along the same lines, stored human milk changes in quality over time, as demonstrated by many of the referenced articles included in this protocol. The effect of stored human milk versus fresh human milk on the health of a child should be studied.

There is also no agreed-upon definition of unsafe milk. Several studies describe the degree of milk contamination over a period of time under certain temperature and storage time conditions, typically described as the number of colony-forming units per milliliter. There is no accepted limit at which point milk should not be consumed, although 1×10^4 colony-forming units/mL has been suggested. Other studies have investigated the bactericidal capacity of stored human milk, which would reflect its immunologic effectiveness for the infant and the risk of the milk becoming contaminated over time during storage. The percentage loss of bactericidal activity that would render human milk unfit has not been determined. A definition for adequate milk quality should be established, with guidelines on what would constitute unsafe milk or lower-quality milk that would necessitate discarding of stored milk.

There is only one study investigating human milk quality after 6 months of freezing. This is particularly concerning, given that a few very small studies have demonstrated a decline in some vitamins after 3 months of freezing. Because some infants rely entirely on frozen human milk for nutrition, studies should be done to confirm that this is nutritionally safe.

REFERENCES

1. Labiner-Wolfe J, Fein SB. How US mothers store and handle their expressed breast milk. *J Hum Lact.* 2013;29:54–58.
2. Gharaibeh H, Al-Sheyab N, Malkawi S. Breast milk collection and storage in the neonatal intensive care unit: Nurses' knowledge, practice, and perceived barriers. *J Contin Educ Nurs.* 2016;47:551–557.

3. Sosa R, Barness L. Bacterial growth in refrigerated human milk. *Am J Dis Child.* 1987;141:111—112.

4. Pardou A, Serruys E, Mascart-Lemone F, et al. Human milk banking: Influence of storage processes and of bacterial contamination on some milk constituents. *Biol Neonate.* 1994;65:302—309.

5. Eteng M, Ebong P, Eyong E, et al. Storage beyond three hours at ambient temperature alters the biochemical and nutritional qualities of breastmilk. *Afr J Reprod Health.* 2001;5:130—134.

6. Haiden N, Pimpel B, Assadian O, et al. Comparison of bacterial counts in expressed breast milk following standard or strict infection control regimens in neonatal intensive care units: Compliance of mothers does matter. *J Hosp Infect.* 2016;92:226—228.

7. Shekelle P, Woolf S, Eccles M, et al. Developing guidelines. *Br Med J.* 1999;318:593—596.

8. Pittard 3rd WB, Geddes K, Brown S, et al. Bacterial contamination of human milk: Container type and method of expression. *Am J Perinatol.* 1991;8:25—27.

9. Boo N, Nordiah A, Alfizah H, et al. Contamination of breast milk obtained by manual expression and breast pumps in mothers of very low birthweight infants. *J Hosp Infect.* 2001;49:274—281.

10. Chang Y-C, Chen C-H, Lin M-C. The macronutrients in human milk change after storage in various containers. *Pediatr Neonatol.* 2012;53:205—209.

11. Garza C, Johnson C, Harrist R, et al. Effects of methods of collection and storage on nutrients in human milk. *Early Hum Dev.* 1982;6:295—303.

12. Goldblum R, Garza C, Johnson C, et al. Human milk banking I. Effects of container upon immunologic factors in human milk. *Nutr Res.* 1981;1:449—459.

13. Takci S, Gulmez D, Yigit S, et al. Effects of freezing on the bactericidal activity of human milk. *J Pediatr Gastroenterol Nutr.* 2012;55:146—149.

14. Manohar A, Williamson M, Koppikar G. Effect of storage of colostrum in various containers. *Indian Pediatr.* 1997;34:293—295.

15. Williamson M, Murti P. Effect of storage, time, temperature, and composition of containers on biologic components of human milk. *J Hum Lact.* 1996;12:31—35.

16. Hopkinson J, Garza C, Asquith M. Human milk storage in glass containers. *J Hum Lact.* 1990;6:104—105.

17. Janjindamai W, Thatrimontrichai A, Maneenil G, et al. Soft plastic bag instead of hard plastic container for long-term storage of breast milk. *Indian J Pediatr.* 2013;80:809—813.

18. Vom Saal F, Hughes C. An extensive new literature concerning low dose effects of bisphenol A shows the need for a new risk assessment. *Environ Health Perspect.* 2005;113:926—933.

19. Blouin M, Coulombe M, Rhainds M. Specimen plastic containers used to store expressed breast milk in neonatal care units: A case of precautionary principle. *Can J Public Health.* 2014;105:e218—e220.

20. Price E, Weaver G, Hoffman P, et al. Decontamination of breast pump milk collection kits and related items at home and in hospital: Guidance from a Joint Working Group of the Healthcare Infection Society and Infection Prevention Society. *J Hosp Infect.* 2016;92:213—221.

21. Hamosh M, Ellis L, Pollock D, et al. Breastfeeding and the working mother: Effect of time and temperature of shortterm storage on proteolysis, lipolysis, and bacterial growth in milk. *Pediatrics.* 1996;97:492—498.

22. Nwankwo M, Offor E, Okolo A, et al. Bacterial growth in expressed breast milk. *Ann Trop Paediatr.* 1988;8:92—95.

23. Pittard 3rd WB, Anderson D, Cerutti E, et al. Bacteriostatic qualities of human milk. *J Pediatr.* 1985;107:240—243.

24. Igumbor E, Mukura R, Makandiramba B, et al. Storage of breast milk: Effect of temperature and storage duration on microbial growth. *Cent Afr J Med.* 2000;46:247—251.

25. Ajusi J, Onyango F, Mutanda L, Wamola. Bacteriology of unheated expressed breastmilk stored at room temperature. *East Afr Med J.* 1989;66:381—387.

26. Martínez-Costa C, Silvestre M, López M, et al. Effects of refrigeration on the bactericidal activity of human milk: A preliminary study. *J Pediatr Gastroenterol Nutr.* 2007;45:275—277.

27. Silvestre D, López M, March L, et al. Bactericidal activity of human milk: Stability during storage. *Br J Biomed Sci.* 2006;63:59—62.

28. Ogundele M. Effects of storage on the physicochemical and antibacterial properties of human milk. *Br J Biomed Sci.* 2002;59:205—211.

29. Slutzah M, Codipilly C, Potak D, et al. Refrigerator storage of expressed human milk in the neonatal intensive care unit. *J Pediatr.* 2010;156:26—28.

30. Bertino E, Giribaldi M, Baro C, et al. Effect of prolonged refrigeration on the lipid profile, lipase activity, and oxidative status of human milk. *J Pediatr Gastroenterol Nutr.* 2013;56:390—396.

31. Raoof NA, Adamkin DH, Radmacher PG, et al. Comparison of lactoferrin activity in fresh and stored human milk. *J Perinatol.* 2016;36:207—209.

32. Rollo DE, Radmacher PG, Turcu RM, et al. Stability of lactoferrin in stored human milk. *J Perinatol.* 2014;34:284—286.

33. Ramírez-Santana C, Pérez-Cano FJ, Audí C, et al. Effects of cooling and freezing storage on the stability of bioactive factors in human colostrum. *J Dairy Sci.* 2012;95:2319—2325.

34. Marín ML, Arroyo R, Jiménez E, et al. Cold storage of human milk: Effect on its bacterial composition. *J Pediatr Gastroenterol Nutr.* 2009;49:343—348.

35. USDA. Freezing and food storage. 2013. Available at https://www.fsis.usda.gov/wps/portal/fsis/topics/food-safety-education/get-answers/food-safety-fact-sheets/safe-food-handling/freezing-and-food-safety/ct-index/!ut/p/a1/jVFtT8IwEP417Nto55CgSWMWDCoiaFAZ-7IUetuajHa2h4K-3g4kEQNKm1zu5Xnae-5IQmKSKP4uc45SK17WcdJO6RNtBxdd2h9dBD16N3x9Gt13u7QzPneA6R-AYXgi-8iJ6H-8-gkfnJmH7kNOkopj4UuVaRLngD5X9gOMJXGmtfAtzwDX-fsbn6NsCAF2hzvmbasGVKKXKHdgAfDrP0YX-g0niOaZ-SCViRCUn2u6KBu3fDcNy67Q9DOmr9BhwY2xZwfC5Oe-F7q2WZH00jNwo5TaCADA6a5NC5dIFb2skEb1AI386JZ-d7tttpnr9136603tNHkzVDfNFaNbZ-3tsPE (Accessed April 2, 2017).

36. García-Lara NR, Escuder-Vieco D, García-Algar O, et al. Effect of freezing time on macronutrients and energy content of breastmilk. *Breastfeed Med.* 2012;7:295—301.

37. Vázquez-Román S, Escuder-Vieco D, García-Lara NR, et al. Impact of freezing time on dornic acidity in three types of milk: Raw donor milk, mother's own milk, and pasteurized donor milk. *Breastfeed Med.* 2016;11:91—93.

38. Romeu-Nadal M, Castellote A, Lopez-Sabater M. Effect of cold storage on vitamins C and E and fatty acids in human milk. *Food Chem.* 2008;106:65—70.

39. Buss I, McGill F, Darlow B, et al. Vitamin C is reduced in human milk after storage. *Acta Paediatr.* 2001;90:813−815.

40. Bank MR, Kirksey A, West K, et al. Effect of storage time and temperature on folacin and vitamin C levels in term and preterm human milk. *Am J Clin Nutr.* 1985;41:235−242.

41. Ahrabi A, Handa D, Codipilly C, et al. Effects of extended freezer storage on the integrity of human milk. *J Pediatr.* 2016;177:140−143.

42. Spitzer J, Klos K, Buettner A. Monitoring aroma changes during human milk storage at +4°C by sensory and quantification experiments. *Clin Nutr.* 2013;32:1036−1042.

43. Sandgruber S, Much D, Amann-Gassner U, et al. Sensory and molecular characterisation of the protective effect of storage at −80°C on the odour profiles of human milk. *Food Chem.* 2012;130:236−242.

44. Handa D, Ahrabi AF, Codipilly CN, et al. Do thawing and warming affect the integrity of human milk? *J Perinatol.* 2014;34:863−866.

45. Lönnerdal B. Bioactive proteins in breast milk. *J Paediatr Child Health.* 2013;49(Suppl 1):1−7.

46. Akinbi H, Meinzen-Derr J, Auer C, et al. Alterations in the host defense properties of human milk following prolonged storage or pasteurization. *J Pediatr Gastroenterol Nutr.* 2010;51:347−352.

47. Thatrimontrichai A, Janjindamai W, Puwanant M. Fat loss in thawed breast milk: Comparison between refrigerator and warm water. *Indian Pediatr.* 2012;49:877−880.

48. Bransburg-Zabary S, Virozub A, Mimouni FB. Human milk warming temperatures using a simulation of currently available storage and warming methods. *PLoS One.* 2015;10:e0128806.

49. Ovesen L, Jakobsen J, Leth T, et al. The effect of microwave heating on vitamins B1 and E, and linoleic and linolenic acids, and immunoglobulins in human milk. *Int J Food Sci Nutr.* 1996;47:427−436.

50. Quan R, Yang C, Rubinstein S, et al. Effects of microwave radiation on anti-infective factors in human milk. *Pediatrics.* 1992;89:667−669.

51. Sigman M, Burke K, Swarner O, et al. Effects of microwaving human milk: Changes in IgA content and bacterial count. *J Am Diet Assoc.* 1989;89:690−692.

52. Hernandez J, Lemons P, Lemons J, et al. Effect of storage processes on the bacterial growth-inhibiting activity of human breast milk. *Pediatrics.* 1979;63:597−601.

53. CDC. Are special precautions required for handling breast milk? 2015. Available at https://www.cdc.gov/breastfeeding/faq/#Precautions (accessed June 26, 2017).

54. Delgado S, Arroyo R, Jimenez E, et al. Mastitis infecciosas durante la lactancia: Un problema infravalorado. *Acta Pediatr Esp.* 2009;67:564−571.

55. Heikkilä M, Saris P. Inhibition of Staphylococcus aureus by the commensal bacteria of human milk. *J Appl Microbiol.* 2003;95:471−478.

ABM protocols expire 5 years from the date of publication.

Content of this protocol is up-to-date at the time of publication. Evidence-based revisions are made within 5 years or sooner if there are significant changes in the evidence.
The 2004 and 2010 editions of this protocol were authored by Anne Eglash.
The Academy of Breastfeeding Medicine Protocol Committee:
Wendy Brodribb, MBBS, PhD, FABM, Chairperson
Sarah Reece-Stremtan, MD, Co-Chairperson
Larry Noble, MD, FABM, Translations Chairperson
Nancy Brent, MD
Maya Bunik, MD, MSPH, FABM,
Cadey Harrel, MD
Ruth A. Lawrence, MD, FABM
Yvonne LeFort, MD,
FABM Kathleen A. Marinelli, MD, FABM
Casey Rosen-Carole, MD, MPH, MSEd
Susan Rothenberg, MD
Tomoko Seo, MD, FABM
Rose St. Fleur, MD
Michal Young, MD
For correspondence: abm@bfmed.org

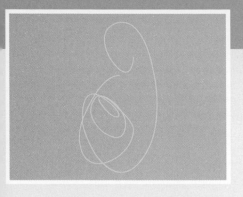

ABM Clinical Protocol #9
Use of Galactagogues in Initiating or Augmenting Maternal Milk Production, Second Revision 2018*

Wendy Brodribb and the Academy of Breastfeeding Medicine

ABSTRACT

A central goal of the Academy of Breastfeeding Medicine is the development of clinical protocols for managing common medical problems that may impact breastfeeding success. These protocols serve only as guidelines for the care of breastfeeding mothers and infants and do not delineate an exclusive course of treatment or serve as standards of medical care. Variations in treatment may be appropriate according to the needs of an individual patient.

BACKGROUND

GALACTOGOGUES (OR LACTAGOGUS) are medications or other substances believed to assist initiation, maintenance, or augmentation of maternal milk supply. Because perceived or actual low milk supply is one of the most common reasons given for discontinuing breastfeeding,[1–4] both mothers and health professionals have sought medication(s), in addition to other nonpharmacological interventions, to address this concern.

Human milk production is a complex physiological process involving physical and emotional factors and the interaction of multiple hormones, the most important of which is believed to be prolactin. Despite the fact that prolactin is required for lactation, once lactation is established, there is no direct correlation between serum prolactin levels (either baseline levels or percentage increase after suckling) and the volume of milk produced in lactating women.[5,6] However, most lactating women have a higher baseline prolactin level than nonlactating women for a number of months and continue to experience suckling-induced peaks when breastfeeding.

Lactation is initiated with parturition, expulsion of the placenta, and falling progesterone levels in the presence of very high prolactin levels. Systemic endocrine control of other supporting hormones (estrogen, progesterone, oxytocin, growth hormone, glucocorticoids, and insulin) is also important.[7] These hormonal changes trigger secretory activation (lactogenesis II) of the mammary secretory epithelial cells, also called lactocytes. Prolactin secretion functions in a negative feedback system in which dopamine serves as an inhibitor. Therefore, when dopamine concentration decreases, prolactin secretion from the anterior pituitary increases.[7]

Once secretory activation has occurred and the mother's milk supply has been established, the rate of milk synthesis is mainly controlled locally in the mammary gland by autocrine control. Lactating breasts are never completely empty of milk, so the terms drain, drainage, and draining are more appropriate. If the breasts are not drained regularly and thoroughly, milk production declines. Alternatively, more frequent and thorough drainage of the breasts typically results in an increased rate of milk secretion, with both immediate (per feeding) and delayed (several days) effects.[8,9]

POTENTIAL INDICATIONS FOR GALACTOGOGUES

Galactogogues have commonly been used to increase low (or perceived low) milk supply. Physiologically, low milk supply is often related to suboptimal milk removal with reasons including problems with infants draining the breast, inappropriate breastfeeding management, maternal or infant illness and hospitalization, and regular mother–infant separation, for example, work or school. In addition, galactogogues have frequently been used in the neonatal intensive care unit in mothers with preterm infants, where the aim has been to stimulate initial secretory activation or augment declining milk secretion. Mothers who are not breastfeeding, but are expressing milk by hand or with a pump, often experience a decline in milk production after several weeks. Galactogogues have also been used in women inducing lactation when they have not been pregnant with the current child, in women relactating after weaning, or in transgender women.[10]

Many breastfeeding medicine specialists and lactation consultants have recommended various drugs and herbs when other nonpharmacological measures have not resulted

* Courtesy of the Academy of Breastfeeding Medicine. Please go to https://www.bfmed.org/protocols for complete protocols, translations, and the most up-to-date information (protocols are updated every 5–7 years).

in an increase in milk volume. However, some providers may inappropriately recommend galactogogues before emphasizing the primary means of increasing the overall rate of milk synthesis (i.e., frequent and effective milk drainage at regular intervals) or evaluating other medical factors that may potentially be involved (see point 1 in the Practice Recommendations section).

PHARMACEUTICAL GALACTOGOGUES

Human growth hormone[11–13] (lB, llA) (quality of evidence [levels of evidence IA, IB, IIA, IIB, III, and IV] is based on levels of evidence used for the National Guidelines Clearing House[14] and is noted in parentheses), sulpride[15,16] (llB), and thyrotropin-releasing hormone[17,18] (lB) may be helpful as galactogogues in some populations, but are not currently used in most countries. Domperidone and metoclopramide are the most commonly used pharmaceutical galactogogues at present. Both are dopamine antagonists that increase prolactin secretion. A number of older mainly observational or controlled studies documented increased baseline prolactin levels in lactating women who took metoclopramide or domperidone and provide some evidence for their effectiveness.[19,20] (llA, lll)

However, high-quality evidence is lacking. The numbers of women in randomized, placebo-controlled blinded studies (RCTs) with each of these agents are small. Studies also tended to have high dropout rates, differed in patient selection (i.e., some were expressing for preterm infants, not all women had documented low milk supply), and differed in dose and duration of the galactogogue and application of other nonpharmacological measures before starting the galactogogue. Most studies also had limited follow-up.

Domperidone

A Cochrane systematic review[21] (lA) published in 2012 included two studies with a total of 59 mothers with preterm infants and found a moderate benefit (mean increase of 99 mL per day) when using domperidone, 30 mg per day, for 7 or 14 days. Other systematic reviews have similar findings,[22] with the most recent review that included one finding a mean increase of 88.3 mL per day (95% confidence interval 56.8–119.8).[23] (lA) There have been four RCTs using domperidone since the Cochrane review. In one study of 45 women, 22 were given domperidone, 30 mg per day, for 4 days postcesarean section and were found to have increased milk production during that time compared with the control group.[24] (lB)

In a second study of only 15 women with low milk supply who were expressing for preterm infants, there was a 300-mL per day difference in milk production for women given domperidone, 60 mg per day, for 4 weeks compared with women given domperidone, 30 mg per day, for a similar length of time.[25] (lB) A third trial in the United Kingdom compared the effects of domperidone, 30 mg per day, with metoclopramide, 30 mg per day. Women had 24-hour milk production measured from 10 days before the commencement of

medication administration and during the 10 days of medication administration.[26] The 51 women were expressing for their preterm infants and had documented low milk supply. They all received high-quality breastfeeding assistance throughout the study. Milk production almost doubled from the steady premedication level with both medications and plateaued after about 7 days of treatment.[26] (lB)

The fourth and largest trial to date (EMPOWER) included 90 women who had low milk supply when expressing for preterm infants. They were randomized between 8 and 21 days postpartum to receive domperidone, 30 mg per day, for 28 days or a placebo for 14 days and then domperidone, 30 mg per day, from day 15 to 28.[27] At 14 days, 77.8% of women in the first group had increased their milk production by 50% compared with 57.8% in the second group. By 28 days, there were no significant differences between the two groups, nor were there differences at term or at 6 weeks postterm.[27] (lB) The results of one older very small study ($n = 6$) suggested that individual women may be responders or nonresponders and that primiparas may respond to domperidone with higher prolactin levels than multiparas.[28] (lB)

With respect to potential risks, there is evidence that domperidone increases the QTc interval and it has been implicated in ventricular arrhythmias and sudden cardiac death, particular in older and unwell adults.[29,30] (lA, IV) The risk for domperidone to increase the incidence of arrhythmias in postpartum women with no other risk factors appears to be very small, but may increase with other factors such as a past history of ventricular arrhythmias, high BMI, higher dosages, and concomitant use of medications that inhibit CYP3A4.[31] (lll) In this large study of more than 225,532 postpartum women, the only women who developed ventricular arrhythmias while taking domperidone had a past history of ventricular arrhythmias.[32] See Table 1 for further information.

Metoclopramide

Five randomized, placebo-controlled blinded studies researching the effect of metoclopramide have been published between 1980 and 2011.[33–37] (lB) Of these, participants in three studies commenced metoclopramide within 4 days of birth without a diagnosis of low milk supply,[33,34,37] one study investigated women who were relactating,[36] and one recruited women whose infants had not gained 500 g within the first month of life.[35] None of these studies found differences in milk volumes and/or breastfeeding duration between metoclopramide and placebo groups, even with optimal breast expression and counseling.[37] However, as mentioned above, Ingram et al.[26] found similar positive effects with metoclopramide and domperidone.

In addition, a number of older randomized controlled trials,[38–41] (lB, llA) controlled trials,[42,43] (llB) and observational studies[20,44–46] (lll) reported a significant increase in milk yield using metoclopramide, 5–20 mg, three times a day for periods of 5 days to 4 weeks. The one study that compared different doses of metoclopramide found no response with 15 mg per day, but similar responses with 30 and 45 mg per day. The scientific rigor of these older studies may not be

TABLE 1   Commonly Used Galactogogues

	Domperidone	Fenugreek	Metoclopramide	Silymarin[a]
References	21,24–27,29–31,47,61	56,62–66	20,26,33–37,39–41,45	67–70
Chemical class or properties	Dopamine antagonist	A commonly used spice; active constituents are trigonelline, 4-hydroxyisoleucine, and sotolon.	Dopamine antagonist	Flavolignans (presumed active ingredient)
Level of evidence	Five Level 1B studies; others have inadequate methodology or excessive dropout rates	IIA–IIB (three studies in lactating women) most not of high quality; mixed results	IB–IIB high-quality and low-quality studies give mixed results; effect on overall rate of milk secretion is unclear, but may be effective	IIB (one study in lactating women)
Suggested dosage	10 mg, orally, 3 times per day used in most of the Level IB studies; one Level 1B study compared 10 mg 3 times per day with 20 mg 3 times per day and found higher milk production using the higher dose. Doses >60 mg per day have not been studied in this context.	Herbal tea (200 ml 3 times per day); 570–600 mg 3 times per day.	10 mg, orally, 3 to 4 times per day	Micronized silymarin, 420 mg, orally, per day in the study by Di Pierro et al.[67]; silymarin-phosphatidylserine and galega (5 g per day); anecdotal, strained tea (simmer 1 tsp of crushed seeds in 8 oz of water for 10 minutes), 2–3 cups per day[71]
Length/duration of therapy	Various commencement times from 2 days to 3 to 4 weeks postpartum in Level 1B studies. Duration of therapy between 7 and 28 days. Maximum effect usually reached by 7–14 days.	1–3 weeks	7–14 days in various studies	Micronized silymarin was studied for 63 days; silymarinphosphatidylserine and galega were used for 28 days
Herbal considerations	—	Need reliable source of standard preparation without contaminants	—	Need reliable source of standard preparation without contaminants
Effects on lactation	Increased rate of milk secretion in both pump-dependent mothers of preterm infants and other mothers with low milk supply.	Insufficient evidence; likely a significant placebo effect	Possible increased rate of milk secretion; possible responders versus nonresponders	Inconclusive. Possible increase in milk secretion in the short term
Potential side effects	Maternal: Dry mouth, headache (resolved with decreased dosage), and abdominal cramps. One case reported	Generally well tolerated. Diarrhea (most common), unusual body odor similar to maple syrup; cross-allergy	Reversible CNS effects with short-term use, including sedation, anxiety, depression/agitation, motor restlessness, dystonic	Generally well tolerated; occasional mild gastrointestinal side effect; cross-allergy with Asteraceae/Compositae

(Continued)

TABLE 1   Commonly Used Galactogogues—cont'd

Domperidone	Fenugreek	Metoclopramide	Silymarin[a]
of psychomotor withdrawal symptoms from a dose of 160 mg per day.[72] Although not reported in studies of lactation, rare complications (1.3/ 10,000 postpartum women) of cardiac arrhythmias due to a prolonged QTc interval have been reported, but all these women had a past history of ventricular arrhythmias.[31] Risk may increase with a previous history of cardiac arrhythmias, high doses, high BMI, or concurrent use of drugs that inhibit domperidone's metabolism (see Interactions, immediately below). Neonatal: Very low levels in milk and no QTc prolongation in premature infants who had ingested breast milk of mothers on domperidone.[73] In the United States, the FDA has issued an advisory against the use of domperidone in lactating women.[47]	with Asteraceae/ Compositae family (ragweed and related plants), peanuts, and Fabaceae family such as chickpeas, soybeans, and green peas— possible anaphylaxis. Theoretically, asthma, bleeding, dizziness, flatulence, hypoglycemia, loss of consciousness, skin rash, or wheezing—but no reports in lactating women.	reactions, and extrapyramidal symptoms. Rare reports of tardive dyskinesia (usually irreversible), causing the FDA to place a black box warning on this drug in the United States.	family (ragweed and related plants) possible anaphylaxis
Interactions	Increased blood levels of domperidone when combined with some substrates metabolized by CYP3A4 enzyme inhibitors, for example, fluconazole, macrolide antibiotics, grapefruit juice, cannabinoids, antipsychotics, and others	Hawthorne, hypoglycemics, including insulin, antiplatelet drugs, aspirin, heparin, warfarin, feverfew, primrose oil, and many other herbals	Monoamine oxidase inhibitors, tacrolimus, antihistamines, any drugs with CNS effects (including antidepressants)	Caution with CYP2C9 substrates—may increase levels of the drugs. Possible increased clearance of estrogens (decreased blood levels). Possible increased levels of statins.

(Continued)

TABLE 1 Commonly Used Galactogogues—cont'd				
Domperidone		**Fenugreek**	**Metoclopramide**	**Silymarin[a]**
Comments	a. Do not advise exceeding maximum recommended dosage	If patient develops diarrhea, reducing the dose is often helpful.	Some studies suggest tapering off the dose at the end of treatment.	No prescription required
	b. Generally licensed for use as a drug for gastrointestinal dismotility where doses of 20 mg 3 or 4 times per day may be recommended if no response to lower doses. Some areas use this dose initially to stimulate prolactin. However, there is only one study using this dose in lactating women.			
	c. Tapering of dose usually recommended.			

CNS, central nervous system; CYP, cytochrome c; FDA, Food and Drug Administration.
[a]Silymarin (micronized silymarin) or *Silybum marianum* (milk thistle).

as strong as more recent studies, so their results should be interpreted with caution. As for potential risks, metoclopramide may cause neurological side effects in the mother. Further information can be found in Table 1.

SUMMARY

Despite the widespread use of these pharmaceutical galactogogues, there are important issues to consider:

1. Pharmaceutical galactogogues do increase baseline serum prolactin, and there is evidence for increased milk production with domperidone use (and perhaps metoclopramide). However, the population that would most benefit from this treatment is still uncertain as it is unknown if all women with low milk supply have low levels of prolactin and whether increasing prolactin increases milk supply in women with both low and normal prolactin levels. In addition, there does not appear to be a direct correlation between baseline prolactin levels and rates of milk synthesis or measured volumes of milk production.

2. Potential side effects (minor and significant) should be weighed carefully against any potential benefit.

3. Prescription medications used as galactogogues constitute off-label use in most countries (they are not approved by regulatory agencies for this indication). Domperidone is not approved by the Food and Drug Administration (FDA) for use in the United States, except for some specific circumstances. The FDA has explicitly recommended against the use of Domperidone to increase milk production.[47,48]

HERBALS, FOODS, AND BEVERAGES AS GALACTOGOGUES

In non-Western cultures, postpartum women are assisted in a number of ways that are intended to ease their transition to motherhood and to optimize breastfeeding. Many cultures keep new mothers very warm and insist on a period of rest of ~1 month. Many also have traditional foods and herbs for postpartum women that are meant to increase the mother's strength and enhance lactation.[49–52] (IV)

Many of these herbal remedies have been used throughout history to enhance milk supply. Some herbs commonly mentioned as galactogogues include fenugreek, goat's rue, milk thistle (*Silybum marianum*), oats, dandelion, millet, seaweed, anise, basil, blessed thistle, fennel seeds, marshmallow, moringa leaf, shatavari, and torbangun among others.[22,53] (IA) LactMed (https://toxnet.nlm.nih.gov/newtoxnet/lactmed.htm) has further information about the effect on lactation of some of these herbs. Although beer is used in some cultures to increase milk supply, hops appear to be the active ingredient, while alcohol may actually reduce milk production.[54] (IA) A barley component of beer (even nonalcoholic beer) can also increase prolactin secretion.[55]

While the fact that these herbs have been used for centuries without apparent harm is reassuring, there is also little or no scientific evidence for their effectiveness or safety.[56] The mechanisms of action for most herbals are unknown, and available studies for herbs, herbal medicines, or herbal galactogogues suffer from the same deficiencies as the studies for pharmacologic agents: small numbers of subjects, lack of information regarding breastfeeding advice, and lack of randomization, controls, or blinding. The placebo effect when taking herbal preparations may be the reason for widespread anecdotal experience of their effectiveness. Because of the limited data available, only two herbal preparations have been included in Table 1.

It is important to note that caution is required for the use of herbal preparations because of the lack of standardized dosing preparations (other than in research settings), possible contaminants, allergic potential, and drug interactions. Adverse effects for both mother and infant from several herbs have been reported,[56] (IV) and some will increase patient blood levels of warfarin, heparin, and other anticoagulants, while others may affect insulin resistance and blood sugars. There are several reports of severe maternal allergic reactions to fenugreek.[57] (lll)

PRACTICE RECOMMENDATIONS

The following recommendations, based upon current evidence, apply to women experiencing difficulties with a low rate of milk production (e.g., the infant is not gaining weight normally or supplementation is being used because of low milk production during either the initiation or maintenance of milk supply). It is always important to ensure that low weight gain is due to insufficient calories from low milk supply and not other infant causes.

Specific information about individual drugs and herbs is summarized at the end of these recommendations in Table 1.

1. Evaluate the mother for medical causes of low milk supply: pregnancy, medications, primary mammary glandular insufficiency, breast surgery, polycystic ovarian syndrome, hypothyroidism, retained placenta, ingestion of placenta capsules, theca lutein cyst, loss of prolactin secretion following postpartum hemorrhage, heavy smoking or alcohol use, or other pertinent conditions. Treat the condition as indicated if treatment is available.[58] For many of these women, a galactogogue should not be recommended or prescribed.

2. Assess and increase the frequency and effectiveness of milk removal. Use nonpharmacologic measures to increase the overall rate of breast milk synthesis. For women whose infants are not effective at milk removal or are unable to feed at the breast (e.g., premature, hospitalized, hypotonic, and anatomical problems), regularly expressing by hand and/or breast pump is necessary. Ensure that the expressing technique and any breast pumps used are effective. Galactogogues will not increase the milk supply if there is infrequent or inadequate breast drainage.

3. Although there are more high-quality studies of domperidone and some studies of herbal galactogogues since the last revision of this protocol, current research of both pharmaceutical and herbal galactogogues is still relatively inconclusive and all agents have potential adverse effects. Therefore, ABM cannot recommend any specific galactogogue at this time.

4. If the healthcare provider chooses to prescribe a galactogogue after weighing potential risks versus potential benefits of these agents, they should follow the guidelines below.[56,59,60] (IV)
   a. Inform women about available data concerning efficacy, timing of use, and duration of therapy of galactogogues.
   b. Inform women about available data concerning potential adverse effects of galactogogues.
   c. Screen the mother for contraindications to, allergies to, or drug interactions with the chosen medication or other substance.
      If prescribing domperidone:
      i. It is particularly important to screen mothers for a past history of cardiac arrhythmias and concomitant use of medications such as fluconazole, erythromycin, and other macrolide antibiotics (Table 1).
      ii. While no studies have been undertaken, some practitioners perform an electrocardiogram on women of concern before commencement of the medication and at 48 hours. If there is prolongation of the QTc interval, the medication is ceased.
   d. Provide ongoing care to, supervise ongoing care of, or transfer care of both mother and infant to ensure appropriate follow-up and attention to any side effects.
   e. Prescribe galactogogues at the lowest possible doses for the shortest period of time; do not exceed recommended therapeutic doses.
   f. Consider gradually discontinuing the drug (tapering the dose) rather than abruptly discontinuing the therapy; some studies simply stop the drug at the conclusion of therapy and others gradually discontinue the drug, with no clear advantage to either method.
   g. If milk production wanes after stopping the drug and improves again with resumption of medication, attempt to gradually decrease the drug to the lowest effective dose and then discontinue the drug at a later date if possible.
   h. Consider documenting that there has been a discussion about contraindications and that the mother has been provided with information about the benefits and risks of any galactogogue being prescribed.

CONCLUSIONS

Before the use of a galactogogue, a lactation expert should thoroughly evaluate the entire feeding process and maximize nongalactogogue management. In the absence of evidence for low milk supply, the mother should be reassured. When intervention is indicated, modifiable factors should be addressed: maternal anxiety and mental health issues, comfort and relaxation for the mother, frequency and effectiveness of milk removal, and any underlying medical conditions.

Medication should never replace evaluation and counseling on modifiable factors. There remain selected indications for the use of galactogogues, but the current data are insufficient to make any definitive recommendations. A number of high-quality studies have found domperidone to be useful in mothers of preterm infants (Table 1), although there is concern about rare, but significant, adverse effects. Herbal galactogogues are problematic because of lack of regulation of preparations and insufficient evidence of efficacy and safety.

Clinicians should prescribe galactogogues with appropriate caution with regard to drug-to-drug (or drug-to-herb) interactions as well as an overall risk-to-benefit approach and complete informed consent. Close follow-up of both mother and infant is essential to monitor the status of lactation as well as any adverse effects of the drug(s) on the mother or infant.

RECOMMENDATIONS FOR FURTHER RESEARCH

At present, there are ongoing studies investigating the effects of insulin resistance on milk supply and whether metformin can act as a galactogogue in women with insulin resistance and low milk supply. We await with interest the outcome of these studies.

However, existing studies about galactogogues cannot be considered conclusive, and many of the recommendations are based primarily on expert opinion, small studies, and studies in which nonpharmacologic breastfeeding support was suboptimal and not standardized. Most studies have been conducted on mothers of preterm infants using mechanical breast pumps rather than on mothers of term infants whose problems usually arise in the first few days to weeks postpartum. There is a clear need for well-designed, adequately powered, randomized controlled trials using adequate doses of galactogogues in populations of women in which both the experimental and control groups receive up-to-date, appropriate lactation support.

These studies need to be done in mothers of both term and preterm infants and need to measure clinically relevant outcomes such as infant weight gain, need for artificial feeding (supplements other than mother's own milk), quantification of maternal milk production, and adverse drug effects. In addition, research should be undertaken investigating cultural practices and foods that have been used to stimulate and maintain milk production over many centuries.

ACKNOWLEDGMENTS

Stephanie Omage and Sara Whitburn assisted in updating the annotated bibliography for this protocol.

REFERENCES

1. Li R, Fein SB, Chen J, et al. Why mothers stop breastfeeding: Mothers' self-reported reasons for stopping during the first year. *Pediatrics*. 2008;122(Suppl 2):S69—S76.
2. Robert E, Coppieters Y, Swennen B, et al. The reasons for early weaning, perceived insufficient breast milk, and maternal dissatisfaction: Comparative studies in two belgian regions. *Int Sch Res Not*. 2014;2014:678564.
3. Hauck Y, Fenwick J, Dhaliwal SS, et al. A Western Australian survey of breastfeeding initiation, prevalence and early cessation patterns. *Matern Child Health J*. 2011;15:260—268.
4. Gatti L. Maternal perceptions of insufficient milk supply in breastfeeding. *J Nurs Scholarsh*. 2008;40:355—363.
5. Kent JC. How breastfeeding works. *J Midwifery Womens Health*. 2007;52:564—570.
6. Cox D, Owens R, Hartmann P. Blood and milk prolactin and the rate of milk synthesis in women. *Exp Physiol*. 1996;81:1007—1020.
7. Czank C, Henderson JL, Kent JC, et al. Hormonal control of the lactation cycle. In: Hale TW, Hartmann PE, eds. *Hale & Hartmann's Textbook of Human Lactation*. Amarillo, TX: Hale Publishing; 2007:89—111.
8. Daly S, Hartmann P. Infant demand and milk supply. Part 1: Infant demand and milk production in lactating women. *J Hum Lact*. 1995;11:21—26.
9. Daly S, Hartmann P. Infant demand and milk supply. Part 2: The short-term control of milk synthesis in lactating women. *J Hum Lact*. 1995;11:27—37.
10. Reisman T, Goldstein Z. Case report: Induced lactation in a trans gender woman. *Transgend Health*. 2018;3:24—26.
11. Milsom S, Breier B, Gallaher B, et al. Growth hormone stimulates galactopoiesis in healthy lactating women. *Acta Endocrinol*. 1992;127:337—343.
12. Gunn A, Gunn T, Rabone D, et al. Growth hormone increases breast milk volumes in mothers of preterm infants. *Pediatrics*. 1996;98:279—282.
13. Milsom S, Rabone D, Gunn A, et al. Potential role for growth hormone in human lactation insufficiency. *Horm Res*. 1998;50:147—150.
14. Shekelle P, Woolf S, Eccles M, et al. Developing guidelines. *Br Med J*. 1999;318:593—596.
15. Aono T, Aki T, Koike K, et al. Effect of sulpiride on poor puerperal lactation. *Am J Obstet Gynecol*. 1982;143:927—932.
16. Ylikorkala O, Kauppila A, Kivinen S, et al. Sulpiride improves inadequate lactation. *Br Med J*. 1982;285:249—251.
17. Peters R, Schulze-Tollert J, Schuth W. Thyrotrophin releasing hormone—A lactation-promoting agent? *Br J Obstet Gynaecol*. 1982;98:880—885.
18. Tyson J, Perez A, Zanartu J. Human lactational response to oral thyrotropin releasing hormone. *J Clin Endocrinol Metab*. 1976;43:760—768.
19. da Silva OP, Knoppert DC, Angelini MM, et al. Effect of domperidone on milk production in mothers of premature newborns: A randomized, double-blind, placebo-controlled trial. *Can Med Assoc J*. 2001;164:17—21.
20. Kauppila A, Kivinen S, Ylikorkala O. Metoclopramide increases prolactin release and milk secretion in puerperium without stimulating the secretion of thyrotropin and thyroid hormones. *J Clin Endocrinol Metab*. 1981;52:436—439.
21. Donovan TJ, Buchanan K. Medications for increasing milk supply in mothers expressing breastmilk for their preterm hospitalised infants. *Cochrane Database Syst Rev*. 2012;3: CD005544.
22. Bazzano A, Hofer R, Thibeau S, et al. A review of herbal and pharmaceutical galactagogues for breast-feeding. *Ochsner J*. 2016;16:511—524.
23. Grzeskowiak L, Smithers L, Amir L, et al. Domperidone for increasing breast milk volume in mothers expressing breast

milk for their preterm infants: A systematic review and meta-analysis. *BJOG*. 2018. [Epub ahead of print]; DOI:10.1111/1471-0528.15177.

24. Jantarasaengaram S, Sreewapa P. Effects of domperidone on augmentation of lactation following cesarean delivery at full term. *Int J Gynaecol Obstet*. 2012;116:240–243.

25. Knoppert DC, Page A, Warren J, et al. The effect of two different domperidone doses on maternal milk production. *J Hum Lact*. 2013;29:38–44.

26. Ingram J, Taylor H, Churchill C, et al. Metoclopramide or domperidone for increasing maternal breast milk output: A randomised controlled trial. *Arch Dis Child Fetal Neonatal Ed*. 2012;97:F241–F245.

27. Asztalos EV, Campbell-Yeo M, da Silva OP, et al. Enhancing human milk production with domperidone in mothers of preterm infants. *J Hum Lact*. 2017;33:181–187.

28. Wan EWX, Davey K, Page-Sharp M, et al. Dose-effect study of domperidone as a galactagogue in preterm mothers with insufficient milk supply, and its transfer into milk. *Br J Clin Pharmacol*. 2008;66:283–289.

29. Doggrell SA, Hancox JC. Cardiac safety concerns for domperidone, an antiemetic and prokinetic, and galactogogue medicine. *Expert Opinion On Drug Safety*. 2014;13:131–138.

30. Leelakanok N, Holcombe A, Schweizer ML. Domperidone and risk of ventricular arrhythmia and cardiac death: A systematic review and meta-analysis. *Clin Drug Investig*. 2016;36:97.

31. Smolina K, Mintzes K, Hanley GE, et al. The association between domperidone and ventricular arrhythmia in the postpartum period. *Pharmacoepidemiol Drug Saf*. 2016;25:1210–1214.

32. Grzeskowiak LE. Domperidone for lactation: What healthcare providers really should know. *Obstet Gynecol*. 2017;130:913.

33. Lewis PJ, Devenish C, Kahn C. Controlled trial of metoclopramide in the initiation of breast feeding. *Br J Clin Pharmacol*. 1980;9:217–219.

34. Hansen W, McAndrew S, Harris L, et al. Metoclopramide effect on breastfeeding the preterm infant: A randomized trial. *Obstet Gynecol*. 2005;105:383–389.

35. Sakha K, Behbahan A. Training for perfect breastfeeding or metoclopramide: Which one can promote lactation in nursing mothers? *Breastfeed Med*. 2008;3:120–123.

36. Seema Patwari AK, Satyanarayana L. Relactation: An effective intervention to promote exclusive breastfeeding. *J Trop Pediatr*. 1997;43:213–216.

37. Fife S, Gill P, Hopkins M, et al. Metoclopramide to augment lactation, does it work? A randomized trial. *J Matern Fetal Neonatal Med*. 2011;24:1317–1320.

38. Kauppila A, Anunti P, Kivinen S, et al. Metoclopramide and breast feeding: Efficacy and anterior pituitary responses of the mother and child. *Eur J Obstet Gynecol*. 1985;19:19–22.

39. Ertl T, Sulyok E, Ezer E, et al. Metoclopramide on the composition of human breast milk. *Acta Paediatr Hung*. 1991;31:415–422.

40. de Gezelle H, Ooghe W, Thiery M, et al. Metoclopramide and breast milk. *Eur J Obstet Gynecol*. 1983;15:31–36.

41. Guzman V, Toscano G, Canales E, et al. Improvement of defective lactation by using oral metoclopramide. *Acta Obstet Gynecol Scand*. 1979;58:53–55.

42. Kauppila A, Kivinen S, Ylikorkala O. A dose response relation between improved lactation and metoclopramide. *Lancet*. 1981;1:1175–1177.

43. Toppare M, Laleli Y, Senses D, et al. Metoclopramide for breast milk production. *Nutr Res*. 1994;14:1019–1029.

44. Ehrenkrantz R, Ackerman B. Metoclopramide effect on faltering milk production by mothers of premature infants. *Pediatrics*. 1986;78:614.

45. Gupta AP, Gupta PK. Metoclopramide as a lactogogue. *Clin Pediatr*. 1985;24:269–272.

46. Tolino A, Tedeschi A, Farace R, et al. The relationship between metoclopramide and milk secretion in puerperium. *Clin Exp Obstet Gynecol*. 1981;8:93–95.

47. Sewell CA, Chang CY, Chehab MM, et al. Domperidone for lactation: What health care providers need to know. *Obstet Gynecol*. 2017;129:1054–1058.

48. US Food and Drug Administration. How to request domperidone for expanded access use. 2018. Available at www.fda.gov/Drugs/DevelopmentApprovalProcess/HowDrugsareDevelopedandApproved/ApprovalApplications/InvestigationalNewDrugINDApplication/ucm368736.htm (accessed April 21, 2018).

49. Kim-Godwin Y. Postpartum beliefs and practices among non-Western cultures. *MCN Am J Matern Child Nurs*. 2003;28:74–78.

50. Kim M-K, Shin J-S, Patel RA, et al. The effects of pigs' feet consumption on lactation. *Ecol Food Nutr*. 2013;52:223–238.

51. Thaweekul P, Thaweekul Y, Sritipsukho P. The efficacy of hospital-based food program as galactogogues in early period of lactation. *J Med Assoc Thai*. 2014;97:478–482.

52. Özalkaya E, Aslandoğdu Z, Özkoral A, et al. Effect of a galactagogue herbal tea on breast milk production and prolactin secretion by mothers of preterm babies. *Niger J Clin Pract*. 2018;21:38–42.

53. Mortel M, Mehta SD. Systematic review of the efficacy of herbal galactogogues. *J Hum Lact*. 2013;29:154–162.

54. Haastrup MB, Pottegård A, Damkier P. Alcohol and breastfeeding. *Basic Clin Pharmacol Toxicol*. 2014;114:168–173.

55. Koletzko B, Lehner F. Beer and breastfeeding. *Adv Exp Biol*. 2000;478:23–38.

56. Anderson PO. Herbal use during breastfeeding. *Breastfeed Med*. 2017;12:507–509.

57. Tiran D. The use of fenugreek for breast feeding women. *Complement Ther Nurs Midwifery*. 2003;9:155–156.

58. Lawrence R, Lawrence R. *Breastfeeding: A Guide for the Medical Profession*. 8th ed. Philadelphia, PA: Elsevier Mosby; 2015.

59. Anderson PO. The galactogogue bandwagon. *J Hum Lact*. 2013;29:7–10.

60. Grzeskowiak LE, Amir LH. Pharmacological management of low milk supply with domperidone: Separating fact from fiction. *Med J Aust*. 2014;201:257–258.

61. Campbell-Yeo ML, Allen AC, Joseph KS, et al. Effect of domperidone on the composition of preterm human breast milk. *Pediatrics*. 2010;125:e107–e114.

62. Turkyılmaz C, Onal E, Hirfanoglu IM, et al. The effect of galactagogue herbal tea on breast milk production and short-term catch-up of birth weight in the first week of life. *J Altern Complement Med*. 2011;17:139–142.

63. Damanik R, Wahlqvist ML, Wattanapenpaiboon N. Lactagogue effects of Torbangun, a Bataknese traditional cuisine. *Asia Pac J Clin Nutr*. 2006;15:267–274.

64. Khan TM, Wu DB-C, Dolzhenko AV. Effectiveness of fenugreek as a galactagogue: A network meta-analysis. *Phytother Res*. 2018;32:402–412.

65. Reeder C, Legrand A, O'Connor-Von SK. The effect of fenugreek on milk production and prolactin levels in mothers of preterm infants. *Clin Lact*. 2013;4:159–165.

66. Fenugreek. Lactmed 2018. Available at https://toxnet.nlm.nih. gov/cgi-bin/sis/search2/f?./temp/ ~jReBbc:1 (accessed March 13, 2018).

67. Di Pierro F, Callegari A, Carotenuto D, Tapia MM. Clinical efficacy, safety and tolerability of BIO-C (micronized Silymarin) as a galactagogue. *Acta Biomed.* 2008;79:205—210.

68. Jellin J, Gregory P, Batz F, et al. *Natural Medicines Comprehensive Database.* Stockton, CA: Therapeutic Research Faculty; 2009.

69. Serrao F, Corsello M, Romagnoli C, et al. The long-term efficacy of a galactagogue containing Sylimarin-Phosphatidylserine and Galega on milk production of mothers of preterm infants. *Breastfeed Med.* 2018;13:67—69.

70. Zecca E, Zuppa A, D'Antuono A, et al. Efficacy of a galactogogue containing silymarin-phosphatidylserine and galega in mothers of preterm infants: A randomized controlled trial. *Eur J Clin Nutr.* 2016;70:1151—1154.

71. Low Dog T. The use of botanicals during pregnancy and lactation. *Altern Ther Health Med.* 2009;15:54—58.

72. Doyle M, Grossman M. Case report: Domperidone use as a galactagogue resulting in withdrawal symptoms upon discontinuation. *Arch Womens Ment Health.* 2017. [Epub ahead of print]; DOI:10.1007/s00737-017-0796-8.

73. Djeddi D, Kongola G, Lefaix C, et al. Effect of domperidone on QT interval in neonates. *J Pediatr.* 2008;153: 663—666.

ABM protocols expire 5 years from the date of publication.

The content of this protocol is up to date at the time of publication. Evidence-based revisions are made within 5 years or sooner if there are significant changes in the evidence.
Previous versions of this protocol were authored by Nancy Powers and Anne Montgomery.
The Academy of Breastfeeding Medicine Protocol Committee
Sarah Reece-Stremtan, MD, Chairperson
Larry Noble, MD, FABM, Translations Chairperson
Melissa Bartick, MD
Wendy Brodribb, MD, FABM
Maya Bunik, MD, MSPH, FABM
Sarah Dodd, MD
Megan Elliott-Rudder, MD
Cadey Harrel, MD
Ruth A. Lawrence, MD, FABM
Kathleen A. Marinelli, MD, FABM
Katrina Mitchell, MD
Casey Rosen-Carole, MD, MPH, MSEd
Susan Rothenberg, MD
Tomoko Seo, MD, FABM
Rose St. Fleur, MD
Adora Wonodi, MD
Michal Young, MD, FABM
For correspondence: abm@bfmed.org

APPENDIX I

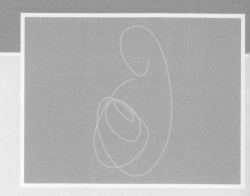

ABM Clinical Protocol #10
Breastfeeding the Late Preterm (34–36 6/7 Weeks of Gestation) and Early Term Infants (37–38 6/7 Weeks of Gestation), Second Revision 2016*

Cyd G. Boies, Yvonne E. Vaucher and the Academy of Breastfeeding Medicine

ABSTRACT

A central goal of the Academy of Breastfeeding Medicine is the development of clinical protocols for managing common medical problems that may impact breastfeeding success. These protocols serve only as guidelines for the care of breastfeeding mothers and infants and do not delineate an exclusive course of treatment or serve as standards of medical care. Variations in treatment may be appropriate according to the needs of an individual patient.

HIGHLIGHTS OF NEW INFORMATION SINCE THE 2010 REVISION INCLUDE

1. Increased risk for breastfeeding-related problems in the early term infant similar to those of the late preterm infant.
2. Importance of proactive lactation management strategies for many late preterm infants and some early term infants.
3. Importance of early expression of colostrum within the first hour after delivery.
4. Role of hand expression with or without mechanical expression in the initial postpartum hours and days.
5. Risk for iron insufficiency and iron-deficient anemia in the late preterm breastfed infant.
6. Increased risk for long-term developmental problems in the late preterm infant.

---

* Courtesy of the Academy of Breastfeeding Medicine. Please go to https://www.bfmed.org/protocols for complete protocols, translations, and the most up-to-date information (protocols are updated every 5–7 years).
Department of Pediatrics, University of California, San Diego, California.

PURPOSE

The purpose of this protocol is to:
1. Assist the late preterm and early term infant to breastfeed and/or breast milk feed to the greatest extent possible.
2. Heighten awareness of difficulties that late preterm and early term infants and their mothers may experience with breastfeeding.
3. Offer strategies to anticipate, identify promptly, and manage breastfeeding problems that the late preterm and early term infant and their mothers may experience in the inpatient and outpatient settings.
4. Prevent problems such as dehydration, hypoglycemia, hyperbilirubinemia, hospital readmission, and failure to thrive in the late preterm and early term infant.

BACKGROUND

The initial Academy of Breastfeeding Medicine protocol was written for the "near term infant" born from 35 0/7 to 36 6/7 weeks of gestation. In 2005, the National Institute of Child Health and Human Development designated infants born between 340/7 and 366/7 weeks of gestation as *late preterm* to establish a standard terminology and to emphasize the fact that these infants are really "preterm" and not "almost term."[1]

Over the past 10 years, a growing body of literature has documented an increased risk of morbidity and mortality in the late preterm infant that is often related to feeding problems, especially when there is inadequate support of breastfeeding. In addition, hospital readmission of these infants within the first 7–10 days after hospital discharge is almost always due to feeding-related problems (hyperbilirubinemia, failure to thrive, hypernatremia, and/or dehydration).[2,3]

Establishing breastfeeding in the late preterm infant is often more difficult compared with the full-term infant born at ≥ 39 weeks of gestation. Because of their immaturity, late preterm infants are less alert, have less stamina, and have greater difficulty with latch, suck, and swallow than full-term infants. The sleepiness and inability to suck vigorously may be misinterpreted as sepsis, leading to unnecessary separation, investigation and treatment, as well as poor nutrition. Conversely, some infants appear deceptively vigorous, and physically large preterm newborns (e.g., infants of diabetic mothers) are often mistakenly thought to be more developmentally mature than their actual gestational age. As a result, these infants may receive less attention than they need. Although some infants appear to have a good latch, suck, and swallow, they often do not transfer adequate breast milk volume when checked with test weights.

Late preterm infants are at greater risk for a number of transitional and breastfeeding-related morbidities (Table 1).

Late preterm infants are often separated from their mothers for evaluation and treatment and are discharged home before secretory activation (lactogenesis II)[4] is fully established. Problems with latch and milk transfer are often not identified or adequately addressed. Furthermore, mothers of late preterm and early term infants are more likely to give birth to multiples or have medical conditions such as diabetes, pregnancy-induced hypertension, chorioamnionitis, or a Cesarean-section birth that may adversely affect the onset of lactation and the success of breastfeeding.[5] Parents may go home without adequate knowledge and appropriate expectations regarding establishing breastfeeding.

It is now recognized that some early term infants, born between 37 0/7 and 38 6/7 weeks of gestation, are also at higher risk compared with term infants, born between 39 0/7 and 41 6/7 weeks of gestation, for problems including hyperbilirubinemia, hospital readmission, and reduced breastfeeding initiation and duration.[2,6] Early term infants, especially when born via elective Cesarean section, are also at increased risk for respiratory problems, Neonatal Intensive Care Unit (NICU) admission, sepsis, and hypoglycemia requiring treatment.[7-9]

Although term infants have a greater chance of successfully breastfeeding when hospitals adhere to the Ten Steps to Successful Breastfeeding of the Baby Friendly Hospital Initiative, these guidelines alone are insufficient to overcome challenges that late preterm and some early term infants and their mothers face in the immediate postpartum period and after discharge from the hospital.[10,11] Breastfeeding management of the late preterm and some early term infants requires a paradigm shift from that used with full-term infants, where an effective latch, suck, and swallow is the cornerstone for successful lactation and nutrition for the infant. Recognizing that effective suckling often takes some time to become established, management should ensure the infant is adequately nourished and that the maternal milk supply is developed and protected.[12-14] Breastfeeding adjuncts (e.g., nipple shields, supplementation, milk expression, breast compressions) are more likely to be required for the late preterm and even some early term dyads.

Given the increased risk of medical problems of the late preterm and early term infants compared with term infants, close observation and monitoring are required, especially in the first 12–24 hours after birth when the risk of inadequate adaptation to extra-uterine life is the highest. Late preterm infants born at 34 0/7 to 34 6/7 weeks of gestation have a 50% risk for morbidity during the birth hospitalization.[5,15] Transfer to a higher level of care for appropriate care and monitoring may be needed.

Late preterm and early term infants also require timely evaluation soon after hospital discharge. These follow-up services must be able to assist with breastfeeding problems

TABLE 1 Morbidities of the Late Preterm Infant[2,3,5,8,9,15,57,59–63]
Hypothermia
Hypoglycemia
Excessive weight loss
Dehydration
Slow weight gain
Failure to thrive
Prolonged infant formula supplementation
Exaggerated jaundice
Kernicterus
Dehydration
Fever secondary to dehydration
Sepsis
Apnea
Re-hospitalization
Breastfeeding failure

TABLE 2   Principles of Care for the Late Preterm Infant

1. Develop specific policies/pathways for lactation management
2. Ensure communication among all care providers and parents
3. Assure appropriate assessment and reassessment of the mother and infant
4. Provide timely inpatient and outpatient lactation support
5. Avoid or minimize separation of mother and infant
6. Prevent and promptly recognize problems
7. Educate parents, nurses, lactation consultants, and physicians about vulnerabilities and challenges that are specific to the care of these infants
8. Develop specific discharge/follow-up guidelines
9. Monitor care through quality improvement projects

---

or questions from the first post-discharge visit. For more complicated breastfeeding problems, mothers and infants should be seen by a lactation consultant, a breastfeeding medicine specialist, or a healthcare professional who is experienced with managing lactation issues as soon as possible.

RECOMMENDATIONS

Principles of care

These principles are guidelines for optimal care of the late preterm and early term infant and are presented to help guide policy development. Each provider and newborn unit should use these recommendations, where applicable to their institution and practice. All but principle #8 are applicable to both the in-patient and out-patient settings (Table 2).

Implementation of principles of care: inpatient
Initial steps

a. Develop and communicate in writing to hospital staff a standard feeding plan for late preterm infants that can be easily implemented and modified as needed.[16,17] (IV) (Quality of evidence [levels of evidence IA, IB, IIA, IIB, III, and IV] is based on levels of evidence used for the National Guidelines Clearing House[18] and is noted in parentheses.)

b. Facilitate extended skin-to-skin contact immediately after birth when the mother is alert to improve postpartum stabilization of heart rate, respiratory effort, temperature control, blood glucose, metabolic stability, and early breastfeeding.[19–21] (IV, I, and llA)

c. Determine gestational age by obstetrical estimate and Ballard/modified Dubowitz scoring.[22] (III)

d. Observe the infant closely for 12–24 hours after birth to rule out physiologic instability (e.g., hypothermia, apnea, tachypnea, oxygen desaturation, hypoglycemia, poor feeding). Where the infant is observed will depend on the local conditions, facilities and staffing available, and how the mother–infant dyad can be supported to breastfeed.[16,17,19] Close observation must be continued during skin-to-skin care, breastfeeding, and rooming-in.

e. Encourage rooming-in 24 hours a day, with frequent extended periods of skin-to-skin contact when the mother is awake. If the infant is physiologically stable and healthy, allow the infant to remain with the mother while receiving intravenous antibiotics or phototherapy.[20]

f. Allow free access to the breast, encouraging initiation of breastfeeding within 1 hour after birth.[23,24] (l, IIA) If the mother and infant are separated, the mother should begin hand expression of colostrum within the first hour of birth[25] (IB) and at ~3 hourly intervals. Some, but not all, studies demonstrate that hand expression is as good or better than breast pump expression in establishing milk supply immediately after birth.[23,24,26–29] Even if the mother and infant are not separated, many of these infants will not effectively suckle when first offered the breast, so consider hand expression and feeding expressed colostrum to the infant with a spoon, dropper, or other device after the first attempted breastfeed.[26] (III)

g. Encourage breastfeeding ad libitum and on demand. It may be necessary to wake the infant if he or she does not indicate hunger cues within 4 hours of the previous feed, which is not unusual in the late preterm infant.[12] (IV) The infant should be breastfed (or breast milk fed) 8–12 times per 24-hour period. Instruct and help initiate milk expression by pump or hand in mothers whose infant is smaller, sleepier, or unable to successfully latch in the first 24 hours. These infants, especially if they have intrauterine growth retardation (IUGR), may need supplemental feeds (preferably of expressed breast milk) for low blood glucose levels, or excessive weight loss.

h. Show the mother techniques to facilitate effective latch with careful attention to adequate support of the jaw and head.[10,30] (IV)

Ongoing care

a. Communicate any changes in the feeding plan to parents and hospital staff directly and/or in writing as appropriate depending on the local procedures and protocols.[16,17]

b. Evaluate breastfeeding, preferably within 24 hours of birth, by a lactation consultant or other healthcare professional with expertise in lactation management of late preterm and early term infants.[16,19]

c. Assess and document breastfeeding at least twice daily by two different healthcare professionals, preferably by using a standardized tool (e.g., LATCH Score, IBFAT, Mother/Baby Assessment Tool).[31–34] (III)

d. Educate the mother about breastfeeding her late preterm infant (e.g., position, latch, duration of feeds, early feeding cues, breast compressions, etc.).[12,17,19] Provide written information as well as oral instruction about breastfeeding the late preterm infant.

e. Monitor vital signs every 6–8 hours, weight change, stool and urine output, and milk transfer.[16,17,19]

f. Monitor for frequently occurring problems (e.g., hypoglycemia, hypothermia, poor feeding, hyperbilirubinemia, hypotonia).[30,31,35,37] (l) Late preterm and early term infants should be followed closely with a low threshold for checking bilirubin levels. Many healthcare facilities determine bilirubin levels and plot them on an appropriate curve according to age in hours (e.g., Bhutani chart) before the infant is discharged.[1,32,36,37] (IV, III, and IV) Some infants may need to be transferred to a higher level of care for medically appropriate management and monitoring.

g. Avoid excessive weight loss or dehydration. Losses greater than 3% of birth weight by 24 hours of age or greater than 7% by day 3 merit evaluation and may require further monitoring and adjustment of medical and breastfeeding support.[16,17,19]

   i. If there is evidence of ineffective milk transfer, breast compressions while the infant suckles may be helpful,[26,38,39] (III, IV) and the use of an ultrathin silicone nipple shield could be considered.[12,39] If a nipple shield is used, the mother and infant should be followed closely by a lactation consultant or a knowledgeable healthcare professional until the nipple shield is no longer needed. (IV)

   ii. Consider pre- and post-feeding test weights daily or after some (but not all) breastfeeds to assess the quantity of milk transferred.[12,40] Infants are weighed immediately before the feed on an electronic scale with accuracy at minimum ± 5 g, and then reweighed immediately after the feed under the exact same circumstances.

   iii. The infant may need to be supplemented after breastfeeding with small quantities (5–10 mL per feeding on day1, 10–30 mL per feeding thereafter) of the mother's expressed milk, donor human milk, or infant formula.[16,17] Choice of methods of supplementation includes cup, syringe, supplemental device, or bottle and depends on the clinical situation, the mother's preference, and the experience of the healthcare professionals assisting the mother. Cup feedings have demonstrated safety in late preterm and term infants, with careful attention to appropriate technique allowing infants to "lap up" the feeding at their own pace.[41] (IV) Some investigators found that cup feeding takes longer with less intake compared with bottle feeds.[42] (IB) There is little evidence about the safety or efficacy of other alternative feeding methods or their effect on breastfeeding. A recent study, however, found no difference in weight gain, feeding times, and length of hospital stays in the cup versus bottle-fed infants; cup feeding was associated with a significant protective effect on any and exclusive breastfeeding at hospital discharge, 3 and 6 months post-discharge.[43] (IB) Smaller IUGR or immature late preterm infants may not have regular sleep/wake periods. For these infants, consider offering expressed breast milk (by bottle, cup, etc) when sleepy and breastfeeds when more alert.[12]

   iv. If supplementing with expressed breast milk or infant formula, the mother should express by pump or hand after breastfeeding at least six times per 24 hours to help establish and maintain her milk supply until the infant is breastfeeding well.[12,16,17,19]

   If the infant is not feeding at the breast at all, mothers should express at least 8 times per 24 hours. Milk production may be increased by hand massage of the breasts while pumping.[26]

h. Avoid hypothermia by using skin-to-skin contact, that is, kangaroo care[20] as much as possible when the mother is awake or by double wrapping if necessary and dressing the baby in a shirt and hat or cap. Intermittent use of an incubator may be required to maintain normothermia.[16]

Discharge planning

a. Assess readiness for discharge, including physiologic stability and intake exclusively at breast, or with supplemental feedings.[12,16,19,44] (IV) The physiologically stable late preterm infant should be able to maintain body temperature for at least 24 hours without assistance and have a normal respiratory rate. Preferably, weight should be no more than 7% below birth weight, although all aspects of the mother/infant dyad should be taken into account. Adequate intake should be documented by feeding volume (e.g., test weights) or infant weight (e.g., stable or increasing).[12,16]

b. Develop a discharge-feeding plan. Consider method of feeding (breast, cup, supplemental device, bottle etc.), type of feeding (i.e., breast milk, donor human milk, or infant formula), and volume of milk intake (mL/kg/day), especially if being supplemented. If required, determine the most practical and acceptable method of supplementation for the mother.[12,16,17,19]

c. Communicate the discharge-feeding plan to mother and the healthcare professional/s involved in following up the infant. Written communication is preferable.[16]

d. When breast milk transfer is low, it may be appropriate to send the mother home with a scale to do test weights to confirm milk transfer during breastfeeds, or arrange for the infant to have frequent weight checks.[12] Parents should also be asked to monitor and record urine and stool output.

Implementation of principles of care: outpatient or community follow-up
Initial visit

a. Although timing of the length of hospital stay may vary, late preterm and early term infants require close follow-up in the early postpartum period and the first follow up appointment or home health visit should normally occur 1 or 2 days after hospital discharge.[17,45,46] (IV)

b. Relevant information, including prenatal, perinatal, infant, and feeding history (e.g., need for supplement in the hospital, problems with latch, need for phototherapy, etc.), should be recorded. Gestational age and birth weight should be specifically noted. Electronic medical record templates with breastfeeding-specific queries are useful in recording this information.

c. Review feeding since discharge with specific attention to frequency and approximate duration of feeding at the breast and if needed, method and type (expressed breast milk, infant formula) of supplementation. Obtain information about stool and urine output, color of stools, and the infant's behavior (e.g., crying, not satisfied after a feed, sleepy and difficult to keep awake at the breast during a feed, etc.). If the parents have a written feeding record, it should be reviewed.[17,46,47] (IV)

d. Examine the infant, noting state of alertness and hydration. Obtain an accurate infant weight without clothing. Calculate percentage change in weight from birth and change in weight from discharge. Assess for jaundice, preferably with a transcutaneous bilirubin screening device and/or serum bilirubin determination if indicated.[17,46]

e. Assess the mother's breasts for nipple shape, pain, trauma, engorgement, and mastitis. The mother's emotional state and degree of fatigue should be taken into account, especially when considering supplemental feeding routines. Whenever possible, observe the baby feeding at the breast, evaluating the latch, suck, and swallow.[46]

f. Review the mother's goals and expectations regarding breastfeeding her late preterm or early term infant. She may need encouragement and education regarding the process of transitioning from expressing and giving supplemental feeds to exclusive breastfeeding. Mothers should be cautioned not to taper expressing sessions too rapidly to ensure the maintenance of a generous milk supply that will allow for more effective milk transfer.[12]

g. Review with the parents where their infant is sleeping and educate about safe sleeping practices. Asking, "where did you and your baby sleep last night?" may give a more accurate picture of actual sleeping practice.

Problem solving

a. Poor weight gain (<20 g/day) is almost always the result of inadequate milk intake. The median daily weight gain of a healthy newborn is 28–34 g/day.[48] (IV) The healthcare provider must determine whether the problem is insufficient milk production, inability of the infant to transfer sufficient milk, or a combination of both. The infant who is getting enough breast milk should have at least six voids and three to four sizable yellow seedy stools daily by day 4, be satisfied after 20–40 minutes of breastfeeding, and have an age appropriate weight loss/gain.[46] Although a 10% weight loss may be acceptable in the larger, healthy late preterm or early term infant who is effectively breastfeeding and whose mother is achieving secretory activation, in many situations a maximum of 7% weight loss is more appropriate for the smaller and/or IUGR infant. The following strategies may be helpful to increase weight gain:

 i. The infant should be observed breastfeeding with attention to the latch, suck, and swallow. Test weights may be useful to evaluate the quantity of milk transferred (see 2gii).

 ii. Increase the frequency of breastfeeds.

 iii. Start supplementing (preferably with expressed breast milk or donor human milk) after breastfeeding or increase the amount of supplement already being given.

 iv. Offer the supplement if the infant is awake and not satisfied after ~30–40 minutes at the breast. Additional time suckling may tire the infant without significantly increasing intake. Newborns need to rest between feeds rather than suckling continuously.

 v. Institute or increase frequency of expressing (hand or pump), especially after a breastfeed if the breasts are not well drained. If already using a breast pump appropriately, switch to a more effective type (e.g., hand to mechanical, mechanical to hand, or a more efficient mechanical pump). Expressing more than six times a day may not be feasible for many mothers once their infant is home, whereas expressing eight or more times a day may be necessary to maximize milk removal. (IV)

 vi. Explore ways for the mother to relax while expressing: Arrange for help with other chores and to get more sleep.

 vii. Triple feeding regimens (breastfeeding, followed by supplementation and then expressing) for every feed are effective, but they may not be sustainable for some mothers, especially if they have limited support at home. The mother's ability to cope and manage breastfeeding and expressing must be taken into account when devising a feeding plan. (IV)

 viii. In conjunction with the mother, consider the use of a galactogogue (a medicine or herb to increase her milk supply) if there is documented low breast milk supply and for whom other efforts to increase milk production have failed (see ABM Clinical Protocol #9).[49]

ix. Consider referral to a lactation consultant or breastfeeding medicine specialist.

b. For infants with difficulties in latching, the infant's mouth should be examined for anatomical abnormalities (e.g., ankyloglossia [tongue-tie], cleft palate), and it may be helpful for a digital suck examination to be performed by a suitably trained healthcare professional. The mother's nipples and breasts should be examined to assess breast development, an atomic configuration, plugged or blocked ducts, mastitis, engorgement, nipple trauma, or postfeeding nipple compression. A referral to a lactation consultant or breastfeeding medicine specialist or in the case of ankyloglossia, referral to a healthcare professional trained in frenotomy may be indicated.[50] (III)

c. Jaundice and hyperbilirubinemia are more common in late preterm and early term infants. Although all risk factors should be considered, if the principal causative factor is lack of milk, the primary treatment is to provide more milk to the infant, preferably through improved breastfeeding or supplementation with expressed breast milk or donor milk. If home or hospital-based phototherapy is indicated, breast milk production and intake should not be compromised.[51,52] (IV) If the mother's own milk or donor milk is not available, small amounts of cow's milk-based infant formula should be used. Hydrolyzed casein formulas may be considered for this purpose, as there is evidence that these formulas are more effective in lowering serum bilirubin than standard infant formula.[53] (IIB)

Ongoing care

a. Infants who are not gaining weight well and for whom adjustments are being made to the feeding plan must be evaluated by a suitably trained healthcare professional frequently (e.g., daily or every 2–3 days depending on the situation) after each feeding adjustment either in the clinic or in the office or by a home healthcare provider with feedback to the primary care provider. (III)

b. The late preterm infant should have weekly weight checks until 40 weeks of post-conceptual age or until he or she is thriving. Weight gain should average 20–30 g/day, and length and head circumference should each increase by an average of 0.5 cm/week.[48]

c. Breastfed late preterm infants are at increased risk for iron deficiency and iron deficiency anemia compared with term infants, and routine iron supplementation is recommended.[54–56] (IV, III, and IB)

d. Late preterm infants are also more likely to sleep in unsafe situations as compared with term infants,[57] thus adding to the established increased risk of sudden infant death syndrome (SIDS) in preterm infants. Therefore, regular inquiry into sleep position and location is also warranted.

e. The diagnosis of late preterm birth should remain on the primary care giver's problem list for several years, as these children are at increased risk for pulmonary and mild neurodevelopmental problems.[8,58]

Multiples

a. Multiple gestations (twins, triplets etc.) more often result in preterm or late preterm birth. The issues of having enough breast milk for two or more infants and feeding two at the breast are more challenging than when managing a singleton dyad.

b. Supplemental feeds are more frequently required. Consider donor human milk if available, at least in the first few weeks of life, if the mother is not producing enough milk.

c. Help the mother of multiples in managing her time. This includes how best to use the help of family, friends, and even hiring help.

d. The mother of late preterm twins will usually not be able to feed them in tandem until they are older and are each effectively feeding at the breast alone due to their immaturity and need for more help with positioning, latch, and continued attention during a feed.

e. Some mothers will never produce enough milk to exclusively breastfeed more than one infant, and those infants will need supplementation with donor human milk or infant formula.

RECOMMENDATIONS FOR FUTURE RESEARCH

1. Evaluation of care in the first 12–24 hours while the infant is transitioning to the extra-uterine environment, as there is no uniform approach at present.
2. Determination of discharge readiness and optimal post-discharge care.
3. Best practices for optimizing maternal breast milk volume.
4. Best practices for transitioning the infant to full breastfeeding.
5. Best practices for helping the mother cope with time consuming pumping and breastfeeding regimens.

REFERENCES

1. Engle WA. A recommendation for the definition of "late preterm" (near-term) and the birth weight-gestational age classification system. *Semin Perinatol*. 2006;30:2–7.
2. Young PC, Korgenski K, Buchi KF. Early readmission of newborns in a large health care system. *Pediatrics*. 2013;131: e1538–e1544.
3. Ray KN, Lorch SA. Hospitalization of early preterm, late preterm, and term infants during the first year of life by gestational age. *Hosp Pediatr*. 2013;3:194–203.
4. Pang WW, Hartmann PE. Initiation of human lactation: Secretory differentiation and secretory activation. *J Mammary Gland Biol Neoplasia*. 2007;12:211–221.

5. Shapiro-Mendoza CK, Tomashek KM, Kotelchuck M, et al. Effect of late-preterm birth and maternal medical conditions on newborn morbidity risk. *Pediatrics.* 2008;121: e223—e232.

6. Norman M, Åberg K, Holmsten K, et al. Predicting nonhemolytic neonatal hyperbilirubinemia. *Pediatrics.* 2015;136:1087—1094.

7. Tita ATN, Landon MB, Spong CY, et al. Timing of elective repeat cesarean delivery at term and neonatal outcomes. *N Engl J Med.* 2009;360:111—120.

8. Seikku L, Gissler M, Andersson S, et al. Asphyxia, neurologic morbidity, and perinatal mortality in early-term and postterm birth. *Pediatrics.* 2016;137:e20153334.

9. Reddy UM, Bettegowda VR, Dias T, et al. Term pregnancy: A period of heterogeneous risk for infant mortality. *Obstet Gynecol.* 2011;117:1279—1287.

10. Eidelman AI. The challenge of breastfeeding the late preterm and the early-term infant. *Breastfeed Med.* 2016;11. 99—99.

11. Philipp BL. ABM Clinical Protocol #7: Model Breastfeeding Policy (Revision 2010). *Breastfeeding Med.* 2010;5:173—177.

12. Meier P, Patel AL, Wright K, et al. Management of breastfeeding during and after the maternity hospitalization for late preterm infants. *Clin Perinatol.* 2013;40:689—705.

13. Morton J. Perfect storm or perfect time for a bold change? *Breastfeed Med.* 2014;9:180—183.

14. Neifert M, Bunik M. Overcoming clinical barriers to exclusive breastfeeding. *Pediatr Clin North Am.* 2013;60:115—145.

15. Pulver LS, Denney JM, Silver RM, et al. Morbidity and discharge timing of late preterm newborns. *Clin Pediatr.* 2010;49:1061—1067.

16. UC San Diego Health Supporting Premature Infant Nutrition (SPIN). Protocol for late preterm infants. 2016. Available at https://health.ucsd.edu/specialties/obgyn/maternity/newborn/nicu/spin/staff/Pages/late-preterm.aspx (accessed August 25, 2016).

17. California Perinatal Quality Care Collaborative. Care and management of the late preterm infants toolkit. 2013. Available at www.cpqcc.org/sites/default/files/LatePretermInfantToolkitFINAL2-13.pdf (accessed August 25, 2016).

18. Shekelle PG, Woolf SH, Eccles M, et al. Developing guidelines. *BMJ.* 1999;318:593—596.

19. Phillips RM, Goldstein M, Hougland K, et al. Multidisciplinary guidelines for the care of late preterm infants. *J Perinatol.* 2013;33(Suppl 2):S5—S22.

20. Moore ER, Anderson GC, Bergman N, et al. Early skin-to-skin contact for mothers and their healthy newborn infants. *Cochrane Database Syst Rev.* 2012;CD003519.

21. Righard L, Alade MO. Effect of delivery room routines on success of first breast-feed. *Lancet.* 1990;336:1105—1107.

22. Ballard JL, Khoury JC, Wedig K, et al. New Ballard Score, expanded to include extremely premature infants. *J Pediatr.* 1991;119:417—423.

23. Becker GE, Smith HA, Cooney F. Methods of milk expression for lactating women. *Cochrane Database Syst Rev.* 2015; CD006170.

24. Maastrup R, Hansen BM, Kronborg H, et al. Factors associated with exclusive breastfeeding of preterm infants. *Results from a prospective national cohort study. PLoS One.* 2014;9:e89077.

25. Parker LA, Sullivan S, Krueger C, et al. Effect of early milk expression on milk volume and timing of lactogenesis stage II among mothers of very low birthweight infants: A pilot study. *J Perinatol.* 2012;32:205—209.

26. Morton J, Hall JY, Wong RJ, et al. Combining hand techniques with electric pumping increases milk production in mothers of preterm infants. *J Perinatol.* 2009;29: 757—764.

27. Ohyama M, Watabe H, Hayasaka Y. Manual expression and electric breast pumping in the first 48h after delivery. *Pediatr Int.* 2010;52:39—43.

28. Lussier MM, Brownell EA, Proulx TA, et al. Daily breastmilk volume in mothers of very low birth weight neonates: A repeated-measures randomized trial of hand expression versus electric breast pump expression. *Breastfeed Med.* 2015;10:312—317.

29. Slusher TM, Slusher IL, Keating EM, et al. Comparison of maternal milk (breastmilk) expression methods in an African nursery. *Breastfeed Med.* 2012;7:107—111.

30. Thomas J, Marinelli KA. ABM Clinical Protocol #16: Breastfeeding the Hypotonic Infant, Revision 2016. *Breastfeed Med.* 2016;11:271—276.

31. Jensen D, Wallace S, Kelsay P. LATCH: A breastfeeding charting system and documentation tool. *J Obstet Gynecol Neonatal Nurs.* 1994;23:27—32.

32. Matthews MK. Developing an instrument to assess infant breastfeeding behaviour in the early neonatal period. *Midwifery.* 1988;4:154—165.

33. Mulford C. The Mother-Baby Assessment (MBA): An "Apgar score" for breastfeeding. *J Hum Lact.* 1992;8:79—82.

34. Ingram J, Johnson D, Copeland M, et al. The development of a new breast feeding assessment tool and the relationship with breast feeding self-efficacy. *Midwifery.* 2015;31:132—137.

35. Wight N, Marinelli KA. ABM Clinical Protocol #1: Guidelines for blood glucose monitoring and treatment of hypoglycemia in term and late-preterm neonates, revised 2014. *Breastfeed Med.* 2014;9:173—179.

36. Bhutani VK, Stark AR, Lazzeroni LC, et al. Predischarge screening for severe neonatal hyperbilirubinemia identifies infants who need phototherapy. *J Pediatr.* 2013;162. 477—482. e471.

37. Maisels MJ, Bhutani VK, Bogen D, et al. Hyperbilirubinemia in the newborn infant $>$ or $=$ 35 weeks' gestation: An update with clarifications. *Pediatrics.* 2009;124:1193—1198.

38. Morton J, Wong RJ, Hall JY, et al. Combining hand techniques with electric pumping increases the caloric content of milk in mothers with preterm infants. *J Perinatol.* 2012;32:791—796.

39. Walker M. Breastfeeding the late preterm infant. *J Obstet Gynecol Neonatal Nurs.* 2008;37:692—701.

40. Haase B, Barreira J, Murphy P, et al. The development of an accurate test weighing technique for preterm and high-risk hospitalized infants. *Breastfeed Med.* 2009;4:151—156.

41. Lang S, Lawrence CJ, Orme RL. Cup feeding: An alternative method of infant feeding. *Arch Dis Child.* 1994;71:365—369.

42. Marinelli KA, Burke GS, Dodd VL. A comparison of the safety of cupfeedings and bottlefeedings in premature infants whose mothers intend to breastfeed. *J Perinatol.* 2001;21:350—355.

43. Yilmaz G, Caylan N, Karacan CD, et al. Effect of cup feeding and bottle feeding on breastfeeding in late preterm infants: A randomized controlled study. *J Hum Lact.* 2014;30:174—179.

44. American Academy of Pediatrics Committee on Fetus and Newborn. Hospital discharge of the high-risk neonate. *Pediatrics.* 2008;122:1119—1126.

45. American Academy of Pediatrics Section on Breastfeeding. Breastfeeding and the use of human milk. *Pediatrics*. 2012;129: e827–e841.

46. Neifert MR. Prevention of breastfeeding tragedies. *Pediatr Clin North Am*. 2001;48:273–297.

47. Neifert MR. Breastmilk transfer: Positioning, latch-on, and screening for problems in milk transfer. *Clin Obstet Gynecol*. 2004;47:656–675.

48. Grummer-Strawn LM, Reinold C, Krebs NF. Use of World Health Organization and CDC growth charts for children aged 0–59 months in the United States. *MMWR Recomm Rep*. 2010;59:1–15.

49. Academy of Breastfeeding Medicine Protocol Committee. ABM Clinical Protocol #9: Use of galactogogues in initiating or augmenting the rate of maternal milk secretion (First Revision January 2011). *Breastfeed Med*. 2011;6:41–49.

50. Geddes DT, Langton DB, Gollow I, et al. Frenulotomy for breastfeeding infants with ankyloglossia: Effect on milk removal and sucking mechanism as imaged by ultrasound. *Pediatrics*. 2008;122:e188–e194.

51. American Academy of Pediatrics Subcommittee on Hyperbilirubinemia. Management of hyperbilirubinemia in the newborn infant 35 or more weeks of gestation. *Pediatrics*. 2004;114:297–316.

52. Academy of Breastfeeding Medicine Protocol Committee. ABM Clinical Protocol #22: Guidelines for management of jaundice in the breastfeeding infant equal to or greater than 35 weeks' gestation. *Breastfeed Med*. 2010;5:87–93.

53. Gourley GR, Kreamer B, Cohnen M, et al. Neonatal jaundice and diet. *Arch Pediatr Adolesc Med*. 1999;153:184–188.

54. Baker RD, Greer FR. Diagnosis and prevention of iron deficiency and iron-deficiency anemia in infants and young children (0–3 years of age). *Pediatrics*. 2010;126:1040–1050.

55. Yamada RT, Leone CR. Hematological and iron content evolution in exclusively breastfed late-preterm newborns. *Clinics (São Paulo, Brazil)*. 2014;69:792–798.

56. Berglund SK, Westrup B, Domellöf M. Iron supplementation until 6 months protects marginally low-birth-weight infants from iron deficiency during their first year of life. *J Pediatr Gastroenterol Nutr*. 2015;60:390–395.

57. Hwang SS, Barfield WD, Smith RA, et al. Discharge timing, outpatient follow-up, and home care of late-preterm and early-term infants. *Pediatrics*. 2013;132:101–108.

58. Kugelman A, Colin AA. Late preterm infants: Near term but still in a critical developmental time period. *Pediatrics*. 2013;132:741–751.

59. Leone A, Ersfeld P, Adams M, Schiffer PM, et al. Neonatal morbidity in singleton late preterm infants compared with full-term infants. *Acta Paediatr*. 2012;101:e6–e10.

60. Loftin RW, Habli M, Snyder CC, et al. Late preterm birth. *Rev Obstet Gynecol*. 2010;3:10–19.

61. Morag I, Okrent AL, Strauss T, et al. Early neonatal morbidities and associated modifiable and non-modifiable risk factors in a cohort of infants born at 34–35 weeks of gestation. *J Matern Fetal Neonatal Med*. 2015;28: 876–882.

62. Nagulesapillai T, McDonald SW, Fenton TR, et al. Breastfeeding difficulties and exclusivity among late preterm and term infants: Results from the all our babies study. *Can J Public Health*. 2013;104:e351–e356.

63. Radtke JV. The paradox of breastfeeding-associated morbidity among late preterm infants. *J Obstet Gynecol Neonatal Nurs*. 2011;40:9–24.

ABM protocols expire 5 years from the date of publication.

Content of this protocol is up-to-date at the time of publication. Evidence based revisions are made within 5 years or sooner if there are significant changes in the evidence.

The first and second versions of this protocol were authored by Eyla G Boies and Yvonne E Vaucher.

The Academy of Breastfeeding Medicine Protocol Committee:
Wendy Brodribb, MBBS, PhD, FABM, Chairperson
Larry Noble, MD, FABM, Translations Chairperson
Nancy Brent, MD
Maya Bunik, MD, MSPH, FABM
Cadey Harrel, MD
Ruth A. Lawrence, MD, FABM
Kathleen A. Marinelli, MD, FABM
Kate Naylor, MBBS, FRACGP
Sarah Reece-Stremtan, MD
Casey Rosen-Carole, MD, MPH
Tomoko Seo, MD, FABM
Rose St. Fleur, MD
Michal Young, MD
For correspondence: abm@bfmed.org

ABM Clinical Protocol #11

Guidelines for the Evaluation and Management of Neonatal Ankyloglossia and Its Complications in the Breastfeeding Dyad: The Academy of Breastfeeding Medicine*: ABM Protocols

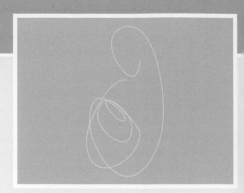

ABSTRACT

A central goal of **The Academy of Breastfeeding Medicine** *is the development of clinical protocols for managing common medical problems that may impact breastfeeding success. These protocols serve only as guidelines for the care of breastfeeding mothers and infants and do not delineate an exclusive course of treatment or serve as standards of medical care. Variations in treatment may be appropriate according to the needs of an individual patient.*

DEFINITION

Ankyloglossia, partial: The presence of a sublingual frenulum that changes the appearance or function of the infant's tongue because of its decreased length, lack of elasticity, or attachment too distal beneath the tongue or too close to or onto the gingival ridge. In this document we will refer to partial ankyloglossia as simply "ankyloglossia." "True" or "complete ankyloglossia," extensive fusion of the tongue to the floor of the mouth, is extremely rare and is not within the scope of this discussion.

BACKGROUND

At birth, the infant's tongue is normally able to extend over and past the mandibular gum pad. Significant ankyloglossia prevents an infant from anteriorly extending and elevating the tongue, and many breastfeeding experts believe that these limitations alter the normal peristaltic motion of the tongue during feeding, resulting in the potential for nipple trauma and problems with effective milk transfer and infant weight gain.

Ankyloglossia, commonly known as tongue-tie, occurs in approximately 3.2% to 4.8% of consecutive term infants at birth[1,2] and in 12.8% of infants with breastfeeding problems.[2]

The condition has been associated with an increased incidence of breastfeeding difficulties: 25% in affected versus 3% in unaffected infants.[1]

Various methods have been suggested to diagnose and evaluate the severity of ankyloglossia[3,4] and to determine the criteria for intervention.[5,6] Short- and long-term consequences of ankyloglossia may include feeding and speech difficulties,[7,8] as well as orthodontic and mandibular abnormalities[9–12] and psychological problems.[13]

In the 1990s a number of case reports and observational studies were published that documented an association between ankyloglossia and breastfeeding problems.[14–18] There is considerable controversy regarding the significance of ankyloglossia and its management, both within and among medical specialty groups.[19,20] Both the diagnosis of ankyloglossia and the use of frenotomy, an incision or "snipping" of the frenulum, to treat ankyloglossia vary widely. The frenotomy procedure, carefully performed, has recently been shown to decrease maternal nipple pain to improve infant latch,[2] and to improve milk transfer (personal communication, J. Ballard, July 27, 2004). There is a growing tendency among breastfeeding medicine specialists to favor releasing the tongue of the infant to facilitate breastfeeding and to protect the breastfeeding experience. To date, no randomized trials exist to demonstrate frenotomy for ankyloglossia is effective in treating infant or maternal breastfeeding problems.

ASSESSMENT OF ANKYLOGLOSSIA

All newborn infants, whether healthy or ill, should have a thorough examination of the oral cavity that assesses function as well as anatomy. This examination should include palpation of the hard and soft palate, gingivae, and sublingual areas in addition to the movements of the tongue, and the length, elasticity, and points of insertion of the sublingual frenulum.

When breastfeeding difficulties are encountered and a short or tight sublingual frenulum is noted, the appearance and function of the tongue may be semi-quantified using a scoring system such as the Hazelbaker[3] (Table 1). The Hazelbaker scale has been tested for interrater reliability (personal communication, J Ballard, July 27, 2004) and

---

* Courtesy of the Academy of Breastfeeding Medicine. Please go to https://www.bfmed.org/protocols for complete protocols, translations, and the most up-to-date information (protocols are updated every 5–7 years).

TABLE 1   Hazelbaker assessment tool for lingual frenulum function*

Appearance Items	Function Items
Appearance of tongue when lifted	*Lateralization*
2: Round or square	2: Complete
1: Slight cleft in tip apparent	1: Body of tongue but not tongue tip
0: Heart- or V-shaped	0: None
Elasticity of frenulum	*Lift of tongue*
2: Very elastic	2: Tip to mid-mouth
1: Moderately elastic	1: Only edges to mid-mouth
0: Little or no elasticity	0: Tip stays at lower alveolar ridge or rises to mid-mouth only with jaw closure
Length of lingual frenulum when tongue lifted	*Extension of tongue*
2: > 1 cm	2: Tip over lower lip
1: 1 cm	1: Tip over lower gum only
0: <1 cm	0: Neither of the above, or anterior or mid-tongue humps AND/OR dimples
Attachment of lingual frenulum to tongue	*Spread of anterior tongue*
2: Posterior to tip	2: Complete
1: At tip	1: Moderate or partial
0: Notched tip	0: Little or none
Attachment of lingual frenulum to inferior	*Cupping alveolar ridge*
2: Entire edge, firm cup	2: Attached to floor of mouth or well below ridge
1: Side edges only, moderate cup	1: Attached just below ridge
0: Poor or no cup	0: Attached at ridge
	Peristalsis
	2: Complete, anterior to posterior
	1: Partial, originating posterior to tip
	0: None or reverse motion
	Snapback
	2: None
	1: Periodic
	0: Frequent or with each suck

*The infant's tongue is assessed using the 5 appearance items and the 7 function items. Significant ankyloglossia is diagnosed when the appearance score total is 8 or less and/or the function score total is 11 or less. (2;3)
Adapted with permission from Hazelbaker AK: The assessment tool for lingual frenulum function (ATLFF): Use in a lactation consultant private practice Masters thesis, Pacific Oaks College, 1993.

validated in a sample of term neonates.[2] Hazelbaker scores consistent with significant ankyloglossia have been shown to be highly correlated with difficulty with latching the infant onto the breast and maternal complaints of sore nipples.[2] Alternatively, ankyloglossia may be qualified as mild, moderate, or severe by the appearance of the tongue and of the frenulum.

ASSESSMENT OF THE BREASTFEEDING DYAD

Breastfeeding complications caused by ankyloglossia can generally be placed into broad categories of those caused by maternal nipple trauma or failure of the infant to breastfeed effectively. Specific complaints include difficulty latching or sustaining a latch, infant becoming frustrated or falling asleep at breast, prolonged feedings, a dissatisfied baby, gumming or chewing at the breast, poor weight gain, or failure to thrive. Maternal complaints include traumatized nipples, severe unrelenting pain with feeding, inability to let down because of

pain, incomplete breast drainage, breast infections, and plugged ducts.

The physician should interview the mother to ascertain her degree of confidence and comfort while breastfeeding. This can be done semi-quantitatively by using a scoring system such as the LATCH score or a similar tool.[21] The LATCH score has been shown to correlate with breastfeeding duration but only due to subscores for breast comfort.[22]

If the mother describes nipple pain, the physician may wish to use a pain scale in order to semiquantify her perception of the degree of her pain. This serves to follow trends in the severity of pain, which may help in determining the effectiveness of an intervention.

The infant should be weighed, and the rate of weight gain since birth should be assessed. The physician should observe the mother and infant while breastfeeding to assess the effectiveness of the feeding and provide assistance as appropriate. Problems including an inadequate or nonsustained latch and ineffective feedings should be noted. Test weights may be useful in assessing milk transfer. The infant should be weighed prior to and after breastfeeding without a change in clothing or diaper; the difference between the weights in grams indicates the amount of breast milk consumed in milliliters.

The mother's nipples should be examined carefully for creases, bruises, blisters, cracks, or bleeding. Areolar edema and erythema should be noted as possible signs of nipple infection. A family history of bleeding diatheses should be elicited.

RECOMMENDATIONS

Conservative management of tongue-tie may be sufficient, requiring no intervention beyond breastfeeding assistance, parental education, and reassurance.[19] For partial ankyloglossia, if a tongue-tie release is deemed appropriate, the procedure should be performed by a physician or pedodontist experienced with the procedure; otherwise a referral should be made to an ear, nose, and throat specialist or oral surgeon. Release of the tongue-tie appears to be a minor procedure, but it may be ineffective in solving the immediate clinical problem and may cause complications such as infant pain and distress and postoperative bleeding, infection, or injury to Wharton's duct.[19] Complications are rare, however.[1,2,5,9]

Frenotomy, or simple incision or "snipping," of a tongue-tie is the most common procedure performed for partial ankyloglossia. It should be recognized that postoperative scarring may further limit tongue movement.[19] Excision with lengthening of the ventral surface of the tongue or a z-plasty release is a procedure with less postoperative scarring, but it carries the additional risks of general anesthesia.[19]

THE FRENOTOMY PROCEDURE

Instruments: Iris scissors and grooved retractor
Supplies: Clean gloves and gauze; gelatin foam.
Method: Parents should be counseled about risks, benefits, and alternatives of the procedure and informed consent should be obtained. This counseling should include a discussion of the possibility that the clinical breastfeeding problem will not improve.

The frenulum may be transilluminated to check for translucency and lack of vasculature. The frenulum is usually a thin, translucent hypovascular membrane, where a simple frenotomy results in an almost bloodless procedure. Rarely, it may be thick and fibrous or muscular and relatively vascular. Thicker frenula are best incised by an otolaryngologist or oral surgeon under controlled conditions.

The frenulum is almost devoid of sensory innervation. Infants under 4 months of age can usually tolerate the frenotomy very well without any local anesthesia. Alternatively, topical anesthetic (e.g., benzocaine gel or paste) may be applied with cotton applicators to both sides of the frenulum in the area to be incised. This, however, may have the undesirable effect of numbing the mouth, such that the baby may not be able to suck effectively after the frenotomy is completed.

The infant is placed supine on the examining table or mother's lap. An assistant holds the baby's elbows firmly against the ears and stabilizes the chin with one index finger. Alternatively, the infant

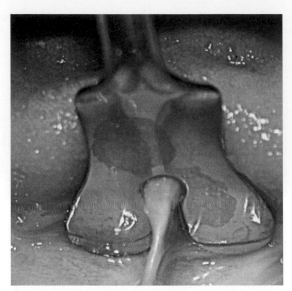

Figure 1 Using a Lorenz tongue elevator, the lingual frenum is exposed. Pulling upward on the tongue stretches and allows visualization of the frenum and the floor of the mouth. In this infant an 8 mm incision was needed to allow sufficient movement of the tongue for effective breastfeeding to occur. Picture courtesy of Dr. Larry Kotlow.

may be swaddled with a receiving blanket to immobilize the arms while the assistant stabilizes the head. Slight extension of the infant's neck allows better visualization of the tongue and frenulum. Using the grooved retractor or physician's fingers, the physician lifts the tongue to expose the frenulum. With the tips of the iris scissors an incision is made in the thinnest portion of the frenulum, close to the retractor and parallel to the tongue. Care is taken not to incise the tongue, the genioglossus muscle, or the gingival tissue. The incision should extend into the sulcus between the tongue and the genioglossus muscle, just beyond the level of the muscle, carefully avoiding the floor of the mouth. This ensures complete detachment of the tongue from the gingiva, without causing damage to the sublingual mucosa or to the salivary duct (Figure 1).

The site beneath the tongue is blotted with gauze until little or no blood is seen. In the event of unexpected bleeding beyond 2 to 3 minutes, a strip of gelatin foam may be used to achieve rapid hemostasis. The infant may be returned to the mother immediately to be breastfed. Infant latch and maternal nipple pain should be reassessed at this time. There is no specific aftercare required except for breastfeeding. A small white patch or eschar is seen in some infants for 1 or 2 weeks during the healing process. Infection of the site is exceedingly rare if clean technique is used as described.

See Figure 1, picture courtesy of Dr. Larry Kotlow.

Medical equipment used in this procedure should be sterilized or disinfected in accordance with the guidelines of the Centers for Disease Control.[23]

MANAGEMENT OF MATERNAL AND INFANT COMPLICATIONS OF ANKYLOGLOSSIA

If nipple damage or infection is present, a problem-specific treatment program should be instituted. Mastitis and yeast infections should be treated according to established guidelines.[24]

Some mothers may need nipple rest for one to several days to allow healing to occur before reinstituting feedings at the breast. These mothers should be encouraged to express their breast milk in order to maintain their milk supply and to feed their milk to the baby by an alternate method.

Suppressed lactation should be addressed and every attempt made to reestablish the mother's milk supply. Infants who have been gaining weight slowly or failing to thrive may need to receive supplements of expressed breast milk or formula temporarily.

Follow-up for resolution of maternal and infant complications of ankyloglossia should take place by the mother's or infant's primary health care provider within 3 or 4 days of the frenotomy.

FURTHER RESEARCH

This protocol was developed by the Academy of Breastfeeding Medicine to provide clinicians with guidance about the assessment and treatment of ankyloglossia and associated breastfeeding problems. More definitive recommendations await future research in this area. The Academy of Breastfeeding Medicine urges that more research be undertaken so that the benefits and risks of frenotomy for ankyloglossia and its effectiveness in treating breastfeeding concerns can be better understood. We specifically recognize that the Hazelbaker and LATCH instruments cited in this document require further interrater and intrarater reliability and validity testing. We recognize that a critical need exists for clinical tools to assess breastfeeding performance as well as the degree of ankyloglossia and function of the tongue. In addition, a randomized investigator-blinded clinical trial is needed to assess the effectiveness of frenotomy in treating infant and maternal breastfeeding problems associated with ankyloglossia.

Copyright protected © 2004 The Academy of Breastfeeding Medicine, Inc.

Approved August 3, 2004

The Academy of Breastfeeding Medicine Protocol Committee

*Jeanne Ballard, MD

Caroline Chantry MD, FABM, Co-Chairperson

Cynthia R. Howard MD, MPH, FABM, Co-Chairperson

Development supported in part by a grant from the Maternal and Child Health Bureau, Department of Health and Human Services

*lead author(s)

REFERENCES

1. Messner AH, Lalakea ML. Ankyloglossia: controversies in management. *Int J Pediatr Otorhinolaryngol.* 2000;54:123–131.
2. Ballard JL, Auer CE, Khoury JC. Ankyloglossia: assessment, incidence, and effect of frenuloplasty on the breastfeeding dyad. *Pediatrics.* 2002;110:e63.
3. Hazelbaker, AK: The assessment tool for lingual frenulum function (ATLFF): Use in a lactation consultant private practice. Master's Thesis, Pacific Oaks College, 1993.
4. Kotlow LA. Ankyloglossia (tongue-tie): a diagnostic and treatment quandary. *Quintessence Int.* 1999;30:259–262.
5. Masaitis NS, Kaempf JW. Developing a frenotomy policy at one medical center: A case study approach. *J Hum Lact.* 1996;12:229–232.
6. Sanchez-Ruiz I, Gonzalez Landa G, Perez, Gonzalez V, et al. [Section of the sublingual frenulum. Are the indications correct?] [Spanish]. *Cir Pediatr.* 1999;12:161–164.
7. Garcia Pola MJ, Gonzalez Garcia M, Garcia Martin JM, Gallas M, Seoane Leston J. A study of pathology associated with short lingual frenum. *ASDC J Dent Child.* 2002;69(59–62):12.
8. Messner AH, Lalakea ML. The effect of ankyloglossia on speech in children. *Otolaryngol Head Neck Surg.* 2002;127:539–545.
9. Wright JE. Tongue-tie. *J Paediatr Child Health.* 1995;31:276–278.
10. Williams WN, Waldron CM. Assessment of lingual function when ankyloglossia (tongue-tie) is suspected. *J Am Dent Assoc.* 1985;110:353–356.
11. Yoel J. [Tongue tie and speech disorders]. *Trib Odontol (B Aires).* 1976;60(195–196):198. 200.
12. Hasan N. Tongue tie as a cause of deformity of lower central incisor. *J Pediatr Surg.* 1973;8:985.
13. Ketty N, Sciullo PA. Ankyloglossia with psychological implications. *ASDC J Dent Child.* 1974;41:43–46.
14. Jain E. Tongue-tie: its impact on breastfeeding. *AARN News Lett.* 1995;18.
15. Notestine GE. The importance of the identification of ankyloglossia (short lingual frenulum) as a cause of breastfeeding problems. *J Hum Lact.* 1990;6:113–115.
16. Berg KL. Tongue-tie (ankyloglossia) and breastfeeding: A review. *J Hum Lact.* 1990;6:109–112.
17. Marmet C, Shell E, Marmet R. Neonatal frenotomy may be necessary to correct breastfeeding problems. [Review]. *J Hum Lact.* 1990;6:117–121.
18. Nicholson WL. Tongue-tie (ankyloglossia) associated with breastfeeding problems. *J Hum Lact.* 1991;7:82–84.
19. Canadian Paediatric Society, Community Paediatrics Committee. Canadian Paediatric Society Statement: Ankyloglossia and breastfeeding. *Paediatr Child Health.* 2002;7:269–270.
20. Messner AH, Lalakea ML, Aby J, Macmahon J, Bair E. Ankyloglossia: Incidence and associated feeding difficulties. *Arch Otolaryngol Head Neck Surg.* 2000;126:36–39.
21. Jensen D, Wallace S, Kelsay P. LATCH: a breastfeeding charting system and documentation tool. *J Obstet Gynecol Neonatal Nurs.* 1994;23:27–32.
22. Riordan J, Bibb D, Miller M, Rawlins T. Predicting breastfeeding duration using the LATCH breastfeeding assessment tool. *J Hum Lact.* 2001;17:20–23.
23. Centers for Disease Control: Sterilization or disinfection of medical devices: General principles. Available at: www.cdc.gov/ncidod/hip/Sterile/Sterilgp.htm. 8-20-2002.
24. Protocol Committee Academy of Breastfeeding Medicine, Amir LH, Chantry C, Howard C R: Clinical Protocol Number 4: Mastitis. Available at: www.bfmed.org. Academy of Breastfeeding Medicine, 2002.

ABM Clinical Protocol #12
*Transitioning the Breastfeeding Preterm Infant from the Neonatal Intensive Care Unit to Home, Revised 2018**

Lawrence M. Noble[1], Adora C. Okogbule-Wonodi[2], Michal A. Young[2] and The Academy of Breastfeeding Medicine

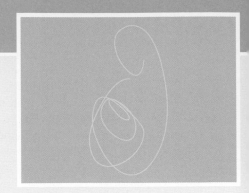

ABSTRACT

A central goal of the Academy of Breastfeeding Medicine is the development of clinical protocols, free from commercial interest or influence, for managing common medical problems that may impact breastfeeding success. These protocols serve only as guidelines for the care of breastfeeding mothers and infants and do not delineate an exclusive course of treatment or serve as standards of medical care. Variations in treatment may be appropriate according to the needs of an individual patient.

INTRODUCTION AND BACKGROUND

THE PRACTICE OF breastfeeding or providing expressed mother's milk to preterm infants is promoted because of the considerable benefits to their health and well-being.[1-3] Ideally, preterm infants in the neonatal intensive care unit (NICU) are fed their own mothers' milk or donor human milk fortified with multiple nutrients and calories to optimize growth and development.[4] Breastfeeding at the breast in the NICU before discharge should be encouraged as it may increase the breastfeeding duration.[5] Near the time of discharge, a decision must be made as to how preterm infants should feed in the postdischarge period.

Growth faltering has been observed in some preterm infants in the NICU and in the postdischarge period if they receive exclusive human milk feedings without nutrient and caloric fortification.[4,6-10] Of concern, evidence also suggests that such a nutritional deficit may adversely affect the head circumference,[7,10,11] a finding that is associated with poorer neurodevelopmental outcomes.[11,12] In addition, these infants are at risk for developing metabolic bone disease osteopenia or even rickets.[7,10,13]

Unfortunately, there are few systematic studies on the impact of postdischarge fortification for preterm infants.[8-11,13,14] A 2011 Cochrane review of published studies stated that there is not enough evidence to conclude that fortification improves infant growth.[15] In addition, studies suggest that overly rapid early growth may be detrimental for NICU graduates, increasing the risk of long-term health problems such as obesity, diabetes, heart disease, and metabolic syndrome.[16]

As such, the following guidelines are a consensus of best practices that include recommendations for monitoring and providing optimal nutritional support for preterm infants after they are discharged from the hospital. This protocol addresses the care of preterm infants born at a gestational age less than 34 weeks who are discharged home after a stay in the NICU. The American Academy of Pediatrics has recommended that preterm infants be discharged after achieving three physiologic competencies: oral feeding sufficient to support appropriate growth, the ability to maintain normal body temperature in a home environment, and sufficiently mature respiratory control.[17] These competencies are achieved by most preterm infants at a postmenstrual age (PMA) between 36 and 37 weeks, but may take longer. This protocol does not distinguish infants born appropriate for gestational age from small for gestational age, but bases decisions on current nutritional status and body weight. Quality of evidence [levels of evidence IA, IB, IIA, IIB, III, and IV] is based on levels of evidence used for the National Guidelines Clearing House and is noted in parentheses.[18]

---

* Courtesy of the Academy of Breastfeeding Medicine. Please go to https://www.bfmed.org/protocols for complete protocols, translations, and the most up-to-date information (protocols are updated every 5–7 years).

[1] Department of Pediatrics, Icahn School of Medicine at Mount Sinai, New York, New York.

[2] Department of Pediatrics and Child Health, Howard University College of Medicine, Washington, District of Columbia.

GENERAL STRATEGIES

A. The goal of the discharge feeding plan recommendations for preterm infants is to enable the mother to exclusively breastfeed or provide as much human milk as possible while protecting and supporting the mothers' decisions. Specific recommendations on supporting breastfeeding in mothers of premature infants are given in the Support for Breastfeeding Mothers of Premature Infants section.

B. In addition, the feeding plan should correct deficits that arose during the NICU stay and minimize further nutrient deficits after discharge. As the nutritional status of preterm infants varies widely, creating individualized feeding plans is the best approach.

C. All preterm infants should be routinely supplemented with iron, 2–4 mg/kg/day.[19] Vitamin D supplementation of 400 IU per day is recommended by the American Academy of Pediatrics,[20] while 800–1,000 IU/day is recommended by the European Society for Paediatric Gastroenterology Hepatology and Nutrition.[20] Higher doses of iron are recommended, up to 5 mg/kg/day, if hemoglobin is <11 g/dL (Table 1), and higher doses of vitamin D, up to 1,000 IU/day, are recommended in infants with evidence of metabolic bone disease, with an alkaline phosphatase >500[21] (IIA).

D. Enriched formula or human milk fortifier is used when fortification is necessary because it provides greater nutrient intake than human milk alone or term infant formula. Although the current published studies on postdischarge supplementation utilized human milk fortifiers,[8,9,11,14] fortifiers are usually not given at home due to lack of availability and expense. The new liquid human milk fortifiers derived from human milk can be tailored more and could potentially be useful in this population; however, they are not readily available and are very expensive.

Therefore, enriched formula mixed with expressed human milk generally is a more practical plan to provide fortification in the postdischarge period (IIA).

PREDISCHARGE FEEDING ASSESSMENT

Before the actual day of discharge, a general plan for feeding at home should be developed. Rooming-in by the mother for a few days before discharge during this transition period is strongly recommended[17] (IV). Feeding plans should reflect shared decision-making by the mother, the infant's clinician, and any others involved in feeding support (nursing, lactation consultant, and dietitian). Appropriate plans may include exclusive breastfeeding, breastfeeding combined with expressed human milk (fortification may be necessary) or formula, or a combination of all. This shared decision must consider parental perceptions and preferences, which address work and family needs, as maternal satisfaction can increase breastfeeding duration.[22] Whenever unfortified human milk is stated in this protocol, it includes breastfeeding and/or the feeding of expressed human milk.

Assessment of the following parameters should be considered when making discharge feeding plans (IV).

A. Current nutrition
1. Diet: unfortified human milk, fortified human milk, formula, or a combination
2. Milk intake (mL/kg/day) should be assessed, if not at or close to ad libitum on demand with adequate weight gain

TABLE 1 Biochemical and Growth Monitoring for Premature Infants in the Postdischarge Period

Parameters	Goal	Action values
A. Growth		
1. Weight gain	20 g/day	<15 g/day
2. Length increase	0.5–0.8 cm/week	<0.5 cm/week
3. Head circumference increase[a]	0.5–0.8 cm/week	<0.5 cm/week or >1 cm/week
4. Weight/length	>85%[c]	
B. Biochemical markers		
1. Alkaline phosphatase[b]	<450 IU/L	>500 IU/L
2. Blood urea nitrogen	>10 mg/dL	<8 mg/dL
3. Phosphorus	>5 mg/dL	<5 mg/dL
4. Vitamin D level	>30 ng/mL	<25 ng/mL
5. Hemoglobin	>11.5 g/dL	<11 g/dL

Modified from Hall[44] and Schanler[45] Conversion factors for biochemical markers: 1. Milligrams/deciliter (mg/dL) to millimoles/liter—divide by 18. 2. Nanograms/milliliter (ng/mL) to nanomoles/liter—multiply by 2.5 (i.e., 1 ng/mL = 2.5 nmol/L). 3. International units to micrograms—divide by 40.
[a]Changes in head circumference require cranial imaging, such as a cranial ultrasound.
[b]High alkaline phosphatase levels may indicate a need for bone imaging, such as a bone x-ray.
[c]This is an indication of overnutrition and a cue to stop supplementation.

TABLE 2   Assessment of Breastfeeding Adequacy and Troubleshooting Problems

Parameter of adequacy	Suggestions
1. Latch and milk transfer 2. Volume of milk production	Assess for a proper latch and for evidence of infant swallowing and improve as necessary. (a) If the supply is low, interventions may be necessary to increase milk volume. (b) If baby is not adequately draining the breast, recommend expressing milk after feeding and/or triple feeding to augment or maintain the mother's milk supply. Triple feeding is a three-step process in which the mother breastfeeds, supplements with expressed breast milk, and pumps to remove any remaining milk. Triple feeding or pumping after every feeding requires careful follow-up as it is difficult to sustain for many mothers, especially during the night (c) Consider the use of galactogogues.[46] (d) If the frequency of feeds at the breast is too low, the infant may be a sleepy preemie who requires to be woken more often or that the mother may be missing subtle feeding cues and not putting the baby to the breast enough
3. Optimize any breastfeeding that is occurring	(a) Instruct the mother to massage the breast and express some milk to begin letdown before the infant begins the feed. (b) Instruct the mother to massage the breast and employ breast compression during the feeding to increase the fat composition and volume of milk consumed.[47,48]
4. Volume of milk intake	(a) Nipple shields: Conflicting data report improved milk transfer[41] and, more recently, an association with decreased exclusive breastfeeding.[42,43] A mother who is discharged using a nipple shield should be monitored closely by a trained lactation professional and its use should be discontinued as soon as possible due to the risk of decreased supply, insufficient emptying, and other breastfeeding problems[49] (IIB). (b) Nursing supplementer/feeding tube device while at the breast. (c) Some have used a nipple shield and nursing supplementer together effectively (IV).
5. Weight gain	Consider pre- and postfeeding test weights after some breastfeeds to assess the quantity of milk transferred.[35] Infants are weighed immediately before the feed on an electronic scale, with accuracy at minimum of ± 5 g, and then reweighed immediately after the feed under the exact same circumstances, including the same diaper.

3. Oral (breastfeeding, bottle, cup, nursing supplementer [also known as supplemental nursing system], or other method).

Note: there are some facilities that supplement discharged breastfeeding preterm infants with tube feedings and report improved breastfeeding rates.[23–25]

B. Nutritional assessment: optimal versus suboptimal. Parameters for growth and biochemical measures are listed in Table 1.
1. Optimal (includes ALL the following)
   (a) Infant can feed orally, minimally 160 mL/kg/day (or growing well on exclusive breastfeeding at the breast).
   (b) In-hospital growth is normal or improving as per daily rate of weight gain and weekly rate of length and head circumference gain is calculated and/or plotted on appropriate growth charts (Table 1).
   (c) Biochemical measures of nutritional status are normal or normalizing and not indicative of ongoing protein or mineral insufficiency (Table 1).
2. Suboptimal (includes ANY one or more of the following)
   (a) Infant's intake is <160 mL/kg/day.
   (b) Growth is less than adequate as per growth standards (Table 1).
   (c) Biochemical measures of nutritional status are abnormal, not normalizing, and are indicative

of ongoing protein or mineral insufficiency (Table 1).

DISCHARGE FEEDING PLAN (IV)

A. For infants with optimal assessment
1. If the infant has been receiving fortified human milk, consider the following two options and ensure that the follow-up clinician understands the rationale for the approach prescribed:
   (a) Option 1: Change the diet to unfortified human milk, ad libitum about 1 week before discharge.
       (1) Monitor growth and milk intake (if not exclusively breastfeeding) during these days.
       (2) If intake and growth are adequate, continue this diet after discharge.
   (b) Option 2: If discharge follow-up can be arranged to assess the infant quickly (within a day or 2) and repeatedly, consider changing the diet to unfortified human milk ad libitum any time before discharge (without the need to monitor in the hospital for 1 week), and monitor growth and milk intake (if not exclusively breastfeeding) carefully after discharge.
2. If the infant has been receiving unfortified human milk, continue this diet after discharge.

B. For infants with suboptimal assessment

1. If the infant has been receiving fortified human milk, consider the following three options and ensure that the follow-up clinician understands the rationale for the approach prescribed:

   (a) Option 1: Change to unfortified human milk for most feedings, but add three feedings a day of preterm discharge formula prepared as per manufacturer's instructions (22 kcal/30 mL)[26] or one feeding of a 30-kcal/30 mL calorie formula per day (Table 3). This option allows for breastfeeding at the breast except for the formula feeds. It is important for mothers to express milk when the infant is receiving these feedings to maintain her milk supply.

   (b) Option 2: Add powdered preterm discharge formula to expressed human milk feedings to enrich it to 22 kcal/30 mL[27] (Table 3). This option will provide human milk with each feeding.

   (c) Option 3: Change to breastfeeding at the breast for all feedings while supplementing with 15 mL of preterm discharge formula (22 kcal/ 30 mL) for all feeds using a nursing supplementer (Table 3). This option will allow a baby to breastfeed at the breast for all feedings. Mothers should consider expressing milk after feedings if there is a concern that the infant is not adequately emptying the breast.

   (d) Nutritional information for the three options is given in Table 4.

   (e) For some mothers, a combination of different options may be preferable and more sustainable. For example, another caregiver gives one to two feedings of preterm discharge formula, then the mother breastfeeds with a nursing supplementer for most feedings, while breastfeeding without a supplementer for one to two of the feedings.

   (f) Assess adequacy of breastfeeding and address problems or potential problems. Optimize any breastfeeding that is occurring and consider the use of feeding devices to improve the volume of intake (Table 2).

   (g) Initiate these changes at least 1 week before anticipated discharge and monitor milk intake and growth during this week. If intake and growth are adequate during this week after changing the feeding plan, continue this diet after discharge.

   (h) If intake and growth continue to be suboptimal after 1 week, enhance fortification as per Table 3.

2. If the infant has been receiving unfortified human milk at the breast and/or by another feeding method, consider the following:

   (a) Assess the adequacy of breastfeeding, address problems or potential problems, optimize any breastfeeding that is occurring, and consider the use of feeding devices to improve the volume of intake (Table 2).

   (b) If addressing any existing breastfeeding problems does not result in optimal assessment, start fortification (Table 3). Initiate this at least 1 week before anticipated discharge and monitor milk intake and growth during this week.

   (c) If intake and growth are adequate during this week after changing the feeding plan, continue this diet after discharge.

   (d) If intake and growth continue to be suboptimal after 1 week, increase fortification (Table 3).

3. Special situation: An infant with chronic lung disease, especially on oxygen, will likely require fortification.[28]

TABLE 3   Three Options for Fortification of Human Milk

Option	Initial fortification	Enhanced fortification
1: Some formula feeds	Unfortified human milk for most feedings, with three feedings per day of preterm discharge formula (22 kcal/30 mL) or one feeding of a 30-calorie formula per day.	Increase the number of feedings a day of preterm discharge formula and/or increase formula concentration to 24 kcal/30 mL or higher.
2: Enriching feeds	Add powdered preterm discharge formula to expressed human milk feedings to enrich it to 22 kcal/30 mL.	Increase the amount of powdered preterm discharge formula added to expressed human milk to enrich it to 24 kcal/30 mL or higher.
3: Nursing supplementer	Change to breastfeeding at the breast for all feedings while supplementing with 15 mL of preterm discharge formula (22 kcal/30 mL) in all feeds using a nursing supplementer.	Increase the amount of preterm discharge formula given through the nursing supplementer during breastfeeding.

For each option, start with initial fortification. If the infant does not improve, enhance the fortification. We recommend an unfortified human milk diet for infants with an optimal nutritional assessment.

TABLE 4   **Comparisons of Nutritional Intake for Selected Nutrients (per kg/day) Based on Total Daily Volume of 180 mL/kg/day**

Feeding type	Calories, kcal/kg/day	Protein, mg/kg/day	Ca, mg/kg/day	Ph, mg/kg/day
HM[50]	126	1.9	58	25
Option 1: HM +3 feedings/day of 22 kcal/30 mL preterm discharge formula[50,51]	129	2.6	89	47
Option 1: HM +1 feed a day of 30 kcal/30 mL preterm formula[50,52]	133	2.3	91	45
Option 2: HM enriched to 22 kcal/30 mL with preterm discharge formula[53]	132	2.3	67	34
Option 2: HM Enriched to 24 kcal/30 mL with preterm discharge formula[54]	144	2.6	78	42
Option 3: Breastfeeding +15 mL of 22 kcal/30 mL preterm discharge formula in all feeds using a nursing supplementer[50,51]	128	2.5	85	45

Calculations assume a volume of 180 mL/kg/day and 8 equal feeds a day. The option 3 calculation is based on a 2-kg infant. *HM*, human milk.

POSTDISCHARGE ASSESSMENT (IV)

A. Nutrition monitoring as early as possible, preferably within 72 hours.[29] Again, ensure that the follow-up clinician understands the rationale for the approach prescribed.
  1. Assess intake
    (a) Take a detailed feeding history on what the mother has been feeding her infant since discharge, including details on providing expressed human milk versus direct breast-feeding, a full pumping history, and the use of fortified human milk or formula. Ask the mother how she is coping with caring for the infant and discuss revising the feeding plan if it is not sustainable. Consider screening for postpartum depression as bringing a preterm infant home may be a difficult time for mothers.[30]
    (b) Measure weight, length, and head circumference. Length should be measured with a stadiometer. These growth data should be plotted on appropriate growth curves, preferably the new INTERGROWTH-21st Postnatal Growth of Preterm Infants Charts,[31–33] until 64 weeks' PMA. Other acceptable growth charts are the Fenton Preterm Infant Growth Charts[30] and the Olsen Intrauterine Growth Curves[34] until 50 weeks' PMA. After 64 or 50 weeks, use the World Health Organization (WHO) growth charts.
    (c) Observation of a feeding.
    (d) Consider test weighing to assess the quantity of milk transferred.[35]
  2. Infants with adequate growth should be followed at 1 month following discharge.

  3. For infants with inadequate growth since discharge (Table 1), consider the following:
    (a) Assess the adequacy of breastfeeding, address problems or potential problems, optimize any breastfeeding that is occurring, and consider the use of feeding devices to improve the volume of intake (Table 2).
    (b) If addressing any existing breastfeeding problems does not improve growth, increase fortification (Table 3).
    (c) Weekly follow-up until the infant has demonstrated appropriate growth on the feeding plan (Table 1).
B. Nutrition monitoring 1 month after discharge
  1. Assess intake by following the same protocol as the first postpartum visit.
  2. Draw laboratories and assess growth and biochemical measures of nutritional status (Table 1).
  3. For infants with a suboptimal assessment in growth or biochemical measures, consider the following:
    (a) Assess and address breastfeeding problems or potential problems, optimize any breastfeeding that is occurring, and consider the use of feeding devices to improve the volume of intake (Table 2).
    (b) Consider starting or increasing fortification (Table 3).
    (c) Weekly follow-up until the infant has demonstrated appropriate growth on the feeding plan.
C. Frequency of nutrition monitoring
    For all preterm infants, growth monitoring is recommended every month[25] until 6 months' corrected age, then every 2 months till 1 year. Biochemical markers should be followed 1 month after discharge and at 4 months' corrected age. Infants with abnormal laboratories may require more frequent monitoring.

D. How long to continue the use of enriched formula
   1. Randomized trials showing benefits of fortification discontinued supplementation at 3 months[7,9] (1B). At a minimum, enriched formula supplementation should be continued until nutritional monitoring on the fortified diet has been adequate for several months.
   2. In addition, it is important to prevent over nutrition. If the infant's growth is rapidly increasing such that the weight/length percentile is >85% (Table 1), revise dietary supplementation.
E. When to start complementary feeds

Most experts recommend starting complementary feedings at ~6 months' corrected age.

SUPPORT FOR BREASTFEEDING MOTHERS OF PREMATURE INFANTS

Both pre- and postdischarge

A. Optimal feeding, for preterm as well as term infants, is exclusive breastfeeding at the breast. With appropriate support, this goal is attainable for most premature infants.
B. Sustained suckling with swallowing for 5 minutes is one indicator that the infant may be ready to transition from the nasogastric tube to breastfeeding[36,37] (IB). Other studies suggest that early introduction of oral feeding hastens the development of oral motor skills[38–40] (IB). Nursing supplementers may provide additional volume.[38]
C. Monitor mothers for nipple soreness. If present, this may be an indication of a shallow latch. Temporary use of silicone nipple shields can be a helpful adjunct for milk transfer and more efficient latch-on for preterm infants with shallow latch,[41] although studies report an association with decreased exclusive breastfeeding[42,43] (IIB).
D. Refer and coordinate care, such as providing a written discharge summary for the parents and primary care physician that includes detailed nutrition support recommendations, community support referrals, visiting nurse, skilled lactation consultant visits, and social services.
E. Ideally, all mothers discharged from the NICU with a breastfeeding or human milk feeding infant should have follow-up examinations with a trained, skilled lactation professional within 2 to 3 days after discharge for ongoing support and troubleshooting.

RECOMMENDATIONS FOR FUTURE RESEARCH

1. A survey of neonatologists and NICU dieticians is necessary to understand the global heterogeneity of fortification plans and breastfeeding postdischarge.
2. Comparative effectiveness studies of the different post-discharge feeding regimens are needed. We do acknowledge that the challenge in compiling and following growth parameters for at least 6 months using various protocols will be arduous and expensive.
3. Data on growth and follow-up of IUGR preterm infants need to be evaluated separately to measure the effectiveness of feeding regimens in this special subset of preterm infants.
4. QI evaluations are needed to determine the effectiveness of patient discharge instructions and communication to the outpatient follow-up team.

REFERENCES

1. Eidelman AI. Breastfeeding and the use of human milk: Analysis of the American Academy of Pediatrics 2012 Breastfeeding Policy Statement. *Breastfeed Med.* 2012;7:323–324.
2. Maffei D, Schanler RJ. Human milk is the feeding strategy to prevent necrotizing enterocolitis!. *Semin Perinatol.* 2017;41:36–40.
3. Lechner BE, Vohr BR. Neurodevelopmental outcomes of preterm infants fed human milk. *Clin Perinatol.* 2017;44:69–83.
4. Brown JVE, Embleton ND, Harding JE, et al. Multinutrient fortification of human milk for preterm infants. *Cochrane Database Syst Rev.* 2016;5:CD000343.
5. Briere CE, McGrath MJ, Cong X, et al. Direct-breastfeeding in the neonatal intensive care unit and breast-feeding duration for premature infants. *Appl Nurs Res.* 2016;32:47–51.
6. Stevens TP, Shields E, Campbell D, et al. Variation in enteral feeding practices and growth outcomes among very premature infants: A report from the New York State Perinatal Quality Collaborative. *Am J Perinatol.* 2016;33:009–019.
7. Wheeler RE, Hall RT. Feeding of premature infant formula after hospital discharge of infants weighing less than 1800 grams at birth. *J Perinatol.* 1996;16:111–116.
8. O'Connor DL, Khan S, Weishuhn K, et al. Growth and nutrient intakes of human milk-fed preterm infants provided with extra energy and nutrients after hospital discharge. *Pediatrics.* 2008;121:766–776.
9. Aimone A, Rovet J, Ward W, et al. Growth and body composition of human milk-fed premature infants provided with extra energy and nutrients early after hospital discharge: 1-year follow-up. *J Pediatr Gastroenterol Nutr.* 2009;49:456–466.
10. Chotigeat U, Vongpakorn J. Comparative growth outcome of preterm neonate fed post-discharge formula and breast milk after discharge. *J Med Assoc Thai.* 2014;97(Suppl 6):S33–S39.
11. O'Connor DL, Weishuhn K, et al. Post-Discharge Feeding Study Group. Visual development of human milk-fed preterm infants provided with extra energy and nutrients after hospital discharge. *JPEN J Parenter Enteral Nutr.* 2012;36:349–353.
12. Ghods E, Kreissl A, Brandstetter S, et al. Head circumference catch-up growth among preterm very low birth weight infants: Effect on neurodevelopmental outcome. *J Perinat Med.* 2011;39:579–586.

13. Kurl S, Heinonen K, Länsimies E. Pre- and post-discharge feeding of very preterm infants: Impact on growth and bone mineralization. *Clin Physiol Funct Imaging.* 2003;23:182–189.

14. Zachariassen G, Faerk J, Grytter C, et al. Nutrient enrichment of mother's milk and growth of very preterm infants after hospital discharge. *Pediatrics.* 2011;127:e995–e1003.

15. Young L, Embleton ND, McCormick FM, et al. Multinutrient fortification of human breast milk for preterm infants following hospital discharge. *Cochrane Database Syst Rev.* 2013;2: CD004866.

16. Kerkhof GF, Willemsen RH, Leunissen RWJ, et al. Health profile of young adults born preterm: Negative effects of rapid weight gain in early life. *J Clin Endocrinol Metab.* 2012;97:4498–4506.

17. Committee on Fetus and Newborn. Hospital discharge of the high-risk neonate. *Pediatrics.* 2008;122:1119–1126. Reaffirmed by the AAP in Pediatrics 2012;129:e1103.

18. Shekelle PG, Woolf SH, Eccles M, et al. Clinical guidelines: Developing guidelines. *BMJ.* 1999;318:593–596.

19. Baker RD, Greer FR. The Committee On Nutrition. Diagnosis and prevention of iron deficiency and iron-deficiency anemia in infants and young children (0–3 years of age). *Pediatrics.* 2010;126:1040–1050.

20. Abrams SA, the Committee On Nutrition. Calcium and vitamin D requirements of enterally fed preterm infants. *Pediatrics.* 2013;131:e1676–e1683.

21. Agostoni C, Buonocore G, Carnielli VP, et al. Enteral nutrient supply for preterm infants: Commentary from the European Society of Paediatric Gastroenterology, Hepatology and Nutrition Committee on Nutrition. *J Pediatr Gastroenterol Nutr.* 2010;50:85–91.

22. Fenton TR, Tough SC, Belik J. Breast milk supplementation for preterm infants: Parental preferences and postdischarge lactation duration. *Am J Perinatol.* 2000;17:329–333.

23. Meerlo-Habing ZE, Kosters-Boes EA, Klip H, et al. Early discharge with tube feeding at home for preterm infants is associated with longer duration of breast feeding. *Arch Dis Child Fetal Neonatal Ed.* 2009;94:F294–F297.

24. Ahnfeldt AM, Stanchev H, Jorgensen HL, et al. Age and weight at final discharge from an early discharge programme for stable but tube-fed preterm infants. *Acta Paediatr.* 2015;104:377–383.

25. Brodsgaard A, Zimmermann R, Petersen M. A preterm lifeline: Early discharge programme based on family-centred care. *J Spec Pediatr Nurs.* 2015;20:232–243.

26. Cohen RS, Mayer O, Fogleman AD. Managing the human-milk-fed, preterm, VLBW infant at NICU discharge: A simpler algorithm? *Infant Child Adolesc Nutr.* 2015;7:177–179.

27. Japakasetr S, Sirikulchayanonta C, Suthutvoravut U, et al. Implementation of a nutrition program reduced postdischarge growth restriction in Thai very low birth weight preterm infants. *Nutrients.* 2016;8. pii:E820.

28. Guimarães H, Rocha G, Guedes M, et al. Nutrition of preterm infants with bronchopulmonary dysplasia after hospital discharge—Part I. *J Pediatr Neonat Individual Med.* 2014;3: e030116.

29. Kuo DZ, Lyle RE, Casey PH, et al. Care system redesign for preterm children after discharge from the NICU. *Pediatrics.* 2017;139. pii:e20162969.

30. Sriraman NK, Melvin K, Meltzer-Brody S. ABM Clinical Protocol #18: Use of antidepressants in breastfeeding mothers. *Breastfeed Med.* 2015;10:290–299.

31. Villar J, Giuliani F, Bhuttaet ZA, et al. Postnatal growth standards for preterm infants: The Preterm Postnatal Follow-up Study of the INTERGROWTH-21st Project. *Lancet Glob Health.* 2015;3:e681–e691.

32. INTERGROWTH-21st. Postnatal growth of preterm infants. The Global Health Network. Available at: https://intergrowth21.tghn.org/postnatal-growth-preterm-infants/#pg1 (accessed February 1, 2018).

33. Fenton TR, Kim JH. A systematic review and meta-analysis to revise the Fenton growth chart for preterm infants. *BMC Pediatr.* 2013;13:59.

34. Olsen IE, Groveman SA, Lawson ML, et al. New intrauterine growth curves based on United States data. *Pediatrics.* 2010;125:e214–24.

35. Rankin MW, Jimenez EY, Caraco M, et al. Validation of test weighing protocol to estimate enteral feeding volumes in preterm infants. *J Pediatr.* 2016;178:108–112.

36. Kliethermes PA, Cross ML, Lanese MG, et al. Transitioning preterm infants with nasogastric tube supplementation: Increased likelihood of breastfeeding. *J Obstet Gynecol Neonatal Nurs.* 1999;28:264–273.

37. Park J, Knafl G, Thoyre S, et al. Factors associated with feeding progression in extremely preterm infants. *Nurs Res.* 2015;64:159–167.

38. Edwards TM, Spatz DL. An innovative model for achieving breast-feeding success in infants with complex surgical anomalies. *J Perinat Neonatal Nurs.* 2010;24:246–253.

39. Bache M, Pizon E, Jacobs J, et al. Effects of pre-feeding oral stimulation on oral feeding in preterm infants: A randomized clinical trial. *Early Hum Dev.* 2014;90:125–129.

40. Medeiros AM, Oliveira AR, Fernandes AM, et al. Characterization of the transition technique from enteral tube feeding to breastfeeding in preterm newborns. *J Soc Bras Fonoaudiol.* 2011;23:57–65.

41. Meier PP, Brown LP, Hurst NM, et al. Nipple shields for preterm infants: Effect on milk transfer and duration of breastfeeding. *J Hum Lact.* 2000;16:106–114.

42. Maastrup R, Hansen BM, Kronborg H, et al. Factors associated with exclusive breastfeeding of preterm infants. Results from a Prospective National Cohort Study. *PLoS One.* 2014;9: e89077.

43. Kronborg H, Foverskov E, Ingrid N, et al. Why do mothers use nipple shields and how does this influence duration of exclusive breastfeeding? *Matern Child Nutr.* 2017;13:e12251.

44. Hall RA. Nutritional follow-up of the breastfeeding premature infant after hospital discharge. *Pediatr Clin North Am.* 2001;48:453–460.

45. Schanler RJ. Nutrition support of the low birth weight infant. In: Walker A, Watkins JB, Duggan C, eds. *Nutrition in pediatrics: basic science and clinical applications.* 3rd edition Hamilton, Canada: BC Decker, Inc; 2003:392–412.

46. Academy of Breastfeeding Medicine Protocol Committee. ABM Clinical Protocol #9: Use of galactogogues in initiating or augmenting the rate of maternal milk secretion. *Breastfeed Med.* 2011;6:41–49.

47. Morton J, Hall JY, Wong RJ, et al. Combining hand techniques with electric pumping increases milk production in mothers of preterm infants. *J Perinatol.* 2009;29: 757–764.

48. Fouad G, Korraa A, Zaglol G, et al. The effect of different techniques of breast milk expression in its fat content in mothers of preterm infants. *Med J Cairo Univ.* 2014;82:893—899.

49. McKechnie AC, Eglash A. Nipple shields: A review of the literature. *Breastfeed Med.* 2010;5:309—314.

50. Australian National Health and Medical Research Council. Infant Feeding guidelines: Information for health workers. 2012. Table 2.1: Composition of mature human milk, cow's milk and infant formula. Available at: https://www.nhmrc.gov.au/guidelines-publications/n56 (accessed February 27, 2018).

51. Abbott Nutrition Abbott Laboratories. Product information: Similac NeoSure. 2016. Available at: http://static.abbottnutrition.com/cms-prod/abbottnutrition.com/img/Similac-NeoSure.pdf (accessed February 27, 2018).

52. Abbott Nutrition Abbott Laboratories. Product information: Similac Special Care 30. 2018. Available at: https://abbottnutrition.com/similac-special-care-30 (accessed February 27, 2018).

53. El Sakka A, El Shimi MS, Salama K, et al. Post discharge formula fortification of maternal human milk of very low birth weight preterm infants: An Introduction of a feeding protocol in a university hospital. *Pediatr Rep.* 2016;8:6632.

54. Adler A, Groh-Wargo S. Transitioning the preterm neonate from hospital to home: Nutritional discharge criteria. *NICUCurrents.* 2012;3:1—11.

ABM protocols expire 5 years from the date of publication.

The content of this protocol is up-to-date at the time of publication. Evidence-based revisions are made within 5 years or sooner if there are significant changes in the evidence.

The 2004 edition of this protocol was authored by Lori Feldman-Winter and Richard Schanler.

The Academy of Breastfeeding Medicine Protocol Committee:

Sarah Reece-Stremtan, MD, Chairperson

Larry Noble, MD, FABM, Translations Chairperson

Melissa Bartick, MD

Maya Bunik, MD, MSPH, FABM

Megan Elliott-Rudder, MD

Cadey Harrel, MD

Ruth A. Lawrence, MD, FABM

Kathleen A. Marinelli, MD, FABM

Katrina Mitchell, MD

Casey Rosen-Carole, MD, MPH, MSEd

Susan Rothenberg, MD

Tomoko Seo, MD, FABM

Rose St. Fleur, MD

Adora Wonodi, MD

Michal Young, MD, FABM

For correspondence: abm@bfmed.org

ABM Clinical Protocol #13
*Contraception During Breastfeeding, Revised 2015**

Pamela Berens[1], Miriam Labbok[2] and The Academy of Breastfeeding Medicine

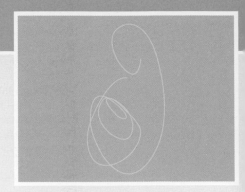

ABSTRACT

A central goal of The Academy of Breastfeeding Medicine is the development of clinical protocols for managing common medical problems that may impact breastfeeding success. These protocols serve only as guidelines for the care of breastfeeding mothers and infants and do not delineate an exclusive course of treatment or serve as standards of medical care. Variations in treatment may be appropriate according to the needs of an individual patient.

PURPOSE

THE PURPOSE OF THIS PROTOCOL is to outline considerations in assisting breastfeeding families to achieve optimal birth spacing by selecting a contraceptive method that is effective, unlikely to disrupt lactation, and satisfactory for the mother and her partner. The protocol covers the use of contraceptive methods during breastfeeding and provides guidance on the lactational amenorrhea method (LAM).

This protocol assumes that the practitioner is well versed in the risks and benefits of different types of contraception, including all pharmaceutical, permanent, and periodic abstinence/natural family planning methods.

ISSUES IN COUNSELING AND SELECTION OF CONTRACEPTIVES DURING BREASTFEEDING

1. Considerations for clinician counselling and method use

Postpartum contraception, like breastfeeding, should be discussed with women during their own obstetric prenatal and postpartum visits and the infant's pediatric well baby visits. A woman's contraceptive choice depends on many factors such as previous experience with contraceptives, future childbearing plans, husband or partner's attitude, level of user attention required for use, medical considerations, return of menses, and the woman's lactation status. If a woman is not comfortable with a method, she may not use it effectively.

2. Advantages and disadvantages of available options

Contraceptive counseling during breastfeeding extends beyond issues of efficacy, because the selected method must be appropriate for a woman's breastfeeding expectations.

Table 1 provides useful information for counseling the breastfeeding mother Considerations include the potential for hormonal methods to either disrupt milk synthesis or expose the infant to synthetic hormones. Because a falling progesterone level after birth is necessary for onset of milk production, initiation of hormonal contraception before lactation is established is of particular concern. Published evidence is insufficient to exclude these risks. At the same time, long-acting reversible hormonal methods have high contraceptive efficacy. Healthcare providers should discuss the limitations of the available data within the context of a mother's desire to breastfeed, her risk of low milk production, and her risk of unplanned pregnancy, so that she can make an autonomous and informed decision.

LAM FOR CONTRACEPTION IN THE EARLY POSTPARTUM PERIOD AND FOR INTRODUCTION OF OTHER METHODS

A. Background

Data published in the 1970s showed that women who breastfed were less likely to ovulate early postpartum and that if breastfeeding were more intensive, they were less likely than partial or nonbreastfeeders to experience a normal ovulation prior to the first menstrual-like bleed.[1] In 1988, at a Bellagio Conference, a group of expert scientists proposed three criteria as sufficient to predict fertility return. This

---

* Courtesy of the Academy of Breastfeeding Medicine. Please go to https://www.bfmed.org/protocols for complete protocols, translations, and the most up-to-date information (protocols are updated every 5–7 years).
[1] Department of Obstetrics and Gynecology, University of Texas, Houston, Texas.
[2] Carolina Global Breastfeeding Institute, Department of Maternal and Child Health, Gillings School of Global Public Health, University of North Carolina, Chapel Hill, North Carolina.

TABLE 1   General Principles for Counseling Breastfeeding Women Concerning Contraceptive Selection and Birth Spacing

Issues	Considerations
1. Breastfeeding patterns, status, and plans	Consider both short- and long-term breastfeeding intent as well as well birth spacing plans. There is the potential for hormonal methods to have an impact depending on when they are started.
	Mothers may plan to exclusively breastfeed; some may do so to use LAM, others may use LAM because they are already fully breastfeeding. LAM users should be counseled to have another method in hand for when menses return or breastfeeding patterns change. Effectiveness of LAM in exclusively breastmilk pumping mothers may not be equivalent to direct breastfeeding.
	Many women who intend to breastfeed exclusively are not able to achieve their goals.
2. Child's age/time postpartum	Many methods should not be introduced until breastfeeding is well established (i.e., at 4–6 weeks), as there may be potential for hormonal methods to directly impact lactogenesis and/or to impact the infant.
3. Maternal age and future childbearing plans	Choices depend on desire to space births or desire to limit family size. Globally recommended interpregnancy intervals are at least 18 months to 2 + years for maternal health, depending on the setting, and about 3–5 years for child health outcomes.
4. Previous contraceptive experience	Discussion of previous contraceptive experience, including compliance, satisfaction, side effects, and social issues, is essential. These issues can influence compliance and satisfaction, particularly as they pertain to prior lactation experiences.
5. Partners/interactions	Partner's experiences and opinions may impact compliance, particularly for barrier methods, LAM, and natural family planning.
	The woman's social and behavioral considerations, such as number of partners and sexual activity, should be explored. A woman's history of unplanned pregnancy and short interpregnancy interval should be reviewed and discussed.
6. Previous lactation experience/ medical conditions	Prior insufficient milk supply or inadequate infant growth
	Prior breastfeeding experience did NOT meet goals (either exclusivity or duration), AND supply was a potential reason
	Physical examination suggestive of insufficient glandular tissue
	Prior breast surgery
	Medical conditions potentially adversely affecting supply (polycystic ovary syndrome, infertility, obesity)
	Multiple gestation
	Preterm infant(s)

LAM, lactational amenorrhea method.

three-criteria approach described in further detail below as the "Lactational Amenorrhea Method" was subsequently tested.[2,3] Studies of the acceptability and contraceptive efficacy of active LAM use continue to confirm the original findings, demonstrating that LAM is acceptable, learn-able, user-friendly, and as effective as many other alternatives.[4–9] (II-2) (Quality of evidence [levels of evidence I, II-1, II-2, II-3, and III] is based on the U.S. Preventive Services Task Force Appendix A Task Force Ratings[10] and is noted throughout this protocol in parentheses.)

B. Method: what is LAM?

LAM is presented as an algorithm (Fig. 1) and includes three criteria for defining the period of lowest pregnancy risk. If one of these criteria is not met, women should immediately initiate another method. Clinically, the mother is asked these three questions:

"Are you amenorrheic?" meaning that you have you not had a menstrual bleed, or any bleed of >2 days in duration (discounting any bleed in the first 2 months).

"Are you fully or nearly fully breastfeeding?" This includes not giving your baby any supplementary foods or fluids in addition to breastfeeding (greater than once or twice a week)?

"Is your infant less than 6 months of age?"

If she answers "yes" to all three questions, she meets the requirements for LAM. If *any* of the above three questions is answered "no," then her chance of pregnancy is increased, and she should be advised to initiate another form of contraception to prevent pregnancy. If the mother is interested in and qualifies for LAM, she should review these three questions regularly. Clinicians should ensure that she has chosen her next method of contraception and either has it on hand or knows how to obtain it if it is an implant or intrauterine device (IUD).

C. Definitions for LAM use

To use LAM correctly, it is important that the patient understand each of the three criteria, which can be remembered using the letters "LAM" to indicate Lactation, Amenorrhea, and the number of Months:

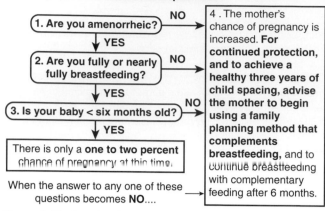

The Lactational Amenorrhea Method – LAM
Ask the mother, or advise her to ask herself,
these three questions:

1. Are you amenorrheic? — **NO** →
↓ **YES**
2. Are you fully or nearly fully breastfeeding? — **NO** →
↓ **YES**
3. Is your baby < six months old? — **NO** →
↓ **YES**
There is only a **one to two percent** chance of pregnancy at this time.

When the answer to any one of these questions becomes **NO**.... →

4. The mother's chance of pregnancy is increased. **For continued protection, and to achieve a healthy three years of child spacing, advise the mother to begin using a family planning method that complements breastfeeding,** and to continue breastfeeding with complementary feeding after 6 months.

Figure 1. The lactational amenorrhea method.

1. *Lactation.* Full or nearly full breastfeeding includes exclusive, nearly exclusive, and some irregularly provided supplements, as long as they do not disrupt the frequency of feeds.[11]
2. *Amenorrhea.* For the purposes of LAM use, menses return is defined as any bleeding that occurs after 56 days postpartum that is perceived by the patient as a menses, or any two consecutive days of bleeding.
3. *Months.* The "6 months" criterion is added primarily because this is the time that complementary feeding should begin. If breastfeeding continues at the same frequency and complementary foods are offered after the breastfeed, efficacy apparently remains high as long as amenorrhea continues. In Rwanda, the method was used up to 9 months, by maintaining the breastfeeding frequency experienced during month 6.[12] This was achieved by feeding before each complementary feeding. Another study in Pakistan found a continued high efficacy under these conditions for up to 12 months.[13] (II-2)

D. Efficacy

A Cochrane literature review[14] (and assessed as up to date in 2008) concluded that fertility rates are low among fully breastfeeding, amenorrheic women. In controlled studies of LAM, pregnancy rates for 6 months ranged from 0.45% to 2.45%. In six uncontrolled studies of LAM users, pregnancy ranged from 0% to 7.5%. The World Health Organization (WHO) carried out a prospective trial on lactational amenorrhea and fertility return; although this was not a study of women selecting and using LAM, the findings confirmed the physiological potential for high efficacy as seen in the LAM trials.[4,5] Subsequently, studies of method use have consistently found a 6-month pregnancy rate averaging 2%.[15] (I, II-2)

E. LAM management issues

Suggested behaviors contributing to method success and duration include:
1. Number of feedings. One controlled study found exclusively breastfeeding women using LAM are more

likely to be amenorrheic at 6 months than exclusively breastfeeding controls (84% vs. 69.7%, respectively).[16] Women using LAM had a higher feeding frequency and a shorter interfeeding interval than other exclusive breastfeeding women.
2. LAM can be used beyond the sixth month. The two studies mentioned above in Rwanda[12] and Pakistan[13] have indicated that the efficacy of LAM can be maintained during the 6—12-month period, provided the mother continues to breastfeed before giving complementary foods at less than 4-hour intervals during the day and 6-hour intervals at night while remaining amenorrheic. (II-2)
3. LAM effectiveness has not as yet been adequately tested to offer the method with confidence to women who are giving supplemental feedings daily or expressing milk by hand or pump instead of breastfeeding.[17] (II-2) Women who are expressing milk more than a few times per week should be counseled to initiate an additional contraceptive method. (III)

F. Transition to other methods

LAM may also be used as an introductory method to inform the user when it is time to initiate use of another method. Of note is that fully breastfeeding women are very unlikely to conceive in the first 56 days postpartum so secondary methods can be delayed until at least 8 weeks postpartum. When LAM criteria no longer apply or whenever a breastfeeding woman wishes to use an alternate family planning method, she should have an alternative method readily available. Alternative methods are discussed in terms of advantages and disadvantages and special issues related to breastfeeding.

ADDITIONAL COMMENTS ON INDIVIDUAL METHODS

Table 2 provides additional specific information for many individual methods, including advantages, disadvantages, and potential issues related to breastfeeding for each.

NATURAL FAMILY PLANNING

Four methods of "fertility awareness" natural family planning include the Billings ovulation method (OM), the Creighton model system, the symptothermal method, and the Marquette method. Each of these methods can be used even when a woman's menses has not yet returned because of breastfeeding. These methods rely on observation of various combinations of cervical mucus, temperature, and/or hormonal monitoring, and then couples abstain during fertile periods. All of these methods have specific protocols for women to use during the postpartum period so they may plan accordingly if they wish to delay another pregnancy. The Marquette model has a recent peer-reviewed study to show the efficacy of its postpartum protocol.[18]

These methods may require significant periods of abstinence. Research on the use of the Billings OM during the

TABLE 2   Use of Contraceptive Methods During Lactation: Advantages, Disadvantages, and Impact on Lactation

Method	Advantages	Disadvantages	Effects related to breastfeeding
Lactational amenorrheic method Natural family planning • Billings ovulation • Creighton model • Marquette • Symptothermal	• No side effects • Effectiveness rates comparable with other user-directed methods of birth control (i.e., pills or barriers) • Low cost for most methods	• Requires special instruction for use during breastfeeding • ClearBlue fertility monitor expense with Marquette • May require long periods of abstinence	• None
Barrier methods • Diaphragm/cap • Spermicide • Condoms	• Few side effects • Effective with diligent and appropriate use • Easily accessible as "backup" • Low cost • Also provide protection from sexually transmitted infection	• Potential for user error • Allergy possible • May be inconvenient and limit spontaneity • Cervical cap and diaphragm require fitting.	• None • Use of lubricant may be beneficial with condoms in setting of vaginal atrophy.
Other contraceptive options IUDs • Copper IUD (ParaGard T380A), 10 years • Levonorgestrel IUD (Mirena), 5 years • Levonorgestrel IUD (Skyla), 3 years	• Highly effective • Reversible • Long-term contraceptives • Little user attention required (typical use and perfect use are similar)	• Small risk of infection, perforation, expulsion • Requires provider insertion and removal • Copper contraindicated with Wilson's disease and copper allergy • Short-term use costly; long-term use cost-effective	• Copper IUD: no known impact on lactation • Possible risk of perforation at insertion requiring surgical removal, which may necessitate short interruption in breastfeeding • Levonorgestrel IUD (Mirena) placed immediately postpartum may be associated with shorter duration of breastfeeding. No adverse effect on breastfeeding reported when placed 6 weeks postpartum or later
Sterilization • Male (vasectomy) • Female: postpartum; laparoscopic; hysteroscopic • Male vasectomy and female hysteroscopic occlusion may be performed on an outpatient basis.	• Highly effective	• Permanent; risk of regret • Surgical procedural risks • Cost related to surgery • Requires surgeon • Risk of ectopic pregnancy with female procedures	• Male sterilization: none • Female sterilization: postpartum procedure separates mother and infant and may require use of maternal narcotics (ideally avoid procedures in first 1–2 hours to allow skin to skin, initial breastfeeding, etc.).
Progestin-only hormonal options[a] • Injectable (DMPA) every 3 months • Oral daily pills (norethindrone) • Progestin-releasing IUD (see above): LNG IUD (Mirena), 5 years; LNG IUD (Skyla), 3 years • Progestin vaginal rings • Implants: etonogestrel (Implanon/ Nexplanon), 3 years (Jadelie), 5 years	• Long-term options highly reliable	• Common side effect of irregular bleeding may be less problematic in breastfeeding mothers. • Potential for user failure with daily pills • Other progestin side effects: headache, acne, weight gain, bloating, depressed mood • DMPA may have delayed return to fertility	• Theoretical potential to adversely impact milk supply when started in the early postpartum period prior to establishing a milk supply. Insufficient data to determine risk at this time • If milk supply decreases with DMPA, cannot be discontinued or removed • LNG IUD (Mirena) placed immediately postpartum may be associated with shorter duration of breastfeeding (single study). No adverse effect on breastfeeding

(Continued)

TABLE 2 Use of Contraceptive Methods During Lactation: Advantages, Disadvantages, and Impact on Lactation—cont'd

Method	Advantages	Disadvantages	Effects related to breastfeeding
		• Implant and IUDs require provider insertion and removal.	reported when placed 6 weeks postpartum or later
Estrogen-containing combined hormonal options • COC pills, daily • Estrogen-containing vaginal ring (NuvaRing), monthly • Estrogen-containing transdermal patch (Ortho Evra), weekly	• Options can be self-administered. • Regular menstrual cycles (extended cycle options have more breakthrough bleeding) • Non-contraceptive benefits: decreased bleeding, less anemia, improved acne, improved dysmenorrhea	• Potential for user failure (especially with COCs) • Increased risk of blood clots • Potential for drug interactions • Multiple medical contraindications	• Ideally avoid until lactation/milk supply well established • Potential for adverse effect on milk supply. Risk appears more pronounced with higher estrogen levels than used in contemporary products. • If used by a breastfeeding mother, begin lowest possible dose as late as possible into well-established breastfeeding
• Emergency contraceptives • Combined estrogen/ progestin pills (Preven, Yuzpe method) • Progestin-only pills—LNG (Plan B) • Mifepristone • Ulipristal • Copper IUD	• Most effective within 72 hours of exposure • LNG options appear to have superior efficacy to COC with fewer side effects • Copper IUD most effective and provides continued contraception • Mifepristone similar or superior to LNG in efficacy	• Estrogen-containing options cause nausea/ vomiting and often require use of antiemetics. • No data for ulipristal in lactation currently available • Limited data on mifepristone in lactation	• LNG preferred over estrogen-containing options in breastfeeding mothers owing to previously described concerns related to estrogen and milk supply

COC, combined oral contraceptive; DMPA, depo-medroxyprogesterone acetate; IUD, intrauterine device; LNG, levonorgestrel.
aConclusive research regarding the clinical implications of progestin contraceptive administration in the early postpartum period is contradictory and insufficient.

postpartum period found that those who were using OM and were breastfeeding had a lower pregnancy rate than those using OM but not breastfeeding. The rate of unplanned pregnancy was less than 1% during the first 6 months of lactational amenorrhea. However, OM-associated pregnancy rates were elevated among breastfeeders after menses returned (36% vs. 13% for nonlactating women) and when infant feeding supplementation was started. This increase in unplanned pregnancies was not directly attributable to OM nonadherence. Special emphasis on both the need for improved breastfeeding support to delay menses return and the increased potential for method failure among new users during this period of time should be incorporated into OM training and support programs.[19]

Hormonal contraceptive method: general comments

Controversy exists in the literature regarding hormonal contraceptive effects on milk supply. Although Koetsawang[20] reported an increase, Tankeyoon et al.[21] noted a 12% decline in milk supply with progestin-only contraception compared with placebo. Other studies have not found an effect. A recent study quantified the effect of hormonal contraception on infant's milk ingestion between Days 42 and 63 using deuterium as a marker.[22] Forty women who had previously breastfed began contraception at 42 days postpartum with an estrogen-containing pill (150 μg of levonorgestrel [LNG] and 30 μg of ethinyl-estradiol), the LNG-IUD (Mirena®; Bayer Pharmaceuticals, Leverkeusen, Germany), the etonorgestrel implant (Implanon®; Merck & Co., Whitehouse Station, NJ), or the copper-containing IUD (ParaGard®; Teva Women's Health, Inc., North Wales, PA). No difference in the infants' milk intake was noted among groups in this study. A Cochrane review indicated that evidence from randomized controlled trials on the effect of hormonal contraceptives during lactation is limited and of poor quality: "The evidence is inadequate to make evidence-based recommendations regarding hormonal contraceptive use for lactating women."[23] Until better evidence exists, it is prudent to advise women that hormonal contraceptive methods may decrease milk supply especially in the early postpartum period. Hormonal methods should be discouraged in some circumstances (III):

1. existing low milk supply or history of lactation failure
2. history of breast surgery
3. multiple birth (twins, triplets)
4. preterm birth
5. compromised health of mother and/or baby

Hormonal contraceptive method: progestin-only options

There is theoretical concern related to milk supply when progesterone options are initiated in the initial 48 hours after delivery[24] as a drop in progesterone levels after birth is necessary for secretory differentiation/lactogenesis II to occur. Progestin-containing contraceptives include the progestogen-only pill ("minipill") as well as contraceptive implants such as Nexplanon® (Merck & Co.), DepoProvera® (depot medroxyprogesterone acetate [DMPA]; Pfizer, New York, NY), and the Mirena intrauterine system. A 2010 systematic review of the effects of progestin-only contraceptive options when initiated *after* the initial postpartum period found five randomized controlled trials and 38 observational trials addressing the topic.[25] No adverse effects on breastfeeding through 12 months of age, infant immunoglobulins, or infant sex hormones were noted. Research regarding the clinical implications of progestin contraceptive administration in the early postpartum period is contradictory.

Particularly controversial in clinical practice is the effect of DMPA. Prior studies of DMPA did not account for infant weight, milk supply, and the amount of supplement used. A systematic review of prospective studies on the effects of early postpartum DMPA use in lactating mothers by Brownell et al.[26] found all studies to be of low quality with inadequate control of confounders. Another study of low-income new mothers found that of the 31.3% who received DMPA, 62.6% received it prior to hospital discharge,[27] indicating that early postpartum use is common in some settings. This study team quantified the association between postpartum DMPA and early breastfeeding cessation among 183 women and concluded that if there is a causal effect of DMPA on breastfeeding duration, it is minimal. A prospective case control study of 150 women receiving DMPA after initiation of lactation but prior to hospital discharge (Days 2–10) compared with 100 women not receiving hormonal contraception followed up for 6 months found no difference in satisfaction with their breastfeeding experience or infant growth, although it is unclear how the breastfeeding patterns compared.[28]

A study by Brito et al.[29] compared either insertion of an etonogestrel-releasing implant within 1–2 days after delivery or DMPA given at 6 weeks postpartum. Forty women were then followed up through 12 weeks postpartum. Newborns of those in the implant group had a trend toward more weight gain in the first 6 weeks, but the overall duration of exclusive breastfeeding was not statistically different. Gurtcheff et al.[30] similarly studied early (1–3 days) versus delayed (4–8 weeks) insertion of the contraceptive implant. This noninferiority study found no difference in breastfeeding failure rates with early insertion compared with the delayed group.

Estrogen-containing combined hormonal options

Estrogen-containing options include combination oral contraceptive (COC) pills (taken daily using monthly cyclic, extended cyclic, or continuous options), transdermal patch (weekly), or combined contraceptive vaginal rings (monthly).

Estrogen-containing options are not ideal for early postpartum breastfeeding mothers because of the potential adverse impact on milk supply. The potential for estrogen to cause milk suppression is exemplified by the historical use of large estrogen doses immediately postpartum for lactation suppression prior to our understanding of the elevated thrombogenic risk during that time period. A Cochrane review on methods of lactation suppression noted seven trials using four different estrogen preparations and found a significant reduction in lactation within 7 days postpartum; of note is that the doses and estrogen preparations used differ from those currently used in hormonal contraceptives.[31]

A 2010 systematic review on COCs and breastfeeding found only three randomized controlled trials and four observational studies; the three randomized controlled trials found a decreased mean breastfeeding duration in COC users and an increased use of supplement.[32] No other documented adverse effects on infant health were noted.

If an estrogen-containing contraceptive is chosen, it is prudent to start the lowest estrogen-containing options as late as possible and after milk supply and lactation are well established (III). Additionally, estrogen-containing options should not be initiated in the first few weeks postpartum because of the elevated risk of deep venous thrombosis and pulmonary embolism. Absolute and relative contraindications are otherwise the same for lactating women as for nonlactating women.

Contemporary COCs have estrogen doses ranging from 10 to 35 μg daily. No significant difference in contraceptive efficacy has been found in a Cochrane review of COCs containing < 20 μg of estrogen compared with those with > 20 μg.[33] This information should provide reassurance regarding anticipated efficacy when choosing lower estrogen dose options in a breastfeeding mother in order to minimize potential adverse effects.

Direct comparison of progestin-only pills and COCs

A WHO task force study done in the 1980s found a 41.9% decrease in supply in women using COCs within 6 weeks of initiation.[21] However, a recent randomized controlled trial compared 63 women using a 35-μg progestin-only pill (POP) with 64 women using a COC containing 35 μg of ethinylestradiol from 2 through 8 weeks postpartum; the authors found no difference in continued breastfeeding at 8 weeks (63.5% POP vs. 64.1% COC).[34] Forty-four percent of those in the POP group stopped breastfeeding because of perceived insufficient milk supply compared with 55% in the COC group. Twenty-three percent of women who stopped their pills in the POP group and 21% in the COC groups reported that they did so because of a perceived negative impact on milk supply.

Emergency contraception

Emergency contraception is most effective when initiated within 72 hours after unprotected sexual intercourse, although it is still useful up to 120 hours. Postcoital copper IUD placement, mifepristone, COC, and progesterone options (LNG) are potentially available choices. Postcoital copper IUD placement would be unlikely to impact lactation (see section on IUDs) and has the advantage of providing continued contraception. LNG options are slightly more effective than the COC and also are less likely to cause significant nausea and vomiting.[35] Furthermore, in theory, LNG options would be less likely to impact lactation. A pharmacologic study of 12 breastfeeding mothers found the estimated infant exposure to the maternal treatment of 1.5 mg of LNG was 1.6 μg on the day of therapy.[36] A single observational study comparing progestin-only with estrogen-containing options for postcoital contraception found that an adverse effect on breastfeeding was uncommon and similar in both groups.[37] Based on similar efficacy, less propensity to nausea, and the absence of exposure to estrogen, it appears that the use of LNG is likely the preferred option over a COC in a breastfeeding mother. There are limited data on mifepristone and ulipristal in lactation. The use of postcoital mifepristone (an antiprogesterone) is similar to or superior in efficacy to LNG depending on dosage. Based on a small study, mifepristone transfers into milk in low levels (relative infant doses $\leq$ 1.5%) and would not be anticipated to have adverse effects on the breastfeeding infant.[38] Ulipristal is a selective progesterone receptor modulator. There are currently no data available on its use in breastfeeding mothers.

Postcoital contraception has also been evaluated as a backup to lactational amenorrhea. Although this may not be a practical option, one study found a lower pregnancy rate for the group that was provided with a postcoital contraceptive during counseling regarding lactational amenorrhea at the postpartum visit.[39]

Barrier methods

There are no known adverse effects on lactation with the use of barrier methods of contraception. Patients should be counseled regarding the reduced efficacy of these methods compared with other hormonal, intrauterine, or permanent options.

IUDs

The IUD is one of the most frequently used contraceptives in the world. Prevalence rates range from 6% in the United States and in other countries up to 80% of contraceptive users.[40,41] Hormonal and nonhormonal IUDs are available and have different side effect profiles.

Progestin-releasing IUDs are associated with reduced menstrual blood flow, although around the time of insertion, women frequently experience irregular bleeding. This side effect is most pronounced during the initial 6 months and typically improves with time. Other progestin-related side effects are also possible. The copper IUD is associated with increased dysmenorrhea and menorrhagia.

In a study comparing breastfeeding outcomes in women randomized to receive a copper or progestin IUD at 6−8 weeks postpartum, the authors found no difference in full breastfeeding duration, infant growth, or development through 1 year postpartum.[42] However, in a secondary analysis of a randomized controlled trial comparing women who had an LNG-IUD placed immediately postpartum versus 6−8 weeks postpartum, early LNG-IUD placement was associated with lower breastfeeding rates[43]; in the delayed placement group, four women received DMPA prior to their 6-week visit. Studies of the copper-containing IUD have found no change in milk or serum copper levels.[44]

Complications related to the device itself include uterine perforation, failure (pregnancy), inability to visualize strings, vaginal discharge, infection, pain, the partner feeling the strings, malpositioning (which may require a surgical procedure to remove the IUD), and expulsion (2−10% within the first year). Data do suggest that there is an increased risk of perforation when either IUD is inserted in breastfeeding women.[45] A recent systematic review suggested that IUDs remain a long-acting reversible contraceptive option for breastfeeding women with cesarean birth.[46]

Irreversible options (sterilization)

Multiple methods of surgical sterilization are available, including male vasectomy, postpartum tubal ligation, laparoscopic tubal ligation, and hysteroscopic tubal occlusion. These procedures involve different technologies, surgical techniques, anesthesia, and procedural settings.

Important considerations for breastfeeding dyads include the potential to impact early maternal−infant interaction. Ideally, procedures should not be performed during the initial hours postpartum to allow skin-to-skin contact between the mother and infant and initiation of breastfeeding. Early maternal−infant contact should not, however, prevent breastfeeding mothers from undergoing postpartum tubal ligation. To minimize disruption, the infant should be kept skin-to-skin with the mother in the preoperative area and be reunited with her as soon as the mother is awake and alert in the recovery room. This interruption should be managed in a breastfeeding-supportive way, and the provider should remain cognizant of the implications of anesthesia and analgesia on the breastfeeding dyad.[47]

Unfortunately, women who do not have the postpartum tubal sterilization procedure performed during their maternity stay are at risk for ultimately not having the procedure performed and subsequent pregnancy.[48−50] This risk should be considered. Such considerations may warrant early maternal−infant separation in order for the procedure to be completed prior to discharge.

THE MEDICAL ELIGIBILITY CRITERIA

Medical Eligibility Criteria provide guidance on the level of safety of contraception in relation to specific medical conditions and other demographic variables. Risks are divided into four categories as outlined in Table 3, although the categories are sometimes divided into two categories: generally use and generally do not use. The current recommendations from WHO and the Centers for Disease Control and Prevention (CDC) differ. Table 4 shows the categories for the use of

TABLE 3   Medical Eligibility Criteria

WHO category	With clinical judgment	With limited clinical judgment
1	Use the method in any circumstances	Use the method
2	Generally use the method	Use the method
3	Use of the method not usually recommended unless other, more appropriate methods are not available or acceptable	Do not use the method
4	Method not to be used	Do not use the method

Where a doctor or nurse is not available to make clinical judgments, the four categories can be simplified into a two-category system (third column) by combining World Health Organization (WHO) Categories 1 with 2 and 3 with 4.

TABLE 4   World Health Organization and Centers for Disease Control and Prevention Medical Eligibility Categories

	WHO		CDC	
	Timing postpartum	MEC level	Timing postpartum	MEC level
Combined oral contraceptive	0–6 weeks	4	<1 month	3
	6 weeks–6 months	3	≥1 month	2
	>6 months	2		
Progestin only contraceptive (oral and implants)	0–6 weeks	3	<1 month	2
	6 weeks–6 months	1	≥1month	1
	>6 months	1		
LNG-IUD	<48 hours	3	<10 minutes	2
	48 hours–4 weeks	3	10 minutes to <4 weeks	2
	>4 weeks	1	≥4 weeks	1
Cu-IUD	<48 hours	1	<10 minutes	1
	48 hours–4 weeks	3	10 minutes to <4 weeks	2
	>4 weeks	1	≥4 weeks	1

Adapted from the World Health Organization (WHO) Medical Eligibility Criteria (MEC) and the Centers for Disease Control and Prevention (CDC) Summary Chart of U.S. Medical Eligibility Criteria for Contraceptive Use Updated June 2012 (www.cdc.gov/reproductivehealth/unintendedpregnancy/USMEC.htm). See Table 3 for MEC categories. *IUD*, intrauterine device; *LNG*, levonorgestrel.

several methods during lactation as presented by WHO and revised by CDC. CDC recently revised recommendations to include reducing the postpartum period from 6 weeks to 4 weeks and no longer contraindicating immediate postpartum use of progesterone-only contraception.

There are limited data from well-conducted scientific studies that adequately take into consideration the effect on the infant or exclusive breastfeeding, especially in the immediate postpartum period when the establishment of lactation and adequate milk production is essential. (III) Moreover, exclusively breastfeeding women are very unlikely to become pregnant in the first 6 weeks after birth as described above. In this setting, hormonal contraception has minimal benefit, and early initiation may derail a woman's exclusive breastfeeding intentions. Unless the risk of unplanned pregnancy or loss to follow-up is high, early initiation of hormonal contraception in breastfeeding women is not recommended.

FUTURE RESEARCH

There is need for more detailed prospective research regarding the impact of all hormonal contraception on breastfeeding and on the potential long-term impact on the infant due to exposure to exogenous hormones. Such information will enable women to make informed decisions regarding the risk of unplanned pregnancy versus the risks of disrupted breastfeeding. Prior research has often not adequately accounted for maternal breastfeeding goals, the importance of breastfeeding exclusivity, and amount of supplement used. Until research has addressed these concerns and focused on women's intentions to exclusively breastfeed, it is not possible to exclude adverse potential effects on milk supply, on long-term breastfeeding success, or on the infant, especially if any is a rare occurrence. This is particularly true when initiating hormonal contraception in the initial postpartum period.

Research is needed to evaluate the impact of contemporary contraceptive options, which include lower estrogen doses and progestin-only agents, on both breastfeeding in the short term and on the infant in the long term. Further research is also needed on the effectiveness of LAM given the widespread availability of breast pumps and the growing number of mothers who are choosing to exclusively express and feed their infants expressed breastmilk. In sum, rare or long-term adverse outcomes are often not detected, and method efficacy has not been evaluated under a wide variety of conditions. Both of these issues demand study of large populations over time. For the individual breastfeeding family, this lack of sufficient data regarding the impact of hormonal contraception may have significant negative consequences.

CONCLUSIONS

Every woman should be offered full information and support about contraception options so she can make an optimal decision for her individual situation. Physicians and other healthcare providers should not "pre-decide" which method is most appropriate; rather, in discussion with the patient, clinicians should discuss the risks, benefits, availability, and affordability of all methods. This discussion should address contraceptive efficacy and possible impact on breastfeeding outcomes, within the context of each woman's desire to breastfeed, risk of breastfeeding difficulties, and risk of unplanned pregnancy.

ACKNOWLEDGMENTS

This work was supported in part by a grant from the Maternal and Child Health Bureau, U.S. Department of Health and Human Services and through the resources of the Carolina Global Breastfeeding Institute.

REFERENCES

1. Perez A, Vela P, Masnick GS, et al. First ovulation after childbirth: The effect of breast-feeding. *Am J Obstet Gynecol.* 1972;114:1041–1047.
2. Perez A, Labbok M, Queenan J. A clinical study of the lactational amenorrhea method for family planning. *Lancet.* 1992;339:968–970.
3. Labbok M, Perez A, Valdes V, et al. The lactational amenorrhea method: A new postpartum introductory family planning method with program and policy implications. *Adv Contraception.* 1994;10:93–109.
4. The World Health Organization multinational study of breast-feeding and lactational amenorrhea. IV. Postpartum bleeding and lochia in breast-feeding women. World Health Organization Task Force on Methods for the Natural Regulation of Fertility. *Fertil Steril.* 1999;72:441–447.
5. The World Health Organization multinational study of breast-feeding and lactational amenorrhea. III. Pregnancy during breast-feeding. World Health Organization Task Force on Methods for the Natural Regulation of Fertility. *Fertil Steril.* 1999;72:431–440.
6. Labbok M, Hight-Laukaran V, Peterson A, et al. Multicenter study of the lactational amenorrhea method (LAM) I. Efficacy, duration, and implications for clinical application. *Contraception.* 1997;55:327–336.
7. Peterson AE, Peréz-Escamilla R, Labbok MH, et al. Multicenter study of the lactational amenorrhea method (LAM) III: Effectiveness, duration, and satisfaction with reduced client-provider contact. *Contraception.* 2000;62:221–230.
8. Hight-Laukaran V, Labbok M, Peterson A, et al. Multicenter study of the lactational amenorrhea method (LAM) II. Acceptability, utility, and policy implications. *Contraception.* 1997;55:337–346.
9. Kennedy KI. Efficacy and effectiveness of LAM. *Adv Exp Med Biol.* 2002;503:207–216.
10. Appendix A Task Force Ratings. Guide to Clinical Preventive Services: Report of the U.S. Preventive Services Task Force, 2nd edition. Available at: www.ncbi.nlm.nih.gov/books/NBK15430 (accessed December 19, 2014).
11. Labbok M, Krasovec K. Towards consistency in breastfeeding definitions. *Stud Fam Plann.* 1990;21:226–230.
12. Cooney KA, Nyirabukeye T, Labbok MH, et al. An assessment of the nine-month lactational amenorrhea method (MAMA-9) in Rwanda. *Stud Fam Plann.* 1996;27:102–171.
13. Kazi A, Kennedy KI, Visness CM, et al. Effectiveness of the lactational amenorrhea method in Pakistan. *Fertil Steril.* 1995;64:717–723.
14. Van der Wijden C, Kleijnen J, Van den Berk T. Lactational amenorrhea for family planning. *Cochrane Database Syst Rev.* 2003;4:CD001329.
15. Hatcher RA, Trussell J, Stewart F, et al. *Contraceptive Technology.* 17th ed. New York: Contraceptive Technology Communications, Inc., Ardent Media, Inc.; 2011.
16. Labbok MH, Starling A. Definitions of breastfeeding: Call for the development and use of consistent definitions in research and peer-reviewed literature. *Breastfeed Med.* 2012;7:397–402.
17. Valde's V, Labbok MH, Pugin E, et al. The efficacy of the lactational amenorrhea method (LAM) among working women. *Contraception.* 2000;62:217–219.
18. Bouchard T, Fehring RJ, Schneider M. Efficacy of a new postpartum transition protocol for avoiding pregnancy. *J Am Board Fam Med.* 2013;26:35–44.
19. Labbok MH, Stallings RY, Shah F, et al. Ovulation method use during breastfeeding: Is there increased risk of unplanned pregnancy? *Am J Obstet Gynecol.* 1991;165:2031–2036.
20. Koetsawang S. The effects of contraceptive methods on the quality and quantity of breast milk. *Int J Gynaecol Obstet.* 1987;25(Suppl):115–127.
21. Tankeyoon M, Dusitsin N, Chalapati S, et al. Effects of hormonal contraceptives on milk volumes and infant growth. WHO Special Programme of Research, Development and Research Training in Human Reproduction Task force on oral contraceptives. *Contraception.* 1984;30:505–522.
22. Bahamondes L, Bahamondes MV, Modesto W, et al. Effect of hormonal contraceptives during breastfeeding on infant's milk ingestion and growth. *Fertil Steril.* 2013;100:445–450.
23. Truitt ST, Fraser AB, Grimes DA, et al. Combined hormonal versus nonhormonal versus progestin-only contraception in lactation. *Cochrane Database Syst Rev.* 2003;2:CD003988.
24. Kennedy KI, Short RV, Tully MR. Premature introduction of progestin-only contraceptive methods during lactation. *Contraception.* 1997;55:347–350.

25. Kapp N, Curtis K, Nanda K. Progestogen-only contraceptive use among breastfeeding women: A systematic review. *Contraception.* 2010;82:17−37.

26. Brownell EA, Fernandez ID, Howard CR, et al. A systematic review of early postpartum medroxyprogesterone receipt and early breastfeeding cessation: Evaluating the methodological rigor of the evidence. *Breastfeed Med.* 2012;7:10−18. Erratum in *Breastfeed Med* 2012;7:129.

27. Dozier AM, Nelson A, Brownell EA, et al. Patterns of postpartum depot medroxyprogesterone administration among low-income mothers. *J Womens Health (Larchmt).* 2014;23:224−230.

28. Singhal S, Sarda N, Gupta S, et al. Impact of injectable progestogen contraception in early puerperium on lactation and infant health. *J Clin Diagn Res.* 2014;8:69−72.

29. Brito MB, Ferriani RA, Quintana SM, et al. Safety of the etonogestrel-releasing implant during the immediate postpartum period: A pilot study. *Contraception.* 2009;80:519−526.

30. Gurtcheff SE, Turok DK, Stoddard G, et al. Lactogenesis after early postpartum use of the contraceptive implant: A randomized controlled trial. *Obstet Gynecol.* 2011;117:1114−1121.

31. Oladapo OT, Fawole B. Treatments for suppression of lactation. *Cochrane Database Syst Rev.* 2012;9:CD005937.

32. Kapp N, Curtis KM. Combined oral contraceptive use among breastfeeding women: A systematic review. *Contraception.* 2010;82:10−16.

33. Gallo MF, Grimes DA, Lopez LM, et al. Combination injectable contraceptives for contraception. *Cochrane Database Syst Rev.* 2008;4:CD004568.

34. Espey E, Ogburn T, Leeman L, et al. Effect of progestin compared with combined oral contraceptive pills on lactation: A randomized controlled trial. *Obstet Gynecol.* 2012;119:5−13.

35. Cheng L, Che Y, Gulmezoglu AM. Interventions for emergency contraception. *Cochrane Database Syst Rev.* 2012;8:CD001324.

36. Gainer E, Massai R, Lillo S, et al. Levonorgestrel pharmacokinetics in plasma and milk of lactating women who take 1.5 mg for emergency contraception. *Hum Reprod.* 2001;22:1578−1584.

37. Polakow-Farkash S, Gilad O, Merlob P, et al. Levonorgestrel used for emergency contraception during lactation—A prospective observational cohort study on maternal and infant safety. *J Matern Fetal Neonatal Med.* 2013;26:219−221.

38. Saav I, Fiala C, Hamalainen JM, et al. Medical abortion in lactating women—Low levels of mifepristone in breast milk. *Acta Obstet Gynecol Scand.* 2010;89:618−622.

39. Shaaban OM, Hassen SG, Nour SA, et al. Emergency contraceptive pills as a backup for lactational amenorrhea method (LAM) of contraception: A randomized controlled trial. *Contraception.* 2013;87:363−369.

40. Jones J, Mosher WD, Daniels K. Current contraceptive use in the United States, 2006−2010, and changes in patterns of use since 1995. *Natl Health Stat Rep.* 2012;(60)1−25. Available at: www.cdc.gov/nchs/data/nhsr/nhsr060.pdf (accessed March 20, 2013).

41. The ESHRE Capri Workshop Group. Intrauterine devices and intrauterine systems. *Hum Reprod Update.* 2008;14:197−208.

42. Shaamash AH, Sayed GH, Hussien MM, et al. A comparative study of the levonorgestrel-releasing intrauterine system Mirena versus the Copper T380A intrauterine device during lactation: Breast-feeding performance, infant growth and infant development. *Contraception.* 2005;72:346−351.

43. Chen BA, Reeves MF, Creinin MD, et al. Postplacental or delayed levonorgestrel intrauterine device insertion and breast-feeding duration. *Contraception.* 2011;84:499−504.

44. Rodrigues da Cunha AC, Dorea JG, Cantuaria AA. Intrauterine device and maternal copper metabolism during lactation. *Contraception.* 2001;63:37−39.

45. Heinemann K, Westhoff CL, Grimes DA, et al. Intrauterine devices and the risk of uterine perforations: Final results from the EURAS-IUD Study. *Obstet Gynecol.* 2014;123(Suppl 1):3S.

46. Goldstuck ND, Steyn PS. Intrauterine contraception after cesarean section and during lactation: A systematic review. *Int J Womens Health.* 2013;5:811−818.

47. Montgomery A, Hale T. Academy of Breastfeeding Medicine. ABM Clinical Protocol #15: Analgesia and anesthesia for the breastfeeding mother, revised 2012. *Breastfeed Med.* 2012;7:547−553.

48. Committee on Health Care for Underserved Women. Committee opinion no. 530: Access to postpartum sterilization. *Obstet Gynecol.* 2012;120:212−215.

49. Zite N, Wuellner S, Gilliam M. Failure to obtain desired postpartum sterilization: Risk and predictors. *Obstet Gynecol.* 2005;105:794−799.

50. Thurman AR, Janecek T. One-year follow-up of women with unfulfilled postpartum sterilization requests. *Obstet Gynecol.* 2010;116:1071−1077.

ABM protocols expire 5 years from the date of publication. Evidence-based revisions are made within 5 years or sooner if there are significant changes in the evidence.

The Academy of Breastfeeding Medicine Protocol Committee
Kathleen A. Marinelli, MD, FABM, Chairperson
Maya Bunik, MD, MSPH, FABM, Co-Chairperson
Larry Noble, MD, FABM, Translations Chairperson
Nancy Brent, MD
Amy E. Grawey, MD
Ruth A. Lawrence, MD, FABM
Sarah Reece-Stremtan, MD
Tomoko Seo, MD, FABM
Michal Young, MD
For correspondence: abm@bfmed.org

ABM Clinical Protocol #14
Breastfeeding-Friendly Physician's Office: Optimizing Care for Infants and Children, Revised 2013*

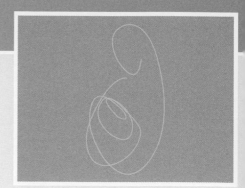

Amy E. Grawey[1], Kathleen A. Marinelli[2,3], Alison V. Holmes[4] and the Academy of Breastfeeding Medicine

ABSTRACT

A central goal of The Academy of Breastfeeding Medicine is the development of clinical protocols for managing common medical problems that may impact breastfeeding success. These protocols serve only as guidelines for the care of breastfeeding mothers and infants and do not delineate an exclusive course of treatment or serve as standards of medical care. Variations in treatment may be appropriate according to the needs of an individual patient.

DEFINITIONS

Breastfeeding-Friendly physician's office

A PHYSICIAN'S PRACTICE that enthusiastically promotes and supports breastfeeding through the combination of a conducive office environment and education of healthcare professionals, office staff, and families. (For the purposes of this document "physician" refers to anyone who is rendering the primary medical care to the breastfeeding dyad, both the mother antepartum and the dyad postpartum. In different countries and cultures that could be a doctor, a midwife, or another healthcare professional. All should strive for a "Breastfeeding-Friendly Practice" in which to care for these families.)

---

* Courtesy of the Academy of Breastfeeding Medicine. Please go to https://www.bfmed.org/protocols for complete protocols, translations, and the most up-to-date information (protocols are updated every 5–7 years).
[1] Little Flower Family Medicine, O'Fallon, Missouri.
[2] Division of Neonatology, Connecticut Children's Medical Center, Hartford, Connecticut;
[3] Department of Pediatrics, University of Connecticut School of Medicine, Farmington, Connecticut.
[4] Department of Pediatrics, The Geisel School of Medicine at Dartmouth, New Hampshire.

Breastmilk substitutes

Infant formula, glucose water, or other liquids given in place of human milk.

BACKGROUND

A mother's prenatal intention to breastfeed is influenced to a great extent by the opinion and support of the healthcare providers she encounters.[1–5] Ongoing parental support through in-person visits and phone contacts with healthcare providers usually results in increased breastfeeding duration.[6–12] Healthcare providers who interact with mothers and babies are in a unique position to contribute to the initial and ongoing support of the breastfeeding dyad.[3–5,11–15] Practices that employ a healthcare professional trained in lactation have significantly higher breastfeeding initiation and maintenance rates, with mothers experiencing fewer problems related to breastfeeding.[16–20] The World Health Organization's Baby-Friendly Hospital Initiative describes Ten Steps for Successful Breastfeeding.[21,22] These Ten Steps are based on scientific evidence and the experience of respected authorities. The scientific basis of many of these recommendations can also be extended to outpatient practices caring for infants and young children.[14,16,17] Even initiating incremental changes to improving breastfeeding support is of value because there is a "dose–response" relationship between the number of steps achieved and breastfeeding outcomes.[23]

Recommendations

Quality of evidence (levels of evidence I, II-1, II-2, II-3, and III) for each recommendation, as defined in the U.S. Preventive Services Task Force guideline for "Quality of Evidence,"[24] is noted in parentheses.

1. Establish a written breastfeeding-friendly office policy.[16,17,21] Collaborate with colleagues and office staff during development. Inform all new staff about the policy. Provide copies of your practice's policy to hospitals, physicians, and all healthcare professionals covering your practice for you. (III)

2. Offer culturally and ethnically competent care.[25] Understand that families may follow cultural practices regarding discarding of colostrum, maternal diet during lactation, and early introduction of solid foods. Provide access to a multilingual staff, medical interpreters, and ethnically diverse educational material as needed within your practice. (III)

3. If providing antenatal care for the mother, introduce the subject of infant feeding in the first trimester and continue to express your support of breastfeeding throughout the course of the pregnancy. If you are a physician providing postnatal care for the infant, you can offer a prenatal visit to become acquainted with the family during which your commitment to breastfeeding can be shown.[2,7,8] Use open-ended questions, such as "What have you heard about breastfeeding?," to inquire about a feeding plan for this child. Provide educational material that highlights the many ways in which breastfeeding is superior to formula feeding. Encourage attendance of both parents at prenatal breastfeeding classes. Direct education and educational material to all family members involved in childcare (father, grand-parents, etc.).[1,13,26] The father of the infant is particularly important in support of the mother.[26] Identify patients with lactation risk factors (such as flat or inverted nipples, history of breast surgery, no increase in breast size during pregnancy, previous unsuccessful breastfeeding experience) to enable individual breastfeeding care for her particular situation. (I, II-1, II-2, II-3, III)

4. Physician interaction with the breastfeeding dyad in the immediate postpartum period depends on the system of healthcare and insurance systems in his or her country. For example, if you are in a system in which you can see the infants while in-hospital, you can collaborate with local hospitals and maternity care professionals in your community,[16,23,25] providing your office policies on breastfeeding initiation within the first hour after birth to delivery rooms and newborn units. Leave orders in the hospital or birthing facility not to give formula/sterile water/glucose water to a breastfeeding infant without specific medical orders and not to dispense commercial discharge bags containing infant formula, formula coupons, and/or feeding bottles to mothers.[27,28] Show support for breastfeeding during hospital rounds. Help mothers initiate and continue breastfeeding. Counsel mothers to follow their infant's states of alertness as they relate to hunger and satiety cues and ensure that the infant breastfeeds eight to 12 times in 24 hours.[29] Encourage rooming-in and breastfeeding on demand. (I, II-2, III) If you are in a system in which hospital staff members are responsible for the care of the newborns in the hospital and outside physicians do not give orders to hospital staff, you will not be able to see babies and offer support to the mothers until after discharge (see point 6 below). However, in many countries hospitals will have received Baby-Friendly Hospital training where mothers should receive good support while inpatients.

5. Encourage breastfeeding mothers to feed newborns only human milk and to avoid offering supplemental formula, glucose water, or other liquids unless medically indicated.[25,30] Advise the mother not to offer a bottle or a pacifier/dummy until breastfeeding is well established.[31,32] (I, III)

6. In many areas of the world, the first follow-up visit will be done by non—physician healthcare workers.[33] In most European countries midwives care for the mother and infant in the days and weeks after discharge from the hospital. In Germany, for example, every mother and infant has the right to a midwife (often up to 8 weeks of daily visits) covered by insurance. Mothers contact their pediatrician within the first 3 weeks of delivery for the infant's first check-up, which is covered by insurance. In this system, this is the first opportunity the pediatrician has to support breastfeeding. In other countries, such as Australia and New Zealand, routine medical care of infants is undertaken by general practitioners (family physicians), and infants may never visit a pediatrician. In countries such as the United States, where the postpartum care of the mother and infant is done by physicians or physician extenders (for example, physician assistants, nurse practitioners), schedule a first infant follow-up visit 48—72 hours after hospital discharge or earlier if breastfeeding-related problems, such as excessive weight loss ($>7\%$) or jaundice, are present at the time of hospital discharge.[25,30,34] (In cultures or medical situations in which the dyad has remained hospitalized for long enough that weight gain and parental confidence are established prior to hospital discharge, follow-up may be deferred until 1—2 weeks of age if otherwise appropriate. For example, in Japan the dyad usually stays in hospital for 5—6 days after childbirth. The Japanese Pediatric Society recommends the first visit to the pediatrician 1 week after discharge, when the infant is about 2 weeks old.) Ensure there is access to a lactation consultant/educator or other healthcare professional trained to address breastfeeding questions or concerns during this visit. Advise the mother that feeding will be observed during the visit so that she can let staff know if the infant is ready to breastfeed while she is waiting. Provide comfortable seating, privacy, and a nursing pillow as needed for the breastfeeding dyad to facilitate an adequate evaluation.

7. Begin by asking parents open-ended questions, such as "How is breastfeeding going?," and then focus on their concerns. Take the time to address the many questions that a mother may have. Assess latch and successful and adequate milk transfer at the early follow-up visit. Identify lactation risk factors and assess the infant's weight, hydration, jaundice, feeding activity, and output. Provide medical help for women with sore

nipples or other maternal health problems that may impact breastfeeding. Provide close follow-up until the parents feel confident and the infant is doing well with adequate weight gain by the World Health Organization Child Growth Standards.[35] (III)

8. Ensure availability of appropriate educational resources for parents. In accordance with the World Health Organization International Code of Marketing of Breastmilk Substitutes,[36] educational material should be noncommercial and should not advertise human milk substitutes, bottles, or nipples/teats.[28] Educational resources may be in the form of handouts, pictures, books, and DVDs. Recommended topics for educational material can include growth patterns, feeding and sleep patterns of breastfed babies, management of growth spurts, recognition of hunger and satiety cues, positioning and attachment, management of sore nipples, mastitis, low supply, blocked ducts, engorgement, reflux, normal stool and voiding patterns, maintaining lactation when separated from the infant (for example, during illness, prematurity, or return to work), breastfeeding in public, postpartum depression, maternal medication use, and maternal illness during breastfeeding). (I)

9. Allow and encourage breastfeeding in the waiting room. Display signs in the waiting area encouraging mothers to breastfeed (Figs. 1 and 2). Provide a comfortable private area to breastfeed for those mothers who prefer privacy.[2,10,14,17] Do not interrupt or discourage breastfeeding in the office. (II-2, II-3)

10. Ensure an office environment that demonstrates breastfeeding promotion and support. Eliminate the practice of distribution of free formula and baby items from formula companies to parents.[27,28] In accordance with the World Health Organization Code,[36] store formula supplies out of view of parents. Display noncommercial posters, pamphlets, pictures, and photographs of breastfeeding mothers in your office.[1,14,17] Do not display images of infants bottle-feeding. Do not accept gifts (including writing pads, pens, or calendars) or personal samples from companies manufacturing infant formula, feeding bottles, or pacifiers/dummies.[36] Specifically target educational material to populations with low breastfeeding rates in your practice. (II-2, II-3)

11. Develop and follow telephone triage protocols to address breastfeeding concerns and problems.[10,12,37] Conduct follow-up phone calls to assist breastfeeding mothers. Provide readily accessible resources like books and protocols to triage nurses. (See Table 1.) (I)

12. Commend breastfeeding mothers during each visit for choosing and continuing breastfeeding. Provide breastfeeding anticipatory guidance, give educational handouts, and discuss breastfeeding goals at routine periodic health maintenance visits. Encourage fathers of infants and other infant caregivers to accompany the mother and infant to office visits.[3–5,11,26] (I, II-1, II-2, II-3)

13. Encourage mothers to exclusively breastfeed for 6 months and to continue breastfeeding with complementary foods until at least 24 months and thereafter

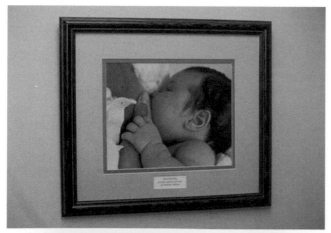

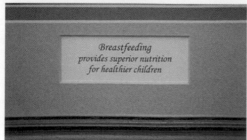

Figure 1. Breastfeeding-friendly graphic in a family physician's office in the United States. Printed with permission of Tim Tobolic, MD, FABM.

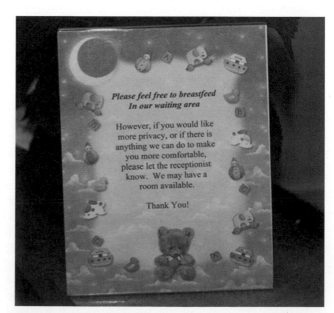

Figure 2. Breastfeeding-friendly graphic in a family physician's office in the United States. Printed with permission of Tim Tobolic, MD, FABM.

TABLE 1	Examples of Telephone Triage Resources	
Organization	**Audience**	**Web site**
World Health Organization	Health professionals	www.emro.who.int/health-topics/breastfeeding (accessed February 9, 2013)
Academy of Breastfeeding Medicine	Health professionals	www.bfmed.org/Resources/protocols.aspx (accessed February 9, 2013)
American Academy of Pediatrics Section on Breastfeeding	Healthcare professionals and families	www2.aap.org/breastfeeding/ (accessed February 9, 2013)
International Lactation Consultants Association	Lactation consultants and health professionals	www.ILCA.org (accessed February 9, 2013)
La Leche League International American Academy of Pediatrics	General information	www.llli.org (accessed February 9, 2013)
	Health professionals	Bunik,[37] "Breastfeeding Telephone Triage and Advice"
Australian Breastfeeding Association	Health professionals	https://www.breastfeeding.asn.au/ (accessed February 9, 2013)
e-lactancia	Health professionals	www.e-lactancia.org/ingles/inicio.asp (accessed February 9, 2013)
Toxnet US National Library of Medicine	Health professionals	http://toxnet.nlm.nih.gov/cgi-bin/sis/htmlgen?LACT (accessed February 9, 2013)

as long as mutually desired. Discuss the introduction of solid food at 6 months of age, emphasizing the need for high-iron solids and recommend supplementing vitamins (for example, vitamin D, K, or A) in accordance with published standards,[25] which vary depending on recommendations of the medical society of the country of practice. (III)

14. Set an example for your patients and community. Have a written breastfeeding employee policy and provide a lactation room with supplies for your employees who breastfeed or express milk at work.[16,38,39] (II-2, III) For countries with long paid maternity leaves (for example, 12 months in Germany), this may not be as relevant as for countries with no or short paid maternity leaves.

15. Acquire or maintain a list of community resources (for example, breast pump rental locations) and be knowledgeable about referral procedures. Refer expectant and new parents to peer, community support, and resource groups. Identify local breastfeeding specialists, know their background and training, and develop working relationships for additional assistance. Support local breastfeeding support groups.[6,19,33,40,41] (I, II-3, III)

16. Support and advocate for health policy that incorporates the costs of breastfeeding care into routine health services in those countries in which it is not. These costs also include consultation and equipment that may be needed for particular clinical situations.

17. Where laws exist, enforce workplace laws that support breastfeeding. Where laws do not exist, encourage employers and daycare providers to support breastfeeding.[38,39] Web sites are available to provide material to help motivate and guide employers in providing lactation support in the workplace.[38] (II-2, III)

18. All clinical physicians should receive education regarding breastfeeding, beginning in the preclinical years.[13,42–46] Areas of suggested education include the risks of artificial feeding, the physiology of lactation, management of common breastfeeding problems, and medical contraindications to breastfeeding. Make available educational resources for quick reference by healthcare professionals in your practice (books, protocols, Web links, etc. [Table 1]). Staff education and training should be provided to all, including front office staff, nurses, and medical assistants. Identify one or more breastfeeding resource personnel on staff. In countries where the practice model makes it possible, consider employing a lactation consultant or a nurse trained in lactation. If this is not possible, network with other professionals and participate in local perinatal networks as available and appropriate to your location.[6,19,33] (I, II-2, II-3)

19. Volunteer to let medical students and residents rotate in your practice. Participate in medical student and resident physician education. Encourage establishment of formal training programs in lactation for current and future healthcare providers.[42–46] (II-2, II-3)

20. Track breastfeeding initiation and duration rates in your practice and learn about breastfeeding rates in your community.

OBSTACLES TO PROVIDING BREASTFEEDING CARE

Establishing a Breastfeeding-Friendly office will present some challenges. In the United States and some other nations, primary care services have traditionally received reimbursement based primarily on numbers of patients seen rather than the quality of care delivered.[47]

Breastfeeding management and counseling are often labor intensive. In systems in which the finances of the office are dependent on numbers of patients seen, without reassurance that the practice will be reimbursed for time invested in caring for the breastfeeding dyad, the provider will be under considerable pressure to forego or abbreviate such care. Even if reimbursement is not an issue, the time constraints of scheduling as many patients as possible during the day tend to preclude labor-intensive interventions. Complicated breastfeeding problems will often require immediate attention and may result in disruption of efficient patient flow; patients with previously scheduled appointments will be kept waiting too long.

Although the physician may have a staff member to assist dyads experiencing breastfeeding difficulties, the time spent by a nonprovider lactation specialist in the United States is usually poorly reimbursed, if reimbursed at all. Referral to other breastfeeding support services will likely be an extra expense requiring payment by the family.

These obstacles, while daunting, are not insurmountable. For example, advocacy in the United States has led to strong public health recommendations and recent legislation requiring insurance coverage of breastfeeding services; implementation is in the early phases.[46,47] Insurance coverage for lactation consultant services would greatly enhance breastfeeding care at many levels. Because of the uniqueness and complexity of the U.S. healthcare system, some suggestions specific to current U.S. financial and care policy are listed in the Appendix.

RECOMMENDATIONS FOR FUTURE RESEARCH

1. A large, multicenter, prospective, randomized study should evaluate the routine use of an International Board Certified Lactation Consultant (IBCLC) versus nonuse in the outpatient setting. The control group will have "usual breastfeeding support." Outcomes assessed should include the duration of exclusive breastfeeding and duration of non—formula feeding after the introduction of complementary foods, ideally following breastfeeding rates until at least 1 year of age. A retrospective study of this intervention at a single site showed an improvement in non—formula feeding,[6] but a multicenter trial will evaluate effectiveness in other settings. As many physicians themselves outside the United States also have the IBCLC designation, this may not be a helpful study in these settings.

2. A large multicenter trial should evaluate the effectiveness of having mothers set breastfeeding goals. A very small pilot study showed that an intervention that included educational handouts and mothers setting breastfeeding goals increased breastfeeding duration and exclusivity.[15] A larger study could use the intervention at each prenatal and well-infant visit up to 1 year, even if prenatal care and well-infant care are delivered at separate sites (i.e., an obstetrics office and a pediatric office). The intervention could be evaluated in different populations, with greater ethnic and socioeconomic diversity and specifically including high-risk populations. Should this intervention prove effective across varied populations, the surveys and handouts could be used to develop a standard tool that could be easily reproduced and distributed, analogous to those used to assess developmental milestones.

3. A large pre- and post-intervention trial could evaluate the impact of continuing medical education concerning breastfeeding for practicing physicians. Outcomes assessed should include rates of breastfeeding initiation and exclusivity and non-formula feeding after the introduction of complementary foods.

4. More studies regarding the cost-effectiveness of steps related to making an outpatient practice breastfeeding-friendly are needed.

ACKNOWLEDGMENTS

This work was supported in part by a grant from the Maternal and Child Health Bureau, U.S. Department of Health and Human Services.

REFERENCES

1. Bentley M, Caulfield L, Gross S, et al. Sources of influence on intention to breastfeed among African-American women at entry to WIC. *J Hum Lact*. 1999;15:27—34.
2. Lu M. Provider encouragement of breastfeeding: Evidence from a national survey. *Obstet Gynecol*. 2001;97:290—295.
3. Taveras EM, Capra AM, Braveman PA, et al. Clinical support and psychosocial risk factors associated with breastfeeding discontinuation. *Pediatrics*. 2003;112:108—115.
4. Taveras EM, Li R, Grummer-Strawn L, et al. Opinions and practices of clinicians associated with continuation of exclusive breastfeeding. *Pediatrics*. 2004;113:e283—e290.
5. Taveras EM, Li R, Grummer-Strawn L, et al. Mothers' and clinicians' perspectives on breastfeeding counseling during routine preventive visits. *Pediatrics*. 2004;113:e405—e411.
6. Witt AM, Smith S, Mason MJ, Flocke SA. Integrating routine lactation consultant support into a pediatric practice. *Breastfeed Med*. 2012;7:38—42.
7. Szucs KA, Miracle DJ, Rosenman MB. Breastfeeding knowledge, attitudes, and practices among providers in a medical home. *Breastfeed Med*. 2009;4:31—42.
8. de Oliveira M, Camacho L, Tedstone A. A method for the evaluation of primary health care units' practice in the promotion, protection, and support of breastfeeding: Results from the State of Rio de Janeiro, Brazil. *J Hum Lact*. 2003;19:365—373.

9. Chung M, Raman G, Trikalinos T, et al. Interventions in primary care to promote breastfeeding: An evidence review for the U.S. Preventive Services Task Force. *Ann Intern Med*. 2008;149:565–582.

10. Bunik M, Shobe P, O'Connor ME, et al. Are 2 weeks of daily breastfeeding support insufficient to overcome the influences of formula? *Acad Pediatr*. 2010;10:21–28.

11. Renfrew MJ, McCormick FM, Wade A, et al. Support for healthy breastfeeding mothers with healthy term babies. *Cochrane Database Syst Rev*. 2012;5:CD001141.

12. Pugh LC, Serwint JR, Frick KD, et al. A randomized controlled community-based trial to improve breastfeeding rates among urban low-income mothers. *Acad Pediatr*. 2010;10:14–20.

13. Labarere J, Gelbert-Baudino N, Ayral A-S, et al. Efficacy of breastfeeding support provided by trained clinicians during an early, routine, preventive visit: A prospective, randomized, open trial of 226 mother-infant pairs. *Pediatrics*. 2005;115:139–146.

14. Shariff F, Levitt C, Kaczorowski J, et al. Workshop to implement the Baby-Friendly Office Initiative. Effect on community physicians' offices. *Can Fam Physician*. 2000;46:1090–1097.

15. Betzold C, Laughlin K, Shi C. A family practice breastfeeding education pilot program: An observational, descriptive study. *Int Breastfeed J*. 2007;2:4.

16. ABM clinical protocol #7. Model breastfeeding policy (revisions 2010). *Breastfeed Med*. 2010;5:173–177.

17. Cardoso LO, Vicente AS, Damião JJ, et al. The impact of implementation of the Breastfeeding Friendly Primary Care Initiative on the prevalence rates of breastfeeding and causes of consultations at a basic healthcare center. *J Pediatr (Rio J)*. 2008;84:147–153.

18. Lawlor-Smith C, McIntyre E, Bruce J. Effective breastfeeding support in a general practice. *Aust Fam Physician*. 1997;26 (573–575):578–580.

19. Thurman S, Allen P. Integrating lactation consultants into primary health care services: Are lactation consultants affecting breastfeeding success? *Pediatr Nurs*. 2008;34:419–425.

20. Mattar C, Chong Y, Chan Y, et al. Simple antenatal preparation to improve breastfeeding practice: A randomized controlled trial. *Obstet Gynecol*. 2007;109:73–80.

21. UNICEF Breastfeeding Initiatives Exchange. The Baby Friendly Hospital Initiative. Available at: www.unicef.org/programme/breastfeeding/baby.htm (accessed February 9, 2013).

22. Baby-Friendly Hospital Initiative Revised, Updated and Expanded for Integrated Care. Section 2. Strengthening and Sustaining the Baby-Friendly Hospital Initiative: A Course for Decision-Makers. Available at: www.unicef.org/nutrition/files/BFHI_section_2_2009_eng.pdf (accessed February 9, 2013).

23. DiGirolamo AM, Grummer-Strawn LM, Fein SB. Effect of maternity-care practices on breastfeeding. *Pediatrics*. 2008;122 (Suppl 2):S43–S49.

24. Appendix A Task Force Ratings. Available at: www.ncbi.nlm.nih.gov/books/NBK15430 (accessed February 9, 2013).

25. Section on Breastfeeding. Breastfeeding and the use of human milk. *Pediatrics*. 2012;129:e827–e841.

26. Wolfberg AJ, Michels KB, Shields W, et al. Dads as breastfeeding advocates: Results from a randomized controlled trial of an educational intervention. *Am J Obstet Gynecol*. 2004;191:708–712.

27. Rosenberg KD, Eastham CA, Kasehagen LJ, et al. Marketing infant formula through hospitals: The impact of commercial hospital discharge packs on breastfeeding. *Am J Public Health*. 2008;98:290–295.

28. Howard C, Howard F, Lawrence R, et al. Office prenatal formula advertising and its effect on breastfeeding patterns. *Obstet Gynecol*. 2000;95:296–303.

29. Kandiah J, Burian C, Amend V. Teaching new mothers about infant feeding cues may increase breastfeeding duration. *Food Nutr Sci*. 2011;2:259–264.

30. ABM clinical protocol #3. Hospital guidelines for the use of supplementary feedings in the healthy, term breastfed neonate, revised 2009. *Breastfeed Med*. 2009;4:175–182.

31. Howard CR, Howard FM, Lanphear B, et al. Randomized clinical trial of pacifier use and bottle-feeding or cup feeding and their effect on breastfeeding. *Pediatrics*. 2003;111:511–518.

32. O'Connor NR, Tanabe KO, Siadaty MS, et al. Pacifiers and breastfeeding: A systematic review. *Arch Pediatr Adolesc Med*. 2009;163:378–382.

33. Paul IM, Beiler JS, Schaefer EW, et al. A randomized trial of single home nursing visits vs. office-based care after nursery/maternity discharge: The Nurses for Infants Through Teaching and Assessment After the Nursery (NITTANY) Study. *Arch Pediatr Adolesc Med*. 2012;166:263–270.

34. American Academy of Pediatrics Subcommittee on Hyperbilirubinemia. Management of hyperbilirubinemia in the newborn infant 35 or more weeks of gestation. *Pediatrics*. 2004;114:297–316.

35. World Health Organization Child Growth Standards. Available at: www.who.int/childgrowth/standards/technical_report/en/index.html (accessed February 9, 2013).

36. World Health Organization. International Code of Marketing of Breast-milk Substitutes. 1981. Available at: www.unicef.org/nutrition/files/nutrition_code_english.pdf (accessed February 9, 2013).

37. Bunik M. Breastfeeding Telephone Triage and Advice. American Academy of Pediatrics, Elk Grove Village, IL, 2012.

38. U.S. Department of Health and Human Services. The Business Case for Breastfeeding. Available at: www.womenshealth.gov/breastfeeding/government-in-action/business-case-forbreastfeeding/ (accessed February 9, 2013).

39. Ortiz J, McGilligan K, Kelly P. Duration of breast milk expression among working mothers enrolled in an employer-sponsored lactation program. *Pediatr Nurs*. 2004;30:111–119.

40. World Health Assembly. The Global Strategy for Infant and Young Child Feeding. 2003. Available at: www.who.int/nutrition/topics/global_strategy/en/index.html (accessed February 9, 2013).

41. Chapman DJ, Morel K, Anderson AK, et al. Breastfeeding peer counseling: From efficacy through scale-up. *J Hum Lact*. 2010;26:314–332.

42. Freed G, Clark S, Sorenson J, et al. National assessment of physicians' breastfeeding knowledge, attitudes, training, and experience. *JAMA*. 1995;273:472–476.

43. O'Connor M, Brown E, Orkin Lewin L. An Internet-based education program improves breastfeeding knowledge of maternal–child healthcare providers. *Breastfeed Med*. 2011;6:421–427.

44. Hillenbrand K, Larsen P. Effect of an educational intervention about breastfeeding on the knowledge, confidence, and behaviors of pediatric resident physicians. *Pediatrics*. 2002;110:e59.

45. Feldman-Winter LB, Shanler RJ, O'Connor KG, et al. Pediatricians and the promotion and support of breastfeeding. *Arch Pediatr Adolesc Med.* 2008;162:1142–1149.

46. Feldman-Winter L, Barone L, Milcarek B, et al. Residency curriculum improves breastfeeding care. *Pediatrics.* 2010;126:289–297.

47. Miller HD. From volume to value: Better ways to pay for health care. *Health Aff (Millwood).* 2009;28:1418–1428.

48. GovTrack.us. H.R. 3590 (111th): Patient Protection and Affordable Care Act. 2009. Available at: www.govtrack.us/congress/bill.xpd?bill = h111-3590&tab = reports (accessed February 9, 2013).

49. American Academy of Pediatrics. Building Your Medical Home Toolkit. www.pediatricmedhome.org (accessed February 5, 2013).

50. Title XIII—Health Information Technology for Economic and Clinical Health Act (HITECH). Available at: http://waysandmeans.house.gov/media/pdf/111/hitech.pdf (accessed February 9, 2013).

51. Dlugacz YD. *Value-Based Health Care: Linking Finance to Quality.* San Francisco: John Wiley and Sons; 2010.

ABM protocols expire 5 years from the date of publication. Evidence-based revisions are made within 5 years or sooner if there are significant changes in the evidence.

Academy of Breastfeeding Medicine Protocol Committee
Kathleen A. Marinelli, MD, FABM, Chairperson
Maya Bunik, MD, MSPH, FABM, Co-Chairperson
Larry Noble, MD, FABM, Translations Chairperson
Nancy Brent, MD
Amy E. Grawey, MD
Alison V. Holmes, MD, MPH, FABM
Ruth A. Lawrence, MD, FABM
Nancy G. Powers, MD, FABM
Tomoko Seo, MD, FABM
Julie Scott Taylor, MD, MSc, FABM
For correspondence: abm@bfmed.org

APPENDIX I

ABM Clinical Protocol #15
Analgesia and Anesthesia for the Breastfeeding Mother, Revised 2017*

Sarah Reece-Stremtan[1], Matilde Campos[2], Lauren Kokajko[1] and The Academy of Breastfeeding Medicine

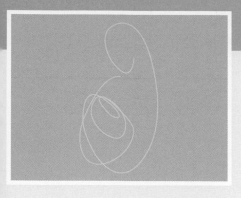

ABSTRACT

A central goal of The Academy of Breastfeeding Medicine is the development of clinical protocols, free from commercial interest or influence, for managing common medical problems that may impact breastfeeding success. These protocols serve only as guidelines for the care of breastfeeding mothers and infants and do not delineate an exclusive course of treatment or serve as standards of medical care. Variations in treatment may be appropriate according to the needs of an individual patient.

BACKGROUND

THERE IS LITTLE RIGOROUS INFORMATION in the scientific literature about anesthesia or procedural sedation in breastfeeding mothers. Recommendations in this area typically focus on pharmacologic properties of anesthetic agents, limited studies of milk levels, and rare infant effects. In addition to medication concerns, additional perioperative considerations may impact a breastfeeding dyad's continued breastfeeding success when a mother undergoes anesthesia or sedation. Despite the lack of controlled studies regarding outcomes of breastfeeding in mothers receiving anesthesia, multiple review articles conclude that most mothers may safely breastfeed immediately following anesthesia.[1−8] (IV) (Quality of evidence [levels of evidence IA, IB, IIA, IIB, III, and IV] is based on levels of evidence used for the National Guidelines Clearing House and is noted in parentheses.)[9] Most recommendations for breastfeeding in the perioperative setting come from expert opinion rather than from extensive studies or trials. Up-to-date information on specific

medications can be found on the United States National Library of Medicine website LactMed,[10] with additional resources listed in Table 1.

Medication guidelines discussed in this protocol may be extended to mothers in the immediate postpartum period; however, specific considerations for this population are detailed in ABM Protocol #28, Peripartum Anesthesia and Analgesia for the Breastfeeding Mother. The focus of this protocol is on anesthesia and analgesia for breastfeeding mothers outside the postpartum period.

RECOMMENDATIONS

General principles
Medications
The implications of medications used in breastfeeding mothers depend on numerous factors, including the amount of medication that passes into breast milk, the oral absorption of medication, the gestational and postpartum age of the child, and the potential for adverse effects on the breastfeeding infant.[11] Anesthetic agents cause little or no effects for older infants, but could potentially cause problems in neonates, particularly those who are preterm and/or suffer from preexisting apnea.

- Mothers with healthy term or older infants can generally resume breastfeeding as soon as they are awake, stable, and alert.[1−8] (IV) Resumption of normal mentation is a hallmark that medications have redistributed from the plasma compartment (and thus generally the milk compartment) and entered adipose and muscle tissue where they are slowly released.
- Infants at risk for apnea, hypotension, or hypotonia may benefit from a brief interruption of breastfeeding (6−12 hours) after maternal anesthesia. In this situation, mothers can express and store her milk in small amounts to be used when the infant is older, or it can be mixed with fresh milk containing no medications to dilute the milk with medications present.
- The most concerning class of medications used for anesthesia and analgesia in breastfeeding mothers is opioids, as these medications transfer into breast milk and may

---

* Courtesy of the Academy of Breastfeeding Medicine. Please go to https://www.bfmed.org/protocols for complete protocols, translations, and the most up-to-date information (protocols are updated every 5−7 years).

[1] Division of Anesthesiology, Pain, and Perioperative Medicine, Children's National Health System, Washington, District of Columbia.

[2] Division of Anesthesiology, Centro Hospitalar do Porto, Porto, Portugal.

TABLE 1	Resources of Information About Medications	
Resource	Sponsor	Website and contact information
LactMed	U.S. National Library of Medicine	https://toxnet.nlm.nih.gov/newtoxnet/lactmed.htm
E-Lactancia	Association for Promotion and Cultural and Scientific Research of Breastfeeding, Spain	www.e-lactancia.org
Infant Risk Center	Texas Tech University Health Sciences Center, TX	www.infantrisk.org and +1 806-352-2519
Breastfeeding and Human Lactation Study Center	University of Rochester, NY	+1 585-275-0088
Mother to Baby	Organization of Teratology Information Specialists	https://mothertobaby.org and +1 866-626-6847
Motherisk	Hospital for Sick Children, Toronto Canada	www.motherisk.org and +1 877-439-2744

cause infant sedation or apnea. Judicious use of opioids for short periods is likely to be safe for most breastfeeding mothers and infants.[6,12–14] (IV)

Brief procedures

Mothers who have undergone dental extractions or other short procedures requiring the use of single doses of medication for sedation and analgesia can breastfeed as soon as they are awake and stable. Although shorter-acting agents such as fentanyl and midazolam may be preferred, single doses of meperidine/pethidine or diazepam are unlikely to affect the breastfeeding infant.[15] (III) Local anesthetics given by injection or topical application are considered safe for breastfeeding mothers.[2,3] (IV)

Regional anesthesia

Regional anesthesia, including spinal, epidural, or peripheral nerve block, should be considered whenever possible, whether for intraoperative anesthesia or postoperative analgesia.[3] (IV) Regional anesthesia reduces the need for intraoperative medications and may also decrease the amount of pain medication needed postoperatively. In addition, the mother will be more awake and alert in the immediate postoperative period and will therefore be able to resume breastfeeding sooner.

Perioperative considerations

Breastfeeding mothers undergoing anesthesia or sedation should be scheduled as the first case of the day when possible to allow for minimal fasting times. Mothers should breastfeed or express milk immediately before surgery; a pump or help with hand expression must be available in the recovery room after surgery if infants are not allowed in this area. Hospital policies and procedures vary, but preventing engorgement and protecting a mother's milk supply and her confidence with breastfeeding should be prioritized. A more comprehensive perioperative breastfeeding plan is included at the end of this protocol.

INFORMATION ABOUT SPECIFIC AGENTS USED FOR ANESTHESIA AND ANALGESIA

Local anesthetics

Local anesthetics are given during a variety of procedures and are used in varying modalities. Medications may be used in spinal or epidural anesthesia, injected as a peripheral nerve block, infiltrated into the surgical field, or used as a topical application. Use of these medications typically helps minimize the need for additional systemic medications, and their use should be encouraged in breastfeeding mothers to decrease the need for opioids. Local anesthetics such as lidocaine, bupivacaine, and ropivacaine can be safely used in breastfeeding mothers. These and other local anesthetics are poorly absorbed orally and the large polarized molecules do not easily transfer into milk.[2,3] (IV)

Anesthetic agents

- Drugs used for anesthetic induction such as propofol, midazolam, etomidate, or thiopental enter the milk compartment only minimally, as they have very brief plasma distribution phases (only minutes), and hence their transport to milk is low to nil.[16–19] (III)
- Little or nothing has been reported about the use of anesthetic gases in breastfeeding mothers. However, they too have brief plasma distribution phases, and milk levels are likely to be nil. A series of case reports suggests that xenon maintenance after propofol induction allows for breastfeeding immediately after surgery.[20] (III)
- A study of low-dose ketamine for pain treatment after cesarean section has demonstrated no effects in the newborn, namely on the duration on breastfeeding.[21] (III) There is no information available on its use at anesthetic doses in breastfeeding mothers; it may be prudent to avoid large doses of this medication in breastfeeding mothers and monitor exposed infants afterward.[22] (IV)
- Dexmedetomidine is an alpha-2 agonist that acts centrally to reduce sympathetic outflow, producing sedation and

analgesia. It has low oral availability and is usually administered through the intravenous route. A single study of milk levels following infusion used during cesarean delivery determined that a breastfeeding infant would receive a relative infant dose (RID) of 0.04–0.098%.[23] (III)

- The United States Federal Drug Administration (FDA) in 2016 issued a Drug Safety Communication warning of the risk of using general anesthesia and some sedative medications in young children and pregnant women.[24] This advisory focused on the risk of possible effects on brain development when these agents are used repeatedly or for more than 3 hours. Note that there is no evidence to suggest a similar concern over use of anesthetic agents and medications in a breastfeeding mother.

- Neuromuscular blocking agents are safe for the breastfeeding infant, as they have low lipid solubility and are largely distributed in the extracellular fluid volume.[3] Although there are no data on the pharmacokinetics of these drugs in breast milk, based on their physical characteristics and their poor oral availability, they are considered safe for use in the breastfeeding mother. (IV)

- Reversal agents and anticholinergics used together to act against neuromuscular blockers appear to be generally safe for use, although there are no data on breast milk pharmacokinetics related to pyridostigmine or edrophonium. The anticholinesterase neostigmine could not be found in the breast milk of a mother with myasthenia whose infant appeared to have abdominal cramps after administration of the drug to the mother.[25] (III) Pyridostigmine was found in a very small amount in breast milk of mothers receiving the drug for treatment of myasthenia gravis, and was considered safe for the infant.[26] (III) Sugammadex is known to be excreted in small concentrations in breast milk in animal studies, although there are no studies in humans.[27–29] (III) Oral absorption of cyclodextrins in general is low and no effect on the breastfeeding child is anticipated. Of the anticholinergic agents, atropine is found in trace amounts in breast milk. Glycopyrrolate is not expected to be found in breast milk and is poorly absorbed through the gastrointestinal tract.[5]

- Antiemetics are used commonly in the perioperative period, and most of these medications are considered safe during breastfeeding. Ondansetron, dexamethasone, and metoclopramide may be preferred because of their lack of sedating side effects.[3] (IV) Prochlorperazine, promethazine, and scopolamine are likely safe, but may lead to maternal sedation; promethazine and scopolamine may also adversely affect milk supply if given repeatedly.[30–32] (III)

Analgesics
Opioid analgesics

Opioids are frequently used during surgery as part of a balanced anesthetic technique, and they may be continued postoperatively for pain. All opioids transfer into breast milk in varying amounts, and differences in breast milk concentration along with variation in oral availability make certain types of these medications more or less safe for a breastfeeding mother. In general, opioids of any type should be used with caution and for the shortest reasonable course in a breastfeeding mother.[12,13]

Opioids are given intravenously during surgery and may be administered as oral pain medications once mothers are tolerating oral intake postoperatively. Two specific medications used frequently during the perioperative period, morphine and hydromorphone, may be given through the intravenous or oral route. Because their oral availability is rather poor, the American Academy of Pediatrics (AAP) has identified them as possible safer choices for breastfeeding mothers over other opioids.[11] Intravenous opioids used during surgery are generally considered safe for immediate resumption of breastfeeding as soon as mothers are awake in the recovery room.

Intravenous medications

- Morphine. Morphine is still considered a reasonable option for breastfeeding mothers due to its limited transport to milk and its poor oral availability.[11,33,34] (III) It may be given through the intravenous or oral route.

- Fentanyl. Fentanyl levels in breast milk have been studied and are extremely low after 2 hours and generally below the limit of detection.[35,36] (III) Fentanyl also demonstrates very low oral availability and it is unlikely to cause any appreciable effects by its low levels in breast milk. Its use is typically restricted in the hospital to the operating room, emergency department, or critical care areas because of its potency and rapid onset of action.

- Hydromorphone. There are two reports available regarding hydromorphone and breastfeeding, neither of which evaluates its use through the intravenous route. One study evaluating a single intranasal dose of hydromorphone 2 mg found that infants would receive an RID of 0.67%.[37] A more recent single case report discusses the course of a 6-day-old infant who presented to the emergency room with sedation and poor feeding, and who required naloxone after episodes of apnea and bradycardia. Mother had been receiving hydromorphone 4 mg orally every 4 hours around the clock since her cesarean delivery 6 days before.[38] (III) Remifentanil. Although there are no published data on remifentanil, this esterase-metabolized opioid has a brief half-life even in infants (<10 minutes) and has been documented to produce no fetal sedation even in utero. Although its duration of action is limited, it could be used safely and indeed may be ideal in breastfeeding mothers for short painful procedures.

- Sufentanil. Sufentanil transfer into milk has not been published, but its safety profile is likely similar to fentanyl.[36] This opioid is most commonly used during general anesthesia, or as an additive in epidural anesthesia and analgesia.

- Meperidine. The transfer of meperidine/pethidine into breast milk is low (1.7–3.5% of maternal weight-adjusted dose). However, meperidine/pethidine and its metabolite (normeperidine) are consistently associated with dose-related neonatal sedation. Transfer into milk and neonatal sedation have been documented for even up to 36 hours after a single dose.[33] (III) Infants of mothers who have been exposed to repeated doses of meperidine/pethidine should be closely monitored for sedation, cyanosis, bradycardia, and possibly seizures, and the AAP recommends against its use in breastfeeding mothers.[11] (IV)

- Nalbuphine and butorphanol. Nalbuphine and butorphanol are partial opioid agonists, with nalbuphine administered intravenously and butorphanol usually through the nasal route. Levels of both these medications in breast milk are very low, although they are not typically used as part of perioperative analgesic regimens. However, the AAP has recommended butorphanol as a reasonable choice if opioid analgesics are required for a breastfeeding mother.[11] (IV)

Oral medications given for postoperative pain. All oral opioids used for postoperative pain should be limited to the shortest reasonable course, and infants should be watched closely for sedation when mothers require these medications. Analgesic effects from codeine and tramadol derive from metabolites that are dependent upon the CYP2D6 activity. Interindividual variation in the CYP2D6 activity may cause ultrarapid metabolizers to receive excessively high amounts of active metabolites, leading to potential for sedation or respiratory depression from typical dosing. Although hydrocodone and oxycodone also partially undergo metabolism by CYP2D6 to more potent metabolites, the parent drug also exerts an analgesic effect and there is less concern over the clinical effects of variation in metabolism.

- Hydrocodone. Hydrocodone has been used frequently in breastfeeding mothers. Occasional cases of neonatal sedation have been documented, but these are rare and generally dose related.[39,40] Doses in breastfeeding mothers should be limited to 30 mg per day.[40] (III)
- Oxycodone. Oxycodone levels in milk have been studied, with a range of 5–226 μg/L (RID up to 8%).[41] One retrospective study showed that one in five breastfed infants with mothers taking oxycodone experienced central nervous system depression. The strong concordance between maternal and infant symptoms may be used to identify infants at higher risk. It is important to monitor these infants carefully for drowsiness.[42] (III) LactMed recommends a maximum total daily dose of 30 mg,[43] and the AAP advises against the use of the medication in breastfeeding mothers.[11] (IV)
- Codeine. A report of a neonatal death following the maternal use of codeine suggests that the use of codeine in breastfeeding mothers should be limited.[44] Although rare, rapid metabolizers of codeine exist, and levels of morphine following the use of codeine may be unexpectedly and significantly elevated, thus putting a breastfeeding infant at risk. The FDA in 2017 issued an advisory against the use of the medication in breastfeeding mothers in the United States[45]; (IV) it continues to be prescribed in other areas of the world, but other medications are preferred when available.[12,46]

- Tramadol. Tramadol is a weak opioid with an additional activity at central norepinephrine and serotonin receptors. Like codeine, it needs to be metabolized by CYP2D6 to an active metabolite to exert its analgesic effects. With an RID of <1% of the active metabolite and no reported effects in breastfed infants, it has previously been considered a safe choice for breastfeeding mothers.[47–49] However, the FDA has advised against the use of this medication in breastfeeding mothers in the United States.[45] (IV)

Regardless of the opioid chosen, the dose needs to be carefully considered. Virtually any opioid may be used transiently, but infants should be monitored for sedation,[13] especially when these medications are used for more than 4 days.[6] Note that mothers on chronic opioid therapy may be using exceedingly high doses of hydrocodone, oxycodone, methadone, and other opioid analgesics that were started before or during pregnancy. Safety of breastfeeding for these patients should be considered on an individual basis.

Nonsteroidal anti-inflammatory drug analgesics

Use of nonsteroidal anti-inflammatory drugs (NSAIDs) alone or in combination with opioids after surgery can improve pain control due to their anti-inflammatory properties. NSAIDs are generally safe for breastfeeding and can help minimize the total dose of opioid needed to control pain.[50,51] (III) In addition, due to their low lipid solubility and high protein binding, NSAIDs have limited transfer into breast milk (milk to plasma ratios <1).[52] While transfer of NSAIDs to breast milk is low, this class of medications should be avoided in mothers with infants who have ductal-dependent cardiac lesions.[11]

- Ibuprofen. Ibuprofen is considered an ideal, moderately effective analgesic. Its transfer to milk is low to nil.[53] (III) Ketorolac. Ketorolac is a potent analgesic in breastfeeding mothers and increasingly popular when used postoperatively. Its primary benefit is excellent analgesia, with no sedative properties. In addition, the transfer of ketorolac into milk is extremely low.[54] However, its use in postsurgical patients with hemorrhage may be risky as it inhibits platelet function, although this is somewhat controversial. It should not be used in patients with a history of gastritis, aspirin allergy, or renal insufficiency. If there is no risk of hemorrhage, it carries few complications for breastfeeding mothers and their infants. (III)
- Celecoxib. Celecoxib transfer into milk is extraordinarily low (<0.3% of the weight-adjusted maternal dose).[55] Its short-term use is safe in breastfeeding mothers. (III)
- Naproxen. Naproxen transfer into milk is low, but gastrointestinal disturbances have been reported in some infants following prolonged therapy. Short-term use (1 week) is likely to be safe.[56] (III)

Other analgesics

- Acetaminophen/paracetamol. Acetaminophen/paracetamol has been used for postoperative analgesia as well as maternal fever. Transfer into the milk is low and appears to be less than the usual dosage given to infants. One study showed that infants would only receive a maximum of 2% of the maternal weight-adjusted dose.[57] Hepatotoxicity is thought to be less common in newborns given the low levels of specific cytochrome P-450 enzymes that convert the drug to its toxic metabolites.[11]

- Gabapentin. Gabapentin is one of the first-line drugs for treatment of neuropathic pain and is also used as part of a multimodal analgesia regimen in the perioperative period. Limited studies indicate low serum concentrations in infants of mothers taking up to 2 g a day.[58−60] (III) It is suggested to monitor the infant for weight gain and drowsiness. Gabapentin is likely safe, especially in single or short-term doses.[61]

- Pregabalin. Pregabalin is also used in the treatment of neuropathic and postoperative pain. There is limited information about the passage of this medication into the breast milk, but the RID is 7−8%.[62] (III) LactMed recommends monitoring infants for drowsiness and suggests using possible alternative medications if available.[63]

PERIOPERATIVE BREASTFEEDING PLAN

Preoperatively

- Consider postponing elective procedures until child is older and milk supply and breastfeeding relationship are well established.
- Breastfeeding mothers should be encouraged to express milk ahead of the surgical date, to have milk available for their child in case of extended separation at the time of surgery.
- A responsible adult other than the mother should be identified to care for and observe the child postoperatively if opioids are required for postoperative pain.
- Breastfeeding mothers should be scheduled for first case or early in the day to minimize fasting times, and may use a 2-hour window for clear fluids if there are no risk factors for aspiration.
- Mothers should breastfeed or express milk just before the start of the procedure.

Intraoperatively

- Consider regional anesthetic technique to minimize use of systemic sedative medications.
- Aggressive postoperative nausea and vomiting prophylaxis should be utilized.
- Fluid management strategies should focus on maintaining euvolemia without overhydration that may cause edema.
- Employ multimodal pain management strategies to minimize need for opioids.

Postoperatively

- Mothers with term, healthy children may breastfeed as soon as they are awake in the recovery room.

- If children are not allowed in the recovery room, a breast pump or assistance with hand expression must be available for mothers immediately after surgery.
- For vulnerable infants who should be protected by a brief interruption from breastfeeding postoperatively, milk should be expressed as soon as the mother is awake. The milk does not necessarily need to be discarded. It can be frozen for use when the child is at lower risk in the future. Alternatively, the milk can be used diluted with other breast milk not containing anesthetic (expressed either before or 1 day after the procedure).
- The mother should be encouraged to express during the interruption from breastfeeding, at least as often as she would normally breastfeed to maintain supply (around every 2−4 hours depending on child's age).
- Opioids should be used judiciously, at the lowest dose and for the shortest period of time that provides adequate analgesia. The breastfed child should be cared for and observed by an adult other than the mother, when opioids are used.

RECOMMENDATIONS FOR FUTURE RESEARCH

More study of specific breastfeeding outcomes after surgical anesthesia in breastfeeding mothers is needed. Common-sense recommendations to avoid prolonged fasting times in breastfeeding mothers and encourage frequent expressing or breastfeeding in the immediate perioperative period have not been rigorously explored in controlled settings. The effect of fluid management strategies and hemodynamic variation and need for vasoactive medications on milk supply should be investigated. In addition, breastfeeding-friendly policies in hospitals and outpatient surgery centers should be prioritized and studied, and may be reasonable options for quality improvement processes.

As is the case for many medications used during breastfeeding, more information on medication transfer into breast milk and infant effects is urgently needed. Case reports of negative outcomes may help to delineate where significant concern is warranted, but reports of single dyads or small series with apparently uneventful breastfeeding courses do not necessarily assure safety. More study in particular is required of the special needs of premature and unstable infants, including how their ability to clear maternal anesthetic and analgesic drugs may differ from healthy, term newborns. In addition, thoughtful investigation into the implications of maternal anesthesia on neurobehavioral outcomes in breastfeeding infants may help allay concerns over this theoretical small risk.[64]

REFERENCES

1. Chu TC, McCallum J, Yii MF. Breastfeeding after anaesthesia: A review of the pharmacological impact on children. *Anaesth Intensive Care.* 2013;41:35−40.

2. Cobb B, Liu R, Valentine E, et al. Breastfeeding after anesthesia: A review for anesthesia providers regarding the transfer of medications into breast milk. *Transl Perioper Pain Med.* 2015;1:1−7.

3. Dalal PG, Bosak J, Berlin C. Safety of the breast-feeding infant after maternal anesthesia. *Paediatr Anaesth.* 2014;24:359−371.

4. Kundra S, Kundra S. Breastfeeding in the perioperative period. *J Obstet Anaesth Crit Care.* 2011;1:46−47.

5. Hale TW. Anesthetic medications in breastfeeding mothers. *J Hum Lact.* 1999;15:185−194.

6. Allegaert K, van den Anker J. Maternal analgosedation and breastfeeding: Guidance for the pediatrician. *J Pediatr Neonat Individual Med.* 2015;4:1−6.

7. Dumphy D. The breastfeeding surgical patient. *AORN J.* 2008;87:759−766. quiz 767−770.

8. Smathers AB, Collins S, Hewer I. Perianesthetic considerations for the breastfeeding mother. *J Perianesth Nurs.* 2016;31:317−329.

9. Shekelle PG, Woolf SH, Eccles M, et al. Clinical guidelines: Developing guidelines. *BMJ.* 1999;318:593−596.

10. National Library of Medicine. Drugs and lactation database (LactMed). Updated 2017. Available at https://toxnet.nlm.nih.gov/newtoxnet/lactmed.htm (accessed May 18, 2017).

11. Sachs HC. Committee on Drugs. The transfer of drugs and therapeutics into human breast milk: An update on selected topics. *Pediatrics.* 2013;132:e796−e809.

12. van den Anker JN. Is it safe to use opioids for obstetric pain while breastfeeding? *J Pediatr.* 2012;160:4−6.

13. Hendrickson RG, McKeown NJ. Is maternal opioid use hazardous to breast-fed infants? *Clin Toxicol (Phila).* 2012;50:1−14.

14. Spigset O, Hagg S. Analgesics and breast-feeding: Safety considerations. *Paediatr Drugs.* 2000;2:223−238.

15. Grimm D, Pauly E, Pöschl J, et al. Buprenorphine and norbuprenorphine concentrations in human breast milk samples determined by liquid chromatography-tandem mass spectrometry. *Ther Drug Monit.* 2005;27:526−530.

16. Andersen LW, Qvist T, Hertz J, et al. Concentrations of thiopentone in mature breast milk and colostrum following an induction dose. *Acta Anaesthesiol Scand.* 1987;31:30−32.

17. Matheson I, Lunde PK, Bredesen JE. Midazolam and nitrazepam in the maternity ward: Milk concentrations and clinical effects. *Br J Clin Pharmacol.* 1990;30:787−793.

18. Dailland P, Cockshott ID, Lirzin JD, et al. Intravenous propofol during cesarean section: Placental transfer, concentrations in breast milk, and neonatal effects. A preliminary study. *Anesthesiology.* 1989;71:827−834.

19. Schmitt JP, Schwoerer D, Diemunsch P, et al. [Passage of propofol in the colostrum. *Preliminary data]. Ann Fr Anesth Reanim.* 1987;6:267−268.

20. Stuttmann R, Schäfer C, Hilbert P, et al. The breast feeding mother and xenon anaesthesia: Four case reports. Breast feeding and xenon anaesthesia. *BMC Anesthesiol.* 2010;10. 1−1.

21. Suppa E, Valente A, Catarci S, et al. A study of low-dose ketamine infusion as "preventive" pain treatment for cesarean section with spinal anesthesia: Benefits and side effects. *Minerva Anestesiol.* 2012;78:774−781.

22. National Library of Medicine. Ketamine. Drugs and lactation database (LactMed). Updated 2017. Available at https://toxnet.nlm.nih.gov/cgi-bin/sis/search2/f?./temp/∼BojiMV:1 (accessed May 17, 2017).

23. Nakanishi R, Yoshimura M, Suno M, et al. Detection of dexmedetomidine in human breast milk using liquid chromatography-tandem mass spectrometry: Application to a study of drug safety in breastfeeding after cesarean section. *J Chromatogr B Analyt Technol Biomed Life Sci.* 2017;1040:208−213.

24. U.S. Food and Drug Administration. FDA drug safety communication: FDA review results in new warnings about using general anesthetics and sedation drugs in young children and pregnant women. Updated 2016. Available at: www.fda.gov/Drugs/DrugSafety/ucm532356.htm (accessed May 20, 2017).

25. Fraser D, Turner JW. Myasthenia gravis and pregnancy. *Proc R Soc Med.* 1963;56:379−381.

26. Hardell LI, Lindstrom B, Lonnerholm G, et al. Pyridostigmine in human breast milk. *Br J Clin Pharmacol.* 1982;14:565−567.

27. Merck & Co. I. Sugammadex prescribing information. Available at: www.merck.com/product/usa/pi_circulars/b/bridion/bridion_pi.pdf (accessed May 17, 2017).

28. Cada DJ, Levien TL, Baker DE. Sugammadex. *Hosp Pharm.* 2016;51:585−596.

29. Sokol-Kobielska E. Sugammadex—Indications and clinical use. *Anaesthesiol Intensive Ther.* 2013;45:106−110.

30. National Library of Medicine. Prochlorperazine. In: Drugs and lactation database (LactMed). Updated 2015. Available at: https://toxnet.nlm.nih.gov/cgi-bin/sis/search2/f?./temp/∼7SuYzf:1 (accessed May 17, 2017).

31. National Library of Medicine. Promethazine. In: Drugs and lactation database (LactMed). Updated 2015. Available at: https://toxnet.nlm.nih.gov/cgi-bin/sis/search2/f?./temp/∼vcQMox:1 (accessed May 17, 2017).

32. National Library of Medicine. Scopolamine. In: Drugs and lactation database (LactMed). Updated 2015. Available at: https://toxnet.nlm.nih.gov/cgi-bin/sis/search2/f?./temp/∼HqD17Y:1 (accessed May 17, 2017).

33. Wittels B, Scott DT, Sinatra RS. Exogenous opioids inhuman breast milk and acute neonatal neurobehavior: A preliminary study. *Anesthesiology.* 1990;73:864−869.

34. Wittels B, Glosten B, Faure EA, et al. Postcesarean analgesia with both epidural morphine and intravenous patient-controlled analgesia: Neurobehavioral outcomes among nursing neonates. *Anesth Analg.* 1997;85:600−606.

35. Leuschen MP, Wolf LJ, Rayburn WF. Fentanyl excretion in breast milk. *Clin Pharm.* 1990;9:336−337.

36. Madej TH, Strunin L. Comparison of epidural fentanyl with sufentanil. Analgesia and side effects after a single bolus dose during elective caesarean section. *Anaesthesia.* 1987;42:1156−1161.

37. Edwards JE, Rudy AC, Wermeling DP, et al. Hydromorphone transfer into breast milk after intranasal administration. *Pharmacotherapy.* 2003;23:153−158.

38. Schultz ML, Kostic M, Kharasch S. A case of toxic breastfeeding? *Pediatr Emerg Care.* 2017;. Available from: https://doi.org/10.1097/PEC.0000000000001009.

39. Anderson PO, Sauberan JB, Lane JR, et al. Hydrocodone excretion into breast milk: The first two reported cases. *Breastfeed Med.* 2007;2:10−14.

40. Sauberan JB, Anderson PO, Lane JR, et al. Breast milk hydrocodone and hydromorphone levels in mothers using hydrocodone for postpartum pain. *Obstet Gynecol.* 2011;117:611−617.

41. Marx CM, Pucino F, Carlson JD, et al. Oxycodone excretion in human milk in the puerperium. *Drug Intell Clin Pharm.* 1986;20:474.

42. Lam J, Kelly L, Ciszkowski C, et al. Central nervous system depression of neonates breastfed by mothers receiving oxycodone for postpartum analgesia. *J Pediatr.* 2012;160:33–37. e2.

43. National Library of Medicine. Oxycodone. In: Drugs and lactation database (LactMed). Updated 2017. Available at: https://toxnet.nlm.nih.gov/cgi-bin/sis/search2/f?./temp/∼r97Ebu:1 (accessed May 17, 2017).

44. Koren G, Cairns J, Chitayat D, et al. Pharmacogenetics of morphine poisoning in a breastfed neonate of a codeine-prescribed mother. *Lancet.* 2006;368. 704–704.

45. U.S. Food and Drug Administration. FDA drug safety communication: FDA restricts use of prescription codeine pain and cough medicines and tramadol pain medicines in children; recommends against use in breastfeeding women. Updated 2017. Available at: www.fda.gov/Drugs/DrugSafety/ucm549679.htm (accessed May 17, 2017).

46. Madadi P, Moretti M, Djokanovic N, et al. Guidelines for maternal codeine use during breastfeeding. *Can Fam Physician.* 2009;55:1077–1078.

47. Ilett KF, Paech MJ, Page-Sharp M, et al. Use of a sparse sampling study design to assess transfer of tramadol and its O-desmethyl metabolite into transitional breast milk. *Br J Clin Pharmacol.* 2008;65:661–666.

48. Salman S, Sy SK, Ilett KF, et al. Population pharmacokinetic modeling of tramadol and its O-desmethyl metabolite in plasma and breast milk. *Eur J Clin Pharmacol.* 2011;67:899–908.

49. National Library of Medicine. Tramadol. In: Drugs and lactation database (LactMed). Updated 2017. Available at: https://toxnet.nlm.nih.gov/cgi-bin/sis/search2/f?./temp/∼1vlzLz:1 (accessed May 18, 2017).

50. Gadsden J, Hart S, Santos AC. Post-cesarean delivery analgesia. *Anesth Analg.* 2005;101:S62–S69.

51. Sutton CD, Carvalho B. Optimal pain management after cesarean delivery. *Anesthesiol Clin.* 2017;35:107–124.

52. Bloor M, Paech M. Nonsteroidal anti-inflammatory drugs during pregnancy and the initiation of lactation. *Anesth Analg.* 2013;116:1063–1075.

53. Weibert RT, Townsend RJ, Kaiser DG, et al. Lack of ibuprofen secretion into human milk. *Clin Pharm.* 1982;1:457–458.

54. Wischnik A, Manth SM, Lloyd J, et al. The excretion of ketorolac tromethamine into breast milk after multiple oral dosing. *Eur J Clin Pharmacol.* 1989;36:521–524.

55. Hale TW, McDonald R, Boger J. Transfer of celecoxib into human milk. *J Hum Lact.* 2004;20:397–403.

56. Jamali F, Stevens DR. Naproxen excretion in milk and its uptake by the infant. *Drug Intell Clin Pharm.* 1983;17:910–911.

57. National Library of Medicine. Acetaminophen. In: Drugs and lactation database (LactMed). Updated 2017. Available at: https://toxnet.nlm.nih.gov/cgi-bin/sis/search2/f?./temp/*T8KYDk:1 (accessed May 18, 2017).

58. Kristensen JH, Ilett KF, Hackett LP, et al. Gabapentin and breastfeeding: A case report. *J Hum Lact.* 2006;22:426–428.

59. Ohman I, Vitols S, Tomson T. Pharmacokinetics of gabapentin during delivery, in the neonatal period, and lactation: Does a fetal accumulation occur during pregnancy? *Epilepsia.* 2005;46:1621–1624.

60. Ohman I, Tomson T. Gabapentin kinetics during delivery, in the neonatal period, and during lactation. *Epilepsia.* 2009;50 (Suppl 10):108.

61. National Library of Medicine. Gabapentin. In: Drugs and lactation database (LactMed). Updated 2017. Available at: https://toxnet.nlm.nih.gov/cgi-bin/sis/search2 (accessed May 18, 2017).

62. Lockwood PA, Pauer L, Scavone JM, et al. The pharmacokinetics of pregabalin in breast milk, plasma, and urine of healthy postpartum women. *J Hum Lact.* 2016;.

63. National Library of Medicine. Pregabalin. In: Drugs and lactation database (LactMed). Updated 2017. Available at: https://toxnet.nlm.nih.gov/cgi-bin/sis/search2/f?./temp/*38kYuD:1 (accessed May 18, 2017).

64. Camporesi A, Silvani P. Comment on 'Safety of the breastfeeding infant after maternal anesthesia' Dalal PG, Bosak J, Berlin C. *Pediatr Anesth.* 2014;24:453.

ABM protocols expire 5 years from the date of publication. Content of this protocol is up-to-date at the time of publication. Evidence based revisions are made within 5 years or sooner if there are significant changes in the evidence.

The 2012 edition of this protocol was authored by Anne Montgomery and Thomas W. Hale.
The Academy of Breastfeeding Medicine Protocol Committee:
Wendy Brodribb, MBBS, PhD, FABM, Chairperson
Sarah Reece-Stremtan, MD, Co-Chairperson
Larry Noble, MD, FABM, Translations Chairperson
Nancy Brent, MD
Maya Bunik, MD, MSPH, FABM
Cadey Harrel, MD
Ruth A. Lawrence, MD, FABM
Yvonne LeFort, MD, FABM
Kathleen A. Marinelli, MD, FABM
Casey Rosen-Carole, MD, MPH, MSEd
Susan Rothenberg, MD
Tomoko Seo, MD, FABM
Rose St. Fleur, MD
Michal Young, MD
For correspondence: abm@bfmed.org

ABM Clinical Protocol #16
Breastfeeding the Hypotonic Infant, Revision 2016*

Jennifer Thomas[1], Kathleen A. Marinelli[2,3] and the Academy of Breastfeeding Medicine

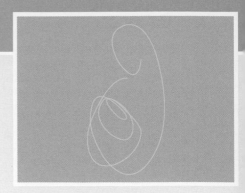

ABSTRACT

A central goal of The Academy of Breastfeeding Medicine is the development of clinical protocols for managing common medical problems that may impact breastfeeding success. These protocols serve only as guidelines for the care of breastfeeding mothers and infants and do not delineate an exclusive course of treatment or serve as standards of medical care. Variations in treatment may be appropriate according to the needs of an individual patient.

GOAL

TO PROMOTE, SUPPORT, and sustain breastfeeding in infants and young children with hypotonia.

DEFINITION

Muscle tone, the muscle's resistance to passive stretch during resting state, is distinct from muscle strength and can be affected by many factors. Hypotonia, a condition of diminished muscle tone, may occur with or without muscle weakness. There are diverse etiologies including abnormalities of the central or peripheral nervous systems; neuromuscular junction; muscle, metabolic, endocrine, or nutritional disorders; connective tissue diseases; and chromosomal abnormalities. Perinatal hypoxia and hypotonic cerebral palsy may result in central hypotonia. In addition, benign congenital hypotonia, a diagnosis of exclusion, improves or disappears entirely with age.[1]

---

* Courtesy of the Academy of Breastfeeding Medicine. Please go to https://www.bfmed.org/protocols for complete protocols, translations, and the most up-to-date information (protocols are updated every 5–7 years).

[1] Department of Pediatrics, Aurora Health Care, Franklin, Wisconsin.

[2] Division of Neonatology, Connecticut Human Milk Research Center, Connecticut Children's Medical Center, Hartford, Connecticut.

[3] School of Medicine, University of Connecticut, Farmington, Connecticut.

BACKGROUND

Hypotonic infants often have breastfeeding problems that result from abnormal or underdeveloped control of the oropharyngeal structures, contributing to an uncoordinated and/or weak suck, similar to those experienced by premature infants. Despite the many etiologies for hypotonia, little research has been specifically undertaken on the feeding problems of the hypotonic infant. However, interventions used for infants with important causes of hypotonia, such as Trisomy 21 (Down syndrome) and prematurity, can be applied to the care of these infants.

Trisomy 21, a genetic disorder where more than 90% of infants have hypotonia, shares many of the same feeding risks and complicating morbidities as other causes of hypotonia. Associated oral abnormalities characteristically include malocclusion and a small mouth with a relatively large protruding tongue, which when coupled with hypotonia result in significant feeding difficulties in some of these children.[2]

In many countries premature infants, who may also have hypotonia-related difficulties, are often separated from their mothers shortly after birth, which can increase breastfeeding difficulties. Premature infants also struggle with small and underdeveloped oral structures and difficulties with suck–swallow coordination.[3]

The Academy of Breastfeeding Medicine, the American Academy of Pediatrics, the World Health Organization, and other international organizations recommend that all infants should be breastfed unless there is a medical contraindication.[4,5] It is particularly important that infants and young children with hypotonia, including those with Trisomy 21, be breastfed because of their increased risk of morbidities associated with artificial feeding. For example, children with Trisomy 21 are more susceptible to ear, respiratory, and other infections, have developmental delay, and an increased incidence of other congenital anomalies such as heart and gastrointestinal malformations in addition to oral abnormalities and malocclusion.

A systematic review examining the effects of breastfeeding on these problems in a healthy population found that breastfeeding is protective against the development of ear and respiratory infections.[6,7] It is also associated with a significantly lower risk of malocclusion (odds ratio 0.34; 95% confidence interval 0.24—0.48),[8] which suggests that breastfeeding promotes oral motor strength, and, therefore, has potential benefit to children with Trisomy 21 and other causes of hypotonia.[2] Breastfeeding helps with normal mouth and tongue coordination.

Studies indicate that there is a positive neurocognitive advantage of breastfeeding,[6,9] which is most pronounced in children with low birth weight or who were small for gestational age.[10] As hypotonic infants may have disorders associated with neurocognitive impairment, this advantage of human milk over infant formula could make an important difference to their long-term outcome.

Children with congenital heart disease who breastfeed have better growth, shorter hospital stays, and higher oxygen saturations than children with congenital heart disease who are formula fed.[11] Again, these findings suggest a potential advantage for breastfeeding hypotonic infants with congenital heart disease, such as can occur in infants with Trisomy 21. Thus, although children with hypotonia have not been specifically studied, based on information from studies in the general population, they would be expected to benefit from breastfeeding and/or being fed expressed human milk.

Sucking behavior in hypotonic infants, specifically those with Trisomy 21, is less efficient than in normal term infants with multiple parameters affected, including the pressure, frequency, and duration of sucking and smooth peristaltic tongue movement.[12] (II-2) (Quality of evidence [Levels of evidence I, II-1, II-2, II-3, and III] is based on the U.S. Preventive Services[13] Task Force Appendix A Task Force Ratings and is noted in parentheses.) When followed longitudinally over the first year, sucking pressure increased significantly by 4 months and again by 8 months and sucking frequency increased by 4 months. Sucking duration did not increase over time, and peristalsis only normalized in the minority of infants who were restudied at 8 months. However, the overall result was an improvement in sucking efficiency over the first year.

Mothers tended to report that feeding problems improved substantially by 3—4 months of age. Understanding this time frame allows practitioners to effectively support mothers and their hypotonic infants to improve breastfeeding skills and reach and maintain a sufficient milk supply that may enable them to successfully breastfeed, despite the presence of significant difficulties at the beginning.

Breastfeeding the hypotonic infant is challenging, but many can successfully feed at the breast. There is no evidence that infants with Trisomy 21 or other hypotonic infants feed better with the bottle than at the breast and no evidence suggests that these children need to feed from a bottle before attempting to breastfeed.

Whenever possible, a team of professionals with expertise in assisting infants with special needs to breastfeed should work together to help the mother—infant dyad. The importance of knowledgeable health professionals is highlighted in studies that found some mothers of children with Trisomy 21 felt they were not given important support for breastfeeding.

Instead, they expressed feeling "helpless"[14] or were frustrated that they were not able to meet their breastfeeding goals. Had these mothers received support that enabled them to breastfeed their infants, they would likely have felt empowered rather than discouraged or frustrated.

PROCEDURES

A. Prenatal care:
1. Healthcare providers should encourage all mothers to breastfeed, whether the infant has a high risk of hypotonia or not. Encouragement can make a significant difference as to whether a mother decides to breastfeed or not.[15,16] (II-2, II-2)
2. A breastfeeding history should be obtained as part of prenatal care, and identified concerns and risk factors for breastfeeding difficulties should be communicated to the infant's healthcare provider(s).[17] (III)
3. If it is known during pregnancy that the infant will have hypotonia, mothers should be referred to breastfeeding medicine specialists and/or lactation consultants with expertise with hypotonic infants.

B. Education:
1. All mothers should be educated about the advantages for themselves and their infants of breastfeeding and of providing human milk. A significant proportion of hypotonic infants can feed at the breast without difficulty.
2. Infants with hypotonia should be followed closely both before and after discharge from the hospital to assess further needs.

C. Facilitation and assessment of feeding at the breast in the immediate postpartum period:
1. The first feed should be initiated as soon as the infant is stable. There is no reason this cannot occur early, for example, in the delivery room, if the infant is physiologically stable. Extra support and supervision may be required.
2. Kangaroo (skin-to-skin) care should be strongly encouraged. As with all infants, when infants with hypotonia are being held skin-to-skin, care should be taken to ensure the mother is fully awake and infant's face is visible and airway remains open. If the infant does not feed well, the touching may be stimulating so that the infant is easier to arouse for feedings. Skin-to-skin care has also been shown to help increase mother's milk supply,[18,19] (II-2, II-2) and, in addition to eye contact and touching, can assist with bonding that may be especially important for these families.
3. Assessment of the infant's ability to latch, suck, and transfer milk should involve personnel specifically trained in breastfeeding evaluation and management.
4. For attempts at breastfeeding, particular attention should be given to providing good head and body support for the infant since he/she needs to spend

effort sucking, not supporting body position. Use of a sling or pillows to support the infant in a flexed position allows the mother to use her hands to support both her breast and the infant's jaw simultaneously (Dancer hand position). Skin-to-skin contact will facilitate frequent attempts at breast.

5. The "Dancer hand" position (Fig. 1) may be helpful for the mother to try as it supports both her breast and her infant's chin and jaw while the infant is breastfeeding. The mother cups her breast in the palm of her hand (holding her breast from below), with the third, fourth, and fifth fingers curling up toward the side of her breast to support it, while simultaneously allowing the infant's chin to rest on the web space between her thumb and index finger. The thumb and index finger can then give gentle pressure to the masseter muscle, which stabilizes the jaw.[20,21] (II-2, II-2) In addition, pulling the jaw slightly forward may allow the infant to better grasp the breast and form a seal. The other hand is free to support the infant's neck and shoulders

6. Other strategies to help the infant latch and transfer milk may also be effective. Some mothers facilitate milk transfer by using hand compression in conjunction with breastfeeding. Instead of placing the thumb and index finger on the infant's jaw for support (Dancer hand position), the fingers are kept proximal to the areola, and milk is hand expressed as the infant suckles. A thin silicone nipple shield may be useful if milk production is generous (> 500 mL/day) and mothers learn how to keep the reservoir filled by synchronizing breastfeeding with hand compression or using a nursing supplementation device simultaneously inside the shield.[22] (II-3)

   By making the mother aware of various techniques, aids, and ideas, she can experiment and discover the best ways to fit her and her infant's individual needs.

7. More time may be necessary in the early weeks to complete a feeding. Mothers, and the family that supports them, should also know that in many cases the infant's ability to feed will improve over the first weeks to months.

8. Trained personnel should reassess the infant frequently (a minimum of once every 8 hours) as these infants must be considered at high risk of breastfeeding difficulties, similar to the late preterm infant (see ABM Protocol #10: Breastfeeding the Late Preterm Infant).[23] Encourage frequent breastfeeding throughout the day as the ability to sustain suck may be impaired. Infants should go to breast as often as possible, aiming for at least 8 to 12 times per 24 hours.[5] Prolonged periods of skin-to-skin contact will facilitate these frequent attempts at breast. Assessments should include state

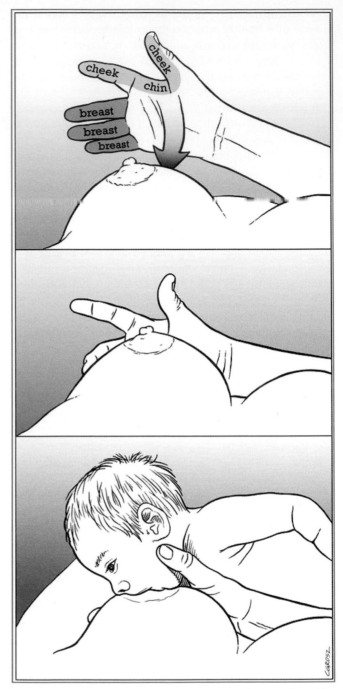

Figure 1. Dancer hand position from the mother's view. Illustration by Claudia Grosz, MFA.

of hydration and jaundice to identify possible complications of poor oral intake.

9. Once transitional milk is present, test weighing with an appropriate digital scale may be an option to assess adequate milk transfer for these infants. Infants are weighed immediately before the feed on an electronic scale with accuracy at minimum ± 5 g, and then reweighed immediately after the feed under the exact same circumstances: diaper (nappy), clothing, blankets, etc. Intake during the

breastfeed is reflected by weight gain, 1 g = 1 mL. Infants with Trisomy 21 may gain weight more slowly than normal full-term infants.[24] (II-3) New growth charts for infants with Trisomy 21, introduced in 2015, are designed to more accurately reflect normal growth for these infants.[24]

10. Consider alternative modes of feeding such as a cup,[25] (I) spoon, or syringe, if the infant is unable to breastfeed or sustain adequate suckling. The use of a nursing supplementation aid alone (without a nipple shield—see C6) may not be as helpful, as it works best with an infant who has an effective latch and infants with hypotonia often have difficulties with latch.

11. If supplementation is necessary, see Academy of Breastfeeding Medicine Protocol #3 (Hospital Guidelines for the Use of Supplementary Feedings in the Healthy Term Breastfed Infant).[26] If the infant is attempting to suckle, follow each breastfeeding encounter with breastmilk expression (see D) and then feed expressed milk to the infant by spoon, cup, or other device. This provides more stimulation to the breasts and more milk to the infant.

12. At times, some of these infants may have issues with dysphagia and aspiration of feedings of any type. There is some evidence that thickening of feedings in these circumstances can decrease the risks. Close communication with the team managing these feeds is crucial for the breastfeeding mother who will be providing breastmilk to be used with the thickening substance.[27,28] (I, III)

D. Preventive measures to protect a milk supply:

1. If the infant is unable to successfully and fully breastfeed, or if the mother is separated from her infant (e.g., NICU admission), lactation should be initiated and/or maintained through milk expression by hand or pump. Mothers should be encouraged to express milk shortly after the birth, ideally within the first hour,[29] (I) and approximately every 3 hours thereafter. Older recommendations suggested expressing within the first 6 hours of birth.[30] (II-3) The mother should aim to remove milk at least eight times in a 24 hour period, mimicking the stimulation of a vigorous term breastfeeding infant. Even if the infant shows some ability to go to breast, latch, and transfer milk, the mother will benefit from expressing extra milk in the early weeks to build and maintain her milk supply.

2. Most of the research on initiating and maintaining milk supply by expressing milk has been conducted on mothers of preterm infants. The strongest determinant of duration and exclusivity of breastfeeding the preterm infant is the volume of milk produced by the pump-dependent mother, whereas insufficient milk production is the most common reason for cessation of efforts to provide milk for these infants.[30–32] (II-3, II-3)

As milk transfer begins to improve with the infant developing sucking rhythms, and showing feeding cues, expressing can be tailored to these signs (i.e., breast emptying by expression after each attempt at breast). This pattern should continue until the dyad is reunited and/or the infant is able to sustain full breastfeeding. It is critical that mothers be instructed on effective milk removal, including expressing with the use of a hospital-grade electric pump, if available, and hand expression. Combining mechanical pumping and hand expression can increase both milk volume[33] (III) and the caloric content.[34] (I)

3. Extrapolating from preterm research for guidance in feeding the hypotonic infant, breastmilk production of 500 mL/day is commonly cited as the minimum volume enabling premature infants of less than 1,500 g to transition from tube or bottle feeding to successful, exclusive breastfeeding.[35] (III) Until studies are done in infants with hypotonia, this is a minimum volume from which mothers can start to reduce any supplementation and can be adjusted based on calculations of intake necessary for growth.

4. When an electric breast pump is used, simultaneous expression of both breasts with a hospital-grade pump is more effective than single breast expression. Hand expression while pumping improves expressed milk volume and milk caloric content in pump-dependent women. Thus, in contrast to the usual practice of passively depending on the pump to remove milk from the breast, hand expression, massage, and compression, used in conjunction with mechanical expression, enable mothers to enhance breast emptying.[33,36,37] (II-2, I)

5. Mothers should consider keeping an accurate expressing/feeding log to enable her and her healthcare providers to track milk supply and intervene if there is concern about milk volume.[38] (III)

E. At discharge and in the neonatal period:

1. If the infant remains hospitalized, the mother's milk supply should be assessed daily. That assessment should include time at the breast, expression frequency, 24 hour milk total by expression, and any signs of breast discomfort. The infant's weight gain should be carefully monitored and supplementation considered as necessary.

2. Monitor the length of breastfeeds (e.g., limit to1 hour) to ensure the infant is not becoming overtired from feeding.

3. Inform mothers that sucking efficiency frequently continues to improve over the first year, so that the breastfeeding experience may "normalize" and expressing, supplementation, diary keeping, and other interventions may no longer be necessary.

4. If breastfeeding does not continue to improve, assess the infant for other causes of breastfeeding difficulties (e.g., ankyloglossia).

5. Provide information about local support groups for breastfeeding and for specific diagnoses such as Trisomy 21. Because of the additional patience and time that are sometimes required to breastfeed these infants, support and encouragement are particularly important for mothers and families.

6. If maternal milk supply does not equal or exceed the infant's needs, or begins to slow despite optimal breastfeeding and/or expressing, the use of galactogogues to enhance maternal milk supply may be considered. See Academy of Breastfeeding Medicine Protocol #9 (Use of Galactogogues in Initiating or Augmenting Maternal Milk Supply).[39] (III) Supplementation with pasteurized donor milk is an option if supplementation becomes necessary and donor milk is available.[26]

FURTHER RESEARCH

This protocol was developed for the Academy of Breastfeeding Medicine to give clinicians guidance based on the expert opinion of practitioners who have worked extensively with infants with hypotonia. It is also one of only a handful addressing breastfeeding and children with special needs. Although this population especially has need of evidence-based breastfeeding practices, there is little scientific evidence upon which to base recommendations. Little new research exists for this revision and we continue to extrapolate best practice from other vulnerable patient populations. Specific areas recommended for further research include the following:

1. Research into best practices for breastfeeding infants with special needs is scarce and needs to become a priority. These mothers and children stand to gain much from a successful breastfeeding experience and we require better information on how to support the family in that effort.

2. Methods of optimizing the hypotonic infant's suck and milk transfer require further study.

3. Use of pacifiers in premature infants as "practice" oral feeding during gavage feeds has assisted with the transition to breast in preterm infants, and merits evaluation in hypotonic infants when needed.[40]

4. Accurate means to evaluate normal growth in breastfed versus formula-fed hypotonic infants, especially those with Trisomy 21, once breastfeeding has been established, should be developed.

5. Evidence of the efficacy of different methods available to supplement hypotonic infants (cup, bottle, and spoon) to help determine best practice should be explored.

6. Information on how modifiable factors such as positioning, labor analgesia/anesthesia, skin-to-skin contact, and counseling in the perinatal period may compound or ameliorate the difficulties with breastfeeding in these infants should be available to assist in developing best practice standards.

7. Research into the risk of aspiration while breastfeeding compared with bottle feeding breastmilk (thickened or not) or formula in this population should be conducted, as this is a common concern for the hypotonic infant and may lead to premature and possibly preventable cessation of breastfeeding.

REFERENCES

1. Bodensteiner JB. The evaluation of the hypotonic infant. *Semin Pediatr Neurol.* 2008;15:10–20.

2. Aumonier ME, Cunningham CC. Breast feeding in infants with Down's syndrome. *Child Care Health Dev.* 1983;9:247–255.

3. Lau C. Development of infant oral feeding skills. What do we know? *Am J Clin Nutr.* 2016;103:616S–621S.

4. World Health Organization. *Global Strategy for Infant and Young Child Feeding.* Geneva, Switzerland: WHO; 2003.

5. Section on Breastfeeding. Breastfeeding and the use of human milk. *Pediatrics.* 2012;129:e827–e841.

6. Victora CG, Bahl R, Barros AJD, et al. Breastfeeding in the 21st century: Epidemiology, mechanisms, and lifelong effect. *Lancet.* 2016;387:475–490.

7. Bowatte G, Tham R, Allen KJ, et al. Breastfeeding and childhood acute otitis media: A systematic review and meta-analysis. *Acta Paediatr.* 2015;104:85–95.

8. Peres KG, Cascaes AM, Nascimento GG, et al. Effect of breastfeeding on malocclusions: A systematic review and meta-analysis. *Acta Paediatr.* 2015;104:54–61.

9. Horta BL, Loret de Mola C, Victora CG. Breastfeeding and intelligence: A systematic review and meta-analysis. *Acta Paediatr.* 2015;104:14–19.

10. Vohr BR, Wright LL, Dusick AM, et al. Beneficial effect of breast milk in the neonatal intensive care unit on the development outcomes of extremely low birth weight infants at 18 months of age. *Pediatrics.* 2006;118:e115–e123.

11. Marino BL, O'Brien P, LoRe H. Oxygen saturations during breast and bottle feedings in infants with congenital heart disease. *J Pediatr Nurs.* 1995;10:360–364.

12. Mizuno K, Ueda A. Development of sucking behavior in infants with Down's syndrome. *Acta Paediatr.* 2001;90:1384–1388.

13. Guide to Clinical Preventive Services. *Report of the U.S. Preventive Services Task Force. US Preventive Services Task Force.* 2nd edition Washington, DC: US Department of Health and Human Services; 1996. Available from: www.ncbi.nlm.nih.gov/books/NBK15430/ (accessed January 4, 2016).

14. Skotko B. Mothers of children with Down Syndrome reflect on their postnatal support. *Pediatrics.* 2005;115:64–77.

15. Taveras EM, Capra AM, Braveman PA, et al. Clinician support and psychosocial risk factors associated with breastfeeding discontinuation. *Pediatrics.* 2003;112:108–115.

16. Taveras EM, Li R, Grummer-Strawn L, et al. Opinions and practices of clinicians associated with continuation of exclusive breastfeeding. *Pediatrics.* 2004;113:e283–e290.

17. ACOG. Optimizing support for breastfeeding as part of obstetric practice. 2016 Available at: www.acog.org/Resources-And-Publications/Committee-Opinions/Committeeon-Obstetric-Practice/Optimizing-Support-for-Breastfeedingas-Part-of-Obstetric-Practice (accessed March 13, 2016).

18. Hung KJ, Berg O. Early skin-to-skin after cesarean to improve breastfeeding. *MCN Am J Matern Child Nurs.* 2011;36:318–324.

19. Hurst NM, Valentine CJ, Renfro L, et al. Skin-to-skin holding in the neonatal intensive care unit influences maternal milk volume. *J Perinatol.* 1997;17:213–217.

20. Danner SC. Breastfeeding the neurologically impaired infant. *NAACOGS Clin Issu Perinat Womens Health Nurs.* 1992;3:640–646.

21. McBride MC, Danner SC. Sucking disorders in neurologically impaired infants: Assessment and facilitation of breastfeeding. *Clin Perinatol.* 1987;14:109–130.

22. Meier PP, Brown LP, Hurst NM, et al. Nipple shields for preterm infants: Effect on milk transfer and duration of breastfeeding. *J Hum Lact.* 2000;16:106–114.

23. Academy of Breastfeeding Medicine. ABM clinical protocol #10: Breastfeeding the late preterm infant (340/7 to 366/7 Weeks Gestation) (First Revision June 2011). *Breastfeed Med.* 2011;6:151–156.

24. Zemel B, Pipan M, Stallings V, et al. Growth charts for children with Down Syndrome in the United States. *Pediatrics* 136:e1204–e1211.

25. Marinelli KA, Burke GS, Dodd VL. A comparison of the safety of cupfeedings and bottlefeedings in premature infants whose mothers intend to breastfeed. *J Perinatol.* 2001;212:350–355.

26. Academy of Breastfeeding Medicine Protocol Committee. ABM Clinical Protocol #3: Hospital guidelines for the use of supplementary feedings in the healthy term breastfed neonate, Revised 2009. *Breastfeed Med.* 2009;4:175–182.

27. Gosa M, Schooling T, Coleman J. Thickened liquids as a treatment for children with dysphagia and associated adverse effects: A systematic review. *ICAN.* 2011;3:344–350.

28. Tutor JD, Gosa MM. Dysphagia and aspiration in children. *Pediatr Pulmonol.* 2011;47:321–337.

29. Parker LA, Sullivan S, Krueger C, et al. Effect of early milk expression on milk volume and timing of lactogenesis stage II among mothers of very low birthweight infants: A pilot study. *J Perinatol.* 2012;32:205–209.

30. Furman L, Minich N, Hack M. Correlates of lactation in mothers of very low birth weight infants. *Pediatrics.* 2002;109:e57.

31. Sisk PM, Lovelady CA, Dillard RG, et al. Lactation counselling for mothers of very low birth weight infants: Effect on maternal anxiety and infant intake of human milk. *Pediatrics.* 2006;117:e67–e75.

32. Killersreiter B, Grimmer I, Bührer C, et al. Early cessation of breast milk feeding in very low birthweight infants. *Early Hum Dev.* 2001;60:193–205.

33. Morton J, Hall JY, Wong RJ, et al. Combining hand techniques with electric pumping increases milk production in mothers of preterm infants. *J Perinatol.* 2009;29:757–764.

34. Flaherman VJ, Gay B, Scott C, et al. Randomised trial comparing hand expression with breast pumping for mothers of term newborns feeding poorly. *Arch Dis Child.* 2012;97: F18–F23.

35. Meier PP. Supporting lactation in mothers with very low birth weight infants. *Pediatr Ann.* 2003;32:317–325.

36. Morton J, Wong RJ, Hall JY, et al. Combining hand techniques with electric pumping increases the caloric content of milk in mothers with preterm infants. *J Perinatol.* 2012;32:791–796.

37. Jones E, Dimmock PW, Spencer SA. A randomised controlled trial to compare methods of milk expression after preterm delivery. *Arch Dis Child.* 2001;85:F91–F95.

38. Meier PP, Engstrom JL. Evidence-based practices to promote exclusive feeding of human milk in very low-birthweight infants. *Neuroreviews.* 2007;8:e467–e477.

39. Academy of Breastfeeding Medicine Protocol Committee. ABM Clinical Protocol #9: Use of galactogogues in initiating or augmenting the rate of maternal milk secretion (First revision January 2011). *Breastfeed Med.* 2011;6:41–46.

40. McCain GC, Gartside PS, Greenberg JM, et al. A feeding protocol for healthy preterm infants that shortens time to oral feeding. *J Pediatr.* 2001;139:374–379.

ABM protocols expire 5 years from the date of publication. Content of this protocol is up-to-date at the time of publication. Evidence-based revisions are made within 5 years or sooner if there are significant changes in the evidence.

The first version of this protocol was authored by Jennifer Thomas, Kathleen Marinelli, and Margaret Hennessy. The Academy of Breastfeeding Medicine Protocol Committee
Wendy Brodribb, MBBS, PhD, FABM, Chairperson
Larry Noble, MD, FABM, Translations Chairperson
Nancy Brent, MD
Maya Bunik, MD, MSPH, FABM
Cadey Harrel, MD
Ruth A. Lawrence, MD, FABM
Kathleen A. Marinelli, MD, FABM
Kate Naylor, MBBS, FRACGP
Sarah Reece-Stremtan, MD
Casey Rosen-Carole, MD, MPH
Tomoko Seo, MD, FABM
Rose St. Fleur, MD
Michal Young, MD
For correspondence: abm@bfmed.org

ABM Clinical Protocol #17
Guidelines for Breastfeeding Infants with Cleft Lip, Cleft Palate, or Cleft Lip and Palate—Revised 2019*

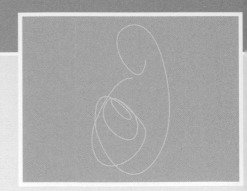

Jessica O. Boyce[1,2,†], Sheena Reilly[2,3,†], Jemma Skeat[1], Petrea Cahir[4] and the Academy of Breastfeeding Medicine

ABSTRACT

A central goal of the Academy of Breastfeeding Medicine is the development of clinical protocols for managing common medical problems that may impact breastfeeding success. These protocols serve only as guidelines for the care of breastfeeding mothers and infants and do not delineate an exclusive course of treatment or serve as standards of medical care. Variations in treatment may be appropriate according to the needs of an individual patient.

BACKGROUND

WHEN A CLEFT LIP (CL) occurs, the lip is not contiguous, and when a cleft palate (CP) occurs, there is communication between the oral and nasal cavities (see Fig. 1 for a completely formed lip and palate).[1] CL may involve the lip only; lip and alveolus; or lip, alveolus, and a notch in the hard palate. The notch in the hard palate may extend all the way to the incisive foramen (Fig. 2).[2] Similarly, a CP may involve only the uvula (e.g., bifid uvula), the uvula and soft palate, or extend through both the hard and soft palates (Fig. 3).[1] In a complete cleft of hard and soft palates, there is no bone or muscle separating the oral and nasal cavities. A CP may be submucosal and not immediately detected intraorally if there are subtle or no corresponding clinical signs or symptoms.[1] Therefore, it is essential that health professionals check for palatal clefting (both overt and submucosal) on initial presentation, by visually inspecting and palpating the palate. This should be done using a tongue depressor and flashlight to allow for inspection of the entire palate, including the uvula. An oral examination is of relevance if an infant is presenting with feeding difficulties or not gaining weight.

Surgical cleft repairs can involve multiple procedures, depending on the nature and extension of the cleft (i.e., unilateral CL versus bilateral cleft lip and palate [CLP]). The primary repair(s) are generally completed within 18 months of life, with the lip being repaired before the palate at 3—9 months of age.[3,4]

Incidence

The worldwide prevalence of CL and/or CP (CL/P) ranges from 0.8 to 2.7 cases per 1,000 live births.[5,6] There are differences in incidence rates across racial groups and geographical locations, with the lowest reported incidence among populations of African ($\sim 0.5/1,000$)[6—8] and European descent ($\sim 1/1,000$ births)[5] and higher incidence among Native American ($\sim 3.5/1,000$) and Asian ($\sim 1.7/1,000$) populations.[6,7]

Although reports vary considerably, it is estimated that out of the total number of infants with CL/P, $\sim 50\%$ have combined cleft lip and palate (CLP) (Fig. 4), 30% have isolated CP, and 20% have isolated CL; CL extending to include the alveolus occurs in $\sim 5\%$ of cases.[9] Clefts are more commonly unilateral, but can also occur bilaterally.[10] Approximately 30% of cases are part of identified syndromes or multiple congenital anomaly disorders, such as 22q11 deletion syndrome, Van der Woude syndrome, or Pierre Robin sequence.[6,7] The remaining 70% are nonsyndromic and occur in isolation of identified syndromes.[6,7]

Breastfeeding and CL/P

In these guidelines, *breastfeeding* refers to direct placement of the infant to the breast for feeding, and *breast milk feeding* refers to delivery of breast milk to the infant through bottle, cup, spoon, or any other means except the breast. Babies use suction to breastfeed successfully. The ability to generate suction is necessary for attachment to the breast, maintenance of a stable feeding position, and, together with the let-down reflex, milk extraction. Normally, when babies are feeding,

---

* Courtesy of the Academy of Breastfeeding Medicine. Please go to https://www.bfmed.org/protocols for complete protocols, translations, and the most up-to-date information (protocols are updated every 5—7 years).

[1] Department of Audiology and Speech Pathology, The University of Melbourne, Melbourne, Australia.

[2] Speech and Language Group, Murdoch Children's Research Institute, Melbourne, Australia.

[3] Menzies Health Institute Queensland, Griffith University, Southport, Australia.

[4] Intergenerational Health, Murdoch Children's Research Institute, Parkville, Victoria, Australia.

[†] Joint first authors.

their lips flange firmly against the areola, sealing the oral cavity anteriorly. The soft palate rises up to contact the pharyngeal walls and seal the oral cavity posteriorly. As the tongue and jaw drop during sucking, the oral cavity increases in size, and negative pressure is generated, drawing milk from the breast.[11] Suction and wave-like movement of the tongue help milk transfer and delivery during breastfeeding.[11–13]

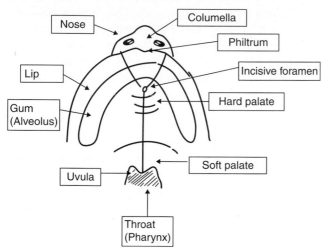

Fig. 1 Completely formed lip and palate (no cleft). This illustration shows an intact inferior view of the nose, upper lip, and hard and soft palates. Note the y-shaped suture lines where the lip, alveolus, and palate fused during gestation. During gestation, the suture lines fuse from the incisive foramen toward the philtrum area of the lip (just below the nose) and from the incisive foramen toward the uvula. A cleft of the lip and/or palate occurs when this fusion is incomplete or does not occur. (Illustration courtesy of Aiden Farrow, copyright 2018).

There is a relationship between the size and type of cleft, maturity of the infant, and amount of oral pressure generated during feeding.[13] Younger infants with larger clefts can be expected to generate less oral pressure. Most infants with isolated CL are often able to successfully breastfeed because they can generate suction and negative pressure. This is achieved when the nipple is compressed between the tongue and maxilla leading to milk being expelled into the oral cavity.[14] Some infants with small soft palate clefts can generate adequate negative pressure, but others with larger soft and/or hard palate clefts may not.[15,16] In addition, term and preterm newborns may generate lower suction pressure than older infants.[17,18] In general, infants with CP or CLP have difficulty creating suction and negative pressure because the oral cavity cannot be adequately separated from the nasal cavity during feeding.[19,20] For these infants, negative consequences may include fatigue during breastfeeding, prolonged feeding times, nasal regurgitation, reflux, insufficient milk transfer, and impaired growth and nutrition.[21,22]

The literature describing breastfeeding outcomes in infants with CL/P is limited. Available evidence is anecdotal and sometimes contradictory, making it challenging to develop appropriate recommendations.[23] Recommendations are outlined below, and answers to frequently asked questions are detailed in Appendix A1.

RECOMMENDATIONS

Quality of evidence for each recommendation is noted in parentheses. Levels of evidence are listed as 1-5, with level 1 being the highest, as defined in the Oxford Centre for Evidence-Based Medicine 2011 Levels of Evidence.[24]

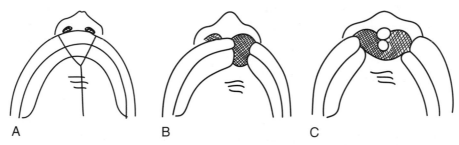

Fig. 2 Clefts of the lip. This figure illustrates **(A)** completely formed lip and palate (no cleft), **(B)** unilateral CL and **(C)** bilateral CL. The CLs in **(B)** and **(C)** involve the lip, alveolus, and a small notch in the hard palate. (Illustration courtesy of Aiden Farrow, copyright 2018). CL, cleft lip.

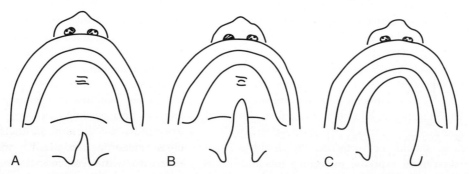

Fig. 3 Clefts of the palate. This figure illustrates three presentations of a CP. **(A)** cleft of the soft palate, **(B)** cleft of the hard and soft palate, and **(C)** a wide U-shaped cleft, typical of PRS. (Illustration courtesy of Aiden Farrow, copyright 2018). CP, cleft palate; PRS, Pierre Robin sequence.

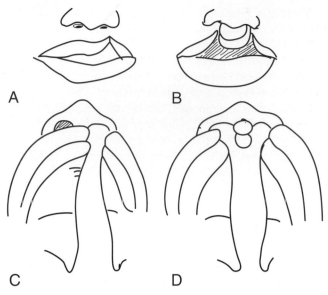

Fig. 4 Unilateral and bilateral CLP. This illustration shows **(A)** unilateral CL (*left*), **(C)** accompanying **(A)** unilateral CP (*left*), **(B)** bilateral complete cleft of the lip and gum with the columella present, and **(D)** accompanying **(B)** complete cleft of the palate. (Illustration courtesy of Aiden Farrow, copyright 2018). CLP, cleft lip and palate.

Recommendations for clinical practice

Based on the reviewed evidence, the following recommendations are made:

A. Encourage parents to breastfeed and provide breast milk when possible

1. Parents should be educated about the protective benefits of breast milk. Evidence suggests that breastfeeding protects against acute otitis media, which is highly prevalent in this population[25–27] (level 2). Breast milk feeding has also been shown to have long-term health and developmental benefits above that of artificial breast milk substitutes for both infants and their breastfeeding parents.[28–30] Breast milk feeding (through cup, spoon, bottle, syringe, etc.) should be promoted in preference to artificial breast milk substitutes if breastfeeding is not possible.[21] Bottles that facilitate milk flow may be necessary for short- or long-term use if compensatory techniques are not sufficient for growth. These bottles may have specially designed teats, be squeezable, or use one-way valves to control milk flow. There are various brands available. Parents should be provided with anticipatory guidance regarding effective techniques for milk expression, alongside the quantity of milk needed and storage methods.[31,32]

2. Parents of infants with CL/P should be advised of expected feeding outcomes based on the infant's cleft type and what has been documented in the available literature.[31,33] This guidance should be provided during the antenatal and postnatal periods.[34] Consistent and expert counseling should be provided by health professionals with clinical expertise in feeding infants with CL/P[31,33–35] (levels 4 and 5).

3. There is moderate evidence to suggest that infants with CL may be able to generate sufficient suction[19]

(level 4), and descriptive reports suggest that these infants are often able to breastfeed successfully[36–38] (levels 4–5). There is moderate evidence that infants with CP or CLP have difficulty generating sufficient intraoral suction[15] (level 2) and may have inefficient sucking patterns[16] (level 3) compared with noncleft infants. Overall, infants with CP or CLP are observed to have lower success rates for breastfeeding than infants with CL or no cleft. This applies even after surgical repair[39] (level 3). Nonetheless, breastfeeding attempts may still be beneficial for maintaining milk supply if a mother is also expressing breast milk.[15,16] Breastfeeding may also provide comfort and bonding opportunities for infants and mothers, while allowing infants to experience feeding from the breast.[40,41]

4. Evidence suggests that breastfeeding can commence/recommence immediately after CL repair[3,4,42] (levels 2–3). Breastfeeding can commence/recommence 1 day after CP repair without complication to the wound.[4] In a survey of surgeons regarding postoperative care after palatoplasty, two-thirds of surgeons allowed mothers to breastfeed immediately after surgery[43] (level 4). However, as cleft repairs do not occur immediately after birth, infants may require additional support to be taught how to breastfeed with their newly repaired clefts. Therefore, parents should be counseled that alternative means of feeding may still be required postsurgically to meet growth and nutritional goals.[35] Personal and social supports are also important during this time.[31,32]

B. Provide timely assessment and support

1. Parental education and supports should be provided in a timely manner. Surveys have indicated that parents of a child with CL, CLP, or CP desire more instruction on feeding challenges as early as possible; this commences in the antenatal period and should be ongoing[32] (level 4). Involving partners and other caregivers in the feeding process is also recommended.[31]

2. Several studies have suggested that there are benefits from having access to a health professional who specializes in CL/P and breastfeeding, such as a clinical nurse specialist or lactation specialist (including International Board Certified Lactation Consultants [IBCLC]), during the newborn and later periods. Specialists can determine the feasibility of breastfeeding and advise about managing milk supply and expressing for supplemental feeds. Early advice is key, as mothers may be encouraged to initiate milk expression within the first few hours of birth.[44] Specialists can also assist with suitable supportive techniques (outlined in the "Implement Strategies to Support Breastfeeding" section).[31,33,45] It is important to consider the size and location of the infant's cleft, breast anatomy, the parent's wishes, and previous experience with breastfeeding.

3. Families may benefit from peer support around breastfeeding or breast milk feeding found through local support groups and associations, such as Wide

Smiles,[46] in addition to routine referral to breastfeeding support groups.

4. An infant's hydration and weight gain should be monitored while a feeding method is being established. If breast milk feeding alone is inadequate, supplemental feeding should be implemented or increased if indicated (see "ABM clinical protocol #3: Hospital guidelines for the use of supplementary feedings in the healthy term breastfed neonate, revised 2017"[47]). Infants with CL/P may require supplemental feeds for adequate growth and nutrition[20,38] (level 4). Evidence from a single study demonstrated that additional maternal support by a clinical nurse specialist can both improve weight gain and facilitate early referral to appropriate services[48] (level 4).

5. When CL/P occurs as part of a syndrome/sequence, the potential for breastfeeding should be assessed on a case-by-case basis, taking into account any additional features of the syndrome that may impact breastfeeding success.

6. If a palatal prosthesis is used for orthopedic alignment before surgery, caution should be taken in advising parents to use such a device to facilitate breastfeeding. Rather, parents should be informed that the device likely will not significantly increase breastfeeding efficiency or effectiveness (levels 1–4).[49,50]

C. Implement strategies to support breastfeeding

1. Modified breastfeeding positions may increase the efficiency and effectiveness of breastfeeding. There are many recommendations about physical positioning of the infant to support breastfeeding. However, they are supported by weak evidence (clinical experience or expert opinion). Specific recommendations that require future evaluation include:

- For infants with CL.
  - The infant should be held so that the CL is oriented toward the top of the breast[50,51] (level 4). For example, an infant with a right CL may feed more efficiently in a crosscradle position at the right breast and a "football/twin style" position (i.e., the body of the infant positioned alongside the mother, rather than across the mother's lap, with the infant's shoulders higher than his or her body) at the left breast (Fig. 5).
  - For bilateral CL, a "face on" straddle position may be more effective than other breastfeeding positions[51] (level 4).
- For infants with CP or CLP.
  - Positioning should be semi-upright to reduce nasal regurgitation and flow of breast milk into the eustachian tubes (Fig. 6)[51–55] (level 4).
    - A "football/twin style" position may be more effective than a cross-cradle position[54,55] (level 4).

2. In addition to modifying positioning of the infant, parents can implement the following strategies. These strategies are supported by similarly weak evidence (clinical experience or expert opinion):

- For infants with CL.
  - The parent may occlude the CL with a thumb or finger[51,52] and/or support the infant's cheeks to decrease the width of the cleft and increase closure around the nipple[56] (level 4).

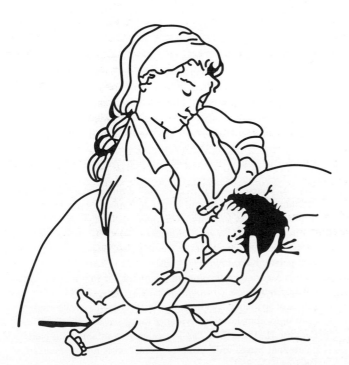

Fig. 5 "Football Hold" feeding position. This illustration shows the "Football Hold" breastfeeding position that may be used for infants with CL, CP, or CLP. (Illustration courtesy of Children's Minnesota Hospital).

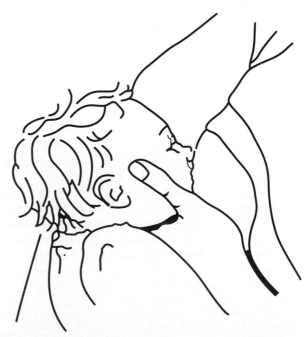

Fig. 6 Supporting the infant's chin during breastfeeding. This illustration demonstrates how a mother may use her free hand to support an infant's chin and/or breast to maintain a semi-upright position. This can help to stabilize the jaw during breastfeeding and ensure that the breast remains in the infant's mouth. (Illustration courtesy of Children's Minnesota Hospital).

- For infants with CP or CLP.
  - For infants with CP, it may be useful to position the breast toward the "greater segment" of the palate. That is, the side of the palate that has the most intact bone. This may facilitate better generation of negative pressure and thus milk extraction, while preventing the nipple from being pushed into the cleft site[57] (level 4).
  - If the cleft is large, some experts suggest that the breast be positioned downward to stop the nipple being pushed into the cleft[51] (level 4).
  - Some experts suggest supporting the infant's chin to stabilize the jaw during sucking[52] and/or supporting the breast so that it remains in the infant's mouth (Fig. 6)[56,58] (level 4).
  - Mothers may need to manually express breast milk into the baby's mouth to compensate for absent suction and compression and to stimulate the let-down reflex[15] (level 4).

Recommendations for future research

The most pressing issue for health care professionals working with parents who wish to breastfeed their infants with CL/P is the lack of evidence on which to base clinical recommendations. Well-designed data-driven investigations are imperative to generate high-level evidence and inform future guidelines. Future research is needed, covering the areas of feeding rates, management strategies, economic outcomes for breastfeeding infants with clefts, and health and developmental outcomes for infants with CL/P (e.g., communication, parent satisfaction, and rates of upper respiratory tract infections). Furthermore, investigators must clearly describe their sample of infants and intervention techniques so that the research outcomes can be generalized. Differentiation between cleft types and sizes is particularly important in this cohort.

ACKNOWLEDGMENTS

We thank international reviewers, Dr. Sandra Massry, Dr. Makiko Ohyama, and Aiden Farrow, BSc, Cert PPH, IBCLC, for their valuable input toward the revision of this protocol. We extend our gratitude to Aiden Farrow and Children's Minnesota Hospital for permission to use their illustrations.

REFERENCES

1. Allori AC, Mulliken JB, Meara JG, et al. Classification of cleft lip/palate: Then and now. *Cleft Palate Craniofac J.* 2017;54:175–188.
2. Fogh-Andersen P. *Inheritance of Harelip and Cleft Palate: Contribution to the Elucidation of the Etiology of the Congenital Clefts of the Face.* Copenhagen: Munksgaard; 1942.
3. de Ladeira PR, Alonso N. Protocols in cleft lip and palate treatment: Systematic review. *Plast Surg Int.* 2012;2012:1–9.
4. Bessell A, Hooper L, Shaw WC, et al. Feeding interventions for growth and development in infants with cleft lip, cleft palate or cleft lip and palate. *Cochrane Database Syst Rev.* 2011; CD003315.
5. Conway H, Wagner KJ. Incidence of clefts in New York City. *Cleft Palate Craniofac J.* 1996;33:284–290.
6. WHO. *Global Registry and Database on Craniofacial Anomalies: Report of a WHO Registry Meeting on Craniofacial Anomalies.* Baru, Brazil: World Health Organization, Programme HG; 2001.
7. IPDTOC Working Group. Prevalence at birth of cleft lip with or without cleft palate: Data from the International Perinatal Database of Typical Oral Clefts (IPDTOC). *Cleft Palate Craniofac J.* 2011;48:66–81.
8. Croen LA, Shaw GM, Wasserman CR, et al. Racial and ethnic variations in the prevalence of orofacial clefts in California, 1983–1992. *Am J Med Genet.* 1998;79:42–47.
9. Mulliken JB. Repair of bilateral complete cleft lip and nasal deformity—State of the art. *Cleft Palate Craniofac J.* 2000;37:342–347.
10. Mossey PA, Modell B. Epidemiology of oral clefts 2012: An international perspective. *Front Oral Biol.* 2012;16:1–18.
11. Brake SC, Fifer WP, Alfasi G, et al. The first nutritive sucking responses of premature newborns. *Infant Behav Dev.* 1988;11:1–19.
12. Weber F, Woolridge MW, Baum JD. An ultrasonographic study of the organisation of sucking and swallowing by newborn infants. *Dev Med Child Neurol.* 1986;28:19–24.
13. Reid J. *Feeding Babies with Cleft Lip and/or Palate: An Overrated Problem or a Neglected Aspect of Care?* Melbourne: La Trobe University; 2004.
14. Reid J, Reilly S, Kilpatrick N. Sucking performance of babies with cleft conditions. *Cleft Palate Craniofac J.* 2007;44:312–320.
15. Masarei AG, Sell D, Habel A, et al. The nature of feeding in infants with unrepaired cleft lip and/or palate compared with healthy noncleft infants. *Cleft Palate Craniofac J.* 2007;44:321–328.
16. Mizuno K, Ueda A, Kani K, et al. Feeding behaviour of infants with cleft lip and palate. *Acta Paediatr.* 2002;91:1227–1232.
17. Mizuno K, Ueda A. Development of sucking behavior in infants who have not been fed for 2 months after birth. *Pediatr Int.* 2001;43:251–255.
18. Choi BH, Kleinheinz J, Joos U, et al. Sucking efficiency of early orthopaedic plate and teats in infants with cleft lip and palate. *Int J Oral Maxillofac Surg.* 1991;20:167–169.
19. Smedegaard L, Marxen D, Moes J, et al. Hospitalization, breast-milk feeding, and growth in infants with cleft palate and cleft lip and palate born in Denmark. *Cleft Palate Craniofac J.* 2008;45:628–632.
20. Abbott MA. Cleft lip and palate. *Pediatr Rev.* 2014;35:177–181.
21. Kaye A, Thaete K, Snell A, et al. Initial nutritional assessment of infants with cleft lip and/or palate: Interventions and return to birth weight. *Cleft Palate Craniofac J.* 2017;54:127–136.
22. Gottschlich MM, Mayes T, Allgeier C, et al. A retrospective study identifying breast milk feeding disparities in infants with cleft palate. *J Acad Nutr Diet.* 2018;11:2154–2161.
23. Reid J. A review of feeding interventions for infants with cleft palate. *Cleft Palate Craniofac J.* 2004;41:268–278.
24. Levels of Evidence. 2011. Available at: https://www.cebm.net/2016/05/ocebm-levels-of-evidence (accessed March 22, 2019).
25. Paradise JL, Elster BA, Tan L. Evidence in infants with cleft palate that breast milk protects against otitis media. *Pediatrics.* 1994;94:853–860.
26. Kuo CL, Tsao YH, Cheng HM, et al. Grommets for otitis media with effusion in children with cleft palate: A systematic review. *Pediatrics.* 2014;134:983–994.

27. Garcez LW, Giugliani ER. Population-based study on the practice of breastfeeding in children born with cleft lip and palate. *Cleft Palate Craniofac J.* 2005;42:687—693.

28. Victora CG, Bahl R, Barros AJD, et al. Breastfeeding in the 21st century: Epidemiology, mechanisms, and lifelong effect. *Lancet.* 2016;387:475—490.

29. Bernard JY, De Agostini M, Forhan A, et al. Breastfeeding duration and cognitive development at 2 and 3 years of age in the EDEN mother-child cohort. *J Pediatr.* 2013;163:36—42.

30. Kramer MS, Kakuma R. Optimal duration of exclusive breastfeeding. *Cochrane Database Syst Rev.* 2012;8:1—139.

31. Lindberg N, Berglund AL. Mothers' experiences of feeding babies born with cleft lip and palate. *Scand J Caring Sci.* 2014;28:66—73.

32. Owens J. Parents' experiences of feeding a baby with cleft lip and palate. *Br J Midwifery.* 2008;16:778—784.

33. Alperovich M, Frey JD, Shetye PR, et al. Breast milk feeding rates in patients with cleft lip and palate at a north American craniofacial center. *Cleft Palate Craniofac J.* 2017;54:334—337.

34. Kaye A, Cattaneo C, Huff HM, et al. A pilot study of mothers' breastfeeding experiences in infants with cleft lip and/or palate. *Adv Neonatal Care.* 2018;1—11.

35. McGuire E. Cleft lip and palates and breastfeeding. *Breastfeed Rev.* 2017;25:17—23.

36. Merrow JM. Feeding management in infants with craniofacial anomalies. *Facial Plast Surg Clin North Am.* 2016;24:437—444.

37. Goyal A, Jena AK, Kaur M. Nature of feeding practices among children with cleft lip and palate. *J Indian Soc Pedod Prev Dent.* 2012;30:47—50.

38. Gil-Da-Silva-Lopes VL, Xavier AC, Klein-Antunes D, et al. Feeding infants with cleft lip and/or palate in Brazil: Suggestions to improve health policy and research. *Cleft Palate Craniofac J.* 2013;50:577—590.

39. Burianova I, Kulihova K, Vitkova V, et al. Breastfeeding after early repair of cleft lip in newborns with cleft lip or cleft lip and palate in a baby-friendly designated hospital. *J Hum Lact.* 2017;33:504—508.

40. Dieterich CM, Felice JP, O'Sullivan E, et al. Breastfeeding and health outcomes for the mother-infant dyad. *Pediatr Clin North Am.* 2013;60:31—48.

41. Liu J, Leung P, Yang A. Breastfeeding and active bonding protects against children's internalizing behavior problems. *Nutrients.* 2013;6:76—89.

42. Lazarou S. Comparison of neonatal cleft lip repair to standard time repair done by same surgeon. *Cleft Palate Craniofac J.* 2016;53:e107.

43. Darzi MA, Chowdri NA, Bhat AN. Breast feeding or spoon feeding after cleft lip repair: A prospective, randomised study. *Br J Plast Surg.* 1996;49:24—26.

44. Burca ND, Gephart SM, Miller C. A nurse's guide to promoting breast milk nutrition in infants with cleft lip and/or palate. *Adv Neonatal Care.* 2016;16:345—346.

45. Chuacharoen R, Ritthagol W, Hunsrisakhun J, et al. Felt needs of parents who have a 0- to 3-month-old child with a cleft lip and palate. *Cleft Palate Craniofac J.* 2009;46:252—257.

46. Wide Smiles. Wide Smiles Website 2018. Available at: http://widesmiles.org; Last accessed 22 Mar 2019.

47. Kellams A, Harrel C, Omage S, et al. ABM clinical protocol #3: Supplementary feeding in healthy term breastfed neonate, revised 2017. *Breastfeed Med.* 2017;12:1—8.

48. Danner SC. Breastfeeding the infant with a cleft defect. *NAACOGS Clin Issu Perinat Womens Health Nurs.* 1992;3:634—639.

49. Prahl C, Kuijpers-Jagtman AM, Van 't Hof MA, et al. Infant orthopedics in UCLP: Effect on feeding, weight, and length: A randomized clinical trial (Dutchcleft). *Cleft Palate Craniofac J.* 2005;42:171—177.

50. Cohen M, Marschall MA, Schafer ME. Immediate unrestricted feeding of infants following cleft lip and palate repair. *J Craniofac Surg.* 1992;3:30—32.

51. Helsing E, King FS. Breastfeeding under special conditions. *Nurs J India.* 1985;76:46—47.

52. Bardach J, Morris HL. *Multidisciplinary Management of Cleft Lip and Palate.* Philadelphia: WB Saunders Co; 1990.

53. Dunning Y. Child nutrition. Feeding babies with cleft lip and palate. *Nurs Times.* 1986;82:46—47.

54. McKinstry RE. Presurgical management of cleft lip and palate patients. In: McKinstry RE, ed. *Cleft Palate Dentistry.* Arlington: ABI Professional Publications; 1998:33—66.

55. Burca ND, Gephart SM, Miller C, et al. Promoting breast milk nutrition in infants with cleft lip and/or palate. *Adv Neonatal Care.* 2016;16:337—344.

56. Arvedson JC. Feeding with craniofacial anomalies. In: Arvedson JC, Brodsky LB, eds. *Pediatric Swallowing and Feeding: Assessment and Management.* 2nd ed. Albany, NY: Singular Publishing Group; 2002:527—561.

57. Glass RP, Wolf LS. Feeding management of infants with cleft lip and palate and micrognathia. *Infants Young Child.* 1999;12:70—81.

58. Masarei AG. *An Investigation of the Effects of Pre-surgical Orthopaedics on Feeding in Infants with Cleft Lip and/or Palate.* London: University College; 2003.

Jessica O. Boyce, PhD, lead author
Sheena Reilly, PhD
Jemma Skeat, PhD
Petrea Cahir, M (Sp Path)
Protocol Committee Members 2019:
Michal Young, MD, FABM, Chairperson
Larry Noble, MD, FABM, Translations Chairperson
Sarah Reece-Stremtan, Secretary
Melissa Bartick, MD, FABM
Sarah Calhoun, MD
Sarah Dodd, MD
Megan Elliott-Rudder, MD
Laura Rachael Kair, MD, FABM
Susan Lappin, MD
Ilse Larson, MD
Ruth A. Lawrence, MD, FABM
Yvonne Lefort, MD, FABM
Kathleen A. Marinelli, MD, FABM
Nicole Marshall, MD, MCR
Katrina Mitchell, MD, FABM
C. Murak, MD
Eliza Myers, MD
Adora Okogbule-Wonodi, MD
Casey Rosen-Carole, MD, MPH, MSEd
Susan Rothenberg, MD, FABM
Tricia Schmidt, MD
Tomoko Seo, MD, FABM
Natasha Sriraman, MD
Elizabeth K. Stehel, MD
Rose St. Fleur, MD
Nancy Wight, MD
Lori Winter, MD
For correspondence: abm@bfmed.org

APPENDIX A1. FREQUENTLY ASKED QUESTIONS

Breastfeeding infants with cleft lip (CL), cleft palate (CP), or CL and CP (CLP)

Except where noted, the literature reviewed relates to infants with nonsyndromic CL/P.

1. Can infants with CL breastfeed successfully?

   There was no strong evidence with regard to breastfeeding infants with CL. There was moderate (levels 2−3) evidence that babies with CL can create suction during feeding.[A1,A2] Descriptive studies (level 4) have demonstrated successful breastfeeding at rates approaching the general population.[A3] Expert opinion (level 4) suggested that infants with CL may find breastfeeding relatively easy compared with bottle feeding because the breast tissue molds to the cleft and occludes the defect more successfully than an artificial nipple.[A4,A5] Expert opinion also suggested that modifications to positioning can facilitate breastfeeding for these infants.[A6−A8]

2. Can infants with CP breastfeed successfully?

   There was no strong evidence with regard to breastfeeding infants with CP. There was moderate (levels 2−3) evidence that infants with CP do not create adequate suction when bottle feeding.[A1,A2] Some infants with clefts of the soft palate only may be able to create suction, although this is not usually the case.[A1,A9] Descriptive studies and a systematic review indicated that breastfeeding success for infants with CP was much lower than for infants with CL.[A7,A10−A16] There was weak evidence (level 4) to suggest that partial breastfeeding (with supplementation) can be achieved and that the size and location of the cleft are determining factors for breastfeeding success.[A5,A17,A18] As with infants with CL, supportive and compensatory strategies are reported to increase breastfeeding success (level 4)[A6,A7,A17,A18]

3. Can infants with cleft lip and palate (CLP) breastfeed successfully?

   There was no strong evidence with regard to breastfeeding infants with CLP. There was moderate evidence that infants with CLP are unable to create suction when fed using a bottle[A1,A2,A9] (levels 2−3) and moderate to weak evidence that infants with CLP are sometimes able to breastfeed successfully.[A14] Descriptive studies suggested breastfeeding success rates ranging from 0% to 40%.[A3,A13,A19] Supportive and compensatory strategies recommended by experts may increase breastfeeding success[A6,A8,A17,A18,A20,A21] (level 4). There was weak evidence that suggests breastfeeding rates for infants with CLP decrease sharply after 6 months of age.[A20]

4. Is there evidence to guide assessment and management of breastfeeding in infants with CL/P?

   There is moderate evidence that lactation education is important to facilitate successful feeding in infants with CL/P[A4,A22−A25] (levels 3−4). This support should be provided by professionals with knowledge and expertise specific to feeding infants with CL/P. The remaining evidence is weak and focuses on (a) areas for monitoring, (b) recommendations for supplementation, (c) compensatory and supportive strategies, and (d) the importance of counseling to encourage breast milk feeding[A23] (level 4).

5. Is there evidence that palatal obturators facilitate breastfeeding success with infants with CLP or CP?

   Breastfeeding outcomes may be affected by the use of feeding plates (which obturate some of the cleft and attempt to "normalize" the oral cavity for feeding)[A26] or presurgical orthopedic devices (prostheses used to reposition the cleft segments before surgery). These are collectively referred to as "obturators" for this report. There was strong evidence that obturators do not facilitate feeding or weight gain in breastfed babies with CLP[A27] and that they do not improve the infant's ability to efficiently bottle feed[A6] (levels 1−2). There was moderate evidence that obturators do not facilitate suction during bottle feeding[A28] (level 3). This is because obturators do not enable complete closure of the soft palate against the walls of the throat during feeding. Contradictory evidence exists, supporting the use of obturators to facilitate breastfeeding in infants with CP or CLP, but it is from much weaker sources[A4,A21,A29] (levels 3−4).

6. Is there evidence for additional benefits of breastfeeding for infants with CL/P compared with the noncleft population?

   Several moderate to weak studies (levels 3−4) exist, with the majority of evidence representing expert opinion (level 4). It is well accepted that breastfeeding and breast milk feeding convey positive benefits to both mother and infant. With regard to infants with CP, there was moderate to weak evidence that feeding with breast milk protects against otitis media.[A4,A30] These infants are more prone to otitis media than the general population because of the abnormal soft palate musculature.[A30] There was moderate to weak evidence that breast milk can promote intellectual development and academic outcomes in individuals with clefts.[A31] In addition, experts have suggested that breastfeeding facilitates the development of oral facial musculature,[A21] speech,[A18,A21] bonding,[A18] and pacifying infants after surgery.[A4,A21]

7. Is there evidence to indicate when it is safe to commence/recommence breastfeeding after lip or palate surgery?

   CL repair (cheiloplasty) is generally carried out within a few months of birth, and CP repair (palatoplasty) often takes place between 6 and 12 months of age.[A32] There are several studies that have yielded strong evidence to inform this area. There was moderate to strong evidence (levels 2−3) that it is safe to commence/recommence breastfeeding immediately after CL repair[A33,A34] (levels 2−3), and there was moderate evidence for initiating breastfeeding 1 day after CP repair[A34] (level 3). There was strong evidence that breastfeeding immediately after surgery is more effective for weight gain than spoon feeding, with associated lower hospital costs[A34] (levels 1−2). Contradictory evidence exists, but it is from weaker sources and is divided as to recommendations[A8,A35] (level 4).

8. Is there evidence to indicate whether infants with CP as part of a syndrome/sequence can breastfeed?

There are > 340 syndromes in which CL/P appears. It is beyond the scope of this protocol to review and make recommendations for them all in detail. However, some key data are presented to guide breastfeeding practice. Moderate to weak evidence suggested that, as well as the cleft, additional oral facial anomalies associated with these syndromes (e.g., hypotonia, micrognathia, and glossoptosis) impact feeding success.[A13,A15,A17,A36] It is important to examine the influence of additional structural and functional anomalies on feeding and design individualized treatment accordingly.

APPENDIX REFERENCES

A1. Masarei AG, Sell D, Habel A, et al. The nature of feeding in infants with unrepaired cleft lip and/or palate compared with healthy noncleft infants. *Cleft Palate Craniofac J.* 2007;44:321–328.

A2. Smedegaard L, Marxen D, Moes J, et al. Hospitalization, breast-milk feeding, and growth in infants with cleft palate and cleft lip and palate born in Denmark. *Cleft Palate Craniofac J.* 2008;45:628–632.

A3. Garcez LW, Giugliani ER. Population-based study on the practice of breastfeeding in children born with cleft lip and palate. *Cleft Palate Craniofac J.* 2005;42:687–693.

A4. Paradise JL, Elster BA, Tan L. Evidence in infants with cleft palate that breast milk protects against otitis media. *Pediatrics.* 1994;94:853–860.

A5. Gopinath VK, Muda WA. Assessment of growth and feeding practices in children with cleft lip and palate. *Southeast Asian J Trop Med Public Health.* 2005;36:254–258.

A6. Cohen M, Marschall MA, Schafer ME. Immediate unrestricted feeding of infants following cleft lip and palate repair. *J Craniofac Surg.* 1992;3:30–32.

A7. Helsing E, King FS. Breastfeeding under special conditions. *Nurs J India.* 1985;76:46–47.

A8. Bardach J, Morris HL. *Multidisciplinary Management of Cleft Lip and Palate. Philadelphia: WB.* Saunders Co; 1990.

A9. Reid J, Reilly S, Kilpatrick N, eds. Breastmilk consumption in babies with clefts. In: 63rd Annual meeting of the American Cleft Palate-Craniofacial Association, Vancouver, 2006.

A10. Kaye A, Thaete K, Snell A, et al. Initial nutritional assessment of infants with cleft lip and/or palate: Interventions and return to birth weight. *Cleft Palate Craniofac J.* 2017;54:127–136.

A11. Gottschlich MM, Mayes T, Allgeier C, et al. A retrospective study identifying breast milk feeding disparities in infants with cleft palate. *J Acad Nutr Diet.* 2018;11:2154–2161.

A12. Gil-Da-Silva-Lopes VL, Xavier AC, Klein-Antunes D, et al. Feeding infants with cleft lip and/or palate in Brazil: Suggestions to improve health policy and research. *Cleft Palate Craniofac J.* 2013;50:577–590.

A13. Burianova I, Kulihova K, Vitkova V, et al. Breastfeeding after early repair of cleft lip in newborns with cleft lip or cleft lip and palate in a baby-friendly designated hospital. *J Hum Lact.* 2017;33:504–508.

A14. Chuacharoen R, Ritthagol W, Hunsrisakhun J, et al. Felt needs of parents who have a 0- to 3-month-old child with a cleft lip and palate. *Cleft Palate Craniofac J.* 2009;46:252–257.

A15. de Vries IA, Breugem CC, van der Heul AM, et al. Prevalence of feeding disorders in children with cleft palate only: A retrospective study. *Clin Oral Investig.* 2014;18:1507–1515.

A16. Galvao D, Lopes A, Martins C, et al. Breastfeeding children with cleft LIP and/or palate. *Atencion Primaria.* 2014;46 (Supplement 5):26.

A17. Dunning Y. Child nutrition. Feeding babies with cleft lip and palate. *Nurs Times.* 1986;82:46–47.

A18. McKinstry RE. Presurgical management of cleft lip and palate patients. In: McKinstry RE, ed. *Cleft Palate Dentistry.* Arlington: ABI Professional Publications; 1998:33–66.

A19. Aniansson G, Svensson H, Becker M, et al. Otitis media and feeding with breast milk of children with cleft palate. *Scand J Plast Reconstr Surg Hand Surg.* 2002;36:9–15.

A20. Goyal A, Jena AK, Kaur M. Nature of feeding practices among children with cleft lip and palate. *J Indian Soc Pedod Prev Dent.* 2012;30:47–50.

A21. Danner SC. Breastfeeding the infant with a cleft defect. *NAACOGS Clin Issu Perinat Womens Health Nurs.* 1992;3:634–639.

A22. Lindberg N, Berglund AL. Mothers' experiences of feeding babies born with cleft lip and palate. *Scand J Caring Sci.* 2014;28:66–73.

A23. Alperovich M, Frey JD, Shetye PR, et al. Breast milk feeding rates in patients with cleft lip and palate at a north american craniofacial center. *Cleft Palate Craniofac J.* 2017;54:334–337.

A24. Kaye A, Cattaneo C, Huff HM, et al. A pilot study of mothers' breastfeeding experiences in infants with cleft lip and/or palate. *Adv Neonatal Care.* 2018;1–11.

A25. McGuire E. Cleft lip and palates and breastfeeding. *Breastfeed Rev.* 2017;25:17–23.

A26. Masarei AG. *An Investigation of the Effects of Presurgical Orthopaedics on Feeding in Infants with Cleft Lip and/or Palate.* London: University College,; 2003.

A27. Prahl C, Kuijpers-Jagtman AM, Van 't Hof MA, et al. Infant orthopedics in UCLP: Effect on feeding, weight, and length: A randomized clinical trial (Dutchcleft). *Cleft Palate Craniofac J.* 2005;42:171–177.

A28. Choi BH, Kleinheinz J, Joos U, et al. Sucking efficiency of early orthopaedic plate and teats in infants with cleft lip and palate. *Int J Oral Maxillofac Surg.* 1991;20:167–169.

A29. Goyal M Chopra R, Bansal K, et al. Role of obturators and other feeding interventions in patients with cleft lip and palate: A review. *Eur Arch Paediatr Dent.* 2014;15:1–9.

A30. Erkkila AT, Isotalo E, Pulkkinen J, et al. Association between school performance, breast milk intake and fatty acid profile of serum lipids in ten-year-old cleft children. *J Craniofac Surg.* 2005;16:764–769.

A31. World Health Organization Health. Health factors which may interfere with breast-feeding. *Bull World Health Organ.* 1989;67(Suppl:):41–54.

A32. Abbott MA. Cleft lip and palate. *Pediatr Rev.* 2014;35:177–181.

A33. de Ladeira PR, Alonso N. Protocols in cleft lip and palate treatment: Systematic review. *Plast Surg Int.* 2012;2012:1–9.

A34. Bessell A, Hooper L, Shaw WC, et al. Feeding interventions for growth and development in infants with cleft lip, cleft palate or cleft lip and palate. *Cochrane Database Syst Rev.* 2011; Cd003315.

A35. Arvedson JC. Feeding with craniofacial anomalies. In: Arvedson JC, Brodsky LB, eds. *Pediatric Swallowing and Feeding: Assessment and Management.* 2nd ed. Albany, NY: Singular Publishing Group; 2002:527–561.

A36. Pandya AN, Boorman JG. Failure to thrive in babies with cleft lip and palate. *Br J Plast Surg.* 2001;54:471–475.

ABM Clinical Protocol #18
*Use of Antidepressants in Breastfeeding Mothers**

Natasha K. Sriraman[1], Kathryn Melvin[2], Samantha Meltzer-Brody[2,3] and the Academy of Breastfeeding Medicine

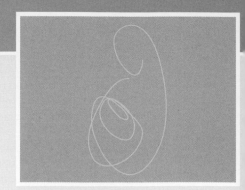

ABSTRACT

A central goal of The Academy of Breastfeeding Medicine is the development of clinical protocols for managing common medical problems that may impact breastfeeding success. These protocols serve only as guidelines for the care of breastfeeding mothers and infants and do not delineate an exclusive course of treatment or serve as standards of medical care. Variations in treatment may be appropriate according to the needs of an individual patient.

BACKGROUND

POSTPARTUM DEPRESSION (PPD) (sometimes referred to as pregnancy-related mood disorder) is one of the most common and serious postpartum conditions, affecting 10—20% of mothers within the first year of childbirth.[1] Studies have found that up to 50% of women with PPD are undiagnosed.[2] Risk factors include a prior history of depression (approximately 25—30% risk of recurrence),[3,4] including PPD, and depression during pregnancy. Other risk factors include recent stressful life events, lack of social support, unintended pregnancy,[5] and women who are economically stressed, disadvantaged, low income, or black.[6] Moreover, studies of economically disadvantaged families have shown that approximately 25% of women will have ongoing depressive symptoms that last well beyond the initial postpartum year.[7]

Treatment approaches include nonpharmacological therapies such as interpersonal psychotherapy or cognitive behavioral therapy, pharmacological therapies, or a combination of both. Antidepressant medications are one of the most commonly prescribed pharmacologic treatments of PPD. The mother and her provider should work together to make an individually tailored choice. Breastfeeding mothers may be concerned about continuing and/or starting medication for PPD. Some providers are reluctant to prescribe for lactating mothers due to lack of information about antidepressants and breastfeeding. The risks of untreated depression, the risks of the medication to the breastfeeding dyad, and the benefits of treatment must be fully considered when making treatment decisions.

This protocol will discuss the spectrum of disease, emphasize the importance of screening, and provide evidence-based information recommendations for treatment of PPD in breastfeeding mothers.

Spectrum of disease

There has been controversy about whether PPD is a distinct entity. In the *Diagnostic and Statistical Manual of Mental Disorders*, 4th and 5th editions (DSM-IV and V, respectively), PPD is considered a subtype of major depression, and there is an associated specifier to denote onset in the postpartum period.[8] The newer DSM-V expanded the definition of PPD to include onset of symptoms during pregnancy through 4 weeks postpartum.[9] Diagnosis may be further complicated by other comorbid conditions, including anxiety and bipolar disorder. Postpartum mood disorders are common in the postpartum period but differ according to timing and severity of symptoms and encompass a wide range of disorders.[2,8,10]

"Postpartum blues" is a condition characterized by emotional changes, insomnia, appetite loss, and feelings of being overwhelmed that can affect 30—80% of women.[7,8] It is a transient condition that usually peaks on postpartum Day 5 and resolves by Day 10. Unlike PPD, postpartum blues does not adversely affect infant care.

"Postpartum depression" is a major depressive episode that impairs social and occupational functioning. Symptoms cause significant distress and can include suicidal ideation. If untreated, symptoms may persist beyond 14 days and can last several months to a year.[1]

---

* Courtesy of the Academy of Breastfeeding Medicine. Please go to https://www.bfmed.org/protocols for complete protocols, translations, and the most up-to-date information (protocols are updated every 5—7 years).

[1] Department of Pediatrics, Children's Hospital of The King's Daughters/Eastern Virginia Medical School, Norfolk, Virginia.

[2] Department of Psychiatry, University of North Carolina Chapel Hill School of Medicine, Chapel Hill, North Carolina.

[3] Perinatal Psychiatry Program, University of North Carolina Chapel Hill Center for Women's Mood Disorders, Chapel Hill, North Carolina.

"Postpartum psychosis" is a psychiatric emergency and is characterized by paranoia, hallucinations, delusions, and suicidal ideation, with the potential risk of suicide and/or infanticide. It can occur in one to three of every 1,000 deliveries and usually has a rapid onset (within hours to a few weeks) after delivery.[7,8] Women with postpartum psychosis may have a prior history of postpartum psychosis or bipolar disorder, but in some women there is no prior psychiatric history.[11,12] Approximately 25–50% of women with bipolar disorder are at risk of developing postpartum psychosis.[13]

"Postpartum intrusive thoughts" and "obsessive compulsive disorder" commonly occur in women, but with a wide range of severity of symptoms they are concerns for postpartum women. Intrusive or obsessive thoughts are unwelcome and involuntary thoughts, images, or unpleasant ideas that may become obsessions. These thoughts are usually upsetting or distressing to the woman, and they can be difficult to manage or eliminate.[14,15]

Screening for PPD

Research confirms that most mothers (80%) are comfortable with the idea of being screened for depression.[1] Internationally, guidelines and authorities recommend screening for PPD.[16–18]

Although definitive evidence of benefit is limited, the American College of Obstetricians and Gynecologists recommends that clinicians screen patients at least once during the perinatal period for depression and anxiety symptoms using a standardized, validated tool.[19] For the first time, a large U.S. multicenter study of screening and follow-up care for PPD in a family practice setting has shown improved maternal outcomes at 12 months.[20] (I) (Quality of evidence [levels of evidence I, II-1, II-2, II-3, and III] is based on the U.S. Preventive Services Task Force Appendix A Task Force Ratings[21] and is noted throughout this protocol in parentheses.)

Most physicians and maternal/child healthcare providers recognize the detrimental effects of PPD and agree that screening new mothers is within the scope of their practice.[22,23] The American Academy of Pediatrics and the U.S. Surgeon General's Office recognize and call for the early identification and treatment of mental health disorders, including PPD.[24,25] It is important that screening for PPD be done systematically globally as detection and treatment have been shown to be beneficial in many countries.[26] (I)

Screening instruments

The screening instrument that has been most studied throughout the world is the Edinburgh Postnatal Depression Scale (EPDS).[7,27] The EPDS is free, considered to be in the public domain, and available in many languages and has cross-cultural validity. It has 10 questions to be completed by the mother based on symptoms over the past 7 days and takes approximately 5 minutes to complete.[27] There are multiple points of contact in which screening can occur. In well-childcare visits, EPDS screening could occur during the 1-, 2-, 4-, and 6-month visits.[7,16–18,28–30] The cesarean section incision check at 2 weeks and the postpartum visit at 4–8 weeks are also important screening opportunities. The EPDS can be readily administered and has demonstrated validity to detect postpartum mood disorders at as early as 4–8 weeks postpartum.[30,31] (II-3) Either a score of 10 or higher or a positive response to Question 10 about suicidal thoughts is considered positive and indicates that the mother may be suffering from a depressive illness of varying severity.[32] (II-3) Providers caring for the infant must refer a mother with a positive screen for appropriate care.

Effects of PPD

In addition to the obvious adverse effects on the mother, PPD affects the child, spouse and/or partner, and other family members. It can cause family dysfunction, prevent effective mother–baby bonding, lead to early cessation of breastfeeding, and adversely affect infant growth and brain development.[7,33–36] Rates of paternal depression are higher when the mother has PPD, which can compound the negative effects of depression on children. Infants of depressed mothers show less engagement and eye contact with their mother and are at risk for failure to thrive, attachment disorder, and development delay.[2]

A shared neuroendocrine mechanism among maternal mood, oxytocin levels, and maternal affect during breastfeeding has been demonstrated.[37] This strengthens the position that women with depression would benefit from early and sustained support with breastfeeding. Likewise, women with negative early breastfeeding experiences may be more likely to have depressive symptoms at 2 months postpartum; thus women experiencing breastfeeding difficulties should be screened for depressive symptoms.[33]

CLINICAL APPROACH TO TREATING PPD

Once a woman is identified as being at risk for PPD, treatment choices must be considered and offered to her. For mild to moderate depression in the breastfeeding mother, psychology/cognitive behavioral therapy, if available, should be considered as first-line therapy.[38] (II-2)

TREATMENT

Nonpharmacological
Psychological therapy

Psychological therapy is effective for the treatment of major depressive disorder in the postpartum period, and different types of therapy seem equally effective.[39–41] (I) There are three approaches to administration of psychological therapy in the postpartum period, including interpersonal therapy, cognitive behavioral therapy, and psychodynamic psychotherapy (nondirective therapy).[39–47] Nonpharmacological treatment is not harmful to the infant and is often acceptable to mothers with PPD.

Infant feeding considerations

Breastfeeding difficulties and perinatal depression symptoms often present together, and management of depression should include a discussion of the mother's experience of breastfeeding. Some mothers with depression find that breastfeeding enhances bonding and improves their mood, whereas others find breastfeeding to be difficult. For dyads struggling with milk production and latch issues, efforts should be undertaken to simplify feeding plans to ensure that mother and infant have time to enjoy one another. The demands of nighttime breastfeeding can be challenging for mothers for whom interruption of sleep is a major trigger for mood symptoms. In these cases, it may be helpful to arrange for another caregiver to feed the infant once at night, allowing the mother to receive 5—6 hours of uninterrupted sleep. A caregiver may also bring the infant to the mother to feed at the breast and then assume responsibility for settling the baby back to sleep, thereby minimizing maternal sleep disruption. (III)

Medications

If psychological/cognitive behavioral therapy is unavailable, symptoms are severe, or mothers refuse this therapy, antidepressants are an effective option. Many factors must be considered when choosing an antidepressant during breastfeeding. All antidepressants are present in human milk to some extent. Data to inform clinical decisions are derived primarily from case reports or case series. Therefore, the initial treatment choice should be based on an informed clinical approach that takes into account the patient's previous treatments for depression, especially use during the pregnancy, the targeted symptoms, family history of depression and their experiences with antidepressants, current and past medical disorders, current medications, allergies, side effects of the medications, and maternal wishes. An individualized risk—benefit analysis of the treatments must be conducted (Table 1).[48] (I)

CLINICAL FACTORS AFFECTING ANTIDEPRESSANT CHOICE

- Obtain a psychiatric history with a focus on previous episodes of mood and anxiety disorders and effective treatment interventions. If psychotropic medications were used, determine what treatments were effective with a tolerable side effect profile. Past treatment response is often the best predictor of future response.[48] (II-2)
- Obtain a family history of psychiatric illness and treatment response. An immediate family member's history may be indicative of the mother's treatment response.[48] (II-2)
- Consider the primary symptoms that the medication will be targeting and its potential side effect profile.
- Choose psychotropic medications with an evidence base in lactating women. Older medications with available data are preferred over newer antidepressants with limited safety information.

CHOOSING AN ANTIDEPRESSANT DURING LACTATION

When considering the use of any medication in a lactating woman, providers must consider both maternal and infant safety factors. The medication must be both efficacious for the mother and safe for the infant. Although infant serum levels of psychotropic medication are the most accurate measure of infant exposure, it is often difficult to measure infant serum levels in routine clinical practice. However, factors affecting the passage of medication into human milk must be considered, including the following:

1. Route of drug administration and pharmacokinetics[49]:
   - absorption rate
   - half-life and peak serum time
   - dissociation constant
   - volume of distribution
   - molecular size
   - degree of ionization
   - pH of plasma (7.4) and milk (6.8)
   - solubility of the drug in water and in lipids
   - binding to plasma protein
2. Amount of drug received by the infant in human milk[49]:
   - milk yield
   - colostrum versus mature milk
   - concentration of the drug in the milk
   - how well the breast was emptied during the previous feeding
   - the infant's ability to absorb, detoxify, and excrete the drug.

Up-to-date information about medication use during lactation is easily available from the Internet on TOXNET LACTMED (http://toxnet.nlm.nih.gov/newtoxnet/lactmed.htm) (available in English) and e-lactancia (http://e-lactancia.org/) (available in both English and Spanish).

Most antidepressant studies provide milk levels, or milk to mother's plasma ratio, that are not constant and depend on factors such as dose, frequency, duration of dosing, maternal variation in drug disposition, drug interactions, and genetic background. Few studies provide infant serum levels, although they are the best measure of infant exposure.[49]

SPECIFIC ANTIDEPRESSANTS

Data from a recent meta-analysis indicated that all antidepressants were detected in milk but that not all were found in infant serum.[50] Infant serum levels of nortriptyline, paroxetine, and sertraline were undetectable in most cases. Infant serum levels of citalopram and fluoxetine exceeded the recommended 10% maternal level in 17% and 22% of cases, respectively. Few adverse outcomes were reported for any of the antidepressants. Conclusions could not be drawn for other antidepressants due to an insufficient number of cases. There is little or no evidence that ethnic or regional "medicines" are safe or effective; thus their use by healthcare providers is strongly cautioned. (II-2) For specific antidepressant medications, see Table 1.

TABLE 1 Specific Antidepressants

Class	Drug	Dosage/day	Indications	Maternal side effects	Infant exposure effects	Comments
SSRIs	Citalopram[52–54] Escitalopram[55,56] Fluoxetine[56–64] Fluvoxamine[65–70] Paroxetine[67,71–73] Sertraline[3,67,74–78]	10–60 mg 10–20 mg 10–80 mg 50–300 mg 10–60 mg 25–200 mg (usually a daily dose). Start at 25 mg for 5–7 days, then increase to 50 mg.	Depressive or anxiety disorders; may be prescribed for fibromyalgia, neuropathic pain, premenstrual symptoms and disorders	Gastrointestinal distress, headaches, sexual dysfunction, nervousness, or sedation	All SSRIs have been detected in human milk. Paroxetine[71,72] and sertraline[74–73] have not exceeded the recommended 10% maternal level and are usually undetectable in infant serum.[75] Fluoxetine[57–61] and citalopram[52,53] have exceeded the 10% maternal level.[79] The infant adverse events reported include uneasy sleep, colic, irritability, poor feeding, and drowsiness.[56,63,64,80–82] The FDA indicated that fluoxetine should not be use by nursing mothers.[64]	Sertraline is the most likely SSRI to be prescribed, low to undetectable in milk and relative safety profile in pregnancy. Long-term effects on neurobehavior and development from exposure to any SSRI during pregnancy and lactation have a limited evidence base, but more recent studies are relatively reassuring.[56,63,80,81]
SNRIs	Venlafaxine[51,83] Duloxetine[84] Desvenlafaxine[82]	37.5–225 mg 20–120 mg 50–100 mg	Depression	Galactorrhea	Venlafaxine and its active metabolite are in milk, and its metabolite can be found in the plasma of most breastfed infants, but no proven drug-related side effects. Monitor for sedation and adequate weight gain.	Sporadic case reports for these medications.[82–84] Limited number to report significant outcomes for nursing infants.
Other antidepressants (norepinephrine/dopamine/serotonin reuptake block)	Bupropion[85–88]	150–450 mg	Depression	Dose-dependent drowsiness, dry mouth, increased appetite, weight gain, and dizziness	Very limited data, ranging from asymptomatic with undetectable infant serum levels to concerns with irritability and seizures	Use not a reason to discontinue breastfeeding. However, another drug may be preferred.
	Mirtazapine[89]	15–30 mg			Limited infant data; no adverse side effects noted	
TCAs/heterocyclics	Amitriptyline, amoxapine, clomipramine, desipramine, doxepin, maprotiline,	Nortriptyline, 30–50 mg/day, in 3–4 divided doses, or the total daily dosage may be given once a day.	Depression and anxiety disorders; often used in low doses for sleep and chronic pain	Hypotension, sedation, dry mouth, urinary retention, weight gain, sexual dysfunction, and constipation. In an	Only nortriptyline has a sufficient number of reported cases to comment on its use during lactation; it is generally undetectable in infant serum; no adverse events have been	One of the older classes

(Continued)

TABLE 1   Specific Antidepressants—cont'd

Class	Drug	Dosage/day	Indications	Maternal side effects	Infant exposure effect	Comments
	nortriptyline, protriptyline, and trimipramine			overdose, these medications can cause cardiac arrhythmias and death.	reported.[90–92] Use of doxepin is often cautioned because of a case report of hypotonia, poor feeding, emesis, and sedation in a breastfeeding infant that resolved after discontinuation of nursing.[93]	
Herbal/natural	St. John's wort (*Hypericum perforatum*) contains hypericin and hyperforin as well as flavonoids such as quercetin.	300 mg	Depression	One study found a slightly increased frequency of colic, drowsiness, and lethargy among breastfed infants but none required treatment.[95]	Both hypericin and hyperforin are poorly excreted into human milk.	Has been used for the treatment of mild to moderate depression for many years, especially in Europe. Its use as a treatment for depression is controversial in the United States.
	Omega-3 fatty acids		Depression during pregnancy and the postpartum period[94]	Appears to be of little risk to mothers and infants. The primary negative side effect is the "fishy smell."		Lack of sufficient evidence at this time to consider it a treatment for depression.
Antipsychotic	Quetiapine	Start at 25 mg, titrate. Maximum dose, 600 mg	Bipolar disorder, schizophrenia	Sedation	Sedation	
Mood stabilizer	Lithium	Start at 300 mg, titrate as per LI levels. Maximum dose, 900–1,200 mg		Diarrhea, vomiting	Elevated TSH	Dosing is dictated by lithium blood levels in the mother, which need to be regularly checked.

[a]Best safety profile of selective serotonin reuptake inhibitors (SSRIs) in lactation. *FDA*, Food and Drug Administration; *LI*, lithium, *SNRI*, serotonin-norepinephrine reuptake inhibitors; *TCA*, tricyclic antidepressant; *TSH*, thyroid-stimulating hormone.

RECOMMENDATIONS FOR ANTIDEPRESSANT TREATMENT IN LACTATING WOMEN

- Current evidence suggests that untreated maternal depression can have serious and long-term effects on mothers and infants and that treatment may improve outcomes for mothers and infants. Therefore treatment is strongly preferred. (II-2)
- However, it is important not to label mothers who are only suffering from mild cases of postpartum blues as "depressed." We must make a distinction. For women with mild symptoms who are in the first 2 weeks postpartum, close follow-up, rather than initiation of antidepressant medication, is suggested. (II-2)
- When available and when symptoms are in the mild to moderate range, psychological/cognitive behavioral therapy is the first line of treatment for lactating women as it carries no known risk for the infant. Mothers must be monitored and reevaluated. If they are not improving or their symptoms are worsening, antidepressant drug treatment should be considered. (II-2)
- Both psychological/cognitive behavioral therapy and antidepressant medication are recommended for women with moderate to severe symptoms or for whom there are current stressors or interpersonal issues that psychological therapy may help address. Maternal lactation status should not delay treatment. (II-2)
- Women with moderate to severe symptoms may require only antidepressant drug treatment. In the setting of moderate to severe depression, the benefits of treatment likely outweigh the risks of the medication to the mother or infant.
- There is no widely accepted algorithm for antidepressant medication treatment of depression in lactating women. An individualized risk–benefit analysis must be conducted in each situation and take into account the mother's clinical history and response to treatment, the risks of untreated depression, the risks and benefits of breastfeeding, the benefits of treatment, the known and unknown risks of the medication to the infant, and the mother's wishes.
- If a mother has no history of antidepressant treatment, an antidepressant such as sertraline that has evidence of lower levels in human milk and infant serum and few side effects is an appropriate first choice. (II-2) Sertraline has the best safety profile during lactation. The recommended starting dose is 25 mg for 5–7 days to avoid side effects, which then can be increased to 50 mg/day.
- If a mother has been successfully treated with a particular selective serotonin reuptake inhibitor, tricyclic antidepressant, or serotonin–norepinephrine uptake inhibitor in the past, the data regarding this particular antidepressant should be reviewed, and it should be considered as a first line treatment if there are no contraindications.
- Mothers who were being treated with a selective serotonin reuptake inhibitor, tricyclic antidepressant, or serotonin–norepinephrine uptake inhibitor during pregnancy with good symptom control should continue on the same agent during breastfeeding. It is important to reassure the mother that exposure to the antidepressant in breastmilk is far less than exposure to the antidepressant during pregnancy. Moreover, ongoing treatment of the mood disorder is critical for the health of both mother and baby. Mothers should be provided information regarding the known and unknown risks and benefits of the treatment to make an informed decision.
- Mothers should be monitored carefully in the initial stages of treatment for changes in symptoms, including worsening of symptoms. Specifically, women with histories of bipolar disorder, which may be undiagnosed, are at increased risk of developing an episode of depression, mania, or psychosis in the postpartum period. Although this situation is rare, mothers and partners should be made aware of the symptoms to watch for such as increased insomnia, delusions, hallucinations, racing thoughts, and talking/moving fast. Women experiencing such symptoms should contact their mental health provider immediately.
- The mother's provider should communicate with the infant's provider to facilitate monitoring and follow-up. Infants should be monitored carefully by the physician/health care worker, including carefully following growth. Serum levels are not indicated on a regular basis without a clinical indication or concern. In addition, in most cases, the serum level would not provide helpful information unless it is a psychotropic that has a documented therapeutic window and laboratory norms (i.e., tricyclic antidepressants).
- A strategy that may be used to decrease infant exposure based on breastfeeding pharmacokinetic reports is medication administration immediately after feedings. (III)
- There are several Web-based and book references available for professionals and mothers to assist in gaining knowledge and help regarding these issues (Table 2).

CONCLUSIONS AND SUGGESTIONS FOR FUTURE RESEARCH

Despite many publications about antidepressants and breastfeeding, the scientific literature continues to lack the depth of robust large-scale studies for clinicians and mothers to make confident decisions about individual medications. Multiple reviews of the literature broadly suggest tricyclic antidepressants and selective serotonin reuptake inhibitors are relatively safe, and all recommend individual risk–benefit assessments.[51]

Future research that would help guide clinical practice includes:

1. Randomized clinical trials in lactating women for any class of antidepressant that include the following:
   a. Sufficient control for level of depression

TABLE 2   Resources for Women's Mental Health and Postpartum Depression Help

Resource	Description	URL
Web sites		
International Marcé Society for Perinatal Mental Health	Primarily a multidisciplinary group of healthcare providers interested in promoting, facilitating, and communicating about research in all aspects of the mental health of women, their infants and partners around the time of childbirth.	www.marcesociety.com
Maternal and Child Health Bureau, U.S. Health Resources and Services Administration	Handbook entitled *"Depression During and After Pregnancy: A Resource for Women, Their Families, and Friends"*	www.mchb.hrsa.gov/ pregnancyandbeyond/ depression
National Suicide Prevention Lifeline, U.S. Substance Abuse and Mental Health Services Administration	1–800–273–TALK (8255)	www. suicidepreventionlifeline. org
Postpartum Support International	Information and resources on postpartum depression for providers, mothers, fathers, and families. Includes live chats and help for new parents. Access help according to state. PSI Warmline (weekdays only) 800–944-4PPD (4773)	www.postpartum.net
Postpartum Depression Online Support Group	A privately funded online support group that offers information, support, and assistance to those dealing with postpartum mood disorders and their families, friends, physicians, and counselors	www.ppdsupportpage.com
Mental Health America	The nonprofit Mental Health America is concerned with fathers' mental health as well as mothers.	www.mentalhealthamerica. net/conditions/ postpartumdisorders
Beyond Blue	A national initiative in Australia to raise awareness of anxiety and depression, providing resources for recovery, management and resilience	www.beyondblue.org.au
Books	Bennett SS, Indman P. *Beyond the Blues: Understanding and Treating Prenatal and Postpartum Depression & Anxiety.* Moodswings, San Jose, CA, 2011.	
	Cooper PJ, Murray L, eds. *Postpartum Depression and Child Development.* Guilford, New York, 1999.	
	Kendall-Tackett KA. *A Breastfeeding-Friendly Approach to Postpartum Depression.* Praeclarus Press, Amarillo, TX, 2015.	
	Kendall-Tackett KA. *Depression in New Mothers*, 2nd ed. Routledge, London, 2010.	
	Kleiman K. *Therapy and the Postpartum Woman: Notes on Healing Postpartum Depression for Clinicians and the Women Who Seek Their Help.* Routledge, Abingdon, United Kingdom, 2008.	
	Kleiman KR. *The Postpartum Husband: Practical Solutions for Living with Postpartum Depression.* Xlibris, Bloomington, IN, 2001.	
	Shields B. *Down Came the Rain: My Journey Through Postpartum Depression.* Hyperion, New York, 2006	
	Wiegartz PS, Gyoerkoe KL, Miller LJ. *The Pregnancy and Postpartum Anxiety Workbook: Practical Skills to Help You Overcome Anxiety, Worry, Panic Attacks, Obsessions, and Compulsions.* New Harbinger Publications, Oakland, CA, 2009.	

b. Provision of drug, information on infant serum levels, the amount detected in human milk, maternal serum levels, and the timing of sampling

c. Information on infant consumption in the milk

d. Information on infant behavioral outcomes

e. Evaluation of impact of continued breastfeeding on mitigating infant withdrawal symptoms for those mothers treated antenatally.

2. Study reasons mothers and clinicians elect to defer treatment in lactating mothers and follow-up behavioral outcomes of these infants.

REFERENCES

1. Gjerdingen DK, Yawn BP. Postpartum depression screening: Importance, methods, barriers, and recommendations for practice. *J Am Board Fam Med*. 2007;20:280–288.

2. Chaudron LH, Szilagyi PG, Tang W, et al. Accuracy of depression screening tools for identifying postpartum depression among urban mothers. *Pediatrics*. 2010;125: e609–e617.

3. Wisner KL, Perel JM, Peindl KS, et al. Prevention of recurrent postpartum depression: A randomized clinical trial. *J Clin Psychiatry*. 2001;62:82–86.

4. Marcus SM. Depression during pregnancy: Rates, risks, and consequences—Motherisk Update 2008. *Can J Clin Pharmacol*. 2009;16:e15–e22.

5. Oppo A, Mauri M, Ramacciotti D, et al. Risk factors for postpartum depression: The role of the Postpartum Depression Predictors Inventory-Revised (PDPI-R). Results from the Perinatal Depression-Research and Screening Unit (PNDReScU) study. *Arch Womens Ment Health*. 2009;12:239–249.

6. Cutler CB, Legano LA, Dreyer BP, et al. Screening for maternal depression in a low education population using a two item questionnaire. *Arch Womens Ment Health*. 2007;10:277–283.

7. Earls MF, Committee on Psychosocial Aspects of Child and Family Health American Academy of Pediatrics. Incorporating recognition and management of perinatal and postpartum depression into pediatric practice. *Pediatrics*. 2010;126:1032–1039.

8. Mishina H, Takayama JI. Screening for maternal depression in primary care pediatrics. *Curr Opin Pediatr*. 2009;21:789–793.

9. American Psychiatric Association. *Diagnostic and Statistical Manual of Mental Disorders (DSM-V)*. Arlington, VA: American Psychiatric Publishing; 2013.

10. Sriraman NK. Postpartum depression: Why paediatricians should screen new moms. *Cont Pediatr*. 2012;29:40–46.

11. Sharma V. Treatment of postpartum psychosis: Challenges and opportunities. *Curr Drug Saf*. 2008;3:76–81.

12. Chaudron LH, Pies RW. The relationship between postpartum psychosis and bipolar disorder: A review. *J Clin Psychiatry*. 2003;64:1284–1292.

13. Jones I, Craddock N. Familiarity of the puerperal trigger in bipolar disorder: Results of a family study. *Am J Psychiatry*. 2001;158:913–917.

14. Abramowitz JS, Meltzer-Brody S, Leserman J, et al. Obsessional thoughts and compulsive behaviors in a sample of women with postpartum mood symptoms. *Arch Womens Ment Health*. 2010;13:523–530.

15. Russell EJ, Fawcett JM, Mazmanian D. Risk of obsessive-compulsive disorder in pregnant and postpartum women: A meta-analysis. *J Clin Psychiatry*. 2013;74:377–385.

16. National Institute for Health and Clinical Excellence. *Postnatal Care: Routine Postnatal Care of Women and Their Babies (CG37)*. London: National Institute for Health and Clinical Excellence; 2006.

17. Royal Australian College of General Practitioners. *Guidelines for Preventive Activities in General Practice*. East Melbourne, Australia: Royal Australian College of General Practitioners; 2012.

18. Scottish Intercollegiate Guidelines Network. *Management of Perinatal Mood Disorder*. Edinburgh: Scottish Intercollegiate Guidelines Network; 2012.

19. Screening for perinatal depression. Committee Opinion No. 630. American College of Obstetricians and Gynecologists. *Obstet Gynecol* 2015;125:1268–1271. Available at: www.acog. org/Resources-And-Publications/Committee-Opinions/ Committee-on-Obstetric-Practice/Screening-for-PerinatalDepression (accessed June 1, 2015).

20. Yawn BP, Dietrich AJ, Wollan P, et al. TRIPPD: A practice based network effectiveness study of postpartum depression screening and management. *Ann Fam Med*. 2012;10:320–329.

21. Appendix A Task Force Ratings. *Guide to Clinical Preventive Services: Report of the U.S. Preventive Services Task Force*, 2nd ed. Available at: www.ncbi.nlm.nih.gov/books/NBK15430/ (accessed May 27, 2015).

22. Olson AL, Kemper KJ, Kelleher KJ, et al. Primary care pediatricians' roles and perceived responsibilities in the identification and management of maternal depression. *Pediatrics*. 2002;110:1169–1176.

23. Chaudron LH, Szilagyi PG, Campbell AT, et al. Legal and ethical considerations: Risks and benefits of postpartum depressions screening at well-child visits. *Pediatrics*. 2007;119:123–128.

24. U.S. Public Health Service. Report of the Surgeon General's Conference on Children's Mental Health: A National Action Agenda. U.S. Department of Health and Human Services, Washington, DC, 2000. Available at: www.ncbi.nlm.nih.gov/ books/NBK44233/ (accessed May 27, 2015).

25. Committee on the Psychosocial Aspects of Child and Family Health and Task Force on Mental Health. Policy statement— The future of pediatrics: Mental health competencies for pediatric primary care. *Pediatrics*. 2009;124:410–421.

26. Myers ER, Aubuchon-Endsley N, Bastian LA, et al. *Efficacy and Safety of Screening for Postpartum Depression. Comparative Effectiveness Reviews, No. 106*. Rockville, MD: Agency for Healthcare Research and Quality; 2013. Available at: www.ncbi.nlm.nih.gov/books/NBK137724/ (accessed May 27, 2015).

27. Cox JL, Holden JM, Sagovsky R. Detection of postnatal depression. Development of the 10-item Edinburgh Postnatal Depression Scale. *Br J Psychiatry*. 1987;150:782–786. Available at: http://pesnc.org/wp-content/uploads/EPDS.pdf (accessed May 27, 2015).

28. Hagan JF Jr, Shaw JS, Duncan P, eds. *Bright Futures: Guidelines for Health Supervision of Infants, Children, and Adolescents*. 3rd ed. Elk Grove Village, IL: American Academy of Pediatrics; 2008.

29. Sheeder J, Kabir K, Stafford B. Screening for postpartum depression at well-child visits: Is once enough during the first 6 months of life? *Pediatrics*. 2009;123:e982–e988.

30. Freeman MP, Wright R, Watchman M, et al. Postpartum depression assessments at well-baby visits: Screening feasibility, prevalence, and risk factors. *J Womens Health (Larchmt)*. 2005;14:929–935.

31. Dennis CL. Can we identify mothers at risk for postpartum depression in the immediate postpartum period using the

Edinburgh Postnatal Depression Scale? *J Affect Disord.* 2004;78:163–169.

32. Jardri R, Pelta J, Maron M, et al. Predictive validation study of the Edinburgh Postnatal Depression Scale in the first week after delivery and risk analysis for postnatal depression. *J Affect Disord.* 2006;93:169–176.

33. Watkins S, Meltzer-Brody S, Zolnoun D, Stuebe A. Early breastfeeding experiences and postpartum depression. *Obstet Gynecol.* 2011;118:214–221.

34. Trapolini T, McMahon CA, Ungerer JA. The effect of maternal depression and marital adjustment on young children's internalizing and externalizing behaviour problems. *Child Care Health Dev.* 2007;33:794–803.

35. Minkovitz CS, O'Campo PJ, Chen YH, et al. Associations between maternal and child health status and patterns of medical care use. *Ambul Pediatr.* 2002;2:85–92.

36. Kavanaugh M, Halterman JS, Montes G, et al. Maternal depressive symptoms are adversely associated with prevention practice and parenting behaviors for preschool children. *Ambul Pediatr.* 2006;6:32–37.

37. Stuebe AM, Grewen K, Meltzer-Brody S. Association between maternal mood and oxytocin response to breastfeeding. *J Womens Health (Larchmt).* 2013;22:352–361.

38. Office of Disease Prevention and Health Promotion, U.S. Department of Health and Human Services. Healthy People 2020. Maternal, Infant, and Child Health. Available at: http://healthypeople.gov/2020/topicsobjectives2020/overview.aspx?topicid = 26 (accessed May 27, 2015).

39. Dennis CL, Ross LE, Grigoriadis S. Psychosocial and psychological interventions for treating antenatal depression. *Cochrane Database Syst Rev.* 2007;3:CD006309.

40. Brandon AR, Freeman MP. When she says "no" to medication: Psychotherapy for antepartum depression. *Curr Psychiatry Rep.* 2011;13:459–466.

41. Cuijpers P, Brannmark JG, van Straten A. Psychological treatment of postpartum depression: A meta-analysis. *J Clin Psychol.* 2008;64:103–118.

42. O'Hara MW, Schlechte JA, Lewis DA, et al. Prospective study of postpartum blues. Biologic and psychosocial factors. *Arch Gen Psychiatry.* 1991;48:801–806.

43. Dekker JJ, Koelen JA, Van HL, et al. Speed of action: The relative efficacy of short psychodynamic supportive psychotherapy and pharmacotherapy in the first 8 weeks of a treatment algorithm for depression. *J Affect Disord.* 2008;109:183–188.

44. O'Hara MW, Stuart S, Gorman LL, et al. Efficacy of interpersonal psychotherapy for postpartum depression. *Arch Gen Psychiatry.* 2000;57:1039–1045.

45. Brandon AR, Ceccotti N, Hynan LS, et al. Proof of concept: Partner-assisted interpersonal psychotherapy for perinatal depression. *Arch Womens Ment Health.* 2012;15:469–480.

46. Mulcahy R, Reay RE, Wilkinson RB, et al. A randomised control trial for the effectiveness of group interpersonal psychotherapy for postnatal depression. *Arch Womens Ment Health.* 2010;13:125–139.

47. Grote NK, Swartz HA, Geibel SL, et al. A randomized controlled trial of culturally relevant, brief interpersonal psychotherapy for perinatal depression. *Psychiatr Serv.* 2009;60:313–321.

48. Burt VK, Suri R, Altshuler L, et al. The use of psychotropic medications during breast-feeding. *Am J Psychiatry.* 2001;158:1001–1009.

49. Hale T. *Medications and Mothers Milk.* 16th ed. Plano, TX: Hale Publishing; 2014.

50. Weissman AM, Levy BT, Hartz AJ, et al. Pooled analysis of antidepressant levels in lactating mothers, breast milk, and nursing infants. *Am J Psychiatry.* 2004;161:1066–1078.

51. Molyneaux E, Howard LM, McGeown HR, et al. Antidepressant treatment for postnatal depression. *Cochrane Database Syst Rev.* 2014;9:CD002018.

52. Heikkinen T, Ekblad U, Kero P, et al. Citalopram in pregnancy and lactation. *Clin Pharmacol Ther.* 2002;2:184–191.

53. Lee A, Woo J, Ito S. Frequency of infant adverse events that are associated with citalopram use during breastfeeding. *Am J Obstet Gynecol.* 2004;190:218–221.

54. Schmidt K, Olesen OV, Jensen PN. Citalopram and breastfeeding: Serum concentration and side effects in the infant. *Biol Psychiatry.* 2000;47:164–165.

55. Bellantuono C, Bozzi F, Orsolini L, et al. The safety of escitalopram during pregnancy and breastfeeding: A comprehensive review. *Hum Psychopharmacol.* 2012;27:534–539.

56. Brent NB, Wisner KL. Fluoxetine and carbamazepine concentrations in a nursing mother/infant pair. *Clin Pediatr (Phila).* 1998;37:41–44.

57. Kristensen JH, Ilett KF, Hackett LP, et al. Distribution and excretion of fluoxetine and norfluoxetine in human milk. *Br J Clin Pharmacol.* 1999;48:521–527.

58. Epperson CN, Jatlow PI, Czarkowski K, et al. Maternal fluoxetine treatment in the postpartum period: Effects on platelet serotonin and plasma drug levels in breastfeeding mother-infant pairs. *Pediatrics.* 2003;112:e425.

59. Heikkinen T, Ekblad U, Palo P, Laine K. Pharmacokinetics of fluoxetine and norfluoxetine in pregnancy and lactation. *Clin Pharmacol Ther.* 2003;73:330–337.

60. Hendrick V, Stowe ZN, Altshuler LL, et al. Fluoxetine and norfluoxetine concentrations in nursing infants and breast milk. *Biol Psychiatry.* 2001;50:775–782.

61. Suri R, Stowe ZN, Hendrick V, Hostetter A, et al. Estimates of nursing infant daily dose of fluoxetine through breast milk. *Biol Psychiatry.* 2002;52:446–451.

62. Lester BM, Cucca J, Andreozzi L, et al. Possible association between fluoxetine hydrochloride and colic in an infant. *J Am Acad Child Psychiatry.* 1993;32:1253–1255.

63. Chambers CD, Anderson PO, Thomas RG, et al. Weight gain in infants whose mothers take fluoxetine. *Pediatrics.* 1999;104:e61.

64. Nightingale SL. Fluoxetine labeling revised to identify phenytoin interaction and to recommend against use in nursing mothers. *JAMA.* 1994;271:106.

65. Arnold LM, Suckow RF, Lichtenstein PK. Fluvoxamine concentrations in breast milk and in maternal and infant sera. *J Clin Psychopharmacol.* 2000;20:491–493.

66. Hagg S, Granberg K, Carleborg L. Excretion of fluvoxamine into breast milk. *Br J Clin Pharmacol.* 2000;49:286–288.

67. Hendrick V, Fukuchi A, Altshuler L, et al. Use of sertraline, paroxetine and fluvoxamine by nursing women. *Br J Psychiatry.* 2001;179:163–166.

68. Piontek CM, Wisner KL, Perel JM, Peindl KS. Serum fluvoxamine levels in breastfed infants. *J Clin Psychiatry.* 2001;62:111–113.

69. Yoshida K, Smith B, Kumar RC. Fluvoxamine in breastmilk and infant development. *Br J Clin Pharmacol.* 1997;44:210–211.

70. Wright S, Dawling S, Ashford JJ. Excretion of fluvoxamine in breast milk. *Br J Clin Pharmacol.* 1991;31:209.

71. Misery S, Kim J, Riggs KW, Kostaras X. Protein levels in postpartum depressed women, breast milk, and infant serum. *J Clin Psychiatry.* 2000;61:828—832.

72. Stowe ZN, Cohen LS, Hostettler A, et al. Paroxetine in human breast milk and nursing infants. *Am J Psychiatry.* 2000;157:185—189.

73. Merlob P, Stahl B, Sulkes J. Paroxetine during breastfeeding: Infant weight gain and maternal adherence to counsel. *Eur J Pediatr.* 2004;163:135—139.

74. Epperson CN, Anderson GM, McDougle CJ. Sertraline and breast-feeding. *N Engl J Med.* 1997;336:1189—1190.

75. Stowe ZN, Owens MJ, Landry JC, et al. Sertraline and desmethylsertraline in human breast milk and nursing infants. *Am J Psychiatry.* 1997;154:1255—1260.

76. Epperson N, Czarkowski KA, Ward-O'Brien D, et al. Maternal sertraline treatment and serotonin transport in breast-feeding mother-infant pairs. *Am J Psychiatry.* 2001;158:1631—1637.

77. Wisner KL, Perel JM, Blumer J. Serum sertraline and N-desmethylsertraline levels in breast-feeding mother-infant pairs. *Am J Psychiatry.* 1998;155:690—692.

78. Dodd S, Stocky A, Buist A, et al. Sertraline analysis in the plasma of breast-fed infants. *Aust N Z J Psychiatry.* 2001;35:545—546.

79. Ito S, Koren G. Antidepressants and breast-feeding. *Am J Psychiatry.* 1997;154:1174.

80. Olivier JD, Akerud H, Kaihola H, et al. The effects of maternal depression and maternal selective serotonin reuptake inhibitor exposure on offspring. *Front Cell Neurosci.* 2013;7:73.

81. Austin MP, Karatas JC, Mishra P, et al. Infant neurodevelopment following in utero exposure to antidepressant medication. *Acta Paediatr.* 2013;102:1054—1059.

82. Rampono J, Teoh S, Hackett LP, et al. Estimation of desvenlafaxine transfer into milk and infant exposure during its use in lactating women with postnatal depression. *Arch Womens Ment Health.* 2011;14:49—53.

83. Ilett KF, Kristensen JH, Hackett LP, et al. Distribution of venlafaxine and its O-desmethyl metabolite in human milk and their effects in breastfed infants. *Br J Clin Pharmacol.* 2002;53:17—22.

84. Boyce PM, Hackett LP, Ilett KF. Duloxetine transfer across the placenta during pregnancy and into milk during lactation. *Arch Womens Ment Health.* 2011;14:169—172.

85. Baab SW, Peindl KS, Piontek CM, et al. Serum bupropion levels in two breastfeeding mother-infant pairs. *J Clin Psychiatry.* 2002;63:910—911.

86. Neuman G, Colantonio D, Delaney S, et al. Bupropion and escitalopram during lactation. *Ann Pharmacother.* 2014;48:928—931.

87. Chaudron LH, Schoenecker CJ. Bupropion and breastfeeding: A case of a possible infant seizure. *J Clin Psychiatry.* 2004;65:881—882.

88. Davis MF, Miller HS, Nolan PE Jr. Bupropion levels in breast milk for four mother-infant pairs: More answers to lingering questions. *J Clin Psychiatry.* 2009;70:297—298.

89. Aichhorn WMD, Whitworth ABM, Weiss UMD, et al. Mirtazapine and breast-feeding. *Am J Psychiatry.* 2004;161:2325.

90. Wisner KL, Perel JM. Nortriptyline treatment of breastfeeding women. *Am J Psychiatry.* 1996;153:295.

91. Wisner KL, Perel JM. Serum nortriptyline levels in nursing mothers and their infants. *Am J Psychiatry.* 1991;148:1234—1236.

92. Wisner KL, Perel JM, Findling RL, Hinnes RL. Nortriptyline and its hydroxymetabolites in breastfeeding mothers and newborns. *Psychopharmacol Bull.* 1997;33:249—251.

93. Frey OR, Scheidt P, von Brenndorff AI. Adverse effects in a newborn infant breast-fed by a mother treated with doxepin. *Ann Pharmacother.* 1999;33:690—693.

94. Freeman MP, Hibbeln JR, Wisner KL, et al. Randomized dose-ranging pilot trial of omega-3 fatty acids for postpartum depression. *Acta Psychiatr Scand.* 2006; 113:31—35.

95. Lee A, Minhas R, Matsuda N, et al. The safety of St. John's wort (*Hypericum perforatum*) during breast-feeding. *J Clin Psychiatry.* 2003;64:966—968.

ABM protocols expire 5 years from the date of publication. Evidence-based revisions are made within 5 years or sooner, if there are significant changes in the evidence.

Academy of Breastfeeding Medicine Protocol Committee
Kathleen A. Marinelli, MD, FABM, Chairperson
Maya Bunik, MD, MSPH, FABM, Co-Chairperson
Larry Noble, MD, FABM, Translations Chairperson
Nancy Brent, MD
Ruth A. Lawrence, MD, FABM
Sarah Reece-Stremtan, MD
Casey Rosen-Carole, MD
Tomoko Seo, MD, FABM
Rose St. Fleur, MD
Michal Young, MD
For correspondence: abm@bfmed.org

ABM Clinical Protocol #19
*Breastfeeding Promotion in the Prenatal Setting, Revision 2015**

Casey Rosen-Carole[1], Scott Hartman[2] and the Academy of Breastfeeding Medicine

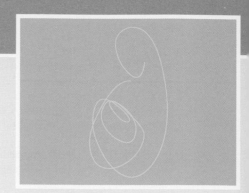

ABSTRACT

A central goal of the Academy of Breastfeeding Medicine is the development of clinical protocols for managing common medical problems that may impact breastfeeding success. These protocols serve only as guidelines for the care of breastfeeding mothers and infants and do not delineate an exclusive course of treatment or serve as standards of medical care. Variations in treatment may be appropriate according to the needs of an individual patient.

BACKGROUND

BREASTFEEDING PROVIDES IDEAL INFANT nutrition and is physiologic for mothers and children.[1-4] Pregnant women often make a decision regarding breastfeeding early in pregnancy, and many have already decided whether to breastfeed prior to conception.[5-7] Encouragement and education from healthcare providers result in increased breastfeeding initiation, exclusivity, and duration.[8-16] Yet, healthcare providers consistently overestimate the amount and adequacy of counseling and support that pregnant women receive.[17-24] Although the focus of this protocol is on the prenatal setting, programs or interventions that include preconception, prenatal, and postnatal components should be strongly considered as they appear to yield larger positive results on breastfeeding duration and exclusivity.[8,10,25-27]

The quality of evidence (levels of evidence I, II-1, II-2, II-3, and III) is based on the U.S. Preventive Services Task Force Appendix A Task Force Ratings[28] and is noted throughout this protocol in parentheses.

* Courtesy of the Academy of Breastfeeding Medicine. Please go to https://www.bfmed.org/protocols for complete protocols, translations, and the most up-to-date information (protocols are updated every 5–7 years).
[1] Departments of General Pediatrics, University of Rochester, Rochester, New York.
[2] Departments of Family Medicine, University of Rochester, Rochester, New York.

RECOMMENDATIONS

1. Create a breastfeeding friendly office and community.
   A. Breastfeeding friendly office[9]:
      - The primary healthcare provider should be involved in each of the following steps, in cooperation with a multidisciplinary team that includes other healthcare professionals and healthcare workers (e.g., including, but not limited to, doctors, nurses, midwives, medical assistants, various lactation specialists/consultants [International Board Certified Lactation Consultants, in particular when their expertise is needed], nutritionists, doulas, health and breastfeeding educators, and peer support).
      - Educate staff to promote, protect, and support breastfeeding.
      - Have a written breastfeeding policy to facilitate such support.[9] (III)
      - Literature and samples provided by artificial infant formula companies should not be used in healthcare settings, as this advertising has been demonstrated to decrease breastfeeding initiation and shorten duration, and it constitutes a breach of the World Health Organization's International Code of Marketing of Breast-milk Substitutes.[29-33] (I, II-2, II-3, III)
      - Intention to breastfeed should be included as part of all transfer-of-care materials, including prenatal records and hospital and birth center discharge summaries.
      - Create breastfeeding friendly office spaces, including safe, clean, and comfortable spaces for patients and staff to breastfeed or express milk, as well as posters and artwork supporting breastfeeding. For more details see the Academy of Breastfeeding Medicine's Protocol #14: "Breastfeeding Friendly Physician's Office."[9] (III)
   B. Breastfeeding friendly community:
      - Community-based interventions have shown significant success in improving breastfeeding outcomes.[34-38] (I, II-1, II-2, III)

- Partner with local and regional organizations in order to maximize patient services and support (e.g., local, regional, and national maternal—child organizations, local La Leche League International groups, community health workers, health departments, local or regional maternity hospitals or birth centers, not-for-profit organizations, breast-feeding peer counseling programs; supplemental food programs [such as the Special Supplemental Nutrition Program for Women, Infant and Children in the United States], and home visiting programs).
- Be aware of local community and professional breastfeeding support services and understand the particular content and services provided. Make available current listings of such support to women throughout their pregnancy.
- Consider the use of prenatal home-visiting programs, particularly in underserved areas or populations, while ensuring that providers have been adequately trained.[34,36,39–46] (I, II-1, III)

2. Consider the background, ethnicity, and culture of individual women, families, and communities.
   - Learn about patients' family and community structure. Social support, or the lack thereof, is likely to play a large role in feeding decisions of many women, particularly adolescents.[7,47] (I, II-2)
   - Understand that perspectives and beliefs of partners and support persons may affect breastfeeding success and educate where appropriate.[45,48–51] Attention to gender dynamics and targeted behavioral interventions (e.g., education, counseling, sharing housework) may improve breastfeeding duration and exclusivity.[48] (I, II-2, III)
   - In some cultures, enlisting the cooperation of an important family member may greatly assist in the promotion of breastfeeding.[51] (I)
   - Ensure that parents from diverse cultures understand the importance of exclusive breastfeeding to their children's growth and development.[51] (I) Acculturation or assimilation of immigrant populations should be considered with respect to a family's current feeding choices.[52] (I)
   - Cultural traditions and taboos associated with lactation should be respected, adapting cultural beliefs to facilitate optimal breastfeeding, while sensitively educating about traditions that may be detrimental to breastfeeding.[52,53] (I, II-1)
   - Whenever possible, provide all information and instructions in patients' native language and assess for literacy level when appropriate. Instructional photos and pictures can also be used where literacy is a concern.
   - Understand the specific financial, work, time, and sociocultural obstacles to breastfeeding and work with families to overcome them.
   - Healthcare providers should be aware of their own personal cultural attitudes when interacting with patients.[2] (III)

3. Consider behavioral and psycho-educational approaches to breastfeeding support.
   - Self-efficacy and breastfeeding confidence play a large role in women's breastfeeding initiation, duration, and exclusivity.[50,54–57] (I, II-2)
   - Cognitive-behavioral counseling, social-cognitive theory—based influential models, competence theory, and workbook-based or group self-efficacy interventions can be considered and have shown to improve breastfeeding outcomes.[7,52,58–63] (I, II-1, II-2)
   - Whenever possible, healthcare providers should use motivational and self-efficacy supporting techniques when discussing breastfeeding, for example:
     1. Guiding a pregnant woman to consider her own knowledge of and reasons for breastfeeding: "What do you know about breastfeeding?" and "What are your reasons for breastfeeding your baby?"
     2. Helping to think through barriers: "Can you think of anything that might get in the way of you reaching your goal?" or
     3. Helping to associate breastfeeding with other successes in a woman's life: "Are there other areas in your life when you have been successful in reaching a goal you set out to achieve?"[64,65] (II-3)
   - Consider strengthening routine prenatal education on postpartum symptoms (bleeding, mood changes, pain, hair loss, incontinence, infant colic, breastfeeding, etc.) and opportunities for social support and self-management, as qualitative work shows insufficient maternal preparation,[66] and this behavioral intervention has been shown to improve breastfeeding duration in one minority population.[67] (I, III)

4. Integrate breastfeeding promotion, education, and support throughout prenatal care.
   - Support of breastfeeding should be actively stated in the preconception period,[68] or as early as possible in prenatal care, with acknowledgement that there are risks to artificial infant formula feeding.[2] Consider a statement such as "As your healthcare provider, I want you to know that I recommend breastfeeding. Formula feeding has many health risks for mothers and babies." (I, III)
   - Use of electronic medical record prompts may be used to improve consistency of healthcare provider support statements.[69,70] (I, III)
   - Strongly consider integrating lactation consultant support and education into the prenatal office visits,[71] as it is noted for its effect on improving breastfeeding initiation and exclusivity.[69,70,72] (I, III)
   - Strongly consider offering group prenatal care or connecting women with a group prenatal care program as these groups have been noted for their positive impact on breastfeeding initiation.[73,74] (I, II-3)
   - At this point, there is no evidence to determine what role Internet education can play in breastfeeding support.[75] However, many mothers will seek information on the Internet and may find Web sites

with little medical oversight and factual errors. Patients should be directed to appropriate online sources of support and information, such as the World Health Organization's Web site on breastfeeding: www.who.int/topics/breastfeeding (II-2)

- Consider using novel technological approaches such as education and networking through text-messaging/mobile phones as preliminary international data suggest improved breastfeeding duration and exclusivity with this approach.[76,77] (I)

5. Take a detailed breastfeeding history as a part of the prenatal history.[2,9,78] (III)

- For each previous child, ask about breastfeeding initiation, duration of exclusive/any breastfeeding, sources of prior breastfeeding support, perceived benefits and challenges, and reason(s) for weaning.
- For women who did not breastfeed, consider asking about the perceived advantages of artificial infant formula feeding, as well as the perceived disadvantages. Inquiry should be made regarding what may have helped her breastfeed previous children.
- It is also important to determine any family medical history that may make breastfeeding especially helpful for this child (e.g., asthma, eczema, diabetes, and obesity) and/or mother (e.g., obesity, diabetes, depression, and breast or ovarian cancer).[1-3] (I)

6. Incorporate breastfeeding as an important component of the initial prenatal breast examination.[79] (II-3)

- Observe for appropriate breast development and anatomy.
- Note whether the history or physical exam findings suggest that a pregnant woman is at high risk for breastfeeding problems (e.g., maternal history of failure to breastfeed a previous child, chronic medication or supplement use, infertility, breast surgery or trauma, cranial or chest irradiation, or domestic or intimate partner violence; physical exam suggestive of flat or inverted nipples, glandular hypoplasia, or obesity; history or physical exam suggestive of diabetes, thyroid conditions, or polycystic ovarian syndrome).[1] (I)
- Consider a prenatal lactation referral to a physician who specializes in breastfeeding medicine or a lactation consultant (International Board Certified Lactation Consultant where possible) if concerns are identified.

7. Discuss breastfeeding at each prenatal visit.[1,2] (I)

- Consider the use of the Best Start 3-Step Counseling Strategy[64,79] by:
  1. Encouraging open dialogue about breastfeeding by beginning with open-ended questions.
  2. Affirming the patient's feelings.
  3. Providing targeted education.[64,80] (II-4, II-1)
- Address concerns and dispel misconceptions at each visit.
- Provide information on medication safety during pregnancy and breastfeeding.

- Consider using a set of educational materials in your practice, such as "Ready, Set, Baby" (www.tinyurl.com/readysetbaby), which includes materials for patients and guidance for educators.

During the first trimester

- If there are no contraindications, make a clear recommendation to exclusively breastfeed for 6 months and then with complementary foods for 1–2 years or as long thereafter as the mother and infant desire. Making this recommendation alone has shown to improve breastfeeding rates.[81] (II-2)
- Incorporate and educate partners and support persons about the benefits of breastfeeding for mothers and infants.[82] (II-2)
- Address known common barriers such as lack of self-confidence, embarrassment, time and social constraints, dietary and health concerns, lack of social support, employment and childcare concerns, and fear of pain.[65,79] (I, II-3) Addressing social and lifestyle factors can play a particularly pivotal role for adolescent[7,45] (I), obese[83,84] (I), and ethnic minority[25,37,44,47,85] women. (I, II-2, II-3, III)

During the second trimester

- Encourage women to identify breastfeeding role models by talking with family, friends, and colleagues who have breastfed successfully.
- Recommend that pregnant women and their partners or support persons attend a breastfeeding course, peer support group, and/or group prenatal care in addition to routine office-based education.[73,74,85-90] (I, II-1, II-3)
- Review breastfeeding basics, such as the importance of exclusive breastfeeding, the relationship of supply and demand, feeding on demand, frequency of feedings, cues of hunger and satiety, avoiding artificial nipples (teats) until the infant is breastfeeding well, and the importance of a good latch.
- For women who plan to return to school or work outside of the home after birth, encourage consideration of what facilities are available for expressing and storing mother's milk, how much time will be taken for maternity leave, and what worksite/school policies and legislation provide support.[1,2] (III)
- Encourage women to engage the support of a trained birth assistant (doula) for labor, birth, and postpartum care, as this significantly improves breastfeeding outcomes.[90,91] (I)

During the third trimester

- Consider demonstrating with dolls and props the mechanics of a good latch and common breastfeeding positions, such as laid-back breastfeeding, cradle, cross-cradle, and the clutch (football) hold.[92] (I)

- Review the physiology of breastfeeding initiation and the impact of supplementation.[1,2,65] (II-3, III)
- Recommend the purchase of properly fitting nursing bras and clothes that will facilitate breastfeeding, as culturally appropriate.
- Encourage another visit to a breastfeeding support group as women's interest and goals of attending may be different than earlier in the pregnancy.[3,26,32,36,79] (I, II-3)
- Review potential options for pain management during labor and their possible impacts on breastfeeding, as many pain medications can negatively impact breastfeeding outcomes.[93–95] (I, III)
- Discuss the importance of early skin-to-skin contact after birth (regardless of delivery mode) and during the postpartum period for optimal breastfeeding outcomes and general newborn health.[93,96–98] (I, II-3) Discuss the biologically normal first latch, including the "breast crawl," and how to facilitate this in the birthing room.[99,100] (III)
- Recommend that pregnant women discuss plans for their infant's health care and breastfeeding support with their infant's healthcare provider.[101] (I)
- Stress the need for early follow-up postpartum if there are any concerns that a woman, infant, or both are at high risk for breastfeeding problems.
8. Empower women and their families to have the birth experience most conducive to breastfeeding.
- Inform patients about the Ten Steps to Successful Breastfeeding and how to advocate for breastfeeding friendly hospital care.[101] (I)
- Discuss support of breastfeeding in the event of a cesarean delivery.[96–98] (I, II-3)
- Encourage mothers to ask for help from a lactation specialist in the birth hospital and/or soon after discharge, particularly if they are having any breastfeeding difficulties.
- Recommend the infant see a healthcare provider soon after hospital discharge to ensure infant health and optimal breastfeeding (III), particularly for infants discharged in the first 1–3 days of life.
- Ensure the mother has an adequate support system in place during the postpartum period and knows how to get help.
- Provide anticipatory guidance on topics such as engorgement, frequent feedings, and nighttime feedings.

RECOMMENDATIONS FOR FURTHER RESEARCH

1. Although many studies have demonstrated efficacy of specific prenatal interventions, cost-effectiveness studies are needed to determine which of these interventions should receive the greatest emphasis in routine clinical practice.
2. Studies examining the cost-effectiveness of making an outpatient practice breastfeeding friendly are needed.

3. Additional research is needed on the effect of prenatal breastfeeding interventions on multiple populations, such as women of different socioeconomic status and cultural backgrounds. For instance, outcomes of father and partner studies vary significantly by geography; the sociocultural factors affecting the impact of these interventions deserve attention.
4. Studies are needed examining the role of technology (electronic medical record, mobile texting, online resources and groups, etc.) in improving the breastfeeding outcomes and experiences of women.
5. Many studies have been published in the past 5 years on prenatal interventions with substantial success. Translational research investigating implementation and advocacy among healthcare organizations, community organizations, and political systems should be undertaken.

ACKNOWLEDGMENTS

This work was supported in part by a grant from the Maternal and Child Health Bureau, U.S. Department of Health and Human Services.

REFERENCES

1. Eidelman A, Schanler R. AAP executive summary: Breastfeeding and the use of human milk. *Pediatrics.* 2012;129:600–603.
2. AAFP Breastfeeding Advisory Committee. Position paper: Breastfeeding, family physicians supporting. Updated 2014. Available at: www.aafp.org/about/policies/all/breastfeedingsupport.html (accessed November 2, 2015).
3. Ip S, Chung M, Raman G, et al. Breastfeeding and maternal and infant health outcomes in developed countries. *Evid Rep Technol Assess (Full Rep).* 2007;153:1–186.
4. Horta B, Victora C. *Long-Term Effects of Breastfeeding: A Systematic Review.* Geneva: World Health Organization; 2013.
5. Izatt SD. Breastfeeding counseling by health care providers. *J Hum Lact.* 1997;13:109–113.
6. Gurka KK, Hornsby PP, Drake E, et al. Exploring intended infant feeding decisions among low-income women. *Breastfeed Med.* 2014;9:377–384.
7. Wambach KA, Aaronson L, Breedlove G, et al. A randomized controlled trial of breastfeeding support and education for adolescent mothers. *West J Nurs Res.* 2011;33:486–505.
8. Guise JM, Palda V, Westhoff C, et al. The effectiveness of primary care-based interventions to promote breastfeeding: Systematic evidence review and meta-analysis for the US Preventive Services Task Force. *Ann Fam Med.* 2003;1:70–78.
9. Grawey AE, Marinelli KA, Holmes AV. ABM clinical protocol #14: Breastfeeding-friendly physician's office: Optimizing care for infants and children, revised 2013. *Breastfeed Med.* 2013;8:237–242.
10. Mansbach IK, Palti H, Pevsner B, et al. Advice from the obstetrician and other sources: Do they affect women's breast feeding practices? A study among different Jewish groups in Jerusalem. *Soc Sci Med.* 1984;19:157–162.
11. Hannula L, Kaunonen M, Tarkka MT. A systematic review of professional support interventions for breastfeeding. *J Clin Nurs.* 2008;17:1132–1143.

12. Lu MC, Lange L, Slusser W, et al. Provider encouragement of breast-feeding: Evidence from a national survey. *Obstet Gynecol*. 2001;97:290–295.

13. Taveras EM, Li R, Grummer-Strawn L, et al. Opinions and practices of clinicians associated with continuation of exclusive breastfeeding. *Pediatrics*. 2004;113:e283–e290.

14. Taveras EM, Capra AM, Braveman PA, et al. Clinician support and psychosocial risk factors associated with breastfeeding discontinuation. *Pediatrics*. 2003;112:108–115.

15. Mekuria G, Edris M. Exclusive breastfeeding and associated factors among mothers in Debre Markos, Northwest Ethiopia: A cross-sectional study. *Int Breastfeed J*. 2015;10:1.

16. Jahan K, Roy SK, Mirshahi S, et al. Short-term nutrition education reduces low birthweight and improves pregnancy outcomes among urban poor women in Bangladesh. *Food Nutr Bull*. 2014;35:414–421.

17. Cross-Barnet C, Augustyn M, Gross S, et al. Long-term breastfeeding support: Failing mothers in need. *Matern Child Health J*. 2012;16:1926–1932.

18. Pound CM, Williams K, Grenon R, et al. Breastfeeding knowledge, confidence, beliefs, and attitudes of Canadian physicians. *J Hum Lact*. 2014;30:298–309.

19. Demirci JR, Bogen DL, Holland C, et al. Characteristics of breastfeeding discussions at the initial prenatal visit. *Obstet Gynecol*. 2013;122:1263–1270.

20. Archabald K, Lundsberg L, Triche E, et al. Women's prenatal concerns regarding breastfeeding: Are they being addressed? *J Midwifery Womens Health*. 2011;56:2–7.

21. Szucs KA, Miracle DJ, Rosenman MB. Breastfeeding knowledge, attitudes, and practices among providers in a medical home. *Breastfeed Med*. 2009;4:31–42.

22. Miracle DJ, Fredland V. Provider encouragement of breast-feeding: Efficacy and ethics. *J Midwifery Womens Health*. 2007;52:545–548.

23. Dusdieker LB, Dungy CI, Losch ME. Prenatal office practices regarding infant feeding choices. *Clin Pediatr (Phila)*. 2006;45:841–845.

24. Taveras EM, Li R, Grummer-Strawn L, et al. Mothers' and clinicians' perspectives on breastfeeding counseling during routine preventive visits. *Pediatrics*. 2004;113: e405–e411.

25. Wong KL, Tarrant M, Lok KY. Group versus individual professional antenatal breastfeeding education for extending breastfeeding duration and exclusivity: A systematic review. *J Hum Lact*. 2015;31:354–366.

26. de Oliveira MI, Camacho LA, Tedstone AE. Extending breastfeeding duration through primary care: A systematic review of prenatal and postnatal interventions. *J Hum Lact*. 2001;17:326–343.

27. Renfrew MJ, McCormick FM, Wade A, et al. Support for healthy breastfeeding mothers with healthy term babies. *Cochrane Database Syst Rev*. 2012;5:CD001141.

28. Appendix A Task Force Ratings. Guide to clinical preventive services: Report of the U.S. Preventive Services Task Force, 2nd ed. Available at: www.ncbi.nlm.nih.gov/books/NBK15430/ (accessed November 2, 2015).

29. Howard C, Howard F, Lawrence R, et al. Office prenatal formula advertising and its effect on breast-feeding patterns. *Obstet Gynecol*. 2000;95:296–303.

30. Donnelly A, Snowden HM, Renfrew MJ, et al. Commercial hospital discharge packs for breastfeeding women. *Cochrane Database Syst Rev*. 2000;(2)CD002075.

31. Rosenberg KD, Eastham CA, Kasehagen LJ, et al. Marketing infant formula through hospitals: The impact of commercial hospital discharge packs on breastfeeding. *Am J Public Health*. 2008;98:290–295.

32. Feldman-Winter L, Grossman X, Palaniappan A, et al. Removal of industry-sponsored formula sample packs from the hospital: Does it make a difference? *J Hum Lact*. 2012;28:380–388.

33. World Health Organization. International Code of Marketing of Breast-milk Substitutes, 1981, Resolution WHA34. 22. Available at: www.who.int/nutrition/publications/code_english.pdf (accessed September 10, 2015).

34. Memon ZA, Khan GN, Soofi SB, et al. Impact of a community-based perinatal and newborn preventive care package on perinatal and neonatal mortality in a remote mountainous district in Northern Pakistan. *BMC Pregnancy Childbirth*. 2015;15:106.

35. Brunton G, O'Mara-Eves A, Thomas J. The 'active ingredients' for successful community engagement with disadvantaged expectant and new mothers: A qualitative comparative analysis. *J Adv Nurs*. 2014;70:2847–2860.

36. Lassi ZS, Das JK, Salam RA, et al. Evidence from community level inputs to improve quality of care for maternal and newborn health: Interventions and findings. *Reprod Health*. 2014;11(Suppl 2):S2.

37. Bentley ME, Caulfield LE, Gross SM, et al. Sources of influence on intention to breastfeed among African-American women at entry to WIC. *J Hum Lact*. 1999;15(1):27–34.

38. Muhajarine N, Ng J, Bowen A, et al. Understanding the impact of the Canada Prenatal Nutrition Program: A quantitative evaluation. *Can J Public Health*. 2012;103(7 Suppl 1): eS26–eS31.

39. Edwards RC, Thullen MJ, Korfmacher J, et al. Breastfeeding and complementary food: Randomized trial of community doula home visiting. *Pediatrics*. 2013;132(Suppl 2):S160–S166.

40. Khan AI, Hawkesworth S, Ekstrom EC, et al. Effects of exclusive breastfeeding intervention on child growth and body composition: The MINIMat trial, Bangladesh. *Acta Paediatr*. 2013;102:815–823.

41. Karp SM, Howe-Heyman A, Dietrich MS, et al. Breastfeeding initiation in the context of a home intervention to promote better birth outcomes. *Breastfeed Med*. 2013;8:381–387.

42. Kirkwood BR, Manu A, ten Asbroek AH, et al. Effect of the Newhints home-visits intervention on neonatal mortality rate and care practices in Ghana: A cluster randomised controlled trial. *Lancet*. 2013;381:2184–2192.

43. Ochola SA, Labadarios D, Nduati RW. Impact of counselling on exclusive breast-feeding practices in a poor urban setting in Kenya: A randomized controlled trial. *Public Health Nutr*. 2013;16:1732–1740.

44. Gogia S, Sachdev HS. Home visits by community health workers to prevent neonatal deaths in developing countries: A systematic review. *Bull World Health Organ*. 2010;88:658–666B.

45. Ingram J, Johnson D. Using community maternity care assistants to facilitate family-focused breastfeeding support. *Matern Child Nutr*. 2009;5:276–281.

46. Sandy JM, Anisfeld E, Ramirez E. Effects of a prenatal intervention on breastfeeding initiation rates in a Latina immigrant sample. *J Hum Lact*. 2009;25:404–411.

47. Apostolakis-Kyrus K, Valentine C, DeFranco E. Factors associated with breastfeeding initiation in adolescent mothers. *J Pediatr*. 2013;163:1489–1494.

48. Kraft JM, Wilkins KG, Morales GJ, et al. An evidence review of gender integrated interventions in reproductive and maternal-child health. *J Health Commun.* 2014;19 (Suppl 1):122–141.

49. Chapman DJ, Perez-Escamilla R. Breastfeeding among minority women: Moving from risk factors to interventions. *Adv Nutr.* 2012;3:95–104.

50. Inoue M, Binns CW, Otsuka K, et al. Infant feeding practices and breastfeeding duration in Japan: A review. *Int Breastfeed J.* 2012;7:15.

51. Clifford J, McIntyre E. Who supports breastfeeding? *Breastfeed Rev.* 2008;16:9–19.

52. Schlickau JM. *Prenatal Breastfeeding Education: An Intervention for Pregnant Immigrant Hispanic Women.* Lincoln, NE: University of Nebraska Medical Center; 2005.

53. Bevan G, Brown M. Interventions in exclusive breastfeeding: A systematic review. *Br J Nurs.* 2014;23:86–89.

54. Meedya S, Fahy K, Kable A. Factors that positively influence breastfeeding duration to 6 months: A literature review. *Women Birth.* 2010;23:135–145.

55. Otsuka K, Dennis CL, Tatsuoka H, et al. The relationship between breastfeeding self-efficacy and perceived insufficient milk among Japanese mothers. *J Obstet Gynecol Neonatal Nurs.* 2008;37:546–555.

56. Blyth R, Creedy DK, Dennis CL, et al. Effect of maternal confidence on breastfeeding duration: An application of breastfeeding self-efficacy theory. *Birth.* 2002;29:278–284.

57. Hundalani SG, Irigoyen M, Braitman LE, et al. Breastfeeding among inner-city women: From intention before delivery to breastfeeding at hospital discharge. *Breastfeed Med.* 2013;8:68–72.

58. Sikander S, Maselko J, Zafar S, et al. Cognitive-behavioral counseling for exclusive breastfeeding in rural pediatrics: A cluster RCT. *Pediatrics.* 2015;135:e424–e431.

59. Hildebrand DA, McCarthy P, Tipton D, et al. Innovative use of influential prenatal counseling may improve breastfeeding initiation rates among WIC participants. *J Nutr Educ Behav.* 2014;46:458–466.

60. Otsuka K, Taguri M, Dennis CL, et al. Effectiveness of a breast feeding self-efficacy intervention: Do hospital practices make a difference? *Matern Child Health J.* 2014;18:296–306.

61. Nichols J, Schutte NS, Brown RF, et al. The impact of a self-efficacy intervention on short-term breast-feeding outcomes. *Health Educ Behav.* 2009;36:250–258.

62. Olenick P. *The Effect of Structured Group Prenatal Education on Breastfeeding Confidence, Duration and Exclusivity to Twelve Weeks Postpartum [PhD thesis].* Toronto: Toronto University International; 2006.

63. Kronborg H, Maimburg RD, Vaeth M. Antenatal training to improve breast feeding: A randomised trial. *Midwifery.* 2012;28:784–790.

64. Best Start Social Marketing. Using Loving Support to Implement Best Practices in Peer Counseling. Updated 2004. Available at: www.nal.usda.gov/wicworks/Learning_Center/research_brief.pdf (accessed July 3, 2015).

65. Hartley BM, O'Connor ME. Evaluation of the 'Best Start' breast-feeding education program. *Arch Pediatr Adolesc Med.* 1996;150:868–871.

66. Martin A, Horowitz C, Balbierz A, et al. Views of women and clinicians on postpartum preparation and recovery. *Matern Child Health J.* 2014;18:707–713.

67. Howell EA, Bodnar-Deren S, Balbierz A, et al. An intervention to extend breastfeeding among black and Latina mothers after delivery. *Am J Obstet Gynecol.* 2014;210:239–248.

68. Dean SV, Lassi ZS, Imam AM, et al. Preconception care: Closing the gap in the continuum of care to accelerate improvements in maternal, newborn and child health. *Reprod Health.* 2014;11(Suppl 3):S1.

69. Andaya E, Bonuck K, Barnett J, et al. Perceptions of primary care-based breastfeeding promotion interventions: Qualitative analysis of randomized controlled trial participant interviews. *Breastfeed Med.* 2012;7:417–422.

70. Bonuck K, Stuebe A, Barnett J, et al. Effect of primary care intervention on breastfeeding duration and intensity. *Am J Public Health.* 2014;104(Suppl 1):S119–S127.

71. Committee on Health Care for Underserved Women, American College of Obstetricians and Gynecologists. ACOG committee opinion no. 361: Breastfeeding: Maternal and infant aspects. *Obstet Gynecol.* 2007;109:479–480.

72. Hartman S, Barnett J, Bonuck K. Implementing international board-certified lactation consultants intervention into routine care: Barriers and recommendations. *Clin Lact.* 2012;3–4:131–137.

73. Ickovicks JR, Kershaw TS, Westdahl C. Group prenatal care and perinatal outcomes: A randomized, controlled trial. *Obstet Gynecol.* 2007;110:330–339.

74. Tanner-Smith E, Steinka-Fry K, Lipsey M. Effects of Centering Pregnancy group prenatal care on breastfeeding outcomes. *J Midwifery Womens Health.* 2013;58:389–395.

75. Giglia R, Binns C. The effectiveness of the internet in improving breastfeeding outcomes: A systematic review. *J Hum Lact.* 2014;30:156–160.

76. Gallegos D, Russell-Bennett R, Previte J, et al. Can a text message a week improve breastfeeding? *BMC Pregnancy Childbirth.* 2014;14:374.

77. Flax VL, Negerie M, Ibrahim AU, et al. Integrating group counseling, cell phone messaging, and participant generated songs and dramas into a microcredit program increases Nigerian women's adherence to international breastfeeding recommendations. *J Nutr.* 2014;144:1120–1124.

78. American Academy of Pediatrics, American College of Obstetricians and Gynecologists. *Breastfeeding Handbook for Physicians.* 2nd ed. Elk Grove Village, IL: American Academy of Pediatrics; 2013:337.

79. Issler H, de Sa MB, Senna DM. Knowledge of new born health care among pregnant women: Basis for promotional and educational programs on breastfeeding. *Sao Paulo Med J.* 2001;119:7–9.

80. Humenick SS, Hill PD, Spiegelberg PL. Breastfeeding and health professional encouragement. *J Hum Lact.* 1998;14:305–310.

81. Lu MC, Lange L, Slusser W, et al. Provider encouragement of breast-feeding: Evidence from a national survey. *Obstet Gynecol.* 2001;97:290–295.

82. Ingram J, Johnson D. A feasibility study of an intervention to enhance family support for breast feeding in a deprived area in Bristol, UK. *Midwifery.* 2004;20:367–379.

83. Martin J, MacDonald-Wicks L, Hure A, et al. Reducing postpartum weight retention and improving breastfeeding outcomes in overweight women: A pilot randomised controlled trial. *Nutrients.* 2015;7:1464–1479.

84. Chapman DJ, Morel K, Bermudez-Millan A, et al. Breastfeeding education and support trial for overweight and obese women: A randomized trial. *Pediatrics*. 2013;131: e162–e170.

85. Pitcock N. *Evaluation of an Initiative to Increase Rates of Exclusive Breastfeeding Among Rural Hispanic Immigrant Women [PhD thesis]*. Charlottesville, VA: University of Virginia; 2013.

86. Reifsnider E, Eckhart D. Prenatal breastfeeding education: Its effect on breastfeeding among WIC participants. *J Hum Lact*. 1997;13:121–125.

87. Wong KL, Fong DY, Lee IL, et al. Antenatal education to increase exclusive breastfeeding: A randomized controlled trial. *Obstet Gynecol*. 2014;124:961–968.

88. Lumbiganon P, Martis R, Laopaiboon M, et al. Antenatal breastfeeding education for increasing breastfeeding duration. *Cochrane Database Syst Rev*. 2012;9:CD006425.

89. Chapman DJ, Damio G, Perez-Escamilla R. Differential response to breastfeeding peer counseling within a low-income, predominantly Latina population. *J Hum Lact*. 2004;20:389–396.

90. Chapman DJ, Damio G, Young S, et al. Effectiveness of breastfeeding peer counseling in a low-income, predominantly Latina population: A randomized controlled trial. *Arch Pediatr Adolesc Med*. 2004;158:897–902.

91. Hodnett ED, Gates S, Hofmeyr GJ, et al. Continuous support for women during childbirth. *Cochrane Database Syst Rev*. 2013;7:CD003766.

92. Duffy EP, Percival P, Kershaw E. Positive effects of an antenatal group teaching session on postnatal nipple pain, nipple trauma and breast feeding rates. *Midwifery*. 1997;13:189–196.

93. Holmes AV, McLeod AY, Bunik M. ABM clinical protocol#5: Peripartum breastfeeding management for the healthy mother and infant at term, revision 2013. *Breastfeed Med*. 2013;8:469–473.

94. American College of Obstetricians and Gynecologists. Committee opinion: Breastfeeding in underserved women: Increasing initiation and continuation of breastfeeding. *Obstet Gynecol*. 2013;122:423–428.

95. Montgomery A, Hale TW, Academy of Breastfeeding Medicine. ABM clinical protocol #15: Analgesia and anesthesia for the breastfeeding mother, revised 2012. *Breastfeed Med*. 2012;7:547–553.

96. Thukral A, Sankar MJ, Agarwal R, et al. Early skin-to-skin contact and breast-feeding behavior in term neonates: A randomized controlled trial. *Neonatology*. 2012;102:114–119.

97. Hung KJ, Berg O. Early skin-to-skin after cesarean to improve breastfeeding. *MCN Am J Matern Child Nurs*. 2011;36:318–324.

98. Mahmood I, Jamal M, Khan N. Effect of mother-infant early skin-to-skin contact on breastfeeding status: A randomized controlled trial. *J Coll Physicians Surg Pak*. 2011;21:601–605.

99. Henderson A. Understanding the breast crawl: Implications for nursing practice. *Nurs Womens Health*. 2011;15:296–307.

100. Klaus M. Mother and infant: Early emotional ties. *Pediatrics*. 1998;102(5 Suppl E):1244–1246.

101. Loh NR, Kelleher CC, Long S, et al. Can we increase breast feeding rates? *Ir Med J*. 1997;90:100–101.

ABM protocols expire 5 years from the date of publication. Evidence-based revisions are made within 5 years or sooner, if there are significant changes in the evidence.

The Academy of Breastfeeding Medicine Protocol Committee:
Kathleen A. Marinelli, MD, FABM, Chairperson
Maya Bunik, MD, MSPH, FABM, Co-chairperson
Larry Noble, MD, FAMB, Protocols Committee
Translations Chairperson
Nancy Brent, MD
Cadey Harrel, MD
Ruth A. Lawrence, MD, FABM
Kate Naylor, MBBS, FRACGP
Sarah Reece-Stremtan, MD
Casey Rosen-Carole, MD, MPH
Tomoko Seo, MD, FABM
Rose St. Fleur, MD
Michal Young, MD
For correspondence: abm@bfmed.org

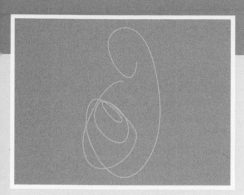

ABM Clinical Protocol #20
Engorgement, Revised 2016

Pamela Berens[1], Wendy Brodribb[2] and the Academy of Breastfeeding Medicine*

ABSTRACT

A central goal of The Academy of Breastfeeding Medicine is the development of clinical protocols for managing common medical problems that may impact breastfeeding success. These protocols serve only as guidelines for the care of breastfeeding mothers and infants and do not delineate an exclusive course of treatment or serve as standards of medical care. Variations in treatment may be appropriate according to the needs of an individual patient.

PURPOSE

The Purpose of this protocol is to evaluate the state of evidence as to the prevention, recognition, and management of breast engorgement to encourage successful breastfeeding.

BACKGROUND

Engorgement has been defined as "the swelling and distension of the breasts, usually in the early days of initiation of lactation, caused by vascular dilation as well as the arrival of the early milk."[1] The concept put forward by Newton and Newton[2] in 1951 suggested that alveolar distension from milk then led to compression of surrounding ducts, which subsequently led to secondary vascular and lymphatic compression. Some degree of breast fullness in the second stage of lactogenesis (secretory activation)[3] is considered physiologic and should be reassuring for the mother and healthcare provider that milk is present. A recent study suggested considering distinguishing between "breast engorgement" and "breast edema" although both may cause significant issues for mothers and infants in the postpartum period.[4] (II-2) (Quality of evidence [Levels of evidence I, II-1, II-2, II-3, and III] is based on the U.S. Preventive Services[5] Task Force

Appendix A Task Force Ratings and is noted in parentheses.) Breast edema is fluid accumulation in the interstitial space caused by generalized fluid accumulation late in pregnancy or as a result of large amounts of intravenous fluids during labor and may be responsible for edema around the areola and nipple.[6,7] (III, III).

Engorgement symptoms occur most commonly between days 3 and 5 postpartum, with more than two-thirds of women experiencing tenderness by day 5, but the onset may be as late as days 9–10.[4,8,9] (II-2, III) In the 2008 Infant Feeding Practices Survey, 36.6% of women reported overly full breasts within the first 2 weeks postpartum,[10] while other studies indicate that up to two-thirds of women experience at least moderate symptoms of engorgement.[9,11] (III) The incidence of engorgement may depend on breastfeeding management within the first few days following birth. Engorgement occurs less commonly when infants spend more time breastfeeding in the first 48 hours[12] (III) and when mother and infant are rooming in. One difficulty when evaluating incidence and treatment options for this condition involves the spectrum of engorgement, from expected physiologic breast fullness through to severely symptomatic engorgement. In addition, more optimal lactation management and support that are available in some healthcare facilities may reduce the frequency of significant symptoms compared to less supportive environments.

ASSESSMENT OF ENGORGEMENT

Tools

No standardized reliable tool for assessing breast engorgement has yet been established. Various methods of subjectively rating engorgement have been utilized, such as visual descriptions, cup size, hardness or firmness scales, skin tension measurements, and thermography, but none has become clinically useful.[2,9,13–16]

Predictors

1. The onset of lactogenesis II (secretory activation) occurs sooner in multiparous compared to primiparous women[17,18] (II-2, II-2) and tends to resolve more rapidly than in primiparous women.[9,19] (II-2)

[1] Department of Obstetrics and Gynecology, University of Texas Health Sciences Center at Houston, Houston, Texas.

[2] Discipline of General Practice, University of Queensland, Brisbane, Australia.

* Courtesy of the Academy of Breastfeeding Medicine. Please go to https://www.bfmed.org/protocols for complete protocols, translations, and the most up-to-date information (protocols are updated every 5–7 years).

2. In one study, women who underwent cesarean section typically experienced peak engorgement 24—48 hours later than those who gave birth vaginally.[12] Women in this study also initiated breastfeeding significantly later than their vaginally delivered counterparts and the impact of this delay has not been adequately explored. This finding appears consistent with other research that has found that a cesarean birth may correlate with a higher likelihood of delayed onset of lactogenesis.[17,18]

3. Large amounts of intravenous fluids given during labor appear to be associated with an earlier and more prolonged maternal perception of breast fullness and tenderness as well as increased levels of breast edema extending beyond day 9 postpartum.[4]

4. One study suggests that women who experience premenstrual breast tenderness and engorgement may be more likely to develop more severe engorgement postpartum.[20] (II-2)

5. It is not uncommon for women who have undergone any breast surgery or lumpectomy to experience engorgement, and so, they should be given anticipatory guidance regarding these potential complications.[21,22] (III, III)

6. The influence of length of labor, premature delivery, and anesthetic options remain unclear.[23—25] (III, III, III)

Differential diagnosis

Differentiating engorgement from these other causes of breast swelling is key.

1. Mastitis. Engorgement may be associated with a slight elevation of maternal temperature, but significant fever, especially when associated with breast erythema and systemic symptoms such as myalgias, suggests the diagnosis of mastitis. Typically, mastitis affects only one breast with a segmental pattern of redness.[26] Engorgement is usually diffuse, bilateral, and not associated with breast erythema.[1]

2. Gigantomastia. Gigantomastia is a diffuse bilateral process that occurs very rarely and does not typically present in the postpartum period. The reported incidence is ~1:100,000, but some feel that it is more common with a rate as high as 1:8,000.[27] It is usually regarded as bilateral, benign but progressive massive breast enlargement to an extent that respiratory depression or tissue necrosis may occur. Infection and sepsis may result. Histologic findings suggest marked lobular hypertrophy and ductal proliferation. No clear etiology for this condition has been elicited, although hormonal changes may be involved.[27—30]

PREVENTION AND TREATMENT

Prevention

There has been a great deal of research into medical therapies to suppress lactation, but limited research into prevention and treatment strategies for lactating women who may develop engorgement. Focused education given to mothers regarding breastfeeding positioning and attachment has shown no difference in subsequent incidence of engorgement.[31,32] (III, III) However, some breastfeeding techniques have been specifically associated with less engorgement, including emptying one breast at each feeding and alternating which breast is offered first.[33,34] (II-1, II-2) Limited evidence suggests breast massage after feeds performed for the first 4 days postpartum may reduce the extent of engorgement.[32] Although it appears that, in observational studies, frequent, effective feeding patterns help prevent engorgement,[12] this management option has not been studied in detail.[33] One recent study found a reduction in engorgement in women who expressed colostrum once or twice for 25—30 minutes in the first 1—2 days (vaginal birth) or 2—3 days (cesarean birth) postpartum. Infants of the women in this study did not have free access to the breast and were limited to six to eight breastfeeds per day.[20] However, these findings do suggest that early and frequent breast emptying in this population may prevent engorgement.

Treatment

While one study found an increase in milk production on day 4 for primiparous women with marked engorgement,[19] adequate management of engorgement is important for successful long-term lactation.[35,36] (III, III) Experiencing engorgement is temporarily uncomfortable for mothers and appears to be associated with an increase in the likelihood of early weaning.[37] (III) Failure to effectively resolve prolonged symptomatic engorgement may also have a negative impact on continued production of an adequate milk supply. Suckling problems in the infant should be considered at the same time. Moreover, pain control is an important consideration in managing a woman with symptomatic engorgement.

Both pharmacologic and nonpharmacologic therapies have been considered to be beneficial for the treatment of engorgement. A Cochrane Systematic Review of both randomized and quasirandomized controlled studies assessing the effectiveness of treatments for breast engorgement was done by Mangesi and Dowswell in 2010.[38] (I) This analysis identified eight studies, including 744 women who evaluated acupuncture, cabbage leaves, protease complex, therapeutic ultrasound, oxytocin (subcutaneous), and cold packs. Meta-analyses could not be performed because of the differences in the study designs. Overall, the authors concluded that there was insufficient evidence to recommend any particular treatment regimen.[38] However, they did find the following.

1. Acupuncture resulted in significantly fewer women having engorgement symptoms on day 4 and 5, but not day 6 postpartum.

2. Although the study investigating cold packs found a reduction in pain intensity in the intervention group, problems with the study design make results difficult to interpret.

3. Enzyme therapy using a protease complex enteric-coated tablet containing 20,000 of bromelain and 2,500 U of crystalline trypsin, another anti-inflammatory agent

taken orally, was compared to a placebo. However, this study is now 50 years old and it is not certain that the preparation is in general use.[39] (I)

4. Treatments such as cabbage leaves may be soothing, are inexpensive, and are unlikely to be harmful although evidence for their use is not conclusive.

5. For many treatments (ultrasound, cabbage leaves, and oxytocin), the interventions did not result in more rapid resolution of symptoms than occurred in the comparison groups (engorgement symptoms often resolve over time).

Another later systematic review conducted by the Joanna Briggs Institute[40] (I) specifically looked at the effect of the application of cabbage leaves on engorgement and found that, although women who used cabbage leaves had a reduction in pain scores, there was not sufficient evidence to indicate that they were more effective than other treatments for reduction in engorgement.[40] Researchers continue to explore the effect of cabbage leaves.[41] (I) In Japan, grated potatoes are used for the same purpose, although there is no evidence for its use. (III)

It may be that some treatments help a mother's discomfort without relieving the actual engorgement but could still have an effect on preventing early weaning.

Other treatment considerations

1. Breast massage. Two studies of trials of different types of breast massage, Gua-Sha Therapy[42] (I) and Oketani breast massage[43] (II-2), compared to conventional breast massage in control groups found that there was a reduction in pain, engorgement, and discomfort in the control and intervention groups in both studies, but the intervention groups had a significantly greater reduction in symptoms.

Another observational study performed in breastfeeding women with symptomatic pain, engorgement, plugged ducts, or mastitis evaluated therapeutic breast massage during lactation (TBML) by a trained provider combined with consultation with a lactation professional. TBML included an average of 30 minutes (range 15–60 minutes) of gentle breast massage toward the axilla alternating with hand expression. Breast pain, tenderness, and engorgement severity were significantly reduced following treatment. Periareolar swelling decreased from 93% to 7% ($p < 0.001$) and engorgement severity using the 6-point Humenick scale decreased from 5.31 before treatment to 3.48 after TBML.[34]

1. Herbal remedies. At the present time, herbal remedies for breast engorgement and oversupply have been described, but evidence regarding their effectiveness is limited. One randomized trial of the application of Hollyhock compresses in conjunction with hot and cold compresses found a significant reduction in engorgement severity compared to hot and cold compresses alone.[44] (II-I)

2. Hot and cold packs. A number of intervention trials have used the application of warm/hot packs before a breastfeed[42] and cold packs following a breastfeed in their control groups. These studies found a reduction in engorgement symptoms in both the control and intervention groups suggesting that hot and cold packs may be as effective as other treatments.[42–45] (II-3) There are no trials that compared hot and cold packs with no treatment.

3. Hand expression or pumping. If the infant cannot successfully attach to the breast or breastfeed, measures should be undertaken to assist the mother with milk expression for a few minutes to allow sufficient softening of the breast so that the infant can latch well. If the infant cannot breastfeed, the milk may be given to the infant by cup, spoon, or other suitable method, and the mother should be encouraged to breastfeed more frequently before the recurrence of severe breast engorgement. All new mothers should be instructed in the technique of hand breast expression.[46] Handpumps should not be introduced unnecessarily at this point in time.

4. The reverse pressure softening technique is especially useful for breast edema and uses gentle positive pressure to soften an area ($\sim$ 3–4 cm [1–2 inches]) near the areola surrounding the base of the nipple. The goal is to temporarily move some swelling slightly backward and upward into the breast. Moving the edema away from the areola has been shown to improve the latch of the infant during engorgement.[6] The physiologic basis for this technique is the presence of increased resistance in the subareolar tissues during engorgement.

5. Anticipatory guidance regarding the occurrence of breast engorgement should be given to all breastfeeding mothers before birth center or hospital discharge. In countries where women may have longer hospital stays, engorgement may occur in the birth hospital. However, many women are discharged before the expected time of peak symptomatic engorgement. Mothers should be counselled about symptomatic treatment options for pain control. Acetaminophen (or paracetamol) and ibuprofen are both safe options for breastfeeding mothers to take in appropriate doses. In addition, contact information for breastfeeding supportive advice should be provided. Healthcare personnel seeing either the newborn or mother after discharge should routinely inquire about breast fullness and engorgement.

RECOMMENDATIONS FOR FUTURE RESEARCH

Currently, there is inadequate research into both the physiologic process of engorgement and effective prevention and treatment strategies.

- A uniform measurement system for the severity of the engorgement should be developed to allow standardized measures and comparison of results among studies.
- Once an objective noninvasive bedside measure of breast engorgement has been developed, then clinical trials

correlating objective measures of engorgement and treatment of engorgement and the subsequent effect on breastfeeding duration and problems can be conducted.

- Knowledge about the influence of labor interventions and patient characteristics predisposing to the development of significant engorgement would be useful in identifying patients at risk for engorgement and those who could benefit from counseling, surveillance, and a closer follow-up.
- More evidence-based investigation of nonpharmacologic remedies for the management of engorgement is needed because these tend to be popular especially in non-US sites.
- Double-blinded placebo controlled studies of medications known to be safe during lactation and with the potential to relieve symptomatic engorgement should be prioritized.

REFERENCES

1. Lawrence RA, Lawrence RM. Practical management of the mother-infant nursing couple. In: Lawrence RA, Lawrence RM, eds. *Breastfeeding: A Guide for the Medical Profession*. 8th ed Philadelphia: Elsevier; 2015:250–252.
2. Newton M, Newton N. Postpartum engorgement of the breast. *Am J Obstet Gynecol*. 1951;61:664–667.
3. Pang WW, Hartmann PE. Initiation of human lactation: Secretory differentiation and secretory activation. *J Mammary Gland Biol Neoplasia*. 2007;12:211–221.
4. Kujawa-Myles S, Noel-Weiss J, Dunn S, et al. Maternal intravenous fluids and postpartum breast changes: A pilot observational study. *Int Breastfeed J*. 2015;10:18.
5. Guide to Clinical Preventive Services, 2nd ed.; Report of the U.S. Preventive Services Task Force. US Preventive Services Task Force Washington (DC). US Department of Health and Human Services. 1996. Available at: www.ncbi.nlm.nih.gov/books/NBK15430 (accessed January 4, 2016).
6. Cotterman KJ. Reverse pressure softening: A simple tool to prepare areola for easier latching during engorgement. *J Hum Lact*. 2004;20:227–237.
7. Miller V, Riordan J. Treating postpartum breast edema with areolar compression. *J Hum Lact*. 2004;20:223–226.
8. Swift K, Janke J. Breast binding.is it all that it's wrapped up to be? *J Obstet Gynecol Neonatal Nurs*. 2003;32:332–339.
9. Hill PD, Humenick S. The occurrence of breast engorgement. *J Hum Lact*. 1994;10:79–86.
10. DNPAO. National Centre for Chronic Disease Prevention and Health Promotion. Infant feeding practices survey II: Results. 2009. Available at: www.cdc.gov/ifps/results/ch2/table2-38.htm (accessed January 4, 2016).
11. Spitz A, Lee N, Peterson H. Treatment of lactation suppression: Little progress in one hundred years. *Am J Obstet Gynecol*. 1998;179:1485–1490.
12. Moon J, Humenick S. Engorgement: Contributing variables and variables amenable to nursing intervention. *J Obstet Gynecol Neonatal Nurs*. 1989;18:309–315.
13. Humenick S, Hill PD, Anderson M. Breast engorgement: Patterns and selected outcomes. *J Hum Lact*. 1994;10:87–93.
14. Neifert MR, DeMarzo S, Seacat JM, et al. The influence of breast surgery, breast appearance, and pregnancy-induced breast changes on lactation sufficiency as measured by infant weight gain. *Birth*. 1990;17:31–38.
15. Heberle A, de Moura M, de Souza M, et al. Assessment of techniques of massage and pumping in the treatment of breast engorgement by thermography. *Rev Lat Am Enfermagem*. 2014;22:277–285.
16. Ferris C. Hand-held instrument for evaluation of breast engorgement. *Biomed Sci Instrum*. 1996;32:299–304.
17. Dewey KG, Nommsen-Rivers LA, Heinig MJ, et al. Risk factors for suboptimal infant breastfeeding behavior, delayed onset of lactation, and excess neonatal weight loss. *Pediatrics*. 2003;112:607–619.
18. Scott J, Binns C, Oddy W. Predictors of delayed onset of lactation. *Matern Child Nutr*. 2007;3:186–193.
19. Bystrova K, Widstrom A-M, Matthiesen A-S, et al. Early lactation performance in primiparous and multiparous women in relation to different maternity home practices. A randomised trial in St. Petersburg. *Int Breastfeed J*. 2007;2:9.
20. Alekseev N, Vladimir I, Nadezhada T. Pathological postpartum breast engorgement: Prediction, prevention and resolution. *Breastfeed Med*. 2015;10:203–208.
21. Brzozowski D, Niessen M, Evans H, et al. Breast-feeding after inferior pedicle reduction mammoplasty. *Plast Reconstr Surg*. 2000;105:530–534.
22. Acarturk S, Gencel E, Tuncer I. An uncommon complication of secondary augmentation mammoplasty: Bilaterally massive engorgement of breasts after pregnancy attributable to postinfection and blockage of mammary ducts. *Aesthetic Plast Surg*. 2005;29:274–279.
23. Lurie S, Rotmensch N, Glezerman M. Breast engorgement and galactorrhea during magnesium sulfate treatment for preterm labor. *Am J Perinatol*. 2002;19:239–240.
24. Shalev J, Frankel Y, Eshkol A, et al. Breast engorgement and galactorrhea after preventing premature contractions with ritodrine. *Gynecol Obstet Invest*. 1983;17:190–193.
25. Hardwick-Smith S, Mastrobattista J, Nader S. Breast engorgement and lactation associated with thyroid-releasing hormone administration. *Obstet Gynecol*. 1998;92:717.
26. Amir L. Academy of Breastfeeding Medicine. ABM Clinical Protocol #4: Mastitis, Revised March 2014. *Breastfeed Med*. 2014;9:239–243.
27. Antevski B, Smilevski D, Stojovski M, et al. Extreme gigantomastia in pregnancy: Case report and review of literature. *Arch Gynecol Obstet*. 2007;275:149–153.
28. Antevski B, Jovkovski O, Filipovski V, et al. Extreme gigantomastia in pregnancy: Case report—my experience with two cases in last 5 years. *Arch Gynecol Obstet*. 2011;284:575–578.
29. Rezai S, Nakagawa J, Tedesco J, et al. Gestational gigantomastia complicating pregnancy: A case report and review of the literature. *Case Rep Obstet Gynecol*. 2015;2015:892369.
30. Swelstad M, Swelstad B, Rao V, et al. Management of gestation gigantomastia. *Plast Reconstr Surg*. 2006;118:840–848.
31. de Oliveira L, Giugliani E, do Espírito Santo L, et al. Effect of intervention to improve breastfeeding technique on the frequency of exclusive breastfeeding and lactation-related problems. *J Hum Lact*. 2006;22:315–321.
32. Storr G. Prevention of nipple tenderness and breast engorgement in the postpartal period. *J Obstet Gynecol Neonatal Nurs*. 1988;17:203–209.
33. Evans K, Evans R, Simmer K. Effect of the method of breast feeding on breast engorgement, mastitis and infantile colic. *Acta Paediatr*. 1995;84:849–852.

34. Witt A, Bolman M, Kredit S, et al. Therapeutic breast massage in lactation for the management of engorgement, plugged ducts, and mastitis. *J Hum Lact*. 2016;32:123–131.

35. Li R, Fein SB, Chen J, et al. Why mothers stop breastfeeding: Mothers' self-reported reasons for stopping during the first year. *Pediatrics*.. 2008;122(Suppl 2):S69–S76.

36. Stamp G, Casanova H. A breastfeeding study in a rural population in South Australia. *Rural Remote Health*. 2006;6:495.

37. Odom E, Li R, Scanlon K, et al. Reasons for earlier than desired cessation of breastfeeding. *Pediatrics*. 2013;131: e726–e732.

38. Mangesi L, Dowswell T. Treatments for breast engorgement during lactation. *Cochrane Database Syst Rev*. 2010;9: CD006946.

39. Murata T, Hanzawa M, Nomura Y. The clinical effects of "protease complex" on postpartum breast engorgement. *J Jpn Obstet Gynecol Soc*. 1965;12:139–147.

40. Wong B, Koh S, Hegney D, et al. The effectiveness of cabbage leaf application (treatment) on pain and hardness in breast engorgement and its effect on the duration of breastfeeding. *JBI Libr Syst Rev*. 2012;10:1185–1213.

41. Lim A-R, Song J-A, Hur M-H, et al. Cabbage compression early breast care on breast engorgement in primiparous women after cesarean birth: A controlled clinical trial. *Int J Clin Exp Med*. 2015;8:21335–21342.

42. Chiu J-Y, Gau M-L, Kuo S-Y, et al. Effects of Gua-Sha therapy on breast engorgement: A randomized controlled trial. *J Nurs Res*. 2010;18:1–10.

43. Cho J, Hy A, Ahn S, et al. Effects of Oketani breast massage on breast pain, the breast milk pH of mothers, and the sucking speed of neonates. *Korean J Women Health Nurs*. 2012;18:149–158.

44. Khosravan S, Mohammadzadeh-Moghadam H, Mohammadzadeh F, et al. The effect of Hollyhock (Althaea officinalis L) leaf compresses combined with warm and cold compress on breast engorgement in lactating women: A randomized clinical trial. *J Evid Based Complementary Altern Med*. 2015;. pii:2156587215617106.

45. Arora S, Vatsa M, Dadhwal V. A comparison of cabbage leaves vs hot and cold compresses in the treatment of breast engorgement. *Indian J Community Med*. 2008;33:160–162.

46. Morton J. Hand expression of breastmilk. Available at: http://newborns.stanford.edu/Breastfeeding/HandExpression.html (accessed January 4, 2016).

ABM protocols expire 5 years from the date of publication. Evidenced-based revisions are made within five years or sooner if there are significant changes in the evidence.

The Academy of Breastfeeding Medicine Protocol Committee:
Wendy Brodribb, MBBS, PhD, FABM, Chairperson
Larry Noble, MD, FABM, Translations Chairperson
Nancy Brent, MD
Maya Bunik, MD, MSPH, FABM
Cadey Harrel, MD
Ruth A. Lawrence, MD, FABM
Kathleen A. Marinelli, MD, FABM
Kate Naylor, MBBS, FRACGP
Sarah Reece-Stremtan, MD
Casey Rosen-Carole, MD, MPH
Tomoko Seo, MD, FABM
Rose St. Fleur, MD
Michal Young, MD
For correspondence: abm@bfmed.org

With Gratitude to Our Global Protocol Reviewers 2012–2015 Kathleen A. Marinelli, MD, FABM Chair, ABM Protocol Committee

The Academy of Breastfeeding Medicine Clinical Protocols are the work of the ABM Protocol Committee and subject expert authors. We also send each protocol to the ABM Board for review and final vote, and to global content expert reviewers as well to ensure global content applicability.

The Protocol Committee would like to extend our thanks and gratitude to all our global expert reviewers of 2012–2015. Without their invaluable assistance, our protocols would not attain the level of excellence and international applicability we strive for. Thank you for your time and expertise, many of you for more than one protocol!

Australia:
Ju Lee Oei, MBBS, FRACP, MD
Australia:
Gudrun Boëhm, MD
Brazil:
Sonia Isoyama Venancio, MD, PhD
Chile:
Verónica Valdés, MD
France:
Marie-Claude Marchand, MD
Georgia:
Ketevan Nemsadze, MD
Germany:
Elien Rouw, MD
Skadi Springer, MD
Iran:
Maryam Kashanian, MD
Italy:
Marcia Bettinelli, MD
Japan:
Makiko Ohyama, MD, PhD
Toshihiko Nishida, MD
Tomoko Seo, MD
Slovenia:
Andreja Tekauc Golob, MD
Spain:
Leonardo Landa Rivera, MD
United Kingdom:
Jane Hawdon, MBBS, PhD
United States:
Debra Bogen, MD
Sydney Butts, MD
Linda Dahl, MD
Nancy Danoff, MD, MPH
John Girotto, MD

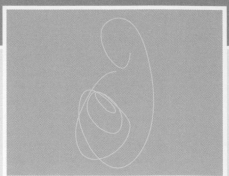

ABM Clinical Protocol #21
*Guidelines for Breastfeeding and Substance Use or Substance Use Disorder, Revised 2015**

*Sarah Reece-Stremtan[1,2], Kathleen A. Marinelli[3,4] and The Academy of Breastfeeding Medicine**

ABSTRACT

A central goal of The Academy of Breastfeeding Medicine is the development of clinical protocols for managing common medical problems that may impact breastfeeding success. These protocols serve only as guidelines for the care of breastfeeding mothers and infants and do not delineate an exclusive course of treatment or serve as standards of medical care. Variations in treatment may be appropriate according to the needs of an individual patient.

PURPOSE

The choice of breastfeeding by a pregnant or newly postpartum woman with a history of past or current illegal/illicit drug abuse or legal substance use or misuse is challenging for many reasons. The purpose of this protocol is to provide literature-based guidelines for the evaluation and management of the woman with substance use or a substance use disorder who is considering breastfeeding.

BACKGROUND

Illicit drug use and legal substance use/abuse remain a significant problem among women of childbearing age. The 2013 National Survey on Drug Use and Health revealed that among pregnant women 15—44 years of age in the United States, 5.2% had used illicit drugs in the past month, 9.4% reported current alcohol use, 2.3% reported binge drinking, 0.4% reported heavy drinking during the pregnancy, and 15.4% reported cigarette use in the past month.[1]

The healthcare provider presented with a pregnant or recently postpartum woman with a history of current or past illegal drug abuse or legal drug use or misuse who desires to breastfeed often faces multiple significant challenges. Substance use disorders frequently engender behaviors or conditions that independently signify risk for the breastfed infant, in addition to the drug exposure per se. These mothers may have coexisting risk factors such as low socioeconomic status (although substance use crosses all socioeconomic lines), low levels of education, poor nutrition, and little to no prenatal care. Multiple drug use is common, in addition to the use of other harmful legal substances, including tobacco and alcohol. Illicit drugs are frequently mixed and extended with dangerous adulterants that can pose additional threats to the health of the mother and the infant. Drug users are at high risk for infections such as human immunodeficiency virus and/or hepatitis B and C. Psychiatric disorders that require pharmacotherapeutic intervention are more prevalent with substance use, making breastfeeding an even more complicated choice, as breastfeeding may not be recommended for women taking some psychotropic medications.

Despite the myriad factors that may make breastfeeding a difficult choice for women with substance use disorders, drug-exposed infants, who are at a high risk for an array of medical, psychological, and developmental issues, as well as their mothers, stand to benefit significantly from breastfeeding. Although many of the factors listed above may pose a risk to the infant, the documented benefits of human milk and breastfeeding must be carefully and thoughtfully weighed against the risks associated with the substance that the infant may be exposed to during lactation. Confounding many efforts to examine longer-term developmental outcomes in infants exposed to some substances is the lack of data evaluating infants who were not exposed during pregnancy but only during lactation.

Ideally, women with substance use disorders delivering an infant and desiring to breast feed are engaged incomprehensive

[1] Divisions of Pain Medicine and of Anesthesiology, Sedation, and Perioperative Medicine, Children's National Health System, Washington, D.C.

[2] The George Washington University, Washington, D.C.

[3] Division of Neonatology and The Connecticut Human Milk Research Center, Connecticut Children's Medical Center, Hartford, Connecticut.

[4] University of Connecticut School of Medicine, Farmington, Connecticut.

* Courtesy of the Academy of Breastfeeding Medicine. Please go to https://www.bfmed.org/protocols for complete protocols, translations, and the most up-to-date information (protocols are updated every 5—7 years).

healthcare and substance abuse treatment during pregnancy, but this is not always the case. Substance abuse treatment for these women is often not available, not gender specific, and not comprehensive, forcing the mother's healthcare provider during and after pregnancy to rely on maternal self-report and a "best guess" at adequacy of services, compliance to treatment, length of "clean" time, community support systems, etc. In a recent retrospective study in the United Kingdom, significantly lower rates of breastfeeding initiation occurred in mothers who used illicit substances or opioid maintenance therapy during pregnancy (14% versus 50% of the general population).[2] In Norway, among opioid-dependent women on opioid maintenance therapy, 77% (compared with 98% in the general population) initiated breastfeeding after delivery.[3]

The specific terms used to describe use and misuse of various legal and illegal substances continue to evolve and may vary from country to country and among different organizations. The 5th edition of the *Diagnostic and Statistical Manual of Mental Disorders* combines the previous categories of substance abuse and substance dependence into the category single substance use disorder, which is measured on a continuum from mild to severe.[4] Of important note is that we would like to make it clear that drugs of any type should be avoided in pregnant and breastfeeding women, unless prescribed for specific medical conditions. The casual use of drugs—legal, illegal, illicit, dose appropriate or not—still may have ramifications for the developing fetus and infant that we have yet to determine, and hence, in general, drugs of all types should be avoided unless medically necessary.

SPECIFIC SUBSTANCES

Perhaps the most critical challenge facing the healthcare provider for the woman with a substance use disorder who wishes to breastfeed is the lack of research leading to evidence-based guidelines. Table 1 gives two online Web sites, one in English and one in both English and Spanish, that are kept updated and are easily accessible for current information on drugs and breastfeeding. There have been several comprehensive reviews of breastfeeding among substance-using women, essentially concluding that breastfeeding is generally contraindicated in mothers who use illegal drugs.[5–8] (III) (Quality of evidence [levels of evidence I, II-1, II-2, II-3,

and III] is based on the U.S. Preventive Services Task Force Appendix A Task Force Ratings[9] and is noted throughout this protocol in parentheses.) Yet, research on individual drugs of abuse remains lacking and difficult to perform. Pharmacokinetic data for most drugs of abuse in lactating women are sparse and based on small numbers of subjects and case reports.[7] Most illicit drugs are found in human milk, with varying degrees of oral bioavailability.[7] Phencyclidine hydrochloride has been detected in human milk in high concentrations,[10] as has cocaine,[11] leading to infant intoxication.[12] There is little to no evidence to describe the effects of even small amounts of other drugs of abuse and/or their metabolites in human milk on infant development aside from those discussed further below.

Methadone

For pregnant and postpartum women with opioid dependence in treatment, methadone maintenance has been the treatment of choice in the United States, Canada,[13] and many other countries. In contrast to other substances, concentrations of methadone in human milk and the effects on the infant have been studied. The concentrations of methadone found in human milk are low, and all authors have concluded that women on stable doses of methadone maintenance should be encouraged to breastfeed if desired, irrespective of maternal methadone dose.[3,14–22] (II-1, II-2, II-3) Previously, no apparent effects of methadone exposure prenatally and in human milk were reported on infant neurobehavior at 30 days.[19] Recently an ongoing longitudinal follow-up study of methadone-exposed infants with 200 methadone-exposed and nonexposed, demographically matched families has shown neurocognitive delays in methadone-exposed 1-month-old infants compared with nonexposed infants. When retested at 7 months, methadone-exposed infants were similar to nonexposed, comparison infants. At 9 months of age, 37.5% of this sample of methadone-exposed infants showed clinically significant motor delays ($\geq$ 1.5 standard deviation) compared with low but typical development in the comparison group.[21] Exposed infants typically have high environmental risk profiles, which continue at birth, posing ongoing risk to the developing child.

The current thought is that environmental risk factors combine with prenatal exposures to promote epigenetic changes in

TABLE 1   Online Web Sites with Updated Breastfeeding and Drug Information

Web Site	URL	Language
U.S. National Library of Health, National Institute of Health, U.S. Department of Health and Human Services, "LactMed"	http://toxnet.nlm.nih.gov/newtoxnet/lactmed.htm	English
e-Lactancia	http://e-lactancia.org/	English
Association for Promotion and Cultural and Scientific Research of Breastfeeding Under a Creative Commons International License	(Also contains medical prescriptions, phytotherapy, homeopathy and other alternative products, cosmetic and medical procedures, contaminants, maternal and infant diseases and more)	Spanish

gene expression and methylation patterns that have both immediate and long-term implications related to developmental programming.[22] Note that these findings relate to infants exposed to methadone both prenatally and after birth via breastfeeding, and there is little information available on infants with chronic methadone exposure via breastfeeding alone.

In addition, about 70% of infants born to women prescribed methadone during pregnancy will experience neonatal abstinence syndrome (NAS),[23] the constellation of signs and symptoms often presenting following in utero opioid exposure. Infants with significant NAS can experience difficulties with attaching and sucking/swallowing during breastfeeding that can impact their ability to breastfeed.

However, given that there is increasing evidence supporting the conclusion that there is a reduction in the severity and duration of treatment of NAS when mothers on methadone maintenance therapy breastfeed, breastfeeding for these dyads should be encouraged.[3,17–19] (II-1, II-3) Unfortunately, the rate of breastfeeding initiation in this cohort is generally low, less than half that reported in the U.S. general population.[24] A small recent qualitative study demonstrated that lack of support from the healthcare community and misinformation about the dangers of breastfeeding while on methadone therapy are significant, yet modifiable, barriers to breastfeeding success in these women.[25] Given the benefits to these mothers and infants to remain on methadone maintenance therapy and breastfeed, it is important for us to provide robust ongoing support for this vulnerable group.

Buprenorphine

Buprenorphine is a partial opioid agonist used for treatment of opioid dependency during pregnancy in some countries and increasingly in the United States. Multiple small case series have examined maternal buprenorphine concentrations in human milk. All concur that the amounts of buprenorphine in human milk are small and are unlikely to have short-term negative effects on the developing infant.[26–31] In one study, 76% of 85 maternal–infant pairs breastfed, with 66% still breastfeeding 6–8 weeks postpartum. The breastfed infants had less severe NAS and were less likely to require pharmacological intervention than the formula-fed infants, similar to methadone discussed above, although this did not reach statistical significance with the size of the sample studied.[31]

Other opioids

Use of opioids in the United States has increased substantially over the last decade. A retrospective cross-sectional analysis of NAS in hospital births in the years from 2000 to 2009 found an increase in incidence from 1.2 to 3.39 per 1,000 births. Antepartum maternal opioid use was also found to have risen from 1.19 to 5.63 per 1,000 hospital births from 2000 to 2009; any use of opioids was included in data collection.[32] A recent Centers for Disease Control and Prevention *Morbidity and Mortality Weekly Report* highlighted data demonstrating that approximately one-third of women of reproductive age filled a prescription for opioids each year between 2008 and 2012.[33]

When use of narcotics during pregnancy is determined to be consistent with an opioid use disorder rather than a modality for short-term pain relief, consideration of initiation of maintenance methadone or buprenorphine as previously discussed is strongly encouraged,[13,34,35] and these mothers should be supported in breastfeeding initiation. (III) Short courses of most other low-dose prescription opioids can be safely used by a breastfeeding mother,[36,37] but caution is urged with codeine, as *CYP2D6* ultra-rapid metabolizers may experience high morphine (metabolite) blood levels, and there has been a single case report of a breastfeeding neonatal death after maternal use.[38] (III) Information is lacking on the safety of breastfeeding when moderate to high doses of opioids are used for long periods of time. There is also a lack of information available about transitioning mothers from short-acting opioids to opioid maintenance therapy while breastfeeding rather than during pregnancy.

Marijuana

Uniform guidelines regarding the varied use of marijuana by breastfeeding mothers are difficult to create and cannot hope to cover all situations. The legality of possessing and using marijuana varies greatly from country to country; in the United States, there are increasing numbers of states where it is legal for "medicinal use" with a prescription, and a few states where it is legal for "recreational use," but under federal law, it remains illegal in all states. Therefore, basing recommendations on marijuana use and concurrent breastfeeding from a purely legal standpoint becomes inherently complex, problematic, and impossible to apply uniformly across all settings and jurisdictions. As laws shift and marijuana use becomes even more common in some areas, it becomes increasingly important to carefully weigh the risks of initiation and continuation of breastfeeding while using marijuana with the risks of not breastfeeding while also considering the wide range of occasional, to regular medical, to heavy exposure to marijuana.

In addition to the potential legal risk, the health risks to the infant from the mother's marijuana use must be carefully considered. Δ^9-Tetrahydrocannabinol (THC), the main compound in marijuana, is present in human milk up to eight times that of maternal plasma levels, and metabolites are found in infant feces, indicating that THC is absorbed and metabolized by the infant.[39] It is rapidly distributed to the brain and adipose tissue and stored in fat tissues for weeks to months. It has a long half-life (25–57 hours) and stays positive in the urine for 2–3 weeks,[40] making it impossible to determine who is an occasional versus a chronic user at the time of delivery by urine toxicology screening. Evidence regarding the effects of THC exposure on infant development via breastfeeding alone is sparse and conflicting,[41,42] and there are no data evaluating neurodevelopmental outcomes beyond the age of 1 year in infants who are only exposed after birth. Also notable in this discussion of risk is that the potency of marijuana has been steadily increasing, from about 3% in the 1980s to 12% in 2012, so data from previous studies may no longer even be relevant.[43] Additionally, current concern over marijuana use during lactation stems from possible infant sedation and maternal inability to safely care for her infant while directly under its influence; however, this remains a theoretical problem and has not been well established in the literature.[44]

Human and animal evidence examining the behavioral and neurobiological effects of exposure to cannabinoids during pregnancy and lactation shows that the endocannabinoid system plays a crucial role in the ontogeny of the central nervous system and its activation, during brain development. As Campolongo et al.[45] concluded, cannabinoid exposure during critical periods of brain development can induce subtle and long-lasting neurofunctional alterations. Several preclinical studies highlight how even low to moderate doses during particular periods of brain development can have profound consequences for brain maturation, potentially leading to long-lasting alterations in cognitive functions and emotional behaviors.[45] Exposure to second-hand marijuana smoke by infants has been associated with an independent two times possible risk of sudden infant death syndrome (SIDS)[46] (III); because breastfeeding reduces risk of SIDS, this needs to be additionally considered. Thus careful contemplation of these issues should be fully incorporated into the care plans of the lactating woman in the setting of THC use. Breastfeeding mothers should be counseled to reduce or eliminate their use of marijuana to avoid exposing their infants to this substance and advised of the possible long-term neurobehavioral effects from continued use. (III)

Alcohol

Use of alcohol during pregnancy is strongly discouraged, as it can cause fetal alcohol syndrome, birth defects, spontaneous abortion, and premature births, among other serious problems.[47,48] (III) Many women who significantly decrease or eliminate their alcohol intake during pregnancy may choose to resume consuming alcohol after giving birth, with approximately half of breastfeeding women in Western countries reported to consume alcohol at least occasionally.[49] Alcohol interferes with the milk ejection reflex, which may ultimately reduce milk production through inadequate breast emptying.[50] (III) Human milk alcohol levels generally parallel maternal blood alcohol levels, and studies evaluating infant effects of maternal alcohol consumption have been mostly mixed, with some mild effects seen in infant sleep patterns, amount of milk consumed during breastfeeding sessions, and early psychomotor development.[50] (III) Possible long-term effects of alcohol in maternal milk remain unknown. Most sources advise limiting alcohol intake to the equivalent of 8 ounces of wine or two beers, and waiting 2 hours after drinking to resume breastfeeding.[5–7,35] (III) To ensure complete elimination of alcohol from breastmilk, mothers may consult a nomogram devised by the Canadian Motherisk program to determine length of time needed based on maternal weight and amount consumed.[51] (III)

Tobacco

Approximately two-thirds as many pregnant women as non-pregnant women smoke tobacco, with decreasing numbers of women smoking as pregnancy progresses.[1] Many mothers quit during pregnancy. but postpartum relapse is common. with about 50% resuming tobacco use in the first few months after birth.[52–54] Data on the epidemiology of breastfeeding mothers who smoke cigarettes remains complex, and smoking in many series has been found to be associated with reduced rates of breastfeeding.[55,56] Nicotine and other compounds are known to transfer to the infant via milk, and considerable transfer of chemicals via second-hand smoke also occurs when infants are exposed to environmental tobacco smoke. Increases in the incidence of respiratory allergy in infants and in SIDS are just two significant well-known risks of infant exposure to environmental tobacco smoke.[8] (III) Most sources endorse promotion of breastfeeding in the setting of maternal smoking while vigorously supporting smoking cessation.[57] (III) Some smoking cessation modalities (nicotine patch, nicotine gum, and possibly bupropion) are compatible with breastfeeding and can be encouraged in many circumstances.[6,7,58] (III)

RECOMMENDATIONS

General (Circumstances favorable with consideration)

Infants of women with substance use disorders, at risk for multiple health and developmental difficulties, stand to benefit substantially from breastfeeding and human milk, as do their mothers. A prenatal plan preparing the mother for parenting, breastfeeding, and substance abuse treatment should be formulated through individualized, patient-centered discussions with each woman. This care plan should include instruction in the consequences of relapse to drug or excessive alcohol use during lactation, as well as teaching regarding potential for donor milk, formula preparation, and bottle handling and cleaning should breastfeeding be or become contraindicated. In the perinatal period each mother—infant dyad should be carefully and individually counseled on breastfeeding prior to discharge from maternity care. This evaluation must consider several factors, including (III)

- drug use and substance abuse treatment histories, including medication-assisted treatment with methadone or buprenorphine
- medical and psychiatric status
- other maternal medication needs
- infant health status (to include ongoing evaluation for NAS and impact on ability to breastfeed)
- the presence or absence and adequacy of maternal family and community support systems
- plans for postpartum care and substance abuse treatment for the mother and pediatric care for the child.

Optimally, the woman with a substance use disorder who presents a desire to breastfeed should be engaged in treatment pre- and postnatally. Maternal written consent for communication with her substance abuse treatment provider should be obtained prior to delivery if possible. (III)

Any discussion with mothers who use substances with sedating effects should include counseling on safely caring for her infant and instruction on safe sleep practices. (III)

Encourage women under the following circumstances to breastfeed their infants (III):

- Engaged in substance abuse treatment; provision of maternal consent to discuss progress in treatment and plans for postpartum treatment with substance abuse treatment counselor; counselor recommendation for breastfeeding
- Plans to continue in substance abuse treatment in the postpartum period
- Abstinence from drug use for 90 days prior to delivery; ability to maintain sobriety demonstrated in an outpatient setting
- Toxicology testing of maternal urine negative at delivery
- Engaged in prenatal care and compliant.

Opioids/narcotics

- Encourage stable methadone- or buprenorphine-maintained women to breastfeed regardless of dose
- Management of mothers who use chronic opioid therapy for pain should be closely supervised by a chronic pain physician who is familiar with pregnancy and breastfeeding (III):
  a. Length of time on these medications, total dose, and whether the medications were used during pregnancy should all help inform the decision of whether breastfeeding may be safely undertaken in certain cases.
  b. Judicious amounts of oral narcotic pain medication, when used in a time-limited situation for an acute pain problem, are generally compatible with continued breastfeeding if supervision and monitoring of the breastfeeding infant are adequate.[36,37]
- Rapidly increasing narcotic dosing in a breastfeeding mother should prompt further evaluation and reconsideration of the safety of continued breastfeeding.

Nicotine

- Counsel mothers who smoke cigarettes after giving birth to reduce their intake as much as possible, and not to smoke around their infant, to reduce infant exposure to second-hand smoke. Smoking cessation and nicotine replacement modalities such as nicotine patches and gum may be useful for some mothers. (III)
- Give mothers who smoke tobacco additional support, as maternal smoking appears to be an independent and associated risk factor for noninitiation and early cessation of breastfeeding, to help ensure its success. (III)

Alcohol

- Counsel mothers who wish to drink occasional alcohol that alcohol easily transfers into human milk. Recommendations from the American Academy of Pediatrics, the World Health Organization, and others

advise waiting 90–120 minutes after ingesting alcohol before breastfeeding, or expressing and discarding milk within that time frame.[5–7,35] (III)

Cannabis (THC)

- Information regarding long-term effects of marijuana use by the breastfeeding mother on the infant remains insufficient to recommend complete abstention from breastfeeding initiation or continuation based on the scientific evidence at this time. However, extrapolation from in utero exposure and the limited data available helps to inform the following recommendations (III):
  a. Counsel mothers who admit to occasional or rare use to avoid further use or reduce their use as much as possible while breastfeeding, advise them as to its possible long-term neurobehavioral effects, and instruct them to avoid direct exposure of the infant to marijuana and its smoke.
  b. Strongly advise mothers found with a positive urine screen for THC to discontinue exposure while breastfeeding and counsel them as to its possible long-term neurobehavioral effects.
  c. When advising mothers on the medicinal use of marijuana during lactation, one must take into careful consideration and counsel on the potential risks of exposure of marijuana and benefits of breastfeeding to the infant.
  d. The lack of long-term follow-up data on infants exposed to varying amounts of marijuana via human milk, coupled with concerns over negative neurodevelopmental outcomes in children with in utero exposure, should prompt extremely careful consideration of the risks versus benefits of breastfeeding in the setting of moderate or chronic marijuana use. A recommendation of abstaining from any marijuana use is warranted.
  e. At this time, although the data are not strong enough to recommend not breastfeeding with any marijuana use, we urge caution.

General (Circumstances contraindicated or requiring more caution)

Counsel women under any of the following circumstances not to breastfeed (III):

- Not engaged in substance abuse treatment, or engaged in treatment and failure to provide consent for contact with counselor
- Not engaged in prenatal care
- Positive maternal urine toxicology screen for substances other than marijuana at delivery [see (b) above] No plans for postpartum substance abuse treatment or pediatric care
- Women relapsing to illicit drug use or legal substance misuse in the 30-day period prior to delivery
- Any behavioral or other indicators that the woman is actively abusing substances
- Chronic alcohol use.

Evaluate carefully women under the following circumstances, and determine appropriate advice for breastfeeding by discussion and coordination among the mother, maternal care providers, and substance abuse treatment providers (III):

- Relapse to illicit substance use or legal substance misuse in the 90–30-day period prior to delivery
- Concomitant use of other prescription medications deemed to be incompatible with lactation
- Engaged later (after the second trimester) in prenatal care and/or substance abuse treatment
- Attained drug and/or alcohol sobriety only in an inpatient setting
- Lack of appropriate maternal family and community support systems
- Report that they desire to breastfeed their infant in order to either retain custody or maintain their sobriety in the postpartum period.

In the United States, women who have established breastfeeding and subsequently relapse to illegal drug use are counseled not to breastfeed, even if milk is discarded during the time period surrounding relapse. There are no known pharmacokinetic data to establish the presence and/or concentrations of most illicit substances and/or their metabolites in human milk and effects on the infant, and this research is unlikely to occur given the ethical dilemmas it presents. The lack of pharmacokinetic data for most drugs of abuse in recently postpartum women with substance use disorders precludes the establishment of a "safe" interval after use when breastfeeding can be reestablished for individual drugs of abuse. Additionally, women using illicit substances in the postnatal period may exhibit impaired judgment and secondary behavioral changes that may interfere with the ability of the mother to care for her infant or to breastfeed adequately. Passive drug exposures may pose additional risks to the infant. Therefore, any woman relapsing to illicit drug use or legal substance misuse after the establishment of lactation should be provided an appropriate human milk substitute (donor milk, formula) and intensified drug treatment, along with guidance on how to taper milk production to prevent mastitis. (III)

The woman with a substance use disorder who has successfully initiated breastfeeding should be carefully monitored, along with her infant, in the postpartum period. Ongoing substance abuse treatment, postpartum care, psychiatric care when warranted, and pediatric care are important for women with substance use disorders. Lactation support is particularly important for infants experiencing NAS and their mothers. Communication among all care providers involved with the health, welfare, and substance abuse support of the mother and the child should provide an interactive network of supportive care for the dyad. (III)

RECOMMENDATIONS FOR FUTURE RESEARCH

1. Long-term randomized controlled trials or paired cohort evaluations of infants exposed to methadone or buprenorphine via human milk, including infant developmental assessments
2. Further evaluations of maternal milk and plasma and infant plasma pharmacokinetic data regarding prescription opioids and lactation, especially for mothers who were on chronic high-dose medications during pregnancy that are continued when breastfeeding
3. Long-term controlled evaluations of infants exposed to marijuana via human milk, to include infants and later neurodevelopmental outcomes, including those exposed to marijuana in a controlled manner, such as with legalized medical marijuana
4. Evaluation of nicotine replacement patches, gum, and vaporized cigarettes as substitutes for tobacco smoking in pregnant and lactating women, to determine if these can or should be widely recommended in place of tobacco products.

ACKNOWLEDGMENTS

This work was supported in part by a grant from the Maternal and Child Health Bureau, U.S. Department of Health and Human Services.

REFERENCES

1. Results from the 2013 National Survey on Drug Use and Health: National findings. Available at: www.samhsa.gov/data/sites/default/files/NSDUHresultsPDFWHTML2013/Web/NSDUHresults2013.pdf (accessed February 18, 2015).
2. Goel N, Beasley D, Rajkumar V, et al. Perinatal outcome of illicit substance use in pregnancy—Comparative and contemporary socio-clinical profile in the UK. *Eur J Pediatr.* 2011;170:199–205.
3. Welle-Strand GK, Skurtveit S, Jansson LM, et al. Breastfeeding reduces the need for withdrawal treatment in opioid-exposed infants. *Acta Paediatr.* 2013;102:1060–1066.
4. *Diagnostic and Statistical Manual of Mental Disorders*, 5th ed. American Psychiatric Association, Washington, DC, 2013.
5. D'Apolito K. Breastfeeding and substance abuse. *Obstet Clin Gynecol.* 2013;56:202–211.
6. Sachs HC. American Academy of Pediatrics Committee on Drugs. The transfer of drugs and therapeutics into human breast milk: An update on selected topics. *Pediatrics.* 2013;132:e796–e809..
7. Rowe H, Baker T, Hale TW. Maternal medication, drug use, and breastfeeding. *Pediatr Clin North Am.* 2013;60:275–294.
8. Eidelman AI, Schanler R. Section on Breastfeeding. Breastfeeding and the use of human milk. *Pediatrics.* 2012;129:e827–e841.
9. Appendix A Task Force Ratings. Guide to clinical preventive services: Report of the U.S. Preventive Services Task Force, 2nd edition. Available at: www.ncbi.nlm.nih.gov/books/NBK15430/ (accessed February 27, 2015).
10. Kaufman R, Petrucha RA, Pitts FN, et al. PCP in amniotic fluid and breast milk: Case report. *J Clin Psychiatry.* 1983;44:269–270.

11. Winecker RE, Goldberger BA, Tebbett IR, et al. Detection of cocaine and its metabolites in breast milk. *J Forensic Sci.* 2001;46:1221–1223.

12. Chasnoff I, Lewis DE, Squires L. Cocaine intoxication in a breast fed infant. *Pediatrics.* 1987;80:836–838.

13. Wong S, Ordean A, Kahan M, et al. Substance use in pregnancy. *J Obstet Gynaecol Can.* 2011;33:367–384.

14. Wojnar-Horton RE, Kristensen JH, Yapp P, et al. Methadone distribution and excretion into breast milk of clients in a methadone maintenance programme. *Br J Clin Pharmacol.* 1997;44:543–547.

15. McCarthy JJ, Posey BL. Methadone levels in human milk. *J Hum Lact.* 2000;16:115–120.

16. Begg EJ, Malpas TJ, Hackett LP, et al. Distribution of R and S-methadone into human milk during multiple, medium to high oral dosing. *Br J Clin Pharmacol.* 2001;52:681–685.

17. Bogen DL, Perel JM, Helsel JC, et al. Estimated infant exposure to enantiomer-specific methadone levels in breastmilk. *Breastfeed Med.* 2011;6:377–384.

18. Abdel-Latif ME, Pinner J, Clews S, et al. Effects of breast milk on the severity and outcome of NAS among infants of drug-dependent mothers. *Pediatrics.* 2006;117:1163–1169.

19. Jansson LM, Choo R, Velez ML, et al. Methadone maintenance and breastfeeding in the neonatal period. *Pediatrics.* 2008;121:106–114.

20. McQueen KA, Murphy-Oikonen J, Gerlach K, et al. The impact of infant feeding method on neonatal abstinence scores of methadone-exposed infants. *Adv Neonatal Care.* 2011;11:282–290.

21. Logan BA, Brown MS, Hayes MJ. Neonatal abstinence syndrome: Treatment and pediatric outcomes. *Clin Obstet Gynecol.* 2013;56:186–192.

22. Jansson LM, Choo R, Velez ML, et al. Methadone maintenance and long-term lactation. *Breastfeed Med.* 2008;3:34–37.

23. Kocherlakota P. Neonatal abstinence syndrome. *Pediatrics.* 2014;134:e547–e561.

24. Wachman EM, Byun J, Philipp BL. Breastfeeding rates among mothers of infants with neonatal abstinence syndrome. *Breastfeed Med.* 2010;5:159–164.

25. Demirci JR, Bogen DL, Klionsky Y. Breastfeeding and methadone therapy: The maternal experience. *Subst Abus.* 2014 April 4 [Epub ahead of print]. doi: 10.1080/08897077.2014.902417.

26. Ilett KF, Hackett LP, Gower S, et al. Estimated dose exposure of the neonate to buprenorphine and its metabolite norbuprenorphine via breastmilk during maternal buprenorphine substitution treatment. *Breastfeed Med.* 2012;7:269–274.

27. Grimm D, Pauly E, Poschl J, et al. Buprenorphine and norbuprenorphine concentrations in human breastmilk samples determined by liquid chromatography-tandem mass spectrometry. *Ther Drug Monit.* 2005;27:526–530.

28. Marquet P, Chevral J, Lavignasse P, et al. Buprenorphine withdrawal syndrome in a newborn. *Clin Pharmacol Ther.* 1997;62:569–571.

29. Johnson RE, Jones HE, Jasinski DR, et al. Buprenorphine treatment of pregnant opioid dependent women: Maternal and neonatal outcomes. *Drug Alcohol Depend.* 2001;63:97–103.

30. Gower S, Bartu A, Ilett KF, et al. The wellbeing of infants exposed to buprenorphine via breast milk at 4 weeks of age. *J Hum Lact.* 2014;30:217–223.

31. O'Connor AB, Collett A, Alto WA, et al. Breastfeeding rates and the relationship between breastfeeding and neonatal abstinence syndrome in women maintained on buprenorphine during pregnancy. *J Midwifery Womens Health.* 2013;58:383–388.

32. Patrick SW, Schumacher RE, Benneyworth BD, et al. Neonatal abstinence syndrome and associated health care expenditures. *JAMA.* 2012;307:1934–1940.

33. Centers for Disease Control and Prevention. Opioid painkillers widely prescribed among reproductive age women [press release]. January 2015. Available at: www.cdc.gov/media/releases/2015/p0122-pregnancy-opioids.html (accessed February 23, 2015).

34. ACOG Committee on Health Care for Underserved Women; American Society of Addiction Medicine. ACOG Committee Opinion No. 524: Opioid abuse, dependence, and addiction in pregnancy. *Obstet Gynecol.* 2012;119:1070–1076.

35. World Health Organization. Guidelines for the identification and management of substance use and substance use disorders in pregnancy. 2014. Available at: www.who.int/substance_abuse/publications/pregnancy_guidelines/en/ (accessed February 18, 2015).

36. Montgomery A, Hale TW. The Academy of Breastfeeding Medicine. ABM Clinical Protocol #15: Analgesia and anesthesia for the breastfeeding mother, revised 2012. *Breastfeed Med.* 2012;7:547–553.

37. Hendrickson RG, McKeown NJ. Is maternal opioid use hazardous to breast-fed infants? *J Toxicol.* 2012;50:1–14.

38. Madadi P, Koren G, Cairns J, et al. Safety of codeine during breastfeeding. *Fatal morphine poisoning in the breastfed neonate of a mother prescribed codeine. Can Fam Physician.* 2007;53:33–35.

39. Perez-Reyes M, Wall ME. Presence of D9-tetrahydrocannabinol in human milk. *N Engl J Med.* 1982;307:819–820.

40. Hale TW, Rowe HE. *Medications and Mothers' Milk.* 16th ed. Plano, TX: Hale Publishing LP; 2014.

41. Astley SJ, Little RE. Maternal marijuana use during lactation and infant development at one year. *Neurotoxicol Teratol.* 1990;12:161–168.

42. Tennes K, Avitable N, Blackard C, et al. Marijuana: Prenatal and postnatal exposure in the human. *NIDA Res Monogr.* 1985;59:48–60.

43. Volkow ND, Baler RD, Compton WM, et al. Adverse health effects of marijuana use. *N Engl J Med.* 2014;370:2219–2227.

44. Hill M, Reed K. Pregnancy, breast-feeding, and marijuana: A review article. *Obstet Gynecol Surv.* 2013;68:710–718.

45. Campolongo P, Trezza V, Palmery M, et al. Developmental exposure to cannabinoids causes subtle and enduring neurofunctional alterations. *Int Rev Neurobiol.* 2009;85:117–133.

46. Klonoff-Cohen H, Lam-Kruglick P. Maternal and paternal recreational drug use and sudden infant death syndrome. *Arch Pediatr Adolesc Med.* 2001;155:765–770.

47. American Academy of Pediatrics. Joint Call to Action on Alcohol and Pregnancy. 2012. Available at: www.aap.org/en-us/advocacy-and-policy/aap-health-initiatives/fetalalcohol-spectrum-disorders-toolkit/Pages/Joint-Call-toAction-on-Alcohol-and-Pregnancy.aspx (accessed February 18, 2015).

48. Carson G, Cox LV, Crane J, et al. Alcohol use and pregnancy consensus clinical guidelines. *J Obstet Gynaecol Can.* 2010;32(8 Suppl 3):S1–S32.

49. Haastrup MB, Pottegard A, Damkier P. Alcohol and breastfeeding. *Basic Clin Pharmacol Toxicol.* 2014;114:168–173.

50. Lactmed. Alcohol Monograph. Available at: http://toxnet.nlm.nih.gov/ (accessed February 11, 2015).

51. Koren G. Drinking alcohol while breastfeeding. *Will it harm my baby? Can Fam Physician.* 2002;48:39–41.

52. Yang I, Hall L. Smoking cessation and relapse challenges reported by postpartum women. *MCN Am J Matern Child Nurs.* 2004;39:375–380.

53. Levitt C, Shaw E, Wong S, et al. Systematic review of the literature on postpartum care: Effectiveness of interventions for smoking relapse prevention, cessation, and reduction in postpartum women. *Birth.* 2007;34:341–347.

54. Texas Tech University Health Sciences Center, Infant Risk Center. Tobacco Use. Available at: www.infantrisk.com/content/tobacco-use (accessed February 20, 2015).

55. Horta BL, Victora CG, Menezes AM, et al. Environmental tobacco smoke and breastfeeding duration. *Am J Epidemiol.* 1997;146:128–133.

56. Myr R. Promoting, protecting, and supporting breastfeeding in a community with a high rate of tobacco use. *J Hum Lact.* 2014;20:415–416.

57. Dorea JG. Maternal smoking and infant feeding: Breastfeeding is better and safer. *Matern Child Health J.* 2007;11:287–291.

58. Heydari G, Masjedi M, Ahmady AE, et al. A comparative study on tobacco cessation methods: A quantitative systematic review. *Int J Prev Med.* 2014;5:673–678.

ABM protocols expire 5 years from the date of publication. Evidence-based revisions are made within 5 years or sooner if there are significant changes in the evidence.

Academy of Breastfeeding Medicine Protocol Committee
Kathleen A. Marinelli, MD, FABM, Chairperson
Larry Noble, MD, FABM, Translations Chairperson
Nancy Brent, MD
Ruth A. Lawrence, MD, FABM
Sarah Reece-Stremtan, MD
Casey Rosen-Carole, MD
Tomoko Seo, MD, FABM
Rose St. Fleur, MD
Michal Young, MD
For correspondence: abm@bfmed.org

ABM Clinical Protocol #22
Guidelines for Management of Jaundice in the Breastfeeding Infant 35 Weeks or More of Gestation—Revised 2017*

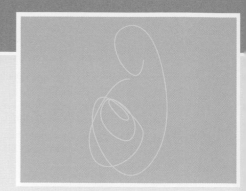

*Valerie J. Flaherman[1], M. Jeffrey Maisels[2] and The Academy of Breastfeeding Medicine**

ABSTRACT

A central goal of The Academy of Breastfeeding Medicine is the development of clinical protocols free from commercial interest or influence for managing common medical problems that may impact breastfeeding success. These protocols serve only as guidelines for the care of breastfeeding mothers and infants and do not delineate an exclusive course of treatment or serve as standards of medical care. Variations in treatment may be appropriate according to the needs of an individual patient.

PURPOSE

1. To provide guidance in determining whether and how breastfeeding may or may not be contributing to infant jaundice.
2. To review evidence-based strategies for ameliorating jaundice in the breastfeeding infant.
3. To provide protocols for supporting breastfeeding while infants are being evaluated and/or treated for jaundice.

BIOLOGIC BASIS FOR JAUNDICE IN THE NEWBORN AND ITS RELATIONSHIP TO BREASTFEEDING

Some comprehensive reviews of bilirubin metabolism and jaundice in the newborn are listed in the references for a more complete discussion of the biology and pathobiology of jaundice in the newborn and its relationship to breastfeeding.[1-3]

[1] Department of Pediatrics, School of Medicine, University of California, San Francisco, California

[2] Department of Pediatrics, William Beaumont School of Medicine, Oakland University, Royal Oak, Michigan

* Courtesy of the Academy of Breastfeeding Medicine. Please go to https://www.bfmed.org/protocols for complete protocols, translations, and the most up-to-date information (protocols are updated every 5–7 years).

Although the management of breastfeeding and jaundice varies in different countries,[4] the following principles and recommendations should apply universally.

Hyperbilirubinemia of the newborn

Virtually all newborns have some elevation of their total serum bilirubin (TSB) ($>90\%$ of which is unconjugated or indirect reacting) relative to normal adult values, which are ≤ 17 μmol/L (≤ 1.0 mg/dL).[5] The catabolism of heme by heme oxygenase (HO) produces biliverdin. Biliverdin is reduced by biliverdin reductase to unconjugated bilirubin, which is conjugated in the liver and excreted through the gut. Newborns have higher TSB levels because of a combination of three factors: increased production of bilirubin due to postnatal heme degradation; decreased uptake and conjugation of bilirubin due to developmental hepatic immaturity; and increased intestinal reabsorption of bilirubin. In the first week of life, more than 80% of newborns appear jaundiced[6,7] and, depending on the racial and sociocultural population mix, about 75% have a transcutaneous bilirubin (TcB) of $>100-150$ μmol/L ($>6-9$ mg/dL) by 96 hours.[8-10] Bilirubin is antioxidant and may protect infants from the relatively hyperoxygenic environment after birth. The term physiologic jaundice is often used to describe newborns with a TSB well above normal adult levels, but not attributable to a specific cause such as hemolytic disease; however, such terminology may be inappropriate because having an unknown etiology does not necessarily mean that a condition is physiologic.[11]

Breastfeeding and jaundice

Although some early studies[12,13] reported no differences in TSB concentrations between breastfed and formula-fed infants, subsequent studies using larger sample sizes and more robust research design demonstrated a strong association between hyperbilirubinemia and breastfeeding compared with formula feeding, especially when breastfeeding was exclusive.[14-22] Nonetheless, in comparison with previous data,[23] Buiter et al.'s[24] study of the relationship between stool production and jaundice in healthy breastfed or formula-fed newborns found significantly less stool production in formula-fed infants and no difference in stool production or TcB concentrations in the first 4 days between breastfed and formula-fed infants. Based on this body of evidence, two broad categories of the association between breastfeeding and jaundice have been described. Jaundice, which occurs in the first week in association with ongoing weight loss, has been termed breastfeeding jaundice, breastfeeding-associated jaundice, breast-nonfeeding jaundice, or starvation jaundice.[25] However, as this jaundice is almost always associated with low enteral intake rather than breastfeeding per se, in this protocol, it will be called suboptimal intake jaundice. Jaundice that persists past the onset of robust weight gain is known as breast milk jaundice or the breast milk jaundice syndrome. Although this protocol focuses on breastfeeding and jaundice, it is important to note that early onset jaundice occurring within 24—48 hours of birth is unlikely to be related to breastfeeding and should be assessed and treated promptly without interruption of breastfeeding.

Suboptimal intake jaundice of the newborn

During the first days after birth, it is normal for colostrum volumes to be small; appropriate for the infant's stomach size and physiologic need. In the first 24 hours of life, exclusively breastfed infants may receive no more than 1—5 mL of milk per feeding[26—29] or 5—37 mL in total.[30,31] Encouraging breastfeeding with in the first hour of birth and frequently there after maximizes caloric and fluid intake and stimulates breast milk production.

In normal adults, the absence of caloric intake, even for as brief a period as 24 hours and with good hydration, results in a small increase in unconjugated hyperbilirubinemia of about 17—34 μmol/L (1—2 mg/dL),[32—34] an effect due to an increase in the enterohepatic circulation of bilirubin.[35] Similarly, in newborns, breastfeeding difficulties or a delay in the onset of secretory activation (lactogenesis II)[36] may result in lower caloric intake, which may lead to an increase in enterohepatic circulation[35] and the development of hyperbilirubinemia. In addition, the mechanism for an increase in TSB is likely to include other developmental limitations in bilirubin metabolism and transport in the newborn.[37—39] Because formula-fed infants are typically given volumes of milk much greater than physiologically normal (27 mL formula per feeding or about 150 mL/day), during that same period,[40] it is uncommon for them to become jaundiced. Oral intake equalizes for the groups once maternal secretory activation occurs around 2—5 days of age, and copious milk production begins.

The interaction between low enteral intake and other factors related to neonatal hyperbilirubinemia is the subject of recent investigation.[18,24,41,42] Sato et al. found that the hyperbilirubinemia associated with the G71R mutation of UDP glucuronosyltransferase family 1 member A1 (*UGT1A1*) gene could be prevented by adequate enteral intake.[41,42] People with Gilbert's syndrome have lower activity of UDP glucuronosyltransferase and develop significantly higher TSB with fasting than the normal population.

Breast milk jaundice (prolonged jaundice associated with breast milk feeding)

Many breastfed infants have unconjugated hyperbilirubinemia that extends into the second and third week, but can continue for as long as 2—3 months.[43,44] At 28 days, 21% of predominantly breastfed infants were still visibly jaundiced and 34% had a TcB $\geq$ 85 μmol/L ($\geq$5 mg/dL).[43] Prolonged jaundice beyond the second to third week in healthy breastfeeding newborns has been called breast milk jaundice to distinguish it from suboptimal intake jaundice, which should resolve by 1—2 weeks.[45]

The precise mechanism of breast milk jaundice remains unknown despite much investigation. Multiple factors appear to contribute to whether bilirubin is eliminated together with fecal fat[46] or reabsorbed into the blood stream (the enterohepatic circulation). The development of breast milk jaundice has been attributed to numerous processes involved in bilirubin excretion, including enhanced intestinal reabsorption of unconjugated bilirubin[43]; increased concentrations of cytokines (including IL-1, IL-10, and TNF-) in human milk[47]; low total antioxidant capacity in human milk[48]; variations in the HO-1 gene promoter[49]; variations in the UGT1A1 gene[18,41,42,50,51]; lower serum and milk levels of epidermal growth factor[52]; higher serum alpha-fetoprotein levels[53]; higher cholesterol levels[54]; and lower abundance of *Bifidobacterium adolescentis*, *Bifidobacterium longum* and *Bifidobacterium bifidum*[55] in human milk and stool. The relative contribution of each of these factors, their potential interaction, and their precise mechanism of action remain unknown. Over time, the jaundice and elevated TSB decline at varying rates to normal adult values even while breastfeeding continues. Features that may distinguish suboptimal intake jaundice from breast milk jaundice are summarized in Table 1.

Whenever jaundice in a breastfed newborn is prolonged beyond the third week, it is important to rule out cholestasis by measuring the direct or conjugated bilirubin level and to evaluate for other causes of prolonged indirect hyperbilirubinemia such as congenital hypothyroidism. For indirect hyperbilirubinemia that extends beyond 2 months, conditions such as ongoing undiagnosed hemolysis, Gilbert's syndrome, or the very rare Crigler—Najjar syndrome (with an incidence of 1 per million births) should be considered.[56]

Interaction of suboptimal intake jaundice and breast milk jaundice

Strong evidence suggests that increased serum bilirubin in the first few days is highly correlated with suboptimal enteral intake; serum bilirubin concentrations are highly associated with greater weight loss in breastfed infants.[41,42,57—62] Ineffective suckling with inadequate caloric intake during the first days of life increases TSB levels because of relative starvation.[32,35,37,38] If jaundice continues beyond the second and third weeks, despite adequate milk intake and weight gain, it is likely that one or more of the factors listed above are contributing to the hyperbilirubinemia. Early optimizing of

TABLE 1 Characteristics Distinguishing Suboptimal Intake Jaundice from Breast Milk Jaundice

	Typical time frame	Weight	Stool output	Urine output	Clinical findings
Suboptimal intake jaundice	Onset 2–5 days of age and usually resolved by 2 weeks	Ongoing weight loss	<5/day with color black, brown, or green	<5/day with uric acid crystals (brick color)	Commonly <38 weeks and rarely ≥40 weeks gestation. May be fussy and difficult to settle between feedings or sleepy and difficult to wake for feeding
Breast milk jaundice	Onset 2–5 days and may last up to 3 months	Gaining ≥30 g/day[107]	≥8/day with yellow color	≥8/day with yellow or clear color	Waking to feed 8–12 ×/day

breastfeeding and consideration of additional enteral intake when there is clinical or laboratory evidence that breastfeeding is compromised might mitigate the development of subsequent hyperbilirubinemia. Options for additional enteral intake are discussed below.

Kernicterus and bilirubin encephalopathy

The most recent studies in high-resource countries suggest that in the absence of significant comorbidities such as sepsis or Rh hemolytic disease, kernicterus or chronic bilirubin encephalopathy occurs in about 1 in 200,000 live births and only when TSB levels exceeded 600 μmol/L (35 mg/dL).[63–65] In lower resource countries, bilirubin encephalopathy and comorbidities are much more common so that kernicterus can and does occur more frequently and at lower bilirubin levels.[66] Even in high-resource countries, extreme hyperbilirubinemia in apparently healthy breastfeeding infants can cause kernicterus.[67,68] In the U.S. Kernicterus Registry, a database of 125 cases of kernicterus in infants discharged as healthy newborns, 98% of these infants were fully or partially breastfed, highlighting the importance of appropriate breastfeeding support and follow-up from the prenatal period through to the early postpartum months. Whether hyperbilirubinemia, in the absence of the classic symptoms of bilirubin toxicity, produces subtle neurologic deficits is a controversial topic beyond the scope of this protocol. Recent studies suggest, however, if severe hyperbilirubinemia does cause subtle neurologic deficits, it is a rare occurrence.[63–65]

EVIDENCE-BASED STRATEGIES FOR PREVENTING OR AMELIORATING JAUNDICE IN THE BREASTFEEDING INFANT

Management of jaundice once treatment thresholds for TSB are reached is discussed in the next section. The following measures are recommended to maintain TSB levels below those proposed for treatment while supporting the successful establishment of breastfeeding:

1. Initiate early breastfeeding.

a. Initiate breastfeeding as early as possible, preferably in the first hour after birth[69–72] (I) (quality of evidence [levels of evidence IA, IB, IIA, IIB, III, and IV] is based on levels of evidence used for the National Guidelines Clearing House[73] and is noted in parentheses) even for infants delivered by cesarean section. In the vast majority of births, breastfeeding should be initiated in the first hour.

2. Encourage frequent exclusive breastfeeding.

a. Frequent breastfeeding (8–12 times or more in 24 hours) is crucial both to increase infant enteral intake and to maximize breast emptying, which is essential for the establishment of milk supply. Feeding anything before the onset of breastfeeding delays the establishment of good breastfeeding practices and may hinder milk production, increasing the risk of reduced enteral intake and exaggerated hyperbilirubinemia. There is a positive association between the number of breastfeeds a day and lower TSB.[74] (III) It is unnecessary to give glucose water to test the infant's ability to swallow or avoid aspiration.

b. Hand expression or pumping of colostrum or breastmilk can provide extra milk to support intake in some infants at risk for suboptimal intake jaundice and exaggerated hyperbilirubinemia and assist in establishing a good milk supply. Although pumping is commonly used, it is noteworthy that hand expression may be better tolerated by mothers in the immediate postpartum period. Randomized trials have shown that the initiation of pumping may reduce milk transfer and eventual breastfeeding duration for some populations of infants.[26,27] (IB)

3. Optimize early breastfeeding management.

a. Ensure comfortable positioning (that avoids nipple compression or rubbing), effective latch, and adequate milk transfer (swallowing) from the outset by having a healthcare provider trained in breastfeeding management (e.g., nurse, lactation consultant, midwife, or physician) and evaluate position and latch, providing recommendations as necessary.

b. Support skin-to-skin contact for all mothers and infants (in a safe manner when the mother is awake and alert), but particularly for those breastfeeding, starting immediately after birth and throughout the postpartum period as it helps with milk supply and makes mother's milk easily available to the infant in the first days and weeks of life.[72] (I)

4. Provide education on early feeding cues.

a. Teach the mother to respond to the earliest cues of infant hunger, such as moving about or restlessness, lip smacking, hand movements toward the mouth, and vocalizing. Most newborns need to be fed every 2 ½ to 3 hours. Infants should be put to the breast before the onset of crying as crying is a late sign of hunger and often results in a poor start to the breastfeeding episode. Attention should also be paid to infants who are sleepy or do not show signs of hunger.

5. Identify mothers and infants at risk for hyperbilirubinemia.

a. Some maternal factors (e.g., diabetes, Rh sensitization, and past family history of jaundiced infants) increase the risk of hyperbilirubinemia in the newborn. Primiparous mothers are at risk for delayed secretory activation as are those who give birth through cesarean section or have a maternal body—mass index over 27 kg/m^2. Infants of these mothers are therefore at risk for suboptimal intake.[75] (III)

b. With the exception of infants with pathologic conditions such as Rh or ABO hemolytic disease and glucose-6-phosphate dehydrogenase (G6PD) deficiency, the single most important clinical risk factor for hyperbilirubinemia in newborns is decreasing gestational age. For each week of gestation below 40 weeks, the odds of developing a TSB ≥ 428 μmol/ L (25 mg/dL) increase by a factor of 1.7 (95% CI 1.4—2.5).[19] Management of 34—37-week late preterm and early term infants who are not breastfeeding well can be found in the relevant ABM Clinical Protocol.[76] (IV)

c. Significant bruising or cephalohematoma can increase the risk of hyperbilirubinemia due to the increased breakdown of heme. East Asian newborns also have a higher risk of jaundice, perhaps related to their ethnic or genetic background.[59] (III)

d. The above factors can be additive with suboptimal intake jaundice and/or breast milk jaundice and produce even higher bilirubin levels than would otherwise be seen. When risk factors are identified, it is prudent to seek assistance with breastfeeding in the early hours after birth to ensure optimal breastfeeding management. Mothers may benefit from early instruction about milk expression by hand or pump to protect the milk supply.

6. Do not supplement infants with anything other than mother's own expressed milk in the absence of a specific clinical indication. Indications for supplementation are discussed briefly below. Full details on indications for supplementation, choice of supplement, and methods of supplementation are available in ABM Clinical Protocol #3: Supplementary Feedings in the Healthy Term Breastfed Neonate, Revised 2017.[77] (IV)

7. While management of newborns varies from country to country, most infants discharged before 72 hours of age should be seen by a healthcare provider within 2 days of discharge from birth hospitalization. This is especially important for exclusively breastfed infants. Close follow-up of the breastfeeding newborn both facilitates prevention of excess weight loss that may contribute to hyperbilirubinemia[17,20,57—60] (III) and ensures that elevated bilirubin concentrations are promptly treated.[21] (IV) Individual clinical judgment regarding follow-up can be used, such as in the case of an experienced multiparous mother who has breastfed previous infants and is going home with an infant who has no hyperbilirubinemia risk factors.[21] Protocols for monitoring bilirubin vary from country to country and within countries. While the U.K. guidelines do not recommend measuring bilirubin levels at follow-up unless the infant is visibly jaundiced, frequent monitoring using a TcB meter is recommended by the Japanese Society for Neonatal Health and Development.

MANAGEMENT OF BREASTFEEDING IN THE NEWBORN WITH JAUNDICE

Consensus-based guidelines for the management of hyperbilirubinemia, including monitoring procedures, recommended treatment, and thresholds for treatment, have been developed in the United States, Canada, Norway, the United Kingdom, and some 14 other countries.[1,21,78,79] (IV) For monitoring, guidelines from the United States,[21] Canada,[80] and several other countries recommend a measurement of the TSB or TcB in every infant before discharge from the birth hospitalization, although this is not specifically recommended in the U.K. guidelines. Universal TcB measurement is also standard practice in Japan. Combining the TcB measurement with the infant's gestational age and plotting on an appropriate graph provide a prediction of the risk of hyperbilirubinemia that is as accurate as the combination of all other nonpathologic risk factors. When TSB levels rise above the thresholds stated in guidelines, despite adequate lactation support, phototherapy is recommended as the most effective treatment. Other therapeutic options, which may be used either alone or in combination with phototherapy, depending on clinical circumstance, include (1) temporary additional feedings with expressed breast milk; (2) temporary supplementation with donor human milk if available; (3) temporary supplementation with infant formula; or (4) very rarely, temporary interruption of breastfeeding and replacement feeding with infant formula. These options are described in more detail below.

When discussing any treatment options with parents, healthcare providers should emphasize that all treatments are compatible with continuation of breastfeeding. Because parents may associate breastfeeding with the development of jaundice requiring special treatment or hospitalization, they may be reluctant to continue breastfeeding, particularly if infant formula supplementation or interrupting breastfeeding is suggested as treatment. Healthcare providers should offer special assistance to these mothers to ensure that they understand the importance of continuing to breastfeed and know how to maintain their milk supply if temporary interruption is necessary. Special care should be taken to address and discuss any guilt parents have about their feeding decisions, both because such guilt can be counterproductive to continued breastfeeding[81–84] (III) and because many factors contribute to jaundice and the relative contribution of each factor is often unknown.[85–88] (III, IV)

Treatment options

1. Phototherapy. Phototherapy is the most frequently used treatment option when TSB concentrations exceed treatment thresholds, especially when levels are rising rapidly. Phototherapy can be used while continuing full breastfeeding or it can be combined with supplementation of expressed breast milk or infant formula if maternal supply is insufficient. Only in extenuating circumstances is temporary interruption of breastfeeding with replacement feeding necessary.[1,21,89] (IV) Phototherapy can be done in the hospital or at home. Home phototherapy is acceptable for low-risk infants provided TSB levels are monitored.[90] (IV) In the hospital, it is best done in the mother's room or a hospital room where the mother can also reside to minimize mother–infant separation and so that breastfeeding can be continued. Interruption of phototherapy for durations of up to 30 minutes or longer to permit breastfeeding without eye patches does not alter the effectiveness of the treatment.[91–93] (III, IB) Although phototherapy increases insensible water loss to some degree, infants under phototherapy do not routinely require extra oral or intravenous fluids.[90] (IV) However, if newborns receiving phototherapy are too sleepy to breastfeed vigorously, or if breastfeeding appears ineffective, mothers should express milk to feed by syringe, bottle, or gavage until newborns are vigorous enough to transfer milk effectively. The routine provision of intravenous fluids is discouraged because they may inhibit thirst and diminish oral intake. However, they may be indicated in cases of infant dehydration, hypernatremia, or inability to ingest adequate milk.

2. In settings where phototherapy is not readily available, results in significant mother–infant separation, or has other potential negative consequences, physicians may consider recommending supplementary feedings at levels of bilirubin approaching those recommended for initiating phototherapy. Such decisions should be individualized with the goal of keeping mother and infant together as well as preserving and optimizing breastfeeding while effectively preventing or treating the hyperbilirubinemia.

   a. First and best supplement is expressed own mother's milk. It can be hand expressed into a small cup or spoon and directly fed to the infant with help from staff who are knowledgeable in this technique. In this way, breastfeeding is best supported.

   b. If own mother's milk is not available, supplementing with donor human milk will increase enteral intake. Breastfeeding infants supplemented only with donor milk meet the World Health Organization definition of exclusive breastfeeding. The specific effect of donor milk supplementation on bilirubin levels has not been studied.

   c. It may be necessary to supplement with infant formula if neither own mothers' milk nor donor human milk is available. The impact of introducing formula to an exclusively breastfed infant must be considered. The effect of supplementation with donor human milk versus infant formula is not well studied.

   d. Supplementation with water or glucose water is contraindicated because it does not reduce serum bilirubin,[94,95] (IIA, III) interferes with breastfeeding, and might cause hyponatremia.

   e. Supplementation of breastfeeding should preferably be undertaken using a cup, spoon, syringe, or supplemental nursing system (if infant is latching) simultaneously with or immediately following each breastfeed. Nipples/teats and bottles should be avoided where possible. However, there is no evidence that any of these methods are unsafe or that one is necessarily better than the other.[77,96] (IA)

3. When TSB levels are very high or associated with evidence of poor breast milk intake despite appropriate intervention, supplementation with infant formula can eliminate the deleterious effect of *UGT1A1* polymorphisms on serum bilirubin and is a reasonable addition if it can be done in a way that is supportive of breastfeeding.[51] (IIA) Depending on the TSB level, follow-up TSB measurements within 4–24 hours are needed. Supplementation cannot be substituted for phototherapy in the treatment of infants with hemolytic hyperbilirubinemia.

   a. Supplementation of breastfeeding with infant formula. As infant formula inhibits the intestinal reabsorption of bilirubin,[97] (IV) it may sometimes be used to lower TSB in breastfeeding infants.[77] Small-volume (10–15 mL) feedings of formula immediately following a breastfeeding may be preferred to intermittent large-volume (30–60 mL) supplementation so as to maintain frequent breastfeeding and preserve maternal milk production at a high level.[98] (IA) Larger volumes may be required if the infant is not receiving sufficient milk at the breast (i.e., low milk supply or poor milk transfer).

   b. Temporary interruption of breastfeeding. Temporary interruption of breastfeeding is very rarely needed, but may be considered for specific clinical scenarios in which rapid reduction in TSB is urgently needed or if phototherapy is unavailable.[99] (IIA) If urgent clinical needs necessitate the temporary interruption of breastfeeding, it is critical to maintain maternal milk production by teaching the mother to effectively and frequently express milk by hand or pump. The infant needs to return to a good supply of milk when breastfeeding resumes, or poor milk supply may result in a return of higher TSB concentrations.

Post-treatment follow-up and evaluation

Infants who have had any of the above treatments for excessive hyperbilirubinemia need to be carefully followed with repeat TSB determinations and support of breastfeeding because suboptimal breast milk intake may result in recurrence of hyperbilirubinemia.

Encouragement to continue breastfeeding is of the greatest importance since many parents will be fearful that continued breastfeeding may result in more jaundice or other problems. Parents can be reassured that almost all hyperbilirubinemia requiring treatment resolves within the first 5 days after birth. Even those infants with more prolonged breast milk jaundice who required and received treatment rarely have sufficient rise in bilirubin with continued breastfeeding to require further intervention.

SUMMARY AND CONCLUSIONS

Breastfeeding and some degree of hyperbilirubinemia are normal and expected aspects of neonatal development.[45] Managing the confluence of jaundice and breastfeeding in a physiologic and supportive manner to ensure optimal health, growth, and development of the infant is the responsibility of all healthcare providers. A complete understanding of normal and abnormal states of both bilirubin and breastfeeding is essential if optimal care is to be provided and the best outcome achieved for the child. We provide guidelines for managing this problem while recognizing the need for adjusting the guidelines to the individual needs of each infant.

RESEARCH NEEDS

The recommendations above are based on the most current research and clinical experience available. Identifying the components in human milk that increase total serum bilirubin and whether and to what extent these components interact with genetic variation to increase jaundice might substantially improve risk-based strategies to prevent and treat hyperbilirubinemia. Because both commercial and noncommercial sources of banked donor milk are increasingly available,[100–104] further research on the effect of supplementing breastfed infants with banked donor milk on TSB levels is urgently needed. Small volumes of L-aspartic acid, enzymatically hydrolyzed casein or whey/casein, immediately after breastfeeding show potential promise in reducing TSB without interfering with breastfeeding or milk supply, but such interventions need further evaluation before they can be recommended for use.[105] In addition, widely generalizable research is also needed to evaluate specific strategies for feeding management of the breastfed infant with hyperbilirubinemia that allow uninterrupted breastfeeding while

reducing serum bilirubin concentrations to safe levels. Additional strategies to maximize maternal milk intake and shorten the duration of phototherapy need to be further explored and considered.[106]

ACKNOWLEDGMENT

The authors are grateful to Heather Molnar, MD, for her review of the manuscript.

REFERENCES

1. American Academy of Pediatrics Subcommittee on Hyperbilirubinemia. Management of hyperbilirubinemia in the newborn infant 35 or more weeks of gestation. *Pediatrics.* 2004;114:297–316.
2. Maisels MJ. Managing the jaundiced newborn: A persistent challenge. *CMAJ.* 2015;187:335–343.
3. Preer GL, Philipp BL. Understanding and managing breast-milk jaundice. *Arch Dis Child Fetal Neonatal Ed.* 2011;96: F461–F466.
4. Olusanya BO, Osibanjo FB, Slusher TM. Risk factors for severe neonatal hyperbilirubinemia in low and middle-income countries: A systematic review and meta-analysis. *PLoS One.* 2015;10:e0117229.
5. VanWagner LB, Green RM. Evaluating elevated bilirubin levels in asymptomatic adults. *JAMA.* 2015;313:516–517.
6. Bhutani VK, Stark AR, Lazzeroni LC, et al. Predischarge screening for severe neonatal hyperbilirubinemia identifies infants who need phototherapy. *J Pediatr.* 2013;162. 477–482 e471.
7. Keren R, Luan X, Friedman S, et al. A comparison of alternative risk-assessment strategies for predicting significant neonatal hyperbilirubinemia in term and near-term infants. *Pediatrics.* 2008;121:e170–e179.
8. Fouzas S, Mantagou L, Skylogianni E, et al. Transcutaneous bilirubin levels for the first 120 postnatal hours in healthy neonates. *Pediatrics.* 2010;125:e52–e57.
9. De Luca D, Romagnoli C, Tiberi E, et al. Skin bilirubin nomogram for the first 96h of life in a European normal healthy newborn population, obtained with multiwavelength transcutaneous bilirubinometry. *Acta Paediatr.* 2008;97:146–150.
10. Bhutani VK, Vilms RJ, Hamerman-Johnson L. Universal bilirubin screening for severe neonatal hyperbilirubinemia. *J Perinatol.* 2010;30(Suppl):S6–S15.
11. Maisels MJ. What's in a name? Physiologic and pathologic jaundice: The conundrum of defining normal bilirubin levels in the newborn. *Pediatrics.* 2006;118:805–807.
12. Bertini G, Dani C, Tronchin M, et al. Is breastfeeding really favoring early neonatal jaundice? *Pediatrics.* 2001;107:E41.
13. Dahms BB, Krauss AN, Gartner LM, et al. Breast feeding and serum bilirubin values during the first 4 days of life. *J Pediatr.* 1973;83:1049–1054.
14. Jangaard KA, Fell DB, Dodds L, et al. Outcomes in a population of healthy term and near-term infants with serum bilirubin levels of >or = 325 micromol/L (> or = 19 mg/dL) who were born in Nova Scotia, Canada, between 1994 and 2000. *Pediatrics.* 2008;122:119–124.
15. Kaplan M, Herschel M, Hammerman C, et al. Neonatal hyperbilirubinemia in African American males: The importance of glucose-6-phosphate dehydrogenase deficiency. *J Pediatr.* 2006;149:83–88.

16. Kuzniewicz MW, Escobar GJ, Wi S, et al. Risk factors for severe hyperbilirubinemia among infants with borderline bilirubin levels: A nested case-control study. *J Pediatr.* 2008;153:234–240.

17. Chen CF, Hsu MC, Shen CH, et al. Influence of breastfeeding on weight loss, jaundice, and waste elimination in neonates. *Pediatr Neonatol.* 2011;52:85–92.

18. Yang H, Wang Q, Zheng L, et al. Multiple genetic modifiers of bilirubin metabolism involvement in significant neonatal hyperbilirubinemia in patients of Chinese descent. *PLoS One.* 2015;10:e0132034.

19. Newman TB, Xiong B, Gonzales VM, et al. Prediction and prevention of extreme neonatal hyperbilirubinemia in a mature health maintenance organization. *Arch Pediatr Adolesc Med.* 2000;154:1140–1147.

20. Huang MS, Lin MC, Chen HH, et al. Risk factor analysis for late-onset neonatal hyperbilirubinemia in Taiwanese infants. *Pediatr Neonatol.* 2009;50:261–265.

21. Maisels MJ, Bhutani VK, Bogen D, et al. Hyperbilirubinemia in the newborn infant > or = 35 weeks' gestation: An update with clarifications. *Pediatrics.* 2009;124:1193–1198.

22. Itoh S, Kondo M, Kusaka T, et al. Differences in transcutaneous bilirubin readings in Japanese term infants according to feeding method. *Pediatr Int.* 2001;43:12–15.

23. De Carvalho M, Robertson S, Klaus M. Fecal bilirubin excretion and serum bilirubin concentrations in breastfed and bottle-fed infants. *J Pediatr.* 1985;107:786–790.

24. Buiter HD, Dijkstra SS, Oude Elferink RF, et al. Neonatal jaundice and stool production in breast- or formula-fed term infants. *Eur J Pediatr.* 2008;167:501–507.

25. Gartner LM. Breastfeeding and jaundice. *J Perinatol.* 2001;21 (Suppl 1):S25–S29.

26. Flaherman VJ, Gay B, Scott C, et al. Randomised trial comparing hand expression with breast pumping for mothers of term newborns feeding poorly. *Arch Dis Child Fetal Neonatal Ed.* 2012;97:F18–F23.

27. Chapman DJ, Young S, Ferris AM, et al. Impact of breast pumping on lactogenesis stage II after cesarean delivery: A randomized clinical trial. *Pediatrics.* 2001;107:E94.

28. Evans KC, Evans RG, Royal R, et al. Effect of caesarean section on breast milk transfer to the normal term newborn over the first week of life. *Arch Dis Child Fetal Neonatal Ed.* 2003;88:F380–F382.

29. Santoro W Jr, Martinez FE, Ricco RG, et al. Colostrum ingested during the first day of life by exclusively breastfed healthy newborn infants. *J Pediatr.* 2010;156:29–32.

30. Aaltonen T, Alvarez Gonzalez B, Amerio S, et al. Measurement of b hadron lifetimes in exclusive decays containing a J/psi in pp collisions at radicals = 1.96 TeV. *Phys Rev Lett.* 2011;106:121804.

31. Saint L, Smith M, Hartmann PE. The yield and nutrient content of colostrum and milk of women from giving birth to 1 month post-partum. *Br J Nutr.* 1984;52:87–95.

32. Whitmer DI, Gollan JL. Mechanisms and significance of fasting and dietary hyperbilirubinemia. *Semin Liver Dis.* 1983;3:42–51.

33. White GL Jr, Nelson JA, Pedersen DM, et al. Fasting and gender (and altitude?) influence reference intervals for serum bilirubin in healthy adults. *Clin Chem.* 1981;27:1140–1142.

34. Bloomer JR, Barrett PV, Rodkey FL, et al. Studies on the mechanism of fasting hyperbilirubinemia. *Gastroenterology.* 1971;61:479–487.

35. Fevery J. Fasting hyperbilirubinemia: Unraveling the mechanism involved. *Gastroenterology.* 1997;113:1798–1800.

36. Pang WW, Hartmann PE. Initiation of human lactation: Secretory differentiation and secretory activation. *J Mammary Gland Biol Neoplasia.* 2007;12:211–221.

37. De Carvalho M, Klaus MH, Merkatz RB. Frequency of breastfeeding and serum bilirubin concentration. *Am J Dis Child.* 1982;136:737–738.

38. Yamauchi Y, Yamanouchi I. Breast-feeding frequency during the first 24 hours after birth in full-term neonates. *Pediatrics.* 1990;86:171–175.

39. Wu PY, Hodgman JE, Kirkpatrick BV, et al. Metabolic aspects of phototherapy. *Pediatrics.* 1985;75(2 Pt 2):427–433.

40. Davila-Grijalva H, Troya AH, King E, et al. How much do formula-fed infants take in the first 2 days? *Clin Pediatr.* 2016;. pii: 0009922816637647.

41. Sato H, Uchida T, Toyota K, et al. Association of neonatal hyperbilirubinemia in breast-fed infants with UGT1A1 or SLCOs polymorphisms. *J Hum Genet.* 2015;60:35–40.

42. Sato H, Uchida T, Toyota K, et al. Association of breast-fed neonatal hyperbilirubinemia with UGT1A1 polymorphisms: 211G > A (G71R) mutation becomes a risk factor under inadequate feeding. *J Hum Genet.* 2013;58:7–10.

43. Maisels MJ, Clune S, Coleman K, et al. The natural history of jaundice in predominantly breastfed infants. *Pediatrics.* 2014;134:e340–e345.

44. Kivlahan C, James EJ. The natural history of neonatal jaundice. *Pediatrics.* 1984;74:364–370.

45. American Academy of Pediatrics. Breastfeeding and the use of human milk. *Pediatrics.* 2012;129:e827–e841.

46. Verkade HJ. A novel hypothesis on the pathophysiology of neonatal jaundice. *J Pediatr.* 2002;141:594–595.

47. Apaydin K, Ermis B, Arasli M, et al. Cytokines in human milk and late-onset breast milk jaundice. *Pediatr Int.* 2012;54:801–805.

48. Uras N, Tonbul A, Karadag A, et al. Prolonged jaundice in newborns is associated with low antioxidant capacity in breast milk. *Scand J Clin Lab Invest.* 2010;70:433–437.

49. Bozkaya OG, Kumral A, Yesilirmak DC, et al. Prolonged unconjugated hyper bilirubinaemia associated with the haemoxygenase-1 gene promoter polymorphism. *Acta Paediatr.* 2010;99:679–683.

50. Zaja O, Tiljak MK, Stefanovic M, et al. Correlation of UGT1A1 TATA-box polymorphism and jaundice in breastfed newborns-early presentation of Gilbert's syndrome. *J Matern Fetal Neonatal Med.* 2014;27:844–850.

51. Chou HC, Chen MH, Yang HI, et al. 211G to a variation of UDP-glucuronosyl transferase 1A1 gene and neonatal breast-feeding jaundice. *Pediatr Res.* 2011;69:170–174.

52. Kumral A, Ozkan H, Duman N, et al. Breast milk jaundice correlates with high levels of epidermal growth factor. *Pediatr Res.* 2009;66:218–221.

53. Manganaro R, Marseglia L, Mami C, et al. Serum alpha fetoprotein (AFP) levels in breastfed infants with prolonged indirect hyperbilirubinemia. *Early Hum Dev.* 2008;84:487–490.

54. Nagao Y, Ohsawa M, Kobayashi T. Correlation between unconjugated bilirubin and total cholesterol in the sera of 1-month-old infants. *J Paediatr Child Health.* 2010;46:709–713.

55. Tuzun F, Kumral A, Duman N, et al. Breast milk jaundice: Effect of bacteria present in breast milk and infant feces. *J Pediatr Gastroenterol Nutr.* 2013;56:328–332.

56. Watchko JF, Lin Z. Genetics of neonatal jaundice. In: Stevenson DK, Maisels MJ, Watchko JF, eds. *Care of the Jaundiced Neonate.* New York, NY: McGraw Hill; 2012:1–27.

57. Chang RJ, Chou HC, Chang YH, et al. Weight loss percentage prediction of subsequent neonatal hyperbilirubinemia in exclusively breastfed neonates. *Pediatr Neonatol.* 2012;53:41–44.

58. Chen YJ, Chen WC, Chen CM. Risk factors for hyperbilirubinemia in breastfed term neonates. *Eur J Pediatr.* 2012;171:167–171.

59. Huang A, Tai BC, Wong LY, et al. Differential risk for early breastfeeding jaundice in a multi-ethnic Asian cohort. *Ann Acad Med Singapore.* 2009;38:217–224.

60. Huang HC, Yang HI, Chang YH, et al. Model to predict hyperbilirubinemia in healthy term and near-term newborns with exclusive breast feeding. *Pediatr Neonatol.* 2012;53:354–358.

61. Salas AA, Salazar J, Burgoa CV, et al. Significant weight loss in breastfed term infants readmitted for hyperbilirubinemia. *BMC Pediatr.* 2009;9:82.

62. Yang WC, Zhao LL, Li YC, et al. Bodyweight loss in predicting neonatal hyperbilirubinemia 72 hours after birth in term newborn infants. *BMC Pediatr.* 2013;13:145.

63. Ebbesen F, Bjerre JV, Vandborg PK. Relation between serum bilirubin levels >/= 450 mumol/L and bilirubin encephalopathy; a Danish population-based study. *Acta Paediatr.* 2012;101:384–389.

64. Kuzniewicz MW, Wickremasinghe AC, Wu YW, et al. Incidence, etiology, and outcomes of hazardous hyperbilirubinemia in newborns. *Pediatrics.* 2014;134:504–509.

65. Newman TB, Kuzniewicz MW. Follow-up of extreme neonatal hyperbilirubinaemia: More reassuring results from Denmark. *Dev Med Child Neurol.* 2015;57:314–315.

66. Bhutani VK, Zipursky A, Blencowe H, et al. Neonatal hyperbilirubinemia and Rhesus disease of the newborn: Incidence and impairment estimates for 2010 at regional and global levels. *Pediatr Res.* 2013;74(Suppl 1):86–100.

67. Bhutani VK, Johnson LH, Jeffrey Maisels M, et al. Kernicterus: Epidemiological strategies for its prevention through systems-based approaches. *J Perinatol.* 2004;24:650–662.

68. Maisels MJ, Newman TB. Kernicterus in otherwise healthy, breast-fed term newborns. *Pediatrics.* 1995;96(4 Pt 1):730–733.

69. Righard L, Alade MO. Effect of delivery room routines on success of first breast-feed. *Lancet.* 1990;336:1105–1107.

70. Mikiel-Kostyra K, Mazur J, Boltruszko I. Effect of early skin-to-skin contact after delivery on duration of breastfeeding: A prospective cohort study. *Acta Paediatr.* 2002;91:1301–1306.

71. Bramson L, Lee JW, Moore E, et al. Effect of early skin-to-skin mother–infant contact during the first 3 hours following birth on exclusive breastfeeding during the maternity hospital stay. *J Hum Lact.* 2010;26:130–137.

72. Moore ER, Bergman N, Anderson GC, et al. Early skin-to-skin contact for mothers and their healthy newborn infants. *Cochrane Database Syst Rev.* 2016. Available from: https://doi.org/10.1002/14651858.CD003519.pub4.

73. Shekelle PG, Woolf SH, Eccles M, et al. Developing guidelines. *BMJ.* 1999;318:593–596.

74. Boskabadi H, Zakerihamidi M. The correlation between frequency and duration of breastfeeding and the severity of neonatal hyperbilirubinemia. *J Matern Fetal Neonatal Med.* 2017. Available from: http://doi.org/10.1080/14767058.2017.1287897.

75. Dewey KG, Nommsen-Rivers LA, Heinig MJ, et al. Risk factors for suboptimal infant breastfeeding behavior, delayed onset of lactation, and excess neonatal weight loss. *Pediatrics.* 2003;112(3 Pt 1):607–619.

76. Boies EG, Vaucher YE. The Academy of Breastfeeding Medicine. ABM Clinical Protocol #10: Breastfeeding the late preterm (34–36 6/7 weeks of gestation) and early term infants (37–38 6/7 weeks of gestation), second revision 2016. *Breastfeed Med.* 2016;11:494–500.

77. Kellams A, Harrel C, Omage S, et al. ABM clinical protocol #3: Supplementary feedings in the healthy term breastfed neonate. *Breastfeed Med.* 2017;12:188–198.

78. National Institute for Health and Care Excellence (NICE). *Jaundice in Newborn Babies Under 28 Days.* London: NICE; 2016.

79. Bratlid D, Nakstad B, Hansen TW. National guidelines for treatment of jaundice in the newborn. *Acta Paediatr.* 2011;100:499–505.

80. Guidelines for detection, management and prevention of hyperbilirubinemia in term and late preterm newborn infants (35 or more weeks' gestation)—Summary. *Paediatr Child Health* 2007;12:401–418.

81. Flaherman VJ, Hicks KG, Cabana MD, et al. Maternal experience of interactions with providers among mothers with milk supply concern. *Clin Pediatr.* 2012;51:778–784.

82. Kair LR, Flaherman VJ, Newby KA, et al. The experience of breastfeeding the late preterm infant: A qualitative study. *Breastfeed Med.* 2015;10:102–106.

83. Hill PD. Insufficient milk supply syndrome. *NAACOGS Clin Issu Perinat Womens Health Nurs.* 1992;3:605–612.

84. Hill PD. The enigma of insufficient milk supply. *MCN Am J Matern Child Nurs.* 1991;16:312–316.

85. Lauer BJ, Spector ND. Hyperbilirubinemia in the newborn. *Pediatr Rev.* 2011;32:341–349.

86. Maisels MJ. Screening and early postnatal management strategies to prevent hazardous hyperbilirubinemia in newborns of 35 or more weeks of gestation. *Semin Fetal Neonatal Med.* 2010;15:129–135.

87. Schwartz HP, Haberman BE, Ruddy RM. Hyperbilirubinemia: Current guidelines and emerging therapies. *Pediatr Emerg Care.* 2011;27:884–889.

88. Watchko JF. Identification of neonates at risk for hazardous hyperbilirubinemia: Emerging clinical insights. *Pediatr Clin North Am.* 2009;56:671–687.

89. Gulcan H, Tiker F, Kilicdag H. Effect of feeding type on the efficacy of phototherapy. *Indian Pediatr.* 2007;44:32–36.

90. Maisels MJ, Newman TB, Watchko J, et al. Phototherapy and other treatments. In: Stevenson DK, Maisels MJ, Watchko JF, eds. *Care of the Jaundiced Neonate.* New York: McGraw Hill; 2012:195–227.

91. Lau SP, Fung KP. Serum bilirubin kinetics in intermittent phototherapy of physiological jaundice. *Arch Dis Child.* 1984;59:892–894.

92. Vogl TP, Hegyi T, Hiatt IM, et al. Intermediate phototherapy in the treatment of jaundice in the premature infant. *J Pediatr.* 1978;92:627–630.

93. Sachdeva M, Murki S, Oleti TP, et al. Intermittent versus continuous phototherapy for the treatment of neonatal non-hemolytic moderate hyperbilirubinemia in infants more than 34 weeks of gestational age: A randomized controlled trial. *Eur J Pediatr.* 2015;174:177–181.

94. de Carvalho M, Hall M, Harvey D. Effects of water supplementation on physiological jaundice in breast-fed babies. *Arch Dis Child.* 1981;56:568—569.

95. Nicoll A, Ginsburg R, Tripp JH. Supplementary feeding and jaundice in newborns. *Acta Paediatr Scand.* 1982;71:759—761.

96. Howard CR, Howard FM, Lanphear B, et al. Randomized clinical trial of pacifier use and bottle-feeding or cupfeeding and their effect on breastfeeding. *Pediatrics.* 2003;111:511—518.

97. Gartner LM, Lee KS, Moscioni AD. Effect of milk feeding on intestinal bilirubin absorption in the rat. *J Pediatr.* 1983;103:464—471.

98. Flaherman VJ, Aby J, Burgos AE, et al. Effect of early limited formula on duration and exclusivity of breastfeeding in at-risk infants: An RCT. *Pediatrics.* 2013;131:1059—1065.

99. Martinez JC, Maisels MJ, Otheguy L, et al. Hyperbilirubinemia in the breast-fed newborn: A controlled trial of four interventions. *Pediatrics.* 1993;91:470—473.

100. Updegrove KH. Donor human milk banking: Growth, challenges, and the role of HMBANA. *Breastfeed Med.* 2013;8:435—437.

101. U.S. Food and Drug Administration. Use of Donor Human Milk. 2014. Available at: www.fda.gov/scienceresearch/specialtopics/pediatrictherapeuticsresearch/ucm235203.htm (accessed January 25, 2014).

102. Kair LR, Colaizy TT, Hubbard D, et al. Donor milk in the newborn nursery at the University of Iowa Children's Hospital. *Breastfeed Med.* 2014;9:547—550.

103. Bulpitt DW, Elmore KE, Catterton LJ. Implementing use of donor breast milk in the well baby population: It's not just for the NICU any more. *J Obstet Gynecol Neonatal Nurs.* 2014;43(Suppl 1):S56.

104. Brownell EA, Lussier MM, Herson VC, et al. Donor human milk bank data collection in North America: An assessment of current status and future needs. *J Hum Lact.* 2014;30:47—53.

105. Gourley GR, Li Z, Kreamer BL, et al. A controlled, randomized, double-blind trial of prophylaxis against jaundice among breastfed newborns. *Pediatrics.* 2005;116:385—391.

106. Samra N, El Taweel A, Cadwell K. The effect of kangaroo mother care on the duration of phototherapy of infants readmitted for neonatal jaundice. *J Matern Fetal Neonatal Med.* 2012;25:1354—1357.

107. Paul IM, Schaefer EW, Miller JR, et al. Weight change nomograms for the first month after birth. *Pediatrics.* 2016;138. pii: e20162625.

ABM protocols expire 5 years from the date of publication.

Content of this protocol is up-to-date at the time of publication. Evidence-based revisions are made within 5 years or sooner if there are significant changes in the evidence. The first version of this protocol was authored by Lawrence Gartner.

The Academy of Breastfeeding Medicine Protocol Committee:

Wendy Brodribb, MBBS, PhD, FABM, Chairperson

Larry Noble, MD, FABM, Translations Chairperson

Nancy Brent, MD

Maya Bunik, MD, MSPH, FABM

Cadey Harrel, MD

Ruth A. Lawrence, MD, FABM

Kathleen A. Marinelli, MD, FABM

Sarah Reece-Stremtan, MD

Casey Rosen-Carole, MD, MPH

Tomoko Seo, MD, FABM

Rose St. Fleur, MD

Michal Young, MD

For correspondence: abm@bfmed.org

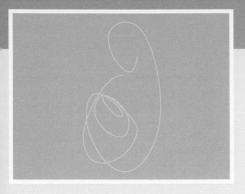

ABM Clinical Protocol #23
Nonpharmacological Management of Procedure-Related Pain in the Breastfeeding Infant, Revised 2016*

Sarah Reece-Stremtan[1], Larry Gray[2] and The Academy of Breastfeeding Medicine*

ABSTRACT

A central goal of The Academy of Breastfeeding Medicine is the development of clinical protocols for managing common medical problems that may impact breastfeeding success. These protocols serve only as guidelines for the care of breastfeeding mothers and infants and do not delineate an exclusive course of treatment or serve as standards of medical care. Variations in treatment may be appropriate according to the needs of an individual patient. These guidelines are not intended to be all-inclusive, but to provide a basic framework for physician education regarding breastfeeding.

PURPOSE

THE INTERNATIONAL EVIDENCE-BASED GROUP for Neonatal Pain and the American Academy of Pediatrics recommends that all neonatal units develop strategies to minimize the number of minor painful or stressful procedures and to provide effective nonpharmacological and/or pharmacological pain relief for newborns.[1,2] The purpose of this protocol is to provide healthcare professionals with evidence-based guidelines on how to incorporate nonpharmacological or behavioral interventions to relieve procedure-induced pain in the breastfeeding infant.

BACKGROUND

Newborns and young infants routinely experience pain associated with commonly used invasive procedures such as blood sampling and intramuscular injections (e.g., vaccinations and vitamin K) and, in some countries, circumcision (the removal of some or all of the foreskin [prepuce] from the penis).[1] Reduction of pain is both a professional imperative and an ethical expectation because untreated pain has detrimental consequences[2] such as greater pain sensitivity in later childhood[3–6] and may lead to permanent neuroanatomical and behavioral abnormalities as demonstrated in animal models.[3,7]

Moreover, pain is a source of concern and distress for new parents and may disturb mother–infant bonding.[8] Pain reduction therapies are often underused for the numerous minor procedures that are part of routine medical and nursing care for neonates.[9,10] Growing scientific and clinical evidence from both animal and human newborns points to the efficacy of natural, nonpharmacological interventions to reduce pain due to minor procedures. Parents should be educated about the benefits of using breastfeeding and human milk in these situations.[11]

SOOTHING THE NEWBORN INFANT

There are several techniques that have been shown to provide pain relief for newborns (0–28 days of age) undergoing painful procedures. In breastfed newborns, breastfeeding itself is the preferred method to alleviate procedural pain. In addition to being safe, effective, natural, and without added cost, it provides an additional opportunity to promote and support breastfeeding. The individual components of breastfeeding (sucking, sweet taste, and warm contact) may be used separately or in combination when breastfeeding itself is not possible.

Breastfeeding or human milk

1. Breastfeeding should be the first choice to alleviate procedural pain in neonates undergoing a single painful procedure, such as venipuncture or heel lance (IA).[12–14] (Quality of evidence [levels of evidence IA, IB, IIA, IIB, III, and IV] is based on levels of evidence used for the National Guidelines Clearing House[15] and is noted in

* Courtesy of the Academy of Breastfeeding Medicine. Please go to https://www.bfmed.org/protocols for complete protocols, translations, and the most up-to-date information (protocols are updated every 5–7 years).
[1] Division of Anesthesiology, Pain, and Perioperative Medicine, Children's National Health System, Washington, District of Columbia.
[2] Department of Pediatrics, University of Chicago, Chicago, Illinois.

parentheses.) Breastfeeding should not be discontinued before the procedure (IB). Studies show that when breastfeeding is stopped shortly before a painful procedure, there was no significant difference in the infant's orogustatory, emotional, tactile, or thermal experience compared with a control group that was not breastfed at all.[16] When breastfeeding is not possible, whether because of the unavailability of the mother or difficulties with breastfeeding, expressed human milk given by dropper, syringe, or bottle has been shown to soothe newborns experiencing procedural pain (IA).[17-20] Administration of human milk can also be combined with sucking, by dipping a pacifier (dummy) in the milk, as described hereunder for sucrose.

2. Although some studies have demonstrated the efficacy of human milk alone,[18,21] human milk may not be equivalent to breastfeeding because of breastfeeding's multicomponent experience. Breastfeeding throughout the painful procedure is likely to be superior to human milk alone on the basis of synergism between the components of breastfeeding (IB).[16,21] One study that used near-infrared spectroscopy to evaluate brain activity in infants undergoing heel prick found generalized cortical activation in breastfed infants that was lacking in infants receiving glucose for analgesia. It was theorized that breastfeeding's multisensory experience helped to overwhelm the pain sensation.[22]

Skin-to-skin contact

1. Coordinating a breastfeeding session with the timing of the procedure is best, but, if this is not possible, skin-to-skin contact with the mother or other caregiver can comfort infants undergoing a procedure such as a heel lance (IA).[22] Skin-to-skin contact also gives the mother a caretaking role during the procedure that is unobtrusive and, by diminishing infant stress, can increase maternal confidence as to her importance in all aspects of her newborn's care.[23] At least one study has found that breastfeeding performed in conjunction with skin-to-skin contact provided superior analgesia during a painful procedure than with sucrose alone or with only skin-to-skin contact.[24]

2. Parental contact and sucrose may act synergistically to reduce pain in neonates. Therefore, if feasible, this combination can be employed (IB).[25] Sucrose taste—first studied in 1991[26]—is readily available for increasing the efficacy of other nonpharmacological techniques.[15] Sucrose administration is covered in more detail in the following section. The use of sucrose and a pacifier can be combined with the skin-to-skin contact.

Warmth and scent

1. Two studies evaluating the effects of warmth on infant pain associated with immunization found a significant analgesic effect when used as the sole intervention and when used in concert with administration of a sucrose solution.[23,24] Infants received 2 minutes of radiant warmer exposure, which was shown not to affect infant core temperature. This maneuver may be a safe and easy intervention if skin-to-skin contact or breastfeeding is not available (IB).

2. The scent of human milk and various other substances such as lavender, vanilla, formula, and amniotic fluid has been evaluated as possible analgesics for painful procedures in preterm and full-term infants, with human milk consistently found to be effective at reducing pain (IB).[25-29]

SUCROSE AND SUCKING (IN COMBINATION OR SEPARATELY)

Sucrose taste has been shown to be an effective analgesia for newborns and young infants for many minor procedures[30,31] but not for more lengthy or invasive procedures such as circumcision[32] or bladder catheterizations in infants older than 30 days.[33] When breastfeeding infants are undergoing painful procedures without mother available for direct breastfeeding and when expressed human milk is not available to use as a supplement, use of sucrose and sucking may be considered (IA).

1. *Sucrose and pacifier.* The combination of oral sucrose and pacifier or non-nutritive sucking is remarkably soothing.[34] This technique offers consistent pain reduction to infants undergoing heel lance, venipuncture, and intramuscular injection. Evidence for pain reduction in procedures such as arterial puncture, subcutaneous injection, insertion of nasogastric or orogastric tubes, bladder catheterization, and eye examinations is less conclusive though most trials demonstrate at least some benefit of sucrose use.[1,31,35] Because pain reduction achieved when using both sucrose and non-nutritive sucking is similar to that with breastfeeding, using a pacifier dipped in 24% sucrose (by weight) solution whenever breastfeeding is not possible is an effective option (IB).[36,37] Sucrose administration should begin 2 minutes before the procedure (IB). If use of a pacifier is not an available or acceptable option, sucrose can also be combined with sucking by dipping a clean, gloved (or nongloved parental) finger in the sucrose solution. When parents are present, they should be educated that sweet substances other than human milk and pacifiers are recommended in the newborn period only for procedural pain.

2. *Sucrose by syringe.* If sucking a pacifier or finger is not an option, 0.5—2 mL of a 24% sucrose solution can be administered orally through syringe 2 minutes before the painful procedure (IB).[1,38] Several 24% sucrose solutions are commercially available. Sucrose administered by oro- or nasogastric tube is not analgesic.

3. *Glucose versus sucrose.* Glucose has also been shown to be an acceptable and effective alternative analgesic (IB).[32,33] Taste difference is not a factor. Studies in rat[39]

and human[40] newborns have not shown a preference for sucrose over glucose. The commercial availability of sucrose (table sugar) may have increased its use.

4. *Sucrose better than human milk?* At least one small study indicates that sucrose is significantly more effective than human milk, when both are administered orally through syringe, at reducing infants' cry time, recovery time (heart rate peak returns to baseline), and change in heart rate (IB).[30] The sugar in human milk is lactose, which has been shown to be an ineffective analgesic.[36] The analgesic component of human milk may be attributed to its fat content or other constituents.

5. *Pacifier alone.* Although pacifiers alone may decrease crying associated with painful procedures, they do not have the same effect on physiological parameters such as heart rate or vagal tone.[41,42] Moreover, sucking a pacifier has been found to reduce pain only when the suck rate exceeds 30 sucks/minute.[31] A pacifier (or clean gloved or parental finger) should be used as the sole soothing intervention only if breastfeeding, human milk, sucrose (or glucose), and skin-to-skin contact are unavailable (IB). Non-nutritive sucking has consistently been found to be better than no intervention at all.[43]

SOOTHING THE PRETERM NEWBORN

Less research has been undertaken for preterm than term newborns, but there are several techniques that can be used to relieve pain in this population. Breastfeeding may be difficult secondary to the medical status of the infant. Preterm infants may be medically compromised and/or may be developmentally unable to suck or swallow. In such cases, individual components of breastfeeding or a combination of the components (e.g., contact and sweet taste) is available (IB). There are concerns about prolonged sucrose exposure in the preterm infant.[39] One study documented infants born at <31 weeks who were given a higher number of sucrose doses had lower scores in motor development and attention when assessed at term.[44] There are no uniform gestational age criteria for studies on analgesia used in preterm infants. The following recommendations are based on studies of infants with an average gestational age of 30 weeks or greater. Not all studies have included infants between 28 and 30 weeks gestational age, and it is unclear whether the following recommendations are generalizable to that age range. Available data do not allow us to extrapolate these recommendations to the smallest preterm infants (<27 weeks).

1. Skin-to-skin contact provides effective pain reduction for preterm newborns (IB).[38,45]

2. In very-low-birth-weight neonates (27–31 weeks gestation) undergoing consecutive heel lances, a pacifier dipped in sucrose or water significantly reduced pain compared with infants who did not receive any intervention (IB).[46]

3. The value of sucrose as a pain reducer in the preterm infant is well established (IB).[40,44,47,48] The recommended dosage in this population is 0.1–0.4 mL of 24% sucrose solution.[1,47] Further pain reduction can be achieved when preterm infants receive 24% sucrose as three doses (0.1 mL, 2 minutes apart given 2 minutes and immediately before heel lance and 2 minutes after lance) rather than as a single dose (IB).[48]

4. The efficacy of breastfeeding and human milk as a pain reducer for the preterm or low-birth-weight infant is less well established; a single study has shown comparable analgesic effects between human milk and breastfeeding with sucrose administration in a population of infants aged 32–37 weeks gestation.[43] Certainly if a mother wishes to breastfeed or provide her preterm infant with human milk instead of using other interventions, this should not be discouraged (IB).

5. Scent of human milk has been found to be an effective analgesic in the preterm infant undergoing venipuncture and heel lance procedures and may be considered in conjunction with other analgesic techniques (IB).[26,27,29]

6. Skin-to-skin contact plus sucrose has not been formally evaluated in preterm infants, but may provide pain reduction for the preterm or low-birth-weight neonates (IV).

SOOTHING THE OLDER INFANT (1 MONTH TO 1 YEAR)

Breastfeeding or its components as an analgesic technique has not been fully researched across this older population. For children older than 1 year, the focus of published literature is on the use of distraction techniques, which falls outside the scope of this protocol.[49] Discussion of additional non-pharmacological techniques such as acupressure, topical vapocoolant spray, and vibration-based devices is also beyond the scope of this protocol.

1. *Sucrose.* Two meta-analyses of 10 and 14 randomized clinical trials on infant pain[50,51] found sucrose to be an effective pain management strategy for infants up to 12 months of age (IA). Two mL of 25% sucrose was effective during vaccination up to 6 months of age[52]; however, 2 mL of 24% sucrose was not effective for more invasive procedures such as bladder catheterization in children older than 1 month.[53] Increasing the concentration of sucrose solution may be more effective as the infant ages.[51] One study explored the pain-relieving qualities of sucrose in children up to 48 months of age[54] and found it was effective compared with no treatment. Others, however, report lack of effectiveness with lower concentrations and younger ages.[52,55] Sucrose taste alone was effective for one vaccination up to 12 months of age,[56] but did not demonstrate similar analgesia for multiple (three) vaccinations.[57] The higher concentrations of sucrose solutions may be more effective at older ages.[58] However, the majority of studies used differing concentrations, therefore, precluding recommendations on the optimal concentration and dose.[50,51]

2. *Maternal/caretaker behavior.* Maternal behavior during a painful procedure accounts for up to 26% of infant pain behavior during both the procedure and the recovery period.[59] Maternal distress was an especially important determinant of pain behavior in infants with low vagal tone compared with infants with high vagal tone.[60] Giving parents a caretaking role, such as securing or distracting the child, can reduce parental sense of helplessness. When parents are unavailable or unable to play a caretaking role, consider enlisting another healthcare provider to help secure and/or distract the child (IV).[61]

3. *Breastfeeding.* Although the efficacy of breastfeeding and human milk as a pain reducer for older infants has not been extensively studied, there is potential benefit/minimal risk. Therefore, mothers who are breastfeeding should be invited to breastfeed the infant during painful procedures (IV).

4. *Older than 12 months.* The upper age limit of effectiveness of sucrose as a pain reducer has not been fully studied, and sucrose, therefore, cannot be recommended as a pain reducer in children older than 12 months at this time (IA).[50,52,61] A publication of workshop proceedings reviewing the evidence for other techniques such as physical, psychological, and pharmacological interventions shows a range of nonpharmacological treatments to be effective at reducing older childhood vaccine injection pain (IA).[50,62-64]

RECOMMENDATIONS FOR FURTHER RESEARCH

Further research is needed to establish the most effective nonpharmacological methods to treat procedural pain for both preterm newborns and infants out of the newborn period. In particular, research should focus on the potential of breastfeeding and human milk to reduce pain for preterm newborns, newborns experiencing multiple painful procedures, and the older breastfeeding infant. Research is also needed on the effectiveness and effect of increasing concentrations of sweet tastes across different ages in early childhood, as well as the comparison of different combinations of analgesic treatments for older infants/toddlers experiencing procedure-induced pain.

REFERENCES

1. Anand KJ. Consensus statement for the prevention and management of pain in the newborn. *Arch Pediatr Adolesc Med.* 2001;155:173–180.

2. Committee on Fetus and Newborn and Section on Anesthesiology and Pain Medicine. Prevention and Management of Procedural Pain in the Neonate: An Update. *Pediatrics.* 2016;137. e20154271–e20154271.

3. Ruda MA, Ling QD, Hohmann AG, et al. Altered nociceptive neuronal circuits after neonatal peripheral inflammation. *Science.* 2000;289:628–631.

4. Grunau RE, Oberlander TF, Whitfield MF, et al. Demographic and therapeutic determinants of pain reactivity in very low birth weight neonates at 32 Weeks' postconceptional Age. *Pediatrics.* 2001;107:105–112.

5. Taddio A, Shah V, Gilbert-MacLeod C, et al. Conditioning and hyperalgesia in newborns exposed to repeated heel lances. *JAMA.* 2002;288:857–861.

6. Oberlander TF, Grunau RE, Whitfield MF, et al. Biobehavioral pain responses in former extremely low birth weight infants at four months' corrected age. *Pediatrics.* 2000;105:e6.

7. Anand KJ, Coskun V, Thrivikraman KV, et al. Long-term behavioral effects of repetitive pain in neonatal rat pups. *Physiol Behav.* 1999;66:627–637.

8. Franck LS, Cox S, Allen A, et al. Parental concern and distress about infant pain. *Arch Dis Child Fetal Neonatal Ed.* 2004;89: F71–F75.

9. Carbajal R, Rousset A, Danan C, et al. Epidemiology and treatment of painful procedures in neonates in intensive care units. *JAMA.* 2008;300:60–70.

10. Simons S, van Dijk M, Anand K, et al. Do we still hurt newborn babies?: A prospective study of procedural pain and analgesia in neonates. *Arch Pediatr Adolesc Med.* 2003;157:1058–1064.

11. Taddio A, Parikh C, Yoon EW, et al. Impact of parent directed education on parental use of pain treatments during routine infant vaccinations: A cluster randomized trial. *Pain.* 2015;156:185–191.

12. Codipietro L, Ceccarelli M, Ponzone A. Breastfeeding or oral sucrose solution in term neonates receiving heel lance: A randomized, controlled trial. *Pediatrics.* 2008;122: e716–e721.

13. Carbajal R, Veerapen S, Couderc S, et al. Analgesic effect of breast feeding in term neonates: Randomised controlled trial. *BMJ.* 2003;326. 13–13.

14. Gray L, Miller LW, Philipp BL, et al. Breastfeeding is analgesic in healthy newborns. *Pediatrics.* 2002;109:590–593.

15. Shekelle P, Woolf S, Eccles M, et al. Developing guidelines. *BMJ.* 1999;318:593–596.

16. Gradin M, Finnström O, Schollin J. Feeding and oral glucose—Additive effects on pain reduction in newborns. *Early Hum Dev.* 2004;77:57–65.

17. Mathew PJ, Mathew JL. Assessment and management of pain in infants. *Postgrad Med J.* 2003;79:438–443.

18. Upadhyay A, Aggarwal R, Narayan S, et al. Analgesic effect of expressed breast milk in procedural pain in term neonates: A randomized, placebo-controlled, double-blind trial. *Acta Paediatr.* 2004;93:518–522.

19. Taddio A, Shah V, Hancock R, et al. Effectiveness of sucrose analgesia in newborns undergoing painful medical procedures. *CMAJ.* 2008;179:37–43.

20. Shah P, Herbozo C, Aliwalas L, et al. Breastfeeding or breast milk for procedural pain in neonates. *Cochrane Database Syst Rev.* 2012;12:CD004950.

21. Shah P, Aliwalas L, Shah V. Breastfeeding or breastmilk to alleviate procedural pain in neonates: A systematic review. *Breastfeed Med.* 2007;2:74–82.

22. Bembich S, Davanzo R, Brovedani P, et al. Functional neuroimaging of breastfeeding analgesia by multichannel near-infrared spectroscopy. *Neonatology.* 2013;104:255–259.

23. Gray L, Lang CW, Porges SW. Warmth is analgesic in healthy newborns. *Pain.* 2012;153:960–966.

24. Gray L, Garza E, Zageris D, et al. Sucrose and warmth for analgesia in healthy newborns: An RCT. *Pediatrics*. 2015;135: e607—e614.

25. Nishitani S, Miyamura T, Tagawa M, et al. The calming effect of a maternal breast milk odor on the human newborn infant. *Neurosci Res*. 2009;63:66—71.

26. Badiee Z, Asghari M, Mohammadizadeh M. The calming effect of maternal breast milk odor on premature infants. *Pediatr Neonatol*. 2013;54:322—325.

27. Jebreili M, Neshat H, Seyyedrasouli A, et al. Comparison of breastmilk odor and vanilla odor on mitigating premature infants' response to pain during and after venipuncture. *Breastfeed Med*. 2015;10:362—365.

28. Akcan E, Polat S. Comparative effect of the smells of amniotic fluid, breast milk, and lavender on newborns' pain during heel lance. *Breastfeed Med*. 2016;11:309—314.

29. Neshat H, Jebreili M, Seyyedrasouli A, et al. Effects of breast milk and vanilla odors on premature neonate's heart rate and blood oxygen saturation during and after venipuncture. *Pediatr Neonatol*. 2016;57:225—231.

30. Ors R, Ozek E, Baysoy G, et al. Comparison of sucrose and human milk on pain response in newborns. *Eur J Pediatr*. 1999;158:63—66.

31. Stevens B, Yamada J, Lee GY, et al. Sucrose for analgesia in newborn infants undergoing painful procedures. *Cochrane Database Syst Rev*. 2016;CD001069.

32. Axelin A, Salanterä S, Kirjavainen J, et al. Oral glucose and parental holding preferable to opioid in pain management in preterm infants. *Clin J Pain*. 2009;25:138—145.

33. Idam-Siuriun DI. Zhirkova IV, Mikhel'son VA, et al. [Prevention of pain during finger prick in neonatal infants]. *Anesteziol Reanimatol*. 2008;14—17.

34. Blass EM, Watt LB. Suckling- and sucrose-induced analgesia in human newborns. *Pain*. 1999;83:611—623.

35. Stevens B, Yamada J, Beyene J, et al. Consistent management of repeated procedural pain with sucrose in preterm neonates: Is it effective and safe for repeated use over time? *Clin J Pain*. 2005;21:543—548.

36. Blass EM, Shide DJ. Some comparisons among the calming and pain-relieving effects of sucrose, glucose, fructose and lactose in infant rats. *Chem Senses*. 1994;19:239—249.

37. Akman I, Ozek E, Bilgen H, et al. Sweet solutions and pacifiers for pain relief in newborn infants. *J Pain*. 2002;3:199—202.

38. Ludington-Hoe SM, Hosseini R, Torowicz DL. Skin-to-skin contact (Kangaroo Care) analgesia for preterm infant heel stick. *AACN Clin Issues*. 2005;16:373—387.

39. Holsti L, Grunau RE. Considerations for using sucrose to reduce procedural pain in preterm infants. *Pediatrics*. 2010;125:1042—1047.

40. Ramenghi LA, Wood CM, Griffith GC, et al. Reduction of pain response in premature infants using intraoral sucrose. *Arch Dis Child Fetal Neonatal Ed*. 1996;74:F126—F128.

41. Taddio A. Pain management for neonatal circumcision. *Paediatr Drugs*. 2001;3:101—111.

42. Porges S, Lipsitt L. Neonatal responsivity to gustatory stimulation: The gustatory-vagal hypothesis. *Infant Behav Dev*. 1993;16:487—494.

43. Simonse E, Mulder PGH, van Beek RHT. Analgesic effect of breast milk versus sucrose for analgesia during heel lance in late preterm infants. *Pediatrics*. 2012;129:657—663.

44. Johnston CC, Filion F, Snider L, et al. Routine sucrose analgesia during the first week of life in neonates younger than 31 weeks' postconceptional age. *Pediatrics*. 2002;110: 523—528.

45. Johnston CC, Stevens B, Pinelli J, et al. Kangaroo care is effective in diminishing pain response in preterm neonates. *Arch Pediatr Adolesc Med*. 2003;157:1084—1088.

46. Stevens B, Johnston C, Franck L, et al. The efficacy of developmentally sensitive interventions and sucrose for relieving procedural pain in very low birth weight neonates. *Nurs Res*. 1999;48:35—43.

47. Abad F, Díaz NM, Domenech E, et al. Oral sweet solution reduces pain-related behaviour in preterm infants. *Acta Paediatr*. 1996;85:854—858.

48. Johnston CC, Stremler R, Horton L, et al. Effect of repeated doses of sucrose during heel stick procedure in preterm neonates. *Biol Neonate*. 1999;75:160—166.

49. Felt BT, Mollen E, Diaz S, et al. Behavioral interventions reduce infant distress at immunization. *Arch Pediatr Adolesc Med*. 2000;154:719—724.

50. Shah V, Taddio A, Rieder MJ. Effectiveness and tolerability of pharmacologic and combined interventions for reducing injection pain during routine childhood immunizations: Systematic review and meta-analyses. *Clin Ther*. 2009;31(Suppl 2): S104—S151.

51. Harrison D, Stevens B, Bueno M, et al. Efficacy of sweet solutions for analgesia in infants between 1 and 12 months of age: A systematic review. *Arch Dis Child*. 2010;95:406—413.

52. Lewindon PJ, Harkness L, Lewindon N. Randomised controlled trial of sucrose by mouth for the relief of infant crying after immunisation. *Arch Dis Child*. 1998;78:453—456.

53. Rogers AJ, Greenwald MH, Deguzman MA, et al. A randomized, controlled trial of sucrose analgesia in infants younger than 90 days of age who require bladder catheterization in the pediatric emergency department. *Acad Emerg Med*. 2006;13:617—622.

54. Dilli D, Küçük IG, Dallar Y. Interventions to reduce pain during vaccination in infancy. *J Pediatr*. 2009;154:385—390.

55. Barr RG, Young SN, Wright JH, et al. "Sucrose analgesia" and diphtheria-tetanus-pertussis immunizations at 2 and 4 months. *J Dev Behav Pediatr*. 1995;16:220—225.

56. Thyr M, Sundholm A, Teeland L, et al. Oral glucose as an analgesic to reduce infant distress following immunization at the age of 3, 5 and 12 months. *Acta Paediatr*. 2007;96:233—236.

57. Mowery B. *Effects of sucrose on immunization injection pain in Hispanic infants [PhD Thesis]*. Charlottesville: University of Virginia; 2007.

58. Ramenghi LA, Webb AV, Shevlin PM, et al. Intra-oral administration of sweet-tasting substances and infants' crying response to immunization: A randomized, placebo-controlled trial. *Biol Neonate*. 2002;81:163—169.

59. Sweet SD, McGrath PJ. Relative importance of mothers' versus medical staffs' behavior in the prediction of infant immunization pain behavior. *J Pediatr Psychol*. 1998;23:249—256.

60. Sweet SD, McGrath PJ, Symons D. The roles of child reactivity and parenting context in infant pain response. *Pain*. 1999;80:655—661.

61. Schechter NL, Zempsky WT, Cohen LL, et al. Pain reduction during pediatric immunizations: Evidence-based review and recommendations. *Pediatrics*. 2007;119: e1184—e1198.

62. Taddio A, Chambers CT, Halperin SA, et al. Inadequate pain management during routine childhood immunizations: The nerve of it. *Clin Ther.* 2009;31(Suppl 2):S152−S167.

63. Taddio A, Ilersich AL, Ipp M, et al. Physical interventions and injection techniques for reducing injection pain during routine childhood immunizations: Systematic review of randomized controlled trials and quasi-randomized controlled trials. *Clin Ther.* 2009;31(Suppl 2):S48−S76.

64. Chambers CT, Taddio A, Uman LS, et al. Psychological interventions for reducing pain and distress during routine childhood immunizations: A systematic review. *Clin Ther.* 2009;31 (Suppl 2):S77−S103.

ABM protocols expire 5 years from the date of publication. Content of this protocol is up-to-date at the time of publication. Evidence-based revisions are made within 5 years or sooner if there are significant changes in the evidence. The first version of this protocol was authored by Larry Gray, Patel Tanvi, and Elizabeth Garza.

The Academy of Breastfeeding Medicine Protocol Committee:
Wendy Brodribb, MBBS, PhD, FABM, Chairperson
Larry Noble, MD, FABM, Translations Chairperson
Nancy Brent, MD
Maya Bunik, MD, MSPH, FABM
Cadey Harrel, MD
Ruth A. Lawrence, MD, FABM
Kathleen A. Marinelli, MD, FABM
Kate Naylor, MBBS, FRACGP
Sarah Reece-Stremtan, MD
Casey Rosen-Carole, MD, MPH
Tomoko Seo, MD, FABM
Rose St. Fleur, MD
Michal Young, MD
For correspondence: abm@bfmed.org

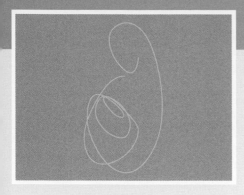

ABM Clinical Protocol #24:
Allergic Proctocolitis in the Exclusively Breastfed Infant*

The Academy of Breastfeeding Medicine

ABSTRACT

A central goal of The Academy of Breastfeeding Medicine is the development of clinical protocols for managing common medical problems that may impact breastfeeding success. These protocols serve only as guidelines for the care of breastfeeding mothers and infants and do not delineate an exclusive course of treatment or serve as standards of medical care. Variations in treatment may be appropriate according to the needs of an individual patient. These guidelines are not intended to be all-inclusive, but to provide a basic framework for physician education regarding breastfeeding.

PURPOSE

THE PURPOSE OF THIS clinical protocol is to explore the scientific basis, pathologic aspects, and clinical management of allergic proctocolitis in the breastfed infant as we currently understand the condition and to define needs for further research in this area. Although there can be a variety of allergic responses to given foods, this protocol will focus on those that occur in the gastrointestinal tract of the breastfed infant, specifically allergic proctocolitis.

DEFINITIONS

- Exclusive breastfeeding: The infant has received only breastmilk from the mother or expressed breastmilk, and no other liquids or solids with the exception of drops or syrups consisting of vitamins, mineral supplements, or medicines.[1,2]
- Food allergy: An adverse health effect arising from a specific immune response that occurs reproducibly on exposure to a given food.[3]

---

* Courtesy of the Academy of Breastfeeding Medicine. Please go to https://www.bfmed.org/protocols for complete protocols, translations, and the most up-to-date information (protocols are updated every 5—7 years).

BACKGROUND

Over recent decades, a group of exclusively breastfed infants has been described that develop bloody stools but are otherwise well appearing. This entity has carried a number of titles ranging from allergic colitis to benign dietary protein proctitis to eosinophilic proctitis to breastmilk-induced proctocolitis.[4] Herein this appearance is referred to as allergic proctocolitis in the exclusively breastfed infant, and knowledge of the clinical course and factors associated with the development of this entity are essential to optimize breastfeeding success and to support the growth and overall health of the infant.

Incidence

The incidence of adverse reactions to food proteins in the exclusively breastfed infant is poorly defined. Prospective data indicate approximately 0.5—1% of exclusively breastfed infants develop allergic reactions to cow's milk proteins excreted in the mother's milk.[5] Given that cow's milk protein is the offending antigen in 50—65% of cases,[4,6] the total incidence of food allergy in the exclusively breastfed infant appears slightly higher than 0.5—1%. Comparatively, infants fed human milk appear to have a lower incidence of allergic reactions to cow's milk protein than those fed cow's milk—based formula.[7] This may be attributable to the relatively low level of cow's milk protein excreted in human milk,[8] immunomodulatory substances present in human milk, and/or differences in the intestinal flora between breastfed and formula-fed infants.[9—12]

Clinical presentation

The most common symptoms associated with food-induced allergic disorders in the exclusively breastfed infant are cutaneous reactions (eczema) and gastrointestinal symptoms.[5] Severe manifestations of food allergy are extremely rare. The most common gastrointestinal symptom is the development of bloody stools.[13—15] This usually occurs between 2 and 6 weeks of age,[6] although some have reported symptoms beginning as early as the first day of life.[16,17] Dietary proteins excreted in the mother's milk are responsible for the majority of cases and induce an inflammatory response of the rectum and distal sigmoid colon referred to as allergic proctocolitis.[18] It should be emphasized that breastfed infants with allergic proctocolitis are generally "well appearing" other than the presence of blood within the stool. Blood loss is typically modest but can occasionally produce anemia and/or hypoalbuminemia. In very rare cases, symptoms may lead to failure to thrive.[19–21] Systemic manifestations such as emesis, dramatic diarrhea, or abdominal distention are rare and may suggest other allergic disorders of the gastrointestinal tract such as food protein–induced enterocolitis or enteropathy (not reviewed in this protocol).

Additional laboratory studies may be considered but are often unnecessary to make the diagnosis of allergic proctocolitis. Peripheral eosinophil counts may be elevated; however, this is poorly indicative in an individual patient.[21,22] A fecal smear looking for an increased number of eosinophils is often reported negative.[18] If the fecal smear does not contain detectable leukocytes, it is not suitable for mucosal cytology, and the report of no eosinophilia is not reliable (T. Takamasu, personal communication, June 9, 2011). Stool cultures are negative for pathogenic bacteria, and radiographic studies exclude necrotizing enterocolitis.[6,24] Total and antigen-specific serum immunoglobulin E concentrations are similar to those of non-affected infants and thus need not be measured.[13] In severe or protracted cases unresponsive to dietary modification, endoscopic evaluation may be warranted.

Pathophysiology

The symptoms and severity of food hypersensitivity vary according to the mechanism of immune response (immunoglobulin E vs. cell-mediated) and location of intestinal involvement.[6,25] Allergic proctocolitis in the breastfed infant is a cell-mediated hypersensitivity disorder of the distal large bowel characterized by mucosal edema, focal epithelial erosions, and eosinophilic infiltration of the epithelium and lamina propria.[14,18,19,26,27] Biopsy specimens typically demonstrate eosinophil counts of greater than 20 per high-powered field.[21,28,29] The passage of dietary proteins into maternal milk is responsible for the majority of cases,[30] and elimination of the offending agent from the maternal diet usually results in cessation of symptoms within 72–96 hours.[6] In some cases, dietary restriction for up to 2–4 weeks may be required to notice improvement.[12,31] In a published series of 95 breastfed infants with bloody stools, 65% were determined to be attributable to maternal ingestion of cow's milk, 19% to egg, 6% to corn, and 3% to soy.[4,6]

It remains unclear when the sensitization phase of allergic proctocolitis occurs. Some infants have been reported to respond adversely to food proteins excreted in the mother's milk within the first day of life.[16,17] It is apparent that dietary and environmental antigens are capable of crossing the placental barrier[32] or entering the amniotic fluid,[33] which is swallowed by the fetus. These findings suggest the possibility of in utero sensitization following maternal antigen exposure during pregnancy.[34] Alternatively, variations in the concentration of several immunomodulatory substances in human milk appear to influence the protective effect of breastfeeding against allergy.[35–38] Human milk contains viable leukocytes that may play a role in antigen processing and presentation to neonatal lymphocytes in the intestine.[39,40] Thus, it is possible that ingestion of dietary food proteins excreted in the mother's milk, accompanied by physiologic conditions favoring immunogenic responses (in the neonate or maternal milk), may result in allergic sensitization. At present, however, there are insufficient data to recommend dietary restriction during pregnancy and/or lactation as a means of allergy prevention.[3,41] Breastfeeding should be encouraged in all neonates, even though small quantities of food allergens may be present within the milk. Indeed, recent data in animal models suggest that ingesting small quantities of allergens excreted in the mother's milk in the presence of the anti-inflammatory cytokine transforming growth factor-b may actually protect offspring against subsequent allergic responses to that same allergen later in life.[42–44]

MATERNAL ELIMINATION DIET

When an exclusively breastfed baby has clinical evidence of allergic colitis, the first line of treatment is the maternal elimination diet, avoiding food containing the most likely allergen, cow's milk protein. Having a rigorous diet imposed can be extremely hard for a new mother, who is dealing not only with being a new mother and breastfeeding, but also with her concerns for her baby's symptoms.

Elimination diet plan

Several different methods are proposed:

1. To make it as simple as possible, one can start by eliminating the most likely suspects for allergies one at a time (i.e., cow's milk [and products made with cow's milk like cheese, butter, ice cream, and other dairy products], soy, citrus fruits, eggs, nuts, peanuts, wheat, corn, strawberries, and chocolate). Mothers are instructed to eliminate one food or food group (e.g., dairy products) at a time and wait a minimum of 2 weeks and up to 4 weeks. Most cases will improve within 72–96 hours.[6]

2. If there have been no changes with the infant's symptoms in that time, the mother can usually add this food back into her diet and eliminate another food or food group from the list. This continues until she has eliminated all of the foods listed. When eliminating a food, she also needs to remember to eliminate any other foods that contain this product (i.e., when eliminating cow's milk, eliminate anything made with cow's milk, not forgetting the specific protein components like casein, whey, lactoglobulin, etc.; it is important to read labels for these other component ingredients). Often mothers don't think about the fact that other foods contain these products. The Summary of the United States Expert Panel suggests that individuals with food allergy and their caregivers receive education and training on how to interpret ingredient lists on food labels and how to recognize labeling of the food allergens used as ingredients in foods; the Expert Panel also suggests that products with precautionary labeling, such as "this product may contain

trace amounts of allergen," be avoided.[3] Don't forget that some medications, vitamins, and even vaccines may have allergenic ingredients.

3. If eliminating each of these foods does not solve the problem, the next step could be to have the mother keep a very complete food diary for 2 weekdays and 1 weekend to see what her usual eating habits are. By carefully reviewing her food diary, one may be able to pinpoint the offending food.

Geographic differences

Others recommend eliminating the most likely causes of allergies, cow's milk protein, and any other likely allergens based on the region in which the baby lives.[12] For example, in some regions, hen's eggs are the second most common cause of allergy, whereas in others, like the United States, the United Kingdom, and some areas of Europe, peanuts are a common allergen.[12]

DIFFICULT CASES

Moving further to a diet that also excludes fish, wheat, and other gluten-containing grain products is very difficult for a mother to follow and may increase her risk of consuming an unhealthy diet. The maternal risks of an extensively restrictive elimination diet must be weighed against the potential infant benefits. In a secondary approach, the additional elimination of wheat and fish and/or other significant parts of a mother's diet should require the advice of an experienced dietician to ensure that an adequate nutritional intake is maintained.[12]

For babies with more significant symptoms, one can place the mother on a very low-allergen diet of foods like lamb, pears, squash, and rice. Again, this approach requires ongoing consultation with an experienced dietician. When the baby's symptoms resolve, other foods are added back to the mother's diet one at a time, with sufficient time between additions (minimum of 1 week) to look for recurrence of symptoms in the baby. If symptoms recur, that recently added food is removed again and is likely the offending food. Other foods may also be incriminated. Continuing to add foods in one at a time allows the mother to liberalize her diet if the baby tolerates it.

USE OF PANCREATIC ENZYMES

There have been a few published reports[45,46] and some anecdotal discussions of a novel treatment for allergic colitis—the use of pancreatic enzymes by the mother. The theory is that by giving the mother exogenous pancreatic enzyme, the protease component will help further break down the potential protein allergens in the mother's gastrointestinal tract, before they are absorbed into her bloodstream and secreted into her milk. Specific dosing has yet to be defined, but generally one starts with the lowest dose of pancreatic enzyme (e.g., pancrelipase Creon 6 [in United States]/Kreon [Europe], Abbott Laboratories, Abbott Park, IL) (the strength is based on the lipase content, in this case 6,000 USP units of lipase; it also contains 19,000 USP units of protease and 30,000 USP units

of amylase) so as to minimize, although rare, any side effect to the mother. The dose can begin as two capsules with meals and one with snacks and be doubled if the desired effect is not achieved. The use of proprietary enzymes that are pork-derived should be avoided in persons allergic to this allergen. There are alternative plant-derived enzymes, but the dosing is less clear as their comparative potency is difficult to ascertain (A. Repucci, personal communication, May 1, 2011). Reports are generally positive with this approach. This is usually in addition to the elimination diet and can be used in situations where food ingredients may not be known for sure, as in foods consumed at a restaurant.

EVALUATION AND MANAGEMENT

Quality of evidence for each recommendation, as defined in the U.S. Preventive Task Force guideline,[47] is noted in parentheses (I, II-2, and III).

The initial evaluation of the exclusively breastfed infant with bloody or occult heme-positive stools should include a comprehensive history and physical examination:

- Particular emphasis should be directed towards a strong family history of allergy (biological parent or sibling), which places the infant at high risk for developing allergy.[3,12,41]
- Assurance of the exclusive nature of human milk feeding is important because the management strategies differ for breastfed and formula-fed infants.
- Evaluation for additional symptoms of food-induced allergic disorders is necessary. Many infants with allergic proctocolitis will also exhibit cutaneous reactions (eczema).[5]
- Accurate assessment of growth (weight and length gain), heart rate, and respiratory rate should be undertaken.
- Performance of a thorough abdominal examination. Infants with allergic proctocolitis are generally "well appearing," non-distended, and non-tender.
- Inspection for a perianal fissure or significant rash.
- Laboratory evaluations are generally unnecessary; however, in cases of suspected moderate to severe allergic proctocolitis, one may consider obtaining a hemoglobin level to screen for blood loss and serum albumin, which decreases in protein-losing enteropathy.

RECOMMENDATIONS

1. If severe allergic proctocolitis is suspected based on any of the following:
   - Failure to thrive
   - Moderate to large amounts of blood in the stool with decreasing hemoglobin
   - Protein-losing enteropathy
     i. The infant should be referred to a pediatric subspecialist (allergist or pediatric gastroenterologist) for diagnosis and treatment. (III)[47]
     ii. While awaiting the appointment, begin an elimination diet in the mother, continuing her

daily vitamins as suggested for all breastfeeding mothers and adding calcium supplementation (1,000 mg/day divided into several doses).[12] (See Maternal Elimination Diet, above). (II-2)[47]

   iii. In the majority of patients, it is reasonable and safe to continue breastfeeding through the elimination process while awaiting the appointment and thus to protect breastfeeding. However, if the hemoglobin or albumin level is significantly low (based on age-dependent published norms), the use of a hypoallergenic formula may be considered (III).[47]

2. If mild to moderate allergic proctocolitis is suspected based on the following.
- Blood-positive stool or small amounts of visible blood in stool).
- Weight gain and growth are normal.
- Abdominal exam is benign; no abdominal distention or recurrent vomiting.
- Stable hemoglobin and albumin levels (if measured).
   i. The infant should continue breastfeeding. The mother should be started on an elimination diet, continue her daily vitamins as suggested for all breastfeeding mothers, and add calcium supplementation (1,000 mg/day divided into several doses).[12] (II-2)[47]
   ii. The elimination diet trial for any given food or food group should be continued for a minimum of 2 weeks and up to 4 weeks. Most cases will improve within 72—96 hours.[6] (II-2)[47]

3. In cases of suspected mild to moderate allergic proctocolitis with improvement in response to maternal elimination diet:
- Consider reintroducing the allergen back into the mother's diet. (I)[47]
- If symptoms recur, the suspected food should be eliminated from the mother's (and infant's) diet until 9—12 months of age and for at least 6 months.[12,13,48] (II-2)[47] Most babies/children will tolerate the offending allergen in the diet after 6 months "from the time of diagnosis" if at least 9 months old. For example, if a baby is diagnosed at 2 weeks, the food should be avoided until 9—12 months of age. If in the rare circumstance that a baby develops allergic colitis at 5—6 months of age, the caregivers should wait a full 6 months (after diagnosis) to re-introduce, therefore at least 12 months of age, not at 9 months of age, or until the mother decides to wean, whichever comes first.[12,13,48] (II-2)[47]

4. In cases of suspected mild to moderate allergic proctocolitis with no improvement in response to maternal elimination diet:
- Consider eliminating other allergens. (II-2)[47]
- Breastfeeding may continue with monitoring of weight gain and growth. (II-2)[47]
- Consider following hemoglobin and albumin levels if continued moderate degree of blood loss (blood is visible) in stools. (II-2)[47]

- Consider use of pancreatic enzymes for the mother. Dosage is generally one or two capsules with snacks and two to four with meals as needed dependent on the baby's symptoms (see Use of Pancreatic Enzymes above).[45,46] (III)[47]
- In severe cases with impaired growth, decreasing hemoglobin level, or decreasing serum albumin level, the use of a hypoallergenic formula may be considered; however, one should consider referral to a specialist. (III)

SUGGESTIONS FOR AREAS OF FUTURE RESEARCH

Determine the current incidence of allergic colitis in exclusively breastfed infants

Most available epidemiologic data are from over 20 years ago, and we know the incidence of other atopic diseases (e.g., asthma) has increased over the past few decades. In addition, the results of many studies on allergic colitis in breastfed infants are complicated by the inclusion of infants who received cow's milk formula in addition to breastmilk. It would also be interesting to look at familial patterns such as what is the risk of this happening with the same mother in a subsequent pregnancy.

Determine the influence of maternal or neonatal immunity on development of allergic proctocolitis

It is clear that antigens ingested by the mother and transferred via the milk to breastfeeding infants are responsible for the clinical manifestations of allergic proctocolitis. However, it is uncertain if the fetus is sensitized to these antigens during pregnancy or as a newborn through repeated exposure within human milk. The precise contribution of maternal immune factors transmitted to progeny during pre- and/or postnatal life on the development of allergic responses in the neonate is also unclear. Additional investigation is needed to define the immunologic mechanisms involved in the context of specific genetic, developmental, and environmental factors in the mother and infant. Further insight into these factors would allow more focused efforts at prevention.

Determine the safety and efficacy of maternal pancreatic enzyme use in alleviating the symptoms of allergic colitis, and if efficacious, under what circumstances they should be used

Current data are either anecdotal or in a small case study that maternal pancreatic enzyme use is both safe and efficacious. If this is shown in larger-scale studies, one would want to determine if this adjunct to maternal elimination diet should be used only as the last resort, when the elimination diet is not efficacious, or possibly as an earlier adjunct, to make the diet less onerous for the mother to follow.

Should breastfed infants with a history of allergic proctocolitis delay or avoid exposure to other major food allergens in an attempt to prevent the development of additional food allergies?

Because young children with allergic reactions to cow's milk protein have an increased risk of developing other food allergies,[49] it was previously recommended that major food allergens such as peanuts, tree nuts, fish, and shellfish be avoided until at least 3 years of age.[50] At present, there is no evidence to conclude that this approach will be successful in preventing future allergy. Thus, consistent with recent published guidelines for the diagnosis and management of food allergy in the United States,[3,41] breastfed infants with a history of allergic proctocolitis should not be limited in their exposure to other major food allergens. Infants and breastfeeding mothers should only avoid the allergen identified during maternal elimination diets until 9–12 months of age and for at least 6 months. This is an active area of current research, and additional studies may provide more substantial evidence to support or change these recommendations. (III)[47]

Determine the utility of additional laboratory tests for the diagnosis of allergic proctocolitis

Laboratory tests may be considered but are often unnecessary to make the diagnosis of allergic proctocolitis. In one recent case report, an infant who developed hematochezia associated with the feeding of cow's milk formula was found to have selective elevation of serum interleukin 5 (a T-helper cell type 2 cytokine).[51] At present, it remains unclear if serum measurements of inflammatory cytokines would be helpful for the diagnosis of allergic colitis in the exclusively breastfed infant.

ACKNOWLEDGMENTS

This work was supported in part by a grant from the Maternal and Child Health Bureau, U.S. Department of Health and Human Services. Thanks to Lisa H. Akers, M.S., and Jeanne Blankenship, M.S., from the American Dietetic Association for helpful suggestions and insights.

REFERENCES

1. Labbok MH, Krasovec K. Towards consistency in breastfeeding definitions. *Stud Fam Plan.* 1990;21:226–230.
2. WHO Division of Child Health and Development. Indicators for Assessing Breastfeeding Practices. Report of an Informal Meeting in June 1991, Geneva. Available at: www.who.int/nutrition/databases/infantfeeding/data_source_inclusion_criteria/en/index.html (accessed October 25, 2011).
3. Boyce JA, Assa'ad A, Burks AW, et al. Guidelines for the diagnosis and management of food allergy in the United States: Summary of the NIAID-Sponsored Expert Panel Report. *J Allergy Clin Immunol.* 2010;126:1105–1118.
4. Lake AM. Food-induced eosinophilic proctocolitis. *J Pediatr Gastroenterol Nutr.* 2000;30(Suppl):S58–S60.
5. Host A, Husby S, Osterballe O. A prospective study of cow's milk allergy in exclusively breast-fed infants. Incidence, pathogenetic role of early inadvertent exposure to cow's milk formula, and characterization of bovine milk protein in human milk. *Acta Paediatr Scand.* 1988;77:663–670.
6. Lake AM. Dietary protein enterocolitis. *Immunol Allergy Clin North Am.* 1999;19:553–561.
7. Muraro A, Dreborg S, Halken S, et al. Dietary prevention of allergic diseases in infants and small children. Part III: Critical review of published peer-reviewed observational and interventional studies and final recommendations. *Pediatr Allergy Immunol.* 2004;15:291–307.
8. Host A, Husby S, Hansen LG, et al. Bovine beta-lactoglobulin in human milk from atopic and non-atopic mothers. Relationship to maternal intake of homogenized and unhomogenized milk. *Clin Exp Allergy.* 1990;20:383–387.
9. Walker WA. The dynamic effects of breastfeeding on intestinal development and host defense. *Protecting Infants Through Human Milk.* 2004;554:155–170.
10. Newburg DS, Ruiz-Palacios GM, Morrow AL. Human milk glycans protect infants against enteric pathogens. *Annu Rev Nutr.* 2005;25:37–58.
11. Penders J, Vink C, Driessen C, et al. Quantification of *Bifidobacterium* spp., *Escherichia coli* and *Clostridium difficile* in faecal samples of breast-fed and formula-fed infants by real-time PCR. *FEMS Microbiol Lett.* 2005;243:141–147.
12. Vandenplas Y, Koletzko S, Isolauri E, et al. Guidelines for the diagnosis and management of cow's milk protein allergy in infants. *Arch Dis Child.* 2007;92:902–908.
13. Lake AM. Food Protein-Induced Proctitis, Enteropathy, and Enterocolitis of Infancy. UptoDate® 3.1. 2010. Available at: www.uptodate.com (accessed October 25, 2011).
14. Dupont C, Badoual J, Le Luyer B, et al. Rectosigmoidoscopic findings during isolated rectal bleeding in the neonate. *J Pediatr Gastroenterol Nutr.* 1987;6:257–264.
15. Goldman H, Proujansky R. Allergic proctitis and gastroenteritis in children. Clinical and mucosal biopsy features in 53 cases. *Am J Surg Pathol.* 1986;10:75–86.
16. Kumar D, Repucci A, Wyatt-Ashmead J, et al. Allergic colitis presenting in the first day of life: report of three cases. *J Pediatr Gastroenterol Nutr.* 2000;31:195–197.
17. Feiterna-Sperling C, Rammes S, Kewitz G, et al. A case of cow's milk allergy in the neonatal period—evidence for intrauterine sensitization? *Pediatr Allergy Immunol.* 1997;8:152–155.
18. Odze RD, Bines J, Leichtner AM, et al. Allergic proctocolitis in infants: A prospective clinicopathologic biopsy study. *Hum Pathol.* 1993;24:668–674.
19. Sampson HA. 9. Food allergy. *J Allergy Clin Immunol.* 2003;111(2 Suppl):S540–S547.
20. Sampson HA. Update on food allergy. *J Allergy Clin Immunol.* 2004 May;113:805–819.
21. Machida HM, Catto Smith AG, Gall DG, et al. Allergic colitis in infancy: Clinical abnd pathologic aspects. *J Pediatr Gastroenterol Nutr.* 1994;19:22–26.

22. Winter HS, Antonioli DA, Fukagawa N, et al. Allergy-related proctocolitis in infants: Diagnostic usefulness of rectal biopsy. *Mod Pathol.* 1990;3:5–10.

23. Chang JW, Wu TC, Wang KS, et al. Colon mucosal pathology in infants under three months of age with diarrhea disorders. *J Pediatr Gastroenterol Nutr.* 2002;35:387–390.

24. Arvola T, Ruuska T, Keranen J, et al. Rectal bleeding in infancy: Clinical, allergological, and microbiological examination. *Pediatrics.* 2006;117:e760–e768.

25. Sampson HA. Food allergy. Part 2: Diagnosis and management. *J Allergy Clin Immunol.* 1999;103:981–989.

26. Sierra Salinas C, Blasco Alonso J, Olivares, Sánchez L, et al. [Allergic cilitis in exclusively breast-fed infants]. *An Pediatr (Barc).* 64. 2006158–161.

27. Hwang JB, Park MH, Kang YN, et al. Advanced criteria for clinicopathological diagnosis of food protein-induced proctocolitis. *J Korean Med Sci.* 2007;22:213–217.

28. Sampson HA, Anderson JA. Summary and recommendations: Classification of gastrointestinal manifestations due to immunologic reactions to foods in infants and young children. *J Pediatr Gastroenterol Nutr.* 2000;30(Suppl):S87–S94.

29. Kumagai H, Masuda T, Maisawa S, et al. Apoptotic epithelial cells in biopsy specimens from infants with streaked rectal bleeding. *J Pediatr Gastroenterol Nutr.* 2001;32:428–433.

30. Kilshaw PJ, Cant AJ. The passage of maternal dietary proteins into human breast milk. *Int Arch Allergy Appl Immunol.* 1984;75:8–15.

31. Jakobsson I. Food antigens in human milk. *Eur J Clin Nutr.* 1991;45(Suppl 1):29–33.

32. Szepfalusi Z, Loibichler C, Pichler J, et al. Direct evidence for transplacental allergen transfer. *Pediatr Res.* 2000;48:404–407.

33. Holloway JA, Warner JO, Vance GH, et al. Detection of house-dust-mite allergen in amniotic fluid and umbilical cord blood. *Lancet.* 2000;356:1900–1902.

34. Sicherer SH, Wood RA, Stablein D, et al. Maternal consumption of peanut during pregnancy is associated with peanut sensitization in atopic infants. *J Allergy Clin Immunol.* 2010;126:1191–1197.

35. Duchen K, Gu Y, Bjorksten B. Atopic sensitization during the first year of life in relation to long chain polyunsaturated fatty acid levels in human milk. *Pediatr Res.* 1998;44:478–484.

36. Bottcher MF, Jenmalm MC, Garofalo RP, et al. Cytokines in breast milk from allergic and nonallergic mothers. *Pediatr Res.* 2000;47:157–162.

37. Laitinen K, Arvola T, Moilanen E, et al. Characterization of breast milk received by infants with gross blood in stools. *Biol Neonate.* 2005;87:66–72.

38. Jarvinen KM, Laine ST, Jarvenpaa AL, et al. Does low IgA inhuman milk predispose the infant to development of cow's milk allergy? *Pediatr Res.* 2000;48:457–462.

39. Jarvinen KM, Juntunen-Backman K, Suomalainen H. Relation between weak HLA-DR expression on human breast milk macrophages and cow milk allergy (CMA) in suckling infants. *Pediatr Res.* 1999;45:76–81.

40. Järvinen KM, Suomalainen H. Leucocytes in human milk and lymphocyte subsets in cow's milk-allergic infants. *Pediatr Allergy Immunol.* 2002;13:243–254.

41. Greer FR, Sicherer SH, Burks AW. Effects of early nutritional interventions on the development of atopic disease in infants and children: The role of maternal dietary restriction, breast-feeding, timing of introduction of complementary foods, and hydrolyzed formulas. *Pediatrics.* 2008;121:183–191.

42. Verhasselt V, Milcent V, Cazareth J, et al. Breast milk-mediated transfer of an antigen induces tolerance and protection from allergic asthma. *Nat Med.* 2008;14:170–175.

43. Mosconi E, Rekima A, Seitz-Polski B, et al. Breast milk immune complexes are potent inducers of oral tolerance in neonates and prevent asthma development. *Mucosal Immunol.* 2010;3:461–474.

44. Puddington L, Matson A. Breathing easier with breast milk. *Nat Med.* 2008;14:116–118.

45. Repucci A. Resolution of stool blood in breast-fed infants with maternal ingestion of pancreatic enzymes [abstract]. *J Pediatr Gastroenterol Nutr.* 1999;29:500A.

46. Schach B, Haight M. Colic and food allergy in the breastfed infant: Is it possible for an exclusively breastfed infant to suffer from food allergy? *J Hum Lact.* 2002;18:50–52.

47. U.S. Preventive Services Task Force. Quality of Evidence. Available at: www.ncbi.nlm.nih.gov/books/NBK15430 (accessed October 25, 2011).

48. Bock SA. Prospective appraisal of complaints of adverse reactions to foods in children during the first 3 years of life. *Pediatrics.* 1987;79:683–688.

49. Host A, Halken S. A prospective study of cow milk allergy in Danish infants during the first 3 years of life. Clinical course in relation to clinical and immunological type of hypersensitivity reaction. *Allergy.* 1990;45:587–596.

50. American Academy of Pediatrics, Committee on Nutrition. Hypoallergenic infant formulas. *Pediatrics.* 2000;106:346–349.

51. Koike Y, Takahashi N, Yada Y, et al. Selectively high level of serum interleukin 5 in a newborn infant with cow's milk allergy. *Pediatrics.* 2011;127:e231–e234.

ABM protocols expire 5 years from the date of publication. Evidence-based revisions are made within 5 years or sooner if there are significant changes in the evidence.

Contributors
*Adam P. Matson, M.D.
*Kathleen A. Marinelli, M.D., FABM
Academy of Breastfeeding Medicine Protocol Committee
Maya Bunik, M.D., MSPH, FABM
Caroline J. Chantry, M.D., FABM
Cynthia R. Howard, M.D., M.P.H., FABM
Ruth A. Lawrence, M.D., FABM
*Kathleen A. Marinelli, M.D., FABM, Chairperson
Larry Noble, M.D., FABM, Translations Chairperson
Nancy G. Powers, M.D., FABM
Julie Scott Taylor, M.D., M.Sc., FABM
*Primary contributors
For correspondence: abm@bfmed.org

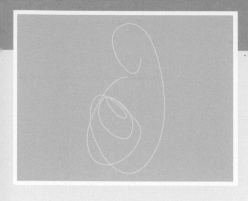

ABM Clinical Protocol #25
Recommendations for Preprocedural Fasting for the Breastfed Infant: "NPO" Guidelines*

The Academy of Breastfeeding Medicine

ABSTRACT

A central goal of The Academy of Breastfeeding Medicine is the development of clinical protocols for managing common medical problems that may impact breastfeeding success. These protocols serve only as guidelines for the care of breastfeeding mothers and infants and do not delineate an exclusive course of treatment or serve as standards of medical care. Variations in treatment may be appropriate according to the needs of an individual patient. These guidelines are not intended to be all-inclusive, but to provide a basic framework for physician education regarding breastfeeding.

PURPOSE

This protocol will help define the minimum fasting requirements for breastfed infants and provide suggestions to avoid unnecessary fasts while improving the infant's safety and comfort during the required fasting periods. When providing guidance for breastfeeding mothers of nil per os (NPO) infants in the preprocedure period, the main goals are to:

- Prevent pulmonary aspiration of gastric contents during anesthesia or sedation
- Prevent hypoglycemia intraoperatively and during the NPO period
- Prevent volume depletion and maximize hemodynamics Minimize stress or anxiety in the NPO infant
- Support optimal breastfeeding of the dyad before and after the procedure

Both general anesthesia and moderate sedation require adherence to the same fasting guidelines that will be discussed in this protocol. For further information about sedation please refer to the guidelines created by the American Society of Anesthesiologists (ASA) Task Force on Sedation and Analgesia by Non-Anesthesiologists. As defined by these guidelines, "sedation and analgesia comprise a continuum of states ranging from minimal sedation (anxiolysis) through general anesthesia."[1] For the purposes of discussing fasting guidelines in this protocol, the term anesthesia is used to encompass the continuum of moderate sedation to general anesthesia.

BACKGROUND

Requiring a breastfed infant to fast for any period of time can be stressful for both the infant and the mother.[2] Hence, it is appropriate to minimize unnecessary fasting while maximizing the safety of diagnostic examinations, surgeries, and procedures with the patient under anesthesia.

Consequences of feeding prior to sedation or general anesthesia

The most serious sequela of noncompliance with fasting guidelines is pulmonary aspiration.[3] Regurgitation and aspiration have been documented concerns of physicians providing sedation since the early 19th and 20th centuries[4-6] and a leading cause of death under anesthesia in both adults and children. When this was established, all patients had to be NPO or nothing by mouth after midnight to avoid pulmonary aspiration syndrome.[7,8] The fasting guidelines have developed through the years to be more reasonable for breastfeeding infants[3] and are still evolving. Although potentially uncomfortable for the infant, the safest practice and most effective prevention of pulmonary aspiration is adherence to current fasting guidelines.

Mechanism

Upon initiation of sedation or induction of anesthesia, the gag and cough reflexes are inhibited; therefore, any remaining stomach contents can regurgitate and trickle into the open larynx that would have otherwise closed upon contact with acidic gastric fluid.[9-11] This can cause aspiration of solid food particulates and acidic gastric juices into the unprotected airway, which can then lead to pneumonitis or pneumonia. While the incidence of aspiration is low with proper fasting (anywhere from 3 to 10 out of every 10,000 anesthetics performed on children),[3,12] the consequences of pulmonary aspiration of residual gastric contents can be serious.[5-8,12] Aspiration pneumonitis may necessitate mechanical ventilation and/or a prolonged hospital course.[3]

* Courtesy of the Academy of Breastfeeding Medicine. Please go to https://www.bfmed.org/protocols for complete protocols, translations, and the most up-to-date information (protocols are updated every 5–7 years).

Infants with multiple co-morbidities are placed in a higher risk stratification by the ASA, and they have a higher incidence of aspiration.[12]

Animal models

Animal models of pulmonary aspiration of gastric contents containing human breastmilk (HBM) are characterized by airway irritability from inflammatory mediators, increased alveolar-to-arterial oxygen gradients, and decreased dynamic compliance. This leads to poor oxygenation and difficulty with ventilation[13] and is especially evident when HBM is acidified. Death is more likely with gastric contents that have a pH of less than 2.5,[11] with other studies showing increased death and severity with decreasing pH and increasing volume. Assuming that aspiration of HBM in an infant would have similar consequences as compared with animal studies, this could potentially affect adequate ventilation and oxygenation in the infant. Aspiration of larger volumes or concentrated particulate matter from HBM mixed with gastric juices further increases the severity of lung injury, including respiratory distress syndrome, alveolitis, atelectasis, and/or postobstructive pneumonia.[13,14]

Gastric emptying

Increased fat and protein content of a liquid correlates to increased gastric clearance times and heightened risk for aspiration. Acidified formula and casein formula empty from the stomach over a 3−4-hour period or more,[15,16] but some formulas may take up to 6 hours to empty from the stomach. Gastric emptying time for cow's milk can also take up to 6 hours, similar to that of solids, although some studies show that it can empty almost as fast as HBM.[17] Although some studies have demonstrated that HBM empties within 2−3 hours,[15,17−20] gastric emptying times of HBM vary from infant to infant, and fat content of HBM is not consistent.[21] The ASA perioperative task force on sedation recommends a four-hour fast from HBM due to individual variation in gastric emptying and human milk content, though this may differ from international recommendations.[1] Of note is that emptying time of liquids has not been proven to be altered by the presence of gastroesophageal reflux.[18]

Use of clear liquids

The only intake that is proven to empty from the stomach quickly is clear liquid, which can serve as a temporary substitute for HBM in the fasting period. Gastric volume and pH are not affected by unlimited ingestion of clear fluids up to 2 hours prior to anesthesia in healthy patients.[17,19,21,22] Ad libitum ingestion of clear liquids 2−3 hours prior to anesthesia induction in high-risk populations, such as pediatric patients undergoing elective cardiac surgery, does not demonstrate additional risk when compared with healthy patients.[22,23] Fast absorption of clear liquid minimizes the risk of residual gastric contents and pulmonary aspiration. Furthermore, the lack of particulate matter decreases the extent of lung injury if the clear liquid is aspirated.

Clear liquids, addressed below in our recommendations, may maintain electrolyte balance and can provide sugars to replete glycogen stores in the fasting breastfed infant. Newborns have impaired gluconeogenesis, so it is important to offer frequent feeding.[24,25] Up to 2 hours prior to anesthesia, a clear sucrose/electrolyte-based solution can be provided to the newborn. Aside from providing a safer form of volume and calories during a preprocedure fast from HBM, clear liquids ad libitum up to 2 hours prior to a procedure allow for greater infant comfort and less irritability.[22,23]

Infant comfort

When an infant is not required to fast, breastfeeding can provide comfort during a painful procedure.[26] Otherwise, when the infant is fasting for a procedure and unable to access the breast for 4 hours, he or she may experience separation anxiety, frustration from hunger, and crying. In full-term healthy neonates, extensive crying causes oxygen desaturation, which can occasionally lead to cyanosis and bradycardia.[27] Nonnutritive sucking on a pacifier (dummy), when used as a temporary comfort measure, has been shown to reduce crying.[28,29] Relief of anxiety is also potentially beneficial for improvement of gastric motility and increasing clearance of any residual gastric volume.[30]

Prolonged fasting times

Although we cannot ask infants if they are anxious, hungry or thirsty, older children have stated that they are very hungry or "starving" in the perioperative period.[31] The fasting period in pediatrics is sometimes prolonged beyond recommendations. Engelhardt et al.[31] recently suggested that fasting times are commonly in excess of the recommended guidelines in a study of 1,350 healthy children 2−16 years old. Children are fasting 12 hours from solids instead of 6−8 hours and fasting from fluids for 7 hours instead of 2−4 hours.[31] The fasting times for newborn breastfeeding infants may also exceed the recommended 4-hour period, causing unnecessary hypoglycemia, discomfort, and anxiety.

RECOMMENDATIONS

Quality of evidence for each recommendation, as defined in the U.S. Preventive Task Force guideline,[32] is noted in parentheses (I, II-1, II-3, and III).

1. *Minor painless procedures or procedures requiring local anesthesia for pain control that do not require sedation or fasting.* Minor procedures such as circumcision with a local block, diagnostic examinations, placement of peripheral intravenous lines, and drawing blood can be performed without sedation or general anesthesia. A procedure that is considered minor should cause minimal physical trauma and psychological impact, therefore not requiring sedation. Without sedation, the infant can protect his or her airway with an intact cough/gag reflex, and thus fasting is not required (I).[10,11] The need for sedation should be decided upon at the physician's discretion based on the intensity and

duration of the procedure as well as the infant's medical history.[1] If sedation is not necessary, the need for oral analgesics or other means for comfort should be determined by the practitioner.

- *If it is a minor procedure not requiring sedation or general anesthesia, then feed normally.* Infants are more likely to tolerate minor procedures when the usual feeding pattern is maintained. They will be more comfortable when they have eaten in a normal routine. Without anesthesia, even if the patient is sleeping during the procedure, the upper airway reflexes are intact, and infants will be able to naturally protect their airways (I).[9,10]

- *If possible, consider breastfeeding for comfort during the minor procedure without sedation.* Breastfeeding while receiving a heel stick, intravenous placement, or drawing blood has been shown to be an effective means of pain relief and should be an option made available to mothers and infants (III).[26] Please refer to the Academy of Breastfeeding Medicine Clinical Protocol #23 for more information.[26]

- *Exceptions for the active patient.* The child who is unable to follow instructions or cooperate because of age or level of development may require sedation for minor procedures after efforts to perform the procedure without it have failed. Under these circumstances, the procedure may need to be postponed so that the patient can follow strict fasting guidelines.

2. *Diagnostic examinations or invasive procedures requiring pharmacologic immobilization or sedation.* Procedures that are more painful or stressful, such as bone marrow biopsies or lumbar puncture with intrathecal chemotherapy administration, require sedation (III).[2] Other procedures may require a motionless patient, such as central line placement or magnetic resonance imaging/computed tomography exams. In these situations, a licensed anesthesia provider may need to perform a general anesthetic, but these procedures can possibly be performed under sedation if a strict sedation protocol is followed and the provider is well trained (III).[1,33]

- *When should the infant fast?* When an infant undergoes a surgery or diagnostic examination under anesthesia, the mother must withhold breastfeeding for at least 4 hours prior to anesthesia (see Table 1) (III).[1,3,21,34,35] Conditions such as gastroesophageal reflux disease have not been shown to change the gastric emptying times versus controls, so recommendations for these patients do not differ (I).[18]

- *If the infant needs to fast, provide clear instructions to the caregiver.* The physician providing or supervising the sedation or anesthesia at the hospital, clinic, or surgery center must provide strict fasting instructions to minimize adverse outcomes such as pulmonary aspiration, hypoglycemia, and volume depletion (I). These instructions are often provided in a preprocedure office visit and/or by phone the day before the scheduled procedure. The mother can be reassured that adherence to fasting guidelines is for the safety of her child.

- Consider the infant's daily medications. Vital prescriptions such as antiepileptics, reflux, and cardiac medications should be taken as scheduled. If the prescription in the form of a clear sugar-based syrup, then the volume of the medication and its rapid absorption[17] make the risk of aspiration of the medication lower than the risk of missing the needed prescription drug (I). This is also true of oral liquid acetaminophen/paracetamol, which may be given to the child prior to the procedure for analgesia. When possible, the dose can be timed a little earlier or a little later to separate the ingestion from the time of anesthesia. Whenever possible, nonprescription medications, multivitamins, or any medications that are opaque or alkaline should be avoided for 8 hours before a procedure because they are considered equivalent to solids (III).[34,35]

- *It is best to finish breastfeeding at 4 hours prior to fasting and anesthesia.* Per ASA guidelines, the mother (or other caretaker) should be advised to finish breastfeeding or providing breastmilk to the infant approximately 4 hours prior to the scheduled surgery time, even if the infant needs to be awakened. Waking the child to feed 4 hours prior to the scheduled procedure decreases the risk for hypoglycemia and hemodynamic instability, especially in children less than 3 months old (II-1).[24,25] This optimizes the

TABLE 1   Summary of Fasting Recommendations to Reduce the Risk of Pulmonary Aspiration[35]

Ingested material	Minimum fasting period (hours)[a]
Clear liquids[b]	2
Human breastmilk	4
Infant formula	6
Non-human milks[c]	6
Light meal[d]	6

These recommendations apply to healthy patients who are undergoing elective procedures. They are not intended for women in labor. Following the guidelines does not guarantee complete gastric emptying.

[a]The fasting periods noted above apply to all ages.

[b]Examples of clear liquids include water, fruit juices without pulp, carbonated beverages, clear tea, and black coffee.

[c]Because non-human milk is similar to solids in gastric emptying time, the amount ingested must be considered when determining an appropriate fasting period.

[d]A light meal typically consists of toast and clear liquids. Meals that include fried or fatty foods or meat may prolong gastric emptying time. Both the amount and type of foods ingested must be considered when determining an appropriate fasting period.

infant's glycogen stores and volume status because the infant might otherwise sleep through the night and not receive optimal nutrition or hydration prior to the scheduled surgery or procedure.

- *Continue clear liquids until 2 hours prior to anesthesia.* Ad libitum clear liquids up to 2 hours prior to anesthesia or sedation are recommended (III).[17,19−23,25,34−36] They are considered safe up to 2 hours prior because they empty from the stomach much more rapidly than HBM. They can prevent volume depletion, improve glycogen stores, and maximize hemodynamics by hydrating the infant. The most common clear liquids provided to breastfeeding patients are apple juice, water, sucrose-based solutions, clear broth (nonfat commercially prepared only—homemade will have fat in it), and electrolyte solutions. Water is least preferred because of the absence of a glucose source. If the mother prefers to avoid the bottle, the clear liquid can be offered via a small cup, syringe, or spoon (III).[26] Clear liquids can help to soothe an anxious infant while fasting and separated from the mother's breast. This can help to maximize satisfaction of the patient and parent and allow for a more pleasant perioperative experience.[22,23]

- *Do not give formula and other HBM supplements for at least 6 hours prior to the anesthesia.* Enriched feedings include additives or supplements to expressed HBM,[37] like formula,[15] protein powder, vitamins, or minerals. These empty more slowly from the stomach and worsen the lung injury if aspirated.[13] Some fortifications to HBM may not change the gastric emptying (II1),[38] but to avoid confusion, HBM given to an infant 4 hours prior to surgery must be "non-enriched."

- *Do not give non-human milk for 6−8 hours prior to the anesthesia.* Gastric emptying times of soy, rice, or cow's milk vary, and volume ingested must be considered. Thus, it is safest to recommend that all nonhuman milk be held for 6−8 hours (III).[17,34,35]

- *Solid food must be avoided for at least 8 hours prior to the anesthesia.* An 8-hour fast is recommended for fatty or proteinaceous solids such as meat or any fried food (III).[34,35] This is suggested for children who are at the stage of development when they are concurrently eating solid foods and breastfeeding. To avoid confusion, most physicians recommend a fast from all heavy solid meals, which would include most foods fed to babies, for an 8-hour period.[3,34,35]

- *Postpone sedation or anesthesia if fasting requirements are not met.* If an infant has breastfed within 4 hours prior to an elective sedation or anesthetic, the risk of aspiration of acidic contents or particulate matter is greatly increased (III).[3] Attempts to allow "non-nutritive" suckling of the breast for infant comfort within the 4 hours prior to anesthesia may increase gastric contents and should not occur (III). Also, if clear liquids have been ingested in the 2 hours prior to sedation, the patient can have residual gastric contents. Thus, if the procedure is not an emergency,

the case should be cancelled or postponed until the minimum fasting period is met.

3. *Comfort for the infant and mother during a fast.* Infant comfort during the fasting period can be addressed with a pacifier (dummy) or other measures such as swaddling, rocking, and holding by caregivers or nursing staff.[26] The mother holding the infant may send signals consistent with an impending meal; thus some mothers find that the infant may need to be held by another adult during the fasting period.

   - *Use of a pacifier (dummy) in the NPO period.* Non-nutritive sucking on a pacifier (or a gloved clean finger)[76] has been shown to reduce crying spells and can be considered a temporary measure in the preoperative NPO period prior to the start of sedation or induction of anesthesia. Sucrose should be treated as a clear liquid if used with the pacifier for comfort. Therefore the use of sucrose should cease 2 hours prior to sedation per ASA guidelines (III).[35] Introducing a pacifier for the first time, with or without sucrose, may prove to be unrealistic in infants accustomed to breastfeeding. Also, mothers may try to avoid pacifiers (dummies) to prevent premature weaning. Studies on this have mixed results (I).[39,40] If accepted by the infant and allowed by the mother, pacifiers (dummies) are an inexpensive and temporary way to relieve anxiety and improve the infant's comfort and physiologic status (I).[25−29] Please refer to the Academy of Breastfeeding Medicine Clinical Protocol #23 for further information on comforting an infant with a pacifier and sucrose.[26]

   - *If possible, express and store breastmilk during the NPO period.* Until the time the mother can breastfeed again, she should be encouraged to express and store HBM for her own comfort and to avoid feedback inhibition of milk synthesis. Mothers should be advised of lactation rooms or other private spaces to express milk.

4. *Breastfeed immediately after the procedure.* After a minor procedure under anesthesia, if her child is stable, otherwise healthy, and the type of surgery does not prevent oral intake, a mother can immediately begin to breastfeed her infant as soon as he or she is awake (II3).[41] This increases comfort, reduces pain in the child, and is widely practiced and evidence-based, even following cleft lip and palate repairs.[41−43]

SUMMARY

The recommendations exist to protect the infant from pulmonary aspiration of gastric contents and to educate clinicians and parents of the risks associated with improper fasting. A summary of the current guidelines from the ASA Task Force for fasting periods for other foods or liquids a nonexclusively breastfed infant can ingest are provided in Table 1. Following the ASA guidelines helps prevent untoward events and decreases the risk of morbidity and mortality (III).[3,35]

Current practice and evidence suggests that the safety of performing anesthesia is increased when a mother withholds breastfeeding for 4 hours, but no longer than this, prior to sedation or anesthesia. This is a general consensus in Western medicine (III).[20,34,35] Hospitals and clinics are encouraged to review and revise their preprocedural instructions for care-givers, in order to integrate the current preprocedural fasting recommendations. Alternatives to comfort the infant during the fasting period improve patient, clinician, and parent satisfaction. By following the recommendations outlined in this protocol, the stress of the breastfeeding mother can be reduced, and the well-being of the NPO breastfeeding infant can be maintained.

SUGGESTED AREAS FOR FUTURE RESEARCH

Consistency of HBM and gastric emptying time

There is insufficient evidence to determine if the variable consistency and components of HBM (i.e. fat content, protein, etc.) alter gastric emptying times. The contents of breastmilk in the first week are clearly different than the milk produced at 1 year. Some believe that breastmilk is similar in emptying times to clear liquids. Although studies have shown that it is safe to provide HBM up to 2 hours prior to a procedure, others report that the gastric emptying time can match that of 3% fat milk.[17] This discrepancy could be due to the varying components of the HBM. Studies should be conducted with gastric ultrasound to determine the emptying time of an infant's meal of HBM that has been sampled throughout the meal for measurements of fat content and protein content. The gastric emptying time of a fat-rich HBM meal may be much longer than a mostly clear, lactose-rich meal of HBM that has a low fat content. In general it is safer to recommend that an infant not be fed HBM within 4 hours of sedation or anesthesia because it is undetermined if breastmilk will clear faster than this time period.

Co-morbidities in breastfeeding infants

There is insufficient published evidence to define whether gastric acidity or volume has a clear relationship to gastro-esophageal reflux disease, dysphasia symptoms, gastrointestinal motility disorders, cardiac disease, and metabolic disorders such as diabetes mellitus in breastfed infants. The risk of regurgitation and pulmonary aspiration may be increased in such disorders.[23] Although one study suggests that pediatric patients having elective cardiac surgeries share equal risk of aspiration with non-cardiac patients, there are not enough published scientific studies to support this hypothesis. More studies need to be performed on fasting infants with significant co-morbidities who are fed HBM.

Effect of non-nutritive sucking on gastric contents

It is difficult to find studies regarding measurement of gastric contents after an infant has been suckling on the mother's breast or a pacifier. It is well known that stimulation of the nipple causes milk let down in breastfeeding mothers, so "nonnutritive" suckling on the breast is likely impossible. This is even true if the mother has "prepumped" to make the beast more empty—even a small amount of breastmilk in the infant's stomach can have untoward consequences if aspirated. It almost certainly would increase the infant's gastric contents and delay the procedure. Sucking on a pacifier may have similar effects to chewing gum, which is known to increase gastric contents, but one study found the opposite to be true. Widström et al.[30] showed that sucking on a pacifier decreases gastric retention in tube-fed premature infants. Thus, aside from reducing anxiety and crying, pacifiers may also speed gastric emptying time and reduce the risk for aspiration. Effects of nonnutritive sucking on gastric contents need further investigation.

Pacifier use and weaning from breastfeeding

Pacifiers are an inexpensive means to reducing anxiety in an infant; however, pacifiers may contribute to early weaning from breastfeeding. Studies are inconclusive. If pacifiers are only used temporarily in the perioperative period, this risk of early weaning from the breast should be minimized.[39,40]

Excessive fasting times

It is suggested that NPO guidelines are excessive and that the time from the last meal to the time of the procedures exceeds the amount of time required by fasting guidelines. The study of Engelhardt et al.[31] demonstrated that fasting children 2–16 years old report significant hunger and thirst. No studies have addressed excessive fasting in breastfeeding infants. It is difficult to assess hunger and thirst in infants, but it is well known that their glycogen stores are used quickly and a fasting period of longer than 4 hours for a newborn infant can be detrimental.[24,25] More evidence needs to be obtained pertaining to the actual fasting times of breastfeeding infants.

ACKNOWLEDGMENTS

This work was supported in part by a grant from the Maternal and Child Health Bureau, U.S. Department of Health and Human Services.

REFERENCES

1. American Society of Anesthesiology Task Force. Practice guidelines for sedation and analgesia by non-anesthesiologists. *Anesthesiology.* 2002;96:1004–1017.
2. Lawrence R. Lactation support when the infant will require general anesthesia: Assisting the breastfeeding dyad in remaining content through the preoperative fasting period. *J Hum Lact.* 2005;21:355–357.
3. Warner MA, Warner ME, Warner DO, et al. Perioperative pulmonary aspiration in infants and children. *Anesthesiology.* 1999;90:66–71.
4. Cote CJ. NPO after midnight for children—A reappraisal. *Anesthesiology.* 1990;72:589–592.

5. Bannister WK, Sattilaro AJ. Vomiting and aspiration during anesthesia. *Anesthesiology*. 1962;23:251–264.

6. Mendelson CL. The aspiration of stomach contents into the lungs during obstetric anesthesia. *Am J Obstet Gynecol*. 1946;52:191–205.

7. Weaver DC. Preventing aspiration deaths during anesthesia. *JAMA*. 1964;188:971–975.

8. Winternitz MC, Smith GH, McNamara FP. Effect of intrabronchial insufflations of acid. *J Exp Med*. 1920;32:199–204.

9. St-Hilaire M, Nseqbe E, Gagnon-Gervais K, et al. Laryngeal chemoreflexes induced by acid, water, and saline in nonsedated newborn lambs during quiet sleep. *J Appl Physiol*. 2005;98:2197–2203.

10. Murphy PJ, Langton JA, Barker P, et al. Effect of oral diazepam on the sensitivity of upper airway reflexes. *Br J Anaesth*. 1993;70:131–134.

11. Szekely SM, Vickers MD. A comparison of the effects of codeine and tramadol on laryngeal reactivity. *Eur J Anaesthesiol*. 1992;9:111–120.

12. Borland LM, Sereika SM, Woelfel SK, et al. Pulmonary aspiration in pediatric patients during general anesthesia: Incidence and outcome. *J Clin Anesth*. 1998;10:95–102.

13. O'Hare B, Lerman J, Endo J, et al. Acute lung injury after instillation of human breast milk or infant formula into rabbits' lungs. *Anesthesiology*. 1996;84:1386–1391.

14. O'Hare B, Chin C, Lerman J, et al. Acute lung injury after installation of human breast milk into rabbits' lungs: Effects of pH and gastric juice. *Anesthesiology*. 1999;90:1112–1118.

15. Van Den Driessche M, Peeters K, Marien P, et al. Gastric emptying in formula-fed and breast-fed infants measures with the ^{13}C-octanoic acid breath test. *J Pediatr Gastronenterol Nutr*. 1999;29:46–51.

16. Lauro HV. Counterpoint: Formula before surgery: Is there evidence for a new consensus on pediatric NPO guidelines? *Soc Pediatr Anesth Newslett*. 2003;16(3). Available at: www.pedsanesthesia.org/newsletters/2003summer/counterpoint.iphtml (accessed May 3, 2012).

17. Sethi AK, Chatterji C, Bhargava SK, et al. Safe pre-operative fasting times after milk or clear fluid in children—A preliminary study using real-time ultrasound. *Anaesthesia*. 1999;54:51–59.

18. Billeaud C, Guillet J, Sandler B. Gastric emptying in infants with or without gastro-oesophageal reflux according to the type of breast milk. *Eur J Clin Nutr*. 1990;44:577–583.

19. Litman RS, Wu CL, Quinlivan JK. Gastric volume and pH in infants fed clear liquids and breast milk prior to surgery. *Anesth Analg*. 1994;79:482–485.

20. Cook-Sather SD, Litman RS. Modern fasting guidelines in children. *Best Pract Res Clin Anaesthesiol*. 2006;20:471–481.

21. Splinter WM, Schreiner MS. Preoperative fasting in children. *Anesth Analg*. 1999;89:80–89.

22. Brady M, Kinn S, Ness V, et al. Preoperative fasting for preventing perioperative complications in children. *Cochrane Database Syst Rev*. 2009;(4)CD005285.

23. Nicholson SC, Dorsey AT, Schreiner MS. Shortened preanesthetic fasting interval in pediatric cardiac surgical patients. *Anesth Analg*. 1992;74:694–697.

24. Girard J, Ferre P, Gilbert M. Energy metabolism in the perinatal period (author's transl) [in French]. *Diabete Metab*. 1975;1:241–257.

25. Van der Walt JH, Foate JA, Murrell D, et al. A study of preoperative fasting in infants aged less than three months. *Anaesth Intensive Care*. 1990;18:527–531.

26. Academy of Breastfeeding Medicine Protocol Committee. ABM clinical protocol #23: Non-pharmacologic management of procedure-related pain in the breastfeeding infant. *Breastfeed Med*. 2010;5:315–319.

27. Treloar DM. The effect of nonnutritive sucking on oxygenation in healthy, crying full-term infants. *Appl Nurs Res*. 1994;7:52–58.

28. Curtis SJ, Jou H, Ali S, et al. A randomized controlled trial of sucrose and/or pacifier as analgesia for infants receiving venipuncture in a pediatric emergency department. *BMC Pediatr*. 2007;7:27.

29. Phillips RM, Chantry CJ, Gallagher MP. Analgesic effects of breast-feeding or pacifier use with maternal holding in term infants. *Ambul Pediatr*. 2005;5:359–364.

30. Widström AM, Marchini G, Matthiesen AS. Nonnutritive sucking in tube-fed preterm infants: Effects on gastric motility and gastric contents of somatostatin. *J Pediatr Gastroenterol Nutr*. 1988;7:517–523.

31. Engelhardt T, Wilson G, Horne L, et al. Are you hungry? Are you thirsty?—Fasting times in elective outpatient pediatric patients. *Paediatr Anaesth*. 2011;21:964–968.

32. U.S. Preventive Task Force. Quality of Evidence. Available at: www.ncbi.nlm.nih.gov/books/NBK15430 (accessed April 19, 2012).

33. Cravero JP. Risk and safety of pediatric sedation/anesthesia for procedures outside the operating room. *Curr Opin Anaesthesiol*. 2009;22:509–513.

34. Ferrari LR, Rooney FM, Rockoff MA. Preoperative fasting practices in pediatrics. *Anesthesiology*. 1999;90:978–980.

35. American Society of Anesthesiologists Committee. Practice guidelines for preoperative fasting and the use of pharmacologic agents to reduce the risk of pulmonary aspiration: Application to healthy patients undergoing elective procedures: An updated report by the American Society of Anesthesiologists Committee on Standards and Practice Parameters. *Anesthesiology*. 2011;114:495–511.

36. Green CR. Preoperative fasting time: Is the traditional policy changing? Results of a national survey. *Anesth Analg*. 1996;83:123–128.

37. Academy of Breastfeeding Medicine Protocol Committee. ABM clinical protocol #3: Hospital guidelines for the use of supplementary feedings in the healthy term breastfed neonate, revised 2009. *Breastfeed Med*. 2009;4:175–182.

38. Gathwala G, Shaw C, Shaw P, et al. Human milk fortification and gastric emptying in the preterm neonate. *Int J Clin Pract*. 2008;62:1039–1043.

39. Benis MM. Are pacifiers associated with early weaning from breastfeeding? *Adv Neonatal Care*. 2002;2:259–266.

40. Kramer MS, Barr RG, Dagenais S, et al. Pacifier use, early weaning, and cry/fuss behavior: A randomized controlled trial. *JAMA*. 2001;286:322–326.

41. Cohen M, Marschall MA, Schafer ME. Immediate unrestricted feeding of infants following cleft lip and palate repair. *J Craniofac Surg*. 1992;3:30–32.

42. Johnson HA. The immediate postoperative care of a child with cleft lip: time-proven suggestions. *Ann Plast Surg*. 1983;11:87.

43. Darzi MA, Chowdri NA, Bhat AN. Breast feeding or spoon-feeding after cleft lip repair: A prospective, randomized study. *Br J Plast Surg.* 1996;49:24–26.

ABM protocols expire 5 years from the date of publication. Evidence-based revisions are made within 5 years or sooner if there are significant changes in the evidence.

Lead Contributors
Geneva B. Young, M.D. Cathy R. Lammers, M.D.
Academy of Breastfeeding Medicine Protocol Committee

Kathleen A. Marinelli, M.D., FABM, Chairperson
Caroline J. Chantry, M.D., FABM, Co-Chairperson
Maya Bunik, M.D., MSPH, FABM, Co-Chairperson
Larry Noble, M.D., FABM, Translations Chairperson
Nancy Brent, M.D.
Alison V. Holmes, M.D., M.P.H., FABM
Ruth A. Lawrence, M.D., FABM
Nancy G. Powers, M.D., FABM
Tomoko Seo, M.D., FABM
Julie Scott Taylor, M.D., M.Sc., FABM
For correspondence: abm@bfmed.org

ABM Clinical Protocol #26
*Persistent Pain with Breastfeeding**

*Pamela Berens[1], Anne Eglash[2], Michele Malloy[2],
Alison M. Steube[3,4] and the Academy of Breastfeeding Medicine*

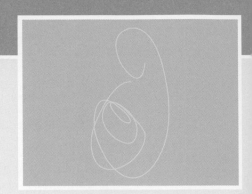

ABSTRACT

A central goal of The Academy of Breastfeeding Medicine is the development of clinical protocols for managing common medical problems that may impact breastfeeding success. These protocols serve only as guidelines for the care of breastfeeding mothers and infants and do not delineate an exclusive course of treatment or serve as standards of medical care. Variations in treatment may be appropriate according to the needs of an individual patient.

PURPOSE

TO PROVIDE EVIDENCE-BASED GUIDANCE in the diagnosis, evaluation, and management of breastfeeding women with persistent nipple and breast pain.

DEFINITIONS

Among breastfeeding women, it can be challenging to distinguish pathologic pain from discomfort commonly reported in the first few weeks of breastfeeding. In this protocol, we define persistent pain as breastfeeding-associated pain lasting longer than 2 weeks. We are not addressing acute or recurrent mastitis as it is covered in ABM Protocol #4 Mastitis, Revised March 2014.[1]

---

* Courtesy of the Academy of Breastfeeding Medicine. Please go to https://www.bfmed.org/protocols for complete protocols, translations, and the most up-to-date information (protocols are updated every 5–7 years).

[1] Department of Obstetrics and Gynecology, University of Texas Health Sciences Center at Houston, Houston, Texas.

[2] Department of Family and Community Medicine, University of Wisconsin School of Medicine and Public Health, Madison, Wisconsin.

[3] Department of Obstetrics and Gynecology, University of North Carolina School of Medicine, Chapel Hill, North Carolina.

[4] Carolina Global Breastfeeding Institute, Department of Maternal and Child Health, Gillings School of Global Public Health, Chapel Hill, North Carolina.

BACKGROUND

Pain and discomfort associated with breastfeeding are common in the first few weeks postpartum.[2] (II-2) (Quality of evidence [levels of evidence I, II-1, II-2, II-3, and III] is based on the U.S. Preventive Services Task Force Appendix A Task Force Ratings[3] and is noted in parentheses.) Since this is a common cause for early breastfeeding cessation,[4] the mother–baby dyad should be evaluated by a lactation specialist. Beyond this early period, reports of pain generally decline, but as many as one in five women report persistent pain at 2 months postpartum.[5] While initial discomfort with early latch may be considered physiological, pain severe enough to cause premature weaning should not. In one study of 1323 mothers who stopped breastfeeding during the first month postpartum, 29.3% cited pain and 36.8% identified sore, cracked, or bleeding nipples as an important reason.[6] Several authors have found a relationship between breastfeeding-associated pain and postpartum depression.[7,8] (II-2, III)

These studies suggest that breastfeeding-associated pain is linked with significant psychological stress; thus, mothers presenting with pain should be evaluated for mood symptoms and followed closely for resolution or treatment as needed. Timely identification and appropriate management of persistent breastfeeding-associated pain are crucial to enable women to achieve their infant feeding goals.

Although the literature on persistent nipple and/or breast pain is limited and the differential diagnosis is extensive, a number of etiologies and management strategies are emerging, most of which are based on expert opinion (Table 1). The highly individual nature of the breastfeeding relationship combined with the complexity of the lactating breast, including its anatomy, physiology, and dynamic microbiome, adds challenges to the clinicians' efforts.

HISTORY AND EXAMINATION

Assessment of persistent pain begins with a careful history and physical examination of both mother and infant, with particular attention to the following:

- Breastfeeding history
  - Previous breastfeeding experiences/problems/pain
  - Nipple/breast sensitivity before pregnancy

TABLE 1   Conditions, Symptoms, and Management of Persistent Nipple/Breast Pain

Condition	Symptoms/signs	Management
Infant ankyloglossia	Ongoing nipple damage and an infant with restricted tongue movement due to a tight lingual frenulum	• Frenulotomy/frenulectomy using scissors or laser by a trained health professional[44–46] (I, II-2, 1).
Breast pump trauma/ misuse	Nipple or soft tissue injury/bruising	• Observe a pumping session.
Eczematous conditions	Erythematous skin *Acute* episodes: blisters, erosions, weeping/oozing, and crust formation *Chronic* eruptions: dry, scaling, and lichenified (thickened) areas. Lesions can be pruritic, painful, or even burning.[18,20]	• Reduce identifiable triggers. • Apply an emollient • Apply low/medium-strength steroid ointment twice daily for 2 weeks (immediately after a breastfeed to maximize contact time before the next breastfeed).[20] • Use second-generation antihistamines for pruritus.[20] • Consider a short course (less than 3 weeks) of oral prednisolone or prednisone in resistant cases.[20,47]
Psoriasis	Erythematous plaques Clearly demarcated borders Fine silvery overlying scale	• Apply an emollient.[20,48] (I) • Apply low/medium-strength steroid ointment twice daily (immediately after a breastfeed) as first-line treatment.[20,48] • Avoid prolonged topical steroid use to prevent thinning of the nipple epithelium and delayed healing. • Topical vitamin D creams or gels and phototherapy (UVB) are safe to use.[20,48] • Immunomodulating agents should not be used on the nipple due to the risk of infant oral absorption.[47]
Superficial bacterial infection associated with skin trauma	Persistent cracks, fissures Weeping, yellow crusted lesions especially in conjunction with other skin conditions Cellulitis	• Topical mupirocin or bacitracin ointment • Oral antibiotics such as a cephalosporin or penicillinase-resistant penicillin[18,49] (I)
Bacterial dysbiosis	Bilateral dull, deep aching bilateral breast pain ± burning Pain during and after breastfeeds Breast tenderness (especially lower quadrants)[29]	• Consider oral antibiotics such as a cephalosporin, amoxicillin/clavulanate, dicloxacillin, or erythromycin for 2–6 weeks.[20,29] • Indirect evidence to support that breast probiotics may assist the restoration of normal breast flora.[50,51]
Candida infection	Pink nipple/areola area Shiny or flaky appearance of the nipple Nipple pain out of proportion to the clinical findings Burning nipple pain and pain radiating into the breast[20,23]	• Topical azole antifungal ointment or cream (miconazole and clotrimazole also inhibit the growth of *Staphylococcus sp*) on nipples.[20] • Nystatin suspension or miconazole oral gel for infant's mouth.[20] • Gentian violet (less than 0.5% aqueous solution) may be used daily for no more than 7 days. Longer durations and higher concentrations may cause ulcerations and skin necrosis.[20,52] • Oral fluconazole (200 mg once, then 100 mg daily for 7–10 days) may be used for resistant cases. • Before prescribing fluconazole, review all maternal medications and assess for drug interactions. Do not use fluconazole in combination with domperidone or erythromycin due to concern of prolonged QT intervals.
Herpes simplex	Small, clustered exquisitely tender vesicles with an erythematous, edematous base Solitary small ulcer[20,53]	• Oral antiviral therapy such as acyclovir or valacyclovir should be used in doses recommended

(Continued)

TABLE 1 Conditions, Symptoms, and Management of Persistent Nipple/Breast Pain—cont'd

Condition	Symptoms/signs	Management
	Axillary lymphadenopathy[53]	for treating primary or recurrent Herpes simplex infections. • Prevent contact between lesions and the infant. • Avoid breastfeeding or feeding expressed breast milk to infants from an affected breast/nipple until the lesions are healed to prevent neonatal herpes infection.
Herpes zoster	Pain and vesicular rash following a dermatome	• Oral antiviral therapy such as acyclovir or valacyclovir should be used in doses recommended for treating Herpes zoster • Avoid breastfeeding or feeding expressed breast milk to infants from an affected breast/nipple until the lesions are healed
Vasospasm	Shooting or burning breast pain with blanching and other color changes (purple or red) of the nipple associated with pain[38,39]	• Warmth (compresses, heat pads) following a breastfeed or whenever the mother experiences pain. • Avoid cold on the breasts and nipples. • Nifedipine 30–60 mg sustained release daily or immediate release 10–20 mg thrice a day for 2 weeks initially if pain persists.[54] (I) Longer treatment may be necessary for some women.
Allodynia/functional pain	Pain to light touch Clothing brushing against the nipple causes excruciating pain, or that drying their breasts with a towel is painful History of other pain disorders	• Round-the-clock nonsteroidal anti-inflammatory medications. • Propranolol starting at 20 mg thrice a day if not responding.[55] (I based on treatment of TMJ pain) • Antidepressants may also be effective (see ABM Protocol #18 Use of Antidepressants in Breastfeeding Mothers). • Consider evaluation for trigger points and treatment with massage therapy.[56]
Recurrent plugged (blocked) ducts	Localized tender cord of tissue, usually a few centimeters in size, which is usually reversible with expression	• Heat, direct pressure, and milk expression usually offer relief
Oversupply	Breast fullness, milk leakage	• Stop any overstimulation by not pumping or hand expressing between breastfeeds. Only hand express or pump in lieu of breastfeeding or if breasts are overfull before bedtime. • Block feeding is a strategy that many lactation consultants endorse, but is controversial with limited evidence. This involves feeding from one breast for a block of time, typically 3 hours. The other breast rests, allowing the fullness to provide feedback to the breast to reduce milk supply.[57] • Medication such as pseudoephedrine[58] and sage extract have been used to reduce milk supply as has the oral contraceptive pill containing estrogen.

Data to support management of persistent breastfeeding-associated pain are limited and based largely on expert opinion. Recommendations below are therefore based on Level III evidence, unless otherwise indicated. *TMJ*, temporomandibular joint pain.

- Milk supply (ongoing engorgement, high supply versus low supply)
- Pattern of breastfeeding (frequency, duration, one, or both breasts)
- Expression of milk, frequency, hand expression, and or type of pump
- Mother's attitudes toward breastfeeding and her breastfeeding goals
- Pain history
  - Early nipple trauma (abrasions, cracks, bleeding)
  - Context (with latch, during breastfeeding, between breastfeeds, with milk expression)
  - Location (nipple and/or breast; superficial versus deep)
  - Duration (timing, intermittent, or constant)
  - Character (burning, itching, sharp, shooting, dull, aching)

- Pain severity using rating scale, such as 0–10
- Associated signs and symptoms (skin changes, nipple color change, nipple shape/appearance after feeding, fever)
- Exacerbating/ameliorating factors (cold, heat, light touch, deep pressure)
- Treatment thus far (analgesia, including nonsteroidal anti-inflammatory drugs and/or narcotic preparations), antibiotics, antifungals, steroids, herbs, lubricants, other supplements
- Maternal history
  - Complications during pregnancy, labor, and birth (medical conditions, interventions)
  - Medical conditions (especially Raynaud's phenomenon, cold sensitivity, migraines, dermatitis, eczema, chronic pain syndromes, candida infection, family history of ankyloglossia)
  - History of breast surgery and reason
  - Medications
  - Allergies
  - Depression, anxiety
  - History of herpes simplex or zoster in the nipple/breast region
  - History of recent breast infections
- Infant history
  - Birth trauma or abnormalities on examination
  - Current age and gestational age at birth
  - Birth weight, weight gain, and general health
  - Behavior at the breast (pulling, squirming, biting, coughing, shortness of breath, excessive sleepiness)
  - Fussiness
  - Gastrointestinal problems (reflux symptoms, bloody stools, mucous stools)
  - Medical conditions/syndromes
  - Previous diagnosis of ankyloglossia; frenotomy
  - Medications
  Examination should include the following:
- Mother
  - General appearance (pale [anemia], exhaustion)
  - Assessment of nipples (skin integrity, sensitivity, purulent drainage, presence/absence of rashes, coloration, lesions)
  - Breast examination (masses, tenderness to light/deep pressure)
  - Sensitivity to light or sharp touch on body of breast, areola, and nipple
  - Manual expression of milk (assess for pain with maneuver)
  - Assessment of maternal mood using a validated instrument, such as the Edinburgh Postnatal Depression Scale
- Infant
  - Symmetry of head and facial features (including jaw angle, eye/ear position)
  - Oral anatomy (presence/absence of lingual frenulum, evidence of thrush, palate abnormality, submucosal cleft)
  - Airway (looking for nasal congestion)
  - Head and neck range of motion

- Infant muscle tone
- Other infant behavior that may give clues to underlying neurologic problems, for example, nystagmus

A breastfeeding session should be directly observed to assess the following:
- Maternal positioning
- Infant positioning and behavior at the breast
- Latch (wide-open mouth with lips everted)
- Suck dynamics—pattern of feeding, nutritive and nonnutritive sucking, sleeping
- Shape and color of nipple after feeding

If the mother is expressing milk, the clinician should directly observe an expressing session to assess the following:
- Hand expressing technique
- Breast shield/flange fit
- Breast pump dynamics, including suction and cycle frequency with the pump the mother is using
- Evidence of trauma from the breast pump

Laboratory studies, such as milk and nipple cultures (Table 2), may be considered based on the history and physical exam findings such as the following:
- Acute mastitis or mastitis that is not resolving with antibiotics
- Persistent nipple cracks, fissures, or drainage
- Erythema or rashes suggesting viral or fungal infection
- Breast pain out of proportion to examination (appear normal, but very tender, breasts or nipples)

DIFFERENTIAL DIAGNOSIS

The potential causes of persistent breast and nipple pain are numerous, may occur concurrently or sequentially, and include the following:
- Nipple damage
- Dermatosis
- Infection
- Vasospasm/Raynaud's phenomenon
- Allodynia/functional pain

Table 1 lists symptoms and management of the different diagnoses described below.

Nipple damage

Epidermal compromise increases the risk of developing infection and pain. Breastfeeding or using a breast pump to express milk can induce an inflammatory response in nipple skin, which may result in erythema, edema, fissures, and/or blisters.
1. Abnormal latch/suck dynamic
   - *Suboptimal positioning.* Often cited as the most common cause of sore nipples, suboptimal positioning of the infant during a breastfeed can lead to a shallow latch and abnormal compression of the nipple between the tongue and palate.[9–11] (II-2, III, III)
   - *Disorganized or dysfunctional latch/suck*: The ability of an infant to properly latch and breastfeed is dependent, among other factors, on prematurity, oral and mandibular anatomy, muscle tone, neurological maturity, and reflux or congenital abnormities, as well as maternal

TABLE 2   Culture Methods (Nipple, Breast Milk) (III)

Methods for culture[59]

For all cultures, ensure that the person collecting the sample has clean hands and applied gloves and that the sample is labeled correctly (with right or left side) and transported appropriately.

Nipple swab (intact skin)

Moisten tip of a dry swab in culture tube media.

Sweep the swab in a zigzag pattern (reaching 10 different points) over the areola (avoid touching swab to breast skin).

Replace swab in culturette (holder for swab).

Label culturette with patient label and nipple side (left or right).

Repeat for contralateral nipple.

Nipple/areola fissure or open wound culture

Dry wound: Moisten tip of swab in culture media.

Rotate the swab in the wound for 5 seconds.

Place swab in culturette.

Milk culture

Ask patient if she would prefer to hand express milk herself or have the provider do so.

Cleansing the nipple

Place a towel in the patient's lap before irrigation.

Before milk expression, irrigate the nipple with sterile saline.

Blot the nipple with sterile gauze after irrigation.

Cleanse each nipple with an alcohol wipe. Allow alcohol to dry.

Remove gloves and clean hands.

Apply clean gloves.

Position dominant hand in a "C" shape, with pads of the thumb and fingers ~1.5 inches behind the nipple.

Push straight back into the chest wall.

Roll thumb and fingers forward to express milk without touching nipple directly.

Allow the first few drops of milk to fall onto the towel.

Express 5–10 mL of milk into a sterile cup without touching cup to nipple.

Repeat for contralateral breast.

---

issues such as milk flow, breast/nipple size, and engorgement. Infants who are premature, have low oral tone, and reflux/aspiration or congenital anomalies that may be at risk for disorganized suckling.[12] (III) Evaluation of the infant for difficulty coordinating sucking and swallowing may be indicated.

- *Ankyloglossia* (tongue-tie), recognized in 0.02–10.7% of newborns, involves the restriction of tongue movement (projection) beyond the lower gum[13] due to an abnormally short or thickened lingual frenulum. Poor tongue movement may lead to difficulty attaining a deep latch and is frequently associated with maternal nipple pain.[14,15] (II-3, I) Factors such as breast fullness, milk flow, nipple size and elasticity, infant palate shape, and height affect the impact of ankyloglossia on the mother's nipples. Not all infants with ankyloglossia cause problems for the breastfeeding dyad.
- *Infant biting or jaw clenching at the breast:* Infants who bite or clench their jaws while breastfeeding may cause nipple damage and breast pain. Conditions that may lead to this behavior include clavicle fractures, torticollis, head/neck or facial trauma, mandibular asymmetry,[16] oral defensiveness or aversion (e.g., infants force-fed with ridged nipples [teats]), tonic

bite reflex, nasal congestion, a response to an overactive milk ejection reflex, and teething. (III)

2. Breast pump trauma/misuse

Because of the widespread use of breast pumps in many countries and the variability of consumer education, literacy, and support, there is significant potential for harm from breast pump use. In a survey in the United States, 14.6% of 1844 mothers reported injuries related to pump use.[17] (II-2) Injury may be either a direct result of pump misuse or failure or an exacerbation of pre-existing nipple damage or pathology. Observing the mother while using the breast pump may clarify the cause(s) of trauma (i.e., improper flange fit, excessive high-pressure suction, or prolonged duration).

Dermatoses

Breast dermatoses such as eczematous conditions or, less commonly, psoriasis and mammary Paget's disease may be responsible for nipple and/or breast pain in lactating women. Any of these conditions may be secondarily infected with *Staphylococcus aureus*, causing impetiginous changes such as weeping, yellow crusting, and blisters.[18] (III)

1. Eczematous conditions

These conditions can affect any skin, but are commonly seen on and around the areola in breastfeeding women. Attention to the distribution of skin irritation and lesions may help identify the underlying cause/trigger. Eczematous rashes vary considerably.

- *Atopic dermatitis (eczema):* This condition occurs in women with an atopic tendency and may be triggered by skin irritants and other factors such as weather and temperature change.[19]
- *Irritant contact dermatitis:* Common offending agents include friction, infant (oral) medications, solid foods (consumed by the infant), breast pads, laundry detergents, dryer sheets, fabric softeners, fragrances, and creams used for nipple soreness.[18]
- *Allergic contact dermatitis:* Common offending agents include lanolin, antibiotics (topical), chamomile, vitamins A and E, and fragrances.[18,20] (III)

2. Psoriasis

Flares can occur during lactation sporadically (usually 4—6 weeks after the birth[21] (III) or as a response to skin injury (koebnerization) from latch, suckling, or biting.

3. Mammary Paget's disease (Paget's disease of the nipple)

More common in postmenopausal women (60—80% of cases), but observed in younger women, this slow-growing intraductal carcinoma mimics eczema of the nipple. A unilateral, slowly advancing nipple eczema that begins on the face of the nipple is unresponsive to usual treatment, persists longer than 3 weeks, or is associated with a palpable mass should increase suspicion for Paget's disease.[18] Other findings consistent with the diagnosis are ulceration, moist erythema, vesicles, and/or granular erosions.[22] (II-2) Skin biopsy and referral for specialist treatment are necessary.

Infection

Although a number of studies have attempted to identify what, if any, microbe may cause persistent nipple/breast pain during lactation, the roles of bacteria and yeast remain unclear. Both *Staphylococcus sp* and Candida can be found on nipples and in breast milk of women with no symptoms.[23] (II-2) Additional theories suggest a role for virulence traits that make detection and elimination of potentially causative microbes extremely difficult. These include biofilm formation, consisting of bacteria alone[24,25] (III, III animal/in vitro studies) or mixed species of *Staphylococcus sp* and Candida,[26,27] (III, III animal/in vitro studies), as well as intracellular infection by small colony variants.[28] (III animal/in vitro studies)

1. Bacterial
- *Superficial bacterial infection in setting of skin trauma:* Infection secondary to damaged skin, especially around the nipple—areolar complex, is a common occurrence. Impetigo and cellulitis may occur alone or concurrent with an underlying dermatitis.[18]
- *Bacterial dysbiosis and lactiferous duct infection:* Bacterial overgrowth combined with biofilm formed by bacteria (possibly in conjunction with *Candida sp*)

may lead to narrowed lactiferous ducts and inflamed epithelium. (III) A relatively constant, dull, deep aching pain in both breasts is characteristic of this inflammation as well as tenderness to palpation on breast examination.[29] (II-3) Milk flow and ejection cause increased pressure and sharp shooting pain during milk ejection and breastfeeding. Recurrent blocked ducts, engorgement and oversupply, and nipple cracks and fissures may also be associated with this condition.[30] (III)

Factors that are thought to predispose a woman to developing dysbiosis and ductal infection include the following:
- History of similar symptoms during prior lactations[29]
- Previous episodes of acute mastitis
- Nipple cracks or lesions[29]
- Recent treatment with antifungals and/or antibiotics Judicious use of antibiotics is encouraged and so the workup should include[29] (Table 2) the following:
- Nipple and breast milk cultures
- Wound culture if crack/fissure present

2. Candida infection
- The association of Candida with nipple/breast pain remains controversial. Human milk does not inhibit growth of Candida in fungal cultures.[31] (II-2) Some authors have not found a correlation between symptoms and *Candida sp* identification,[32,33] (II-2, II-2) while others have,[34,35] (II2, II-2) including one study using PCR technology.[23] (II-2)
- Factors that are thought to predispose a woman to develop Candida infection include the following:
- A predisposition to Candida infections
- Thrush in the infant's mouth or in the diaper (nappy) area (monilial rash)
- Recent use of antibiotics in mother or child

3. Viral infection
- Herpes simplex: Herpes simplex infection (HSV) that either predates lactation or is acquired from a breastfeeding child can infect the breast or nipples. HSV infection of the breast or nipple skin can result in neonatal transmission during breastfeeding, putting the infant at significant risk for morbidity and mortality.[36] (III) Culturing the blisters to confirm the diagnosis is optimal. Mothers should not breastfeed on the affected side and expressed milk should be discarded until the lesions have healed.[19,37] (III)
- Herpes zoster: Herpes zoster may erupt along a dermatome that involves the breast. The rash often starts close to the spinal column on the posterior thorax and migrates peripherally along the dermatome toward the breast. Exposure to these lesions can result in chicken pox (varicella zoster) in unimmunized infants. In most situations, it should be treated similarly to a Herpes simplex infection and women should not breastfeed or use expressed breast milk from an affected breast until the lesions have healed.[19] Infants may be given Zoster immunoglobulin if appropriate.

Vasospasm

Vasospasm presents with blanching or purple color changes of the nipple accompanied by sharp, shooting, or burning pain.[38,39] (II-3, II-3) Women may report pain after breastfeeding, on getting out of a warm shower, or in the setting of cold temperatures, such as in the frozen food section of the grocery store. Symptoms may be bilateral or unilateral in the setting of current or past nipple trauma. Some mothers report a history of cold hands and feet, such as needing to wear socks to sleep or gloves in mild weather, or a formal diagnosis of Raynaud's syndrome. Women with a history of connective tissue disorders such as rheumatoid arthritis or prior diagnosis of Raynaud's phenomenon are at risk for vasospasm of the nipple.

Allodynia/functional pain

Allodynia is defined as sensation of pain in response to a stimulus, such as light touch, which would not normally elicit pain. Breast allodynia can occur in isolation or in the context of other pain disorders, such as irritable bowel syndrome, fibromyalgia, interstitial cystitis, migraines, temporomandibular joint disorders (TMJ), and pain with intercourse. Taking a careful history to assess for other pain disorders is important for informing treatment.

In the chronic pain literature, pain disorders are associated with catastrophization,[40] reduced psychological acceptance,[41] depression, and anxiety, and these psychological factors are associated with diminished treatment response.[42] (II-2) This literature suggests that mothers who present with breast allodynia, particularly in the setting of other chronic pain syndromes, may benefit from psychological therapy designed to treat chronic pain, given findings from studies of other chronic pain conditions.[43] (I)

Other etiologies

1. Recurrent plugged (blocked) ducts

    Plugged (blocked) ducts are very common among breastfeeding women and can be associated with persistent pain. Reducing an excessive milk supply is paramount in reducing plugged ducts. Reliance on expressing rather than breastfeeding can increase the risk of block ages due to insufficient breast drainage. If there is redness, an infection should be ruled out, while an abscess should be ruled out if symptoms persist for more than 3 days.

2. Maternal oversupply

    Oversupply of milk can cause persistent breast and nipple pain. Mothers will typically complain of sharp breast pain or dull breast aching and breast tenderness when their breasts are quite full. Oversupply is very common in the first few weeks postpartum as the body adapts to the infant's milk supply needs. Milk expression should be minimized because it can lead to continued oversupply issues.

RECOMMENDATIONS FOR FUTURE RESEARCH

There continue to be many controversies on management of persistent breast pain.

- More scientific study is needed on assessment and management of almost all potential causes, including infection, neuropathic pain issues, breast pump technology (e.g., proper fitting of breast shields), and management of lip-ties/posterior tongue-ties.
- Standardized assessment of breast pain is lacking to compare studies on severity and management.
- The role of central pain sensitivity and mood disorders in breastfeeding-associated pain also requires further study. Future studies should quantify maternal mood, pain catastrophization, and comorbid dysautonomias among women presenting with chronic breastfeeding-associated pain.
- There is still no consensus among lactation specialists regarding whether deep aching and sharp pain is attributable to a *Candida* infection, dysbiosis of typical bacteria present in breast milk, or a noninfectious etiology. Block feeding as a treatment for oversupply also deserves further study.
- Further research is needed to elucidate the causes of persistent pain and understand the complex interactions inherent in breastfeeding/lactation, including the principles of biofilms.

REFERENCES

1. Amir LH. ABM clinical protocol #4: Mastitis, revised March 2014. *Breastfeed Med.* 2014;9:239—243.
2. Division of Nutrition Physical Activity and Obesity. National Center for Chronic Disease Prevention and Health Promotion. Infant Feeding Practices Survey II: Results. Centers for Disease Control and Prevention. 2009. Available at: www.cdc.gov/ifps/results/ch2/table2-37.html (accessed November 11, 2015).
3. US Department of Health and Human Services. *Guide to Clinical Preventive Services: Report of the U.S. Preventive Services Task Force.* 2nd edition Washington (DC): US Preventive Services Task Force; 1996. Available at: http://www.ncbi.nlm.nih.gov/books/NBK15430/ (accessed January 4, 2016).
4. Odom E, Li R, Scanlon K, et al. Reasons for earlier than desired cessation of breastfeeding. *Pediatrics.* 2013;131: e726—e732.
5. Buck ML, Amir LH, Cullinane M, et al. Nipple pain, damage, and vasospasm in the first 8 weeks postpartum. *Breastfeed Med.* 2014;9:56—62.
6. Li R, Fein SB, Chen J, et al. Why mothers stop breastfeeding: Mothers' self-reported reasons for stopping during the first year. *Pediatrics.* 2008;122(Suppl 2):S69—S76.
7. Amir LH, Dennerstein L, Garland SM, et al. Psychological aspects of nipple pain in lactating women. *J Psychosom Obstet Gynaecol.* 1996;17:53—58.
8. Watkins S, Meltzer-Brody S, Zolnoun D, et al. Early breast-feeding experiences and postpartum depression. *Obstet Gynecol.* 2011;118:214—221.
9. Blair A, Cadwell K, Turner-Maffei C, et al. The relationship between positioning, the breastfeeding dynamic, the latching process and pain in breastfeeding mothers with sore nipples. *Breastfeed Rev.* 2003;11:5—10.
10. Morland-Schultz K, Hill P. Prevention of and therapies for nipple pain: A systematic review. *J Obstet Gynecol Neonatal Nurs.* 2005;34:428—437.

11. Woolridge MW. Aetiology of sore nipples. *Midwifery*. 1986;2:172–176.

12. Lau C, Smith EO, Schanler RJ. Coordination of sucks-wallow and swallow respiration in preterm infants. *Acta Paediatr*. 2003;92:721–727.

13. Power RF, Murphy JF. Tongue-tie and frenotomy in infants with breastfeeding difficulties: Achieving a balance. *Arch Dis Child*. 2015;100:489–494.

14. Ballard JL, Auer CE, Khoury JC. Ankyloglossia: Assessment, incidence, and effect of frenuloplasty on the breastfeeding dyad. *Pediatrics*. 2002;110:e63.

15. Segal LM, Stephenson R, Dawes M, et al. Prevalence, diagnosis, and treatment of ankyloglossia: Methodologic review. *Can Fam Physician*. 2007;53:1027–1033.

16. Wall V, Glass R. Mandibular asymmetry and breastfeeding problems: Experience from 11 cases. *J Hum Lact*. 2006;22:328–334.

17. Qi Y, Zhang Y, Fein S, et al. Maternal and breast pump factors associated with breast pump problems and injuries. *J Hum Lact*. 2014;30:62–72.

18. Barankin B, Gross MS. Nipple and areolar eczema in the breastfeeding woman. *J Cutan Med Surg*. 2004;8:126–130.

19. Schalock P, Hsu J, Arndt K. *Lippincott's Primary Care Dermatology*. Philadelphia: Wolter Kluwer Health/Lippincott Williams & Wilkins; 2010. pp. 29, 146–147, 174–175, 232–236.

20. Barrett ME, Heller MM, Fullerton Stone H, et al. Dermatoses of the breast in lactation. *Dermatol Ther*. 2013;26:331–336.

21. Mervic L. Management of moderate to severe plaque psoriasis in pregnancy and lactation in the era of biologics. *Acta Dermatovenerol Alp Pannonica Adriat*. 2014;23:27–31.

22. Kollmorgen DR, Varanasi JS, Edge SB, Carson 3rd WE. Paget's disease of the breast: A 33-year experience. *J Am Coll Surg*. 1998;187:171–177.

23. Amir LH, Donath SM, Garland SM, et al. Does Candida and/or Staphylococcus play a role in nipple and breast pain in lactation? A cohort study in Melbourne, Australia. *BMJ Open*. 2013;3:e002351.

24. von Eiff C, Proctor RA, Peters G. Coagulase-negative staphylococci. Pathogens have major role in nosocomial infections. *Postgrad Med*. 2001;110. 63–64, 69–70, 73–66.

25. Melchior MB, Vaarkamp H, Fink-Gremmels J. Biofilms: A role in recurrent mastitis infections? *Vet J*. 2006;171:398–407.

26. Harriott MM, Noverr MC. Candida albicans and Staphylococcus aureus form polymicrobial biofilms: Effects on antimicrobial resistance. *Antimicrob Agents Chemother*. 2009;53:3914–3922.

27. Adam B, Baillie GS, Douglas LJ. Mixed species biofilms of Candida albicans and Staphylococcus epidermidis. *J Med Microbiol*. 2002;51:344–349.

28. Proctor RA, von Eiff C, Kahl BC, et al. Small colony variants: A pathogenic form of bacteria that facilitates persistent and recurrent infections. *Nat Rev Microbiol*. 2006;4:295–305.

29. Eglash A, Plane MB. Mundt M. History, physical and laboratory findings, and clinical outcomes of lactating women treated with antibiotics for chronic breast and/or nipple pain. *J Hum Lact*. 2006;22:429–433.

30. Delgado S, Arroyo R, Jiménez E, et al. Mastitis infecciosas durante la lactancia: Un problem a infravalorado. *Acta Pediatr Esp*. 2009;67:77–84.

31. Hale TW, Bateman TL, Finkelman MA, et al. The absence of Candida albicans in milk samples of women with clinical symptoms of ductal candidiasis. *Breastfeed Med*. 2009;4:57–61.

32. Graves S, Wright W, Harman R, et al. Painful nipples in nursing mothers: Fungal or staphylococcal? *Aust Fam Physician*. 2003;32:570–571.

33. Hale T, Bateman T, Finkelman M, et al. The absence of Candida albicans in milk samples of women with clinical symptoms of ductal candidiasis. *Breastfeed Med*. 2009;4:57–61.

34. Andrews JI, Fleener D, Messer S, et al. The yeast connection: Is Candida linked to breastfeeding associated pain? *Am J Obstet Gynecol*. 2007;197:e421–e424.

35. Francis-Morrill J, Heinig MJ, Pappagianis D, et al. Diagnostic value of signs and symptoms of mammary candidosis among lactating women. *J Hum Lact*. 2004;20:288–295.

36. Parra J, Cneude F, Huin N, et al. Mammary herpes: A little known mode of neonatal herpes contamination. *J Perinatol*. 2013;33:736–737.

37. Jaiyeoba O, Amaya MI, Soper DE, et al. Preventing neonatal transmission of herpes simplex virus. *Clin Obstet Gynecol*. 2012;55:510–520.

38. Anderson JE, Held N, Wright K. Raynaud's phenomenon of the nipple: A treatable cause of painful breastfeeding. *Pediatrics*. 2004;113:e360–e364.

39. Barrett ME, Heller MM, Stone HF, et al. Raynaud phenomenon of the nipple in breastfeeding mothers: An underdiagnosed cause of nipple pain. *JAMA Dermatol*. 2013;149:300–306.

40. de Boer MJ, Struys MM, Versteegen GJ. Pain-related catastrophizing in pain patients and people with pain in the general population. *Eur J Pain*. 2012;16:1044–1052.

41. de Boer MJ, Steinhagen HE, Versteegen GJ, et al. Mindfulness, acceptance and catastrophizing in chronic pain. *PLoS One*. 2014;9:e87445.

42. Bergbom S, Boersma K, Overmeer T, et al. Relationship among pain catastrophizing, depressed mood, and outcomes across physical therapy treatments. *Phys Ther*. 2011;91:754–764.

43. Williams AC, Eccleston C, Morley S. Psychological therapies for the management of chronic pain (excluding headache) in adults. *Cochrane Database Syst Rev*. 2012;11:CD007407.

44. Buryk M, Bloom D, Shope T. Efficacy of neonatal release of ankyloglossia: A randomized trial. *Pediatrics*. 2011;128:280–288.

45. Geddes DT, Langton DB, Gollow I, et al. Frenulotomy for breastfeeding infants with ankyloglossia: Effect on milk removal and sucking mechanism as imaged by ultrasound. *Pediatrics*. 2008;122:e188–e194.

46. Dollberg S, Botzer E, Grunis E, et al. Immediate nipple pain relief after frenotomy in breast-fed infants with ankyloglossia: A randomized, prospective study. *J Pediatr Surg*. 2006;41:1598–1600.

47. Butler DC, Heller MM, Murase JE. Safety of dermatologic medications in pregnancy and lactation: Part II. Lactation. *J Am Acad Dermatol*. 2014;70(417):e1–e10.

48. Bae YS, Van Voorhees AS, Hsu S, et al. Review of treatment options for psoriasis in pregnant or lactating women: From the Medical Board of the National Psoriasis Foundation. *J Am Acad Dermatol*. 2012;67:459–477.

49. Livingstone V, Stringer LJ. The treatment of *Staphylococcus aureus* infected sore nipples: A randomized comparative study. *J Hum Lact*. 1999;15:241–246.

50. Arroyo R, Martin V, Maldonado A, et al. Treatment of infectious mastitis during lactation: Antibiotics versus oral administration of Lactobacilli isolated from breast milk. *Clin Infect Dis.* 2010;50:1551−1558.

51. Fernández L, Arroyo R, Espinosa I, et al. Probiotics for human lactational mastitis. *Benef Microbes.* 2014;5:169−183.

52. Kayama C, Goto Y, Shimoya S, et al. Effects of gentian violet on refractory discharging ears infected with methicillin-resistant *Staphylococcus aureus. J Otolaryngol.* 2006;35:384−386.

53. Dekio S, Kawasaki Y, Jidoi J. Herpes simplex on nipples inoculated from herpetic gingivostomatitis of a baby. *Clin Exp Dermatol.* 1986;11:664−666.

54. Thompson AE, Pope JE. Calcium channel blockers for primary Raynaud's phenomenon. A meta analysis. *Rheumatology.* 2005;44:145−150.

55. Tchivileva IE, Lim PF, Smith SB, et al. Effect of catechol-O-methyltransferase polymorphism on response to propranolol therapy in chronic musculoskeletal pain: A randomized, double-blind, placebo-controlled, crossover pilot study. *Pharmacogenet Genomics.* 2010;20:239−248.

56. Kernerman E, Park E. Severe breast pain resolved with pectoral muscle massage. *J Hum Lact.* 2014;30:287−291.

57. van Veldhuizen-Staas CG. Overabundant milk supply: An alternative way to intervene by full drainage and block feeding. *Int Breastfeed J.* 2007;2:11.

58. Aljazaf K, Hale TW, Ilett KF, et al. Pseudoephedrine: Effects on milk production in women and estimation of infant exposure via breastmilk. *Br J Clin Pharmacol.* 2003;56:18−24.

59. UNC protocol. UNC School of Medicine at Chapel Hill staff. Health Care Professionals: OB Algorithms: Breastfeeding: Culture Collection Protocol. 2014. Available at: http://momba-by.org/PDF/culture_protocol.2.0.pdf (accessed November 1, 2014).

ABM protocols expire 5 years from the date of publication. Evidenced based revisions are made within 5 years or sooner if there are significant changes in the evidence.

The Academy of Breastfeeding Medicine Protocol Committee:
Wendy Brodribb, MBBS, PhD, FABM, Chairperson
Larry Noble, MD, FABM, Translations Chairperson
Nancy Brent, MD
Maya Bunik, MD, MSPH, FABM
Cadey Harrel, MD
Ruth A Lawrence, MD, FABM
Kathleen A. Marinelli, MD, FABM
Sarah Reece-Stremtan, MD
Casey Rosen-Carole, MD, MPH
Tomoko Seo, MD, FABM
Rose St. Fleur, MD
Michal Young, MD
For correspondence: abm@bfmed.org

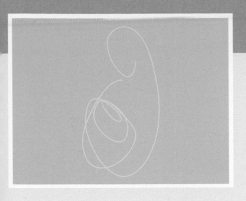

ABM Clinical Protocol #27
*Breastfeeding an Infant or Young Child with Insulin-Dependent Diabetes**

Diana Miller[1], Leena Mamilly[1], Shannon Fourtner[1],
Casey Rosen-Carole[2] and the Academy of Breastfeeding Medicine

ABSTRACT

A central goal of The Academy of Breastfeeding Medicine is the development of clinical protocols for managing common medical problems that may impact breastfeeding success. These protocols serve only as guidelines for the care of breastfeeding mothers and infants and do not delineate an exclusive course of treatment or serve as standards of medical care. Variations in treatment may be appropriate according to the needs of an individual patient.

PURPOSE

TO PROVIDE GUIDANCE for the care of breastfeeding infants or young children with insulin-dependent diabetes mellitus (called diabetes in this protocol) and their families, describing:

1. The basis of insulin dosing for carbohydrate intake for breastfeeding infants
2. The basis of assessing the amount of carbohydrate for expressed breast milk
3. Insulin dosing in infants who have the style of small volume, frequent feeds
4. Goals and methods for glycemic control in breastfeeding infants and young children with diabetes
5. Guidance on counseling parents of breastfeeding infants and young children with diabetes, addressing the guilt associated with poor glycemic control and providing support to continue breastfeeding after diagnosis

BACKGROUND

Breastfeeding provides ideal infant nutrition and is the physiologic norm for mothers and children.[1,2] Families with infants or young children with diabetes may wish to breastfeed but struggle with the challenges of glycemic control in the setting of unpredictable feeding quantities and patterns. Following the diagnosis of diabetes in their infant or young child, families often infer that they should not continue to breastfeed because of these challenges.[3]

This frequently occurs despite the evidence of maternal and child health benefits of human milk and breastfeeding.[4] The incidence of type 1 diabetes has been rising overall, with about 4% of patients being diagnosed younger than the age of 2 years in one Finnish study.[5] It is important to note that diabetes diagnosed in neonates and young infants is more likely to be of the monogenic form[a] (usually diagnosed before 9 months of age)[6] rather than the autoimmune type 1 diabetes seen in older infants and children, and management of these infants can be different.[7] For the purpose of treatment of diabetes requiring insulin, the same principles are used for both types of diabetes in infants.

PRINCIPLES OF MANAGEMENT

The goal of management of diabetes in the pediatric population is to maintain blood glucose levels within a target range with the least amount of variability to prevent complications of both hypo- and hyperglycemia. Achieving that goal in a very young child is challenging regardless of whether they are breast- or formula-fed, even for the most diligent caregivers.

---

* Courtesy of the Academy of Breastfeeding Medicine. Please go to https://www.bfmed.org/protocols for complete protocols, translations, and the most up-to-date information (protocols are updated every 5—7 years).
[1] Pediatric Endocrinology, University at Buffalo School of Medicine, Buffalo, New York.
[2] Divisions of Neonatology, Maternal Fetal Medicine and General Pediatrics, University of Rochester, School of Medicine, Rochester, New York.

[a] Monogenic diabetes is caused by a single gene variant, and includes neonatal diabetes and Maturity Onset Diabetes of the Young (MODY). Although insulin is often used for the treatment of monogenic forms of diabetes, occasionally oral sulfonylureas are used after initial diagnosis and stabilization. In addition, infants with neonatal diabetes often have multiple other organ systems impacted, including severe neurologic manifestations making breastfeeding more difficult to initiate at birth. Expressed breast milk is an excellent alternative to breastfeeding in these rare cases.

This is, in part, attributable to the continuously changing feeding needs and patterns of infants and young children.

Conventionally, caregivers are instructed to perform capillary (finger stick) glucose levels in young children before meals and snacks, occasionally after meals, at bedtime, and before exercise in older children, when they suspect low blood glucose and after treating low blood glucose until they are normoglycemic (6–10 times/day).[8]

In addition, caregivers are instructed to give insulin for all meals and snacks containing more than 10–15 g of carbohydrates or for blood glucose levels outside of a target range (typically >14 mmol/L [250 mg/dL]) via injection or insulin pump. Total daily insulin requirements are mainly determined by weight and in conjunction with the family and the diabetes team. To mimic the normative patterns of pancreatic insulin secretion, total insulin requirements for patients with type 1 diabetes are divided into two parts: basal insulin and insulin for blood glucose level corrections. Both intermediate (insulin isophane or human neutral protamine Hagedorn [NPH]) and long acting preparations (insulin detemir and insulin glargine) are used to cover the basal insulin component. Intermediate insulin preparations are characterized by having a peak of action about 4–6 hours after the injection is given. This peak can be used to cover a meal or snack within that time period while that carbohydrate consumption is necessary to prevent hypoglycemia associated with the peak. Long acting insulin preparations, on the contrary, lack that peak of action, providing more flexibility with meal times and carrying a smaller risk of hypoglycemia.[9] Despite being widely used in clinical practice for children younger than 6 years of age, insulin detemir and glargine are not approved by the U.S. Food and Drug Administration in children younger than 6 years. They are, however, approved by the European Medicines Agency for children older than 2 years of age.

About a half (insulin detemir and insulin glargine) to two thirds (NPH) of the total insulin requirements are usually covered by the basal preparations. The rest of those requirements are given in the form of a short (rapid)-acting insulin (insulin aspart, lispro, or glulisine) to be given before meals and large snacks and for corrections of elevated blood glucose values. Families are usually provided with calculations or scales that can be used to determine short-acting insulin doses based on blood glucose level (insulin sensitivity factor) and the carbohydrates consumed by the child (carbohydrate ratio). An alternative management method is by continuous subcutaneous insulin infusion (insulin pump) that uses only short-acting insulin. The pump delivers insulin both as a continuous infusion replacing basal insulin and as boluses based on the same principles discussed above. In addition, families can be taught how to dilute insulin for administration via syringe or pump to provide more precise doses of insulin.

Perhaps the most challenging part of insulin dosing in infants and young children with diabetes is the calculation of the amount of carbohydrate consumed. This is, in part, due to the normal variability in appetite and food intake at this age. In infants consuming significant breast milk volumes, it is important for the clinician and family to attempt to quantify the breast milk intake and the carbohydrate content, when possible, for optimum insulin dosing.

Carbohydrate content of breast milk

Coppa et al.[10] previously observed that the lactose content in breast milk increased from 56 ± 6 g/L on day 4 of lactation to 68.9 ± 8 g/L on day 120. Given that most infants with Type 1 diabetes are diagnosed beyond the age of 6 months, using a carbohydrate count of 70 g/L would be applicable to most infants. Those carbohydrates are predominantly in the form of lactose, although there are several other oligosaccharides that contribute insignificantly to carbohydrate counts. Therefore, 100 mL of breast milk would contain ~7 g of carbohydrate.

Carbohydrate content of breast milk compared with commercial infant formulas

The predominant carbohydrate found in cow's milk-based infant formulas is lactose. The content is roughly equivalent to that of breast milk (70 g/L). What differs substantially between infant formulas and breast milk is the fat content. Infant formulas have an average of about 10 g/L less fat than that of equivalent volumes of breast milk.[11] This may be an important consideration as fat modulates the absorption rate of glucose into the bloodstream. Therefore, though not formally studied yet, one might conjecture that infants consuming breast milk have a more steady and mild postprandial glycemic variability than infants consuming infant formula.

Quantifying consumed breast milk

In the case of the infants provided with expressed breast milk or donor human milk, the calculations of carbohydrate content can be used to determine the required insulin dose. When the infant is breastfeeding, utilizing normative data for quantities of breast milk produced in a 24-hour period and dividing by the average number of breastfeeds would work well for most mother–infant dyads (Table 1). The average volume of breast milk produced in 24 hours

TABLE 1   Summary of Methods of Estimating Carbohydrate Intake

Method of carbohydrate calculation	Formula to derive grams of carbohydrate intake
Average breast milk volume in 24 hours @ 70 g/L of carbohydrate/number of feeds (for 7–12-month-old infants)	52 g lactose/number of feeds in 24 hours = x g carbohydrate per feed (estimated)
Pre- and postfeed weight calculation	Weight in grams = mL of milk intake × 7 g/100 mL = x g of carbohydrate consumption (estimated)

TABLE 2   Average Milk Volumes/Day of Well-Nourished Women Who Exclusively Breastfed Their Infants

			MONTHS OF LACTATION											
			<1		1–2		2–3		3–4		4–5		5–6	
Country	No. days measured	Sex	n	mL/ 24 hour	n	mL/ 24 hour	n	mL/ 24 hour	n	mL/ 24 hour	n	mL/ 24 hour	n	8mL/ 24 hour
United States	2	M, F	—	—	3	691	5	655	3	750	—	—	—	—
United States	1–2	M, F	46	681	—	—	—	—	—	—	—	—	—	—
Canada	?	M, F	—	—	—	—	—	—	33	793	31	856	28	925
Sweden	?	M, F	15	558	11	724	12	752	—	—	—	—	—	—
United States	3	M, F	—	—	11	600	—	—	2	833	—	—	3	682
United States	3	M, F	—	—	26	606	26	601	20	626	—	—	—	—
United Kingdom	4	M, F	—	—	—	—	23	820	18	829	5	790	1	922
		F	—	—	20	677	17	742	14	775	6	814	4	838
United States	1	M, F	16	673 ± 192	19	756 ± 170	16	782 ± 172	13	810 ± 142	11	805 ± 117	11	896 ± 122
Months of lactation			7		8		9		10		11		12	
United States	1	M, F	875 ± 142		834 ± 99		774 ± 180		691 ± 233		516 ± 215		759 ± 28	

Modified from Ferris and Jensen.[30] Reproduced with permission from Breastfeeding: A Guide to the Medical Profession, 7th ed.

across ages 7–12 months is about 740 mL (Table 2). This is on an average 52 g of lactose in 24 hours. Therefore, a 7-month-old infant who is breastfeeding six times a day would consume ~8.5 g of carbohydrate per breastfeed.[12] Alternatively, a 12-month-old infant breastfeeding three times a day may consume 8.5–17 g per breastfeed if it continues to consume ~740 mL per day. A more recently performed study of infants of younger ages (1–6 months) demonstrates similar breast milk production in a 24-hour period as noted in the prior study; infants fed on an average of 11 ± 3 times in 24 hours (range of 6–18) consuming 76 ± 12.6 mL each feed with a range of 0–240 mL.[13] It was noted that there tended to be higher volumes in the morning feedings compared with the evening feedings, and there was often a discrepancy in production between the left and right breasts.[13] Parents should be encouraged to notice if there are particular patterns to the carbohydrate estimates resulting in hyper- or hypoglycemia after breastfeeding and adjust their estimates accordingly as the aforementioned factors may be the cause rather than physiologic variation in insulin sensitivity.

These rough calculations may not be applicable for infants who have small volume frequent feeds rather than consuming more discrete "meals" at regular intervals. In this case, it is important to keep in mind that most blood glucose measurements will reflect the postprandial state[14] and that infants tend to consume small, hard-to-measure amounts of nutrients that would require very small doses of insulin, which cannot be given with the delivery systems (syringes, pens) presently available. In this situation it may be more practical to measure the infant's capillary glucose level every 3 hours and give insulin for correction of blood glucose levels without measuring the infant's carbohydrate intake. However, the goal should be to use the conventional insulin dosing methods as soon as the child starts to consume food at regular intervals (meals).

Pre- and postfeed weights

Weighing the infant before and immediately after a breastfeed may provide a more precise calculation of breast milk volume and thus carbohydrate intake for determining insulin doses (Table 1). An accurate digital scale should be used. The difference in weight in grams between the two measurements equals the amount of milk ingested in milliliters. A simple calculation can then be performed given that there are ~7 g of carbohydrate in 100 mL of human milk. Families do not always have access to a digital scale, nor is it recommended as a daily method as it is burdensome for parents. However, obtaining pre- and postfeed measurements at well-child checks every 2–3 months, or performing this procedure over a 24-hour period every few months would allow for an approximation of the proper dose of insulin for a full feed. This is also a strategy that could be more easily used while the infant is being stabilized in hospital following the initial diagnosis to help establish the quantities consumed and fine-tune the insulin dose. Every effort should be made by the medical team to give the parents a message of support and acceptance that breastfeeding is the optimal form of nutrition for the infant.

Insulin pumps

The use of continuous subcutaneous insulin infusion (insulin pump) provides optimum insulin dosing in infants and young children with diabetes. Because of the factors mentioned above, the amount of insulin that infants need is sometimes very small. Insulin syringes with half unit markings are often used to deliver a dose as little as a half a unit. However, that may not be small enough in some cases. Insulin pumps, on the contrary, have the capability of delivering tenths to hundredths of a unit of insulin. The use of insulin pumps has been shown to improve the quality of life for families and infants, young children, and preschool children compared with multiple daily injections.[15] A systematic meta-analysis of six randomized control trials found better effectiveness of insulin pumps compared with multiple daily injection in improving metabolic control in children with type 1 diabetes mellitus.[16]

Solid foods

Older infants and young children are routinely offered solid foods that often comprise the majority of their carbohydrate consumption. At that time, quantifying carbohydrates in infrequent breastfeeding sessions may not be as important for improving glycemic control. Parents can estimate the carbohydrates in solid foods with or without breast milk with rounding the insulin dose to the nearest half unit.

THE IMPACT OF HYPO- AND HYPERGLYCEMIA

The goal of management in infants and very young children with diabetes is to avoid frequent hypoglycemia associated with neurocognitive sequelae while also aiming to reduce sustained hyperglycemia.

Hypoglycemia

Early childhood is a critical time for growth and brain development. Studies have shown that exposure to hypoglycemia is associated with a decline in neurodevelopmental outcomes in children.[17,18] Very young children with diabetes are particularly at risk of severe hypoglycemia due to their small insulin requirements, marked sensitivity to exogenous insulin, variability in oral intake and inability to express symptoms of hypoglycemia. These factors create anxiety in both healthcare providers and the parents/caretakers who often tend to aim for higher glucose levels to avoid the detrimental effects of

hypoglycemia. In addition, the practice of postmeal dosing of insulin in the face of unpredictable amount of food ingested at meals, and the style of small volume frequent feeds results in higher blood glucose levels after meals.

Hyperglycemia

Regional changes noted in brain growth of very young children with diabetes suggest that hyperglycemia and perhaps glycemic variability also play a role in brain development.[19] Furthermore, while there is evidence to suggest that the progression toward microvascular complications begins with the onset of puberty, glycemic control in the first few years following the diagnosis of diabetes sets the risk pattern, a form of metabolic memory, and trajectory for an individual toward developing microvascular and macrovascular complications.[20] It has also been found that good glycemic control, even during the first few years following the diagnosis of diabetes, is associated with delay in microvascular complications, particularly diabetic retinopathy.[21,22]

Achieving the balance between good glycemic control and minimal hypoglycemic episodes would provide the best outcomes with regard to brain growth and neurocognitive function. This requires vigilance, collaboration, and support among the family, other caretakers, and the medical team.

FAMILY DYNAMICS AND THE IMPORTANCE OF BREASTFEEDING

As in the general population, breastfeeding is superior to other forms of nutrition in infants and young children with diabetes. Families of those children should be provided with support and understanding from their medical team, which will foster lifelong collaboration toward the health of the child.

The stress of diagnosis and healthcare provider attitudes

Following the diagnosis of diabetes in their infant or young child, many parents feel tremendous guilt over abnormal blood glucose levels and find the intensive management of diabetes stressful. Mothers of infants and very young children who are breastfeeding at the time of diagnosis may perceive that healthcare providers are frustrated by the difficulty of quantifying carbohydrate intake from breastfeeds.[3] This adds to the psychological burden of the parents and also implies that breastfeeding is detrimental to the health of their child, which has no scientific basis. Although there is a lack of literature supporting improved outcomes for infants or young children with diabetes who were breastfed, there is good evidence that breastfeeding improves cognitive function, irrespective of socioeconomic status, and increases brain white matter development.[23,24]

Other benefits of breastfeeding

Breastfeeding represents the normative standard in infant feeding and nutrition,[4] and should be there commended method of infant feeding in the case of diabetic infants as well. The benefits of breastfeeding in decreasing the risk of infections and hospitalizations,[25] decreasing the future risk of obesity,[26] and other chronic health outcomes in addition to improving bonding between mother and child may be especially beneficial in improving the health outcomes for children with diabetes. Infants who directly breastfeed instead of being bottle-fed expressed breast milk exhibit an increased ability to self-regulate their milk intake during late infancy.[27] The duration of breastfeeding demonstrates a potential link to satiety responsiveness in older children.[28] The ability to make healthy food choices later in life is likely to aid in achieving better glycemic control in adolescents and adults with diabetes.

SUMMARY OF THE RECOMMENDATIONS

1. Breastfeeding is the optimal form of infant nutrition for infants and it should be promoted as such by healthcare providers for infants with diabetes.
2. When calculation of carbohydrate intake is utilized for insulin dosing, a carbohydrate count of 70 g/L can be used for breast milk. (IA) (Quality of evidence [levels of evidence IA, IB, IIA, IIB, III, and IV] is based on levels of evidence used for the National Guidelines Clearing House[29] and is noted in parentheses.)
3. The norms for 24-hour total volumes of breast milk can be used in determining the amount of breast milk consumed by the infant at a single feed. (IIB, IV)
4. For infants who have a small volume frequent style of food consumption, blood glucose levels should be measured every 3 hours and insulin doses given for correction of levels above the glycemic target. (IV)
5. When feasible, infant weights before and after a breastfeed can be used to determine the amount of milk usually consumed by the infant at each feed. (IV)
6. The use of continuous subcutaneous insulin infusion (insulin pumps) should be considered for infants and young children with diabetes as desired by their caregivers. (III)
7. Support should be provided to the families of infants and young children diagnosed with diabetes along with tailoring the diabetes management plan to the patterns of breastfeeding and the needs of the mother–infant dyad. (III/IV)

RECOMMENDATIONS FOR FUTURE RESEARCH

The lack of information on the feeding trends and breastfeeding rates of infants and young children with type 1 diabetes is concerning. We, therefore, propose the following to begin to improve our understanding of breastfeeding infants or young children with diabetes:

1. There is a need for a prospective longitudinal data base to track breastfeeding rates and monitor for outcomes of infants with diabetes. Existing databases such as T1D Exchange Registry or other comprehensive diabetes registries could be used to track this information and carry out studies. This would allow for the systematic evaluation of the preventative role of breastfeeding an infant with diabetes, as well as guide the management of diabetes in these infants. To our knowledge, there is currently no information being collected in the T1D Exchange or other diabetes registries with respect to breastfeeding.
2. Studies evaluating the feasibility and benefit of current technologies (insulin pumps and continuous glucose monitoring systems [CGMs]) in infants and young children with diabetes are needed. In the United States and European Union, CGMs are only approved for use in children older than 2 years of age. The use of these systems could potentially bring insulin management closer to the goal of achieving the balance between the avoidance of hypoglycemia and achieving optimal glycemic control. In addition, it would allow the study of the glycemic profile differences of breast milk compared with infant formula in infants with diabetes.

REFERENCES

1. American Academy of Pediatrics Section on Breastfeeding. Breastfeeding and the use of human milk. *Pediatrics*. 2012;129:827–841.
2. World Health Organization. *Global Strategy for Infant and Young Child Feeding*. Geneva: WHO; 2003.
3. Hayden-Baldauf E. Breastfeeding the type 1 diabetic child. *Kelly Mom*. 2014. Available at: http://kellymom.com/health/baby-health/breastfeeding-type-1-diabetes-child (accessed September 13, 2016).
4. Victora CG, Bahl R, Barros AJD, et al. Breastfeeding in the 21st century: Epidemiology, mechanisms, and lifelong effect. *Lancet*. 2016;387:475–490.
5. Komulainen J, Kulmala P, Savola K, et al. Clinical, autoimmune, and genetic characteristics of very young children with type 1 diabetes. Childhood Diabetes in Finland (DiMe) Study Group. *Diabetes Care*. 1999;22:1950–1955.
6. Støy J, Greeley SAW, Paz VP, et al. Diagnosis and treatment of neonatal diabetes: A United States experience. *Pediatr Diabetes*. 2008;9:450–459.
7. Iafusco D, Stazi MA, Cotichini R, et al. Permanent diabetes mellitus in the first year of life. *Diabetologia*. 2002;45:798–804.
8. American Diabetes Association. Standards of medical care in diabetes-2016. *Diabetes Care*. 2016;39(Suppl 1):S86–S94.
9. Mullins P, Sharplin P, Yki-Jarvinen H, et al. Negative binomial meta-regression analysis of combined glycosylated hemoglobin and hypoglycemia outcomes across eleven Phase III and IV studies of insulin glargine compared with neutral protamine Hagedorn insulin in type 1 and type 2 diabetes mellitus. *Clin Ther*. 2007;29:1607–1619.
10. Coppa GV, Gabrielli O, Pierani P, et al. Changes in carbohydrate composition in human milk over 4 months of lactation. *Pediatrics*. 1993;91:637–641.
11. Institute of Medicine Committee on the Evaluation of the Addition of Ingredients New to Infant Formula. *Composition*

of infant formulas and human milk for feeding term infants in the United States. Infant Formula: Evaluating the Safety of New Ingredients. Washington, DC: National Academies Press; 2004.

12. Lawrence RA, Lawrence RM. *Breastfeeding: A Guide for the Medical Profession.* 8th ed. Philadelphia: Elsevier; 2015.

13. Kent JC, Mitoulas LR, Cregan MD, et al. Volume and frequency of breastfeedings and fat content of breast milk throughout the day. *Pediatrics.* 2006;117:e387—e395.

14. Cody D. Infant and toddler diabetes. *Arch Dis Child.* 2007;92:716—719.

15. Weinzimer SA, Swan KL, Sikes KA, et al. Emerging evidence for the use of insulin pump therapy in infants, toddlers, and preschool-aged children with type 1 diabetes. *Pediatr Diabetes.* 2006;7(Suppl 4):15—19.

16. Pankowska E, Blazik M, Dziechciarz P, et al. Continuous subcutaneous insulin infusion vs multiple daily injections in children with type 1 diabetes: A systematic review and meta-analysis of randomized control trials. *Pediatr Diabetes.* 2009;10:52—58.

17. Hannonen R, Tupola S, Ahonen T, et al. Neurocognitive functioning in children with type-1 diabetes with and without episodes of severe hypoglycaemia. *Dev Med Child Neurol.* 2003;45:262—268.

18. Hershey T, Perantie D, Warren S, et al. Frequency and timing of severe hypoglycemia affects spatial memory in children with type 1 diabetes. *Diabetes Care.* 2005;28:2372—2377.

19. Mazaika PK, Weinzimer SA, Mauras N, et al. Variations in brain volume and growth in young children with type 1 diabetes. *Diabetes.* 2016;65:476—485.

20. Svensson M, Eriksson JW, Dahlquist G. Early glycemic control, age at onset, and development of microvascular complications in childhood-onset type 1 diabetes: A population-based study in northern Sweden. *Diabetes Care.* 2004;27:955—962.

21. Salardi S, Porta M, Maltoni G, et al. Infant and toddler type 1 diabetes: Complications after 20 years' duration. *Diabetes Care.* 2012;35:829—833.

22. Holl RW, Lang GE, Grabert M, et al. Diabetic retinopathy in pediatric patients with type-1 diabetes: Effect of diabetes duration, prepubertal and pubertal onset of diabetes, and metabolic control. *J Pediatr.* 1998;132:790—794.

23. Deoni SCL, Dean 3rd DC, Piryatinsky I, et al. Breastfeeding and early white matter development: A cross-sectional study. *Neuroimage.* 2013;82:77—86.

24. Horta BL, Loret de Mola C, Victora CG. Breastfeeding and intelligence: A systematic review and meta-analysis. *Acta Paediatr.* 2015;104:14—19.

25. Bowatte G, Tham R, Allen KJ, et al. Breastfeeding and childhood acute otitis media: A systematic review and meta-analysis. *Acta Paediatr.* 2015;104:85—95.

26. Horta BL, Loret de Mola C, Victora CG. Long-term consequences of breastfeeding on cholesterol, obesity, systolic blood pressure and type 2 diabetes: A systematic review and meta-analysis. *Acta Paediatr.* 2015;104:30—37.

27. Li R, Fein SB, Grummer-Strawn LM. Do infants fed from bottles lack self-regulation of milk intake compared with directly breastfed infants? *Pediatrics.* 2010;125:e1386—e1393.

28. Brown A, Lee M. Breastfeeding during the first year promotes satiety responsiveness in children aged 18—24 months. *Pediatr Obes.* 2012;7:382—390.

29. Shekelle PG, Woolf SH, Eccles M, Grimshaw J. Developing guidelines. *BMJ.* 1999;318:593—596.

30. Ferris AM, Jensen RG. Lipids in human milk: A review. *J Pediatr Gastroenterol Nutr.* 1984;3:108.

ABM protocols expire 5 years from the date of publication. Content of this protocol is up-to-date at the time of publication. Evidence-based revisions are made within five years or sooner if there are significant changes in the evidence.

The Academy of Breastfeeding Medicine Protocol Committee:
Wendy Brodribb, MBBS, PhD, FABM, Chairperson
Larry Noble, MD, FABM, Translations Chairperson
Nancy Brent, MD
Maya Bunik, MD, MSPH, FABM
Cadey Harrel, MD
Ruth A. Lawrence, MD, FABM
Kathleen A. Marinelli, MD, FABM
Sarah Reece-Stremtan, MD
Casey Rosen-Carole, MD, MPH, MSEd
Tomoko Seo, MD, FABM
Rose St. Fleur, MD
Michal Young, MD
For correspondence: abm@bfmed.org

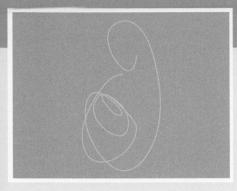

ABM Clinical Protocol #28
*Peripartum Analgesia and Anesthesia for the Breastfeeding Mother**

*Erin Martin[1], Barbara Vickers[2], Ruth Landau[3], Sarah Reece-Stremtan[4]
and The Academy of Breastfeeding Medicine**

ABSTRACT

A central goal of the Academy of Breastfeeding Medicine is the development of clinical protocols, free from commercial interest or influence, for managing common medical problems that may impact breastfeeding success. These protocols serve only as guidelines for the care of breastfeeding mothers and infants and do not delineate an exclusive course of treatment or serve as standards of medical care. Variations in treatment may be appropriate according to the needs of an individual patient.

BACKGROUND

THE WORLD HEALTH ORGANIZATION recommends exclusive breastfeeding for 6 months followed by a continuation of breastfeeding with the introduction of complementary foods for 2 years or longer as mutually desired by mother and infant.[1] This recommendation is supported by a growing body of evidence for both the short- and long-term health benefits to infants and mothers.[2] Despite its large public health impact, the study of breastfeeding initiation and continuation beginning in the peripartum phase is methodologically complex, lacking in scientific rigor, and sparse. There are several external factors such as maternal intention to breastfeed, community traditions and support, level of education, maternal age, race, and social class that influence breastfeeding outcomes.[3,4] Many intrapartum interventions also have the potential to impact breastfeeding outcomes.[5] Oxytocin, endorphins, and adrenaline produced in response to the physiological pain of labor may play significant roles in maternal and neonatal responses to birth and early breastfeeding.[6] The use of pharmacologic and nonpharmacologic agents for pain relief in labor and postpartum may improve outcomes by relieving suffering during labor; however, some of these methods may affect the course of labor and the neurobehavioral state of the neonate.

Few studies directly address the impact of various approaches to peripartum anesthesia and analgesia on breastfeeding outcomes. While a Cochrane review evaluated 38 studies published before 2011 on epidural analgesia compared with other pain management options, it is notable that only one assessed breastfeeding outcomes.[7]

This protocol will examine the evidence currently available, make recommendations for prudent practice regarding peripartum analgesia and anesthesia for the breastfeeding mother and offer suggestions for future research. Quality of evidence (levels of evidence: IA, IB, IIA, IIB, III, and IV) is based on levels of evidence used for the National Guidelines Clearinghouse and is noted in parentheses.[8] The first part of the protocol will discuss the use of analgesia during labor and anesthesia for operative deliveries, and the second half will discuss specific medications used for postpartum pain relief. Note that some medications will be mentioned in both situations as infant effects may be different with medication through placental transfer versus colostrum and milk intake.

RECOMMENDATIONS

Analgesia for labor pain

Women experience labor pain in different ways and have differing levels of pain tolerance. Labor pain may exceed a woman's ability to cope or be magnified by fear and anxiety. Suffering in labor may lead to dysfunctional labors, poorer psychological outcomes, delayed secretory activation, and increased risk of postpartum depression, all of which may have negative effects on breastfeeding.[9–11] In addition, severe maternal physiologic stress in labor also causes in utero fetal stress as well as increased physiologic stress for infants, which may affect their readiness to breastfeed at birth[3] (III).

* Courtesy of the Academy of Breastfeeding Medicine. Please go to https://www.bfmed.org/protocols for complete protocols, translations, and the most up-to-date information (protocols are updated every 5–7 years).

[1] Department of Anesthesiology, University of California, San Diego, California.

[2] Department of Anesthesiology and Critical Care Medicine, Johns Hopkins University, Baltimore, Maryland.

[3] Department of Anesthesiology, Columbia University, New York City, New York.

[4] Division of Anesthesiology, Pain, and Perioperative Medicine, Children's National Health System, Washington, District of Columbia.

Maternity care providers should discuss labor pain management options during the prenatal period, before the onset of labor. This discussion should include what is known about the association of various modalities on the progress of labor, risk of instrumented and cesarean delivery, effects on the newborn, and possible breastfeeding effects (IV).

Regardless of the modality used for labor analgesia, comprehensive patient and provider education, early and uninterrupted initiation of maternal—infant skin-to-skin contact, continuing lactation support in the postpartum phase, and identifying and actively addressing barriers to breastfeeding improve outcomes[12–14] (IIA-IV).

Neuraxial labor analgesia

- Neuraxial analgesia continues to be the most commonly used modality in many countries and the most effective pain management option available to parturients.[5,7] There are no studies comparing breastfeeding outcomes according to neuraxial technique (i.e., epidural, combined spinal-epidural, spinal, and continuous spinal), therefore these will all be discussed together under the method of neuraxial analgesia.

- The effect of neuraxial analgesia on breastfeeding outcomes continues to be inconclusive due to inconsistent reporting, differences in study design and end points, and mixed results. A 2016 systematic review found 23 studies examining the association between neuraxial analgesia and breastfeeding outcomes. These were mostly observational studies. Twelve found negative associations, 10 found no effect, and 1 found positive association between neuraxial analgesia and breastfeeding success[5] (IIA-III). In addition, Lee et al. in 2017 reported no association between the cumulative fentanyl dose and rate of breastfeeding at 3 months postpartum[15] (IB).

- Opioids are commonly used in combination with local anesthetics in neuraxial solutions for labor analgesia. There are three prospective randomized studies evaluating the effect of epidural fentanyl dose on breastfeeding success, and the results differ. Beilin et al. reported that in mothers who had previously breastfed a child, those randomized to receive a high dose of epidural fentanyl (cumulative dose greater than or equal to 150 mcg) were more likely to stop breastfeeding 6 weeks postpartum when compared with mothers receiving no fentanyl or low dose of fentanyl (cumulative dose less than 150 mcg)[16] (IB). Wilson et al. reported that neuraxial analgesia, with or without epidural fentanyl, did not impact breastfeeding up to 12 months postpartum[17] (IIA). The third study was that by Lee et al., a randomized controlled trial (RCT) with objective measures of maternal and umbilical cord venous fentanyl and bupivacaine concentrations in multiparous mothers with previous breastfeeding experience. Of note, only 19% of participants in this trial received greater than or equal to 150 mcg cumulative dose of epidural fentanyl, which has been the suggested cutoff for breastfeeding effects[15] (IB).

- The association between neuraxial analgesia and neonatal neurobehavioral organization is also controversial and inconclusive in its long-term effects on breastfeeding outcomes. There may be depressed hand massage and suckling behavior in neonates exposed to neuraxial analgesia, but some of the neonates studied were also exposed to oxytocin and/or meperidine/pethidine during the course of labor, which were not accounted for in statistical analysis. There were no long-term differences in breastfeeding outcomes or these outcomes were not reported[18–20] (III).

- Like many other aspects of breastfeeding, neuraxial labor analgesia likely has minimal effects on women who strongly intend to breastfeed and have good support but may present one more subtle challenge to women whose intention to breastfeed is more vulnerable.

  - When neuraxial labor analgesia has been used, particular care should be taken to provide mothers with good breastfeeding support and close postpartum follow-up. Zuppa et al., in a retrospective cohort study, reported that in the case of partial rooming-in, the rate of exclusive or predominant breastfeeding was higher in mothers who did not receive epidural analgesia, although this may be a casual association rather than a causal one; in the case of full rooming-in, there was no difference in breastfeeding rates between mothers who did or did not receive neuraxial labor analgesia[21] (III).

  - While there is currently no recommendation to encourage intrapartum fluid administration before neuraxial analgesia placement,[22] intravenous fluids are still often provided as a bolus to mothers receiving epidural analgesia as a way to increase the intravascular volume and offset sympathetic blockade. Excessive fluid can potentially lead to maternal engorgement and affect birth weight and newborn weight loss[23,24] (IIA).

Systemic pain medications in labor

- All opioids easily cross the placenta. In utero, this may affect fetal heart rate variability. Once delivered, opioids are associated with varying degrees of neonatal respiratory depression and neurobehavioral changes that may impact latching. Long-term effects are unclear.[25] When a mother has received intravenous or intramuscular narcotics for labor, mother and infant should be given more skin-to-skin time to encourage early breastfeeding, with appropriate supervision if any concerns exist over maternal or infant sedation (IV).

- Short-acting opioids such as fentanyl or remifentanil may be preferred when compared with longer-acting opioids with active metabolites. Remifentanil is potent and has rapid onset and offset, but can be associated with a high incidence of maternal apnea, requiring increased monitoring[26] (IIB-III). Remifentanil has also been shown to result in a number of cases of neonatal depression in a recent survey in academic centers across the United States.[27] Evidence on breastfeeding outcomes is lacking.

- Longer-acting opioids with active metabolites such as meperidine/pethidine or morphine should be used with caution and administered less than 1 hour or more than 4 hours before anticipated delivery because of greater incidence and duration of respiratory depression, cyanosis, and bradycardia in neonates. When compared with intranasal or subcutaneous fentanyl, mothers receiving intramuscular meperidine/pethidine reported greater difficulties in establishing breastfeeding at 6 weeks postpartum[28,29] (IIB).
- Partial opioid agonists such as nalbuphine, butorphanol, and pentazocine are used during labor at some institutions, particularly for patients with certain opioid allergies or for other indications. Data on breastfeeding outcomes for exposed dyads are lacking.

Nitrous oxide for labor analgesia

- There are minimal data concerning the effects on the neonate of inhaled nitrous oxide. In some institutions, where nitrous oxide is available, it may serve as an alternative to parenteral opioids or neuraxial analgesia for labor. One recent study reported a positive relationship between its use and breastfeeding rates at 7 days and 1 and 3 months postpartum, and a review article reported no apparent adverse effect on suckling[30,31] (III-IV).

Other nonopioid systemic medications for labor analgesia

- Nonopioid medications such as nonsteroidal anti-inflammatory drugs (NSAIDs), acetaminophen/paracetamol, antispasmodics, sedatives, and antihistamines have insufficient evidence to support their role in managing labor pain. There is little to no evidence on breastfeeding outcomes.[32-34] Further study is needed (III-IV).

Nonpharmacologic pain relief

- In a 2016 Cochrane review, when compared with other care models, midwife-led continuity models led to decreased use of regional analgesia and instrumental vaginal birth and led to increased length of labor and rate of spontaneous vaginal birth. There were no differences in cesarean births, induction of labor, augmentation/oxytocin in labor, opioid analgesia, postpartum hemorrhage, 5-minute Apgar score less than or equal to seven, and admission of infant to special care or the neonatal intensive care unit. There were no differences in breastfeeding initiation and no data on long-term breastfeeding outcomes[35] (IIA-III).
- Continuous support in labor, ideally by a doula, reduces the need for pharmacologic pain management in labor and decreases the rates of instrumented delivery and

cesarean section. The most recent review did not find statistical differences in breastfeeding outcomes, which were neither comprehensive nor consistent in their reporting[36] (IIA-III). In socially disadvantaged mothers, those who worked with a certified doula in the antenatal period was more likely to initiate breastfeeding compared with matched controls. No longevity data on breastfeeding were reported[37,38] (III).

- Nonpharmacologic methods for pain management in labor such as hypnosis, massage, psychoprophylaxis, intradermal/subcutaneous water injections, and acupuncture have varying results in reducing labor pain.[39-41] These methods appear to be safe and have no known adverse neonatal effects. In reviews of hypnosis for pain management in labor, there were no significant differences in breastfeeding at hospital discharge in hypnosis groups compared with control groups[39,42] (III). Additional study of breastfeeding outcomes in various nonpharmacologic methods is needed.

Anesthesia for cesarean delivery

- The decision to use a particular anesthetic technique for cesarean delivery (i.e., neuraxial versus general anesthesia) should be individualized based on anesthetic, obstetric, maternal, and fetal risk factors. There is a preference for neuraxial anesthesia over general anesthesia for most cesarean deliveries, but general anesthesia may be most appropriate in certain circumstances such as profound fetal bradycardia, ruptured uterus, severe maternal hemorrhage, and severe placental abruption[22] (IB-IV). These recommendations do not address implications for breastfeeding initiation or outcomes in these emergent situations. Note that neuraxial anesthesia allows for administration of neuraxial preservative-free morphine, which will reduce postoperative systemic opioid consumption.
- Separation of a mother and her infant should be minimized and skin-to-skin contact should be initiated in the operating room as soon as feasible. The infant may go to the breast in the operating room during abdominal closure with supervision and support after maternal and infant stability is established[43,44] (III).
- General anesthesia may be associated with delayed secretory activation and greater reported difficulties with breastfeeding,[45,46] although confounding medical factors related to the underlying need for general anesthesia may impact breastfeeding too (III). A mother who has had general anesthesia may breastfeed postoperatively as soon as she is alert enough to hold the infant and is not sedated[47,48] (III-IV). Please refer to ABM clinical protocol #15: Analgesia and Anesthesia for the Breastfeeding Mother, Revised 2017, and the U.S. National Library of Medicine website LactMed for greater details on specific medications for breastfeeding mothers.[48,49] Small doses of intravenous ketamine, opioids, and midazolam used to supplement regional

anesthesia during cesarean delivery should not preclude breastfeeding once the mother is stable and alert (IV).

- Multimodal analgesic modalities with opioid-sparing effects, such as a transverse abdominis plane block, particularly if the cesarean delivery required general anesthesia, or the use of wound infiltration with a local anesthetic, may decrease systemic opioid consumption, provide better comfort during breastfeeding, and decrease time to first breastfeed[50,51] (IIA).

Postpartum pain management

In addition to evaluating the effects of analgesia used during labor—or in the subset of women who may have had an intrapartum cesarean delivery after neuraxial labor analgesia was provided—on the establishment and continuation of breastfeeding, the safety of analgesic medications used during breastfeeding immediately postpartum needs to be considered.

Most medications transfer easily into colostrum because the intracellular junctions between lactocytes only start to close during the first 48–72 hours after delivery. However, because colostrum volume and initial milk intake are low, total medication dose ingested by neonates is typically minimal until milk volume increases.[52] Intracellular junctions do not fully close until ~7–10 days postpartum,[53] however, indicating that infant exposure to maternal medications may actually be highest during days 3–10 of life.

Opioids are the most concerning class of medication that may be used in the postpartum period, and medication dosing and requirements may vary considerably between patients. Concerns over breastfeeding safety need to be weighed with opioid effects because when maternal pain is adequately treated, breastfeeding outcomes improve[54–56] (III-IV).

Current recommendations insist on multimodal analgesia being offered in a tiered manner after delivery. Nonopioid analgesics should be the first choice for pain management in breastfeeding postpartum women as they do not impact maternal or infant alertness or respiratory drive.

- Acetaminophen/paracetamol is widely used for analgesia. It may be given orally, rectally, and through the intravenous route; transfer into milk is low and appears to be less than the dosage given to infants[57] (III).
- NSAIDs are commonly used for postpartum analgesia. While transfer of these medications into breast milk is low, this class of medications should be avoided in mothers of infants with ductal-dependent cardiac lesions[57] (IV).
  - Aspirin in a dose of 81 mg daily results in undetectable levels in human milk, with subclinical levels of its metabolite.[58] Its use as chronic antiplatelet therapy is considered safe (III), but variable transfer into milk with higher analgesic dosing may reflect nonlinear metabolism; other medications are preferred when chronic higher dosing is required[49] (IV).
  - Ibuprofen has a very short half-life with little to no milk transfer[59] (III).

- Ketorolac is commonly used for postpartum analgesia, especially after cesarean delivery or when stronger analgesia is required (IV). Milk levels after oral administration are quite low, but levels have not been measured after parenteral administration.[60]
- Diclofenac is administered as a suppository, orally, intramuscularly, and intravenously. There are limited studies on breast milk levels and effects on the infant. Available studies show undetectable levels following intramuscular or oral administration[49] (III).
- Naproxen transfer into milk is low, but gastrointestinal disturbances have been reported in some infants after prolonged maternal therapy. Short-term use (1 week) is likely safe[61] (III).
- Indomethacin demonstrates low transfer into milk and is considered a safe option for pain in the postpartum period[49] (III).

Postvaginal delivery analgesia

Nonopioid analgesics should be the first choice for pain management in breastfeeding postpartum women as they do not impact maternal or infant alertness or respiratory drive. These medications alone are sufficient analgesia for most women after uncomplicated vaginal delivery and they can be safely dosed on an as-needed basis or as scheduled around-the-clock medications for more significant pain.

After uncomplicated vaginal delivery in women who delivered with labor epidural analgesia, postpartum administration of a single epidural dose of preservative-free morphine has been shown to reduce the use of oral pain medication[62] (IB), which may be very useful after severe perineal tear.

Postcesarean delivery analgesia

Most women will have received neuraxial anesthesia for their cesarean delivery, which allows for administration of single or repeated dosing of neuraxial opioids and/or the maintenance of epidural infusion of local anesthesia solution. This forms the basis of multimodal analgesia as it should provide some pain relief for 18–24 hours and will reduce systemic opioid consumption.

Neuraxial (epidural/spinal) medications

- Continuous postcesarean epidural infusion may be an effective form of pain relief that minimizes systemic maternal use and hence opioid exposure. A randomized study that compared combined spinal-epidural anesthesia for elective cesarean with or without the use of postoperative epidural continuous bupivacaine found that the continuous group had lower pain scores and a higher volume of milk fed to their infants.[54] This option may limit postpartum mobility and increase healthcare costs, but its use may be considered in mothers with chronic pain or for whom systemic opioids should be limited (IV).
- Local anesthetics are large polarized molecules that do not cross easily into milk. They also have a low oral bioavailability. The transfer of epidural local anesthetics

and their metabolites to breast milk is low and they can be safely administered during breastfeeding.[47,48,63]

- Single-dose, long-acting opioid medications (e.g., neuraxial morphine or hydromorphone) have minimal effects on breastfed infants because of negligible maternal plasma levels achieved. Extremely low doses are effective and may be repeated if epidural catheters are kept in place postpartum. These opioids typically last ∼24 hours, and this approach has become standard of care at many hospitals.[64,65]

In addition to neuraxial analgesia and the use of acetaminophen and NSAIDs, a short course of systemic opioids may be required for pain relief. As with opioids needed for any acute problem, their use should be limited to the lowest effective dose for the shortest possible duration. When opioids are needed, a multimodal approach is suggested and the use of other analgesic medications such as acetaminophen,[64,65] paracetamol, and NSAIDs should be maximized (IV).

All opioids are present in human milk. Information on risks of various opioid medications is largely derived from case reports, skewing comparisons between more commonly and less commonly prescribed opioids. Regardless of the opioid prescribed, it is recommended that patients be counseled about the risk of sedation for both the mother and the breastfed infant. If the mother is experiencing central nervous system (CNS) depression symptoms, the infant should be evaluated for CNS depression as well. At least one article recommends limiting opioid medications to 4 days for breastfeeding mothers to minimize risk to the breastfeeding infant[66] (IV).

- Parenteral (IV/IM) opioids may be required for women with severe pain or who are not tolerating oral intake. Patient-controlled analgesia using a pump may be used for dosing convenience in some institutions, although there are no clear advantages or risks identified for breastfeeding mothers with this modality.
  - Meperidine/pethidine should be avoided where possible due to reported neonatal sedation when given to breastfeeding mothers postpartum[67] (IV). Meperidine and its metabolite normeperidine have variable half-lives, which make estimating breast milk levels difficult, and the American Academy of Pediatrics (AAP) recommends against use of this medication in breastfeeding mothers[57] (IV).
  - Morphine remains a reasonable option for use when intravenous medications are required. Administration of moderate to low doses of intravenous or intramuscular morphine is preferred to meperidine/pethidine as passage to milk and oral bioavailability are low.[57,67] Its oral dose is approximately three times greater than the intravenous dose, indicating low oral availability.
  - Fentanyl transfer into breast milk is quite low and it has very limited oral availability. One study showed peak colostrum levels of 0.4 mcg/L after a maternal 2 mcg/kg intravenous dose.[68] This is a negligible infant

dose for oral intake. These attributes make it an ideal opioid for use in breastfeeding mothers, but it is often restricted in the hospital to the critical care unit, operating room, and emergency room settings because of its rapid onset and short duration of action.

- There are no data available regarding intravenous hydromorphone use, although one report of its use through intranasal administration noted a relative infant dose (RID) of 0.67% after a single maternal dose of 2 mg.[69] Oral availability of this medication is low, with the equianalgesic oral dose approximately five times greater than the intravenous dose.
- Levels of nalbuphine in human milk are quite low and its metabolites are inactive. In one study, the levels of nalbuphine in milk average only 42 lg/L with an estimated RID of 0.59%[70] (III).
- Levels of butorphanol in human milk following an intramuscular dose were reported as very low, with an RID of 0.08% to 0.11%[71] (III). It has inactive metabolites and poor oral bioavailability, and there are limited data on prolonged or higher dosages. The AAP has identified this as a reasonable choice when mothers require opioids.[57]

- Oral opioids are generally preferred over intravenous formulations when mothers are tolerating oral intake.
  - Codeine is no longer recommended for use in breastfeeding mothers.[72] As a prodrug, its analgesic effect is dependent upon metabolism to morphine through the CYP2D6 pathway, and it may variably cause either inadequate pain relief or a relative overdose of the active metabolite morphine. There have been case reports of significant infant sedation and one report of infant death after routine maternal intake; the mother was subsequently identified to be an ultrarapid metabolizer and infant an extensive metabolizer after the breastfeeding infant's death.[73]
  - Tramadol is another weak opioid that is no longer recommended in the United States for use in breastfeeding mothers. While there are no reports of ill effects in breastfeeding infants, the U.S. Food and Drug Administration has issued a warning against its use, similar to codeine, based on its CYP2D6 metabolism.[72] It continues to be used frequently in other areas of the world where it is considered safe for breastfeeding mothers.[56,74]
  - Hydrocodone has been used frequently in breastfeeding mothers worldwide. Like all opioids, it should be used with caution and breastfeeding babies should be observed for sedation and respiratory depression. The recommended maximum daily dose of 30 mg should not be exceeded[49] (IV).
  - Oxycodone is the most commonly used opioid for cesarean delivery pain in North America. Up to 8.5% of the weight-adjusted maternal dose (RID) transfers into human milk.[75] Prolonged and frequent administration may lead to neonatal sedation, and a maximum daily dose of 30 mg should not be exceeded[49] (IV).

- Hydromorphone and morphine may be used for oral opioid analgesia, although they have relatively poor oral availability and there is little data available on breastfeeding when mothers use these medications orally. The AAP recommends cautious use of these medications instead of other opioid options[57] (IV). Subsequent to publication of AAP recommendations, there has been one case report of a 6-day-old infant exposed to hydromorphone through breast milk who presented to the emergency room with respiratory depression that required naloxone. The mother had been taking oral hydromorphone, 4 mg, every 4 hours around the clock since birth.[76]
- Chronic opioid therapy
  - In the United States, in particular, pregnant women may be prescribed methadone or buprenorphine for maintenance as part of the medication-assisted treatment for opioid use disorder. Some women may be taking high doses of oxycodone or other opioids for chronic pain issues. Infants of these patients are at significant risk of developing opioid withdrawal syndrome (OWS) shortly after birth. Labor and postpartum analgesic approaches should be tailored to the woman's specific condition and infants closely observed for development of symptoms of withdrawal. Breastfeeding is encouraged for patients on stable doses of methadone or buprenorphine[77] (IV), and safety of breastfeeding should be determined on an individual basis for patients chronically taking other opioids (IV).
- Analgesic adjuncts
  - Ketamine has not been well examined with regard to breastfeeding. A single study on its use as a low-dose infusion for 24 hours postcesarean delivery did not demonstrate any effects on duration of breastfeeding[78] (III). However, transfer of ketamine into milk is relatively unknown, and concerns exist over its use during anesthesia for infants and young children based on some evidence of neurotoxicty[79] (III). There is insufficient evidence of long-term safety to the infant for this medication to be used as an infusion for pain control for breastfeeding mothers (IV).
  - Gabapentin and pregabalin may be useful additions to pain management strategies for certain mothers with chronic pain syndromes or for whom opioid use should be minimized. Gabapentin likely has less transfer to milk and is considered the safer option[48,49] (IV).
  - Dexmedetomidine has been examined in a single study in which it was used as an adjunct infusion during cesarean delivery. It was determined that a breastfeeding infant would receive an RID of 0.04—0.098%, a negligible dose[80] (III).
  - Clonidine used as a neuraxial adjunct may decrease the use of systemic opioids immediately postpartum. Specific effects on breastfeeding have not been examined, but its use as a single neuraxial dose is unlikely to affect breastfeeding (IV).

- Other medications may be needed to treat side effects of opioids. Antinausea medications are considered safe, with ondansetron and other 5HT-3 blockers, dexamethasone, and metoclopramide preferred over more sedating medications, although prochlorperazine and promethazine are likely to be safe as well[48,49] (III-IV). Stool softeners and laxatives, such as docusate, senna, and bisacadoyl, are minimally absorbed from the gastrointestinal tract and are also considered safe for breastfeeding mothers[49] (III-IV).

RECOMMENDATIONS FOR FUTURE RESEARCH

Research on evaluating labor analgesia, anesthesia for cesarean delivery and postcesarean analgesia, and nonobstetric pain management in the breastfeeding mother needs to include breastfeeding outcomes more consistently. Greater standardization is required in the way we measure breastfeeding out-comes as many studies do not address the same breastfeeding end points. For example, the time to first breastfeed, number of feeds in the first 24 hours, rate of exclusive breastfeeding at discharge, exclusive breastfeeding at 6 weeks, and any breastfeeding at 6 and 12 months are all important indicators of breastfeeding attainment, yet each may be a separate outcome measured in different studies; it remains unclear which end point may be most important in determining effects of labor interventions on overall breastfeeding success.

Much of the literature on systemic opioid use, especially fentanyl and remifentanil, in labor does not include breastfeeding outcomes. Research on ketamine use, both intra- and postoperatively, and its implications for neonatal safety and breastfeeding outcomes is lacking and requires further investigation. Breast milk levels of ketamine after maternal administration have not been measured or reported to date, which would be an important starting point for guidelines on its use in lactating women. Additional gaps in knowledge exist with medication adjuncts, such as gabapentin, clonidine, and dexmedetomidine, as well as in more comprehensive evaluation of milk levels of different opioids that are commonly used postdelivery in breastfeeding patients. In addition to specific medications, research on postpartum pain control should also include evaluation of patient counseling approaches that support women to both attain adequate pain control and minimize adverse effects of opioid medication on themselves and their infants. With better data and consistent reporting, practitioners will be able to provide more comprehensive and informed consent regarding peripartum pain management.

REFERENCES

1. WHO exclusive breastfeeding. Available at: www.who.int/nutrition/topics/exclusive_breastfeeding/en (accessed January 22, 2018).

2. Anonymous. Breastfeeding and the use of human milk. *Pediatrics.* 2012;129:e841.

3. Reynolds F. Labour analgesia and the baby: Good news is no news. *Int J Obstet Anesth.* 2011;20:38−50.

4. Fleming N, Ng N, Osborne C, et al. Adolescent pregnancy outcomes in the province of Ontario: A cohort study. *J Obstet Gynaecol Can.* 2013;35:234−245.

5. French CA, Cong X, Chung KS. Labor epidural analgesia and breastfeeding. *J Hum Lact.* 2016;32:507−520.

6. Smith L. *Impact of Birthing Practices on Breastfeeding.* 2nd ed. Sudbury, MA: Jones & Bartlett Learning; 2010.

7. Anim-Somuah M, Smyth RM, Jones L. Epidural versus non-epidural or no analgesia in labour. *Cochrane Database Syst Rev.* 2011;12:CD000331.

8. Shekelle PG, Woolf SH, Eccles M, et al. Clinical guidelines: Developing guidelines. *BMJ.* 1999;318:593−596.

9. Ferber SG, Granot M, Zimmer EZ. Catastrophizing labor pain compromises later maternity adjustments. *Am J Obstet Gynecol.* 2005;192:826−831.

10. Hiltunen P, Raudaskoski T, Ebeling H, et al. Does pain relief during delivery decrease the risk of postnatal depression? *Acta Obstet Gynecol Scand.* 2004;83:257−261.

11. Dimitraki M, Tsikouras P, Manav B, et al. Evaluation of the effect of natural and emotional stress of labor on lactation and breast-feeding. *Arch Gynecol Obstet.* 2016;293:317−328.

12. Moore ER, Anderson GC, Bergman N, et al. Early skin-to-skin contact for mothers and their healthy newborn infants. *Cochrane Database Syst Rev.* 2012;5:CD003519.

13. McFadden A, Gavine A, Renfrew MJ, et al. Support for healthy breastfeeding mothers with healthy term babies. *Cochrane Database Syst Rev.* 2017;2:CD001141.

14. Meek Joan Younger, Hatcher Amy J. The breastfeeding-friendly pediatric office practice. *Pediatrics.* 2017;139: E20170647.

15. Lee A, McCarthy R, Toledo P, et al. Epidural labor analgesia—fentanyl dose and breastfeeding success: A randomized clinical trial. *Anesthesiology.* 2017;127:614−624.

16. Beilin Y, Bodian CA, Weiser J, et al. Effect of labor epidural analgesia with and without fentanyl on infant breast-feeding: A prospective, randomized, double-blind study. *Anesthesiology.* 2005;103:1211−1217.

17. Wilson MJA, MacArthur C, Cooper GM, et al. Epidural analgesia and breastfeeding: A randomised controlled trial of epidural techniques with and without fentanyl and a non-epidural comparison group. *Anaesthesia.* 2010;65:145−153.

18. Ransjö-Arvidson AB, Matthiesen AS, Lilja G, Nissen E, Widström AM, Uvnäs-Moberg K. Maternal analgesia during labor disturbs newborn behavior: Effects on breast-feeding. *temperature, and crying. Birth.* 2001;28:5−12.

19. Brimdyr K, Cadwell K, Widström A, et al. The association between common labor drugs and suckling when skin-to-skin during the first hour after birth. *Birth.* 2015;42:319−328.

20. Riordan J, Gross A, Angeron J, et al. The effect of labor pain relief medication on neonatal suckling and breast-feeding duration. *J Hum Lact.* 2000;16:7−12.

21. Zuppa AA, Alighieri G, Riccardi R, et al. Epidural analgesia, neonatal care and breastfeeding. *Ital J Pediatr.* 2014;40:82.

22. Apfelbaum J, Hawkins J, Agarkar M, et al. Practice guidelines for obstetric anesthesia: An updated report by the american society of anesthesiologists' task force on obstetric anesthesia and the society for obstetric anesthesia and perinatology. *Anesthesiology.* 2016;124:270−300.

23. Chantry CJ, Nommsen-Rivers L, Peerson JM, et al. Excess weight loss in first-born breastfed newborns relates to maternal intrapartum fluid balance. *Pediatrics.* 2011;127: e179.

24. Kujawa-Myles S, Noel-Weiss J, Dunn S, et al. Maternal intravenous fluids and postpartum breast changes: A pilot observational study. *Int Breastfeed J.* 2015;10:18.

25. Phillips SN, Fernando R, Girard T. Parenteral opioid analgesia: Does it still have a role? *Best Pract Res Clin Anaesthesiol.* 2017;31:3−14.

26. Jelting Y, Weibel S, Afshari A, et al. Patient-controlled analgesia with remifentanil vs. alternative parenteral methods for pain management in labour: A cochrane systematic review. *Anaesthesia.* 2017;72:1016−1028.

27. Aaronson J, Abramovitz S, Smiley R, et al. A survey of intravenous remifentanil uses for labor analgesia at academic medical centers in the United States. *Anesth Analg.* 2017;124:1208−1210.

28. Fleet J, Jones M, Belan I. The influence of intrapartum opioid use on breastfeeding experience at 6 weeks postpartum: A secondary analysis. *Midwifery.* 2017;50:106−109.

29. Fleet J, Belan I, Jones M, et al. A comparison of fentanyl with pethidine for pain relief during childbirth: A randomised controlled trial. *BJOG.* 2015;122:983−992.

30. Zanardo V, Volpe F, Parotto M, et al. Nitrous oxide labor analgesia and pain relief memory in breastfeeding women. *J Matern Fetal Neonatal Med.* 2017:1−6. [Epub ahead of print]; DOI:10.1080/14767058.2017.1368077.

31. Rooks JP. Safety and risks of nitrous oxide labor analgesia: A review. *J Midwifery Womens Health.* 2011;56:557−565.

32. Othman M, Jones L, Neilson JP. Non-opioid drugs for pain management in labour. *Cochrane Database Syst Rev.* 2012;7: CD009223.

33. Bloor M, Paech M. Nonsteroidal anti-inflammatory drugs during pregnancy and the initiation of lactation. *Anesth Analg.* 2013;116:1063−1075.

34. Bloor M, Paech MJ, Kaye R. Tramadol in pregnancy and lactation. *Int J Obstet Anesth.* 2012;21:163−167.

35. Sandall J, Soltani H, Gates S, et al. Midwife-led continuity models versus other models of care for childbearing women. *Cochrane Database Syst Rev.* 2016;4:CD004667.

36. Hodnett ED, Gates S, Hofmeyr GJ, et al. Continuous support for women during childbirth. *Cochrane Database Syst Rev.* 2012;10:CD003766.

37. Gruber KJ, Cupito SH, Dobson CF. Impact of doulas on healthy birth outcomes. *J Perinat Educ.* 2013;22:49−58.

38. Kozhimannil KB, Attanasio LB, Hardeman RR, et al. Doula care supports Near-Universal breastfeeding initiation among diverse, Low-Income women. *J Midwifery Womens Health.* 2013;58:378−382.

39. Madden K, Middleton P, Cyna AM, et al. Hypnosis for pain management during labour and childbirth. *Cochrane Database Syst Rev.* 2012;11:CD009356.

40. Derry S, Straube S, Moore RA, et al. Intracutaneous or subcutaneous sterile water injection compared with blinded controls for pain management in labour. *Cochrane Database Syst Rev.* 2012;1:CD009107.

41. Jones L, Othman M, Dowswell T, et al. Pain management for women in labour: An overview of systematic reviews. *Cochrane Database Syst Rev.* 2012;3:CD009234.

42. Werner A, Uldbjerg N, Zachariae R, et al. Effect of self-hypnosis on duration of labor and maternal and neonatal

outcomes: A randomized controlled trial. *Acta Obstet Gynecol Scand.* 2013;92:816—823.

43. Mathur GP, Pandey PK, Mathur S, et al. Breastfeeding in babies delivered by cesarean section. *Indian Pediatr.* 1993;30:1285—1290.

44. Guala A, Boscardini L, Visentin R, et al. Skin-to-skin contact in cesarean birth and duration of breastfeeding: A cohort study. *Sci World J.* 2017;2017. Available from: https://doi.org/10.1155/2017/1940756, Article ID 1940756. Available from: https://www.hindawi.com/journals/tswj/2017/1940756/cta/.

45. Kutlucan L, Seker IS, Demiraran Y, et al. Effects of different anesthesia protocols on lactation in the postpartum period. *J Turk Ger Gynecol Assoc.* 2014;15:233—238.

46. Alus Tokat M, Serçekuxs P, Yenal K, et al. Early postpartum breast-feeding outcomes and breastfeeding self efficacy in turkish mothers undergoing vaginal birth or cesarean birth with different types of anesthesia. *Int J Nurs Knowl.* 2015;26:73—79.

47. Chu TC, McCallum J, Yii MF. Breastfeeding after anaesthesia: A review of the pharmacological impact on children. *Anaesth Intensive Care.* 2013;41:35—40.

48. Reece-Stremtan S, Campos M, Kokajko L. ABM clinical protocol #15: Analgesia and anesthesia for the breastfeeding mother, revised 2017. *Breastfeed Med.* 2017;12:5—506..

49. National Library of Medicine. Drugs and lactation database (LactMed). Updated 2017. Available at: https://toxnet.nlm.nih.gov/newtoxnet/lactmed.htm (accessed February 10, 2018).

50. Jolly C, Jathières F, Keïta H, et al. Cesarean analgesia using levobupivacaine continuous wound infiltration: A randomized trial. *Eur J Obstet Gynecol Reprod Biol.* 2015;194:125—130.

51. Simavli S, Kaygusuz I, Kafali H. Effect of bupivacaine-soaked spongostan in cesarean section wound on postoperative maternal health. *Arch Gynecol Obstet.* 2014;290:249—256.

52. Lawrence RA, Lawrence RM. *Breastfeeding: A Guide for the Medical Professional.* 8th ed. Philadelphia: Elsevier; 2016.

53. Hale TW, Rowe HE. *Medications and Mothers' Milk 2017.* 17th ed. New York: Springer Publishing Company; 2016.

54. Hirose M, Hara Y, Hosokawa T, et al. The effect of post-operative analgesia with continuous epidural bupivacaine after cesarean section on the amount of breast feeding and infant weight gain. *Anesth Analg.* 1996;82:1166—1169.

55. Gadsden J, Hart S, Santos AC. Post-cesarean delivery analgesia. *Anesth Analg.* 2005;101:S69.

56. Yefet E, Taha H, Salim R, et al. Fixed time interval compared with on-demand oral analgesia protocols for post-caesarean pain: A randomised controlled trial. *BJOG.* 2017;124:1063—1070.

57. Sachs HC. Committee On Drugs. The transfer of drugs and therapeutics into human breast milk: An update on selected topics. *Pediatrics.* 2013;132:796.

58. Datta P, Rewers-Felkins K, Kallem RR, et al. Transfer of low dose aspirin into human milk. *J Hum Lact.* 2017;33:296—299.

59. Weibert RT, Townsend RJ, Kaiser DG, et al. Lack of ibuprofen secretion into human milk. *Clin Pharm.* 1982;1:457—458.

60. Wischnik A, Manth SM, Lloyd J, et al. The excretion of ketorolac tromethamine into breast milk after multiple oral dosing. *Eur J Clin Pharmacol.* 1989;36:521—524.

61. Jamali F, Stevens DR. Naproxen excretion in milk and its uptake by the infant. *Drug Intell Clin Pharm.* 1983;17:910—911.

62. Goodman SR, Drachenberg AM, Johnson SA, et al. Decreased postpartum use of oral pain medication after a single dose of epidural morphine. *Reg Anesth Pain Med.* 2005;30:134—139.

63. Dalal PG, Bosak J, Berlin C. Safety of the breast-feeding infant after maternal anesthesia. *Paediatr Anaesth.* 2014;24:359—371.

64. Sutton CD, Carvalho B. Optimal pain management after cesarean delivery. *Anesthesiol Clin.* 2017;35:107—124.

65. Carvalho B, Butwick A. Postcesarean delivery analgesia. *Best Pract Res Clin Anaesthesiol.* 2017;31:69—79.

66. Allegaert K, van den Anker J. Maternal analgosedation and breastfeeding: Guidance for the pediatrician. *J Pediatr Neonatal Individ Med.* 2015;4:1—6.

67. Wittels B, Scott DT, Sinatra RS. Exogenous opioids in human breast milk and acute neonatal neurobehavior: A preliminary study. *Anesthesiology.* 1990;73:864—869.

68. Steer PL, Biddle CJ, Marley WS, et al. Concentration of fentanyl in colostrum after an analgesic dose. *Can J Anaesth.* 1992;39:231—235.

69. Edwards JE, Rudy AC, Wermeling DP, et al. Hydromorphone transfer into breast milk after intranasal administration. *Pharmacotherapy.* 2003;23:153—158.

70. Jacqz-Aigrain E, Serreau R, Boissinot C, et al. Excretion of ketoprofen and nalbuphine in human milk during treatment of maternal pain after delivery. *Ther Drug Monit.* 2007;29:815—818.

71. Pittman KA, Smyth RD, Losada M, et al. Human perinatal distribution of butorphanol. *Am J Obstet Gynecol.* 1980;138 (7 Pt 1):797—800.

72. U.S. Food and Drug Administration. FDA drug safety communication: FDA restricts use of prescription codeine pain and cough medicines and tramadol pain medicines in children; recommends against use in breastfeeding women. Updated 2017. Available at: https://www.fda.gov/Drugs/DrugSafety/ucm549679.htm (accessed February 10, 2018).

73. Koren G, Cairns J, Chitayat D, et al. Pharmacogenetics of morphine poisoning in a breastfed neonate of a codeine-prescribed mother. *Lancet.* 2006;368:704.

74. Palmer G, Anderson B, Allegaert K, et al. SPANZA advisory on tramadol—use of tramadol during breastfeeding and in the neonate. Updated 2017. Available at: www.anzca.edu.au/documents/policy_spanza-tramadol_20170624.pdf (accessed February 17, 2018).

75. Marx CM, Pucino F, Carlson JD, et al. Oxycodone excretion in human milk in the puerperium. *Drug Intell Clin Pharm.* 1986;20:474.

76. Schultz ML, Kostic M, Kharasch S. A case of toxic breast-feeding? *Pediatr Emerg Care.* 2017;. Available from: https://doi.org/10.1097/PEC.0000000000001009. Epub ahead of print].

77. Reece-Stremtan S, Marinelli KA. ABM clinical protocol #21: Guidelines for breastfeeding and substance use or substance use disorder, revised 2015. *Breastfeed Med.* 2015;10:135—141.

78. Suppa E, Valente A, Catarci S, et al. A study of low-dose S-ketamine infusion as "preventive" pain treatment for cesarean section with spinal anesthesia: Benefits and side effects. *Minerva Anestesiol.* 2012;78:774.

79. Yan J, Li Y, Zhang Y, et al. Repeated exposure to anesthetic ketamine can negatively impact neurodevelopment in infants. *J Child Neurol.* 2014;29:1333—1338.

80. Nakanishi R, Yoshimura M, Suno M, et al. Detection of dexmedetomidine in human breast milk using liquid chromatography-tandem mass spectrometry: Application to a study of drug safety in breastfeeding after cesarean section. *J Chromatogr B Analyt Technol Biomed Life Sci.* 2017;1040:208—213.

ABM protocols expire 5 years from the date of publication. Content of this protocol is up-to-date at the time of publication. Evidence-based revisions are made within 5 years or sooner if there are significant changes in the evidence.

This protocol is a new expansion of the previous 2012 protocol on Analgesia and Anesthesia for the Breastfeeding Mother, authored by Anne Montgomery and Thomas Hale.
The Society for Obstetric Anesthesia and Perinatology (SOAP) fully endorses the content of this ABM Clinical Protocol #28 entitled "ABM Clinical Protocol #28, Peripartum Analgesia and Anesthesia for the Breastfeeding Mother."

The Academy of Breastfeeding Medicine Protocol Committee:
Sarah Reece-Stremtan, MD, Chairperson
Larry Noble, MD, FABM, Translations Chairperson
Melissa Bartick, MD
Maya Bunik MD, MSPH, FABM
Megan Elliott-Rudder, MD
Cadey Harrel, MD
Ruth A. Lawrence, MD, FABM
Kathleen A. Marinelli, MD, FABM
Katrina Mitchell, MD
Casey Rosen-Carole, MD, MPH, MSEd
Susan Rothenberg, MD
Tomoko Seo, MD, FABM
Rose St. Fleur, MD
Adora Wonodi, MD
Michal Young, MD, FABM
For correspondence: abm@bfmed.org

I APPENDIX

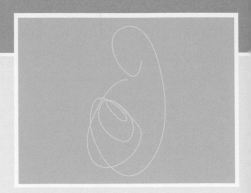

ABM Clinical Protocol #29
Iron, Zinc, and Vitamin D Supplementation During Breastfeeding*

Sarah N. Taylor and The Academy of Breastfeeding Medicine

ABSTRACT

A central goal of The Academy of Breastfeeding Medicine is the development of clinical protocols, free from commercial interest or influence, for managing common medical problems that may impact breastfeeding success. These protocols serve only as guidelines for the care of breastfeeding mothers and infants and do not delineate an exclusive course of treatment or serve as standards of medical care. Variations in treatment may be appropriate according to the needs of an individual patient.

HUMAN MILK is designed to deliver comprehensive nutrition through the first 6 months of age and complementary nutrition through the early years. However, micronutrient supplementation may be appropriate, especially when a mother is deficient or an infant has special needs such as prematurity. In contemporary high- and low-resource settings, concern has been raised regarding iron, zinc, and vitamin D status of human milk-fed infants. This protocol reviews the available evidence regarding iron, zinc, and vitamin D supplementation of the breastfeeding dyad. Quality of evidence (levels of evidence [LOE] IA, IB, IIA, IIB, III, and IV) is provided and based on levels of evidence used for the National Guidelines Clearing House.[1] From currently available evidence, recommendations are provided and areas for future study are identified. A brief summary of recommendations is presented first, followed by more in-depth discussion of the three micronutrients.

RECOMMENDATIONS

Iron

Iron supplementation is not required for the non-anemic breastfeeding mother. Iron supplementation to the 4-month-old full-term, exclusively breastfed infant is associated with improved

hematological indices. However, the long-term benefit of improved hematologic indices at 4–6 months is not known. If iron supplementation is given before 6 months, it should be given as a 1 mg/kg/day distinct iron supplement until iron-fortified cereals (7–7.5 mg ferrous sulfate/day) or other iron-rich foods such as meat, tofu, beans, and others are initiated at 6 months of age with other complementary foods. (LOE IB)

Zinc

Zinc supplementation, above dietary intake, to the lactating mother or breastfeeding infant is not associated with improved outcomes and, therefore, is not recommended. (LOE IB)

Vitamin D

The breastfeeding infant should receive vitamin D supplementation shortly after birth in doses of 10–20 μg/day (400–800 IU/day) (LOE IB). This supplement should be cholecalciferol, vitamin D_3, because of superior absorption unless a vegetable source such as ergocaliferol vitamin D_2, is desired (LOE IIA). Randomized trials demonstrate that safe vitamin D supplementation may be provided to a nursing mother to achieve healthy vitamin D status in her breastfeeding infant, when there is objection or contraindication to direct infant supplementation. A maternal dose of 160 μg/day (6,400 IU/day) is suggested.

IRON

Background section

Iron is a mineral critical to infant somatic growth and neurodevelopment. It is most commonly recognized for its role in iron-deficiency anemia, but it importantly has direct effects on brain maturation. Iron deficiency during infancy is associated with poor cognitive and behavioral outcomes that may persist after iron repletion. Therefore, ensuring adequate iron stores in infancy is essential.

Infants born at term have transplacentally acquired hepatic iron stores that are mobilized and utilized over the first 4–6 months. Preterm infants, term infants born growth-restricted, and infants born to mothers with iron deficiency during pregnancy may have smaller iron stores. The iron in

---

* Courtesy of the Academy of Breastfeeding Medicine. Please go to https://www.bfmed.org/protocols for complete protocols, translations, and the most up-to-date information (protocols are updated every 5–7 years).
Department of Pediatrics, Yale School of Medicine, New Haven, Connecticut.

human milk has high bioavailability ($\sim$50%) to complement the infant's iron stores.[2] Research has investigated whether these two sources, fetal accretion and human milk iron concentration, provide adequate supply and for how long this supply alone is adequate. Studies have also examined the role of iron-containing or fortified complementary foods in protecting iron stores, especially in the second half of the first year when the fetal supply is diminished.

Iron is a pro-oxidant and some studies have shown supplemental iron to negatively affect immune function. In fact, iron may mitigate the antipathogenic actions of human milk.[3–5]

Iron-deficiency anemia is diagnosed by abnormal hematological values. Studies of iron supplementation in infants have used serum iron, ferritin, iron binding capacity, mean corpuscular volume (MCV), and hemoglobin as indicators of sufficient iron to avoid the risk of anemia. Other potential markers of adequate iron supplementation include anthropometric growth and neurodevelopment. Randomized controlled trials (LOE IB) of iron supplementation to the lactating mother or to the infant have included serum and milk iron concentrations, ferritin and iron binding capacity, hematologic indices, growth, and neurodevelopment as outcomes.

There are few studies investigating iron supplementation directly to the breastfeeding mother to support infant iron status. One study recruited 168 healthy, nonanemic mothers in the first 10–20 postnatal days if they planned to exclusively breastfeed for at least 4 months. These mothers were randomized to receive 80 mg elemental iron daily or placebo. No difference was seen in maternal or infant iron studies, rate of iron-deficiency anemia, or infant growth. In the intervention group, both mother and infant had significantly increased serum iron binding capacity but the significance of this single difference is not known (LOE IB).[6]

When evaluating the evidence of direct infant supplementation, it is necessary to consider the age at which supplementation occurred—in the first 4 months, starting at 4–6 months, or starting at 6 months of age. Two small randomized controlled trials have evaluated iron supplementation initiated before 4 months of age. The first study included 77 term breastfed infants who were randomized to receive either 7.5 mg elemental iron as ferrous sulfate or placebo from 1 to 6 months of age (LOE IB).[7] At 6 months, the supplemented group had significantly higher hemoglobin (124 versus 116 g/L) and MCV (81 versus 77 fL). Forty-six of the 77 study subjects had neurodevelopmental assessment at 12–18 months; the intervention group exhibited higher Bayley psychomotor development indexes and visual acuity. No significant differences were seen in mental development indices.

A second study of early iron supplementation specifically focused on the term low birth weight ($<$2,500 g) infant. Healthy infants ($n = 62$) who were predominantly breastfed at 50–80 days were randomized to iron 3 mg/kg/day (25 mg Fe/mL ferric ammonia citrate) or placebo for 8 weeks (LOE IB).[8] Infant hemoglobin levels were significantly higher in the iron-supplemented group at 2 months of therapy (117 versus

107 g/L). No difference was found between groups in serum ferritin, infant growth, or morbidity. These two studies of early iron supplementation suggest that early iron may lead to higher hemoglobin levels, but the studies are too small to promote a specific recommendation for the breastfed term infant. Given small sample size and significant methodologic limitations, we cannot draw conclusions about the effect of early iron supplementation for term newborns on neurodevelopmental outcomes.

Large randomized controlled trials have examined iron supplementation at 4–9 months of age. Some studies have specifically compared iron initiation at 4 or 6 months. Others have compared iron drops and iron-fortified foods. In one study of 609 infants in Thailand, both iron and zinc supplementation were evaluated with initiation at 4–6 months. Infants receiving 10 mg iron as iron sulfate (with or without zinc) exhibited significantly higher hemoglobin and ferritin concentrations at 6 months of therapy compared with infants receiving only zinc or placebo. When controlling for gender and birth weight, infants receiving iron had significantly higher Ponderal weight growth and weight-for-length z-score (LOE IB).[9]

One double-blinded randomized placebo-controlled trial, occurring in Honduras and Sweden, evaluated iron supplementation alone. In this study, 232 near-exclusive or exclusively breastfeeding infants at 4 months of age were randomized to receive (1) placebo until 9 months of age, (2) placebo for 4–6 months followed by iron (1 mg/kg/day) for 6–9 months, or (3) iron (1 mg/kg/day) until at least 9 months.[10,11] The primary aim, to detect a difference in hemoglobin, was demonstrated for the infants receiving iron supplementation starting at 4 months. When iron supplementation started at 6 months, the infants in Honduras demonstrated significantly higher hemoglobin while the Swedish infants did not (LOE IB).[11] In evaluation of growth, the Swedish infants supplemented with iron had significantly lower length and head circumference gains than those infants receiving placebo from 4 to 9 months (LOE IB).[10] In Honduras, a negative effect on linear growth was evident at 4–6 months only among iron-sufficient infants (with an initial Hb $\geq$110 g/L). In addition, in both sites, iron supplementation increased the likelihood of diarrhea among iron-sufficient infants.

The question as to whether iron should be provided as a daily or weekly dose has been evaluated by one randomized trial without study blinding. No difference in iron deficiency or iron-deficiency anemia was observed with ferrous sulfate suspension dosed at 1 mg/kg daily, 7 mg/kg weekly, versus no supplement provided to breastfeeding infants at 4–10 months of age ($n = 79$) (LOE IB).[12]

Studies of whether iron should be provided as a distinct dose or instead through fortified cereal are open-label studies. In 2004 in Honduras, 4-month-old, exclusively breastfeeding infants were randomized to iron-fortified cereal or no cereal until 6 months of age (LOE IB).[13] In this study, infants who exhibited anemia at study initiation (58% of the iron-fortified group and 47% of exclusively breastfeeding group) also received iron drops. Of the infants who were not anemic at study initiation, those receiving iron-fortified cereal had significantly higher hemoglobin and lower prevalence of anemia than those exclusively breastfed. However, when analysis also included infants receiving iron drops for preexisting anemia, hemoglobin was higher in the exclusively breastfed group. This study raises concern that iron-fortified cereals may hinder the action of iron drops to improve hemoglobin.

Further study of iron-fortified cereal has occurred in the United States. The first study was an open-label randomized trial comparing iron drops (7—7.5 mg ferrous sulfate/day), iron-fortified cereal (7—7.5 mg ferrous sulfate/day), and no intervention from 4 to 9 months of age in 93 infants who were exclusively breastfeeding at 1 month (LOE IB).[14] In this study, the group with no intervention demonstrated significantly lower plasma ferritin concentrations throughout the intervention period and up to 15 months of age. There was no significant difference in serum ferritin levels between the group receiving iron drops and iron-fortified cereal. The iron-fortified cereal was well tolerated. Of interest, the infants receiving iron drops demonstrated significantly lower length growth during the intervention, although this difference dissipated in the second year. Further study of iron-fortified cereal compared electrolytic iron (54.5 mg Fe/100 g cereal) and ferrous fumarate (52.2 mg Fe/100 g cereal) from 4 to 9 months and demonstrated no difference in iron deficiency or iron-deficiency anemia between groups ($n = 95$) (LOE IB).[15]

One further randomized controlled trial evaluated whether iron supplementation of the breastfeeding infant at 4—9 months of age had an effect on copper status and showed that infants receiving iron supplementation had significantly lower copper-zinc oxide dismutase when compared with controls at 9 months. In addition to the negative effect on growth parameters exhibited in the iron supplementation trials mentioned previously, this potential negative effect on copper status warrants further investigation.[16]

Both the European Society for Pediatric Gastroenterology, Hepatology, and Nutrition (ESPGHAN) and the American Academy of Pediatrics (AAP) have reviewed the existing literature up to 2014 and 2010, respectively, and have published a position article or clinical report, respectively.[17,18] ESPGHAN reports that "there is insufficient evidence to support general iron supplementation of healthy European infants and toddlers of normal birth weight." In contrast, the AAP Committee on Nutrition concludes that breastfeeding infants should be "supplemented with 1 mg/kg per day of oral iron beginning at 4 months of age until appropriate iron-containing complementary foods (including iron containing cereals) are introduced in the diet." Of note, when the AAP Section on Breastfeeding reviewed the evidence, they concluded that studies demonstrating benefit of iron supplementation before 6 months of age were inadequate both in number and in the clinical importance of the outcomes.[19]

In summary of the literature regarding direct infant supplementation, two small studies demonstrate potential for hematologic and neurodevelopmental benefit with supplementation as early as 1 month of age. Specifically, one small study of 77 term breastfed newborns who were supplemented at some time between 1 and 6 months of age showed improved psychomotor, but not cognitive, development at 13 months. Larger studies with initiation of iron supplementation at 4 or 6 months of age demonstrate improved hematologic indices. Both iron drops and iron-fortified cereal appear to increase laboratory indices of iron deficiency and iron-deficiency anemia but, when given together, the fortified cereal may hinder the action of the drops. Of note, iron supplementation is not only associated with improved weight for length measurements but also shows a negative association with both length and head circumference parameters.

Recommendations

Iron supplementation is not required for the nonanemic breastfeeding mother. Iron supplementation to the 4-month-old full-term, exclusively breastfed infant is associated with improved hematological indices. However, the long-term benefit of improved hematologic indices at 4—6 months is not known. There are potential harms of iron supplementation, especially on immune function and in possibly decreasing the bioavailability of iron contained in human milk. In addition, there is potential harm in infant growth and morbidity when iron supplementation is provided to iron-sufficient infants. If iron supplementation is given before 6 months, it should be given as a 1 mg/kg/day distinct iron supplement until iron-fortified cereals (7—7.5 mg ferrous sulfate/day) or other iron-rich foods such as meat, tofu, beans, and the like are initiated at 6 months of age with other complementary foods. (LOE IB)

Recommendations for future research

Future research is essential to evaluate the neurodevelopmental outcomes associated with iron supplementation. Moreover, the process of delayed cord clamping at birth may also have significant effects on iron stores.[20,21] Other areas of potential evaluation include earlier supplementation (as early as one postnatal month), the potential for positive or negative effects on growth, potential for negative effects on immune function, and potential for positive or negative effect on the homeostasis of other minerals such as zinc and copper.

ZINC

Background

Zinc is involved in many functions of human health including enzymatic; cell differentiation; protein, lipid, and carbohydrate metabolism; gene transcription; and immunity. Zinc deficiency is associated with growth failure and increased susceptibility to infection and skin inflammation, diarrhea, alopecia, and behavioral disturbances. Randomized controlled trials (LOE IB) of zinc supplementation to lactating mothers or to infants have evaluated serum and milk zinc concentrations, growth, infection, neurodevelopment, hematologic indices, and copper levels as outcomes.

A blinded randomized controlled trial of zinc supplementation (zinc sulfate 10 mg/day) to lactating mothers demonstrated increased maternal zinc concentrations and increased milk zinc concentrations[22] (LOE IB). In contrast, another study of supplementation of mothers with preterm infants with 50 mg/day zinc chelate showed no difference in maternal serum zinc levels (LOE IIA).[23] Neither study showed a difference in infant zinc levels or in infant growth when compared with infants whose mothers did not receive zinc supplementation.[22,23]

Double-blind randomized controlled trials of direct zinc supplementation to the breastfed infant in Thailand have evaluated 4–10 month-old infants receiving 5 mg elemental zinc sulfate for 10 months[24] (LOE IB) and 4–6 month old infants receiving 10 mg zinc either with or without iron for 6 months (LOE IB).[9] Of note, these infants also received complementary foods. Wasantwisut et al. studied infants who received zinc alone and demonstrated significantly higher zinc levels than those who received iron alone (no zinc) (LOE IB).[9] In both studies, no difference in growth was observed. The Heinig et al. study that also monitored for diarrhea, otitis media, respiratory illness, fever, total illness, and motor development found no difference between groups.[24]

Of note, though only case series are published, infant zinc deficiency has been reported in breastfeeding infants. This rare disorder is called Transient Neonatal Zinc Deficiency and is due to a maternal mutation in the zinc transporter gene.[25,26] When a breastfeeding infant develops zinc deficiency, mother should be evaluated for this rare genetic disorder.

Recommendations

Zinc supplementation, above dietary intake, to the lactating mother or breastfeeding infant is not associated with improved outcomes and, therefore, is not recommended. (LOE IB)

Recommendations for future research

Evidence regarding the role of zinc in susceptibility to infection or in the severity of infection requires further investigation in the breastfed infant population. Studies specifically evaluating these health outcomes, and studies in populations at risk for deficiency or at increased risk for infection, such as preterm infants, are warranted.

VITAMIN D

Background

Vitamin D is a hormone involved in calcium absorption, bone mineralization, and immune function. In its most severe form, vitamin D deficiency appears as rickets—bony abnormalities including bowed legs, splayed wrists, and associated muscle weakness. In the past three decades, both high and low resource countries have experienced a resurgence in rickets associated with dark skin pigmentation, living at higher latitude, practices of body covering, and exclusive breastfeeding.[27] The breast milk of a mother receiving a vitamin D dose of 10 μg/day (400 IU/day) will contain $\sim$ 80 IU/ L, thereby putting her infant at risk for vitamin D deficiency.[28] Vitamin D supplementation is therefore routinely recommended for the breastfeeding infant.

Vitamin D deficiency currently is defined by the Institute of Medicine and ESPGHAN as a 25-hydroxyvitamin D [25(OH)D] concentration less than 50 nmol/L (20 ng/mL).[29,30] Some authors choose to define vitamin D sufficiency, the threshold associated with optimal function of vitamin D-dependent processes. Vitamin D sufficiency definitions range from 75 to 110 nmol/L (30–44 ng/mL) based mostly on studies in the adult population. Further investigation defining vitamin D sufficiency for infants is warranted.

Recent research has investigated the vitamin D needs of both mother and infant, seeking to identify a maternal vitamin D dose that is both efficacious and safe for mother and infant. The majority of randomized trials have compared the vitamin D levels, as measured by 25(OH)D, achieved by specific doses. Additionally, studies have evaluated whether a vitamin D dose is associated with avoidance of vitamin D deficiency. A few trials have measured infant bone health as an outcome.

Randomized trials of direct supplementation to the exclusively breastfeeding infant have compared doses up to 40 μg/day (1,600 IU/day). Some of these studies have a placebo arm. Others provide at least 5 μg/day (200 IU/day) vitamin D. One study compared the efficacy of vitamin D_2 or ergocalciferol (from plants) and vitamin D_3 or cholecalciferol (from animals) given as 10 μg/day (400 IU/day) to 52, 1 month-old, breastfeeding infants for 3 months. The change in 25(OH)D levels from baseline to study end was not significantly different between groups (change of 56 and 44 nmol/L, respectively). However, 25% of the infants in the vitamin D_2 group and only 4% of infants in the vitamin D_3 exhibited vitamin D deficiency after 3 months (LOE IB).[31]

Randomized trials with a true placebo control have evaluated doses of 5 μg/day (200 IU/day) in Korea and 10 μg/day (400 IU/day) in Italy. In the study of 5 μg/day (200 IU/day), the supplemented infants demonstrated significantly higher mean 25(OH)D status at both 6 and 12 months. However, lumbar spine bone mineral density was not significantly different between groups (LOE IIA).[32] In the study of 10 μg/day (400 IU/day), bone strength was measured by ultrasound and found to be significantly higher in vitamin D supplemented group (LOE IIA).[33] Of note, the utility of ultrasound measurement of bone strength has not been established.

Randomized trials without a true placebo have compared 5, 10, 15, and 20 μg/day (200, 400, 600, and 800 IU/day);[34] 10, 20, 30, and 40 μg/day (400, 800, 1,200, and 1,600 IU/day);[35] and 6.25 and 12.5 μg/day (125 and 250 IU/day).[36] For the comparison of 6.25 and 12.5 μg/day (125 and 250 IU/day) in Greece, no significant difference in vitamin D outcomes was observed (LOE IB).[36] For the comparison of 5 up to 20 μg/ day (200 up to 800 IU/day) beginning at one postnatal month and continued for 9 months, at the end of winter (average of 7 months of therapy) in the United States, the four doses achieved mean serum 25(OH)D levels ranging 78 to 107 nmol/L and were not significantly different. Of note, the infants receiving 20 μg/day (800 IU/day) had no vitamin D deficiency through the study time period (LOE IB).[34] In the double-blind randomized trial of doses ranging from 10 to 40 μg/day (400 to 1,600 IU/day), 97% of infants in all dose groups achieved 25(OH)D >50 nmol/L by 3 months of age (LOE IB).[35] The study's primary aim for 97.5% of infants to achieve 25(OH)D >75 nmol/L was only achieved by the 40 μg/day (1,600 IU/day) group. However, this dosing was discontinued early due to concern that the 25(OH)D levels achieved were too high. Additionally, no difference in bone mineral content was seen between dosing groups during the study or at 3 years of age.[35,37]

In addition to study of direct infant supplementation with vitamin D, recent investigation has focused on methods to provide vitamin D to the infant by supplementing the mother and thereby augmenting the level of vitamin D in her breast milk. These studies have addressed the question—is there a maternal vitamin D dose that is efficacious and safe for both the mother and infant? Two studies, based on previous research,[28,38] were designed and performed to address this question. One randomized, blinded clinical trial compared maternal intake of 10, 60, and 160 μg/day (400, 2,400, and 6,400 IU/day) in 334 mother/infant dyads.[39] For the group with maternal dose of 10 μg/day (400 IU/day), the infant also received 10 μg/day (400 IU/day). For the other two groups, no vitamin D was provided to the infant. The maternal 60 μg/day (2,400 IU/day) dose group was discontinued early due to vitamin D deficiency in the infant, demonstrating that maternal 60 μg/day (2,400 IU/day) was not sufficient to provide adequate vitamin D to the breastfeeding infant. In the remaining two dose groups, 148 mothers were exclusively breastfeeding at 4 months and 95 at 7 months. At both visits, for the mothers receiving 160 μg/day (6,400 IU/day), the infants' mean 25(OH)D status was similar to the status of infants receiving 10 μg/day (400 IU/day) directly (at 7 months, 109 nmol/L in each group). Mothers in the 160 μg/day (6,400 IU/day) group had significantly higher 25(OH)D levels than mothers in the 10 μg/day (400 IU/day) group (151.2 and 79 nmol/L, respectively). No vitamin D toxicity was observed.

A second study to address maternal supplementation to achieve vitamin D—replete milk compared maternal and infant vitamin D status for 28 days with either a daily oral dose of 125 μg/day (5,000 IU/day) or a one-time oral dose of 3,750 μg (150,000 IU). In both groups, the 40 infants achieved mean 25(OH)D levels of 97.5nmol/L. For mothers, the 3,750 μg (150,000 IU) group, demonstrated a mean peak 25(OH)D concentration of 125 nmol/L on day 3. At day 28, mothers receiving the 3,750 μg (150,000 IU) dose and those receiving 125 μg/day (5,000 IU/day) exhibited mean 25(OH)D of 103 and 110 nmol/L, respectively. Vitamin D status remained in the normal range for all mothers in the study. However, four mothers in the one-dose group and three mothers in the daily-dose group demonstrated urinary calcium excretion above the acceptable range defined by the study.[40]

One further study evaluated the effect of maternal supplementation initiated in pregnancy (13—24 weeks' gestation) in 100 women who exclusively breastfed through 8 weeks.[41] With maternal doses of 10, 25, and 50 μg/day (400, 1,000, 2,000 IU/day), rates of infant vitamin D deficiency (<50 nmol/L) at 8 weeks were 59%, 48%, and 13%, respectively. This study demonstrates improved vitamin D status with maternal supplementation, but, as observed in the previous dose of 60 μ/day (2,400 IU/day),[39] 50 μg/day (2,000 IU/day) may not be an adequate maternal dose to avoid vitamin D deficiency in all infants.

In summary, randomized trials have not shown a specific dose of vitamin D, to the breastfeeding infant, to be associated with optimal bone mineralization. Therefore, vitamin D supplementation recommendations are based on the amount of supplementation needed to achieve an infant 25(OH)D >50 nmol/L, the level associated with a reduced risk of rickets. In studies evaluating the ability of infant vitamin D dosing to achieve 25(OH)D >50 nmol, one study in the United States in winter found a dose of 20 μg/day (800 IU/day) to achieve this goal. In a second study in Canada, avoidance of vitamin D deficiency was achieved only with the 40 μg/day (1,600 IU/day) dose, but this dose also was associated with abnormally high vitamin status as defined by the authors.

For vitamin D supplementation of the mother to provide vitamin D in her milk to achieve adequate vitamin D status in the infant, a maternal dose of 160 μg/day (6,400 IU/day) maintained adequate status in the infant for 7 months and maternal doses of 125 μg/day (5,000 IU/day) and a single dose of 3,750 μg (150,000 IU) maintained infant status for 28 days. Maternal doses as high as 60 μg/day (2,400 IU/day) were not adequate to support the infant. This research demonstrates the ability for mother's milk to be replete with vitamin D with adequate supplementation to mother.

Recommendations

The breastfeeding infant should receive vitamin D supplementation for a year, beginning shortly after birth in doses of 10—20 μg/day (400—800 IU/day) (LOE IB). This supplement should be cholecalciferol, vitamin D_3, because of superior absorption unless a vegetable source such as ergocaliferol vitamin D_2, is desired (LOE IIA).

Randomized trials demonstrate that safe vitamin D supplementation may be provided to a nursing mother to achieve healthy vitamin D status in her breastfeeding infant, when there is objection or contraindication to direct infant supplementation. Current studies point to 160 μg/day (6,400 IU/day) for 7 months and 125 μg/day (5,000 IU/day) for 28 days or 3,750 μg (150,000 IU) in a single dose (lasting at least 28 days) as appropriate to achieve 25(OH)D status in the normal range for both mother and infant (LOE IB), although infant outcomes beyond those time periods were not evaluated. Data are lacking as to which option, infant versus mother supplementation, may result in greater maternal adherence to recommendations.

Recommendations for future research

The amount of vitamin D supplementation required to avoid vitamin D deficiency likely varies due to differences in baseline vitamin D status and sun exposure in populations around the world. Further study to assess the role of skin pigmentation, seasons, latitude, and sun exposure to ensure healthy vitamin D status for all populations is warranted. Currently, the 25(OH)D status associated with toxicity is not defined. Identifying this upper limit of healthy vitamin D status is critical to future research. In addition, identifying infant vitamin D sufficiency, the 25(OH)D status associated with optimal outcomes, is needed. Further research is also needed to determine the extent to which maternal vitamin D supplementation will produce levels of Vitamin D in human milk that meet infant needs.

PRETERM INFANTS

Preterm infants are known to be deficient in zinc and iron compared with term-born infants. Their vitamin D status at birth is similar to term infants, but, like term infants, they require vitamin D supplementation. Human milk fortifier delivers zinc, vitamin D, and sometimes iron. Randomized controlled trials specific to the human milk-fed preterm infants are mostly studies of multi-component fortifier, including zinc and vitamin D, and demonstrate improved infant weight and length gain, head growth, and neurodevelopmental outcome.[42] Further research is required, but, at this point, AAP and World Health Organization recommendations for iron (2–4 mg/kg/day) and vitamin D supplementation (at least 400–800 IU/day) and also supplementation with a zinc-containing fortifier should be followed.[18,43–45] Routine iron and vitamin D supplementation for the late preterm infant is also recommended.[46]

SUMMARY

Current evidence points to sufficiency in iron, zinc, and vitamin D for the exclusively breastfeeding infant in the first 6 months when mother is sufficient in these nutrients. Current research shows that human milk delivers adequate zinc and iron at least through the first 4–6 months. The need for supplemental iron may overlap with the introduction of iron-containing foods at 6 months, but current published studies demonstrate that initiating iron drops at 4 months is associated with better hematological outcomes. However, it is not clear that universal direct iron supplementation starting at 4 months and continued until receiving iron-containing feeds should be considered. For zinc, human milk delivers a sufficient supply. Vitamin D also may be delivered adequately through human milk. Maternal vitamin D deficiency is common enough, however, that routine supplementation is recommended for the breastfeeding infant. The randomized controlled trials described in this protocol demonstrate that this risk is mitigated by maternal vitamin D supplementation at a dose that is both safe for her and efficacious for the infant.

REFERENCES

1. Shekelle PG, Woolf SH, Eccles M, et al. Clinical guidelines: Developing guidelines. *BMJ.* 1999;318:593–596.
2. Saarinen UM, Siimes MA, Dallman PR. Iron absorption in infants: High bioavailability of breast milk iron as indicated by the extrinsic tag method of iron absorption and by the concentration of serum ferritin. *J Pediatr.* 1977;91:36–39.
3. Chan GM. Effects of powdered human milk fortifiers on the antibacterial actions of human milk. *J Perinatol.* 2003;23:620–623.
4. Ovali F, Ciftci I, Cetinkaya Z, et al. Effects of human milk fortifier on the antimicrobial properties of human milk. *J Perinatol.* 2006;26:761–763.
5. Campos LF, Repka JC, Falcao MC. Effects of human milk fortifier with iron on the bacteriostatic properties of breast milk. *J Pediatr.* 2013;89:394–399.
6. Baykan A, Yalcin SS, Yurdakok K. Does maternal iron supplementation during the lactation period affect iron status of exclusively breast-fed infants? *Turk J Pediatr.* 2006;48:301–307.
7. Friel JK, Aziz K, Andrews WL, et al. A double-masked, randomized control trial of iron supplementation in early infancy in healthy term breast-fed infants. *J Pediatr.* 2003;143:582–586.
8. Aggarwal D, Sachdev HP, Nagpal J, et al. Haematological effect of iron supplementation in breast fed term low birth weight infants. *Arch Dis Child.* 2005;90:26–29.
9. Wasantwisut E, Winichagoon P, Chitchumroonchokchai C, et al. Iron and zinc supplementation improved iron and zinc status, but not physical growth, of apparently healthy, breast-fed infants in rural communities of northeast Thailand. *J Nutr.* 2006;136:2405–2411.
10. Dewey KG, Domellof M, Cohen RJ, et al. Iron supplementation affects growth and morbidity of breast-fed infants: Results of a randomized trial in Sweden and Honduras. *J Nutr.* 2002;132:3249–3255.
11. Domellof M, Cohen RJ, Dewey KG, et al. Iron supplementation of breast-fed Honduran and Swedish infants from 4 to 9 months of age. *J Pediatr.* 2001;138:679–687.
12. Yurdakok K, Temiz F, Yalcin SS, et al. Efficacy of daily and weekly iron supplementation on iron status in exclusively breast-fed infants. *J Pediatr Hematol Oncol.* 2004;26:284–288.
13. Dewey KG, Cohen RJ, Brown KH. Exclusive breast-feeding for 6 months, with iron supplementation, maintains adequate micronutrient status among term, low-birthweight, breast-fed infants in Honduras. *J Nutr.* 2004;134:1091–1098.
14. Ziegler EE, Nelson SE, Jeter JM. Iron status of breastfed infants is improved equally by medicinal iron and iron-fortified cereal. *Am J Clin Nutr.* 2009;90:76–87.
15. Ziegler EE, Fomon SJ, Nelson SE, et al. Dry cereals fortified with electrolytic iron or ferrous fumarate are equally effective in breast-fed infants. *J Nutr.* 2011;141:243–248.
16. Domellof M, Dewey KG, Cohen RJ, et al. Iron supplements reduce erythrocyte copper-zinc superoxide dismutase activity in term, breastfed infants. *Acta Paediatr.* 2005;94:1578–1582.
17. Domellof M, Braegger C, Campoy C, et al. Iron requirements of infants and toddlers. *J Pediatr Gastroenterol Nutr.* 2014;58:119–129.

18. Baker RD, Greer FR. Diagnosis and prevention of iron deficiency and iron-deficiency anemia in infants and young children (0−3 years of age). *Pediatrics*. 2010;126:1040−1050.

19. AAP Section on Breastfeeding SREC, Feldman-Winter L, Landers S, Noble L, Szucs KA, Viehmann L. Concerns with early universal iron supplementation of breastfeeding infants. *Pediatrics*. 2011;127:e1097.

20. Committee on Obstetric Practice. Committee opinion no. 684: Delayed umbilical cord clamping after birth. *Obstet Gynecol*. 2017;129:e5−e10.

21. McDonald SJ, Middleton P, Dowswell T, et al. Effect of timing of umbilical cord clamping of term infants on maternal and neonatal outcomes. *Cochrane Database Syst Rev*. 2013; Cd004074.

22. Shaaban SY, Azzel-Hodhod MA, Nasou MT, et al. Zinc status of lactating Egyptian mothers and their infants: Effect of maternal zinc supplementation. *Nutr Res*. 2005;25:45−53.

23. de Figueiredo CS, Palhares DB, Melnikov P, et al. Zinc and copper concentrations in human preterm milk. *Biol Trace Elem Res*. 2010;136:1−7.

24. Heinig MJ, Brown KH, Lonnerdal B, et al. Zinc supplementation does not affect growth, morbidity, or motor development of US term breastfed infants at 4−10 mo of age. *Am J Clin Nutr*. 2006;84:594−601.

25. Krieger I, Alpern BE, Cunnane SC. Transient neonatal zinc deficiency. *Am J Clin Nutr*. 1986;43:955−958.

26. Miletta MC, Bieri A, Kernland K, et al. Transient neonatal zinc deficiency caused by a heterozygous G87R mutation in the zinc transporter ZnT-2 (SLC30A2) gene in the mother highlighting the importance of Zn (2 +) for normal growth and development. *Int J Endocrinol*. 2013;2013:259189.

27. Holick MF. Resurrection of vitamin D deficiency and rickets. *J Clin Invest*. 2006;116:2062−2072.

28. Hollis BW, Wagner CL. Vitamin D requirements during lactation: High-dose maternal supplementation as therapy to prevent hypovitaminosis D for both the mother and the nursing infant. *Am J Clin Nutr*. 2004;80(6 Suppl):1752s−1758s.

29. Review Institute of Medicine (US) Committee. *Dietary Reference Intakes for Calcium and Vitamin D*. Washington, DC: National Academies Press (US); 2011.

30. Braegger C, Campoy C, Colomb V, et al. Vitamin D in the healthy European paediatric population. *J Pediatr Gastroenterol Nutr*. 2013;56:692−701.

31. Gallo S, Phan A, Vanstone CA, et al. The change in plasma 25-hydroxyvitamin D did not differ between breast-fed infants that received a daily supplement of ergocalciferol or cholecalciferol for 3 months. *J Nutr*. 2013;143:148−153.

32. Kim MJ, Na B, No SJ, et al. Nutritional status of vitamin D and the effect of vitamin D supplementation in Korean breast-fed infants. *J Korean Med Sci*. 2010;25:83−89.

33. Bagnoli F, Casucci M, Toti S, et al. Is vitamin D supplementation necessary in healthy full-term breastfed infants? A follow-up study of bone mineralization in healthy full-term infants with and without supplemental vitamin D. *Minerva Pediatr*. 2013;65:253−260.

34. Ziegler EE, Nelson SE, Jeter JM. Vitamin D supplementation of breastfed infants: A randomized dose-response trial. *Pediatr Res*. 2014;76:177−183.

35. Gallo S, Comeau K, Vanstone C, et al. Effect of different dosages of oral vitamin D supplementation on vitamin D status in healthy, breastfed infants: A randomized trial. *JAMA*. 2013;309:1785−1792.

36. Siafarikas A, Piazena H, Feister U, et al. Randomised controlled trial analysing supplementation with 250 versus 500 units of vitamin D3, sun exposure and surrounding factors in breastfed infants. *Arch Dis Child*. 2011;96:91−95.

37. Gallo S, Hazell T, Vanstone CA, et al. Vitamin D supplementation in breastfed infants from Montreal, Canada: 25-hydroxyvitamin D and bone health effects from a follow-up study at 3 years of age. *Osteoporos Int*. 2016;27:2459−2466.

38. Wagner CL, Hulsey TC, Fanning D, et al. High-dose vitamin D3 supplementation in a cohort of breastfeeding mothers and their infants: A 6-month follow-up pilot study. *Breastfeed Med*. 2006;1:59−70.

39. Hollis BW, Wagner CL, Howard CR, et al. Maternal versus infant vitamin D supplementation during lactation: A randomized controlled trial. *Pediatrics*. 2015;136:625−634.

40. Oberhelman SS, Meekins ME, Fischer PR, et al. Maternal vitamin D supplementation to improve the vitamin D status of breast-fed infants: A randomized controlled trial. *Mayo Clin Proc*. 2013;88:1378−1387.

41. March KM, Chen NN, Karakochuk CD, et al. Maternal vitamin D(3) supplementation at 50 mug/d protects against low serum 25-hydroxyvitamin D in infants at 8 wk of age: A randomized controlled trial of 3 doses of vitamin D beginning in gestation and continued in lactation. *Am J Clin Nutr*. 2015;102:402−410.

42. Brown JV, Embleton ND, Harding JE, et al. Multi-nutrient fortification of human milk for preterm infants. *Cochrane Database Syst Rev*. 2016;Cd000343.

43. Wagner CL, Greer FR. Prevention of rickets and vitamin D deficiency in infants, children, and adolescents. *Pediatrics*. 2008;122:1142−1152.

44. Noble L, Okogbule-Wonodi A, Young M. ABM Clinical Protocol #12: Transitioning the breastfeeding preterm infant from the neonatal intensive care unit to home, revised 2018. *Breastfeed Med*. 2018;13:230−236.

45. WHO Guidelines Approved by the Guidelines Review Committee. Copyright (c) World Health Organization 2016 *Guideline: Daily Iron Supplementation in Infants and Children*. Geneva: World Health Organization; 2016.

46. Boies E, Vaucher Y. ABM Clinical Protocol #10: Breastfeeding the late preterm (34−36 6/7 weeks of gestation) and early term infants (37−38 6/7 weeks of gestation), second revision 2016. *Breastfeed Med*. 2016;11:494−500.

ABM protocols expire 5 years from the date of publication.

The content of this protocol is up-to-date at the time of publication. Evidence-based revisions are made within 5 years or sooner if there are significant changes in the evidence.
The Academy of Breastfeeding Medicine Protocol Committee:
Sarah Reece-Stremtan, MD, Chairperson
Larry Noble, MD, FABM, Translations Chairperson
Melissa Bartick, MD, FABM
Wendy Brodribb, MD, FABM
Maya Bunik, MD, MSPH, FABM
Sarah Calhoun, MD
Sarah Dodd, MD

Megan Elliott-Rudder, MD
Cadey Harrel, MD
Susan Lappin, MD
Ilse Larson, MD
Ruth A. Lawrence, MD, FABM
Kathleen A. Marinelli, MD, FABM
Nicole Marshall, MD

Katrina Mitchell, MD
Casey Rosen-Carole, MD, MPH, MSEd
Susan Rothenberg, MD
Tomoko Seo, MD, FABM
Adora Wonodi, MD
Michal Young, MD, FABM
For correspondence: abm@bfmed.org

ABM Clinical Protocol #30
*Breast Masses, Breast Complaints, and Diagnostic Breast Imaging in the Lactating Woman**

Katrina B. Mitchell[1], Helen M. Johnson[2], Anne Eglash[3] and the Academy of Breastfeeding Medicine*

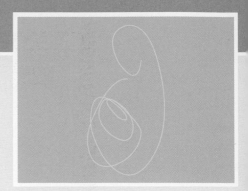

ABSTRACT

A central goal of The Academy of Breastfeeding Medicine is the development of clinical protocols, free from commercial interest or influence, for managing common medical problems that may impact breastfeeding success. These protocols serve only as guidelines for the care of breastfeeding mothers and infants and do not delineate an exclusive course of treatment or serve as standards of medical care. Variations in treatment may be appropriate according to the needs of an individual patient.

INTRODUCTION

BREASTFEEDING WOMEN MAY develop breast masses or complaints at any point during lactation. Symptoms may be related to lactation, such as a lactating adenoma, or may be due to a condition that coincidentally has manifested during the postpartum period. Understanding the importance of appropriate workup and imaging, as well as indications for referral to breast surgery, is essential to establishing a diagnosis and avoiding delay in care.

Breast symptoms require evaluation by physicians and/or lactation consultants and may also require diagnostic breast imaging and/or biopsy. The American College of Radiology (ACR) released new guidelines in 2018 regarding breast imaging of pregnant and lactating women.[1] These guidelines state that all breast imaging studies and biopsies are safe for women to undergo while breastfeeding, and also provide recommendations for maximizing examination sensitivity and minimizing biopsy-related complications in this patient population.

When approaching a breastfeeding woman with breast symptomatology, it is helpful for providers to frame the workup based on the presence or absence of a palpable mass on examination (Fig. 1). Some conditions always present as a mass, whereas others rarely have a palpable finding. However, several conditions have variable presentations and may manifest as a mass and/or another sign/symptom such as nipple discharge (Fig. 2).

Quality of evidence is based on the Oxford Centre for Evidence-Based Medicine 2011 Levels of Evidence[2] (levels I–IV) and is noted in parentheses.

BREAST MASSES

The majority of persistent breast masses warrant diagnostic imaging. Although several breast masses may occur in the setting of lactation and are benign, imaging generally is required to distinguish these from non-lactation-specific breast masses. Both benign and malignant masses unrelated to lactation also may present during the postpartum period. Thus, clinicians should perform axillary and supraclavicular lymph node examinations on all women presenting with a breast mass. Specific masses and/or associated symptomatology may warrant referral to a breast surgeon for biopsy or intervention. The most common breast masses diagnosed during lactation are highlighted in Table 1.

Lactation-specific masses

When history and examination by an experienced breastfeeding medicine physician are consistent with a lactation-related condition that the provider is comfortable managing, imaging can be deferred. If the condition presents atypically or does not resolve with standard treatment, diagnostic imaging is indicated. Examples of such conditions include the following:

- **Accessory breast tissue** occurs in 2–6% of women, most commonly in the axilla, with bilaterality in about one-third of cases. Although this tissue is congenital, women

* Courtesy of the Academy of Breastfeeding Medicine. Please go to https://www.bfmed.org/protocols for complete protocols, translations, and the most up-to-date information (protocols are updated every 5–7 years).

[1] Breast Surgical Oncology, Presbyterian Healthcare Services-MD Anderson Cancer Network, Albuquerque, New Mexico.

[2] Department of Surgery, Brody School of Medicine, East Carolina University, Greenville, North Carolina.

[3] Department of Family and Community Medicine, University of Wisconsin School of Medicine and Public Health, Madison, Wisconsin.

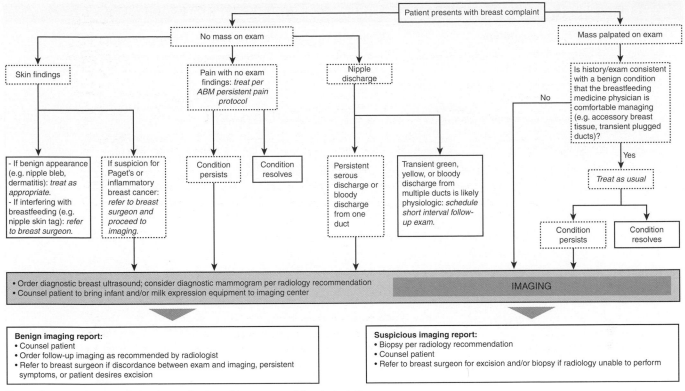

Fig. 1 Suggested approach for the evaluation of breast complaints in lactating women.

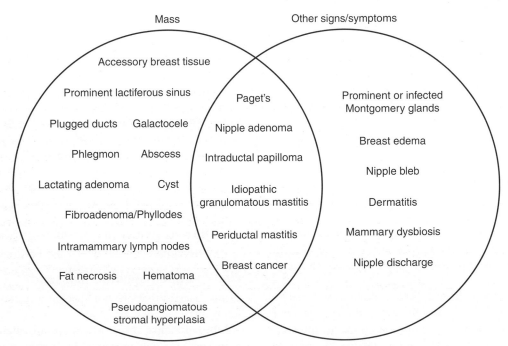

Fig. 2 Presenting signs/symptoms of common breast conditions that may affect lactating women.

may not notice its presence until they experience physiologic breast growth during pregnancy and lactation[3] (IV). Women may describe fullness during pregnancy and engorgement, and the tissue may be irritating while wearing a bra. If engorgement of this tissue does not resolve after several weeks postpartum, diagnostic imaging is indicated to rule out an alternative diagnosis.

- **Plugged ducts** occur in areas of milk stasis usually localized to a specific quadrant of the breast and resulting

TABLE 1   Most Common Breast Masses Diagnosed During Lactation

Condition	Clinical presentation	Diagnostic considerations	Treatment options
Lactating adenoma	Painless rubbery mobile mass. Often in upper outer quadrant. Grows rapidly due to hormonal stimulation.	Core needle biopsy recommended to establish diagnosis	Observation (mass spontaneously regresses after weaning)
Galactocele	Painless lump, may be single or multiple, unilateral or bilateral. Somewhat more common in the retroareolar region.	Aspiration of milky fluid can confirm the diagnosis. At risk for infection due to milk stasis, so may mimic abscess.	Observation (mass spontaneously resolves) versus serial aspirations and or/drainage catheter for symptomatic control
Phlegmon	Tender persistent mass in ductal distribution	May or may not have antecedent and/or concomitant infectious symptoms (e.g., erythema)	Conservative measures (e.g., ice), antibiotic therapy, and surveillance to monitor for progression to abscess
Abscess	Fluctuant tender mass with overlying erythema and induration	Aspiration or drainage of purulent material can confirm the diagnosis	Drainage +/− antibiotic therapy
Fibroadenoma	Rubbery smooth mobile mass. More common in upper outer quadrant. May be asymptomatic or tender. Growth during pregnancy and/or lactation.	Core needle biopsy is recommended for lesions >2–3 cm to rule out Phyllodes tumor, significant growth rate, and/or discordance between clinical and radiographic findings	Surveillance versus surgical excision for symptomatic control
Breast cancer	Variable. May be occult, present as a mass (usually nontender), present as skin/soft tissue changes such as dimpling or nipple retraction, or present with spontaneous bloody or serous nipple discharge.	Core needle biopsy, image guided in the case of nonpalpable cancers, is required for diagnosis and treatment selection. In the case of an equivocal percutaneous biopsy, surgical biopsy may be required.	Treatment varies according to stage and tumor characteristics such as histologic subtype and hormonal receptor expression

from milk that has remained unemptied. Plugs generally are self-limited and resolve with conservative measures such as increasing feeding frequency and gentle massage[4] (IV). Recurrent or persistent plugging in a ductal distribution that does not resolve with conservative measures is an indication for diagnostic imaging.

Lactation-specific masses that require imaging for diagnosis include the following:

- **Galactocele**, also known as a milk retention cyst, results from a persistent plugged duct. Galactocele is the most common benign breast mass in lactating women[5] (IV). Large galactoceles may require referral to a breast surgeon for serial aspirations for symptomatic control. In addition, galactoceles are at risk for infection due to stasis and may warrant intervention such as drainage[6] (IV).
- **Phlegmon**, a poorly defined fluid collection that results from obstruction and inflammation with or without infection, is well described in the surgical literature on perforated appendicitis and diverticulitis. A similar inflammatory phenomenon occurs in the lactating breast and may present as a tender mass in a ductal distribution, often associated with a recent or concurrent history of mastitis. It may have an irregular, heterogeneous, and vascular appearance on imaging and, therefore, may warrant biopsy to rule out malignancy[7] (IV).
- **Abscess** is a well-defined fluid collection that progresses from unresolved mastitis in ~3% of cases[8] (II). A

galactocele also may undergo conversion to an infected galactocele, and a phlegmon may develop into a drainable fluid collection. Treatment options include antibiotics, aspiration, and catheter drainage. Surgical drainage no longer represents first-line treatment[9,10] (IV, I).

- **Lactating adenomas** are painless benign masses that often present in the upper outer quadrant of breast tissue in pregnant and lactating patients, and likely are a result of hormonal stimulation. They can grow large quickly, and involute spontaneously with cessation of lactation[11] (IV). Biopsy is recommended to establish the diagnosis.
- **Lactiferous sinuses** may be more prominent in breastfeeding women and present as a subareolar mass[12] (IV).

Non-lactation-specific masses

Benign masses that are not specific to lactation include the following:

- **Fibroadenoma**, the most common benign breast mass to present in the reproductive years, is highlighted in Table 1.
- **Phyllodes tumor**, a fibroepithelial lesion similar to a fibroadenoma, has the potential for malignant transformation. Any suspicion of phyllodes requires surgical excision to rule out malignancy[13] (IV).
- **Cysts** are particularly common in women with fibrocystic breasts and are readily classified as simple or complex by ultrasonography. Complex cysts require aspiration

for cytologic analysis, whereas simple cysts can be observed[14] (IV).

- **Pseudoangiomatous stromal hyperplasia is a benign**, often irregular, firm mobile mass that can grow large but does not require surgical excision if proven on biopsy[15] (IV).
- **Intramammary lymph nodes**, although uncommon to palpate, are sometimes discovered by patients. Imaging can distinguish between benign versus malignant appearance[16] (I).
- **Fat necrosis** is common after previous breast surgery or trauma; although benign, this condition may present as an irregular palpable mass that may be tender or asymptomatic[17] (IV).
- **Hematoma** can also develop after trauma, such as a motor vehicle accident involving seat belt injury, or vigorous massage in the setting of lactation[18] (IV). In addition to a mass, transient nipple discharge may occur.
- **Periductal mastitis** is an uncommon condition that generally presents in smokers and results from squamous metaplasia of the lactiferous ducts. Patients experience chronic, persistent abscesses, and fistulae in the superficial periareolar region. Optimal treatment Is controversial and may include smoking cessation, antibiotic therapy, and/or drainage, with surgical excision reserved for refractory cases[19] (IV).
- **Idiopathic granulomatous mastitis** is an inflammatory disorder of the breast with unclear etiology that results in erythema, abscess, and fistula formation. It most often occurs in young women of Hispanic descent within several years of pregnancy or lactation[20] (IV). The presentation is variable and can mimic other conditions such as bacterial mastitis or inflammatory breast cancer. Diagnosis is made by exclusion, including negative cultures to rule out infectious mastitis and biopsy to rule out malignancy and to confirm histopathologic evidence of noncaseating granulomas.

Breast cancer (Table 1) is the most commonly diagnosed malignancy among women in their reproductive years and thus may present during lactation. In addition, breastfeeding women are at risk for postpartum breast cancer, which has higher risk of metastatic spread than other forms of breast cancer. Women with postpartum breast cancer have markedly lower 5-year overall survival when compared with nulliparous cases, even adjusting for biologic subtype and stage at diagnosis[21] (III). Breast cancer is a broad term that includes preinvasive disease and invasive disease. Diagnosis is established histologically. Management is multidisciplinary in nature and is complex, tailored to the individual patient.

NON-MASS BREAST COMPLAINTS

Breastfeeding women seeking medical evaluation of breast symptoms who do not have a palpable mass on examination may present with a variety of conditions, some of which require diagnostic imaging. These conditions can be categorized into skin conditions, nipple discharge, and breast pain.

Skin conditions

A number of skin conditions can be diagnosed by history and physical examination and thus do not require diagnostic imaging. Benign lesions that are interfering with breastfeeding, such as a skin tag on the nipple—areolar complex (NAC), warrant referral to a breast surgeon. Lesions that raise suspicion for Paget's disease, inflammatory breast cancer, or other malignancy require both diagnostic imaging and referral to a breast surgeon.

Examples of skin conditions for which breastfeeding women may seek care include the following:

- **Montgomery glands** serve to lubricate the areola and nipple and attract the infant to the breast through olfactory signals. They naturally enlarge during lactation and pregnancy and may not have been noticeable before this time[22] (IV). They may become obstructed and/or infected like any other sebaceous gland and require treatment with warm compresses and/or topical antibiotics.
- **Breast edema** is common in women with larger breasts. It may become more pronounced during pregnancy and lactation, particularly in the immediate postpartum period associated with engorgement. Reassuring features include bilaterality, edema confined only to the dependent portion of the breast, and improvement with supportive bras. If the patient or provider is concerned, referral can be made for diagnostic imaging and breast surgery evaluation.
- **Nipple bleb** an inflammatory lesion of the surface of one or multiple nipple orifices is often white or yellow. Blebs can cause significant latch pain and/or ductal obstruction despite their small size. They may resolve spontaneously. Management for more tenacious blebs includes warm compresses, steroid cream, or procedural unroofing[23] (IV). If persistent and/or causing plugging and mass-like obstruction, imaging may be warranted in certain patients.
- **Dermatitis** may be localized to the NAC or involves the skin of the breast. The risk of dermatitis may be increased in a breastfeeding patient with a history of atopy and allergy: the mother may have an allergy to ingredients in nipple creams such as lanolin, or allergic to substances the child is touching or ingesting[24] (IV).
- **Subacute mastitis, or mammary dysbiosis**, also may cause nipple flaking, erythema, blebs, and scabbing of the nipple and areola with associated deep breast pain. This condition has been termed "mammary candidiasis" in this past, but newer research is disproving the causative agent as yeast and implicating bacterial imbalance instead[25] (IV).
- **Paget's disease** is an eczematous oozing itching lesion of the NAC usually associated with underlying breast malignancy. It arises on the nipple and progresses to the areola; this develops in contrast to dermatitis, which generally behaves oppositely. If Paget's disease is suspected, referral to a breast surgeon for punch biopsy and diagnostic imaging is required[26] (III).

- **Nipple adenoma**, also known as erosive adenomatosis of the nipple, nipple papillomatosis, or papillary adenoma of the nipple, presents with a nipple nodule, nipple erosion, and/or nipple discharge and can mimic Paget's disease. Nipple adenomas are benign lesions, although they may be associated with preinvasive or invasive lesions[27] (IV).

Nipple discharge

Although breastfeeding women experience physiologic milk expression from their nipple orifices, they also may note other colors of **nipple discharge** during lactation. Bilateral multiduct discharge that is yellow or green is generally not concerning and considered physiologic[28] (IV). Serous nipple discharge is more concerning for malignancy and should be evaluated with diagnostic imaging.

Bloody discharge may be due to several conditions including the following:

- **"Rusty pipe syndrome"** is the term for transient bilateral multiduct rusty brown or bloody discharge seen in the first few weeks of lactation that resolves spontaneously[29] (IV).
- In addition, bloody nipple discharge may occur in up to 24% of women at any point during lactation[30] (IV). This phenomenon is related to proliferative epithelial changes and increased vascularity in the breast, and is usually self-limited. Persistent bloody nipple discharge presenting after the immediate postpartum period should be evaluated with diagnostic imaging.
- **Papillary** lesions of the breast, which represent a spectrum of disease from benign **intraductal papilloma** to **papillary carcinoma**, often present with bloody nipple discharge. Persistent unilateral bloody nipple discharge, particularly from a single duct and/or if associated with a subareolar mass, warrants imaging[31] (IV).
- Although pink- or red-tinged expressed milk may raise concern for bloody nipple discharge, this phenomenon may be due to colonization with the pigment-producing bacterium *Serratia marcescens* and should resolve with antibiotic therapy[32] (IV).

Breast pain

The workup and treatment for breast pain in lactating women with no mass or other physical examination findings to suggest a diagnosis have been previously described and are beyond the scope of this protocol[33] (IV). Women with pain that does not resolve with appropriate intervention should undergo diagnostic imaging.

DIAGNOSTIC BREAST IMAGING AND BREAST BIOPSY DURING LACTATION

Few international organizations report specific recommendations regarding breast imaging during lactation. The ACR recommends that diagnostic breast imaging in lactating women follow the same guidelines as for nonlactating women[1] (IV), with the exception of ductography that is not recommended in lactation[34] (IV). As shown in Fig. 1, we recommend diagnostic breast imaging of almost all breast masses and for several specific non-mass breast complaints.

For diagnostic imaging in a breastfeeding woman, ultrasonography is recommended as the initial imaging modality. If ultrasonography shows suspicious findings or is discordant with clinical examination, additional imaging with mammography or digital breast tomosynthesis (DBT, or "3D mammography") may be indicated.[1] This is related to the fact that mammogram or DBT can visualize architectural distortion and/or calcifications not seen on ultrasonography, as well as delineate extent of disease in the setting of malignancy[35] (IV).

Core needle biopsy rather than fine needle aspiration should be performed after a full diagnostic imaging workup has been completed. Core needle biopsy generally can be performed under ultrasound guidance for a palpable mass. However, if the mass does not have an ultrasound correlate, a woman may be recommended to undergo a stereotactic core needle biopsy with mammographic guidance or a magnetic resonance imaging (MRI)-guided biopsy. Although there is a small but rare risk of milk fistula, this risk should not preclude biopsy of any suspicious lesion[36] (IV). Lactating women should also be counseled about a theoretical small increased risk of postprocedural bleeding secondary to hypervascularity[37] (IV). We do not recommend discontinuation of breastfeeding before biopsy in an effort to minimize these risks. In fact, the inflammation related to abrupt weaning[38] (IV) could increase the risk of fistula formation, and lack of alternative drainage routes (e.g., through the nipple) could promote fistula formation through the biopsy tract.

If a woman is diagnosed with a breast malignancy on initial imaging and biopsy, she may be recommended to undergo additional biopsy of suspicious lymph nodes in her regional nodal basins (axillary, internal mammary, and supra- and infraclavicular). Breast radiology and breast surgical oncology also may recommend breast MRI to rule out multifocal or multicentric tumors, contralateral disease, or pectoralis and/or skin involvement. Although MRI is less sensitive in the setting of lactation due to increased parenchymal density and vascularity, it nevertheless is not contraindicated and may provide diagnostic and treatment planning benefit.[1]

RECOMMENDATIONS FOR FUTURE RESEARCH

Although there is strong evidence for the safety and feasibility of nearly all breast imaging studies in lactating women, the data on the relative sensitivities of each modality are limited. There is a growing body of literature that describes normal imaging findings in the lactating breast compared with the nonlactating breast, but there is a paucity of data on the radiologic differences between lactating women with specific pathologies and lactating women without breast lesions. Another area for further study is the management of breast masses and breast complaints of transgender individuals who are chestfeeding. In the absence of specific data, it is reasonable to follow the algorithms described herein for lactating women.

REFERENCES

1. Expert Panel on Breast Imaging, diFlorio-Alexander RM, Slanetz PJ, Moy L, et al. ACR Appropriateness Criteria® Breast imaging of pregnant and lactating women. *J Am Coll Radiol.* 2018;15:S263–S275.

2. OCEBM Levels of Evidence Working Group. The Oxford2011 Levels of Evidence. Oxford Centre for Evidence Based Medicine. Available at: http://www.cebm.net/index.aspx? o = 5653 (accessed January 30, 2019).

3. Lesavoy MA, Gomez-Garcia A, Nejdl R, et al. Axillary breast tissue: Clinical presentation and surgical treatment. *Ann Plast Surg.* 1995;35:356–360.

4. World Health Organization. Mastitis: Causes and management. 2000. Available at: http://apps.who.int/iris/bitstream/ handle/10665/66230/WHO_FCH_CAH_00.13_eng.pdf? sequence=1 (accessed January 30, 2019).

5. Couto LS, Glassman LM, Batista Abreu DC, et al. Chronic galactocele. *Breast J.* 2016;22:471–472.

6. Ghosh K, Morton MJ, Whaley DH, et al. Infected galactocele: A perplexing problem. *Breast J.* 2004;10:159.

7. Johnson HM, Mitchell KB. Lactational phlegmon: a distinct clinical entity within the mastitis-abscess spectrum. Accepted for presentation at the American Society of Breast Surgeon's 20th Annual Meeting on May 4, 2019, in Dallas, TX. Ann Surg Oncol (in press).

8. Amir LH, Forster D, McLachlan H, et al. Incidence of breast abscess in lactating women: Report from an Australian cohort. *BJOG.* 2004;111:1378–1381.

9. Amir LH. the Academy of Breastfeeding Medicine. ABM Clinical Protocol #4: Mastitis, revised March 2014. *Breastfeed Med.* 2014;9:239–243.

10. Irusen H, Rohwer AC, Steyn DW, et al. Treatments for breast abscess in breastfeeding women. *Cochrane Database Syst Rev.* 2015;17:CD010490.

11. Barco Nebreda I, Vidal MC, Fraile M, et al. Lactating adenoma of the breast. *J Hum Lact.* 2016;32:559–562.

12. Nicholson BT, Harvey JA, Cohen MA. Nipple-areolar complex: Normal anatomy and benign and malignant processes. *Radiographics.* 2009;29:509–523.

13. Tan BY, Acs G, Apple SK, et al. Phyllodes tumours of the breast: A consensus review. *Histopathology.* 2016;68:5–21.

14. Langer A, Mohallem M, Berment H, et al. Breast lumps in pregnant women. *Diagn Interv Imaging.* 2015;96:1077–1087.

15. Virk RK, Khan A. Pseudoangiomatous stromal hyperplasia: An overview. *Arch Pathol Lab Med.* 2010;134:1070–1074.

16. Abdullgaffar B, Gopal P, Abdulrahim M, et al. The significance of intramammary lymph nodes in breast cancer: A systematic review and meta-analysis. *Int J Surg Pathol.* 2012;20:555–563.

17. Tan PH, Lai LM, Carrington EV, et al. Fat necrosis of the breast—A review. *Breast.* 2006;15:313–318.

18. Madden B, Phadtare M, Ayoub Z, et al. Hemorrhagic shock from breast blunt trauma. *Int J Emerg Med.* 2015;8:83.

19. Taffurelli M, Pellegrini A, Santini D, et al. Recurrent periductal mastitis: Surgical treatment. *Surgery.* 2016;160:1689–1692.

20. Barreto DS, Sedgwick EL, Nagi CS, et al. Granulomatous mastitis: Etiology, imaging, pathology, treatment, and clinical findings. *Breast Cancer Res Treat.* 2018;171:527–534.

21. Callihan EB, Gao D, Jindal S, et al. Postpartum diagnosis demonstrates a high risk for metastasis and merits and expanded definition of pregnancy-associated breast cancer. *Breast Cancer Res Treat.* 2013;138:549–559.

22. Doucet S, Soussignan R, Sagot P, et al. The secretion of areolar (Montgomery's) glands from lactating women elicits selective, unconditional responses in neonates. *PLoS One.* 2009;4:37579.

23. Tait P. Nipple pain in breastfeeding women: Causes, treatment, and prevention strategies. *J Midwifery Womens Health.* 2000;45:212–215.

24. Barrett ME, Heller MM, Fullerton Stone H, et al. Dermatoses of the breast in lactation. *Dermatol Ther.* 2013;26:331–336.

25. Eglash A, Plane MB, Mundt M. History, physical and laboratory findings, and clinical outcomes of lactating women treated with antibiotics for chronic breast and/or nipple pain. *J Hum Lact.* 2006;22:429–433.

26. Kothari AS, Beechey-Newman N, Hamed H, et al. Paget disease of the nipple: A multifocal manifestation of higher-risk disease. *Cancer.* 2002;95:1–7.

27. Lee C, Boughey J. Case report of a synchronous nipple adenoma and breast carcinoma with current multi-modality radiologic imaging. *Breast J.* 2016;22:105–110.

28. Stone K, Wheeler A. A review of anatomy, physiology, and benign pathology of the nipple. *Ann Surg Oncol.* 2015;22:3236–3240.

29. Silva JR, Carvalho R, Maia C, et al. Rusty pipe syndrome, a cause of bloody nipple discharge: Case report. *Breastfeed Med.* 2014;9:411–412.

30. Kline TS, Lash SR. The bleeding nipple of pregnancy and postpartum period: A cytologic and histologic study. *Acta Cytol.* 1964;8:336–340.

31. de Paula IB, Campos AM. Breast imaging in patients with nipple discharge. *Radiol Bras.* 2017;50:383–388.

32. Quinn L, Ailsworth M, Matthews E, et al. *Serratia marcescens* colonization causing pink breast milk and pink diapers: A case report and literature review. *Breastfeed Med.* 2018;13:388–394.

33. Berens P, Eglash A, Malloy M, et al. the Academy of Breastfeeding Medicine. ABM Clinical Protocol #26: Persistent pain with breastfeeding. *Breastfeed Med.* 2016;11:46–53.

34. Expert Panel on Breast Imaging, Lee SJ, Trikha S, Moy L, et al. ACR Appropriateness Criteria Evaluation of nipple discharge. *J Am Coll Radiol.* 2017;14:S138–S153.

35. Expert Panel on Breast Imaging, Moy L, Heller SL, Bailey L, et al. ACR Appropriateness Criteria Palpable breast masses. *J Am Coll Radiol.* 2017;14:S203–S224.

36. Larson KE, Valente SA. Milk fistula: Diagnosis, prevention, and treatment. *Breast J.* 2016;22:111–112.

37. Sabate JM, Clotet M, Torrubia S, et al. Radiologic evaluation of breast disorders related to pregnancy and lactation. *Radiographics.* 2007;27(Suppl 1):S101–S124.

38. Silanikove N. Natural and abrupt involution of the mammary gland affects differently the metabolic and health consequences of weaning. *Life Sci.* 2014;102: 10–15.

ABM protocols expire 5 years from the date of publication.

Content of this protocol is up-to-date at the time of publication.
Evidence-based revisions are made within 5 years or sooner if
there are significant changes in the evidence.

Katrina B. Mitchell, MD, lead author
Helen M. Johnson, MD
Anne Eglash, MD
The Academy of Breastfeeding Medicine
Protocol Committee
Michal Young, MD, FABM, Chairperson
Larry Noble, MD, FABM, Translations Chairperson
Sarah Reece-Stremtan, MD, Secretary
Melissa Bartick, MD, FABM
Sarah Calhoun, MD
Sarah Dodd, MD
Megan Elliott-Rudder, MD
Laura Rachel Kair, MD, FABM
Susan Lappin, MD

Ilse Larson, MD
Ruth A. Lawrence, MD, FABM
Yvonne Lefort, MD, FABM
Kathleen A. Marinelli, MD, FABM
Nicole Marshall, MD, MCR
C. Murak, MD
Eliza Myers, MD
Casey Rosen-Carole, MD, MPH, MSEd
Susan Rothenberg, MD, FABM
Audrey Roberts, MD
Tricia Schmidt, MD, IBCLC
Tomoko Seo, MD, FABM
Natasha Sriraman, MD
Elizabeth K. Stehel, MD
Rose St. Fleur, MD
Lori Winter, MD
Adora Wonodi, MD
For correspondence: abm@bfmed.org

ABM Clinical Protocol #31
*Radiology and Nuclear Medicine Studies in Lactating Women**

Katrina B. Mitchell[1], Margaret M. Fleming[2], Philip O. Anderson[3],
Jamie G. Giesbrandt[4] and the Academy of Breastfeeding Medicine*

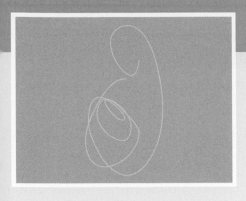

ABSTRACT

A central goal of the Academy of Breastfeeding Medicine is the development of clinical protocols for managing common medical problems that may impact breastfeeding success. These protocols serve only as guidelines for the care of breastfeeding mothers and infants and do not delineate an exclusive course of treatment or serve as standards of medical care. Variations in treatment may be appropriate according to the needs of an individual patient.

INTRODUCTION

BREASTFEEDING WOMEN MAY be required to undergo diagnostic imaging and/or nuclear medicine procedures at any point during lactation. Many women report being incorrectly instructed to discard ("pump and dump") their breast milk or stop breastfeeding after procedures. We seek to provide guidelines and recommendations regarding the safety of common imaging and nuclear medicine procedures performed during lactation. Although the vast majority of circumstances do not require interruption of breastfeeding, certain exceptions do exist and will be reviewed. A summary of recommendations is provided in Table 1.

It should be noted that breastfeeding mothers involved in the care of patients undergoing nuclear medicine procedures and/or imaging studies and procedures should take standard precautions. However, due to the fact that these health care workers are not directly ingesting, inhaling, or receiving intravenous radiopharmaceuticals and/or contrast, no

---

* Courtesy of the Academy of Breastfeeding Medicine. Please go to https://www.bfmed.org/protocols for complete protocols, translations, and the most up-to-date information (protocols are updated every 5—7 years).
[1] Presbyterian Healthcare Services-MD Anderson Cancer Network, Albuquerque, New Mexico.
[2] Emory University School of Medicine, Atlanta, Georgia.
[3] Division of Clinical Pharmacy, Skaggs School of Pharmacy and Pharmaceutical Sciences, University of California, San Diego, La Jolla, California.
[4] X-Ray Associates of New Mexico, Albuquerque, New Mexico.

interruption in breastfeeding is required. Should a mother have an unexpected exposure, the institutional Radiology Safety Officer (RSO) should be contacted. Other sources for recommendations regarding unintended health care exposures include MotherToBaby.org and Infantrisk.com

RECOMMENDATIONS

Breast imaging

Several organizations, including the American College of Radiology (ACR), have made recommendations regarding breast imaging in pregnant and lactating women.[1–11]

Screening

The ACR states that initiation or continuation of screening mammography should be considered dependent on the patient's individual risk and expected duration of lactation. This includes average risk women of age ≥ 40 years as well as some intermediate- to high-risk women of age <40 years.

There is no contraindication to obtaining a mammogram during lactation. Nursing or expressing milk before mammography is recommended to decrease parenchymal density, thereby improving the sensitivity of mammography. Ultrasound may also be used as a supplemental screening modality in conjunction with mammography. The physiologic increased vascularity caused by lactation results in marked increase in background parenchymal enhancement of the breast on magnetic resonance imaging (MRI). For high-risk women breastfeeding for short periods of time, MRI should be performed 3 months after cessation of lactation. For high-risk women who plan to breastfeed for longer periods of time, MRI may be considered in addition to mammography for screening.

Diagnostic

Diagnostic breast imaging during lactation is the same as that for nonlactating women. For diagnostic evaluation of an area of palpable concern or persistent bloody nipple discharge, ultrasound is often the initial imaging modality. If ultrasound is either negative or demonstrates suspicious findings, additional imaging with mammography may be indicated.

TABLE 1   Common Nuclear Medicine Imaging Agents and Recommendations for Breastfeeding

Imaging agent	Breastfeeding interruption
Noncontrast radiographs	No
Nonvascular administration of iodinated contrast	No
CT with iodinated intravenous contrast	No
MRI with gadolinium-based intravenous contrast	No
Nuclear medicine imaging	
PET	No
Bone scan	No
Thyroid imaging	
I-131	Cessation for this infant
I-123	Recommendations vary, up to 3 weeks
Technetium-99m pertechnetate	Up to 24 hours, depending on dose
Renal imaging	
Tc-99m DTPA	No[a]
Tc-99m MAG3	No[a]
Tc-99m DMSA	No[a]
Tc-99m glucoheptonate	No[a]
Cardiac imaging	
Tc-99m Sestamibi	No[a]
Tc-99m Tetrofosmin	No[a]
MUGA	
Tc-99m RBCs in vitro	No[a]
Tc-99m RBCs in vivo	Up to 12 hours, depending on dose
VQ scan	
Tc-99m MAA	12 hours
Breast imaging	
Screening or diagnostic mammography	No
Ultrasound	No
MRI with gadolinium-based intravenous contrast	No

CT, computed tomography; MRI, magnetic resonance imaging; MUGA, multigated acquisition scan; Tc-99m MAA, technetium-99m macroaggregated albumin; PET, positron emission tomography; Tc-99m MAG3, technetium-99m mertiatide; Tc-99m DMSA, technetium-99m succimer; VQ, ventilation-perfusion.
[a]The International Atomic Energy Administration recommends withholding breastfeeding for 4 hours or one feeding to account for any external radiation and free Tc99m pertechnetate in the product.

Noncontrast enhanced radiographic imaging

The radiation associated with image acquisition in radiography has no effect on the breastmilk itself. This includes plain film radiography, fluoroscopy, mammography, and computed tomography (CT). Do not interrupt breastfeeding for any of these procedures.

Nonvascular administration of iodinated contrast

When iodinated contrast is administered through nonvascular routes, systemic absorption of these contrast agents is low and has few known adverse reactions. However, there are reports of anaphylactoid-like reactions with these agents, so some degree of systemic absorption can occur. With enteral administration (e.g., oral or rectal), excretion is through the fecal route and is dependent on bowel transit time. Intracavity (e.g., hysterosalpingography) or intravesical (e.g., cystography) administration may result in small amounts being absorbed and excreted through the kidneys; however, most contrast drains from the cavity after the conclusion of the procedure. There is a paucity of information regarding concentration of nonvascularly administered contrast agents in breast milk and guidelines on breastfeeding after such procedures are not available.[12,13] However, based on very low systemic absorption rates and known low excretion of intravenously administered contrast into breast milk, we do not recommend routine interruption of breastfeeding for these types of procedures.

CT with iodinated intravenous contrast

CT uses a form of intravenous contrast containing highly bound iodine that helps visualize vascular structures and organs. Less than 1% of the administered maternal dose is excreted into the breast milk,[14,15] and <1% of the contrast ingested by the child is absorbed by the gastrointestinal (GI) tract.[16] Therefore, the systemic dose to the child is <0.01% of the intravenous dose given to the mother. The ACR states in its published manual on contrast media that it is safe for the mother to continue breastfeeding after the administration of intravenous iodinated contrast.[12] This recommendation is based on multiple studies that have demonstrated the safety and efficacy of iodinated contrast in the breastfeeding patient.[14–18] The taste of the breast milk may be altered slightly after administration of intravenous iodinated contrast, but it is not harmful to the breastfeeding child.

MRI with gadolinium-based intravenous contrast

Gadolinium is a heavy metal incorporated into intravenous contrast agents to enhance vascular structures and organs during MRI. Less than 0.04% of the administered maternal dose is excreted into the breast milk,[17,19,20] and <1% of the contrast ingested by the child is absorbed from the GI tract.[20,21] Therefore, the systemic dosage to the child is <0.0004% of the intravenous dose given to the mother. The ACR states in its published manual on contrast media that it is safe for the mother to continue breastfeeding after the administration of intravenous gadolinium-based contrast.[12] This recommendation is based on numerous studies that have shown the safety of gadolinium-based contrast in the breastfeeding patient.[15-21] The taste of the breast milk may be altered slightly after intravenous gadolinium-based contrast, but it is not harmful to the breastfeeding child.

Nuclear medicine imaging

Nuclear medicine imaging involves the use of radioactive materials called radionuclides or radiopharmaceuticals to produce functional imaging of the body. Depending on the study, these materials may be inhaled, injected intravenously, or ingested orally. Images are then obtained to document sites of accumulation within the body.

When advising the breastfeeding patient, consideration must be given to the fact that a child may be exposed to radiation through two routes. The most common route of exposure is radioactivity within the ingested milk itself. The other possible route to consider is external exposure while in proximity to the mother. This second situation occurs when metabolically active lactating breast tissue concentrates the administered radioactivity. This second route of exposure is only a concern with fludeoxyglucose-F18 (FDG), the agent used for positron emission tomography (PET). The other agents discussed do not accumulate within active breast tissue.[22] The risks involved with specific agents are discussed hereunder.

Estimated radiation doses to the child from ingested radioactivity have been reported for the most common radiopharmaceuticals used in diagnostic nuclear medicine. As a general rule, no interruption of breastfeeding is required for radiation doses <100 mrem (1 mSV).[23] Both the Nuclear Regulatory Commission (NRC) and International Commission on Radiological Protection (ICRP) have published guidelines for the most commonly used radiopharmaceuticals. Note that recommendations for some agents differ between the NRC and ICRP, and the International Atomic Energy Agency (IAEA) recommends an interruption of breastfeeding for four hours or one feeding to account for any external radiation and free Tc99m pertechnetate in the product.[22-31]

Positron emission tomography

PET is one of the most commonly ordered nuclear medicine studies and is often used in cancer diagnosis and staging.

FDG is chemically similar to glucose, but with the positron-emitting radionuclide fluorine-18 substituted on the molecule allowing identification of metabolically active lesions in the body.

FDG is not excreted into breast milk. Contact between the mother and child, however, should be limited for 12 hours after the injection of FDG due to radioactivity concentrated within the breast tissue itself. Milk can be expressed and safely given to the child during this time. The milk does not need to be discarded.

Bone scan

Bone scans can be used to detect osseous metastatic disease and most commonly use technetium 99 m medronate (Tc-99m MDP). Very littleTc-99m MDP is excreted into breast milk. No interruption in breastfeeding is required.

Thyroid imaging

There are three radionuclides used in nuclear thyroid imaging: 1−131, I-123, and pertechnetate Tc 99 m. I-131 is most commonly used for the treatment of thyroid cancer or Graves' disease. Although it is sometimes used to assess metastases in the setting of thyroid cancer, I-131 is generally not used for routine thyroid imaging due to its high principle gamma energy (364 keV), high beta emission (resulting in large dose to the thyroid), and long half-life (8.04 days). Use of I-131 requires complete cessation of breastfeeding this child. It is recommended that breastfeeding is stopped at least 4 weeks before receiving a therapeutic dose of I-131. This reduces radiation dose to the breast and reduces the risk of contaminating clothing with milk leakage of radioactive iodine.[32]

I-123 and pertechnetate Tc 99 m are the preferred radionuclides for routine thyroid imaging. I-123 results in a lower dose to the thyroid than I-131 and also has a shorter half-life than I-131 (13 hours versus 8 days). Recommendations with regard to breastfeeding after I-123 administration vary. Some sources cite no interruption required, whereas others recommend up to 3 weeks interruption. We recommend discussion with your local nuclear medicine physician regarding approach to individual patients, as the previous concern for I-124 contamination has likely been resolved.[32] In addition, milk can be measured for radioactivity before being given to the child.[33]

Technetium-99m pertechnetate has a short half-life (6 hours) but higher background levels than radioiodine. It is the preferred agent when the patient has recently received thyroid-blocking agents (such as iodinated contrast media). Breastfeeding recommendations regarding Tc-99m pertechnetate depend on the dose administered, as it does have higher concentrations in breast milk than other radiopharmaceuticals.[34] Owing to potential for differences in radiopharmaceutical production, the length of interruption recommended ranges from 12 to 24 hours, and may be as short as 4 hours for 185 Mbq (5 mCi).[23] The milk expressed can be stored refrigerated and given to the infant after 10 physical half-lives, or about ∼ 60 hours, have elapsed.[34]

Renal imaging

There are four radiopharmaceuticals that are commonly used in renal imaging. Technetium-99m pentetate (Tc-99m DTPA) is used to evaluate glomerular filtration rate (GFR). Technetium-99m mertiatide (Tc-99m MAG3) is used to estimate effective renal plasma flow. Technetium-99m succimer (Tc-99m DMSA) is used to evaluate the renal cortex. Technetium Tc-99m glucoheptonate allows assessment of renal perfusion, renal collecting system/ureters, and renal cortex. No interruption in breastfeeding is required for any of these agents because their free pertechnetate is negligible.

Cardiac imaging

The two most common aspects of cardiac function that may need to be evaluated in the lactating patient include evaluation of myocardial perfusion and assessment of left ventricular function.

A "stress test" is the study used for the evaluation of myocardial perfusion. Stress tests were initially obtained using thallium-201. This radionuclide has since been largely replaced by Tc-99m sestamibi and Tc-99m tetrofosmin. These newer radiopharmaceuticals are now preferred for assessing myocardial perfusion. No interruption in breastfeeding is required when Tc-99m sestamibi or Tc-99m tetrofosmin is used, because lower doses of these Tc-99m compounds are excreted into breast milk.[34,35] The recommendations for thallium vary from a 48-hour to 3-week interruption period. We recommend discussion with your local nuclear medicine physician regarding the approach to individual patients, and consider testing breast milk for radioactivity.[23]

A multigated acquisition scan (MUGA) can be used to assess left ventricular ejection fraction, and technetium-99m pertechnetate is the radionuclide used to label autologous RBCs for this test. The recommendations for MUGA depend on whether in vivo or in vitro labeling of the RBCs was performed. No breastfeeding interruption is required for in vitro labeling, which occurs outside of the patient. However, a 6–12-hour interruption is recommended for in vivo labeling, as Tc-99m pertechnetate is directly injected into the patient using this protocol. The milk expressed can be stored, refrigerated, and given to the infant after 10 physical half-lives, or ~ 60 hours, have elapsed.[34] In breastfeeding patients, an echocardiogram should be strongly considered as an alternative to MUGA, because it is not associated with any radiation.

Ventilation-perfusion scan

A ventilation-perfusion (VQ) scan can be used to evaluate for pulmonary embolism in patients with iodinated contrast allergy or renal insufficiency. Imaging of both perfusion and ventilation is obtained. A mismatched defect in perfusion imaging can indicate the presence of a pulmonary embolism. The perfusion agent used is technetium-99m macroaggregated albumin (Tc-99m MAA). The ventilation agents include Tc-99m DTPA and xenon-133.

For Tc-99m MAA, 12-hour interruption is recommended. Although no interruption is required for the ventilation agents Tc-99m DTPA or xenon gas, a 12-hour interruption is recommended for all VQ scans because these agents are always used in conjunction with the perfusion agent Tc-99m MAA.[34,36,37] During interruption, patients should express breast milk every 3–4 hours for 10–15 minutes or until minimal milk flows. The milk expressed can be stored refrigerated and given to the infant after 10 physical half-lives, or ~ 60 hours, have elapsed.[34,38–40]

It should be noted that CT angiography is the preferred imaging modality for the evaluation of suspected pulmonary embolism in all patients without contraindication to iodinated contrast. In the setting of contrast allergy or renal insufficiency (GFR <30), VQ scan can be performed with the already noted guidelines regarding interruption for Tc-99m MAA.

RECOMMENDATIONS FOR FUTURE RESEARCH

The safety of intravenous contrast agents and commonly used radionuclides has been well studied. As new agents are introduced, further research will need to be performed.

ANNOTATED BIBLIOGRAPHY

For more information on radiology and nuclear medicine protocols for lactating women, please see the Supplementary Data.

SUPPLEMENTARY MATERIAL

Supplementary Data

REFERENCES

1. Boivin G, de Korvin B, Marion J, et al. Is a breast MRI possible and indicated in case of suspicion of breast cancer during lactation? *Diagn Interv Imaging.* 2012;93:823–827.
2. Espinosa LA, Daniel BL, Vidarsson L, et al. The lactating breast: Contrast-enhanced MR imaging of normal tissue and cancer. *Radiology.* 2005;237:429–436.
3. Expert Panel on Breast Imaging, diFlorio-Alexander RM, Slanetz PJ, et al. ACR appropriateness criteria: Breast imaging of pregnant and lactating women. *J Am Coll Radiol.* 2018;15 (11S):S263–S275.
4. Helewa M, Levesque P, Provencher D, et al. Breast cancer, pregnancy, and breastfeeding. *J Obstet Gynaecol Can.* 2002;24:164–180. quiz 181–184.
5. National Comprehensive Cancer Network Inc. NCCN Clinical Practice Guidelines in Oncology: Breast Cancer Screening and Diagnosis. 2018; Version 3.2018. Available at: https://www.nccn.org/professionals/physician_gls/pdf/breast-screening.pdf (accessed November 1, 2018).
6. Newman J. Breastfeeding and radiologic procedures. *Can Fam Physician.* 2007;53:630–631.
7. Obenauer S, Dammert S. Palpable masses in breast during lactation. *Clin Imaging.* 2007;31:1–5.

8. Robbins J, Jeffries D, Roubidoux M, et al. Accuracy of diagnostic mammography and breast ultrasound during pregnancy and lactation. *AJR Am J Roentgenol.* 2011;196:716−722.

9. Sabate JM, Clotet M, Torrubia S, et al. Radiologic evaluation of breast disorders related to pregnancy and lactation. *Radiographics.* 2007;27(Suppl 1):S101−S124.

10. Talele AC, Slanetz PJ, Edmister WB, et al. The lactating breast: MRI findings and literature review. *Breast J.* 2003;9:237−240.

11. Vashi R, Hooley R, Butler R, et al. Breast imaging of the pregnant and lactating patient: Physiologic changes and common benign entities. *AJR Am J Roentgenol.* 2013;200:329−336.

12. American College of Radiology. ACR Manual on Contrast Media. Administration of contrast media to women who are breast-feeding. 2018 (Version 10.3), 99−100. Available at: https://www.acr.org/-/media/ACR/Files/Clinical-Resources/Contrast_Media.pdf (accessed November 1, 2018).

13. Davis PL. Anaphylactoid reactions to the nonvascular administration of water-soluble iodinated contrast media. *AJR Am J Roentgenol.* 2015;204:1140−1145.

14. Bettmann MA. Frequently asked questions: Iodinated contrast agents. *Radiographics.* 2004;24(Suppl 1):S3−S10.

15. Webb JA, Thomsen HS, Morcos SK. Members of Contrast Media Safety Committee of European Society of Urogenital Radiology (ESUR). The use of iodinated and gadolinium contrast media during pregnancy and lactation. *Eur Radiol.* 2005;15:1234−1240.

16. Tremblay E, Therasse E, Thomassin-Naggara I, et al. Quality initiatives: Guidelines for use of medical imaging during pregnancy and lactation. *Radiographics.* 2012;32:897−911.

17. Wang PI, Chong ST, Kielar AZ, et al. Imaging of pregnant and lactating patients: Part 1, evidence-based review and recommendations. *AJR Am J Roentgenol.* 2012;198:778−784.

18. Tirada N, Dreizin D, Khati NJ, et al. Imaging pregnant and lactating patients. *Radiographics.* 2015;35:1751−1765.

19. Rofsky NM, Weinreb JC, Litt AW. Quantitative analysis of gadopentetate dimeglumine excreted in breast milk. *J Magn Reson Imaging.* 1993;3:131−132.

20. Kubik-Huch RA, Gottstein-Aalame NM, Frenzel T, et al. Gadopentetate dimeglumine excretion into human breast milk during lactation. *Radiology.* 2000;216:555−558.

21. Lin SP, Brown JJ. MR contrast agents: Physical and pharmacologic basics. *J Magn Reson Imaging.* 2007;25:884−899.

22. Siegel J. Guide for Diagnostic Nuclear Medicine. Nuclear Regulatory Commission Regulation of Nuclear Medicine; 2002. Available at: https://www.nrc.gov/materials/miau/miaureg-initiatives/guide_2002.pdf (accessed November 1, 2018).

23. Stabin MG, Breitz HB. Breast milk excretion of radiopharmaceuticals: Mechanisms, findings, and radiation dosimetry. *J Nucl Med.* 2000;41:863−873.

24. International Commission on Radiological Protection. Radiation Dose to Patients from Radiopharmaceuticals. Annex D. Recommendations on breastfeeding interruptions. ICRP Publication 106. *Annals of the ICRP.* 2008;38:163−165.

25. Alexander EK, Pearce EN, Brent GA, et al. 2017 Guidelines of the American Thyroid Association for the diagnosis and management of thyroid disease during pregnancy and the postpartum. *Thyroid.* 2017;27:315−389.

26. Howe DB, Beardsley M, Bakhsh S. Consolidated Guidance About Materials Licenses: Program-Specific Guidance About Medical Use Licenses. Vol. 9; 2008. Available at: https://www.nrc.gov/docs/ML0734/ML073400289.pdf (accessed November 1, 2018).

27. Jamar F, Buscombe J, Chiti A, et al. EANM/SNMMI guideline for 18F-FDG use in inflammation and infection. *J Nucl Med.* 2013;54:647−658.

28. Mettler F, Guiberteau M. *Essentials of Nuclear Medicine Imaging.* 6th ed. Philadelphia, PA: Saunders Elsevier; 2012:565−567.

29. Society of Nuclear Medicine. The SNM Procedure Guideline for General Imaging 6.0. 2010 (Version 6.0). Available at: http://snmmi.files.cms-plus.com/docs/General_Imaging_Version_6.0.pdf (accessed November 1, 2018).

30. Mandel SJ, Shankar LK, Benard F, et al. Superiority of iodine-123 compared with iodine-131 scanning for thyroid remnants in patients with differentiated thyroid cancer. *Clin Nucl Med.* 2001;26:6−9.

31. International Atomic Energy Agency. Radiation Protection and Safety in Medical Uses of Ionizing Radiation, IAEA Safety Standards Series No. SSG-46, IAEA, Vienna. 2018. Available at: https//www.iaea.org/publications/11102/radiation-protectionand-safety-in-medical-uses-of-ionizing-radiation (accessed April 26, 2019).

32. Drugs and Lactation Database (LactMed) [Internet]. Bethesda (MD): National Library of Medicine (US); 2006. Sodium Iodide I 131. Updated October 31, 2018. Available at: https://www.ncbi.nlm.nih.gov/books/NBK501563 (accessed April 22, 2019).

33. Romney B, Nickoloff EL, Esser PD. Excretion of radioiodine in breast milk. *J Nucl Med.* 1989;30:124−126.

34. Leide-Svegborn S, Ahlgren L, Johansson L, et al. Excretion of radionuclides in human breast milk after nuclear medicine examinations. Biokinetic and dosimetric data and recommendations on breastfeeding interruption. *Eur J Nucl Med Mol Imaging.* 2016;43:808−821.

35. Drugs and Lactation Database (LactMed) [Internet]. Bethesda (MD): National Library of Medicine (US); 2006-. Technetium Tc 99m Sestamibi. Updated October 31, 2018). Available at: https://www.ncbi.nlm.nih.gov/books/NBK501581 (accessed April 22, 2019).

36. Howe DB, Beardsley M, Bakhsh S. Appendix U. Model Procedure for Release of Patients or Human Research Subjects Administered Radioactive Materials. NUREG1556. Consolidated guidance about materials licenses. Program-specific guidance about medical use licenses. Final report. U.S. Nuclear Regulatory Commission Office of Nuclear Material Safety and Safeguards. 2008;9, Rev. 2. Available at: www.nrc.gov/reading-rm/doc-collections/nuregs/staff/sr1556/v9/r2 (accessed April 22, 2019).

37. Mattsson S, Johansson L, Leide Svegborn S, et al. Radiation dose to patients from radiopharmaceuticals: A compendium of current information related to frequently used substances. *Ann ICRP.* 2015;44(2 Suppl):7−321.

38. Mountford PJ, Coakley AJ. A review of the secretion of radioactivity in human breast milk: Data, quantitative analysis and recommendations. *Nucl Med Commun.* 1989;10:15−27.

39. Early PJ, Sodee DB. *Principles and Practice of Nuclear Medicine.* 2nd ed. St. Louis: Mosby-Year Book, Inc; 1995:1380−1381.

40. Administration of Radioactive Substances Advisory Committee. Notes for guidance on the clinical administration of radiopharmaceuticals and use of sealed radioactive sources. 2006;25−27. Available at: www.arsac.org.uk (accessed April 22, 2019).

Katrina B. Mitchell, MD, lead author
Margaret M. Fleming, MD, MSc
Philip O. Anderson, PharmD, FASHP
Jamie G. Giesbrandt, MD
The Academy of Breastfeeding Medicine Protocol Committee:
Michal Young, MD, Chairperson
Larry Noble, MD, Translations Chairperson
Sarah Reece-Stremtan, MD, Secretary
Melissa Bartick, MD, MSc
Sarah Calhoun, MD
Sarah Dodd, MD
Megan Elliott-Rudder, PhD, MBBS
Laura Rachel Kair, MD
Susan Lappin, MD

Ilse Larson, MD
Ruth A. Lawrence, MD
Yvonne LeFort, MD
Kathleen A. Marinelli, MD
Nicole Marshall, MD
Catherine Murak, MD
Eliza Myers, MD
Adora Okogbule-Wonodi, MD
Audrey Roberts, MD
Casey Rosen-Carole, MD, MPH, MSEd
Susan Rothenberg, MD
Tricia Schmidt, MD
Tomoko Seo, MD
Natasha Sriraman, MD, MPH
Elizabeth K. Stehel, MD
Rose St. Fleur, MD
Nancy Wight, MD
Lori Winter, MD, MPH
For correspondence: abm@bfmed.org

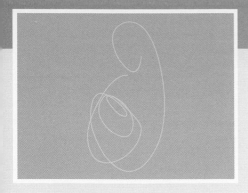

ABM Clinical Protocol #32
*Management of Hyperlactation**

Helen M. Johnson[1], Anne Eglash[2], Katrina B. Mitchell[3],
Kathy Leeper[4], Christina M. Smillie[5], Lindsay Moore-Ostby[6],
Nadine Manson[7], Liliana Simon[8] and
the Academy of Breastfeeding Medicine

ABSTRACT

A central goal of the Academy of Breastfeeding Medicine is the development of clinical protocols for managing common medical problems that may impact breastfeeding success. These protocols serve only as guidelines for the care of breast-feeding mothers and infants and do not delineate an exclusive course of treatment or serve as standards of medical care. Variations in treatment may be appropriate according to the needs of an individual patient.

INTRODUCTION

THE AIM OF THIS PROTOCOL is to review the diagnosis of hyperlactation and describe management recommendations. Throughout this protocol, the quality of evidence based on the Oxford Centre for Evidence-Based Medicine 2011 Levels of Evidence (Levels 1–5)[1] is noted in parentheses.

Hyperlactation, also termed hypergalactia or "oversupply," is the production of breast milk in excess of the volume required for growth of healthy infant(s) based on international standards. No precise definition for this term exists, so reported cases constitute a wide spectrum of excess volumes. An average term infant consumes 450–1,200 mL daily (Level 4),[2] and production volumes higher than this may represent hyperlactation.

Multiple factors regulate milk production homeostasis (Levels 3 and 4).[3,4] These include the following:
- Amount of mammary glandular tissue in an individual breast
- Alveolar distension in the breast
- Degree and frequency of milk emptying
- Complex neuroendocrine pathways

In addition, the complex signaling of serotonin and possibly other bioactive factors may mediate some of the actions previously attributed to a single substance termed "Feedback Inhibitor of Lactation" (Level 4).[5]

Patients with hyperlactation may experience multiple breast-feeding complications, including breast pain, plugged ducts, and mastitis. Dyads are at risk for early weaning and/or exclusive pumping due to latch difficulties and/or forceful letdown. Maternal and infant signs and symptoms of hyperlactation are summarized in Table 1. If medical complications and/or psychological distress occur, women with hyperlactation may be advised to decrease their milk production. Behavioral interventions, herbal therapies, and prescription medications have been used to treat hyperlactation, with varying success rates and levels of evidence. As the effect of each intervention may vary between individuals, determination of optimal therapy regimens, such as dosage and frequency, remains challenging.

DIFFERENTIAL DIAGNOSIS

Hyperlactation may be self-induced, iatrogenic, or idiopathic.
- *Self-induced hyperlactation* occurs when the mother stimulates production of more milk than the infant requires. This may occur from excessive pumping in addition to breastfeeding. Mothers may fear not having sufficient milk in the future, desire to donate milk, or misunderstand that they do not need to store high volumes of milk for return to work. Women who exclusively pump may produce more milk than needed for the infant(s). Women also may self-induce a rate of milk production higher than needed by their infant(s) by taking herbal substances and/or prescription medications that may increase milk production.

* Courtesy of the Academy of Breastfeeding Medicine. Please go to https://www.bfmed.org/protocols for complete protocols, translations, and the most up-to-date information (protocols are updated every 5–7 years).
[1] Department of Surgery, Brody School of Medicine, East Carolina University, Greenville, North Carolina.
[2] Department of Family and Community Medicine, University of Wisconsin School of Medicine and Public Health, Madison, Wisconsin.
[3] Surgical Oncology, Ridley Tree Cancer Center at Sansum Clinic, Santa Barbara, California.
[4] MilkWorks Breastfeeding Center, Lincoln and Omaha, Nebraska.
[5] Breastfeeding Resources, Stratford, Connecticut.
[6] Internal Medicine and Pediatrics - Primary Care, HealthNet, Indianapolis, Indiana.
[7] Department of Family Medicine, McMaster University, Hamilton, Ontario, Canada.
[8] Department of Pediatrics, University of Maryland Medical Center, Baltimore, Maryland.

TABLE 1   Signs and Symptoms That May Be Associated with Hyperlactation in the Breastfeeding Dyad

Maternal signs/symptoms	Infant signs/symptoms
Excessive breast growth during pregnancy >2 cup sizes	Excessive weight gain
Persistent or frequent breast fullness	Difficulty achieving a sustained, deep latch
Breast and/or nipple pain	Fussiness at the breast
Copious milk leakage	Choking, coughing, or unlatching during feeds
Recurrent plugged ducts	Breast refusal
Recurrent mastitis	Clamping down on the nipple/areola
Nipple blebs	Short feedings
Vasospasm	Gastrointestinal symptoms (e.g., spitting up, gas, reflux, or explosive green stools)

- *Iatrogenic hyperlactation* occurs when health professionals contribute to excessive milk production. Providers may advise women to take galactogogues (i.e., substances that increase the rate of human milk synthesis) without close follow-up and/or guidance regarding cessation. In addition to prescribing metoclopramide and/or domperidone, other medications such as metformin may increase the rate of milk synthesis (Level 4).[6] Health professionals also may advise expressing milk in addition to direct breastfeeding. While this may be appropriate in certain situations, it also may lead to persistent overproduction of milk if not closely monitored.
- *Idiopathic hyperlactation* is a term reserved for mothers who struggle with high rates of milk production with no clear etiology. It is normal for healthy mothers to experience breast fullness in the first several weeks postpartum, as their milk production adjusts to the demands of their infant(s). However, if fullness and high production persist, idiopathic hyperlactation represents a diagnostic consideration.

Although hyperprolactinemia has been suggested as a cause of hyperlactation, no evidence exists that correlates prolactin level with rate of milk production (Levels 3 and 4).[7,8] In fact, mothers with a history of pituitary adenomas have been reported to have insufficient milk production (Level 4).[9]

No consensus exists regarding how early in the postpartum period a diagnosis of hyperlactation can be made. Hyperlactation can be distinguished from engorgement by lack of interstitial edema and persistence of symptoms beyond 1–2 weeks postpartum (Level 4).[10] Mild cases of hyperlactation may never be formally diagnosed, as they may resolve spontaneously within a few months as prolactin levels decline and regulation of milk synthesis shifts from predominantly hormonal to local control (Level 3).[7,11]

MANAGEMENT

General principles

Laboratory testing or pituitary imaging tests are not recommended in the setting of hyperlactation. An algorithm for the suggested management of hyperlactation is presented in Fig. 1. In the absence of data on the relative efficacies of different interventions, we recommend using low-risk, low-cost management strategies before progressing to substances or medications with potential adverse drug reactions (Level 5). Specifically, we recommend the following:

- Behavioral interventions and anticipatory counseling to prevent and treat self-induced and iatrogenic hyperlactation.
- For idiopathic hyperlactation, first line therapy should be block feeding under close supervision by a breastfeeding medicine expert, as detailed below.
- For persistent cases of idiopathic hyperlactation that do not respond adequately to block feeding, herbal therapies and/or prescription medications may be considered. Selection of second line and subsequent therapies should be individualized to the dyad, based on factors such as number of weeks postpartum, potential adverse drug reactions, potential medication interactions, patient preferences, and cultural beliefs.
- Dopamine agonists should be reserved for the most refractory cases of idiopathic hyperlactation, due to risks of serious adverse drug reactions and the potential for complete cessation of milk production.

Until the rate of milk production is normalized, mothers can try using the laid-back/biological nursing position to decrease flow rate and maintain a positive direct breastfeeding relationship. To maximize the fat content of the milk—particularly if there is clinical concern for significant foremilk-hindmilk imbalance—mothers can perform gentle breast massage (Level 3)[12] before feeds and prioritize hand expression over mechanical expression (Level 2)[13] when milk expression is needed. No evidence exists to support the use of cabbage leaves or breast binding in hyperlactation.

Behavioral interventions
Prevention of self-induced and iatrogenic hyperlactation

To avoid a scenario of self-induced or iatrogenic hyperlactation, we recommend counseling breastfeeding mothers and family about the following:

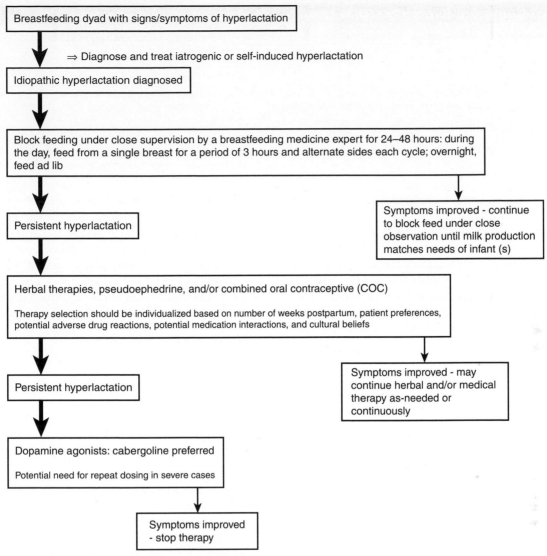

Fig. 1 Algorithm for the diagnosis and management of idiopathic hyperlactation.

- Individualized, rather than prescriptive, recommendations for frequency and duration of direct breastfeeding and expressing milk.
- Avoiding unnecessary consumption of galactogogues, including traditional foods that may contain galactogogues (e.g., herbal teas, curry sauces spiced with fenugreek, soups containing moringa) (Levels 4 and 1).[6,14,15]
- Misconception that healthy term infant feeding volumes will increase significantly beyond the initial 6 weeks of life.
- Cultural expectations about normal infant feeding and sleeping patterns.
- Appropriate quantities of stored milk needed for emergency and/or return to work, according to the specific needs of the dyad.
- Prior challenges with breastfeeding, including fear/anxiety or lower production volumes than desired by mother.
- Misinterpretation of infant feeding cues and fussing as a sign of insufficient milk production.

- Block feeding. Most cases of self-induced and iatrogenic hyperlactation should resolve with removal of external stimuli such as excessive expressing and/or galactogogues. Dyads who exhibit persistent signs and symptoms of hyperlactation or those who experience idiopathic hyperlactation may benefit first from intervention with block feeding.

Block feeding—breastfeeding or expressing milk from one breast for a specific period of time—can decrease overproduction of milk by engaging local breast autocrine regulatory mechanisms. The literature describes several variations of this technique (Level 4).[16,17] We recommend direct breastfeeding or expressing milk from a single breast during a period of 3 hours, alternating breasts each cycle (Level 5). Feeding by time blocks should be performed during the day (e.g., 09:00—18:00) and ad lib feeding from both breasts should be performed overnight (Level 4).[18] If the contralateral breast becomes too full, the mother can express small volumes of milk for comfort. If effective for the dyad, these

TABLE 2   Common Herbal Therapies Used for Hyperlactation Management

Herb	Dosing/ administration	Potential adverse drug reactions
Peppermint oil	No consensus	Heartburn, nausea, vomiting
Sage	1—3 g dried leaves in one cup of hot water, or one dose of sage extract per manufacturer's recommendations	Nausea, vomiting, dizziness, wheezing, agitation, hypoglycemia, seizures
Jasmine	No consensus	Allergic reaction
Chasteberry	No consensus	Nausea, headache, gastrointestinal symptoms, menstrual irregularity, acne, pruritis, exanthema

cycles should result in clinical improvement within 24 to 48 hours.

Due to risks of plugged ducts, mastitis, poor infant weight gain, infant reluctance to cooperate with the block schedule, or too great a decrease in milk production, block feeding requires close supervision by a physician knowledgeable in breastfeeding care. Given differences in response to block feeding, providers should modify management for individual dyads and follow patients throughout the course of block feeding (Level 4).[19] Close monitoring on an individualized daily or weekly basis can help ensure adequate infant growth and reduce maternal complications. Block feeding must be discontinued in the event that milk production falls below the infant's needs.

Herbal therapies

Peppermint, sage, jasmine flowers, and chasteberry commonly have been used to reduce milk production (Table 2).

- No published literature has reported the use of peppermint (Level 4)[20] in the treatment of hyperlactation. Anecdotal evidence supports oral ingestion and topical application to the breast, but infant toxicity (e.g., apnea, muscle weakness) may result from the latter (Level 4).[18]
- There are no scientific studies on the impact of sage (Level 4)[21] on milk production. If a dose of sage is ingested, it is advisable to monitor for effect on milk production for 8—12 hours before repeating the dose (Level 4).[18]
- Jasmine flowers placed on the breast and replaced every 24 hours for 5 days was shown in an older study to be as effective as bromocriptine 2.5 mg three times daily to suppress lactation (Level 2).[22]

- Chasteberry has phytoestrogenic and phytoprogesteronic activity and traditionally has been used to treat gynecologic conditions. The effect of chasteberry (*Vitex agnus castus*) on milk synthesis is controversial (Level 1)[23] and some advise against its use during lactation due to lack of safety data (Level 1).[24]
- Other less widely used herbs, but which are utilized more regionally, include basil, caraway, and parsley (Level 4).[15]

Prescription medications

Pseudoephedrine is a nonprescription decongestant medication that can decrease milk production, although the mechanism of action remains unknown. Aljazaf et al. found that a 60 mg dose decreased milk production by 24% (Level 2).[25] We recommend starting with 30 mg once and observing for infant and maternal adverse drug events for 8—12 hours (Table 3); if no adverse events or decrease in milk production is observed, increase to 60 mg (Level 5). Mothers can continue dosing every 12 hours as needed. The dyad must be followed closely: most mothers will require only as-needed dosing or otherwise risk a too great drop in production. However, a select few may require more scheduled dosing.

Estrogen may significantly decrease milk production in some women (Level 1),[26] particularly at high doses in the early postpartum period (Level 4).[27] The World Health Organization recommends against the use of estrogen-containing oral contraceptives in breastfeeding women in the first 6 weeks after delivery and cautions against use before 6 months postpartum (Level 4).[28] For the treatment of hyperlactation, we recommend prescribing a combined oral contraceptive (COC) that contains 20—35 micrograms (mcg) of

TABLE 3   Common Prescription Medications Used for Hyperlactation Management

Medication	Dosing/ administration	Potential adverse drug reactions
Pseudoephedrine	30—60 mg once to twice daily	Jitteriness, insomnia, irritability, hypertension, tachycardia, arrhythmia
Estrogen	Combined oral contraceptive with 20—35 μg estradiol	Venous thromboembolism, pulmonary embolism
Cabergoline	0.25—0.5 mg every 3—5 days as needed	Headache, nausea, depressed mood, dizziness, drowsiness or nervousness
Bromocriptine	2.5 mg daily for 3 days	Stroke, seizure, severe hypertension, myocardial infarction, psychosis

estradiol, no sooner than 6 weeks postpartum (Level 5). Milk production may significantly decrease within 7 days, at which point the COC could be stopped to prevent further decline (Level 4).[18] For some mothers, continual use of COC maintains milk production at a reasonable rate. Close monitoring is essential given the variability in individual responses.

If hyperlactation persists despite all other interventions, dopamine agonists such as bromocriptine or cabergoline can be utilized. The more ideal side effect profile of cabergoline makes it preferred over bromocriptine in lactating women (Level 4).[29,30] Cabergoline is a long-acting medication with a half-life of ∼68 hours (Level 4).[29] We recommend starting with a single dose of 0.25 milligrams (mg) (Level 5). If the mother experiences no decline in milk production by 72 hours, repeat this dose. If this low dose has no effect, increase the dose to 0.5 mg 3 to 5 days later. If cabergoline is unavailable, bromocriptine may be dosed at 0.25 mg daily for 3 days (Level 2).[31]

RECOMMENDATIONS FOR FUTURE RESEARCH

As current knowledge of physiologic factors associated with endocrine and autocrine control of lactation is largely based on bovine and other animal studies, further research is needed to determine whether similar pathways regulate human milk production. There is a particular need for human lactation research on factors that cause idiopathic hyperlactation and development of dramatic pathology such as gigantomastia. Targeted therapies, such as an upregulator of local inhibitory mediators, can be identified through translational research.

In addition, as limited data exist regarding the methods used to manage hyperlactation, further studies are needed to evaluate the relative efficacies of different management strategies for hyperlactation. Prospective studies would provide high-level data on the effect of specific therapies on milk production. Case series of women treated with a single therapy would improve our understanding of the natural range of responses as well as side effects. Clinical research studies comparing various treatment approaches would provide evidence on relative efficacies. In addition, observational studies could be done to compare different doses of a single therapy.

ANNOTATED BIBLIOGRAPHY

For more information on management of hyperlactation, please see the Supplementary Data.

DISCLOSURE STATEMENT

No competing financial interests exist.

FUNDING INFORMATION

No funding was received.

SUPPLEMENTARY MATERIAL

Supplementary Data

REFERENCES

1. OCEBM Levels of Evidence Working Group. The Oxford 2011 Levels of Evidence. Oxford Centre for Evidence Based Medicine. Available at: www.cebm.net/index.aspx?o = 5653 (accessed May 15, 2019).
2. Lawrence RA, Lawrence RM. *Breastfeeding: A Guide for the Medical Profession.* 8th ed. Philadelphia, PA: Elsevier; 2016.
3. Stull MA, Pai V, Vomachka AJ, et al. Mammary gland homeostasis employs serotonergic regulation of epithelial tight junctions. *Proc Natl Acad Sci U S A.* 2007;104:16708−16713.
4. Collier RJ, Hernandez LL, Horseman ND. Serotonin as a homeostatic regulator of lactation. *Domest Anim Endocrinol.* 2012;43:161−170.
5. Weaver SR, Hernandez LL. Autocrine-paracrine regulation of the mammary gland. *J Dairy Sci.* 2016;99:842−853.
6. Brodribb W. ABM Clinical Protocol #9: Use of galactogogues in initiating or augmenting maternal milk production, second revision 2018. *Breastfeed Med.* 2018;13:307−314.
7. Stuebe AM, Meltzer-Brody S, Pearson B, et al. Maternal neuroendocrine serum levels in exclusively breastfeeding mothers. *Breastfeed Med.* 2015;10:197−202.
8. Saleem M, Martin H, Coates P. Prolactin biology and laboratory measurement: An update on physiology and current analytical issues. *Clin Biochem Rev.* 2018;39:3−16.
9. Laws ER, Ezzat S, Asa SL, Rio LM, et al. *Pituitary Disorders, Diagnosis and Treatment.* West Sussex, UK: Wiley Blackwell; 2013:236.
10. Berens P, Brodribb W. ABM Clinical Protocol #20: Engorgement, revised 2016. *Breastfeed Med.* 2016;11:159−163.
11. Cox DB, Owens RA, Hartmann PE. Blood and milk prolactin and the rate of milk synthesis in women. *Exp Physiol.* 1996;81:1007−1020.
12. Foda MI, Kawashima T, Nakamura S, Kobayashi M, Oku T. Composition of milk obtained from unmassaged versus massaged breasts of lactating mothers. *J Pediatr Gastroenterol Nutr.* 2004;38:484−487.
13. Mangel L, Ovental A, Batscha N, et al. Higher fat content in breastmilk expressed manually: A randomized trial. *Breastfeed Med.* 2015;10:352−354.
14. Budzynska K, Gardner ZE, Dugoua JJ, Low Dog T, Gardiner P. Systematic review of breastfeeding and herbs. *Breastfeed Med.* 2012;7:489−503.
15. Kabiri M, Kamalinejad M, Sohrabvand F, et al. Management of breast milk oversupply in traditional Persian medicine. *J Evid Based Complementary Altern Med.* 2017;22:1044−1050.
16. Livingstone V. Too much of a good thing. Maternal and infant hyperlactation syndromes. *Can Fam Physician.* 1996;42:89−99.
17. van Veldhuizen-Staas CG. Overabundant milk supply: An alternative way to intervene by full drainage and block feeding. *Int Breastfeed J.* 2007;2:11.
18. Eglash A. Treatment of maternal hypergalactia. *Breastfeed Med.* 2014;9:423−425.
19. Smillie CM, Campbell SH, Iwinski S. Hyperlactation: How left-brained 'Rules' for breastfeeding can wreak havoc with a natural process. *Newborn Infant Nurs Rev.* 2005;5:49−58.

20. Drugs and Lactation Database (LactMed) [Internet]. Bethesda (MD): National Library of Medicine (US), 2006-. Peppermint. [Updated 2019]. Available at: www.ncbi.nlm.nih.gov/books/NBK501851 (accessed June 4, 2019).

21. Drugs and Lactation Database (LactMed) [Internet]. Bethesda (MD): National Library of Medicine (US), 2006-. Sage. [Updated 2018]. Available at: www.ncbi.nlm.nih.gov/books/NBK501816 (accessed June 4, 2019).

22. Shrivastav P, George K, Balasubramaniam N, et al. Suppression of puerperal lactation using jasmine flowers (Jasminum sambac). *Aust N Z J Obstet Gynaecol.* 1988;28:68−71.

23. Dugoua JJ, Seely D, Perri D, et al. Safety and efficacy of chastetree (Vitex agnus-castus) during pregnancy and lactation. *Can J Clin Pharmacol.* 2000;15:e74−e79.

24. Daniele C, Thompson Coon J, Pittler MH, et al. Vitex agnus castus: A systematic review of adverse events. *Drug Saf.* 2005;28:319−332.

25. Aljazaf K, Hale TW, Ilett KF, et al. Pseudoephedrine: Effects on milk production in women and estimation of infant exposure via breastmilk. *Br J Clin Pharmacol.* 2003;56:18−24.

26. Lopez LM, Grey TW, Stuebe AM, et al. Combined hormonal versus nonhormonal versus progestin-only contraception in lactation. *Cochrane Database Syst Rev.* 2015;CD003988.

27. Berens P, Labbok M. ABM Clinical Protocol #13: Contraception during breastfeeding, revised 2015. *Breastfeed Med.* 2015;10:3−12.

28. World Health Organization Department of Reproductive Health and Research. *Medical Eligibility Criteria for Contraceptive Use: Executive Summary.* 5th ed. Geneva: World Health Organization; 2015.

29. Drugs and Lactation Database (LactMed) [Internet]. Bethesda (MD): National Library of Medicine (US), 2006. Cabergoline. [Updated 2018]. Available at: www.ncbi.nlm.nih.gov/books/NBK501327 (accessed June 4, 2019).

30. Drugs and Lactation Database (LactMed) [Internet]. Bethesda (MD): National Library of Medicine (US), 2006. Bromocriptine. [Updated 2018]. Available at: www.ncbi.nlm.nih.gov/books/NBK501306 (accessed June 4, 2019).

31. Peters F, Geisthovel F, Breckwoldt M. Serum prolactin levels in women with excessive milk production. Normalization by transitory prolactin inhibition. *Acta Endocrinol (Copenh).* 1985;109:463−466.

ABM protocols expire 5 years from the date of publication. Content of this protocol is up-to-date at the time of publication. Evidence-based revisions are made within 5 years or sooner if there are significant changes in the evidence.

Helen M. Johnson, MD, lead author
Anne Eglash, MD, FABM
Katrina B. Mitchell, MD
Kathy Leeper, MD, FABM
Christina M. Smillie, MD, FABM
Lindsay Moore-Ostby, MD
Nadine Manson, MD, FABM
Liliana Simon, MD, FABM
Academy of Breastfeeding Medicine Protocol Committee
Members:
Michal Young, MD, FABM, Chairperson
Larry Noble, MD,
FABM, Translations Chairperson
Melissa Bartick, MD, MSc, FABM
Sarah Calhoun, MD
Megan Elliott-Rudder, MD
Lori Feldman-Winter, MD, MPH
Laura Rachael Kair, MD, FABM Susan Lappin, MD
Ilse Larson, MD
Ruth A. Lawrence, MD, FABM
Yvonne Lefort, MD, FABM
Kathleen A. Marinelli, MD, FABM
Nicole Marshall, MD, MCR
Katrina Mitchell, MD, FABM
Catherine Murak, MD
Eliza Myers, MD
Sarah Reece-Stremtan, MD
Casey Rosen-Carole, MD, MPH, MSEd
Susan Rothenberg, MD, IBCLC, FABM
Tricia Schmidt, MD
Tomoko Seo, MD, FABM
Natasha Sriraman, MD
Elizabeth K. Stehel, MD
Nancy Wight, MD
Adora Wonodi, MD
For correspondence: abm@bfmed.org

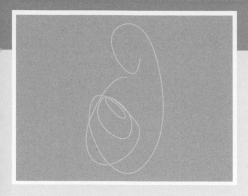

Educational Objectives and Skills for the Physician with Respect to Breastfeeding, Revised 2018*

Joan Younger Meek and The Academy of Breastfeeding Medicine

ABSTRACT

The Academy of Breastfeeding Medicine is a worldwide organization of physicians dedicated to the promotion, protection and support of breastfeeding and human lactation. Our mission is to unite into one association members of the various medical specialties with this common purpose.

INTRODUCTION

THE SCIENCE OF BREASTFEEDING and human lactation requires that physicians from many different specialties have a collaborative forum to promote progress in physician education. To optimize breastfeeding practices globally, physicians must incorporate the attitudes and skills needed to practice evidence-based breastfeeding medicine. The study of breastfeeding and human lactation is not currently recognized as a medical subspecialty, so the maintenance of a multispecialty organization dedicated to physician education and expansion of knowledge in this field has been vital.

BACKGROUND

The numerous benefits of breastfeeding for mothers and children have been well documented.[1–3] Physicians (medical doctors) play a key role in supporting breastfeeding, and they interact with women, children, and families throughout the life span. To advocate for breastfeeding, educate families about breastfeeding, and provide optimal clinical management of breastfeeding, these physicians must be educated about and skilled in breastfeeding establishment, maintenance, and support, as well as how to diagnose and treat breastfeeding complications.[4–8] Lack of sufficient education to provide breastfeeding support and guidance by physicians has been well documented in the medical literature.[9,10]

---

* Courtesy of the Academy of Breastfeeding Medicine. Please go to https://www.bfmed.org/protocols for complete protocols, translations, and the most up-to-date information (protocols are updated every 5–7 years).
Department of Clinical Sciences, Florida State University College of Medicine, Orlando, Florida.

The World Health Organization (WHO) and United Nations Children's Fund (UNICEF) "Ten Steps to Successful Breastfeeding," (Ten Steps), revised in 2018, called for all health care staff to have sufficient knowledge, competence, and skills to support breastfeeding.[11] The *Innocenti Declaration on the Protection, Promotion and Support of Breastfeeding*[12] identified four key goals in breastfeeding support: establishing national committees for oversight, ensuring maternity facilities practice the Ten Steps, enforcing the International Code of Marketing of Breast-milk Substitutes,[13] and enacting legislation that protects the breastfeeding rights of working women. Where national committees exist, many have an objective to educate all health care providers regarding appropriate breastfeeding and lactation support (e.g., the Australian National Breastfeeding Strategy,[14] the German Breastfeeding Committee,[15] Breastfeeding Promotion Network of India,[16] Kenya's National Infant and Young Child Feeding Committee, and the United States Breastfeeding Committee,[17]). The United States Breastfeeding Committee published "Core Competencies in Breastfeeding Care and Services for All Health Professionals."[18]

The Academy of Breastfeeding Medicine was founded to promote physician education and has a central goal to develop and disseminate the standard for physician education around breastfeeding and human lactation.[19] Guidance for the integration of breastfeeding medicine throughout the undergraduate, graduate, and postgraduate medical education of physicians is provided in this statement. While this guidance may be applicable to other health care disciplines, the competencies are aimed at physicians specifically. ABM protocols are useful in teaching evidence-based practices throughout the medical education continuum. ABM recognizes that terminology used to describe levels of medical education in various medical education systems around the globe differs. In this statement, the term "undergraduate medical education" is used to describe education received before obtaining a medical doctor degree; "graduate medical education" refers to clinical education received after the medical degree has been conferred and before the independent practice of medicine (i.e., doctors training during residency and/or fellowship); and "postgraduate education" refers to continuing medical education (CME) and maintenance of certification activities completed during ongoing professional development and/or as a requirement to maintain licensure/registration after the training phases have been completed.

GUIDELINES

Undergraduate medical education

a. All physicians, regardless of discipline, should have basic knowledge and skills in breastfeeding initiation, maintenance, diagnosis, and treatment.[20] Therefore, the theory and practice of breastfeeding should be incorporated routinely into the medical school curricula.[21]

Medical students should learn the anatomy of the breast, the physiology of lactation (including milk production), hormonal impact on mother and child, fertility changes, and the biochemical and immunological properties of human milk. Students should be able to explain the biological, sociological, and cultural aspects involved in protecting, promoting, and supporting breastfeeding. They should recognize the disparities that exist among different groups,[22] and that structural, institutional, and systemic barriers, as well as exposure to racism and implicit biases, pose challenges to Black, Indigenous, People of Color (BIPOC) receiving equitable breastfeeding and lactation support.[23] They should have opportunities to take a maternal history, obtain a feeding history of a newborn or child, and observe breastfeeding mothers and children in a variety of settings. Students need to recognize the value of breastfeeding and human milk feeding, as well as the risk of less than optimal breastfeeding. Ideally, this education should be integrated longitudinally throughout the curriculum, incorporated into block rotations, systems-based curricula, or case-based learning in the preclinical education, and be reinforced during maternal/child health clinical rotations, including obstetrics and gynecology, pediatrics, and family medicine.[24] All students, regardless of specialty choice, should receive this basic education.

All applicable examinations, whether standardized subject matter, written or oral examinations, or observed structured clinical examinations, should assess knowledge base and clinical decision-making skills in breastfeeding. Examinations for licensure or board certification, as applicable, should also include breastfeeding knowledge and skills assessment. At a basic level, all medical students, and therefore, all physicians, should understand the scientific evidence for breastfeeding, evidence-based clinical management of mothers and newborns, and the societal context of lactation to provide health care that supports breastfeeding initiation and maintenance, avoids creating barriers for breastfeeding women, and enables women to meet their breastfeeding goals.[25] Online courses are available for medical student education.[26] Additional

resources may be helpful in developing a breastfeeding curriculum.[24,25,27–29]

b. Preclinical medical school training in breastfeeding should address the following objectives[8,20,24,25,30]:
   • List the health risks of not breastfeeding for children, mothers, families, and society.
   • Recognize that most infants, even those with special health care needs, can breastfeed.
   • Diagram anatomy of the mammary gland and supportive breast structures and identify normal and abnormal histology.
   • Describe the physiology of milk production and secretion.
   • Describe the hormones of lactation and their multiple effects on mother and child.
   • Explain the biochemical and immunologic properties of human milk.
   • Describe the physiology of lactation-related fertility suppression.
   • Discuss the biological, sociological, psychological, and cultural aspects of supporting breastfeeding.
   • Identify structural, institutional, and systemic barriers that contribute to disparities in breastfeeding initiation and duration experienced by BIPOC or based on education level and socioeconomic status.
   • Identify national and/or international goals for breastfeeding rates and goals for breastfeeding practices, as appropriate.
   • Compare latch (attachment) and suckling dynamics of breastfeeding to bottle-feeding mechanics.
   • Describe evidence-based practices for maternity care providers shown to increase rates of initiation, duration, and exclusivity of breastfeeding.

c. Clinical training in medical school (clerkship rotations in obstetrics and gynecology, pediatrics, family medicine, maternal/child health, preventive medicine or public health, etc.) should address relevant objectives related to clinical management of breastfeeding, as follows[8,20,24,25,30]:
   • Identify factors that contribute to parental decision making about breastfeeding.
   • Apply the principles of shared decision-making to engage families in discussions about breastfeeding initiation and continuation.
   • Obtain a detailed breastfeeding history and perform a breastfeeding-related examination of the mother and infant.
   • Describe the association between labor and delivery interventions and initiation of breastfeeding.
   • Describe the impact of intrapartum and immediate postpartum procedures and medications on lactation.
   • Observe and be prepared to facilitate the first feeding in the delivery room.
   • Recognize correct attachment and effective suckling at the breast.
   • Counsel mothers about the importance of exclusive breastfeeding.

- Counsel a breastfeeding mother about basic nutritional needs for herself and her child.
- Counsel mothers about establishing and maintaining milk supply during separation due to illness or return to school or employment.
- Provide anticipatory guidance for breastfeeding mothers and children.
- Access evidence-based resources to recommend medications and treatment options that are compatible with lactation.
- Apply the principles of shared decision-making to discuss family planning options with the lactating woman.
- Discuss causes, prevention, and management of common breastfeeding problems (e.g., sore nipples, low milk supply, poor weight gain, and jaundice).
- Describe normal growth patterns for breastfed infants and children.
- Describe appropriate timing, introduction, and selection of complementary foods.
- Coordinate services with, and provide appropriate referral to, other health professionals, laypersons, and community groups to provide support for breastfeeding.
- Support policies and procedures across all specialty services that promote breastfeeding.

Graduate medical education

a. Residents (postmedical school training) in obstetrics and gynecology, pediatrics, family medicine, and preventive medicine residency training programs report a lack of education in breastfeeding, lack of knowledge and clinical experience in breastfeeding skills, and lack of competence or confidence in providing breastfeeding support to patients.[31-35] Inconsistencies also exist among breastfeeding training received in various training programs in pediatrics.[36] Resident physicians report a need for more direct patient interaction with regard to breastfeeding. Residents also note a lack of experience in counseling breastfeeding mothers and developing problem-solving skills during their training.[37] Residents have demonstrated deficits in interpreting growth patterns of breastfed babies.[38] Program directors also report that training programs do not provide adequate training or experience in breastfeeding.[39]

b. Several specific activities to achieve resident competency in breastfeeding management have resulted in an increase in knowledge of residents and improved breastfeeding management and behaviors. Examples include[40-42]:
  - Didactic presentations and small group discussions about breastfeeding recommendations, benefits, resources, and maternal medication use.
  - Role playing of breastfeeding counseling skills.
  - Videos on breastfeeding initiation, assessing latch on, and adequacy of breastfeeding.

- Panel discussion with breastfeeding mothers and individuals who provide support services.
- Participation on postpartum rounds with a physician with expertise in breastfeeding support and/or with an international board-certified lactation consultant (IBCLC).
- Supervised assessment of latch and breastfeeding technique with mother/infant dyads.
- Supervised management of maternal problems and maintenance of breastfeeding after return to work, including knowledge of applicable legal protections for lactating women in the workplace and training in use of hand expression or breast pumps.
- Observation of breastfeeding consults.
- Participation in outpatient breastfeeding or lactation consultant/specialist clinics.
- Attendance at peer counselor meetings (e.g., La Leche League International) or at peer support provided at other volunteer or government-supported programs (e.g., Australian Breastfeeding Association, National Childbirth Trust [United Kingdom], or Special Supplemental Nutrition Program for Women, Infants, and Children [United States], and hospital-based groups).

c. For primary care disciplines, resident competencies in breastfeeding build on those established for medical students.[8,10,20,24,25,30,32,42-44] The residency competencies are classified below according to the Accreditation Council for Graduate Medical Education[45] (ACGME) competency domains. The ACGME is the organization responsible for the accreditation of postmedical degree medical training programs within the United States and some international sites. The competencies are relevant worldwide.

Medical knowledge

- Identify risks of not breastfeeding for infants, mothers, and society.
- Identify anatomic structures of the breast.
- Describe physiology of milk production and removal.
- Describe the physiology of lactational fertility suppression and its use and limitations as a method of family planning.
- Describe the hormones of lactation and their multiple effects on mother and child.
- Explain the biochemical and immunologic properties of human milk.
- Describe the importance of breastfeeding in the establishment of microbiome.
- Describe breastfeeding recommendations.
- Discuss the importance of exclusive breastfeeding.
- Describe differences in the rates of breastfeeding initiation and duration based on factors, such as race/ethnicity, socioeconomic status, and maternal education.
- Describe suckling and compare breastfeeding and bottle-feeding mechanics.

- Recognize the impact of intrapartum and postpartum medications and procedures on lactation.
- Describe the importance of skin-to-skin care for the initiation of breastfeeding.
- Describe signs of adequate milk intake by the infant.
- Describe the normal growth pattern of breastfed infants.
- List absolute contraindications to breastfeeding.
- Describe the lactational amenorrhea method of family planning.
- Identify indications for maternal milk expression.
- Describe how to maintain breastfeeding during maternal/infant separation.
- List the specific benefits of human milk for premature infants.
- Identify the late preterm infant as being at higher risk of complications and breastfeeding failure compared with the term infant.
- Describe the interactions between jaundice, breastfeeding, and breast milk with appropriate diagnostic and management strategies.
- Describe the role of human milk banking and the appropriate indications and utilization of donor human milk.

Patient care

- Obtain a relevant medical history of breastfeeding mothers and babies.
- Perform a maternal breast assessment, including nipple configuration and assessment for scars.
- Facilitate skin-to-skin care in the delivery room or operating room.
- Provide assistance with the first feeding after delivery as needed.
- Perform infant oral assessment and general health assessment.
- Evaluate breastfeeding latch and attachment for the breastfeeding mother and infant.
- Evaluate effective nutritive suckling pattern.
- Identify mothers and infants at risk for inadequate milk transfer.
- Weigh the benefits of exclusive breastfeeding against a potential need for supplementation.
- Counsel mothers about the perception of inadequate milk.
- Counsel mothers on techniques for hand expression.[46]
- Counsel mothers about breastfeeding multiples.
- Counsel mothers about maternal nutrition during lactation.
- Recommend supplementation of vitamin D, iron, and other nutrients as appropriate.
- Counsel mothers and families about safe sleep practices for breastfeeding newborns and infants.[47,48]
- Identify common causes, prevention, and treatment of engorgement.[49]
- Develop a differential diagnosis for sore nipples or breast pain.
- Evaluate and manage sore nipples and breast pain.

- Diagnose and treat plugged ducts, mastitis, and abscess.[50]
- Evaluate maternal infections and potential risk of transmission to the breastfed infant.
- Counsel families on the risks and benefits of informal milk sharing.[51]
- Develop a differential diagnosis for neonatal hypoglycemia and manage newborn blood sugars in a manner that supports breastfeeding.[52]
- Evaluate and manage infants with neonatal jaundice in a manner that supports breastfeeding.[53]
- Monitor for inadequate milk production or milk transfer and implement supplementation when medically necessary.[54]
- Identify and manage newborns at risk for excessive weight loss and dehydration.
- Evaluate and manage infants with ankyloglossia.[55]
- Measure, plot, monitor, and interpret infant growth patterns using the WHO growth standards.
- Evaluate and manage infants with poor weight gain.
- Develop management plans that incorporate the use of expressed maternal milk and/or donor human milk when supplementation is necessary.
- Support nontraditional family units in breastfeeding support (e.g., same sex couples, transgender).
- Counsel families about breastfeeding adopted or surrogate children.
- Counsel families about vaccination practices during breastfeeding.
- Counsel families about family planning and the potential impact on breastfeeding.
- Counsel mothers about maintaining breastfeeding during separation from the infant.
- Counsel mothers about storage of expressed human milk.
- Counsel mothers about returning to work or school.
- Evaluate medication risk during lactation by referring to appropriate evidence-based resources (e.g., LactMed).[56]
- Counsel breastfeeding mothers on the use of recreational drugs.
- Evaluate and manage infants born to mothers with substance abuse who desire to breastfeed.[57]
- Support breastfeeding in special circumstances (e.g., prematurity, infant congenital anomalies, cleft lip/palate,[58] congenital heart disease, trisomy 21, maternal diabetes, and delayed lactogenesis stage II).
- Provide appropriate introduction and progression of breastfeeding for premature infants according to gestational age.
- Counsel mothers about introduction of complementary feedings.
- Counsel mothers about weaning.

Communication and interpersonal skills

- Apply shared decision-making principles to counseling mothers and families about optimal infant feeding decision for health outcomes, child spacing, and nutrition.

- Demonstrate sensitivity to cultural and ethnic differences and practices related to breastfeeding and infant care.
- Demonstrate sensitivity to the spectrum of family configurations and the impact on breastfeeding.

Systems-based practice

- Identify and help implement policies that support breastfeeding in maternity care facilities (e.g., the Ten Steps),[11] managed by Baby-Friendly USA,[59] in the United States and other appropriate country specific agencies, such as ministries of health.
- Identify barriers to successful breastfeeding and suggest strategies to overcome them.
- Describe structural, institutional, and systemic barriers that contribute to disparities in breastfeeding initiation and duration experienced by BIPOC, or based on education level and socioeconomic status.
- Describe how exposure to racism and implicit biases pose challenges to families of color receiving equitable breastfeeding and lactation support.
- Identify cultural and psychosocial factors that impact breastfeeding rates.
- Refer breastfeeding mothers and babies for expert assistance as needed.
- List ways in which the community can support breastfeeding.
- Identify community resources to assist breastfeeding mothers, including breastfeeding-friendly practitioners, prenatal or postpartum classes, drop in breastfeeding services, mother-to-mother support, and internet resources.
- Describe the role of IBCLCs, other levels of professional and lay breastfeeding support, as well as other members of the health care team in caring for mothers and babies.
- Be able to identify current laws protecting breastfeeding mothers with regard to maternity leave, breastfeeding or pumping/expressing breast milk at work, and breastfeeding in public.
- Advocate for legislative policies to enable families to meet their breastfeeding goals.
- Facilitate follow-up visits for breastfeeding mothers and babies.

Practice-based learning and improvement

- Locate resources for CME.
- Assess current breastfeeding knowledge base and identify gaps in knowledge and clinical skills.
- Perform evidence-based review of breastfeeding educational topics or clinical issues.
- Investigate program or hospital-specific breastfeeding initiation and duration rates.
- Participate in or develop quality improvement plans to improve breastfeeding rates and support in the local clinic, practice, or hospital environment.

d. Lactation education should be integrated longitudinally throughout the curriculum and should occur in a variety of clinical settings: outpatient continuity clinic and practices; inpatient settings (e.g., labor and delivery, newborn nursery, mother/baby units or postpartum units, neonatal intensive care units, inpatient general pediatrics, and adult medical and surgical wards); and community settings such as public health department clinics or government-funded community health centers. In addition, breastfeeding-specific curricula should be presented through a variety of teaching modalities, to include didactics, case presentations and discussions, daily attending rounds, and journal "clubs" in which peer-reviewed journal articles are reviewed critically. Residents may attend live presentations or discussions, review online resources (e.g., videos), read breastfeeding textbooks or periodicals (e.g., *Breastfeeding Medicine*, the *Journal of Human Lactation*, or specialty-specific literature), and complete online web-based training modules.[60–62] In the United States, a multidisciplinary, competency-based curriculum in breastfeeding education that provides multiple activities for integration throughout the residency program is available on the American Academy of Pediatrics website.[63] Use of this curriculum has been associated with better care of lactating mothers and infants and improved breastfeeding rates when implemented in residency programs.[64] In each country, resident participation in public clinics would provide an important exposure to common breastfeeding problems in a diverse patient population.

e. The knowledge, skills, and attitudes of residents are important in supporting breastfeeding in patients. It is equally important that residents in training are supported themselves when they are breastfeeding parents. Residents report lack of support for breastfeeding, and their need to express milk after return to work, from their faculty and peer colleagues.[65,66] Residency directors, faculty, deans and department chairs, and administrative support personnel need to advocate for program and human resource policies that support breastfeeding for residents, as well as for medical students, faculty, and staff.

f. The need for physician leadership in residency training to make the human lactation curriculum an ongoing sustainable component of medical education has been described.[24] Physician administrators (e.g., department chairs, residency program directors) either need to identify and support or develop this expertise within the local training program, institution, or hospital.

g. Breastfeeding medicine electives in the form of block rotations devoted to breastfeeding, occurring in a variety of clinical settings, have been described in family medicine and pediatric residency training programs.[37,67] These electives may include more advanced topics (e.g., relactation, induced lactation) and should stimulate more sophisticated clinical problem solving skills and/or provide an experience in clinical research or advocacy. Faculty oversight by individuals with a high degree of knowledge and skills in breastfeeding and human lactation is essential. The ABM has a peer-reviewed process for review of the credentials and background of physicians in breastfeeding with the Fellow of the Academy of Breastfeeding Medicine award.[19] Fellowship in the ABM is one, but not the only, means of identifying those individuals with a high degree of specialization in breastfeeding medicine. The emergence of breastfeeding medicine practices provides an additional opportunity for education of residents in an intensive setting and should assist in encouraging participating residents to make the practice of breastfeeding medicine an integral part of their professional practices.[68]

h. Subspecialty training programs (e.g., fellowship program in subspecialty disciplines, such as maternal/fetal medicine or neonatology) require additionally structured didactic and experiential education, as well as research opportunities, to further the science and advance the understanding of the role and importance of breastfeeding and human milk.

Postgraduate/In-Service/CME

a. Practicing physicians, especially those in the disciplines of obstetrics and gynecology,[69] pediatrics, and family medicine,[70] require ongoing CME in breastfeeding medicine to maintain and enhance their clinical skills and expertise. Key components of ongoing education should encompass the importance of breastfeeding and, especially, the risks of not breastfeeding, lactation management, and counseling skills.[71,72] Practicing physicians acknowledge that they do not understand clearly the health outcomes related to breastfeeding.[73] Patients have reported not receiving routine prenatal or postpartum counseling about breastfeeding by their physicians.[74] Physician attitudes about counseling mothers have been shown to be a significant factor in the mother's infant feeding decisions. Breastfeeding education of physicians can increase breastfeeding initiation rates.[75,76] Physicians' lack of knowledge has led patients to seek guidance elsewhere. Some physicians are not proactive about supporting breastfeeding, are neutral, or may not provide appropriate advice.[77,78] Mothers who report receiving encouragement from their physician are more likely to continue breastfeeding.[79] The role of the physician in encouraging breastfeeding has been shown to be especially important in those patient populations less likely to initiate breastfeeding.[80] Surveys of practicing physicians indicate that many are either not aware of policy statements on breastfeeding or are not following these policies in counseling patients.[6,81–83] Requirements to maintain specialty or subspecialty certification should incorporate breastfeeding-related materials into activities required for ongoing certification.

b. Practicing physicians have the following areas of need in terms of CME regarding breastfeeding:
- Skills in teaching breastfeeding techniques.
- Clinical management and problem solving skills in breastfeeding.[84]
- Awareness about maternal concerns such as weight loss, contraception during lactation, and maternal medications.
- Training in evaluating latch and attachment.[85]
- Identification and treatment of maternal complications such as mastitis and engorgement.[86]
- Evaluating problems with nipple or breast pain.
- Applying evidence-based strategies for assessment and monitoring to support exclusive breastfeeding.
- Addressing maternal perception of not enough breast milk.[79]
- Advising mothers about returning to work and continued breastfeeding.
- Availability of referral services existing for breastfeeding support.[87]
- More practical training and self-study materials.[88]
- Interactive training sessions.[89,90]
- Recognition of the role of family support.[89]
- Importance of avoiding routine provision of infant formula, infant formula samples, or educational materials that bear infant formula logos or product information.[91]

c. The ABM course, "What Every Physician Needs to Know about Breastfeeding," offered annually, provides CME at an introductory level for physicians and other health care practitioners. The ABM also sponsors an annual international conference that provides education for physicians about the current state-of-the-art of breastfeeding knowledge and research.[19] Many national organizations also offer CME in breastfeeding medicine for practicing physicians. A growing number of sources that provide breastfeeding CME for physicians are available, including online resources and web-based seminars.

d. The residency competencies for resident physicians are equally applicable to practicing physicians. Many practicing physicians are in positions of authority and may be able to affect health policy, so additional educational objectives for CME relate to breastfeeding advocacy[6–8]:
- Promote hospital policies and procedures that facilitate breastfeeding.
- Develop the hospital policies indicated in the Ten Steps and implement those policies and practices.
- Collaborate with other primary care disciplines, appropriate subspecialties (e.g., neonatologists, maternal/fetal medicine specialists), and dental health professionals to ensure optimal outcomes.
- Provide space for breastfeeding or milk expression and private lactation areas for all breastfeeding mothers, both patient and staff, in hospital and office settings.
- Develop office practices that promote and support breastfeeding.
- Advocate for reimbursement for breastfeeding services provided by physicians and/or lactation specialists

from government payers and third-party health insurance companies.

- Promote governmental policies and legislation that support breastfeeding mothers and children and increase breastfeeding rates.
- Increase availability of lactation consultants and other skilled breastfeeding support personnel in inpatient and outpatient settings.
- Monitor breastfeeding rates in the practice and/or hospital to include initiation and duration, as well as exclusive breastfeeding rates.
- Develop quality improvement practices that have a positive impact on breastfeeding rates.
- Advocate for dismantling of structural, institutional, and systemic barriers and take steps to mitigate racism and implicit biases that contribute to racial inequities in breastfeeding.
- Incorporate practices that acknowledge cultural differences in the local breastfeeding community.
- Achieve a positive image of breastfeeding as normative behavior in the media.
- Encourage support of breastfeeding and the use of expressed milk in childcare settings.
- Implement evidence-based protocols addressing breastfeeding policy and management, such as those available from the ABM.

SUMMARY

The medical community plays a critical role in promoting, protecting, and supporting breastfeeding for optimal outcomes for all families. Implementation of high-quality breastfeeding education throughout the continuum of medical education is critical to ensure that physicians-in-training develop appropriate knowledge, skills, and attitudes and that practicing physicians maintain their skills and competency to protect every parent's human right to breastfeed and the right of every child to be breastfed.[92]

ACKNOWLEDGMENT

The author acknowledges Dr. Abigail Adair-Dimmick for her contribution to conducting the literature review for this revised statement.

REFERENCES

1. Victora CG, Bahl R, Barros AJ, et al. Breastfeeding in the21st century: Epidemiology, mechanisms, and lifelong effect. *Lancet*. 2016;387:475—490.
2. Grummer-Strawn LM, Rollins N. Summarising the health effects of breastfeeding. *Acta Paediatr*. 2015;104:1—2.
3. Feltner C, Weber RP, Stuebe A, et al. Breastfeeding Programs and Policies, Breastfeeding Uptake, and Maternal Health Outcomes in Developed Countries. Comparative Effectiveness Review No. 210. (Prepared by the RTI International—University of North Carolina at Chapel Hill Evidence-based Practice Center under Contract No. 2902015-00011-I.) AHRQ

Publication No. 18-EHC014-EF. Rockville, MD: Agency for Healthcare Research and Quality, July 2018. Available at: https://effectivehealthcare.ahrq.gov/topics/breastfeeding/research (accessed November 2, 2018).

4. U.S. Department of Health and Human Services. *The Surgeon General's Call to Action to Support Breastfeeding*. Washington, DC: U.S. Department of Health and Human Services, Office of the Surgeon General; 2011. Available at: www.surgeongeneral.gov/library/calls/breastfeeding/index.html (accessed November 2, 2018).
5. How Doctors Can Help, The Surgeon General's Call to Action to Support Breastfeeding. Available at: www.cdc.gov/breastfeeding/pdf/actionguides/doctors_in_action.pdf (accessed November 2, 2018).
6. Eidelman AI, Schanler RJ, Johnston M, et al. Breastfeeding and the use of human milk. *Pediatrics*. 2012;129:e827—e841.
7. American College of Obstetricians and Gynecologists. Optimizing support for breastfeeding as part of obstetric practice. Committee Opinion No. 756. *Obstet Gynecol*. 2018;132:e187—e196.
8. American Academy of Family Physicians. Breastfeeding, family physicians supporting (position paper). June17, 2017. Available at: www.aafp.org/about/policies/all/breastfeedingsupport.html (accessed November 2, 2018).
9. Freed GL, Clark SJ, Sorenson J, et al. National assessment of physicians' breast-feeding knowledge, attitudes, training, and experiences. *JAMA*. 1995;273:472—476.
10. Williams EL, Hammer LD. Breastfeeding attitudes and knowledge of pediatricians-in-training. *Am J Prev Med*. 1995;11:26—33.
11. Baby Friendly Hospital Initiative Global Criteria, revised 2018. Ten steps to successful breastfeeding. Available at: www.who.int/nutrition/bfhi/ten-steps/en (accessed November 2, 2018).
12. WHO/UNICEF Innocenti Declaration on the Protection, Promotion and Support of Breastfeeding. Spedale degli Innocenti, Florence, Italy, July 30—August 1, 1990. Available at: www.unicef.org/nutrition/index_24807.html (accessed November 2, 2018).
13. International Code of Marketing of Breast-milk Substitutes. Available at: www.who.int/nutrition/publications/code_english.pdf (accessed November 2, 2018).
14. Australian Government Department of Health Enduring Australian National Breastfeeding Strategy. Available at: www.health.gov.au/breastfeeding (accessed November 2, 2018).
15. NSK Praämbel. 1994. Available at: www.bfr.bund.de/cd/2404 (accessed November 2, 2018).
16. Breastfeeding Promotion Network of India. Available at: www.bpni.org (accessed November 2, 2018).
17. United States Breastfeeding Committee Strategic Framework. Available at: www.usbreastfeeding.org/strategicframework (accessed November 2, 2018).
18. United States Breastfeeding Committee. *Core Competencies in Breastfeeding Care and Services for All Health Professionals*. Revised ed. Washington, DC: United States Breastfeeding Committee; 2010.
19. Academy of Breastfeeding Medicine. Available at: www.bfmed.org (accessed November 2, 2018).
20. American Academy of Pediatrics, The American College of Obstetricians and Gynecologists. The scope of breastfeeding. In: Schanler R, ed. *Breastfeeding Handbook for Physicians*. 2nd ed. Elk Grove Village, IL: American Academy of Pediatrics; 2014:1—26.

21. Anjum Q, Ashfaq T, Siddiqui H. Knowledge regarding breast-feeding practices among medical students of Ziauddin University Karachi. *J Pak Med Assoc*. 2007;57:480–483.

22. Anstey EH, Chen J, Elam-Evans LD, et al. Racial and geographic differences in breastfeeding—United States, 2011–2015. *MMWR Morb Mortal Wkly Rep*. 2017;66:723–727.

23. Asiodu IV, Waters CW, Laydon A. Infant feeding decision-making and the influences of social support persons among first-time African American mothers. *Matern Child Health J*. 2017;21:863–872.

24. Lawrence RA, Lawrence RM. Educating and training the medical professional. In: Lawrence RA, Lawrence RM, eds. *Breastfeeding: A Guide for the Medical Profession*. 8th ed. Philadelphia, PA: Elsevier; 2016:751–765.

25. Naylor A, Cataldo J, Creer E, et al. *Lactation Management Curriculum: A Faculty Guide for Schools of Medicine, Nursing, and Nutrition*. 4th ed San Diego: Wellstart International, in collaboration with the University of California; 1999.

26. Wellstart International. *Lactation Management Self-Study Modules, Level I*. Fourth Edition Shelburne, Vermont: Wellstart International; 2013. Available at: www.wellstart.org/Self-Study-Module.pdf (accessed November 2, 2018).

27. Turner-Maffei C. Lactation resources for clinicians. *J Midwifery Womens Health*. 2007;52:e57–e65.

28. Labbok, M, Glob. librt.women's med. (ISSN: 1756-2228) 2008; https:doi.org/10.3843/GLOWM.10397. Available at: http://www.glowm.com/section_view/item/396/recordset/71685/value/396 (accessed December 17, 2018).

29. Dozier AM. Quick reference breastfeeding guide available for medical students and residents. *Breastfeed Med*. 2012;7:320.

30. Ogburn T, Espey E, Leeman L, et al. A breastfeeding curriculum for residents and medical students: A multidisciplinary approach. *J Hum Lact*. 2005;21:458–464.

31. Freed GL, Clark SJ, Cefalo RC, et al. Breast-feeding education of obstetrics-gynecology residents and practitioners. *Amer J Obstet Gynecol*. 1995;173:1607–1613.

32. Freed GL, Clark SJ, Curtis P, et al. Breast-feeding education and practice in family medicine. *J Fam Pract*. 1995;40:297–298.

33. Goldstein AO, Freed GL. Breast-feeding counseling practices of family practice residents. *Fam Med*. 1993;25:524–529.

34. Leavitt G, Martinez S, Ortiz N, et al. Knowledge about breastfeeding among a group of primary care physicians and residents in Puerto Rico. *J Community Health*. 2009;34:1–5.

35. Pound CM, Moreau KA, Hart F, et al. The planning of a national breastfeeding educational intervention for medical residents. *Med Educ Online*. 2015;20:26380.

36. Osband YB, Altman RL, Patrick PA, et al. Breastfeeding education and support services offered to pediatric residents in the US. *Acad Pediatr*. 2011;11:75–79.

37. Freed GL, Clark SJ, Lohr JA, et al. Pediatrician involvement in breast-feeding promotion: A national study of residents and practitioners. *Pediatrics*. 1995;96:490–494.

38. Guise J-M, Freed G. Resident physicians' knowledge of breastfeeding and infant growth. *Birth*. 2000;27:49–53.

39. Eden A, Mir M. Breastfeeding education of pediatric residents: A national survey. *Arch Pediatr Adolesc Med*. 2000;154:1271–1272.

40. Saenz RB. A lactation management rotation for family medicine residents. *J Hum Lact*. 2000;16:342–345.

41. Hillenbrand KM, Larsen PG. Effect of an educational intervention about breastfeeding on the knowledge, confidence, and behaviors of pediatric resident physicians. *Pediatrics*. 2002;110:e59.

42. Bunik M, Gao D, Moore L. An investigation of the field trip model as a method for teaching breastfeeding to pediatric residents. *J Hum Lact*. 2006;22:195–202.

43. Baldwin C, Kittredge D, Bar-on M, et al. Academic Pediatric Association Educational Guidelines for Pediatric Residency. MedEdPORTAL; 2009. Available at: http://services.aamc.org/30/mededportal/servlet/s/segment/mededportal/?subid = 1736 (accessed November 2, 2018).

44. Howett M, Spangler A, Cannon RB. Designing a university based lactation course. *J Hum Lact*. 2006;22:104–107.

45. Accreditation Council for Graduate Medical Education. Available at: www.acgme.org (accessed November 2, 2018).

46. Stanford Medicine Newborn Nursery. Available at https://med.stanford.edu/newborns/professional-education/breastfeeding/hand-expressing-milk.html (accessed November 2, 2018).

47. AAP Task Force on Sudden Infant Death Syndrome. SIDS and other sleep-related infant deaths: Updated 2016 recommendations for a safe infant sleeping environment. *Pediatrics*. 2016;138. e20162938.

48. Feldman-Winter L, Goldsmith JP. AAP Committee on Fetus and Newborn, AAP Task Force on Sudden Infant Death Syndrome. Safe sleep and skin-to-skin care in the neonatal period for healthy term newborns. *Pediatrics*. 2016;138: e20161889.

49. Berens P. Brodribb, Academy of Breastfeeding Medicine. ABM clinical protocol #20: Engorgement, revised 2016. *Breastfeed Med*. 2016;11:159–163.

50. Amir LH, Academy of Breastfeeding Medicine Protocol Committee. ABM clinical protocol #4: Mastitis, revised March 2014. *Breastfeed Med*. 2014;9:239–243.

51. Sriraman NK, Evans AE, Lawrence R, et al. Academy of Breastfeeding Medicine's 2017 position statement on informal breast milk sharing for the term healthy infant. *Breastfeed Med*. 2018;13:2–4.

52. Wight N, Marinelli KA. The Academy of Breastfeeding Medicine. ABM clinical protocol #1: Guidelines for blood glucose monitoring and treatment of hypoglycemia in term and late-preterm neonates, Revised 2014. *Breastfeed Med*. 2014;9:173–179.

53. Flaherman VJ, Maisels MJ. The Academy of Breastfeeding Medicine. ABM clinical protocol #22: Guidelines for management of jaundice in the breastfeeding infant 35 weeks or more of gestation, Revised 2017. *Breastfeed Med*. 2017;12:250–257.

54. Kellams A, Harrel C, Omage S, et al. ABM clinical protocol #3: Supplementary feedings in the healthy term breastfed neonate, Revised 2017. *Breastfeed Med*. 2017;12:1–11.

55. Academy of Breastfeeding Medicine Protocol #11: Guidelines for the evaluation and management of neonatal ankyloglossia and its complications in the breastfeeding dyad. Available at: https://abm.memberclicks.net/assets/DOCUMENTS/PROTOCOLS/11-neonatal-ankyloglossiaprotocol-english.pdf (accessed November 2, 2018).

56. Drugs and Lactation Database, LactMed. Available at: https://toxnet.nlm.nih.gov/newtoxnet/lactmed.htm (accessed November 2, 2018).

57. Reece-Stremtan S, Marinelli KA. The Academy of Breastfeeding Medicine. ABM clinical protocol #21: Guidelines

for breastfeeding and substance use or substance use disorder, Revised 2015. *Breastfeed Med.* 2015;10:135–141.

58. Reilly S, Reid J, Skeat J, et al. ABM clinical protocol #17: Guidelines for breastfeeding infants with cleft lip, cleft palate, or cleft lip and palate, revised 2013. *Breastfeed Med.* 2013;8:349–353.

59. Baby-Friendly USA. Available at Available at: www.babyfriendlyusa.org (accessed September 7, 2018).

60. Lasarte Velillas JJ, Hernandez-Aguilar MT, Pallas Alonso CR, et al. A breastfeeding e-learning project based on a web forum. *Breastfeed Med.* 2007;2:219–228.

61. O'Connor ME, Brown EW, Lewin LO. An Internet-based education program improves breastfeeding knowledge of maternal-child healthcare providers. *Breastfeed Med.* 2011;6:421–427.

62. Tender JA, Cuzzi S, Kind T, et al. Educating pediatric residents about breastfeeding: Evaluation of 3 time efficient teaching strategies. *J Hum Lact.* 2014;30:458–465.

63. American Academy of Pediatrics Breastfeeding Residency Curriculum. Available at: www.aap.org/en-us/advocacy-andpolicy/aap-health-initiatives/Breastfeeding/Pages/ResidencyCurriculum.aspx (accessed September 7, 2018).

64. Feldman-Winter L, Barone L, Milcarek B, et al. Residency curriculum improves breastfeeding care. *Pediatrics.* 2010;126:289–297.

65. Miller NH, Miller DJ, Chism M. Breastfeeding practices among resident physicians. *Pediatrics.* 1996;98:434–437.

66. Dixit A, Feldman-Winter L, Szucs KA. "Frustrated," "depressed," and "devastated" pediatric trainees: US academic medical centers fail to provide adequate workplace breastfeeding support. *J Hum Lact.* 2015;31:240–248.

67. Meek JY. An Integrated Approach to Breastfeeding Education in Pediatric Residency Training. *Academy of Breastfeeding Medicine News and Views.* 1999;5(4).

68. Shaikh U, Smillie CM. Physician-led outpatient breastfeeding medicine clinics in the United States. *Breastfeed Med.* 2008;3:28–33.

69. Mass SB. Educating the obstetrician about breastfeeding. *Clin Obstet Gynecol.* 2015;58:936–943.

70. Srinivasan A, Graves L, D'Souza V. Effectiveness of a 3-hour breastfeeding course for family physicians. *Can Fam Physician.* 2014;60:e601–e606.

71. Naylor AJ, Creer AE, Woodward-Lopez G, et al. Lactation management education for physicians. *Semin Perinatol.* 1994;18:525–531.

72. Sigman-Grant M, Kim Y. Breastfeeding knowledge and attitudes of nevada health care professionals remain virtually unchanged over 10 years. *J Hum Lact.* 2016;32:350–354.

73. McFadden A, Renfrew MJ, Dykes F, et al. Assessing learning needs for breastfeeding: Setting the scene. *Matern Child Nutr.* 2006;2:196–203.

74. Izatt S. Breastfeeding counseling by health care providers. *J Hum Lact.* 1997;13:109–113.

75. Grossman X, Chaudhuri J, Feldman-Winter L, et al. Hospital Education in Lactation Practices (Project HELP): Does clinician education affect breastfeeding initiation and exclusivity in the hospital? *Birth.* 2009;36:54–59.

76. Holmes AV, McLeod AY, Thesing C, et al. Physician breastfeeding education leads to practice changes and improved clinical outcomes. *Breastfeed Med.* 2012;7:403–408.

77. DiGirolamo AM, Grummer-Strawn LM, Fein SB. Do perceived attitudes of physicians and hospital staff affect breastfeeding decisions? *Birth.* 2003;30:94–100.

78. Dillaway HE, Douma ME. Are pediatric offices "supportive" of breastfeeding? Discrepancies between mothers' and healthcare professionals' reports. *Clin Pediatr.* 2004;43:417–430.

79. Taveras EM, Capra AM, Braveman PA, et al. Clinical support and psychosocial risk factors associated with breastfeeding discontinuation. *Pediatrics.* 2003;112:108–115.

80. Lu MC, Lange L, Slusser W, Hamilton J, Halfon N. Provider encouragement of breast-feeding: Evidence from a national survey. *Obstet Gynecol.* 2001;97:290–295.

81. Schanler RJ, O'Connor KG, Lawrence RA. Pediatricians' practices and attitudes regarding breastfeeding promotion. *Pediatrics.* 1999;103:e35.

82. Feldman-Winter L, Szucs K, Milano A, et al. National trends in pediatricians' practices and attitudes about breastfeeding: 1995 to 2014. *Pediatrics.* 2017;140:e20171229.

83. Meek JY. Pediatrician competency in breastfeeding support has room for improvement. *Pediatrics.* 2017;140:e20172509.

84. Krogstrand KS, Parr K. Physicians ask for more problem solving information to promote and support breastfeeding. *J Am Diet Assoc.* 2005;105:1943–1947.

85. Okolo SN, Ogbonna C. Knowledge, attitude and practice of health workers in Keffi local government hospitals regarding Baby-Friendly Hospital Initiative (BFHI) practices. *Eur J Clin Nutr.* 2002;56:438–441.

86. Bagwell JE, Kendrick OW, Stitt KR, et al. Knowledge and attitudes toward breastfeeding: Differences among dietitians, nurses, and physicians working with WIC clients. *J Am Diet Assoc.* 1993;93:801–804.

87. Taveras EM, Ruowei L, Grummer-Strawn L, et al. Opinions and practices of clinicians associated with continuation of exclusive breastfeeding. *Pediatrics.* 2004;113:283–290.

88. Wallace LM, Kosmala-Anderson J. A training needs survey of doctors' breastfeeding support skills in England. *Matern Child Nutr.* 2006;2:217–231.

89. Burt S, Whitmore M, Vearncombe D, et al. The development and delivery of a practice-based breastfeeding education package for general practitioners in the UK. *Matern Child Nutr.* 2006;2:91–102.

90. Ingram J. Multiprofessional training for breastfeeding management in primary care in the UK. *Int Breastfeed J.* 2006;1:9.

91. Valaitis RK, Sheeshka JD, O'Brien MF. Do consumer infant feeding publications and products available in physicians' offices protect, promote, and support breastfeeding? *J Hum Lact.* 1997;13:203–208.

92. Joint statement by the UN Special Rapporteurs on the Right to Food, Right to Health, the Working Group on Discrimination against Women in law and in practice, and the Committee on the Rights of the Child in support of increased efforts to promote, support and protect breastfeeding. Available at: www.ohchr.org/EN/NewsEvents/Pages/DisplayNews.aspx?NewsID = 20871 (accessed November 2, 2018).

Joan Younger Meek, MD, MS, FABM
Lead Author
The Academy of Breastfeeding Medicine Protocol Committee:
Michal Young, MD, FABM, Chairperson
Larry Noble, MD, FABM, Translations Chairperson
Sarah Calhoun, MD

Sarah Dodd, MD
Megan Elliott-Rudder, MD
Susan Lappin, MD
Ilse Larson, MD
Ruth A. Lawrence, MD, FABM
Kathleen A. Marinelli, MD, FABM
Nicole Marshall, MD

Katrina Mitchell, MD
Sarah Reece-Stremtan, MD
Casey Rosen-Carole, MD, MPH, MSEd
Susan Rothenberg, MD
Tomoko Seo, MD, FABM
Adora Wonodi, MD
For correspondence: abm@bfmed.org

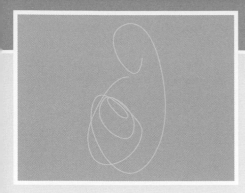

Medical Education for Basic Proficiency in Breastfeeding

Casey Rosen-Carole

LEARNING OBJECTIVE/TRANSFER GOAL

By the end of medical school, medical students should have a basic understanding of the histology, anatomy, physiology, pathology, pharmacology, public health, and clinical issues surrounding breastfeeding; be able to understand relevance of this knowledge to clinical scenarios; and begin to apply this knowledge in clinical decision-making (see Chapter 26).

The following topics should be included:

1. *Histology:* The histology of the breast, including the acinar cells, ductal cells, and hormonal stimuli of milk release. Histology of newborn gut cells to comprehend the impact of breast milk against foreign substances.

2. *Anatomy:* Basic breast anatomy, including blood supply, innervation, and lymphatic drainage. Location of the milk ducts, their proximity to surgical incision sites. Surgeries and surgical sites with varying effects on breastfeeding. Suspension ligaments. Role of the interstitial spaces that fill with fluid during engorgement to prevent release ("let down") of milk. Locations of adiposity.

3. *Physiology:* Seeing the newborn and mother as a "dyad" biophysically during the first year of life. Normal hormonal stimulation of milk ejection, mechanisms of milk expression by mechanics of neonatal tongue/lips/gums, and differences with milk ejection by artificial methods (hand expression and pumps). Impact of breast milk on the newborn gut, biomes, hormones, digestion, and infant and maternal genetics.

4. *Pathology:* Mastitis causes and prevention, and appropriate management of breast abscess while not interrupting ductal tissue. Few contraindications to breastfeeding. Infant malformations associated with difficulty breastfeeding. Diseases affected by breastfeeding. Genetic and epigenetic influences of breastfeeding.

5. *Pharmacology:* Impact of artificial infant formula on newborn gut, especially premature gut. Risks of artificial infant formula and proposed mechanisms (e.g., changed microbiota leading to increased inflammation, increased permeability of mucosal membranes, decreased host defenses, and increased infection). Breast-milk fortifiers and their role in growth and nutrition of premature babies (both human- and cow milk–based fortifiers). Considerations of the transfer of medications into human milk. Determining the safety of medications for breastfeeding. Role of certain medications in altering breast milk production.

6. *Nutrition and immunology:* Nutritional impact of breastfeeding and breast milk as species-specific. Co-factors for absorption, presence of cells, and immunoglobulins for immunologic support. Colostrum as first nutrition and first vaccine.

7. *Public health:* Breastfeeding as a human right, health disparities, and equity issue. Low rates of breastfeeding and impact on cost of health care and burden of disease.

8. *Primary care clerkship preparation:* How to discuss breastfeeding in a supportive manner with families, the importance of breastfeeding education and physician recommendation. The basics of a good latch and positioning.

CURRICULUM DESIGN CONSIDERATIONS

- Material included should meet the highest standards of evidence-based medicine. Involving a physician with advanced training in breastfeeding medicine is recommended, if available, for this process.
- Curricula should be designed by a multidisciplinary team, including basic science and clinical faculty (obstetric, pediatric, family medicine, surgical, etc.), medical student leaders, patients, and administrators. This is likely to improve buy-in, humanism, and integration with other parts of the curriculum.
- Each area of the medical school curriculum should include some information on breastfeeding: basic science, preclinical, and clinical years. Material should be considered for inclusion in an integrated manner with other course topics (e.g., a discussion of the role of breastfeeding in breast cancer prevention could be included in a problem-based learning cancer case or in a traditional lecture on breast cancer).

- Dedicated sessions on breastfeeding should be used to focus on the clinical skills necessary for the clinical years (e.g., latch, positioning, motivational interviewing, physician's role).
- In schools that use a systems-based integrative model, or modular, problem-based learning, a case or unit on breastfeeding should be strongly considered or should be included as a teaching point of a related case (e.g., bronchiolitis, diabetes, etc.).

The Reference list is available at www.expertconsult.com.

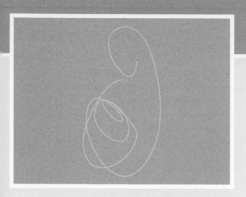

A

Acinus The tube leading to the smallest lobule of a compound gland; it is characterized by a narrow lumen.

ACNM American College of Nurse-Midwives.

ACOG American Congress of Obstetricians and Gynecologists.

ACOP American College of Osteopathic Pediatricians.

Acquired immune system The collection of cells and cellular products that contribute to antigen recognition and cell differentiation into memory cells for subsequent encounters with the same antigen(s). The system is characterized by high antigen specificity and enhanced and accelerated immune response on reencountering the specific antigen(s).

Adipose tissue See *Panniculus adiposus.*

Afferent Conducting inward to, or toward, the center of an organ, gland, or other structure or area. Applies to sensory nerves, arteries, and lymph vessels.

AHRQ The Agency for Healthcare Research and Quality (AHRQ) is the lead federal agency charged with improving the safety and quality of America's health care system. The AHRQ develops the knowledge, tools, and data needed to improve the health care system and help Americans, health care professionals, and policy makers make informed health decisions. It exists within the Department of Health and Human Services (DHHS).

Alactogenesis Familial puerperal alactogenesis is a genetically transmitted, isolated prolactin deficiency.

Allergy The inappropriate and sometimes excessive response of the immune system to common antigens (allergens) in the environment. Examples of such allergens include foods (milk, egg, fish, nuts), pollen, dust mites, bee venom, etc.

ALPP Academy of Lactation Policy and Practice.

Alveolus A glandular acinus or terminal portion of the alveolar gland, where milk is secreted and stored, that measures approximately 0.12 mm in diameter. From 10 to 100 alveoli, or tubulosaccular secretory units, make up a lobulus.

Amastia Congenital absence of the breast—breast tissue, areola, and nipple.

Amazia Congenital absence of breast tissue but with a nipple and areola.

Ampulla Elastic portion of the duct, just proximal to the nipple, that expands as milk fills the breast.

Ankyloglossia A tight lingual frenulum (the membrane attaching the tongue to the bottom of the mouth). This condition is also referred to as *tongue-tie*. When the frenulum is tight, it can restrict the movement of the tongue, which on occasion can result in difficulty with breastfeeding for some mothers (nipple pain) and babies (poor latch and milk transfer).

Apocrine A term descriptive of a gland cell that loses part of its protoplasmic substance in the process of excretion.

Apoptosis The occurrence of cell death without inflammation, as a programmed and controlled part of growth and development of an organ or organism.

Apt test A test, named after its developer, performed on fresh blood to distinguish between adult and fetal hemoglobin. The blood is suspended in saline, and an equal amount of 10% sodium hydroxide (NaOH) is added and mixed; adult hemoglobin turns brown, and fetal hemoglobin remains red. A control sample of known adult blood also should be tested for comparison.

Arborization Development of a branched arrangement or structure.

Areola mammae Areola. The pigmented area surrounding the papilla mammae, or nipple.

Artificial nipple or teat An artificial object used in place of and therefore often shaped like a mammary nipple used with a bottle to feed an infant formula or used by itself for an infant to suck on instead of a bottle or breast.

Australian posture or position A breastfeeding position in which the baby is above the mother (or the mother is "down under" the baby), the reason for the name of the posture. The mother is supine while the infant is usually prone with its legs straddling one of the mother's legs and the infant's face aligned with the breast.

Autophagic vacuole Autophagosome. A membrane-bound body within a cell containing degenerating cell organelles.

Available milk The amount of milk present in a breast that is removed by a suckling infant or expressed from the breast by hand or pump. This volume is the "storage" capacity of the breast in the interval between emptying the breast.

B

Baby Friendly Hospital Initiative (BFHI or BFI) An international program of the World Health Organization and United Nations International Children's Education Fund (UNICEF). The initiative is a global effort for improving the role of maternity services to enable mothers to successfully breastfeed their infants. Its main goals are improving the care of pregnant women, mothers, and newborns at any health facilities that provide maternity services and for protecting, promoting, and supporting breastfeeding, in alignment with the International Code of Marketing of Breastmilk Substitutes.

Baby-led weaning The concept that infants as young as 6 months can play a role in their own food intake. Infant behavior contributes to choosing the complementary foods, amounts of food, and timing or rhythm of eating, making weaning a gradual and manageable adjustment for both mother and infant.

BALT Bronchus-associated immunocompetent lymphoid tissue, to which the mammary gland may act as an extension. See *GALT* and *MALT.*

Basal lamina The layer of material, 50 to 100 nm thick, that lies adjacent to the plasma membrane of the basal surfaces of epithelial cells. The basal lamina is visualized by electron microscopy. It contains collagen and certain carbohydrates. It is often called the *basement* membrane when visualized by light microscopy.

Bifidobacteria Gram-positive anaerobic bacteria found in breast milk and often common in the gastrointestinal tract (and stools) of breastfed infants. They ferment sugars (oligosaccharides) into fatty acids (acetate, butyrate, propionate). Human milk oligosaccharides (HMOs) are a readily used source of oligosaccharides.

Bioactive component A component of food characterized as nonnutritive. It exerts an effect on nutrition and health by a chemical or regulatory process. There are many bioactive components in human milk, some of which have both a nutritive and nonnutritive function.

Bleb A milk-filled, blocked nipple pore often manifesting as a white, yellow, or clear dot or blister on the nipple or areola.

Blocked milk duct A relative obstruction of a milk duct as a result of stasis or impaired drainage leading to a local swelling in the breast. The swelling can vary in size and shape from a small nodule to a large wedge-shaped area. It should be distinguished from engorgement, mastitis, and breast abscess and is not associated with systemic signs of inflammation.

Block nursing Nursing on the same breast for two or more feedings without nursing or otherwise releasing milk from the other breast. This strategy is often used to decrease an overly abundant milk supply.

Bottle-feeding The act of feeding an infant through a bottle regardless of the liquid being fed.

Breast A common term for mammary gland. The breast is rudimentary in males but evolves through developmental stages in females (embryogenesis, puberty, mammogenesis, pregnancy, lactogenesis/lactation, involution). The breast's primary function is the synthesis and secretion of milk to feed an infant; it subsequently involutes to a quiescent period after weaning.

Breast abscess An inflammatory swelling within the breast with pain and swelling, often with redness, warmth, and fluctuance as it evolves to a fluid-filled mass. Systemic signs of inflammation occur in some instances. It should be distinguished from engorgement, a blocked duct and mastitis.

Breast crawl Refers to the innate behavior of a newborn infant after being placed on the mother's abdomen (skin to skin or tummy to tummy), moving up to the mother's breast, latching on, and suckling if unimpeded.

Breast cyst A fluid-filled mass within breast tissue. It is often characterized as smooth, firm, lobulated, and mobile. It should be distinguished from a galactocele (fluid within the mass is milk), abscess, tumor, or cancer.

Breast hypoplasia The underdevelopment of the breast.

Breast massage The manipulation of the breast in a pattern or technique of kneading or rubbing the breast. During lactation, it is often useful for relieving blocked ducts, stimulating secretion, or as a comfort measure.

Breast pump A piece of equipment for removing milk from a breast. It can be manual or electric and usually removes the milk by suction.

Breast refusal When an infant does not attach to the breast and suckle well after a period of prior effective breastfeeding. The infant will turn its head away from the breast or side to side, arching its back, crying, and even flailing its arms as if avoiding the breast. This may be a temporary behavior or lead to weaning.

Breast shell A plastic device worn to manage inverted nipples or protect damaged nipples.

The breast side of the device surrounds the nipple, and the outer piece is often dome shaped to separate the nipple from the pressure of the bra or clothing.

Breast shield One component of a breast pump. It is the funnel-shaped portion covering the areola and creating a tunnel that encircles the nipple, creating space for milk flow into the collection container.

Breastfeed The removal of milk from a breast by an infant suckling on the breast.

Breastfeeding The action of an infant removing milk from a breast by sucking (nursing).

Breastfeeding positions The various positions in which a mother holds herself and her infant to facilitate an effective latch and successful breastfeeding. A few of those positions include lying back, side-lying, cradle, cross-cradle, and football hold position.

Breast milk The fluid produced in the mammary gland after the birth of an infant, during the period of lactation. Lactocytes produce this fluid as nutrition for the infant; composed of fats, carbohydrates, proteins, vitamins, nutrients, and biologically active components contributing to the growth, development, and maturation of the infant. Breast milk is usually specifically human milk, because the milk of other animals is not called breast milk. (*Colostrum, transitional breast milk*, and *mature breast milk* are associated terms.)

Breast-milk expression The removal of milk from a breast. It occurs by a breast pump or hand expression.

Breast-milk feeding When the infant is fed breast milk by some other manner besides directly removing it from the breast. The infant is fed breast milk by finger, cup, syringe, bottle, etc.

Breast-milk substitute Any fluid or food produced and marketed to replace breast milk. The World Health Organization determines the relative nutritional suitability of such foods. Infant formula is the most recognized example of a breast milk substitute produced by modification of other animal milks or food sources (soy).

Breast-milk transfer The active movement of human milk from the breast to the infant during a breastfeed.

Breastsleeping Breastsleeping refers to bed-sharing (mother and infant) along with breastfeeding. The term, coined by James McKenna and Lee Gettler, is meant to highlight the benefits of ongoing breastfeeding in combination with bed-sharing in the absence of known hazardous factors related to formula- or bottle-sharing and bedsharing.

C

Casein A group of milk-specific proteins and derivatives of caseinogen, characterized by ester-bound phosphate, high-protein content, and low solubility. The fraction of milk protein that forms the curd in milk. The human caseins form a micellar structure, which facilitates the high availability of calcium in

human milk compared with other animal caseins.

CGBI Carolina Global Breastfeeding Institute.

CLC Certified lactation counselor. Breastfeeding care provider who has completed a course of study resulting in certification as a lactation counselor.

Cleft lip and palate A continuum of birth defects resulting from incomplete fusion of tissue in the midline of the face during the normal embryonic process. Clefts vary as unilateral or bilateral and can be as mild as a small notch in the upper lip to the complete opening in the lip through the hard and soft palate into the nasal cavity.

Closet nursing Nursing privately at home, in secret, as a result of insensitive, uninformed relatives and friends and even health care providers.

Cluster feeding A cycle of short, closely spaced feedings, usually in less than 30 minutes, interspersed with periods of rest or sleep.

Colic The behavior of an infant characterized by recurrent and usually prolonged crying, fussiness, and irritability without an obvious cause. It is benign and self-resolving and is without an apparent easy solution. It most commonly occurs between 2 and 5 months of age. There is no known cause.

Colostrum The first milk. This yellow, sticky fluid is secreted by the breast during the first few days postpartum and provides nutrition and protection against infectious disease with its high level of immune globulins. It contains more protein, less sugar, and much less fat than mature breast milk. It comes in small volumes, estimated at 30 mL in the first day.

Columnar secretory cell A type of secretory cell in the shape of a hexagonal prism; it appears rectangular when sectioned across the long axis, the length being considerably greater than the width.

Cooper ligaments Triangular ligaments stretching between the mammary gland, the skin, the retinacula cutis, the pectineal ligament, and the chorda obliqua. These ligaments underlie and support the breasts.

Corpus mammae The mammary gland; breast mass after freeing breast from deep attachments and removal of skin, subcutaneous connective tissue, and fat.

Co-sleeping When a baby or young child sleeps close to one or both parents, as opposed to in a separate room. Usually, this means within an arm's length of one another, but sometimes it is meant to imply sleeping in the same room.

Creamatocrit Measurement for estimating the fat content and therefore the caloric content of a milk sample. A microhematocrit tube is filled with milk (usually a mix of foremilk and hind milk) and spun in a microcentrifuge for 15 min. The layer of fat is measured as a percentage, as one measures a blood hematocrit.

Cross nursing When a lactating woman breastfeeds a baby that is not her own, often temporarily, in the role of a childcare arrangement. A wet nurse is an old term for such a lactating woman who breastfeeds a child besides her own for some form of remuneration.

Cuboidal secretory cell   A secretory cell that has similar height and breadth measurements.

Cytokines   A generic term for small nonantibody proteins produced by a broad range of cells that are then involved in cell signaling without entering the cytoplasm. Cytokines include chemokines, interferons, interleukins, and lymphokines but not growth factors or hormones. They are an important part of the immune system.

Cytosol   Cell fluid.

D

DHHS   The Department of Health and Human Services (DHHS) in the United States is a US governmental agency tasked with protecting the health of all Americans and providing human services.

Donor human milk   Excess milk produced by lactating women and voluntarily donated to a milk bank for use for other infants besides their own. Mothers are screened for health and social risk factors (not dissimilar from blood donors), and the milk is processed and pasteurized before providing it to a recipient infant.

Doula   An individual who supports, interacts with, and aids the mother at any time within the period that includes pregnancy, birth, and lactation; this may be a relative, friend, or neighbor and is usually, but not necessarily, a woman. One who gives psychological encouragement and physical assistance to a new mother. These are lay individuals who train to assist the mother during labor and delivery.

Dummy (pacifier)   An artificial nipple made of plastic, rubber, or silicone for use by an infant to suck in place of a breast or bottle. Its shape usually includes the "nipple" and a mouth shield and handle attached to prevent choking or swallowing of the nipple.

Dyad (breastfeeding dyad, mother–infant dyad)   A social relationship between two individuals. The breastfeeding dyad refers to all that is involved in such a relationship between a mother and her breastfeeding infant.

Dysphoric milk ejection reflex   The negative emotions and experience of a breastfeeding woman just before and during the stimulation of the milk ejection reflex. The dysphoric milk ejection reflex (D-MER) usually occurs suddenly and the mother is happy or without dysphoria between episodes.

E

Efferent   Carrying impulses away from a nerve center.

Ejection reflex   A reflex initiated by the suckling of the infant at the breast, which triggers the pituitary gland to release oxytocin into the bloodstream. The oxytocin causes the myoepithelial cells to contract and eject the milk from the collecting ductules. Also called *let-down reflex* or *draught*.

Embryogenesis   The first stage of mammary development, beginning with the mammary band about the 35th embryonic day.

Engorgement   The swelling and distention of the breasts, usually in the early days of initiation of lactation, caused by vascular dilatation and the arrival of the early milk. This can occur normally in the first 2 to 3 days after birth. It may become a problem when the swelling increases, becomes firm or hard or painful with warmth and sometimes a low-grade fever. Obstruction of the breast lymphatics can lead to secondary edema. The treatment and prevention of engorgement is through the frequent and adequate drainage of milk from the breast.

Enteromammary pathway   The system through which lactogenic hormones or cytokines lead to the migration of lymphocytes from the intestine to the mammary glands. These transported lymphocytes produce secretory immunoglobulin A antibodies, which enter the breast milk and provide added protection of the infant to antigens in the mother and infant's environs, which the mother was exposed to in her respiratory tree and intestine.

Ever breastfed   A term sometimes used to "quantify" the relative amount of breast milk an infant received. It is applied to an infant who has ever been put to the breast. That includes if the infant was put to the breast only once or 100 times, so it is a poor term and inaccurate quantification.

Exclusive breastfeeding   When an infant is fed only breast milk and no other foods or liquids. This means not even water. The breast milk can be by breastfeeding, expressed mother's own milk, donor human milk, or milk from a wet nurse or milk sharing. Drops or syrups of vitamins, minerals, or medicines are "allowed."

Expressed breast milk   Breast milk removed by expression, although sometimes includes pumped breast milk.

F

Familial puerperal alactogenesis   Primary lactation failure caused by an isolated prolactin deficiency occurring genetically in families.

Finger feeding   Stimulation of an infant's tongue with a finger to initiate sucking. A feeding tube attached to a syringe of milk along the finger will provide milk to the infant when suckling is correct.

Foremilk   The first milk obtained at the onset of suckling or expression. It contains less fat than later milk of that same feeding (i.e., the hind milk).

Formula   The generic term for infant or artificial formula. It is a liquid food processed from other animal milks or plants (soy) as a substitute for human breast milk. The *Codex Alimentarius* maintains standards, guidelines, and codes of practice for preparation and content of infant formulas intended for use in infants under 1 year of age. Infant formula is made up of nutrients, micronutrients, vitamins, and minerals intended to support normal growth and development of infants.

Frenulum   A fold of mucous membrane extending from the floor of the mouth to the underside of the tongue. This anchors the tongue to the floor of the mouth in various degrees of tightness and/or limitation of the movement of the tongue.

Frenulotomy   A very simple procedure removing the frenulum. (Other procedures are frenectomy, frenotomy, and frenulectomy.)

G

Galactocele   A cystic tumor (benign) in the ducts of the breast that contains a milky fluid.

Galactagogue   A food or drug that stimulates the production of milk.

Galactopoiesis   The development of milk in the mammary gland and maintenance of established lactation, also known as stage III lactogenesis. The maintenance of established lactation requires the autocrine system and ongoing demand (removal of milk).

Galactorrhea   Abnormal or inappropriate lactation.

Galactose   A simple sugar ($C_6H_{12}O_6$) that is a component of the disaccharide lactose, or milk sugar.

Galactosemia   A congenital metabolic disorder in which there is an inability to metabolize galactose because of a deficiency in one of several enzymes—galactose-1-phosphate uridyltransferase, galactokinase, or galactose-6-phosphate epimerase. There is a spectrum of illness in the infant depending on the deficient enzyme and the degree of enzyme deficiency. It can cause failure to thrive, hepatomegaly, and splenomegaly.

GALT   Gut-associated lymphoid tissue to which the mammary gland may act as an extension. See *BALT* and *MALT*.

Genome   All of the genetic material of an organism, including coding, noncoding, and mitochondrial DNA. It can include RNA in RNA viruses or chloroplast DNA in photosynthetic plants.

Gigantomastia   The excessive enlargement of the breast beyond physiologic needs during pregnancy and lactation, usually of unknown cause. When it occurs in association with medications that cause galactorrhea (calcium-channel blockers), it can be reversed by stopping the drug.

Glandular hypoplasia   Lack of breast growth during pregnancy. Nipples point downward, and there is a tubular shape to the breast and little palpable glandular tissue. This occurs with failure of lactogenesis.

Golgi apparatus   A specialized region of the cytoplasm, often close to the nucleus, composed of flattened cisternae, numerous vesicles, and some larger vacuoles. In secretory cells, it is concerned with packaging the secretory product(s). It is also probably concerned with the secretion of polysaccharides in some cells, but its full range of functions has not yet been elucidated.

H

Hand expression A means of removing human milk manually from the breast using one's hands that requires no equipment or apparatus.

Hind milk Milk obtained later during the nursing period, that is, the end of the feeding. This milk is usually high in fat compared with foremilk.

Hirschsprung's disease A congenital abnormality of the colon resulting from failure of migration of ganglion cells throughout the colon. Lack of these cells and the missing innervation limits the normal movement of intestinal contents through the colon. The level of the colon (proximal to distal) where there are missing ganglion cells determines the severity of the defect and level of blockage of the colon.

Homocystinuria A rare inborn error of amino acid metabolism that can lead to subsequent complications, including mental deficiency, epilepsy, dislocation of the lens, growth disturbance, thromboses, and defective hair growth.

Human milk bank An organization that collects, processes, stores, and dispenses human milk. Most milk banks are nonprofit and collect donated breast milk from women without remuneration. The organizations do recruit and screen donors for health concerns and social issues that could place a woman at greater risk for illness (most commonly infection).

Human milk cells Cells that routinely are in human milk. Cells derived from the breast include lactocytes, myoepithelial cells, progenitor cells, and stem cells. Cells derived from the blood that can enter human milk include immune cells, hematopoietic stem cells, and other cells of blood origin.

Human milk fortifiers Milk-based modified supplements added to human milk to provide additional nutrients and minerals to premature infants (primarily) for normal growth and development. They can be derived from human breast milk or bovine milk and contain predominantly proteins and minerals with some sugars and fats.

Human milk oligosaccharides (HMOs) See *Oligosaccharides*.

Hyperadenia The existence of mammary tissue without nipples.

Hyperbilirubinemia The presence of an abnormally large amount of bilirubin in the blood. This condition can involve conjugated and/or unconjugated bilirubin and be due to a long list of potential causes that may need to be specifically identified to be effectively treated.

Hypergalactia The excessive, uncontrolled production of milk over and above the needs of a suckling infant.

Hyperlactation An oversupply of milk beyond the needs or capacity of the infant.

Hypermastia The existence of accessory mammary glands.

Hyperthelia The existence of abundant, more or less developed nipples without accompanying mammary tissue.

I

Immunoglobulin The protein fraction of globulin, which has been demonstrated to have immunologic properties. Immunoglobulins are produced by B cells (called plasma cells when fully matured to produce immunoglobulins) and include IgA, secretory IgA, IgD, IgE, IgG, and IgM. They can be in breast milk and protect against infection. IgA is usually present in the largest amount in breast milk followed by IgG.

Induced lactation Process by which non-puerperal females (or males) are stimulated to lactate.

Innate immune system The complex of cells that are activated by molecules associated with pathogenic microorganisms (pathogen associated molecular patterns [PAMPs]) or released in the process of tissue damage (damage associated molecular patterns [DAMPs]). The recognition of these patterns (by pattern recognition receptors [PRRs]) on cells leads to an immediate and non—antigen-specific immune response.

Intraductal papilloma A benign breast tumor within the milk ducts of the breast. They are often located near the nipple and can grow to be 1 to 2 cm in size. On occasion they are associated with a serous or bloody fluid from the nipple.

Inverted nipple The nipple is not normally everted, protruding out from the surface of the areola. It projects into the breast often creating an indentation in the areola. It can occur bilaterally or unilaterally and may cause difficulties with latch and breastfeeding.

Involution (of the breast) The two-part postlactational process of secretory epithelial cells' apoptosis and mammary gland membrane degradation and remodeling.

J

Jaundice A yellowish color to the skin, mucous membranes, and conjunctiva as a result of hyperbilirubinemia (elevated bilirubin in the blood). It should be distinguished between orangish skin color caused by carotenemia, an excess of dietary carotenoids that does not cause discoloration of the conjunctiva.

K

Kangaroo Mother Care (KMC) A standardized, protocol-based system for preterm and/or low-birth-weight infants in which an infant is held skin to skin against a mother's or father's chest inside her/his clothing. An important constituent of the support program for milk production by mothers who are pumping to produce milk without the benefit of the infant suckling at the breast.

L

Lactation The period of ongoing milk synthesis after birth to provide breast milk for an infant. Maintenance of the ongoing breast milk synthesis requires both hormonal stimulation within the mother and the frequent, effective removal of milk.

Lactational Amenorrhea Method (LAM) A recognized method of family planning for the exclusively breastfeeding women in the first 6 months of lactation. Exclusive breastfeeding for LAM includes limited amounts of time between breastfeeds (4 hours or maximum 6 hours at night), increased number of breastfeeds during 24 hours (>8) and that the mother is amenorrheic. After 6 months, the risk for pregnancy increases (without another form of birth control) as the episodes of menses increases and the number of ovulatory cycles increases.

Lactation dysfunction An alteration in the normal process of lactation. This can be due to a variety of anatomic or physiologic problems associated with breastfeeding and lactation. Nipple or breast pain, difficulty with latch, or perceived low milk supply often lead to inadequate removal of milk effectively from the breast leading to diminishing milk synthesis. These all can be reasons for undesired early weaning.

Lactation failure The inability to produce sufficient breast milk to support an infant's ongoing nutritional needs. Lactation failure can be primary (uncommon) or secondary (relatively common).

Lactiferous ducts The main ducts of the mammary gland, which number from 15 to 30 and open onto the nipple. They carry milk to the nipple and are very elastic.

Lactobacillus bifidus A gram-positive anaerobic bacterium (also known as *Bifidobacterium*) found in breast milk and the intestinal tract of breastfed infants. It is considered normal flora in breastfed infants and a probiotic bacteria.

Lactocele Cystic tumor of the breast caused by the dilatation and obstruction of a milk duct that is usually filled with milk.

Lactocyte The mammary secretory cell responsible for synthesizing and secreting breast milk. The lactocyte uses multiple pathways to secrete milk: exocytosis for protein and lactose, secretion of fat in the milk fat globule, transmembrane secretion of ions and water, exocytosis of immunoglobulins and cells, and movement of plasma proteins via the paracellular pathway into the milk.

Lacto-engineering The process of enhancing the nutrient value of human milk by adding nutrients obtained by drying and separating out specific nutrients, such as protein, from pooled human milk. It is also known as adjustable fortification to provide individual infants with specific nutrients and micronutrients to optimize protein and nutrient content and infant growth.

Lactoferrin An iron-binding protein of external secretions, including human milk. It inhibits the growth of iron-dependent microorganisms in the gut.

Lactogenesis Initiation of milk secretion.

Lactoglobulin (β-lactoglobulin) A major protein occurring naturally in the whey fraction of most animals' milk, but not human milk. β-Lactoglobulin in human milk has been associated with cow's milk allergy in the infant.

Lactose The primary disaccharide in human milk. It is made up of glucose and galactose molecules.

Latch The positioning of the infant's face to the breast with the mouth directly attached to the nipple and areola of the breast to facilitate coordinated suck-swallow-breathe movements of the lips, mouth, tongue, and palate and effective milk transfer.

Let-down reflex See *Ejection reflex*.

Ligand A low-molecular-weight substance that binds trace elements loosely for ready availability (e.g., zinc ligands in human milk).

Lobulus A subunit of the parenchymal structure of the breast made up of 10 to 100 alveoli or tubulosaccular secretory units. From 20 to 40 lobuli make up a lobus.

Lobus A subunit of the parenchymal structure of the breast made up of 20 to 40 lobuli. From 15 to 25 lobi are arranged like the spokes of a wheel with the nipple as the central point.

Lymphocyte A mature leukocyte derived through the intermediate stage of lymphoblast from the reticuloendothelium found in lymphatic tissue.

Lyophilization The process of rapidly freezing and drying a fluid in a vacuum, resulting in a solid.

M

MALT Mucosal-associated lymphoid tissue, which includes gut, lung, mammary gland, salivary and lacrimal glands, and genital tract. There is traffic of cells between mucosal and lymphoid sites. Immune recognition and response at one site can be effectively transferred by activated cells to distant sites. See *GALT* and *BALT*.

Mamilla The nipple; any teat-like structure.

Mammary gland The secretory organ in women that normally produces human milk. The mammary gland is rudimentary in males but evolves through developmental stages in females (embryogenesis, puberty, mammogenesis, pregnancy, lactogenesis/lactation, involution). The breast's primary function is the synthesis and secretion of milk to feed an infant, and it subsequently involutes to a quiescent period after weaning.

Mammogenesis Growth of the mammary gland, primarily during pregnancy. Cellular proliferation leads to ongoing formation of terminal buds, ducts, and alveoli in preparation for milk production.

Mammoplasty A general term for surgery performed on the mammary gland to change its shape, size, appearance, and/or position. It includes augmentation (increase in size), reduction (decrease in size), and reconstruction to change shape, volume, and appearance, most often after a mastectomy.

Mastalgia Painful breasts.

Mastectomy This is the surgical removal of some or all the breast tissue, unilateral or bilateral.

Mastitis Inflammation of the breast, including cellulitis and, occasionally, abscess formation. Generically, it can be due to a range of inflammatory disorders besides infection. Disruption of the breast microbiome (dysbiosis), with decreased microbial diversity and increased numbers of some recognized bacterial pathogens (*Aeromonas*, *Staphylococcus*, *Ralstonia*, *Klebsiella*, *Serratia*, *Enterococcus*, and *Pseudomonas*) is one of the proposed mechanisms of lactational mastitis.

Matrescence The state of becoming a mother or motherhood as a new event in an individual's life.

Megaloblastic anemia Defective red blood cell formation caused by megaloblastic hyperplasia of the marrow; there are often megaloblasts, or primitive nucleated red blood cells, in the peripheral blood.

Meconium This is the first stool passed by a mammalian infant. It is made up of materials ingested while the infant is in utero: cells, mucus, amniotic fluid, and water. It is viscous and tar-like in consistency and dark olive green—black in color.

Merocrine Pertaining to the type of secretion in which the active cell remains intact while forming and discharging its secretory product(s).

Metabolome Constitutes all the metabolic products associated with the pathways of a specific organism or organ. Human milk metabolome relates to all the metabolic products related to human milk synthesis produced by the mammary gland.

Methylmalonic acidemia A group of inherited conditions related to more than five different genes leading to a build-up of methylmalonic acid in blood and urine. Without treatment and preventive measures, it can cause varying degrees of growth delay, intellectual disability, kidney disease, and pancreatitis.

Microbiome The aggregate of all microorganisms that reside in a specific location or environment (mouth, nose, skin, gastrointestinal tract, breast, uterus, vagina, etc.). The human microbiome is all the microorganisms contained in or on a human body.

Micronutrients Chemical substances present in very small amounts in foods that ensure the health and growth of a living organism. Examples include vitamins and trace elements (copper, zinc, selenium, iron, etc.).

Milk-fat globule membrane (MFGM) A complex membrane structure of lipids and proteins surrounding the milk fat globule released by exocytosis from a lactocyte into human milk. The MFGM is composed of bioactive factors, including glycolipids, phospholipids, glycoproteins, and carbohydrates.

Milk fever A syndrome of fever and general malaise associated with early engorgement of the breasts or engorgement associated with sudden weaning from the breast.

Milk sharing The sharing of excess breast milk by one woman with others for use with their infants (by wet nursing, donor human milk and milk banks, and informal milk sharing). Donor human milk and milk banks rely on informed choice/decision making, donor screening, safe handling and processing of milk, and pasteurization to ensure the safety of donor human milk. Wet nursing or informal milk sharing should rely on these same principles to safely share human milk. Informal milk sharing is the exchange of breast milk from one woman to another without involving some other organization or group or an official agreement to share the milk.

Milk-to-plasma ratio (M/P) The concentration of a drug in mother's milk divided by its concentration in mother's plasma at the same time. A higher M/P ratio indicates that a higher amount of drug will reach the milk for a given concentration. The overall amount of drug reaching the milk is primarily determined by the concentration of the drug in the plasma.

Mitogen A substance capable of stimulating cells to enter mitosis.

Montgomery glands Small prominences, sebaceous glands in the areola of the breast, that become more marked in pregnancy and lactation. They number 20 to 24 and secrete a fluid that lubricates the nipple and areola.

Morgagni's tubercle Small sinuses into which the miniature ducts of the Montgomery glands open in the epidermis of the areola.

Myoepithelial cell An epithelial cell with contractile capability, surrounding each alveolus. Oxytocin causes these cells to contract, expressing milk into the milk ducts.

N

Necrotizing enterocolitis A pathologic inflammatory process within the gastrointestinal tract (primarily the colon) leading to damage and necrosis of the mucosal surface and often full-thickness damage of the intestinal tract in infants. It is a multifactorial disease that includes risk factors such as prematurity, intestinal immaturity, infection, dysbiosis, discoordinated inflammatory reaction, and tissue hypoxia.

Neonatal galactorrhea Milk-like secretion produced in male and female infant breasts, occurring relatively soon after birth because of the withdrawal of maternal hormones.

Nipple The central pigmented protuberance of the mammary gland. It is usually surrounded by the areola (larger pigmented flat circle) and contains multiple milk duct openings.

Nipple-areolar complex (NAC) This is the anatomically and physiologically related collection of nipple, areola, Montgomery glands, and terminal milk ducts of the breast. It includes the involved skin, nerves, muscle components, blood vessels, Cooper ligaments, and lymphatics.

Nonnutritive sucking The act of suckling the breast with little or no secretion of milk. Infant may suckle when distressed or to be calmed or quieted.

Nonpuerperal lactation The production of milk in a woman who has not given birth.

Nucleotides Compounds derived from nucleic acid by hydrolysis and consisting of phosphoric acid combined with a sugar and a purine or pyrimidine derivative. The milk nucleotides are secreted from glandular epithelial cells.

Nursing strike The sudden onset of—and temporary—refusal to nurse, often taken by mothers to mean that there is not enough milk or that something is wrong with their milk. The various causes associated with this abrupt infant behavior include onset of menses in the mother; dietary indiscretion by the mother; change in maternal soap, perfume, or deodorant; stress in the mother; earache or nasal obstruction in the infant; teething; episode of biting with startle and pain reaction by the mother.

Nutritive sucking When the infant is suckling at the breast and effectively removing and swallowing breast milk.

O

Oligosaccharides Complex sugars that provide protective and early-life immune programming and prevention functions. They are the third largest solid component in milk, also known as human milk oligosaccharides (HMOs). They are not absorbed from the intestine and function as "prebiotics" favoring the growth of specific bacteria that can metabolize the specific HMOs.

Organogenesis The ductal and lobular growth that begins before and continues through puberty, resulting in growth of the breast parenchyma with its surrounding fat pad.

Oxytocin This is a nonapeptide that is synthesized in the cell bodies of neurons, located mainly in the paraventricular nucleus and, in smaller amounts, in the supraoptic nucleus of the hypothalamus. Oxytocin stimulates the ejection reflex by the stimulation of the myoepithelial cells in the mammary gland and contraction of the uterus.

P

Panniculus adiposus Adipose tissue. The superficial fascia, which contains fatty pellicles.

Papilla mammae Mamilla. The nipple of the breast.

Pasteurization The process of heating food or drink to inactivate or destroy any microorganisms present. The specific process, relative to time and temperature of treating the food/liquid are variable but have been "standardized" for human milk banks to provide safe pasteurized donor human milk (PDHM).

Perinatal The time around birth and delivery. It is commonly considered from the 28th week of pregnancy until 1 week after birth.

Plasma cell Cell derived from the B-cell series, which manufactures and secretes antibodies.

Poland syndrome Chest wall and breast hypoplasia. It is an uncommon congenital condition involving absence of chest musculature and webbed fingers on the same side as the affected breast.

Polycystic ovary syndrome (PCOS) A hormonal disorder of women of child-bearing age. It commonly involves lack of ovulation, abnormal menses, an excess of male hormones, and potential long-term complications of insulin resistance and heart disease.

Polythelia Supernumerary nipples. Usually arising along the embryonic "milk line."

Postpartum The period after childbirth.

Postpartum depression The prolonged presence of depressive symptoms in a postpartum woman. It persists longer than a week or two and interferes with normal functioning and caring for her infant. This is different from "baby blues," which are common in the first week postpartum. Depressive symptoms should be screened for routinely in the postpartum period using a screening questionnaire or clinical tool for that purpose.

Prebiotic A nondigestible food ingredient that benefits the host by selectively favoring growth and activity of one or more indigenous probiotic bacteria.

Probiotic Beneficial bacteria that colonize specific anatomic locations of the human body.

Prolactin (hPRL) A hormone present in both males and females and at all ages produced in the anterior pituitary gland. During pregnancy, it stimulates and prepares the mammary alveolar epithelium for secretory activity. During lactation, it stimulates synthesis and secretion of milk. At other ages and in males, it interacts with other steroids.

Prostaglandins Any of a class of physiologically active lipid molecules derived from arachidonic acid, producing effects including vasodepression, stimulation of intestinal smooth muscle, uterine stimulation, aggregation of blood platelets, and antagonism to hormones influencing lipid metabolism.

Puerperium or puerperal The period from childbirth until the mother's uterus returns to its normal, nonpregnant size (commonly 6 weeks).

R

Rachitic Relating to, characterized by, or affected by rickets. Rickets is the softening or weakening of bones, most commonly because of insufficient vitamin D.

Raynaud's phenomenon of the nipple The occurrence of intermittent ischemia of the nipple after exposure to cold or some other stimuli. It is characterized by biphasic or triphasic color changes of the nipple (white, red, blue) and severe nipple (and sometimes breast) pain throughout the episode. The ischemia can manifest during pregnancy and even when not breastfeeding.

Re-lactation Process by which a woman who has given birth but did not initially breastfeed is stimulated to lactate (also applies to reinstituting lactation after it has been discontinued).

Relative infant dose (RID) An estimate of the "relative" amount of a medication an infant receives by breast milk compared with the daily maternal dose of the medication. It is calculated by dividing the estimated absolute infant dose of medication (mg/kg/day) by the maternal dose (mg/kg/day) times 100. Experts generally recommend an RID of less than 10% as acceptable for maternal use of a medication during breastfeeding.

Retained placenta When the placenta is not expelled from the uterus within 30 minutes of the birth. The partial separation of the placenta without complete expulsion leads to continued hemorrhage and may interfere with lactogenesis.

Rooming in The placement of the newborn infant in the mother's hospital room instead of in the nursery.

Rooting reflex Newborn reflex that occurs when the infant's mouth is stroked or touched and the infant turns his or her head and opens the mouth to follow in the direction of the stroking and ideally finds the object on which to suckle. This reflex is present at birth and usually disappears by 4 months of age.

S

Secretory activation The initiation of copious milk secretion associated with major changes in the concentrations of many milk constituents, triggered by the withdrawal of progesterone naturally after pregnancy.

Secretory differentiation The stage of pregnancy when the mammary epithelial cells differentiate into lactocytes with the capacity to synthesize unique milk constituents such as lactose, also known as stage I lactogenesis.

Squamous epithelium A sheet of flattened, scale-like epithelial cells adhering edge to edge.

Stroma The connective tissue basis or framework of an organ.

Suck training A special technique developed to help an infant who cannot coordinate the undulating (peristaltic) motion of the tongue. See *Finger feeding*.

Sucking reflex Sucking in response to a stimulus that occurs when the roof of the mouth (hard palate) is touched by anything the infant tries to suck. It is connected to the rooting reflex, and is present at about 32 weeks' gestational age but is not well-developed until about 36 weeks. Premature infants may have a weak or immature sucking ability.

Suckling The physical process of taking nourishment at the breast.

Suck-swallow-breathe reflex (SSwB) The coordinated activity an infant must develop to effectively suck, swallow, and breathe during breastfeeding or bottle-feeding. There is usually a pause in breathing to swallow.

Supplemental nursing system A device consisting of a thin feeding tube connected to a container of breast milk, positioned such that the end of the tube extends just beyond the breast nipple facilitating the transfer of breast milk through the tubing when the infant suckles the breast.

Supplementary feeding Providing an infant with another nutrient-rich fluid in addition to what it receives by breastfeeding. This can be expressed breast milk, donor human milk, or infant formula.

Swaddling The practice of wrapping an infant in a blanket or cloth with only the head protruding so that movement of the limbs is restricted without interfering with breathing.

Switch nursing Nursing in which the mother moves the baby from one breast to the other and back again during the feeding with the hope that this will stimulate the milk supply.

Symmastia Abnormal ectodermal webbing across the midline between the breasts, which are usually symmetric.

T

Tail of Spence The axillary tail of breast tissue that can extend into the axilla.

Tandem breastfeeding This is continuing to breastfeed an older infant after the birth of a sibling and breastfeeding both infants.

Tanner staging System to classify the stages of pubertal development, based on observational data on physical changes in the breasts and male or female genitalia.

Thelarche The development of breast buds in females that commonly occurs between the ages of 8 and 13 years of age.

Therapeutic Breast Massage in Lactation (TBML) A hand expression technique for the purposes of relieving engorgement, plugged ducts, and mastitis, facilitated by rolling the breasts between both hands or kneading the breasts with one or both hands.

Tight junctions These are connections that join the apical borders of adjacent secretory cells in the lactating mammary gland. They function to limit the transfer of milk or serum components between the interstitial space and the milk space.

Tongue extrusion reflex (tongue thrust) A normal reflex in infants from 0 to 4 months of age, in which they forcibly push their tongue forward when the lips are touched, or the tongue depressed. It does not usually interfere with suckling but does limit feeding with a spoon or cup at this earlier age.

Torticollis The twisted position of the neck resulting from tightening and shortening of the sternocleidomastoid (SCM) muscle. This shortening of the SCM muscle leads to tilting of the ear on the same side as the muscle shortens toward the shoulder, and the nose and face rotate in the opposite direction.

Transitional breast milk The milk produced early in the postpartum period as the colostrum diminishes and the mature milk develops. It is commonly described as extending from about 36 to 40 hours after birth to 2 to 3 weeks postpartum. It is characterized by decreasing concentrations of immunoglobulins and protein and increasing lactose, fat, and total caloric content.

Tubuloalveolar Having both tubular and alveolar qualities.

Tubulosaccular Having both tubular and saccular character.

Turgescence The swelling up of a part. The unusual turgid feeling that results from swelling with fluid.

U

Ultrasonic homogenization The process of dispersion of minute droplets of fat in expressed human milk by ultrasonic wave treatment to limit the separation and potential loss of fat from the milk in processing, storing, or administering it.

W

Weaning Complex process by which an infant is transitioned from exclusive breastfeeding to additional or other nutrient-rich and caloric-rich solids and liquid while maintaining optimal nutrition, growth, and development of the infant. The process involves nutritional, microbiologic, immunologic, biochemical, and psychologic adjustments.

Wet nurse A woman who breastfeeds an infant who is not her own, usually for some remuneration.

Whey protein The protein remaining when casein curds have been removed. The mixture of proteins present in human milk is complex and includes hundreds of proteins and specifically lactoferrin, α-lactalbumin, and numerous enzymes.

Witch's milk Product of neonatal galactorrhea or neonatal breast secretion caused by placental prolactin in the infant's circulation (neonatal galactorrhea).

Note: Page numbers followed by *b* indicate boxes, *f* indicate figures and *t* indicate tables.